United States Pharmacopeia
DRUG INFORMATION FOR THE CONSUMER

1988 Edition

By authority of the United States Pharmacopeial Convention, Inc.

Consumers Union   **Mount Vernon, New York**

Library of Congress Catalog Card Number: 81-640842
ISBN: 0-89043-210-4

First printing, January 1988

Printed by Mack Printing Company, Easton, Pennsylvania   18042

Published simultaneously by USPC, Inc., under the title *USP DI, Volume II (Advice for the Patient)*, Eighth Edition, 1988.

United States Pharmacopeia Drug Information for the Consumer, 1988 Edition, is a Consumer Reports Book published by Consumers Union, the nonprofit organization that publishes *Consumer Reports*, the monthly magazine of test reports, product Ratings, and buying guidance. Established in 1936, Consumers Union is chartered under the Not-For-Profit Corporation Law of the State of New York.

The purposes of Consumers Union, as stated in its charter, are to provide consumers with information and counsel on consumer goods and services, to give information on all matters relating to the expenditure of the family income, and to initiate and to cooperate with individual and group efforts seeking to create and maintain decent living standards.

Consumers Union derives its income solely from the sale of *Consumer Reports* and other publications. In addition, expenses of occasional public service efforts may be met, in part, by nonrestrictive, noncommercial contributions, grants, and fees. Consumers Union accepts no advertising or product samples and is not beholden in any way to any commercial interest. Its Ratings and reports are solely for the use of the readers of its publications. Neither the Ratings nor the reports nor any Consumers Union publications, including this book, may be used in advertising or for any commercial purpose. Consumers Union will take all steps open to it to prevent such uses of its material, its name, or the name of *Consumer Reports*.

NOTICE AND WARNING

Contents

United States Pharmacopeia
Drug Information for the Consumer

Consumers Union Foreword

For more than 160 years, the United States Pharmacopeial Convention (USPC) has set official standards of strength, quality, purity, packaging, and labeling for medical products in the United States. And for more than 50 years, Consumers Union through its publication, *Consumer Reports*, has served as this country's foremost source for authoritative, reliable, and unbiased product testing and buying guidance. It seems only natural then that these two organizations, both holding the consumer's perspective as the most important, should join forces to publish a layman's guide to prescription and over-the-counter drugs.

At one time or another, most of us will find it necessary to use some sort of drug. The common perception is that these medications, whether prescribed by a health practitioner, or obtained over the counter (prescription not required), will make us feel better if not cure us entirely. Many people feel that in order to be effective, medical treatment must include drug therapy. Last year, over $18.8 billion were spent on prescription drugs, and another $8.5 billion on nonprescription drugs. And studies show that up to 50 percent of all prescriptions are taken incorrectly, and as many as 70 percent of all patients receive little or no counseling about drug usage, interactions with food or other drugs, and side effects. There is a grave need for a straightforward objective guide to drugs that cautions and informs the consumer about prescription drugs as part of medical care.

United States Pharmacopeia Drug Information for the Consumer lists almost every medicine, prescription and nonprescription, available in the United States and Canada and provides consumers with up-to-date information about drug usage and side effects. It is organized alphabetically by generic or family name, and each entry includes different dosage forms and common brand names as well—over 5,000 in all. It is well indexed according to both generic and brand names, making it easy to look up any medication. What CU considers the most important feature of this book is the fact that it is put together by experts—physicians, pharmacists, pharmacologists, dentists, nurses, chemists, microbiologists, and other individuals particularly qualified to judge drugs—95 people in all, supported by 26 advisory panels representing differing medical specialties, health professionals, and consumers. Unlike other drug information books available to the consumer, notably the *Physicians' Desk Reference*, the information presented in this guide is not controlled by drug manufacturers or anyone connected with the drug industry. Instead, it is a consensus book put together by the people who prescribe and use the drugs out on today's market. Because it is a work that is constantly in revision and reviewed by so many experts, information about precautions and side effects may be found here that is not readily available elsewhere.

Consumers Union believes that the therapeutic use of drugs deserves much closer scrutiny than is usual, by physicians, pharmacists, and patients. There is no question that drug breakthroughs in several areas have given us new tools to combat a wide variety of diseases, disorders, and complaints. But even the exacting approval process undertaken by the Food and Drug Administration (FDA) cannot possibly guarantee that drugs that reach the market are totally safe and effective. Post-marketing surveillance by physician and patient must be an integral part of drug usage. Reporting the side effects of drugs, by patients to physicians and by physicians to the FDA is important so that future editions of *Drug Information for the Consumer* can reflect new knowledge and experience.

The material in this book is presented in a straightforward, factual manner—there is no editorial opinion and no biased discussion about the relative merits of one drug over another. Each medication profile lists indications, precautions, proper usage, and side effects. The language is intelligible, straight to the point, and targeted specifically to the patient. *Drug Information for the Consumer* is the most comprehensive drug information book available to the public and we are proud to present it to our readers.

To The Reader

When purchasing a medicine, whether over-the-counter (nonprescription) or with a doctor's prescription, you may have questions about its usefulness to you, the best way to take it, possible side effects, and precautions to take to avoid complications. For instance, some medicines should be taken with meals, others between meals. Some may make you drowsy while others may tend to keep you awake. Alcoholic or other beverages, other medicines, certain foods, or smoking may affect the way your medicine works. As for side effects, some are merely bothersome and may go away while others may require medical attention.

Drug Information for the Consumer contains information which may provide general answers to some of your questions as well as suggestions for the correct use of your medicine. *It is important to remember, however, that the human body is very complex and medicines may act differently on different people—and even in the same person at different times. If you want additional information about your medicine or its possible side effects, ask your doctor, nurse, or pharmacist. They are there to help you.*

How To Use This Book:

Drug Information for the Consumer contains a section of general information about the correct use of any medicine, as well as individual discussions of a wide variety of commonly and not so commonly used medicines. *You should read both the general information and the information specific to the medicine you are taking.* See Appendix II for this general information.

Each medicine has a generic name that all manufacturers who make that medicine must use. Some manufacturers also create a brand name to put on the label and to use in advertising. *Look in the index* for the generic name or the brand name of the medicine about which you have questions. We have put the generic names and common brand names in the same index, so you do not have to know whether the name you have is a generic name or a brand name. However, it is a good idea for you to learn both the generic and the brand names of the medicines you are using and even to write them down and keep them for future use.

Although the informational monographs generally appear in alphabetical order by generic name, there are numerous occasions when closely related medicines are grouped under a family name. Therefore, the surest way to find the page number of the information about each medicine is to *look in the index first.*

The information for each medicine is presented according to the area of the body which is affected. As a general rule, information for one type of use will not be the same as for other types of use. Thus, if you take tetracycline capsules by mouth for their systemic effect in treating an infection, the information will not be the same as for tetracycline ointment, which is applied directly to the skin for its topical effects. And both of these will be different from the information for tetracyclines used in the eye. The common divisions used in this publication are:

- *SYSTEMIC*—For general effects throughout the body; applies to most medicines when taken by mouth or given by injection.
- *TOPICAL*—For local effects when applied directly to the skin.
- *MUCOSAL*—For local effects when applied directly to mucous membranes (for example, the inside of the mouth).
- *NASAL*—For local effects when used in the nose.
- *INHALATION*—For local, and in some cases systemic, effects when inhaled into the lungs.
- *OPHTHALMIC*—For local effects when applied directly to the eyes.
- *OTIC*—For local effects when used in the ear.
- *DENTAL*—For local effects when applied to the teeth or gums.
- *RECTAL*—For local, and in some cases systemic, effects when used in the rectum.
- *VAGINAL*—For local, and in some cases systemic, effects when used in the vagina.

Notice:

The information about the drugs contained herein is general in nature and is intended to be used in consultation with your health care providers. It is not intended to replace specific instructions or directions or warnings given to you by your physician or other prescriber or accompanying a particular product. The information is selective and it is not claimed that it includes all known precautions, contraindications, effects, or interactions possibly related to the use of a drug. The information may differ from that contained in the product labeling which is required by law. The information is not sufficient to make an evaluation as to the risks and benefits of taking a particular drug in a particular case and is not medical advice for individual problems and should not alone be relied upon for these purposes. Since the inclusion or exclusion of particular information about a drug is judgmental in nature and since opinion as to drug usage may differ, you may wish to consult additional sources. Should you desire additional information or if you have any questions as to how this information may relate to you in particular, ask your doctor, nurse, pharmacist, or other health care provider.

Since new drugs are constantly being marketed and since previously unreported side effects, newly recognized precautions, or other new information for any given drug may come to light at any time, continuously updated drug information sources should be consulted as necessary.

There are many brands of drugs on the market. The listing of selected brand names is intended only for ease of reference. The inclusion of a brand name does not mean the USPC or Consumers Union has any particular knowledge that the brand listed has properties different from other brands of the same drug, nor should it be interpreted as an endorsement by the USPC or Consumers Union. Similarly, the fact that a brand name has not been included does not indicate that that particular brand has been judged to be unsatisfactory or unacceptable.

If any of the information in this book causes you special concern, do not decide against taking any medicine prescribed for you without first checking with your doctor.

About USPC:

The information in this volume is prepared by the United States Pharmacopeial Convention, Inc. (USPC), the organization that sets the official standards of strength, quality, purity, packaging, and labeling for medical products used in the United States.

The United States Pharmacopeial Convention is an independent, nonprofit corporation composed of delegates from the accredited colleges of medicine and pharmacy in the U.S.; state medical and pharmaceutical associations; many national associations concerned with medicines, such as the American Medical Association, the American Nurses Association, the American Dental Association, the National Association of Retail Druggists, and the American Pharmaceutical Association; and various departments of the federal government, including the Food and Drug Administration. In addition, four members of the Convention have been appointed by the Board of Trustees specifically to represent the public. USPC was established over 160 years ago, and is the only national body that represents the professions of both pharmacy and medicine.

The first convention came into being on January 1, 1820, and within the year published the first national drug formulary of the United States. The *U.S. Pharmacopeia* of 1820 contained 217 drug names, divided into two groups according to the level of general acceptance and usage.

When Congress passed the first major drug safety law in 1906, the standards recognized by that statute were those set forth in the *United States Pharmacopeia* and in the *National Formulary*. Today, the *USP* continues to be the official U.S. compendium for standards for drugs and for the inactive ingredients in drug dosage forms. The *United States Pharmacopeia* is the world's oldest regularly revised national pharmacopeia and is generally accepted as being the most influential.

USP DI was first published in 1980. It is a continuously reviewed and revised base of drug information intended for use by prescribers, dispensers, and consumers of medications. The information is developed by the consensus of the USP Committee of Revision and its Advisory Panels and anyone, including users of medicines, may contribute through review and comment. Committee and Panel members serve without pay and are assisted by other outside reviewers and USPC staff.

The United States Pharmacopeial Convention 1985–1990

USP Advisory Panels 1985–1990

Members who serve as Chairmen are listed first.

The information presented in this text represents an ongoing review of the drugs contained herein and represents a consensus of various viewpoints expressed. The individuals listed below are currently on the USP Advisory Panels and have contributed to the development of the 1988 USP DI data base. Such listing does not imply that these individuals have reviewed all of the material in this text or that they individually agree with all statements contained herein.

Panel on Anesthesiology
Walter L. Way, M.D., San Francisco, CA; Frederic Berry, M.D., Charlottesville, VA; Roy Cronnelly, M.D., Ph.D., Somerset, CA; Betty Grundy, M.D., Gainesville, FL; Dennis Mangano, M.D., Ph.D., San Francisco, CA; Carl Rosow, M.D., Ph.D., Boston, MA; Bradley Smith, M.D., Nashville, TN; Paul White, M.D., Ph.D., Palo Alto, CA

Panel on Biological Tests and Assays
Terry E. Munson, B.S., Fairfax, VA; Robert L. Amos, Indianapolis, IN; Janet C. Curry, New York, NY; Herbert N. Prince, Ph.D., Fairfield, NJ

Panel on Bulk Packaging
Garnet E. Peck, Ph.D., West Lafayette, IN; Terry Benney, Ph.D., Philadelphia, PA; Gregory Haines, Union, NJ; Gordon E. Mallett, Ph.D., Indianapolis, IN

Panel on Cardiovascular and Renal Drugs
Edward D. Frohlich, M.D., New Orleans, LA; Emmanuel L. Bravo, M.D., Cleveland, OH; Aram V. Chobanian, M.D., Boston, MA; James E. Doherty, M.D., Little Rock, AR; Garabed Eknoyan, M.D., Houston, TX; Ruth Eshleman, Ph.D., Kingston, RI; Thomas M. Glenn, Ph.D., Summit, NJ; Norman K. Hollenberg, M.D., Ph.D., Boston, MA; John L. Juergens, M.D., Rochester, MN; Michael Lesch, M.D., Chicago, IL; Benjamin F. McGraw, Pharm.D., Kansas City, MO; Patrick A. McKee, M.D., Oklahoma City, OK; Bernard L. Mirkin, Ph.D., M.D., Minneapolis, MN; Burton E. Sobel, M.D., St. Louis, MO; W. David Watkins, M.D., Ph.D., Durham, NC

Panel on Clinical Immunology
Albert L. Sheffer, M.D., Boston, MA; John Baum, M.D., Rochester, NY; Jonathan S. Coblyn, M.D., Brookline, MA; Elliot F. Ellis, M.D., Buffalo, NY; Patricia A. Fraser, M.D., Boston, MA; Thomas Gilman, Pharm.D., Los Angeles, CA; Stephen R. Kaplan, M.D., Providence, RI; Sandra Koehler, Milwaukee, WI; Floyd Malveaux, M.D., Ph.D., Washington, DC; Edward B. Nelson, M.D., Ph.D., Houston, TX; Robert E. Reisman, M.D., Buffalo, NY; Daniel J. Stechschulte, M.D., Kansas City, KS; Martin D. Valentine, M.D., Baltimore, MD

Panel on Consumer Interest
James Rankin, B.S., Taos, NM; Byllye Avery, Atlanta, GA; Judith Brown, B.A., Washington, DC; Jose Camacho, Austin, TX; Margaret A. Charters, Ph.D., Syracuse, NY; Jennifer Cross, San Francisco, CA; Gabriel Daniel, Washington, DC; John Forbes, Rio Piedras, PR; Jerome Halperin, Edison, NJ; Anita M. LeValdo, Window Rock, AZ; Janice Lieberman, Buffalo, NY; Esther Peterson, Washington, DC; Ruth Richards, M.A., M.P.H., Los Angeles, CA; T. Donald Rucker, Ph.D., Chicago, IL; Gordon Schiff, M.D., Chicago, IL

Panel on Dentistry
Sebastian G. Ciancio, D.D.S., Buffalo, NY; Donald F. Adams, D.D.S., Portland, OR; Karen Baker, M.S., Iowa City, IA; Priscilla C. Bourgault, Ph.D., Maywood, IL; Frederick A. Curro, D.M.D., Ph.D., Jersey City, NJ; Phyllis Eliasberg, Boston, MA; Tommy W. Gage, D.D.S., Ph.D., Dallas, TX; Stephen F. Goodman, D.D.S., New York, NY; Zack Kasloff, D.D.S., Winnipeg, Manitoba, Canada; Joseph Margarone, D.D.S., Buffalo, NY; Michael Newman, D.D.S., Los Angeles, CA; James W. Smudski, D.M.D., Ph.D., Pittsburgh, PA; Clarence L. Trummel, D.D.S., Ph.D., Farmington, CT; Raymond P. White, Jr., D.D.S., Ph.D., Chapel Hill, NC

Panel on Dermatology
Robert S. Stern, M.D., Boston, MA; Richard D. Baughman, M.D., Hanover, NH; Michael Bigby, M.D., Brookline, MA; Henry Jolly, M.D., New Orleans, LA; W. Stuart Maddin, M.D., F.R.C.P., Vancouver, British Columbia, Canada; Milton Orkin, M.D., Minneapolis, MN; Edgar Benton Smith, M.D., Galveston, TX; John Strauss, M.D., Iowa City, IA; Dennis West, M.S., Chicago, IL; Gail Zimmerman, B.A., Portland, OR

Panel on Diagnostic Agents—Nonradioactive
Harry W. Fischer, M.D., Rochester, NY; James A. Nelson, M.D., Seattle, WA; Robert L. Siegle, M.D., San Antonio, TX; Jovitas Skucas, M.D., Rochester, NY; William M. Thompson, M.D., Minneapolis, MN; Gerald L. Wolf, Ph.D., M.D., Pittsburgh, PA

Panel on Endocrinology
Dean H. Lockwood, M.D., Rochester, NY; Louis V. Avioli, M.D., St. Louis, MO; Edwin D. Bransome, Jr., M.D., Augusta, GA; P. Reed Larsen, M.D., Boston, MA; Marvin E. Levin, M.D., St. Louis, MO; Marvin M. Lipman, M.D., Mt. Vernon, NY; Walter J. Meyer, III., M.D., Galveston, TX; Rita Nemchik, R.N., M.S., Philadelphia, PA; Maria New, M.D., New York, NY; John A Owen, M.D., Charlottesville, VA; Robert W. Rebar, M.D., Chicago, IL; Thomas H. Wiser, Pharm.D., Buies Creek, NC

Panel on Family Practice
Donald R. Bennett, M.D., Ph.D., Chicago, IL; Paul C. Brucker, M.D., Philadelphia, PA; Allan H. Bruckheim, M.D., Hoboken, NJ; Robert E. Davis, Pharm.D., Englewood, CO; Robert Guthrie, M.D., Columbus, OH; Marlene Haffner, M.D., Rockville, MD; Edward L. Langston, M.D., R.Ph. Flora, IN; Jack M. Rosenberg, Pharm.D., Ph.D., Brooklyn, NY; John Thornburg, D.O., Ph.D., East Lansing, MI

Panel on Gastroenterology
James D. Finkelstein, M.D., Washington, DC; Rosemary R. Berardi, Pharm.D., Ann Arbor, MI; James J. Cerda, M.D., Gainesville, FL; Gerald Friedman, M.D., New York, NY; Donald J. Glotzer, M.D., Boston, MA; Louis Y. Korman, M.D., Washington, DC; Suzanne Rosenthal, New York, NY

Paul A. Palmisano, M.D., Birmingham, AL; Albert W. Pruitt, M.D., Augusta, GA; Philip D. Walson, M.D., Columbus, OH; Sumner J. Yaffe, M.D., Bethesda, MD

Panel on Pharmacy Practice

William F. Appel, D.Sc., Minneapolis, MN; Henry Cade, B.S., Chicago, IL; Herbert S. Carlin, D.Sc., Chappaqua, NY; Olya Duzey, M.S., Reed City, MI; Frances Hall Grogan, B.S., Wickliffe, KY; Ned Heltzer, M.S., Taos, NM; James E. Hosch, B.S., Kansas City, KS; Patricia A. Kramer, B.S., Bismarck, ND; Shirley P. McKee, B.S., Houston, TX; Thomas P. Reinders, Pharm.D., Richmond, VA; Lorie G. Rice, B.A., M.P.H., Sacramento, CA; Al Sebok, B.S., Twinsburg, OH; Stephen M. Sleight, M.S., Jackson, MS; William E. Smith, Pharm.D., M.P.H., Long Beach, CA; Thomas C. Snader, Pharm.D., Doylestown, PA; J. Richard Wuest, Pharm.D., Cincinnati, OH

Panel on Radiopharmaceuticals

Edward B. Silberstein, M.D., Cincinnati, OH; Neil M. Abel, M.B.A., M.S., Rockville, MD; William H. Briner, Capt., B.S., Durham, NC; Henry Chilton, Pharm.D., Winston-Salem, NC; Jan M. Ellerhorst-Ryan, R.N., M.S.N., C.S., Cincinnati, OH; Richard Holmes, M.D., Columbia, MO; William Kaplan, M.D., Boston, MA; David L. Laven, C.R.Ph., F.A.S.C.P., Bay Pines, FL; Merle K. Loken, M.D., Ph.D., Minneapolis, MN; Norman L. McElroy, M.A., Washington, DC; William B. Nelp, M.D., Seattle, WA; Buck A. Rhodes, Ph.D., Albuquerque, NM; Barry A. Siegel, M.D., St. Louis, MO; Guy Simmons, Ph.D., Lexington, KY; Dennis P. Swanson, R.Ph., M.S., Detroit, MI; David A. Weber, Ph.D., Upton, NY; Henry N. Wellman, M.D., Indianapolis, IN

Panel on Radiopharmaceuticals Standards

William H. Briner, Capt., B.S., Durham, NC; Jacqueline M. Calhoun, Gaithersburg, MD; Paul Early, Cleveland, OH

Panel on Sterility and Microbial Attributes

Murray S. Cooper, Ph.D., Islamarada, FL; Frank W. Adair, Ph.D., Summit, NJ; William C. Alegnani, Ph.D., Rochester, MI; R. Michael Enzinger, Ph.D., Kalamazoo, MI; Henry Jarocha, R.Ph., Rochester, NJ; Eugene A. Timm, Ph.D., Rochester, MI; C. Searle Wadley, North Chicago, IL

Panel on Sterilization Indicators

Virginia C. Ross, Silver Spring, MD; Henry L. Avallone, North Brunswick, NJ; David Bekus, Somerville, NJ; Robert Berube, Ph.D., St. Paul, MN; Frank B. Engley, Jr., Ph.D., Columbia, MO; Gary S. Graham, Ph.D., Erie, PA; Lois A. Jones, Research Triangle Park, NC; Karl Kereluk, Ph.D. (deceased), Rouses Point, NY; Ruth B. Kundsin, Sc.D., Boston, MA; Patrick McCormick, Ph.D., Rochester, NY; Gregg A. Mosley, Belgrade, MT; Theron E. Odlaug, Ph.D., Elkhart, IN; Gordon S. Oxborrow, Minneapolis, MN

Panel on Surgical Drugs and Devices

James W. Pate, M.D., Memphis, TN; C. Andrew Bassett, M.D., New York, NY; Terry Baumann, Pharm.D., Detroit, MI; Peter J. Fabri, M.D., Tampa, FL; Susan Bartlett Foote, J.D., Berkeley, CA; Jack Hirsh, M.D., Hamilton, Ontario, Canada; Larry R. Pilot, Esq., Washington, DC; Lary A. Robinson, M.D., Omaha, NE; H. Harlan Stone, M.D., Cleveland, OH; Clark Watts, M.D., Columbia, MO

Panel on Urology

Saul Boyarsky, M.D., St. Louis, MO; John Belis, M.D., Hershey, PA; Michael Boileau, M.D., Bend, OR; Culley C. Carson, M.D., Durham, NC; Warren Heston, Ph.D., New York, NY; Mark V. Jarowenko, M.D., Hershey, PA, Marguerite Lippert, M.D., Charlottesville, VA; Penelope A. Longhurst, Ph.D., Rockford, IL; Michael G. Mawhinney, Ph.D., Morgantown, WV; Harris Nagler, M.D., New York, NY; Randall H. Rowland, M.D., Ph.D., Indianapolis, IN; J. Patrick Spirnak, M.D., Cleveland, OH; William F. Tarry, M.D., Morgantown, WV; Alan J. Wein, M.D., Philadelphia, PA; Robert Weiss, M.D., New Haven, CT

Panel on Veterinary Medicine

Lloyd E. Davis, D.V.M., Ph.D., Urbana, IL; Arthur L. Aronson, D.V.M., Ph.D., Raleigh, NC; Nicholas H. Booth, D.V.M., Ph.D., Jacksonville, FL; Gordon L. Coppoc, D.V.M., Ph.D., West Lafayette, IN; George T. Edds, D.V.M., Ph.D., Waco, TX; Sidney A. Ewing, D.V.M., Ph.D., Stillwater, OK; Stuart D. Forney, M.S., Fort Collins, CO; William G. Huber, D.V.M., Blacksburg, VA; William L. Jenkins, D.V.M., Ph.D., College Station, TX; Robert W. Phillips, D.V.M., Ph.D., Fort Collins, CO; Thomas E. Powers, D.V.M., Ph.D., Columbus, OH; Charles R. Short, D.V.M., Ph.D., Baton Rouge, LA; Richard H. Teske, D.V.M., Rockville, MD; Jeffrey R. Wilcke, D.V.M., M.S., Blacksburg, VA

Drug Information Division
Additional Contributors

In addition to individuals, many schools, associations, pharmaceutical companies, and governmental agencies have provided comment or otherwise contributed to the development of USP DI.

Jonathan Abrams, M.D., Albuquerque, NM
John Ackerly, M.D., Ph.D., Charleston, SC
Lindsay Allen, Ph.D., Storrs, CT
Sherman Alter, M.D., Dayton, OH
Mason Andrews, M.D., Norfolk, VA
David P. Aucoin, Raleigh, NC
Rudolph Baer, M.D., New York, NY
Danial E. Baker, Pharm.D., Pullman, WA
Patsy Barnett, Pharm.D., Bay Pines, FL
Nunzio Barone, Vancouver, British Columbia, Canada
Robert W. Beightol, Pharm.D., Roanoke, VA
Reina Bejar, Miami Beach, FL
John Bennett, M.D., Bethesda, MD
Jack H. Bernstein, M.D., Dayton, OH
Karen Bertch, Pharm.D., Chicago, IL
Martin Black, M.D., Philadelphia, PA
Robert Blizzard, M.D., Charlottesville, VA
Rebecca E. Boehne, R.N., M.S.N., Portland, OR
H. Bone, M.D., Summit, NJ
Robert Borgatti, Jr., Vienna, VA
Robert Borgatti, Sr., Vienna, VA
Robert Braun, D.D.S., Buffalo, NY
Goodwin Breinin, M.D., New York, NY
Kenneth Bridges, M.D., Boston, MA
Benjamin R. Brooks, M.D., Madison, WI
Estela N. Brown, Miami, FL
Spencer Brudno, M.D., Augusta, GA
Ronald J. Callahan, Ph.D., Boston, MA
Col. Frank A. Cammarata, M.D., Falls Church, VA
Bruce Canaday, Pharm.D., Wilmington, NC
Kelli A. Caprile, Pharm.D., Baton Rouge, LA
Paul P. Carbone, M.D., Madison, WI
Albert A. Carr, M.D., Augusta, GA
M. Catalano, M.D., Summit, NJ
Kenneth R. Chapman, M.D., Toronto, Ontario, Canada
Alan Cheung, Pharm.D., M.P.H., Washington, DC
Allan Coates, M.D., Montreal, Quebec, Canada
Arthur Cocco, M.D., Baltimore, MD
Jay D. Coffman, M.D., Boston, MA
Betsy J. Cooper, M.D., Falls Church, VA
Clinton N. Corder, Ph.D., M.D., Oklahoma City, OK
Fred F. Cowan, Ph.D., Portland, OR
Joseph W. Cranston, Ph.D., Chicago, IL
William F. Crowley, M.D., Boston, MA
Josephine S. Daigle, Ph.D., New Orleans, LA
Ernest A. Daigneault, M.D., Johnson City, TN
Terry Davies, M.D., New York, NY
Carol A. Davis, M.D., Urbana, IL
Robin L. Davis, Pharm.D., Albuquerque, NM
Thomas D. DeCillis, North Port, FL
B. L. Decker, M.D., Townshend, VT
David Decker, M.D., Troy, MI
Olga DeTorres, Pharm.D., Chicago, IL
Virgil Dias, Pharm.D., Kansas City, MO
Richard P. Dickey, M.D., Ph.D., New Orleans, LA
Joyce Dienger, R.N., B.S.N., Cincinnati, OH
C. A. DiFazio, M.D., Charlottesville, VA

Nicholay Dimitrov, M.D., East Lansing, MI
Thomas R. Dirksen, D.D.S., Ph.D., Augusta, GA
L. Dolan, M.D., Cincinnati, OH
F. Douglas, M.D., Ph.D., Summit, NJ
Fritz Dreifuss, M.D., Charlottesville, VA
William Duncan, M.D., Ph.D., Washington, DC
Jacob Eisen, R.Ph., Mountainside, NJ
Rhonda Eldridge, Connersville, IN
Marc Ernstoff, M.D., Pittsburgh, PA
P. Etienne, Ph.D., Summit, NJ
Paula Eugenio, R.Ph., Taunton, MA
R. Mark Evans, Ph.D., Chicago, IL
Donald A. Falace, D.D.S., Lexington, KY
Linda Felver, M.A., R.N., Sedro Woolley, WA
James R. Fenno, R.Ph., Chippewa Falls, WI
Robert Feroli, Baltimore, MD
Anne Feuer, B.S., Cincinnati, OH
Melanie A. Fisher, M.D., Morgantown, WV
Greg C. Flaker, M.D., Columbia, MO
William Foye, Boston, MA
Robert Fragen, M.D., Chicago, IL
Michael M. Frank, M.D., Bethesda, MD
Carl J. Friedman, M.D., Philadelphia, PA
William H. Frishman, M.D., Scarsdale, NY
J. Gallardo, Iowa City, IA
Lawrence A. Gans, M.D., St. Louis, MO
Margery Garbin, R.N., Ph.D., New York, NY
Daniel E. Garcia, R.Ph., Houston, TX
Janice A. Gaska, Pharm.D., Philadelphia, PA
Winston Gaum, M.D., Cincinnati, OH
Barbara George, M.D., Los Angeles, CA
Ray W. Gifford, Jr., M.D., Cleveland, OH
Robert L. Gold, M.D., Worcester, MA
David Goldstein, M.D., Durham, NC
Cpt. John D. Grabenstein, R.Ph., Bremerhaven, West
  Germany
Allan M. Greenspan, M.D., Philadelphia, PA
Donald L. Greer, Ph.D., New Orleans, LA
Donald P. Griffith, M.D., Houston, TX
Jack S. Gruber, M.D., Dayton, OH
Melvin Grumbach, M.D., San Francisco, CA
Luz M. Gutiérrez, Ph.D., San Juan, PR
Nortin M. Hadler, M.D., Chapel Hill, NC
H. Hakkarainen, M.D., Summit, NJ
Richard E. Hall, D.D.S., Ph.D., Buffalo, NY
Thomas G. Hall, Pharm.D., Iowa City, IA
George W. Hambrick, Jr., M.D., New York, NY
Philip Hanno, M.D., Philadelphia, PA
David Hannon, M.D., Cincinnati, OH
John P. Hanson, Jr., M.D., Milwaukee, WI
Jerry M. Hartleip, Waterloo, IA
Edward A. Hartshorn, Ph.D., Charleston, SC
Patricia Hausman, M.S., Silver Spring, MD
Maria Hayes, M.D., Detroit, MI
David L. Helgeland, R.Ph., Yankton, SD
William M. Henderson, Ph.D., Fargo, ND
M. Henis, M.D., Summit, NJ

Victor Herbert, M.D., J.D., Bronx, NY
Freya Hermann, M.S., Corvallis, OR
William Hines, R.Ph., M.S., Washington, DC
Raymond Hintz, M.D., Stanford, CA
M. E. Hoar, M.S., Springfield, MA
William Hoffman, M.D., Augusta, GA
Albert F. Holthuis, Winnipeg, Manitoba, Canada
William A. Hopkins, Jr., Pharm.D., Atlanta, GA
Nancy Hoskins, B.S., Cincinnati, OH
Peter C. Hoyle, Ph.D., Point of Rocks, MD
Mary H. Huett, Hattiesburg, MS
Thomas A. Huff, M.D., Augusta, GA
Bess Hughes, M.D., Boston, MA
William A. Humphrey, Memphis, TN
Christina Israel, Pharm.D., Richmond, VA
Marc K. Israel, Pharm.D., Hampton, VA
Laurence S. Jacobs, M.D., Rochester, NY
Robert M. Jacobson, M.D., Carville, LA
Kenneth M. James, Ph.D., Halifax, Nova Scotia, Canada
Ann L. Janer, M.S., Auburn, AL
Michael W. Jann, Pharm.D., San Antonio, TX
M. J. Javid, M.D., Madison, WI
James W. Jefferson, M.D., Madison, WI
John Jenne, M.D., Hines, IL
Peter Jewesson, Ph.D., Vancouver, British Columbia, Canada
Marcus Jordin, Ph.D., Little Rock, AR
Hugh F. Kabat, Ph.D., Albuquerque, NM
Vicky Kahiwat, M.D., Brooklyn, NY
Selna Kaplan, M.D., San Francisco, CA
George H. Karam, M.D., New Orleans, LA
R. Kartzinel, M.D., Summit, NJ
Carol Kasper, M.D., Los Angeles, CA
Michael A. Kass, M.D., St. Louis, MO
Michael Katz, M.D., New York, NY
John J. Kavanagh, M.D., Tampa, FL
R. Allen Kayser, Jr., M.D., Huntington, WV
Susan Kelley, M.D., New Haven, CT
Charles P. Kellner, M.D., Charleston, SC
N. D. Kennedy, Easton, MD
Kimberly Kill, St. Louis, MO
William D. King, B.S., Birmingham, AL
Rachel Kleiman-Wexler, Iowa City, IA
Juha Kokko, M.D., Atlanta, GA
Mary Ellen Kosman, Ph.D., Chicago, IL
Edward Krenzelok, Pharm.D., Pittsburgh, PA
Robert Krigel, M.D., Philadelphia, PA
Paul B. Kuehn, Ph.D., Woodinville, WA
Ming-Liang Lai, M.D., Charleston, SC
Kenneth F. Lampe, Ph.D., Chicago, IL
Karen Landsberg, Vancouver, British Columbia, Canada
Robert Larsen, M.D., Los Angeles, CA
Robert A. Larson, M.D., Los Angeles, CA
Elliott Lasser, M.D., San Diego, CA
John Laszlo, M.D., New York, NY
Leo B. Lathroum, Ph.D., San Juan, PR
Francis E. LeBlanc, M.D., Ph.D., Calgary, Alberta, Canada
Mark Lebwohl, M.D., New York, NY
J. Lee, M.D., Summit, NJ
Mary Lee, Pharm.D., Chicago, IL
Jerold Lerman, M.D., Toronto, Ontario, Canada
Leonard J. Lerner, Ph.D., Philadelphia, PA
Fidelita Levy, Fort Mead, SD
Michael Levy, M.D., Ph.D., Philadelphia, PA
Mary Jane Lewis, R.Ph., M.S., Bay Pines, FL
Charles Liebow, D.M.D., Ph.D., Buffalo, NY
Anne Lin, Pharm.D., Whitestone, NY
Michael D. Lockshin, M.D., New York, NY
Dan L. Longo, M.D., Frederick, MD
Larry M. Lopez, Pharm.D., Gainesville, FL
Nicholas J. Lowe, M.D., Los Angeles, CA
Tom F. Lue, M.D., San Francisco, CA
Jeanne Lusher, M.D., Detroit, MI

Paul Magalian, R.Ph., Ph.D., North Miami Beach, FL
Howard I. Maibach, M.D., San Francisco, CA
Claude Mailhot, Montreal, Quebec, Canada
Dennis G. Maki, M.D., Madison, WI
Frank Marcus, M.D., Tucson, AZ
Domingo R. Martinez, Birmingham, AL
Mirza D. Martínez, Ph.D., San Juan, PR
Ralph Mastrocola, D.D.S., Buffalo, NY
Richard Matthay, M.D., New Haven, CT
Alice J. Matuszak, Ph.D., Stockton, CA
Harry R. Maxon, III, M.D., Cincinnati, OH
Christiane Mayer, Boucherville, Quebec, Canada
John N. McCormick, Memphis, TN
J. McCullough, Ph.D., Summit, NJ
M. McNab, M.D., Summit, NJ
Rafaela Mena de Giraldi, San Juan, PR
Angela Meyer, Point Pleasant, NJ
John Patrick Mihelic, R.Ph., Shawnee, KS
Penny Miller, Vancouver, British Columbia, Canada
Gladys Miró de Rivera, San Juan, PR
Charles Moertel, M.D., Rochester, MN
Gilles Monif, M.D., Omaha, NE
Gayle Monnig, R.N., M.S.N., San Antonio, TX
H. Morris, M.D., Summit, NJ
John J. Mulcahy, M.D., Ph.D., Indianapolis, IN
K. Mullane, Ph.D., Summit, NJ
William J. Murray, M.D., Ph.D., Durham, NC
Robert Nakagawa, Vancouver, British Columbia, Canada
Robert P. Nelson, Jr., M.D., Charleston, SC
Eugene J. Nordby, M.D., Madison, WI
Gary M. Oderda, Pharm.D., Baltimore, MD
H. Oei, Ph.D., Summit, NJ
Richard I. Ogilvie, M.D., Toronto, Ontario, Canada
Richard M. Oksas, Pharm.D., Torrance, CA
Karen S. Oles, Pharm.D., Winston-Salem, NC
Gretchen Oley, M.D., Huntington, WV
James R. Oster, M.D., Miami, FL
Judith Ozbun, R.Ph., M.S., Fargo, ND
Henry A. Palmer, Ph.D., Storrs, CT
A. Patterson, Pharm.D., Cincinnati, OH
Albert Patterson, Milwaukee, WI
Angela I. Pérez, Ph.D., San Juan, PR
Georges Peter, M.D., Providence, RI
Marie Pineau, B.Pharm., D.P.H., Montreal, Quebec, Canada
Carl Pinsky, Frederick, MD
Philip A. Pizzo, M.D., Bethesda, MD
Philip A. Podrid, M.D. Boston, MA
Therese Poirier, Pharm.D., Pittsburgh, PA
Lynn Pollock, Vancouver, British Columbia, Canada
James Ponto, R.Ph., Iowa City, IA
Steven I. Present, D.D.S., Meadowbrook, PA
Carol M. Proudfit, Ph.D., Chicago, IL
Carol B. Pugh, Pharm.D., Philadelphia, PA
F. Quagliata, M.D., Summit, NJ
Cynthia Raehl, Pharm.D., Madison, WI
Jeffrey Ramirez, Pharm.D., Washington, DC
Nixa Ramos, Manatí, PR
Norbert P. Rapoza, Ph.D., Chicago, IL
Peter A. Ratto, Ph.D., Weatherford, OK
Anthony Reback, M.D., Toronto, Ontario, Canada
Terry D. Rees, D.D.S., M.S.D., Dallas, TX
Robert M. Refowitz, M.D., Ph.D., New York, NY
Jeffrey A. Reitz, Pharm.D., Columbus, OH
Alfred J. Remillard, Pharm.D., Saskatoon, Saskatchewan, Canada
Marilyn Resurreccion, M.D., Brooklyn, NY
Joseph G. Reves, M.D., Durham, NC
L. Ribeiro, M.D., Summit, NJ
Jim E. Riviere, Raleigh, NC
Daniel Robinson, Pharm.D., Los Angeles, CA
Donald S. Robinson, M.D., Wallingford, CT
Ian M. Rollo, Ph.D., Winnipeg, Manitoba, Canada

Headquarters Staff

DRUG INFORMATION DIVISION

KEITH W. JOHNSON, *Director, Research and Development*

Senior Pharmacy Associates:
GEORGIE M. CATHEY (Pharmacy Staff Coordinator)
ESTHER KLEIN

Pharmacy Associates:
NANCY L. DASHIELL
WANDA J. JANICKI
ANGELA MÉNDEZ MAYO (Spanish Publications Coordinator)
BENJAMÍN PÉREZ-DEGRACIA

Pharmacy Consultants:
SANDRA LEE BOYER
GORDON K. WURSTER

Publications Development:
DIANA M. BLAIS (Coordinator)
DOROTHY RAYMOND

Medical Information Specialist:
MARTHA A. D. WOLLAM

Editorial Consultant:
JOHN MORRIS

Office Staff:
LANETTE FLEMING
MICHELINE TRANQUILLE

DRUG STANDARDS DIVISION

LEE T. GRADY, *Director*

Assistant Directors:
CHARLES H. BARNSTEIN (Revision)
ROBERT H. KING (Technical Support)

Senior Scientists:
ROGER DABBAH
AUBREY S. OUTSCHOORN (Ret.)
WILLIAM W. WRIGHT

Scientists:
JOSEPH J. BELSON
FATIMA N. JOHNSON
V. SRINIVASAN

Senior Scientific Associates:
BARBARA B. HUBERT
LARRY W. PAUL
EDGAR E. THEIMER

Hazard Communications:
ROBERT C. MOORE (Coordinator)
DANNY B. BAKER
KIM MARTINELLI

Office Staff:
ANN K. FERGUSON
THERESA H. LEE

PUBLICATION SERVICES

MARY C. GRIFFITHS, *Director*

Managing Editor, USP DI:
A. V. PRECUP

Editorial Associates:
MARGARET C. AVERY
NANCY E. FARLEY
CAROL M. GRIFFIN
ELIZABETH C. HOROWITZ
ELLEN R. LOEB

Database Management:
LINDA S. McCARTY

Typesetters:
DEBORAH R. CONNELLY
JANE D. RIGHTER

Typesetting Systems Coordinator:
JEAN E. DALE

Graphics Coordinator:
GAIL M. ORING

Also Contributing: Emmy Kolodny and Melissa Smith, Proofreaders; Diane Visceglia, Indexing; Tia Calomeris, Graphics.

Managing Editor, USP-NF:
PATRICIA H. MORGENSTERN

Editorial Associates:
JESUSA D. CORDOVA
CAROLYN A. FLEEGER
MARILYN B. GENTHER
SUZANNE LASSANDRO

Typesetter:
MARIE MICKLE

USPC ADMINISTRATIVE STAFF

WILLIAM M. HELLER, Executive Director
WENDY M. AUSTIN
ALICE E. KIMBALL
SALVATORE A. SALEME
J. ROBERT STRANG
JOSEPH G. VALENTINO

Members of the United States Pharmacopeial Convention and the Institutions and Organizations Represented as of July 1, 1987

Current Officers and Board of Trustees

President: Arthur Hull Hayes, Jr., M.D.,* President and Chief Executive Officer, EM Industries, Inc., 5 Skyline Drive, Hawthorne, NY 10532

Vice President: Joseph M. Benforado, M.D.,* 730 Seneca Place, Madison, WI 53711

Past President: Frederick E. Shideman, M.D., Ph.D.,* Department of Pharmacology, 3-260 Millard Hall, University of Minnesota, 435 Delaware Street, S.E., Minneapolis, MN 55455

Treasurer: Paul F. Parker, D.Sc.,* 917 Celia Lane, Lexington, KY 40504

Representing Medicine: J. Richard Crout, M.D.,* Boehringer Mannheim Corporation, 1301 Piccard Drive, Rockville, MD 20850
Leo E. Hollister, M.D., 5100 San Felipe Boulevard #393, West Houston, TX 77056

Representing Pharmacy: Joseph P. Buckley, Ph.D.,* College of Pharmacy, 141 SR2, University of Houston, 4800 Calhoun, Houston, TX 77004
James T. Doluisio, Ph.D.,* College of Pharmacy, University of Texas at Austin, Austin, TX 78712

Public Member: Estelle G. Cohen, M.A.* 5813 Greenspring Avenue, Baltimore, MD 21209

At Large: John V. Bergen, Ph.D.,* National Committee for Clinical Laboratory Standards, 771 E. Lancaster Avenue, Villanova, PA 19085
John T. Fay, Jr., Ph.D.,* Bergen Brunswig Corporation, 4000 Metropolitan Drive, Orange, CA 92668

Executive Director and Secretary: William M. Heller, Ph.D.,* 12601 Twinbrook Parkway, Rockville, MD 20852

United States Government Services

Food and Drug Administration: Peter H. Rheinstein, M.D., J.D.,* Director, Office of Drug Standards, Center for Drugs and Biologics, 5600 Fishers Lane, HFN-200, Rockville, MD 20857

National Bureau of Standards: Stanley D. Rasberry,* Chemistry, B311, National Bureau of Standards, Gaithersburg, MD 20899

Office of the Chief of Naval Operations, U.S. Navy: Robert D. Tackitt, Captain,* Medical Services Corp, U.S. Navy, Defense Personnel Support Center, Attn: DPSC-RS, 2800 S. 20th Street, Philadelphia, PA 19101

Office of the Surgeon General, U.S. Air Force: Lt. Col. John M. Hammond,* USAF/SCB, Bolling AFB, DC 20332

United States Public Health Service: Richard R. Ashbaugh,* 18413 Queen Elizabeth Drive, Olney, MD 20832

U.S. Office of Consumer Affairs: Robert F. Steeves, J.D.,* Dep. Spec. Adv. to the President for Consumer Affairs, 1725 I Street, N.W., Suite 1003, Washington, DC 20201

Veterans Administration, Central Office: Stephen M. Sleight, M.Sc.,* Director of Pharmacy Services, Pharmacy Service (119), Jackson Veterans Administration Medical Center, Jackson, MS 39216

National Organizations

American Chemical Society: Samuel M. Tuthill, Ph.D.,* Mallinckrodt, Inc., Mallinckrodt and Second Streets, St. Louis, MO 63147

American Dental Association: Edgar W. Mitchell, Ph.D.,* American Dental Association, 211 E. Chicago Avenue, Chicago, IL 60611

American Hospital Association: William R. Reid, Community Hospital of Roanoke Valley, 101 Elm Avenue, S.E., Box 12946, Roanoke, VA 24029

American Medical Association: John C. Ballin, Ph.D.,* American Medical Association, 535 N. Dearborn Street, Chicago, IL 60610

American Nurses' Association, Inc.: Jean Marshall, B.A., R.N.,* Employee Relations Coordinator, Paul Kimball Hospital, 600 River Avenue, Lakewood, NJ 08701

American Pharmaceutical Association: John F. Schlegel, Pharm.D.,* President, American Pharmaceutical Association, 2215 Constitution Avenue, N.W., Washington, DC 20037

American Society for Clinical Pharmacology & Therapeutics: William B. Abrams, M.D.,* Merck Sharp & Dohme Research Laboratories, West Point, PA 19486

American Society of Hospital Pharmacists: R. David Anderson,* Director of Pharmacy Services, Waynesboro Community Hospital, 501 Oak Avenue, Waynesboro, VA 22980

American Society for Pharmacology & Experimental Therapeutics: Marilyn E. Hess, Ph.D.,* School of Medicine, University of Pennsylvania, Philadelphia, PA 19104

American Society for Quality Control: Theodore C. Fleming,* 7125 Monterrey Drive, Fort Worth, TX 76112

American Veterinary Medical Association: L. Meyer Jones, D.V.M., Ph.D.,* 1225 St. Andrews Drive, Pinehurst, NC 28374

Association of Food and Drug Officials: David R. Work, J.D.,* Executive Director, North Carolina State Board of Pharmacy, P. O. Box H, Carrboro, NC 27510

Association of Official Analytical Chemists: James B. Kottemann,* Food and Drug Administration, 200 C Street, S.W., HFN-004, Washington, DC 20204

Chemical Manufacturers Association: Andrew J. Schmitz, Jr.,* Pfizer, Inc., 235 East 42nd Street, New York, NY 10017

Cosmetic, Toiletry & Fragrance Association, Inc.: Richard M. Bednarz, Cosmetic, Toiletry & Fragrance Association, Inc., 1110 Vermont Avenue, N.W., Suite 800, Washington, DC 20005

Health Industry Manufacturers Association: James F. Jorkasky, Director,* Manufacturing & Quality Programs, Health Industry Manufacturers Association, 1030 15th Street, N.W., Washington, DC 20005

National Association of Boards of Pharmacy: Fred T. Mahaffey, D.Sc.,* Executive Director, National Association of Boards of Pharmacy, O'Hare Corporate Center, 1300 Higgins Road, Suite 103, Park Ridge, IL 60068

National Association of Chain Drug Stores, Inc.: Donald Bell,* Thrift Drug Company, 615 Alpha Drive, Pittsburgh, PA 15230

National Association of Retail Druggists: William N. Tindall, Ph.D.,* 205 Daingerfield Road, Alexandria, VA 22314

National Wholesale Druggists' Association: Ronald J. Streck, Vice President,* Government Affairs, National Wholesale Druggists' Association, 105 Oronoco Street, P. O. Box 238, Alexandria, VA 22313

Parenteral Drug Association, Inc.: Sol Motola, Ph.D.,* Bausch & Lomb, Personal Products Division, 1400 North Goodman Street, Rochester, NY 14692

Pharmaceutical Manufacturers Association: John Jennings, M.D.,* Pharmaceutical Manufacturers Association, 1100 Fifteenth Street, N.W., Washington, DC 20005

The Proprietary Association: R. William Soller, Ph.D.,* Vice President, Scientific Affairs, The Proprietary Association, 1150 Connecticut Avenue, N.W. Washington, DC 20036

Other Organizations and Institutions

ALABAMA

University of Alabama, School of Medicine: Robert B. Diasio, M.D.,* School of Medicine, University of Alabama, Birmingham, AL 35294

Auburn University, School of Pharmacy: Kenneth N. Barker, Ph.D.,* Department of Pharmacy Care Systems, School of Pharmacy, Auburn University, Auburn, AL 36849

Samford University, School of Pharmacy: Stanley V. Susina, Ph.D.,* School of Pharmacy, Samford University, 800 Lakeshore Drive, Birmingham, AL 35229

Medical Association of the State of Alabama: Paul A. Palmisano, M.D.,* Professor of Pediatrics, University of Alabama in Birmingham, University Station, Birmingham, AL 35294

---

*Present at the 1985 Quinquennial Meeting.

ALASKA

Alaska Pharmaceutical Association: Jacqueline L. Warren, 2200 Chinook, Anchorage, AK 99516

ARIZONA

University of Arizona, College of Medicine: Kenneth A. Conrad, M.D., Department of Internal Medicine, College of Medicine, University of Arizona, 1501 North Campbell Avenue, Tucson, AZ 85724

University of Arizona, College of Pharmacy: Samuel H. Yalkowsky, Ph.D.,* College of Pharmacy, University of Arizona, Tucson, AZ 85721

Arizona Pharmacy Association: Richard J. Hammel, Ph.D.,* 8110 E. Del Tiburon Drive, Scottsdale, AZ 85258

ARKANSAS

University of Arkansas for Medical Sciences, College of Medicine: James E. Doherty, III, M.D., VA Hospital, 4300 West 7th Street, Little Rock, AR 72205

University of Arkansas for Medical Sciences, College of Pharmacy: James R. McCowan, Ph.D., College of Pharmacy, University of Arkansas for Medical Sciences, 4301 W. Markham Street, Slot 522, Little Rock, AR 72205

Arkansas Pharmacists Association: Marcus W. Jordin, Ph.D.,* 309 Brookside Drive, Little Rock, AR 72205

CALIFORNIA

University of California, Davis, School of Medicine: Larry Stark, Ph.D.,* Department of Pharmacology, School of Medicine, University of California, Davis, CA 95616

University of California, Los Angeles, School of Medicine: Don H. Catlin,* Department of Pharmacology, School of Medicine, CHS, University of California, Los Angeles, CA 90024

University of California, San Francisco, School of Medicine: Walter L. Way, M.D.,* Department of Anesthesia, Rm. S-436, University of California, San Francisco, CA 94143

University of California, San Francisco, School of Pharmacy: Jack Cooper, Ph.D.,* School of Pharmacy, University of California, San Francisco, CA 94143

University of Southern California, School of Pharmacy: Robert T. Koda, Pharm.D., Ph.D.,* School of Pharmacy, University of Southern California, 1985 Zonal Avenue, Los Angeles, CA 90033

University of the Pacific, School of Pharmacy: Alice Jean Matuszak, Ph.D., 751 Brookside Road, Stockton, CA 95207

Loma Linda University, School of Medicine: Ralph E. Cutler, M.D.,* Department of Medicine, Loma Linda School of Medicine, Anderson and Barton, Loma Linda, CA 92354

California Pharmacists Association: Max Stollman,* 8314 Wilshire Boulevard, Beverly Hills, CA 90211

COLORADO

University of Colorado, School of Pharmacy: Duane C. Bloedow, Ph.D.,* 3630 Silver Plume Lane, Boulder, CO 80303

Colorado Pharmacal Association: Thomas G. Arthur,* 9852 Corsair Drive, Conifer, CO 80433

CONNECTICUT

University of Connecticut, School of Medicine: Paul F. Davern,* Director of Pharmacy, University of Connecticut Health Center, 261 Farmington Avenue, Farmington, CT 06032

University of Connecticut, School of Pharmacy: Max W. Miller, Ph.D.,* School of Pharmacy, University of Connecticut, Storrs, CT 06268

Connecticut Pharmaceutical Association: Henry A. Palmer, Ph.D.,* 26 Timber Drive, Storrs, CT 06268

Connecticut State Medical Society: James E. O'Brien, M.D., 31 Surrey Drive, Wethersfield, CT 06109

DELAWARE

Delaware Pharmaceutical Society: Hazen L. Richardson, Biomedical Products Department, DuPont, Barley Mill Plaza, Building #25, Wilmington, DE 19898

Medical Society of Delaware: Jeffry I. Komins, M.D.,* 2323 Pennsylvania Avenue, Wilmington, DE 19806

DISTRICT OF COLUMBIA

Georgetown University, School of Medicine: Arthur Raines, Ph.D., 3900 Reservoir Road, N.W., Washington, DC 20007

Howard University, College of Medicine: Robert E. Taylor, M.D., Ph.D., Department of Medicine, Howard University Hospital, 2041 Georgia Avenue, N.W., Washington, DC 20060

Howard University, College of Pharmacy & Pharmacal Sciences: Wendell T. Hill, Jr., Pharm.D.,* 2300 Fourth Street, N.W., Washington, DC 20059

Medical Society of the District of Columbia: Michael D. Abramowitz, M.D.,* 111 Michigan Avenue, N.W., Washington, DC 20010

FLORIDA

Florida A & M University, College of Pharmacy and Pharmaceutical Sciences: Henry Lewis, III, Pharm.D.,* College of Pharmacy and Pharmaceutical Sciences, Florida A & M University, Tallahassee, FL 32307

University of Florida, College of Medicine: Thomas F. Muther, Ph.D.,* Department of Pharmacology & Therapeutics, College of Medicine, University of Florida, Box J-267, J. Hillis Miller Health Center, Gainesville, FL 32610

University of Florida, College of Pharmacy: Michael A. Schwartz, Ph.D.,* Box J-4, J. Hillis Miller Health Center, Gainesville, FL 32610

University of South Florida, College of Medicine: Joseph J. Krzanowski, Jr., Ph.D.,* 12901 N. 30th Street, Box 9, Tampa, FL 33612

Florida Pharmacy Association: George Browning,* 8552 Sylvan Drive, Melbourne, FL 32901

GEORGIA

Medical College of Georgia, School of Medicine: Merle W. Riley, Ph.D.,* Department of Pharmacology & Toxicology, Medical College of Georgia, 1120 Fifteenth Street, Augusta, GA 30912

Mercer University, Southern School of Pharmacy: A. Vincent Lopez, Ph.D.,* Southern School of Pharmacy, Mercer University, 345 Boulevard, N.E., Atlanta, GA 30312

Morehouse School of Medicine: Ralph W. Trottier, Ph.D.,* Morehouse School of Medicine, 720 Westview Drive, S.W., Atlanta, GA 30310

University of Georgia, College of Pharmacy: Howard C. Ansel, Ph.D.,* Dean, College of Pharmacy, University of Georgia, Athens, GA 30602

Georgia Pharmaceutical Association: Charles L. Braucher, Ph.D., College of Pharmacy, University of Georgia, Athens, GA 30602

Medical Association of Georgia: E. D. Bransome, Jr., M.D.,* Professor of Medicine, Medical College of Georgia, Augusta, GA 30912

IDAHO

Idaho State University, College of Pharmacy: Eugene I. Isaacson, Ph.D.,* 1619 East Terry, Pocatello, ID 83201

ILLINOIS

Chicago Medical School/University of Health Sciences: Seymour Ehrenpreis, Ph.D.,* Department of Pharmacology, University of Health Sciences/The Chicago Medical School, 3333 N. Green Bay Road, N. Chicago, IL 60064

Southern Illinois University, School of Medicine: Ronald A. Browning, Ph.D.,* Department of Medical Physiology and Pharmacology, Southern Illinois University School of Medicine, Carbondale, IL 62901

University of Illinois, College of Medicine: Marten M. Kernis, Ph.D., College of Medicine, University of Illinois, 1853 West Polk Street, 131 CMW (M/C 784), Chicago, IL 60612

University of Illinois, College of Pharmacy: Martin I. Blake, Ph.D.,* 9023 Kenton Avenue, Skokie, IL 60076

Illinois Pharmacists Association: Ronald W. Gottrich,* 3161 Elmhurst, Springfield, IL 62704

Illinois State Medical Society: Vincent A. Costanzo, Jr., M.D.,* 18304 Maple, Lansing, IL 60438

INDIANA

Butler University, College of Pharmacy: Margaret A. Shaw, Ph.D.,* College of Pharmacy, Butler University, 4600 Sunset Avenue, Indianapolis, IN 46208

Indiana University, School of Medicine: George R. Aronoff, M.D., Department of Medicine, Indiana University, School of Medicine, 1120 South Drive, Fesler Hall 108, Indianapolis, IN 46223

Purdue University, School of Pharmacy and Pharmacal Sciences: Adelbert M. Knevel, Ph.D.,* School of Pharmacy & Pharmacal Sciences, Purdue University, West Lafayette, IN 47907

Indiana State Medical Association: Edward Langston, M.D., 203 North Division, Flora, IN 46924

IOWA

Drake University, College of Pharmacy: Wendell Southard, Ph.D.,* College of Pharmacy, Drake University, Des Moines, IA 50311

---

*Present at the 1985 Quinquennial Meeting.

University of Iowa, College of Pharmacy: Robert A. Wiley, Ph.D.,* Dean, College of Pharmacy, University of Iowa, Iowa City, IA 52242

Iowa Pharmacists Association: Robert Osterhaus,* 124 S. Main, Maquoketa, IA 52060

KANSAS

University of Kansas, School of Medicine: Edward J. Walaszek, Ph.D.,* School of Medicine, University of Kansas Medical Center, 39th and Rainbow Boulevard, Kansas City, KS 66103

University of Kansas, School of Pharmacy: Siegfried Lindenbaum, Ph.D.,* 1025 Holiday Drive, Lawrence, KS 66044

Kansas Pharmacists Association: John Owen,* 1202 Eastmoor, Wichita, KS 67207

KENTUCKY

University of Kentucky, College of Pharmacy: Patrick P. DeLuca, Ph.D.,* 3292 Nantucket Drive, Lexington, KY 40502

University of Louisville, School of Medicine: Peter P. Rowell, Ph.D.,* Department of Pharmacology & Toxicology, School of Medicine, University of Louisville, Louisville, KY 40292

Kentucky Medical Association: Ellsworth C. Seeley, M.D.,* 820 South Limestone, Annex 4, Lexington, KY 40536

Kentucky Pharmacists Association: Chester L. Parker, Pharm.D.,* 1816 Darien Drive, Lexington, KY 40504

LOUISIANA

Northeast Louisiana University, School of Pharmacy: Robert D. Kee, Ph.D.,* Turtledove Drive, Monroe, LA 71203

Tulane University, School of Medicine: Floyd R. Domer, Ph.D.,* Department of Pharmacology, School of Medicine, Tulane University, 1430 Tulane Avenue, New Orleans, LA 70112

Xavier University of Louisiana, College of Pharmacy: Josephine Daigle, Ph.D.,* 7325 Palmetto Street, New Orleans, LA 70125

Louisiana Pharmacists Association: William G. Day,* 13114 Country Manor, Baton Rouge, LA 70816

Louisiana State Medical Society: John Adriani, M.D.,* 67 N. Park Place, New Orleans, LA 70124

MARYLAND

Johns Hopkins University, School of Medicine: E. Robert Feroli, Pharm.D.,* Johns Hopkins Hospital, 600 N. Wolfe Street (526 Osler), Baltimore, MD 21205

Uniformed Services University of the Health Sciences, F. Edward Hebert School of Medicine: Jeffrey D. Lazar, M.D., Department of Pharmacology, USUHS, 4301 Jones Bridge Road, Bethesda, MD 20814

University of Maryland, School of Medicine: James I. Hudson, M.D.,* Dean's Office, School of Medicine, University of Maryland, 655 W. Baltimore Street, Baltimore, MD 21201

University of Maryland, School of Pharmacy: Larry L. Augsburger, Ph.D.,* 20 North Pine Street, Baltimore, MD 21201

Maryland Pharmacists Association: Paul Freiman,* 7405 Monita Road, Baltimore, MD 21208

MASSACHUSETTS

Boston University, School of Medicine: Edward W. Pelikan, M.D.,* Department of Pharmacology, Boston University School of Medicine, 80 East Concord Street, Boston, MA 02118

Harvard Medical School: Peter Goldman, M.D., Harvard Medical School, 25 Shattuck Street, Boston, MA 02115

Massachusetts College of Pharmacy & Allied Health Sciences: William O. Foye, Ph.D.,* 179 Longwood Avenue, Boston, MA 02115

Northeastern University, College of Pharmacy and Allied Health Professions: Larry N. Swanson, Pharm.D.,* 124 Cobble Hill Road, Warwick, RI 02886

University of Massachusetts Medical School: Brian Johnson, M.D.,* University of Massachusetts Medical Center, 55 Lake Avenue, North, Worcester, MA 01605

Massachusetts Medical Society: Edward J. Khantzian, M.D., Cambridge Hospital, 1493 Cambridge Street, Cambridge, MA 02139

Massachusetts State Pharmaceutical Association: Bertram A. Nicholas, M.Sc.,* 179 Longwood Avenue, Boston, MA 02115

MICHIGAN

Ferris State College, School of Pharmacy: Gerald W. A. Slywka, Ph.D.,* 7630 Crestview Drive, Reed City, MI 49677

University of Michigan, College of Pharmacy: Ara G. Paul, Ph.D., Dean, College of Pharmacy, University of Michigan, Ann Arbor, MI 48109-1065

Wayne State University, College of Pharmacy and Allied Health Professions: Martin Barr, Ph.D., Dean, College of Pharmacy and Allied Health Professions, Wayne State University, 105 Health Sciences Building, Detroit, MI 48201

Wayne State University, School of Medicine: Ralph E. Kauffman, M.D.,* 3901 Beaubien, Detroit, MI 48201

Michigan Pharmacists Association: Salvador Pancorbo, Ph.D., Pharm.D.,* College of Pharmacy & Allied Health Professions, Wayne State University, Detroit, MI 48202

MINNESOTA

University of Minnesota, College of Pharmacy: Edward G. Rippie, Ph.D.,* 2 N. Mallard Road, St. Paul, MN 55110

University of Minnesota Medical School, Minneapolis: Jack W. Miller, Ph.D.,* University of Minnesota Medical School, 3-260 Millard Hall, 435 Delaware Street, S.E., Minneapolis, MN 55455

Minnesota State Pharmaceutical Association: Arnold D. Delger,* 1533 Grantham Street, St. Paul, MN 55108

MISSISSIPPI

University of Mississippi, School of Medicine: Richard L. Klein, Ph.D.,* Department of Pharmacology & Toxicology, University of Mississippi Medical Center, Jackson, MS 39216-4504

University of Mississippi, School of Pharmacy: Robert W. Cleary, Ph.D.,* Department of Pharmaceutics, University of Mississippi, University, MS 38677

Mississippi Pharmacists Association: Phylliss M. Moret,* Mississippi Pharmacists Association, 401 E. Capitol Street, Suite 504, Jackson, MS 39201

MISSOURI

St. Louis College of Pharmacy: John W. Zuzack, Ph.D.,* St. Louis College of Pharmacy, 4588 Parkview Place, St. Louis, MO 63110

St. Louis University, School of Medicine: Alvin H. Gold, Ph.D.,* 1402 S. Grand Boulevard, St. Louis, MO 63104

University of Missouri, Columbia, School of Medicine: John W. Yarbro, M.D., Ph.D.,* N408 Health Sciences Center, Columbia, MO 65212

University of Missouri, Kansas City, School of Medicine: David Rush, Pharm.D.,* Truman Medical Center-East, Little Blue & Lee's Summit Roads, Kansas City, MO 64139

University of Missouri, Kansas City, School of Pharmacy: Wayne M. Brown, Ph.D.,* School of Pharmacy, University of Missouri-Kansas City, 5005 Rockhill Road, Kansas City, MO 64110-2499

Washington University, School of Medicine: H. Mitchell Perry, Jr., M.D.,* School of Medicine, Washington University, Box 8048, 660 S. Euclid Avenue, St. Louis, MO 63110

Missouri Pharmaceutical Association: James R. Boyd, P.D.,* 215 Shirley Ridge Drive, St. Charles, MO 63303

MONTANA

Montana State Pharmaceutical Association: Robert H. Likewise, Executive Director, Montana State Pharmaceutical Association, 472 Russell, #2, Helena, MT 59601

NEBRASKA

Creighton University, School of Medicine: Michael C. Makoid, Ph.D.,* School of Medicine, Creighton University, 2500 California Street, Omaha, NE 68178

Creighton University, School of Pharmacy and Allied Health Professions: James M. Crampton, Ph.D., School of Pharmacy and Allied Health Professions, Creighton University, California and 24th Streets, Omaha, NE 68178

University of Nebraska, College of Medicine: Manuchair Ebadi, Ph.D., Professor and Chairman, Department of Pharmacology, University of Nebraska, College of Medicine, 42nd Street and Dewey Avenue, Omaha, NE 68105

University of Nebraska, College of Pharmacy: Clarence T. Ueda, Pharm.D., Ph.D., Int. Dean, College of Pharmacy, University of Nebraska, 42nd and Dewey Avenues, Omaha, NE 68105

Nebraska Pharmacists Association: Rex C. Higley, R.P.,* 3110 South 42nd, Lincoln, NE 68506

NEVADA

University of Nevada, Reno, School of Medicine: Iain L. O. Buxton, D.Ph.,* Department of Pharmacology, School of Medicine, University of Nevada, Reno, NV 89557

NEW HAMPSHIRE

Dartmouth Medical School: James J. Kresel, Ph.D.,* Dartmouth-Hitchcock Medical Center, Hanover, NH 03756

---

*Present at the 1985 Quinquennial Meeting.

New Hampshire Pharmaceutical Association: William J. Lancaster,* 4 Woodmore Drive, Hanover, NH 03755

NEW JERSEY

University of Medicine and Dentistry of New Jersey, New Jersey Medical School: Sheldon B. Gertner, Ph.D.,* New Jersey Medical School, UMDNJ, 100 Bergen Street, Newark, NJ 07103

Rutgers, The State University of New Jersey, College of Pharmacy: Thomas Medwick, Ph.D.,* College of Pharmacy, Rutgers, The State University of New Jersey, P. O. Box 789, Piscataway, NJ 08854

New Jersey Pharmaceutical Association: Stephen J. Csubak, Ph.D.,* 4 Decision Way East, Washington Crossing, PA 18977

NEW MEXICO

University of New Mexico, College of Pharmacy: William M. Hadley, Ph.D., Dean, College of Pharmacy, University of New Mexico, Albuquerque, NM 87131

New Mexico Pharmaceutical Association: Hugh Kabat, Ph.D.,* College of Pharmacy, University of New Mexico, Albuquerque, NM 87131

NEW YORK

Albert Einstein College of Medicine of Yeshiva University: Dr. Walter G. Levine,* Albert Einstein College of Medicine, 1300 Morris Park Avenue, New York, NY 10461

City University of New York, Mt. Sinai School of Medicine: Joel S. Mindel, M.D., Ph.D.,* Department of Ophthalmology, Annenberg Bldg. 22-14, Mt. Sinai School of Medicine, 1 Gustave L. Levy Place, New York, NY 10029

Columbia University College of Physicians and Surgeons: Dr. Norman Kahn,* Department of Pharmacology, Columbia University, 630 West 168th Street, New York, NY 10032

Cornell University Medical College: W. Y. Chan, Ph.D.,* Cornell University Medical College, New York, NY 10021

Long Island University, Arnold and Marie Schwartz College of Pharmacy and Health Sciences: John J. Sciarra, Ph.D.,* 8 Allen Drive, Locust Valley, NY 11560

New York Medical College: Mario A. Inchiosa, Jr., Ph.D.,* Department of Pharmacology, New York Medical College, Valhalla, NY 10595

State University of New York, Buffalo, School of Medicine: Robert J. McIsaac, Ph.D.,* Department of Pharmacology and Therapeutics, School of Medicine, 127 Farber Hall, SUNY at Buffalo, Buffalo, NY 14214

State University of New York, Buffalo, School of Pharmacy: Walter D. Conway, Ph.D., School of Pharmacy, SUNY at Buffalo, H565 Hochstetter Hall, Buffalo, NY 14260

St. John's University, College of Pharmacy and Allied Health Professions: Andrew J. Bartilucci, Ph.D.,* Dean, College of Pharmacy and Allied Health Professions, St. John's University, Grand Central and Utopia Parkways, Jamaica, NY 11439

Union University, Albany College of Pharmacy: Barry S. Reiss, Ph.D.,* Albany College of Pharmacy, Union University, 106 New Scotland Avenue, Albany, NY 12208

University of Rochester, School of Medicine and Dentistry: Michael Weintraub, M.D.,* University of Rochester Medical Center, Box 644, Rochester, NY 14642

Medical Society of the State of New York: Michael L. Friedland, M.D., Dean of Clinical Affairs, New York Medical College, Elmwood Hall, Valhalla, NY 10595

Pharmaceutical Society of the State of New York: Walter Singer, Ph.D., Pharmaceutical Society of the State of New York, Pine West Plaza IV, Washington Avenue Extension, Albany, NY 12205

NORTH CAROLINA

Bowman Gray School of Medicine, Wake Forest University: Jack W. Strandhoy, Ph.D.,* Department of Physiology/Pharmacology, Bowman Gray School of Medicine, Wake Forest University, 300 S. Hawthorne Road, Winston-Salem, NC 27103

Duke University, School of Medicine: William J. Murray, M.D., Ph.D.,* Box 3061, Duke University Medical Center, Durham, NC 27710

University of North Carolina, Chapel Hill, School of Medicine: Tai-Chan Peng, M.D.,* Department of Pharmacology, School of Medicine, Faculty Laboratory Office Building 231H, University of North Carolina, Chapel Hill, NC 27514

University of North Carolina, Chapel Hill, School of Pharmacy: Richard J. Kowalsky, Pharm.D.,* School of Pharmacy, 24 Beard Hall 200H, University of North Carolina, Chapel Hill, NC 27514

North Carolina Pharmaceutical Association: George H. Cocolas, Ph.D.,* Beard Hall 200H, Chapel Hill, NC 27514

NORTH DAKOTA

North Dakota State University, College of Pharmacy: William M. Henderson, Ph.D.,* College of Pharmacy, North Dakota State University, Fargo, ND 58105

North Dakota Pharmaceutical Association: William H. Shelver, Ph.D., College of Pharmacy, North Dakota State University, Fargo, ND 58105

OHIO

Case Western Reserve University, School of Medicine: Kenneth A. Scott, Ph.D.,* School of Medicine, Case Western Reserve University, 2119 Abington Road, Cleveland, OH 44106

Medical College of Ohio: Robert D. Wilkerson, Ph.D.,* Department of Pharmacology, Medical College of Ohio, 3000 Arlington Avenue, Toledo, OH 43699

Ohio State University, College of Medicine: Gopi A. Tejwani, Ph.D., Department of Pharmacology, College of Medicine, Ohio State University, 5086 Graves Hall, 333 West 10th Avenue, Columbus, OH 43210-1239

Ohio State University, College of Pharmacy: Michael C. Gerald, Ph.D.,* College of Pharmacy, Ohio State University, 500 West 12th Avenue, Columbus, OH 43210

University of Cincinnati, College of Medicine: Leonard T. Sigell, Ph.D.,* College of Medicine, University of Cincinnati, Rm. 7701, 231 Bethesda Avenue, Mail Location No. 144, Cincinnati, OH 45267-0144

University of Cincinnati, College of Pharmacy: Henry S. I. Tan, Ph.D.,* College of Pharmacy, University of Cincinnati, 136 Health Professions Building, 3223 Eden Avenue, Mail Location No. 4, Cincinnati, OH 45267

University of Toledo, College of Pharmacy: Norman F. Billups, Ph.D., Dean, College of Pharmacy, University of Toledo, Toledo, OH 43606

Wright State University, School of Medicine: John O. Lindower, M.D., Ph.D.,* 3301 Stonebridge Road, Kettering, OH 45419

Ohio State Medical Association: Ray W. Gifford, Jr., M.D.,* 3479 Glen Allen Drive, Cleveland, OH 44121

Ohio State Pharmaceutical Association: J. Richard Wuest, Pharm.D.,* 2720 Topichills Drive, Cincinnati, OH 45211

OKLAHOMA

Oral Roberts University, School of Medicine: Jimmie L. Valentine, Ph.D.,* 8181 South Lewis, Tulsa, OK 74137

Southwestern Oklahoma State University, School of Pharmacy: William G. Waggoner, Ph.D.,* School of Pharmacy, Southwestern Oklahoma State University, 100 Campus Drive, Weatherford, OK 73096

University of Oklahoma, College of Pharmacy: Loyd V. Allen, Jr., Ph.D.,* College of Pharmacy, University of Oklahoma, 1110 N. Stonewall, P. O. Box 26901, Oklahoma City, OK 73190

Oklahoma Pharmaceutical Association: Carl D. Lyons,* Skyline Terrace Nursing Center, 6202 E. 61st, Tulsa, OK 74136

Oklahoma State Medical Association: Clinton Nicholas Corder, M.D., Ph.D.,* 1000 N. Lee, P. O. Box 205, Oklahoma City, OK 73101

OREGON

Oregon Health Sciences University, School of Medicine: Hall Downes, M.D., Ph.D., Pharmacology (SM) L221, Oregon Health Sciences University, Portland, OR 97201

Oregon State University, College of Pharmacy: Freya F. Hermann, College of Pharmacy, Oregon State University, Corvallis, OR 97331

Oregon Medical Association: Richard E. Lahti, M.D.,* 2350 S.W. Multnomah Boulevard, Portland, OR 97219

Oregon State Pharmacists Association: Mrs. Hallie L. Lahti,* 1601 S.E. Oak Shore Lane, Milwaukie, OR 97222

PENNSYLVANIA

Duquesne University, School of Pharmacy: Lawrence H. Block, Ph.D., School of Pharmacy, Mellon Hall of Science, Room 441, Duquesne University, Pittsburgh, PA 15282

Medical College of Pennsylvania: Athole G. McNeil Jacobi, M.D., FFARCS,* Medical College of Pennsylvania, 3300 Henry Avenue, Philadelphia, PA 19129

---

*Present at the 1985 Quinquennial Meeting.

Pennsylvania State University, College of Medicine: John D. Connor, Ph.D.,* Milton S. Hershey Medical Center, Pennsylvania State University, P. O. Box 850, Hershey, PA   17033

Philadelphia College of Pharmacy and Science: Alfonso R. Gennaro, Ph.D.,* Philadelphia College of Pharmacy and Science, 43rd Street and Kingsessing Mall, Philadelphia, PA   19104

Temple University, School of Medicine: Charles A. Papacostas, Ph.D.,* Department of Pharmacology, Temple University School of Medicine, 3400 North Broad Street, Philadelphia, PA   19140

Temple University, School of Pharmacy: Murray Tuckerman, Ph.D.,* School of Pharmacy, Temple University, 3307 N. Broad Street, Philadelphia, PA   19140

Thomas Jefferson University, Jefferson Medical College: C. Paul Bianchi, Ph.D.,* Jefferson Medical College, Thomas Jefferson University, 1020 Locust Street, Philadelphia, PA   19107

University of Pennsylvania, School of Medicine: George B. Koelle, M.D., Ph.D., Department of Pharmacology, School of Medicine, University of Pennsylvania, 36th and Hamilton Walk, Philadelphia, PA   19104-6084

University of Pittsburgh, School of Medicine: Robert H. McDonald, Jr., M.D.,* School of Medicine, University of Pittsburgh, 448 Scaife Hall, 3550 Terrace Street, Pittsburgh, PA   15261

Pennsylvania Medical Society: Benjamin Calesnick, M.D.,* 646 W. Springfield Road, Springfield, PA   19064

Pennsylvania Pharmaceutical Association: Joseph A. Mosso,* 319 Carolyn Avenue, Latrobe, PA   15650

PUERTO RICO

Universidad Central del Caribe School of Medicine: Jesús Santos-Martínez, Ph.D., Department of Physiology, School of Medicine, Universidad Central del Caribe, P.O. Box 935, Cayey, PR   00634

University of Puerto Rico, College of Pharmacy: Andrés Malavé, Ph.D., Dean, College of Pharmacy, University of Puerto Rico, G.P.O. Box 5067, San Juan, PR   00936-5067

RHODE ISLAND

Brown University Program in Medicine: Michael C. Wiemann, M.D.,* Roger Williams General Hospital, 825 Chalkstone Avenue, Providence, RI   02908

University of Rhode Island, College of Pharmacy: Christopher Rhodes, Ph.D.,* Department of Pharmaceutics, University of Rhode Island, Kingston, RI   02881

SOUTH CAROLINA

Medical University of South Carolina, College of Medicine: James F. Cooper, Pharm.D., College of Pharmacy, Medical University of South Carolina, 171 Ashley Avenue, Charleston, SC   29425

Medical University of South Carolina, College of Pharmacy: Paul J. Niebergall, Ph.D.,* Department of Pharmaceutical Sciences, Medical University of South Carolina, 171 Ashley Avenue, Charleston, SC   29425

University of South Carolina, College of Pharmacy: Robert L. Beamer, Ph.D.,* College of Pharmacy, University of South Carolina, Columbia, SC   29208

SOUTH DAKOTA

South Dakota State University, College of Pharmacy: Gary S. Chappell, Ph.D., College of Pharmacy, South Dakota State University, Box 2201, Brookings, SD   57007

TENNESSEE

East Tennessee State University, Quillen-Dishner College of Medicine: Ernest A. Daigneault, Ph.D.,* 104 Hillside Road, Johnson City, TN   37601

Meharry Medical College, School of Medicine: Dolores C. Shockley, Ph.D.,* Meharry Medical College, 1005 D. B. Todd Boulevard, Nashville, TN   37208

University of Tennessee, College of Medicine: Murray Heimberg, M.D., Ph.D.,* University of Tennessee Center for Health Sciences, 874 Union Avenue, Room 100, Memphis, TN   38163

University of Tennessee, College of Pharmacy: Michael R. Ryan, Ph.D., Dean, College of Pharmacy, University of Tennessee, Center for the Health Sciences, 874 Union Avenue, Room 109, Memphis, TN   38163

TEXAS

Texas Southern University, College of Pharmacy and Health Sciences: Mary Ann Galley, Pharm.D.,* College of Pharmacy and Health Sciences, Texas Southern University, 3100 Cleburne Street, Houston, TX   77004

Texas Tech University, School of Medicine: Thomas W. Hale, Ph.D.,* Texas Tech University Health Science Center, Regional Academic Health Center at Amarillo, 1400 Wallace Boulevard, Amarillo, TX   79106

University of Houston, College of Pharmacy: Joseph P. Buckley, Ph.D.,* College of Pharmacy, University of Houston, 4800 Calhoun Boulevard, Houston, TX   77004

University of Texas, Austin, College of Pharmacy: James T. Doluisio, Ph.D.,* College of Pharmacy, University of Texas at Austin, Austin, TX   78712

University of Texas, Medical School, Galveston: Wayne R. Snodgrass, M.D., Ph.D., Professor of Pediatrics and Pharmacology-Toxicology, University of Texas Medical Branch, Galveston, TX   77550

University of Texas Medical School, Houston: Larry K. Pickering, M.D.,* Medical School at Houston, University of Texas, 6431 Fannin, P. O. Box 20708, Houston, TX   77030

University of Texas Medical School, San Antonio: Arthur H. Briggs, M.D.,* University of Texas Health Science Center at San Antonio, 7703 Floyd Curl Drive, San Antonio, TX   78284

Texas Pharmaceutical Association: Shirley McKee,* P. O. Box 1971, Houston, TX   77251

UTAH

University of Utah, College of Pharmacy: James D. McMahon, Ph.D.,* 3421 El Serrito Circle, Salt Lake City, UT   84109

University of Utah, School of Medicine: Douglas E. Rollins, M.D., Ph.D.,* Department of Pharmacology, School of Medicine, University of Utah, 50 N. Medical Drive, Salt Lake City, UT   84132

Utah Pharmaceutical Association: Robert V. Petersen, Ph.D.,* College of Pharmacy, University of Utah, Salt Lake City, UT   84112

VIRGINIA

Eastern Virginia Medical School: Desmond R. H. Gourley, Ph.D.,* Department of Pharmacology, Eastern Virginia Medical School, 700 Olney Road, Norfolk, VA   23501

Medical College of Virginia/Virginia Commonwealth University, School of Medicine: Albert J. Wasserman, M.D., Box 565, MCV Station, Richmond, VA   23298

Medical College of Virginia/Virginia Commonwealth University, School of Pharmacy: William H. Barr, Pharm.D., Ph.D.,* MCV School of Pharmacy, Virginia Commonwealth University, MCV Station Box 581, Richmond, VA   23298-0001

University of Virginia, School of Medicine: Peyton E. Weary, M.D.,* Chairman, Department of Dermatology, School of Medicine, University of Virginia, Box 134-Medical Center, Charlottesville, VA   22908

Medical Society of Virginia: William J. Hagood, Jr., M.D.,* P. O. Box 158, Clover, VA   24534

Virginia Pharmaceutical Association: Elmer R. Deffenbaugh, Jr.,* 1407 Cummings Drive, Richmond, VA   23220

WASHINGTON

University of Washington, School of Pharmacy: Lynn R. Brady, Ph.D.,* Asst. Dean, School of Pharmacy, T-341 Health Sciences, SC-69, University of Washington, Seattle, WA   98195

Washington State University, College of Pharmacy: William E. Johnson, Ph.D.,* College of Pharmacy, Washington State University, Pullman, WA   99164-6510

WEST VIRGINIA

Marshall University, School of Medicine: Timothy G. Saxe, M.D.,* School of Medicine, Marshall University, 1801 Sixth Avenue, Huntington, WV   25701

West Virginia University Medical Center, School of Pharmacy: Sidney A. Rosenbluth, Ph.D.,* Dean, School of Pharmacy, West Virginia University Medical Center, Morgantown, WV   26506

West Virginia Pharmacists Association: Art Jacknowitz, Pharm.D.,* 329 Wagner Road, Morgantown, WV   26505

WISCONSIN

Medical College of Wisconsin: Richard I. H. Wang, M.D., Ph.D.,* VA Medical Center, 5000 W. National Avenue, Wood, WI   53193

University of Wisconsin, Madison, School of Pharmacy: Chester A. Bond, Pharm.D., School of Pharmacy, University of Wisconsin, Madison, 425 N. Charter Street, Madison, WI   53706

University of Wisconsin Medical School, Madison: Joseph M. Benforado, M.D.,* 730 Seneca Place, Madison, WI   53711

Wisconsin Pharmacists Association: Dennis Dziczkowski,* 11330 W. Woodside Drive, Hales Corners, WI   53130

ACETAMINOPHEN (Systemic)

This information applies to the following medicines:

Acetaminophen (a-seat-a-MIN-oh-fen)
Acetaminophen and Caffeine (KAF-een)
Buffered Acetaminophen

Some commonly used brand names or other names are:

For Acetaminophen†

A'Cenol	Liquiprin
Acephen	Meda Cap
Aceta	Meda Tab
Ace-Tabs*	Myapap
Acetaminophen Uniserts	Neopap
Actamin	Oraphen-PD
Anacin-3	Panadol
Anuphen	Panasorb*
Apacet	Panex
APAP	Paracetamol
Apo-Acetaminophen*	Paraphen*
Aspirin Free Pain Relief	Pedric
Atasol*	Phenaphen (U.S.)
Banesin	Robigesic*
C2A*	Rounox*
Campain*	St. Joseph Aspirin-Free
Conacetol	Suppap
Dapa	Tapanol
Datril	Tempra
Dolanex	Tenol
Dorcol Children's Fever and Pain Reducer	Ty Caplets
	Tylenol
Exdol*	Ty Pap
Genapap	Ty Tab
Genebs	Valadol
Genetabs	Valorin
Halenol	

For Acetaminophen and Caffeine	
Cafadol*	Summit

For Buffered Acetaminophen
Bromo-Seltzer

*Not available in the U.S.
†Generic name product may also be available in the U.S.

To the Reader: If you do not recognize the names of medical conditions or medicines referred to in this information, check with your doctor, nurse, or pharmacist. Definitions for selected medical terms may be found in the Glossary. Brand names for the generic drug names listed can be found in the Index. In addition, selected brand names commonly associated with the generic name have been included in the text to help you recognize medicine you may be taking. The fact that a brand name product is not mentioned does not mean the information does not apply. It is a good idea for you to learn both the generic and brand names of your medicines and to write them down for future use.

Acetaminophen is used to relieve pain and reduce fever. Unlike aspirin, it does not relieve the redness, stiffness, or swelling caused by rheumatoid arthritis. However, it may relieve the pain caused by mild forms of arthritis. Acetaminophen can be taken by mouth or used rectally in the form of suppositories.

Buffered acetaminophen is used to relieve pain occurring together with an upset stomach.

This medicine is available without a prescription; however, your physician or dentist may have special instructions on the proper dose of acetaminophen for your medical condition.

Remember:
- **Keep all medicines out of the reach of children.**

- In order for this medicine to work, it must be used as directed. **If you are using this medicine without a prescription, it is very important to follow the directions on the label.**

- **It is also very important that you read and understand the following information.** If any of the information causes you special concern, check with your doctor before using this medicine without a prescription.

- Before you begin using any new medicine (prescription or nonprescription) or if you develop any new medical problem while you are using this medicine, check with your doctor, nurse, or pharmacist.

- **If you have any questions** about the following information or if you want more information about this medicine or your medical problem, **ask your doctor, nurse or pharmacist.**

Before Using This Medicine

Before you use acetaminophen, check with your doctor or pharmacist:

—if you have ever had any unusual or allergic reaction to acetaminophen or aspirin.

—if you are on a low-salt, low-sugar, or any other special diet, or if you are allergic to any substance, such as foods, sulfites or other preservatives, or dyes. Most medicines contain more than their active ingredient, and many liquid medicines contain alcohol. Your doctor, nurse, or pharmacist can help you avoid products that may cause a problem.

—if you are **pregnant** or if you may become pregnant. Acetaminophen has not been shown to cause birth defects or other problems in humans. However, studies on birth defects have not been done in humans.

—if you are **breast-feeding**. Although acetaminophen passes into the breast milk in small amounts, it has not been shown to cause problems in nursing babies.

—if you have any of the following medical problems:
Alcoholism
Kidney disease (severe)
Hepatitis or other liver disease

—if you regularly drink large amounts of alcoholic beverages.

—if you are taking **any** other prescription or nonprescription (OTC) medicine, especially if you are taking buffered acetaminophen effervescent granules and are also taking adrenocorticoids (cortisone-like medicines).

Proper Use of This Medicine

For patients taking buffered acetaminophen effervescent granules:

- Pour the amount of granules directed on the package into a glass.

- Add ½ glass (4 ounces) of cool water.

© 1988   The United States Pharmacopeial Convention, Inc.

• Drink all of the liquid in order to be sure you get the full dose of medicine.

• You may drink the liquid while it is still fizzing or after the fizzing stops.

For patients using the suppository dosage form of acetaminophen:

• If the suppository is too soft to insert because of storage in a warm place, before removing the foil wrapper chill the suppository in the refrigerator for 30 minutes or run cold water over it.

• How to insert the suppository: First remove the foil wrapper and moisten the suppository with water. Lie down on one side and push the suppository well up into the rectum with a finger.

Unless otherwise directed by your physician or dentist:

• **Do not take more of this medicine than is recommended on the package label.** If too much is taken, liver damage may occur.

• **Children up to 12 years of age should not take this medicine more than 5 times a day or for more than 5 days in a row.**

• **Adults should not take this medicine for more than 10 days in a row.**

If you have been directed to take this medicine for a longer period of time, especially in large doses, it is important that your doctor check your progress at regular visits.

This medicine will not relieve the redness, stiffness, or swelling that may occur with rheumatoid arthritis. If you plan to take this medicine for arthritic (rheumatic) conditions, check with your doctor first.

How to store this medicine:

• **Keep out of the reach of children.**

• Store away from heat and direct light.

• Do not store acetaminophen tablets, capsules, or effervescent granules in the bathroom, near the kitchen sink, or in other damp places. Heat or moisture may cause the medicine to break down.

• Keep the liquid and suppository forms of this medicine from freezing.

• Do not keep outdated medicine or medicine no longer needed. Be sure that any discarded medicine is out of the reach of children.

Precautions While Using This Medicine

Check with your physician or dentist:

—if your symptoms do not improve or if they get worse.

—if you are taking this medicine to bring down a fever, and the fever lasts for more than 3 days or returns.

Check the labels of all over-the-counter (OTC), nonprescription, and prescription medicines you now take. If any contain acetaminophen be especially careful, since taking them while taking this medicine may lead to overdose. If you have any questions about this, check with your physician, dentist, or pharmacist.

Do not drink alcoholic beverages while taking acetaminophen. To do so may increase the chance of liver damage, especially if you drink large amounts of alcoholic beverages regularly, if you take more acetaminophen than is recommended on the package label, or if you take it regularly for a long period of time.

Too much use of acetaminophen together with certain other medicines may increase the chance of kidney problems. Therefore, do not regularly take acetaminophen with any of the following, unless directed to do so by your physician or dentist:

    Aspirin or other salicylates
    Diclofenac (e.g., Voltaren)
    Diflunisal (e.g., Dolobid)
    Fenoprofen (e.g., Nalfon)
    Flurbiprofen, oral (e.g., Ansaid)
    Ibuprofen (e.g., Advil; Motrin; Nuprin)
    Indomethacin (e.g., Indocid; Indocin)
    Ketoprofen (e.g., Orudis)
    Meclofenamate (e.g., Meclomen)
    Mefenamic acid (e.g., Ponstan; Ponstel)
    Naproxen (e.g., Anaprox; Naprosyn)
    Phenylbutazone (e.g., Azolid; Butazolidin)
    Piroxicam (e.g., Feldene)
    Sulindac (e.g., Clinoril)
    Tiaprofenic acid (e.g., Surgam)
    Tolmetin (e.g., Tolectin)

For patients taking buffered acetaminophen effervescent granules:

• If you are also taking a tetracycline antibiotic, do not take the two medicines within 1 to 2 hours of each other. Taking them together may prevent the tetracycline from being absorbed by your body. If you have any questions about this, check with your doctor or pharmacist.

• **If you have heart or blood vessel disease or if you are on a sodium-restricted (low salt) diet, do not take the buffered acetaminophen effervescent granules without first checking with your doctor.** This medicine contains a large amount of sodium.

If you think that you or anyone else may have taken an overdose of acetaminophen, get emergency help at once, even if there are no signs of poisoning. Signs of severe poisoning may not appear for 2 to 4 days after the overdose is taken, but treatment to prevent liver damage or death must be started within 24 hours or less after the overdose is taken.

Side Effects of This Medicine

Along with its needed effects, a medicine may cause some unwanted effects. Although not all of these side effects may occur, if they do occur they may need medical attention.

Check with your doctor immediately if any of the following side effects occur:

Rare

Yellow eyes or skin

Signs of overdose

Diarrhea
Increased sweating
Loss of appetite
Nausea or vomiting
Stomach cramps or pain
Swelling, pain, or tenderness in the upper abdomen or stomach area

Also check with your doctor as soon as possible if any of the following side effects occur:

Rare

Bloody or cloudy urine
Difficult or painful urination
Skin rash, hives, or itching

Sudden decrease in amount of urine
Unexplained sore throat and fever
Unusual bleeding or bruising
Unusual tiredness or weakness

For elderly patients: Many medicines have not been tested in older people. Therefore, it is not known whether the medicine acts the same way it does in younger adults. Check with your doctor or pharmacist if you notice any ususual effects while taking this medicine or if you think it is not working as it should.

Other side effects not listed above may also occur in some patients. If you notice any other effects, check with your doctor.

December 1987

ACETAMINOPHEN AND SALICYLATES
(Systemic)

This information applies to the following medicines:
Acetaminophen and Aspirin (a-seat-a-MIN-oh-fen and AS-pir-in)
Acetaminophen, Aspirin, and Salicylamide (sal-i-SILL-a-mide)
Acetaminophen and Salicylamide
Acetaminophen and Sodium Salicylate (SOE-dee-um sa-LI-si-late)

Some commonly used brand names are:	Generic names:
Gemnisyn	Acetaminophen and Aspirin
APAP Fortified Duradyne Excedrin (U.S.) Goody's Extra Strength Tablets Goody's Headache Powders Pain Reliever Salatin Trigesic	Acetaminophen, Aspirin, and Caffeine
Buffets II Supac Vanquish	Buffered Acetaminophen, Aspirin, and Caffeine
Tri-Pain	Acetaminophen, Aspirin, and Salicylamide
Saleto Salocol	Acetaminophen, Aspirin, Salicylamide, and Caffeine
Presalin	Buffered Acetaminophen, Aspirin, and Salicylamide
Arthralgen Banesin Doan's Pills (Canada) Duoprin Salimeph Forte	Acetaminophen and Salicylamide
Accurate Forte* 445 Anti-Pain Compound* Rid-A-Pain Compound S-A-C	Acetaminophen, Salicylamide, and Caffeine
Tisma	Acetaminophen, Sodium Salicylate, and Caffeine

*Not available in the U.S.

To the Reader: If you do not recognize the names of medical conditions or medicines referred to in this information, check with your doctor, nurse, or pharmacist. Definitions for selected medical terms may be found in the Glossary. Brand names for the generic drug names listed can be found in the Index. In addition, selected brand names commonly associated with the generic name have been included in the text to help you recognize medicine you may be taking. The fact that a brand name product is not mentioned does not mean the information does not apply. It is a good idea for you to learn both the generic and brand names of your medicines and to write them down for future use.

Acetaminophen and salicylate combination medicines are taken by mouth to relieve pain and reduce fever. They may be used to relieve occasional pain caused by mild inflammation or arthritis (rheumatism). However, neither acetaminophen nor salicylamide is as effective as aspirin or sodium salicylate for treating chronic or severe pain, or other symptoms, caused by inflammation or arthritis.

Some of these combination medicines do not contain any aspirin or sodium salicylate. Even those that do contain aspirin or sodium salicylate may not contain enough to be effective in treating these conditions.

A few reports have suggested that acetaminophen and salicylates may work together to cause kidney damage or cancer of the kidney or urinary bladder. This may occur if large amounts of both medicines are taken together for a very long period of time. However, taking usual amounts of these combination medicines for short periods of time has not been shown to cause these unwanted effects. Also, these effects have not been reported with either acetaminophen or a salicylate used alone, even if large amounts have been taken for a long time. Therefore, for long-term use, it may be best to use either acetaminophen or a salicylate, but not both, unless you are under a doctor's care.

Before giving any of these combination medicines to a child, check the package label very carefully. Some of these medicines are too strong for use in children. If you are not certain whether a specific product can be given to a child, or if you have any questions about the amount to give, check with your doctor, nurse, or pharmacist.

These medicines are available without a prescription. However, your doctor may have special instructions on the proper dose of these medicines for your medical condition.

Remember:
- **Keep all medicines out of the reach of children.**

- In order for this medicine to work, it must be used as directed. **If you are using this medicine without a prescription, it is very important to follow the directions on the label.**

- **It is also very important that you read and understand the following information.** If any of the information causes you special concern, check with your doctor before using this medicine without a prescription.

- Before you begin using any new medicine (prescription or nonprescription) or if you develop any new medical problem while you are using this medicine, check with your doctor, nurse, or pharmacist.

- **If you have any questions** about the following information or if you want more information about this medicine or your medical problem, **ask your doctor, nurse, or pharmacist.**

Before Using This Medicine

Before you use an acetaminophen and salicylate combination medicine, check with your doctor or pharmacist:

—if you have ever had any unusual or allergic reaction to acetaminophen, to aspirin or other salicylates, including methyl salicylate (oil of wintergreen), or to any of the following medicines:

Diclofenac (e.g., Voltaren)
Diflunisal (e.g., Dolobid)
Fenoprofen (e.g., Nalfon)
Flurbiprofen, oral (e.g., Ansaid)
Ibuprofen (e.g., Advil; Motrin; Nuprin)
Indomethacin (e.g., Indocid; Indocin)

Ketoprofen (e.g., Orudis)
Meclofenamate (e.g., Meclomen)
Mefenamic acid (e.g., Ponstan; Ponstel)
Naproxen (e.g., Anaprox; Naprosyn)
Oxyphenbutazone (e.g., Oxalid; Tandearil)
Phenylbutazone (e.g., Azolid; Butazolidin)
Piroxicam (e.g., Feldene)
Sulindac (e.g., Clinoril)
Suprofen (e.g., Suprol)
Tiaprofenic acid (e.g., Surgam)
Tolmetin (e.g., Tolectin)
Zomepirac (e.g., Zomax)

—if you are on a low-salt, low-sugar, or any other special diet, or if you are allergic to any substance, such as foods, sulfites or other preservatives, or dyes. Most medicines contain more than their active ingredient, and many liquid medicines contain alcohol. Your doctor, nurse, or pharmacist can help you avoid products that may cause a problem.

—if you are **pregnant** or if you may become pregnant. Although acetaminophen has not been shown to cause birth defects or other problems, the chance always exists. Studies have not been done in humans.

Salicylates have not been shown to cause birth defects in humans. Studies on birth defects in humans have been done with aspirin, but not with salicylamide or sodium salicylate. However, salicylates have been shown to cause birth defects in animals.

Some reports have suggested that too much use of aspirin late in pregnancy may cause a decrease in the newborn's weight and possible death of the fetus or newborn infant. However, the mothers in these reports had been taking much larger amounts of aspirin than are usually recommended. Studies of mothers taking aspirin in the doses that are usually recommended did not show these unwanted effects. However, there is a chance that regular use of salicylates late in pregnancy may cause unwanted effects on the heart or blood flow in the fetus or newborn infant.

Use of salicylates, especially aspirin, during the last 2 weeks of pregnancy may cause bleeding problems in the fetus before or during delivery, or in the newborn infant. Also, too much use of salicylates during the last 3 months of pregnancy may increase the length of pregnancy, prolong labor, cause other problems during delivery, or cause severe bleeding in the mother before, during, or after delivery.

Studies in humans have not shown that caffeine (contained in some of these combination medicines) causes birth defects. However, studies in animals have shown that caffeine causes birth defects when given in very large doses (amounts equal to the amount of caffeine in 12 to 24 cups of coffee a day).

—if you are **breast-feeding**. Although acetaminophen and salicylates have not been shown to cause problems in nursing babies, these medicines pass into the breast milk. Also, caffeine (contained in some of these combination medicines) passes into the breast milk in small amounts.

—if you are taking any of these combination medicines and have any of the following medical problems:

Anemia
Gout
Hepatitis or other liver disease
Kidney disease
Stomach ulcer or other stomach problems

—if you are taking one of the combination medicines containing aspirin and have a history of asthma, allergies, and nasal polyps.

—if you are taking one of the combination medicines containing aspirin or sodium salicylate and have hemophilia or other bleeding problems.

—if you are taking one of the combination medicines containing caffeine and have heart disease.

—if you regularly take large amounts of antacids.

—if you are taking **any** other medicine or type of medicine, especially:

Anticoagulants (blood thinners)
Antidiabetic agents, oral (diabetes medicine you take by mouth)
Dipyridamole [e.g., Persantine]
Heparin
Methotrexate [e.g., Folex; Mexate]
Other medicine for pain and/or inflammation
Probenecid [e.g., Benemid]
Sulfinpyrazone [e.g., Anturan; Anturane]
Urinary alkalizers (medicine that makes the urine less acid, such as acetazolamide [e.g., Diamox], dichlorphenamide [e.g., Daranide], methazolamide [e.g., Neptazane], potassium or sodium citrate and/or citric acid)
Valproic acid [Depakene; Depakote]

Proper Use of This Medicine

Take this medicine with food or a full glass (8 ounces) of water to lessen the chance of stomach upset.

There have been reports suggesting that use of aspirin in children with fever caused by a viral infection (especially flu or chickenpox) may cause a serious illness called Reye's syndrome. **Do not give a medicine containing aspirin or other salicylates to a child with flu or chickenpox without first discussing this with your child's doctor.**

Unless otherwise directed by your doctor:

• **Do not take more of this medicine than directed on the package label.** Taking too much acetaminophen may cause liver damage or lead to other medical problems because of an overdose. Also, taking too much of a salicylate can cause stomach problems or lead to other medical problems because of an overdose.

• **Children up to 12 years of age should not take this medicine more often than 5 times a day or for more than 5 days in a row.**

• **Adults should not take this medicine for more than 10 days in a row.**

• Elderly patients should probably not take this medicine for longer than 5 days in a row.

If you have been directed to take this medicine for a longer period of time or in high doses, **it is important that your doctor check your progress at regular visits.**

Check with your doctor before taking one of these combination medicines to treat severe or chronic inflammation or arthritis (rheumatism). These combination medicines may not relieve the severe pain, redness, swelling, or stiffness caused by these conditions unless very large amounts are taken for a long period of time. **It is best not to take acetaminophen and salicylate combination medicines in large amounts for a long period of time** unless you are under a doctor's care.

If a combination medicine containing aspirin has a strong vinegar-like odor, do not use it. This means the medicine is breaking down. If you have any questions about this, check with your pharmacist.

How to store this medicine:

• **Keep out of the reach of children** because overdose of the salicylates in these combination medicines is very dangerous in young children.

• Store away from heat and direct light.

• Do not store tablets, capsules, or powders in the bathroom, near the kitchen sink, or in other damp places. Heat or moisture may cause the medicine to break down.

• Do not keep outdated medicine or medicine no longer needed. Be sure that any discarded medicine is out of the reach of children.

Precautions While Using This Medicine

Check with your doctor:

—if your symptoms do not improve or if they become worse.

—if you are taking this medicine for a fever, and the fever lasts for more than 3 days or returns.

Diabetics—False urine sugar test results may occur if you take 8 or more 325-mg (5-grain) doses of aspirin or sodium salicylate every day for several days in a row. Smaller doses or occasional use of aspirin or sodium salicylate usually will not affect urine sugar tests. If you have any questions about this, check with your doctor, nurse, or pharmacist, especially if your diabetes is not well controlled.

Do not take any of the combination medicines containing aspirin for 5 days before any surgery, including dental surgery, unless otherwise directed by your physician or dentist. Taking aspirin during this time may cause bleeding problems.

Check the label of all over-the-counter (OTC), nonprescription, and prescription medicines you now take. If any contain acetaminophen or aspirin or other salicylates, including bismuth subsalicylate (e.g., Pepto-Bismol), be especially careful. Also, be careful if you regularly apply a shampoo or other medicine containing salicylic acid to your skin or scalp. Taking or using

any of these medicines together with this combination medicine may lead to overdose. If you have any questions about this, check with your doctor or pharmacist.

Do not drink alcoholic beverages while taking this medicine. Stomach problems may be more likely to occur if you drink alcoholic beverages while you are taking a salicylate. Also, liver damage may be more likely to occur if you drink large amounts of alcoholic beverages while you are taking acetaminophen.

Too much use of any of these combination medicines together with certain other medicines may increase the chance of stomach or kidney problems. Therefore, do not regularly take any of these combination medicines together with any of the following medicines, unless directed to do so by your physician or dentist:

Diclofenac (e.g., Voltaren)
Diflunisal (e.g., Dolobid)
Fenoprofen (e.g., Nalfon)
Flurbiprofen, oral (e.g., Ansaid)
Ibuprofen (e.g., Advil; Motrin; Nuprin)
Indomethacin (e.g., Indocid; Indocin)
Ketoprofen (e.g., Orudis)
Meclofenamate (e.g., Meclomen)
Mefenamic acid (e.g., Ponstan; Ponstel)
Naproxen (e.g., Anaprox; Naprosyn)
Phenylbutazone (e.g., Azolid; Butazolidin)
Piroxicam (e.g., Feldene)
Sulindac (e.g., Clinoril)
Tiaprofenic acid (e.g., Surgam)
Tolmetin (e.g., Tolectin)

If you are taking one of the buffered acetaminophen and salicylate combination medicines, and you are also taking a tetracycline antibiotic, do not take the two medicines within 1 to 2 hours of each other. Taking them together may prevent the tetracycline from being absorbed by your body. If you have any questions about this, check with your doctor or pharmacist.

If you are taking a laxative containing cellulose, do not take it within 2 hours of taking this medicine. Taking them close together may make this medicine less effective by preventing the salicylate in it from being absorbed by your body.

If you think that you or anyone else may have taken an overdose of this medicine, get emergency help at once. Taking an overdose of a salicylate may cause unconsciousness or death. The first sign of overdose of a salicylate may be ringing or buzzing in the ear. Other signs include convulsions (seizures), hearing loss, confusion, severe drowsiness or tiredness, severe excitement or nervousness, and unusually fast or deep breathing. Signs of severe acetaminophen overdose may not appear until 2 to 4 days after the overdose is taken, but treatment to prevent liver damage or death must be started within 24 hours or less after the overdose is taken.

Side Effects of This Medicine

Along with its needed effects, a medicine may cause some unwanted effects. Although not all of these side effects may occur, if they do occur they may need medical attention.

Check with your doctor immediately if any of the following side effects occur:

Less common or rare

Shortness of breath, troubled breathing, tightness in chest, or wheezing (for medicines containing aspirin only)
Sudden decrease in amount of urine

Signs of overdose

Any loss of hearing
Bloody urine
Confusion
Convulsions (seizures)
Diarrhea (severe or continuing)
Dizziness or lightheadedness
Drowsiness (severe)
Fast or deep breathing
Hallucinations (seeing, hearing, or feeling things that are not there)
Headache (severe or continuing)
Increased sweating
Loss of appetite
Nausea or vomiting (continuing)
Nervousness, excitement, or confusion (severe)
Ringing or buzzing in ear (continuing)
Shortness of breath or troubled breathing
Stomach cramps or pain (severe or continuing)
Swelling, pain, or tenderness in the upper abdomen or stomach area
Uncontrollable flapping movements of the hands, especially in elderly patients
Unexplained fever
Unusual thirst
Vision problems

Signs of overdose in children

Changes in behavior
Drowsiness or tiredness (severe)
Fast or deep breathing

Also, check with your doctor as soon as possible if any of the following side effects occur:

More common

Nausea, vomiting, or stomach pain (mild, especially with medicines containing aspirin)

Less common or rare

Bloody or black tarry stools
Cloudy urine
Difficult or painful urination

Skin rash, hives, or itching
Swelling of face, feet, or lower legs
Unexplained sore throat and fever
Unusual bleeding or bruising
Unusual tiredness or weakness
Unusual weight gain
Vomiting of blood or material that looks like coffee grounds
Yellow eyes or skin

Other side effects may occur that usually do not require medical attention. These side effects may go away during treatment as your body adjusts to the medicine. However, check with your doctor if any of the following side effects continue or are bothersome:

More common

Heartburn or indigestion (especially with medicines containing aspirin)

Less common

Drowsiness (only for medicines containing salicylamide)
Sleeplessness, nervousness, or jitters (only for medicines containing caffeine)

Some side effects may occur after you have stopped taking these combination medicines, especially if you have taken large amounts of them for a long time. **Check with your doctor immediately** if any of these side effects occur after you have stopped taking this medicine:

Rare

Bloody or cloudy urine
Difficult or decreased urination
Swelling of face, feet, or lower legs
Unusual weight gain

For children or elderly patients: Some of the above side effects are more likely to occur in children, especially those who have a fever or are dehydrated (those who have lost large amounts of body fluid because of vomiting, diarrhea, or sweating), and in the elderly (60 years of age or older). These patients are usually more sensitive to the effects of salicylates.

Other side effects not listed above may also occur in some patients. If you notice any other effects, check with your doctor.

_____
December 1987

ACETOHYDROXAMIC ACID (Systemic)

A commonly used brand name is Lithostat.

To the Reader: If you do not recognize the names of medical conditions or medicines referred to in this information, check with your doctor, nurse, or pharmacist. Definitions for selected medical terms may be found in the Glossary. Brand names for the generic drug names listed can be found in the Index. In addition, selected brand names commonly associated with the generic name have been included in the text to help you recognize medicine you may be taking. The fact that a brand name product is not mentioned does not mean the information does not apply. It is a good idea for you to learn both the generic and brand names of your medicines and to write them down for future use.

Acetohydroxamic acid (a-SEE-toe-hye-drox-AM-ik AS-id) is used to keep kidney stones from forming and to stop the growth of existing stones. Such stone build-up is often caused by certain bacterial infections.

The bacteria produce an enzyme that makes the urine too alkaline. Under such conditions, kidney stones tend to form and continue to grow in size. Acetohydroxamic acid stops the enzyme action and so reduces the chance for stones to form. This medicine is not used to dissolve existing stones and is not used in place of surgery. It is sometimes used to make antibiotics or similar medicine work better when treating kidney or urinary tract infections.

Acetohydroxamic acid is available only with your doctor's prescription.

Remember:

• **This medicine has been prescribed for your current medical problem only.** It must not be given to other people or used for other problems unless you are directed to do so by your doctor.

• **Keep all medicines out of the reach of children.**

• In order for this medicine to work, it must be used as directed.

• **It is very important that you read and understand the following information.** If any of the information causes you special concern, do not decide against using this medicine without first checking with your doctor.

• Before you begin using any new medicine (prescription or nonprescription) or if you develop any new medical problem while you are using this medicine, check with your doctor, nurse, or pharmacist.

• **If you have any questions** about the following information or if you want more information about this medicine or your medical problem, **ask your doctor, nurse, or pharmacist.**

Before Using This Medicine

In order to decide on the best treatment for your medical problem, your doctor should be told:

—if you have ever had any unusual or allergic reaction to acetohydroxamic acid.

—if you are on a low-salt, low-sugar, or any other special diet, or if you are allergic to any substance, such as foods, sulfites or other preservatives, or dyes. Most medicines contain more than their active ingredient. Your doctor, nurse, or pharmacist can help you avoid products that may cause a problem.

—if you are **pregnant** or if you may become pregnant. Acetohydroxamic acid is not recommended during pregnancy since it has been shown to cause serious birth defects in animals. Effective methods of contraception (birth control) must be used during treatment with this medicine in order to avoid a pregnancy that could result in birth defects. Be sure you have discussed this with your doctor.

—if you are **breast-feeding**. It is not known whether acetohydroxamic acid passes into the breast milk. This medicine has not been shown to cause problems in nursing babies. However, its use in breast-feeding mothers is not recommended.

—if you have any of the following medical problems:
  Anemia or other blood disorder
  Blood clots (history of)
  Other kidney disorder
  Phlebitis (vein inflammation)

—if you are now taking an iron supplement or other medicine containing iron.

Proper Use of This Medicine

Acetohydroxamic acid works best when taken on an empty stomach. Take the medicine one hour before or two hours after meals whenever possible.

Take this medicine exactly as ordered by your doctor. This is especially important because it is used along with antibiotics or other medicine to clear up the infection.

Do not miss any doses. Skipped doses may delay treatment progress and your recovery. When too many doses are missed, stone formation and growth may start again. Remember that this medicine is intended to prevent kidney stones and the surgery that is sometimes required to remove them.

If you do miss a dose of this medicine, take it as soon as possible. Then go back to your regular dosing schedule. Do not double doses.

How to store this medicine:

• **Keep out of the reach of children.**

• Store away from heat and direct light.

• Do not store in the bathroom, near the kitchen sink, or in other damp places. Heat or moisture may cause the medicine to break down.

• Do not keep outdated medicine or medicine no longer needed. Be sure that any discarded medicine is out of the reach of children.

Precautions While Using This Medicine

Your doctor should check your progress at regular visits to make sure that this medicine is working properly and does not cause unwanted effects.

Do not take any form of iron by mouth at the same time as acetohydroxamic acid. Neither medicine will work well in the body if they are taken together.

Do not drink alcoholic beverages while you are taking acetohydroxamic acid. To do so may cause a rash to appear on the arms and face about 30 to 45 minutes after drinking the alcohol. Also, the skin may become flushed with a feeling of warmth and tingling. This reaction lasts about 30 minutes and can be very strong in some patients.

Side Effects of This Medicine

Along with its needed effects, a medicine may cause some unwanted effects. The following side effects may be caused by blood clots, but rarely occur; however, if they do occur, they need immediate medical attention. **Stop taking this medicine and get emergency help immediately** if any of the following side effects occur:

Less common or rare
    Headache (severe or sudden)
    Loss of coordination (sudden)
    Pains in chest, groin, or legs (especially in calves of legs)
    Shortness of breath (sudden)
    Slurred speech (sudden)
    Vision change (sudden)

Other side effects may occur that require medical attention. Check with your doctor as soon as possible if any of the following side effects occur:

More common
    Anxiety
    Loss of appetite
    Mental depression

    Nausea or vomiting
    Nervousness
    Shakiness
    Unusual tiredness or weakness

Other side effects may occur which usually do not require medical attention. These side effects may go away during treatment as your body adjusts to the medicine. However, check with your doctor if any of the following side effects continue or are bothersome:

More common
    Headache (mild)
Less common
    Hair loss
    Skin rash (non-itching) on arms and face

For elderly patients: Many medicines have not been tested in older people. Therefore, it is not known whether the medicine acts the same way it does in younger adults. Check with your doctor or pharmacist if you notice any unusual effects while taking this medicine or if you think it is not working as it should.

Other side effects not listed above may also occur in some patients. If you notice any other effects, check with your doctor at once.

December 1987

ACETYLCYSTEINE (Inhalation)

Some commonly used brand names are Airbron*, Mucomyst, and Mucosal.

*Not available in the U.S.

To the Reader: If you do not recognize the names of medical conditions or medicines referred to in this information, check with your doctor, nurse, or pharmacist. Definitions for selected medical terms may be found in the Glossary. Brand names for the generic drug names listed can be found in the Index. In addition, selected brand names commonly associated with the generic name have been included in the text to help you recognize medicine you may be taking. The fact that a brand name product is not mentioned does not mean the information does not apply. It is a good idea for you to learn both the generic and brand names of your medicines and to write them down for future use.

Acetylcysteine (a-se-teel-SIS-teen) belongs to the group of medicines called mucolytics (medicines that destroy or dissolve mucus). It is usually given by inhalation but may be given in other ways in a hospital.

Acetylcysteine is used to help make breathing easier in conditions such as bronchitis, emphysema, tuberculosis, and other lung diseases. It may also be used in patients with a tracheostomy. Acetylcysteine liquefies (thins) or dissolves mucus so that it may be coughed up. Sometimes the mucus may have to be removed by suction.

This medicine is available only with your doctor's prescription.

Remember:

• **This medicine has been prescribed for your current medical problem only.** It must not be given to other people or used for other problems unless you are directed to do so by your doctor.

• **Keep all medicines out of the reach of children.**

• In order for this medicine to work, it must be used as directed.

• **It is very important that you read and understand the following information.** If any of the information causes you special concern, do not decide against using this medicine without first checking with your doctor.

• Before you begin using any new medicine (prescription or nonprescription) or if you develop any new medical problem while you are using this medicine, check with your doctor, nurse, or pharmacist.

• **If you have any questions** about the following information or if you want more information about this medicine or your medical problem, **ask your doctor, nurse, or pharmacist.**

Before Using This Medicine

In order to decide on the best treatment for your medical problem, your doctor should be told:

—if you have ever had any unusual or allergic reaction to acetylcysteine.

—if you are allergic to any substance, such as certain preservatives or dyes. Most medicines contain more than their active ingredient. Your doctor, nurse, or pharmacist can help you avoid products that may cause a problem.

—if you are **pregnant** or if you may become pregnant. Studies have not been done in humans. However, acetylcysteine has not been shown to cause birth defects or other problems in animal studies when given in doses many times the recommended human dose.

—if you are **breast-feeding**. It is not known whether acetylcysteine passes into the breast milk. This medicine has not been shown to cause problems in nursing babies.

—if you have asthma.

Proper Use of This Medicine

Use acetylcysteine only as directed. Do not use more of it and do not use it more often than your doctor ordered. To do so may increase the chance of side effects.

If you are using this medicine at home, make sure you understand exactly how to use it. If you have any questions about this, check with your doctor.

After using acetylcysteine, try to cough up the loosened or thinned mucus. If this does not work, it may have to be suctioned out. This will prevent too much mucus from accumulating in the lungs. If you have any questions about this, check with your doctor.

If you miss a dose of this medicine, use it as soon as possible. Then use any remaining doses for that day at regularly spaced intervals.

How to store this medicine:

• **Keep out of the reach of children.**

• Before container is opened, store away from heat and direct light.

• After container is opened, store in the refrigerator. However, keep the medicine from freezing.

• Do not keep outdated medicine or medicine no longer needed. Be sure that any discarded medicine is out of the reach of children.

Precautions While Using This Medicine

If your symptoms do not improve or if your condition gets worse, check with your doctor.

If you are using a face mask for inhalation of acetylcysteine, there may be a stickiness on the face after use. This can be removed by washing with water.

Side Effects of This Medicine

Along with its needed effects, a medicine may cause some unwanted effects. Although not all of these side effects may occur, if they do occur they may need medical attention.

Check with your doctor as soon as possible if any of the following side effects occur:

Less common
  Spitting up blood
  Wheezing, tightness in chest, or difficulty in breathing (especially in asthma patients)
Rare
  Skin rash

Other side effects may occur that usually do not require medical attention. These side effects may go away during treatment as your body adjusts to the medicine. However, check with your doctor if any of the following side effects continue or are bothersome:

Less common
> Clammy skin
> Fever
> Increase in bronchial secretions
> Irritation or soreness of mouth, throat, or lungs
> Nausea or vomiting
> Runny nose

When using acetylcysteine, you may notice the medicine having an unpleasant odor at first. However, this will soon disappear.

For elderly patients: Difficulty in breathing may be more likely to occur in elderly patients who have respiratory or breathing problems.

Other side effects not listed above may also occur in some patients. If you notice any other effects, check with your doctor.

_____

December 1987

ACRISORCIN (Topical)*

*Not commercially available in the U.S.

To the Reader: If you do not recognize the names of medical conditions or medicines referred to in this information, check with your doctor, nurse, or pharmacist. Definitions for selected medical terms may be found in the Glossary. Brand names for the generic drug names listed can be found in the Index. In addition, selected brand names commonly associated with the generic name have been included in the text to help you recognize medicine you may be taking. The fact that a brand name product is not mentioned does not mean the information does not apply. It is a good idea for you to learn both the generic and brand names of your medicines and to write them down for future use.

Acrisorcin (ak-ri-SOR-sin) belongs to the general family of medicines called antifungals. Acrisorcin is used on the skin to treat tinea versicolor, sometimes called "sun fungus." It will not work for other fungal infections.

Acrisorcin is available only with your doctor's prescription.

Remember:

• **This medicine has been prescribed for your present infection only.** Another infection later on may require a different medicine. Also, even though other people may have the same symptoms as you, they may have a different kind of infection. Your medicine may not work for them and may even cause them harm. Therefore, **your medicine must not be given to other people or used for other infections** unless you are otherwise directed by your doctor.

• **Keep all medicines out of the reach of children.**

• In order for this medicine to work, it must be used as directed.

• **It is very important that you read and understand the following information.** If any of the information causes you special concern, do not decide against using this medicine without first checking with your doctor.

• Before you begin using any new medicine (prescription or nonprescription) or if you develop any new medical problem while you are using this medicine, check with your doctor, nurse, or pharmacist.

• **If you have any questions** about the following information or if you want more information about this medicine or your medical problem, **ask your doctor, nurse, or pharmacist.**

Before Using This Medicine

In order to decide on the best treatment for your medical problem, your doctor should be told:

—if you have ever had any unusual or allergic reaction to acrisorcin.

—if you are allergic to any substance, such as certain foods or preservatives or dyes. Most medicines contain more than their active ingredient. Your doctor, nurse, or pharmacist can help you avoid products that may cause a problem.

—if you are **pregnant** or if you may become pregnant. Studies have not been done in either humans or animals.

—if you are **breast-feeding**. It is not known whether acrisorcin passes into the breast milk. However, this medicine has not been shown to cause problems in nursing babies.

Proper Use of This Medicine

Do not use this medicine in or around the eyes.

Before applying this medicine at night, wash the affected areas with warm, soapy water. Rinse the areas thoroughly to remove all the soap. If any soap is left on the skin, it may keep this medicine from working as well. Then dry areas completely with a towel.

Apply a small amount of this medicine to the affected areas and rub in well, but gently.

After using this medicine, wash your hands thoroughly with soap and water. This will keep you from getting the medicine in your eyes.

When acrisorcin is used to treat "sun fungus," an airtight covering or occlusive dressing (for example, kitchen plastic wrap) should *not* be applied over the medicine. To do so may cause irritation of the skin. **Do not apply an airtight covering over this medicine unless you have been directed to do so by your doctor.**

To help clear up your infection completely, **it is very important that you keep using acrisorcin for the full time of treatment** even if your symptoms begin to clear up after a few days. Since fungal infections may be very slow to clear up, you may have to continue using this medicine every day for as long as 6 weeks or more. If you stop using this medicine too soon, your symptoms may return. **Do not miss any doses.**

If you do miss a dose of this medicine, apply it as soon as possible. Then go back to your regular dosing schedule.

How to store this medicine:

• **Keep out of the reach of children.**

• Store away from heat and direct light.

• Keep the medicine from freezing.

• Do not keep outdated medicine or medicine no longer needed. Be sure that any discarded medicine is out of the reach of children.

Precautions While Using This Medicine

If your skin problem does not improve within 2 to 3 weeks, or if it becomes worse, check with your doctor.

Some people who use acrisorcin on the skin may notice itching of the treated areas when they are exposed to sunlight or ultraviolet (UV) light. **When you first begin** using this medicine, avoid too much sun or overuse of a sunlamp until you see how you react. If the itching is severe, continues, or is bothersome, check with your doctor.

Side Effects of This Medicine

Along with its needed effects, a medicine may cause some unwanted effects. Although not all of these side effects may occur, if they do occur they may need medical attention.

Check with your doctor as soon as possible if any of the following side effects occur:

Skin rash, hives, blistering, burning, itching, redness, or other sign of irritation not present before using this medicine

Other side effects not listed above may also occur in some patients. If you notice any other effects, check with your doctor.

_____

December 1987

ACYCLOVIR (Systemic)

Some commonly used brand names or other names are Acycloguanosine and Zovirax.

To the Reader: If you do not recognize the names of medical conditions or medicines referred to in this information, check with your doctor, nurse, or pharmacist. Definitions for selected medical terms may be found in the Glossary. Brand names for the generic drug names listed can be found in the Index. In addition, selected brand names commonly associated with the generic name have been included in the text to help you recognize medicine you may be taking. The fact that a brand name product is not mentioned does not mean the information does not apply. It is a good idea for you to learn both the generic and brand names of your medicines and to write them down for future use.

Acyclovir (ay-SYE-kloe-veer) belongs to the general family of medicines called antivirals. Antivirals are used to treat infections caused by viruses. Usually they work for only one kind or group of virus infections.

Acyclovir is taken by mouth to treat the symptoms of herpes virus infections of the genitals (sex organs). It is also given by injection to treat herpes infections of the skin, mucous membranes, and genitals. Although acyclovir will not cure herpes, it does help relieve the pain and discomfort and helps the sores (if any) heal faster.

Acyclovir may also be used for other virus infections as determined by your doctor. However, it does not work in treating certain viruses, such as the common cold.

Acyclovir is available only with your doctor's prescription.

Remember:
• **This medicine has been prescribed for your present infection only.** Another infection later on may require a different medicine. Also, even though other people may have the same symptoms as you, they may have a different kind of infection. Your medicine may not work for them and may even cause them harm. Therefore, **your medicine must not be given to other people or used for other infections** unless you are otherwise directed by your doctor.

• **Keep all medicines out of the reach of children.**

• In order for this medicine to work, it must be used as directed.

• If you are receiving this medicine by injection, some of the information about this medicine may not apply.

• **It is very important that you read and understand the following information.** If any of the information causes you special concern, do not decide against using this medicine without first checking with your doctor.

• Before you begin using any new medicine (prescription or nonprescription) or if you develop any new medical problem while you are using this medicine, check with your doctor, nurse, or pharmacist.

• **If you have any questions** about the following information or if you want more information about this medicine or your medical problem, **ask your doctor, nurse, or pharmacist**.

Before Using This Medicine

In order to decide on the best treatment for your medical problem, your doctor should be told:

—if you have ever had any unusual or allergic reaction to acyclovir.

—if you are on a low-salt, low-sugar, or any other special diet, or if you are allergic to any substance, such as foods, sulfites or other preservatives, or dyes. Most medicines contain more than their active ingredient. Your doctor, nurse, or pharmacist can help you avoid products that may cause a problem.

—if you are **pregnant** or if you may become pregnant. Studies have not been done in humans. However, acyclovir has not been shown to cause birth defects or other problems in mice given many times the usual human dose, or in rats or rabbits given several times the usual human dose.

—if you are **breast-feeding**. It is not known whether acyclovir passes into the breast milk. However, acyclovir has not been shown to cause problems in nursing babies.

—if you are receiving acyclovir by injection and have any of the following medical problems:
  Kidney disease
  Liver disease
  Nerve disease

—if you are receiving acyclovir by injection and are also receiving **any** other prescription or nonprescription (OTC) medicine, especially:
  Aminoglycosides by injection or topical application (amikacin, gentamicin, kanamycin, neomycin, netilmicin, streptomycin, tobramycin)
  Amphotericin B by injection (e.g., Fungizone)
  Capreomycin (e.g., Capastat)
  Captopril (e.g., Capoten)
  Carmustine (e.g., BiCNU)
  Cisplatin (e.g., Platinol)
  Cyclosporine (e.g., Sandimmune)
  Gold salts
  Interferon (e.g., Intron A, Roferon-A) or methotrexate (e.g., Mexate) by injection into spinal canal
  Lithium (e.g., Lithane)
  Medicine for inflammation or pain (diclofenac, diflunisal, fenoprofen, flurbiprofen [oral], ibuprofen, indomethacin, ketoprofen, meclofenamate, mefenamic acid, naproxen, oxyphenbutazone, phenylbutazone, piroxicam, sulindac, suprofen, tolmetin)
  Neomycin by mouth (e.g., Mycifradin)
  Penicillamine (e.g., Cuprimine)
  Plicamycin (e.g., Mithracin)
  Rifampin (e.g., Rifadin)
  Streptozocin (e.g., Zanosar)
  Sulfonamides (sulfa medicine)
  Tetracyclines, except doxycycline and minocycline
  Vancomycin by injection (e.g., Vancocin)

—if you regularly take large amounts of combination pain medicine containing acetaminophen and aspirin (e.g., Excedrin) or other salicylates.

—if you are receiving acyclovir by injection and have ever taken cancer medicines that caused nerve problems.

Proper Use of This Medicine

Patient information about the treatment of herpes is available with this medicine. Read this information carefully.

Acyclovir is best used as soon as possible after the symptoms of herpes infection (for example, pain, burning, blisters) begin to appear.

Acyclovir capsules and tablets may be taken with meals.

To help clear up your herpes infection, **keep taking acyclovir for the full time of treatment,** even if your symptoms begin to clear up after a few days. **Do not miss any doses.** However, **do not use this medicine more often or for a longer period of time than your doctor ordered.**

If you do miss a dose of this medicine, take it as soon as possible. However, if it is almost time for your next dose, skip the missed dose and go back to your regular dosing schedule. Do not double doses.

How to store this medicine:
- **Keep out of the reach of children.**
- Store away from heat and direct light.
- Do not store the capsule or tablet form of this medicine in the bathroom, near the kitchen sink, or in other damp places. Heat or moisture may cause the medicine to break down.
- Do not keep outdated medicine or medicine no longer needed. Be sure that any discarded medicine is out of the reach of children.

Precautions While Using This Medicine

Women with genital herpes may be more likely to get cancer of the cervix (mouth of the womb). Therefore, it is very important that Pap smears be taken at least once a year to check for cancer. Cervical cancer can be cured if found and treated early.

If there is no improvement in your herpes infection after you have taken this medicine for a few days, or if it becomes worse, check with your doctor.

The areas affected by herpes should be kept as clean and dry as possible. Also, wear loose-fitting clothing to avoid irritating the sores (blisters).

The capsule and tablet forms of this medicine may cause some people to become dizzy. **Make sure you know how you react to this medicine before you drive, use machines, or do other jobs that require you to be alert.** If this reaction is especially bothersome, check with your doctor.

Herpes infection of the genitals can be caught from or spread to your partner during any sexual activity. Even though you may get herpes if your partner has no symptoms, it is more likely to be spread if sores are present. This is true until the sores are completely healed and the scabs have fallen off. **Therefore, it is**
best to avoid any sexual activity if either of you has any signs of herpes. The use of a condom (prophylactic) probably will help prevent the spread of herpes. However, spermicidal (sperm-killing) jelly or a diaphragm will probably not help. **It is important to remember that acyclovir will not keep you from spreading herpes to others.**

In some patients (usually younger patients), tenderness, swelling, or bleeding of the gums may appear soon after starting treatment with acyclovir. Brushing and flossing your teeth carefully and regularly and massaging your gums may help prevent this. **See your dentist regularly to have your teeth cleaned. Check with your physician or dentist if you have any questions about how to take care of your teeth and gums, or if you notice any tenderness, swelling, or bleeding of your gums.**

Side Effects of This Medicine

Along with its needed effects, a medicine may cause some unwanted effects. Although not all of these side effects may occur, if they do occur they may need medical attention.

Check with your doctor immediately if any of the following side effects occur:
For acyclovir capsules only
  Less common
    Changes in menstrual periods (with long-term use)
    Skin rash
For acyclovir injection only
  More common
    Skin rash or hives
  Less common
    Blood in urine
    Confusion
    Hallucinations (seeing, hearing, or feeling things that are not there)
    Trembling
  Rare (more common with rapid injection)
    Abdominal or stomach pain
    Convulsions (seizures)
    Difficulty in breathing
    Greatly decreased frequency of urination or amount of urine
    Increased thirst
    Loss of appetite
    Nausea or vomiting
    Unusual tiredness or weakness

Other side effects may occur that usually do not require medical attention. These side effects may go away during treatment as your body adjusts to the medicine. However, check with your doctor if any of the following side effects continue or are bothersome:
For acyclovir capsules only
  More common (less common with short-term use)
    Diarrhea
    Dizziness
    Headache
    Joint pain
    Nausea or vomiting

Less common
   Acne (with long-term use)
   Loss of appetite (with short-term use)
   Trouble in sleeping (with long-term use)
For acyclovir injection only
   More common
      Lightheadedness
   Less common
      Headache
      Increased sweating

Other side effects not listed above may also occur in some patients. If you notice any other effects, check with your doctor.

December 1987

ACYCLOVIR (Topical)

Some commonly used brand names or other names are Acycloguanosine and Zovirax.

To the Reader: If you do not recognize the names of medical conditions or medicines referred to in this information, check with your doctor, nurse, or pharmacist. Definitions for selected medical terms may be found in the Glossary. Brand names for the generic drug names listed can be found in the Index. In addition, selected brand names commonly associated with the generic name have been included in the text to help you recognize medicine you may be taking. The fact that a brand name product is not mentioned does not mean the information does not apply. It is a good idea for you to learn both the generic and brand names of your medicines and to write them down for future use.

Acyclovir (ay-SYE-kloe-veer) belongs to the general family of medicines called antivirals. Antivirals are used to treat infections caused by viruses. Usually they work for only one kind or group of virus infections.

Acyclovir ointment is used on the skin and mucous membranes to treat the symptoms of herpes virus infections of the skin, mucous membranes, and genitals (sex organs). Although acyclovir will not cure herpes, it does help relieve the pain and discomfort and helps the sores (if any) heal faster.

Acyclovir is available only with your doctor's prescription.

Remember:

• **This medicine has been prescribed for your present infection only.** Another infection later on may require a different medicine. Also, even though other people may have the same symptoms as you, they may have a different kind of infection. Your medicine may not work for them and may even cause them harm. Therefore, **your medicine must not be given to other people or used for other infections** unless you are otherwise directed by your doctor.

• **Keep all medicines out of the reach of children.**

• In order for this medicine to work, it must be used as directed.

• **It is very important that you read and understand the following information.** If any of the information causes you special concern, do not decide against using this medicine without first checking with your doctor.

• Before you begin using any new medicine (prescription or nonprescription) or if you develop any new medical problem while you are using this medicine, check with your doctor, nurse, or pharmacist.

• **If you have any questions** about the following information or if you want more information about this medicine or your medical problem, **ask your doctor, nurse, or pharmacist.**

Before Using This Medicine

In order to decide on the best treatment for your medical problem, your doctor should be told:

—if you have ever had any unusual or allergic reaction to acyclovir.

—if you are allergic to any substance, such as certain foods or preservatives or dyes. Most medicines contain more than their active ingredient. Your doctor, nurse, or pharmacist can help you avoid products that may cause a problem.

—if you are **pregnant** or if you may become pregnant. Studies have not been done in humans. However, studies in rabbits have shown that acyclovir given by injection may keep the fetus from becoming attached to the lining of the uterus (womb). In other animal studies, acyclovir given by mouth or by injection has not been shown to cause birth defects or other problems.

—if you are **breast-feeding**. It is not known whether acyclovir passes into the breast milk. However, acyclovir ointment has not been shown to cause problems in nursing babies, even though small amounts of acyclovir are absorbed through the skin and mucous membranes.

Proper Use of This Medicine

Patient information about the treatment of herpes is available with this medicine. Read it carefully before using this medicine.

Do not use this medicine in the eyes.

Acyclovir is best used as soon as possible after the symptoms of herpes infection (for example, pain, burning, blisters) begin to appear.

Use a finger cot or rubber glove when applying this medicine. This will help keep you from spreading the infection to other areas of your body or to other people. Apply enough medicine to completely cover all the sores (blisters). A 1.25-cm (approximately ½-inch) strip of ointment applied to each area measuring 5 × 5 cm (approximately 2 × 2 inches) is usually enough, unless otherwise directed by your doctor.

To help clear up your herpes infection, **keep using acyclovir for the full time of treatment,** even if your symptoms begin to clear up after a few days. **Do not miss any doses.** However, **do not use this medicine more often or for a longer period of time than your doctor ordered.**

If you do miss a dose of this medicine, apply it as soon as possible. However, if it is almost time for your next dose, skip the missed dose and go back to your regular dosing schedule.

How to store this medicine:

• **Keep out of the reach of children.**

• Store away from heat and direct light.

• Keep the medicine from freezing.

• Do not keep outdated medicine or medicine no longer needed. Be sure that any discarded medicine is out of the reach of children.

Precautions While Using This Medicine

Women with genital herpes may be more likely to get cancer of the cervix (mouth of the womb). Therefore, it is very important that Pap smears be taken at least once a year to check for cancer. Cervical cancer can be cured if found and treated early.

If your herpes infection does not improve within 1 week, or if it becomes worse, check with your doctor.

The areas affected by herpes should be kept as clean and dry as possible. Also, wear loose-fitting clothing to avoid irritating the sores (blisters).

Herpes infection of the genitals can be caught from or spread to your partner during any sexual activity. Even though you may get herpes if your partner has no symptoms, the infection is more likely to be spread if sores are present. This is true until the sores are completely healed and the scabs have fallen off. **Therefore, it is best to avoid any sexual activity if either of you has any signs of herpes.** The use of a condom (prophylactic) probably will help prevent the spread of herpes. However, spermicidal (sperm-killing) jelly or a diaphragm will probably not help. **It is important to remember that acyclovir will not keep you from spreading herpes to others.**

Side Effects of This Medicine

Along with its needed effects, a medicine may cause some unwanted effects. The following side effects may go away during treatment as your body adjusts to the medicine. However, check with your doctor if any of these effects continue or are bothersome:

More common
    Mild pain, burning, or stinging
Less common or rare
    Itching
    Skin rash

Other side effects not listed above may also occur in some patients. If you notice any other effects, check with your doctor.

_____

December 1987

ADRENOCORTICOIDS (Dental)

This information applies to the following medicines:

Betamethasone (bay-ta-METH-a-sone)*
Hydrocortisone (hye-droe-KOR-ti-sone)
Triamcinolone (trye-am-SIN-oh-lone)

Some commonly used brand names are:	Generic names:
Betnesol*	Betamethasone*
Orabase-HCA	Hydrocortisone
Adcortyl in Orabase* Kenalog in Orabase	Triamcinolone

*Not available in the U.S.

To the Reader: If you do not recognize the names of medical conditions or medicines referred to in this information, check with your doctor, nurse, or pharmacist. Definitions for selected medical terms may be found in the Glossary. Brand names for the generic drug names listed can be found in the Index. In addition, selected brand names commonly associated with the generic name have been included in the text to help you recognize medicine you may be taking. The fact that a brand name product is not mentioned does not mean the information does not apply. It is a good idea for you to learn both the generic and brand names of your medicines and to write them down for future use.

This medicine is an adrenocorticoid (a-dree-noe-KOR-ti-koid) (cortisone-like medicine). It belongs to the general family of medicines called steroids. These cortisone-like medicines are used in the mouth to relieve the discomfort and redness of some mouth and gum problems.

Dental adrenocorticoids may be absorbed through the lining of the mouth and if used too often or too long may interfere with growth in children. Before using this medicine in children, you should discuss its use with your physician or dentist.

Dental adrenocorticoids are available only with your physician's or dentist's prescription.

Remember:

• **This medicine has been prescribed for your current medical problem only.** It must not be given to other people or used for other problems unless you are directed to do so by your doctor.

• **Keep all medicines out of the reach of children.**

• In order for this medicine to work, it must be used as directed.

• **It is very important that you read and understand the following information.** If any of the information causes you special concern, do not decide against using this medicine without first checking with your doctor.

• Before you begin using any new medicine (prescription or nonprescription) or if you develop any new medical problem while you are using this medicine, check with your doctor, nurse, or pharmacist.

• **If you have any questions** about the following information or if you want more information about this medicine or your medical problem, **ask your doctor, nurse, or pharmacist.**

Before Using This Medicine

In order to decide on the best treatment for your medical problem, your physician or dentist should be told:

—if you have ever had any unusual or allergic reaction to dental adrenocorticoids, or to topical (applied to the skin) adrenocorticoids.

—if you are allergic to any substance, such as certain preservatives or dyes. Most medicines contain more than their active ingredient. Your doctor, nurse, or pharmacist can help you avoid products that may cause a problem.

—if you are **pregnant** or if you may become pregnant. These medicines have not been shown to cause problems in humans. Studies on birth defects with topical adrenocorticoids have not been done in humans. However, studies in animals have shown that topical adrenocorticoids, such as the hydrocortisone or triamcinolone in this medicine, when applied to the skin in large amounts or for a long period of time, cause birth defects. Studies with dental paste have not been done in animals.

—if you are **breast-feeding.** Dental adrenocorticoids have not been shown to cause problems in nursing babies. However, other adrenocorticoids pass into breast milk and may interfere with the infant's growth.

—if you have any of the following medical problems:

Diabetes mellitus (sugar diabetes)
Herpes sores
Infection or ulceration of the mouth or throat
Tuberculosis

Proper Use of This Medicine

How to use hydrocortisone or triamcinolone:

• Using a cotton swab, press (do not rub) a small amount of paste onto the area to be treated until the paste sticks and a smooth, slippery film forms. Do not try to spread the medicine because it will become crumbly and gritty. Apply the paste at bedtime so the medicine can work overnight. The other applications of the paste should be made following meals.

How to use betamethasone:

• Place the pellet as close as possible to the sore (or sores) in your mouth and keep it there until it dissolves.

Do not use adrenocorticoids more often or for a longer period of time than your physician or dentist ordered. To do so may increase the chance of absorption through the lining of the mouth and the chance of side effects.

Do not use any leftover medicine for future mouth problems without first checking with your physician or dentist. This medicine should *not* be used on many kinds of bacterial, viral, or fungal infections.

If your physician or dentist has ordered you to use this medicine according to a regular schedule and you miss a dose, use it as soon as you remember. However, if it is almost time for your next dose, skip the missed dose and go back to your regular dosing schedule.

How to store this medicine:

- **Keep out of the reach of children.**
- Store away from heat and direct light.
- Do not store betamethasone pellets in the bathroom, near the kitchen sink, or in other damp places. Heat or moisture may cause the medicine to break down.
- Keep the medicine from freezing.
- Do not keep outdated medicine or medicine no longer needed. Be sure that any discarded medicine is out of the reach of children.

Precautions While Using This Medicine

Children who must use this medicine should be followed closely by their doctor. This medicine may be absorbed through the lining of the mouth and can affect growth or cause other unwanted effects.

Check with your physician or dentist:
—**if your symptoms do not improve within 1 week.**
—**if your condition gets worse.**

Side Effects of This Medicine

Along with its needed effects, a medicine may cause some unwanted effects. Although not all of these side effects may occur, if they do occur they may need medical attention.

Check with your physician or dentist as soon as possible if the following side effects occur:

> Signs of infection or irritation such as burning, itching, blistering, or peeling not present before using this medicine

Other side effects not listed above may also occur in some patients. If you notice any other effects, check with your physician or dentist.

_____

December 1987

ADRENOCORTICOIDS (Inhalation)

This information applies to the following medicines:

Beclomethasone (be-kloe-METH-a-sone)
Dexamethasone (dex-a-METH-a-sone)
Flunisolide (floo-NISS-oh-lide)
Triamcinolone (trye-am-SIN-oh-lone)

Some commonly used brand names are:	Generic names:
Beclovent Beclovent Rotacaps* Becotide* Vanceril	Beclomethasone
Decadron Respihaler	Dexamethasone
AeroBid	Flunisolide
Azmacort	Triamcinolone

*Not available in the U.S.

To the Reader: If you do not recognize the names of medical conditions or medicines referred to in this information, check with your doctor, nurse, or pharmacist. Definitions for selected medical terms may be found in the Glossary. Brand names for the generic drug names listed can be found in the Index. In addition, selected brand names commonly associated with the generic name have been included in the text to help you recognize medicine you may be taking. The fact that a brand name product is not mentioned does not mean the information does not apply. It is a good idea for you to learn both the generic and brand names of your medicines and to write them down for future use.

Inhalation adrenocorticoids (a-dree-noe-KOR-ti-koids) are cortisone-like medicines. They belong to the general family of medicines called steroids. These medicines are inhaled (breathed in) through the mouth to help prevent asthma attacks. However, they will not relieve an asthma attack that has already started.

Adrenocorticoids may slow or stop growth in children when used for long periods of time. Before this medicine is given to a child, you and your child's doctor should talk about the good this medicine will do as well as the risks of using it. Follow the doctor's directions very carefully in order to lessen the chance that these unwanted effects will occur.

Inhalation adrenocorticoids are available only with your doctor's prescription.

Remember:
• **This medicine has been prescribed for your current medical problem only.** It must not be given to other people or used for other problems unless you are directed to do so by your doctor.

• **Keep all medicines out of the reach of children.**

• In order for this medicine to work, it must be used as directed.

• **It is very important that you read and understand the following information.** If any of the information causes you special concern, do not decide against using this medicine without first checking with your doctor.

• Before you begin using any new medicine (prescription or nonprescription) or if you develop any new medical problem while you are using this medicine, check with your doctor, nurse, or pharmacist.

• **If you have any questions** about the following information or if you want more information about this medicine or your medical problem, **ask your doctor, nurse, or pharmacist.**

Before Using This Medicine

In order to decide on the best treatment for your medical problem, your doctor should be told:

—if you have ever had any unusual or allergic reaction to adrenocorticoids or aerosol spray inhalation medicines.

—if you are allergic to any substance, such as certain foods or preservatives or dyes. Most medicines contain more than their active ingredient. Your doctor, nurse, or pharmacist can help you avoid products that may cause a problem.

—if you are **pregnant** or if you may become pregnant. In one study, use of beclomethasone inhalation by pregnant women did not cause birth defects or other problems. Studies on birth defects with dexamethasone, flunisolide, or triamcinolone inhalations have not been done in humans. However, too much use of an adrenocorticoid during pregnancy may cause the baby to have problems after birth, such as slower growth and reduced adrenal gland function. Also, studies in animals have shown that adrenocorticoids cause birth defects affecting the mouth, tongue, or bones, or other unwanted effects.

—if you are **breast-feeding**. Many adrenocorticoids pass into the breast milk and cause problems with growth or other unwanted effects in nursing babies.

It is not known whether beclomethasone, flunisolide, or triamcinolone passes into the breast milk. However, these medicines have not been shown to cause problems in nursing babies.

Dexamethasone passes into the breast milk and may cause problems in nursing babies. It may be necessary for you to take another medicine or to stop breast-feeding during treatment. Be sure you have discussed the risks and benefits of this medicine with your doctor.

—if you are using any inhalation adrenocorticoid and have an infection of the mouth, throat, or lungs, or if you have ever had tuberculosis (TB).

—if you are using dexamethasone or triamcinolone inhalation aerosol and have any of the following medical problems:

Bone disease
Colitis
Diabetes mellitus (sugar diabetes)
Diverticulitis
Fungal infection
Glaucoma
Heart disease
Herpes simplex (virus) infection of the eye
High blood pressure
High cholesterol levels

Kidney disease or kidney stones
Liver disease
Myasthenia gravis
Stomach ulcer or other stomach problems
Underactive thyroid

—if you are using any inhalation adrenocorticoid and are also using another aerosol spray inhalation for asthma.

—if you are taking **any** other prescription or nonprescription (OTC) medicine, especially:

Antidiabetic agents, oral (diabetes medicine you take by mouth)
Insulin

Proper Use of This Medicine

Inhalation adrenocorticoids are used with a special inhaler and usually come with patient directions. **Read the directions carefully before using.** If you do not understand the directions, or if you are not sure how to use the inhaler, check with your doctor, nurse, or pharmacist.

Do not use more of this medicine, and do not use it more often, than your doctor ordered. To do so may increase the chance of absorption into the body and the chance of unwanted effects.

In order for this medicine to help prevent asthma attacks, it must be taken every day in regularly spaced doses as ordered by your doctor. Up to four weeks may pass before you feel its full effects. However, this may take less time if you have been taking certain other medicines for your asthma.

Do not use this medicine to treat an asthma attack that has already started, because it will not work. However, continue to take this medicine at the usual time, even if you use another medicine to relieve the asthma attack.

The inhaler should be cleaned every day as directed. If you do not receive instructions with the inhaler, or if you are not certain how to clean it, check with your pharmacist.

Gargling and rinsing your mouth with water after each dose may help prevent hoarseness, throat irritation, and infection in the mouth.

If you miss a dose of this medicine, use it as soon as possible. However, if it is almost time for your next dose, skip the missed dose and go back to your regular dosing schedule. Do not double doses.

Check with your pharmacist to see if you should save the inhaler piece that comes with this medicine. Refill units may be available at lower cost. However, remember that the inhaler is meant to be used only for the medicine that comes with it. Do not use the inhaler for any other inhalation aerosol medicine, even if the cartridge fits.

How to store this medicine:

• **Keep out of the reach of children.**

• Store away from heat and direct light.

• Keep the medicine from freezing.

• Do not puncture, break, or burn the aerosol container, even after it is empty.

• Do not keep outdated medicine or medicine no longer needed. Be sure that any discarded medicine is out of the reach of children.

Precautions While Using This Medicine

Check with your doctor:

—**if you go through a period of unusual stress.**

—**if you have an asthma attack** that does not improve after you take a bronchodilator medicine.

—**if signs of mouth, throat, or lung infection occur.**

—**if your symptoms do not improve.**

—**if your condition gets worse.**

Also, **check with your doctor immediately if any of the following side effects occur** while you are using this medicine:

Abdominal or back pain
Dizziness or fainting
Fever
Muscle or joint pain
Nausea or vomiting
Prolonged loss of appetite
Shortness of breath
Unusual tiredness or weakness
Unusual weight loss

Your doctor may want you to carry a medical identification card stating that you are using this medicine and may need additional medicine during times of emergency, a severe asthma attack or other illness, or unusual stress.

Before you have any kind of surgery (including dental surgery) or emergency treatment, tell the physician or dentist in charge that you are using this medicine.

For patients who are also using a bronchodilator inhalation aerosol:

• Unless otherwise directed by your doctor, **use the bronchodilator aerosol first, then wait about 5 minutes before using this medicine.** In order to lessen the chance of unwanted effects, it is best not to use the two kinds of aerosols too close together.

For patients who are also regularly taking an adrenocorticoid in tablet or liquid form:

• **Do not stop taking the other adrenocorticoid without your doctor's advice, even if your asthma seems better.** Your doctor may want you to reduce gradually the amount you are taking before stopping completely, in order to lessen the chance of unwanted effects.

• When your doctor tells you to reduce the dose, or to stop taking the other adrenocorticoid, follow the directions carefully. Your body may need time to adjust to the change. The length of time this takes may depend on the amount of medicine you were taking and how long you took it. **It is especially important that your doctor check your progress at regular visits during this period of time.** Also, ask your doctor if there are special directions you should follow if you have a severe asthma attack, if you need any other medical or surgical treatment, or if certain side effects occur. Be certain that you understand these directions, and follow them carefully.

Side Effects of This Medicine

Along with its needed effects, a medicine may cause some unwanted effects. Although not all of these side effects may occur, if they do occur they may need medical attention.

Check with your doctor immediately if any of the following side effects occur just after you use this medicine:

Rare

   Shortness of breath, troubled breathing, tightness in chest, or wheezing

Also, check with your doctor as soon as possible if any of the following side effects occur:

More common

   Any sign of possible infection, such as chest pain, chills, fever, cough, congestion, ear pain, eye pain, red or teary eyes, runny nose, sneezing, or sore throat
   Creamy white, curd-like patches inside the mouth
   Increased susceptibility to infection
   Nausea or vomiting
   Skin rash or itching
   Unusually fast or pounding heartbeat

Less common or rare

   Decreased or blurred vision
   Difficulty in swallowing
   Hives
   Increased blood pressure
   Increased thirst
   Mental depression or other mood or mental changes
   Swelling of face
   Swelling of feet or lower legs
   Unusual weight gain

Additional side effects may occur after you have been using this medicine for a long period of time. Check with your doctor as soon as possible if any of the following side effects occur:

   Acne or other skin problems
   Back or rib pain
   Bloody or black tarry stools

Filling or rounding out of the face (moon face)
   Frequent urination
   Increased thirst
   Irregular heartbeats
   Menstrual problems
   Muscle weakness, cramps, or pains
   Stomach pain or burning (severe and continuing)
   Unusual tiredness or weakness
   Wounds that will not heal

Other side effects may occur that usually do not require medical attention. These side effects may go away during treatment as your body adjusts to the medicine. However, check with your doctor if any of the following side effects continue or are bothersome:

More common

   Abdominal or stomach pain (mild)
   Bloated feeling or gas
   Constipation
   Diarrhea
   Dizziness or lightheadedness
   Headache
   Heartburn or indigestion
   Loss of appetite
   Loss of smell or taste sense
   Nervousness or restlessness
   Unpleasant taste

Less common or rare

   Cough without other signs of infection
   Dry or irritated nose, mouth, tongue, or throat
   False sense of well-being
   General feeling of discomfort, illness, shakiness, or faintness
   Hoarseness or other voice changes without other signs of infection
   Increase in appetite
   Trouble in sleeping
   Unexplained nosebleeds
   Unusual increase in sweating

Some of the above side effects have been reported for dexamethasone or flunisolide, but not for beclomethasone or triamcinolone. However, all of the inhalation adrenocorticoids are similar. Therefore, the chance always exists that these side effects may occur with beclomethasone or triamcinolone also, especially if large amounts are used for a long time.

Other side effects not listed above may also occur in some patients. If you notice any other effects, check with your doctor.

December 1987

ADRENOCORTICOIDS (Nasal)

This information applies to the following medicines:

Beclomethasone (be-kloe-METH-a-sone)
Dexamethasone (dex-a-METH-a-sone)
Flunisolide (floo-NISS-oh-lide)

Some commonly used brand names are:	Generic names
Beconase Vancenase	Beclomethasone
Decadron Turbinaire	Dexamethasone
Nasalide Rhinalar* Syntaris*	Flunisolide

*Not available in the U.S.

To the Reader: If you do not recognize the names of medical conditions or medicines referred to in this information, check with your doctor, nurse, or pharmacist. Definitions for selected medical terms may be found in the Glossary. Brand names for the generic drug names listed can be found in the Index. In addition, selected brand names commonly associated with the generic name have been included in the text to help you recognize medicine you may be taking. The fact that a brand name product is not mentioned does not mean the information does not apply. It is a good idea for you to learn both the generic and brand names of your medicines and to write them down for future use.

Nasal adrenocorticoids (a-dree-noe-KOR-ti-koids) are cortisone-like medicines. They belong to the family of medicines called steroids. These medicines are sprayed into the nose to help relieve the stuffy nose, irritation, and discomfort of hay fever, other allergies, and other nasal problems. These medicines are also used to prevent nasal polyps from growing back after they have been removed by surgery.

Nasal adrenocorticoids may be absorbed through the lining of the nose into the body and may interfere with growth in children. Therefore, children using this medicine should have their progress checked by their doctor at regular visits.

These medicines are available only with your doctor's prescription.

Remember:
• **This medicine has been prescribed for your current medical problem only.** It must not be given to other people or used for other problems unless you are directed to do so by your doctor.

• **Keep all medicines out of the reach of children.**

• In order for this medicine to work, it must be used as directed.

• **It is very important that you read and understand the following information.** If any of the information causes you special concern, do not decide against using this medicine without first checking with your doctor.

• Before you begin using any new medicine (prescription or nonprescription) or if you develop any new medical problem while you are using this medicine, check with your doctor, nurse, or pharmacist.

• **If you have any questions** about the following information or if you want more information about this medicine or your medical problem, **ask your doctor, nurse, or pharmacist.**

Before Using This Medicine

In order to decide on the best treatment for your medical problem, your doctor should be told:

—if you have ever had any unusual or allergic reaction to beclomethasone, dexamethasone, flunisolide, or other adrenocorticoids, aerosol sprays or inhalations, or other medicines for the nose.

—if you are allergic to any substance, such as propylene glycol, polyethylene glycol, or certain preservatives or dyes. Most medicines contain more than their active ingredient. Your doctor, nurse, or pharmacist can help you avoid products that may cause a problem.

—if you are **pregnant** or if you intend to become pregnant while using this medicine. In a few studies, use of beclomethasone by pregnant women did not cause birth defects or other problems. Studies on birth defects with dexamethasone or flunisolide have not been done in humans. However, too much use of an adrenocorticoid during pregnancy may cause the baby to have problems after birth, such as slower growth and reduced adrenal gland function. Also studies in animals have shown that adrenocorticoids cause birth defects affecting the mouth, tongue, or bones, or other unwanted effects.

—if you are **breast-feeding**. Use of dexamethasone is not recommended in nursing mothers since dexamethasone passes into the breast milk and may affect the infant's growth. Although it is not known whether beclomethasone or flunisolide pass into the breast milk, the chance always exists.

—if you have any of the following medical problems:
Glaucoma
Herpes simplex (virus) infection of the eye
Infections
Injury to the nose (recent)
Nose surgery (recent)
Tuberculosis, active or history of
Ulcers in the nose

Proper Use of This Medicine

This medicine usually comes with patient directions. **Read them carefully before using the medicine.** Beclomethasone and dexamethasone are used with a special inhaler. If you do not understand the directions, or if you are not sure how to use the inhaler, check with your doctor, nurse, or pharmacist.

In order for this medicine to help you, it must be used regularly as ordered by your doctor. This medicine usually begins to work in about 1 week, but up to 3 weeks may pass before you feel its full effects.

Use this medicine only as directed. Do not use more of it and do not use it more often than your doctor ordered. To do so may increase the chance of absorption through the lining of the nose and the chance of unwanted effects.

Check with your doctor before using this medicine for nasal problems other than the one for which it was prescribed, since it should not be used on many bacterial, viral, or fungal nasal infections.

Save the inhaler that comes with beclomethasone or dexamethasone, since refill units may be available at lower cost.

If you miss a dose of this medicine and remember within an hour or so, use it right away. However, if you do not remember until later, skip the missed dose and go back to your regular dosing schedule. Do not double doses.

How to store this medicine:

• **Keep out of the reach of children.**

• Store away from heat and direct light.

• Keep the medicine from freezing.

• Do not puncture, break, or burn the beclomethasone or dexamethasone aerosol container, even after it is empty.

• Do not keep outdated medicine or medicine no longer needed. Also, discard any unused flunisolide 3 months after you open the package. Be sure that any discarded medicine is out of the reach of children.

Precautions While Using This Medicine

If you will be using this medicine for more than a few weeks, your doctor should check your progress at regular visits.

Check with your doctor:

—**if signs of a nose, sinus, or throat infection occur.**

—**if your symptoms do not improve within 7 days (for dexamethasone) or within 3 weeks (for beclomethasone or flunisolide).**

—**if your condition gets worse.**

Side Effects of This Medicine

Along with its needed effects, a medicine may cause some unwanted effects. Although not all of these side effects may occur, if they do occur they may need medical attention.

Check with your doctor as soon as possible if any of the following side effects occur:
Less common or rare
   Bloody mucus or unexplained nosebleeds
   Crusting inside the nose
   Headache
   Hives
   Loss of sense of taste or smell
   Nausea or vomiting
   Shortness of breath, troubled breathing, tightness in chest, or wheezing
   Skin rash
   Sore throat
   Stuffy nose (continuing)
   Swellings on face
Sign of overdose
   Fullness or rounding of the face

Other side effects may occur that usually do not require medical attention. These side effects may go away during treatment as your body adjusts to the medicine. However, check with your doctor if any of the following side effects continue or are bothersome:
More common
   Burning, dryness, or other irritation inside the nose
   Unusual increase in sneezing

Although not all of the side effects listed above have been reported for all of the nasal adrenocorticoids, they have been reported for at least one of them. However, since all of these medicines are very similar, it is possible that any of the above side effects may occur with any of these medicines.

Other side effects not listed above may also occur in some patients. If you notice any other effects, check with your doctor.

December 1987

ADRENOCORTICOIDS (Ophthalmic)

This information applies to the following medicines:

Betamethasone (bay-ta-METH-a-sone)
Dexamethasone (dex-a-METH-a-sone)
Fluorometholone (flure-oh-METH-oh-lone)
Hydrocortisone (hye-droe-KOR-ti-sone)
Medrysone (ME-dri-sone)
Prednisolone (pred-NISS-oh-lone)

Some commonly used brand names and other names are:	Generic names:
Betnesol*	Betamethasone
Ak-Dex Decadron Dexair I-Methasone Maxidex Ocu-Dex	Dexamethasone†
Fluor-Op FML* FML Forte FML Liquifilm FML S.O.P.	Fluorometholone
Cortamed* Cortisol	Hydrocortisone
HMS Liquifilm	Medrysone
Ak-Pred Ak-Tate Econopred Econopred Plus Inflamase Inflamase Forte I-Pred I-Prednicet Metreton Ocu-Pred Ocu-Pred-A Ocu-Pred Forte Predair Predair-A Predair Forte Pred Forte Pred Mild Predsol*	Prednisolone†

*Not available in the U.S.
†Generic name product may also be available in the U.S.

To the Reader: If you do not recognize the names of medical conditions or medicines referred to in this information, check with your doctor, nurse, or pharmacist. Definitions for selected medical terms may be found in the Glossary. Brand names for the generic drug names listed can be found in the Index. In addition, selected brand names commonly associated with the generic name have been included in the text to help you recognize medicine you may be taking. The fact that a brand name product is not mentioned does not mean the information does not apply. It is a good idea for you to learn both the generic and brand names of your medicines and to write them down for future use.

Ophthalmic adrenocorticoids (a-dree-noe-KOR-ti-koids) (cortisone-like medicines) are used in the eye in the form of drops or ointment to prevent permanent damage to the eye, which may occur with certain eye problems. They also provide relief from redness, irritation, and other discomfort.

This medicine may be especially likely to cause unwanted effects in young children, especially those less than 2 years of age. If this medicine has been ordered for a young child, you should discuss its use with your child's doctor. Be sure that you follow all of the doctor's instructions very carefully.

Adrenocorticoids for use in the eye are available only with your doctor's prescription.

Remember:
• **This medicine has been prescribed for your current medical problem only.** It must not be given to other people or used for other problems unless you are directed to do so by your doctor.

• **Keep all medicines out of the reach of children.**

• In order for this medicine to work, it must be used as directed.

• **It is very important that you read and understand the following information.** If any of the information causes you special concern, do not decide against using this medicine without first checking with your doctor.

• Before you begin using any new medicine (prescription or nonprescription) or if you develop any new medical problem while you are using this medicine, check with your doctor, nurse, or pharmacist.

• **If you have any questions** about the following information or if you want more information about this medicine or your medical problem, **ask your doctor, nurse, or pharmacist.**

Before Using This Medicine

In order to decide on the best treatment for your medical problem, your doctor should be told:

—if you have ever had any unusual or allergic reaction to adrenocorticoids.

—if you are allergic to any substance, such as certain preservatives or dyes. Most medicines contain more than their active ingredient. Your doctor, nurse, or pharmacist can help you avoid products that may cause a problem.

—if you are **pregnant** or if you may become pregnant. Although studies on birth defects with ophthalmic adrenocorticoids have not been done in humans, these medicines have not been reported to cause birth defects or other problems in humans. However, in animal studies, dexamethasone, fluorometholone, hydrocortisone, and prednisolone caused birth defects when applied to the eyes of pregnant animals. Also, fluorometholone and medrysone caused other unwanted effects in the fetus.

—if you are **breast-feeding.** Ophthalmic adrenocorticoids have not been shown to cause problems in nursing babies.

—if you have any of the following medical problems:
　Cataracts
　Diabetes mellitus (sugar diabetes)
　Glaucoma or a family history of glaucoma

Herpes infection of the eye
Tuberculosis of the eye (active or history of)
Any other eye infection

—if you are now taking or using any of the following medicines or types of medicine:

Antimuscarinics (medicine for abdominal or stomach spasms or cramps)
Medicine for glaucoma

Proper Use of This Medicine

For patients who wear contact lenses:

• Use of ophthalmic adrenocorticoids while you are wearing contact lenses (either hard lenses or soft lenses) may increase the chance of infection. Therefore, do not apply this medicine while you are wearing contact lenses. Also, check with an ophthalmologist (eye doctor) for advice on how long to wait after applying this medicine before inserting your contact lenses. It is possible that you may be directed not to wear contact lenses at all during the entire time of treatment and for a day or two after treatment has been stopped.

For patients using an eye drop form of this medicine:
• If you are using a suspension form of this medicine, always shake the container very well just before applying the eye drops.

• How to apply this medicine: First, wash your hands. With the middle finger, apply pressure to the inside corner of the eye (and continue to apply pressure for 1 or 2 minutes after the medicine has been placed in the eye). Tilt the head back and with the index finger of the same hand, pull the lower eyelid away from the eye to form a pouch. Drop the medicine into the pouch and gently close your eyes. Do not blink. Keep your eyes closed for 1 or 2 minutes to allow the medicine to come into contact with the irritation. If you think you did not get the drop of medicine into your eye properly, use another drop.

• Remove any excess solution around the eye with a clean tissue, being careful not to touch the eye.

• Immediately after applying the eye drops, wash your hands to remove any medicine that may be on them.

• To prevent contamination of the eye drops, do not touch the dropper or the applicator tip to any surface (including the eye). Always keep the container tightly closed.

For patients using an ointment form of this medicine:
• How to apply this medicine: First, wash your hands. Then pull the lower eyelid away from the eye to form a pouch. Squeeze a thin strip of ointment into the pouch. A 1-cm (approximately ⅓ inch) strip of ointment is usually enough unless otherwise directed by your doctor. Gently close the eyes and keep them closed for 1 or 2 minutes to allow the medicine to spread over the surface of the eye and come into contact with the irritation.

• To prevent contamination of the eye ointment, do not touch the applicator tip to any surface (including the eye). After using the eye ointment, wipe the tip of the ointment tube with a clean tissue. Do not wash the tip with water. Always keep the tube tightly closed.

Do not use adrenocorticoids more often or for a longer period of time than your doctor ordered. To do so may increase the chance of side effects, especially in children 2 years of age or younger.

Do not use any leftover medicine for future eye problems without first checking with your doctor. This medicine should not be used if certain kinds of infections are present. To do so may make the infection worse and possibly lead to eye damage.

If you miss a dose of this medicine, apply it as soon as possible. But if it is almost time for your next dose, skip the missed dose and go back to your regular dosing schedule.

How to store this medicine:

• **Keep out of the reach of children.**

• Store away from heat and direct light.

• Keep the medicine from freezing.

• Do not keep outdated medicine or medicine no longer needed. Be sure that any discarded medicine is out of the reach of children.

Precautions While Using This Medicine

If you will be using this medicine for more than a few weeks, an ophthalmologist (eye doctor) should examine your eyes at regular visits to make sure it does not cause unwanted effects.

If your symptoms have not improved after 5 to 7 days, or if your eye condition becomes worse, check with your doctor.

Side Effects of This Medicine

Along with its needed effects, a medicine may cause some unwanted effects. Although not all of these side effects may occur, if they do occur they may need medical attention. Check with your doctor as soon as possible if any of the following side effects occur:

Less common or rare
Blurred vision (other than temporary blurring after use of ointment)
Drooping of the eyelids
Eye pain
Headache
Seeing halos around lights
Unusually large pupils

Other side effects may occur that usually do not require medical attention. These side effects may go away during treatment as your body adjusts to the medicine. However, check with your doctor if any of the following side effects continue or are bothersome:

Less common or rare
Burning, stinging, or watering of the eyes

After application, eye ointments may be expected to cause your vision to blur for a few minutes.

Some of the side effects listed above may be more likely to occur in very young children, who are usually more sensitive to the effects of these medicines.

Other side effects not listed may also occur in some patients, especially children 2 years of age or younger. If you notice any other effects, check with your doctor.

_____

December 1987

ADRENOCORTICOIDS (Otic)

This information applies to the following medicines:

Betamethasone (bay-ta-METH-a-sone)
Dexamethasone (dex-a-METH-a-sone)
Hydrocortisone (hye-droe-KOR-ti-sone)
Prednisolone (pred-NISS-oh-lone)

Some commonly used brand names or other names are:	Generic names:
Betnesol*	Betamethasone
Decadron	Dexamethasone
Cortamed* Cortisol	Hydrocortisone
Metreton Predsol*	Prednisolone

*Not available in the U.S.

To the Reader: If you do not recognize the names of medical conditions or medicines referred to in this information, check with your doctor, nurse, or pharmacist. Definitions for selected medical terms may be found in the Glossary. Brand names for the generic drug names listed can be found in the Index. In addition, selected brand names commonly associated with the generic name have been included in the text to help you recognize medicine you may be taking. The fact that a brand name product is not mentioned does not mean the information does not apply. It is a good idea for you to learn both the generic and brand names of your medicines and to write them down for future use.

Otic adrenocorticoids (a-dree-noe-KOR-ti-koids) (cortisone-like medicines) are used in the ear to relieve the redness, itching, and swelling caused by certain ear problems.

Adrenocorticoids for use in the ear are available only with your doctor's prescription.

Remember:

• **This medicine has been prescribed for your current medical problem only.** It must not be given to other people or used for other problems unless you are directed to do so by your doctor.

• **Keep all medicines out of the reach of children.**

• In order for this medicine to work, it must be used as directed.

• **It is very important that you read and understand the following information.** If any of the information causes you special concern, do not decide against using this medicine without first checking with your doctor.

• Before you begin using any new medicine (prescription or nonprescription) or if you develop any new medical problem while you are using this medicine, check with your doctor, nurse, or pharmacist.

• **If you have any questions** about the following information or if you want more information about this medicine or your medical problem, **ask your doctor, nurse, or pharmacist.**

Before Using This Medicine

In order to decide on the best treatment for your medical problem, your doctor should be told:

—if you have ever had any unusual or allergic reaction to adrenocorticoids.

—if you are allergic to any substance, such as certain preservatives or dyes. Most medicines contain more than their active ingredient. Your doctor, nurse, or pharmacist can help you avoid products that may cause a problem.

—if you are **pregnant** or if you may become pregnant. Otic adrenocorticoids have not been shown to cause birth defects or other problems in humans.

—if you are **breast-feeding.** Otic adrenocorticoids have not been shown to cause problems in humans.

—if you have any of the following medical problems:

Any other ear infection or condition
Punctured ear drum

Proper Use of This Medicine

How to apply ear drops: Lie down or tilt the head so that the infected ear faces up. Gently pull the ear lobe up and back for adults (down and back for children) to straighten the ear canal. Drop the medicine into the ear canal. Keep the ear facing up for several (about 5) minutes to allow the medicine to run to the bottom of the ear canal. A sterile, soft cotton plug may be gently inserted into the ear opening to prevent the medicine from leaking out.

How to apply ear ointment: Apply a small amount of ointment to the area just inside the ear canal, using a clean finger or a piece of sterile gauze. Do not use a cotton-tipped swab unless your doctor has directed you to do so and has explained exactly how to use it.

To prevent contamination of the drops or ointment, do not touch the dropper or applicator tip to any surface (including the ear). Also, always keep the container tightly closed.

Do not use adrenocorticoids more often or for a longer period of time than your doctor ordered. To do so may increase the chance of side effects.

Do not use any leftover medicine for future ear problems without first checking with your doctor. This medicine should not be used if certain kinds of infections are present. To do so may make the infection worse.

If you miss a dose of this medicine, use it as soon as you remember. However, if it is almost time for your next dose, skip the missed dose and go back to your regular dosing schedule. Do not double doses.

How to store this medicine:

• **Keep out of the reach of children.**

• Store away from heat and direct light.

• Keep the medicine from freezing.

• Do not keep outdated medicine or medicine no longer needed. Be sure that any discarded medicine is out of the reach of children.

Precautions While Using This Medicine

If your symptoms have not improved after 5 to 7 days, or if your ear problem becomes worse, check with your doctor.

Side Effects of This Medicine

Along with its needed effects, a medicine may cause some unwanted effects. The following side effects usually do not need medical attention and may go away during treatment as your body adjusts to the medicine. However, check with your doctor if either of the following side effects continues or is bothersome:

Less common
   Burning or stinging of the ear

There have not been any other common or important side effects reported with this medicine. However, if you notice any unusual effects, check with your doctor.

December 1987

ADRENOCORTICOIDS (Systemic— Mineralocorticoid Effects)

This information applies to the following medicines:

Desoxycorticosterone (des-ox-i-kor-ti-koe-STER-one)
Fludrocortisone (floo-droe-KOR-ti-sone)

Some commonly used brand names and other names are:	Generic names:
DOCA Percorten	Desoxycorticosterone†
Florinef	Fludrocortisone

†Generic product may be available in the U.S.

To the Reader: If you do not recognize the names of medical conditions or medicines referred to in this information, check with your doctor, nurse, or pharmacist. Definitions for selected medical terms may be found in the Glossary. Brand names for the generic drug names listed can be found in the Index. In addition, selected brand names commonly associated with the generic name have been included in the text to help you recognize medicine you may be taking. The fact that a brand name product is not mentioned does not mean the information does not apply. It is a good idea for you to learn both the generic and brand names of your medicines and to write them down for future use.

This medicine is an adrenocorticoid (a-dree-noe-KOR-ti-koid) (cortisone-like medicine). It belongs to the family of medicines called steroids. Your body naturally produces certain cortisones which are necessary in order to maintain good health. If your body does not produce enough, your doctor may have prescribed this medicine to help make up the difference. Fludrocortisone may also be used to treat other medical conditions as determined by your doctor.

Fludrocortisone is taken by mouth. Desoxycorticosterone is given by injection or placed under the skin in pellet form.

These medicines are available only with your doctor's prescription.

Remember:

• **This medicine has been prescribed for your current medical problem only.** It must not be given to other people or used for other problems unless you are directed to do so by your doctor.

• **Keep all medicines out of the reach of children.**

• In order for this medicine to work, it must be used as directed.

• If you are receiving this medicine by injection, some of the information about this medicine may not apply.

• **It is very important that you read and understand the following information.** If any of the information causes you special concern, do not decide against using this medicine without first checking with your doctor.

• Before you begin using any new medicine (prescription or nonprescription) or if you develop any new medical problem while you are using this medicine, check with your doctor, nurse, or pharmacist.

• **If you have any questions** about the following information or if you want more information about this medicine or your medical problem, **ask your doctor, nurse, or pharmacist.**

Before Using This Medicine

In order to decide on the best treatment for your medical problem, your doctor should be told:

—if you have ever had any unusual or allergic reaction to adrenocorticoids.

—if you are allergic to sesame seeds or sesame oil (for desoxycorticosterone injection only).

—if you are **pregnant** or if you intend to become pregnant while using this medicine. Too much use of these adrenocorticoids during pregnancy may cause the baby to have an underactive adrenal gland after birth. Although desoxycorticosterone has not been shown to cause birth defects in humans, the chance always exists. Studies on birth defects in humans or animals have not been done with fludrocortisone.

—if you are **breast-feeding**. Adrenocorticoids pass into the breast milk and may cause problems with growth or other unwanted effects in the nursing baby.

—if you have any of the following medical problems:
Edema (swelling of feet or lower legs)
Heart disease
High blood pressure
Kidney disease
Liver disease

—if you regularly take any medicine that contains sodium (salt).

—if you are taking **any** other prescription or nonprescription (OTC) medicine, especially:
Amphotericin B by injection
Barbiturates
Carbamazepine
Digitalis glycosides (heart medicine)
Diuretics (water pills)
Divalproex
Griseofulvin
Oxyphenbutazone
Phenylbutazone
Phenytoin
Potassium supplements
Primidone
Rifampin
Valproic acid

Proper Use of This Medicine

For patients taking fludrocortisone tablets:

• **Take this medicine only as directed by your doctor.** Do not take more or less of it, do not take it more often, and do not take it for a longer period of time than your doctor ordered. To do so may increase the chance of side effects.

• If you miss a dose of this medicine, take it as soon as you remember. However, if it is almost time for your next dose, skip the missed dose and go back to your regular dosing schedule. Do not double doses.

How to store this medicine:
- **Keep out of the reach of children.**

- Store away from heat and direct light.

- Do not store in the bathroom, near the kitchen sink, or in other damp places. Heat or moisture may cause the medicine to break down.

- Do not keep outdated medicine or medicine no longer needed. Be sure that any discarded medicine is out of the reach of children.

Precautions While Using This Medicine

Your doctor should check your progress at regular visits to make sure this medicine does not cause unwanted effects.

If you will be using this medicine for a long time, your doctor may want you to carry a medical identification card stating that you are using this medicine.

For patients receiving desoxycorticosterone acetate pellets:
- If a pellet comes out from under your skin, see your doctor as soon as possible for replacement.

Side Effects of This Medicine

Along with its needed effects, a medicine may cause some unwanted effects. Although not all of these side effects may occur, if they do occur they may need medical attention.

Check with your doctor as soon as possible if any of the following side effects occur:

Less common or rare
    Dizziness
    Headaches (severe or continuing)
    Increase in blood pressure
    Swelling of feet or lower legs
    Unusual weakness in arms or legs
    Unusual weight gain

Other side effects not listed above may also occur in some patients. If you notice any other effects, check with your doctor.

December 1987

ADRENOCORTICOIDS (Topical)

This information applies to the following medicines:

Amcinonide (am-SIN-oh-nide)
Betamethasone (bay-ta-METH-a-sone)
Clobetasol (kloe-BAY-ta-sol)
Clocortolone (kloe-KOR-toe-lone)
Desonide (DESS-oh-nide)
Desoximetasone (des-ox-i-MET-a-sone)
Dexamethasone (dex-a-METH-a-sone)
Diflorasone (dye-FLOR-a-sone)
Flumethasone (floo-METH-a-sone)
Fluocinolone (floo-oh-SIN-oh-lone)
Fluocinonide (floo-oh-SIN-oh-nide)
Flurandrenolide (flure-an-DREN-oh-lide)
Halcinonide (hal-SIN-oh-nide)
Hydrocortisone (hye-droe-KOR-ti-sone)
Methylprednisolone (meth-ill-pred-NISS-oh-lone)
Triamcinolone (trye-am-SIN-oh-lone)

Some commonly used brand names or other names are:

For Amcinonide
    Cyclocort

For Betamethasone†

Alphatrex	Diprolene
Beben*	Diprosone
Benisone	Ectosone*
Betacort Scalp Lotion*	Ectosone Scalp Lotion*
Betaderm*	Metaderm*
Betaderm Scalp Lotion*	Novobetamet*
Betatrex	Uticort
Beta-Val	Valisone
Betnovate*	Valisone Scalp Lotion*
Celestoderm-V*	

For Clobetasol

Dermovate*	Temovate
Dermovate Scalp Application*	

For Clocortolone
    Cloderm

For Desonide

DesOwen	Tridesilon

For Desoximetasone
    Topicort

For Dexamethasone†

Aeroseb-Dex	Decadron
Decaderm	Decaspray

For Diflorasone

Florone	psorcon
Flutone*	psorcon-E
Maxiflor	

For Flumethasone*
    Locacorten*

For Fluocinolone†

Fluoderm*	Flurosyn
Fluolar*	Synalar
Fluonid	Synamol*
Fluonide*	Synandone*
	Synemol

For Fluocinonide

Lidemol*	Lyderm*
Lidex	Metosyn*
Lidex-E	Metosyn FAPG*
	Topsyn*

For Flurandrenolide

Cordran	Drenison*
Cordran SP	

For Halcinonide

Halciderm*	Halog-E
Halog	

For Hydrocortisone†

Acticort	Epifoam
Aeroseb-HC	Gynecort
Barriere-HC*	HC-Jel
CaldeCORT	Hi-Cor
Carmol HC	H_2 Cort
Cetacort	Hyderm*
Cortaid	Hydro-tex
Cortate*	Hytone
Cort-Dome	Lacticare-HC
Cortef	Lanacort
Corticaine	Locoid
Corticreme*	Novohydrocort*
Cortiment*	nutracort
Cortisol	Penecort
Cortizone	Pharma-Cort
Cortoderm	Racet-SE
Cortril	Rectocort*
Delacort	Rhulicort
Dermacort	Stie-Cort
DermiCort	Synacort
Dermolate	Texacort Scalp Lotion
Dermtex HC	Unicort*
Dioderm*	Westcort
Efcortelan*	
Emo-Cort*	

For Methylprednisolone
    Medrol

For Triamcinolone†

Adcortyl*	Kenalog-E*
Aristocort	Kenalog-H
Aristocort A	Triacet
Aristocort C*	Triaderm*
Aristocort D*	Trianide*
Aristocort R*	Triderm
Flutex	Trymex
Kenalog	

* Not available in the U.S.
† Generic name product may also be available.

To the Reader: If you do not recognize the names of medical conditions or medicines referred to in this information, check with your doctor, nurse, or pharmacist. Definitions for selected medical terms may be found in the Glossary. Brand names for the generic drug names listed can be found in the Index. In addition, selected brand names commonly associated with the generic name have been included in the text to help you recognize medicine you may be taking. The fact that a brand name product is not mentioned does not mean the information does not apply. It is a good idea for you to learn both the generic and brand names of your medicines and to write them down for future use.

This medicine is an adrenocorticoid (a-dree-noe-KOR-ti-koid) (cortisone-like medicine). It belongs to the family of medicines called steroids. Topical cortisone-like medicines are applied to the skin to help relieve redness, swelling, itching, and discomfort of many skin problems.

Topical adrenocorticoids are absorbed through the skin and may rarely affect growth in children. Before using this medicine in children, you should discuss its use with your doctor.

Most adrenocorticoids are available only with your doctor's prescription. Some strengths of hydrocortisone are available without a prescription; however, your doctor may have special instructions on the proper use for your medical condition.

Remember:

• If this medicine has been prescribed for you, **it is to be used for your current medical problem only.** It must not be given to other people or used for other problems unless you are directed to do so by your doctor.

• **Keep all medicines out of the reach of children.**

• In order for this medicine to work, it must be used as directed by your doctor or on the package label.

• **It is very important that you read and understand the following information.** If this medicine has been prescribed for you and any of the information causes you special concern, do not decide against using this medicine without first checking with your doctor.

• Before you begin using any new medicine (prescription or nonprescription) or if you develop any new medical problem while you are using this medicine, check with your doctor, nurse, or pharmacist.

• **If you have any questions** about the following information or if you want more information about this medicine or your medical problem, **ask your doctor, nurse, or pharmacist.**

Before Using This Medicine

In order to decide on the best treatment for your medical problem, your doctor should be told:

—if you have ever had any unusual or allergic reaction to adrenocorticoids.

—if you are allergic to any substance, such as certain preservatives or dyes. Most medicines contain more than their active ingredient. Your doctor, nurse, or pharmacist can help you avoid products that may cause a problem.

—if you are **pregnant** or if you intend to become pregnant while using this medicine. Studies on birth defects have not been done in humans. However, studies in animals have shown that topical adrenocorticoids, when applied to the skin in large amounts or for a long period of time, cause birth defects.

—if you are **breast-feeding**. Although topical adrenocorticoids have not been shown to cause problems in nursing babies, the chance always exists. Other adrenocorticoids pass into breast milk and may interfere with the infant's growth.

—if you have any of the following medical problems:
Diabetes mellitus (sugar diabetes)
Infection or ulcers at the place of treatment
Tuberculosis

Proper Use of This Medicine

Be very careful not to get this medicine in your eyes. If you are using this medicine on your face, it may be best to apply it with a cotton-tipped applicator or a gauze pad.

Do not bandage or otherwise wrap the skin being treated unless directed to do so by your doctor.

If your doctor has ordered an occlusive dressing (for example, kitchen plastic wrap) to be applied over this medicine, make sure you know how to apply it. Since occlusive dressings increase the amount of medicine absorbed through your skin and the possibility of side effects, use them only as directed. If you have any questions about this, check with your doctor.

For patients using the topical aerosol form of this medicine:

• This medicine usually comes with patient directions. Read them carefully before using this medicine.

• It is important to avoid breathing in the vapors from the spray.

• Do not use near heat, near an open flame, or while smoking.

For patients using flurandrenolide tape:

• This medicine usually comes with patient directions. Read them carefully before using this medicine.

Do not use this medicine more often or for a longer period of time than your doctor ordered or than recommended on the package label. To do so may increase the chance of absorption through the skin and the chance of side effects. In addition, too much use, especially on thin skin areas (for example, face, armpits, groin), may result in thinning of the skin and stretch marks or other unwanted effects.

If this medicine has been prescribed for you, it is meant to treat a specific skin problem. **Do not use it for other skin problems, and do not use nonprescription hydrocortisone for skin problems that are not listed on the package label, without first checking with your doctor.** Topical adrenocorticoids should not be used on many kinds of bacterial, viral, or fungal skin infections.

If your doctor has ordered you to use this medicine on a regular schedule and you miss a dose, apply it as soon as possible. But if it is almost time for your next dose, skip the missed dose and apply it at the next regularly scheduled time.

How to store this medicine:

• **Keep out of the reach of children.**

• Store away from heat and direct light.

• Keep the medicine from freezing.

• Do not puncture, break, or burn aerosol containers, even after they are empty.

• Do not keep outdated medicine or medicine no longer needed. Be sure that any discarded medicine is out of the reach of children.

Precautions While Using This Medicine

Children who must use this medicine should be followed closely by their doctor since this medicine may be absorbed through the skin and can affect growth or cause other unwanted effects.

If this medicine is to be used on the diaper area, avoid using tight-fitting diapers or plastic pants on the child. Wearing these may increase the chance of absorption of the medicine through the skin and the chance of side effects.

Side Effects of This Medicine

Along with its needed effects, a medicine may cause some unwanted effects. Although not all of these side effects may occur, if they do occur they may need medical attention.

Check with your doctor as soon as possible if any of the following side effects occur:

> Signs of infection such as pain, redness, or pus-containing blisters
> Signs of irritation such as burning, itching, blistering, or peeling not present before using this medicine

Additional side effects may occur if you use this medicine for a long period of time. Check with your doctor if any of the following side effects occur:

> Acne or oily skin
> Filling or rounding out of the face
> Raised, dark red, wart-like spots on skin
> Reddish purple lines on arms, face, legs, trunk, or groin
> Thinning of skin with easy bruising
> Unusual increase in hair growth, especially on the face
> Unusual loss of hair, especially on the scalp

When the gel, solution, lotion, or aerosol form of this medicine is applied, a mild, temporary stinging may be expected.

Other side effects not listed above may also occur in some patients. If you notice any other effects, check with your doctor.

_____

December 1987

_____

ADRENOCORTICOIDS AND ACETIC ACID (Otic)

This information applies to the following medicines:

Desonide (DESS-oh-nide) and Acetic Acid (a-SEAT-ic AS-id)
Hydrocortisone (hye-droe-KOR-ti-sone) and Acetic Acid

Some commonly used brand names are:	Generic names:
Tridesilon Solution, Otic	Desonide and Acetic Acid
VōSol HC	Hydrocortisone and Acetic Acid

To the Reader: If you do not recognize the names of medical conditions or medicines referred to in this information, check with your doctor, nurse, or pharmacist. Definitions for selected medical terms may be found in the Glossary. Brand names for the generic drug names listed can be found in the Index. In addition, selected brand names commonly associated with the generic name have been included in the text to help you recognize medicine you may be taking. The fact that a brand name product is not mentioned does not mean the information does not apply. It is a good idea for you to learn both the generic and brand names of your medicines and to write them down for future use.

Adrenocorticoid (a-dree-noe-KOR-ti-koid) and acetic acid combinations are used to treat certain infections of the ear canal. They also help relieve the redness, itching, and swelling that may accompany these infections. These medicines may also be used for other conditions as determined by your doctor.

Adrenocorticoid and acetic acid combinations are available only with your doctor's prescription.

Remember:

• **This medicine has been prescribed for your current medical problem only.** It must not be given to other people or used for other problems unless you are directed to do so by your doctor.

• **Keep all medicines out of the reach of children.**

• In order for this medicine to work, it must be used as directed.

• **It is very important that you read and understand the following information.** If any of the information causes you special concern, do not decide against using this medicine without first checking with your doctor.

• Before you begin using any new medicine (prescription or nonprescription) or if you develop any new medical problem while you are using this medicine, check with your doctor, nurse, or pharmacist.

• **If you have any questions** about the following information or if you want more information about this medicine or your medical problem, **ask your doctor, nurse, or pharmacist.**

Before Using This Medicine

In order to decide on the best treatment for your medical problem, your doctor should be told:

—if you have ever had any unusual or allergic reaction to adrenocorticoids.

—if you are allergic to any substance, such as certain preservatives or dyes. Most medicines contain more than their active ingredient. Your doctor, nurse, or pharmacist can help you avoid products that may cause a problem.

—if you are **pregnant** or if you may become pregnant. Adrenocorticoid and acetic acid combinations used in the ear have not been shown to cause birth defects or other problems in humans.

—if you are **breast-feeding.** Otic adrenocorticoid and acetic acid combinations have not been shown to cause problems in nursing babies.

—if you have any of the following medical problems:
   Any other ear infection or condition
   Punctured ear drum

Proper Use of This Medicine

How to apply this medicine: Lie down or tilt the head so that the infected ear faces up. Gently pull the ear lobe up and back for adults (down and back for children) to straighten the ear canal. Drop the medicine into the ear canal. Keep the ear facing up for several (about 5) minutes to allow medicine to run to the bottom of the ear canal. A sterile cotton plug may be gently inserted into the ear opening to prevent the medicine from leaking out.

To prevent contamination of the ear drops, do not touch the dropper or applicator tip to any surface (including the ear). Also, always keep the container tightly closed.

For patients using hydrocortisone and acetic acid ear drops only:

• **Do not wash the dropper or applicator tip,** because water may get into the medicine and make it weaker. If necessary, you may wipe the dropper or applicator tip with a clean tissue.

Do not use adrenocorticoids more often or for a longer period of time than your doctor ordered. To do so may increase the chance of side effects.

Do not use any leftover medicine for future ear problems without first checking with your doctor. This medicine should not be used if certain kinds of infections are present. To do so may make the infection worse.

If you miss a dose of this medicine, apply it as soon as possible. But if it is almost time for your next dose, skip the missed dose and go back to your regular dosing schedule.

How to store this medicine:

• **Keep out of the reach of children.**

• Store away from heat and direct light.

• Keep the medicine from freezing.

• Do not keep outdated medicine or medicine no longer needed. Be sure that any discarded medicine is out of the reach of children.

Precautions While Using This Medicine

If your symptoms have not improved after 5 to 7 days, or if your ear problem becomes worse, check with your doctor.

Side Effects of This Medicine

After this medicine has been applied, occasional stinging, itching, or burning may be expected. If this continues or is bothersome, check with your doctor.

There have not been any other common or important side effects reported with this medicine. However, if you notice any other effects, check with your doctor.

December 1987

ADRENOCORTICOIDS/CORTICOTROPIN
(Systemic—Glucocorticoid Effects)

This information applies to the following medicines:

Betamethasone (bay-ta-METH-a-sone)
Corticotropin (kor-ti-koe-TROE-pin)
Cortisone (KOR-ti-sone)
Dexamethasone (dex-a-METH-a-sone)
Hydrocortisone (hye-droe-KOR-ti-sone)
Methylprednisolone (meth-ill-pred-NISS-oh-lone)
Paramethasone (par-a-METH-a-sone)
Prednisolone (pred-NISS-oh-lone)
Prednisone (PRED-ni-sone)
Triamcinolone (trye-am-SIN-oh-lone)

The following information does *not* apply to desoxycorticosterone or fludrocortisone.

Some commonly used brand names or other names are:

For Betamethasone†

B-S-P	Celestone
Betnelan*	Prelestone
Betnesol*	Selestoject

For Corticotropin†

ACTH	Cortrophin Zinc
Acthar	H P Acthar Gel

For Cortisone†

Cortelan*	Cortone
Cortistab*	

For Dexamethasone†

Ak-Dex	Dexasone
Dalalone	Dexon
Decadrol	Dexone
Decadron	Hexadrol
Decaject	Oradexon*
Decameth	SK-Dexamethasone
Deronil*	Solurex
Dexacen	

For Hydrocortisone†

A-hydroCort	Efcortelan*
Biosone	Efcortesol*
Colifoam*	Hycort*
Cortef	Hydrocortistab*
Cortenema	Hydrocortone
Cortifoam	Lifocort
Cortisol	Solu-Cortef

For Methylprednisolone†

A-methaPred	Medralone
depMedalone	Medrol
Depoject	Medrone
Depo-Medrol	M-Prednisol
Depo-Medrone*	Rep-Pred
Depopred	Solu-Medrol
Depo-Predate	Solu-Medrone*
Duralone	
Durameth	

For Paramethasone
Haldrone

For Prednisolone†

Articulose	Nor-Pred T.B.A.
Codelsol*	Novoprednisolone*
Cortalone	Pediapred
Delta-Cortef	Predaject
Deltastab*	Predate
Hydeltrasol	Predcor
Hydeltra-T.B.A.	Prednisol TBA
Key-Pred	Prelone
Metalone T.B.A.	

For Prednisone†

Apo-Prednisone*	Orasone
Deltasone	Panasol
Liquid Pred	Prednicen-M
Meticorten	SK-Prednisone
Novoprednisone*	Winpred*

For Triamcinolone†

Amcort	Kenalone
Aristocort	Ledercort*
Aristospan	Lederspan*
Articulose-L.A.	Tramacort
Cenocort	Triam
Cinalone	Triamolone
Cinonide	Triamonide
Kenacort	Tri-Kort
Kenaject	Trilog
Kenalog	Trilone
	Tristoject

---

* Not available in the U.S.
† Generic name product may also be available in the U.S.

To the Reader: If you do not recognize the names of medical conditions or medicines referred to in this information, check with your doctor, nurse, or pharmacist. Definitions for selected medical terms may be found in the Glossary. Brand names for the generic drug names listed can be found in the Index. In addition, selected brand names commonly associated with the generic name have been included in the text to help you recognize medicine you may be taking. The fact that a brand name product is not mentioned does not mean the information does not apply. It is a good idea for you to learn both the generic and brand names of your medicines and to write them down for future use.

Adrenocorticoids (a-dree-noe-KOR-ti-koids) (cortisone-like medicines) are used to provide relief for inflamed areas of the body. They lessen swelling, redness, itching, and allergic reactions. They are often used as part of the treatment for a number of different diseases, such as severe allergies or skin problems, asthma, or arthritis. Adrenocorticoids may also be used for other conditions as determined by your doctor.

Your body naturally produces certain cortisone-like hormones that are necessary to maintain good health. If your body does not produce enough, your doctor may have prescribed this medicine to help make up the difference.

Corticotropin is not an adrenocorticoid. It is a hormone that occurs naturally in the body. Corticotropin is known as an adrenocorticotropic hormone, which means it causes the adrenal glands to produce cortisone-like hormones. Corticotropin is used as a test to determine whether your adrenal glands are producing enough hormones. Also, it is sometimes used instead of adrenocorticoids to treat many of the same medical problems.

Adrenocorticoids and corticotropin are very strong medicines. In addition to their helpful effects in treating your medical problem, they have side effects that can be very serious. If your adrenal glands are not producing enough cortisone-like hormones, taking this medicine is not likely to cause problems unless you take too much of it. If you are taking this medicine to treat another medical problem, be sure that you discuss the risks and benefits of this medicine with your doctor.

Adrenocorticoids or corticotropin may slow or stop growth in children and in growing teenagers, especially when they are used for a long time. Before this medicine is given to children or teenagers, you should discuss its use with your doctor and then carefully follow your doctor's instructions.

Adrenocorticoids are taken by mouth, given by injection, or used rectally. Corticotropin is given by injection because it is destroyed by digestion when taken by mouth.

These medicines are available only with your doctor's prescription.

Remember:

• **This medicine has been prescribed for your current medical problem only.** It must not be given to other people or used for other problems unless you are directed to do so by your doctor.

• **Keep all medicines out of the reach of children.**

• In order for this medicine to work, it must be used as directed.

• If you are receiving this medicine by injection, or if you are taking it because your body does not produce enough cortisone-like hormones, some of the information about this medicine may not apply.

• **It is very important that you read and understand the following information.** If any of the information causes you special concern, do not decide against using this medicine without first checking with your doctor.

• Before you begin using any new medicine (prescription or nonprescription) or if you develop any new medical problem while you are using this medicine, check with your doctor, nurse, or pharmacist.

• **If you have any questions** about the following information or if you want more information about this medicine or your medical problem, **ask your doctor, nurse, or pharmacist.**

Before Using This Medicine

In order to decide on the best treatment for your medical problem, your doctor should be told:

—if you have ever had any unusual or allergic reaction to adrenocorticoids or to corticotropin.

—if you are receiving corticotropin and have ever had any unusual or allergic reaction to pork products (corticotropin is often obtained from pigs).

—if you are on a low-salt, low-sugar, or any other special diet, or if you are allergic to any substance, such as sulfites or other preservatives or dyes. Most medicines contain more than their active ingredient, and many liquid medicines contain alcohol. Your doctor or pharmacist can help you avoid products that may cause a problem.

—if you are **pregnant** or if you may become pregnant. Studies on birth defects with adrenocorticoids or with corticotropin have not been done in humans. However, too much use of adrenocorticoids during pregnancy may cause the baby to have problems after birth, such as slower growth. Also, studies in animals have shown that adrenocorticoids cause birth defects and that corticotropin may cause other unwanted effects in the fetus.

—if you are **breast-feeding**. Adrenocorticoids pass into breast milk and may cause problems with growth or other unwanted effects in nursing babies. Depending on the amount of medicine you are taking every day, it may be necessary for you to take another medicine or to stop breast-feeding during treatment. Be sure you have discussed the risks and benefits of the medicine with your doctor.

Corticotropin has not been shown to cause problems in nursing babies.

—if you have an infection at the place of treatment.

—if you have recently had surgery or a serious injury.

—if you have any of the following medical problems:
    Bone disease
    Colitis
    Diabetes mellitus (sugar diabetes)
    Diverticulitis
    Fungus infection or any other infection
    Glaucoma
    Heart disease
    Herpes simplex infection of the eye
    High blood pressure
    High cholesterol levels
    Kidney disease (especially if you are receiving dialysis) or kidney stones
    Liver disease
    Myasthenia gravis
    Overactive thyroid
    Stomach ulcer or other stomach or intestine problems
    Systemic lupus erythematosus (SLE)
    Tuberculosis (active TB, nonactive TB, or past history of)
    Underactive thyroid

—if you regularly take large amounts of antacids.

—if you regularly use any medicine that contains a large amount of sodium (salt).

—if you are now taking or receiving **any** prescription or nonprescription (OTC) medicine, especially:
    Antidiabetic agents, oral (diabetes medicine you take by mouth)
    Barbiturates, except butalbital
    Carbamazepine (e.g., Tegretol)
    Digitalis glycosides (heart medicine)
    Divalproex (e.g., Depakote)
    Diuretics (medicine to increase the amount of urine or to treat high blood pressure)
    Griseofulvin (e.g., Fulvicin)
    Insulin
    Medicine containing potassium
    Phenylbutazone (e.g., Butazolidin)
    Phenytoin (e.g., Dilantin)
    Primidone (e.g., Mysoline)
    Rifampin (e.g., Rifadin)
    Valproic acid (e.g., Depakene)

Proper Use of This Medicine

For patients taking this medicine by mouth:

• **Take this medicine with food** to help prevent stomach upset. If stomach upset, burning, or pain continues, check with your doctor.

• Stomach problems may be more likely to occur if you drink alcoholic beverages while being treated with this medicine. You should not drink alcoholic beverages while taking this medicine, unless you have first checked with your doctor.

For patients using this medicine rectally:

• This medicine usually comes with patient directions. Read them carefully before using this medicine.

• For patients using hydrocortisone enema:

—Each bottle contains a single dose. Use it all, unless otherwise directed by your doctor.

—For best results, use this medicine right after a bowel movement. Lie down on your left side when giving the enema.

—Insert the rectal tip of the enema applicator gently to prevent damage to the rectal wall.

—Stay on your left side for at least 30 minutes after the enema is given so the medicine can work. If you can, keep the enema inside all night.

• For patients using hydrocortisone acetate rectal aerosol foam:

—This medicine is used with a special applicator. Do not insert any part of the aerosol container into the rectum.

• For patients using methylprednisolone acetate for enema:

—Each bottle contains a single dose. Use it all, unless otherwise directed by your doctor.

—Insert the rectal tip of the enema applicator gently to prevent damage to the rectal wall.

—If you have been directed to use this enema slowly (not all at once), shake the bottle once in a while while you are giving the enema.

—Save your applicator. Refill units of this medicine may be available at lower cost.

Use this medicine only as directed by your doctor. Do not use more or less of it, do not use it more often, and do not use it for a longer period of time than your doctor ordered. To do so may increase the chance of side effects.

If you miss a dose of this medicine and your dosing schedule is one dose to be taken:

Every other day—Take the missed dose as soon as possible if you remember it the same morning, then go back to your regular dosing schedule. If you do not remember the missed dose until later, wait and take it the following morning. Then skip a day and start your regular dosing schedule again.

Once a day—Take the missed dose as soon as possible, then go back to your regular dosing schedule. If you do not remember until the next day, skip the missed dose and do not double the next one.

Several times a day—Take the missed dose as soon as possible, then go back to your regular dosing schedule. If you do not remember until your next dose is due, double the next dose.

If you have any questions about this, check with your doctor, nurse, or pharmacist.

How to store this medicine:

• **Keep out of the reach of children.**

• Store away from heat and direct light.

• Do not store tablets in the bathroom, near the kitchen sink, or in other damp places. Heat or moisture may cause the medicine to break down.

• Keep the liquid dosage forms of this medicine, including enemas, and hydrocortisone rectal aerosol foam from freezing.

• Do not puncture, break, or burn the hydrocortisone rectal aerosol foam container, even when it is empty.

• Do not keep outdated medicine or medicine no longer needed. Be sure that any discarded medicine is out of the reach of children.

Precautions While Using This Medicine

Your doctor should check your progress at regular visits. Also, your progress may have to be checked after you have stopped using this medicine, since some of the effects may continue.

Do not stop using this medicine without first checking with your doctor. Your doctor may want you to reduce gradually the amount you are using before stopping completely.

Check with your doctor if your condition reappears or worsens after the dose has been reduced or treatment with this medicine is stopped.

If you will be using adrenocorticoids or corticotropin for a long time:

• **Your doctor may want you to follow a low-salt diet and/or a potassium-rich diet.**

• Your doctor may want you to watch your calories to prevent weight gain.

• Your doctor may want you to add extra protein to your diet.

• Your doctor may want you to have your eyes examined by an ophthalmologist before and also sometime later during treatment.

• Your doctor may want you to carry a medical identification card stating that you are using this medicine.

Tell the doctor in charge that you are using this medicine:

—**before having skin tests.**

—**before having any kind of surgery (including dental surgery) or emergency treatment.**

—**if you get a serious infection or injury.**

While you are being treated with this medicine, and after you stop taking it, **do not have any immunizations without your doctor's approval**. Also, other people living in your home should not receive oral polio vaccine, since there is a chance they could pass the polio virus on to you. In addition, you should avoid close contact with other people at school or work who have recently taken oral polio vaccine.

Diabetics—This medicine may cause your blood sugar levels to rise. If you notice a change in the results of your urine or blood sugar test or if you have any questions, check with your doctor, nurse, or pharmacist.

For patients having this medicine injected into their joints:

• If this medicine is injected into one of your joints, you should be careful not to put too much stress or strain on that joint for a while, even if it begins to feel better. Make sure your doctor has told you how much you are allowed to move this joint while it is healing.

• If redness or swelling occurs at the place of injection, and continues or gets worse, check with your doctor.

For patients using this medicine rectally:

• Check with your doctor if you notice rectal bleeding, pain, burning, itching, blistering, or any other sign of irritation not present before you started using this medicine, or if signs of infection occur.

Side Effects of This Medicine

Adrenocorticoids or corticotropin may lower your resistance to infections. Also, any infection you get may be harder to treat. Always check with your doctor as soon as possible if you notice any signs of a possible infection, such as sore throat, fever, sneezing, or coughing.

Along with its needed effects, a medicine may cause some unwanted effects. Although not all of these side effects may occur, if they do occur they may need medical attention. When this medicine is used for short periods of time, side effects usually are rare. However, check with your doctor as soon as possible if any of the following side effects occur:

Less common
  Decreased or blurred vision
  Decreased or slow growth (in children or growing teen-
    agers)
  Frequent urination
  Increased thirst
  Rectal bleeding, blistering, burning, itching, or pain not
    present before treatment (when used rectally)

Rare
  Burning, numbness, pain, or tingling at or near place of
    injection
  Hallucinations (seeing, hearing, or feeling things that are
    not there)
  Mental depression or other mood or mental changes
  Redness, swelling, or other sign of infection at place of
    injection
  Skin rash or hives

Additional side effects may occur if you take this medicine for a long period of time. Check with your doctor if any of the following side effects occur:
  Abdominal or stomach pain or burning (continuing)
  Acne or other skin problems
  Bloody or black tarry stools
  Filling or rounding out of the face
  Increased blood pressure
  Irregular heartbeats

  Menstrual problems
  Muscle cramps or pain
  Muscle weakness
  Nausea or vomiting
  Pain in back, hips, ribs, arms, shoulders, or legs
  Pitting or depression of skin at place of injection
  Reddish purple lines on arms, face, legs, trunk, or groin
  Swelling of feet or lower legs
  Thin, shiny skin
  Unusual bruising
  Unusual tiredness or weakness
  Unusual weight gain
  Wounds that will not heal

Other side effects may occur that usually do not require medical attention. These side effects may go away during treatment as your body adjusts to the medicine. However, check with your doctor if any of the following side effects continue or are bothersome:

More common
  False sense of well-being
  Increased appetite
  Indigestion
  Loss of appetite (for triamcinolone only)
  Nervousness or restlessness
  Trouble in sleeping

Less common or rare
  Darkening or lightening of skin color
  Dizziness or lightheadedness
  Headache
  Increased joint pain (after injection into a joint)
  Unusual increase in hair growth on body or face

After you stop using this medicine, your body may need time to adjust. The length of time this takes depends on the amount of medicine you were using and how long you used it. If you have taken large doses of this medicine for a long period of time, your body may need one year to adjust. During this period of time, **check with your doctor immediately if any of the following side effects occur:**
  Abdominal or stomach or back pain
  Dizziness or fainting
  Fever
  Loss of appetite (continuing)
  Muscle or joint pain
  Nausea or vomiting
  Shortness of breath
  Unexplained headaches (frequent or continuing)
  Unusual tiredness or weakness
  Unusual weight loss

For children and elderly patients: Some of the above side effects, especially bone problems, may be more likely to occur in children and in the elderly, who are usually more sensitive to some of the effects of these medicines.

Other side effects not listed above may also occur in some patients. If you notice any other effects, check with your doctor.

_____

December 1987

_____

ALCOHOL AND ACETONE (Topical)

Some commonly used brand names are Seba-Nil and tyrosum.

To the Reader: If you do not recognize the names of medical conditions or medicines referred to in this information, check with your doctor, nurse, or pharmacist. Definitions for selected medical terms may be found in the Glossary. Brand names for the generic drug names listed can be found in the Index. In addition, selected brand names commonly associated with the generic name have been included in the text to help you recognize medicine you may be taking. The fact that a brand name product is not mentioned does not mean the information does not apply. It is a good idea for you to learn both the generic and brand names of your medicines and to write them down for future use.

Alcohol and acetone (AL-koe-hol and A-se-tone) combination is used to clean oily or greasy skin associated with acne or other oily skin conditions.

This medicine is available without a prescription; however, your doctor may have special instructions on the proper use of this medicine for your medical condition.

Remember:

• **Keep all medicines out of the reach of children.**

• In order for this medicine to work, it must be used as directed. **If you are using this medicine without a prescription, it is very important to follow the directions on the label.**

• **It is also very important that you read and understand the following information.** If any of the information causes you special concern, check with your doctor or pharmacist.

• Before you begin using any new medicine (prescription or nonprescription) or if you develop any new medical problem while you are using this medicine, check with your doctor or pharmacist.

• **If you have any questions** about the following information or if you want more information about this medicine or your medical problem, **ask your doctor or pharmacist.**

Before Using This Medicine

Before you use alcohol and acetone combination, check with your doctor or pharmacist:

—if you have ever had any unusual or allergic reaction to alcohol or acetone.

—if you are allergic to any substance, such as preservatives or dyes. Most medicine contain more than their active ingredient. Your doctor, nurse, or pharmacist can help you avoid products that may cause a problem.

—if you are **pregnant** or if you may become pregnant, although topical alcohol and acetone combination has not been shown to cause birth defects or other problems in humans.

—if you are **breast-feeding**, although topical alcohol and acetone combination has not been shown to cause problems in nursing babies.

—if you are taking **any** other prescription or nonprescription (OTC) medicine.

Proper Use of This Medicine

Keep this medicine away from the eyes, inside of nose, and lips.

Do not apply this medicine to burns or wounds. To do so may cause severe irritation.

This medicine is flammable. Do not use near heat, near open flame, or while smoking.

Apply this medicine by wiping or rubbing over the face and other affected areas to remove dirt and surface oil.

After applying this medicine, do not rinse the affected areas with water, since this will remove the medicine.

If you are using this medicine on a regular schedule and you miss a dose, apply it as soon as possible. Then go back to your regular dosing schedule.

How to store this medicine:

• **Keep out of the reach of children.**

• Store away from heat and direct light.

• Keep the lotion form of this medicine from freezing.

• Do not keep outdated medicine or medicine no longer needed. Be sure that any discarded medicine is out of the reach of children.

Precautions While Using This Medicine

When using alcohol and acetone combination, do not use any of the following preparations on the same affected area as this medicine, unless otherwise directed by your doctor:

Abrasive soaps or cleaners
Any other topical acne preparation or preparation containing a peeling agent (for example, benzoyl peroxide, resorcinol, salicylic acid, sulfur, or tretinoin [vitamin A acid])
Cosmetics or soaps that dry the skin
Medicated cosmetics
Other alcohol-containing preparations
Other topical medicine for the skin

To use any of the above preparations on the same affected area as this medicine may cause severe irritation of the skin

Side Effects of This Medicine

Along with its needed effects, a medicine may cause some unwanted effects. Although not all of these side effects may occur, if they do occur they may need medical attention.

Check with your doctor as soon as possible if any of the following side effects occur:

Irritation, pain, redness, or swelling of skin
Skin infection

Other side effects may occur that usually do not require medical attention. These side effects may go away during treatment as your body adjusts to the medicine.

© 1988   The United States Pharmacopeial Convention, Inc.

However, check with your doctor or pharmacist if the following side effect continues or is bothersome:
   Burning or stinging of skin

For elderly patients: Many medicines have not been tested in older people. Therefore, it is not known whether the medicine acts the same way it does in younger adults. Check with your doctor or pharmacist if you notice any unusual effects while using this medicine or if you think it is not working as it should.

Other side effects may also occur in some patients. If you notice any other effects, check with your doctor or pharmacist.

December 1987

ALCOHOL AND SULFUR (Topical)

Some commonly used brand names are:

Aknaseb*	Transact
Liquimat	Xerac

*Not available in the U.S.

To the Reader: If you do not recognize the names of medical conditions or medicines referred to in this information, check with your doctor, nurse, or pharmacist. Definitions for selected medical terms may be found in the Glossary. Brand names for the generic drug names listed can be found in the Index. In addition, selected brand names commonly associated with the generic name have been included in the text to help you recognize medicine you may be taking. The fact that a brand name product is not mentioned does not mean the information does not apply. It is a good idea for you to learn both the generic and brand names of your medicines and to write them down for future use.

Alcohol and sulfur (AL-koe-hol and SUL-fur) combination is used in the treatment of acne and oily skin.

This medicine is available without a doctor's prescription; however, your doctor may have special instructions on the proper use of this medicine for your medical condition.

Remember:

• **Keep all medicines out of the reach of children.**

• In order for this medicine to work, it must be used as directed. **If you are using this medicine without a prescription, it is very important to follow the directions on the label.**

• **It is also very important that you read and understand the following information.** If any of the information causes you special concern, check with your doctor or pharmacist.

• Before you begin using any new medicine (prescription or nonprescription) or if you develop any new medical problem while you are using this medicine, check with your doctor, nurse, or pharmacist.

• **If you have any questions** about the following information or if you want more information about this medicine or your medical problem, **ask your doctor, nurse, or pharmacist.**

Before Using This Medicine

Before you use alcohol and sulfur combination, check with your doctor or pharmacist:

—if you have ever had any unusual or allergic reaction to alcohol or sulfur.

—if you are allergic to any substance, such as preservatives or dyes. Most medicines contain more than their active ingredient. Your doctor, nurse, or pharmacist can help you avoid products that may cause a problem.

—if you are **pregnant** or if you may become pregnant, although topical alcohol and sulfur combination has not been shown to cause birth defects or other problems in humans.

—if you are **breast-feeding**, although topical alcohol and sulfur combination has not been shown to cause problems in nursing babies.

—if you are taking **any** other prescription or nonprescription (OTC) medicine.

Proper Use of This Medicine

Before using this medicine, wash or cleanse the affected areas thoroughly and gently pat dry. Then apply a small amount of this medicine to the affected areas and rub in gently.

Keep this medicine away from the eyes, inside of nose, and lips. If you accidentally get some in your eyes, flush them thoroughly with water.

This medicine is flammable. Do not use near heat, near open flame, or while smoking.

Use this medicine only as directed. Do not use it more often than recommended on the label, unless otherwise directed by your doctor.

If you miss a dose of this medicine, apply it as soon as possible. Then go back to your regular dosing schedule.

How to store this medicine:

• **Keep out of the reach of children.**

• Store away from heat and direct light.

• Keep the lotion form of this medicine from freezing.

• Do not keep outdated medicine or medicine no longer needed. Be sure that any discarded medicine is out of the reach of children.

Precautions While Using This Medicine

When using alcohol and sulfur combination, do not use any of the following preparations on the same affected area as this medicine, unless otherwise directed by your doctor.

Abrasive soaps or cleansers
Any other topical acne preparation or preparation containing a peeling agent (for example, benzoyl peroxide, resorcinol, salicylic acid, or tretinoin [vitamin A acid])
Cosmetics or soaps that dry the skin
Medicated cosmetics
Other alcohol-containing preparations
Other topical medicine for the skin

To use any of the above preparations on the same affected area as this medicine may cause severe irritation of the skin.

Do not use any topical mercury-containing preparation, such as ammoniated mercury ointment on the same affected area as this medicine. To do so may cause a foul odor, may be irritating to the skin, and may stain the skin black. If you have any questions about this, check with your doctor or pharmacist.

Side Effects of This Medicine

Along with its needed effects, a medicine may cause some unwanted effects. Although not all of these side effects may occur, if they do occur they may need medical attention.

Check with your doctor as soon as possible if the following side effect occurs:

Skin irritation not present before using this medicine

Other side effects may occur that usually do not require medical attention. These side effects may go away during treatment as your body adjusts to the medicine. However, check with your doctor or pharmacist if any of the following side effects continue or are bothersome:

Burning or stinging of skin
Dryness or peeling of skin (may occur after a few days)

For elderly patients: Many medicines have not been tested in older people. Therefore, it is not known whether the medicine acts the same way it does in younger adults. Check with your doctor or pharmacist if you notice any unusual effects while using this medicine or if you think it is not working as it should.

Other side effects not listed above may also occur in some patients. If you notice any other effects, check with your doctor or pharmacist.

December 1987

ALLOPURINOL (Systemic)

Some commonly used brand names are:

Alloprin*	Purinol*
Aluline*	Roucol*
Apo-Allopurinol*	Zurinol
Caplenal*	Zyloprim
Lopurin	Zyloric*
Novopurol*	

Generic name product may also be available.

---

*Not available in the U.S.

To the Reader: If you do not recognize the names of medical conditions or medicines referred to in this information, check with your doctor, nurse, or pharmacist. Definitions for selected medical terms may be found in the Glossary. Brand names for the generic drug names listed can be found in the Index. In addition, selected brand names commonly associated with the generic name have been included in the text to help you recognize medicine you may be taking. The fact that a brand name product is not mentioned does not mean the information does not apply. It is a good idea for you to learn both the generic and brand names of your medicines and to write them down for future use.

Allopurinol (al-oh-PURE-i-nole) is taken by mouth to treat chronic gout (gouty arthritis). This condition is caused by too much uric acid in the blood.

This medicine works by causing less uric acid to be produced by the body. Allopurinol will not relieve a gout attack that has already started. Also, it does not cure gout, but it will help prevent gout attacks. However, it works only after you have been taking it regularly for a few months. Also, allopurinol will help prevent gout attacks only as long as you continue to take it.

Allopurinol is also used to prevent or treat other medical problems that may occur if too much uric acid is present in the body. These include certain kinds of kidney stones or other kidney problems.

Allopurinol is available only with your doctor's prescription.

Remember:

• **This medicine has been prescribed for your current medical problem only.** It must not be given to other people or used for other problems unless you are directed to do so by your doctor.

• **Keep all medicines out of the reach of children.**

• In order for this medicine to work, it must be used as directed.

• **It is very important that you read and understand the following information.** If any of the information causes you special concern, do not decide against using this medicine without first checking with your doctor.

• Before you begin using any new medicine (prescription or nonprescription) or if you develop any new medical problem while you are using this medicine, check with your doctor, nurse, or pharmacist.

• **If you have any questions** about the following information or if you want more information about this medicine or your medical problem, **ask your doctor, nurse, or pharmacist.**

Before Using This Medicine

In order to decide on the best treatment for your medical problem, your doctor should be told:

—if you have ever had any unusual or allergic reaction to allopurinol.

—if you are on a low-salt, low-sugar, or any other special diet, or if you are allergic to any substance, such as foods, sulfites or other preservatives, or dyes. Most medicines contain more than their active ingredient. Your doctor, nurse, or pharmacist can help you avoid products that may cause a problem.

—if you are **pregnant** or if you may become pregnant. Although studies on birth defects have not been done in humans, allopurinol has not been reported to cause problems in humans. In one study in mice, large amounts of allopurinol caused birth defects and other unwanted effects. However, allopurinol did not cause birth defects or other problems in rats or rabbits given doses up to 20 times the amount usually given to humans.

—if you are **breast-feeding**. Allopurinol passes into the breast milk. However, this medicine has not been shown to cause problems in nursing babies.

—if you have kidney disease.

—if you are now taking **any** other prescription or nonprescription (OTC) medicine, especially:

Anticoagulants (blood thinners)
Azathioprine (e.g., Imuran)
Mercaptopurine (e.g., Purinethol)

Proper Use of This Medicine

If this medicine upsets your stomach, it may be taken after meals. If stomach upset (indigestion, nausea, vomiting, diarrhea, or stomach pain) continues, check with your doctor.

In order for this medicine to help you, it must be taken regularly as ordered by your doctor.

To help prevent kidney stones while taking allopurinol, adults should drink at least 10 to 12 full glasses (8 ounces each) of fluids each day unless otherwise directed by their doctor. Check with the doctor about the amount of fluids that children should drink each day while receiving this medicine. Also, your doctor may want you to take another medicine to make your urine less acid. It is important that you follow your doctor's instructions very carefully.

For patients taking allopurinol for gout:

• After you begin to take allopurinol, gout attacks may continue to occur for a while. However, if you take this medicine regularly as directed by your doctor, the attacks will gradually become less frequent and less painful. After you have been taking allopurinol regularly for several months, they may stop completely.

• Allopurinol is used to help prevent gout attacks. It will not relieve an attack that has already started. **Even if you take another medicine for gout attacks, continue to take this medicine also.**

If you miss a dose of allopurinol and your dosing schedule is one dose to be taken:

Once a day—Take the missed dose as soon as possible. However, if you do not remember the missed dose until the next day, skip the missed dose and go back to your regular dosing schedule. Do not double the next day's dose.

More than once a day—Take the missed dose as soon as possible. However, if it is almost time for your next dose, and each regular dose is one 100-mg tablet, double the next dose. If each regular dose is two 100-mg tablets, take three tablets for the next dose. Then go back to your regular dosing schedule.

How to store this medicine:

• **Keep out of the reach of children.**

• Store away from heat and direct light.

• Do not store this medicine in the bathroom, near the kitchen sink, or in other damp places. Heat or moisture may cause the medicine to break down.

• Do not keep outdated medicine or medicine no longer needed. Be sure that any discarded medicine is out of the reach of children.

Precautions While Using This Medicine

Your doctor should check your progress at regular visits. A blood test may be needed to make sure that this medicine is working properly and is not causing unwanted effects.

Drinking too much alcohol may increase the amount of uric acid in the blood and lessen the effects of allopurinol. Therefore, do not drink alcoholic beverages while taking this medicine, unless you have first checked with your doctor.

Taking too much vitamin C may make the urine more acidic and increase the possibility of kidney stones forming while you are taking allopurinol. Therefore, check with your doctor before you take vitamin C while taking this medicine.

Check with your doctor immediately:

• **if you notice a skin rash, hives, or itching while you are taking allopurinol.**

• **if chills, fever, muscle aches or pains, or nausea or vomiting occur together with or shortly after a skin rash.**

Very rarely, these effects may be the first signs of a serious allergic reaction to the medicine, especially if they occur during the first few months of treatment.

Allopurinol may cause some people to become drowsy or less alert than they are normally. **Make sure you know how you react to this medicine before you drive, use machines, or do other jobs that require you to be alert.**

Side Effects of This Medicine

Along with its needed effects, a medicine may cause some unwanted effects. Although not all of these side effects may occur, if they do occur they may need medical attention.

Stop taking this medicine and check with your doctor immediately if any of the following side effects occur:
More common
Skin rash, hives, or itching
Rare
Bleeding sores on lips
Blood in urine
Chills, fever, muscle aches or pains, nausea, or vomiting occurring with or shortly after a skin rash
Difficult or painful urination
Redness, tenderness, burning, or peeling of skin
Red or irritated eyes
Red, thickened, or scaly skin
Sores, ulcers, or white spots in mouth or on lips
Sore throat and fever
Sudden decrease in amount of urine
Swelling of face, feet, or lower legs
Unusual bleeding or bruising
Unusual tiredness or weakness
Yellow eyes or skin

Also, check with your doctor as soon as possible if any of the following side effects occur:
Rare
Loosening of fingernails
Numbness, tingling, pain, or weakness in hands or feet
Pain in lower back
Unexplained nosebleeds

Other side effects may occur that usually do not require medical attention. These side effects may go away during treatment as your body adjusts to the medicine. However, check with your doctor if any of the following side effects continue or are bothersome:
Less common or rare
Diarrhea
Drowsiness
Headache
Indigestion
Nausea or vomiting occurring without a skin rash
Stomach pain
Unusual hair loss

For elderly patients: Many medicines have not been tested in older people. Therefore, it is not known whether the medicine acts the same way it does in younger adults. Check with your doctor or pharmacist if you notice any ususual effects while taking this medicine or if you think it is not working as it should.

Other side effects not listed above may also occur in some patients. If you notice any other effects, check with your doctor.

December 1987

AMANTADINE (Systemic)

Some commonly used brand names are Symadine and Symmetrel.

Generic name product may also be available in the U.S.

To the Reader: If you do not recognize the names of medical conditions or medicines referred to in this information, check with your doctor, nurse, or pharmacist. Definitions for selected medical terms may be found in the Glossary. Brand names for the generic drug names listed can be found in the Index. In addition, selected brand names commonly associated with the generic name have been included in the text to help you recognize medicine you may be taking. The fact that a brand name product is not mentioned does not mean the information does not apply. It is a good idea for you to learn both the generic and brand names of your medicines and to write them down for future use.

Amantadine (a-MAN-ta-deen) belongs to the general family of medicines called antivirals. It is used to prevent or treat certain flu infections (type A). It is given alone by mouth or may be given along with flu shots. Amantadine will not work for colds, other types of flu, or other virus infections.

Amantadine also belongs to the general family of medicines called antidyskinetics. It is used to treat Parkinson's disease, sometimes called paralysis agitans or shaking palsy. It may be given alone or with other medicines for Parkinson's disease. By improving muscle control and reducing stiffness, this medicine allows more normal movements of the body as the disease symptoms are reduced.

Amantadine is available only with your doctor's prescription.

Remember:

• **This medicine has been prescribed for your present medical problem only.** Another problem later on may require a different medicine. Also, even though other people may have the same symptoms as you, they may have a different kind of problem. Your medicine may not work for them and may even cause them harm. Therefore, **your medicine must not be given to other people or used for other problems** unless you are otherwise directed by your doctor.

• **Keep all medicines out of the reach of children.**

• In order for this medicine to work, it must be used as directed.

• **It is very important that you read and understand the following information.** If any of the information causes you special concern, do not decide against using this medicine without first checking with your doctor.

• Before you begin using any new medicine (prescription or nonprescription) or if you develop any new medical problem while you are using this medicine, check with your doctor, nurse, or pharmacist.

• **If you have any questions** about the following information or if you want more information about this medicine or your medical problem, **ask your doctor, nurse, or pharmacist.**

Before Using This Medicine

In order to decide on the best treatment for your medical problem, your doctor should be told:

—if you have ever had any unusual or allergic reaction to amantadine.

—if you are on a low-salt, low-sugar, or any other special diet, or if you are allergic to any substance, such as foods, sulfites or other preservatives, or dyes. Most medicines contain more than their active ingredient, and many liquid medicines contain alcohol. Your doctor, nurse, or pharmacist can help you avoid products that may cause a problem.

—if you are **pregnant** or if you may become pregnant. Studies have not been done in humans. However, studies in some animals have shown that amantadine taken in high doses causes birth defects and harms the fetus. Lower doses have not been shown to cause problems.

—if you are **breast-feeding.** Use is not recommended in nursing mothers since amantadine passes into the breast milk and may cause vomiting, difficult urination, and skin rash in nursing babies.

—if you have any of the following medical problems:
> Blood vessel disease of the brain
> Eczema (recurring)
> Epilepsy or other seizures (history of)
> Heart disease or other circulation problems
> Kidney disease
> Mental or emotional illness
> Stomach or intestinal ulcers
> Swelling of feet and ankles

—if you are taking **any** other prescription or nonprescription (OTC) medicine, especially:
> Amphetamines
> Appetite suppressants (diet pills), except fenfluramine
> Caffeine (e.g., NoDoz)
> Chlophedianol (e.g., Ulo)
> Medicine for asthma or other breathing problems
> Medicine for colds, sinus problems, or hay fever or other allergies (including nose drops or sprays)
> Methylphenidate (e.g., Ritalin)
> Pemoline (e.g., Cylert)

Proper Use of This Medicine

For patients taking amantadine to prevent or treat flu infections:

• This medicine is best taken before exposure, or as soon as possible after exposure, to people who have the flu.

• To help keep you from getting the flu, **keep taking this medicine for the full time of treatment.** Or if you already have the flu, you should still continue taking this medicine for the full time of treatment even if you begin to feel better after a few days. This will help to clear up your infection completely. If you stop taking this medicine too soon, your symptoms may return.

• This medicine works best when there is a constant amount in the blood. **To help keep this amount constant, do not miss any doses. Also, it is best to take each dose at evenly spaced times day and night.** For example, if you are to take 2 doses a day, the doses should be spaced about 12 hours apart. If this interferes with your sleep or other daily activities, or if you need help in planning the best times to take your medicine, check with your doctor, nurse, or pharmacist.

• If you do miss a dose of this medicine, take it as soon as possible. This will help to keep a constant amount of medicine in the blood. However, if it is almost time for your next dose, skip the missed dose and go back to your regular dosing schedule. Do not double doses.

• If you are using the oral liquid form of amantadine, use a specially marked measuring spoon or other device to measure each dose accurately since the average household teaspoon may not hold the right amount of liquid.

For patients taking amantadine for Parkinson's disease:
• **Take this medicine exactly as directed by your doctor.** Do not miss any doses and do not take more medicine than your doctor ordered.

• If you do miss a dose of this medicine, take it as soon as possible. However, if it is within 4 hours of your next dose, skip the missed dose and go back to your regular dosing schedule. Do not double doses.

• Improvement in the symptoms of Parkinson's disease usually occurs in about 2 days. However, in some patients this medicine must be taken for up to 2 weeks before full benefit is seen.

How to store this medicine:
• **Keep out of the reach of children.**

• Store away from heat and direct light.

• Do not store the capsule form of this medicine in the bathroom, near the kitchen sink, or in other damp places. Heat or moisture may cause the medicine to break down.

• Keep the oral liquid form of this medicine from freezing.

• Do not keep outdated medicine or medicine no longer needed. Be sure that any discarded medicine is out of the reach of children.

Precautions While Using This Medicine

Drinking alcoholic beverages while taking this medicine may cause increased side effects such as circulation problems, dizziness, lightheadedness, fainting, or confusion. Therefore, **you should not drink alcoholic beverages while you are taking this medicine.**

This medicine may cause some people to become dizzy, confused, or lightheaded, or to have blurred vision or trouble concentrating. **Make sure you know how you react to this medicine before you drive, use machines, or do other jobs that require you to be alert or to see clearly.** If these reactions are especially bothersome, check with your doctor.

Getting up suddenly from a lying or sitting position may also be a problem because of the dizziness, lightheadedness, or fainting that may be caused by this medicine. Getting up slowly may help. If this problem continues or gets worse, check with your doctor.

Amantadine may cause dryness of the mouth, nose, and throat. For temporary relief of mouth dryness, use sugarless candy or gum, melt bits of ice in your mouth, or use a saliva substitute. However, if dry mouth continues for more than 2 weeks, check with your physician or dentist. Continuing dryness of the mouth may increase the chance of dental disease, including tooth decay, gum disease, and fungal infections.

This medicine may cause purplish red, net-like, blotchy spots on the skin. This problem occurs more often in females and usually occurs on the legs and/or feet after taking this medicine regularly for a month or more. Although the blotchy spots may remain as long as you are taking this medicine, they usually go away gradually within 2 to 12 weeks after you stop taking this medicine. If you have any questions about this, check with your doctor.

For patients taking amantadine to prevent or treat flu infections:
• If your symptoms do not improve within a few days, or if they become worse, check with your doctor.

For patients taking amantadine for Parkinson's disease:
• **Patients with Parkinson's disease must be careful not to overdo physical activities as their condition improves and body movements become easier** since injuries resulting from falls may occur. Such activities must be gradually increased to give your body time to adjust to changing balance, circulation, and coordination.

• Some patients may notice that this medicine gradually loses its effect while they are taking it regularly for a few months. If you notice this, check with your doctor. Your doctor may want to adjust the dose or stop the medicine for a while and then restart it to restore its effect.

• **Do not suddenly stop taking this medicine without first checking with your doctor** since your Parkinson's disease may get worse very quickly. Your doctor may want you to reduce your dose gradually before stopping the medicine completely.

Side Effects of This Medicine

Along with its needed effects, a medicine may cause some unwanted effects. Although not all of these side effects may occur, if they do occur they may need medical attention.

Check with your doctor immediately if any of the following side effects occur:
More common
    Confusion, especially in elderly patients
    Hallucinations (seeing, hearing, or feeling things that are not there)
    Mood or other mental changes

Less common
    Difficult urination, especially in elderly patients
    Fainting

Rare
    Slurred speech
    Sore throat and fever
    Uncontrolled rolling of eyes

Usually only with long-term therapy
    Swelling of feet or lower legs
    Unexplained shortness of breath
    Weight gain (rapid)

Signs of overdose
    Confusion (severe)
    Convulsions (seizures)
    Mood or other mental changes (severe)
    Trouble in sleeping or nightmares (severe)

Other side effects may occur that usually do not require medical attention. These side effects may go away during treatment as your body adjusts to the medicine. However, check with your doctor if any of the following side effects continue or are bothersome:

More common
    Difficulty concentrating
    Dizziness or lightheadedness
    Irritability
    Loss of appetite
    Nausea
    Nervousness
    Purplish red, net-like, blotchy spots on skin
    Trouble in sleeping or nightmares

Less common or rare
    Blurred vision
    Constipation
    Dry mouth, nose, and throat
    Headache
    Skin rash
    Unusual tiredness or weakness
    Vomiting

For elderly patients: Confusion; difficult urination; blurred vision; constipation; and dry mouth, nose, and throat may be more likely to occur in the elderly, who are usually more sensitive to the effects of amantadine.

Other side effects not listed above may also occur in some patients. If you notice any other effects, check with your doctor.

December 1987

AMINOBENZOATE POTASSIUM
(Systemic)

Some commonly used brand names or other names are:

KPAB	Potassium aminobenzoate
Potaba	Potassium para-aminobenzoate

To the Reader: If you do not recognize the names of medical conditions or medicines referred to in this information, check with your doctor, nurse, or pharmacist. Definitions for selected medical terms may be found in the Glossary. Brand names for the generic drug names listed can be found in the Index. In addition, selected brand names commonly associated with the generic name have been included in the text to help you recognize medicine you may be taking. The fact that a brand name product is not mentioned does not mean the information does not apply. It is a good idea for you to learn both the generic and brand names of your medicines and to write them down for future use.

Aminobenzoate potassium (a-mee-noe-BEN-zoe-ate poe-TAS-ee-um) is taken by mouth to treat fibrosis, a condition in which the skin and underlying tissues tighten and become less flexible. This condition is associated with such diseases as dermatomyositis, morphea, Peyronie's disease, scleroderma, and linear scleroderma.

Aminobenzoate potassium is also used to treat a certain type of inflammation (nonsuppurative inflammation) associated with such diseases as dermatomyositis, pemphigus, and Peyronie's disease.

This medicine is available only with your doctor's prescription.

Remember:

• **This medicine has been prescribed for your current medical problem only.** It must not be given to other people or used for other problems unless you are directed to do so by your doctor.

• **Keep all medicines out of the reach of children.**

• In order for this medicine to work, it must be used as directed.

• **It is very important that you read and understand the following information.** If any of the information causes you special concern, do not decide against using this medicine without first checking with your doctor.

• Before you begin using any new medicine (prescription or nonprescription) or if you develop any new medical problem while you are using this medicine, check with your doctor, nurse, or pharmacist.

• **If you have any questions** about the following information or if you want more information about this medicine or your medical problem, **ask your doctor, nurse, or pharmacist.**

Before Using This Medicine

In order to decide on the best treatment for your medical problem, your doctor should be told:
—if you have ever had any unusual or allergic reaction to aminobenzoate potassium or aminobenzoic acid (PABA).
—if you are on a low-salt, low-sugar, or any other special diet, or if you are allergic to any substance, such as foods, sulfites or other perservatives, or dyes.

Most medicines contain more than their active ingredient. Your doctor, nurse, or pharmacist can help you avoid products that may cause a problem.

—if you are **pregnant** or if you may become pregnant, although aminobenzoate potassium has not been shown to cause birth defects or other problems in humans.

—if you are **breast-feeding**, although aminobenzoate potassium has not been shown to cause problems in nursing babies.

—if you have any of the following medical problems:
   Diabetes mellitus (sugar diabetes)
   Hypoglycemia (low blood sugar)
   Kidney disease

—if you are taking **any** other prescription or nonprescription (OTC) medicine, especially:
   Sulfonamides (sulfa medicine)

Proper Use of This Medicine

Take this medicine after meals or snacks to lessen the possibility of stomach upset. If stomach upset continues, check with your doctor.

For patients taking the capsule or tablet form of aminobenzoate potassium:

• Take each dose with a full glass (8 ounces) of water or milk to lessen the possibility of stomach upset.

• For patients taking aminobenzoate potassium tablets, dissolve them in water before taking. This also will help lessen the possibility of stomach upset.

For patients using the powder form of this medicine:

• This medicine should never be taken in its dry form. Instead, always mix with water or citrus juice, as directed.

• To mask the taste of aminobenzoate potassium, the powder may be dissolved in citrus drinks instead of in water. However, if you do dissolve the powder in water, drinking a citrus juice or a carbonated beverage immediately after each dose of medicine will also help mask the taste.

• The flavor of this medicine is improved if the solution is chilled before you take it.

• For patients using the two-gram individual packets of powder:
   —Dissolve one packet (2 grams) of aminobenzoate potassium in a full glass (8 ounces) of water or citrus juice.
   —Stir well to dissolve powder.

• For patients using the bulk powder form of this medicine:
   —Use a specially marked measuring spoon or other device to measure out the correct amount of medicine. Your doctor or pharmacist can help you with this.
   —To make a 10-percent solution of this medicine:
      Choose a glass, plastic, or stainless steel container large enough to measure one liter (approximately one quart).

Place 100 grams (approximately 3 ounces) of aminobenzoate potassium powder in the container.

Add enough water or citrus juice to make one liter (approximately one quart) of solution and stir well.

Keep the solution refrigerated. Stir well before pouring each dose. Discard the unused portion after one week.

In order for this medicine to be effective, it must be taken every day as ordered by your doctor. It may take 3 or more months before you begin to see an improvement in your condition.

If you miss a dose of this medicine, take it as soon as possible. However, if it is within 2 hours of your next dose, skip the missed dose and go back to your regular dosing schedule. Do not double doses.

How to store this medicine:

• **Keep out of the reach of children.**

• Store away from heat and direct light.

• Do not store the capsules, powder, or tablets in the bathroom, near the kitchen sink, or in other damp places. Heat or moisture may cause the medicine to break down.

• Store the liquid form of this medicine in the refrigerator. However, keep the medicine from freezing.

• Discard the unused portion of the liquid form of this medicine after one week.

• Do not keep outdated medicine or medicine no longer needed. Be sure that any discarded medicine is out of the reach of children.

Precautions While Using This Medicine

While you are taking this medicine, it is important that your doctor check your progress at regular visits.

Check with your doctor right away if you cannot eat normally while taking this medicine because of nausea, loss of appetite, or for any other reason. Taking this medicine when you have not been eating normally for several days may cause low blood sugar (hypoglycemia).

If signs of low blood sugar (hypoglycemia) appear, stop taking this medicine, eat or drink something containing sugar, and check with your doctor right away. Good sources of sugar are table sugar mixed in water, sugar cubes, orange juice, corn syrup, or honey. One popular source of sugar is a glassful of orange juice containing 2 or 3 teaspoonfuls of table sugar.

• **Tell someone ahead of time to take you to your doctor or to a hospital right away if you begin to feel that you may pass out. If you do pass out, emergency help should be gotten at once.**

• Even if the signs of low blood sugar are corrected by eating or drinking something with sugar, it is very important to call your doctor right away. The effects this medicine has on low blood sugar may last for a few days, and the signs may return often during this period of time.

Side Effects of This Medicine

Along with its needed effects, a medicine may cause some unwanted effects. Although not all of these side effects may occur, if they do occur they may need medical attention.

Check with your doctor as soon as possible if any of the following side effects occur:
Less common or rare
   Chills
   Fever
   Skin rash
   Sore throat
Signs of low blood sugar
   Anxiety
   Chills
   Cold sweats
   Confusion
   Cool pale skin
   Difficulty in concentration
   Drowsiness
   Excessive hunger
   Fast heartbeat
   Headache
   Nervousness
   Shakiness
   Unsteady walk
   Unusual tiredness or weakness

Other side effects may occur that usually do not require medical attention. These side effects may go away during treatment as your body adjusts to the medicine. However, check with your doctor if either of the following side effects continues or is bothersome:
More common
   Loss of appetite
   Nausea

For elderly patients: If hypoglycemia occurs in the elderly, some signs of low blood sugar, such as confusion, difficulty in concentration, or headache, are more likely to occur.

Other side effects not listed above may also occur in some patients. If you notice any other effects, check with your doctor.

December 1987

AMINOGLUTETHIMIDE (Systemic)

A commonly used brand name is Cytadren.

To the Reader: If you do not recognize the names of medical conditions or medicines referred to in this information, check with your doctor, nurse, or pharmacist. Definitions for selected medical terms may be found in the Glossary. Brand names for the generic drug names listed can be found in the Index. In addition, selected brand names commonly associated with the generic name have been included in the text to help you recognize medicine you may be taking. The fact that a brand name product is not mentioned does not mean the information does not apply. It is a good idea for you to learn both the generic and brand names of your medicines and to write them down for future use.

Aminoglutethimide (a-mee-noe-gloo-TETH-i-mide) is used to treat some kinds of tumors that affect the adrenal cortex. Also, it is sometimes used when the adrenal cortex is overactive without being cancerous.

In addition, aminoglutethimide is sometimes used to treat certain other conditions as determined by your doctor.

Aminoglutethimide acts on a part of the body called the adrenal cortex. It affects production of steroids and also has some other effects.

Aminoglutethimide is available only with your doctor's prescription.

Remember:

• **This medicine has been prescribed for your current medical problem only.** It must not be given to other people or used for other problems unless you are directed to do so by your doctor.

• **Keep all medicines out of the reach of children.**

• In order for this medicine to work, it must be used as directed.

• **It is very important that you read and understand the following information.** If any of the information causes you special concern, do not decide against using this medicine without first checking with your doctor.

• Before you begin using any new medicine (prescription or nonprescription) or if you develop any new medical problem while you are using this medicine, check with your doctor, nurse, or pharmacist.

• **If you have any questions** about the following information or if you want more information about this medicine or your medical problem, **ask your doctor, nurse, or pharmacist.**

Before Using This Medicine

In order to decide on the best treatment for your medical problem, your doctor should be told:

—if you have ever had any unusual or allergic reaction to glutethimide or aminoglutethimide.

—if you are on a low-salt, low-sugar, or any other special diet, or if you are allergic to any substance, such as foods, sulfites or other preservatives, or dyes. Most medicines contain more than their active ingredient. Your doctor, nurse, or pharmacist can help you avoid products that may cause a problem.

—if you are **pregnant** or if you may become pregnant. Aminoglutethimide has been shown to cause birth defects in humans and animals. However, this medicine may be needed in serious diseases or in other situations which threaten the mother's life. Be sure you have discussed this with your doctor before taking this medicine.

—if you are **breast-feeding**. Aminoglutethimide has not been shown to cause problems in nursing babies.

—if you have any of the following medical problems:

    Chickenpox (including recent exposure)
    Herpes zoster (shingles)
    Infection
    Underactive thyroid

—if you are taking **any** other prescription or nonprescription (OTC) medicine, especially dexamethasone (e.g., Decadron).

Proper Use of This Medicine

Take this medicine only as directed by your doctor. Do not take more or less of it, and do not take it more often than your doctor ordered.

This medicine sometimes causes nausea and vomiting. This effect usually goes away or lessens after you have taken the medicine for a while. It is very important that you continue to use this medicine even if you begin to feel ill. Ask your doctor, nurse, or pharmacist for ways to lessen these effects. **Do not stop taking this medicine without first checking with your doctor.**

If you vomit shortly after taking a dose of aminoglutethimide, check with your doctor. You will be told whether to take the dose again or wait until the next scheduled dose.

If you miss a dose of this medicine and remember within 2 to 4 hours of the missed dose, take it as soon as possible. Then go back to your regular dosing schedule. However, if it is almost time for your next dose, skip the missed dose and go back to your regular dosing schedule. Do not double doses.

How to store this medicine:

• **Keep out of the reach of children.**

• Store away from heat and direct light.

• Do not store in the bathroom, near the kitchen sink, or in other damp places. Heat or moisture may cause the medicine to break down.

• Do not keep outdated medicine or medicine no longer needed. Be sure that any discarded medicine is out of the reach of children.

Precautions While Using This Medicine

It is very important that your doctor check your progress at regular visits to make sure that the medicine is working properly and does not cause unwanted effects.

Your doctor may want you to carry a medical identification card or wear a bracelet stating that you are taking this medicine.

Before having any kind of surgery (including dental surgery) or emergency treatment, tell the physician or dentist in charge that you are taking this medicine.

Check with your doctor right away if you get an injury, infection, or illness of any kind. This medicine may weaken your body's defenses against infection or inflammation.

This medicine may cause some people to become dizzy, drowsy, or less alert than they are normally. **Make sure you know how you react to this medicine before you drive, use machines, or do other jobs that require you to be alert.**

Side Effects of This Medicine

Along with its needed effects, a medicine may cause some unwanted effects. Although not all of these side effects may occur, if they do occur they may need medical attention.

Check with your doctor immediately if any of the following side effects occur:

Rare
   Fever, chills, or sore throat
   Unusual bleeding or bruising
   Yellow eyes and skin

Other side effects may occur that usually do not require medical attention. These side effects may go away during treatment as your body adjusts to the medicine. However, check with your doctor if any of the following side effects continue or are bothersome:

More common
   Clumsiness
   Dizziness or lightheadedness (especially when getting up from a lying or sitting position)
   Drowsiness
   Lack of energy
   Loss of appetite
   Measles-like skin rash or itching on face and/or palms of hands
   Nausea or vomiting
   Uncontrolled eye movements

Less common or rare
   Darkening of skin
   Headache
   Mental depression
   Muscle pain

For elderly patients: Lack of energy is more likely to occur in the elderly, who are usually more sensitive to the effects of aminoglutethimide.

Other side effects not listed above may also occur in some patients. If you notice any other effects, check with your doctor.

December 1987

AMINOGLYCOSIDES (Systemic)

This information applies to the following medicines:

Amikacin (am-i-KAY-sin)
Gentamicin (jen-ta-MYE-sin)
Kanamycin (kan-a-MYE-sin)
Neomycin (nee-oh-MYE-sin)
Netilmicin (ne-til-MYE-sin)
Streptomycin (strep-toe-MYE-sin)
Tobramycin (toe-bra-MYE-sin)

Some commonly used brand names are:	Generic names:
Amikin	Amikacin
Apogen Cidomycin* Garamycin	Gentamicin†
Kantrex Klebcil	Kanamycin†
Mycifradin* Neo-IM	Neomycin
Netromycin	Netilmicin
	Streptomycin†
Nebcin	Tobramycin

*Not available in the U.S.
†Generic name product may also be available in the U.S.

To the Reader: If you do not recognize the names of medical conditions or medicines referred to in this information, check with your doctor, nurse, or pharmacist. Definitions for selected medical terms may be found in the Glossary. Brand names for the generic drug names listed can be found in the Index. In addition, selected brand names commonly associated with the generic name have been included in the text to help you recognize medicine you may be taking. The fact that a brand name product is not mentioned does not mean the information does not apply. It is a good idea for you to learn both the generic and brand names of your medicines and to write them down for future use.

Aminoglycosides (a-mee-noe-GLYE-koe-sides) belong to the general family of medicines called antibiotics. Antibiotics are medicines used in the treatment of infections caused by bacteria. They work by killing bacteria or preventing their growth. Aminoglycosides will not work for colds, flu, or other virus infections.

Aminoglycosides are given by injection into a muscle or vein to treat serious infections in many different parts of the body. In addition, some aminoglycosides may be given by oral inhalation (breathing in the medicine as a fine mist through the mouth) or by irrigation (washing out a body cavity with a solution of the medicine). Streptomycin may also be given for tuberculosis (TB). These medicines may be given with one or more other medicines for infections, or they may be given alone.

Aminoglycosides given by injection are usually used for serious infections in which other medicines may not work. However, these medicines may also cause some serious side effects, including damage to your hearing, balance, and kidneys. These side effects may be more likely to occur in elderly patients and newborn infants. **You and your doctor should talk about the good these medicines will do as well as the risks of receiving them.**

Aminoglycosides are available only with your doctor's prescription.

Remember:
• **This medicine has been prescribed for your present infection only.** Another infection later on may require a different medicine.

• **Keep all medicines out of the reach of children.**

• In order for this medicine to work, it must be used as directed.

• **It is very important that you read and understand the following information.** If any of the information causes you special concern, do not decide against using this medicine without first checking with your doctor.

• Before you begin using any new medicine (prescription or nonprescription) or if you develop any new medical problem while you are using this medicine, check with your doctor, nurse, or pharmacist.

• **If you have any questions** about the following information or if you want more information about this medicine or your medical problem, **ask your doctor, nurse, or pharmacist.**

Before Using This Medicine

In order to decide on the best treatment for your medical problem, your doctor should be told:

—if you have ever had any unusual or allergic reaction to any of the aminoglycosides.

—if you are on a low-salt, low-sugar, or any other special diet, or if you are allergic to any substance, such as foods or sulfites or other preservatives. Most medicines contain more than their active ingredient. Your doctor, nurse, or pharmacist can help you avoid products that may cause a problem.

—if you are **pregnant** or if you may become pregnant. Studies on most of the aminoglycosides have not been done in humans. Some reports have shown that aminoglycosides, especially streptomycin and tobramycin, may cause damage to the infant's hearing, sense of balance, and kidneys. However, this medicine may be needed in serious diseases or other situations that threaten the mother's life. Be sure you have discussed this with your doctor.

—if you are **breast-feeding**. Aminoglycosides have not been shown to cause problems in nursing babies, even though kanamycin, netilmicin, and streptomycin do pass into the breast milk in different amounts. It is not known whether amikacin, gentamicin, or tobramycin passes into the breast milk. However, aminoglycosides are not absorbed very much when taken by mouth. Therefore, this medicine is unlikely to cause serious problems in nursing babies even if they do receive small amounts in the breast milk.

—if you have any of the following medical problems:
Kidney disease
Loss of hearing and/or balance (eighth-cranial-nerve disease)
Myasthenia gravis
Parkinson's disease

—if you are taking **any** other prescription or nonprescription (OTC) medicine, especially:

> Aminoglycosides (used on the skin or mucous membranes and by injection at the same time; or more than one aminoglycoside at a time)
> Amphotericin B by injection (e.g., Fungizone)
> Bacitracin by injection
> Bumetanide by injection (e.g., Bumex)
> Capreomycin (e.g., Capastat)
> Cephalothin (e.g., Keflin)
> Cisplatin (e.g., Platinol)
> Colistimethate (e.g., Coly-Mycin)
> Cyclosporine (e.g., Sandimmune)
> Ethacrynic acid by injection (e.g., Edecrin)
> Furosemide by injection (e.g., Lasix)
> Indomethacin by injection (e.g., Indocin)
> Paromomycin (e.g., Humatin)
> Polymyxin B by injection (e.g., Aerosporin)
> Streptozocin (e.g., Zanosar)
> Vancomycin (e.g., Vancocin)

Proper Use of This Medicine

To help clear up your infection completely, **this medicine must be given for the full time of treatment** even if you begin to feel better after a few days. Also, it works best when there is a constant amount in the blood or urine. To help keep the amount constant, this medicine is given on a regular schedule.

Side Effects of This Medicine

Along with its needed effects, a medicine may cause some unwanted effects. Although not all of these side effects may occur, if they do occur they may need medical attention.

Check with your doctor or nurse immediately if any of the following side effects occur:

More common

> Any loss of hearing
> Blood in urine
> Clumsiness or unsteadiness
> Dizziness
> Greatly increased or decreased frequency of urination or amount of urine
> Increased thirst
> Loss of appetite
> Nausea or vomiting

> Numbness, tingling, or burning of face or mouth (streptomycin only)
> Numbness, tingling, muscle twitching, or convulsions (seizures)
> Ringing or buzzing sound or a feeling of fullness in the ears

Less common

> Any loss of vision (streptomycin only)
> Skin rash, itching, redness, or swelling (may be more common or rare with some aminoglycosides)

Rare

> Difficulty in breathing
> Drowsiness
> Weakness

The above side effects are more likely to occur in elderly patients, or in premature infants and other newborns, who are usually more sensitive to the effects of these medicines. In addition, leg cramps, skin rash, fever, and convulsions (seizures) may occur when gentamicin is given by injection into the muscle or a vein and into the spinal fluid.

For up to several weeks after you stop receiving this medicine, it may still cause some side effects that require medical attention. Check with your doctor if you notice any of the following side effects or if they get worse:

> Any loss of hearing
> Blood in urine
> Clumsiness or unsteadiness
> Difficulty in breathing
> Dizziness
> Drowsiness
> Greatly increased or decreased frequency of urination or amount of urine
> Increased thirst
> Loss of appetite
> Nausea or vomiting
> Ringing or buzzing sound or a feeling of fullness in the ears
> Weakness

Other side effects not listed above may also occur in some patients. If you notice any other effects, check with your doctor.

December 1987

4-AMINOQUINOLINES (Systemic)

This information applies to the following medicines:

Chloroquine (KLOR-oh-kwin)
Hydroxychloroquine (hye-drox-ee-KLOR-oh-kwin)

Some commonly used brand names are:	Generic names:
Aralen	Chloroquine†
Plaquenil	Hydroxychloroquine

†Generic name product may also be available in the U.S.

To the Reader: If you do not recognize the names of medical conditions or medicines referred to in this information, check with your doctor, nurse, or pharmacist. Definitions for selected medical terms may be found in the Glossary. Brand names for the generic drug names listed can be found in the Index. In addition, selected brand names commonly associated with the generic name have been included in the text to help you recognize medicine you may be taking. The fact that a brand name product is not mentioned does not mean the information does not apply. It is a good idea for you to learn both the generic and brand names of your medicines and to write them down for future use.

The 4-aminoquinolines (a-mee-noe-KWIN-oh-leens) belong to the general family of medicines called antiprotozoals. Protozoa are tiny, one-celled animals. Some are parasites that can cause many different kinds of infections in the body.

These medicines are used to prevent and to treat malaria and to treat some conditions such as liver disease caused by protozoa. They are also used in the treatment of arthritis to help relieve inflammation, swelling, stiffness, and joint pain and to help control the symptoms of lupus erythematosus (lupus; SLE).

These medicines are taken by mouth and chloroquine is also given by injection. They may be given alone or with one or more other medicines. They may also be used for other conditions as determined by your doctor.

4-Aminoquinolines are available only with your doctor's prescription.

Remember:

• **This medicine has been prescribed for your present medical problem only.** Another problem later on may require a different medicine. Also, even though other people may have the same symptoms as you, they may have a different kind of problem. Your medicine may not work for them and may even cause them harm. Therefore, **your medicine must not be given to other people or used for other problems** unless you are otherwise directed by your doctor.

• **Keep all medicines out of the reach of children.**

• In order for this medicine to work, it must be used as directed.

• If you are receiving chloroquine by injection, some of the information about this medicine may not apply.

• **It is very important that you read and understand the following information.** If any of the information causes you special concern, do not decide against using this medicine without first checking with your doctor.

• Before you begin using any new medicine (prescription or nonprescription) or if you develop any new medical problem while you are using this medicine, check with your doctor, nurse, or pharmacist.

• **If you have any questions** about the following information or if you want more information about this medicine or your medical problem, **ask your doctor, nurse, or pharmacist.**

Before Using This Medicine

In order to decide on the best treatment for your medical problem, your doctor should be told:

—if you have ever had any unusual or allergic reaction to any of the 4-aminoquinolines.

—if you are on a low-salt, low-sugar, or any other special diet, or if you are allergic to any substance, such as foods, sulfites or other preservatives, or dyes. Most medicines contain more than their active ingredient. Your doctor, nurse, or pharmacist can help you avoid products that may cause a problem.

—if you are **pregnant** or if you may become pregnant. Unless you are taking it for malaria or liver disease caused by protozoa, use of this medicine is not recommended during pregnancy. 4-Aminoquinolines have been shown to cause damage to the central nervous system (brain and spinal cord), including hearing, sense of balance, bleeding inside the eyes, and other eye problems in animals. However, when given in low doses (once a week) to prevent malaria, this medicine has not been shown to cause birth defects or other problems in humans.

—if you are **breast-feeding**. Chloroquine passes into the breast milk. Although 4-aminoquinolines have not been shown to cause problems in nursing babies, the chance always exists. Babies and children are especially sensitive to the effects of 4-aminoquinolines.

—if you have any of the following medical problems:
Alcoholism (active or treated)
Blood disease (severe)
Eye or vision problems
Glucose-6-phosphate dehydrogenase (G6PD) deficiency
Liver disease
Nerve or brain disease (severe), including seizures
Porphyria
Psoriasis
Stomach or intestinal disease (severe)

—if you are taking **any** other prescription or nonprescription (OTC) medicine, especially:
Acetaminophen (e.g., Tylenol) (with long-term, high-dose use)
Amiodarone (e.g., Cordarone)
Anabolic steroids (dromostanolone, ethylestrenol, nandrolone, oxandrolone, oxymetholone, stanozolol)
Androgens (male hormones)
Antithyroid agents (medicine for overactive thyroid)
Azlocillin (e.g., Azlin)
Carbamazepine (e.g., Tegretol)
Carmustine (e.g., BiCNU)
Dantrolene (e.g., Dantrium)
Daunorubicin (e.g., Cerubidine)
Disulfiram (e.g., Antabuse)
Divalproex (e.g., Depakote)

Doxorubicin (e.g., Adriamycin)
Erythromycins
Estrogens (female hormones)
Etretinate (e.g., Tegison)
Furazolidone (e.g., Furoxone)
Gold salts
Isoniazid (e.g., INH, Nydrazid)
Ketoconazole by mouth (e.g., Nizoral)
Mercaptopurine (e.g., Purinethol)
Methotrexate (e.g., Mexate)
Methyldopa (e.g., Aldomet)
Mezlocillin (e.g., Mezlin)
Naltrexone (e.g., Trexan) (with long-term, high-dose use)
Nitrofurantoin (e.g., Furadantin)
Oral contraceptives (birth control pills) containing estrogen
Phenothiazines (acetophenazine, chlorpromazine, fluphenazine, mesoridazine, perphenazine, prochlorperazine, promazine, promethazine, thioridazine, trifluoperazine, triflupromazine, trimeprazine)
Phenytoin (e.g., Dilantin)
Piperacillin (e.g., Pipracil)
Plicamycin (e.g., Mithracin)
Rifampin (e.g., Rifadin)
Sulfonamides (sulfa medicine)
Valproic acid (e.g., Depakene)

Proper Use of This Medicine

Take this medicine with meals or milk to lessen possible stomach upset, unless otherwise directed by your doctor.

Keep this medicine out of the reach of children since children are especially sensitive to the effects of these medicines and overdose is especially dangerous in children. Taking as few as 3 or 4 tablets (250-mg strength) has resulted in death in small children.

It is very important that you **take this medicine only as directed.** Do not take more of it, do not take it more often, and do not take it for a longer period of time than your doctor ordered. To do so may increase the chance of serious side effects.

If you are taking this medicine to help keep you from getting malaria, **keep taking it for the full time of treatment.** If you already have malaria, you should still keep taking this medicine for the full time of treatment even if you begin to feel better after a few days. This will help to clear up your infection completely. If you stop taking this medicine too soon, your symptoms may return.

This medicine works best when you take it on a regular schedule. For example, if you are to take it once a week to prevent malaria, it is best to take it on the same day each week. Or if you are to take 2 doses a day, one dose may be taken with breakfast and the other one with the evening meal. **Make sure that you do not miss any doses.** If you have any questions about this, check with your doctor, nurse, or pharmacist.

If you do miss a dose of this medicine and your dosing schedule is one dose to be taken:

Every seven days—Take the missed dose as soon as possible. Then go back to your regular dosing schedule.

Once a day—Take the missed dose as soon as possible. But if you do not remember until the next day, skip the missed dose and go back to your regular dosing schedule. Do not double doses.

More than once a day—Take it right away if you remember within an hour or so of the missed dose. But if you do not remember until later, skip the missed dose and go back to your regular dosing schedule. Do not double doses.

If you have any questions about this, check with your doctor.

For patients taking this medicine to prevent malaria:

• Your doctor may want you to start taking this medicine 2 weeks before you travel to an area where there is a chance of getting malaria. This will build up a supply of medicine in your body so that you will be protected from malaria at the start of your travels. It will also help you to get used to taking the medicine regularly and to see how you react to it.

• Also, you should keep taking this medicine while you are in the area and for 6 weeks after you leave the area. To protect you completely, **it is important to keep taking this medicine for the full time your doctor ordered.**

For patients taking this medicine for arthritis or lupus:

• This medicine must be taken regularly as ordered by your doctor in order for it to help you. It may take up to several weeks before you begin to feel better. However, it may take up to 6 months before you feel the full benefit of this medicine.

For patients unable to swallow hydroxychloroquine tablets:

• Your pharmacist can crush the tablets and put each dose in a capsule. Contents of the capsules may then be mixed with a teaspoonful of jam, jelly, or jello. Be sure the patient takes all the food in order to get the full dose of medicine.

How to store this medicine:

• **Keep out of the reach of children.**

• Store away from heat and direct light.

• Do not store in the bathroom, near the kitchen sink, or in other damp places. Heat or moisture may cause the medicine to break down.

• Do not keep outdated medicine or medicine no longer needed. Be sure that any discarded medicine is out of the reach of children.

Precautions While Using This Medicine

If you will be taking this medicine for a long period of time:

• Your doctor may want you to have your eyes checked regularly by an ophthalmologist (eye doctor) before, during, and after treatment. This will allow your doctor to check for any unwanted effects that may be caused by this medicine.

If your symptoms do not improve within a few days (or a few weeks or months for arthritis), or if they become worse, check with your doctor.

Liver problems may be more likely to occur if you drink alcoholic beverages while you are taking this medicine. Therefore, **you should not drink alcoholic beverages while you are taking this medicine.**

This medicine may cause blurred vision, difficulty in reading, or other change in vision. It may also cause some people to become dizzy or lightheaded. **Make sure you know how you react to this medicine before you drive, use machines, or do other jobs that require you to be alert or to see clearly.** If these reactions are especially bothersome, check with your doctor.

If you are living in or will be traveling to an area where there is a chance of getting malaria, the following measures will help to prevent malaria or malaria reinfection:

• If possible, sleep under mosquito netting to avoid being bitten by malaria-carrying mosquitoes.

• Wear long-sleeved shirts or blouses and long trousers to protect arms and legs, especially at dusk or during evening hours when mosquitoes are out.

• Apply mosquito repellant to uncovered areas of the skin when mosquitoes are out.

Side Effects of This Medicine

Along with its needed effects, a medicine may cause some unwanted effects. Although not all of these side effects may occur, if they do occur they may need medical attention. When this medicine is used for short periods of time, side effects usually are rare. However, when it is used for long periods of time and/or in high doses, side effects are more likely to occur and may be serious.

Check with your doctor immediately if any of the following side effects occur:

Less common
   Blurred vision, difficulty in reading, or any other change in vision
       Note: The above side effects may also occur or get worse after you stop taking this medicine.

Rare
   Convulsions (seizures)
   Increased muscle weakness
   Mood or other mental changes
   Ringing or buzzing in ears or any loss of hearing
   Sore throat and fever
   Unusual bleeding or bruising
Signs of overdose
   Difficult breathing (severe)
   Drowsiness
   Fainting

Other side effects may occur that usually do not require medical attention. These side effects may go away during treatment as your body adjusts to the medicine. However, check with your doctor if any of the following side effects continue or are bothersome:

More common
   Diarrhea
   Headache
   Loss of appetite
   Nausea or vomiting
   Stomach cramps or pain
Less common
   Bleaching of hair or increased hair loss
   Blue-black discoloration of skin, fingernails, or inside of mouth
   Dizziness or lightheadedness
   Nervousness or restlessness
   Skin rash or itching

Although not all of the side effects listed above have been reported for both of these medicines, they have been reported for at least one of them. However, since chloroquine and hydroxychloroquine are very similar, any of the above side effects may occur with either of these medicines.

The above side effects are more likely to occur in babies and children, who are usually more sensitive to the effects of these medicines. In addition, serious side effects have occurred in children receiving chloroquine by injection.

Other side effects not listed above may also occur in some patients. If you notice any other effects, check with your doctor.

_____

December 1987

AMINOSALICYLATES (Systemic)

This information applies to the following medicines:

Aminosalicylate Calcium (a-mee-noe-sa-LI-si-late KAL-see-um)
Aminosalicylate Sodium (SOE-dee-um)
Aminosalicylic Acid (a-mee-noe-sal-i-SILL-ik AS-id)

Some commonly used brand names are:	Generic names:
	Aminosalicylate Calcium*
P.A.S. Nemasol* Teebacin	Aminosalicylate Sodium
	Aminosalicylic Acid*

*Not commercially available in the U.S.

To the Reader: If you do not recognize the names of medical conditions or medicines referred to in this information, check with your doctor, nurse, or pharmacist. Definitions for selected medical terms may be found in the Glossary. Brand names for the generic drug names listed can be found in the Index. In addition, selected brand names commonly associated with the generic name have been included in the text to help you recognize medicine you may be taking. The fact that a brand name product is not mentioned does not mean the information does not apply. It is a good idea for you to learn both the generic and brand names of your medicines and to write them down for future use.

Aminosalicylates belong to the general family of medicines called anti-infectives. They are taken by mouth, along with one or more other medicines, to help the body overcome tuberculosis (TB).

Aminosalicylates may also be used for other problems as determined by your doctor. They will not work for colds, flu, or other infections.

Aminosalicylates are available only with your doctor's prescription.

Remember:

• **This medicine has been prescribed for your present TB infection only.** Another TB infection later on may require a different medicine. Also, even though other people may have the same symptoms as you, they may have a different kind of TB. Your medicine may not work for them and may even cause them harm. Therefore, **your medicine must not be given to other people or used for other infections** unless you are otherwise directed by your doctor.

• **Keep all medicines out of the reach of children.**

• In order for this medicine to work, it must be used as directed.

• **It is very important that you read and understand the following information.** If any of the information causes you special concern, do not decide against using this medicine without first checking with your doctor.

• Before you begin using any new medicine (prescription or nonprescription) or if you develop any new medical problem while you are using this medicine, check with your doctor, nurse, or pharmacist.

• **If you have any questions** about the following information or if you want more information about this medicine or your medical problem, **ask your doctor, nurse, or pharmacist.**

Before Using This Medicine

In order to decide on the best treatment for your medical problem, your doctor should be told:

—if you have ever had any unusual or allergic reaction to aspirin or other salicylates, including methyl salicylate (oil of wintergreen), or to other related medicines such as sulfonamides (sulfa medicine) or dyes.

—if you are on a low-salt, low-sugar, or any other special diet, or if you are allergic to any substance, such as foods, sulfites or other preservatives, or dyes. Most medicines contain more than their active ingredient. Your doctor, nurse, or pharmacist can help you avoid products that may cause a problem.

—if you are **pregnant** or if you may become pregnant. Aminosalicylates have not been shown to cause birth defects or other problems in humans. However, it is not known whether this medicine causes problems when taken with other TB medicines.

—if you are **breast-feeding**. Aminosalicylates pass into the breast milk. However, aminosalicylates have not been shown to cause problems in nursing babies.

—if you are taking aminosalicylate calcium and have any of the following medical problems:
    Cancer
    Glucose-6-phosphate dehydrogenase (G6PD) deficiency
    Kidney stones or other kidney disease
    Liver disease (severe)
    Overactive parathyroid glands
    Overactive thyroid gland
    Sarcoidosis
    Stomach ulcer
    Underactive adrenal glands (Addison's disease)

—if you are taking aminosalicylate sodium and have any of the following medical problems:
    Glucose-6-phosphate dehydrogenase (G6PD) deficiency
    Heart disease or other circulation problems
    Kidney disease (severe)
    Liver disease (severe)
    Stomach ulcer

—if you are taking **any** other prescription or nonprescription (OTC) medicine, especially (may not apply to all aminosalicylates):
    Aminobenzoic acid (PABA)
    Cellulose sodium phosphate (e.g., Calcibind)
    Demeclocycline (e.g., Declomycin)
    Doxycycline (e.g., Vibramycin)
    Methacycline (e.g., Rondomycin)
    Minocycline (e.g., Minocin)
    Oxytetracycline (e.g., Terramycin)
    Tetracycline (e.g., Achromycin)

Proper Use of This Medicine

Aminosalicylates may be taken with or after meals or with an antacid if they upset your stomach.

For patients taking the dry powder form of this medicine:

- Dissolve the contents of each packet in water immediately before taking. Stir well. Be sure to drink all the liquid in order to get the full dose of medicine.

To help clear up your tuberculosis (TB) completely, **it is important that you keep taking this medicine for the full time of treatment** even if you begin to feel better after a few weeks. Since TB may take a long time to clear up, you may have to take the medicine every day for as long as 1 to 2 years or more. If you stop taking this medicine too soon, your symptoms may return.

This medicine works best when there is a constant amount in the blood. **To help keep the amount constant, do not miss any doses. Also, it is best to take the doses at evenly spaced times day and night.** For example, if you are to take 3 doses a day, doses should be spaced about 8 hours apart. If this interferes with your sleep or other daily activities, or if you need help in planning the best times to take your medicine, check with your doctor, nurse, or pharmacist.

If you do miss a dose of this medicine, take it as soon as possible. This will help to keep a constant amount of medicine in the blood. However, if it is almost time for your next dose, skip the missed dose and go back to your regular dosing schedule. Do not double doses.

How to store this medicine:

- **Keep out of the reach of children.**

- Store away from heat and direct light.

- Do not store in the bathroom, near the kitchen sink, or in other damp places. Heat or moisture may cause the medicine to break down.

- Do not keep outdated medicine or medicine no longer needed. Be sure that any discarded medicine is out of the reach of children.

Precautions While Using This Medicine

If your symptoms do not improve within 2 to 3 weeks, or if they become worse, check with your doctor.

Do not take aminosalicylates within 6 hours of the time you take rifampin since this may keep rifampin from working as well.

For patients taking aminosalicylate calcium:

- Do not take aminosalicylate calcium within 1 to 3 hours of the time you take tetracyclines by mouth since this may keep tetracyclines from working as well.

This medicine may cause your eyes to become more sensitive to light than they are normally. Wearing sunglasses and avoiding too much exposure to bright light may help lessen the discomfort.

This medicine may also cause some people to become drowsy or less alert than they are normally. **Make sure you know how you react to this medicine before you drive, use machines, or do other jobs that require you to be alert.** If these reactions are especially bothersome, check with your doctor.

Diabetics—This medicine may cause false test results with some urine sugar tests. Check with your doctor before changing your diet or the dosage of your diabetes medicine.

Side Effects of This Medicine

Along with its needed effects, a medicine may cause some unwanted effects. Although not all of these side effects may occur, if they do occur they may need medical attention.

Check with your doctor immediately if any of the following side effects occur:

More common

    Chills
    Lower back pain
    Pain or burning while urinating
    Skin rash or itching
    Sore throat and fever
    Unusual tiredness or weakness

Less common

    Blood in urine
    Headache
    Increased sensitivity of eyes to light
    Yellow eyes or skin

Check with your doctor as soon as possible if any of the following side effects occur:

Less common

    Changes in menstrual periods
    Decreased sexual ability in males
    Dry, puffy skin
    Increased weight gain
    Swelling of front part of neck

Also, check with your doctor as soon as possible if you are taking aminosalicylate calcium and the following signs of too much calcium in the body appear:

    Confusion
    Constipation
    Drowsiness
    Greatly increased frequency of urination or amount of urine
    Increased thirst
    Loss of appetite
    Mental depression
    Nausea or vomiting

Other side effects may occur that usually do not require medical attention. These side effects may go away during treatment as your body adjusts to the medicine. However, check with your doctor if either of the following side effects continues or is bothersome:

More common

    Diarrhea
    Stomach pain

This medicine may cause the urine to turn red when it comes into contact with certain chlorine bleaches (such as those used to clean toilet bowls). Red urine may also be caused by blood in your urine, which is a side effect that needs medical attention. If you have questions about this, check with your doctor.

Other side effects not listed above may also occur in some patients. If you notice any other effects, check with your doctor.

December 1987

AMIODARONE (Systemic)

A commonly used brand name is Cordarone.

To the Reader: If you do not recognize the names of medical conditions or medicines referred to in this information, check with your doctor, nurse, or pharmacist. Definitions for selected medical terms may be found in the Glossary. Brand names for the generic drug names listed can be found in the Index. In addition, selected brand names commonly associated with the generic name have been included in the text to help you recognize medicine you may be taking. The fact that a brand name product is not mentioned does not mean the information does not apply. It is a good idea for you to learn both the generic and brand names of your medicines and to write them down for future use.

Amiodarone (am-ee-OH-da-rone) belongs to the group of medicines known as antiarrhythmics. It is taken by mouth to convert irregular heartbeats to a normal rhythm.

Amiodarone produces its helpful effects by slowing nerve impulses in the heart and acting directly on the heart tissues to make them less responsive.

This medicine is available only with your doctor's prescription.

Remember:

• **This medicine has been prescribed for your current medical problem only.** It must not be given to other people or used for other problems unless you are directed to do so by your doctor.

• **Keep all medicines out of the reach of children.**

• In order for this medicine to work, it must be used as directed.

• **It is very important that you read and understand the following information.** If any of the information causes you special concern, do not decide against using this medicine without first checking with your doctor.

• Before you begin using any new medicine (prescription or nonprescription) or if you develop any new medical problem while you are using this medicine, check with your doctor, nurse, or pharmacist.

• **If you have any questions** about the following information or if you want more information about this medicine or your medical problem, **ask your doctor, nurse, or pharmacist.**

Before Using This Medicine

In order to decide on the best treatment for your medical problem, your doctor should be told

—if you have ever had any unusual or allergic reaction to amiodarone.

—if you are on a low-salt, low-sugar, or any other special diet, or if you are allergic to any substance, such as foods, sulfites or other preservatives, or dyes. Most medicines contain more than their active ingredient. Your doctor, nurse, or pharmacist can help you avoid products that may cause a problem.

—if you are **pregnant** or if you may become pregnant. Studies have not been done in humans. However, studies in rats at doses many times the human dose and in some mice at doses of only one-half the human dose have shown that amiodarone causes harm to the fetus. These effects did not occur in rabbits. In addition, there may be a possibility that amiodarone could cause slow heartbeat, thyroid problems, or goiter in the newborn.

—if you are **breast-feeding**. Although amiodarone passes into breast milk, it has not been shown to cause problems in nursing babies. However, amiodarone has been shown to cause growth problems in rats. It may be necessary for you to stop breast-feeding during treatment. Be sure you have discussed the risks and benefits of the medicine with your doctor.

—if you have any of the following medical problems:
   Liver disease
   Thyroid problems

—if you are now taking/using **any** prescription or non-prescription (OTC) medicine, especially:
   Anticoagulants (blood thinners)
   Other heart medicine
   Phenytoin (e.g., Dilantin)

Proper Use of This Medicine

Take amiodarone exactly as directed by your doctor even though you may feel well. Do not take more medicine than ordered and do not miss any doses.

If you do miss a dose of this medicine, do not take the missed dose at all and do not double the next one. Instead, go back to your regular dosing schedule. If you miss two or more doses in a row, check with your doctor.

How to store this medicine:

• **Keep out of the reach of children.**

• Store away from heat and direct light.

• Do not store in the bathroom, near the kitchen sink, or in other damp places. Heat or moisture may cause the medicine to break down.

• Do not keep outdated medicine or medicine no longer needed. Be sure that any discarded medicine is out of the reach of children.

Precautions While Using This Medicine

It is important that your doctor check your progress at regular visits to make sure the medicine is working properly. This will allow for changes to be made in the amount of medicine you are taking, if necessary.

Your doctor may want you to carry a medical identification card or bracelet stating that you are taking this medicine.

Before having any kind of surgery (including dental surgery) or emergency treatment, tell the physician or dentist in charge that you are taking this medicine.

Amiodarone increases the sensitivity of your skin to sunlight; too much exposure could cause a serious burn. Your skin may continue to be sensitive to sunlight for several months after treatment with this medicine is stopped. A burn can occur even through window glass or thin cotton clothing. If you must go out in the sunlight, **cover your skin and wear a wide-brimmed hat. A special sun-blocking cream should also be used**; it must contain zinc or titanium oxide because other sunscreens will not work. **In case of a severe burn, check with your doctor.**

After you have taken this medicine for a long time, it may cause a blue-gray color to appear on your skin, especially in areas exposed to the sun, such as your face, neck, and arms. This color will usually fade after treatment with amiodarone has ended, although it may take several months. However, check with your doctor if this effect occurs.

Side Effects of This Medicine

Along with its needed effects, a medicine may cause some unwanted effects. Although not all of these side effects may occur, if they do occur they may need medical attention. Also, some side effects may not appear until several weeks or months, or even years, after you start taking amiodarone.

Check with your doctor immediately if any of the following side effects occur:

More common
    Cough
    Painful breathing
    Shortness of breath

Check with your doctor as soon as possible if any of the following side effects occur:

More common
    Difficulty in walking
    Fever (slight)
    Numbness or tingling in fingers or toes
    Sensitivity of skin to sunlight
    Trembling or shaking of hands
    Unusual and uncontrolled movements of the body
    Weakness of arms or legs

Less common
    Blue-gray coloring of skin on face, neck, and arms
    Blurred vision or blue-green halos seen around objects
    Coldness
    Dry eyes
    Dry, puffy skin
    Fast or irregular heartbeat
    Nervousness
    Pain and swelling in scrotum

    Sensitivity of eyes to light
    Sensitivity to heat
    Sleeplessness
    Slow heartbeat
    Sweating
    Swelling of feet or lower legs
    Tiredness
    Weight gain or loss

Rare
    Skin rash
    Yellow eyes and skin

Other side effects may occur that usually do not require medical attention. These side effects may go away during treatment as your body adjusts to the medicine. However, check with your doctor if any of the following side effects continue or are bothersome:

More common
    Constipation
    Headache
    Loss of appetite
    Nausea and vomiting

Less common
    Bitter or metallic taste
    Decreased sexual ability in males
    Decrease in sexual interest
    Dizziness
    Flushing of face

After you stop using this medicine, your body may need time to adjust. The length of time this takes depends on the amount of medicine you were using and how long you used it. During this period of time check with your doctor if you notice any of the following side effects:

    Cough
    Fever (slight)
    Painful breathing
    Shortness of breath

For elderly patients: Difficulty in walking, and numbness, tingling, trembling, or weakness in hands or feet, are more likely to occur in the elderly, who may be more sensitive to the effects of amiodarone.

Other side effects not listed above may also occur in some patients. If you notice any other effects, check with your doctor.

December 1987

AMMONIATED MERCURY (Topical)

To the Reader: If you do not recognize the names of medical conditions or medicines referred to in this information, check with your doctor, nurse, or pharmacist. Definitions for selected medical terms may be found in the Glossary. Brand names for the generic drug names listed can be found in the Index. In addition, selected brand names commonly associated with the generic name have been included in the text to help you recognize medicine you may be taking. The fact that a brand name product is not mentioned does not mean the information does not apply. It is a good idea for you to learn both the generic and brand names of your medicines and to write them down for future use.

Ammoniated mercury (a-MOE-nee-ay-ted MER-kyoo-ree) is applied to the skin to treat psoriasis, minor skin infections, and other skin disorders.

Some strengths of these preparations are available only with your doctor's prescription. Others are available without a prescription; however, your doctor may have special instructions on the proper use of this medicine for your medical condition.

Remember:

• **This medicine has been prescribed for your current medical problem only.** It must not be given to other people or used for other problems unless you are directed to do so by your doctor.

• **Keep all medicines out of the reach of children.**

• In order for this medicine to work, it must be used as directed. **If you are using this medicine without a prescription, it is very important to follow the directions on the label.**

• **It is also very important that you read and understand the following information.** If any of the information causes you special concern, check with your doctor or pharmacist.

• Before you begin using any new medicine (prescription or nonprescription) or if you develop any new medical problem while you are using this medicine, check with your doctor, nurse, or pharmacist.

• **If you have any questions** about the following information or if you want more information about this medicine or your medical problem, **ask your doctor, nurse, or pharmacist.**

Before Using This Medicine

Before you use ammoniated mercury, check with your doctor or pharmacist:

—if you have ever had any unusual or allergic reaction to ammoniated mercury.

—if you are allergic to any substance, such as certain preservatives or dyes. Most medicines contain more than their active ingredient. Your doctor or pharmacist can help you avoid products that may cause a problem.

—if you are **pregnant** or if you may become pregnant. Ammoniated mercury may be absorbed through the skin; however, it has not been shown to cause birth defects or other problems in humans.

—if you are **breast-feeding**, since this medicine may be absorbed through the skin. However, ammoniated mercury has not been shown to cause problems in nursing babies.

—if you have any of the following medical problems:
　Deep or open wounds
　Serious burns

—if you are taking **any** other prescription or nonprescription (OTC) medicine.

Proper Use of This Medicine

It is very important that you use this medicine only as directed. Do not use more of it and do not use it more often than recommended on the label, unless otherwise directed by your doctor. To do so may increase the chance of absorption through the skin and the risk of mercury poisoning.

Do not use this medicine on deep or open wounds or serious burns. To do so may cause mercury poisoning.

Keep this medicine away from the eyes.

Apply enough ointment to cover the affected area, and rub in gently.

If you miss a dose of this medicine, apply it as soon as possible. However, if it is almost time for your next dose, skip the missed dose and go back to your regular dosing schedule.

How to store this medicine:

• **Keep out of the reach of children.**

• Store away from heat and direct light.

• Keep the medicine from freezing.

• Do not keep outdated medicine or medicine no longer needed. Be sure that any discarded medicine is out of the reach of children.

Precautions While Using This Medicine

Do not use any topical iodine-containing preparations (for example, iodine solution, iodine tincture, or povidone-iodine) **on the same affected area as this medicine.** To do so may increase the possibility of side effects. If you have any questions about this, check with your doctor or pharmacist.

Do not use any sulfur-containing preparations on the same affected area as this medicine. To do so may cause a foul odor, may irritate the skin, and may stain the skin black. If you have any questions about this, check with your doctor or pharmacist.

Side Effects of This Medicine

Along with its needed effects, a medicine may cause some unwanted effects. Although not all of these side effects may occur, if they do occur they may need medical attention.

Check with your doctor as soon as possible if any of the following side effects occur:

> Skin infection or irritation not present before using this medicine

> *Signs of mercury poisoning*
>> Cloudy urine
>> Dizziness
>> Headache (continuing or severe)
>> Irritation, soreness, or swelling of gums
>> Nausea
>> Skin rash or unusual redness of skin

For elderly patients: Many medicines have not been tested in older people. Therefore, it is not known whether the medicine acts the same way it does in younger adults.

Check with your doctor or pharmacist if you notice any unusual effects while using this medicine or if you think it is not working as it should.

Other side effects not listed above may also occur in some patients. If you notice any other effects, check with your doctor or pharmacist.

December 1987

AMPHETAMINES (Systemic)

This information applies to the following medicines:

Amphetamine (am-FET-a-meen)
Dextroamphetamine (dex-troe-am-FET-a-meen)
Methamphetamine (meth-am-FET-a-meen)

Some commonly used brand names are:	Generic names:
	Amphetamine†
Dexedrine Ferndex Oxydess II Spancap No. 1	Dextroamphetamine†
Desoxyn	Methamphetamine†

†Generic name product may also be available in the U.S.

To the Reader: If you do not recognize the names of medical conditions or medicines referred to in this information, check with your doctor, nurse, or pharmacist. Definitions for selected medical terms may be found in the Glossary. Brand names for the generic drug names listed can be found in the Index. In addition, selected brand names commonly associated with the generic name have been included in the text to help you recognize medicine you may be taking. The fact that a brand name product is not mentioned does not mean the information does not apply. It is a good idea for you to learn both the generic and brand names of your medicines and to write them down for future use.

Amphetamines (am-FET-a-meens) belong to the group of medicines called central nervous system (CNS) stimulants. They are taken by mouth to treat children with attention deficit disorder (ADD). Amphetamines increase attention and decrease restlessness in children who are overactive, unable to concentrate for very long or are easily distracted, and have unstable emotions. These medicines are used as part of a total treatment program that also includes social, educational, and psychological treatment.

One of these medicines, dextroamphetamine, is also used in the treatment of narcolepsy (uncontrollable desire for sleep or sudden attacks of deep sleep).

Amphetamines should not be used for weight loss or weight control. When used for these purposes, they may be dangerous to your health.

These medicines are available only with a doctor's prescription. Prescriptions cannot be refilled. A new prescription must be obtained from your doctor each time you or your child needs this medicine.

Remember:

• **This medicine has been prescribed for your current medical problem only.** It must not be given to other people or used for other problems unless you are directed to do so by your doctor.

• **Keep all medicines out of the reach of children.**

• In order for this medicine to work, it must be used as directed.

• **It is very important that you read and understand the following information.** If any of the information causes you special concern, do not decide against using this medicine without first checking with your doctor.

• Before you begin using any new medicine (prescription or nonprescription) or if you develop any new medical problem while you are using this medicine, check with your doctor, nurse, or pharmacist.

• **If you have any questions** about the following information or if you want more information about this medicine or your medical problem, **ask your doctor, nurse, or pharmacist**.

Before Using This Medicine

In order to decide on the best treatment for your medical problem, your doctor should be told:

—if you have ever had any unusual or allergic reaction to amphetamine, dextroamphetamine, ephedrine, epinephrine, isoproterenol, metaproterenol, methamphetamine, norepinephrine, phenylephrine, phenylpropanolamine, pseudoephedrine, or terbutaline.

—if you are on a low-salt, low-sugar, or any other special diet, or if you are allergic to any substance, such as foods, sulfites or other preservatives, or dyes. Most medicines contain more than their active ingredient, and many liquid medicines contain alcohol. Your doctor, nurse, or pharmacist can help you avoid products that may cause a problem.

—if you are **pregnant** or if you may become pregnant. Studies have not been done in humans. However, animal studies have shown that amphetamines may increase the chance of birth defects if taken during the early months of pregnancy.

In addition, overuse of amphetamines during pregnancy may increase the chances of a premature delivery and of having a baby with a low birth weight. Also, the baby may become dependent on amphetamines and experience withdrawal effects such as agitation and drowsiness.

—if you are **breast-feeding**. Amphetamines pass into breast milk. However, this medicine has not been shown to cause problems in nursing babies.

—if you have any of the following medical problems:
   Anxiety or tension (severe)
   Glaucoma
   Heart or blood vessel disease
   High blood pressure
   Mental illness (severe), especially in children
   Overactive thyroid
   Tourette's disorder (history of)

—if you are now taking **any** other prescription or nonprescription (OTC) medicine, especially:
   Beta-blockers (acebutolol, atenolol, labetalol, levobunolol, metoprolol, nadolol, oxprenolol, pindolol, propranolol, sotalol, timolol)
   Digitalis glycosides (heart medicine)
   Thyroid hormones

—if you are now taking or have taken within the past 2 weeks monoamine oxidase (MAO) inhibitors such as:
   Furazolidone (e.g., Furoxone)
   Isocarboxazid (e.g., Marplan)
   Pargyline (e.g., Eutonyl)
   Phenelzine (e.g., Nardil)
   Procarbazine (e.g., Matulane)
   Tranylcypromine (e.g., Parnate)

Proper Use of This Medicine

If you are taking the short-acting form of this medicine:
- Take the last dose for each day at least 6 hours before bedtime to help prevent trouble in sleeping.

If you are taking the long-acting form of this medicine:
- Take the daily dose about 10 to 14 hours before bedtime to help prevent trouble in sleeping.

- These capsules or tablets are to be swallowed whole. Do not break, crush, or chew them before swallowing.

Take this medicine only as directed by your doctor. Do not take more or less of it, do not take it more often, and do not take it for a longer period of time than your doctor ordered. If too much is taken, it may become habit-forming (causing mental or physical dependence).

If you think this medicine is not working as well after you have taken it for several weeks, **do not increase the dose.** Instead, check with your doctor.

If you miss a dose of this medicine and your dosing schedule is:

One dose a day—Take the missed dose as soon as possible, but not later than stated above, to prevent trouble in sleeping. However, if you do not remember the missed dose until the next day, skip it and go back to your regular dosing schedule. Do not double doses.

Two or three doses a day—If you remember within an hour or so of the missed dose, take the dose right away. However, if you do not remember until later, skip it and go back to your regular dosing schedule. Do not double doses.

How to store this medicine:
- **Keep out of the reach of children.**
- Store away from heat and direct light.
- Do not store the capsule or tablet form of this medicine in the bathroom, near the kitchen sink, or in other damp places. Heat or moisture may cause the medicine to break down.
- Keep the liquid form of this medicine from freezing.
- Do not keep outdated medicine or medicine no longer needed. Be sure that any discarded medicine is out of the reach of children.

Precautions While Using This Medicine

Your doctor should check your progress at regular visits to make sure that this medicine does not cause unwanted effects.

If you will be taking this medicine in large doses for a long period of time, **do not stop taking it without first checking with your doctor.** Your doctor may want you to reduce gradually the amount you are taking before stopping completely.

Amphetamines may cause dryness of the mouth. For temporary relief, use sugarless candy or gum, melt bits of ice in your mouth, or use a saliva substitute. However, if dry mouth continues for more than 2 weeks, check with your physician or dentist. Continuing dryness of the mouth may increase the chance of dental disease, including tooth decay, gum disease, and fungal infections.

This medicine may cause some people to feel a false sense of well-being or to become dizzy, lightheaded, or less alert than they are normally. **Make sure you know how you react to this medicine before you drive, use machines, or do other jobs that require you to be alert.**

If you have been using this medicine for a long time and you think you may have become mentally or physically dependent on it, check with your doctor. Some signs of dependence on amphetamines are:

—a strong desire or need to continue taking the medicine.

—a need to increase the dose to receive the effects of the medicine.

—withdrawal effects (for example, mental depression, nausea or vomiting, stomach cramps or pain, trembling, unusual tiredness or weakness) occurring after the medicine is stopped.

Side Effects of This Medicine

Along with its needed effects, a medicine may cause some unwanted effects. Although not all of these side effects may occur, if they do occur they may need medical attention.

Check with your doctor as soon as possible if any of the following side effects occur:

More common
  Irregular heartbeat

Rare
  Chest pain
  Skin rash or hives
  Uncontrolled movements of head, neck, arms, and legs

With long-term use or high doses
  Mood or mental changes

Other side effects may occur that usually do not require medical attention. These side effects may go away during treatment as your body adjusts to the medicine. However, check with your doctor if any of the following side effects continue or are bothersome:

More common
  False sense of well-being
  Irritability
  Nervousness
  Restlessness
  Trouble in sleeping

Note: After these stimulant effects have worn off, drowsiness, trembling, unusual tiredness or weakness, or mental depression may occur.

Less common

 Blurred vision
 Changes in sexual desire or decreased sexual ability
 Constipation
 Diarrhea
 Dizziness or lightheadedness
 Dryness of mouth or unpleasant taste
 Fast or pounding heartbeat
 Headache
 Increased sweating
 Loss of appetite
 Nausea or vomiting
 Stomach cramps or pain
 Weight loss

After you stop using this medicine, your body may need time to adjust. The length of time this takes depends on the amount of medicine you were using and how long you used it. During this period of time check with your doctor if you notice any of the following side effects:

 Mental depression
 Nausea or vomiting

 Stomach cramps or pain
 Trembling
 Unusual tiredness or weakness

For children: When amphetamines are used for long periods of time in children, they may cause unwanted effects on behavior and growth. Before these medicines are given to a child for a long time, you should discuss their use with your doctor.

For elderly patients: Many medicines have not been tested in older people. Therefore, it is not known whether the medicine acts the same way it does in younger adults. Check with your doctor or pharmacist if you notice any unusual effects while taking this medicine or if you think it is not working as it should.

Other side effects not listed above may also occur in some patients. If you notice any other effects check with your doctor.

———————————

December 1987

———————————————————————————————

AMPHOTERICIN B (Systemic)

A commonly used brand name is Fungizone.

To the Reader: If you do not recognize the names of medical conditions or medicines referred to in this information, check with your doctor, nurse, or pharmacist. Definitions for selected medical terms may be found in the Glossary. Brand names for the generic drug names listed can be found in the Index. In addition, selected brand names commonly associated with the generic name have been included in the text to help you recognize medicine you may be taking. The fact that a brand name product is not mentioned does not mean the information does not apply. It is a good idea for you to learn both the generic and brand names of your medicines and to write them down for future use.

Amphotericin (am-foe-TER-i-sin) B belongs to the family of medicines called antifungals. It is given by injection to help the body overcome serious fungal infections. It may also be used for other problems as determined by your doctor.

Amphotericin B is available only with your doctor's prescription.

Remember:

• **It is very important that you read and understand the following information.** If any of the information causes you special concern, do not decide against using this medicine without first checking with your doctor.

• Before you begin using any new medicine (prescription or nonprescription) or if you develop any new medical problem while you are using this medicine, check with your doctor, nurse, or pharmacist.

• **If you have any questions** about the following information or if you want more information about this medicine or your medical problem, **ask your doctor, nurse, or pharmacist**.

Before Using This Medicine

In order to decide on the best treatment for your medical problem, your doctor should be told:

—if you have ever had any unusual or allergic reaction to amphotericin B. You should not receive this medicine if you are allergic to it unless your doctor decides that you have a life-threatening infection and amphotericin B is the only medicine that will work.

—if you are on a low-salt, low-sugar, or any other special diet, or if you are allergic to any substance, such as foods or sulfites or other preservatives. Most medicines contain more than their active ingredient. Your doctor, nurse, or pharmacist can help you avoid products that may cause a problem.

—if you are **pregnant** or if you may become pregnant. However, amphotericin B has not been shown to cause birth defects or other problems in humans.

—if you are **breast-feeding**. However, amphotericin B has not been shown to cause problems in nursing babies.

—if you have kidney disease.

—if you are taking **any** other prescription or nonprescription (OTC) medicine, especially:

> Adrenocorticoids (cortisone-like medicine)
> Aminoglycosides by injection or topical application (amikacin, gentamicin, kanamycin, neomycin, netilmicin, streptomycin, tobramycin)
> Antineoplastics (cancer medicine)
> Antithyroid agents (medicine for overactive thyroid)
> Azathioprine (e.g., Imuran)
> Capreomycin (e.g., Capastat)
> Captopril (e.g., Capoten)
> Carmustine (e.g., BiCNU)
> Chlorambucil (e.g., Leukeran)
> Chloramphenicol (e.g., Chloromycetin)
> Cisplatin (e.g., Platinol)
> Colchicine
> Corticotropin (ACTH)
> Cyclophosphamide (e.g., Cytoxan)
> Cyclosporine (e.g., Sandimmune)
> Digitalis glycosides (heart medicine)
> Flucytosine (e.g., Ancobon)
> Gold salts
> Interferon (e.g., Intron A, Roferon-A)
> Lithium (e.g., Lithane)
> Medicine for inflammation or pain (diclofenac, diflunisal, fenoprofen, flurbiprofen [oral], ibuprofen, indomethacin, ketoprofen, meclofenamate, mefenamic acid, naproxen, phenylbutazone, piroxicam, sulindac, tolmetin)
> Mercaptopurine (e.g., Purinethol)
> Methotrexate (e.g., Mexate)
> Neomycin by mouth (e.g., Mycifradin)
> Penicillamine (e.g., Cuprimine)
> Plicamycin (e.g., Mithracin)
> Rifampin (e.g., Rifadin)
> Streptozocin (e.g., Zanosar)
> Sulfonamides (sulfa medicine)
> Tetracyclines, except doxycycline and minocycline
> Vancomycin by injection (e.g., Vancocin)
> Zidovudine (e.g., Retrovir)

—if you regularly take large amounts of combination pain medicine containing acetaminophen and aspirin or other salicylates.

—if you have ever been treated with x-rays.

Precautions While Using This Medicine

Amphotericin B by injection may cause bone marrow problems. These problems may result in a greater chance of infection, slow healing, and bleeding of the gums. Therefore, you should be careful when using toothbrushes, dental floss, and toothpicks. Dental work, whenever possible, should be done before you begin receiving this medicine or delayed until your blood counts have returned to normal. Check with your dentist if you have any questions about proper oral hygiene (mouth care) during treatment.

Side Effects of This Medicine

Along with its needed effects, a medicine may cause some unwanted effects. Although not all of these side effects may occur, if they do occur they may need medical attention.

Check with your doctor or nurse immediately if any of the following side effects occur:

With intravenous injection

More common

Fever and chills
Irregular heartbeat
Muscle cramps or pain
Pain at the place of injection
Unusual tiredness or weakness

Less common or rare

Blurred or double vision
Convulsions (seizures)
Increased or decreased urination
Numbness, tingling, pain, or weakness in hands or feet
Ringing or buzzing in ears or any loss of hearing
Shortness of breath, troubled breathing, wheezing, or tightness in chest
Skin rash or itching
Sore throat and fever
Unusual bleeding or bruising

With spinal injection

Less common

Difficult urination
Numbness, tingling, pain, or weakness in hands or feet

Rare

Blurred vision or any change in vision

Other side effects may occur that usually do not require medical attention. These side effects may go away during treatment as your body adjusts to the medicine. However, check with your doctor if any of the following side effects continue or are bothersome:

With intravenous injection

More common

Diarrhea
Headache
Increased weight loss
Indigestion
Loss of appetite
Nausea or vomiting
Stomach pain

With spinal injection

Less common

Back, leg, or stomach pain
Dizziness or lightheadedness
Headache
Nausea or vomiting

Other side effects not listed above may also occur in some patients. If you notice any other effects, check with your doctor.

December 1987

AMPHOTERICIN B (Topical)

A commonly used brand name is Fungizone.

To the Reader: If you do not recognize the names of medical conditions or medicines referred to in this information, check with your doctor, nurse, or pharmacist. Definitions for selected medical terms may be found in the Glossary. Brand names for the generic drug names listed can be found in the Index. In addition, selected brand names commonly associated with the generic name have been included in the text to help you recognize medicine you may be taking. The fact that a brand name product is not mentioned does not mean the information does not apply. It is a good idea for you to learn both the generic and brand names of your medicines and to write them down for future use.

Amphotericin (am-foe-TER-i-sin) B belongs to the family of medicines called antifungals. Amphotericin B topical preparations are used on the skin and mucous membranes to help the body overcome fungal infections.

Amphotericin B is available only with your doctor's prescription.

Remember:

• **This medicine has been prescribed for your present infection only.** Another infection later on may require a different medicine. Also, even though other people may have the same symptoms as you, they may have a different kind of infection. Your medicine may not work for them and may even cause them harm. Therefore, **your medicine must not be given to other people or used for other infections** unless you are otherwise directed by your doctor.

• **Keep all medicines out of the reach of children.**

• In order for this medicine to work, it must be used as directed.

• **It is very important that you read and understand the following information.** If any of the information causes you special concern, do not decide against using this medicine without first checking with your doctor.

• Before you begin using any new medicine (prescription or nonprescription) or if you develop any new medical problem while you are using this medicine, check with your doctor, nurse, or pharmacist.

• **If you have any questions** about the following information or if you want more information about this medicine or your medical problem, **ask your doctor, nurse, or pharmacist.**

Before Using This Medicine

In order to decide on the best treatment for your medical problem, your doctor should be told:

—if you have ever had any unusual or allergic reaction to amphotericin B.

—if you are allergic to any substance, such as certain foods or preservatives or dyes. Most medicines contain more than their active ingredient. Your doctor, nurse, or pharmacist can help you avoid products that may cause a problem.

—if you are **pregnant** or if you may become pregnant. However, amphotericin B topical preparations have not been shown to cause birth defects or other problems in humans.

—if you are **breast-feeding**. However, amphotericin B topical preparations have not been shown to cause problems in nursing babies.

Proper Use of This Medicine

Apply enough amphotericin B to cover the affected areas, and rub in gently.

Do not apply an occlusive dressing or airtight covering (for example, kitchen plastic wrap) over this medicine since it may cause irritation of the skin. If you have any questions about this, check with your doctor.

To help clear up your infection completely, **it is very important that you keep using this medicine for the full time of treatment** even if your symptoms begin to clear up after a few days. Since fungal infections may be very slow to clear up, you may have to continue using this medicine every day for several months or longer. If you stop using this medicine too soon, your symptoms may return. **Do not miss any doses.**

If you do miss a dose of this medicine, apply it as soon as possible. Then go back to your regular dosing schedule.

How to store this medicine:

• **Keep out of the reach of children.**

• Store away from heat and direct light.

• Keep the medicine from freezing.

• Do not keep outdated medicine or medicine no longer needed. Be sure that any discarded medicine is out of the reach of children.

Precautions While Using This Medicine

If your skin problem does not improve within 1 to 2 weeks, or if it becomes worse, check with your doctor.

When amphotericin B is rubbed into the affected skin areas, it may stain the skin slightly, especially if it is applied to areas on or around the nails.

For patients using the cream or lotion form of this medicine:

• If the cream or lotion form of this medicine stains your clothing, the stain may be removed by hand-washing the clothing with soap and warm water.

For patients using the ointment form of this medicine:

• If this form stains your clothing, the stain may be removed with a standard cleaning fluid.

Side Effects of This Medicine

Along with its needed effects, a medicine may cause some unwanted effects. Although not all of these side effects may occur, if they do occur they may need medical attention.

Check with your doctor as soon as possible if any of the following side effects occur:

Less common

    Burning, itching, redness, or other sign of irritation not present before using this medicine

Rare

    Skin rash

Other side effects may occur that usually do not require medical attention. These side effects may go away during treatment as your body adjusts to the medicine.

However, check with your doctor if the following side effect continues or is bothersome:

Less common—for cream dosage form

    Dryness of skin

Other side effects not listed above may also occur in some patients. If you notice any other effects, check with your doctor.

_____

December 1987

AMYL NITRITE (Systemic)

To the Reader: If you do not recognize the names of medical conditions or medicines referred to in this information, check with your doctor, nurse, or pharmacist. Definitions for selected medical terms may be found in the Glossary. Brand names for the generic drug names listed can be found in the Index. In addition, selected brand names commonly associated with the generic name have been included in the text to help you recognize medicine you may be taking. The fact that a brand name product is not mentioned does not mean the information does not apply. It is a good idea for you to learn both the generic and brand names of your medicines and to write them down for future use.

Amyl nitrite (AM-il NYE-trite) is related to the nitrate medicines and is used by inhalation to relieve the pain of angina attacks. It works by relaxing blood vessels and increasing the supply of blood and oxygen to the heart while reducing its work load.

Amyl nitrite may also be used for other conditions as determined by your doctor.

This medicine comes in a glass capsule covered by a protective cloth. The cloth covering allows you to crush the glass capsule between your fingers without cutting yourself.

On the street, this medicine and others like it are sometimes called "poppers." They have been used by some people to cause a "high" or to improve sex. Use in this way is not recommended. Amyl nitrite can cause serious harmful effects if too much is inhaled.

Amyl nitrite is available only with your doctor's prescription.

Remember:

• **This medicine has been prescribed for your current medical problem only.** It must not be given to other people or used for other problems unless you are directed to do so by your doctor.

• **Keep all medicines out of the reach of children.**

• In order for this medicine to work, it must be used as directed.

• **It is very important that you read and understand the following information.** If any of the information causes you special concern, do not decide against using this medicine without first checking with your doctor.

• Before you begin using any new medicine (prescription or nonprescription) or if you develop any new medical problem while you are using this medicine, check with your doctor, nurse, or pharmacist.

• **If you have any questions** about the following information or if you want more information about this medicine or your medical problem, **ask your doctor, nurse, or pharmacist.**

Before Using This Medicine

In order to decide on the best treatment for your medical problem, your doctor should be told:

—if you have ever had any unusual or allergic reaction to amyl nitrite or nitrates.

—if you are **pregnant** or if you may become pregnant while using this medicine. Studies have not been done in either humans or animals.

—if you are **breast-feeding**. It is not known whether amyl nitrite passes into breast milk. This medicine has not been shown to cause problems in nursing babies.

—if you have any of the following medical problems:
Anemia (severe)
Glaucoma
Overactive thyroid

—if you have recently had a stroke, heart attack, or head injury.

—if you are taking/using **any** other prescription or nonprescription (OTC) medicine, especially:
Amantadine (e.g., Symmetrel)
Antidepressants (medicine for depression)
Antihypertensives (high blood pressure medicine)
Beta-blockers (acebutolol, atenolol, esmolol, labetalol, metoprolol, nadolol, oxprenolol, pindolol, propranolol, sotalol, timolol)
Bromocriptine (e.g., Parlodel)
Captopril (e.g., Capoten)
Chlorprothixene (e.g., Taractan)
Diltiazem (e.g., Cardizem)
Diuretics (water pills)
Enalapril (e.g., Vasotec)
Haloperidol (e.g., Haldol)
Hydralazine (e.g., Apresoline)
Levodopa (e.g., Dopar)
Loxapine (e.g., Loxitane)
Molindone (e.g., Moban)
Narcotic pain medicine
Nifedipine (e.g., Procardia)
Nitrates (medicine for angina)
Phenothiazines (acetophenazine, chlorpromazine, fluphenazine, mesoridazine, perphenazine, prochlorperazine, promazine, promethazine, thioridazine, trifluoperazine, triflupromazine, trimeprazine)
Pimozide (e.g., Orap)
Prazosin (e.g., Minipress)
Procainamide (e.g., Pronestyl)
Quinidine (e.g., Quinidex)
Thiothixene (e.g., Navane)
Verapamil (e.g., Calan)

—if you are using either of the following medicines in the eye:
Levobunolol (e.g., Betagan)
Timolol (e.g., Timoptic)

Proper Use of This Medicine

How to use amyl nitrite:

• **When you begin to feel an attack of angina starting (chest pains or a tightness or squeezing in the chest), sit down. Then crush the cloth-covered glass capsule containing amyl nitrite between your finger and thumb. Pass it back and forth close to your nose and inhale the vapor several (1 to 6) times.** Since you may become dizzy, lightheaded, or faint soon after using amyl nitrite, it is best to sit or lie down rather than stand while the medicine is working. If you become dizzy or faint while sitting, take several deep breaths and either bend forward with your head between your knees or lie down with your feet elevated.

• Remain calm and you should feel better in a few minutes.

• **This medicine usually gives relief in 1 to 5 minutes.** However, if the pain is not relieved, crush and inhale from another capsule. **If you still have the chest pains after a total of 2 doses in a 10-minute period, contact your doctor or go to a hospital emergency room without delay.**

Use this medicine exactly as directed by your doctor, and do not use more than your doctor ordered. Using too much amyl nitrite may cause a dangerous overdose. If the medicine does not seem to be working as well after you have used it for a while, check with your doctor. **Do not increase the dose on your own.**

How to store this medicine:

• **Keep out of the reach of children.**

• Store away from heat and direct light.

• Do not store in the bathroom or in the kitchen. Heat may cause the medicine to break down.

• Do not keep outdated medicine or medicine no longer needed. Be sure that any discarded medicine is out of the reach of children.

Precautions While Using This Medicine

Amyl nitrite is extremely flammable. Keep it away from heat or any open flame, especially when crushing the capsule. Amyl nitrite can catch fire very easily and cause serious burns.

Dizziness or lightheadedness may occur, especially when you get up from a lying or sitting position. Getting up slowly may help, but if the problem continues or gets worse, check with your doctor.

Drinking alcohol may make the dizziness or lightheadedness worse and may cause a serious drop in blood pressure. Check with your doctor before drinking alcoholic beverages.

After using a dose of amyl nitrite, you may get a mild headache that lasts for a short time. This is a common side effect and is no cause for alarm. However, if this effect continues, or if the headaches are severe, check with your doctor.

Side Effects of This Medicine

Along with its needed effects, a medicine may cause some unwanted effects. Although not all of these side effects may occur, if they do occur they may need medical attention.

Check with your doctor as soon as possible if any of the following side effects occur:

Rare
   Skin rash

Signs of overdose
   Bluish-colored lips, fingernails, or palms of hands
   Dizziness (extreme) or fainting
   Feeling of extreme pressure in head
   Shortness of breath
   Unusual tiredness or weakness
   Weak and unusually fast heartbeat

Other side effects may occur that usually do not require medical attention. These side effects may go away during treatment as your body adjusts to the medicine. However, check with your doctor if any of the following side effects continue or are bothersome:

More common
   Dizziness or lightheadedness, especially when getting up from a lying or sitting position
   Fast pulse
   Flushing of face and neck
   Headache (mild)
   Nausea or vomiting
   Restlessness

For elderly patients: Dizziness or lightheadedness may be more likely to occur in the elderly, who are usually more sensitive to the effects of amyl nitrite.

Other side effects not listed above may also occur in some patients. If you notice any other effects, check with your doctor.

December 1987

ANABOLIC STEROIDS (Systemic)

This information applies to the following medicines:

Dromostanolone (droe-moe-STAN-oh-lone)
Ethylestrenol (eth-il-ESS-tre-nole)
Nandrolone (NAN-droe-lone)
Oxandrolone (ox-AN-droe-lone)
Oxymetholone (ox-i-METH-oh-lone)
Stanozolol (stan-OH-zoe-lole)

Some commonly used brand names are:	Generic names:
Drolban	Dromostanolone
Maxibolin	Ethylestrenol
Anabolin IM Anabolin LA Androlone Androlone-D Deca-Durabolin Durabolin Hybolin Decanoate Hybolin Improved Kabolin Nandrobolic Nandrobolic L.A. Neo-Durabolic	Nandrolone†
Anavar	Oxandrolone
Anadrol Anapolon*	Oxymetholone
Winstrol	Stanozolol†

*Not available in the U.S.
†Generic name product may also be available.

To the Reader: If you do not recognize the names of medical conditions or medicines referred to in this information, check with your doctor, nurse, or pharmacist. Definitions for selected medical terms may be found in the Glossary. Brand names for the generic drug names listed can be found in the Index. In addition, selected brand names commonly associated with the generic name have been included in the text to help you recognize medicine you may be taking. The fact that a brand name product is not mentioned does not mean the information does not apply. It is a good idea for you to learn both the generic and brand names of your medicines and to write them down for future use.

This medicine belongs to the group of medicines known as anabolic (an-a-BOL-ik) steroids. They are related to testosterone, a male sex hormone. Anabolic steroids help to rebuild tissues that have become weak because of serious injury or illness. A diet high in proteins and calories is necessary with anabolic steroid treatment.

Anabolic steroids are given by injection or taken by mouth for several reasons:

—to help patients gain weight after a severe illness, injury, or continuing infection. They also are used when patients fail to gain or maintain normal weight because of unexplained medical reasons.

—to treat certain types of anemia.

—to help treat weakening of bones and aid in the relief of bone pain.

—to treat certain kinds of breast cancer in some women.

—to treat hereditary angioedema, which causes swelling of the face, arms, legs, throat, windpipe, bowels, or sexual organs.

Anabolic steroids may also be used for other conditions as determined by your doctor.

Anabolic steroids may cause children to stop growing early or to develop sexually too fast. Before this medicine is given to children, you should discuss its use with your doctor.

Use of these medicines by athletes to build muscle tissue and improve performance is not recommended. There is no good medical evidence to support the belief that the use of these medicines by athletes will increase muscle strength. Also, when used for this purpose, they may be dangerous to the health because of unwanted effects such as too much fluid in the body, liver disease, and liver cancer in males and females; reduced fertility and/or swelling of breasts in males; and hoarseness or deepening of voice, unnatural hair growth, or unusual hair loss in females.

Anabolic steroids are available only with your doctor's prescription.

Remember:

• **This medicine has been prescribed for your current medical problem only.** It must not be given to other people or used for other problems unless you are directed to do so by your doctor.

• **Keep all medicines out of the reach of children.**

• In order for this medicine to work, it must be used as directed.

• If you are receiving this medicine by injection, some of the information about this medicine may not apply.

• **It is very important that you read and understand the following information.** If any of the information causes you special concern, do not decide against using this medicine without first checking with your doctor.

• Before you begin using any new medicine (prescription or nonprescription) or if you develop any new medical problem while you are using this medicine, check with your doctor, nurse, or pharmacist.

• **If you have any questions** about the following information or if you want more information about this medicine or your medical problem, **ask your doctor, nurse, or pharmacist.**

Before Using This Medicine

In order to decide on the best treatment for your medical problem, your doctor should be told:

—if you have ever had any unusual or allergic reaction to anabolic steroids or androgens (male hormones).

—if you are on a low-salt, low-sugar, or any other special diet, or if you are allergic to any substance, such as foods, sulfites or other preservatives, or dyes. Most medicines contain more than their active ingredient, and many liquid medicines contain alcohol. Your doctor, nurse, or pharmacist can help you avoid products that may cause a problem.

—if you are **pregnant** or if you intend to become pregnant while using this medicine. Anabolic steroids are not recommended during pregnancy because they may cause the development of male features in the female fetus and premature growth and development of male features in the male fetus.

—if you are **breast-feeding**. Although anabolic steroids have not been shown to cause problems in nursing babies, the chance always exists.

—if you have any of the following medical problems:
Breast cancer (in males and some females)
Diabetes mellitus (sugar diabetes)
Enlarged prostate
Heart or blood vessel disease
Kidney disease
Liver disease
Prostate cancer
Too much calcium in the blood (in females)

—if you are now taking **any** prescription or nonprescription (OTC) medicines, especially:
Adrenocorticoids (cortisone-like medicines)
Anticoagulants, oral (blood thinners you take by mouth)
Antidiabetics, oral (diabetes medicine you take by mouth)
Corticotropin (hormone that stimulates the adrenal gland)
Insulin
Sodium-containing medicines or foods
Somatrem (growth hormone)
Somatropin (growth hormone)

Proper Use of This Medicine

Take this medicine only as directed. Do not take more of it and do not take it more often than your doctor ordered. To do so may increase the chance of side effects.

In order for this medicine to work properly, it is important that you follow a diet high in proteins and calories. If you have any questions about this, check with your doctor, nurse, or pharmacist.

If you miss a dose of this medicine and your dosing schedule is one dose to be taken:
Once a day— Take the missed dose as soon as possible. However, if you do not remember it until the next day, skip the missed dose and go back to your regular dosing schedule. Do not double doses.
More than once a day—Take the missed dose as soon as possible. However, if it is almost time for your next dose, skip the missed dose and go back to your regular dosing schedule. Do not double doses.

How to store this medicine:

• **Keep out of the reach of children.**

• Store away from heat and direct light.

• Do not store the tablet form of this medicine in the bathroom, near the kitchen sink, or in other damp places. Heat or moisture may cause the medicine to break down.

• Keep the liquid form of this medicine from freezing.

• Do not keep outdated medicine or medicine no longer needed. Be sure that any discarded medicine is out of the reach of children.

Precautions While Using This Medicine

Your doctor should check your progress at regular visits to make sure that this medicine does not cause unwanted effects.

Diabetics—This medicine may affect blood sugar levels. If you notice a change in the results of your urine sugar test or if you have any questions about this, check with your doctor.

Side Effects of This Medicine

Tumors of the liver, liver cancer, or peliosis hepatis, a form of liver disease, have occurred during long-term, high-dose therapy with anabolic steroids. Although these effects are rare, they can be very serious and may cause death. Discuss these possible effects with your doctor.

When elderly male patients are treated with anabolic steroids, they may have an increased risk of enlarged prostate or cancer of the prostate. Discuss these possible effects with your doctor.

Along with its needed effects, a medicine may cause some unwanted effects. Although not all of these side effects may occur, if they do occur they may need medical attention.

Check with your doctor immediately if any of the following side effects occur:
For both females and males
Less common
Yellow eyes or skin

Rare (with long-term use)
Black, tarry, or light-colored stools
Dark-colored urine
Purple- or red-colored spots on body or inside the mouth or nose
Sore throat and/or fever
Vomiting of blood

Also, check with your doctor as soon as possible if any of the following side effects occur:
For both females and males
Less common
Bone pain
Nausea or vomiting
Sore tongue
Swelling of feet or lower legs
Unusual bleeding
Unusual weight gain

Rare (with long-term use)
Abdominal or stomach pain
Feeling of discomfort (continuing)
Headache (continuing)
Hives
Loss of appetite (continuing)
Unexplained weight loss
Unpleasant breath odor (continuing)

© 1988   The United States Pharmacopeial Convention, Inc.

For females only
  More common
    Acne or oily skin
    Enlarging clitoris
    Hoarseness or deepening of voice
    Irregular menstrual periods
    Unnatural hair growth
    Unusual hair loss

  Less common
    Mental depression
    Unusual tiredness

For young males (boys) only
  More common
    Acne
    Enlarging penis
    Increased frequency of erections
    Unnatural hair growth

  Less common
    Unexplained darkening of skin

For sexually mature males only
  More common
    Frequent or continuing erections
    Frequent urge to urinate
    Swelling of breasts or breast soreness

For elderly males only
  Less common
    Difficult or frequent urination

Other side effects may occur that usually do not require medical attention. These side effects may go away during treatment as your body adjusts to the medicine. However, check with your doctor if any of the following side effects continue or are bothersome:

For both females and males
  Less common
    Chills
    Diarrhea
    Feeling of abdominal or stomach fullness
    Muscle cramps
    Trouble in sleeping
    Unusual decrease or increase in sexual desire

For males only
  More common
    Acne

  Less common
    Decreased sexual ability

Other side effects not listed above may also occur in some patients. If you notice any other effects, check with your doctor.

_____

December 1987

ANDROGENS (Systemic)

This information applies to the following medicines:

Fluoxymesterone (floo-ox-i-MES-te-rone)
Methyltestosterone (meth-ill-tess-TOSS-te-rone)
Testosterone (tess-TOSS-te-rone)

Some commonly used brand names are:	Generic names:
Android-F Halotestin Ora-Testryl Testolin	Fluoxymesterone†
Android Metandren Metandren Linguets Oreton Methyl Testred Virilon	Methyltestosterone†
Andro Andro-Cyp Android-T Andro-LA Andronaq Andronaq-LA Andronate Andryl Delatestryl depAndro Depotest Depo-Testosterone Duratest Durathate Everone Histerone Malogen* Malogex* T-Cypionate Tesionate Testa-C Testaqua Testex Testoject Testoject-LA Testone L.A. Testrin PA	Testosterone†

*Not available in the U.S.
†Generic name product may also be available.

To the Reader: If you do not recognize the names of medical conditions or medicines referred to in this information, check with your doctor, nurse, or pharmacist. Definitions for selected medical terms may be found in the Glossary. Brand names for the generic drug names listed can be found in the Index. In addition, selected brand names commonly associated with the generic name have been included in the text to help you recognize medicine you may be taking. The fact that a brand name product is not mentioned does not mean the information does not apply. It is a good idea for you to learn both the generic and brand names of your medicines and to write them down for future use.

Androgens (AN-droe-jens) are male hormones. Some are naturally produced in the body and are necessary for the normal sexual development of males.

Androgens are given by injection or taken by mouth and are used for several reasons, such as:

—to replace the hormone when the body is unable to produce enough on its own.

—to stimulate the beginning of puberty in certain boys.

—to treat certain types of breast cancer in females.

—to relieve breast pain and fullness in females who will not be breast-feeding after the birth of a child.

In addition, some of these medicines may be used for other conditions as determined by your doctor.

There is no good medical evidence to support the belief that the use of androgens in athletes will increase muscle strength. When used for this purpose, it may be dangerous to health because of unwanted effects such as too much fluid in the body and liver disease in females and males; swelling of breasts in males; or hoarseness or deepening of voice, unnatural hair growth, or unusual hair loss in females.

Androgens are available only with your doctor's prescription.

Remember:

• **This medicine has been prescribed for your current medical problem only.** It must not be given to other people or used for other problems unless you are directed to do so by your doctor.

• **Keep all medicines out of the reach of children.**

• In order for this medicine to work, it must be used as directed.

• If you are receiving this medicine by injection, some of the information about this medicine may not apply.

• **It is very important that you read and understand the following information.** If any of the information causes you special concern, do not decide against using this medicine without first checking with your doctor.

• Before you begin using any new medicine (prescription or nonprescription) or if you develop any new medical problem while you are using this medicine, check with your doctor, nurse, or pharmacist.

• **If you have any questions** about the following information or if you want more information about this medicine or your medical problem, **ask your doctor, nurse, or pharmacist.**

Before Using This Medicine

In order to decide on the best treatment for your medical problem, your doctor should be told:

—if you have ever had any unusual or allergic reaction to androgens or anabolic steroids.

—if you are on a low-salt, low-sugar, or any other special diet, or if you are allergic to any substance, such as foods, sulfites or other preservatives, or dyes. Most medicines contain more than their active ingredient. Your doctor, nurse, or pharmacist can help you avoid products that may cause a problem.

—if you are **pregnant** or if you may become pregnant. Androgens are not recommended during pregnancy. They have been shown to cause the development of male features in female babies and premature development of male features in male babies in humans.

—if you are an adult male who plans to have children. High doses of androgens may cause infertility.

—if you are **breast-feeding**. Use is not recommended in nursing mothers, since androgens may pass into the breast milk and may cause unwanted effects in the nursing baby, such as premature (too early) sexual development in males and development of male features in female babies.

—if you have any of the following medical problems:
>   Breast cancer (in males)
>   Diabetes mellitus (sugar diabetes)
>   Edema (swelling of face, hands, feet, or lower legs)
>   Enlarged prostate
>   Heart or blood vessel disease
>   Kidney disease
>   Liver disease
>   Prostate cancer

—if you are now taking **any** other prescription or non-prescription (OTC) medicine, especially anticoagulants (blood thinners).

—if you are bedridden.

Proper Use of This Medicine

For patients taking fluoxymesterone or the capsule or regular tablet form of methyltestosterone:
• Take this medicine with food to lessen possible stomach upset, unless otherwise directed by your doctor.

For patients using the buccal tablet form of methyltestosterone:
• **This medicine should not be swallowed whole.** It is meant to be absorbed through the lining of the mouth. Place the tablet in the upper or lower pouch between your gum and the side of your cheek. Let the tablet slowly dissolve there. Do not eat, drink, chew, or smoke while the tablet is dissolving. It is important that you brush your teeth or thoroughly rinse out your mouth after the tablet has completely dissolved and you can no longer taste it. This will help prevent tooth decay and cavities from the sugar in the tablet, as well as mouth irritation or soreness.

Take this medicine only as directed. Do not take more of it and do not take it more often than your doctor ordered. To do so may increase the chance of side effects.

If you miss a dose of this medicine and your dosing schedule is one dose to be taken:

Once a day— Take the missed dose as soon as possible. However, if you do not remember it until the next day, skip the missed dose and go back to your regular dosing schedule. Do not double doses.

More than once a day—Take the missed dose as soon as possible. However, if it is almost time for your next dose, skip the missed dose and go back to your regular dosing schedule. Do not double doses.

How to store this medicine:
• **Keep out of the reach of children.**

• Store away from heat and direct light.

• Do not store in the bathroom, near the kitchen sink, or in other damp places. Heat or moisture may cause the medicine to break down.

• Keep the injection form of this medicine from freezing.

• Do not keep outdated medicine or medicine no longer needed. Be sure that any discarded medicine is out of the reach of children.

Precautions While Using This Medicine

Your doctor should check your progress at regular visits in order to make sure this medicine does not cause unwanted effects.

Diabetics—This medicine may affect blood sugar levels. If you notice a change in the results of your urine sugar test or if you have any quesions about this, check with your doctor.

Side Effects of This Medicine

Discuss these possible effects with your doctor:
• Tumors of the liver, liver cancer, or peliosis hepatis, a form of liver disease, have occurred during long-term, high-dose therapy with androgens. Although these effects are rare, they can be very serious and may cause death.

• When elderly male patients are treated with androgens, they may have an increased risk of enlarged prostate or cancer of the prostate.

• Androgens may cause children to stop growing early or to develop too fast sexually.

• When androgens are used in women, especially in high doses, male-like changes may occur, such as hoarseness or deepening of the voice, unnatural hair growth, or unusual hair loss. Most of these changes will go away if the medicine is stopped as soon as the changes are noticed. However, some changes, such as voice changes, may not go away.

Along with its needed effects, a medicine may cause some unwanted effects. Although not all of these side effects appear very often, when they do occur they may require medical attention.

Check with your doctor immediately if any of the following side effects occur:
For both females and males
> *Less common*
>> Yellow eyes or skin

> *Rare (with long-term use)*
>> Black, tarry, or light-colored stools
>> Dark-colored urine
>> Purple- or red-colored spots on body or inside the mouth or nose
>> Sore throat and/or fever
>> Vomiting of blood

Also, check with your doctor as soon as possible if any of the following side effects occur:

For both females and males
　Less common

　　　Changes in skin color
　　　Confusion
　　　Dizziness
　　　Flushing or redness of skin
　　　Headache (frequent or continuing)
　　　Mental depression
　　　Nausea or vomiting
　　　Shortness of breath
　　　Skin rash or itching
　　　Swelling of feet or lower legs
　　　Unusual bleeding
　　　Unusual tiredness

　Rare (with long-term use)

　　　Abdominal or stomach pain (continuing)
　　　Feeling of discomfort (continuing)
　　　Hives
　　　Loss of appetite (continuing)
　　　Pain, tenderness, or swelling in the upper abdominal or stomach area
　　　Unpleasant breath odor (continuing)

For females only
　More common

　　　Acne or oily skin
　　　Enlarged clitoris
　　　Hair loss
　　　Hoarseness or deepening of voice
　　　Irregular menstrual periods
　　　Unnatural hair growth

For males only
　More common

　　　Frequent or continuing erection
　　　Frequent urge to urinate
　　　Swelling of breasts or breast soreness

For elderly males only
　Less common

　　　Difficult or frequent urination
　　　Unusual increase in sexual desire

Other side effects may occur which usually do not require medical attention. These side effects may go away during treatment as your body adjusts to the medicine. However, check with your doctor if any of the following side effects continue or are bothersome:

For both females and males
　Less common

　　　Constipation
　　　Diarrhea
　　　Hives, infection, redness, pain, or other irritation at the place of injection (for patients receiving testosterone by injection)
　　　Irritation or soreness of mouth or unusual watering of mouth (for patients taking buccal tablet form of methyltestosterone)
　　　Stomach pain
　　　Trouble in sleeping
　　　Unusual decrease or increase in sexual desire

Other side effects not listed above may also occur in some patients. If you notice any other effects, check with your doctor.

December 1987

ANESTHETICS (DENTAL)

This information applies to the following medicines:

Benzocaine (BEN-zoe-kane)
Butacaine (BYOO-ta-kane)
Lidocaine (LYE-doe-kane)

Some commonly used brand names and other names are:	Generic names:
Americaine Ethyl aminobenzoate Hurricaine Orabase with Benzocaine Orajel Rid-A-Pain	Benzocaine
Butyn	Butacaine
Xylocaine Xylocaine Viscous	Lidocaine†

†Generic name product may also be available in the U.S.

To the Reader: If you do not recognize the names of medical conditions or medicines referred to in this information, check with your doctor, nurse, or pharmacist. Definitions for selected medical terms may be found in the Glossary. Brand names for the generic drug names listed can be found in the Index. In addition, selected brand names commonly associated with the generic name have been included in the text to help you recognize medicine you may be taking. The fact that a brand name product is not mentioned does not mean the information does not apply. It is a good idea for you to learn both the generic and brand names of your medicines and to write them down for future use.

Dental anesthetics (an-ess-THET-iks) are used in the mouth to relieve pain or irritation caused by many conditions. Examples include toothache, teething, and sores in the mouth. Also, some of these medicines are used to relieve pain or irritation caused by dentures or other dental appliances, including braces.

One form of lidocaine is also used to relieve pain caused by certain throat conditions.

Benzocaine (present in some of these medicines) may be absorbed into the bodies of young children and cause unwanted effects. Before benzocaine is used for children under 2 years of age, you should discuss its use with your physician or dentist.

Some of these medicines are available only with your doctor's prescription. Others are available without a prescription; however, your physician or dentist may have special instructions on the proper use and dose for your medical problem.

Remember:

• **Keep all medicines out of the reach of children.**

• In order for this medicine to work, it must be used as directed. **If you are using this medicine without a prescription, it is very important to follow the directions on the label.**

• **It is also very important that you read and understand the following information.** If any of the information causes you special concern, check with your doctor before using this medicine without a prescription.

• Before you begin using any new medicine (prescription or nonprescription) or if you develop any new medical problem while you are using this medicine, check with your doctor, nurse, or pharmacist.

• **If you have any questions** about the following information or if you want more information about this medicine or your medical problem, **ask your doctor, nurse, or pharmacist.**

Before Using This Medicine

Before you use a dental anesthetic without a prescription, check with your doctor, nurse, or pharmacist:

—if you have ever had any unusual or allergic reaction to a local anesthetic, especially one that was applied to any part of the body as a liquid, cream, ointment, or spray.

—if you are allergic to any substance, such as certain preservatives or dyes. Most medicines contain more than their active ingredient. Your doctor, nurse, or pharmacist can help you avoid products that may cause a problem.

—if you are **pregnant** or if you may become pregnant. Dental anesthetics have not been shown to cause birth defects or other problems in humans.

—if you are **breast-feeding**. Dental anesthetics have not been shown to cause problems in nursing babies.

—if you have an infection or large sores in your mouth.

—if you taking **any** other prescription or nonprescription (OTC) medicine.

Proper Use of This Medicine

For safe and effective use of this medicine:

• Follow your physician's or dentist's instructions if this medicine was prescribed.

• Follow the manufacturer's package directions if you are treating yourself.

• **Do not use more of this medicine, do not use it more often, and do not use it for a longer period of time than directed.** To do so may increase the chance of absorption into the body and the chance of side effects.

For patients using the viscous (very thick) liquid form of lidocaine:

• This medicine may cause serious side effects, especially in young children, if too much of it is swallowed. Be certain that you understand exactly how you are to use this medicine, and whether or not you are to swallow it. Also, **be very careful to measure the exact amount of medicine that you are to use.**

• If you are using this medicine for a problem in the mouth, you may apply it to the sore places with a cotton-tipped applicator. Or, you may swish the measured amount of medicine around in your mouth until you are certain that it has reached all of the sore places. **Do not swallow the medicine unless your physician or dentist has told you to do so.**

• If you are using this medicine for a problem in the throat, gargle with the measured amount of medicine as directed by your doctor. **Do not swallow the medicine unless your physician or dentist has told you to do so.**

• If you are using this medicine for a young child, be sure that you understand exactly how this medicine should be used. Follow the physician's or dentist's orders very carefully.

For patients using aerosol or spray forms of a dental anesthetic:

• Be very careful not to inhale (breathe in) the medicine, and do not spray the back of your mouth or throat with it, unless your physician or dentist orders you to do so. This helps to prevent unwanted effects.

For patients using benzocaine dental paste:

• Do not rub or try to spread the medicine with your finger while you are applying it, because the medicine will become crumbly and gritty. Use a cotton-tipped applicator to dab small amounts of the medicine onto the sore places.

This medicine should be used only for conditions being treated by your physician or dentist or for problems listed in the package directions. **Do not use it for other problems without first checking with your physician or dentist.** This medicine should not be used if certain kinds of infections are present.

If your physician or dentist has directed you to use this medicine on a regular schedule, and you miss a dose, use it as soon as possible. However, if it is almost time for your next dose, skip the missed dose and go back to your regular dosing schedule. Do not double doses.

How to store this medicine:

• **Keep out of the reach of children.**

• Store away from heat and direct light.

• Keep the medicine from freezing.

• Do not puncture, break, or burn aerosol containers, even when they are empty.

• Do not keep outdated medicine or medicine no longer needed. Be sure that any discarded medicine is out of the reach of children.

Precautions While Using This Medicine

Check with your physician or dentist:

—if your condition does not improve after you have been using this medicine regularly for a few days, or if it becomes worse.

—if you notice any redness, irritation, or sores that were not present before you started using this medicine.

If you are using this medicine in the back of the mouth, or in the throat, **do not eat or drink anything for one hour after using it.** When this medicine is applied to these areas, it may interfere with swallowing and cause choking.

Do not chew gum or food while your mouth or throat feels numb after you use this medicine. To do so may cause an injury. You may accidentally bite your tongue or the inside of your cheeks.

If you are using this medicine to relieve a toothache, remember that it should not be used for a long period of time. It is meant to relieve toothache pain temporarily, until the problem causing the toothache can be corrected. **Call your dentist as soon as possible to arrange for treatment.**

Side Effects of This Medicine

Along with its needed effects, a medicine may cause some unwanted effects. Although not all of these side effects may occur, if they do occur they may need medical attention.

Check with your physician or dentist immediately if any of the following side effects occur:
Less common or rare
Swelling of mouth or throat
Signs of too much medicine being absorbed by the body
Blurred or double vision
Convulsions (seizures)
Dizziness
Drowsiness
Increased sweating
Ringing or buzzing in the ears
Shivering or trembling
Slow or irregular heartbeat
Unusual anxiety, excitement, nervousness, or restlessness
Unusual paleness

Also, check with your physician or dentist as soon as possible if any of the following side effects occur:
Less common or rare
Burning, stinging, swelling, or tenderness not present before treatment
Skin rash, redness, itching, or hives in or around the mouth

For children or elderly patients: Side effects may be more likely to occur in children and the elderly, who are usually more sensitive to the effects of these medicines.

Other side effects not listed above may also occur in some patients. If you notice any other effects, check with your physician or dentist.

December 1987

ANESTHETICS (Ophthalmic)

This information applies to the following medicines:

Proparacaine (proe-PARE-a-kane)
Tetracaine (TET-ra-kane)

Some commonly used brand names are:	Generic names:
Ak-Taine	
Alcaine	
Kainair	
Ocu-Caine	Proparacaine
Ophthaine	
Ophthetic	
Pontocaine	Tetracaine†

†Generic name product may also be available in the U.S.

To the Reader: If you do not recognize the names of medical conditions or medicines referred to in this information, check with your doctor, nurse, or pharmacist. Definitions for selected medical terms may be found in the Glossary. Brand names for the generic drug names listed can be found in the Index. In addition, selected brand names commonly associated with the generic name have been included in the text to help you recognize medicine you may be taking. The fact that a brand name product is not mentioned does not mean the information does not apply. It is a good idea for you to learn both the generic and brand names of your medicines and to write them down for future use.

Proparacaine and tetracaine are local anesthetics that are used in the eye to cause numbness or loss of feeling. They are used before certain procedures such as measuring of eye pressure, removing foreign objects or sutures (stitches) from the eye, and performing certain eye examinations.

These medicines are to be administered only by or under the immediate supervision of your doctor.

Remember:
• If you want more information about this medicine, ask your doctor, nurse, or pharmacist.

• If any of the following information causes you special concern, do not decide against receiving this medicine without first checking with your doctor.

Before Receiving This Medicine

In order to decide on the best treatment for your medical problem, your doctor should be told:

—if you have ever had any unusual or allergic reaction after use of a local anesthetic in the eye. Such a reaction may include severe itching, pain, redness, or swelling of the eye or eyelid, or severe and continuing watering of the eyes.

—if you have ever had any unusual or allergic reaction to tetracaine or other local anesthetics, such as benzocaine, butacaine, butamben, chloroprocaine, procaine, or propoxycaine, when given by injection or applied to the skin.

—if you have ever had any unusual or allergic reaction to para-aminobenzoic acid or PABA (present in some sun screens) or to parabens (preservatives in many foods and medicines).

—if you are allergic to any other substance, such as other preservatives or dyes. Most medicines contain more than their active ingredient. Your doctor can help you avoid products that may cause a problem.

—if you are **pregnant**. Proparacaine and tetracaine have not been shown to cause birth defects or other problems in humans.

—if you are **breast-feeding**. Proparacaine and tetracaine have not been shown to cause problems in nursing babies.

—if you have any of the following medical problems:
Allergies
Heart disease
Overactive thyroid

—if you are now using **any** prescription or nonprescription (OTC) medicine.

Precautions After Receiving This Medicine

After a local anesthetic is applied to the eye, **do not rub or wipe the eye until the anesthetic has worn off or feeling in the eye returns.** To do so may cause injury or damage to the eye. The effects of these medicines usually last for about 20 minutes. However, if more than one dose is applied, the effects may last longer.

If you get one of these medicines on your fingers, it may cause a rash with dryness and cracking of the skin. If you touch your eye after this medicine has been applied, wash your hands as soon as possible.

Side Effects of This Medicine

Along with its needed effects, a medicine may cause some unwanted effects. Although not all of these side effects may occur, if they do occur they may need medical attention.

Tell your doctor immediately if any of the following side effects occur shortly after this medicine has been applied:

Signs of too much medicine being absorbed into the body—very rare
Dizziness or drowsiness
Increased sweating
Irregular heartbeat
Muscle twitching or trembling
Nausea or vomiting
Shortness of breath or troubled breathing
Unusual excitement, nervousness, or restlessness
Unusual tiredness or weakness

Other side effects may occur that usually do not require medical attention. Mild stinging or eye irritation may occur as soon as tetracaine is applied or up to several hours after proparacaine is applied. Although these side effects usually are not serious, **check with your doctor as soon as possible if any of the following side**

effects are severe and continuing, because you may be having an allergic reaction to the medicine. Also, check with your doctor if any of these effects continue or are bothersome:

Less common
   Burning, stinging, redness, or other irritation of eye

Rare
   Itching, pain, redness, or swelling of the eye or eyelid
   Watering of eyes

Other side effects not listed above may also occur in some patients. If you notice any other effects, check with your doctor.

_____

December 1987

_____

ANESTHETICS (Rectal)

This information applies to the following medicines:

Benzocaine (BEN-zoe-kane)
Dibucaine (DYE-byoo-kane)
Pramoxine (pra-MOX-een)
Tetracaine (TET-ra-kane)

Some commonly used brand names and other names are:	Generic names:
Americaine Ethyl aminobenzoate	Benzocaine
Nupercainal	Dibucaine†
Fleet Relief Proctofoam Tronolane Tronothane	Pramoxine
Pontocaine Cream	Tetracaine
Pontocaine Ointment	Tetracaine and Menthol

†Generic name product may also be available in the U.S.

To the Reader: If you do not recognize the names of medical conditions or medicines referred to in this information, check with your doctor, nurse, or pharmacist. Definitions for selected medical terms may be found in the Glossary. Brand names for the generic drug names listed can be found in the Index. In addition, selected brand names commonly associated with the generic name have been included in the text to help you recognize medicine you may be taking. The fact that a brand name product is not mentioned does not mean the information does not apply. It is a good idea for you to learn both the generic and brand names of your medicines and to write them down for future use.

Rectal anesthetics (an-ess-THET-iks) are used to relieve the pain, itching, and swelling of hemorrhoids (piles) and other rectal disorders.

These medicines are available without a prescription; however, your doctor may have special instructions on the proper use and dose for your medical problem.

Remember:
• **Keep all medicines out of the reach of children.**

• In order for this medicine to work, it must be used as directed. **If you are using this medicine without a prescription, it is very important to follow the directions on the label.**

• **It is also very important that you read and understand the following information.** If any of the information causes you special concern, check with your doctor before using this medicine without a prescription.

• Before you begin using any new medicine (prescription or nonprescription) or if you develop any new medical problem while you are using this medicine, check with your doctor, nurse, or pharmacist.

• **If you have any questions** about the following information or if you want more information about this medicine or your medical problem, **ask your doctor, nurse, or pharmacist.**

Before Using This Medicine

Before you use a rectal anesthetic, check with your doctor, nurse, or pharmacist:

—if you have ever had any unusual or allergic reaction to a local anesthetic, especially one that was applied to any part of the body as a liquid, cream, ointment, or spray.

—if you are allergic to any substance, such as certain preservatives or dyes. Most medicines contain more than their active ingredient. Your doctor, nurse, or pharmacist can help you avoid products that may cause a problem.

—if you are **pregnant** or if you may become pregnant. Rectal anesthetics have not been shown to cause birth defects or other problems in humans.

—if you are **breast-feeding**. Rectal anesthetics have not been shown to cause problems in nursing babies.

—if you have hemorrhoids that bleed, especially after bowel movements.

—if you have any of the following medical problems:
  Infection at or near place of treatment
  Large sores, broken skin, or severe injury at or near place of treatment

—if you are using **any** other prescription or nonprescription (OTC) medicine.

Proper Use of This Medicine

For safe and effective use of this medicine:

• Follow your doctor's instructions if this medicine was prescribed.

• Follow the manufacturer's package directions if you are treating yourself.

• **Do not use more of this medicine, do not use it more often, and do not use it for a longer period of time than directed.** To do so may increase the chance of absorption into the body and the chance of unwanted effects.

For patients using the rectal ointment or cream:

• This medicine usually comes with patient directions. Read them carefully before using this medicine.

• This medicine may be applied with a "finger cot" or the applicator that comes in the package.

• If you use the applicator, wash it carefully after each use.

• If you are using the product that comes in pre-filled applicators, each applicator is meant to be used only once. Throw the applicator away after using it.

For patients using pramoxine aerosol rectal foam:

• This medicine usually comes with patient directions. Read them carefully before using this medicine.

• This medicine is used with a special applicator. Do not insert any part of the aerosol container into the rectum.

• Take the applicator apart and wash it carefully after each use.

For patients using the rectal suppository:
- How to insert the suppository: If the suppository is too soft to insert because of storage in a warm place, chill the suppository in the refrigerator for 30 minutes or run cold water over it before removing the wrapper. Remove the wrapper and moisten the suppository with water. Lie down on your side and push the suppository well up into the rectum with a finger.

This medicine should be used only for conditions being treated by your doctor or for problems listed on the package label. **Do not use it for other problems without first checking with your doctor.** This medicine should not be used if certain kinds of infections are present.

If your doctor has directed you to use this medicine on a regular schedule and you miss a dose, use it as soon as possible. However, if it is almost time for your next dose, skip the missed dose and go back to your regular dosing schedule.

How to store this medicine:
- **Keep out of the reach of children.**
- Store away from heat and direct light.
- Keep the medicine from freezing.
- Do not puncture, break, or burn the pramoxine aerosol foam container, even after it is empty.
- Do not keep outdated medicine or medicine no longer needed. Be sure that any discarded medicine is out of the reach of children.

Precautions While Using This Medicine

Check with your doctor:
　　—if your condition does not improve after you have been using this medicine regularly for a few days, or if it becomes worse.

　　—if you notice any rash, redness, or irritation that was not present before you started using this medicine.

Side Effects of This Medicine

Along with its needed effects, a medicine may cause some unwanted effects. Although not all of these side effects may occur, if they do occur they may need medical attention.

Check with your doctor immediately if any of the following side effects occur:
Signs of too much medicine being absorbed by the body
　　Blurred or double vision
　　Convulsions (seizures)
　　Dizziness
　　Drowsiness
　　Increased sweating
　　Ringing or buzzing in ears
　　Shivering or trembling
　　Slow or irregular heartbeat
　　Unusual anxiety, excitement, nervousness, or restlessness
　　Unusual paleness

Also, check with your doctor as soon as possible if any of the following side effects occur:
Less common
　　Burning, stinging, swelling, or tenderness not present before treatment
　　Skin rash, redness, itching, or hives at or near place of application

For children or elderly patients: Some of the side effects listed above may be more likely to occur in the elderly or in children, who are usually more sensitive to the effects of rectal anesthetics.

Other side effects not listed above may also occur in some patients. If you notice any other effects, check with your doctor.

_____

December 1987

ANESTHETICS (Topical)

This information applies to the following medicines:

Benzocaine (BEN-zoe-kane)
Butamben (byoo-TAM-ben)
Dibucaine (DYE-byoo-kane)
Lidocaine (LYE-doe-kane)
Pramoxine (pra-MOX-een)
Tetracaine (TET-ra-kane)

Some commonly used brand names and other names are:	Generic names:
aeroCAINE§	
aeroTHERM§	
Alsinol*§	
Americaine§	
Anbesol§	
Anivy*§	
Bandiseptic*§	
Benzocal	
BiCozene§	
Burntame§	
Chiggerex§	
Chiggertox§	
Dermacoat§	
Derma Medicone§	
Dermoplast§	
Ethyl aminobenzoate	Benzocaine†
First Aid Cream*§	
Foille§	
Histocaine*§	
Ivy-Dry Cream§	
Kreo-Benz§	
Lanacane§	
Medicone Dressing§	
Myoderm*§	
Noivy*§	
Rhulicaine§	
San Cura§	
Solarcaine§	
Tega Caine§	
Unguentine Spray§	

Butesin Picrate Butyl aminobenzoate	Butamben

Nupercainal	Dibucaine†

Bactine§ Lignocaine Medi-Quik§ Unguentine Plus§ Xylocaine	Lidocaine†

Prax Tronothane	Pramoxine

Pontocaine Cream	Tetracaine

Pontocaine Ointment	Tetracaine and Menthol

*Not available in the United States.

†Generic name product may also be available in the U.S. (benzocaine cream, dibucaine, and lidocaine ointment only).

§Contains other active ingredients in addition to the topical local anesthetic.

To the Reader: If you do not recognize the names of medical conditions or medicines referred to in this information, check with your doctor, nurse, or pharmacist. Definitions for selected medical terms may be found in the Glossary. Brand names for the generic drug names listed can be found in the Index. In addition, selected brand names commonly associated with the generic name have been included in the text to help you recognize medicine you may be taking. The fact that a brand name product is not mentioned does not mean the information does not apply. It is a good idea for you to learn both the generic and brand names of your medicines and to write them down for future use.

This medicine belongs to a group of medicines known as topical local anesthetics (an-ess-THET-iks). Topical anesthetics are used to relieve the pain, itching, and redness of minor skin disorders. These include sunburn or other minor burns, insect bites or stings, poison ivy, poison oak, poison sumac, and minor cuts and scratches.

Topical anesthetics deaden the nerve endings in the skin. They do not cause drowsiness or unconsciousness as general anesthetics used for surgery do.

Benzocaine (present in many of these topical medicines) may be absorbed through the skin of young children and cause unwanted effects. Before benzocaine is used for children under 2 years of age, you should discuss its use with your doctor.

Many of the products containing topical anesthetics also contain other ingredients. The following information applies mostly to the local anesthetics contained in these products. However, if you have any questions about the other ingredients, check with your doctor, nurse, or pharmacist.

Most topical anesthetics are available without a prescription; however, your doctor may have special instructions on the proper use and dose for your medical problem.

Remember:

• **Keep all medicines out of the reach of children.**

• In order for this medicine to work, it must be used as directed. **If you are using this medicine without a prescription, it is very important to follow the directions on the label.**

• **It is also very important that you read and understand the following information.** If any of the information causes you special concern, check with your doctor before using this medicine without a prescription.

• Before you begin using any new medicine (prescription or nonprescription) or if you develop any new medical problem while you are using this medicine, check with your doctor, nurse, or pharmacist.

• **If you have any questions** about the following information or if you want more information about this medicine or your medical problem, **ask your doctor, nurse, or pharmacist.**

Before Using This Medicine

Before you use a topical anesthetic, check with your doctor or pharmacist:

—if you have ever had any unusual or allergic reaction to this medicine or to a local anesthetic, especially when applied to the skin or other areas of the body.

—if you have ever had any unusual or allergic reaction to para-aminobenzoic acid (PABA, which is present in some sun screens), to parabens (preservatives in many foods and medicines), or to paraphenylenediamine (a hair dye).

—if you are allergic to any substance, such as other preservatives or dyes. Most medicines contain more than their active ingredient. Your doctor, nurse, or pharmacist can help you avoid products that may cause a problem.

—if you are **pregnant** or if you may become pregnant. Although topical anesthetics have not been shown to cause problems in humans, studies on birth defects have not been done in humans.

—if you are **breast-feeding**. Topical anesthetics have not been shown to cause problems in nursing babies.

—if you have any of the following medical problems:

Infection at or near place of application
Large sores, broken skin, or severe injury at area of application

—if you are taking **any** other prescription or nonprescription (OTC) medicine.

Proper Use of This Medicine

For safe and effective use of this medicine:

• Follow your doctor's instructions if this medicine was prescribed.

• Follow the manufacturer's package directions if you are treating yourself.

• Unless otherwise directed by your doctor, **do not use this medicine on large areas, especially if the skin is broken or scraped. Also, do not use it more often than directed on the package label, or for more than a few days at a time.** To do so may increase the chance of absorption through the skin and the chance of unwanted effects.

This medicine should be used only for problems being treated by your doctor or conditions listed in the package directions. **Check with your doctor before using it for other problems, especially if you think that an infection may be present.** This medicine should not be used to treat certain kinds of skin infections or serious problems, such as severe burns.

Read the package label very carefully to see if the product contains any alcohol. Alcohol is flammable and can catch on fire. **Do not use any product containing alcohol near a fire or open flame, or while smoking. Also, do not smoke after applying one of these products until it has completely dried.**

If you are using this medicine on your face, **be very careful not to get it in your eyes.** If you are using an aerosol or spray form of this medicine, spray it on your hand or an applicator (for example, a sterile gauze pad or a cotton swab) before applying it to your face.

For patients using butamben:

• Butamben may stain clothing. To avoid this, do not touch your clothing while applying the medicine. Also, cover the treated area with a loose bandage after applying butamben, to protect your clothes.

If your doctor has ordered you to use this medicine according to a regular schedule and you miss a dose, use it as soon as possible. However, if it is almost time for your next dose, skip the missed dose and use your next dose at the regularly scheduled time.

How to store this medicine:

• **Keep out of the reach of children.**

• Store away from heat and direct light.

• Keep the medicine from freezing.

• Do not puncture, break, or burn aerosol containers, even when they are empty.

• Do not keep outdated medicine or medicine no longer needed. Be sure that any discarded medicine is out of the reach of children.

Precautions While Using This Medicine

Stop using this medicine and check with your doctor:

—**if your condition does not improve within a few days, or if it gets worse.**

—**if the area you are treating becomes infected.**

—**if you notice a skin rash, burning, stinging, swelling, or any other sign of irritation that was not present when you began using this medicine.**

—**if you swallow any of the medicine.**

Side Effects of This Medicine

Along with its needed effects, a medicine may cause some unwanted effects. Although not all of these side effects may occur, if they do occur they may need medical attention.

Check with your doctor immediately if any of the following side effects occur:

Less common

Swelling of skin, mouth, or throat

Signs of too much medicine being absorbed by the body—very rare

Blurred or double vision
Convulsions (seizures)
Dizziness
Drowsiness
Increased sweating
Ringing or buzzing in the ears
Shivering or trembling
Slow or irregular heartbeat
Unusual anxiety, excitement, nervousness, or restlessness
Unusual paleness

Also, check with your doctor as soon as possible if any of the following side effects occur:

Burning, stinging, or tenderness not present before treatment
Skin rash, redness, itching, or hives

For elderly patients: Many medicines have not been tested in older people. Therefore, it is not known whether the medicine acts the same way it does in younger adults. Check with your doctor or pharmacist if you notice any unusual effects while using this medicine or if you think it is not working as it should.

Other side effects not listed above may also occur in some patients. If you notice any other effects, check with your doctor.

December 1987

ANESTHETICS, GENERAL (Systemic)

This information applies to the following medicines:

Enflurane (EN-floo-rane)
Etomidate (e-TOM-i-date)
Halothane (HA-loe-thane)
Isoflurane (eye-soe-FLURE-ane)
Ketamine (KEET-a-meen)
Methohexital (meth-oh-HEX-i-tal)
Methoxyflurane (meth-ox-ee-FLOO-rane)
Nitrous Oxide
Thiamylal (thye-AM-i-lal)
Thiopental (thye-oh-PEN-tal)

Some commonly used brand names are:	Generic names:
Alyrane* Ethrane	Enflurane
Amidate	Etomidate
Fluothane Somnothane*	Halothane
Aerrane* Forane	Isoflurane
Ketalar	Ketamine
Brevital Brietal*	Methohexital
Penthrane	Methoxyflurane
	Nitrous Oxide
Surital	Thiamylal
Pentothal	Thiopental†

*Not available in the U.S.
†Generic name product may also be available in the U.S.

To the Reader: If you do not recognize the names of medical conditions or medicines referred to in this information, check with your doctor, nurse, or pharmacist. Definitions for selected medical terms may be found in the Glossary. Brand names for the generic drug names listed can be found in the Index. In addition, selected brand names commonly associated with the generic name have been included in the text to help you recognize medicine you may be taking. The fact that a brand name product is not mentioned does not mean the information does not apply. It is a good idea for you to learn both the generic and brand names of your medicines and to write them down for future use.

General anesthetics (an-ess-THET-iks) are normally used to produce loss of consciousness before and during surgery. However, for obstetrics (labor and delivery) or certain minor procedures, an anesthetic may be given in small amounts to relieve pain without causing unconsciousness. Also, some of the anesthetics may be used for certain procedures in a physician's or dentist's office.

Some barbiturate (bar-BI-tyoo-rate) anesthetics (thiamylal and thiopental) are also used to control convulsions (seizures) caused by certain medicines. Thiopental may be used to reduce pressure on the brain in certain conditions. Barbiturate anesthetics may also be used for other conditions as determined by your doctor.

General anesthetics are usually given by inhalation or by injection into a vein. However, certain barbiturate anesthetics may be given rectally to help produce sleep before surgery or certain procedures. Although most general anesthetics can be used by themselves in producing loss of consciousness, some are often used together. This allows for more effective anesthesia in certain patients.

General anesthetics are given only by or under the immediate supervision of a physician or dentist trained to use them. If you will be receiving a general anesthetic during surgery, your doctor or anesthesiologist will give you the medicine and closely follow your progress.

Remember:
• **If you have any questions** about the following information or if you want more information about this medicine or your medical problem, **ask your doctor, nurse, or pharmacist**.

Before Receiving This Medicine

In order to decide on the best anesthetic for you, your doctor should be told:

—if you have ever had any unusual or allergic reaction to barbiturates or general anesthetics.

—if you are **pregnant** or if you may become pregnant shortly after receiving this medicine.

• For barbiturate anesthetics:

Studies on birth defects with methohexital have not been done in humans. However, methohexital has not been shown to cause birth defects or other problems in animal studies. Studies on birth defects with thiamylal and thiopental have not been done in either humans or animals. However, use of barbiturate anesthetics during pregnancy may affect the nervous system in the fetus.

• For etomidate:

Studies on birth defects have not been done in humans. Although studies in animals have not shown etomidate to cause birth defects, this medicine has been shown to cause other unwanted effects in the animal fetus when given in doses usually many times the human dose.

• For inhalation anesthetics:

Studies on birth defects with enflurane, halothane, isoflurane, methoxyflurane, or nitrous oxide have not been done in humans. However, studies in animals have shown that inhalation anesthetics may cause birth defects or other harm to the fetus.

When used as an anesthetic for an abortion, enflurane, halothane, or isoflurane may cause increased bleeding.

When used in small doses to relieve pain during labor and delivery, halothane may slow delivery and increase bleeding in the mother after the baby is born. These effects do not occur with small doses of enflurane, isoflurane, or methoxyflurane. However, they may occur with large doses of these anesthetics.

• For ketamine:

Studies on birth defects with ketamine have not been done in humans. However, studies in animals have not shown that ketamine causes birth defects.

General anesthetics may cause unwanted effects, such as drowsiness, in the newborn baby if large amounts are given to the mother for a long period of time during labor and delivery.

—if you are **breast-feeding**. Barbiturate anesthetics and halothane pass into the breast milk. However, general anesthetics have not been shown to cause problems in nursing babies.

—if you have **any** other medical problems.

—if you or a member of your family has ever had malignant hyperthermia during or shortly after receiving an anesthetic. Signs of malignant hyperthermia include very high fever, fast and irregular heartbeat, muscle spasms or tightness, and breathing problems.

—if you are now taking **any** other prescription or non-prescription (OTC) medicine.

Precautions After Receiving This Medicine

For patients going home within 24 hours after receiving a general anesthetic:

• General anesthetics may cause some people to feel drowsy, tired, or weak for up to a few days after they have been given. They may also cause problems with coordination and one's ability to think. Therefore, for at least 24 hours (or longer if necessary) after receiving a general anesthetic, **do not drive, use machines, or do other jobs that require you to be alert**.

• Unless otherwise directed by your physician or dentist, **do not drink alcoholic beverages or take other CNS depressants (medicines that slow down the nervous system, possibly causing drowsiness) for about 24 hours after you have received a general anesthetic.** To do so may add to the effects of the anesthetic. Some examples of CNS depressants are antihistamines or medicine for hay fever, other allergies, or colds; other sedatives, tranquilizers, or sleeping medicine; prescription pain medicine or narcotics; other barbiturates; medicine for seizures; and muscle relaxants.

Side Effects of This Medicine

Along with its needed effects, a medicine may cause some unwanted effects. Although not all of these side effects may occur, if they do occur they may need medical attention. While you are receiving a general anesthetic, your doctor will closely follow its effects. However, some effects may not be noticed until later.

Check with your doctor as soon as possible if any of the following side effects occur within 2 weeks after you have received an anesthetic:

Rare

Abdominal or stomach pain
Black or bloody vomit
Headache (severe)
Increase or decrease in amount of urine
Loss of appetite
Nausea (severe)
Unusual weight loss
Yellow eyes or skin

Other side effects may occur that usually do not require medical attention. The following side effects may go away as the effects of the anesthetic wear off. However, check with your doctor if any of the following side effects continue or are bothersome:

More common

Shivering or trembling

Less common

Blurred or double vision or other vision problems
Dizziness, lightheadedness, or feeling faint
Drowsiness
Headache
Mood or mental changes
Nausea (mild) or vomiting
Nightmares or unusual dreams

Other side effects not listed above may also occur in some patients. If you notice any other effects, check with your doctor.

December 1987

ANGIOTENSIN-CONVERTING ENZYME (ACE) INHIBITORS (Systemic)

This information applies to the following medicines:

Captopril (KAP-toe-pril)
Enalapril (e-NAL-a-pril)

Some commonly used brand names are:	Generic names:
Capoten	Captopril
Vasotec	Enalapril

To the Reader: If you do not recognize the names of medical conditions or medicines referred to in this information, check with your doctor, nurse, or pharmacist. Definitions for selected medical terms may be found in the Glossary. Brand names for the generic drug names listed can be found in the Index. In addition, selected brand names commonly associated with the generic name have been included in the text to help you recognize medicine you may be taking. The fact that a brand name product is not mentioned does not mean the information does not apply. It is a good idea for you to learn both the generic and brand names of your medicines and to write them down for future use.

ACE inhibitors belong to the general class of medicines called antihypertensives. They are taken by mouth to treat high blood pressure.

High blood pressure adds to the workload of the heart and arteries. If it continues for a long time, the heart and arteries may not function properly. This can damage the blood vessels of the brain, heart, and kidneys, resulting in a stroke, heart failure, or kidney failure. High blood pressure may also increase the risk of heart attacks. These problems may be less likely to occur if blood pressure is controlled.

These medicines are also used to treat congestive heart failure.

The exact way that these medicines work is not known. They block an enzyme in the blood that normally causes blood vessels to tighten. As a result, they probably relax blood vessels. This lowers blood pressure and increases the supply of blood and oxygen to the heart.

These medicines are available only with your doctor's prescription.

Remember:

• **This medicine has been prescribed for your current medical problem only.** It must not be given to other people or used for other problems unless you are directed to do so by your doctor.

• **Keep all medicines out of the reach of children.**

• In order for this medicine to work, it must be used as directed.

• **It is very important that you read and understand the following information.** If any of the information causes you special concern, do not decide against using this medicine without first checking with your doctor.

• Before you begin using any new medicine (prescription or nonprescription) or if you develop any new medical problem while you are using this medicine, check with your doctor, nurse, or pharmacist.

• **If you have any questions** about the following information or if you want more information about this medicine or your medical problem, **ask your doctor, nurse, or pharmacist.**

Before Using This Medicine

In order to decide on the best treatment for your medical problem, your doctor should be told:

—if you have ever had any unusual or allergic reaction to captopril or enalapril.

—if you are on a low-salt, low-sugar, or any other special diet, or if you are allergic to any substance, such as foods, sulfites or other preservatives, or dyes. Most medicines contain more than their active ingredient. Your doctor, nurse, or pharmacist can help you avoid products that may cause a problem.

—if you are **pregnant** or if you may become pregnant.

In humans, captopril has been reported to cause slowed growth of the fetus and difficulty in breathing and low blood pressure in the newborn. In addition, one case of a possible birth defect has been reported. Studies in rabbits and rats at doses up to 400 times the recommended human dose have shown that captopril causes an increase in deaths of the fetus and newborn. Also, captopril has caused deformed skulls in rabbits.

Studies with enalapril have not been done in humans. However, studies in rats at doses many times the recommended human dose have shown that use of enalapril causes the fetus to be smaller than normal. Studies in rabbits have shown that enalapril causes an increase in fetal death. Enalapril has not been shown to cause birth defects in rats or rabbits.

Be sure that you have discussed this with your doctor before taking this medicine.

—if you are **breast-feeding**. Captopril passes into the breast milk. It is not known whether enalapril passes into the breast milk. However, these medicines have not been shown to cause problems in nursing babies.

—if you have any of the following medical problems:
Diabetes mellitus (sugar diabetes)
Heart or blood vessel disease
Kidney disease
Liver disease
Systemic lupus erythematosus (SLE)

—if you have recently had a heart attack or stroke.

—if you have had a kidney transplant.

—if you are now using **any** other prescription or nonprescription (OTC) medicine, especially:
Diuretics (water pills)
Potassium-containing medicines or supplements
Salt substitutes

Proper Use of This Medicine

In order to help you remember to take your medicine, try to get into the habit of taking it at the same time each day.

© 1988   The United States Pharmacopeial Convention, Inc.

For patients taking captopril:

- This medicine is best taken on an empty stomach 1 hour before meals, unless you are otherwise directed by your doctor.

For patients taking this medicine for high blood pressure:

- Importance of diet—When prescribing medicine for your condition, your doctor may also prescribe a personal diet for you. Such a diet may be low in sodium (salt). Most people eat much more sodium than they need and too much sodium in the diet may increase blood pressure. Some foods that contain large amounts of sodium are canned soup, pickles, ketchup, green and ripe olives, relish, frankfurters, soy sauce, and carbonated beverages. Your doctor may want you to limit the amounts of these and other high-sodium foods in your diet. High blood pressure medicine is usually more effective when such a diet is properly followed.

However, too little sodium in the body can also cause problems when this medicine is taken. For example, blood pressure may be lowered more than is wanted. In addition, salt substitutes and low-salt milk may contain potassium, which may cause problems when taken with captopril. Do not use these products unless told to do so by your doctor.

Also, it may be very important for you to go on a reducing diet. However, check with your doctor before changing your diet.

- Many patients who have high blood pressure will not notice any signs of the problem. In fact, many may feel normal. It is very important that you **take your medicine exactly as directed** and that you keep your appointments with your doctor even if you feel well.

- Remember that this medicine will not cure your high blood pressure but it does help control it. Therefore, you must continue to take it as directed if you expect to lower your blood pressure and keep it down. **You may have to take high blood pressure medicine for the rest of your life.** If high blood pressure is not treated, it can cause serious problems such as heart failure, blood vessel disease, stroke, or kidney disease.

If you miss a dose of this medicine, take it as soon as possible. However, if it is almost time for your next dose, skip the missed dose and go back to your regular dosing schedule. Do not double doses.

How to store this medicine:

- **Keep out of the reach of children.**

- Store away from heat and direct light.

- Do not store in the bathroom, near the kitchen sink, or in other damp places. Heat or moisture may cause the medicine to break down.

- Do not keep outdated medicine or medicine no longer needed. Be sure that any discarded medicine is out of the reach of children.

Precautions While Using This Medicine

It is important that your doctor check your progress at regular visits to make sure that this medicine is working properly and to check for unwanted effects.

For patients taking this medicine for high blood pressure:

- **Do not take other medicines unless they have been discussed with your doctor.** This especially includes over-the-counter (nonprescription) medicines for appetite control, asthma, colds, cough, hay fever, or sinus problems, since they may tend to increase your blood pressure.

Dizziness or lightheadedness may occur after the first dose of this medicine, especially if you have been taking a diuretic (water pill). Make sure you know how you react to this medicine before you drive, use machines, or do other jobs that require you to be alert.

Check with your doctor right away if you become sick while taking this medicine, especially with severe or continuing nausea and vomiting or diarrhea. These conditions may cause you to lose too much water and lead to low blood pressure.

Dizziness, lightheadedness, or fainting may also occur if you exercise or if the weather is hot. Heavy sweating can cause loss of too much water and low blood pressure. Use extra care during exercise or hot weather.

Before having any kind of surgery (including dental surgery) or emergency treatment, tell the physician or dentist in charge that you are taking this medicine.

Side Effects of This Medicine

Along with its needed effects, a medicine may cause some unwanted effects. Although not all of these side effects may occur, if they do occur they may need medical attention.

Check with your doctor immediately if any of the following side effects occur:

Rare

Difficult breathing (sudden)
Fever and chills or sore throat
Swelling of face, mouth, hands, or feet

Check with your doctor as soon as possible if any of the following side effects occur:

Less common

Dizziness, lightheadedness, or fainting
Skin rash, with or without itching, fever, or joint pain

Rare

Chest pain

Signs of too much potassium

Confusion
Irregular heartbeat
Numbness or tingling in hands, feet, or lips
Unexplained nervousness
Weakness or heaviness of legs

Other side effects may occur that usually do not require medical attention. These side effects may go away during treatment as your body adjusts to the medicine.

However, check with your doctor if any of the following side effects continue or are bothersome:

Less common

Cough (continuing)
Diarrhea
Headache
Loss of taste
Nausea
Unusual tiredness

For elderly patients: Dizziness and lightheadedness may be more likely to occur in the elderly, who are sometimes more sensitive to the effects of this medicine.

Other side effects not listed above may also occur in some patients. If you notice any other effects, check with your doctor.

_____

December 1987

ANGIOTENSIN-CONVERTING ENZYME (ACE) INHIBITORS AND HYDROCHLOROTHIAZIDE (Systemic)

This information applies to the following medicines:

Captopril (KAP-toe-pril) and Hydrochlorothiazide (hye-droe-klor-oh-THYE-a-zide)

Enalapril (e-NAL-a-pril) and Hydrochlorothiazide

Some commonly used brand names are:	Generic names:
Capozide	Captopril and Hydrochlorothiazide
Vaseretic	Enalapril and Hydrochlorothiazide

To the Reader: If you do not recognize the names of medical conditions or medicines referred to in this information, check with your doctor, nurse, or pharmacist. Definitions for selected medical terms may be found in the Glossary. Brand names for the generic drug names listed can be found in the Index. In addition, selected brand names commonly associated with the generic name have been included in the text to help you recognize medicine you may be taking. The fact that a brand name product is not mentioned does not mean the information does not apply. It is a good idea for you to learn both the generic and brand names of your medicines and to write them down for future use.

This combination belongs to the general class of medicines called antihypertensives. It is used to treat high blood pressure.

High blood pressure adds to the workload of the heart and arteries. If it continues for a long time, the heart and arteries may not function properly. This can damage the blood vessels of the brain, heart, and kidneys, resulting in a stroke, heart failure, or kidney failure. High blood pressure may also increase the risk of heart attacks. These problems may be less likely to occur if blood pressure is controlled.

The exact way in which captopril and enalapril work is not known. They block an enzyme in the blood that normally causes blood vessels to tighten. As a result, they probably relax blood vessels. This lowers blood pressure and increases the supply of blood and oxygen to the heart. Hydrochlorothiazide helps reduce the amount of water in the body by acting on the kidneys to increase the flow of urine; this also helps to lower blood pressure.

This combination may also be used for other conditions as determined by your doctor.

This medicine is available only with doctor's prescription.

Remember:

• **This medicine has been prescribed for your current medical problem only.** It must not be given to other people or used for other problems unless you are directed to do so by your doctor.

• **Keep all medicines out of the reach of children.**

• In order for this medicine to work, it must be used as directed.

• **It is very important that you read and understand the following information.** If any of the information causes you special concern, do not decide against using this medicine without first checking with your doctor.

• Before you begin using any new medicine (prescription or nonprescription) or if you develop any new medical problem while you are using this medicine, check with your doctor, nurse, or pharmacist.

• **If you have any questions** about the following information or if you want more information about this medicine or your medical problem, **ask your doctor, nurse, or pharmacist.**

Before Using This Medicine

In order to decide on the best treatment for your medical problem, your doctor should be told:

—if you have ever had any unusual or allergic reaction to enalapril, captopril, sulfonamides (sulfa medicine), or hydrochlorothiazide or any of the other thiazide diuretics.

—if you are on a low-salt, low-sugar, or any other special diet, or if you are allergic to any substance, such as foods, sulfites or other preservatives, or dyes. Most medicines contain more than their active ingredient. Your doctor, nurse, or pharmacist can help you avoid products that may cause a problem.

—if you are **pregnant** or if you may become pregnant. Studies with this medicine have not been done in humans.

In humans, captopril (contained in this combination medicine) has been reported to cause slowed growth of the fetus and difficult breathing and low blood pressure in the newborn. In addition, one case of a possible birth defect has been reported. Studies in rabbits and rats at doses up to 400 times the recommended human dose have shown that captopril causes an increase in death of the fetus and newborn. Also, captopril has caused deformed skulls in rabbits.

Studies in rats at doses many times the recommended human dose have shown that use of enalapril (contained in this combination medicine) causes the fetus to be smaller than normal. Studies in rabbits have shown that enalapril causes an increase in fetal death. This medicine has not been shown to cause birth defects in rats or rabbits.

Hydrochlorothiazide (contained in this combination medicine) has not been shown to cause birth defects or other problems in animal studies. However, when hydrochlorothiazide is used during pregnancy, it may cause side effects including jaundice, blood problems, and low potassium in the newborn baby.

Be sure that you have discussed this with your doctor before taking this medicine.

—if you are **breast-feeding**. Captopril and hydrochlorothiazide pass into breast milk. It is not known whether enalapril passes into breast milk. However, this medicine has not been shown to cause problems in nursing babies.

—if you have any of the following medical problems:

Diabetes mellitus (sugar diabetes)
Gout (or history of)
Heart or blood vessel disease
Kidney disease

Liver disease
Pancreas disease
Systemic lupus erythematosus (SLE) (or history of)

—if you have recently had a heart attack or stroke.

—if you have had a kidney transplant.

—if you are now using **any** other prescription or non-prescription (OTC) medicine, especially:

Adrenocorticoids (cortisone-like medicine)
Digitalis glycosides (heart medicine)
Diuretics (water pills) or other antihypertensives (high blood pressure medicine)
Lithium (e.g., Lithane)
Methenamine (e.g., Mandelamine)
Potassium-containing medicines or supplements
Salt substitutes

Proper Use of This Medicine

In order to help you remember to take your medicine, try to get into the habit of taking it at the same time each day.

For patients taking captopril and hydrochlorothiazide:

• This medicine is best taken on an empty stomach 1 hour before meals, unless you are otherwise directed by your doctor.

For patients taking this medicine for high blood pressure:

• Importance of diet—When prescribing medicine for your condition, your doctor may also prescribe a personal diet for you. Such a diet may be low in sodium (salt). Most people eat much more sodium than they need and too much sodium in the diet may increase blood pressure. Some foods that contain large amounts of sodium are canned soup, pickles, ketchup, green and ripe olives, relish, frankfurters, soy sauce, and carbonated beverages. Your doctor may want you to limit the amounts of these and other high-sodium foods in your diet. High blood pressure medicine is usually more effective when such a diet is properly followed.

However, too little sodium in the body can also cause problems when this medicine is taken. For example, blood pressure may be lowered more than is wanted.

Also, it may be very important for you to go on a reducing diet. However, check with your doctor before changing your diet.

• Many patients who have high blood pressure will not notice any signs of the problem. In fact, many may feel normal. It is very important that you **take your medicine exactly as directed** and that you keep your appointments with your doctor even if you feel well.

• Remember that this medicine will not cure your high blood pressure but it does help control it. Therefore, you must continue to take it as directed if you expect to lower your blood pressure and keep it down. **You may have to take high blood pressure medicine for the rest of your life.** If high blood pressure is not treated, it can cause serious problems such as heart failure, blood vessel disease, stroke, or kidney disease.

This medicine may cause you to have an unusual feeling or tiredness when you begin to take it. You may also notice an increase in the amount of urine or in your frequency of urination. After you have taken the medicine for a while, these effects should lessen. In general, in order to keep the increase in urine from affecting your nighttime sleep:

• If you are to take a single dose a day, take it in the morning after breakfast.

• If you are to take more than one dose a day, take the last dose no later than 6 p.m., unless otherwise directed by your doctor.

However, it is best to plan your dose or doses according to a schedule that will least affect your personal activities and sleep. Ask your doctor, nurse, or pharmacist to help you plan the best time to take this medicine.

If you miss a dose of this medicine, take it as soon as possible. However, if it is almost time for your next dose, skip the missed dose and go back to your regular dosing schedule. Do not double doses.

How to store this medicine:

• **Keep out of the reach of children.**

• Store away from heat and direct light.

• Do not store in the bathroom, near the kitchen sink, or in other damp places. Heat or moisture may cause the medicine to break down.

• Do not keep outdated medicine or medicine no longer needed. Be sure that any discarded medicine is out of the reach of children.

Precautions While Using This Medicine

It is important that your doctor check your progress at regular visits to make sure that this medicine is working properly and to check for unwanted effects.

Check with your doctor right away if you become sick while taking this medicine, especially with severe or continuing nausea and vomiting or diarrhea. These conditions may cause you to lose too much water and lead to low blood pressure.

Dizziness, lightheadedness, or fainting may also occur if you exercise or if the weather is hot. Heavy sweating can cause loss of too much water and low blood pressure. Use extra care during exercise or hot weather.

Before having any kind of surgery (including dental surgery) or emergency treatment, tell the physician or dentist in charge that you are taking this medicine.

For patients taking this medicine for high blood pressure:

• **Do not take other medicines unless they have been discussed with your doctor.** This especially includes over-the-counter (nonprescription) medicines for appetite control, asthma, colds, cough, hay fever, or sinus problems, since they may tend to increase your blood pressure.

This medicine may cause a loss of potassium from your body.

- To help prevent this, your doctor may want you to:

    —eat or drink foods that have a high potassium content (for example, orange or other citrus fruit juices), or

    —take a potassium supplement, or

    —take another medicine to help prevent the loss of the potassium in the first place.

- It is very important to follow these directions. Also, it is important not to change your diet on your own. This is more important if you are already on a special diet (as for diabetes), or if you are taking a potassium supplement or a medicine to reduce potassium loss. Extra potassium may not be necessary and, in some cases, too much potassium could be harmful. Salt substitutes and low-salt milk may contain potassium, which may cause problems when taken with enalapril. Do not use these products unless told to do so by your doctor.

Diabetics—Hydrochlorothiazide (contained in this combination medicine) may raise blood sugar levels. While you are taking this medicine, be especially careful in testing for sugar in your urine.

Some people who take hydrochlorothiazide (contained in this combination medicine) may become more sensitive to sunlight than they are normally. When you first begin taking this medicine, avoid too much sun and do not use a sunlamp until you see how you react to the sun, especially if you tend to burn easily. If you have a severe reaction, check with your doctor.

Side Effects of This Medicine

Along with its needed effects, a medicine may cause some unwanted effects. Although not all of these side effects may occur, if they do occur they may need medical attention.

Check with your doctor immediately if any of the following side effects occur:

Rare
   Difficult breathing (sudden)
   Fever and chills or sore throat
   Swelling of face, mouth, hands, or feet

Check with your doctor as soon as possible if any of the following side effects occur:

Less common
   Dizziness, lightheadedness, or fainting
   Skin rash, with or without itching or fever

Rare
   Chest pain
   Joint, lower back or side, or stomach pain
   Stomach pain (severe) with nausea and vomiting
   Unusual bleeding or bruising
   Yellow eyes and skin

Signs of too much or too little potassium in the body
   Dryness of mouth
   Increased thirst
   Irregular heartbeats
   Mood or mental changes
   Muscle cramps or pain
   Numbness or tingling in hands, feet, or lips
   Shortness of breath or difficult breathing
   Weak pulse
   Weakness or heaviness of legs

Other side effects may occur that usually do not require medical attention. These side effects may go away during treatment as your body adjusts to the medicine. However, check with your doctor if any of the following side effects continue or are bothersome:

Less common
   Cough (continuing)
   Diarrhea
   Headache
   Increased sensitivity of skin to sunlight
   Loss of taste
   Stomach upset
   Unusual tiredness

For elderly patients: Dizziness or lightheadedness and signs of too much potassium loss may be more likely to occur in the elderly, who are more sensitive to the effects of this medicine.

Other side effects not listed above may also occur in some patients. If you notice any other effects, check with your doctor.

_____

December 1987

_____

ANTACIDS (Oral)

Note: For quick reference the following antacids are numbered to match the corresponding brand names below.

This information applies to the following medicines:

1. Alumina (a-LOO-mi-na) and Magnesia (mag-NEE-zha)
2. Alumina, Magnesia, and Calcium Carbonate (KAL-see-um KAR-boe-nate)
3. Alumina, Magnesia, and Simethicone (si-METH-i-kone)
4. Alumina and Magnesium Carbonate (mag-NEE-zhum KAR-boe-nate)
5. Alumina, Magnesium Carbonate, and Calcium Carbonate
6. Alumina and Magnesium Trisilicate (trye-SILL-i-kate)
7. Alumina, Magnesium Trisilicate, and Sodium Bicarbonate (SOE-dee-um bye-KAR-boe-nate)
8. Aluminum Carbonate (a-LOO-mi-num KAR-boe-nate), Basic
9. Aluminum Hydroxide (hye-DROX-ide)†‡
10. Calcium Carbonate†
11. Calcium Carbonate and Magnesia
11a. Calcium Carbonate, Magnesia, and Simethicone
12. Calcium and Magnesium Carbonates
13. Calcium and Magnesium Carbonates and Magnesium Oxide
14. Dihydroxyaluminum Aminoacetate (dye-hye-DROX-ee-a-LOO-mi-num a-mee-noe-ASS-e-tate)
15. Dihydroxyaluminum Aminoacetate, Magnesia, and Alumina
16. Dihydroxyaluminum Sodium (SOE-dee-um) Carbonate
17. Magaldrate (MAG-al-drate)†
18. Magaldrate and Simethicone
19. Magnesium Carbonate (mag-NEE-zhum KAR-boe-nate) and Sodium Bicarbonate
20. Magnesium Hydroxide†‡
21. Magnesium Oxide (mag-NEE-zhum OX-ide)
22. Magnesium Trisilicate†
23. Magnesium Trisilicate, Alumina, and Magnesia
24. Magnesium Trisilicate, Alumina, and Magnesium Carbonate
25. Simethicone, Alumina, Calcium Carbonate, and Magnesia
26. Simethicone, Alumina, Magnesium Carbonate, and Magnesia

Some commonly used brand names:

Advanced Formula Di-Gel[11a]	Delcid[1]	Maox[21]
Alagel[9]	Dialume[9]	Marblen[12]
Algenic Alka Improved[1]	Dicarbosil[10]	Mi-Acid[3]
Algicon[4]	Di-Gel[3 26]	Mintox[1]
Alka-Mints[10]	Diovol[*3]	M.O.M.[20]
Alkets[13]	Diovol Ex[*1]	Mygel[3]
Almacone[3]	Duracid[5]	Mygel II[3]
Almacone II[3]	Equilet[10]	Mylanta[3]
Alma-Mag Improved[3]	Escot[24]	Mylanta-2[*3]
	Gas-is-gon[7]	Mylanta-II[3]
Alma-Mag #4 Improved[3]	Gaviscon[4 6]	Mylanta-2 Extra Strength[*3]
	Gaviscon-2[6]	
ALternaGEL[9]	Gelamal[1]	Mylanta-2 Plain[*1]
Alu-Cap[9]	Gelusil[3]	Nephrox[9]
Aludrox[1]	Gelusil[*1]	Neutralca-S[*1]
Alumid[1]	Gelusil-II[3]	Newtrogel II[3]
Alumid Plus[3]	Gelusil Extra Strength[*1]	Noralac[12]
Alu-Tab[9]	Gelusil-M[3]	Pama No. 1[10]
Amitone[10]	Gustalac[10]	Par-Mag[21]
Amphojel[9]	Kolantyl[1]	Phillips' Milk of Magnesia[20]
Amphojel 500[*1]	Kudrox[1]	Remegel[4]
Amphojel Plus[*3 26]	Liquimint[4]	Riopan[17]
AntaGel[3]	Lowsium[17]	Riopan Plus[18]
AntaGel-II[3]	Lowsium Plus[18]	Robalate[*14]
Basaljel[8]	Maalox[1]	Rolaids[16]
Bisodol[11 19]	Maalox No. 1[1]	Rolox[1]
Calcilac[10]	Maalox No. 2[1]	Rulox[1]
Calcitrel[11]	Maalox Plus[3]	Rulox No. 1[1]
Calglycine[10]	Maalox TC[1]	Rulox No. 2[1]
Camalox[2]	Magmalin[1]	Silain-Gel[3]
Chooz[10]	Magnagel[4]	Simaal Gel[3]
Creamalin[1]	Magnatril[23]	Simaal 2 Gel[3]
	Mag-Ox 400[21]	Simeco[3]

Spastosed[12]	Tralmag[15]	Univol[*1]
Tempo[25]	Triconsil[7]	Uro-Mag[21]
Titracid[10]	Tums[10]	WinGel[1]
Titralac[10]	Tums E-X[10]	

*Not available in the U.S.
†Generic name product may also be available in U.S.
‡Generic name product available in Canada.

To the Reader: If you do not recognize the names of medical conditions or medicines referred to in this information, check with your doctor, nurse, or pharmacist. Definitions for selected medical terms may be found in the Glossary. Brand names for the generic drug names listed can be found in the Index. In addition, selected brand names commonly associated with the generic name have been included in the text to help you recognize medicine you may be taking. The fact that a brand name product is not mentioned does not mean the information does not apply. It is a good idea for you to learn both the generic and brand names of your medicines and to write them down for future use.

Antacids are taken by mouth to relieve heartburn, sour stomach, or acid indigestion. They work by neutralizing excess stomach acid. Some antacid combinations also contain simethicone, which may relieve the symptoms of excess gas. Antacids alone or in combination with simethicone may also be used to treat the symptoms of stomach or duodenal ulcers.

With larger doses than those used for the antacid effect, magnesium hydroxide (magnesia) and magnesium oxide antacids produce a laxative effect. The information that follows applies only to their use as an antacid.

Some antacids, like aluminum carbonate and aluminum hydroxide, may be prescribed with a low-phosphate diet to treat hyperphosphatemia (too much phosphate in the blood). Aluminum carbonate and aluminum hydroxide may also be used with a low-phosphate diet to prevent the formation of some kinds of kidney stones. Aluminum hydroxide may also be used for other conditions as determined by your doctor.

Antacids should not be given to young children (up to 6 years of age) unless ordered by their doctor. Since children cannot usually describe their symptoms very well, a doctor should first check the child. This is to prevent an unknown condition from getting worse and to avoid causing unwanted effects in the child. In addition, magnesium-containing medicines may cause serious side effects when given to very young children, especially those who have kidney disease or who are dehydrated.

These medicines are available without a prescription; however, your doctor may have special instructions on the proper use and dose for your medical problem.

Remember:
• **Keep all medicines out of the reach of children.**

• In order for this medicine to work, it must be used as directed. **If you are using this medicine without a prescription, it is very important that you follow the directions on the label.**

• **It is also very important that you read and understand the following information.** If any of the information causes you special concern, check with your doctor or pharmacist.

• Before you begin using any new medicine (prescription or nonprescription) or if you develop any new medical problem while you are using this medicine, check with your doctor, nurse, or pharmacist.

• **If you have any questions** about the following information or if you want more information about this medicine or your medical problem, **ask your doctor, nurse, or pharmacist.**

Before Using This Medicine

Before you use this medicine, check with your doctor or pharmacist:

—if you have ever had any unusual or allergic reaction to aluminum-, calcium-, magnesium-, simethicone-, or sodium bicarbonate–containing medicines.

—if you are on a low-salt, low-sugar, or any other special diet, or if you are allergic to any substance, such as foods, sulfites or other preservatives, or dyes. Most medicines contain more than their active ingredient. Your doctor, nurse, or pharmacist can help you avoid products that may cause a problem.

—if you are **pregnant** or if you may become pregnant. Studies have not been done in either humans or animals. However, there have been reports of antacids causing side effects in babies whose mothers took antacids for a long period of time, especially in high doses. Also, sodium-containing medicines should be avoided if you tend to retain (keep) body water.

—if you are **breast-feeding**. These medicines have not been shown to cause problems in nursing babies.

—if you have any of the following medical problems:
   Alzheimer's disease (for aluminum-containing antacids only)
   Appendicitis (or signs of)
   Bone fractures
   Colitis
   Colostomy
   Constipation (severe and continuing)
   Diarrhea (chronic)
   Edema (swelling of feet or lower legs)
   Heart disease
   Hemorrhoids
   Ileostomy
   Inflamed bowel
   Intestinal blockage
   Intestinal or rectal bleeding (of unknown cause)
   Kidney disease
   Liver disease
   Sarcoidosis
   Toxemia of pregnancy
   Underactive parathyroid glands

—if you are now taking **any** other medicines by mouth, especially:
   Adrenocorticoids (cortisone-like medicine)
   Cellulose sodium phosphate (e.g., Calcibind)
   Corticotropin (e.g., ACTH)
   Ketoconazole (e.g., Nizoral)
   Mecamylamine (e.g., Inversine)
   Methenamine (e.g., Mandelamine)
   Sodium polystyrene sulfonate resin (SPSR) (e.g., Kayexalate)
   Tetracyclines

Proper Use of This Medicine

For safe and effective use of this medicine:
   • Follow your doctor's instructions if this medicine was prescribed.

   • Follow the manufacturer's package directions if you are treating yourself.

If you are taking the chewable tablet form of this medicine, chew the tablets well before swallowing. This is to allow the medicine to work faster and be more effective.

For patients taking this medicine for a stomach or duodenal ulcer:
   • **Take it exactly as directed and for the full time of treatment as ordered by your doctor** to obtain maximum relief of your symptoms.

   • Take it 1 and 3 hours after meals and at bedtime for best results, unless otherwise directed by your doctor.

For patients taking aluminum carbonate or aluminum hydroxide to prevent kidney stones:
   • Drink plenty of fluids for best results, unless otherwise directed by your doctor.

For patients taking aluminum carbonate or aluminum hydroxide for hyperphosphatemia (too much phosphate in the blood):
   • Your doctor may want you to follow a low-phosphate diet. If you have any questions about this, check with your doctor.

If this medicine has been ordered by your doctor to be taken on a regular schedule and you miss a dose, take it as soon as possible. However, if it is almost time for your next dose, skip the missed dose and go back to your regular dosing schedule. Do not double doses.

How to store this medicine:
   • **Keep out of the reach of children.**

   • Store away from heat and direct light.

   • Do not store the capsule, tablet, or powder form of this medicine in the bathroom, near the kitchen sink, or in other damp places. Heat or moisture may cause the medicine to break down.

   • Keep the liquid form of this medicine from freezing.

   • Do not keep outdated medicine or medicine no longer needed. Be sure that any discarded medicine is out of the reach of children.

Precautions While Using This Medicine

If this medicine has been ordered by your doctor and if you will be taking it in large doses, or for a long period of time, your doctor should check your progress at regular visits. This is to make sure the medicine does not cause unwanted effects.

Do not take this medicine:

—**if you have any signs of appendicitis or inflamed bowel** (such as stomach or lower abdominal pain, cramping, bloating, soreness, nausea, or vomiting). Instead, check with your doctor as soon as possible.

—**within 1 to 2 hours of taking other medicine by mouth**. To do so may keep the other medicine from working as well.

For patients on a sodium-restricted diet—Some antacids (especially sodium bicarbonate–containing ones) contain a large amount of sodium. If you have any questions about this, check with your doctor or pharmacist.

For patients taking this medicine as an antacid:

• **Do not take for more than 2 weeks unless otherwise directed by your doctor.** Antacids should be used only for occasional relief.

• If your stomach problem is not helped by the antacid or if it keeps on coming back, check with your doctor.

• Using magnesium- or sodium bicarbonate–containing antacids too often, or in high doses, may produce a laxative effect. This happens fairly often and depends on the individual's sensitivity to the medicine.

For patients taking aluminum-containing antacids (including magaldrate):

• Before you have any test in which a radiopharmaceutical will be used, tell the doctor in charge that you are taking this medicine. The results of the test may be affected by aluminum-containing antacids.

For patients taking calcium- or sodium bicarbonate–containing antacids:

• **Do not take with large amounts of milk or milk products.** To do so may increase the chance of side effects.

Side Effects of This Medicine

Along with its needed effects, a medicine may cause some unwanted effects. Although the following side effects occur very rarely when this medicine is taken as recommended, they may be more likely to occur if:

—too much medicine is taken.
—it is taken in large doses.
—it is taken for a long period of time.
—it is taken by patients with kidney disease.

Check with your doctor as soon as possible if any of the following side effects (which may be signs of overdose) occur:
For aluminum-containing antacids (including magaldrate)
   Bone pain
   Constipation (severe and continuing)
   Feeling of discomfort (continuing)

   Loss of appetite (continuing)
   Mood or mental changes
   Muscle weakness
   Swelling of wrists or ankles
   Unusual loss of weight
For calcium-containing antacids
   Constipation (severe and continuing)
   Difficult or painful urination
   Frequent urge to urinate
   Headache (continuing)
   Loss of appetite (continuing)
   Mood or mental changes
   Muscle pain or twitching
   Nausea or vomiting
   Nervousness or restlessness
   Slow breathing
   Unpleasant taste
   Unusual tiredness or weakness
For magnesium-containing antacids (including magaldrate)
   Difficult or painful urination (with magnesium trisilicate)
   Dizziness or lightheadedness
   Irregular heartbeat
   Mood or mental changes
   Unusual tiredness or weakness
For sodium bicarbonate–containing antacids
   Frequent urge to urinate
   Headache (continuing)
   Loss of appetite (continuing)
   Mood or mental changes
   Muscle pain or twitching
   Nausea or vomiting
   Nervousness or restlessness
   Swelling of feet or lower legs
   Slow breathing
   Unpleasant taste
   Unusual tiredness or weakness

Other side effects may occur that usually do not require medical attention. These side effects may go away during treatment as your body adjusts to the medicine. However, check with your doctor if any of the following side effects continue or are bothersome:
More common
   Chalky taste
Less common
   Constipation (mild)
   Diarrhea or laxative effect
   Increase in thirst
   Nausea or vomiting
   Speckling or whitish discoloration of stools
   Stomach cramps

Other side effects not listed above may also occur in some patients. If you notice any other effects, check with your doctor.

December 1987

ANTHRALIN (Topical)

Some commonly used brand names or other names are:

anthra-derm*	Drithocreme HP
Anthraforte*	Drithoscalp
Anthranol*	Lasan
Dithranol	Lasan HP
Drithocreme	Lasan Unguent

Generic name product may also be available in the U.S.

*Not available in the U. S.

To the Reader: If you do not recognize the names of medical conditions or medicines referred to in this information, check with your doctor, nurse, or pharmacist. Definitions for selected medical terms may be found in the Glossary. Brand names for the generic drug names listed can be found in the Index. In addition, selected brand names commonly associated with the generic name have been included in the text to help you recognize medicine you may be taking. The fact that a brand name product is not mentioned does not mean the information does not apply. It is a good idea for you to learn both the generic and brand names of your medicines and to write them down for future use.

Anthralin (AN-thra-lin) is applied to the skin to treat psoriasis. It may also be used to treat other skin conditions as determined by your doctor.

This medicine is available only with your doctor's prescription.

Remember:
• **This medicine has been prescribed for your current medical problem only.** It must not be given to other people or used for other problems unless you are directed to do so by your doctor.

• **Keep all medicines out of the reach of children.**

• In order for this medicine to work, it must be used as directed.

• **It is very important that you read and understand the following information.** If any of the information causes you special concern, do not decide against using this medicine without first checking with your doctor.

• Before you begin using any new medicine (prescription or nonprescription) or if you develop any new medical problem while you are using this medicine, check with your doctor, nurse, or pharmacist.

• **If you have any questions** about the following information or if you want more information about this medicine or your medical problem, **ask your doctor, nurse, or pharmacist.**

Before Using This Medicine

In order to decide on the best treatment for your medical problem, your doctor should be told:
—if you have ever had any unusual or allergic reaction to anthralin.

—if you are allergic to any substance, such as certain preservatives or dyes. Most medicines contain more than their active ingredient. Your doctor, nurse, or pharmacist can help you avoid products that may cause a problem.

—if you are **pregnant** or if you may become pregnant, since anthralin may be absorbed through the skin. Studies on birth defects have not been done in either humans or animals.

—if you are **breast-feeding**, since anthralin may be absorbed through the skin. It is not known whether anthralin passes into the breast milk. However, this medicine has not been shown to cause problems in nursing babies.

—if you are taking **any** other prescription or nonprescription (OTC) medicine.

Proper Use of This Medicine

Keep this medicine away from the eyes and other mucous membranes, such as the mouth and inside of the nose.

Do not apply this medicine to blistered, raw, or oozing areas of the skin or scalp.

Use this medicine only as directed. Do not use more of it, do not use it more often, and do not use it for a longer period of time than your doctor ordered. To do so may increase the chance of side effects.

Anthralin may be used in different ways. In some cases, it is applied at night and allowed to remain on the affected areas overnight, then washed off the next morning or before the next application. In other cases, it may be applied and allowed to remain on the affected areas for a short period of time (usually 20 or 30 minutes), then washed off. (This is called short contact treatment.) Make sure you understand exactly how you are to use this medicine. If you have any questions about this, check with your doctor.

Anthralin may cause irritation of normal skin. If it does, petrolatum may be applied to the skin or scalp around the affected areas for protection before you apply this medicine.

Apply a thin layer of anthralin to only the affected area of the skin or scalp and rub in gently.

Immediately after applying this medicine, wash your hands to remove any medicine that may be on them.

For patients using anthralin for short contact (usually 20 or 30 minutes) treatment:
• After applying anthralin, allow the medicine to remain on the affected area for 20 to 30 minutes or as directed by your doctor. Then remove the medicine by bathing, if the anthralin was applied to the skin, or by shampooing, if it was applied to the scalp.

For patients using the cream form of anthralin for overnight treatment:
• If anthralin cream is applied to the skin, any medicine remaining on the affected areas the next morning should be removed by bathing.

• If anthralin cream is applied to the scalp, shampoo to remove the scales and any medicine remaining on the affected areas from the previous application. Dry the hair and, after parting, rub the cream into the affected areas. Check with your doctor to see when the cream should be removed.

For patients using the ointment form of anthralin for overnight treatment:

• If anthralin ointment is applied to the skin at night, any ointment remaining on the affected areas the next morning should be removed with warm liquid petrolatum followed by bathing.

• If anthralin ointment is applied to the scalp at night, use a shampoo the next morning to clean the scalp.

If you miss a dose of this medicine, apply it as soon as possible. However, if it is almost time for your next dose, skip the missed dose and go back to your regular dosing schedule.

How to store this medicine:

• **Keep out of the reach of children.**

• Store away from heat and direct light.

• Keep the medicine from freezing.

• Do not keep outdated medicine or medicine no longer needed. Be sure that any discarded medicine is out of the reach of children.

Precautions While Using This Medicine

Anthralin may stain the skin, hair, clothing, bed linens, or bathtub or shower:

• Avoid getting the medicine on your clothing or on bed linens. Protective dressings may be used, unless otherwise directed by your doctor.

• The stain on the skin or hair will wear off in several weeks after you stop using this medicine.

• To prevent staining of your hands, plastic gloves may be worn when you apply this medicine.

• If the medicine is applied to the scalp at night, check with your doctor to see if a plastic cap may be worn to prevent staining of the pillow.

• To remove any medicine on the surface of the bathtub or shower, wash it with hot water immediately after bathing or showering. Then use a household cleanser to remove any remaining deposit of the medicine on the bathtub or shower.

Side Effects of This Medicine

Anthralin has been shown to cause tumors (some cancerous) in animals. However, there have been no reports of anthralin causing tumors in humans.

Along with its needed effects, a medicine may cause some unwanted effects. Although not all of these side effects may occur, if they do occur they may need medical attention.

Check with your doctor as soon as possible if any of the following side effects occur:

> Redness or other skin irritation not present before using this medicine
> Skin rash

For elderly patients: Many medicines have not been tested in older people. Therefore, it is not known whether the medicine acts the same way it does in younger adults. Check with your doctor or pharmacist if you notice any unusual effects while using this medicine or if you think it is not working as it should.

Other side effects not listed above may also occur in some patients. If you notice any other effects, check with your doctor.

December 1987

ANTICOAGULANTS (Systemic)

This information applies to the following medicines:

Anisindione (an-iss-in-DYE-one)
Dicumarol (dye-KOO-ma-role)
Warfarin (WAR-far-in)

This information does *not* apply to heparin.

Some commonly used brand names are:	Generic names:
Miradon	Anisindione
	Dicumarol†
Coumadin	
Marevan*	
Panwarfin	Warfarin†
Sofarin	
Warfilone*	

*Not available in the U.S.
†Available by generic name in the U.S.

To the Reader: If you do not recognize the names of medical conditions or medicines referred to in this information, check with your doctor, nurse, or pharmacist. Definitions for selected medical terms may be found in the Glossary. Brand names for the generic drug names listed can be found in the Index. In addition, selected brand names commonly associated with the generic name have been included in the text to help you recognize medicine you may be taking. The fact that a brand name product is not mentioned does not mean the information does not apply. It is a good idea for you to learn both the generic and brand names of your medicines and to write them down for future use.

Anticoagulants decrease the clotting ability of the blood and therefore help to prevent harmful clots from forming in the blood vessels. They are given by mouth; warfarin is also given by injection. These medicines are sometimes called blood thinners, although they do not actually thin the blood. They also will not dissolve clots that already have formed, but they may prevent the clots from becoming larger and causing more serious problems. They are often used as treatment for certain blood vessel, heart, and lung conditions.

In order for an anticoagulant to help you without causing serious bleeding, it must be used properly and all of the precautions concerning its use must be followed exactly. Be sure that you have discussed the use of this medicine with your doctor. It is very important that you understand all of your doctor's orders and that you are willing and able to follow them exactly.

Anticoagulants are available only with your doctor's prescription.

Remember:
• **This medicine has been prescribed for your current medical problem only.** It must not be given to other people or used for other problems unless you are directed to do so by your doctor.

• **Keep all medicines out of the reach of children.**

• In order for this medicine to work, it must be used as directed.

• If you are receiving this medicine by injection, some of the information about this medicine may not apply.

• It is very important that you read and understand the following information. If any of the information causes you special concern, do not decide against using this medicine without first checking with your doctor.

• Before you begin using any new medicine (prescription or nonprescription) or if you develop any new medical problem while you are using this medicine, check with your doctor, nurse, or pharmacist.

• If you have any questions about the following information or if you want more information about this medicine or your medical problem, ask your doctor, nurse, or pharmacist.

Before Using This Medicine

In order to decide on the best treatment for your medical problem, your doctor should be told:

—if you have ever had any unusual or allergic reaction to anticoagulants.

—if you are on a low-salt, low-sugar, or any other special diet, or if you are allergic to any substance, such as foods, sulfites or other preservatives, or dyes. Most medicines contain more than their active ingredient. Your doctor, nurse, or pharmacist can help you avoid products that may cause a problem.

—if you are **pregnant** or if you may become pregnant. Anticoagulants may cause birth defects. They may also cause other problems affecting the physical or mental growth of the fetus or newborn baby. In addition, use of this medicine during the last 6 months of pregnancy may increase the chance of severe, possibly fatal, bleeding in the fetus. If taken during the last few weeks of pregnancy, anticoagulants may cause severe bleeding in both the fetus and the mother before or during delivery and in the newborn infant.

Do not begin taking this medicine during pregnancy, and do not become pregnant while taking this medicine, unless you have first discussed the possible effects of this medicine with your doctor. Also, if you suspect that you may be pregnant and you are already taking an anticoagulant, check with your doctor at once. Your doctor may suggest that you take a different anticoagulant that is less likely to harm the fetus or the newborn infant during all or part of your pregnancy. Anticoagulants may also cause severe bleeding in the mother if taken soon after the baby is born.

—if you are **breast-feeding.** Most anticoagulants pass into the breast milk and may cause bleeding problems in nursing babies.

—if you have **any** other medical problems, or if you are now being treated by any other physician or dentist, since many medical problems and treatments affect the way your body responds to this medicine.

—if you have recently had any of the following conditions or medical procedures:
Childbirth
Falls or blows to the body or head
Fever lasting more than a couple of days
Heavy or unusual menstrual bleeding
Insertion of intrauterine device (IUD)
Medical or dental surgery

Severe or continuing diarrhea
Spinal anesthesia
X-ray (radiation) treatment

—if you are now taking **any** other prescription or non-prescription (OTC) medicine, including aspirin, laxatives, vitamins, or antacids.

Proper Use of This Medicine

Take this medicine only as directed by your doctor. Do not take more or less of it, do not take it more often, and do not take it for a longer period of time than your doctor ordered.

Your doctor should check your progress at regular visits. A blood test must be taken regularly to see how fast your blood is clotting. This will help your doctor decide on the proper amount of anticoagulant you should be taking each day.

If you miss a dose of this medicine, take it as soon as possible. Then go back to your regular dosing schedule. If you do not remember until the next day, do not take the missed dose at all and do not double the next one. **Doubling the dose may cause bleeding.** Instead, go back to your regular dosing schedule. It is recommended that you keep a record of each dose as you take it in order to avoid mistakes. Also, be sure to give your doctor a record of any doses you miss. If you have any questions about this, check with your doctor.

How to store this medicine:

- **Keep out of the reach of children.**

- Store away from heat and direct light.

- Do not store this medicine in the bathroom, near the kitchen sink, or in other damp places. Heat or moisture may cause the medicine to break down.

- Do not keep outdated medicine or medicine no longer needed. Be sure that any discarded medicine is out of the reach of children.

Precautions While Using This Medicine

Tell all physicians, dentists, and pharmacists you go to that you are taking this medicine.

Check with your doctor, nurse, or pharmacist before you start or stop taking any other medicine. This includes any over-the-counter (OTC) or nonprescription medicine, even aspirin or acetaminophen. Many medicines change the way this medicine affects your body. You may not be able to take the other medicine, or the dose of your anticoagulant may need to be changed.

It is recommended that you carry identification stating that you are using this medicine. If you have any questions about what kind of identification to carry, check with your doctor, nurse, or pharmacist.

While you are taking this medicine, it is very important that you avoid sports and activities that may cause you to be injured. Report to your doctor any falls, blows to the body or head, or other injuries, since serious internal bleeding may occur without your knowing about it.

Be careful to avoid cutting yourself. This includes taking special care in brushing your teeth and in shaving. Use a soft toothbrush and floss gently. Also, it is best to use an electric shaver rather than a blade.

Drinking too much alcohol may change the way this anticoagulant affects your body. You should not drink regularly on a daily basis or take more than 1 or 2 drinks at any time. If you have any questions about this, check with your doctor.

The foods that you eat may also affect the way this medicine affects your body. Eat a normal, balanced diet while you are taking this medicine. Do not go on a reducing diet, make other changes in your eating habits, start taking vitamins, or begin using other nutrition supplements unless you have first checked with your doctor, nurse, or pharmacist. Also, check with your doctor if you are unable to eat for several days or if you have continuing stomach upset, diarrhea, or fever.

After you stop taking this medicine, your body will need time to recover before your blood clotting ability returns to normal. Your pharmacist or doctor can tell you how long this will take depending on which anticoagulant you were taking. Use the same caution during this period of time as you did while you were taking the anticoagulant.

Side Effects of This Medicine

Along with its needed effects, a medicine may cause some unwanted effects. Although not all of these side effects may occur, if they do occur they may need medical attention.

Check with your doctor immediately if any of the following side effects occur:
Less common or rare
Blue or purple color of toes and pain in toes
Cloudy or dark urine
Difficult or painful urination
Sores, ulcers, or white spots in mouth or throat
Sore throat and fever or chills
Sudden decrease in amount of urine
Swelling of face, feet, or lower legs
Unusual tiredness or weakness
Unusual weight gain
Yellow eyes or skin

Since many things can affect the way your body reacts to this medicine, you should always watch for signs of unusual bleeding. Unusual bleeding may mean that your body is getting more medicine than it needs. **Check with your doctor immediately if any of the following signs of overdose occur:**
Bleeding from gums when brushing teeth
Unexplained bruising or purplish areas on skin
Unexplained nosebleeds
Unusually heavy bleeding or oozing from cuts or wounds
Unusually heavy or unexpected menstrual bleeding

Signs of bleeding inside the body
> Abdominal or stomach pain or swelling
> Back pain or backaches
> Blood in urine
> Bloody or black tarry stools
> Constipation
> Coughing up blood
> Dizziness
> Headache (severe or continuing)
> Joint pain, stiffness, or swelling
> Vomiting blood or material that looks like coffee grounds

Also, check with your doctor as soon as possible if any of the following side effects occur:

Less common or rare
> Diarrhea (more common with dicumarol)
> Nausea or vomiting
> Skin rash, hives, or itching
> Stomach cramps or pain

For patients taking anisindione tablets:

• Depending on your diet, this medicine may cause your urine to turn orange. Since it may be hard to tell the difference between blood in the urine and this normal color change, check with your doctor if you notice any color change in your urine.

Other side effects may occur that usually do not require medical attention. These side effects may go away during treatment as your body adjusts to the medicine. However, check with your doctor if any of the following side effects continue or are bothersome:

More common
> Bloated feeling or gas (with dicumarol)

Less common
> Blurred vision or other vision problems (with anisindione)
> Loss of appetite
> Unusual hair loss

For very young or elderly patients: Bleeding problems may be especially likely to occur in infants or in elderly patients, who are usually more sensitive to the effects of anticoagulants.

Other side effects not listed above may also occur in some patients. If you notice any other effects, check with your doctor.

December 1987

ANTICONVULSANTS, DIONE (Systemic)

This information applies to the following medicines:
Paramethadione (par-a-meth-a-DYE-one)
Trimethadione (trye-meth-a-DYE-one)

Some commonly used brand names are:	Generic names:
Paradione	Paramethadione
Tridione	Trimethadione

To the Reader: If you do not recognize the names of medical conditions or medicines referred to in this information, check with your doctor, nurse, or pharmacist. Definitions for selected medical terms may be found in the Glossary. Brand names for the generic drug names listed can be found in the Index. In addition, selected brand names commonly associated with the generic name have been included in the text to help you recognize medicine you may be taking. The fact that a brand name product is not mentioned does not mean the information does not apply. It is a good idea for you to learn both the generic and brand names of your medicines and to write them down for future use.

Dione anticonvulsants are used to control certain seizures in the treatment of epilepsy. These medicines act on the central nervous system (CNS) to reduce the number of seizures.

This medicine is available only with your doctor's prescription.

Remember:
• **This medicine has been prescribed for your current medical problem only.** It must not be given to other people or used for other problems unless you are directed to do so by your doctor.

• **Keep all medicines out of the reach of children.**

• In order for this medicine to work, it must be used as directed.

• **It is very important that you read and understand the following information.** If any of the information causes you special concern, do not decide against using this medicine without first checking with your doctor.

• Before you begin using any new medicine (prescription or nonprescription) or if you develop any new medical problem while you are using this medicine, check with your doctor, nurse, or pharmacist.

• **If you have any questions** about the following information or if you want more information about this medicine or your medical problem, **ask your doctor, nurse, or pharmacist.**

Before Using This Medicine

In order to decide on the best treatment for your medical problem, your doctor should be told:
—if you have had any unusual reaction to anticonvulsant medicines in the past.

—if you are on a low-salt, low-sugar, or any other special diet, or if you are allergic to any substance, such as foods, sulfites or other preservatives, or dyes.

Most medicines contain more than their active ingredient, and many liquid medicines contain alcohol. Your doctor, nurse, or pharmacist can help you avoid products that may cause a problem.

—if you are **pregnant** or if you may become pregnant. Although most mothers who take medicine for seizure control deliver normal babies, there have been reports of increased birth defects when dione anticonvulsants were used during pregnancy. This medicine may also cause a bleeding problem in the mother during delivery and in the newborn. Doctors can help prevent this by giving vitamin K to the mother 1 month before and during delivery, and to the baby immediately after birth.

—if you are **breast-feeding**. It is not known whether this medicine passes into breast milk. Dione anticonvulsants have not been shown to cause problems in nursing babies.

—if you have any of the following medical problems:
Blood disease (severe)
Diseases of the eye or optic nerve
Kidney disease (severe)
Liver disease (severe)

—if you are taking **any** other prescription or nonprescription (OTC) medicine, especially:
Central nervous system (CNS) depressants

Proper Use of This Medicine

If you are taking paramethadione capsules:
• Swallow the capsules whole. Do not crush, chew, or break them before swallowing.

If you are taking paramethadione oral solution:
• Take this medicine by mouth even though it comes in a dropper bottle.

• Measure the amount to be taken with the specially marked dropper.

• This medicine may be dropped directly into the mouth or, for small children, mixed with half a glass of water or juice.

If you are taking trimethadione tablets:
• The tablets may be chewed or crushed and dissolved in a small amount of water before swallowing.

If this medicine upsets your stomach, take it with food or milk unless otherwise directed by your doctor.

This medicine must be taken every day in regularly spaced doses as ordered by your doctor.

If you miss a dose of this medicine, take it as soon as possible. However, if it is almost time for your next dose, skip the missed dose and go back to your regular dosing schedule. Do not double doses.

How to store this medicine:

- **Keep out of the reach of children.**

- Store away from heat and direct light.

- Do not store the capsule or tablet form of this medicine in the bathroom, near the kitchen sink, or in other damp places. Heat or moisture may cause the medicine to break down.

- Keep the liquid form of this medicine from freezing.

- Do not keep outdated medicine or medicine no longer needed. Be sure that any discarded medicine is out of the reach of children.

Precautions While Using This Medicine

It is very important that your doctor check your progress at regular visits, especially during the first few months that you take this medicine.

If you have been taking this medicine regularly, do not stop taking it without first checking with your doctor. Your doctor may want you to reduce gradually the amount you are taking before stopping completely, to reduce the possibility of seizures.

This medicine may cause your eyes to become more sensitive to bright light than they are normally, making it difficult for you to see well. Wearing sunglasses and avoiding too much exposure to bright light may help lessen the discomfort. You may also have difficulty seeing in light that changes in brightness. If you notice this effect, be especially careful when driving at night.

This medicine will add to the effects of alcohol and other CNS depressants (medicines that slow down the nervous system, possibly causing drowsiness). Some examples of CNS depressants are antihistamines or medicine for hay fever, other allergies, or colds; sedatives, tranquilizers, or sleeping medicine; prescription pain medicine or narcotics; barbiturates; medicine for seizures; muscle relaxants; or anesthetics, including some dental anesthetics. **Check with your doctor before taking any of the above while you are using this medicine.**

This medicine may cause some people to become drowsy or less alert than they are normally. **Make sure you know how you react to this medicine before you drive, use machines, or do other jobs that require you to be alert.** After you have taken this medicine for a while, this effect may not be so bothersome.

Before having any kind of surgery, dental treatment, or emergency treatment, tell the physician or dentist in charge that you are taking this medicine.

Side Effects of This Medicine

Along with its needed effects, a medicine may cause some unwanted effects. Although not all of these side effects may occur, if they do occur they may need medical attention.

Check with your doctor as soon as possible if any of the following side effects occur:

More common
> Changes in vision, such as glare or snowy image caused by bright light

Rare
> Muscle weakness (severe), especially of the eyes, face, lips, tongue, throat, and neck
> Skin rash
> Sore throat and fever
> Swelling of face, hands, legs, and feet
> Swollen glands
> Unusual bleeding or bruising, such as recurring nosebleeds or bleeding gums
> Yellow eyes or skin

Other side effects may occur that usually do not require medical attention. These side effects may go away during treatment as your body adjusts to the medicine. However, check with your doctor if any of the following side effects continue or are bothersome:

More common
> Dizziness
> Drowsiness (more often with paramethadione)
> Headache
> Increased sensitivity of eyes to light

Less common
> Hair loss
> Itchy skin
> Loss of appetite or weight
> Nausea or vomiting
> Unusual tiredness or weakness

For elderly patients: Many medicines have not been tested in older patients. Therefore, it is not known whether the medicine acts the same way it does in younger adults. Check with your doctor or pharmacist if you notice any unusual effects while taking this medicine or if you think it is not working as it should.

Other side effects not listed above may also occur in some patients. If you notice any other effects, check with your doctor.

December 1987

ANTICONVULSANTS, HYDANTOIN
(Systemic)

This information applies to the following medicines:

Ethotoin (ETH-oh-toyn)
Mephenytoin (me-FEN-i-toyn)
Phenytoin (FEN-i-toyn)

Some commonly used brand names and other names are:	Generic names:
Peganone	Ethotoin
Mesantoin	Mephenytoin
Dilantin Dilantin-125 Dilantin Infatabs Dilantin Kapseals Dilantin-30 Pediatric Diphenylan Diphenylhydantoin	Phenytoin†

†Generic name product may also be available in the U.S.

To the Reader: If you do not recognize the names of medical conditions or medicines referred to in this information, check with your doctor, nurse, or pharmacist. Definitions for selected medical terms may be found in the Glossary. Brand names for the generic drug names listed can be found in the Index. In addition, selected brand names commonly associated with the generic name have been included in the text to help you recognize medicine you may be taking. The fact that a brand name product is not mentioned does not mean the information does not apply. It is a good idea for you to learn both the generic and brand names of your medicines and to write them down for future use.

Hydantoin anticonvulsants (hye-DAN-toyn an-tye-kon-VUL-sants) are used most often to control certain convulsions or seizures in the treatment of epilepsy. Phenytoin may also be used for other conditions as determined by your doctor.

These medicines act on the central nervous system (CNS) to reduce the number and severity of seizures. Hydantoin anticonvulsants may also produce some unwanted effects. These depend on the patient's individual condition, the amount of medicine taken, and how long it has been taken. It is important that you know what the side effects are and when to call your doctor if they occur.

Hydantoin anticonvulsants are available only with your doctor's prescription.

Remember:

• **This medicine has been prescribed for your current medical problem only.** It must not be given to other people or used for other problems unless you are directed to do so by your doctor.

• **Keep all medicines out of the reach of children.**

• In order for this medicine to work, it must be used as directed.

• If you are receiving this medicine by injection, some of the information about this medicine may not apply.

• **It is very important that you read and understand the following information.** If any of the information causes you special concern, do not decide against using this medicine without first checking with your doctor.

• Before you begin using any new medicine (prescription or nonprescription) or if you develop any new medical problem while you are using this medicine, check with your doctor, nurse, or pharmacist.

• **If you have any questions** about the following information or if you want more information about this medicine or your medical problem, **ask your doctor, nurse, or pharmacist**.

Before Using This Medicine

In order to decide on the best treatment for your medical problem, your doctor should be told:

—if you have ever had any unusual or allergic reaction to any hydantoin anticonvulsant medicine.

—if you are on a low-salt, low-sugar, or any other special diet, or if you are allergic to any substance, such as foods, sulfites or other preservatives, or dyes. Most medicines contain more than their active ingredient, and many liquid medicines contain alcohol. Your doctor, nurse, or pharmacist can help you avoid products that may cause a problem.

—if you are **pregnant** or if you may become pregnant. Although most mothers who take medicine for seizure control deliver normal babies, there have been reports of increased birth defects when these medicines were used during pregnancy. It is not definitely known if any of these medicines are the cause of such problems. Also, pregnancy may cause a change in the way hydantoin anticonvulsants are absorbed in your body. You may have more seizures, even though you are taking your medicine regularly. Your doctor may need to increase the anticonvulsant dose during your pregnancy.

In addition, when taken during pregnancy, this medicine may cause a bleeding problem in the mother during delivery and in the newborn. This may be prevented by giving vitamin K to the mother 1 month before and during delivery, and to the baby immediately after birth.

—if you are **breast-feeding**. Phenytoin passes into the breast milk in small amounts. It has not been shown to cause unwanted effects in nursing babies. However, your doctor may want you to take another medicine or to stop breast-feeding during treatment. It is not known whether ethotoin or mephenytoin passes into breast milk. Be sure you have discussed the risks and benefits of the medicine with your doctor.

—if you have any of the following medical problems:
Alcoholism (active or treated)
Blood disease
Diabetes mellitus (sugar diabetes)
Heart disease
Kidney disease
Liver disease
Thyroid disease

—if you are taking **any** other prescription or nonprescription (OTC) medicine, especially:
Adrenocorticoids (cortisone-like medicines)
Aminophylline (e.g., Somophylline)
Amiodarone (e.g., Cordarone)

Anticoagulants (blood thinners)
Caffeine (e.g., Caffedrine; Dexitac; NoDoz)
Central nervous system (CNS) depressants
Chloramphenicol (e.g., Chloromycetin)
Cimetidine (e.g., Tagamet)
Diazoxide (e.g., Proglycem)
Disulfiram (e.g., Antabuse) (medicine for alcoholism)
Estrogens
Folic acid (e.g., Folvite, and also contained in some vitamin formulas)
Isoniazid (INH) (e.g., Nydrazid)
Medicine containing calcium
Methadone (e.g., Dolophine; Methadose)
Oral contraceptives (birth-control pills) containing estrogens
Oxtriphylline (e.g., Choledyl)
Phenylbutazone (e.g., Butazolidin)
Pimozide (e.g., Orap)
Sulfinpyrazone (e.g., Anturane)
Sulfonamides (sulfa drugs)
Theophylline (e.g., Somophylline-T)

Proper Use of This Medicine

For patients taking the liquid form of this medicine:
• Shake the bottle well before using.
• Use a specially marked measuring spoon, a plastic syringe, or a small measuring cup to measure each dose accurately. The average household teaspoon may not hold the right amount of liquid.

For patients taking the chewable tablet form of this medicine:
• Chew or crush the tablet before swallowing it.

For patients taking the capsule form of this medicine:
• Swallow the capsule whole.

If this medicine upsets your stomach, take it with food or milk, unless otherwise directed by your doctor.

In order to control your medical problem, **take this medicine every day** exactly as ordered by your doctor. Do not take more or less of it than your doctor ordered. To help you remember to take the medicine at the correct times, try to get into the habit of taking it at the same time each day.

If you miss a dose of this medicine and your dosing schedule is one dose to be taken:
Once a day—Take the missed dose as soon as possible. However, if you do not remember the missed dose until the next day, skip it and go back to your regular dosing schedule. Do not double doses.
Several times a day—Take the missed dose as soon as possible. However, if it is within 4 hours of your next dose, skip the missed dose and go back to your regular dosing schedule. Do not double doses.
If you miss doses for 2 or more days in a row, check with your doctor.

How to store this medicine:
• **Keep out of the reach of children.**
• Store away from heat and direct light.
• Do not store in the bathroom, near the kitchen sink, or in other damp places. Heat or moisture may cause the medicine to break down.

• Keep the liquid form of this medicine from freezing. Do not refrigerate.

• Do not keep outdated medicine or medicine no longer needed. Be sure any discarded medicine is out of the reach of children.

Precautions While Using This Medicine

Your doctor should check your progress at regular visits, especially during the first few months you take this medicine. During this time the amount of medicine you are taking may have to be changed often to meet your individual needs.

Do not start or stop taking any other medicine without your doctor's advice. Other medicines may affect the way this medicine works.

This medicine will add to the effects of alcohol and other CNS depressants (medicines that slow down the nervous system, possibly causing drowsiness). Some examples of CNS depressants are antihistamines or medicine for hay fever, other allergies, or colds; sedatives, tranquilizers, or sleeping medicine; prescription pain medicine or narcotics; barbiturates; medicine for seizures; muscle relaxants; or anesthetics, including some dental anesthetics. **Check with your doctor before taking any of the above while you are using this medicine.**

Do not change brands or dosage forms of phenytoin without first checking with your doctor. Different products may not work the same way. If you refill your medicine and it looks different, check with your pharmacist.

If you have been taking this medicine regularly for several weeks or more, do not suddenly stop taking it. Your doctor may want you to reduce gradually the amount you are taking before stopping completely.

Your doctor may want you to carry a medical identification card or bracelet stating that you are taking this medicine.

Diabetic patients—This medicine may affect blood sugar levels. If you notice a change in the results of your blood or urine sugar tests or if you have any questions, check with your doctor.

Before having any kind of surgery, dental treatment, or emergency treatment, tell the physician or dentist in charge that you are taking this medicine.

This medicine may cause some people to become dizzy, lightheaded, drowsy, or less alert than they are normally. After you have taken this medicine for a while, this effect may not be so bothersome. However, **make sure you know how you react to this medicine before you drive, use machines, or do other jobs that require you to be alert.**

For patients taking phenytoin or mephenytoin:
• In some patients (usually younger patients), tenderness, swelling, or bleeding of the gums may appear soon after phenytoin treatment is started. To help prevent this, brush and floss your teeth carefully and regularly and massage your gums. Also, **see your dentist**

regularly to have your teeth cleaned. If you have any
questions about how to take care of your teeth and
gums, or if you notice any tenderness, swelling, or
bleeding of your gums, check with your physician or
dentist.

Side Effects of This Medicine

Along with its needed effects, a medicine may cause some
unwanted effects. Although not all of these side effects
may occur, if they do occur they may need medical
attention.

Check with your doctor as soon as possible if any of the
following side effects or signs of overdose occur:

More common
  Behavior changes
  Bleeding, tender, or enlarged gums (rare with ethotoin)
  Clumsiness or unsteadiness of gait (rare with ethotoin)
  Confusion
  Continuous, uncontrolled back-and-forth and/or rolling
    eye movements
  Enlarged glands in neck or underarms
  Fever
  Increase in convulsions (seizures)
  Mood or mental changes
  Muscle weakness
  Skin rash (more common with mephenytoin)
  Slurring of speech
  Sore throat
  Trembling of hands
  Unusual excitement, nervousness, or irritability

Rare
  Unusual bleeding or bruising
  Bone malformations
  Darkening of urine
  Frequent breaking of bones
  Light gray–colored stools
  Loss of appetite
  Restlessness or agitation
  Slowed growth
  Sore throat and fever
  Stomach pain (severe)
  Uncontrolled jerking or twisting movements of hands,
    arms, or legs
  Uncontrolled movements of lips, tongue, or cheeks
  Yellow eyes or skin

Signs of overdose
  Blurred or double vision
  Clumsiness or unsteadiness
  Confusion
  Dizziness or drowsiness (severe)
  Hallucinations (seeing, hearing, or feeling things that are
    not there)
  Nausea
  Slurred speech
  Staggering walk
  Uncontrolled eye movements

Other side effects may occur that usually do not require
medical attention. These side effects may go away
during treatment as your body adjusts to the medicine.
However, check with your doctor if any of the following side effects continue or are bothersome:

More common
  Constipation
  Dizziness (mild)
  Drowsiness (mild)
  Nausea and vomiting

Less common or rare
  Diarrhea (with ethotoin)
  Enlargement of jaw
  Headache
  Muscle twitching
  Swelling of breasts—in males
  Thickening of lips
  Trouble in sleeping
  Unusual and excessive hair growth on body and face (more
    common with phenytoin)
  Widening of nose tip

For elderly patients: The above side effects, especially
the signs of overdose, are more likely to occur in elderly patients and patients with liver disease, who are
usually more sensitive to the effects of hydantoin anticonvulsants.

Some of the above side effects, especially bleeding, tender, or enlarged gums and enlarged facial features are
more likely to occur in young patients. Unusual and
excessive hair growth is more noticeable in young girls.

Other side effects not listed above may also occur in some
patients. If you notice any other effects, check with
your doctor.

_____

December 1987

ANTICONVULSANTS, SUCCINIMIDE
(Systemic)

This information applies to the following medicines:
Ethosuximide (eth-oh-SUX-i-mide)
Methsuximide (meth-SUX-i-mide)
Phensuximide (fen-SUX-i-mide)

Some commonly used brand names are:	Generic names:
Celontin	Methsuximide
Milontin	Phensuximide
Zarontin	Ethosuximide

To the Reader: If you do not recognize the names of medical conditions or medicines referred to in this information, check with your doctor, nurse, or pharmacist. Definitions for selected medical terms may be found in the Glossary. Brand names for the generic drug names listed can be found in the Index. In addition, selected brand names commonly associated with the generic name have been included in the text to help you recognize medicine you may be taking. The fact that a brand name product is not mentioned does not mean the information does not apply. It is a good idea for you to learn both the generic and brand names of your medicines and to write them down for future use.

Succinimide anticonvulsants are used to control certain seizures in the treatment of epilepsy. These medicines act on the central nervous system (CNS) to reduce the number and severity of seizures.

This medicine is available only with your doctor's prescription.

Remember:
• **This medicine has been prescribed for your current medical problem only.** It must not be given to other people or used for other problems unless you are directed to do so by your doctor.

• **Keep all medicines out of the reach of children.**

• In order for this medicine to work, it must be used as directed.

• **It is very important that you read and understand the following information.** If any of the information causes you special concern, do not decide against using this medicine without first checking with your doctor.

• Before you begin using any new medicine (prescription or nonprescription) or if you develop any new medical problem while you are using this medicine, check with your doctor, nurse, or pharmacist.

• **If you have any questions** about the following information or if you want more information about this medicine or your medical problem, **ask your doctor, nurse, or pharmacist.**

Before Using This Medicine

In order to decide on the best treatment for your medical problem, your doctor should be told:
—if you have had any unusual or allergic reactions to anticonvulsant medicines.

—if you are on a low-salt, low-sugar, or any other special diet, or if you are allergic to any substance, such as foods, sulfites or other preservatives, or dyes.

Most medicines contain more than their active ingredient, and many liquid medicines contain alcohol. Your doctor, nurse, or pharmacist can help you avoid products that may cause a problem.

—if you are **pregnant**, or if you may become pregnant. Although succinimide anticonvulsants have not been shown to cause problems in humans, there have been unproven reports of increased birth defects associated with the use of other anticonvulsant medicines.

—if you are **breast-feeding**. It is not known whether succinimide anticonvulsants pass into breast milk. This medicine has not been shown to cause problems in nursing babies.

—if you have any of the following medical problems:
  Blood disease
  Intermittent porphyria
  Kidney disease (severe)
  Liver disease

—if you are now taking **any** other prescription or nonprescription (OTC) medicine, especially:
  Central nervous system (CNS) depressants
  Haloperidol (e.g., Haldol)

Proper Use of This Medicine

This medicine must be taken every day in regularly spaced doses as ordered by your doctor. Do not take more or less of it than your doctor ordered.

If this medicine upsets your stomach, take it with food or milk unless otherwise directed by your doctor.

If you miss a dose of this medicine, take it as soon as possible. However, if it is within 4 hours of your next dose, skip the missed dose and go back to your regular dosing schedule. Do not double doses.

How to store this medicine:
• **Keep out of the reach of children.**

• Store away from heat and direct light.

• Do not store in the bathroom, near the kitchen sink, or in other damp places. Heat or moisture may cause the medicine to break down.

• Keep the medicine from freezing. Do not refrigerate.

• Do not keep outdated medicine or medicine that is no longer needed. Be sure any discarded medicine is out of the reach of children.

Precautions While Using This Medicine

Your doctor should check your progress at regular visits, especially during the first few months you take this medicine. During this time the amount of medicine you are taking may have to be changed often to meet your individual needs.

If you have been taking a succinimide anticonvulsant regularly, do not stop taking it without first checking with your doctor. Your doctor may want you to reduce gradually the amount you are taking before stopping completely. Stopping this medicine suddenly may cause seizures.

This medicine will add to the effects of alcohol and other CNS depressants (medicines that slow down the nervous system, possibly causing drowsiness). Some examples of CNS depressants are antihistamines or medicine for hay fever, other allergies, or colds; sedatives, tranquilizers, or sleeping medicine; prescription pain medicine or narcotics; barbiturates; medicine for seizures; muscle relaxants; or anesthetics, including some dental anesthetics. **Check with your doctor before taking any of the above while you are using this medicine.**

This medicine may cause some people to become drowsy or less alert than they are normally. **Make sure you know how you react to this medicine before you drive, use machines, or do other jobs that require you to be alert.** After you have taken this medicine for a while, this effect may lessen.

Before having any kind of surgery, dental treatment, or emergency treatment, tell the physician or dentist in charge that you are taking this medicine.

Your doctor may want you to carry a medical identification card or bracelet stating that you are taking this medicine.

For patients taking methsuximide:
- Do not use capsules that are not full or in which the contents have melted, because they may not work as well.

Side Effects of This Medicine

Along with its needed effects, a medicine may cause some unwanted effects. Although not all of these side effects may occur, if they do occur they may need medical attention.

Check with your doctor as soon as possible if any of the following side effects occur:

More common
    Skin rash or itching

Less common
    Mood or mental changes
Rare
    Sore throat and fever
    Swollen glands
    Bleeding or bruising

Other side effects may occur that usually do not require medical attention. These side effects may go away during treatment as your body adjusts to the medicine. However, check with your doctor if any of the following side effects continue or are bothersome:

More common
    Headache
    Hiccups
    Loss of appetite
    Nausea and vomiting
    Stomach cramps

Less common
    Dizziness
    Drowsiness
    Irritability
    Tiredness

Phensuximide may cause the urine to turn pink, red, or red-brown. This is harmless and is to be expected while you are taking this medicine.

For elderly patients: Many medicines have not been tested in older people. Therefore, it is not known whether the medicine acts the same way it does in younger adults. Check with your doctor or pharmacist if you notice any unusual effects while taking this medicine or if you do not think it is working as it should.

Other side effects not listed above may also occur in some patients. If you notice any other effects, check with your doctor.

December 1987

ANTIDEPRESSANTS, MONOAMINE OXIDASE (MAO) INHIBITOR (Systemic)

This information applies to the following medicines:
Isocarboxazid (eye-soe-kar-BOX-a-zid)
Phenelzine (FEN-el-zeen)
Tranylcypromine (tran-ill-SIP-roe-meen)
This information does *not* apply to furazolidone, pargyline, or procarbazine.

Some commonly used brand names are:	Generic names:
Marplan	Isocarboxazid
Nardil	Phenelzine
Parnate	Tranylcypromine

To the Reader: If you do not recognize the names of medical conditions or medicines referred to in this information, check with your doctor, nurse, or pharmacist. Definitions for selected medical terms may be found in the Glossary. Brand names for the generic drug names listed can be found in the Index. In addition, selected brand names commonly associated with the generic name have been included in the text to help you recognize medicine you may be taking. The fact that a brand name product is not mentioned does not mean the information does not apply. It is a good idea for you to learn both the generic and brand names of your medicines and to write them down for future use.

MAO inhibitors or MAOIs are taken by mouth to relieve certain types of mental depression. They work by inhibiting an enzyme in the nervous system known as monoamine oxidase (MAO).

Although these medicines are very effective for certain patients, they may also cause some unwanted reactions if not taken in the right way. It is very important to avoid certain foods, beverages, and medicines while you are being treated with an MAOI. Your doctor, nurse, or pharmacist will help you obtain a list of the products you should avoid that you can carry in your wallet or purse as a reminder.

MAO inhibitors are available only with your doctor's prescription.

Remember:

• **This medicine has been prescribed for your current medical problem only.** It must not be given to other people or used for other problems unless you are directed to do so by your doctor.

• **Keep all medicines out of the reach of children.**

• In order for this medicine to work, it must be used as directed.

• **It is very important that you read and understand the following information.** If any of the information causes you special concern, do not decide against using this medicine without first checking with your doctor.

• Before you begin using any new medicine (prescription or nonprescription) or if you develop any new medical problem while you are using this medicine, check with your doctor, nurse, or pharmacist.

• **If you have any questions** about the following information or if you want more information about this medicine or your medical problem, **ask your doctor, nurse, or pharmacist.**

Before Using This Medicine

In order to decide on the best treatment for your medical problem, your doctor should be told:

—if you have ever had any unusual or allergic reaction to any monoamine oxidase inhibitor.

—if you are on a low-salt, low-sugar, or any other special diet, or if you are allergic to any substance, such as foods, sulfites or other preservatives, or dyes. Most medicines contain more than their active ingredient. Your doctor, nurse, or pharmacist can help you avoid products that may cause a problem.

—if you are **pregnant** or if you may become pregnant. Studies have not been done in humans. However, in animal studies, MAO inhibitors caused a slowing of growth and increased excitability in the newborn when very large doses were given to the mother during pregnancy.

—if you are **breast-feeding**. MAO inhibitors have not been shown to cause problems in nursing babies; however, studies in animals have shown that this medicine passes into breast milk.

—if you have any of the following medical problems:
Alcoholism (active or treated)
Angina (chest pain)
Asthma or bronchitis
Diabetes mellitus (sugar diabetes)
Epilepsy
Headaches (severe or frequent)
Heart or blood vessel disease
High blood pressure
Kidney disease
Liver disease
Mental illness (or history of)
Overactive thyroid
Parkinson's disease
Pheochromocytoma (PCC)

—if you have recently had a stroke or heart attack.

—if you are taking **any** other prescription or nonprescription (OTC) medicine, especially:
Amphetamines (e.g., Dexedrine; Desoxyn)
Antidiabetic agents, oral (diabetes medicine you take by mouth)
Antihypertensives (high blood pressure medicine)
Antimuscarinics (medicine for abdominal or stomach spasms or cramps)
Appetite suppressants (diet pills)
Caffeine-containing medicine
Carbamazepine (e.g., Tegretol)
Central nervous system (CNS) depressants
Cyclobenzaprine (e.g., Flexeril)
Insulin
Levodopa (e.g., Dopar)
Maprotiline (e.g., Ludiomil)
Medicine for asthma or other breathing problems
Methylphenidate (e.g., Ritalin)
Nasal decongestants or other cold medicines
Tricyclic antidepressants (amitriptyline, amoxapine, clomipramine, desipramine, doxepin, imipramine, nortriptyline, protriptyline, trimipramine)

—if you are now taking or have taken within the past 2 weeks any *other* monoamine oxidase (MAO) inhibitors, including furazolidone (e.g., Furoxone), pargyline (e.g., Eutonyl), or procarbazine (e.g., Matulane).

—if you use cocaine. Cocaine use by persons taking MAO inhibitors, including furazolidone, pargyline, and procarbazine, may cause a severe increase in blood pressure.

Proper Use of This Medicine

Sometimes this medicine must be taken for several weeks before you begin to feel better. Your doctor should check your progress at regular visits.

Take this medicine only as directed by your doctor. Do not take more of it, do not take it more often, and do not take it for a longer period of time than your doctor ordered.

If you miss a dose of this medicine, take it as soon as possible. However, if it is within 2 hours of your next dose, skip the missed dose and go back to your regular dosing schedule. Do not double doses.

How to store this medicine:

- **Keep out of the reach of children.**

- Store away from heat and direct light.

- Do not store in the bathroom, near the kitchen sink, or in other damp places. Heat or moisture may cause the medicine to break down.

- Do not keep outdated medicine or medicine no longer needed. Be sure that any discarded medicine is out of the reach of children.

Precautions While Using This Medicine

It is very important that your doctor check your progress at regular visits, especially during the first few months of treatment, to make sure that this medicine is working properly and to check for unwanted effects.

When taken with certain foods, drinks, or other medicines, MAO inhibitors can cause very dangerous reactions. To avoid such reactions, **obey the following rules of caution:**

- Do not eat foods that have a high tyramine content (most common in foods that are aged or fermented to increase their flavor), such as cheeses, yeast or meat extracts, fava or broad bean pods, smoked or pickled fish, beef or chicken liver, fermented sausage (bologna, pepperoni, salami, and summer sausage) or other unfresh meat, or any overripe fruit. If a list of these foods and beverages is not given to you, ask your doctor, nurse, or pharmacist to provide one.

- Do not drink alcoholic beverages, including beer and wines (especially chianti and other hearty red wines).

- Do not eat or drink excessive amounts of caffeine-containing food or beverages such as chocolate, coffee, tea, or cola.

- Do not take any other medicine unless approved or prescribed by your doctor. This especially includes over-the-counter (OTC) or nonprescription medicine, such as that for colds (including nose drops or sprays), cough, asthma, hay fever, and appetite control; "keep awake" products; or products that make you sleepy.

This medicine will add to the effects of alcohol and other CNS depressants (medicines that slow down the nervous system, possibly causing drowsiness). Some examples of CNS depressants are antihistamines or medicine for hay fever, other allergies, or colds; sedatives, tranquilizers, or sleeping medicine; prescription pain medicine or narcotics; barbiturates; medicine for seizures; muscle relaxants; or anesthetics, including some dental anesthetics. **Check with your doctor before taking any of the above while you are using this medicine.**

Check with your doctor or hospital emergency room immediately if severe headache, stiff neck, chest pains, fast heartbeat, or nausea and vomiting occur while you are taking this medicine. These may be symptoms of a serious side effect that should have a doctor's attention.

Do not stop taking this medicine without first checking with your doctor. Your doctor may want you to reduce gradually the amount you are using before stopping completely.

Dizziness, lightheadedness, or fainting may occur, especially when you get up from a lying or sitting position. **Getting up slowly may help.** When you get up from lying down, sit on the edge of the bed with your feet dangling for 1 or 2 minutes. Then stand up slowly. If the problem continues or gets worse, check with your doctor.

This medicine may cause some people to become drowsy or less alert than they are normally. **Make sure you know how you react to this medicine before you drive, use machines, or do other jobs that require you to be alert.**

Before having any kind of surgery, dental treatment, or emergency treatment, tell the physician or dentist in charge that you are using this medicine or have used it within the past 2 weeks.

Your doctor may want you to carry an identification card stating that you are using this medicine.

Patients with angina (chest pain)—This medicine may cause you to have an unusual feeling of good health and energy. However, **do not suddenly increase the amount of exercise you get without discussing it with your doctor.** Too much activity could bring on an attack of angina.

Diabetic patients—This medicine may affect blood sugar levels. While you are using this medicine, be especially careful in testing for sugar in your blood or urine. If you have any questions about this, check with your doctor.

After you stop using this medicine, you must continue to obey the rules of caution concerning food, drink, and other medicine for at least 2 weeks since they may continue to react with MAO inhibitors.

Side Effects of This Medicine

Along with its needed effects, a medicine may cause some unwanted effects. Although not all of these side effects may occur, if they do occur they may need medical attention.

Stop taking this medicine and get emergency help immediately if any of the following side effects occur:

Signs of unusually high blood pressure

Chest pain (severe)
Enlarged pupils
Fast or slow heartbeat
Headache (severe)
Increased sensitivity of eyes to light
Increased sweating (possibly with fever or cold, clammy skin)
Nausea and vomiting
Stiff or sore neck

Check with your doctor as soon as possible if any of the following side effects occur:

More common

Dizziness or lightheadedness (severe), especially when getting up from a lying or sitting position

Less common

Diarrhea
Fast or pounding heartbeat
Swelling of feet or lower legs
Unusual excitement or nervousness

Rare

Dark urine
Skin rash
Yellow eyes or skin

Signs of overdose

Anxiety (severe)
Confusion
Cool, clammy skin
Convulsions (seizures)
Dizziness (severe)
Drowsiness (severe)
Fast and irregular pulse
Fever
Hallucinations (seeing, hearing, or feeling things that are not there)
Headache (severe)
High or low blood pressure
Sweating
Trouble in sleeping (severe)
Troubled breathing
Unusual irritability

Other side effects may occur that usually do not require medical attention. These side effects may go away during treatment as your body adjusts to the medicine. However, check with your doctor if any of the following side effects continue or are bothersome:

More common

Blurred vision
Constipation
Decreased sexual ability
Difficult urination
Dizziness or lightheadedness (mild), especially when getting up from a lying or sitting position
Drowsiness
Headache (mild)
Increased appetite (especially for sweets) or weight gain
Muscle twitching during sleep
Restlessness
Shakiness or trembling
Tiredness and weakness
Trouble in sleeping
Weakness

Less common or rare

Chills
Dry mouth

After you stop using this medicine, your body may need time to adjust. The length of time this takes depends on the the amount of medicine you were using and how long you used it. Check with your doctor if any of the following side effects occur:

Agitation, confusion, or irritability
Drowsiness
Fast heartbeat
Hallucinations
Headache
Nausea
Nightmares (severe)
Shivering
Slurred speech
Staggering walk
Sweating

The above side effects are more likely to occur in elderly patients, who are usually more sensitive to the effects of monoamine oxidase inhibitor antidepressants.

Other side effects not listed above may also occur in some patients. If you notice any other effects, check with your doctor.

December 1987

ANTIDEPRESSANTS, TRICYCLIC
(Systemic)

This information applies to the following medicines:

Amitriptyline (a-mee-TRIP-ti-leen)
Amoxapine (a-MOX-a-peen)
Clomipramine (cloe-MIP-ra-meen)
Desipramine (dess-IP-ra-meen)
Doxepin (DOX-e-pin)
Imipramine (im-IP-ra-meen)
Nortriptyline (nor-TRIP-ti-leen)
Protriptyline (proe-TRIP-ti-leen)
Trimipramine (trye-MIP-ra-meen)

Some commonly used brand names are:	Generic names:
Amitril Apo-Amitriptyline* Elavil Emitrip Endep Enovil Levate* Meravil* Novotriptyn*	Amitriptyline†
Asendin	Amoxapine
Anafranil*	Clomipramine*
Norpramin Pertofrane	Desipramine
Adapin Sinequan Triadapin*	Doxepin
Apo-Imipramine* Impril* Janimine Novopramine* Tipramine Tofranil Tofranil-PM	Imipramine†
Aventyl Pamelor	Nortriptyline
Vivactil Triptil*	Protriptyline
Surmontil	Trimipramine

*Not commercially available in the U.S.
†Generic name product may also be available in the U.S.

To the Reader: If you do not recognize the names of medical conditions or medicines referred to in this information, check with your doctor, nurse, or pharmacist. Definitions for selected medical terms may be found in the Glossary. Brand names for the generic drug names listed can be found in the Index. In addition, selected brand names commonly associated with the generic name have been included in the text to help you recognize medicine you may be taking. The fact that a brand name product is not mentioned does not mean the information does not apply. It is a good idea for you to learn both the generic and brand names of your medicines and to write them down for future use.

Tricyclic antidepressants ("mood elevators") are used to relieve mental depression and depression that sometimes occurs with anxiety.

One form of this medicine (imipramine) is also used to treat enuresis (bedwetting). Tricyclic antidepressants may also be used for other conditions as determined by your doctor.

These medicines are available only with your doctor's prescription.

Remember:
• **This medicine has been prescribed for your current medical problem only.** It must not be given to other people or used for other problems unless you are directed to do so by your doctor.

• **Keep all medicines out of the reach of children.**

• In order for this medicine to work, it must be used as directed.

• If you are receiving this medicine by injection, some of the information about this medicine may not apply.

• **It is very important that you read and understand the following information.** If any of the information causes you special concern, do not decide against using this medicine without first checking with your doctor.

• Before you begin using any new medicine (prescription or nonprescription) or if you develop any new medical problem while you are using this medicine, check with your doctor, nurse, or pharmacist.

• **If you have any questions** about the following information or if you want more information about this medicine or your medical problem, **ask your doctor, nurse, or pharmacist**.

Before Using This Medicine

In order to decide on the best treatment for your medical problem, your doctor should be told:

—if you have ever had an unusual or allergic reaction to any tricyclic antidepressant or maprotiline or trazodone.

—if you are on a low-salt, low-sugar, or any other special diet, or if you are allergic to any substance, such as foods, sulfites or other preservatives, or dyes. Most medicines contain more than their active ingredient, and many liquid medicines contain alcohol. Your doctor, nurse, or pharmacist can help you avoid products that may cause a problem.

—if you are **pregnant** or if you may become pregnant. Studies have not been done in humans. However, there have been reports of newborns suffering from heart, breathing, and urinary problems and muscle spasms when their mothers had taken tricyclic antidepressants immediately before delivery. Also, studies in animals have shown that some tricyclic antidepressants may cause unwanted effects in the fetus.

—if you are **breast-feeding**. Some tricyclic antidepressants may pass into the breast milk. However, these medicines have not been shown to cause problems in nursing babies.

—if you have any of the following medical problems:
  Alcoholism, active or treated
  Asthma
  Bipolar disorder (manic-depressive illness)

Blood disorders
Convulsions (seizures)
Difficult urination
Enlarged prostate
Glaucoma or increased eye pressure
Heart disease
High blood pressure
Kidney disease
Liver disease
Overactive thyroid
Schizophrenia
Stomach or intestinal problems

—if you are taking **any** other prescription or nonprescription (OTC) medicine, especially:

Antithyroid agents (medicine for overactive thyroid)
Appetite suppressants (diet pills)
Central nervous system (CNS) depressants
Cimetidine (e.g., Tagamet)
Ephedrine
Epinephrine (e.g., Adrenalin)
Guanadrel (e.g., Hylorel)
Guanethidine (e.g., Ismelin)
Isoproterenol (e.g., Isuprel)
Pemoline (e.g., Cylert)
Phenylephrine (e.g., Neo-Synephrine)

—if you are now taking or have taken within the past 2 weeks monoamine oxidase (MAO) inhibitors such as:

Furazolidone (e.g., Furoxone)
Isocarboxazid (e.g., Marplan)
Pargyline (e.g., Eutonyl)
Phenelzine (e.g., Nardil)
Procarbazine (e.g., Matulane)
Tranylcypromine (e.g., Parnate)

Proper Use of This Medicine

To lessen stomach upset, take this medicine with food, even for a daily bedtime dose, unless your doctor has told you to take it on an empty stomach.

Take this medicine only as directed by your doctor, to benefit your condition as much as possible. Do not take more of it, do not take it more often, and do not take it for a longer period of time than your doctor ordered.

Sometimes this medicine must be taken for several weeks before you begin to feel better. Your doctor should check your progress at regular visits.

For patients taking doxepin oral solution:

• This medicine is to be taken by mouth even though it may come in a dropper bottle. The amount you should take is to be measured with the specially marked dropper and diluted just before you take each dose. Dilute it with about one-half glass (4 ounces) of water, milk, citrus fruit juice, tomato juice, or prune juice. Do not mix this medicine with grape juice or carbonated beverages since these may decrease the medicine's activity.

• Doxepin oral solution must be mixed immediately before taking it. Do not prepare it ahead of time.

If you miss a dose of this medicine and your dosing schedule is:

More than one dose a day—Take the missed dose as soon as possible. However, if it is almost time for your next dose, skip the missed dose, and go back to your regular dosing schedule. Do not double doses.

One dose daily at bedtime—Do not take the missed dose in the morning since it may cause disturbing side effects during waking hours. Instead, check with your doctor.

How to store this medicine:

• **Keep out of the reach of children** since overdose is especially dangerous in young children.

• Store away from heat and direct light.

• Do not store the tablet or capsule form of this medicine in the bathroom, near the kitchen sink, or in other damp places. Heat or moisture may cause the medicine to break down.

• Keep the liquid form of this medicine from freezing.

• Do not keep outdated medicine or medicine no longer needed. Be sure that any discarded medicine is out of the reach of children.

Precautions While Using This Medicine

It is very important that your doctor check your progress at regular visits, in order to allow dosage adjustments and help reduce side effects.

This medicine will add to the effects of alcohol and other CNS depressants (medicines that slow down the nervous system, possibly causing drowsiness). Some examples of CNS depressants are antihistamines or medicine for hay fever, other allergies, or colds; sedatives, tranquilizers, or sleeping medicine; prescription pain medicine or narcotics; barbiturates; medicine for seizures; muscle relaxants; or anesthetics, including some dental anesthetics. **Check with your doctor before taking any of the above while you are taking this medicine.**

This medicine may cause some people to become drowsy or less alert than they are normally. **Make sure you know how you react to this medicine before you drive, use machines, or do other jobs that require you to be alert.**

Dizziness, lightheadedness, or fainting may occur, especially when you get up from a lying or sitting position. Getting up slowly may help. If this problem continues or gets worse, check with your doctor.

This medicine may cause dryness of the mouth. For temporary relief, use sugarless gum or candy, melt bits of ice in your mouth, or use a saliva substitute. However, if your mouth continues to be dry for more than 2 weeks, check with your physician or dentist. Continuing dryness of the mouth may increase the chance of dental disease, including tooth decay, gum disease, and fungal infections.

Before having any kind of surgery, dental treatment, or emergency treatment, tell the physician or dentist in charge that you are using this medicine.

Do not stop taking this medicine without first checking with your doctor. Your doctor may want you to reduce gradually the amount you are using before stopping completely. This may help prevent a possible worsening of your condition and reduce the possibility of withdrawal symptoms such as headache, nausea, and/or an overall feeling of discomfort.

The effects of this medicine may last for 3 to 7 days after you have stopped taking it. Therefore, all the precautions stated here must be observed during this time.

For patients taking protriptyline:
- If taken late in the day, protriptyline may interfere with nighttime sleep.

Side Effects of This Medicine

Along with its needed effects, a medicine may cause some unwanted effects. Although not all of these side effects may occur, if they do occur they may need medical attention.

Stop taking this medicine and get emergency help immediately if any of the following side effects occur:
Rare
    Convulsions (seizures)
    Difficult or fast breathing
    High body temperature with increased sweating
    High or low (irregular) blood pressure
    Loss of bladder control
    Muscle stiffness (severe)
    Pale skin
    Unusual tiredness or weakness

Signs of acute overdose
    Confusion
    Convulsions (seizures) (severe)
    Drowsiness (severe)
    Fast, slow, or irregular heartbeat
    Fever
    Hallucinations
    Restlessness and agitation
    Shortness of breath or troubled breathing
    Unusual tiredness or weakness (severe)
    Vomiting

Check with your doctor as soon as possible if any of the following side effects occur:
Less common
    Blurred vision
    Confusion or delirium
    Constipation (especially in the elderly)
    Decreased sexual ability
    Difficulty in speaking or swallowing
    Eye pain
    Fainting
    Fast or irregular heartbeat (pounding, racing, skipping)
    Hallucinations (seeing, hearing, or feeling things that are not there)
    Loss of balance control
    Mask-like face
    Nervousness or restlessness

    Problems in urinating
    Shakiness or trembling
    Shuffling walk
    Slowed movements
    Stiffness of arms and legs
    Trouble in sleeping
    Uncontrolled movements of hands, mouth, tongue, arms, or legs
Rare
    Anxiety
    Breast enlargement in both males and females (with amoxapine)
    Hair loss
    Increased sensitivity to sunlight
    Irritability
    Muscle twitching
    Ringing, buzzing, or other unexplained sounds in the ears
    Skin rash and itching
    Sore throat and fever
    Swelling of face and tongue
    Swelling of testicles (with amoxapine)
    Trouble with teeth or gums
    Weakness
    Yellow eyes and skin

Other side effects may occur that usually do not require medical attention. These side effects may go away during treatment as your body adjusts to the medicine. However, check with your doctor if any of the following side effects continue or are bothersome:
More common
    Dizziness
    Drowsiness (rare with protriptyline)
    Dry mouth
    Headache
    Increased appetite for sweets
    Nausea
    Tiredness or weakness (mild) (less common with protriptyline)
    Unpleasant taste
    Weight gain
Less common
    Diarrhea
    Excessive sweating
    Heartburn
    Trouble in sleeping (more common with protriptyline, especially when taken late in the day)
    Vomiting

The above side effects, especially drowsiness, dizziness, confusion, vision problems, dry mouth, constipation, and problems in urinating are more likely to occur in elderly patients, who are usually more sensitive to the effects of tricyclic antidepressants.

Side effects in children taking this medicine for bedwetting usually disappear upon continued use. The most common of these are nervousness, sleeping problems, tiredness, and mild stomach upset. However, if these side effects continue or are bothersome, check with your doctor.

Certain side effects of this medicine may occur after you have stopped taking it. Check with your doctor if you notice any of the following effects:
    Chewing movements
    Headache
    Irritability

Lip smacking or puckering
Nausea, vomiting, or diarrhea
Puffing of cheeks
Rapid or worm-like movements of the tongue
Restlessness
Trouble in sleeping, with vivid dreams
Uncontrolled movements of arms or legs
Unusual excitement

Other side effects not listed above also may occur in some patients. If you notice any other effects, check with your doctor.

December 1987

ANTIDIABETICS, ORAL (Systemic)

This information applies to the following medicines:

Acetohexamide (a-set-oh-HEX-a-mide)
Chlorpropamide (klor-PROE-pa-mide)
Glipizide (GLIP-i-zide)
Glyburide (GLYE-byoo-ride)
Tolazamide (tole-AZ-a-mide)
Tolbutamide (tole-BYOO-ta-mide)

Some commonly used brand and other names are:	Generic names:
Dimelor* Dymelor	Acetohexamide
Apo-Chlorpropamide* Diabinese Glucamide Novopropamide*	Chlorpropamide†
Glucotrol	Glipizide
DiaBeta Euglucon* Glibenclamide Micronase	Glyburide
Ronase Tolinase	Tolazamide†
Apo-Tolbutamide* Mobenol* Novobutamide* Oramide Orinase SK-Tolbutamide	Tolbutamide†

*Not available in the U.S.
†Generic name product may also be available in the U.S.

To the Reader: If you do not recognize the names of medical conditions or medicines referred to in this information, check with your doctor, nurse, or pharmacist. Definitions for selected medical terms may be found in the Glossary. Brand names for the generic drug names listed can be found in the Index. In addition, selected brand names commonly associated with the generic name have been included in the text to help you recognize medicine you may be taking. The fact that a brand name product is not mentioned does not mean the information does not apply. It is a good idea for you to learn both the generic and brand names of your medicines and to write them down for future use.

Oral antidiabetes medicines (hypoglycemics) are taken by mouth to help reduce the amount of sugar present in the blood. They are used to treat certain types of diabetes mellitus (sugar diabetes).

Chlorpropamide may also be used for other conditions as determined by your doctor.

Oral antidiabetes medicine can usually be used only by adults who develop diabetes after 30 years of age and who do not require insulin shots (or who usually do not require more than 20 Units of insulin a day) to control their condition. This type of diabetic patient is said to have non–insulin-dependent diabetes mellitus (or NIDDM), sometimes known as maturity-onset or Type II diabetes. Oral antidiabetes medicines do not help diabetic patients who have insulin-dependent diabetes mellitus (or IDDM), sometimes known as juvenile-onset or Type I diabetes.

Patients who are taking oral antidiabetes medicines may have to switch to insulin if they:
—develop diabetic coma or ketoacidosis.
—have a severe injury or burn.
—develop a severe infection.
—are to have major surgery.
—are pregnant.

The use of oral antidiabetes medicines has been reported to increase the risk of death from heart and blood vessel disease. A study (UGDP) compared the use of one of the oral medicines (tolbutamide) to the use of diet alone or diet plus insulin. Although only tolbutamide was studied, other oral antidiabetes medicines may cause a similar effect since they are related chemically and in the way they work. Before you begin treatment with this medicine, you and your doctor should talk about the good the medicine will do as well as the risks of using it. You should also find out about other possible ways to treat your diabetes such as by diet alone or by diet plus insulin.

Oral antidiabetes medicines are available only with your doctor's prescription.

Remember:
• **This medicine has been prescribed for your current medical problem only.** It must not be given to other people or used for other problems unless you are directed to do so by your doctor.

• **Keep all medicines out of the reach of children.**

• In order for this medicine to work, it must be used as directed.

• **It is very important that you read and understand the following information.** If any of the information causes you special concern, do not decide against using this medicine without first checking with your doctor.

• Before you begin using any new medicine (prescription or nonprescription) or if you develop any new medical problem while you are using this medicine, check with your doctor, nurse, or pharmacist.

• **If you have any questions** about the following information or if you want more information about this medicine or your medical problem, **ask your doctor, nurse, or pharmacist.**

Before Using This Medicine

Importance of diet—**Before prescribing medicine for your diabetes, your doctor will probably try to control your condition by prescribing a personal meal plan for you.** Such a diet is low in refined carbohydrates (foods such as sugar and candy used for quick energy). The daily number of calories in this meal plan should equal the number of calories used by your body each day. In addition, meals and snacks are arranged to meet the energy needs of your body at different times of the day.

Many diabetic patients are able to control their condition by carefully following their doctor's orders for proper diet and exercise. **Medicine is prescribed only when additional help is needed and is effective only when a schedule of diet and exercise is properly followed.**

Oral antidiabetes medicines are less effective if you are greatly overweight. It may be very important for you to go on a reducing diet. However, check with your doctor before going on any diet.

In order to decide on the best treatment for your medical problem, your doctor should be told:

—if you have ever had any unusual or allergic reaction to any oral antidiabetes medicine, or to sulfonamide-type (sulfa) medications, including thiazide diuretics.

—if you are on a low-salt, low-sugar, or any other special diet, or if you are allergic to any substance, such as foods, sulfites or other preservatives, or dyes. Most medicines contain more than their active ingredient. Your doctor, nurse, or pharmacist can help you avoid products that may cause a problem.

—if you are **pregnant** or if you may become pregnant while taking this medicine. Oral antidiabetes medicines should not be used during pregnancy. Insulin is needed to maintain blood sugar levels as close to normal as possible. Poor control of blood sugar levels may cause birth defects or death of the fetus. In addition, use of oral antidiabetes medicines during pregnancy may cause the newborn baby to have low blood sugar levels. This may last for several days following birth.

—if you are **breast-feeding**. Chlorpropamide passes into the breast milk and its use is not recommended because it could cause low blood sugar in the baby. Although it is not known if the other oral antidiabetic agents pass into breast milk and these medicines have not been shown to cause problems in humans, the chance always exists.

—if you have any of the following medical problems:
Adrenal disease
Infection (severe)
Kidney disease
Liver disease
Pituitary disease
Thyroid disease

—if you are taking chlorpropamide and have heart disease.

—if you are taking **any** other prescription or nonprescription (OTC) medicine, especially:
Anticoagulants (blood thinners)
Aspirin or other salicylates
Beta-blockers (acebutolol, atenolol, betaxolol, labetalol, levobunolol, metoprolol, nadolol, oxprenolol, pindolol, propranolol, sotalol, timolol)
Chloramphenicol (e.g., Chloromycetin)
Guanethidine (e.g., Ismelin)
Insulin
Sulfonamides (sulfa medicine)

—if you are now taking or have taken within the past 2 weeks monoamine oxidase (MAO) inhibitors such as:
Furazolidone (e.g., Furoxone)
Isocarboxazid (e.g., Marplan)
Pargyline (e.g., Eutonyl)
Phenelzine (e.g., Nardil)
Procarbazine (e.g., Matulane)
Tranylcypromine (e.g., Parnate)

Proper Use of This Medicine

Follow carefully the special meal plan your doctor gave you. This is the most important part of controlling your condition, and is necessary if the medicine is to work properly.

Take your oral antidiabetes medicine only as directed by your doctor. Do not take more or less of it than your doctor ordered, and take it at the same time each day. This will help to control your blood sugar levels.

If you miss a dose of this medicine, take it as soon as possible. However, if it is almost time for your next dose, skip the missed dose and go back to your regular dosing schedule. Do not double doses.

How to store this medicine:

• **Keep out of the reach of children.**

• Store away from heat and direct light.

• Do not store in the bathroom, near the kitchen sink, or in other damp places. Heat or moisture may cause the medicine to break down.

• Do not keep outdated medicine or medicine no longer needed. Be sure that any discarded medicine is out of the reach of children.

Precautions While Using This Medicine

Your doctor should check your progress at regular visits, especially during the first few weeks that you take this medicine.

Test for sugar in your blood or urine as directed by your doctor. This is a convenient way to make sure your diabetes is being controlled and it provides an early warning when it is not.

Do not take any other medicine, unless prescribed or approved by your doctor. This especially includes over-the-counter (OTC) or nonprescription medicine such as that for colds, cough, asthma, hay fever, or appetite control.

Avoid alcoholic beverages until you have discussed their use with your doctor. Some patients who drink alcohol while taking this medicine may suffer stomach pain, nausea, vomiting, dizziness, pounding headache, sweating, or flushing (redness of face and skin). In addition, alcohol may produce hypoglycemia (low blood sugar).

Some people who take oral antidiabetic medicines may become more sensitive to sunlight than they are normally. When you first begin taking this medicine, avoid too much sun and do not use a sunlamp until you see how you react to the sun, especially if you tend to burn easily. **If you have a severe reaction, check with your doctor.**

Eat or drink something containing sugar and check with your doctor right away if symptoms of low blood sugar (hypoglycemia) appear. Good sources of sugar are orange juice, corn syrup, honey, or sugar cubes or table sugar (dissolved in water).

• **Signs of low blood sugar are:**

Anxious feeling
Chills
Cold sweats
Confusion
Cool pale skin
Difficulty in concentration
Drowsiness
Excessive hunger
Fast heartbeat
Headache
Nausea
Nervousness
Shakiness
Unsteady walk
Unusual tiredness or weakness

• **These signs may occur if you:**
—skip or delay meals.
—exercise much more than usual.
—cannot eat because of nausea and vomiting.
—drink a significant amount of alcohol.

• **Instruct someone with you to take you to your doctor or to a hospital right away if you think you are going to pass out.**

Even if you correct these signs by eating sugar, it is very important to call your doctor or hospital emergency service right away. The blood sugar–lowering effects of this medicine may last for days and the signs may return often during this period of time.

Before having any kind of surgery, dental treatment, or emergency treatment, tell the physician or dentist in charge that you are taking this medicine.

Your doctor may want you to carry an identification card or wear a bracelet or necklace stating that you are using this medicine.

Side Effects of This Medicine

Along with their needed effects, oral antidiabetes medicines may cause some unwanted effects. Along with the side effects described below, these medicines have been reported to increase the risks of heart and blood vessel disease. Although not all of these side effects may occur, if they do occur they may need medical attention.

Check with your doctor as soon as possible if any of the following side effects occur:

Rare
Dark urine
Fatigue
Itching of the skin
Light-colored stools
Sore throat and fever
Unusual bleeding or bruising
Weakness and fever
Yellow eyes or skin

Signs of overdose (hypoglycemia)
Anxious feeling
Chills
Cold sweats
Confusion

Cool pale skin
Difficulty in concentration
Drowsiness
Excessive hunger
Fast heartbeat
Headache
Nausea
Nervousness
Shakiness
Unsteady walk
Unusual tiredness or weakness

Other side effects may occur that usually do not require medical attention. These side effects may go away during treatment as your body adjusts to the medicine. However, check with your doctor if any of the following side effects continue or are bothersome:

More common
Diarrhea
Dizziness
Headache
Heartburn
Loss of appetite
Nausea and vomiting
Stomach pain or discomfort

Less common or rare
Increased sensitivity of skin to sun
Skin rash

For patients taking chlorpropamide:
• Some patients who take chlorpropamide may retain (keep) more body water than usual. This may cause more problems in the elderly or in those patients who have heart disease. Check with your doctor as soon as possible if any of the following signs occur:

Breathing difficulty
Convulsions (seizures)
Drowsiness
Muscle cramps
Shortness of breath
Swelling or puffiness of face, hands, or ankles
Weakness

The above side effects are more likely to occur in elderly patients and patients with kidney disease, who are usually more sensitive to the effects of oral antidiabetes medicines.

Other side effects not listed above may also occur in some patients. If you notice any other effects, check with your doctor.

December 1987

Additional Information

For patients taking chlorpropamide for water diabetes:
• Chlorpropamide is sometimes used to treat diabetes insipidus (water diabetes). If you are taking this medicine for water diabetes, the advice listed above that relates to diet and urine testing for patients with *sugar* diabetes *does not apply to you.* However, the advice about hypoglycemia (low blood sugar) does apply to you. Call your doctor right away if you feel any of the signs described.

ANTIDYSKINETICS (Systemic)

This information applies to the following medicines:

Benztropine (BENZ-troe-peen)
Biperiden (bye-PER-i-den)
Ethopropazine (eth-oh-PROE-pa-zeen)
Procyclidine (proe-SYE-kli-deen)
Trihexyphenidyl (trye-hex-ee-FEN-i-dill)

This information does *not* apply to:

Amantadine	Haloperidol
Carbidopa and Levodopa	Levodopa
Diphenhydramine	

Some commonly used brand names are:	Generic names:
Apo-Benztropine* Bensylate* Cogentin PMS Benztropine*	Benztropine†‡
Akineton	Biperiden
Parsidol Parsitan*	Ethopropazine
Kemadrin PMS Procyclidine* Procyclid*	Procyclidine
Aparkane* Apo-Trihex* Artane Artane Sequels Novohexidyl* Trihexane Trihexy	Trihexyphenidyl†

*Not available in the U.S.
†Generic name product may also be available in the U.S.
‡Generic name product may also be available in Canada.

To the Reader: If you do not recognize the names of medical conditions or medicines referred to in this information, check with your doctor, nurse, or pharmacist. Definitions for selected medical terms may be found in the Glossary. Brand names for the generic drug names listed can be found in the Index. In addition, selected brand names commonly associated with the generic name have been included in the text to help you recognize medicine you may be taking. The fact that a brand name product is not mentioned does not mean the information does not apply. It is a good idea for you to learn both the generic and brand names of your medicines and to write them down for future use.

This medicine belongs to the general class of medicines called antidyskinetics. It is used to treat Parkinson's disease, sometimes referred to as "shaking palsy." By improving muscle control and reducing stiffness, this medicine allows more normal movements of the body as the disease symptoms are reduced. It is also used to control the severe reactions to certain medicines such as reserpine (medicine to control high blood pressure) or phenothiazines, chlorprothixene, thiothixene, loxapine, and haloperidol (medicines for nervous, mental, and emotional conditions).

This medicine is available only with your doctor's prescription.

Remember:

• **This medicine has been prescribed for your current medical problem only.** It must not be given to other people or used for other problems unless you are directed to do so by your doctor.

• **Keep all medicines out of the reach of children.**

• In order for this medicine to work, it must be used as directed.

• If you are receiving this medicine by injection, some of the information about this medicine may not apply.

• **It is very important that you read and understand the following information.** If any of the information causes you special concern, do not decide against using this medicine without first checking with your doctor.

• Before you begin using any new medicine (prescription or nonprescription) or if you develop any new medical problem while you are using this medicine, check with your doctor, nurse, or pharmacist.

• **If you have any questions** about the following information or if you want more information about this medicine or your medical problem, **ask your doctor, nurse, or pharmacist**.

Before Using This Medicine

In order to decide on the best treatment for your medical problem, your doctor should be told:

—if you have ever had any unusual or allergic reaction to antidyskinetics.

—if you are on a low-salt, low-sugar, or any other special diet, or if you are allergic to any substance, such as foods, sulfites or other preservatives, or dyes. Most medicines contain more than their active ingredient, and many liquid medicines contain alcohol. Your doctor, nurse, or pharmacist can help you avoid products that may cause a problem.

—if you are **pregnant** or if you may become pregnant. Antidyskinetics have not been shown to cause problems in humans.

—if you are **breast-feeding**. Antidyskinetics have not been shown to cause problems in nursing babies. However, since these medicines tend to decrease the secretions of the body, it is possible that the flow of breast milk may be reduced in some patients.

—if you have any of the following medical problems:
Difficult urination
Enlarged prostate
Glaucoma
Heart or blood vessel disease
High blood pressure
Intestinal blockage
Kidney disease
Liver disease
Myasthenia gravis
Uncontrolled movements of hands, mouth, or tongue

—if you are taking **any** other prescription or nonprescription (OTC) medicine, especially:

    Antacids
    Antimuscarinics (medicine for abdominal or stomach spasms or cramps)
    Central nervous system (CNS) depressants

Proper Use of This Medicine

Take this medicine only as directed by your doctor. Do not take more of it, do not take it more often, and do not take it for a longer period of time than your doctor ordered. To do so may increase the chance of side effects.

To lessen stomach upset, take this medicine with meals or immediately after meals, unless otherwise directed by your doctor.

If you miss a dose of this medicine, take it as soon as possible. However, if it is within 2 hours of your next dose, skip the missed dose and go back to your regular dosing schedule. Do not double doses.

How to store this medicine:

- **Keep out of the reach of children.**

- Store away from heat and direct light.

- Do not store the capsule or tablet form of this medicine in the bathroom, near the kitchen sink, or in other damp places. Heat or moisture may cause the medicine to break down.

- Keep the liquid dosage form of this medicine from freezing.

- Do not keep outdated medicine or medicine no longer needed. Be sure that any discarded medicine is out of the reach of children.

Precautions While Using This Medicine

Your doctor should check your progress at regular visits, especially for the first few months you take this medicine. This will allow your dosage to be changed as necessary to meet your needs.

Your doctor may want you to have your eyes examined by an ophthalmologist before and also sometime later during treatment.

Do not stop taking this medicine without first checking with your doctor. Your doctor may want you to reduce gradually the amount you are taking before stopping completely, in order to prevent side effects or making your condition worse.

This medicine will add to the effects of alcohol and other CNS depressants (medicines that slow down the nervous system, possibly causing drowsiness). Some examples of CNS depressants are antihistamines or medicine for hay fever, other allergies, or colds; sedatives, tranquilizers, or sleeping medicine; prescription pain medicine or narcotics; barbiturates; medicine for seizures; muscle relaxants; or anesthetics, including some dental anesthetics. **Check with your doctor before taking any of the above while you are using this medicine.**

Do not take this medicine within 1 hour of taking antacid or medicine for diarrhea. Taking them too close together will make this medicine less effective.

If you think you have taken an overdose, get emergency help at once. Taking an overdose of this medicine may lead to unconsciousness. Some signs of an overdose are clumsiness or unsteadiness; convulsions (seizures); severe drowsiness; fast heartbeat; hallucinations (seeing, hearing, or feeling things that are not there); mood or mental changes; shortness of breath or troubled breathing; trouble in sleeping; and unusual warmth, dryness, and flushing of skin.

This medicine may cause your eyes to become more sensitive to light than they are normally. Wearing sunglasses and avoiding too much exposure to bright light may help lessen the discomfort.

This medicine may cause some people to have blurred vision or to become drowsy, dizzy, or less alert than they are normally. **Make sure you know how you react to this medicine before you drive, use machines, or do other jobs that require you to be alert.**

Dizziness, lightheadedness, or fainting may occur, especially when you get up from lying or sitting. Getting up slowly may help. If the problem continues or gets worse, check with your doctor.

This medicine will often reduce your tolerance of heat, since it makes you sweat less, causing your body temperature to increase. **Use extra care to avoid becoming overheated during exercise or hot weather while you are taking this medicine as this could cause heat stroke.** Also, hot baths or saunas may make you feel dizzy or faint while you are taking this medicine.

This medicine may cause dryness of the mouth. For temporary relief, use sugarless candy or gum, melt bits of ice in your mouth, or use a saliva substitute. However, if dry mouth continues for more than 2 weeks, check with your physician or dentist. Continuing dryness of the mouth may increase the chance of dental disease, including tooth decay, gum disease, and fungal infections.

Side Effects of This Medicine

Along with its needed effects, a medicine may cause some unwanted effects. Although not all of these side effects may occur, if they do occur they may need medical attention.

Check with your doctor as soon as possible if any of the following side effects occur:

Rare
    Confusion (more common in the elderly or with high doses)
    Eye pain
    Skin rash

Signs of overdose

  Clumsiness or unsteadiness
  Convulsions (seizures)
  Drowsiness (severe)
  Dryness of mouth, nose, or throat (severe)
  Fast heartbeat
  Hallucinations (seeing, hearing, or feeling things that are
    not there)
  Mood or mental changes
  Shortness of breath or troubled breathing
  Trouble in sleeping
  Unusual warmth, dryness, and flushing of skin

Other side effects may occur that usually do not require
  medical attention. These side effects may go away
  during treatment as your body adjusts to the medicine.
  However, check with your doctor if any of the following side effects continue or are bothersome:

More common

  Blurred vision
  Constipation
  Decrease in sweating
  Difficult or painful urination (especially in older men)
  Drowsiness
  Dryness of mouth, nose, or throat
  Increased sensitivity of eyes to light
  Nausea or vomiting

Less common or rare

  Dizziness or lightheadedness when getting up from a lying
    or sitting position
  False sense of well-being (especially in the elderly or with
    high doses)
  Headache
  Loss of memory (especially in the elderly)
  Muscle cramps
  Nervousness
  Numbness or weakness in hands or feet

  Soreness of mouth and tongue
  Stomach upset or pain
  Unusual excitement (more common with large doses of
    trihexyphenidyl)

After you stop using this medicine, your body may need
  time to adjust. The length of time this takes depends
  on the amount of medicine you were using and how
  long you used it. During this period of time check with
  your doctor if you notice any of the following side
  effects:

  Anxiety
  Difficulty in speaking or swallowing
  Dizziness or lightheadedness when getting up from a lying
    or sitting position
  Fast heartbeat
  Loss of balance control
  Mask-like face
  Muscle spasms, especially of face, neck, and back
  Restlessness or desire to keep moving
  Shuffling walk
  Stiffness of arms or legs
  Trembling and shaking of hands and fingers
  Trouble in sleeping
  Twisting movements of body

For children: The above side effects are more likely to
  occur in children since they are usually more sensitive
  to the effects of antidyskinetics.

For elderly patients: Agitation, confusion, disorientation,
  hallucinations, memory loss, and mental changes are
  more likely to occur in elderly patients, who are usually
  more sensitive to the effects of antidyskinetics.

Other side effects not listed above may also occur in some
  patients. If you notice any other effects, check with
  your doctor.

_____

December 1987

ANTIGLAUCOMA AGENTS, CHOLINERGIC, LONG-ACTING
(Ophthalmic)

This information applies to the following medicines:

Demecarium (dem-e-KARE-ee-um)
Echothiophate (ek-oh-THYE-oh-fate)
Isoflurophate (eye-soe-FLURE-oh-fate)

Some commonly used brand names are:	Generic names:
Humorsol	Demecarium
Pholspholine Iodide	Echothiophate
Floropryl	Isoflurophate

To the Reader: If you do not recognize the names of medical conditions or medicines referred to in this information, check with your doctor, nurse, or pharmacist. Definitions for selected medical terms may be found in the Glossary. Brand names for the generic drug names listed can be found in the Index. In addition, selected brand names commonly associated with the generic name have been included in the text to help you recognize medicine you may be taking. The fact that a brand name product is not mentioned does not mean the information does not apply. It is a good idea for you to learn both the generic and brand names of your medicines and to write them down for future use.

Demecarium, echothiophate, and isoflurophate are used in the eye to treat certain types of glaucoma and other eye conditions. They may also be used in the diagnosis of certain eye conditions.

These medicines are available only with your doctor's prescription.

Remember:

• **This medicine has been prescribed for your current medical problem only.** It must not be given to other people or used for other problems unless you are directed to do so by your doctor.

• **Keep all medicines out of the reach of children.**

• In order for this medicine to work, it must be used as directed.

• **It is very important that you read and understand the following information.** If any of the information causes you special concern, do not decide against using this medicine without first checking with your doctor.

• Before you begin using any new medicine (prescription or nonprescription) or if you develop any new medical problem while you are using this medicine, check with your doctor, nurse, or pharmacist.

• **If you have any questions** about the following information or if you want more information about this medicine or your medical problem, **ask your doctor, nurse, or pharmacist.**

Before Using This Medicine

In order to decide on the best treatment for your medical problem, your doctor should be told:

—if you have ever had any unusual or allergic reaction to demecarium, echothiophate, or isoflurophate.

—if you are allergic to any substance, such as preservatives or dyes. Most medicines contain more than their active ingredient. Your doctor, nurse, or pharmacist can help you avoid products that may cause a problem.

—if you are **pregnant** or if you may become pregnant, since this medicine may be absorbed into the body. However, demecarium, echothiophate, and isoflurophate have not been shown to cause birth defects or other problems in humans.

—if you are **breast-feeding**, since this medicine may be absorbed into the body. However, demecarium, echothiophate, and isoflurophate have not been shown to cause problems in humans.

—if you have any of the following medical problems:
Asthma
Down's syndrome (mongolism)
Epilepsy
Eye disease
Heart disease
Parkinsonism
Stomach ulcer or other stomach problems

—if you are taking **any** other prescription or nonprescription (OTC) medicine, especially:
Antimyasthenics (ambenonium, neostigmine, pyridostigmine)
Malathion (topical) (e.g., Prioderm)

Proper Use of This Medicine

For patients using the eye-drop form of this medicine:

• How to apply this medicine: First, wash your hands. With middle finger, apply pressure to the inside corner of the eye (and continue to apply pressure for 1 or 2 minutes after the medicine has been placed in the eye). Tilt the head back and with the index finger of the same hand, pull the lower eyelid away from the eye to form a pouch. Drop the medicine into the pouch and gently close the eyes. Do not blink. Keep the eyes closed for 1 or 2 minutes to allow the medicine to be absorbed.

• Remove any excess solution around the eye with a clean tissue, being careful not to touch the eye.

• Immediately after applying the eye drops, wash your hands to remove any medicine that may be on them.

• To prevent contamination of the eye drops, do not touch the applicator tip to any surface (including the eye). Also, keep the container tightly closed.

For patients using the ointment form of this medicine:

• How to apply this medicine: First, wash your hands. Then pull the lower eyelid away from the eye to form a pouch. Squeeze a thin strip of ointment into the pouch. A ½-cm (approximately ¼-inch) strip of ointment is usually enough unless otherwise directed by your doctor. Gently close the eyes and keep them closed for 1 or 2 minutes to allow the medicine to be absorbed.

• Immediately after applying the eye ointment, wash your hands to remove any medicine that may be on them.

© 1988   The United States Pharmacopeial Convention, Inc.

• Since this medicine loses its effectiveness when exposed to moisture, do not wash the tip of the ointment tube or allow it to touch any moist surface.

• To prevent contamination of the eye ointment, do not touch the applicator tip to any surface (including the eye). After using this eye ointment, wipe the tip of the ointment tube with a clean tissue and keep the tube tightly closed.

It is very important that you use this medicine only as directed. Do not use more of it and do not use it more often than your doctor ordered. To do so may increase the chance of too much medicine being absorbed into the body and the chance of side effects.

If you miss a dose of this medicine and your dosing schedule is one dose to be applied:

Every other day—Apply the missed dose as soon as possible if you remember it on the day it should be applied. However, if you do not remember the missed dose until the next day, apply it at that time. Then skip a day and start your dosing schedule again.

Once a day—Apply the missed dose as soon as possible. However, if you do not remember the missed dose until the next day, skip it and apply your regularly scheduled dose.

More than once a day—Apply the missed dose as soon as possible. However, if it is almost time for your next dose, skip the missed dose and apply your next dose at the regularly scheduled time. Then continue with your regular dosing schedule.

If your dosing schedule is different from any of the above and you miss a dose of this medicine, or if you have any questions, check with your doctor.

How to store this medicine:

• **Keep out of the reach of children.**

• Store away from heat and direct light.

• Keep this medicine from freezing.

• Do not keep outdated medicine or medicine no longer needed. Be sure that any discarded medicine is out of the reach of children.

Precautions While Using This Medicine

If you are using this medicine for glaucoma, your doctor should check your eye pressure at regular visits in order to make sure the medicine is working.

If you will be using this medicine for a long period of time, your doctor should examine your eyes at regular visits to make sure this medicine does not cause unwanted effects.

Your doctor may want you to carry an identification card stating that you are using this medicine.

Before having any kind of surgery (including dental surgery), tell the physician or dentist in charge that you are using this medicine or have used it within the past month.

Avoid breathing in even small amounts of carbamate- or organophosphate-type insecticides or pesticides (for example, carbaryl [Sevin], demeton [Systox], diazinon, malathion, parathion, ronnel [Trolene]). They may add to the effects of this medicine. Farmers, gardeners, residents of communities undergoing insecticide or pesticide spraying or dusting, workers in plants manufacturing such products, or other persons exposed to such poisons should protect themselves by wearing a mask over the nose and mouth, changing clothes frequently, and washing hands often while using this medicine.

After you apply this medicine to your eyes, your pupils may become unusually small. This may cause you to see less well at night or in dim light. **Be especially careful if you drive or do other jobs at night or in dim light that require you to see well.**

After you begin using this medicine, your vision may be blurred or there may be a change in your near or distant vision. This may require a change in your eyeglasses. **Make sure your vision is clear before you drive or do other jobs that require you to see well.**

Side Effects of This Medicine

Along with its needed effects, a medicine may cause some unwanted effects. Although not all of these side effects may occur, if they do occur they may need medical attention.

Check with your doctor immediately if any of the following side effects occur:
Rare
    Veil or curtain appearing across part of vision
Signs of too much medicine being absorbed into the body
    Increase in sweating
    Loss of bladder control
    Muscle weakness
    Nausea, vomiting, diarrhea, or stomach cramps or pain
    Shortness of breath, tightness in chest, or wheezing
    Slow or irregular heartbeat
    Unusual tiredness or weakness
    Watering of mouth

Other side effects may occur that usually do not require medical attention. These side effects may go away during treatment as your body adjusts to the medicine. However, check with your doctor if any of the following side effects continue or are bothersome:
    Blurred vision or change in near or distant vision
    Burning, redness, stinging, or other irritation of eyes
    Eye pain
    Headache or browache
    Twitching of eyelids
    Watering of eyes

For elderly patients: Many medicines have not been tested in older people. Therefore, it is not known whether the medicine acts the same way it does in younger adults. Check with your doctor or pharmacist if you notice any unusual effects while using this medicine or if you think it is not working as it should.

Other side effects not listed above may also occur in some patients. If you notice any other effects, check with your doctor.

December 1987

ANTIHISTAMINES (Systemic)

This information applies to the following medicines:

Azatadine (a-ZA-ta-deen)
Bromodiphenhydramine (broe-moe-dye-fen-HYE-dra-meen)
Brompheniramine (brome-fen-EER-a-meen)
Carbinoxamine (kar-bi-NOX-a-meen)
Chlorpheniramine (klor-fen-EER-a-meen)
Clemastine (KLEM-as-teen)
Cyproheptadine (si-proe-HEP-ta-deen)
Dexchlorpheniramine (dex-klor-fen-EER-a-meen)
Dimenhydrinate (dye-men-HYE-dri-nate)
Diphenhydramine (dye-fen-HYE-dra-meen)
Diphenylpyraline (dye-fen-il-PEER-a-leen)
Doxylamine (dox-ILL-a-meen)
Phenindamine (fen-IN-da-meen)
Pyrilamine (peer-ILL-a-meen)
Terfenadine (ter-FEN-a-deen)
Tripelennamine (tri-pel-ENN-a-meen)
Triprolidine (trye-PROE-li-deen)

This information does *not* apply to Hydroxyzine, Promethazine, or Trimeprazine.

Some commonly used brand names and other names are:	Generic names:
Optimine	Azatadine
	Bromodiphenhydramine#
Bromamine Brombay Bromphen Chlorphed Dehist Dimetane Dimetane Extentabs Dimetane-Ten Histaject Modified Nasahist B ND-Stat Revised Oraminic II Veltane	Brompheniramine†
Clistin	Carbinoxamine
Aller-Chlor Allerid-O.D. Chlo-Amine Chlor-100 Chlor-Mal Chlor-Niramine Chlorphen* Chlor-Pro Chlorspan Chlortab Chlor-Trimeton Chlor-Trimeton Repetabs Chlor-Tripolon* Hal-Chlor Histrey Novopheniram* Phenetron Phenetron Lanacaps T.D. Alermine Teldrin Trymegen	Chlorpheniramine†
Tavist	Clemastine
Periactin	Cyproheptadine†
Polaramine Polaramine Repetabs	Dexchlorpheniramine
Apo-Dimenhydrinate* Calm X Dimentabs Dinate Dommanate Dramamine Dramilin Dramocen Dramoject Dymenate Gravol* Hydrate Marmine Motion-Aid Nauseatol* Novodimenate* PMS-Dimenhydrinate* Reidamine Travamine* Wehamine	Dimenhydrinate†‡
Beldin Bena-D Benadryl Benadryl Children's Allergy Benadryl Complete Allergy Benahist Benoject-10 Benylin Compoz Diahist Dihydrex Diphen Diphenacen Diphenadril Fenylhist Fynex Hydramine Hydril Hyrexin-50 Insomnal* Nervine Nighttime Sleep-Aid Noradryl Nordryl Nytol with DPH Robalyn Sleep-Eze 3 Sominex Formula 2 Tusstat Twilite Valdrene Wehdryl	Diphenhydramine†‡
Hispril	Diphenylpyraline
Unisom Nighttime Sleep-Aid	Doxylamine
Nolahist	Phenindamine
Dormarex Sominex Somnicaps	Pyrilamine†
Seldane	Terfenadine
PBZ PBZ-SR	Tripelennamine†
Actidil Bayidyl	Triprolidine†

*Not available in the U.S.
†Generic name product may also be available in the U.S.
‡Generic name product may also be available in Canada.
#Not available by itself in the United States and Canada. However, it is available in cough/cold combination products.

To the Reader: If you do not recognize the names of medical conditions or medicines referred to in this information, check with your doctor, nurse, or pharmacist. Definitions for selected medical terms may be found in the Glossary. Brand names for the generic drug names listed can be found in the Index. In addition, selected brand names commonly associated with the generic name have been included in the text to help you recognize medicine you may be taking. The fact that a brand name product is not mentioned does not mean the information does not apply. It is a good idea for you to learn both the generic and brand names of your medicines and to write them down for future use.

Antihistamines are used to relieve or prevent the symptoms of hay fever and other types of allergy. They work by preventing the effects of a substance called histamine, which is produced by the body.

Some of the antihistamines are also used to prevent motion sickness, nausea, vomiting, and dizziness. In patients with Parkinson's disease, diphenhydramine may be used to decrease stiffness and tremors. Also, the syrup form of diphenhydramine is used to relieve the cough due to colds or hay fever. In addition, since antihistamines may cause drowsiness as a side effect, some of them may be used to help people go to sleep.

Antihistamines may also be used for other conditions as determined by your doctor.

Some antihistamine preparations are available only with your doctor's prescription. Others are available without a prescription; however, your doctor may have special instructions on the proper dose of the medicine for your medical condition.

Remember:

• **Keep all medicines out of the reach of children.**

• In order for this medicine to work, it must be used as directed. **If you are using this medicine without a prescription, it is very important that you follow the directions on the label.**

• **It is also very important that you read and understand the following information.** If any of the information causes you special concern, check with your doctor before using this medicine without a prescription.

• If you are receiving this medicine by injection, some of the information about this medicine may not apply.

• Before you begin using any new medicine (prescription or nonprescription) or if you develop any new medical problem while you are using this medicine, check with your doctor, nurse, or pharmacist.

• **If you have any questions** about the following information or if you want more information about this medicine or your medical problem, **ask your doctor, nurse, or pharmacist**.

Before Using This Medicine

Before you use this medicine check with your doctor or pharmacist:

—if you have ever had any unusual or allergic reaction to antihistamines.

—if you are on a low-salt, low-sugar, or any other special diet, or if you are allergic to any substance, such as foods, sulfites or other preservatives, or dyes.

Most medicines contain more than their active ingredient, and many liquid medicines contain alcohol. Your doctor, nurse, or pharmacist can help you avoid products that may cause a problem.

—if you are **pregnant** or if you may become pregnant. Antihistamines have not been shown to cause problems in humans. Studies in animals have shown that some other antihistamines, such as meclizine and cyclizine, may cause birth defects.

Studies have not been done in humans with terfenadine. However, studies in animals have shown that terfenadine, when given in doses several times the human dose, lowers the weight of the baby and increases the risk of death of the baby.

—if you are **breast-feeding**. Small amounts of antihistamines pass into the breast milk. Use is not recommended since the chances are greater for most antihistamines to cause side effects, such as unusual excitement or irritability, in the infant. Also, since these medicines tend to decrease the secretions of the body, it is possible that the flow of breast milk may be reduced in some patients. It is not known yet whether terfenadine may cause these same side effects.

—if you have any of the following medical problems:
Asthma (acute)
Enlarged prostate
Glaucoma
Urinary tract blockage or difficult urination

—if you are using **any** other prescription or nonprescription (OTC) medicine, especially:
Antimuscarinics (medicine for abdominal or stomach spasms or cramps)
Central nervous system (CNS) depressants

—if you are now taking or have taken within the past 2 weeks monoamine oxidase (MAO) inhibitors such as:
Furazolidone (e.g., Furoxone)
Isocarboxazid (e.g., Marplan)
Pargyline (e.g., Eutonyl)
Phenelzine (e.g., Nardil)
Procarbazine (e.g., Matulane)
Tranylcypromine (e.g., Parnate)

Proper Use of This Medicine

Antihistamines are used to relieve or prevent the symptoms of your medical problem. Take them only as directed. Do not take more of them and do not take them more often than recommended on the label, unless otherwise directed by your doctor. To do so may increase the chance of side effects.

If you are taking this medicine regularly and you miss a dose, take it as soon as possible. However, if it is almost time for your next dose, skip the missed dose and go back to your regular dosing schedule. Do not double doses.

For patients taking this medicine by mouth:

• Take it with food or a glass of water or milk to lessen stomach irritation if necessary.

• If you are taking the extended-release tablet form of this medicine, swallow the tablets whole. Do not break, crush, or chew before swallowing.

For patients taking dimenhydrinate or diphenhydramine
for motion sickness:
  • Take this medicine at least 30 minutes or, even better,
    1 to 2 hours before you begin to travel.

For patients using the suppository form of this medicine:
  • How to insert suppository: First remove foil wrapper
    and moisten the suppository with water. Lie down on
    side and push the suppository well up into the rectum
    with finger. If the suppository is too soft to insert be-
    cause of storage in a warm place, before removing the
    foil wrapper chill the suppository in the refrigerator
    for 30 minutes or run cold water over it.

For patients using the injection form of this medicine:
  • If you will be giving yourself the injections, make
    sure you understand exactly how to give them. If you
    have any questions about this, check with your doctor,
    nurse, or pharmacist.

How to store this medicine:
  • **Keep out of the reach of children**, since overdose may
    be very dangerous in children.
  • Store away from heat and direct light.
  • Do not store the capsules or tablets in the bathroom
    medicine cabinet, near the kitchen sink, or in other
    damp places. Heat or moisture may cause the medi-
    cine to break down.
  • Keep the liquid form of this medicine from freezing.
  • Do not keep outdated medicine or medicine no longer
    needed. Be sure that any discarded medicine is out of
    the reach of children.

Precautions While Using This Medicine

Tell the doctor in charge that you are taking this medicine
  before you have any skin tests for allergies. The results
  of the test may be affected by this medicine.

When taking antihistamines on a regular basis, make sure
  your doctor knows if you are taking large amounts of
  aspirin at the same time (as in arthritis or rheumatism). Effects of too much aspirin, such as ringing in
  the ears, may be covered up by the antihistamine.

Antihistamines will add to the effects of alcohol and other
  CNS depressants (medicines that slow down the nervous system, possibly causing drowsiness). Some examples of CNS depressants are sedatives, tranquilizers, or sleeping medicine; prescription pain medicine
  or narcotics; barbiturates; medicine for seizures; muscle relaxants; or anesthetics, including some dental
  anesthetics. **Check with your doctor before taking any
  of the above while you are using this medicine.**

This medicine may cause some people to become drowsy
  or less alert than they are normally. Even if taken at
  bedtime, it may cause some people to feel drowsy or
  less alert on arising. Some antihistamines are more
  likely to cause drowsiness than others (terfenadine, for

example, produces this effect rarely). **Make sure you
know how you react to the antihistamine you are taking
before you drive, use machines, or do other jobs that
require you to be alert.**

Antihistamines may cause dryness of the mouth, nose,
  and throat. Some antihistamines are more likely to
  cause dryness of the mouth than others (terfenadine,
  for example, produces this effect rarely). For temporary relief of mouth dryness, use sugarless candy or
  gum, melt bits of ice in your mouth, or use a saliva
  substitute. However, if dry mouth continues for more
  than 2 weeks, check with your physician or dentist.
  Continuing dryness of the mouth may increase the
  chance of dental disease, including tooth decay, gum
  disease, and fungal infections.

For patients using dimenhydrinate or diphenhydramine:
  • This medicine controls nausea and vomiting. For this
    reason, it may cover up the signs of overdose caused
    by other medicines or the symptoms of appendicitis.
    This will make it difficult for your doctor to diagnose
    these conditions. Make sure your doctor knows that
    you are taking this medicine if you have other symp-
    toms of appendicitis such as stomach or lower abdom-
    inal pain, cramping, or soreness. Also, if you think you
    may have taken an overdose of any medicine, tell your
    doctor that you are taking this medicine.

Side Effects of This Medicine

Along with its needed effects, a medicine may cause some
  unwanted effects. Although not all of these side effects
  may occur, if they do occur they may need medical
  attention.

Check with your doctor as soon as possible if any of the
  following side effects occur:
  Less common or rare
      Sore throat and fever
      Unusual bleeding or bruising
      Unusual tiredness or weakness
  Signs of overdose
      Clumsiness or unsteadiness
      Convulsions (seizures)
      Drowsiness (severe)
      Dryness of mouth, nose, or throat (severe)
      Feeling faint
      Flushing or redness of face
      Hallucinations (seeing, hearing, or feeling things that are
        not there)
      Shortness of breath or troubled breathing
      Trouble in sleeping

Other side effects may occur that usually do not require
  medical attention. These side effects may go away
  during treatment as your body adjusts to the medicine.
  However, check with your doctor or pharmacist if any
  of the following side effects continue or are bothersome:

  More common—rare with terfenadine
      Drowsiness
      Thickening of bronchial secretions

Less common or rare

    Blurred vision or any change in vision
    Confusion
    Difficult or painful urination
    Dizziness
    Dryness of mouth, nose, or throat
    Fast heartbeat
    Increased sensitivity of skin to sun
    Increased sweating
    Loss of appetite (increased appetite with cyproheptadine)
    Nightmares
    Ringing or buzzing in ears
    Skin rash
    Stomach upset or stomach pain (more common with pyrilamine and tripelennamine)
    Unusual excitement, nervousness, restlessness, or irritability

For children: Use of antihistamines is not recommended in premature or newborn infants. Serious side effects, such as convulsions (seizures), are more likely to occur in children and would be of greater risk to these infants. Children are usually more sensitive to the effects of antihistamines. Also, nightmares or unusual excitement, nervousness, restlessness, or irritability may be more likely to occur in children.

For elderly patients: Elderly patients are usually more sensitive to the effects of antihistamines. Confusion, difficult or painful urination, dizziness, drowsiness, feeling faint, or dryness of mouth, nose, or throat may be more likely to occur in elderly patients. Also, nightmares or unusual excitement, nervousness, restlessness, or irritability may be more likely to occur in in elderly patients.

Other side effects not listed above may also occur in some patients. If you notice any other effects, check with your doctor or pharmacist.

December 1987

ANTIHISTAMINES AND DECONGESTANTS (Systemic)

Note: For quick reference the following antihistamine and decongestant combinations are numbered to match the corresponding brand names.

This information applies to the following medicines:

1. Azatadine (a-ZA-ta-deen) and Pseudoephedrine (soo-doe-e-FED-rin)
2. Brompheniramine (brome-fen-EER-a-meen), Phenylephrine (fen-ill-EF-rin), and Phenylpropanolamine (fen-ill-proe-pa-NOLE-a-meen)†
2a. Brompheniramine and Phenylpropanolamine
3. Brompheniramine and Pseudoephedrine
4. Carbinoxamine (kar-bi-NOX-a-meen) and Pseudoephedrine
5. Chlorpheniramine (klor-fen-EER-a-meen) and Pseudoephedrine
6. Chlorpheniramine, Pyrilamine (peer-ILL-a-meen), and Phenylpropanolamine
7. Chlorpheniramine, Tripelennamine (tri-pel-ENN-a-meen), Phenylpropanolamine, and Phenylephrine
8. Clemastine (KLEM-as-teen) and Phenylpropanolamine
9. Dexbrompheniramine (dex-brom-fen-EER-a-meen) and Pseudoephedrine†
9a. Diphenhydramine (dye-fen-HYE-dra-meen) and Pseudoephedrine
10. Phenindamine (fen-IN-da-meen), Chlorpheniramine, and Phenylpropanolamine
11. Phenylephrine and Brompheniramine
12. Phenylephrine and Chlorpheniramine
13. Phenylephrine, Chlorpheniramine, and Pyrilamine
14. Phenylephrine, Phenylpropanolamine, and Chlorpheniramine
15. Phenylephrine, Phenylpropanolamine, Pyrilamine, and Chlorpheniramine
16. Phenylpropanolamine and Chlorpheniramine†
17. Phenylpropanolamine, Pheniramine (fen-EER-a-meen), and Pyrilamine
18. Phenylpropanolamine, Phenylephrine, Phenyltoloxamine (fen-ill-toe-LOX-a-meen), and Chlorpheniramine
19. Phenylpropanolamine, Phenyltoloxamine, Pyrilamine, and Pheniramine
20. Promethazine (proe-METH-a-zeen) and Phenylephrine
21. Promethazine and Pseudoephedrine
22. Pseudoephedrine and Chlorcyclizine (klor-SYE-kli-zeen)
23. Triprolidine (trye-PROE-li-deen) and Pseudoephedrine†

Some commonly used brand names are:

Actacin[23]	Bromatap[2a]	Cordamine-PA[2]
Actagen[23]	Bromfed[3]	Corsym[16]
Actamine[23]	Bromfed-PD[3]	Covanamine[15]
Actifed[23]	Bromophen[2a]	Dallergy-D[5 12]
Actifed 12-Hour[23]	Bromophen T.D.[2]	Decohist[12]
Actihist[23]	Bromphen Compound	Deconade[16]
Alamine[16]	T.D.[2]	Deconamine[5]
Allerest[16]	Brompheril[9]	Deconamine SR[5]
Allerest 12 Hour[16]	Children's Allerest[16]	Decongestabs[18]
Allerform[16]	Chlorafed[5]	Dehist[14]
Allerfrin[23]	Chlorafed H.S. Time-	Demazin[12]
Allergesic[16]	celles[5]	Demazin Repetabs[16]
Allergine[16]	Chlorafed Timecelles[5]	Dimetane
Allergy Relief	Chlor-Rest[16]	Decongestant[11]
Medicine[16]	Chlor-Trimeton	Dimetapp[2* 2a]
Amaril D[18]	Decongestant[5]	Dimetapp Extentabs[2 2a]
Amaril D Spantab[18]	Chlor-Trimeton Decon-	Disophrol[9]
Anafed[5]	gestant Repetabs[5]	Disophrol Chronotabs[9]
Anamine[5]	Chlor-Tripolon	Dorcol Liquid Cold
Anamine T.D.[5]	Decongestant*[5 16]	Formula[5]
A.R.M.[16]	Codimal-L.A.[5]	Dristan 12-Hour[12]
Bayaminic[16]	Colrex Decongestant[7]	Drixoral[3 9]
Bayhistine[16]	Coltab[12]	Drixtab*[9]
Benadryl	Condrin-LA[16]	Drize[16]
Decongestant[9a]	Conex D.A.[16]	Duphrene[13]
Benylin D[9a]	Contac[16]	Duralex[5]
Biphetap[2a]	Contac-C*[16]	Efedra P.A.[9]
Brexin L.A.[5]	Cophene No.2[14]	E-Tapp[2]
Bromalix[2]	Co-Pyronil 2[5]	Fedahist[5]

Fedahist Gyrocaps[5]	Prometh VC Plain[20]	Rinade B.I.D.[5]
Fedrazil[22]	Nolamine[10]	Rondec[4]
Genac[23]	Norafed[23]	Rondec-TR[4]
Genamin[16]	Noraminic[16]	Ru-Tuss II[16]
Genaphed[5]	Normatane[2]	Ryna[5]
Genatap[2a]	Novafed A[5]	Rynatan[13]
Gencold[16]	Novahistex*[5]	Sinocon[18]
Histabid Duracaps[16]	Novahistine[12]	S-T Decongest[2]
Histalet[5]	Novahistine LP[12]	Sudafed Plus[5]
Histalet Forte[15]	Novamor[16]	Tagafed[23]
Histamic[18]	Orahist[16]	Tagatap[2]
Histarall[9]	Oraminic Spancaps[16]	Tamine[2]
Histaspan-P*[12]	Ornade*[16]	Tamine SR[2]
Histaspan-Plus[12]	Ornade-A.F.*[16]	Tavist-D[8]
Histatab Plus[12]	Ornade Spansules[16]	Triacin[23]
Histatapp[2a]	Panadyl[17]	Triafed[23]
Hista-Vadrin[14]	PediaCare 2[5]	Triaminic[16 17]
Histor-D[12]	Phenergan-D[21]	Triaminic-12[16]
12 Hour Maximum	Phenergan VC[20]	Triaminic Chewables[16]
Strength Allerest[16]	Phenhist[16]	Triaminic TR[17]
Hournaze[5]	Poly-Histine-D[19]	Trifed[23]
Isoclor[5]	Poly-Histine-DX[3]	Tri-Fed[23]
Isoclor Timesules[5]	Prometh VC Plain[20]	Trilitron[23]
Kronofed-A	Pseudodine[23]	Trinalin Repetabs[1]
Kronocaps[5]	Pseudo-Hist[5]	Trind[16]
Kronohist Kronocaps[6]	Pseudo-Mal[9]	Tri-Nefrin[16]
Midatap[2]	Purebrom[2]	Triphed[23]
Myphetapp[2a]	Purebrom Compound	Tri-Phen-Chlor[18]
Naldecon[18]	T.D.[2]	Triphenyl[16 17]
Naldelate[18]	Quadra Hist[18]	Tripodrine[23]
Napril Plateau[15]	Relemine[15]	Triposed[23]
Nasahist[14]	Resaid T.D.[16]	Tudecon[18]
ND Clear T.D.[5]	Rhinolar-EX[16]	Tussanil[15]
ND-Hist[14]	Rhinosyn[5]	Veltap[2]
Neotep Granucaps[12]	Rhinosyn-PD[5]	Westapp[2]
New-Decongest[18]		

---

*Not available in the U.S.

†Generic name product may also be available in the U.S.

To the Reader: If you do not recognize the names of medical conditions or medicines referred to in this information, check with your doctor, nurse, or pharmacist. Definitions for selected medical terms may be found in the Glossary. Brand names for the generic drug names listed can be found in the Index. In addition, selected brand names commonly associated with the generic name have been included in the text to help you recognize medicine you may be taking. The fact that a brand name product is not mentioned does not mean the information does not apply. It is a good idea for you to learn both the generic and brand names of your medicines and to write them down for future use.

Antihistamine and decongestant combinations are used to treat nasal congestion (stuffy nose), sneezing, and runny nose of colds and hay fever.

Antihistamines work by preventing the effects of a substance called histamine, which is produced by the body. The decongestants, such as phenylpropanolamine (fen-ill-proe-pa-NOLE-a-meen) (also known as PPA), produce a narrowing of blood vessels. This leads to clearing of nasal congestion, but it may also cause an increase in blood pressure in patients who have high blood pressure.

Some of these combinations are available only with your doctor's prescription. Others are available without a prescription; however, your doctor may have special instructions on the proper dose of the medicine for your medical condition.

Remember:

• **Keep all medicines out of the reach of children.**

• In order for this medicine to work, it must be used as directed. **If you are using this medicine without a prescription, it is very important to follow the directions on the label.**

• **It is also very important that you read and understand the following information.** If any of the information causes you special concern, check with your doctor before using this medicine without a prescription.

• Before you begin using any new medicine (prescription or nonprescription) or if you develop any new medical problem while you are using this medicine, check with your doctor, nurse, or pharmacist.

• **If you have any questions** about the following information or if you want more information about this medicine or your medical problem, **ask your doctor, nurse, or pharmacist.**

Before Using This Medicine

Before you use this medicine, check with your doctor, nurse, or pharmacist:

—if you have ever had any unusual or allergic reaction to antihistamines or to amphetamine, dextroamphetamine, ephedrine, epinephrine, isoproterenol, metaproterenol, methamphetamine, norepinephrine, phenylephrine, pseudoephedrine, PPA, or terbutaline.

—if you are on a low-salt, low-sugar, or any other special diet, or if you are allergic to any substance, such as foods, sulfites or other preservatives, or dyes. Most medicines contain more than their active ingredient, and many liquid medicines contain alcohol. Your doctor, nurse, or pharmacist can help you avoid products that may cause a problem.

—if you are **pregnant** or if you may become pregnant. Antihistamines have not been shown to cause problems in humans.

Studies on birth defects have not been done in either humans or animals with decongestants such as phenylephrine or phenylpropanolamine. Studies on birth defects have not been done in humans with the decongestant pseudoephedrine; however, in animal studies pseudoephedrine did not cause birth defects but did cause a reduction in average weight, length, and rate of bone formation in the animal fetus.

Phenothiazines, such as promethazine (contained in one of these combination medicines), have been shown to cause jaundice and muscle tremors in a few newborn infants whose mothers received phenothiazines during pregnancy. To avoid these effects, medicines that contain promethazine should be stopped 1 or 2 weeks before the delivery date.

—if you are **breast-feeding.** Small amounts of antihistamines and decongestants pass into the breast milk. Use is not recommended since the chances are greater for this medicine to cause side effects, such as unusual excitement or irritability, in the nursing baby. Also, since antihistamines tend to decrease the secretions of the body, it is possible that the flow of breast milk may be reduced in some patients.

—if you have any of the following medical problems:

   Asthma attack
   Diabetes mellitus (sugar diabetes)
   Enlarged prostate
   Glaucoma
   Heart or blood vessel disease
   High blood pressure
   Overactive thyroid
   Urinary tract blockage or difficult urination

—if you are taking **any** other prescription or nonprescription (OTC) medicine, especially:

   Antimuscarinics (medicine for abdominal or stomach spasms or cramps)
   Central nervous system (CNS) depressants
   Maprotiline (e.g., Ludiomil)
   Rauwolfia alkaloids (alseroxylon, deserpidine, rauwolfia serpentina, reserpine)
   Tricyclic antidepressants (amitriptyline, amoxapine, clomipramine, desipramine, doxepin, imipramine, nortriptyline, protriptyline, trimipramine)

—if you are taking one of the combinations containing phenylpropanolamine or pseudoephedrine and are also taking:

   Amantadine
   Amphetamines
   Appetite suppressants (diet pills), except fenfluramine
   Beta-blockers (acebutolol, atenolol, labetalol, metoprolol, nadolol, oxprenolol, pindolol, propanolol, sotalol, timolol)
   Caffeine
   Chlophedianol (e.g., Ulo)
   Medicine for asthma or other breathing problems
   Medicine for colds, sinus problems, or hay fever or other allergies (including nose drops or sprays)
   Methylphenidate (e.g., Ritalin)
   Pemoline (e.g., Cylert)

—if you are now taking or have taken within the past 2 weeks monoamine oxidase (MAO) inhibitors, such as:

   Furazolidone (e.g., Furoxone)
   Isocarboxazid (e.g., Marplan)
   Pargyline (e.g., Eutonyl)
   Phenelzine (e.g., Nardil)
   Procarbazine (e.g., Matulane)
   Tranylcypromine (e.g., Parnate)

Proper Use of This Medicine

Take this medicine only as directed. Do not take more of it and do not take it more often than recommended on the label, unless otherwise directed by your doctor. To do so may increase the chance of side effects.

Take this medicine with food or a glass of water or milk to lessen stomach irritation, if necessary.

For patients taking the extended-release capsule or tablet form of this medicine:

• Swallow it whole.

• Do not crush, break, or chew before swallowing.

• If the capsule is too large to swallow, you may mix the contents of the capsule with applesauce, jelly, honey, or syrup and swallow without chewing.

If you are taking this medicine regularly and you miss a dose, take it as soon as possible. However, if it is almost time for your next dose, skip the missed dose and go back to your regular dosing schedule. Do not double doses.

How to store this medicine:

- **Keep out of the reach of children.**

- Store away from heat and direct light.

- Do not store in the bathroom, near the kitchen sink, or in other damp places. Heat or moisture may cause the medicine to break down.

- Keep the liquid form of this medicine from freezing.

- Do not keep outdated medicine or medicine no longer needed. Be sure that any discarded medicine is out of the reach of children.

Precautions While Using This Medicine

Tell the doctor in charge that you are taking this medicine before you have any skin tests for allergies. The results of the test may be affected by the antihistamine in this medicine.

When taking antihistamines (contained in this combination medicine) on a regular basis, make sure your doctor knows if you are taking large amounts of aspirin at the same time (as in arthritis or rheumatism). Effects of too much aspirin, such as ringing in the ears, may be covered up by the antihistamine.

The antihistamine in this medicine will add to the effects of alcohol and other CNS depressants (medicines that slow down the nervous system, possibly causing drowsiness). Some examples of CNS depressants are other antihistamines or medicine for hay fever, other allergies, or colds; sedatives, tranquilizers, or sleeping medicine; prescription pain medicine or narcotics; barbiturates; medicine for seizures; muscle relaxants; or anesthetics, including some dental anesthetics. **Check with your doctor before taking any of the above while you are taking this medicine.**

The antihistamine in this medicine may cause some people to become drowsy, dizzy, or less alert than they are normally. **Make sure you know how you react before you drive, use machines, or do other jobs that require you to be alert.**

The decongestant in this medicine may add to the central nervous system (CNS) stimulant and other effects of phenylpropanolamine (PPA)-containing diet aids. **Do not use medicines for diet or appetite control while taking this medicine unless you have checked with your doctor.**

The decongestant in this medicine may cause some people to be nervous or restless or to have trouble in sleeping. If you have trouble in sleeping, **take the last dose of this medicine for each day a few hours before bedtime.** If you have any questions about this, check with your doctor.

Antihistamines may cause dryness of the mouth, nose, and throat. For temporary relief of mouth dryness, use sugarless candy or gum, melt bits of ice in your mouth, or use a saliva substitute. However, if dry mouth continues for more than 2 weeks, check with your dentist. Continuing dryness of the mouth may increase the chance of dental disease, including tooth decay, gum disease, and fungal infections.

For patients using promethazine-containing medicine:

- This medicine controls nausea and vomiting. For this reason, it may cover up the signs of overdose caused by other medicines or the symptoms of intestinal blockage. This will make it difficult for your doctor to diagnose these conditions. Make sure your doctor knows that you are taking this medicine if you have other symptoms such as stomach or lower abdominal pain, cramping, or soreness. Also, if you think you may have taken an overdose of any medicine, tell your doctor that you are taking this medicine.

Side Effects of This Medicine

Along with its needed effects, a medicine may cause some unwanted effects. Although not all of these side effects may occur, if they do occur they may need medical attention.

Check with your doctor as soon as possible if any of the following side effects occur:

Rare
> Sore throat and fever
> Tightness in chest
> Unusual bleeding or bruising
> Unusual tiredness or weakness

With high doses
> Fast or irregular heartbeat
> Mood or mental changes

Signs of overdose
> Clumsiness or unsteadiness
> Convulsions (seizures)
> Drowsiness (severe)
> Dryness of mouth, nose, or throat (severe)
> Flushing or redness of face
> Hallucinations (seeing, hearing, or feeling things that are not there)
> Headache (continuing)
> Muscle spasms (especially of neck and back)
> Restlessness
> Shortness of breath or troubled breathing
> Shuffling walk
> Slow or fast heartbeat
> Tic-like (jerky) movements of head and face
> Trembling and shaking of hands

Other side effects may occur that usually do not require medical attention. These side effects may go away during treatment as your body adjusts to the medicine. However, check with your doctor or pharmacist if any of the following side effects continue or are bothersome:

More common
> Drowsiness
> Thickening of the bronchial secretions

Less common—more common with high doses
   Blurred vision
   Confusion
   Difficult or painful urination
   Dizziness
   Dryness of mouth, nose, or throat
   Headache
   Loss of appetite
   Nightmares
   Pounding heartbeat
   Ringing or buzzing in ears
   Skin rash
   Stomach upset or pain (more common with pyrilamine
      and tripelennamine)
   Unusual excitement, nervousness, restlessness, or irrita-
      bility

For children: Use of this medicine is not recommended in premature or newborn babies. Serious side effects, such as convulsions (seizures) and fast or irregular heartbeats, are more likely to occur in children and would be of greater risk to these babies.

For children or elderly patients: Children and elderly patients are usually more sensitive to the effects of this medicine. Confusion, difficult and painful urination, dizziness, drowsiness, dryness of mouth, or convulsions (seizures) may be more likely to occur in elderly patients. Nightmares or unusual excitement, nervousness, restlessness, or irritability may be more likely also to occur in children and in elderly patients.

Other side effects not listed above may also occur in some patients. If you notice any other effects, check with your doctor.

_____

December 1987

ANTI-INFLAMMATORY ANALGESICS
(Systemic)

This information applies to the following medicines:

Diflunisal (dye-FLOO-ni-sal)
Fenoprofen (fen-oh-PROE-fen)
Ibuprofen (eye-byoo-PROE-fen)
Meclofenamate (me-kloe-FEN-am-ate)
Mefenamic (me-fe-NAM-ik) Acid
Naproxen (na-PROX-en)
Piroxicam (peer-OX-i-kam)
Sulindac (sul-IN-dak)
Tolmetin (TOLE-met-in)

This information does *not* apply to aspirin or other salicylates, indomethacin, ketoprofen, and phenylbutazone.

Some commonly used brand names are:	Generic names:
Dolobid	Diflunisal
Fenopron* Nalfon Progesic*	Fenoprofen
Advil Amersol* Apo-Ibuprofen* Apsifen* Apsifen-F* Brufen* Haltran Ifen Medipren Midol 200 Motrin Neuvil Novoprofen* Nuprin Pamprin IB Rufen Trendar	Ibuprofen†‡
Meclomen	Meclofenamate†
Ponstan* Ponstel	Mefenamic Acid
Anaprox Apo-Naproxen* Naprosyn Naxen* Novonaprox* Synflex*	Naproxen
Apo-Piroxicam* Feldene Novopirocam*	Piroxicam
Clinoril	Sulindac
Tolectin Tolectin DS	Tolmetin

*Not available in the U.S.
†Generic name product may also be available in the U.S.
‡Generic name product may also be available in Canada.

To the Reader: If you do not recognize the names of medical conditions or medicines referred to in this information, check with your doctor, nurse, or pharmacist. Definitions for selected medical terms may be found in the Glossary. Brand names for the generic drug names listed can be found in the Index. In addition, selected brand names commonly associated with the generic name have been included in the text to help you recognize medicine you may be taking. The fact that a brand name product is not mentioned does not mean the information does not apply. It is a good idea for you to learn both the generic and brand names of your medicines and to write them down for future use.

Anti-inflammatory analgesics are taken by mouth to relieve some symptoms caused by arthritis (rheumatism), such as inflammation, swelling, stiffness, and joint pain. However, this medicine does not cure arthritis and will help you only as long as you continue to take it.

Some of these medicines are also used to relieve other kinds of pain or to treat other painful conditions, such as:

—gout attacks;
—bursitis;
—tendinitis;
—sprains, strains, or other injuries; or
—menstrual cramps.

Ibuprofen is also used to reduce fever.

Anti-inflammatory analgesics may also be used for treating other conditions as determined by your doctor.

Although ibuprofen may be used instead of aspirin to treat many of the same medical problems, it must not be used by people who are allergic to aspirin.

The 200-mg strength of ibuprofen is available without a prescription. However, your physician or dentist may have special instructions on the proper dose of ibuprofen for your medical condition.

Other anti-inflammatory analgesics and other strengths of ibuprofen are available only with your physician's or dentist's prescription.

Remember:
- **If this medicine has been prescribed for you, it should be used to treat your current medical problem only.** It must not be given to other people or used for other problems unless you are directed to do so by your doctor.

- **Keep all medicines out of the reach of children.**

- In order for this medicine to work, it must be used as directed. **If you are using ibuprofen without a prescription, it is very important to follow the directions on the label.**

- **It is very important that you read and understand the following information.** If any of the information causes you special concern, do not decide against using this medicine without first checking with your doctor.

- Before you begin using any new medicine (prescription or nonprescription) or if you develop any new medical problem while you are using this medicine, check with your doctor, nurse, or pharmacist.

- **If you have any questions** about the following information or if you want more information about this medicine or your medical problem, **ask your doctor, nurse, or pharmacist.**

Before Using This Medicine

Before you take this medicine, your physician or dentist should be told:

—if you have ever had any unusual or allergic reaction, such as skin rash, hives, or itching, or breathing problems (wheezing or asthma), to any of the anti-inflammatory analgesics or to any of the following medicines:

    Aspirin or other salicylates
    Diclofenac (e.g., Voltaren)
    Indomethacin (e.g., Indocid; Indocin)
    Ketoprofen (e.g., Orudis)
    Oxyphenbutazone (e.g., Oxalid; Tandearil)
    Phenylbutazone (e.g., Azolid; Butazolidin)
    Suprofen (e.g., Suprol)
    Tiaprofenic acid (e.g., Surgam)
    Zomepirac (e.g., Zomax)

—if you are on a low-salt, low-sugar, or any other special diet, or if you are allergic to any substance, such as foods, sulfites or other preservatives, or dyes. Most medicines contain more than their active ingredient. Your doctor, nurse, or pharmacist can help you avoid products that may cause a problem.

—if you are **pregnant** or if you may become pregnant. Studies on birth defects with these medicines have not been done in humans. However, if taken regularly during the last few months of pregnancy, there is a chance that these medicines may cause unwanted effects on the heart or blood flow of the fetus or newborn baby. Also, studies in animals have shown that these medicines, if taken late in pregnancy, may increase the length of pregnancy, prolong labor, or cause other problems during delivery. Studies in animals have not shown that fenoprofen, ibuprofen, naproxen, piroxicam, or tolmetin causes birth defects. Diflunisal causes birth defects of the spine and ribs in rabbits, but not in mice or rats. Meclofenamate causes unwanted effects on the formation of bones and other unwanted effects in animals. Sulindac causes a lowering of the newborn's weight and, in some animal studies, unwanted effects on the development of bones and organs. Studies on birth defects with mefenamic acid have not been done in animals.

—if you are **breast-feeding**. Although these medicines have not been shown to cause problems in nursing babies, diflunisal, fenoprofen, mefenamic acid, naproxen, piroxicam, and tolmetin pass into the breast milk. Sulindac may pass into the breast milk. Ibuprofen probably does not pass into the breast milk. It is not known whether meclofenamate passes into human breast milk. However, use of meclofenamate by nursing mothers is not recommended because animal studies have shown that it causes unwanted effects on the baby's development. Also, studies in animals have shown that piroxicam may decrease the amount of milk.

—if you have any of the following medical problems:
    Asthma
    Bleeding problems
    Colitis, stomach ulcer, or other stomach problems
    Fluid retention (swelling of feet or lower legs)
    Heart disease

    Hepatitis or other liver disease
    High blood pressure
    Kidney disease or history of

—if you regularly take acetaminophen or aspirin or other salicylates.

—if you are taking **any** other prescription or nonprescription (OTC) medicine, especially:

    Anticoagulants (blood thinners)
    Heparin
    Indomethacin (e.g., Indocid; Indocin)
    Probenecid (e.g., Benemid)

Proper Use of This Medicine

To lessen stomach upset, anti-inflammatory analgesics may be taken with food or antacids. This is especially important when you are taking mefenamic acid or piroxicam. However, your doctor may want you to take other anti-inflammatory analgesics 30 minutes before meals or 2 hours after meals so that they will get into the blood more quickly. An antacid containing magnesium and aluminum hydroxides will not interfere with the way this medicine works and may be the best kind of antacid to use. If stomach upset (indigestion, nausea, vomiting, stomach pain, or diarrhea) continues or if you have any questions about how you should be taking this medicine, check with your doctor, nurse, or pharmacist.

Take this medicine with a full glass (8 ounces) of water. Also, do not lie down for about 15 to 30 minutes after taking it. This helps to prevent irritation that may lead to trouble in swallowing.

For patients taking diflunisal:
• Swallow these tablets whole. Do not break, crush, or chew them before swallowing.

For patients using the suppository form of naproxen:
• If the suppository is too soft to insert because of storage in a warm place, chill the suppository in the refrigerator for 30 minutes or run cold water over it before removing the foil wrapper.

• How to insert the suppository: First remove the foil wrapper and moisten the suppository with water. Lie down on your side and push the suppository well up into the rectum with the finger.

For patients taking 200-mg (nonprescription strength) ibuprofen:
• This medicine comes with a patient information sheet. Read it carefully. If you have any questions about this information, check with your doctor or pharmacist.

For safe and effective use of this medicine, do not take more of it, do not take it more often, and do not take it for a longer period of time than ordered by your physician or dentist or directed on the 200-mg (nonprescription strength) ibuprofen package label. Taking too much of any of these medicines may increase the chance of unwanted effects, especially in elderly patients.

When used for severe or continuing arthritis, this medicine **must be taken regularly as ordered by your doctor** in order for it to help you. These medicines usually begin to work within one week, but in severe cases up to two weeks or even longer may pass before you begin to feel better. Also, several weeks may pass before you feel the full effects of the medicine.

For patients taking mefenamic acid:

• **Always take mefenamic acid with food or antacids**.

• **Do not take mefenamic acid for more than 7 days at a time** unless your doctor tells you to do so. To do so may increase the chance of side effects, especially in elderly patients.

If your doctor has ordered you to take this medicine according to a regular schedule and you miss a dose, take it as soon as you remember. However, if it is almost time for your next dose, skip the missed dose and go back to your regular dosing schedule. Do not double doses.

How to store this medicine:

• **Keep out of the reach of children.**

• Store away from heat and direct light.

• Do not store tablets or capsules in the bathroom, near the kitchen sink, or in other damp places. Heat or moisture may cause the medicine to break down.

• Keep the liquid and suppository forms of naproxen from freezing.

• Do not keep outdated medicine or medicine no longer needed. Be sure that any discarded medicine is out of the reach of children.

Precautions While Using This Medicine

If you will be taking this medicine for a long time, as for arthritis (rheumatism), your doctor should check your progress at regular visits.

Stomach problems may be more likely to occur if you take two or more anti-inflammatory analgesics regularly (for example, every day) or drink alcoholic beverages while being treated with this medicine. Aspirin or other salicylates, diclofenac (e.g., Voltaren), indomethacin (e.g., Indocin), ketoprofen (e.g., Orudis), phenylbutazone (e.g., Butazolidin), and tiaprofenic acid (e.g., Surgam) are also anti-inflammatory analgesics that may cause problems if taken regularly with any of these medicines. Therefore, **do not take other anti-inflammatory analgesics regularly or drink alcoholic beverages while taking this medicine,** unless otherwise directed by your doctor.

Too much use of acetaminophen together with an anti-inflammatory analgesic may increase the chance of kidney problems. Therefore, do not regularly take acetaminophen together with this medicine, unless your physician or dentist has directed you to do so.

Before having any kind of surgery (including dental surgery), tell the physician or dentist in charge that you are taking this medicine.

This medicine may cause some people to become drowsy, dizzy, lightheaded, or less alert than they are normally. **Make sure you know how you react to this medicine before you drive, use machinery, or do other jobs that require you to be alert.**

For patients taking mefenamic acid: If diarrhea occurs while you are using this medicine, **stop taking it and check with your doctor immediately. Do not take it again without first checking with your doctor,** because severe diarrhea may occur each time you take it.

Some people who take anti-inflammatory analgesics may become more sensitive to sunlight than they are normally. These people may become sunburned more easily or break out in a rash after being in the sun. When you first begin taking this medicine, avoid too much sun or too much use of a sunlamp. You may protect yourself against sunlight with clothing or by using a factor-15 sunscreen, until you see how you react, especially if you tend to burn easily. **If you have a severe reaction, check with your doctor.**

Check with your doctor immediately if chills, fever, muscle aches or pains, or other influenza-like symptoms occur shortly before, or together with, a skin rash. Very rarely, these effects may be the first signs of a serious reaction to this medicine.

Anti-inflammatory analgesics may cause a serious type of allergic reaction called anaphylaxis. Although this is rare, it may occur more often in patients who are allergic to aspirin or to any other anti-inflammatory analgesic. **Anaphylaxis requires immediate medical attention.** The most serious signs of this reaction are very fast or irregular breathing, gasping for breath, wheezing, or fainting. Other signs may include very pale, gray, or blue color of the skin of the face; very fast but irregular heartbeat or pulse; hive-like swellings on the skin; and puffiness or swellings of the eyelids or around the eyes. If these effects occur, get emergency help at once. Ask someone to drive you to the nearest hospital emergency room. If this is not possible, do not try to drive yourself. Call an ambulance, lie down, cover yourself to keep warm, and prop your feet higher than your head. Stay in that position until help arrives.

For patients taking ibuprofen without a prescription:

• Check with your physician or dentist:
   —if your symptoms do not improve or if they get worse.
   —if you are using this medicine to bring down a fever and the fever lasts more than 3 days or returns.
   —if the painful area becomes red or swollen.

Side Effects of This Medicine

Along with its needed effects, a medicine may cause some unwanted effects. Although not all of these side effects may occur, if they do occur they may need medical attention.

Stop taking this medicine and check with your doctor immediately if any of the following side effects occur:

Rare

Chest pain
Convulsions (seizures)
Hive-like swellings (large) on face, eyelids, mouth, lips, or tongue
Shortness of breath, troubled breathing, wheezing, or tightness in chest
Sudden decrease in amount of urine

Also, check with your doctor as soon as possible if any of the following side effects occur:

More common

Skin rash

Less common or rare

Abdominal or stomach pain (severe)
Bleeding or crusting sores on lips
Bloody or black tarry stools
Bloody or cloudy urine
Blurred vision or any change in vision
Chills and/or fever
Confusion, mental depression, or other mood or mental changes
Decreased hearing, any other change in hearing, or ringing or buzzing in ears
Difficult, burning, or painful urination
Frequent urge to urinate
Headache (severe) with fever and stiff neck
Hives or itching of skin
Increase in blood pressure
Muscle cramps, pain, or weakness
Rectal bleeding (with naproxen suppositories)
Redness, tenderness, burning, or peeling of skin
Sores, ulcers, or white spots on lips or in mouth
Spitting of blood
Swelling and/or tenderness in upper abdominal or stomach area
Swelling of face, feet, or lower legs
Swollen or painful glands
Thickened or scaly skin
Unexplained nosebleeds
Unexplained sore throat, chills, and fever
Unusual bleeding or bruising
Unusual thirst
Unusual tiredness or weakness
Unusual weight gain
Vomiting of blood or material that looks like coffee grounds
Yellow eyes or skin

Other side effects may occur that usually do not require medical attention. These side effects may go away during treatment as your body adjusts to the medicine. However, check with your doctor if any of the following side effects continue or are bothersome:

More common

Abdominal or stomach pain or discomfort (mild to moderate)
Diarrhea (if taking mefenamic acid, stop taking the medicine and check with your doctor immediately)
Dizziness, drowsiness, or lightheadedness
Headache
Heartburn, indigestion, nausea, or vomiting

Less common or rare

Bloated feeling, gas, or constipation
Decreased appetite or loss of appetite
Fast or pounding heartbeat
General feeling of discomfort or illness
Increased sensitivity of skin to sunlight
Increased sweating
Irritation, dryness, or soreness of mouth
Irritation, dryness, redness, or swelling of eyes
Nervousness or trembling
Numbness, tingling, pain, or weakness in hands or feet
Rectal burning (with naproxen suppositories)
Trouble in sleeping

Although not all of the side effects listed above have been reported for all of these medicines, they have been reported for at least one of them. However, since all anti-inflammatory analgesics are very similar, it is possible that any of the above side effects may occur with any of these medicines.

For elderly patients: Swelling of the face, feet, or lower legs; sudden decrease in the amount of urine; or stomach problems may be especially likely to occur in the elderly, who are usually more sensitive to the effects of these medicines.

Other side effects not listed above may also occur in some patients. If you notice any other effects, check with your doctor.

December 1987

ANTIMUSCARINICS/ANTISPASMODICS
(Systemic)

This information applies to the following medicines:

Anisotropine (an-iss-oh-TROE-peen)
Atropine (A-troe-peen)
Belladonna (bell-a-DON-a)
Clidinium (kli-DI-nee-um)
Dicyclomine (dye-SYE-kloe-meen)
Glycopyrrolate (glye-koe-PYE-roe-late)
Hexocyclium (hex-oh-SYE-klee-um)
Homatropine (hoe-MA-troe-peen)
Hyoscyamine (hye-oh-SYE-a-meen)
Hyoscyamine and Scopolamine (scoe-POL-a-meen)
Isopropamide (eye-soe-PROE-pa-mide)
Mepenzolate (me-PEN-zoe-late)
Methantheline (meth-AN-tha-leen)
Methscopolamine (meth-skoe-POL-a-meen)
Oxyphencyclimine (ox-i-fen-SYE-kli-meen)
Oxyphenonium (ox-i-phe-NOE-nee-um)
Pirenzepine (peer-EN-ze-peen)
Propantheline (proe-PAN-the-leen)
Scopolamine (scoe-POL-a-meen)
Tridihexethyl (trye-dye-hex-E-thill)

Some commonly used brand names are:	Generic names:
Valpin 50	Anisotropine
	Atropine†
	Belladonna†
Quarzan	Clidinium
Antispas A-Spas Bentyl Bentylol* Byclomine Cyclocen Dibent Dicen Di-Cyclonex Dilomine Di-Spaz Formulex* Lomine* Neoquess Or-Tyl Protylol* Spasmoban* Spasmoject Viscerol*	Dicyclomine†
Robinul Robinul Forte	Glycopyrrolate†
Tral Filmtabs	Hexocyclium
Homapin	Homatropine†
Cystospaz	Hyoscyamine
Anaspaz Bellaspaz Cystospaz-M Levsin Levsinex Timecaps Neoquess	Hyoscyamine Sulfate
Bellafoline	Hyoscyamine and Scopolamine
Darbid	Isopropamide

Cantil	Mepenzolate
Banthine	Methantheline
Pamine	Methscopolamine
Daricon	Oxyphencyclimine
Antrenyl	Oxyphenonium
Gastrozepin*	Pirenzepine*
Norpanth Pro-Banthine Propanthel*	Propantheline†
Transderm-Scōp Transderm-V* Triptone	Scopolamine†
Pathilon	Tridihexethyl

*Not commercially available in the U. S.
†Generic name product may also be available.

To the Reader: If you do not recognize the names of medical conditions or medicines referred to in this information, check with your doctor, nurse, or pharmacist. Definitions for selected medical terms may be found in the Glossary. Brand names for the generic drug names listed can be found in the Index. In addition, selected brand names commonly associated with the generic name have been included in the text to help you recognize medicine you may be taking. The fact that a brand name product is not mentioned does not mean the information does not apply. It is a good idea for you to learn both the generic and brand names of your medicines and to write them down for future use.

The antimuscarinics/antispasmodics are a group of medicines that include the natural belladonna alkaloids (atropine, belladonna, hyoscyamine, and scopolamine) and related products. They are taken by mouth or given by injection. Scopolamine is used also by transdermal disk (a small patch that is applied to the skin).

The antimuscarinics/antispasmodics are used to relieve cramps or spasms of the stomach, intestines, and bladder. Some are used together with antacids or other medicine in the treatment of peptic ulcer. Others are used to prevent nausea, vomiting, and motion sickness. These medicines may also be used for other conditions as determined by your doctor.

Antimuscarinics/antispasmodics are also used in certain surgical and emergency procedures. In surgery, some are given by injection before anesthesia to help relax you and to decrease secretions, such as saliva. During anesthesia and surgery, atropine, glycopyrrolate, hyoscyamine, and scopolamine are used to help keep the heartbeat normal. Atropine is also given by injection to help relax the stomach and intestines for certain types of examinations. Some antimuscarinics are also used to treat poisoning caused by medicines such as neostigmine and physostigmine, certain types of mushrooms, and poisoning by "nerve" gases or organic phosphorous pesticides (for example, demeton [Systox], diazinon, malathion, parathion, and ronnel [Trolene]).

The antimuscarinics/antispasmodics are available only with your doctor's prescription.

Remember:

• **This medicine has been prescribed for your current medical problem only.** It must not be given to other people or used for other problems unless you are directed to do so by your doctor.

• **Keep all medicines out of the reach of children.**

• In order for this medicine to work, it must be used as directed.

• If you are receiving this medicine by injection, some of the information about this medicine may not apply.

• **It is very important that you read and understand the following information.** If any of the information causes you special concern, do not decide against using this medicine without first checking with your doctor.

• Before you begin using any new medicine (prescription or nonprescription) or if you develop any new medical problem while you are using this medicine, check with your doctor, nurse, or pharmacist.

• **If you have any questions** about the following information or if you want more information about this medicine or your medical problem, **ask your doctor, nurse, or pharmacist**.

Before Using This Medicine

In order to decide on the best treatment for your medical problem, your doctor should be told:

—if you have ever had any unusual or allergic reaction to any of the natural belladonna alkaloids (atropine, belladonna, hyoscyamine, and scopolamine) or any related products.

—if you are on a low-salt, low-sugar, or any other special diet, or if you are allergic to any substance, such as foods, sulfites or other preservatives, or dyes. Most medicines contain more than their active ingredient, and many liquid medicines contain alcohol. Your doctor, nurse, or pharmacist can help you avoid products that may cause a problem.

—if you are **pregnant** or if you may become pregnant. Studies with antimuscarinics/antispasmodics have not been done in humans. However, the following effects in humans have been noted:

• *Atropine* and *hyoscyamine*—Have been reported to increase the heartbeat of the fetus when given during pregnancy by injection into a vein.

• *Scopolamine*—When given before labor begins, may cause an unusually slow heartbeat, shortness of breath, or troubled breathing, and may also increase the possibility of bleeding in the newborn.

Studies with *belladonna, hyoscyamine, propantheline, or scopolamine* have not been done in animals. However, in animal studies with:

• *Atropine*—Has not been shown to cause birth defects or other problems in animal studies.

• *Clidinium*—Has not been shown to cause birth defects or other problems in animal studies.

• *Glycopyrrolate*—Did not cause birth defects but did cause a decrease in the chance of becoming pregnant and in the newborn's chance of surviving after weaning.

• *Hexocyclium*—Studies in rabbits receiving up to many times the recommended human dose have shown that hexocyclium increases the chance of abortion.

• *Mepenzolate*—Has not been shown to cause birth defects or other problems in animal studies.

—if you are **breast-feeding**. Although these medicines may pass into the breast milk, they have not been shown to cause problems in nursing babies. However, the flow of breast milk may be reduced in some patients.

—if you have any of the following medical problems:

    Bleeding problems (severe)
    Brain damage (in children)
    Colitis (severe)
    Down's syndrome (mongolism)
    Dry mouth (severe and continuing)
    Enlarged prostate
    Fever
    Glaucoma
    Heart disease
    Hernia (hiatal)
    Hypertension (high blood pressure)
    Intestinal blockage or other intestinal problems
    Kidney disease
    Liver disease
    Lung disease (chronic)
    Myasthenia gravis
    Overactive thyroid
    Spastic paralysis (in children)
    Toxemia of pregnancy
    Urinary tract blockage or difficult urination

—if you are taking **any** other prescription or nonprescription (OTC) medicine, especially:

    Antacids
    Central nervous system (CNS) depressants
    Diarrhea medicine containing kaolin or attapulgite
    Ketoconazole (e.g., Nizoral)
    Other antimuscarinics (medicine for abdominal or stomach spasms or cramps)
    Potassium chloride (e.g., Kay Ciel)

—if you are now taking or have taken within the past 2 weeks monoamine oxidase (MAO) inhibitors, such as:

    Furazolidone (e.g., Furoxone)
    Isocarboxazid (e.g., Marplan)
    Pargyline (e.g., Eutonyl)
    Phenelzine (e.g., Nardil)
    Procarbazine (e.g., Matulane)
    Tranylcypromine (e.g., Parnate)

Proper Use of This Medicine

Take this medicine only as directed. Do not take more of it, do not take it more often, and do not take it for a longer period of time than your doctor ordered. To do so may increase the chance of side effects.

For patients taking any of these medicines by mouth:

• Take this medicine 30 minutes to 1 hour before meals unless otherwise directed by your doctor.

For patients using the transdermal disk form of scopolamine:
- This medicine usually comes with patient directions.
Read them carefully before using this medicine.
- Wash and dry your hands thoroughly before and after
handling.
- Apply the disk to the hairless area of skin behind the
ear. Do not place over any cuts or irritations.

If you miss a dose of this medicine, take it as soon as
possible. However, if it is almost time for your next
dose, skip the missed dose and go back to your regular
dosing schedule. Do not double doses.

How to store this medicine:
- **Keep out of the reach of children** since overdose is
especially dangerous in young children.
- Store away from heat and direct light.
- Do not store the capsule or tablet form of this medicine in the bathroom, near the kitchen sink, or in other
damp places. Heat or moisture may cause the medicine to break down.
- Keep the liquid form of this medicine tightly closed
and keep it from from freezing. Do not refrigerate the
syrup form of this medicine.
- Do not keep outdated medicine or medicine no longer
needed. Be sure that any discarded medicine is out of
the reach of children.

Precautions While Using This Medicine

If you think you or someone else may have taken an overdose, get emergency help at once. Taking an overdose
of any of the belladonna alkaloids or taking scopolamine with alcohol or other CNS depressants may lead
to unconsciousness and possibly death. Some signs of
overdose are clumsiness or unsteadiness; dizziness; severe drowsiness; fever; hallucinations (seeing, hearing,
or feeling things that are not there); confusion; shortness of breath or troubled breathing; slurred speech;
unusual excitement, nervousness, restlessness, or irritability; unusually fast heartbeat; and unusual warmth,
dryness, and flushing of skin.

These medicines may make you sweat less, causing your
body temperature to increase. **Use extra care not to
become overheated during exercise or hot weather while
you are taking this medicine,** since overheating may
result in heat stroke.

Antimuscarinics may cause some people to have blurred
vision. **Make sure your vision is clear before you drive
or do other jobs that require you to see well.** These
medicines may also cause your eyes to become more
sensitive to light than they are normally. Wearing sunglasses may help lessen the discomfort from bright
light.

These medicines, especially in high doses, may cause some
people to become dizzy or drowsy. **Make sure you
know how you react to this medicine before you drive,
use machines, or do other jobs that require you to be
alert.**

Dizziness, lightheadedness, or fainting may occur, especially when you get up from a lying or sitting position. Getting up slowly may help lessen this problem.

These medicines may cause dryness of the mouth, nose,
and throat. For temporary relief of mouth dryness, use
sugarless candy or gum, melt bits of ice in your mouth,
or use a saliva substitute. However, if dry mouth continues for more than 2 weeks, check with your physician or dentist. Continuing dryness of the mouth may
increase the chance of dental disease, including tooth
decay, gum disease, and fungal infections.

For patients taking isopropamide:
- Make sure your doctor knows if you are planning to
have any future thyroid tests. The results of the thyroid
test may be affected by the iodine in this medicine.

For patients taking scopolamine:
- This medicine will add to the effects of alcohol and
other CNS depressants (medicines that slow down the
nervous system, possibly causing drowsiness). Some
examples of CNS depressants are antihistamines or
medicine for hay fever, other allergies, or colds; sedatives, tranquilizers, or sleeping medicine; prescription
pain medicine or narcotics; barbiturates; medicine for
seizures; muscle relaxants; or anesthetics, including
some dental anesthetics. **Check with your doctor before
taking any of the above while you are using this medicine.**

For patients taking any of these medicines by mouth:
- Do not take this medicine within 1 hour of taking
antacids or medicine for diarrhea. Taking these types
of medicines too close together may prevent this medicine from working as well.

Side Effects of This Medicine

Along with its needed effects, a medicine may cause some
unwanted effects. Although not all of these side effects
may occur, if they do occur they may need medical
attention.

Check with your doctor as soon as possible if any of the
following side effects occur:
Rare
　Confusion (especially in the elderly)
　Dizziness, lightheadedness (continuing), or fainting
　Eye pain
　Skin rash or hives
Signs of overdose
　Blurred vision (continuing) or changes in near vision
　Clumsiness or unsteadiness
　Confusion
　Convulsions (seizures)
　Difficulty in breathing, muscle weakness (severe), or
　　tiredness
　Dizziness
　Drowsiness (severe)
　Dryness of mouth, nose, or throat (severe)
　Fast heartbeat
　Fever
　Hallucinations (seeing, hearing, or feeling things that are
　　not there)

Shortness of breath or troubled breathing
Slurred speech
Unusual excitement, nervousness, restlessness, or irritability
Unusual warmth, dryness, and flushing of skin

Other side effects may occur that usually do not require medical attention. These side effects may go away during treatment as your body adjusts to the medicine. However, check with your doctor if any of the following side effects continue or are bothersome:

More common

Constipation (less common with hyoscyamine)
Decrease in sweating
Dryness of mouth, nose, throat, or skin

Less common or rare

Bloated feeling
Blurred vision
Decreased flow of breast milk
Difficult urination
Difficulty in swallowing
Drowsiness (more common with high doses of any of these medicines and with usual doses of scopolamine when given by mouth or by injection)
False sense of well-being (for scopolamine only)
Headache
Increased sensitivity of eyes to light
Lightheadedness (with injection)
Loss of memory
Nausea or vomiting
Redness or other signs of irritation at place of injection
Trouble in sleeping (for scopolamine only)
Unusual tiredness or weakness

For patients using scopolamine:

• After you stop using scopolamine, your body may need time to adjust. The length of time this takes depends on the amount of scopolamine you were using and how long you used it. During this period of time check with your doctor if you notice any of the following side effects:

Anxiety
Irritability
Nightmares
Trouble in sleeping

For patients using the transdermal disk of scopolamine:
• While using the disk or even after removing it, your eyes may become more sensitive to light than usual. You may also notice the pupil in one eye is larger than the other. Check with your doctor if this side effect continues or is bothersome.

For children: Children are usually more sensitive to the effects of the antimuscarinics. In infants and children, especially those with spastic paralysis or brain damage, this medicine may be more likely to cause severe side effects. Unusual warmth, dryness, and flushing of skin are more likely to occur in children. Also, when antimuscarinics are given to children during hot weather, a rapid increase in body temperature may occur. In addition, unusual excitement, nervousness, restlessness, or irritability may be more likely to occur in children.

For elderly patients: Elderly patients are usually more sensitive to the effects of antimuscarinics. Confusion, constipation, difficult urination, drowsiness, dryness of mouth, nose, throat, or skin, and memory loss may be more likely to occur. Unusual excitement, nervousness, restlessness, or irritability may also be more likely to occur in elderly patients.

Other side effects not listed above may also occur in some patients. If you notice any other effects, check with your doctor.

December 1987

ANTIMYASTHENICS (Systemic)

This information applies to the following medicines:

Ambenonium (am-be-NOE-nee-um)
Neostigmine (nee-oh-STIG-meen)
Pyridostigmine (peer-id-oh-STIG-meen)

Some commonly used brand names are:	Generic names:
Mytelase	Ambenonium
Prostigmin	Neostigmine†
Mestinon Mestinon Timespans Regonol	Pyridostigmine

†Generic name product may also be available in the U.S.

To the Reader: If you do not recognize the names of medical conditions or medicines referred to in this information, check with your doctor, nurse, or pharmacist. Definitions for selected medical terms may be found in the Glossary. Brand names for the generic drug names listed can be found in the Index. In addition, selected brand names commonly associated with the generic name have been included in the text to help you recognize medicine you may be taking. The fact that a brand name product is not mentioned does not mean the information does not apply. It is a good idea for you to learn both the generic and brand names of your medicines and to write them down for future use.

Antimyasthenics are given by mouth or by injection to treat myasthenia gravis. Neostigmine may also be given by injection as a test for myasthenia gravis. Sometimes neostigmine is given by injection to prevent or treat certain urinary tract or intestinal disorders. In addition, neostigmine or pyridostigmine may be given by injection as an antidote to certain types of muscle relaxants used in surgery.

These medicines are available only with your doctor's prescription.

Remember:

• **This medicine has been prescribed for your current medical problem only.** It must not be given to other people or used for other problems unless you are directed to do so by your doctor.

• **Keep all medicines out of the reach of children.**

• In order for this medicine to work, it must be used as directed.

• If you are receiving this medicine by injection, some of the information about this medicine may not apply.

• **It is very important that you read and understand the following information.** If any of the information causes you special concern, do not decide against using this medicine without first checking with your doctor.

• Before you begin using any new medicine (prescription or nonprescription) or if you develop any new medical problem while you are using this medicine, check with your doctor, nurse, or pharmacist.

• **If you have any questions** about the following information or if you want more information about this medicine or your medical problem, **ask your doctor, nurse, or pharmacist.**

Before Using This Medicine

In order to decide on the best treatment for your medical problem, your doctor should be told:

—if you have ever had any unusual or allergic reaction to ambenonium, bromides, neostigmine, or pyridostigmine.

—if you are on a low-salt, low-sugar, or any other special diet, or if you are allergic to any substance, such as foods, sulfites or other preservatives, or dyes. Most medicines contain more than their active ingredient, and many liquid medicines contain alcohol. Your doctor, nurse, or pharmacist can help you avoid products that may cause a problem.

—if you are **pregnant** or if you may become pregnant while using this medicine. Antimyasthenics have not been shown to cause birth defects or other problems in humans.

—if you are **breast-feeding**. Antimyasthenics have not been shown to cause problems in nursing babies.

—if you are taking any of the antimyasthenics and have any of the following medical problems:
Asthma
Heart disease
Intestinal blockage
Pneumonia
Urinary tract blockage
Urinary tract infection

—if you are now taking or receiving aminoglycoside antibiotics such as amikacin, gentamicin, kanamycin, neomycin, streptomycin, or tobramycin.

—if you are using **any** other prescription or nonprescription (OTC) medicine, especially:
Demecarium (e.g., Humorsol)
Echothiophate (e.g., Phospholine Iodide)
Guanadrel (e.g., Hylorel)
Guanethidine (e.g., Ismelin)
Isoflurophate (e.g., Floropryl)
Malathion (e.g., Prioderm)
Mecamylamine (e.g., Inversine)
Procainamide (e.g., Pronestyl)
Trimethaphan (e.g., Arfonad)

Proper Use of This Medicine

Your doctor may want you to take this medicine with food or milk to help lessen the chance of side effects. If you have any questions about how you should be taking this medicine, check with your doctor.

Take this medicine only as directed. Do not take more of it, do not take it more often, and do not take it for a longer period of time than your doctor ordered. To do so may increase the chance of side effects.

If you are taking this medicine for myasthenia gravis:

• When you first begin taking this medicine, your doctor may want you to keep a daily record of:
—the time you take each dose.
—the period of time you feel better after taking each dose.
—the period of time you feel worse.
—any side effects that occur.

This is to help your doctor decide whether the dose of this medicine should be increased or decreased and how often the medicine should be taken in order for it to be most effective in your condition.

If you miss a dose of this medicine, take it as soon as you remember. However, if it is almost time for your next dose, skip the missed dose and go back to your regular dosing schedule. Do not double doses.

How to store this medicine:

- **Keep out of the reach of children.**

- Store away from heat and direct light.

- Do not store the tablet form of this medicine in the bathroom, near the kitchen sink, or in other damp places. Heat or moisture may cause the medicine to break down.

- Keep the syrup form of pyridostigmine from freezing.

- Do not keep outdated medicine or medicine no longer needed. Be sure that any discarded medicine is out of the reach of children.

Side Effects of This Medicine

Along with its needed effects, a medicine may cause some unwanted effects. Although not all of these side effects may occur, if they do occur they may need medical attention.

Check with your doctor immediately if any of the following side effects occur:

Signs of overdose
  Blurred vision
  Clumsiness or unsteadiness
  Confusion
  Convulsions (seizures)
  Diarrhea (severe)
  Increase in bronchial secretions or salivation (severe)
  Increasing muscle weakness (especially in the arms, neck, shoulders, and tongue)
  Muscle cramps or twitching
  Nausea or vomiting (severe)

  Shortness of breath, troubled breathing, wheezing, or tightness in chest
  Slow heartbeat
  Slurred speech
  Stomach cramps or pain (severe)
  Unusual irritability, nervousness, restlessness, or fear
  Unusual tiredness or weakness

Also, check with your doctor as soon as possible if any of the following side effects occur:
Rare
  Redness, swelling, or pain at place of injection (applies only to pyridostigmine injection)
  Skin rash (does not apply to ambenonium)

Other side effects may occur that usually do not require medical attention. These side effects may go away during treatment as your body adjusts to the medicine. However, check with your doctor if any of the following side effects continue or are bothersome:

More common
  Diarrhea
  Nausea or vomiting
  Stomach cramps or pain
  Unusual increase in sweating
  Unusual watering of mouth

Less common
  Frequent urge to urinate
  Increase in bronchial secretions
  Unusually small pupils
  Unusual watering of eyes

For elderly patients: Many medicines have not been tested in older people. Therefore, it is not known whether the medicine acts the same way it does in younger adults. Check with your doctor or pharmacist if you notice any unusual effects while taking this medicine or if you think it is not working as it should.

Other side effects not listed above may also occur in some patients. If you notice any other effects, check with your doctor.

December 1987

ANTIPYRINE AND BENZOCAINE (Otic)

Some commonly used brand names are:

Auralgan   Auromid
Aurodex   Oto

To the Reader: If you do not recognize the names of medical conditions or medicines referred to in this information, check with your doctor, nurse, or pharmacist. Definitions for selected medical terms may be found in the Glossary. Brand names for the generic drug names listed can be found in the Index. In addition, selected brand names commonly associated with the generic name have been included in the text to help you recognize medicine you may be taking. The fact that a brand name product is not mentioned does not mean the information does not apply. It is a good idea for you to learn both the generic and brand names of your medicines and to write them down for future use.

Antipyrine (an-tee-PYE-reen) and benzocaine (BEN-zoe-kane) combination is used in the ear to help relieve the pain, swelling, and redness of some ear infections. It will not cure the infection itself. This medicine is also used to help remove ear wax.

In the U.S., this medicine is available only with your doctor's prescription. In Canada, this medicine is available without a prescription. However, your doctor may have special instructions on the proper dose for your ear problem.

Remember:

• **This medicine has been prescribed for your current medical problem only.** It must not be given to other people or used for other problems unless you are directed to do so by your doctor.

• **Keep all medicines out of the reach of children.**

• In order for this medicine to work, it must be used as directed.

• **It is very important that you read and understand the following information.** If any of the information causes you special concern, do not decide against using this medicine without first checking with your doctor.

• Before you begin using any new medicine (prescription or nonprescription) or if you develop any new medical problem while you are using this medicine, check with your doctor, nurse, or pharmacist.

• **If you have any questions** about the following information or if you want more information about this medicine or your medical problem, **ask your doctor, nurse, or pharmacist.**

Before Using This Medicine

In order to decide on the best treatment for your medical problem, your doctor should be told:

—if you have had any unusual or allergic reaction to antipyrine or benzocaine or other local anesthetics.

—if you are allergic to any substance, such as certain preservatives or dyes. Most medicines contain more than their active ingredient. Your doctor, nurse, or pharmacist can help you avoid products that may cause a problem.

—if your ear is draining.

—if you are **pregnant** or if you may become pregnant. Although this medicine has not been shown to cause problems, studies have not been done in either humans or animals.

—if you are **breast-feeding.** It is not known whether this medicine passes into the breast milk. However, this medicine has not been shown to cause problems in nursing babies.

Proper Use of This Medicine

You may warm the ear drops to body temperature (37 °C or 98.6 °F) by holding the bottle in your hand for a few minutes before applying.

How to apply this medicine: Lie down or tilt the head so that the affected ear faces up. Gently pull the ear lobe up and back for adults (down and back for children) to straighten the ear canal. Drop the medicine into the ear canal. Keep the ear facing up for about 5 minutes to allow the medicine to run to the bottom of the ear canal. A clean soft cotton plug may be moistened with a few drops of this medicine and gently inserted into the ear opening to prevent the medicine from leaking out.

If you are using this medicine to help remove ear wax, the ear should be flushed with warm water after you have used this medicine for 2 or 3 days. Make sure that you know how to do this. If you have any questions about how to flush the ear with water, check with your doctor.

To prevent contamination of the ear drops, do not touch the dropper to any surface (including the ear).

Do not rinse the dropper after use. Wipe the tip of the dropper with a clean tissue and keep the container tightly closed.

If you miss a dose of this medicine, use it as soon as you remember. However, if it is almost time for your next dose, skip the missed dose and go back to your regular dosing schedule.

How to store this medicine:

• **Keep out of the reach of children.**

• Store away from heat and direct light.

• Keep the medicine from freezing.

• Do not keep outdated medicine or medicine no longer needed. Be sure that any discarded medicine is out of the reach of children.

Side Effects of This Medicine

Along with its needed effects, a medicine may cause some unwanted effects. The following side effects may go away during treatment as your body adjusts to the medicine; however, check with your doctor if either effect continues or is bothersome:

Itching or burning in the ear

For elderly patients: Many medicines have not been tested in older people. Therefore, it is not known whether the medicine acts the same way it does in younger adults. Check with your doctor or pharmacist if you notice any unusual effects while taking this medicine or if you think it is not working as it should.

Other side effects not listed above may also occur in some patients. If you notice any other effects, check with your doctor.

December 1987

ANTITHYROID AGENTS (Systemic)

This information applies to the following medicines:

Methimazole (meth-IM-a-zole)
Propylthiouracil (proe-pill-thye-oh-YOOR-a-sill)

Some commonly used brand names or other names are:	Generic names:
Tapazole Thiamazole	Methimazole
Propyl-Thyracil*	Propylthiouracil†

*Not available in the U.S.
†Generic name product may also be available in the U.S.

To the Reader: If you do not recognize the names of medical conditions or medicines referred to in this information, check with your doctor, nurse, or pharmacist. Definitions for selected medical terms may be found in the Glossary. Brand names for the generic drug names listed can be found in the Index. In addition, selected brand names commonly associated with the generic name have been included in the text to help you recognize medicine you may be taking. The fact that a brand name product is not mentioned does not mean the information does not apply. It is a good idea for you to learn both the generic and brand names of your medicines and to write them down for future use.

Methimazole and propylthiouracil belong to the group of medicines known as antithyroid agents. They are used to treat conditions in which the thyroid gland produces too much thyroid hormone.

These medicines work by making it harder for the body to use iodine to make thyroid hormone. They do not block the effects of thyroid hormone.

Methimazole and propylthiouracil are available only with your doctor's prescription.

Remember:
• **This medicine has been prescribed for your current medical problem only.** It must not be given to other people or used for other problems unless you are directed to do so by your doctor.

• **Keep all medicines out of the reach of children.**

• In order for this medicine to work, it must be used as directed.

• **It is very important that you read and understand the following information.** If any of the information causes you special concern, do not decide against using this medicine without first checking with your doctor.

• Before you begin using any new medicine (prescription or nonprescription) or if you develop any new medical problem while you are using this medicine, check with your doctor, nurse, or pharmacist.

• **If you have any questions** about the following information or if you want more information about this medicine or your medical problem, **ask your doctor, nurse, or pharmacist.**

Before Using This Medicine

In order to decide on the best treatment for your medical problem, your doctor should be told:

—if you have ever had any unusual reaction to methimazole or propylthiouracil.

—if you are on a low-salt, low-sugar, or any other special diet, or if you are allergic to any substance, such as foods, sulfites or other preservatives, or dyes. Most medicines contain more than their active ingredient. Your doctor, nurse, or pharmacist can help you avoid products that may cause a problem.

—if you are **pregnant** or if you may become pregnant. Use of too large a dose during pregnancy may cause blood problems, underactive thyroid, goiter, or birth defects in the baby. However, use of the proper dose, with careful monitoring by the doctor, is not likely to cause problems. Be sure that you have discussed this with your doctor before taking this medicine.

—if you are **breast-feeding**. This medicine passes into breast milk and may cause unwanted effects such as underactive thyroid in nursing babies. It may be necessary for you to take another medicine or to stop breast-feeding during treatment. Be sure you have discussed the risks and benefits of the medicine with your doctor.

—if you have either of the following medical problems:
Infection
Liver disease

—if you are using **any** other prescription or nonprescription (OTC) medicine, especially:
Lithium (e.g., Lithane)
Potassium iodide (e.g., Pima)

Proper Use of This Medicine

Use this medicine only as directed by your doctor. Do not use more or less of it and do not use it more often or for a longer period of time than your doctor ordered. To do so may increase the chance of side effects.

This medicine works best when there is a constant amount in the blood. **To help keep this amount constant, do not miss any doses. Also, it is best to take each dose at evenly spaced times day and night.** For example, if you are to take 3 doses a day, the doses should be spaced about 8 hours apart. If this interferes with your sleep or other daily activities, or if you need help in planning the best times to take your medicine, check with your doctor, nurse, or pharmacist.

Food in your stomach may change the effects of this medicine. To make sure that you always get the same effects, try to take this medicine at the same time in relation to meals every day. That is, always take it with meals or always take it on an empty stomach.

If you miss a dose of this medicine, take it as soon as possible. If it is almost time for your next dose, take both doses together. Then go back to your regular dosing schedule. If you miss more than one dose or if you have any questions about this, check with your doctor.

How to store this medicine:

• **Keep out of the reach of children.**

• Store away from heat and direct light.

• Do not store in the bathroom, near the kitchen sink, or in other high-moisture areas. Heat or moisture may cause the medicine to break down.

• Do not keep outdated medicine or medicine no longer needed. Be sure that any discarded medicine is out of the reach of children.

Precautions While Using This Medicine

It is very important that your doctor check your progress at regular intervals to make sure that this medicine is working properly and to check for unwanted effects.

It may take several days or weeks for this medicine to work. However, **do not stop taking this medicine without first checking with your doctor.** Some medical problems may require several years of continuous treatment.

Before having any kind of surgery (including dental surgery) or emergency treatment, **tell the physician or dentist in charge that you are taking this medicine.**

Check with your doctor right away if you get an injury, infection, or illness of any kind. Your doctor may want you to stop taking this medicine or change the amount you are taking.

Side Effects of This Medicine

Along with its needed effects, a medicine may cause some unwanted effects. Although not all of these side effects may occur, if they do occur they may need medical attention.

Check with your doctor immediately if any of the following side effects occur:
Less common
 Fever, chills, or sore throat
 General feeling of body discomfort or weakness
 Nausea or vomiting (severe)
 Pain, swelling, or redness in joints

Check with your doctor as soon as possible if any of the following side effects occur:
More common
 Skin rash or itching
Rare
 Backache
 Changes in menstrual periods
 Coldness
 Constipation
 Diarrhea
 Dry, puffy skin
 Fast or irregular heartbeat
 Headache
 Increase or decrease in urination
 Irritability
 Listlessness or sleepiness
 Muscle aches
 Swelling of feet or lower legs
 Swollen lymph glands
 Tiredness or weakness
 Unusual bleeding or bruising
 Weight gain
 Yellow eyes and skin

Other side effects may occur that usually do not require medical attention. These side effects may go away during treatment as your body adjusts to the medicine. However, check with your doctor if any of the following side effects continue or are bothersome:
Less common
 Dizziness
 Loss of taste
 Nausea or vomiting
 Numbness or tingling of fingers, toes, or face
 Stomach pain

For elderly patients: Many medicines have not been tested in older people. Therefore, it is not known whether the medicine acts the same way it does in younger adults. Check with your doctor or pharmacist if you notice any unusual effects while taking this medicine or if you think it is not working as it should.

Other side effects not listed above may also occur in some patients. If you notice any other effects, check with your doctor.

December 1987

APOMORPHINE (Systemic)

To the Reader: If you do not recognize the names of medical conditions or medicines referred to in this information, check with your doctor, nurse, or pharmacist. Definitions for selected medical terms may be found in the Glossary. Brand names for the generic drug names listed can be found in the Index. In addition, selected brand names commonly associated with the generic name have been included in the text to help you recognize medicine you may be taking. The fact that a brand name product is not mentioned does not mean the information does not apply. It is a good idea for you to learn both the generic and brand names of your medicines and to write them down for future use.

Apomorphine (a-poe-MOR-feen) is used in the emergency treatment of certain types of poisoning. It is given by injection to cause vomiting of the poison.

Apomorphine is available only on prescription and should be administered only by or under the immediate supervision of a doctor.

Remember:

• **It is very important that you read and understand the following information.** If any of the information causes you special concern, do not decide against receiving this medicine without first checking with your doctor.

• **If you have any questions** about the following information or if you want more information about this medicine or your medical problem, **ask your doctor, nurse, or pharmacist.**

Before Using This Medicine

In order to decide on the best treatment for your medical problem, your doctor should be told:

—if you have ever had any unusual or allergic reaction to codeine, hydromorphone, levorphanol, morphine, opium alkaloids, oxycodone, or oxymorphone.

—if you are **pregnant** or if you intend to become pregnant. Studies have not been done in either humans or animals.

—if you are **breast-feeding**. Apomorphine has not been shown to cause problems in nursing babies.

—if you have heart disease.

—if you tend to vomit easily.

—if you are now taking an antiemetic (medicine for nausea or vomiting).

Proper Use of This Medicine

Before you receive an injection of this medicine, your doctor may want you to drink a full glass (8 ounces) of water. This is to help the medicine cause vomiting of the poison.

Side Effects of This Medicine

Along with its needed effects, a medicine may cause some unwanted effects. Although not all of these side effects may occur, if they do occur they may need medical attention.

Check with your doctor or nurse immediately if any of the following side effects occur:
Shortness of breath or troubled breathing
Slow heartbeat
Vomiting (continuing)

Other side effects may occur that usually do not require medical attention. These side effects may go away during treatment as your body adjusts to the medicine. However, check with your doctor if any of the following side effects continue or are bothersome:

More common
Drowsiness
Nausea
Unusual sweating
Unusual tiredness or weakness
Unusual watering of mouth

Less common or rare
Dizziness or lightheadedness especially when getting up
   from a lying or sitting position
False sense of well-being
Fast heartbeat
Fast or irregular breathing
Restlessness
Trembling

For children or elderly patients: The above side effects are more likely to occur in children or in elderly patients, who are usually more sensitive to the effects of apomorphine.

Other side effects not listed above may also occur in some patients. If you notice any other effects, check with your doctor.

December 1987

APPETITE SUPPRESSANTS (Systemic)

This information applies to the following medicines:

Benzphetamine (benz-FET-a-meen)
Diethylpropion (dye-eth-il-PROE-pee-on)
Mazindol (MAY-zin-dole)
Phendimetrazine (fen-dye-MET-ra-zeen)
Phenmetrazine (fen-MET-ra-zeen)
Phentermine (FEN-ter-meen)

This information does not apply to fenfluramine.

Some commonly used brand names are:	Generic names:
Didrex	Benzphetamine
Nobesine* Propion* Regibon* Tenuate Tenuate Dospan Tepanil Tepanil Ten-Tab	Diethylpropion†
Mazanor Sanorex	Mazindol
Adipost Adphen Anorex Bacarate Bontril PDM Bontril Slow Release Di-Ap-Trol Dyrexan-OD Hyrex Melfiat Metra Obalan Obeval Phenazine-35 Phenzine Plegine Prelu-2 Slyn-LL Statobex Statobex-G Trimcaps Trimstat Trimtabs Wehless Weightrol X-Trozine X-Trozine LA	Phendimetrazine†
Preludin	Phenmetrazine
Adipex-P Dapex Fastin Ionamin Obe-Nix Obephen Obermine Obestin Oby-Trim Parmine Phentrol Span R/D Teramine Unifast Wilpowr	Phentermine†

*Not available in the U.S.
†Generic name product also available.

To the Reader: If you do not recognize the names of medical conditions or medicines referred to in this information, check with your doctor, nurse, or pharmacist. Definitions for selected medical terms may be found in the Glossary. Brand names for the generic drug names listed can be found in the Index. In addition, selected brand names commonly associated with the generic name have been included in the text to help you recognize medicine you may be taking. The fact that a brand name product is not mentioned does not mean the information does not apply. It is a good idea for you to learn both the generic and brand names of your medicines and to write them down for future use.

Appetite suppressants are used in the short-term (a few weeks) treatment of obesity. For a few weeks (6 to 12), these medicines in combination with dieting, exercise, and changes in eating habits can help patients lose weight. However, since their appetite-reducing effect is only temporary, they are useful only for the first few weeks of dieting until new eating habits are established. They are not effective for continuous use in diet control.

These medicines are available only with your doctor's prescription.

Remember:
• **This medicine has been prescribed for your current medical problem only.** It must not be given to other people or used for other problems unless you are directed to do so by your doctor.

• **Keep all medicines out of the reach of children.**

• In order for this medicine to work, it must be used as directed.

• **It is very important that you read and understand the following information.** If any of the information causes you special concern, do not decide against using this medicine without first checking with your doctor.

• Before you begin using any new medicine (prescription or nonprescription) or if you develop any new medical problem while you are using this medicine, check with your doctor, nurse, or pharmacist.

• **If you have any questions** about the following information or if you want more information about this medicine or your medical problem, **ask your doctor, nurse, or pharmacist**.

Before Using This Medicine

In order to decide on the best treatment for your medical problem, your doctor should be told:

—if you have ever had any unusual or allergic reaction to amphetamine, dextroamphetamine, ephedrine, epinephrine, isoproterenol, metaproterenol, methamphetamine, norepinephrine, phenylephrine, phenylpropanolamine, pseudoephedrine, or terbutaline.

—if you are on a low-salt, low-sugar, or any other special diet, or if you are allergic to any substance, such as foods, sulfites or other preservatives, or dyes. Most medicines contain more than their active ingredient. Your doctor, nurse, or pharmacist can help you avoid products that may cause a problem.

—if you are **pregnant** or if you may become pregnant. Benzphetamine is not recommended during pregnancy because it may harm the fetus.

Diethylpropion has not been shown to cause birth defects or other problems in human and animal studies.

Studies in animals have shown that mazindol increases the chance of rib malformations, and also increases the chance of death in the newborn when given in large doses.

Phendimetrazine and phentermine have not been shown to cause birth defects or other problems in humans.

Phenmetrazine has been reported to cause birth defects in humans, although this has not been proven. It has not been shown to cause birth defects in animal studies. However, studies in animals have shown that phenmetrazine may lessen the chance of becoming pregnant.

—if you are **breast-feeding**. Diethylpropion and possibly benzphetamine are excreted in breast milk. It is not known if other appetite suppressants are excreted in breast milk. These medicines have not been shown to cause problems in nursing babies.

—if you have any of the following medical problems:
   Diabetes mellitus (sugar diabetes)
   Epilepsy
   Glaucoma
   Heart or blood vessel disease
   High blood pressure
   Mental illness (severe)
   Overactive thyroid

—if you are taking **any** other prescription or nonprescription (OTC) medicine.

—if you are now taking or have taken within the past 2 weeks monoamine oxidase (MAO) inhibitors such as:
   Furazolidone (e.g., Furoxone)
   Isocarboxazid (e.g., Marplan)
   Pargyline (e.g., Eutonyl)
   Phenelzine (e.g., Nardil)
   Procarbazine (e.g., Matulane)
   Tranylcypromine (e.g., Parnate)

Proper Use of This Medicine

For patients taking the short-acting form of this medicine:
   • Take the last dose for each day about 4 to 6 hours before bedtime to help prevent trouble in sleeping.

For patients taking the long-acting form of this medicine:
   • Take the daily dose about 10 to 14 hours before bedtime to help prevent trouble in sleeping.

   • These capsules or tablets are to be swallowed whole. Do not break, crush, or chew before swallowing.

For patients taking mazindol:
   • To help prevent trouble in sleeping, if you are taking this medicine in a:
      —*1-mg tablet,* take the last dose for each day about 4 to 6 hours before bedtime.

      —*2-mg tablet,* take the dose once each day about 10 to 14 hours before bedtime.

Take this medicine only as directed by your doctor. Do not take more of it, do not take it more often, and do not take it for a longer period of time than your doctor ordered. If too much is taken, it may become habit-forming.

If you think this medicine is not working as well after you have taken it for a few weeks, **do not increase the dose.** Instead, check with your doctor.

How to store this medicine:
   • **Keep out of the reach of children.**

   • Store away from heat and direct light.

   • Do not store in the bathroom, near the kitchen sink, or in other damp places. Heat or moisture may cause the medicine to break down.

   • Do not keep outdated medicine or medicine no longer needed. Be sure that any discarded medicine is out of the reach of children.

Precautions While Using This Medicine

Your doctor should check your progress at regular visits in order to make sure that this medicine does not cause unwanted effects.

This medicine may cause dryness of the mouth. For temporary relief, use sugarless candy or gum, melt bits of ice in your mouth, or use a saliva substitute. However, if dry mouth continues for more than 2 weeks, check with your physician or dentist. Continuing dryness of the mouth may increase the chance of dental disease, including tooth decay, gum disease, and fungal infections.

This medicine may cause some people to feel a false sense of well-being or to become dizzy, lightheaded, drowsy, or less alert than they are normally. **Make sure you know how you react to this medicine before you drive, use machines, or do other jobs that require you to be alert.**

Before having any kind of surgery, dental treatment, or emergency treatment, tell the physician or dentist in charge that you are using this medicine.

If you have been taking this medicine for a long time or in large doses and **you think you may have become mentally or physically dependent on it, check with your doctor.**

Some signs of dependence on appetite suppressants are:
   —a strong desire or need to continue taking the medicine

   —a need to increase the dose to receive the effects of the medicine

   —withdrawal side effects (for example, mental depression, nausea or vomiting, stomach cramps or pain, trembling, unusual tiredness or weakness when you stop taking the medicine)

Diabetic patients—This medicine may affect blood sugar levels. If you notice a change in the results of your urine or blood sugar test or if you have any questions, check with your doctor.

If you have been taking this medicine in large doses for a long period of time, **do not stop taking it without first checking with your doctor**. Your doctor may want you to reduce gradually the amount you are taking before stopping completely.

Side Effects of This Medicine

Along with its needed effects, a medicine may cause some unwanted effects. Although not all of these side effects may occur, if they do occur they may need medical attention.

Check with your doctor as soon as possible if any of the following side effects occur:

Rare
Confusion
Mental depression
Skin rash or hives
Sore throat and fever

Other side effects may occur that usually do not require medical attention. These side effects may go away during treatment as your body adjusts to the medicine. However, check with your doctor if any of the following side effects continue or are bothersome:

More common
False sense of well-being (less common with phentermine)
Irritability
Nervousness or restlessness
Trouble in sleeping
Note: After such stimulant effects have worn off, drowsiness, trembling, unusual tiredness or weakness, or mental depression may occur.

Less common
Blurred vision
Changes in sexual desire or decreased sexual ability
Constipation (more common with mazindol)
Diarrhea
Difficult or painful urination
Dizziness or lightheadedness

Drowsiness (with mazindol)
Dryness of mouth (more common with mazindol)
Fast, pounding, or irregular heartbeat
Frequent urge to urinate or increased urination
Headache
Increased sweating
Nausea or vomiting
Stomach cramps or pain
Unpleasant taste
Unusual tiredness or weakness

Although not all of the side effects listed above have been reported for all of these medicines, they have been reported for at least one of them. However, since all of the appetite suppressants are very similar, any of the above side effects may occur with any of these medicines.

After you stop using this medicine, your body may need time to adjust. The length of time this takes depends on the amount of medicine you were using and how long you used it. During this period of time check with your doctor if you notice any of the following side effects:

Mental depression
Nausea or vomiting
Stomach cramps or pain
Trembling
Unusual tiredness or weakness

For elderly patients: Many medicines have not been tested in older people. Therefore, it is not known whether the medicine acts the same way it does in younger adults. Check with your doctor or pharmacist if you notice any unusual effects while taking this medicine or if you think it is not working as it should.

For children: Appetite suppressants should not be used by children under 12 years of age.

Other side effects not listed above may also occur in some patients. If you notice any other effects, check with your doctor.

December 1987

ASCORBIC ACID (VITAMIN C) (Systemic)

Some commonly used brand names are:

Apo-C*	Cevalin
Arco-Cee	Cevi-Bid
Ascorbicap	Ce-Vi-Sol
Cecon	Cevita
Cemill	Flavorcee
Cenolate	Redoxon*
Cetane	

Generic name product may also be available in the U.S. and Canada.

---

*Not available in the U.S.

To the Reader: If you do not recognize the names of medical conditions or medicines referred to in this information, check with your doctor, nurse, or pharmacist. Definitions for selected medical terms may be found in the Glossary. Brand names for the generic drug names listed can be found in the Index. In addition, selected brand names commonly associated with the generic name have been included in the text to help you recognize medicine you may be taking. The fact that a brand name product is not mentioned does not mean the information does not apply. It is a good idea for you to learn both the generic and brand names of your medicines and to write them down for future use.

Vitamins (VYE-ta-mins) are compounds that you *must* have for growth and health. They are needed in small amounts only and are usually available in the foods that you eat. Ascorbic (a-SKOR-bik) acid, also known as vitamin C, is necessary for healthy bones and teeth as well as the general make-up of the body; it may have other effects as well.

Lack of vitamin C can lead to a condition called scurvy, which causes muscle weakness, swollen and bleeding gums, loss of teeth, and bleeding under the skin, as well as tiredness and depression. Wounds also do not heal easily. Your doctor may treat this by prescribing vitamin C for you.

Ascorbic acid may be used for other conditions as determined by your doctor.

Claims that vitamin C is effective for preventing senility, cancer, and the common cold, and for treating some mental problems, hardening of the arteries, allergy, eye ulcers, blood clots, gum disease, and pressure sores have not been proven.

Most strengths of vitamin C are available without a prescription. However, it may be a good idea to check with your doctor before taking vitamin C on your own.

Remember:
• **Keep all medicines out of the reach of children.**

• In order for this medicine to work, it must be used as directed. **If you are using this medicine without a prescription, it is very important that you follow the directions on the label.**

• **It is also very important that you read and understand the following information.** If any of the information causes you special concern, check with your doctor before using this medicine without a prescription.

• Before you begin using any new medicine (prescription or nonprescription) or if you develop any new medical problem while you are using this medicine, check with your doctor, nurse, or pharmacist.

• **If you have any questions** about the following information or if you want more information about this medicine or your medical problem, **ask your doctor, nurse, or pharmacist**.

Importance of Diet

Vitamin supplements should be taken only if you cannot get enough vitamins in your diet. A balanced diet should provide all the vitamins you normally need.

Nutritionists recommend that you eat:
• Cereal or bread—4 or more servings per day and
• Dairy products (milk, cheese, ice cream, cottage cheese)—3 or more servings per day and
• Meat, fish, or eggs—2 or more servings per day and
• Vegetables and fruits—4 or more servings per day.

If you are not getting all of these foods every day, you may not be getting enough vitamins in your diet. The best way to correct this is to start eating the foods that contain what you need.

Ascorbic acid is found in various foods, including citrus fruits (oranges, lemons, limes, grapefruit), tomatoes, strawberries, cantaloupe, and raw peppers. It is best to eat fresh fruits and vegetables whenever possible since they contain the most vitamins. Food processing may destroy some of the vitamins. For example, drying, salting, or cooking (especially in copper pots), mincing of fresh vegetables, or mashing potatoes may reduce the amount of ascorbic acid in foods. Freezing does not usually cause loss of vitamin C unless foods are stored for very long periods of time.

Vitamins alone will not take the place of a good diet and will not provide energy. Your body also needs other substances found in food such as protein, minerals, carbohydrates, and fat. Vitamins themselves often cannot work without the presence of other foods.

In some cases, it may not be possible for you to get enough food to supply you with the proper vitamins. In other cases, the amount of vitamins you need may be increased above normal. Therefore, a vitamin supplement may be needed.

Experts have developed a list of recommended dietary allowances (RDA) for most of the vitamins. The RDA are not an exact number but a general idea of how much you need. They do not cover amounts needed or problems caused by a serious lack of vitamins.

© 1988   The United States Pharmacopeial Convention, Inc.

The RDA for ascorbic acid are:

Children 4 to 6 years of age—45 mg per day
Adult males—60 mg per day
Adult females—60 mg per day
Pregnant females—80 mg per day
Breast-feeding females—100 mg per day.

Remember:

• The total amount of each vitamin that you get every day includes what you get from the foods that you eat *and* what you may take as a supplement.

• This total amount should not be greater than the RDA, unless ordered by your doctor. Taking too much ascorbic acid over a period of time may cause harmful effects.

Before Using This Medicine

In deciding whether you need additional ascorbic acid, the following should be kept in mind and/or your doctor should be told:

—if you have ever had any unusual or allergic reaction to ascorbic acid.

—if you are **pregnant** or if you may become pregnant. It is especially important that you are receiving enough vitamins when you become pregnant and that you continue to receive the right amount of vitamins throughout your pregnancy. Healthy fetal growth and development depend on a steady supply of nutrients from mother to fetus.

However, taking too much vitamin C may not be good for the fetus and may cause your baby to need more than the usual amount after birth.

—if you are **breast-feeding**. It is especially important that you receive the right amounts of vitamins so that your baby will also get the vitamins needed to grow properly. You should also check with your doctor if you are giving your baby an unfortified formula. In that case, the baby must get the vitamins needed some other way.

—if you are not able to get a diet that contains all of the vitamins you need. This may occur with rapid weight loss, unusual diets (such as some reducing diets in which choice of foods is very limited), prolonged intravenous feeding, or malnutrition.

—if you smoke. You may need more ascorbic acid than usual if you smoke.

—if you do heavy manual labor, if you have been under a lot of stress for a long time, if you have had a long illness or serious injury, or if you have had surgery.

—if you have any of the following medical problems:

Burns
Cancer
Diabetes mellitus (sugar diabetes)
Glucose-6-phosphate dehydrogenase (G6PD) deficiency
Kidney stones (history of)
Overactive thyroid

Sickle cell anemia or other blood problems
Stomach problems (including ulcer, prolonged diarrhea, or stomach or intestinal surgery)
Tuberculosis

—if you are using **any** other prescription or nonprescription (OTC) medicine.

Proper Use of This Medicine

Do not take more than the recommended daily amount. Vitamin C is not stored in the body. If you take more than you need, the extra will pass into your urine. There is a chance that high doses could cause stones to form in your urinary tract. Very large doses may also interfere with tests for sugar in diabetics. Some people believe that taking very large doses of vitamins (called megadoses or megavitamin therapy) is useful for treating certain medical problems. Studies have not proven this. Large doses should be taken only under the direction of your doctor after need has been identified.

For patients taking the oral liquid form of ascorbic acid:
• This preparation is to be taken by mouth even though it comes in a dropper bottle.

• This medicine may be dropped directly into the mouth or mixed with cereal, fruit juice, or other food.

If you miss taking a vitamin for one or more days there is no cause for concern, since it takes some time for your body to become seriously low in vitamins. However, if your doctor has recommended that you take this vitamin, try to remember to take it as directed every day.

How to store this medicine:

• **Keep out of the reach of children.**

• Store away from heat and direct light.

• Do not store in the bathroom, near the kitchen sink, or in other damp places. Heat or moisture may cause the medicine to break down.

• Keep the oral liquid form of this medicine from freezing.

• Do not keep outdated medicine or medicine no longer needed. Be sure that any discarded medicine is out of the reach of children.

Side Effects of This Medicine

Along with its needed effects, a medicine may cause some unwanted effects. Although not all of these side effects may occur, if they do occur, they may need medical attention.

Check with your doctor as soon as possible if the following side effect occurs:
Less common or rare—with high doses
Side or lower back pain

Other side effects may occur that usually do not require medical attention. These side effects may go away during treatment as your body adjusts to the medicine.

However, check with your doctor or pharmacist as soon as possible if any of the following side effects continue or are bothersome:

Less common or rare—with high doses

    Diarrhea
    Dizziness or faintness (with the injection only)
    Flushing or redness of skin
    Headache

    Increase in urination (mild)
    Nausea or vomiting
    Stomach cramps

Other side effects not listed above may also occur in some patients. If you notice any other effects, check with your doctor or pharmacist.

_____

December 1987

ASPARAGINASE (Systemic)

Some commonly used brand names or other names are Colaspase, El-spar, and Kidrolase*.

---

*Not available in the U.S.

To the Reader: If you do not recognize the names of medical conditions or medicines referred to in this information, check with your doctor, nurse, or pharmacist. Definitions for selected medical terms may be found in the Glossary. Brand names for the generic drug names listed can be found in the Index. In addition, selected brand names commonly associated with the generic name have been included in the text to help you recognize medicine you may be taking. The fact that a brand name product is not mentioned does not mean the information does not apply. It is a good idea for you to learn both the generic and brand names of your medicines and to write them down for future use.

Asparaginase (a-SPARE-a-gin-ase) belongs to the group of medicines known as enzymes. It is given by injection to treat some kinds of cancer.

All cells need a chemical called asparagine to stay alive. Normal cells can make this chemical for themselves, while cancer cells cannot. Asparaginase breaks down asparagine in the body. Since the cancer cells cannot make more asparagine, they die.

Before you begin treatment with asparaginase, you and your doctor should talk about the good this medicine will do as well as the risks of using it.

Asparaginase is to be administered only by or under the supervision of your doctor.

Remember:
• **It is very important that you read and understand the following information.** If any of the information causes you special concern, do not decide against using this medicine without first checking with your doctor.

• Before you begin using any new medicine (prescription or nonprescription) or if you develop any new medical problem while you are receiving this medicine, check with your doctor, nurse, or pharmacist.

• **If you have any questions** about the following information or if you want more information about this medicine or your medical problem, **ask your doctor, nurse, or pharmacist.**

Before Using This Medicine

In order to decide on the best treatment for your medical problem, your doctor should be told:

—if you have ever had any unusual or allergic reaction to asparaginase.

—if you are **pregnant** or if you intend to have children. Studies have not been done in humans. However, studies in mice and rats have shown that asparaginase in doses 5 times the usual human dose slows the weight gain of infants and may also increase the risk of birth defects or cause a decrease in successful pregnancies. In addition, doses slightly less than the human dose have caused birth defects in rabbits.

—if you intend to **breast-feed**. Because this medicine may cause serious side effects, breast-feeding is generally not recommended while you are receiving it.

—if you have any of the following medical problems:
Chickenpox (including recent exposure)
Diabetes mellitus (sugar diabetes)
Herpes zoster (shingles)
Gout
Infection
Kidney stones
Liver disease
Pancreatitis (inflammation of the pancreas)

—if you are taking **any** other prescription or nonprescription (OTC) medicine, especially:
Probenecid (e.g., Benemid)
Sulfinpyrazone (e.g., Anturane)

—if you have ever been treated with x-rays or cancer medicines.

Proper Use of This Medicine

This medicine is usually given together with certain other medicines. If you are using a combination of medicines, it is important that you receive each one at the proper time. If you are taking some of these medicines by mouth, ask your doctor, nurse, or pharmacist to help you plan a way to remember to take them at the right time.

While you are using this medicine, your doctor may want you to drink extra fluids so that you will pass more urine. This will help prevent kidney problems and keep your kidneys working well.

This medicine often causes nausea, vomiting, and loss of appetite. However, it is very important that you continue to receive the medicine, even if you begin to feel ill. After several doses, your stomach upset should lessen. Ask your doctor, nurse, or pharmacist for ways to lessen these effects.

Precautions While Using This Medicine

It is very important that your doctor check your progress at regular visits to make sure that this medicine is working properly and to check for unwanted effects.

While you are being treated with asparaginase, and after you stop treatment with it, **do not have any immunizations without your doctor's approval**. Asparaginase lowers your body's resistance and there is a chance you might get the infection the immunization is meant to prevent. In addition, other persons living in your household should not take oral polio vaccine since there is a chance they could pass the polio virus on to you. Also, you should avoid close contact with other persons (for example, at school or work) who have taken oral polio vaccine.

Side Effects of This Medicine

Along with their needed effects, medicines like asparaginase can sometimes cause unwanted effects such as blood problems, allergic reactions, liver problems, and other side effects; these are described below. Also, because of the way these medicines act on the body, there is a chance that they might cause other unwanted effects that may not occur until months or years after the medicine is used. These delayed effects may include certain types of cancer, such as leukemia. Discuss these possible effects with your doctor.

Although not all of these side effects may occur, if they do occur they may need medical attention.

Check with your doctor or nurse immediately if any of the following side effects occur:

More common
> Difficulty in breathing
> Joint pain
> Puffy face
> Skin rash or itching
> Stomach pain (severe) with nausea and vomiting

Less common
> Fever, chills, or sore throat

Rare
> Unusual bleeding or bruising

Check with your doctor or nurse as soon as possible if any of the following side effects occur:

More common
> Yellow eyes and skin

Less common
> Confusion
> Drowsiness
> Frequent urination
> Hallucinations (seeing, hearing, or feeling things that are not there)
> Lower back, side, or stomach pain
> Mental depression
> Nervousness
> Sores in the mouth or on the lips

> Swelling of feet or lower legs
> Tiredness
> Unusual thirst

Rare
> Convulsions (seizures)
> Headache (severe)
> Inability to move arm or leg
> Pain in lower legs

Other side effects may occur that usually do not require medical attention. These side effects may go away during treatment as your body adjusts to the medicine. Also, your doctor or nurse may be able to tell you about ways to prevent or reduce some of these side effects. Check with your doctor or nurse if any of the following side effects continue or are bothersome or if you have any questions about them:

More common
> Headache (mild)
> Loss of appetite
> Nausea or vomiting
> Stomach cramps (mild)
> Weight loss

After you stop receiving asparaginase, it may still produce some side effects that need attention. During this period of time, **check with your doctor or nurse immediately** if you have severe stomach pain with nausea and vomiting.

For elderly patients: Many medicines have not been tested in older people. Therefore, it is not known whether the medicine acts the same way it does in younger adults. Check with your doctor or pharmacist if you notice any unusual effects while taking this medicine or if you think it is not working as it should.

Other side effects not listed above may also occur in some patients. If you notice any other effects, check with your doctor or nurse.

December 1987

ATROPINE (Ophthalmic)

This information applies to the following medicines:

Atropine (A-troe-peen)
Homatropine (hoe-MA-troe-peen)
Scopolamine (skoe-POL-a-meen)

Some commonly used brand names are:	Generic names:
Atropair	
Atropine-Care	
Atropisol	
Isopto Atropine	Atropine†
I-Tropine	
Minims Atropine*	
S.M.P. Atropine*	
AK-Homatropine	
I-Homatrine	
Isopto Homatropine	Homatropine†
Minims Homatropine*	
Isopto Hyoscine	Scopolamine

*Not available in the U.S.
†Generic name product may also be available in the U.S.

To the Reader: If you do not recognize the names of medical conditions or medicines referred to in this information, check with your doctor, nurse, or pharmacist. Definitions for selected medical terms may be found in the Glossary. Brand names for the generic drug names listed can be found in the Index. In addition, selected brand names commonly associated with the generic name have been included in the text to help you recognize medicine you may be taking. The fact that a brand name product is not mentioned does not mean the information does not apply. It is a good idea for you to learn both the generic and brand names of your medicines and to write them down for future use.

Ophthalmic atropine, homatropine, and scopolamine are used in the eye to dilate (enlarge) the pupil. They are used before eye examinations, before and after eye surgery, and to treat certain eye conditions.

These medicines are available only with your doctor's prescription.

Remember:
• **This medicine has been prescribed for your current medical problem only.** It must not be given to other people or used for other problems unless you are directed to do so by your doctor.

• **Keep all medicines out of the reach of children.**

• In order for this medicine to work, it must be used as directed.

• **It is very important that you read and understand the following information.** If any of the information causes you special concern, do not decide against using this medicine without first checking with your doctor.

• Before you begin using any new medicine (prescription or nonprescription) or if you develop any new medical problem while you are using this medicine, check with your doctor, nurse, or pharmacist.

• **If you have any questions** about the following information or if you want more information about this medicine or your medical problem, **ask your doctor, nurse, or pharmacist.**

Before Using This Medicine

In order to decide on the best treatment for your medical problem, your doctor should be told:

—if you have ever had any unusual or allergic reaction to atropine, homatropine, or scopolamine.

—if you are **pregnant** or if you may become pregnant, since this medicine may be absorbed into the body. However, atropine, homatropine, and scopolamine have not been shown to cause birth defects or other problems in humans.

—if you are **breast-feeding**, since this medicine may be absorbed into the body. Atropine passes into the breast milk in very small amounts and may cause unwanted side effects, such as fast pulse, fever, or dry skin, in babies of nursing mothers using ophthalmic atropine. Homatropine and scopolamine have not been shown to cause problems in nursing babies.

—if you have any of the following medical problems:

Brain damage (in children)
Down's syndrome (mongolism)
Glaucoma
Spastic paralysis (in children)

—if you are taking **any** other prescription or nonprescription (OTC) medicine.

Proper Use of This Medicine

For patients using the eye-drop form of this medicine:

• How to apply this medicine: First, wash your hands. With middle finger, apply pressure to the inside corner of the eye (and continue to apply pressure for 1 or 2 minutes after the medicine has been placed in the eye). Tilt the head back and with the index finger of the same hand, pull the lower eyelid away from the eye to form a pouch. Drop the medicine into the pouch and gently close the eyes. Do not blink. Keep the eyes closed for 1 or 2 minutes to allow the medicine to be absorbed.

• Immediately after applying the eye drops, wash your hands to remove any medicine that may be on them.

• To prevent contamination of the eye drops, do not touch the applicator tip to any surface (including the eye). Also, keep the container tightly closed.

For patients using the ointment form of this medicine:

• How to apply this medicine: First, wash your hands. Then pull the lower eyelid away from the eye to form a pouch. Squeeze a thin strip of ointment into the pouch. A ⅓- to ½-cm (approximately ⅛-inch in infants and young children and ¼-inch in older children and adults) strip of ointment is usually enough unless otherwise directed by your doctor. Gently close the eyes and keep them closed for 1 or 2 minutes to allow the medicine to be absorbed.

• Immediately after applying the eye ointment, wash your hands to remove any medicine that may be on them.

• To prevent contamination of the eye ointment, do not touch the applicator tip to any surface (including the eye). After using the eye ointment, wipe the tip of the ointment tube with a clean tissue and keep the tube tightly closed.

Use this medicine only as directed. Do not use more of it and do not use it more often than your doctor ordered. To do so may increase the chance of too much medicine being absorbed into the body and the chance of side effects. **This is especially important when this medicine is used in children, since overdose is very dangerous in children.**

If you miss a dose of this medicine and your dosing schedule is one dose to be applied:

Once a day—Apply the missed dose as soon as possible. However, if you do not remember the missed dose until the next day, skip it and apply your regularly scheduled dose.
More than once a day—Apply the missed dose as soon as possible. However, if it is almost time for your next dose, skip the missed dose and apply your next dose at the regularly scheduled time. Then continue with your regular dosing schedule.

How to store this medicine:

• **Keep out of the reach of children.**

• Store away from heat and direct light.

• Keep this medicine from freezing.

• Do not keep outdated medicine or medicine no longer needed. Be sure that any discarded medicine is out of the reach of children.

Precautions While Using This Medicine

After you apply this medicine to your eyes:

• Your pupils will become unusually large and you will have blurring of vision, especially for close objects. **Make sure your vision is clear before you drive or do other jobs that require you to see well.**

• Your eyes will become more sensitive to light than they are normally. **Wear sunglasses to protect your eyes from sunlight and other bright lights**.

These effects may continue for several days after you stop using this medicine. However, check with your doctor if they continue longer than:
—14 days if you are using atropine.
—3 days if you are using homatropine.
—7 days if you are using scopolamine.

Side Effects of This Medicine

Along with its needed effects, a medicine may cause some unwanted effects. Although not all of these side effects may occur, if they do occur they may need medical attention.

Check with your doctor immediately if any of the following side effects occur:
Signs of too much medicine being absorbed into the body
Clumsiness or unsteadiness
Confusion or unusual behavior
Fever
Flushing or redness of face
Hallucinations (seeing, hearing, or feeling things that are not there)
Increased thirst or unusual dryness of mouth
Skin rash
Slurred speech
Swollen stomach in infants
Unusual drowsiness, tiredness, or weakness
Unusually fast heartbeat

Other side effects may occur that usually do not require medical attention. These side effects may go away during treatment as your body adjusts to the medicine. However, check with your doctor if either of the following side effects continues or is bothersome:
Increased sensitivity of eyes to light
Eye irritation not present before using this medicine

For infants, for children with spastic paralysis, Down's syndrome, or brain damage, and for elderly patients: The above side effects are more likely to occur in infants, in children with spastic paralysis, Down's syndrome, or brain damage, and in elderly patients.

Other side effects not listed above may also occur in some patients. If you notice any other effects, check with your doctor.

December 1987

ATROPINE, HYOSCYAMINE, METHENAMINE, METHYLENE BLUE, PHENYL SALICYLATE, AND BENZOIC ACID (Systemic)

Some commonly used brand names are:

Dolsed	Urinary Antiseptic No. 2
Hexalol	Urised
Prosed	Urisep
Trac Tabs	Uritab
UAA	Urithol
Uridon Modified	Uritin
Urimed	Uroblue
	Uro-Ves

To the Reader: If you do not recognize the names of medical conditions or medicines referred to in this information, check with your doctor, nurse, or pharmacist. Definitions for selected medical terms may be found in the Glossary. Brand names for the generic drug names listed can be found in the Index. In addition, selected brand names commonly associated with the generic name have been included in the text to help you recognize medicine you may be taking. The fact that a brand name product is not mentioned does not mean the information does not apply. It is a good idea for you to learn both the generic and brand names of your medicines and to write them down for future use.

Atropine (A-troe-peen), hyoscyamine (hye-oh-SYE-a-meen), methenamine (meth-EN-a-meen), methylene (METH-i-leen) blue, phenyl salicylate (FEN-ill sa-LI-si-late), and benzoic acid (ben-ZOE-ik AS-id) combination medicine is an antimuscarinic, anti-infective, and analgesic. It is given by mouth to help relieve the discomfort caused by urinary tract infections; however, it will not cure the infection itself. This combination medicine may also be used for other conditions as determined by your doctor.

This medicine is available only with your doctor's prescription.

Remember:

• **This medicine has been prescribed for your current medical problem only.** It must not be given to other people or used for other problems unless you are directed to do so by your doctor.

• **Keep all medicines out of the reach of children.**

• In order for this medicine to work, it must be used as directed.

• **It is very important that you read and understand the following information.** If any of the information causes you special concern, do not decide against using this medicine without first checking with your doctor.

• Before you begin using any new medicine (prescription or nonprescription) or if you develop any new medical problem while you are using this medicine, check with your doctor, nurse, or pharmacist.

• **If you have any questions** about the following information or if you want more information about this medicine or your medical problem, **ask your doctor, nurse, or pharmacist.**

Before Using This Medicine

In order to decide on the best treatment for your medical problem, your doctor should be told:

—if you have ever had any unusual or allergic reaction to any of the belladonna alkaloids such as atropine, hyoscyamine, and scopolamine, or to aspirin or other salicylates.

—if you are on a low-salt, low-sugar, or any other special diet, or if you are allergic to any substance, such as foods, sulfites or other preservatives, or dyes. Most medicines contain more than their active ingredient. Your doctor, nurse, or pharmacist can help you avoid products that may cause a problem.

—if you are **pregnant** or if you may become pregnant while using this medicine. Studies have not been done in either humans or animals.

—if you are **breast-feeding**. This medicine has not been shown to cause problems in nursing babies.

—if you have any of the following medical problems:
Brain damage (in children)
Enlarged prostate
Glaucoma
Heart disease
Intestinal blockage or other intestinal or stomach problems
Kidney disease
Liver disease
Myasthenia gravis
Overactive thyroid
Problems with urination
Urinary tract blockage

—if you are now taking or have taken within the past 2 weeks monoamine oxidase (MAO) inhibitors, such as:
Furazolidone (e.g., Furoxone)
Isocarboxazid (e.g., Marplan)
Pargyline (e.g., Eutonyl)
Phenelzine (e.g., Nardil)
Procarbazine (e.g., Matulane)
Tranylcypromine (e.g., Parnate)

—if you are taking urinary alkalizers (medicine that makes the urine less acid, such as acetazolamide, calcium- and/or magnesium-containing antacids, dichlorphenamide, methazolamide, potassium or sodium citrate and/or citric acid, sodium bicarbonate [baking soda]).

—if you are taking **any** other medicines including over-the-counter (OTC) or nonprescription medicines (for example, antacids or diarrhea medicine). Many medicines change the way belladonna alkaloids (atropine and hyoscyamine) affect your body. Also, the effect of other medicines may be reduced by belladonna alkaloids.

Proper Use of This Medicine

Take this medicine only as directed. Do not take more of it, do not take it more often, and do not take it for a longer period of time than your doctor ordered. To do so may increase the chance of side effects.

Each dose should be taken with a full glass (8 ounces) of water or other liquid (except citrus juices and milk). Drink plenty of water or other liquids every day, unless otherwise directed by your doctor. Drinking enough liquids will help your kidneys work better and lessen your discomfort.

To help clear up your infection completely, **keep taking this medicine for the full time of treatment** even if you begin to feel better after a few days. **Do not miss any doses.**

In order for this medicine to work well, your urine must be acid (pH 5.5 or below).

Before you start taking this medicine, check your urine with phenaphthazine paper or another test to see if it is acid. If you have any questions about this, check with your doctor or pharmacist.

The following changes in your diet may help make your urine more acid; however, check with your doctor first if you are on a special diet (for example, for diabetes). Avoid most fruits (especially citrus fruits and juices), milk and other dairy products, and other foods which make the urine more alkaline. Also, avoid antacids unless otherwise directed by your doctor. Eating more protein and foods such as cranberries (especially cranberry juice with vitamin C added), plums, or prunes may also help. If your urine is still not acid enough, check with your doctor.

If you miss a dose of this medicine, take it as soon as possible. However, if it is almost time for your next dose, skip the missed dose and go back to your regular dosing schedule. Do not double doses.

How to store this medicine:

- **Keep out of the reach of children.**

- Store away from heat and direct light.

- Do not store the tablet form of this medicine in the bathroom, near the kitchen sink, or in other damp places. Heat or moisture may cause the medicine to break down.

- Do not keep outdated medicine or medicine no longer needed. Be sure that any discarded medicine is out of the reach of children.

Precautions While Using This Medicine

If your symptoms do not improve within a few days or if they become worse, check with your doctor.

This medicine may cause some people to have blurred vision. **Make sure you know how you react to this medicine before you drive, use machines, or do other jobs that require you to have clear vision. If your vision continues to be blurred, check with your doctor.**

This medicine may cause dryness of the mouth. For temporary relief, use sugarless candy or gum, melt bits of ice in your mouth, or use a saliva substitute. However, if dry mouth continues for more than 2 weeks, check with your dentist. Continuing dryness of the mouth may increase the chance of dental disease, including tooth decay, gum disease, and fungal infections.

Side Effects of This Medicine

Along with its needed effects, a medicine may cause some unwanted effects. Although not all of these side effects may occur, if they do occur they may need medical attention.

Check with your doctor as soon as possible if any of the following side effects occur:
Less common or rare
  Blurred vision
  Eye pain
  Skin rash or hives
Signs of overdose
  Blood in urine and/or stools
  Diarrhea
  Dizziness
  Drowsiness (severe)
  Fast heartbeat
  Flushing or redness of face
  Headache (severe or continuing)
  Lower back pain
  Pain or burning while urinating
  Ringing or buzzing in the ears
  Shortness of breath or troubled breathing
  Sweating
  Unusual tiredness or weakness

Other side effects may occur that usually do not require medical attention. These side effects may go away during treatment as your body adjusts to the medicine. However, check with your doctor if any of the following side effects continue or are bothersome:
Less common
  Difficult urination (more common with large doses taken over a prolonged period of time)
  Dryness of mouth, nose, and throat
  Nausea or vomiting
  Stomach upset or pain (more common with large doses taken over a prolonged period of time)

For children or elderly patients: The above side effects are more likely to occur in children and the elderly, who are usually more sensitive to the effects of atropine and hyoscyamine (contained in this combination medicine).

This medicine may cause your urine and/or stools to turn blue or blue-green. This is to be expected while you are taking this medicine.

Other side effects not listed above may also occur in some patients. If you notice any other effects, check with your doctor.

December 1987

AZATHIOPRINE (Systemic)

A commonly used brand name is Imuran.

To the Reader: If you do not recognize the names of medical conditions or medicines referred to in this information, check with your doctor, nurse, or pharmacist. Definitions for selected medical terms may be found in the Glossary. Brand names for the generic drug names listed can be found in the Index. In addition, selected brand names commonly associated with the generic name have been included in the text to help you recognize medicine you may be taking. The fact that a brand name product is not mentioned does not mean the information does not apply. It is a good idea for you to learn both the generic and brand names of your medicines and to write them down for future use.

Azathioprine (ay-za-THYE-oh-preen) belongs to the group of medicines known as immunosuppressive agents. It is used to reduce the body's natural immunity in patients who receive organ transplants. It is also used to treat rheumatoid arthritis. Azathioprine may also be used for other conditions as determined by your doctor.

Azathioprine is a very strong medicine. You and your doctor should talk about the need for this medicine and its risks. Even though azathioprine may cause side effects that could be very serious, remember that it may be required in order to treat your medical problem.

Azathioprine is available only with your doctor's prescription.

Remember:

• **This medicine has been prescribed for your current medical problem only.** It must not be given to other people or used for other problems unless you are directed to do so by your doctor.

• **Keep all medicines out of the reach of children.**

• In order for this medicine to work, it must be used as directed.

• If you are receiving this medicine by injection, some of the information about this medicine may not apply.

• **It is very important that you read and understand the following information.** If any of the information causes you special concern, do not decide against using this medicine without first checking with your doctor.

• Before you begin using any new medicine (prescription or nonprescription) or if you develop any new medical problem while you are using this medicine, check with your doctor, nurse, or pharmacist.

• **If you have any questions** about the following information or if you want more information about this medicine or your medical problem, **ask your doctor, nurse, or pharmacist.**

Before Using This Medicine

In order to decide on the best treatment for your medical problem, your doctor should be told:

—if you have ever had any unusual or allergic reaction to azathioprine.

—if you are on a low-salt, low-sugar, or any other special diet, or if you are allergic to any substance, such as foods, sulfites or other preservatives, or dyes.

Most medicines contain more than their active ingredient. Your doctor, nurse, or pharmacist can help you avoid products that may cause a problem.

—if you are **pregnant** or if you may become pregnant. Azathioprine is not recommended during pregnancy. It may cause birth defects if either the male or the female is using it at the time of conception. The use of birth control methods is recommended. If you have any questions about this, check with your doctor.

—if you are **breast-feeding**. Because this medicine may cause serious side effects, breast-feeding is generally not recommended while you are using it.

—if you have any of the following medical problems:
   Chickenpox (including recent exposure)
   Gout
   Herpes zoster (shingles)
   Infection
   Kidney disease
   Liver disease
   Pancreatitis (inflammation of the pancreas)

—if you are taking **any** prescription or nonprescription (OTC) medicine, especially:
   Adrenocorticoids (cortisone-like medicine)
   Allopurinol (e.g., Zyloprim)
   Chlorambucil (e.g., Leukeran)
   Cyclophosphamide (e.g., Cytoxan)
   Cyclosporine (e.g., Sandimmune)
   Mercaptopurine (e.g., Purinethol)
   Muromonab-CD3 (monoclonal antibody) (e.g., Orthoclone OKT3)

—if you have ever been treated with x-rays or cancer medicines.

Proper Use of This Medicine

Use this medicine only as directed by your doctor. Do not use more or less of it, and do not use it more often than your doctor ordered. The exact amount of medicine you need has been carefully worked out. Taking too much may increase the chance of side effects, while taking too little may not improve your condition.

This medicine is sometimes given together with certain other medicines. If you are using a combination of medicines, make sure that you take each one at the proper time and do not mix them. Ask your doctor, nurse, or pharmacist to help you plan a way to remember to take your medicines at the right time.

Do not stop taking this medicine without first checking with your doctor.

Azathioprine sometimes causes nausea or vomiting. Taking this medicine with or after meals may lessen stomach upset. Ask your doctor, nurse, or pharmacist for other ways to lessen these effects.

If you vomit shortly after taking a dose of azathioprine, check with your doctor. You may be told to take the dose again or you may have to wait until the next scheduled dose.

If you miss a dose of this medicine and your dosing schedule is:

Once a day—Do not take the missed dose at all and do not double the next one. Instead, go back to your regular dosing schedule and check with your doctor.

Several times a day—Take the missed dose as soon as you remember it. If it is time for your next dose, take both doses together, then go back to your regular dosing schedule. If you miss more than one dose, check with your doctor.

How to store this medicine:

• **Keep out of the reach of children.**

• Store away from heat and direct light.

• Do not store in the bathroom, near the kitchen sink, or in other damp places. Heat or moisture may cause the medicine to break down.

• Do not keep outdated medicine or medicine no longer needed. Be sure any discarded medicine is out of the reach of children.

Precautions While Using This Medicine

It is very important that your doctor check your progress at regular visits to make sure that this medicine is working properly and to check for unwanted effects.

While you are being treated with azathioprine, and after you stop treatment with it, **do not have any immunizations without your doctor's approval.** Azathioprine lowers your body's resistance and there is a chance you might get the infection the immunization is meant to prevent. In addition, other persons living in your household should not take oral polio vaccine since there is a chance they could pass the polio virus on to you. Also, you should avoid close contact with other persons (for example, at school or work) who have taken oral polio vaccine.

Side Effects of This Medicine

Along with their needed effects, medicines like azathioprine can sometimes cause unwanted effects such as blood problems and other side effects; these are described below. Also, because of the way these medicines act on the body, there is a chance that they might cause other unwanted effects that may not occur until months or years after the medicine is used. These delayed effects may include certain types of cancer, such as leukemia or skin cancer. Discuss these possible effects with your doctor.

Although not all of these side effects may occur, if they do occur they may need medical attention.

Check with your doctor immediately if any of the following side effects occur:

More common
Fever, chills, or sore throat
Unusual tiredness or weakness

Less common
Unusual bleeding or bruising

Rare
Fast heartbeat
Fever (sudden)
Muscle or joint pain
Stomach pain (severe) with nausea and vomiting

Check with your doctor as soon as possible if any of the following side effects occur:

Less common
Yellow eyes and skin

Rare
Cough
Shortness of breath
Sores in the mouth and on the lips

Other side effects may occur that usually do not require medical attention. These side effects may go away during treatment as your body adjusts to the medicine. However, check with your doctor if any of the following side effects continue or are bothersome:

More common
Loss of appetite
Nausea or vomiting

Less common or rare
Skin rash

Signs of blood problems (fever, chills, or sore throat; unusual tiredness or weakness; or unusual bleeding or bruising) are less likely to occur in patients taking azathioprine for rheumatoid arthritis. This is because lower doses are used.

After you stop using this medicine, it may still produce some side effects that need attention. During this period of time **check with your doctor immediately** if you notice any of the following:

Fever, chills, or sore throat
Unusual bleeding or bruising

For elderly patients: Many medicines have not been tested in older people. Therefore, it is not known whether the medicine acts the same way it does in younger adults. Check with your doctor or pharmacist if you notice any unusual effects while taking this medicine or if you think it is not working as it should.

Other side effects not listed above may also occur in some patients. If you notice any other effects, check with your doctor.

December 1987

AZTREONAM (Systemic)

A commonly used brand name is Azactam.

To the Reader: If you do not recognize the names of medical conditions or medicines referred to in this information, check with your doctor, nurse, or pharmacist. Definitions for selected medical terms may be found in the Glossary. Brand names for the generic drug names listed can be found in the Index. In addition, selected brand names commonly associated with the generic name have been included in the text to help you recognize medicine you may be taking. The fact that a brand name product is not mentioned does not mean the information does not apply. It is a good idea for you to learn both the generic and brand names of your medicines and to write them down for future use.

Aztreonam (az-TREE-oh-nam) belongs to the family of medicines called antibiotics. Antibiotics are used in the treatment of infections caused by bacteria. They work by killing bacteria or preventing their growth.

Aztreonam is given by injection to treat bacterial infections in many different parts of the body. It is sometimes given with other antibiotics. This medicine will not work for colds, flu, or other virus infections.

This medicine is available only with your doctor's prescription.

Remember:
- **It is very important that you read and understand the following information.** If any of the information causes you special concern, do not decide against receiving this medicine without first checking with your doctor.

- Before you begin using any new medicine (prescription or nonprescription) or if you develop any new medical problem while you are receiving this medicine, check with your doctor, nurse, or pharmacist.

- **If you have any questions** about the following information or if you want more information about this medicine or your medical problem, **ask your doctor, nurse, or pharmacist.**

Before Using This Medicine

In order to decide on the best treatment for your medical problem, your doctor should be told:

—if you have ever had any unusual or allergic reaction to aztreonam or to any of the penicillins or cephalosporins.

—if you are on a low-salt, low-sugar, or any other special diet, or if you are allergic to any substance, such as foods or sulfites or other preservatives. Most medicines contain more than their active ingredient. Your doctor, nurse, or pharmacist can help you avoid products that may cause a problem.

—if you are **pregnant** or if you may become pregnant. Studies have not been done in humans. However, aztreonam has not been shown to cause birth defects or other problems in studies in rabbits and rats given up to 15 times the highest human daily dose.

—if you are **breast-feeding.** Aztreonam passes into the breast milk in small amounts. However, this medicine is not absorbed when taken by mouth. Therefore, aztreonam is unlikely to cause serious problems in nursing babies.

—if you have any of the following medical problems:
  Cirrhosis (liver disease)
  Drug allergy, general, history of
  Kidney disease

Proper Use of This Medicine

To help clear up your infection completely, **aztreonam must be given for the full time of treatment,** even if you begin to feel better after a few days. Also, this medicine works best when there is a constant amount in the blood or urine. To help keep the amount constant, aztreonam must be given on a regular schedule.

Side Effects of This Medicine

Along with its needed effects, a medicine may cause some unwanted effects. Although not all of these side effects may occur, if they do occur they may need medical attention.

Check with your doctor immediately if any of the following side effects occur:

Less common
  Skin rash, redness, or itching
Rare
  Confusion
  Convulsions (seizures)
  Yellow eyes or skin

Other side effects may occur that usually do not require medical attention. These side effects may go away during treatment as your body adjusts to the medicine. However, check with your doctor if any of the following side effects continue or are bothersome:

Less common or rare
  Abdominal or stomach cramps
  Dizziness
  Double vision
  Itching of the vagina
  Nausea, vomiting, or diarrhea
  Ringing or buzzing sound in the ears

Other side effects not listed above may also occur in some patients. If you notice any other effects, check with your doctor.

December 1987

BACLOFEN (Systemic)

A commonly used brand name is Lioresal.

To the Reader: If you do not recognize the names of medical conditions or medicines referred to in this information, check with your doctor, nurse, or pharmacist. Definitions for selected medical terms may be found in the Glossary. Brand names for the generic drug names listed can be found in the Index. In addition, selected brand names commonly associated with the generic name have been included in the text to help you recognize medicine you may be taking. The fact that a brand name product is not mentioned does not mean the information does not apply. It is a good idea for you to learn both the generic and brand names of your medicines and to write them down for future use.

Baclofen (BAK-loe-fen) is used to help relax certain muscles in your body. It relieves the spasms, cramping, and tightness of muscles caused by medical problems such as multiple sclerosis or certain injuries to the spine. Baclofen does not cure these problems, but it may allow other treatment, such as physical therapy, to be more helpful in improving your condition. Baclofen acts on the central nervous system (CNS) to produce its muscle relaxant effects. Its actions on the CNS may also cause some of the medicine's side effects. Baclofen may also be used to relieve other conditions as determined by your doctor.

This medicine is available only with your doctor's prescription.

Remember:

• **This medicine has been prescribed for your current medical problem only.** It must not be given to other people or used for other problems unless you are directed to do so by your doctor.

• **Keep all medicines out of the reach of children.**

• In order for this medicine to work, it must be used as directed.

• **It is very important that you read and understand the following information.** If any of the information causes you special concern, do not decide against using this medicine without first checking with your doctor.

• Before you begin using any new medicine (prescription or nonprescription) or if you develop any new medical problem while you are using this medicine, check with your doctor, nurse, or pharmacist.

• **If you have any questions** about the following information or if you want more information about this medicine or your medical problem, **ask your doctor, nurse, or pharmacist.**

Before Using This Medicine

In order to decide on the best treatment for your medical problem, your doctor should be told:

—if you have ever had any unusual or allergic reaction to baclofen.

—if you are on a low-salt, low-sugar, or any other special diet, or if you are allergic to any substance, such as foods, sulfites or other preservatives, or dyes. Most medicines contain more than their active ingredient.

—if you are **pregnant** or if you may become pregnant. Studies on birth defects with baclofen have not been done in humans. However, studies in animals have shown that baclofen, when given in doses several times the human dose, increases the chance of hernias and incomplete or slow development of bones in the fetus, and of lower birth weight.

—if you are **breast-feeding**. Although it is not known whether baclofen passes into the breast milk, this medicine has not been shown to cause problems in nursing babies.

—if you have any of the following medical problems:
   Diabetes mellitus (sugar diabetes)
   Epilepsy
   Kidney disease
   Mental or emotional problems
   Stroke or other brain disease

—if you are taking **any** other prescription or nonprescription (OTC) medicine, especially central nervous system (CNS) depressants.

Proper Use of This Medicine

If you miss a dose of this medicine, and you remember within an hour or so of the missed dose, take it as soon as you remember. However, if you do not remember until later, skip the missed dose and go back to your regular dosing schedule. Do not double doses.

How to store this medicine:

• **Keep out of the reach of children.**

• Store away from heat and direct light.

• Do not store in the bathroom, near the kitchen sink, or in other damp places. Heat or moisture may cause the medicine to break down.

• Do not keep outdated medicine or medicine no longer needed. Be sure that any discarded medicine is out of the reach of children.

Precautions While Using This Medicine

Do not suddenly stop taking this medicine. Unwanted effects may occur if the medicine is stopped suddenly. Check with your doctor for the best way to reduce gradually the amount you are taking before stopping completely.

This medicine will add to the effects of alcohol and other CNS depressants (medicines that slow down the nervous system, possibly causing drowsiness). Some examples of CNS depressants are antihistamines or medicine for hay fever, other allergies, or colds; sedatives, tranquilizers, or sleeping medicine; prescription pain medicine or narcotics; barbiturates; medicine for seizures; other muscle relaxants; or anesthetics, including some dental anesthetics. **Check with your doctor before taking any of the above while you are using baclofen.**

This medicine may cause drowsiness, dizziness, vision problems, or clumsiness or unsteadiness in some people. **Make sure you know how you react to this medicine before you drive, use machines, or do other jobs that require you to be alert, well-coordinated, and able to see well.**

Diabetics—This medicine may cause your blood sugar levels to rise. If you notice a change in the results of your urine sugar test or if you have any questions about this, check with your doctor.

Side Effects of This Medicine

Along with its needed effects, a medicine may cause some unwanted effects. Although not all of these side effects may occur, if they do occur they may need medical attention.

Check with your doctor as soon as possible if any of the following side effects occur:

Rare
> Bloody or dark urine
> Chest pain
> Fainting
> Hallucinations (seeing or hearing things that are not there)
> Mental depression or other mood changes
> Ringing or buzzing in the ears
> Skin rash or itching

Signs of overdose
> Blurred or double vision or any change in vision
> Convulsions (seizures)
> Muscle weakness (severe)
> Shortness of breath or unusually slow or troubled breathing
> Vomiting

Other side effects may occur that usually do not require medical attention. These side effects may go away during treatment as your body adjusts to the medicine. However, check with your doctor if any of the following side effects continue or are bothersome:

More common
> Confusion
> Dizziness or lightheadedness
> Drowsiness
> Nausea
> Unusual weakness, especially muscle weakness

Less common or rare
> Abdominal or stomach pain or discomfort
> Clumsiness, unsteadiness, trembling, or other problems with muscle control
> Constipation

> Diarrhea
> Difficult or painful urination or decrease in amount of urine
> False sense of well-being
> Frequent urge to urinate or uncontrolled urination
> Headache
> Loss of appetite
> Low blood pressure
> Muscle pain
> Numbness or tingling in hands or feet
> Pounding heartbeat
> Sexual problems in males
> Slurred speech or other speech problems
> Stuffy nose
> Swelling of ankles
> Trouble in sleeping
> Unexplained muscle stiffness
> Unusual excitement
> Unusual tiredness
> Unusual weight gain

Some side effects may occur after you have stopped taking this medicine, especially if you stop taking it suddenly. **Check with your doctor immediately** if any of the following effects occur:

> Convulsions (seizures)
> Hallucinations (seeing or hearing things that are not there)
> Increase in muscle spasm, cramping, or tightness
> Mood or mental changes
> Unusual nervousness or restlessness

For elderly patients: Some side effects may be more likely to occur in elderly patients, who are usually more sensitive to the effects of baclofen. These include hallucinations, confusion or mental depression, other mood or mental changes, and severe drowsiness.

Other side effects not listed above may also occur in some patients. If you notice any other effects, check with your doctor.

December 1987

BARBITURATES (Systemic)

This information applies to the following medicines:

Amobarbital (am-oh-BAR-bi-tal)
Aprobarbital (a-proe-BAR-bi-tal)
Butabarbital (byoo-ta-BAR-bi-tal)
Mephobarbital (me-foe-BAR-bi-tal)
Metharbital (meth-AR-bi-tal)
Pentobarbital (pen-toe-BAR-bi-tal)
Phenobarbital (fee-noe-BAR-bi-tal)
Secobarbital (see-koe-BAR-bi-tal)
Secobarbital and Amobarbital (see-koe-BAR-bi-tal and am-oh-BAR-bi-tal)
Talbutal (TAL-byoo-tal)

Some commonly used brand names are:	Generic names:
Amytal	Amobarbital†
Alurate	Aprobarbital
Barbased Butalan Buticaps Butisol Day-Barb* Neo-Barb* Sarisol No. 2	Butabarbital†
Mebaral	Mephobarbital
Gemonil	Metharbital
Novopentobarb* Nembutal	Pentobarbital†
Barbita Gardenal* Luminal Solfoton	Phenobarbital†
Novosecobarb* Seconal	Secobarbital†
Tuinal	Secobarbital and Amobarbital
Lotusate	Talbutal

*Not available in the U.S.
†Generic name product may also be available in the U.S.

To the Reader: If you do not recognize the names of medical conditions or medicines referred to in this information, check with your doctor, nurse, or pharmacist. Definitions for selected medical terms may be found in the Glossary. Brand names for the generic drug names listed can be found in the Index. In addition, selected brand names commonly associated with the generic name have been included in the text to help you recognize medicine you may be taking. The fact that a brand name product is not mentioned does not mean the information does not apply. It is a good idea for you to learn both the generic and brand names of your medicines and to write them down for future use.

Barbiturates (bar-BI-tyoo-rates) belong to the group of medicines called central nervous system (CNS) depressants (medicines that slow down the nervous system). They act on the brain and CNS to produce effects that may be helpful or harmful. This depends on the individual patient's condition and response and the amount of medicine taken.

Barbiturates are taken by mouth, given by injection, or used rectally. They may be used to treat insomnia (sleeplessness) by helping patients fall asleep. Also, some of the barbiturates may be used before surgery to relieve anxiety or tension. Some of the barbiturates are used as anticonvulsants to help control seizures in certain disorders or diseases, such as epilepsy. Barbiturates may also be used for other conditions as determined by your doctor.

If barbiturates are used regularly (for example, every day) for insomnia, they usually are not effective for longer than 2 weeks. Also, if too much of a barbiturate is used, it may become habit-forming.

Barbiturates should not be used for anxiety or tension caused by the stress of everyday life.

These medicines are available only with your doctor's prescription.

Remember:
• **This medicine has been prescribed for your current medical problem only.** It must not be given to other people or used for other problems unless you are directed to do so by your doctor.

• **Keep all medicines out of the reach of children.**

• In order for this medicine to work, it must be used as directed.

• If you are receiving this medicine by injection, some of the information about this medicine may not apply.

• **It is very important that you read and understand the following information.** If any of the information causes you special concern, do not decide against using this medicine without first checking with your doctor.

• Before you begin using any new medicine (prescription or nonprescription) or if you develop any new medical problem while you are using this medicine, check with your doctor, nurse, or pharmacist.

• **If you have any questions** about the following information or if you want more information about this medicine or your medical problem, **ask your doctor, nurse, or pharmacist.**

Before Using This Medicine

In order to decide on the best treatment for your medical problem, your doctor should be told:

—if you have ever had any unusual or allergic reaction to barbiturates.

—if you are on a low-salt, low-sugar, or any other special diet, or if you are allergic to any substance, such as foods, sulfites or other preservatives, or dyes. Most medicines contain more than their active ingredient, and many liquid medicines contain alcohol. Your doctor, nurse, or pharmacist can help you avoid products that may cause a problem.

—if you are **pregnant** or if you may become pregnant. Barbiturates have been shown to increase the chance of birth defects in humans. However, this medicine may be needed in serious diseases or other situations that threaten the mother's life. Be sure you have discussed this and the following information with your doctor:

• taking barbiturates regularly during the last 3 months of pregnancy may cause the baby to become dependent on the medicine. This may lead to withdrawal side effects in the baby after birth.

• barbiturates taken for epilepsy during pregnancy may cause bleeding problems in the newborn infant.

• one study in humans has suggested that barbiturates taken during pregnancy may increase the chance of brain tumors in the baby.

• barbiturates taken for anesthesia during labor and delivery may reduce the force and frequency of contractions of the uterus; this may prolong labor and delay delivery.

• use of barbiturates during labor may cause breathing problems in the newborn infant.

—if you are **breast-feeding**. Barbiturates pass into the breast milk and may cause drowsiness, unusually slow heartbeat, shortness of breath, or troubled breathing in babies of nursing mothers taking this medicine.

—if you have any of the following medical problems:
Anemia (severe)
Asthma (history of), emphysema, or other chronic lung disease
Diabetes mellitus (sugar diabetes)
Hyperactivity (in children)
Kidney disease
Liver disease
Mental depression
Overactive thyroid
Pain
Porphyria (or history of)
Underactive adrenal gland

—if you are now taking or receiving **any** other prescription or nonprescripiton (OTC) medicine, especially:
Adrenocorticoids (cortisone-like medicine)
Anticoagulants (blood thinners)
Central nervous system (CNS) depressants
Corticotropin (e.g., ACTH)
Oral contraceptives (birth control pills) containing estrogens

Proper Use of This Medicine

For patients taking the extended-release capsule or tablet form of this medicine:

• These capsules or tablets are to be swallowed whole. Do not break, crush, or chew before swallowing.

For patients taking the pediatric drop form of this medicine:

• Do not use if solution is cloudy.

• This medicine is to be taken by mouth even though it may come in a dropper bottle. Measure the correct amount with the specially marked dropper. Each dose may be taken straight or mixed with water, milk, or fruit juices. Be sure to drink all of the liquid in order to get the full dose of medicine.

For patients using the rectal suppository form of this medicine:

• How to insert suppository: First remove the foil wrapper and moisten the suppository with water. Lie down on side and push the suppository well up into rectum with finger.

Use this medicine only as directed by your doctor. Do not use more of it, do not use it more often, and do not use it for a longer period of time than your doctor ordered. If too much is used, it may become habit-forming (causing mental or physical dependence).

If you think this medicine is not working as well after you have taken it for a few weeks, **do not increase the dose.** To do so may increase the chance of your becoming dependent on the medicine. Instead, check with your doctor.

If you are taking this medicine for epilepsy, it must be taken every day in regularly spaced doses as ordered by your doctor in order for it to control your seizures. This is necessary to keep a constant amount of medicine in the blood. To help keep the amount constant, do not miss any doses.

If you are taking this medicine regularly (for example, every day as in epilepsy) and you do miss a dose, take it as soon as possible. However, if it is almost time for your next dose, skip the missed dose and go back to your regular dosing schedule. Do not double doses.

How to store this medicine:

• **Keep out of the reach of children** since overdose is especially dangerous in children.

• Store away from heat and direct light.

• Do not store the capsule or tablet form of this medicine in the bathroom, near the kitchen sink, or in other damp places. Heat or moisture may cause the medicine to break down.

• Keep the liquid form of this medicine from freezing.

• Store the suppository form of this medicine in the refrigerator.

• Do not keep outdated medicine or medicine no longer needed. Be sure that any discarded medicine is out of the reach of children.

Precautions While Using This Medicine

If you will be using this medicine regularly for a long period of time:

• Your doctor should check your progress at regular visits.

• Do not stop using it without first checking with your doctor. Your doctor may want you to reduce gradually the amount you are using before stopping completely.

This medicine will add to the effects of alcohol and other CNS depressants (medicines that slow down the nervous system, possibly causing drowsiness). Some examples of CNS depressants are antihistamines or medicine for hay fever, other allergies, or colds; sedatives,

tranquilizers, or sleeping medicine; prescription pain medicine or narcotics; barbiturates; medicine for seizures; muscle relaxants; or anesthetics, including some dental anesthetics. **Check with your doctor before taking any of the above while you are using this medicine.**

If you have been using this medicine for a long period of time and you think that you may have become mentally or physically dependent on it, check with your doctor. Some signs of mental or physical dependence on barbiturates are:

—a strong desire or need to continue taking the medicine.

—a need to increase the dose to receive the effects of the medicine.

—withdrawal side effects (for example, anxiety or restlessness, convulsions [seizures], feeling faint, nausea or vomiting, trembling of hands, trouble in sleeping) occurring after the medicine is stopped.

If you think you or someone else may have taken an overdose, get emergency help at once. Taking an overdose of a barbiturate or taking alcohol or other CNS depressants with the barbiturate may lead to unconsciousness and possibly death. Some signs of an overdose are severe drowsiness, severe confusion, severe weakness, shortness of breath or slow or troubled breathing, slurred speech, staggering, and slow heartbeat.

This medicine may cause some people to become dizzy, lightheaded, drowsy, or less alert than they are normally. Even if taken at bedtime, it may cause some people to feel drowsy or less alert on arising. **Make sure you know how you react to this medicine before you drive, use machines, or do other jobs that require you to be alert.**

Side Effects of This Medicine

Along with its needed effects, a medicine may cause some unwanted effects. Although not all of these side effects may occur, if they do occur they may need medical attention.

Check with your doctor immediately if any of the following side effects occur:

Rare
> Bleeding sores on lips
> Chest pain
> Muscle or joint pain
> Red, thickened, or scaly skin
> Skin rash or hives
> Sore throat and/or fever
> Sores, ulcers, or white spots in mouth (painful)
> Swelling of eyelids, face, or lips
> Wheezing or tightness in chest

Also, check with your doctor as soon as possible if any of the following side effects occur:

Less common
> Confusion
> Mental depression
> Unusual excitement

Rare
> Hallucinations (seeing, hearing, or feeling things that are not there)
> Unusual bleeding or bruising
> Unusual tiredness or weakness

With long-term or chronic use
> Bone pain, tenderness, or aching
> Loss of appetite
> Muscle weakness
> Weight loss
> Yellow eyes or skin

Signs of overdose
> Confusion (severe)
> Decrease in or loss of reflexes
> Drowsiness (severe)
> Fever
> Irritability (continuing)
> Low body temperature
> Poor judgment
> Shortness of breath or slow or troubled breathing
> Slow heartbeat
> Slurred speech
> Staggering
> Trouble in sleeping
> Unusual movements of the eyes
> Weakness (severe)

Other side effects may occur that usually do not require medical attention. These side effects may go away during treatment as your body adjusts to the medicine. However, check with your doctor if any of the following side effects continue or are bothersome:

More common
> Clumsiness or unsteadiness
> Dizziness or lightheadedness
> Drowsiness
> "Hangover" effect

Less common
> Anxiety or nervousness
> Constipation
> Feeling faint
> Headache
> Irritability
> Nausea or vomiting
> Nightmares or trouble in sleeping

For children and elderly or very ill patients: Unusual excitement may be more likely to occur in children and in elderly or very ill patients. Also, confusion and mental depression may be more likely to occur in elderly or very ill patients.

After you stop using this medicine, your body may need time to adjust. If you took this medicine in high doses or for a long period of time, this may take up to about 15 days. During this period of time check with your doctor if any of the following side effects occur (usually occur within 8 to 16 hours after medicine is stopped):

> Anxiety or restlessness
> Convulsions (seizures)
> Dizziness or lightheadedness
> Feeling faint
> Hallucinations (seeing, hearing, or feeling things that are not there)

Muscle twitching
Nausea or vomiting
Trembling of hands
Trouble in sleeping, increased dreaming, or nightmares
Vision problems
Weakness

Other side effects not listed above may also occur in some patients. If you notice any other effects, check with your doctor.

December 1987

BELLADONNA ALKALOIDS AND BARBITURATES (Systemic)

This information applies to the following medicines:

Atropine (A-troe-peen), Hyoscyamine (hye-oh-SYE-a-meen), Scopola-
  mine (skoe-POL-a-meen), and Butabarbital (byoo-ta-BAR-bi-tal)
Atropine, Hyoscyamine, Scopolamine, and Phenobarbital (fee-noe-BAR-
  bi-tal)
Atropine and Phenobarbital
Belladonna and Butabarbital
Belladonna and Phenobarbital
Hyoscyamine and Phenobarbital
Hyoscyamine, Scopolamine, and Phenobarbital

Some commonly used brand names are:	Generic names:
Palbar No. 2	Atropine, Hyoscyamime, Scopolamine, and Butabarbital
Barbidonna Barophen Bay-Ase Bellalphen Bellastal Donnapine Donna-Sed Donnatal Donnatal Extentabs Donphen Hybephen Hyosophen Kinesed Malatal Relaxadon Seds Spaslin Spasmolin Spasmophen Spasquid Susano Vanodonnal	Atropine, Hyoscyamine, Scopolamine, and Phenobarbital†
Antrocol	Atropine and Phenobarbital
Butibel	Belladonna and Butabarbital
Belap Bellkatal Chardonna-2 Pheno-Bella	Belladonna and Phenobarbital†
Anaspaz PB Levsinex with Phenobarbital Timecaps Levsin-PB Levsin with Phenobarbital	Hyoscyamine and Phenobarbital
Belladenal Belladenal-S Belladenal Spacetabs*	Hyoscyamine, Scopolamine, and Phenobarbital

*Not available in the U.S.
†Generic name product may also be available in the U.S.

To the Reader: If you do not recognize the names of medical conditions or medicines referred to in this information, check with your doctor, nurse, or pharmacist. Definitions for selected medical terms may be found in the Glossary. Brand names for the generic drug names listed can be found in the Index. In addition, selected brand names commonly associated with the generic name have been included in the text to help you recognize medicine you may be taking. The fact that a brand name

product is not mentioned does not mean the information does not apply. It is a good idea for you to learn both the generic and brand names of your medicines and to write them down for future use.

Belladonna alkaloids and barbiturates are combination medicines taken by mouth to relieve cramping and spasms of the stomach and intestines. They are used also to decrease the amount of acid formed in the stomach.

These medicines are available only with your doctor's prescription.

Remember:

• **This medicine has been prescribed for your current medical problem only.** It must not be given to other people or used for other problems unless you are directed to do so by your doctor.

• **Keep all medicines out of the reach of children.**

• In order for this medicine to work, it must be used as directed.

• **It is very important that you read and understand the following information.** If any of the information causes you special concern, do not decide against using this medicine without first checking with your doctor.

• Before you begin using any new medicine (prescription or nonprescription) or if you develop any new medical problem while you are using this medicine, check with your doctor, nurse, or pharmacist.

• **If you have any questions** about the following information or if you want more information about this medicine or your medical problem, **ask your doctor, nurse, or pharmacist**.

Before Using This Medicine

In order to decide on the best treatment for your medical problem, your doctor should be told:

—if you have ever had any unusual or allergic reaction to any of the belladonna alkaloids (atropine, belladonna, hyoscyamine, and scopolamine) or to barbiturates.

—if you are on a low-salt, low-sugar, or any other special diet, or if you are allergic to any substance, such as foods, sulfites or other preservatives, or dyes. Most medicines contain more than their active ingredient, and many liquid medicines contain alcohol. Your doctor, nurse, or pharmacist can help you avoid products that may cause a problem.

—if you are **pregnant** or if you may become pregnant while taking this medicine. Belladonna alkaloids have not been shown to cause problems in humans. However, barbiturates (contained in this medicine) have been shown to increase the chance of birth defects in humans. Also, when taken during pregnancy, barbiturates may cause bleeding problems in the newborn baby. Be sure that you have discussed this with your doctor before taking this medicine.

—if you are **breast-feeding**. Belladonna alkaloids or barbiturates have not been shown to cause problems in nursing babies. However, traces of the belladonna alkaloids and barbiturates pass into the breast milk.

Also, because the belladonna alkaloids tend to decrease the secretions of the body, it is possible that the flow of breast milk may be reduced in some patients.

—if you have any of the following medical problems:

Asthma, emphysema, or other chronic lung disease
Brain damage (in children)
Down's syndrome (mongolism)
Dry mouth (severe and continuing)
Enlarged prostate
Glaucoma
Heart disease
Hyperactivity (in children)
Intestinal blockage or other intestinal problems
Kidney disease
Liver disease
Spastic paralysis (in children)
Urinary tract blockage or difficult urination

—if you are taking **any** other prescription or nonprescription (OTC) medicine, especially:

Antacids
Anticoagulants, coumarin- or indandione-type (blood thinners)
Antimuscarinics, other (medicine for abdominal or stomach spasms or cramps)
Central nervous system (CNS) depressants
Diarrhea medicine containing kaolin or attapulgite
Digitalis glycosides (heart medicine)
Ketoconazole (e.g., Nizoral)
Potassium chloride (e.g., Kay Ciel)

—if you are now taking or have taken within the past 2 weeks monoamine oxidase (MAO) inhibitors, such as:

Furazolidone (e.g., Furoxone)
Isocarboxazid (e.g., Marplan)
Pargyline (e.g., Eutonyl)
Phenelzine (e.g., Nardil)
Procarbazine (e.g., Matulane)
Tranylcypromine (e.g., Parnate)

Proper Use of This Medicine

Take this medicine about ½ to 1 hour before meals, unless otherwise directed by your doctor.

Take this medicine only as directed. Do not take more or less of it, do not take it more often, and do not take it for a longer period of time than your doctor ordered. To do so may increase the chance of side effects.

If you miss a dose of this medicine, take it as soon as possible. However, if it is almost time for your next dose, skip the missed dose and go back to your regular dosing schedule. Do not double doses.

How to store this medicine:

• **Keep this medicine out of the reach of children** since overdose is especially dangerous in young children.

• Store away from heat and direct light.

• Do not store the capsule or tablet form of this medicine in the bathroom, near the kitchen sink, or in other damp places. Heat or moisture may cause the medicine to break down.

• Keep the liquid form of this medicine from freezing.

• Do not keep outdated medicine or medicine no longer needed. Be sure that any discarded medicine is out of the reach of children.

Precautions While Using This Medicine

This medicine will add to the effects of alcohol and other CNS depressants (medicines that slow down the nervous system, possibly causing drowsiness). Some examples of CNS depressants are antihistamines or medicine for hay fever, other allergies, or colds; sedatives, tranquilizers, or sleeping medicine; prescription pain medicine or narcotics; barbiturates; medicine for seizures; muscle relaxants; or anesthetics, including some dental anesthetics. **Check with your doctor before taking any of the above while you are taking this medicine.**

Do not take this medicine within 1 hour of taking antacids or medicine for diarrhea. Taking them too close together will make the belladonna alkaloids less effective.

Belladonna alkaloids will often make you sweat less, causing your body temperature to increase. **Use extra care not to become overheated during exercise or hot weather while you are taking this medicine,** as overheating could possibly result in heat stroke. This is especially important in children taking belladonna alkaloids.

This medicine may cause your eyes to become more sensitive to light than they are normally. Wearing sunglasses may help lessen the discomfort from bright light.

This medicine may cause some people to have blurred vision or to become drowsy, dizzy, or less alert than they are normally. **Make sure you know how you react to this medicine before you drive, use machines, or do other jobs that require you to be alert or to see well.**

This medicine may cause dryness of the mouth, nose, and throat. For temporary relief of mouth dryness, use sugarless candy or gum, melt bits of ice in your mouth, or use a saliva substitute. However, if dry mouth continues for more than 2 weeks, check with your dentist. Continuing dryness of the mouth may increase the chance of dental disease, including tooth decay, gum disease, and fungal infections.

Side Effects of This Medicine

Along with its needed effects, a medicine may cause some unwanted effects. Although not all of these side effects may occur, if they do occur they may need medical attention.

Check with your doctor as soon as possible if any of the following side effects occur:
Rare
Eye pain
Skin rash or hives
Sore throat and fever
Unusual bleeding or bruising
Yellow eyes or skin

© 1988   The United States Pharmacopeial Convention, Inc.

Signs of overdose
    Blurred vision (continuing) or changes in near vision
    Clumsiness or unsteadiness
    Confusion
    Convulsions (seizures)
    Dizziness (continuing)
    Drowsiness (severe)
    Dryness of mouth, nose, or throat (severe)
    Fast heartbeat
    Fever
    Hallucinations (seeing, hearing, or feeling things that are
        not there)
    Shortness of breath or troubled breathing
    Slurred speech
    Unusual excitement, nervousness, restlessness, or irrita-
        bility
    Unusual warmth, dryness, and flushing of skin

Other side effects may occur that usually do not require
    medical attention. These side effects may go away
    during treatment as your body adjusts to the medicine.
    However, check with your doctor if any of the follow-
    ing side effects continue or are bothersome:

More common
    Constipation
    Decrease in sweating
    Dizziness
    Drowsiness
    Dryness of mouth, nose, throat, or skin

Less common or rare
    Bloated feeling
    Blurred vision
    Decreased flow of breast milk

    Difficult urination
    Difficulty in swallowing
    Headache
    Increased sensitivity of eyes to sunlight
    Loss of memory
    Nausea or vomiting
    Unusual tiredness or weakness

For children: In infants and children, especially those
    with spastic paralysis or brain damage, this medicine
    may be more likely to cause severe side effects. Fever
    or unusual warmth, dryness, and flushing of skin are
    more likely to occur in children. Also, when it is given
    to children during hot weather, a rapid increase in
    body temperature may occur.

For children or elderly patients: Children and elderly pa-
    tients are usually more sensitive to the effects of the
    belladonna alkaloids and barbiturates. Confusion; con-
    stipation; difficult urination; drowsiness; dryness of
    mouth, nose, throat, or skin; and memory loss may be
    more likely to occur in elderly patients. Also, unusual
    excitement, nervousness, restlessness, or irritability may
    be more likely to occur in children and in elderly pa-
    tients.

Other side effects not listed above may also occur in some
    patients. If you notice any other effects, check with
    your doctor.

_____

December 1987

_____

BENTIROMIDE (Systemic)

A commonly used brand name is Chymex.

To the Reader: If you do not recognize the names of medical conditions or medicines referred to in this information, check with your doctor, nurse, or pharmacist. Definitions for selected medical terms may be found in the Glossary. Brand names for the generic drug names listed can be found in the Index. In addition, selected brand names commonly associated with the generic name have been included in the text to help you recognize medicine you may be taking. The fact that a brand name product is not mentioned does not mean the information does not apply. It is a good idea for you to learn both the generic and brand names of your medicines and to write them down for future use.

Bentiromide (ben-TEER-oh-mide) is taken by mouth. It is used to help find out if the pancreas is working the way it should. The pancreas helps break down the bentiromide almost the same way it helps to break down food. After bentiromide is broken down, a part of it appears in the urine. By measuring how much appears in the urine, your doctor can tell how well your pancreas is working.

How the test is done: After you take bentiromide, all of your urine is collected for the next six hours. The total amount is measured and a small sample is saved and examined.

Bentiromide is to be used only under the supervision of a doctor.

Remember:

• **This medicine has been prescribed for your current medical problem only.** It must not be given to other people or used for other problems unless you are directed to do so by your doctor.

• **Keep all medicines out of the reach of children.**

• In order for this medicine to work, it must be used as directed.

• **It is very important that you read and understand the following information.** If any of the information causes you special concern, do not decide against using this medicine without first checking with your doctor.

• **If you have any questions** about the following information or if you want more information about this medicine or your medical problem, **ask your doctor, nurse, or pharmacist.**

Before Having This Test

Before this test is given, your doctor should be told:

—if you have ever had any unusual or allergic reaction to bentiromide.

—if you are on a low-salt, low-sugar, or any other special diet, or if you are allergic to any substance, such as foods, sulfites or other preservatives, or dyes. Most medicines contain more than their active ingredient. Your doctor can help you avoid products that may cause a problem.

—if you are **pregnant** or if you suspect that you may be pregnant. Studies have not been done in humans. However, in animal studies bentiromide has not been shown to cause birth defects or other problems.

—if you are **breast-feeding.** It is not known whether bentiromide passes into the breast milk. However, this medicine has not been shown to cause problems in nursing babies.

—if you have any of the following medical problems:

Disease of the stomach and intestines
Kidney disease
Liver disease (severe)

—if you are using **any** other prescription or nonprescription (OTC) medicine, especially:

Acetaminophen (e.g., Tylenol)
Chloramphenicol (e.g., Chloromycetin)
Local anesthetics (e.g., benzocaine and lidocaine)
Methotrexate (e.g., Mexate)
PABA–containing preparations (e.g., sunscreens and some multivitamins)
Pancreatic supplements (e.g., pancrelipase)
Phenacetin-containing medicines (e.g., APC)
Procainamide (e.g., Pronestyl)
Sulfonamides (sulfa medicines)
Thiazide diuretics (water pills)

—if you have recently had any kind of surgery (including dental surgery) for which you received local anesthesia.

—if you have eaten prunes or cranberries recently.

Preparation For This Test

Your doctor may ask you to avoid certain medicines or foods for at least 72 hours before this test is done. **Follow your doctor's instructions carefully.** Otherwise, this test may not work and will have to be done again.

Unless otherwise directed by your doctor:

• Do not eat anything after midnight the night before the test. Some foods may affect the results of the test.

• Urinate before taking bentiromide. You should have an empty bladder when you take the test.

• After taking bentiromide, drink a large glass of water (at least 8 ounces). Drink another large glass of water in 2 hours and then 2 more glasses of water in the next 4 hours. This will help increase the amount of urine, which is needed for testing.

Side Effects of This Medicine

Along with its needed effects, a medicine may cause some unwanted effects. Although not all of these side effects may occur, if they do occur they may need medical attention.

Check with your doctor or nurse immediately if either of
the following side effects occurs:

Rare

Shortness of breath or troubled breathing

Other side effects may occur that usually do not require
medical attention. These side effects should go away
as the effects of the medicine wear off. However, check
with your doctor if any of the following side effects
continue or are bothersome:

More common

Diarrhea
Headache

Less common or rare

Gas
Nausea and vomiting
Weakness

Other side effects not listed above may also occur in some
patients. If you notice any other effects, check with
your doctor.

December 1987

BENZODIAZEPINES (Systemic)

This information applies to the following medicines:

Alprazolam (al-PRAZ-oh-lam)
Chlordiazepoxide (klor-dye-az-e-POX-ide)
Clonazepam (kloe-NA-ze-pam)
Clorazepate (klor-AZ-e-pate)
Diazepam (dye-AZ-e-pam)
Flurazepam (flure-AZ-e-pam)
Halazepam (hal-AZ-e-pam)
Lorazepam (lor-AZ-e-pam)
Oxazepam (ox-AZ-e-pam)
Prazepam (PRAZ-e-pam)
Temazepam (tem-AZ-e-pam)
Triazolam (trye-AY-zoe-lam)

Some commonly used brand names are:	Generic names:
Xanax	Alprazolam
Apo-Chlordiazepoxide* Libritabs Librium Lipoxide Medilium* Novopoxide* Reposans Sereen SK-Lygen Solium*	Chlordiazepoxide†
Klonopin Rivotril*	Clonazepam
Novoclopate* Tranxene* Tranxene-SD Tranxene T-Tab	Clorazepate†
Apo-Diazepam* E-Pam* Meval* Neo-Calme* Novodipam* Q-Pam Rival* Valium Valrelease Vivol*	Diazepam†
Apo-Flurazepam* Dalmane Durapam Novoflupam* Somnol* Som-Pam*	Flurazepam†
Paxipam	Halazepam
Alzapam Apo-Lorazepam* Ativan Loraz Novolorazem*	Lorazepam†
Apo-Oxazepam* Novoxapam* Ox-Pam* Serax Zapex*	Oxazepam†
Centrax	Prazepam
Razepam Restoril Temaz	Temazepam†
Halcion	Triazolam

*Not available in the U.S.
†Generic name product may also be available in the U.S.

To the Reader: If you do not recognize the names of medical conditions or medicines referred to in this information, check with your doctor, nurse, or pharmacist. Definitions for selected medical terms may be found in the Glossary. Brand names for the generic drug names listed can be found in the Index. In addition, selected brand names commonly associated with the generic name have been included in the text to help you recognize medicine you may be taking. The fact that a brand name product is not mentioned does not mean the information does not apply. It is a good idea for you to learn both the generic and brand names of your medicines and to write them down for future use.

Benzodiazepines (ben-zoe-dye-AZ-e-peens) belong to the group of medicines called central nervous system (CNS) depressants (medicines that slow down the nervous system). They are taken by mouth or given by injection.

Some benzodiazepines are used to relieve nervousness or tension. Others are used in the treatment of insomnia (sleeplessness). However, if used regularly (for example, every day) for insomnia, they are usually not effective for more than a few weeks.

One of the benzodiazepines, diazepam, is also used to relax muscles or relieve muscle spasm. Clonazepam, clorazepate, and diazepam are also used to treat certain convulsive disorders, such as epilepsy. The benzodiazepines may also be used for other conditions as determined by your doctor.

Benzodiazepines should not be used for nervousness or tension caused by the stress of everyday life.

These medicines are available only with your doctor's prescription.

Remember:
- **This medicine has been prescribed for your current medical problem only.** It must not be given to other people or used for other problems unless you are directed to do so by your doctor.

- **Keep all medicines out of the reach of children.**

- In order for this medicine to work, it must be used as directed.

- If you are receiving this medicine by injection, some of the information about this medicine may not apply.

- **It is very important that you read and understand the following information.** If any of the information causes you special concern, do not decide against using this medicine without first checking with your doctor.

- Before you begin using any new medicine (prescription or nonprescription) or if you develop any new medical problem while you are using this medicine, check with your doctor, nurse, or pharmacist.

- **If you have any questions** about the following information or if you want more information about this medicine or your medical problem, **ask your doctor, nurse, or pharmacist**.

Before Using This Medicine

In order to decide on the best treatment for your medical problem, your doctor should be told:

—if you have ever had any unusual or allergic reaction to benzodiazepines.

—if you are on a low-salt, low-sugar, or any other special diet, or if you are allergic to any substance, such as foods, sulfites or other preservatives, or dyes. Most medicines contain more than their active ingredient. Your doctor, nurse, or pharmacist can help you avoid products that may cause a problem.

—if you are **pregnant** or if you may become pregnant. Chlordiazepoxide and diazepam have been reported to increase the chance of birth defects when used during the first 3 months of pregnancy. Although similar problems have not been reported with the other benzodiazepines, the chance always exists since all of the benzodiazepines are related. Also, studies in animals have shown that clonazepam, lorazepam, and temazepam cause birth defects or other problems, including death of the animal fetus.

In addition, too much use of benzodiazepines during pregnancy may cause the baby to become dependent on the medicine. This may lead to withdrawal side effects after birth. Also, use of benzodiazepines during pregnancy, especially during the last weeks, may cause drowsiness, slow heartbeat, shortness of breath, or troubled breathing in the newborn infant.

Benzodiazepines given just before or during labor may cause weakness in the newborn infant. When diazepam is given in high doses (especially by injection) within 15 hours before delivery, it may cause breathing problems, muscle weakness, difficulty in feeding, and body temperature problems in the newborn infant.

—if you are **breast-feeding**. Benzodiazepines may pass into the breast milk and cause drowsiness, unusually slow heartbeat, shortness of breath, or troubled breathing in nursing babies of mothers taking this medicine.

—if you have any of the following medical problems:

Emphysema, asthma, bronchitis, or other chronic lung disease
Epilepsy or history of seizures
Hyperactivity (in children)
Kidney disease
Liver disease
Mental depression
Mental illness (severe)
Myasthenia gravis
Porphyria

—if you are taking **any** other prescription or nonprescription medicine, especially central nervous system (CNS) depressants.

Proper Use of This Medicine

For patients taking diazepam extended-release capsules:

• Swallow capsules whole.

• Do not crush, break, or chew before swallowing.

For patients taking lorazepam sublingual tablets:

• Do not chew or swallow the tablet. This medicine is meant to be absorbed through the lining of the mouth. Place the tablet under your tongue (sublingual) and let it slowly dissolve there. Do not swallow until the tablet has completely dissolved.

Take this medicine only as directed by your doctor. Do not take more of it, do not take it more often, and do not take it for a longer period of time than your doctor ordered. If too much is taken, it may become habit-forming (causing mental or physical dependence).

If you think this medicine is not working as well after you have taken it for a few weeks, **do not increase the dose**. Instead, check with your doctor.

For patients taking this medicine for epilepsy or other seizure disorder:

• **In order for this medicine to control your seizures, it must be taken every day in regularly spaced doses as ordered by your doctor.** This is necessary to keep a constant amount of the medicine in the blood. To help keep the amount constant, do not miss any doses.

For patients taking flurazepam:

• **When you begin to take this medicine, your sleeping problem will improve somewhat the first night. However, 2 or 3 nights may pass before you receive the full effects of this medicine.**

If you are taking this medicine regularly (for example, every day as for epilepsy) and you miss a dose, take it right away if you remember within an hour or so of the missed dose. However, if you do not remember until later, skip the missed dose and go back to your regular dosing schedule. Do not double doses.

How to store this medicine:

• **Keep out of the reach of children** since overdose may be especially dangerous in children.

• Store away from heat and direct light.

• Do not store the capsule or tablet form of this medicine in the bathroom, near the kitchen sink, or in other damp places. Heat or moisture may cause the medicine to break down.

• Keep the liquid form of this medicine from freezing.

• Do not keep outdated medicine or medicine no longer needed. Be sure that any discarded medicine is out of the reach of children.

Precautions While Using This Medicine

If you will be taking this medicine regularly for a long period of time:

• Your doctor should check your progress at regular visits in order to make sure that this medicine does not cause unwanted effects. If you are taking clonazepam, this is also important during the first few months of treatment.

• If you are taking this medicine for nervousness or tension or for insomnia (sleeplessness), check with your doctor at least every 4 months to make sure you need to continue taking this medicine. However, if you are taking flurazepam, temazepam, or triazolam, check with your doctor every month.

If you will be taking this medicine in large doses or for a long period of time, do not stop taking it without first checking with your doctor. Your doctor may want you to reduce gradually the amount you are taking before stopping completely. Stopping this medicine suddenly may cause withdrawal side effects. Also, if you are taking this medicine for epilepsy or other seizure disorder, stopping this medicine suddenly may cause seizures.

For patients taking this medicine for epilepsy or other seizure disorder:
• Your doctor may want you to carry a medical identification card or bracelet stating that you are taking this medicine.

This medicine will add to the effects of alcohol and other CNS depressants (medicines that slow down the nervous system, possibly causing drowsiness). Some examples of CNS depressants are antihistamines or medicine for hay fever, other allergies, or colds; sedatives, tranquilizers, or sleeping medicine; prescription pain medicine or narcotics; barbiturates; medicine for seizures; muscle relaxants; or anesthetics, including some dental anesthetics. This effect may last for a few days after you stop taking this medicine. **Check with your doctor before taking any of the above while you are taking this medicine.**

If you think you or someone else may have taken an overdose, get emergency help at once. Taking an overdose of a benzodiazepine or taking alcohol or other CNS depressants with the benzodiazepine may lead to unconsciousness and possibly death. Some signs of an overdose are continuing slurred speech or confusion, severe drowsiness, severe weakness, and staggering.

This medicine may cause some people, especially older ones, to become drowsy, dizzy, lightheaded, clumsy or unsteady, or less alert than they are normally. Even if taken at bedtime, it may cause some people to feel drowsy or less alert on arising. **Make sure you know how you react to this medicine before you drive, use machines, or do other jobs that require you to be alert.**

Side Effects of This Medicine

When clonazepam is used for long periods of time in children, it may cause unwanted effects on physical and mental development. These effects may not be noticed until after many years. Before this medicine is given to children for long periods of time, you should discuss the use of it with your doctor.

Along with its needed effects, a medicine may cause some unwanted effects. Although not all of these side effects may occur, if they do occur they may need medical attention.

Check with your doctor as soon as possible if any of the following side effects occur:

Less common or rare

    Behavior problems, including difficulty in concentrating and outbursts of anger, especially in children
    Confusion or mental depression
    Hallucinations (seeing, hearing, or feeling things that are not there)
    Muscle weakness
    Skin rash or itching
    Sore throat and fever
    Trouble in sleeping
    Ulcers or sores in mouth or throat (continuing)
    Uncontrolled movements of body, including the eyes
    Unusual bleeding or bruising
    Unusual excitement, nervousness, or irritability
    Unusual tiredness or weakness (severe)
    Yellow eyes or skin

Signs of overdose

    Confusion (continuing)
    Drowsiness (severe)
    Shakiness
    Slow heartbeat, shortness of breath, or troubled breathing
    Slurred speech (continuing)
    Staggering
    Weakness (severe)

Other side effects may occur that usually do not require medical attention. These side effects may go away during treatment as your body adjusts to the medicine. However, check with your doctor if any of the following side effects continue or are bothersome:

More common

    Clumsiness or unsteadiness
    Dizziness or lightheadedness
    Drowsiness

Less common

    Abdominal or stomach cramps or pain
    Blurred vision or other changes in vision
    Constipation
    Diarrhea
    Dryness of mouth or increase in thirst
    False sense of well-being
    Headache
    Increased bronchial secretions or watering of mouth
    Nausea or vomiting
    Problems with urination
    Slurred speech
    Unusual tiredness or weakness

Although not all of the side effects listed above have been reported for all of these medicines, they have been reported for at least one of them. However, since all of the benzodiazepines are very similar, any of the above side effects may occur with any of these medicines.

For children and elderly patients: Most of the above side effects are more likely to occur in children, especially the very young, and in elderly patients. These patients are usually more sensitive to the effects of benzodiazepines.

After you stop using this medicine, your body may need time to adjust. If you took this medicine in high doses or for a long time, this may take up to 3 weeks. During this period of time check with your doctor if you notice any of the following side effects:

More common

Irritability
Nervousness
Trouble in sleeping

Less common or rare

Abdominal or stomach cramps
Confusion
Convulsions (seizures)
Muscle cramps

Nausea or vomiting
Sweating
Trembling

For patients having diazepam or lorazepam injected:
  • Check with your doctor if any of the following side effects occur: redness, swelling, or pain at the place of injection.

Other side effects not listed above may also occur in some patients. If you notice any other effects, check with your doctor.

December 1987

BENZOYL PEROXIDE (Topical)

Some commonly used brand names are:

Acetoxyl*	Cuticura Acne	PanOxyl
Acne-Aid	Dermoxyl*	PanOxyl AQ
Alquam-X*	Dermoxyl Aqua*	Persa-Gel
Ben-Aqua	Desquam-E	Persa-Gel W
Ben-Aqua Mask	Desquam-X	PHisoAc BP
Benoxyl	Dry and Clear	Propa P.H.
benzac	Fostex	Propa P.H. Porox
benzac w	H₂Oxyl*	Stri-Dex
Benzagel	Loroxide	Topex
Buf-Oxal	Neutrogena Acne	Vanoxide
Clearasil	Mask	Xerac BP
Clearasil BP Plus*	Oxy	Zeroxin
Clear By Design	Oxyderm*	

Generic name product may also be available in the U.S.

*Not available in the U.S.

To the Reader: If you do not recognize the names of medical conditions or medicines referred to in this information, check with your doctor, nurse, or pharmacist. Definitions for selected medical terms may be found in the Glossary. Brand names for the generic drug names listed can be found in the Index. In addition, selected brand names commonly associated with the generic name have been included in the text to help you recognize medicine you may be taking. The fact that a brand name product is not mentioned does not mean the information does not apply. It is a good idea for you to learn both the generic and brand names of your medicines and to write them down for future use.

Benzoyl peroxide (BEN-zoe-ill per-OX-ide) is applied to the skin to treat acne. It may also be used for other conditions as determined by your doctor.

Some of these preparations are available only with your doctor's prescription. Others are available without a prescription; however, your doctor may have special instructions on the proper use of benzoyl peroxide for your medical condition.

Remember:
• **Keep all medicines out of the reach of children.**

• In order for this medicine to work, it must be used as directed. **If you are using this medicine without a prescription, it is very important to follow the directions on the label.**

• **It is also very important that you read and understand the following information.** If any of the information causes you special concern, check with your doctor or pharmacist.

• Before you begin using any new medicine (prescription or nonprescription) or if you develop any new medical problem while you are using this medicine, check with your doctor, nurse, or pharmacist.

• **If you have any questions** about the following information or if you want more information about this medicine or your medical problem, **ask your doctor, nurse, or pharmacist.**

Before Using This Medicine

Before you use benzoyl peroxide, check with your doctor or pharmacist:

—if you have ever had any unusual or allergic reaction to benzoyl peroxide.

—if you are **pregnant** or if you may become pregnant, since benzoyl peroxide may be absorbed through the skin. Studies on birth defects have not been done in either humans or animals.

—if you are **breast-feeding**, since benzoyl peroxide may be absorbed through the skin. It is not known whether benzoyl peroxide passes into the breast milk. However, this medicine has not been shown to cause problems in nursing babies.

—if the skin to be treated is very red or raw.

—if you are taking **any** other prescription or nonprescription (OTC) medicine.

Proper Use of This Medicine

For patients using the cream, gel, lotion, or stick form of benzoyl peroxide:

• Before applying, wash the affected area with nonmedicated soap and water or with a degreasing cleanser and then gently pat dry with a towel.

• Apply enough medicine to cover the affected areas, and rub in gently.

For patients using the cleansing bar, cleansing lotion, or soap form of benzoyl peroxide, use to wash the affected areas as directed.

For patients using the facial mask form of benzoyl peroxide:

• Before applying, wash the affected area with a nonmedicated cleanser. Then rinse and pat dry.

• Using a circular motion, apply a thin layer of the mask evenly over the affected area.

• Allow the mask to dry for 15 to 20 minutes.

• Then rinse thoroughly with warm water and pat dry.

Use benzoyl peroxide only as directed. Do not use more of it and do not use it more often than recommended on the label, unless otherwise directed by your doctor.

Keep this medicine away from the eyes, other mucous membranes such as the mouth, lips, and inside of the nose, and sensitive areas of the neck.

Do not apply benzoyl peroxide to raw or irritated skin.

If you miss a dose of this medicine, apply or use it as soon as possible. Then go back to your regular dosing schedule.

How to store this medicine:
• **Keep out of the reach of children.**
• Store away from heat and direct light.
• Keep the cream, gel, or liquid form of this medicine from freezing.

• Do not keep outdated medicine or medicine no longer needed. Be sure that any discarded medicine is out of the reach of children.

Precautions While Using This Medicine

If your skin problem has not improved within 4 to 6 weeks, check with your doctor.

When using benzoyl peroxide, do not use any of the following preparations on the same affected area as this medicine, unless otherwise directed by your doctor:

> Abrasive soaps or cleansers
> Alcohol-containing preparations
> Any other topical acne preparation or preparation containing a peeling agent (for example, resorcinol, salicylic acid, sulfur, or tretinoin [vitamin A acid])
> Cosmetics or soaps that dry the skin
> Medicated cosmetics
> Other topical medicine for the skin

To use any of the above preparations on the same affected area as benzoyl peroxide may cause severe irritation of the skin.

This medicine may bleach hair or colored fabrics.

Side Effects of This Medicine

Along with its needed effects, a medicine may cause some unwanted effects. Although not all of these side effects may occur, if they do occur they may need medical attention.

Check with your doctor as soon as possible if any of the following side effects occur:

Less common or rare
> Painful irritation of skin, including burning, blistering, crusting, itching, severe redness, or swelling
> Skin rash

Signs of overdose
> Burning, itching, scaling, redness, or swelling of skin (severe)

Other side effects may occur that usually do not require medical attention. These side effects may go away during treatment as your body adjusts to the medicine. However, check with your doctor or pharmacist if any of the following side effects continue or are bothersome:

Less common
> Dryness or peeling of skin (may occur after a few days)
> Feeling of warmth, mild stinging, and redness of skin

For elderly patients: Many medicines have not been tested in older people. Therefore, it is not known whether the medicine acts the same way it does in younger adults. Check with your doctor or pharmacist if you notice any unusual effects while using this medicine or if you think it is not working as it should.

Other side effects not listed above may also occur in some patients. If you notice any other effects, check with your doctor or pharmacist.

December 1987

BETA-ADRENERGIC BLOCKING AGENTS
(Systemic)

This information applies to the following medicines:

Acebutolol (a-se-BYOO-toe-lole)
Atenolol (a-TEN-oh-lole)
Labetalol (la-BET-a-lole)
Metoprolol (me-TOE-proe-lole)
Nadolol (NAY-doe-lole)
Oxprenolol (ox-PREN-oh-lole)
Pindolol (PIN-doe-lole)
Propranolol (proe-PRAN-oh-lole)
Sotalol (SOE-ta-lole)
Timolol (TIM-oh-lole)

Some commonly used brand names are:	Generic names:
Monitan* Sectral	Acebutolol
Tenormin	Atenolol
Normodyne Trandate	Labetalol
Apo-Metoprolol* Betaloc* Betaloc Durules* Lopresor* Lopresor SR* Lopressor Novometoprol*	Metoprolol
Corgard	Nadolol
Slow-Trasicor* Trasicor*	Oxprenolol*
Visken	Pindolol
Apo-Propranolol* Detensol* Inderal Inderal LA Novopranol* pms-Propranolol*	Propranolol†‡
Sotacor*	Sotalol*
Blocadren	Timolol

*Not commercially available in the U.S.
†Generic name product may also be available in the U.S.
‡Generic name product may also be available in Canada.

To the Reader: If you do not recognize the names of medical conditions or medicines referred to in this information, check with your doctor, nurse, or pharmacist. Definitions for selected medical terms may be found in the Glossary. Brand names for the generic drug names listed can be found in the Index. In addition, selected brand names commonly associated with the generic name have been included in the text to help you recognize medicine you may be taking. The fact that a brand name product is not mentioned does not mean the information does not apply. It is a good idea for you to learn both the generic and brand names of your medicines and to write them down for future use.

These medicines belong to a group of medicines known as beta-adrenergic blocking agents, beta-blocking agents, or more commonly, beta-blockers. Beta-blockers are used in the treatment of high blood pressure. Some beta-blockers are also used in the relief of angina (heart pain) and in heart attack patients to help prevent additional heart attacks. Beta-blockers have also been found useful in a number of other conditions such as correcting irregular heartbeats and preventing migraine headaches. They may also be used for other conditions as determined by your doctor.

Beta-blockers work by affecting the response to some nerve impulses in certain parts of the body. As a result, they decrease the need for blood and oxygen by the heart by reducing its workload. They also help the heart to beat more regularly.

Beta-adrenergic blocking agents are available only with your doctor's prescription.

Remember:

• **This medicine has been prescribed for your current medical problem only.** It must not be given to other people or used for other problems unless you are directed to do so by your doctor.

• **Keep all medicines out of the reach of children.**

• In order for this medicine to work, it must be used as directed.

• If you are receiving this medicine by injection, some of the information about this medicine may not apply.

• **It is very important that you read and understand the following information.** If any of the information causes you special concern, do not decide against using this medicine without first checking with your doctor.

• Before you begin using any new medicine (prescription or nonprescription) or if you develop any new medical problem while you are using this medicine, check with your doctor, nurse, or pharmacist.

• **If you have any questions** about the following information or if you want more information about this medicine or your medical problem, **ask your doctor, nurse, or pharmacist**.

Before Using This Medicine

In order to decide on the best treatment for your medical problem, your doctor should be told:

—if you have ever had any unusual or allergic reaction to beta-blocker medicine.

—if you are on a low-salt, low-sugar, or any other special diet, or if you are allergic to any substance, such as foods, sulfites or other preservatives, or dyes. Most medicines contain more than their active ingredient. Your doctor, nurse, or pharmacist can help you avoid products that may cause a problem.

—if you are **pregnant** or if you may become pregnant. Adequate studies have not been done in humans. However, use of some beta-blockers during pregnancy has been associated with breathing problems and a lower heart rate in the newborn infant. Some reports have shown no unwanted effects on the newborn infant. Animal studies have shown some beta-blockers to cause problems in pregnancy when used in doses many times the usual human dose.

—if you are **breast-feeding**. Although beta-blockers pass into the breast milk, these medicines have not been shown to cause problems in nursing babies.

—if you have any of the following medical problems:
Allergy, history of (asthma, eczema, hay fever, hives)
Bradycardia (unusually slow heartbeat)
Bronchitis
Diabetes mellitus (sugar diabetes)
Emphysema
Heart or blood vessel disease
Kidney disease
Liver disease
Mental depression (or history of)
Myasthenia gravis (a muscle disease)
Overactive thyroid
Pheochromocytoma (for labetalol only)
Psoriasis

—if you are now taking/using **any** prescription or non-prescription (OTC) medicine, especially:
Aminophylline (e.g., Somophyllin)
Antidiabetic agents, oral (diabetes medicine you take by mouth)
Caffeine (e.g., NoDoz)
Clonidine (e.g., Catapres)
Diltiazem (e.g., Cardizem)
Dyphylline (e.g., Lufyllin)
Insulin
Nifedipine (e.g., Procardia)
Oxtriphylline (e.g., Choledyl)
Theophylline (e.g., Somophyllin-T)
Verapamil (e.g., Calan)

—if you are now taking or have taken within the past 2 weeks monoamine oxidase (MAO) inhibitors such as:
Furazolidone (e.g., Furoxone)
Isocarboxazid (e.g., Marplan)
Pargyline (e.g., Eutonyl)
Phenelzine (e.g., Nardil)
Procarbazine (e.g., Matulane)
Tranylcypromine (e.g., Parnate)

—if you smoke.

Proper Use of This Medicine

For patients taking the extended-release capsule or tablet form of this medicine:

• Swallow the capsule or tablet whole.

• Do not crush, break, or chew before swallowing.

Ask your doctor about checking your pulse rate before and after taking beta-blocking agents. Then, while you are taking this medicine, check your pulse regularly. If it is much slower than your usual rate (or less than 50 beats per minute), check with your doctor. A pulse rate that is too slow may cause circulation problems.

In order to help remember to take your medicine, try to get into the habit of taking it at the same time each day.

For patients taking this medicine for high blood pressure:
• Importance of diet—When prescribing medicine for your condition, your doctor may also prescribe a personal diet for you. Such a diet may be low in sodium

(salt). Most people eat much more sodium than they need. Too much sodium in the diet may increase blood pressure. Some foods that contain large amounts of sodium are canned soup, pickles, ketchup, green and ripe olives, relish, frankfurters, soy sauce, and carbonated beverages. Your doctor may want you to limit the amounts of these and other high-sodium foods in your diet. High blood pressure medicine is usually more effective when such a diet is properly followed.

Also, it may be very important for you to go on a reducing diet. However, check with your doctor before changing your diet.

• Many patients who have high blood pressure will not notice any signs of the problem. In fact, many may feel normal. It is very important that you **take your medicine exactly as directed**. Also, keep your appointments with your doctor even if you feel well.

• Remember that this medicine will not cure your high blood pressure but it does control it. Therefore, you must continue to take it as directed if you expect to lower your blood pressure and keep it down. **You may have to take high blood pressure medicine for the rest of your life.** If high blood pressure is not treated, it can cause serious problems such as heart failure, blood vessel disease, stroke, or kidney disease.

Do not miss any doses. This is especially important when you are taking only one dose per day. Some conditions may become worse when this medicine is not taken regularly.

If you do miss a dose of this medicine, take it as soon as possible. However, if it is within 4 hours of your next dose (8 hours when using atenolol, labetalol, nadolol, sotalol, or extended-release oxprenolol or propranolol), skip the missed dose and go back to your regular dosing schedule. Do not double doses.

How to store this medicine:

• **Keep out of the reach of children.**

• Store away from heat and direct light.

• Do not store in the bathroom, near the kitchen sink, or in other damp places. Heat or moisture may cause the medicine to break down.

• Do not keep outdated medicine or medicine no longer needed. Be sure that any discarded medicine is out of the reach of children.

Precautions While Using This Medicine

It is important that your doctor check your progress at regular visits. This is to make sure the medicine is working for you and to allow the dosage to be changed if needed.

Do not stop taking this medicine without first checking with your doctor. Your doctor may want you to reduce gradually the amount you are taking before stopping completely. Some conditions may become worse when the medicine is stopped suddenly, and danger of heart attack is increased in some patients.

Make sure that you have enough medicine on hand to last through weekends, holidays, or vacations. You may want to carry an extra written prescription in your billfold or purse in case of an emergency. You can then have it filled if you run out of medicine while you are away from home.

Your doctor may want you to carry a medical identification card stating that you are taking this medicine.

Before having any kind of surgery (including dental surgery) or emergency treatment, tell the physician or dentist in charge that you are taking this medicine.

Diabetics—**This medicine may cause your blood sugar levels to fall.** Also, **this medicine may cover up signs of hypoglycemia (low blood sugar),** such as change in pulse rate.

This medicine may cause some people to become dizzy, drowsy, lightheaded, or less alert than they are normally. **Make sure you know how you react to this medicine before you drive, use machines, or do other jobs that require you to be alert.** If the problem continues or gets worse, check with your doctor.

Beta-blockers may make you more sensitive to cold temperatures. They tend to decrease blood circulation in the skin, fingers, and toes. Dress warmly during cold weather and be careful during prolonged exposure to cold, such as in winter sports.

Chest pain resulting from exercise or physical exertion is usually reduced or prevented by this medicine. This may tempt a patient to be overly active. **Make sure you discuss with your doctor a safe amount of exercise for your medical problem.**

For patients taking this medicine for high blood pressure:
- **Do not take other medicines unless they have been discussed with your doctor.** This especially includes over-the-counter (nonprescription) medicines for appetite control, asthma, colds, cough, hay fever, or sinus problems since they may tend to increase your blood pressure.

For patients taking labetalol by mouth:
- **Dizziness, lightheadedness, or fainting may occur, especially when you get up from a lying or sitting position.** This is more likely to occur when you first start taking labetalol or when the dose is increased. **Getting up slowly may help.** When you get up from lying down, sit on the edge of the bed with your feet dangling for 1 to 2 minutes. Then stand up slowly. If the problem continues or gets worse, check with your doctor.

- The dizziness, lightheadedness, or fainting is also more likely to occur if you drink alcohol, stand for long periods of time, exercise, or if the weather is hot. **While you are taking this medicine, be careful in the amount of alcohol you drink. Also, use extra care during exercise or hot weather or if you must stand for long periods of time.**

For patients receiving labetalol by injection:
- It is very important that you lie down flat while receiving labetalol and for up to 3 hours afterward. If you try to get up too soon, you may become dizzy or faint. **Do not try to sit or stand until your doctor tells you to do so.**

Side Effects of This Medicine

Along with its needed effects, a medicine may cause some unwanted effects. Although not all of these side effects may occur, if they do occur they may need medical attention.

Check with your doctor as soon as possible if any of the following side effects occur:
Less common
   Breathing difficulty and/or wheezing
   Cold hands and feet
   Confusion (especially in elderly)
   Hallucinations (seeing, hearing, or feeling things that are not there)
   Irregular heartbeat
   Mental depression
   Nightmares and vivid dreams
   Skin rash
   Slow heartbeat (especially less than 50 beats per minute)—more common with nadolol, propranolol, and sotalol; rare with labetalol and pindolol
   Swelling of ankles, feet, and/or lower legs
Rare
   Back pain or joint pain—more common with pindolol
   Chest pain
   Fever and sore throat
   Red, scaling, or crusted skin
   Unusual bleeding and bruising
Signs of overdose (in the order in which they may occur)
   Slow heartbeat
   Dizziness (severe) or fainting
   Fast or irregular heartbeat
   Difficulty in breathing
   Bluish-colored fingernails or palms of hands
   Convulsions (seizures)

Other side effects may occur that usually do not require medical attention. These side effects may go away during treatment as your body adjusts to the medicine. However, check with your doctor if any of the following side effects continue or are bothersome:
More common
   Decreased sexual ability
   Dizziness or lightheadedness
   Drowsiness (slight)
   Trouble in sleeping
   Unusual tiredness or weakness
Less common or rare
   Anxiety and/or nervousness
   Changes in taste—for labetalol only
   Constipation
   Diarrhea
   Dry, sore eyes
   Frequent urination—for acebutolol only
   Headache
   Itching of skin
   Nausea or vomiting

Numbness and/or tingling of fingers and/or toes
Numbness and/or tingling of skin, especially on scalp—
    for labetalol only
Stomach discomfort
Stuffy nose

Although not all of the side effects listed above have been reported for all of these medicines, they have been reported for at least one of them. Since all of the beta-adrenergic blocking agents are very similar, any of the above side effects may occur with any of these medicines. However, they may be more or less common with some agents than with others.

After you have been taking a beta-blocker for a while, it may cause unpleasant or even harmful effects if you stop taking it too suddenly. After you stop taking this medicine or while you are gradually reducing the amount you are taking, check with your doctor right away if any of the following occur:

Chest pain
Fast or irregular heartbeat
General feeling of body discomfort or weakness

Headache
Shortness of breath (sudden)
Sweating
Trembling

For elderly patients: Some of the above side effects are more likely to occur in the elderly, who are usually more sensitive to the effects of beta-blockers.

You may notice a tingling feeling on your scalp when you first begin to take labetalol. This is to be expected and usually goes away after you have been taking labetalol for a while.

Other side effects not listed above may also occur in some patients. If you notice any other effects, check with your doctor.

December 1987

BETA-ADRENERGIC BLOCKING AGENTS AND THIAZIDE DIURETICS
(Systemic)

This information applies to the following medicines:

Atenolol (a-TEN-oh-lole) and Chlorthalidone (klor-THAL-i-doan)
Labetalol (la-BET-a-lole) and Hydrochlorothiazide (hye-droe-klor-oh-THYE-a-zide)
Metoprolol (me-TOE-proe-lole) and Hydrochlorothiazide
Nadolol (NAY-doe-lole) and Bendroflumethiazide (ben-droe-floo-meth-EYE-a-zide)
Pindolol (PIN-doe-lole) and Hydrochlorothiazide
Propranolol (proe-PRAN-oh-lole) and Hydrochlorothiazide
Timolol (TIM-oh-lole) and Hydrochlorothiazide

Some commonly used brand names are:	Generic names:
Tenoretic	Atenolol and Chlorthalidone
Normozide Trandate HCT	Labetalol and Hydrochlorothiazide
Co-Betaloc* Lopressor HCT	Metoprolol and Hydrochlorothiazide
Corzide	Nadolol and Bendroflumethiazide
Viskazide	Pindolol and Hydrochlorothiazide
Inderide Inderide LA	Propranolol and Hydrochlorothiazide†
Timolide	Timolol and Hydrochlorothiazide

*Not available in the U.S.
†Generic name product may also be available in the U.S.

To the Reader: If you do not recognize the names of medical conditions or medicines referred to in this information, check with your doctor, nurse, or pharmacist. Definitions for selected medical terms may be found in the Glossary. Brand names for the generic drug names listed can be found in the Index. In addition, selected brand names commonly associated with the generic name have been included in the text to help you recognize medicine you may be taking. The fact that a brand name product is not mentioned does not mean the information does not apply. It is a good idea for you to learn both the generic and brand names of your medicines and to write them down for future use.

Beta-blocker and thiazide diuretic combinations belong to the group of medicines known as antihypertensives (blood pressure medicine). Both ingredients of the combination control high blood pressure, but work in different ways. Beta-blockers (atenolol, metoprolol, nadolol, pindolol, propranolol, and timolol) reduce the workload on the heart as well as having other effects. Thiazide diuretics (bendroflumethiazide, chlorthalidone, and hydrochlorothiazide) reduce the amount of fluid pressure in the body by increasing the flow of urine.

High blood pressure adds to the workload of the heart and arteries. If it continues for a long time, the heart and arteries may not function properly. This can damage the blood vessels of the brain, heart, and kidneys resulting in a stroke, heart failure, or kidney failure. High blood pressure may also increase the risk of heart attacks. These problems may be less likely to occur if blood pressure is controlled.

Beta-blocker and thiazide diuretic combinations are available only with your doctor's prescription.

Remember:
• **This medicine has been prescribed for your current medical problem only.** It must not be given to other people or used for other problems unless you are directed to do so by your doctor.

• **Keep all medicines out of the reach of children.**

• In order for this medicine to work, it must be used as directed.

• **It is very important that you read and understand the following information.** If any of the information causes you special concern, do not decide against using this medicine without first checking with your doctor.

• Before you begin using any new medicine (prescription or nonprescription) or if you develop any new medical problem while you are using this medicine, check with your doctor, nurse, or pharmacist.

• **If you have any questions** about the following information or if you want more information about this medicine or your medical problem, **ask your doctor, nurse, or pharmacist**.

Before Using This Medicine

In order to decide on the best treatment for your medical problem, your doctor should be told:

—if you have ever had any unusual or allergic reaction to beta-blockers, sulfonamides (sulfa drugs), bumetanide, furosemide, acetazolamide, dichlorphenamide, methazolamide or to any of the thiazide diuretics.

—if you are on a low-salt, low-sugar, or any other special diet, or if you are allergic to any substance, such as foods, sulfites or other preservatives, or dyes. Most medicines contain more than their active ingredient. Your doctor, nurse, or pharmacist can help you avoid products that may cause a problem.

—if you are **pregnant** or if you may become pregnant. Although adequate studies in humans have not been done, use of some beta-blockers during pregnancy has been associated with breathing problems and a slower heart rate in the newborn infant. However, other reports have shown no unwanted effects in the newborn infant. Animal studies have shown some beta-blockers to cause problems in pregnancy when used in doses many times the usual human dose.

Studies with thiazide diuretics have not been done in humans. However, use during pregnancy may cause side effects such as jaundice, blood problems, and low potassium in the newborn infant. Animal studies have not shown thiazide diuretic medicines to cause birth defects even when used in doses several times the usual human dose.

—if you are **breast-feeding**. Although beta-blockers and thiazide diuretics pass into the breast milk, these medicines have not been shown to cause problems in nursing babies.

—if you have any of the following medical problems:

Allergy, history of (asthma, eczema, hay fever, hives)
Bradycardia (unusually slow heartbeat)
Bronchitis
Diabetes mellitus (sugar diabetes)
Emphysema
Gout (history of)
Heart or blood vessel disease
Kidney disease
Liver disease
Lupus erythematosus (history of)
Mental depression (or history of)
Myasthenia gravis (a muscle disease)
Overactive thyroid
Pancreatitis (inflammation of the pancreas)
Psoriasis

—if you are taking **any** other prescription or nonprescription (OTC) medicine, especially:

Adrenocorticoids (cortisone-like medicines)
Aminophylline (e.g., Somophyllin)
Antidiabetic agents, oral (diabetes medicine you take by mouth)
Caffeine
Clonidine (e.g., Catapres)
Digitalis glycosides (heart medicine)
Diltiazem (e.g., Cardizem)
Dyphylline (e.g., Lufylline)
Insulin
Lithium (e.g., Lithane)
Methenamine (e.g., Mandelamine)
Nifedipine (e.g., Procardia)
Oxtriphylline (e.g., Choledyl)
Theophylline (e.g., Somophyllin-T)
Verapamil (e.g., Calan)

—if you are now taking or have taken within the past 2 weeks monoamine oxidase (MAO) inhibitors such as:

Furazolidone (e.g., Furoxone)
Isocarboxazid (e.g., Marplan)
Pargyline (e.g., Eutonyl)
Phenelzine (e.g., Nardil)
Procarbazine (e.g., Matulane)
Tranylcypromine (e.g., Parnate)

—if you smoke.

Proper Use of This Medicine

Importance of diet—When prescribing medicine for your condition, your doctor may also prescribe a personal diet for you. Such a diet may be low in sodium (salt). Most people eat much more sodium than they need. Too much sodium in the diet may increase blood pressure. Some foods that contain large amounts of sodium are canned soup, pickles, ketchup, green and ripe olives, relish, frankfurters, soy sauce, and carbonated beverages. Your doctor may want you to limit the amounts of these and other high-sodium foods in your diet. High blood pressure medicine is usually more effective when such a diet is properly followed.

Also, it may be very important for you to go on a reducing diet. However, check with your doctor before changing your diet.

Many patients who have high blood pressure will not notice any signs of the problem. In fact, many may feel normal. It is very important that you **take your medicine exactly as directed**. Also, keep your appointments with your doctor even if you feel well.

Remember that this medicine will not cure your high blood pressure but it does help control it. Therefore, you must continue to take it as directed if you expect to lower your blood pressure and keep it down. **You may have to take high blood pressure medicine for the rest of your life.** If high blood pressure is not treated, it can cause serious problems such as heart failure, blood vessel disease, stroke, or kidney disease.

For patients taking the extended-release tablet form of this medicine:

• Swallow the tablet whole.

• Do not crush, break, or chew before swallowing.

In order to help you remember to take your medicine, try to get into the habit of taking it at the same time each day.

Ask your doctor about checking your pulse rate before and after taking beta-blocking agents. Then, while you are taking this medicine, check your pulse regularly. If it is much slower than your usual rate (or less than 50 beats per minute), check with your doctor. A pulse rate that is too slow may cause circulation problems.

The thiazide diuretic (e.g., bendroflumethiazide, chlorthalidone, or hydrochlorothiazide) contained in this combination medicine may cause you to have an unusual feeling of tiredness when you begin to take it. You may also notice an increase in the amount of urine or in your frequency of urination. After taking the medicine for a while, these effects should lessen. In order to keep the increase in urine from affecting your nighttime sleep:

• If you are to take a single dose a day, take it in the morning after breakfast.

• If you are to take more than one dose a day, take the last dose no later than 6 p.m., unless otherwise directed by your doctor.

However, it is best to plan your dose or doses according to a schedule that will least affect your personal activities and sleep. Ask your doctor, nurse, or pharmacist to help you plan the best time to take this medicine.

Do not miss any doses. This is especially important when you are taking only one dose per day. Some conditions may become worse when this medicine is not taken regularly.

If you do miss a dose of this medicine, take it as soon as possible. However, if it is within 4 hours of your next dose (8 hours for atenolol and chlorthalidone, labetalol and hydrochlorothiazide, nadolol and bendroflumethiazide, or extended-release propranolol and hydrochlorothiazide), skip the missed dose and go back to your regular dosing schedule. Do not double doses.

How to store this medicine:

• **Keep out of the reach of children.**

• Store away from heat and direct light.

• Do not store in the bathroom, near the kitchen sink, or in other damp places. Heat or moisture may cause the medicine to break down.

• Do not keep outdated medicine or medicine no longer needed. Be sure that any discarded medicine is out of the reach of children.

Precautions While Using This Medicine

It is important that your doctor check your progress at regular visits. This is to make sure the medicine is properly controlling your blood pressure and to allow the dosage to be changed if needed.

Do not stop taking this medicine without first checking with your doctor. Your doctor may want you to reduce gradually the amount you are taking before stopping completely. Some conditions may become worse when the medicine is stopped suddenly, and the risk of heart attack is increased in some patients.

Make sure that you have enough medicine on hand to last through weekends, holidays, or vacations. You may want to carry an extra written prescription in your billfold or purse in case of an emergency. You can then have it filled if you run out of medicine while you are away from home.

Your doctor may want you to carry a medical identification card stating that you are taking this medicine.

Do not take other medicines unless they have been discussed with your doctor. This especially includes over-the-counter (nonprescription) medicines for appetite control, asthma, colds, cough, hay fever, or sinus problems since they may tend to increase your blood pressure.

Before having any kind of surgery (including dental surgery) or emergency treatment, tell the physician or dentist in charge that you are taking this medicine.

Diabetics—**This medicine may cause your blood sugar levels to rise or to fall.** Also, **this medicine may cover up signs of hypoglycemia (low blood sugar),** such as change in pulse rate. While you are taking this medicine, be especially careful in testing for sugar in your urine. If you have any questions about this, check with your doctor.

The thiazide diuretic contained in this medicine may cause a loss of potassium from your body.

• To help prevent this, your doctor may want you to:
  —eat or drink foods that have a high potassium content (for example, orange or other citrus fruit juices), or
  —take a potassium supplement, or
  —take another medicine to help prevent the loss of the potassium in the first place.

• It is very important to follow these directions. Also, it is important not to change your diet on your own. This is more important if you are already on a special diet (as for diabetes), or if you are taking a potassium supplement or a medicine to reduce potassium loss. Extra potassium may not be necessary and, in some cases, too much potassium could be harmful.

Check with your doctor if you become sick and have severe or continuing vomiting or diarrhea. These problems may cause you to lose additional water and potassium.

This medicine may cause some people to become dizzy, drowsy, lightheaded, or less alert than they are normally. **Make sure you know how you react to this medicine before you drive, use machines, or do other jobs that require you to be alert.** If the problem continues or gets worse, check with your doctor.

The beta-blocker (atenolol, metoprolol, nadolol, pindolol, propranolol, or timolol) contained in this medicine may make you more sensitive to cold temperatures. It tends to decrease blood circulation in the skin, fingers, and toes. Dress warmly during cold weather and be careful during prolonged exposure to cold, such as in winter sports.

Some people who take this medicine may become more sensitive to sunlight than they are normally. When you begin taking this medicine, avoid too much sun and do not use a sunlamp until you see how you react to the sun, especially if you tend to burn easily. If you have a severe reaction, check with your doctor.

Side Effects of This Medicine

Along with its needed effects, a medicine may cause some unwanted effects. Although not all of these side effects may occur, if they do occur they may need medical attention.

Check with your doctor as soon as possible if any of the following side effects occur:

Less common
  Breathing difficulty and/or wheezing
  Cold hands and feet
  Confusion, especially in elderly
  Hallucinations (seeing, hearing, or feeling things that are not there)
  Irregular heartbeat
  Mental depression
  Slow pulse (especially less than 50 beats per minute)

Rare
  Chest pain
  Fever and sore throat
  Joint, side, or stomach pain

© 1988   The United States Pharmacopeial Convention, Inc.   *All rights reserved*

Red, scaling, or crusted skin
Skin rash or hives
Stomach pain (severe) with nausea and vomiting
Unusual bleeding or bruising
Yellow eyes or skin

Signs of too much potassium loss
Dryness of mouth
Increased thirst
Irregular heartbeats
Mood or mental changes
Muscle cramps or pain
Weak pulse

Signs of overdose (in the order in which they may occur)
Slow heartbeat
Dizziness (severe) or fainting
Difficulty in breathing
Bluish-colored fingernails or palms of hands
Convulsions (seizures)

Other side effects may occur that usually do not require medical attention. These side effects may go away during treatment as your body adjusts to the medicine. However, check with your doctor if any of the following side effects continue or are bothersome:

More common
Decreased sexual ability
Dizziness or lightheadedness
Drowsiness (slight)
Trouble in sleeping
Unusual tiredness or weakness

Less common
Anxiety or nervousness
Constipation
Diarrhea
Dry, sore eyes
Headache
Increased sensitivity of skin to sunlight
Itching of skin
Loss of appetite
Nausea or vomiting
Nightmares and vivid dreams

Numbness or tingling of fingers and toes
Stomach discomfort or upset
Stuffy nose

Although not all of the above side effects have been reported for all of these medicines, they have been reported for at least one of the beta-adrenergic blockers or thiazide diuretics. Since all of the beta-adrenergic blocking agents are very similar and the thiazide diuretics are also very similar, any of the above side effects may occur with any of these medicines. However, they may be more common with some combinations than with others.

After you have been taking this medicine for a while, it may cause unpleasant or even harmful effects if you stop taking it too suddenly. After you stop taking this medicine or while you are gradually reducing the amount you are taking, check with your doctor right away if any of the following occur:

Chest pain
Fast or irregular heartbeat
General feeling of body discomfort or weakness
Headache
Shortness of breath (sudden)
Sweating
Trembling

For elderly patients: Some of the above side effects, especially dizziness or lightheadedness and signs of too much potassium loss, may be more likely to occur in the elderly, who are usually more sensitive to the effects of this medicine.

Other side effects not listed above may also occur in some patients. If you notice any other effects, check with your doctor.

_____

December 1987

BETAXOLOL (Ophthalmic)

A commonly used brand name is Betoptic.

To the Reader: If you do not recognize the names of medical conditions or medicines referred to in this information, check with your doctor, nurse, or pharmacist. Definitions for selected medical terms may be found in the Glossary. Brand names for the generic drug names listed can be found in the Index. In addition, selected brand names commonly associated with the generic name have been included in the text to help you recognize medicine you may be taking. The fact that a brand name product is not mentioned does not mean the information does not apply. It is a good idea for you to learn both the generic and brand names of your medicines and to write them down for future use.

Betaxolol (be-TAX-oh-lol) is used in the eye to treat certain types of glaucoma. It appears to work by reducing the production of fluid in the eye to lower pressure in the eye.

This medicine is available only with your doctor's prescription.

Remember:

• **This medicine has been prescribed for your current medical problem only.** It must not be given to other people or used for other problems unless you are directed to do so by your doctor.

• **Keep all medicines out of the reach of children.**

• In order for this medicine to work, it must be used as directed.

• **It is very important that you read and understand the following information.** If any of the information causes you special concern, do not decide against using this medicine without first checking with your doctor.

• Before you begin using any new medicine (prescription or nonprescription) or if you develop any new medical problem while you are using this medicine, check with your doctor, nurse, or pharmacist.

• **If you have any questions** about the following information or if you want more information about this medicine or your medical problem, **ask your doctor, nurse, or pharmacist.**

Before Using This Medicine

In order to decide on the best treatment for your medical problem, your doctor should be told:

—if you have ever had any unusual or allergic reaction to betaxolol or other beta blockers (such as acebutolol, atenolol, labetalol, levobunolol, metoprolol, nadolol, oxprenolol, pindolol, propranolol, sotalol, or timolol).

—if you are allergic to any substance, such as preservatives. Most medicines contain more than their active ingredient. Your doctor, nurse, or pharmacist can help you avoid products that may cause a problem.

—if you are **pregnant** or if you may become pregnant, since ophthalmic betaxolol may be absorbed into the body. Studies on birth defects have not been done in humans. However, studies in animals have not shown that betaxolol causes birth defects.

—if you are **breast-feeding**, since ophthalmic betaxolol may be absorbed into the body. It is not known whether ophthalmic betaxolol passes into the breast milk. This medicine has not been shown to cause problems in nursing babies.

—if you have any of the following medical problems:
  Diabetes mellitus (sugar diabetes)
  Heart disease
  Lung disease
  Overactive thyroid

—if you are taking **any** other prescription or nonprescription (OTC) medicine.

Proper Use of This Medicine

How to apply betaxolol eye drops: First, wash your hands. With the middle finger, apply pressure to the inside corner of the eye (and continue to apply pressure for 1 or 2 minutes after the medicine has been placed in the eye). Tilt the head back and with the index finger of the same hand, pull the lower eyelid away from the eye to form a pouch. Drop the medicine into the pouch and gently close the eyes. Do not blink. Keep the eyes closed for 1 or 2 minutes to allow the medicine to be absorbed.

To prevent contamination of the eye drops, do not touch the applicator tip to any surface (including the eye) and keep the container tightly closed.

Use this medicine only as directed. Do not use more of it and do not use it more often than your doctor ordered. To do so may increase the chance of too much medicine being absorbed into the body and the chance of side effects.

If you miss a dose of this medicine, apply it as soon as possible. However, if it is almost time for your next dose, skip the missed dose and apply your next dose at the regularly scheduled time. Then continue with your regular dosing schedule.

How to store this medicine:

• **Keep out of the reach of children.**

• Store away from heat and direct light.

• Keep this medicine from freezing.

• Do not keep outdated medicine or medicine no longer needed. Be sure that any discarded medicine is out of the reach of children.

Precautions While Using This Medicine

Your doctor should check your eye pressure at regular visits in order to make certain that your glaucoma is being controlled.

Before having any kind of surgery (including dental surgery) or emergency treatment, tell the physician or dentist in charge that you are using this medicine.

Diabetics—**This medicine may cover up some signs of hypoglycemia (low blood sugar),** such as increase in pulse rate or trembling. However, other signs of low

---

© 1988   The United States Pharmacopeial Convention, Inc.

blood sugar, such as sweating, are not affected. If you have any questions about this, check with your doctor.

This medicine may cause your eyes to become more sensitive to light than they are normally. Wearing sunglasses and avoiding too much exposure to bright light may help lessen the discomfort.

Side Effects of This Medicine

Along with its needed effects, a medicine may cause some unwanted effects. Although not all of these side effects may occur, if they do occur they may need medical attention.

Check with your doctor as soon as possible if any of the following side effects occur:

Rare

Eye irritation or inflammation (severe)

Signs of too much medicine being absorbed into the body

Confusion or mental depression
Slow heartbeat
Trouble in sleeping
Unusual tiredness or weakness
Wheezing or troubled breathing

Other side effects may occur that usually do not require medical attention. These side effects may go away during treatment as your body adjusts to the medicine. However, check with your doctor if any of the following side effects continue or are bothersome:

More common

Stinging of eye

Less common or rare

Increased sensitivity of eye to light
Redness, itching, or unusual watering of eye

For elderly patients: Many medicines have not been tested in older people. Therefore, it is not known whether the medicine acts the same way it does in younger adults. Check with your doctor or pharmacist if you notice any unusual effects while using this medicine or if you think it is not working as it should.

Other side effects not listed above may also occur in some patients. If you notice any other effects, check with your doctor.

_____

December 1987

BETHANECHOL (Systemic)

Some commonly used brand names are Duvoid, Myotonachol, and Urecholine.

Generic name product may also be available in the U.S.

To the Reader: If you do not recognize the names of medical conditions or medicines referred to in this information, check with your doctor, nurse, or pharmacist. Definitions for selected medical terms may be found in the Glossary. Brand names for the generic drug names listed can be found in the Index. In addition, selected brand names commonly associated with the generic name have been included in the text to help you recognize medicine you may be taking. The fact that a brand name product is not mentioned does not mean the information does not apply. It is a good idea for you to learn both the generic and brand names of your medicines and to write them down for future use.

Bethanechol (be-THAN-e-kole) is taken by mouth or given by injection to treat certain disorders of the urinary tract or bladder. It helps to cause urination and emptying of the bladder. Bethanechol may also be used for other conditions as determined by your doctor.

Bethanechol is available only with your doctor's prescription.

Remember:

• **This medicine has been prescribed for your current medical problem only.** It must not be given to other people or used for other problems unless you are directed to do so by your doctor.

• **Keep all medicines out of the reach of children.**

• In order for this medicine to work, it must be used as directed.

• If you are receiving this medicine by injection, some of the information about this medicine may not apply.

• **It is very important that you read and understand the following information.** If any of the information causes you special concern, do not decide against using this medicine without first checking with your doctor.

• Before you begin using any new medicine (prescription or nonprescription) or if you develop any new medical problem while you are using this medicine, check with your doctor, nurse, or pharmacist.

• **If you have any questions** about the following information or if you want more information about this medicine or your medical problem, **ask your doctor, nurse, or pharmacist.**

Before Using This Medicine

In order to decide on the best treatment for your medical problem, your doctor should be told:

—if you have ever had any unusual or allergic reaction to bethanechol.

—if you are on a low-salt, low-sugar, or any other special diet, or if you are allergic to any substance, such as foods, sulfites or other preservatives, or dyes. Most medicines contain more than their active ingredient. Your doctor, nurse, or pharmacist can help you avoid products that may cause a problem.

—if you are **pregnant** or if you may become pregnant while taking this medicine. Studies have not been done in humans. However, some studies in animals have shown bethanechol to cause contractions of the uterus.

—if you are **breast-feeding**. It is not known whether bethanechol passes into the breast milk. However, this medicine has not been shown to cause problems in nursing babies.

—if you have any of the following medical problems:
Asthma
Epilepsy
Heart or blood vessel disease
High or low blood pressure
Intestinal blockage or other intestinal problems
Overactive thyroid
Parkinson's disease
Recent bladder or intestinal surgery
Stomach ulcer or other stomach problems
Urinary tract blockage or difficult urination

—if you are using **any** other prescription or nonprescription (OTC) medicine.

Proper Use of This Medicine

Take this medicine on an empty stomach (either 1 hour before or 2 hours after meals) to lessen the possibility of nausea and vomiting, unless otherwise directed by your doctor.

Take this medicine only as directed. Do not take more of it, do not take it more often, and do not take it for a longer period of time than your doctor ordered. To do so may increase the chance of side effects.

If you miss a dose of this medicine and you remember within an hour or so of the missed dose, take it right away. However, if you do not remember until 2 or more hours after, skip the missed dose and go back to your regular dosing schedule. Do not double doses.

How to store this medicine:

• **Keep out of the reach of children.**

• Store away from heat and direct light.

• Do not store the tablet form of this medicine in the bathroom, near the kitchen sink, or in other damp places. Heat or moisture may cause the medicine to break down.

• Do not keep outdated medicine or medicine no longer needed. Be sure that any discarded medicine is out of the reach of children.

Precautions While Using This Medicine

Dizziness, lightheadedness, or fainting may occur, especially when you get up from a lying or sitting position. Getting up slowly may help lessen this problem.

Side Effects of This Medicine

Along with its needed effects, a medicine may cause some unwanted effects. Although not all of these side effects may occur, if they do occur they may need medical attention.

© 1988   The United States Pharmacopeial Convention, Inc.

Check with your doctor as soon as possible if any of the following side effects occur:

Rare—more common with the injection

Shortness of breath, wheezing, or tightness in chest

Other side effects may occur that usually do not require medical attention. These side effects may go away during treatment as your body adjusts to the medicine. However, check with your doctor if any of the following side effects continue or are bothersome:

Less common or rare—more common with the injection

Belching
Blurred vision or change in near or distant vision
Diarrhea
Dizziness or lightheadedness
Feeling faint
Frequent urge to urinate

Headache
Nausea or vomiting
Redness or flushing of skin or feeling of warmth
Stomach discomfort or pain
Unusual increase in salivation or sweating

For elderly patients: Many medicines have not been tested in older people. Therefore, it is not known whether the medicine acts the same way it does in younger adults. Check with your doctor or pharmacist if you notice any unusual effects while taking this medicine or if you think it is not working as it should.

Other side effects not listed above may also occur in some patients. If you notice any other effects, check with your doctor.

December 1987

BLEOMYCIN (Systemic)

A commonly used brand name is Blenoxane.

To the Reader: If you do not recognize the names of medical conditions or medicines referred to in this information, check with your doctor, nurse, or pharmacist. Definitions for selected medical terms may be found in the Glossary. Brand names for the generic drug names listed can be found in the Index. In addition, selected brand names commonly associated with the generic name have been included in the text to help you recognize medicine you may be taking. The fact that a brand name product is not mentioned does not mean the information does not apply. It is a good idea for you to learn both the generic and brand names of your medicines and to write them down for future use.

Bleomycin (blee-oh-MYE-sin) belongs to the general group of medicines called antineoplastics. It is given by injection to treat some kinds of cancer.

Bleomycin seems to act by interfering with the growth of cancer cells, which are eventually destroyed. Since the growth of normal body cells may also be affected by bleomycin, other effects will also occur. Some of these may be serious and must be reported to your doctor. Other effects, like darkening of skin or hair loss, may not be serious but may cause concern. Some effects may not occur for months or years after the medicine is used.

This medicine may also be used for other conditions, as determined by your doctor.

Before you begin treatment with bleomycin, you and your doctor should talk about the good this medicine will do as well as the risks of using it.

Bleomycin is to be administered only by or under the immediate supervision of your doctor.

Remember:

• **It is very important that you read and understand the following information.** If any of the information causes you special concern, do not decide against using this medicine without first checking with your doctor.

• Before you begin using any new medicine (prescription or nonprescription) or if you develop any new medical problem while you are receiving this medicine, check with your doctor, nurse, or pharmacist.

• **If you have any questions** about the following information or if you want more information about this medicine or your medical problem, **ask your doctor, nurse, or pharmacist**.

Before Using This Medicine

In order to decide on the best treatment for your medical problem, your doctor should be told:

—if you have ever had any unusual or allergic reaction to bleomycin.

—if you are **pregnant** or if you intend to have children. Studies have not been done in humans. However, there is a chance that this medicine may cause birth defects if either the male or female is receiving it at the time of conception or if it is used during pregnancy. Studies in mice given large doses of bleomycin have shown that it causes birth defects. In addition, many cancer medicines may cause sterility which could be permanent. Although this has not been reported with this medicine, the possibility should be kept in mind. Be sure that you have discussed this with your doctor before receiving this medicine.

—if you intend to **breast-feed**. Because this medicine may cause serious side effects, breast-feeding is generally not recommended while you are receiving it.

—if you have any of the following medical problems:
  Kidney disease
  Liver disease
  Lung disease

—if you have ever been treated with x-rays or cancer medicines.

—if you are taking **any** other prescription or nonprescription (OTC) medicine.

—if you smoke.

Proper Use of This Medicine

Bleomycin is sometimes given together with certain other medicines. If you are using a combination of medicines, it is important that you receive each medicine at the proper time. If you are taking some of these medicines by mouth, ask your doctor, nurse, or pharmacist to help you plan a way to take them at the right time.

Bleomycin often causes nausea, vomiting, and loss of appetite. However, it is very important that you continue to receive the medicine, even if you begin to feel ill. Ask your doctor, nurse, or pharmacist for ways to lessen these effects.

Precautions While Using This Medicine

It is very important that your doctor check your progress at regular visits to make sure that this medicine is working properly and to check for unwanted effects.

Before having any kind of surgery (including dental surgery) or emergency treatment, **tell the physician or dentist in charge that you are receiving or have received this medicine.**

Side Effects of This Medicine

Along with their needed effects, medicines like bleomycin can sometimes cause unwanted effects such as loss of hair, lung problems, and other side effects; these are described below. Also, because of the way these medicines act on the body, there is a chance that they might cause other unwanted effects that may not occur until months or years after the medicine is used. These delayed effects may include certain types of cancer, such as leukemia. Discuss these possible effects with your doctor.

Although not all of these side effects may occur, if they do occur they may need medical attention.

Check with your doctor or nurse immediately if the following side effects occur:

More common
   Fever and chills (occurring within 3 to 6 hours after a dose)

Less common
   Confusion
   Faintness
   Sweating
   Wheezing

Check with your doctor or nurse as soon as possible if any of the following side effects occur:

More common
   Cough
   Shortness of breath
   Sores in the mouth and on the lips

Other side effects may occur that usually do not require medical attention. These side effects may go away during treatment as your body adjusts to the medicine. Also, your doctor or nurse may be able to tell you about ways to prevent or reduce some of these side effects. Check with your doctor or nurse if any of the following side effects continue or are bothersome or if you have any questions about them:

More common
   Darkening or thickening of the skin
   Itching of skin
   Skin rash or colored bumps on fingertips, elbows, or palms
   Skin redness or tenderness
   Swelling of the fingers
   Vomiting and loss of appetite

Less common
   Changes in fingernails or toenails
   Weight loss

Bleomycin may cause a temporary loss of hair in some people. After treatment has ended, normal hair growth should return, although it may take several months.

Side effects that affect your lungs (for example, cough and shortness of breath) may be more likely to occur if you smoke.

For elderly patients: Lung problems are also more likely to occur in elderly patients (over 70 years of age), who are usually more sensitive to the effects of bleomycin.

After you stop receiving bleomycin, it may still produce some side effects that need attention. During this period of time, check with your doctor or nurse **immediately** if you notice either of the following:
   Cough
   Shortness of breath

Other side effects not listed above may also occur in some patients. If you notice any other effects, check with your doctor or nurse.

_____

December 1987

_____

Additional Information

For patients being treated with bleomycin for warts:

• Bleomycin is used to treat severe cases of warts when other treatments have not worked.

• Bleomycin is injected directly into the wart. Because it is not absorbed into the body, it does not cause loss of hair, lung problems, or other unwanted effects described above. However, it may cause burning or pain at the site of injection.

BROMOCRIPTINE (Systemic)

A commonly used brand name is Parlodel.

To the Reader: If you do not recognize the names of medical conditions or medicines referred to in this information, check with your doctor, nurse, or pharmacist. Definitions for selected medical terms may be found in the Glossary. Brand names for the generic drug names listed can be found in the Index. In addition, selected brand names commonly associated with the generic name have been included in the text to help you recognize medicine you may be taking. The fact that a brand name product is not mentioned does not mean the information does not apply. It is a good idea for you to learn both the generic and brand names of your medicines and to write them down for future use.

Bromocriptine (broe-moe-KRIP-teen) belongs to the group of medicines known as ergot alkaloids. It is used to treat some menstrual problems or as a fertility medicine in some women who are unable to become pregnant. It is also used to stop milk production in some women who have abnormal milk leakage or when mothers do not wish to breast-feed. Bromocriptine blocks release of a hormone called prolactin from the anterior pituitary gland. Prolactin affects the menstrual cycle and milk production.

Bromocriptine is also used to treat some people who have Parkinson's disease. It works by stimulating certain parts of the central nervous system (CNS) which are involved in this disease.

Bromocriptine is also used to treat acromegaly (overproduction of growth hormone) and pituitary prolactinomas (tumors of the pituitary gland).

It may also be used for other conditions as determined by your doctor.

Bromocriptine is available only with your doctor's prescription.

Remember:

• **This medicine has been prescribed for your current medical problem only.** It must not be given to other people or used for other problems unless you are directed to do so by your doctor.

• **Keep all medicines out of the reach of children.**

• In order for this medicine to work, it must be used as directed.

• **It is very important that you read and understand the following information.** If any of the information causes you special concern, do not decide against using this medicine without first checking with your doctor.

• Before you begin using any new medicine (prescription or nonprescription) or if you develop any new medical problem while you are using this medicine, check with your doctor, nurse, or pharmacist.

• **If you have any questions** about the following information or if you want more information about this medicine or your medical problem, **ask your doctor, nurse, or pharmacist.**

Before Using This Medicine

In order to decide on the best treatment for your medical problem, your doctor should be told:

—if you have ever had any unusual or allergic reaction to bromocriptine or other ergot medicines such as ergotamine.

—if you are on a low-salt, low-sugar, or any other special diet, or if you are allergic to any substance, such as foods, sulfites or other preservatives, or dyes. Most medicines contain more than their active ingredient. Your doctor, nurse, or pharmacist can help you avoid products that may cause a problem.

—if you intend to become **pregnant** while taking this medicine. Bromocriptine is not generally recommended during pregnancy because of the possibility that it might worsen certain existing medical problems in the mother. However, bromocriptine can be used during pregnancy in certain patients who are closely monitored by their doctor. In addition, although this medicine has not been shown to cause birth defects in humans, bromocriptine has been shown to increase the risk of cleft lip in rabbits; however, studies in other animals did not show this problem.

—if you intend to **breast-feed**. This medicine stops milk from being produced.

—if you have either of the following medical problems:
Liver disease
Mental problems (history of)

—if you are taking **any** other prescription or nonprescription (OTC) medicine, especially:
Estrogens
Oral contraceptives (birth control pills)
Progestins

Proper Use of This Medicine

If bromocriptine upsets your stomach, it may be taken with meals or milk. If stomach upset continues, check with your doctor.

If you miss a dose of this medicine and remember it within 4 hours, take the missed dose when you remember it. However, if a longer time has passed, skip the missed dose and go back to your regular dosing schedule. Do not double doses.

How to store this medicine:

• **Keep out of the reach of children.**

• Store away from heat and direct light.

• Do not store in the bathroom, near the kitchen sink, or in other damp places. Heat or moisture may cause the medicine to break down.

• Do not keep outdated medicine or medicine no longer needed. Be sure that any discarded medicine is out of the reach of children.

Precautions While Using This Medicine

It is important that your doctor check your progress at regular visits, to make sure that this medicine is working and to check for unwanted effects.

This medicine may cause some people to become drowsy, dizzy, or less alert than they are normally. **Make sure you know how you react to this medicine before you drive, use machines, or do other jobs that require you to be alert.**

Dizziness is more likely to occur after the first dose of bromocriptine. Taking the first dose at bedtime or when you are able to lie down may lessen problems.

It may take several weeks for bromocriptine to work. Do not stop taking this medicine or reduce the amount you are taking without first checking with your doctor.

For females of child-bearing potential taking this medicine for menstrual problems, to stop milk production, for acromegaly, or for pituitary tumors:
• It is best to use some type of birth control while you are taking bromocriptine. However, do not use oral contraceptives ("the Pill") since they may prevent this medicine from working. If you wish to become pregnant, you and your doctor should decide on the best time for you to stop using contraception. Tell your doctor right away if you think you have become pregnant while taking this medicine. You and your doctor should discuss whether or not you should continue to take bromocriptine during pregnancy.
• **Check with your doctor right away** if you get blurred vision, a sudden headache, or severe nausea and vomiting.

For females taking bromocriptine for infertility:
• In general, it is best to use some type of birth control when you start taking bromocriptine. However, do not use oral contraceptives ("the Pill") since they may prevent this medicine from working. When your normal menstrual cycle returns, you and your doctor can decide on the best time for you to stop using contraception. Tell your doctor right away if you think you have become pregnant while taking this medicine. You and your doctor should discuss whether or not you should continue to take bromocriptine during pregnancy.
• **Check with your doctor right away** if you get blurred vision, a sudden headache, or severe nausea and vomiting.

For patients taking bromocriptine for acromegaly or pituitary tumors:
• If you are taking bromocriptine for either of these problems, it may cause you to be unusually sensitive to the effects of alcohol. **Avoid alcoholic beverages until you have discussed their use with your doctor.**

Side Effects of This Medicine

Along with its needed effects, a medicine may cause some unwanted effects. Although not all of these side effects may occur, if they do occur they may need medical attention.

Check with your doctor immediately if any of the following side effects occur:
Rare
    Black tarry stools
    Bloody vomit
    Convulsions (seizures)
    Weakness (sudden)

Check with your doctor as soon as possible if any of the following side effects occur:
Less common—reported more often in patients with Parkinson's disease
    Confusion
    Hallucinations (seeing, hearing, or feeling things that are not there)
    Uncontrolled movements of the body, such as the face, tongue, arms, hands, head, and upper body
Rare
    Fainting
    Runny nose (continuing)

Other side effects may occur that usually do not require medical attention. These side effects may go away during treatment as your body adjusts to the medicine. However, check with your doctor if any of the following side effects continue or are bothersome:
More common
    Dizziness or lightheadedness, especially when getting up from a lying or sitting position
    Headache
    Nausea

Less common
    Constipation
    Diarrhea
    Drowsiness or tiredness
    Dry mouth
    Leg cramps at night
    Loss of appetite
    Mental depression
    Stomach pain
    Stuffy nose
    Tingling or pain in fingers and toes when exposed to cold
    Vomiting

Some side effects may be more likely to occur in the elderly, and in patients who are taking bromocriptine for Parkinson's disease, acromegaly, or pituitary tumors since they may be taking larger doses.

Other side effects not listed above may also occur in some patients. If you notice any other effects, check with your doctor.

December 1987

BRONCHODILATORS, ADRENERGIC
(Inhalation)

This information applies to the following medicines:

Albuterol (al-BYOO-ter-ole)
Bitolterol (bye-TOLE-ter-ole)
Epinephrine (ep-i-NEF-rin)
Fenoterol (fen-OH-ter-ole)
Isoetharine (eye-soe-ETH-a-reen)
Isoproterenol (eye-soe-proe-TER-e-nole)
Metaproterenol (met-a-proe-TER-e-nole)
Racepinephrine (race-ep-i-NEF-rin)
Terbutaline (ter-BYOO-ta-leen)

Some commonly used brand names or other names are:	Generic names:
Proventil Salbutamol Ventolin	Albuterol
Tornalate	Bitolterol
Adrenalin AsthmaHaler Bronitin Mist Bronkaid Mist Bronkaid Mistometer* Bronkaid Mist Suspension Dysne-Inhal* Medihaler-Epi Primatene Mist Solution Primatene Mist Suspension	Epinephrine†
Berotec*	Fenoterol*
Arm-a-Med Isoetharine Beta-2 Bisorine Bronkometer Bronkosol Dey-Dose Isoetharine Dey-Dose Isoetharine S/F Dey-Lute Isoetharine Dispos-a-Med Isoetharine	Isoetharine†
Aerolone Dey-Dose Isoproterenol Dispos-a-Med Isoproterenol Isuprel Isuprel Mistometer Medihaler-Iso Norisodrine Aerotrol Vapo-Iso	Isoproterenol†
Alupent Metaprel	Metaproterenol
AsthmaNefrin Dey-Dose Racepinephrine microNEFRIN S-2 Inhalant Vaponefrin	Racepinephrine
Brethaire	Terbutaline

*Not commercially available in the U.S.
†Generic name product may also be available in the U.S.

To the Reader: If you do not recognize the names of medical conditions or medicines referred to in this information, check with your doctor, nurse, or pharmacist. Definitions for selected medical terms may be found in the Glossary. Brand names for the generic drug names listed can be found in the Index. In addition, selected brand names commonly associated with the generic name have been included in the text to help you recognize medicine you may be taking. The fact that a brand name product is not mentioned does not mean the information does not apply. It is a good idea for you to learn both the generic and brand names of your medicines and to write them down for future use.

Adrenergic bronchodilators are medicines that open up the bronchial tubes (air passages) of the lungs. They are taken by oral inhalation to treat the symptoms of bronchial asthma, chronic bronchitis, emphysema, and other lung diseases. They relieve cough, wheezing, shortness of breath, and troubled breathing by increasing the flow of air through the bronchial tubes.

Albuterol is also taken by oral inhalation to prevent bronchospasm (wheezing or difficulty in breathing) caused by exercise. In addition, some of these medicines are taken by oral inhalation to prevent attacks of bronchial asthma and bronchospasm. Also, racepinephrine may be used in the treatment of croup.

All of these medicines, except some epinephrine preparations, are available only with your doctor's prescription. Although some of the epinephrine preparations are available without a prescription, your doctor may have special instructions on the proper dose of epinephrine for your medical condition.

Remember:
- **If this medicine has been prescribed for you, it should be used to treat your current medical problem only.** It must not be given to other people or used for other problems unless you are directed to do so by your doctor.

- **Keep all medicines out of the reach of children.**

- In order for this medicine to work, it must be used as directed. **If you are using epinephrine without a prescription, it is very important that you follow the directions on the label.**

- **It is also very important that you read and understand the following information.** If any of the information causes you special concern, check with your doctor or pharmacist.

- Before you begin using any new medicine (prescription or nonprescription) or if you develop any new medical problem while you are using this medicine, check with your doctor, nurse, or pharmacist.

- **If you have any questions** about the following information or if you want more information about this medicine or your medical problem, **ask your doctor, nurse, or pharmacist.**

Before Using This Medicine

Before you use this medicine, check with your doctor or pharmacist:

—if you have ever had any unusual or allergic reaction to albuterol, bitolterol, epinephrine, fenoterol, isoetharine, isoproterenol, metaproterenol, racepinephrine, terbutaline, or other inhalation medicines.

—if you are allergic to any substance, such as sulfites or other preservatives. Most medicines contain more than their active ingredient. Your doctor, nurse, or pharmacist can help you avoid products that may cause a problem.

—if you are **pregnant** or if you may become pregnant. Studies on birth defects with isoetharine have not been done in either humans or animals. Studies on birth defects with albuterol, bitolterol, epinephrine, metaproterenol, and terbutaline have not been done in humans. However, studies in animals have shown that albuterol, bitolterol, epinephrine, and metaproterenol cause birth defects when given in doses many times the usual human inhalation dose. Terbutaline has not been shown to cause birth defects in animal studies when given in doses many times the human inhalation dose. Fenoterol and isoproterenol have not been shown to cause birth defects or other problems in humans.

Use of epinephrine during pregnancy may decrease the supply of oxygen to the fetus. Also, terbutaline may delay labor.

—if you are **breast-feeding**. Epinephrine passes into the breast milk and may cause unwanted side effects in babies of mothers using epinephrine. Although terbutaline passes into the breast milk, it has not been shown to cause problems in nursing babies.

Although it is not known whether albuterol, bitolterol, fenoterol, isoetharine, isoproterenol, or metaproterenol passes into the breast milk, these medicines have not been shown to cause problems in nursing babies.

—if you have any of the following medical problems:

Brain damage
Diabetes mellitus (sugar diabetes)
Heart or blood vessel disease
High blood pressure
Mental disease
Overactive thyroid
Parkinson's disease
Seizures (or history of)

—if you are now using **any** other prescription or nonprescription (OTC) medicine, especially:

Beta-blockers (acebutolol [e.g., Sectral], atenolol [e.g., Tenormin], betaxolol [e.g., Betoptic], labetalol [e.g., Normodyne], levobunolol [e.g., Betagan], metoprolol [e.g., Lopressor], nadolol [e.g., Corgard], oxprenolol [e.g., Trasicor], pindolol [e.g., Visken], propranolol [e.g., Inderal], sotalol [e.g., Sotacor], timolol [e.g., Blocadren, Timoptic])
Digitalis glycosides (heart medicine)
Ergoloid mesylates (e.g., Hydergine)
Ergotamine (e.g., Gynergen)
Maprotiline (e.g., Ludiomil)
Tricyclic antidepressants (medicine for depression)

—if you are now taking or have taken within the past 2 weeks monoamine oxidase (MAO) inhibitors, such as:

Furazolidone (e.g., Furoxone)
Isocarboxazid (e.g., Marplan)
Pargyline (e.g., Eutonyl)
Phenelzine (e.g., Nardil)
Procarbazine (e.g., Matulane)
Tranylcypromine (e.g., Parnate)

Proper Use of This Medicine

For patients using epinephrine, isoetharine, or isoproterenol:

• Do not use if the solution turns pinkish to brownish in color or if it becomes cloudy.

Some epinephrine preparations are available without a doctor's prescription. However, **do not use this medicine without a doctor's prescription, unless your medical problem has been diagnosed as asthma by a doctor.**

Some of these preparations may come with patient directions. Read them carefully before using this medicine.

If you are using this medicine in a nebulizer or in a combination nebulizer and respirator, make sure you understand exactly how to use it. If you have any questions about this, check with your doctor or pharmacist.

For patients using the inhalation aerosol form of this medicine:

• **Keep spray away from the eyes because it may cause irritation.**

• **Do not take more than 2 inhalations of this medicine at any one time,** unless otherwise directed by your doctor. Allow 1 to 2 minutes after the first inhalation to make certain that a second inhalation is necessary.

• Save your applicator. Refill units of this medicine may be available.

Use this medicine only as directed. Do not use more of it and do not use it more often than recommended on the label, unless otherwise directed by your doctor. To do so may increase the chance of serious side effects. Inhalation aerosol medicines have been reported to cause death when too much of the medicine was used.

If you are using this medicine regularly and you miss a dose, use it as soon as possible. Then use any remaining doses for that day at regularly spaced intervals. Do not double doses.

How to store this medicine:

• **Keep out of the reach of children.**

• Store away from heat.

• Store the solution form of this medicine away from direct light. Store the inhalation aerosol form of this medicine away from direct sunlight.

• Keep the medicine from freezing.

• Do not puncture, break, or burn the inhalation aerosol container, even if it is empty.

• Do not keep outdated medicine or medicine no longer needed. Be sure that any discarded medicine is out of the reach of children.

Precautions While Using This Medicine

If you still have trouble breathing after using this medicine, or if your condition gets worse, check with your doctor at once.

For patients using epinephrine:

• Diabetics—This medicine may cause your blood sugar levels to rise. If you notice a change in the results of your urine sugar test or if you have any questions, check with your doctor.

Dryness of the mouth and throat may occur after using this medicine. Rinsing the mouth with water after each dose may help prevent the dryness.

For patients using the aerosol form of this medicine:
• If you are also using the inhalation aerosol form of an adrenocorticoid (cortisone-like medicine, such as beclomethasone, dexamethasone, flunisolide, or tri-amcinolone) or ipratropium, **allow 5 minutes between using the isoetharine and an adrenocorticoid or ipratropium,** unless otherwise directed by your doctor. This will help to reduce the possibility of side effects.

For patients using albuterol inhalation aerosol:
• If you use all of the medicine in one canister (container) in less than 2 weeks, check with your doctor. You may be using too much of the medicine.

Side Effects of This Medicine

In some animal studies, albuterol and terbutaline were shown to increase the chance of benign (not cancerous) tumors. Terbutaline was also shown to increase the chance of ovarian cysts. The doses given were many times the inhalation dose of albuterol and the oral dose of terbutaline given to humans. It is not known if al-buterol or terbutaline increases the chance of tumors in humans, or if terbutaline increases the chance of ovarian cysts in humans.

Along with its needed effects, a medicine may cause some unwanted effects. Although not all of these side effects may occur, if they do occur they may need medical attention.

Check with your doctor as soon as possible if any of the following side effects occur:
Rare
Chest discomfort or pain
Increase in wheezing or difficulty in breathing
Irregular heartbeat
With high doses
Hallucinations (seeing, hearing, or feeling things that are not there)
Signs of overdose
Chest discomfort or pain (continuing or severe)
Chills or fever
Convulsions (seizures)
Dizziness or lightheadedness (continuing or severe)
Fast or slow heartbeat (continuing)
Headache (continuing or severe)
Increase or decrease in blood pressure (severe)
Irregular or pounding heartbeat (continuing or severe)
Muscle cramps (severe)
Nausea or vomiting (continuing or severe)
Shortness of breath or troubled breathing (severe)
Trembling (severe)

Unusual anxiety, nervousness, or restlessness
Unusually large pupils or blurred vision
Unusual paleness and coldness of skin
Weakness (severe)

Other side effects may occur that usually do not require medical attention. These side effects may go away during treatment as your body adjusts to the medicine. However, check with your doctor if any of the following side effects continue or are bothersome:
More common
Nervousness or restlessness
Trembling
Less common
Coughing or other bronchial irritation
Dizziness or lightheadedness
Drowsiness
Dryness or irritation of mouth or throat
Fast or pounding heartbeat
Flushing or redness of face or skin
Headache
Increase in blood pressure
Muscle cramps or twitching
Nausea or vomiting
Trouble in sleeping
Unusual increase in sweating
Unusual paleness
Weakness

Although not all of the side effects listed above have been reported for all of these medicines, they have been reported for at least one of them. However, since all of the adrenergic bronchodilators are similar, any of the above side effects may occur with any of these medicines.

While you are using albuterol, bitolterol, fenoterol, met-aproterenol, or terbutaline, you may notice an unusual or bad taste. This may be expected and will go away when you stop using the medicine.

Isoproterenol may cause the saliva to turn pinkish to red. This is to be expected while you are using this medicine.

For elderly patients: Many medicines have not been tested in older people. Therefore, it is not known whether the medicine acts the same way it does in younger adults. Check with your doctor or pharmacist if you notice any unusual effects while taking this medicine or if you think it is not working as it should.

Other side effects not listed above may also occur in some patients. If you notice any other effects, check with your doctor.

_____

December 1987

BRONCHODILATORS, ADRENERGIC
(Oral/Injection)

This information applies to the following medicines:

Albuterol (al-BYOO-ter-ole)
Ephedrine (e-FED-rin)
Epinephrine (ep-i-NEF-rin)
Ethylnorepinephrine (ETH-il-nor-ep-i-NEF-rin)
Fenoterol (fen-OH-ter-ole)
Isoproterenol (eye-soe-proe-TER-e-nole)
Metaproterenol (met-a-proe-TER-e-nole)
Terbutaline (ter-BYOO-ta-leen)

Some commonly used brand names or other names are:	Generic names:
Novosalmol* Proventil Salbutamol Ventolin	Albuterol
Ephed II	Ephedrine†
Adrenalin EpiPen EpiPen Jr. Sus-Phrine	Epinephrine†
Bronkephrine	Ethylnorepinephrine
Berotec*	Fenoterol*
Isuprel	Isoproterenol†
Alupent Metaprel	Metaproterenol
Brethine Bricanyl	Terbutaline

*Not commercially available in the U.S.
†Generic name product may also be available in the U.S.

To the Reader: If you do not recognize the names of medical conditions or medicines referred to in this information, check with your doctor, nurse, or pharmacist. Definitions for selected medical terms may be found in the Glossary. Brand names for the generic drug names listed can be found in the Index. In addition, selected brand names commonly associated with the generic name have been included in the text to help you recognize medicine you may be taking. The fact that a brand name product is not mentioned does not mean the information does not apply. It is a good idea for you to learn both the generic and brand names of your medicines and to write them down for future use.

Adrenergic bronchodilators are medicines that open up the bronchial tubes (air passages) of the lungs. They are taken by mouth or given by injection to treat the symptoms of bronchial asthma, chronic bronchitis, emphysema, and other lung diseases. They relieve cough, wheezing, shortness of breath, and troubled breathing by increasing the flow of air through the bronchial tubes.

Ephedrine may also be used for the relief of nasal congestion in hay fever or other allergies. Ephedrine injection may be used to treat low blood pressure. In addition, ephedrine may be used in the treatment of narcolepsy (uncontrolled desire for sleep or sudden attacks of sleep) and certain types of mental depression.

Epinephrine injection (not including the auto-injector or the sterile suspension) may also be used in certain heart conditions. In addition, epinephrine injection may be used

in eye surgery to stop bleeding, reduce congestion, and dilate the pupil. It may also be applied topically to the skin or mucous membranes to stop bleeding.

Epinephrine injection (including the auto-injector but not the sterile suspension) is used in the emergency treatment of allergic reactions to insect stings, medicines, foods, or other substances. It relieves skin rash, hives, and itching; wheezing; and swelling of the lips, eyelids, tongue, and inside of nose.

Isoproterenol injection and tablets may also be used in the treatment of certain heart disorders.

Adrenergic bronchodilators may be used for other conditions as determined by your doctor.

Ephedrine capsules, syrup, and tablets are available without a prescription. However, your doctor may have special instructions on the proper dose of ephedrine for your medical condition.

All of the other adrenergic bronchodilators are available only with your doctor's prescription.

Remember:

• **If this medicine has been prescribed for you, it should be used to treat your current medical problem only.** It must not be given to other people or used for other problems unless you are directed to do so by your doctor.

• **Keep all medicines out of the reach of children.**

• In order for this medicine to work, it must be used as directed. **If you are using ephedrine without a prescription, it is very important that you follow the directions on the label.**

• If you are receiving this medicine by injection, some of the information about this medicine may not apply.

• **It is also very important that you read and understand the following information.** If any of the information causes you special concern, check with your doctor or pharmacist.

• Before you begin using any new medicine (prescription or nonprescription) or if you develop any new medical problem while you are using this medicine, check with your doctor, nurse, or pharmacist.

• **If you have any questions** about the following information or if you want more information about this medicine or your medical problem, **ask your doctor, nurse, or pharmacist.**

Before Using This Medicine

Before you use this medicine, check with your doctor or pharmacist:

—if you have ever had any unusual or allergic reaction to albuterol, ephedrine, epinephrine, ethylnorepinephrine, fenoterol, isoproterenol, metaproterenol, or terbutaline.

—if you are on a low-salt, low-sugar, or any other special diet, or if you are allergic to any substance, such as foods, sulfites or other preservatives, or dyes. Most medicines contain more than their active ingredient and many liquid medicines contain alcohol. Your doctor, nurse, or pharmacist can help you avoid products that may cause a problem.

—if you are **pregnant** or if you may become pregnant. Studies on birth defects with ephedrine or ethylnorepinephrine have not been done in either humans or animals. Studies on birth defects with albuterol, epinephrine, metaproterenol, and terbutaline have not been done in humans. However, studies in animals have shown that albuterol, epinephrine, and metaproterenol cause birth defects when given in doses many times the usual human dose. Terbutaline has not been shown to cause birth defects in animal studies when given in doses many times the usual human dose. Fenoterol and isoproterenol have not been shown to cause birth defects or other problems in humans.

Also, studies in animals have shown that metaproterenol causes death of the animal fetus when given in doses many times the usual human dose. Use of epinephrine during pregnancy may decrease the supply of oxygen to the fetus. Terbutaline given by injection during pregnancy has been reported to cause an unusually fast heartbeat in the fetus.

Although albuterol has been reported to delay preterm labor when taken by mouth, it has not been shown to stop preterm labor or prevent labor at term. Terbutaline may also delay labor. Epinephrine is not recommended for use during labor since it may delay the second stage of labor. Also, high doses of epinephrine that decrease contractions of the uterus may result in excessive bleeding when used during labor and delivery. When ephedrine is used just before or during labor, its effects on the newborn infant or on the growth and development of the child are not known.

—if you are **breast-feeding**. Epinephrine passes into the breast milk and may cause unwanted side effects in babies of mothers using epinephrine. Although terbutaline passes into the breast milk, it has not been shown to cause problems in nursing babies.

Although it is not known whether albuterol, ephedrine, fenoterol, isoproterenol, or metaproterenol pass into the breast milk, these medicines have not been shown to cause problems in nursing babies.

—if you have any of the following medical problems:

Brain damage
Diabetes mellitus (sugar diabetes)
Enlarged prostate
Heart or blood vessel disease
High blood pressure
Mental disease
Overactive thyroid
Parkinson's disease
Seizures (history of)

—if you are now using **any** other prescription or non-prescription (OTC) medicine, especially:

Beta-blockers (acebutolol [e.g., Sectral], atenolol [e.g., Tenormin], betaxolol [e.g., Betoptic], labetalol [e.g., Normodyne], levobunolol [e.g., Betagan], metoprolol [e.g., Lopressor], nadolol [e.g., Corgard], oxprenolol [e.g., Trasicor], pindolol [e.g., Visken], propranolol [e.g., Inderal], sotalol [e.g., Sotacor], timolol [e.g., Blocadren, Timoptic])
Digitalis glycosides (heart medicine)
Ergoloid mesylates (e.g., Hydergine)

Ergotamine (e.g., Gynergen)
Maprotiline (e.g., Ludiomil)
Tricyclic antidepressants (medicine for depression)

—if you are now taking or have taken within the past 2 weeks monoamine oxidase (MAO) inhibitors, such as:

Furazolidone (e.g., Furoxone)
Isocarboxazid (e.g., Marplan)
Pargyline (e.g., Eutonyl)
Phenelzine (e.g., Nardil)
Procarbazine (e.g., Matulane)
Tranylcypromine (e.g., Parnate)

Proper Use of This Medicine

For patients taking ephedrine:

• To help prevent trouble in sleeping, **take the last dose of ephedrine for each day a few hours before bedtime**. If you have any questions about this, check with your doctor.

For patients taking isoproterenol sublingual tablets:

• Do not chew or swallow the tablet. This medicine is meant to be absorbed through the lining of the mouth. Place the tablet under your tongue (sublingual) and let it slowly dissolve there. Do not swallow until the tablet has dissolved completely.

For patients using the injection form of this medicine:

• Do not use the epinephrine solution or suspension if it turns pinkish to brownish in color or if the solution becomes cloudy.

• **Use this medicine only for conditions as ordered by your doctor.**

• Keep this medicine ready for use at all times. Also, keep the telephone numbers for your doctor and the nearest hospital emergency room readily available.

• Check the expiration date on the injection regularly. Replace the medicine before it expires.

• This medicine is for injection only. If you will be giving yourself the injections, make sure you understand exactly how to give them. If you have any questions about this, check with your doctor.

For patients using epinephrine injection for an allergic reaction emergency:

• If an allergic reaction as described by your doctor occurs, **use the epinephrine injection immediately.**

• Notify your doctor immediately or go to the nearest hospital emergency room. If you have used the epinephrine injection, be sure to tell your doctor.

• If you have been stung by an insect, remove the insect's stinger with your fingernails, if possible. Be careful not to squeeze, pinch, or push it deeper into the skin. Ice packs or sodium bicarbonate (baking soda) soaks, if available, may then be applied to the area stung.

• If you are using the epinephrine auto-injector (automatic injection device):

—It is important that you do not remove the safety cap on the auto-injector until you are ready to use it. This prevents accidental activation of the device during storage and handling.

—Epinephrine auto-injector comes with patient directions. Read them carefully before you actually need to use this medicine. Then, when an emergency arises, you will know how to inject the epinephrine.

—How to use the epinephrine auto-injector:

• Remove the gray safety cap.

• Place the black tip on the thigh, at a right angle to the leg.

• Press hard into the thigh until the auto-injector functions. Hold in place for several seconds. Then remove the auto-injector and discard.

• Massage the injection area for 10 seconds.

Use this medicine only as directed. Do not use more of it and do not use it more often than your doctor ordered, or more than recommended on the label unless otherwise directed by your doctor. To do so may increase the chance of side effects.

If you are using this medicine regularly and you miss a dose, use it as soon as possible. Then use any remaining doses for that day at regularly spaced intervals. Do not double doses.

How to store this medicine:

• **Keep out of the reach of children.**

• Store away from heat and direct light.

• Do not store the capsule or tablet form of this medicine in the bathroom, near the kitchen sink, or in other damp places. Heat or moisture may cause the medicine to break down.

• Keep the injection or syrup form of this medicine from freezing.

• Store the suspension form of epinephrine injection in the refrigerator.

• Do not keep outdated medicine or medicine no longer needed. Be sure that any discarded medicine is out of the reach of children.

Precautions While Using This Medicine

If after using this medicine for asthma or other breathing problems you still have trouble breathing, or if your condition gets worse, check with your doctor at once.

For patients using epinephrine:

• Diabetics—This medicine may cause your blood sugar levels to rise. If you notice a change in the results of your urine sugar test or if you have any questions, check with your doctor.

Side Effects of This Medicine

In some animal studies, albuterol and terbutaline were shown to increase the chance of benign (not cancerous) tumors. Terbutaline was also shown to increase the chance of ovarian cysts. The doses given were many times the oral dose of albuterol or terbutaline given to humans. It is not known if albuterol or terbutaline increases the chance of tumors in humans, or if terbutaline increases the chance of ovarian cysts in humans.

Along with its needed effects, a medicine may cause some unwanted effects. Although not all of these side effects may occur, if they do occur they may need medical attention.

Check with your doctor as soon as possible if any of the following side effects occur:

Rare

    Chest discomfort or pain
    Increase in wheezing or difficulty in breathing
    Irregular heartbeat

With high doses

    Hallucinations (seeing, hearing, or feeling things that are not there)
    Mood or mental changes (reported for ephedrine only)

Signs of overdose

    Bluish coloration of skin
    Chest discomfort or pain (continuing or severe)
    Chills or fever
    Convulsions (seizures)
    Dizziness or lightheadedness (continuing or severe)
    Fast or slow heartbeat (continuing)
    Headache (continuing or severe)
    Increase or decrease in blood pressure (severe)
    Irregular or pounding heartbeat (continuing or severe)
    Muscle cramps (severe)
    Nausea or vomiting (continuing or severe)
    Shortness of breath or troubled breathing (severe)
    Trembling (severe)
    Unusual anxiety, nervousness, or restlessness
    Unusually large pupils or blurred vision
    Unusual paleness and coldness of skin
    Weakness (severe)

Other side effects may occur that usually do not require medical attention. These side effects may go away during treatment as your body adjusts to the medicine. However, check with your doctor if any of the following side effects continue or are bothersome:

More common

    Nervousness or restlessness
    Trembling

Less common

    Difficult or painful urination
    Dizziness or lightheadedness
    Drowsiness
    Fast or pounding heartbeat
    Flushing or redness of face or skin
    Headache
    Heartburn
    Increase in blood pressure
    Loss of appetite
    Muscle cramps or twitching

Nausea or vomiting
Trouble in sleeping
Unusual increase in sweating
Unusual paleness
Weakness

Although not all of the side effects listed above have been reported for all of these medicines, they have been reported for at least one of them. However, since all of the adrenergic bronchodilators are similar, any of the above side effects may occur with any of these medicines.

While you are using albuterol, fenoterol, metaproterenol, or terbutaline, you may notice an unusual or bad taste. This may be expected and will go away when you stop using the medicine.

Isoproterenol sublingual (under-the-tongue) tablets may cause the saliva to turn pinkish to red. This is to be expected while you are using this medicine.

For elderly patients: Many medicines have not been tested in older people. Therefore, it is not known whether the medicine acts the same way it does in younger adults. Check with your doctor or pharmacist if you notice any unusual effects while taking this medicine or if you think it is not working as it should.

Other side effects not listed above may also occur in some patients. If you notice any other effects, check with your doctor.

December 1987

BRONCHODILATORS, XANTHINE-DERIVATIVE (Systemic)

This information applies to the following medicines:

Aminophylline (am-in-OFF-i-lin)
Dyphylline (DYE-fi-lin)
Oxtriphylline (ox-TRYE-fi-lin)
Theophylline (thee-OFF-i-lin)

Some commonly used brand names are:	Generic names:
Aminophyllin	
Amoline	
Corophyllin*	
Palaron*	Aminophylline†
Phyllocontin	
Somophyllin	
Somophyllin-DF	
Truphylline	

Asminyl	
Dilor	
Droxine	
Droxine L.A.	
Droxine S.F.	
Dyflex	Dyphylline†
Dylline	
Dy-Phyl-Lin	
Lufyllin	
Neothylline	
Protophylline*	

Apo-Oxtriphylline*	
Choledyl	
Choledyl SA	Oxtriphylline†
Novotriphyl*	

Accurbron	
Aerolate	
Aquaphyllin	
Asmalix	
Bronkodyl	
Constant-T	
Elixicon	
Elixomin	
Elixophyllin	
Elixophyllin SR	
LaBID	
Lanophyllin	
Liquophylline	
Lixolin	
Lodrane	
PMS Theophylline*	
Pulmophylline*	
Quibron-T*	
Quibron-T Dividose	
Quibron-T/SR Dividose	Theophylline†
Respbid	
Slo-bid Gyrocaps	
Slo-Phyllin	
Slo-Phyllin Gyrocaps	
Somophyllin-12*	
Somophyllin-CRT	
Somophyllin-T	
Sustaire	
Theo-24	
Theobid Duracaps	
Theobid Jr. Duracaps	
Theochron	
Theoclear	
Theoclear L.A. Cenules	
Theo-Dur	
Theo-Dur Sprinkle	
Theolair	
Theolair-SR	
Theon	

Theophyl	
Theophyl-SR	
Theospan SR	
Theostat	Theophylline†
Theo-Time	
Theovent Long-acting	
Uniphyl	

Synophylate	Theophylline Sodium Glycinate

*Not available in the U.S.
†Generic name product may also be available in the U.S.

To the Reader: If you do not recognize the names of medical conditions or medicines referred to in this information, check with your doctor, nurse, or pharmacist. Definitions for selected medical terms may be found in the Glossary. Brand names for the generic drug names listed can be found in the Index. In addition, selected brand names commonly associated with the generic name have been included in the text to help you recognize medicine you may be taking. The fact that a brand name product is not mentioned does not mean the information does not apply. It is a good idea for you to learn both the generic and brand names of your medicines and to write them down for future use.

Xanthine-derivative bronchodilators are used to treat the symptoms of bronchial asthma, chronic bronchitis, and emphysema. These medicines relieve cough, wheezing, shortness of breath, and troubled breathing. They work by opening up the bronchial tubes or air passages of the lungs and increasing the flow of air through them.

Aminophylline and theophylline may also be used for other conditions as determined by your doctor.

Xanthine-derivative bronchodilators are taken by mouth, given by injection, or used rectally. The oral liquid, uncoated or chewable tablet, capsule, and rectal enema dosage forms may be used for treatment of the acute attack and for chronic (long-term) treatment. If rectal enemas are used, they should not be used for longer than 48 hours because they may cause rectal irritation. The enteric-coated tablet and extended-release dosage forms are usually used only for chronic treatment. Sometimes, aminophylline rectal suppositories may be used but they generally are not recommended because of possible poor absorption.

These medicines are available only with your doctor's prescription.

Remember:
• **This medicine has been prescribed for your current medical problem only.** It must not be given to other people or used for other problems unless you are directed to do so by your doctor.

• **Keep all medicines out of the reach of children.**

• In order for this medicine to work, it must be used as directed.

• If you are receiving this medicine by injection, some of the information about this medicine may not apply.

• **It is very important that you read and understand the following information.** If any of the information causes you special concern, do not decide against using this medicine without first checking with your doctor.

- Before you begin using any new medicine (prescription or nonprescription) or if you develop any new medical problem while you are using this medicine, check with your doctor, nurse, or pharmacist.
- **If you have any questions** about the following information or if you want more information about this medicine or your medical problem, **ask your doctor, nurse, or pharmacist.**

Before Using This Medicine

In order to decide on the best treatment for your medical problem, your doctor should be told:

—if you have ever had any unusual or allergic reaction to aminophylline, caffeine, dyphylline, ethylenediamine (contained in aminophylline), oxtriphylline, theobromine, or theophylline.

—if you are on a low-salt, low-sugar, or any other special diet, or if you are allergic to any substance, such as foods, sulfites or other preservatives, or dyes. Most medicines contain more than their active ingredient, and many liquid medicines contain alcohol. Your doctor, nurse, or pharmacist can help you avoid products that may cause a problem.

—if you are **pregnant** or if you may become pregnant. Studies on birth defects have not been done in humans. However, some studies in animals have shown that theophylline (includes aminophylline and oxtriphylline) causes birth defects when given in doses many times the human dose. Also, use of aminophylline, oxtriphylline, or theophylline during pregnancy may cause unwanted effects such as fast heartbeat, jitteriness, irritability, gagging, vomiting, and breathing problems in the newborn infant. Studies on birth defects with dyphylline have not been done in either humans or animals.

—if you are **breast-feeding**. Theophylline passes into the breast milk and may cause irritability, fretfulness, or trouble in sleeping in babies of mothers taking either aminophylline, oxtriphylline, or theophylline. Although dyphylline passes into the breast milk, it has not been shown to cause problems in nursing babies.

—if you have any of the following medical problems:
Diarrhea
Enlarged prostate
Fever
Fibrocystic breast disease
Heart disease
Irritation or infection of the rectum or lower colon (for aminophylline rectal enema only)
Kidney disease
Liver disease
Overactive thyroid
Respiratory infections, such as influenza (flu)
Stomach ulcer (or history of) or other stomach problems

—if you are now using **any** other prescription or nonprescription (OTC) medicine, especially:
Beta-blockers (acebutolol [e.g., Sectral], atenolol [e.g., Tenormin], betaxolol [e.g., Betoptic], labetalol [e.g., Normodyne], levobunolol [e.g., Betagan], metoprolol [e.g., Lopressor], nadolol [e.g., Corgard], oxprenolol [e.g., Trasicor], pindolol [e.g., Visken], propranolol [e.g., Inderal], sotalol [e.g., Sotacor], timolol [e.g., Blocadren, Timoptic])

Cimetidine (e.g., Tagamet)
Erythromycin (e.g., E-Mycin)
Phenytoin (e.g., Dilantin)
Troleandomycin (e.g., TAO)

—if you smoke or have smoked (tobacco or marijuana) regularly within the last 2 years. The amount of medicine you need may vary, depending on how much and how recently you have smoked.

Proper Use of This Medicine

For patients taking this medicine by mouth:

- If you are taking the capsule, tablet, liquid, or extended-release (not including the once-a-day capsule or tablet) form of this medicine, **it works best when taken with a glass of water on an empty stomach** (either 30 minutes to 1 hour before meals or 2 hours after meals). That way the medicine will get into the blood sooner. However, in some cases your doctor may want you to take this medicine with meals or right after meals to lessen stomach upset. If you have any questions about how you should be taking this medicine, check with your doctor.

- If you are taking the once-a-day capsule or tablet form of this medicine, **take one dose each morning after fasting overnight and at least 1 hour before eating**. Try to take the medicine about the same time each day.

- There are several different forms of xanthine-derivative bronchodilator capsules and tablets. If you are taking:

—chewable tablets, chew the tablets before swallowing.

—enteric-coated tablets, swallow the tablets whole. Do not crush, break, or chew before swallowing.

—extended-release capsules, swallow the capsule whole. Do not crush, break, or chew before swallowing.

—extended-release tablets, swallow the tablets whole. Do not break (unless tablet is scored for breaking), crush, or chew before swallowing.

For patients using the aminophylline enema:

- This medicine usually comes with patient directions. Read them carefully before using this medicine.

- If crystals form in the solution, dissolve them by placing the closed container of solution in warm water. If the crystals do not dissolve, do not use the medicine.

Use this medicine only as directed by your doctor. Do not use more of it, do not use it more often, and do not use it for a longer period of time than your doctor ordered. To do so may increase the chance of serious side effects.

In order for this medicine to help your medical problem, it must be taken every day in regularly spaced doses as ordered by your doctor. This is necessary to keep a constant amount of this medicine in the blood. To help keep the amount constant, do not miss any doses.

If you do miss a dose of this medicine, take it as soon as possible. However, if it is almost time for your next dose, skip the missed dose and go back to your regular dosing schedule. Do not double doses.

How to store this medicine:

- **Keep out of the reach of children.**

- Store away from heat and direct light.

- Do not store the capsule or tablet form of this medicine in the bathroom, near the kitchen sink, or in other damp places. Heat or moisture may cause the medicine to break down.

- Keep the liquid form of this medicine from freezing.

- Do not keep outdated medicine or medicine no longer needed. Be sure that any discarded medicine is out of the reach of children.

Precautions While Using This Medicine

Your doctor should check your progress at regular visits, especially for the first few weeks after you begin using this medicine. A blood test may be taken to help your doctor decide whether the dose of this medicine should be changed.

Do not change brands or dosage forms of this medicine without first checking with your doctor. Different products may not work the same way. If you refill your medicine and it looks different, check with your pharmacist.

This medicine may add to the central nervous system stimulant effects of caffeine-containing foods or beverages such as chocolate, cocoa, tea, coffee, and cola drinks. **Avoid eating or drinking large amounts of these foods or beverages while using this medicine.** If you have any questions about this, check with your doctor.

For patients using aminophylline, oxtriphylline, or theophylline:

- Do not eat charcoal-broiled foods every day while using this medicine since these foods may keep the medicine from working as well.

- **Check with your doctor at once if you develop symptoms of influenza (flu) or a fever** since either of these may increase the chance of side effects with this medicine.

- Also, **check with your doctor if diarrhea occurs** because the dose of this medicine may need to be changed.

For patients using the aminophylline enema:

- If burning or other irritation of the rectal area occurs after you use this medicine and if it continues or becomes worse, check with your doctor.

Side Effects of This Medicine

Along with its needed effects, a medicine may cause some unwanted effects. Although not all of these side effects may occur, if they do occur they may need medical attention.

Check with your doctor as soon as possible if any of the following side effects occur:

Less common
　　Heartburn and/or vomiting

Rare
　　Skin rash or hives (with aminophylline only)

Signs of overdose
　　Bloody or black tarry stools
　　Confusion or change in behavior
　　Convulsions (seizures)
　　Diarrhea
　　Dizziness or lightheadedness
　　Fast breathing
　　Fast, pounding, or irregular heartbeat
　　Flushing or redness of face
　　Headache
　　Increased urination
　　Irritability
　　Loss of appetite
　　Muscle twitching
　　Nausea (continuing or severe) or vomiting
　　Stomach cramps or pain
　　Trembling
　　Trouble in sleeping
　　Unusual tiredness or weakness
　　Vomiting blood or material that looks like coffee grounds

Other side effects may occur that usually do not require medical attention. These side effects may go away during treatment as your body adjusts to the medicine. However, check with your doctor if any of the following side effects continue or are bothersome:

More common
　　Nausea
　　Nervousness or restlessness

Less common
　　Burning or irritation of rectum (for rectal enema only)

For elderly patients and newborn infants: The above side effects are more likely to occur in elderly patients and newborn infants, who are usually more sensitive to the effects of these medicines.

Other side effects not listed above may also occur in some patients. If you notice any other effects, check with your doctor.

December 1987

BUSPIRONE (Systemic)

A commonly used brand name is BuSpar.

To the Reader: If you do not recognize the names of medical conditions or medicines referred to in this information, check with your doctor, nurse, or pharmacist. Definitions for selected medical terms may be found in the Glossary. Brand names for the generic drug names listed can be found in the Index. In addition, selected brand names commonly associated with the generic name have been included in the text to help you recognize medicine you may be taking. The fact that a brand name product is not mentioned does not mean the information does not apply. It is a good idea for you to learn both the generic and brand names of your medicines and to write them down for future use.

Buspirone (byoo-SPYE-rone) is taken by mouth. It is used to treat certain anxiety disorders or to relieve the symptoms of anxiety. However, buspirone is usually not used for anxiety or tension caused by the stress of everyday life.

It is not known exactly how buspirone works to relieve the symptoms of anxiety.

Buspirone is available only with your doctor's prescription.

Remember:
• **This medicine has been prescribed for your current medical problem only.** It must not be given to other people or used for other problems unless you are directed to do so by your doctor.

• **Keep all medicines out of the reach of children.**

• In order for this medicine to work, it must be used as directed.

• **It is very important that you read and understand the following information.** If any of the information causes you special concern, do not decide against using this medicine without first checking with your doctor.

• Before you begin using any new medicine (prescription or nonprescription) or if you develop any new medical problem while you are using this medicine, check with your doctor, nurse, or pharmacist.

• **If you have any questions** about the following information or if you want more information about this medicine or your medical problem, **ask your doctor, nurse, or pharmacist.**

Before Using This Medicine

In order to decide on the best treatment for your medical problem, your doctor should be told:

—if you have ever had any unusual or allergic reaction to buspirone.

—if you are on a low-salt, low-sugar, or any other special diet, or if you are allergic to any substance, such as foods, sulfites or other preservatives, or dyes. Most medicines contain more than their active ingredient. Your doctor, nurse, or pharmacist can help you avoid products that may cause a problem.

—if you are **pregnant** or if you may become pregnant. Studies have not been done in humans. However, buspirone has not been shown to cause birth defects or other problems in animal studies.

—if you are **breast-feeding**. It is not known whether buspirone passes into the breast milk of humans.

—if you have any of the following medical problems:
  Drug abuse or dependence (history of)
  Kidney disease
  Liver disease

—if you are now taking or have taken within the past 2 weeks monoamine oxidase (MAO) inhibitors, such as:
  Furazolidone (e.g., Furoxone)
  Isocarboxazid (e.g., Marplan)
  Pargyline (e.g., Eutonyl)
  Phenelzine (e.g., Nardil)
  Procarbazine (e.g., Matulane)
  Tranylcypromine (e.g., Parnate)

—if you are now taking **any** other prescription or nonprescription (OTC) medicine.

Proper Use of This Medicine

Take buspirone only as directed by your doctor. Do not take more of it, do not take it more often, and do not take it for a longer period of time than your doctor ordered. To do so may increase the chance of unwanted effects.

After you begin taking buspirone, 1 to 2 weeks may pass before you feel the full effects of this medicine.

If you are taking this medicine regularly and you miss a dose, take it as soon as possible. However, if it is almost time for your next dose, skip the missed dose and go back to your regular dosing schedule. Do not double doses.

How to store this medicine:
• **Keep out of the reach of children.**

• Store away from heat and direct light.

• Do not store in the bathroom, near the kitchen sink, or in other damp places. Heat or moisture may cause the medicine to break down.

• Do not keep outdated medicine or medicine no longer needed. Be sure that any discarded medicine is out of the reach of children.

Precautions While Using This Medicine

If you will be using buspirone regularly for a long period of time, your doctor should check your progress at regular visits to make sure the medicine does not cause unwanted effects.

Buspirone when taken with alcohol or other CNS depressants (medicines that slow down the nervous system, possibly causing drowsiness) may increase the chance of drowsiness. Some examples of CNS depressants are antihistamines or medicine for hay fever, other allergies, or colds; sedatives, tranquilizers, or sleeping medicine; prescription pain medicine or narcotics; barbiturates; medicine for seizures; muscle relaxants; or anesthetics, including some dental anesthetics. Check with your doctor before taking any of the above while you are taking this medicine.

Buspirone may cause some people to become dizzy, lightheaded, drowsy, or less alert than they are normally. **Make sure you know how you react to this medicine before you drive, use machines, or do other jobs that require you to be alert.**

If you think you or someone else may have taken an overdose of buspirone, get emergency help at once. Some signs of an overdose are severe dizziness or drowsiness; severe stomach upset, including nausea or vomiting; or unusually small pupils.

Side Effects of This Medicine

Along with its needed effects, a medicine may cause some unwanted effects. Although not all of these side effects may occur, if they do occur they may need medical attention.

Check with your doctor as soon as possible if any of the following side effects occur:

Rare
Chest pain
Confusion or mental depression
Fast or pounding heartbeat
Numbness, tingling, pain, or weakness in hands or feet
Sore throat or fever

Signs of overdose
Dizziness (severe)
Drowsiness (severe)
Stomach upset, including nausea or vomiting (severe)
Unusually small pupils

Other side effects may occur that usually do not require medical attention. These side effects may go away during treatment as your body adjusts to the medicine. However, check with your doctor if any of the following side effects continue or are bothersome:

More common
Dizziness or lightheadedness
Headache
Nausea
Restlessness, nervousness, or unusual excitement

Less common or rare
Decreased concentration
Drowsiness (more common with doses of more than 20 mg per day)
Dryness of mouth
Ringing in the ears
Stomach upset
Trouble in sleeping, nightmares, or vivid dreams
Unusual tiredness or weakness

Other side effects not listed above may also occur in some patients. If you notice any other effects, check with your doctor.

December 1987

BUSULFAN (Systemic)

A commonly used brand name is Myleran.

To the Reader: If you do not recognize the names of medical conditions or medicines referred to in this information, check with your doctor, nurse, or pharmacist. Definitions for selected medical terms may be found in the Glossary. Brand names for the generic drug names listed can be found in the Index. In addition, selected brand names commonly associated with the generic name have been included in the text to help you recognize medicine you may be taking. The fact that a brand name product is not mentioned does not mean the information does not apply. It is a good idea for you to learn both the generic and brand names of your medicines and to write them down for future use.

Busulfan (byoo-SUL-fan) belongs to the group of medicines known as alkylating agents. It is used to treat some kinds of cancer.

Busulfan seems to act by interfering with the function of the bone marrow. Since the growth of normal body cells may also be affected by busulfan, other effects will also occur. Some of these may be serious and must be reported to your doctor. Other effects may not be serious but may cause concern. Some effects may not occur for months or years after the medicine is used.

Before you begin treatment with busulfan, you and your doctor should talk about the good this medicine will do as well as the risks of using it.

Busulfan is available only with your doctor's prescription.

Remember:
• **This medicine has been prescribed for your current medical problem only.** It must not be given to other people or used for other problems unless you are directed to do so by your doctor.

• **Keep all medicines out of the reach of children.**

• In order for this medicine to work, it must be used as directed.

• **It is very important that you read and understand the following information.** If any of the information causes you special concern, do not decide against using this medicine without first checking with your doctor.

• Before you begin using any new medicine (prescription or nonprescription) or if you develop any new medical problem while you are using this medicine, check with your doctor, nurse, or pharmacist.

• **If you have any questions** about the following information or if you want more information about this medicine or your medical problem, **ask your doctor, nurse, or pharmacist.**

Before Using This Medicine

In order to decide on the best treatment for your medical problem, your doctor should be told:
—if you have ever had any unusual or allergic reaction to busulfan.

—if you are **pregnant** or if you intend to have children. Although only one case has been reported, there is a chance that this medicine may cause birth defects if either the male or the female is taking it at the time of conception or if it is taken during pregnancy. In addition, many cancer medicines may cause sterility which could be permanent. This may occur with busulfan and the possibility should be kept in mind. Be sure that you have discussed this with your doctor before taking this medicine.

—if you intend to **breast-feed.** Although it is not known whether busulfan passes into breast milk, because this medicine may cause serious side effects, breast-feeding is generally not recommended while you are taking it.

—if you have any of the following medical problems:
Chickenpox (including recent exposure)
Gout (history of)
Herpes zoster (shingles)
Infection
Kidney stones (or history of)

—if you are taking **any** other prescription or nonprescription (OTC) medicine, especially:
Amphotericin B by injection (e.g., Fungizone)
Antithyroid agents (medicine for overactive thyroid)
Azathioprine (e.g., Imuran)
Chloramphenicol (e.g., Chloromycetin)
Colchicine
Flucytosine (e.g., Ancobon)
Interferon (e.g., Intron A; Roferon-A)
Probenecid (e.g., Benemid)
Sulfinpyrazone (e.g., Anturane)

—if you have ever been treated with x-rays or cancer medicines.

Proper Use of This Medicine

Take this medicine only as directed by your doctor. Do not take more or less of it, and do not take it more often than your doctor ordered. The exact amount of medicine you need has been carefully worked out. Taking too much may increase the chance of side effects while taking too little may not improve your condition.

Take each dose at the same time each day to make sure it has the best effect.

While you are taking this medicine, your doctor may want you to drink extra fluids so that you will pass more urine. This will help prevent kidney problems and keep your kidneys working well.

This medicine sometimes causes nausea and vomiting. However, it is very important that you continue to use the medicine, even if you begin to feel ill. **Do not stop taking this medicine without first checking with your doctor.** Ask your doctor, nurse, or pharmacist for ways to lessen these effects.

If you vomit shortly after taking a dose of busulfan, check with your doctor. You will be told whether to take the dose again or wait until the next scheduled dose.

If you miss a dose of this medicine, skip the missed dose and go back to your regular dosing schedule. Do not double doses.

How to store this medicine:

- **Keep out of the reach of children.**

- Store away from heat and direct light.

- Do not store in the bathroom, near the kitchen sink, or in other damp places. Heat or moisture may cause the medicine to break down.

- Do not keep outdated medicine or medicine no longer needed. Be sure that any discarded medicine is out of the reach of children.

Precautions While Using This Medicine

It is very important that your doctor check your progress at regular visits to make sure that this medicine is working properly and to check for unwanted effects.

While you are being treated with busulfan, and after you stop treatment with it, **do not have any immunizations without your doctor's approval**. Busulfan lowers your body's resistance and there is a chance you might get the infection the immunization is meant to prevent. In addition, other persons living in your house should not take oral polio vaccine since they could pass the polio virus on to you. Also, you should avoid close contact with other persons (for example, at school or work) who have taken oral polio vaccine.

Busulfan can lower the number of white blood cells in your body. This may increase the chance of getting an infection. If you can, avoid people with colds or other infections. If you think you are getting a cold or other infection, check with your doctor.

Side Effects of This Medicine

Along with their needed effects, medicines like busulfan can sometimes cause unwanted effects such as lung problems, blood problems, and other side effects; these are described below. Also, because of the way these medicines act on the body, there is a chance that they might cause other unwanted effects that may not occur until months or years after the medicine is used. These delayed effects may include certain types of cancer, such as leukemia. Discuss these possible effects with your doctor.

Although not all of these side effects may occur, if they do occur they may need medical attention.

Check with your doctor immediately if any of the following side effects occur:
More common
    Fever, chills, or sore throat
    Unusual bleeding or bruising

Check with your doctor as soon as possible if any of the following side effects occur:
Less common
    Cough
    Joint pain
    Lower back, side, or stomach pain
    Shortness of breath
    Sores in the mouth and on the lips
    Swelling of feet or lower legs

Other side effects may occur that usually do not require medical attention. These side effects may go away during treatment as your body adjusts to the medicine. Also, your doctor or nurse may be able to tell you about ways to prevent or reduce some of these side effects. Check with your doctor if any of the following side effects continue or are bothersome or if you have any questions about them:
More common
    Darkening of the skin
    Missed or irregular menstrual periods
Less common
    Confusion
    Diarrhea
    Dizziness
    Loss of appetite
    Nausea and vomiting
    Unusual tiredness

After you stop taking busulfan, it may still produce some side effects that need attention. During this period of time, check with your doctor if you notice any of the following:
    Fever, cough, or shortness of breath
    Unusual bleeding or bruising

For elderly patients: Many medicines have not been tested in older people. Therefore, it is not known whether the medicine acts the same way it does in younger adults. Check with your doctor or pharmacist if you notice any unusual effects while taking this medicine or if you think it is not working as it should.

Other side effects not listed above may also occur in some patients. If you notice any other effects, check with your doctor.

December 1987

BUTALBITAL AND ACETAMINOPHEN
(Systemic)

Some commonly used brand names are:	Generic names:
Bancap Bucet Phrenilin Phrenilin Forte Sedapap Triaprin	Butalbital and Acetaminophen
Amaphen Anoquan Butace Endolor Esgic Fioricet G-1 Medigesic Plus Pacaps Repan Triad Two-Dyne	Butalbital, Acetaminophen, and Caffeine†

†Generic name product may also be available in the U.S.

To the Reader: If you do not recognize the names of medical conditions or medicines referred to in this information, check with your doctor, nurse, or pharmacist. Definitions for selected medical terms may be found in the Glossary. Brand names for the generic drug names listed can be found in the Index. In addition, selected brand names commonly associated with the generic name have been included in the text to help you recognize medicine you may be taking. The fact that a brand name product is not mentioned does not mean the information does not apply. It is a good idea for you to learn both the generic and brand names of your medicines and to write them down for future use.

Butalbital (byoo-TAL-bi-tal) and acetaminophen (a-seat-a-MIN-oh-fen) combination is a pain reliever and relaxant. It is used to treat tension headaches. Butalbital belongs to the group of medicines called barbiturates. Barbiturates act in the central nervous system (CNS) to produce their effects. When butalbital is used for a long time, your body may get used to it so that larger amounts are needed to produce its effects. This is called tolerance to the medicine. Also, butalbital may become habit-forming (causing mental or physical dependence) when it is used for a long time or in large doses. Physical dependence may lead to withdrawal side effects when you stop taking the medicine.

Some butalbital and acetaminophen combinations also contain caffeine (Kaf-EEN). Caffeine may help to relieve headache.

Butalbital and acetaminophen combinations are available only with your doctor's prescription.

Remember:
• **This medicine has been prescribed for your current medical problem only.** It must not be given to other people or used for other problems unless you are directed to do so by your doctor.

• **Keep all medicines out of the reach of children.**

• In order for this medicine to work, it must be used as directed.

• It is very important that you read and understand the following information. If any of the information causes you special concern, do not decide against using this medicine without first checking with your doctor.

• Before you begin using any new medicine (prescription or nonprescription) or if you develop any new medical problem while you are using this medicine, check with your doctor, nurse, or pharmacist.

• **If you have any questions** about the following information or if you want more information about this medicine or your medical problem, **ask your doctor, nurse, or pharmacist.**

Before Using This Medicine

In order to decide on the best treatment for your medical problem, your doctor should be told:

—if you have ever had any unusual or allergic reaction to barbiturates or to acetaminophen.

—if you are on a low-salt, low-sugar, or any other special diet, or if you are allergic to any substance, such as foods, sulfites or other preservatives, or dyes. Most medicines contain more than their active ingredient. Your doctor, nurse, or pharmacist can help you avoid products that may cause a problem.

—if you are **pregnant** or if you may become pregnant. Barbiturates such as butalbital have been shown to increase the chance of birth defects in humans. Also, one study in humans has suggested that barbiturates taken during pregnancy may increase the chance of brain tumors in the baby.

Taking a barbiturate regularly during the last 3 months of pregnancy may cause the fetus to become dependent on the medicine. This may lead to withdrawal side effects in the newborn baby. Also, butalbital may cause breathing problems in the newborn baby if taken just before or during delivery.

Although acetaminophen has not been shown to cause birth defects or other problems in humans, studies on birth defects with acetaminophen have not been done in humans.

Studies in humans have not shown that caffeine (contained in some of these combination medicines) causes birth defects. However, studies in animals have shown that caffeine causes birth defects when given in very large doses (amounts equal to those present in 12 to 24 cups of coffee a day).

—if you are **breast-feeding.** Barbiturates such as butalbital pass into the breast milk and may cause drowsiness, unusually slow heartbeat, shortness of breath, or troubled breathing in nursing babies.

Although acetaminophen and caffeine (contained in some of these combination medicines) have not been shown to cause problems in nursing babies, acetaminophen and caffeine pass into the breast milk in small amounts.

—if you have any of the following medical problems:
Anemia (severe)
Asthma (or history of), emphysema, or other chronic lung disease
Diabetes mellitus (sugar diabetes)

© 1988   The United States Pharmacopeial Convention, Inc.

Heart disease
Kidney disease
Hepatitis or other liver disease
Mental depression
Overactive thyroid
Porphyria (or history of)
Underactive adrenal gland

—if you are taking **any** other prescription or nonprescription (OTC) medicine, especially central nervous system (CNS) depressants.

Proper Use of This Medicine

Take this medicine only as directed by your doctor. Do not take more of it, do not take it more often, and do not take it for a longer period of time than your doctor ordered. If too much butalbital is taken, it may become habit-forming (causing mental or physical dependence) or lead to medical problems because of an overdose. Also, too much acetaminophen may cause liver damage.

If you have been taking this medicine regularly for a few weeks and you think it is not working as well as before, **do not increase the dose.** To do so may increase the chance of your becoming dependent on the butalbital. Instead, check with your doctor.

If your doctor has ordered you to take this medicine according to a regular schedule and you miss a dose, take it as soon as you remember. However, if it is almost time for your next dose, skip the missed dose and go back to your regular dosing schedule. **Do not double doses.**

How to store this medicine:

• **Keep out of the reach of children** because overdose is especially dangerous in young children.

• Store away from heat and direct light.

• Do not store this medicine in the bathroom, near the kitchen sink, or in other damp places. Heat or moisture may cause the medicine to break down.

• Do not keep outdated medicine or medicine no longer needed. Be sure that any discarded medicine is out of the reach of children.

Precautions While Using This Medicine

If you will be taking this medicine in high doses or for a long period of time (for example, for several months at a time), your doctor should check your progress at regular visits.

Check the labels of all over-the-counter (OTC) or prescription medicines you now take. If any contain a barbiturate or acetaminophen, be especially careful, since taking them while taking this medicine may lead to overdose. If you have any questions about this, check with your doctor or pharmacist.

The butalbital in this medicine will add to the effects of alcohol and other CNS depressants (medicines that slow down the nervous system, possibly causing drowsiness). Some examples of CNS depressants are antihistamines or medicine for hay fever, other allergies, or colds; sedatives, tranquilizers, or sleeping medicine; other prescription pain medicine; narcotics; other barbiturates; medicine for convulsions (seizures); muscle relaxants; or anesthetics, including some dental anesthetics. Also, drinking large amounts of alcoholic beverages regularly while taking this medicine may increase the chance of liver damage, especially if you take more of this medicine than your doctor ordered or if you take it regularly for a long period of time. **Therefore, do not drink alcoholic beverages, and check with your doctor before taking any of the medicines listed above, while you are using this medicine.**

Too much use of the acetaminophen in this medicine together with certain other medicines may increase the chance of kidney problems. Therefore, do not regularly take this medicine with any of the following, unless directed to do so by your doctor:

Aspirin or other salicylates
Diclofenac (e.g., Voltaren)
Diflunisal (e.g., Dolobid)
Fenoprofen (e.g., Nalfon)
Flurbiprofen, oral (e.g., Ansaid)
Ibuprofen (e.g., Advil; Motrin; Nuprin)
Indomethacin (e.g., Indocid; Indocin)
Ketoprofen (e.g., Orudis)
Meclofenamate (e.g., Meclomen)
Mefenamic acid (e.g., Ponstan; Ponstel)
Naproxen (e.g., Anaprox; Naprosyn)
Phenylbutazone (e.g., Azolid; Butazolidin)
Piroxicam (e.g., Feldene)
Sulindac (e.g., Clinoril)
Suprofen (e.g., Suprol)
Tiaprofenic acid (e.g., Surgam)
Tolmetin (e.g., Tolectin)

This medicine may cause some people to become drowsy, dizzy, or lightheaded. **Make sure you know how you react to this medicine before you drive, use machines, or do other jobs that require you to be alert and clearheaded.**

If you have been taking large amounts of this medicine, or if you have been taking it regularly for several weeks or more, **do not suddenly stop taking it without first checking with your doctor.** Your doctor may want you to reduce gradually the amount you are taking before stopping completely in order to lessen the chance of withdrawal side effects.

If you think you or anyone else may have taken an overdose of this medicine, get emergency help at once. Taking an overdose of this medicine or taking alcohol or CNS depressants with this medicine may lead to unconsciousness or possibly death. Signs of butalbital overdose include severe drowsiness, confusion, severe weakness, shortness of breath or unusually slow or troubled breathing, slurred speech, staggering, and unusually slow heartbeat. Signs of severe acetaminophen poisoning may not occur until 2 to 4 days after the overdose is taken, but treatment to prevent liver damage or death must be started within 24 hours or less after the overdose is taken.

Side Effects of This Medicine

Along with its needed effects, a medicine may cause some unwanted effects. Although not all of these side effects may occur, if they do occur they may need medical attention.

Check with your doctor immediately if any of the following side effects occur:

Rare

> Bleeding sores on lips
> Chest pain
> Muscle or joint pain
> Red, thickened, or scaly skin
> Skin rash or hives
> Sore throat and/or fever
> Sores, ulcers, or white spots in mouth (painful)
> Swelling of eyelids, face, or lips
> Wheezing or tightness in chest
> Yellow eyes or skin

Signs of overdose

> Confusion (severe)
> Diarrhea
> Drowsiness (severe)
> Loss of appetite
> Nausea or vomiting
> Poor judgment
> Shortness of breath or unusually slow or troubled breathing
> Slow heartbeat
> Slurred speech
> Staggering
> Stomach cramps or pain
> Swelling or tenderness in the upper abdomen or stomach area
> Trouble in sleeping
> Unusual increase in sweating
> Unusual irritability (continuing)
> Unusual movements of the eyes
> Weakness (severe)

Also, check with your doctor as soon as possible if any of the following side effects occur:

Less common

> Confusion (mild)
> Mental depression
> Unusual excitement

Rare

> Bloody or cloudy urine
> Difficult or painful urination
> Hallucinations (seeing, hearing, or feeling things that are not there)
> Itching of skin
> Sudden decrease in amount of urine
> Unusual bleeding or bruising
> Unusual tiredness or weakness

With long-term or chronic use

> Bone pain, tenderness, or aching
> Muscle weakness
> Unusual weight loss

Other side effects may occur that usually do not require medical attention. These side effects may go away during treatment as your body adjusts to the medicine. However, check with your doctor if any of the following side effects continue or are bothersome:

More common

> Clumsiness or unsteadiness
> Dizziness or lightheadedness (mild)
> Drowsiness (mild)
> "Hangover" effect

Less common

> Anxiety or nervousness (mild)
> Constipation
> Feeling faint
> Headache
> Nightmares
> Unusual irritability (mild)

For children and elderly patients: Unusual excitement, confusion, and mental depression may be more likely to occur in elderly or very ill patients, who are usually more sensitive to the effects of the butalbital in this combination medicine. Also, some of the side effects listed above may be especially likely to occur in children, who are also usually more sensitive to the effects of the butalbital in this combination medicine.

After you stop using this medicine, your body may need time to adjust. If you took this medicine in high doses or for a long period of time, this may take up to about 15 days. During this period of time check with your doctor if any of the following side effects occur (usually occur within 8 to 16 hours after the medicine is stopped):

> Anxiety or unusual restlessness
> Convulsions (seizures)
> Dizziness or lightheadedness
> Feeling faint
> Hallucinations (seeing, hearing, or feeling things that are not there)
> Increased dreaming or nightmares
> Muscle twitching
> Nausea or vomiting
> Trembling of hands
> Unusual weakness
> Vision problems

Other side effects not listed above may also occur in some patients. If you notice any other effects, check with your doctor.

———————

December 1987

———————————————————————————————————————

BUTALBITAL, ACETAMINOPHEN, AND NARCOTIC ANALGESICS (Systemic)

This information applies to the following medicines:

Butalbital (byoo-TAL-bi-tal), Acetaminophen (a-seat-a-MIN-oh-fen), and Codeine (KOE-deen)

Butalbital, Acetaminophen, Codeine, and Caffeine (kaf-EEN)

Butalbital, Acetaminophen, Hydrocodone (hye-droe-KOE-done), and Caffeine

Some commonly used brand names are:	Generic names:
G-2 G-3 Phrenilin with Codeine Sedapap with Codeine	Butalbital, Acetaminophen, and Codeine
Amaphen with Codeine	Butalbital, Acetaminophen, Codeine, and Caffeine
T-Gesic	Butalbital, Acetaminophen, Hydrocodone, and Caffeine

To the Reader: If you do not recognize the names of medical conditions or medicines referred to in this information, check with your doctor, nurse, or pharmacist. Definitions for selected medical terms may be found in the Glossary. Brand names for the generic drug names listed can be found in the Index. In addition, selected brand names commonly associated with the generic name have been included in the text to help you recognize medicine you may be taking. The fact that a brand name product is not mentioned does not mean the information does not apply. It is a good idea for you to learn both the generic and brand names of your medicines and to write them down for future use.

Butalbital, acetaminophen, and codeine or hydrocodone combinations are used to relieve pain. Codeine and hydrocodone belong to the group of medicines called narcotic analgesics (nar-KOT-ik an-al-JEE-ziks). The use of acetaminophen together with a narcotic analgesic may provide better pain relief than either acetaminophen or a narcotic analgesic used alone. In some cases, relief of pain may come at lower doses of each medicine.

Butalbital belongs to the group of medicines called barbiturates. It helps to reduce the tension that may occur with pain. Both butalbital and narcotic analgesics act in the central nervous system (CNS) to produce their effects. When butalbital or a narcotic analgesic is used for a long time, your body may get used to it so that larger amounts are needed to produce its effects. This is called tolerance to the medicine. Also, butalbital and narcotic analgesics may become habit-forming (causing mental or physical dependence) when they are used for a long time or in large doses. Physical dependence may lead to withdrawal side effects when you stop taking the medicine.

Some of these combination medicines also contain caffeine, which may help to relieve headache.

Butalbital, acetaminophen, and narcotic analgesic combinations are available only with your doctor's prescription.

Remember:

• **This medicine has been prescribed for your current medical problem only.** It must not be given to other people or used for other problems unless you are directed to do so by your doctor.

• **Keep all medicines out of the reach of children.**

• In order for this medicine to work, it must be used as directed.

• **It is very important that you read and understand the following information.** If any of the information causes you special concern, do not decide against using this medicine without first checking with your doctor.

• Before you begin using any new medicine (prescription or nonprescription) or if you develop any new medical problem while you are using this medicine, check with your doctor, nurse, or pharmacist.

• **If you have any questions** about the following information or if you want more information about this medicine or your medical problem, **ask your doctor, nurse, or pharmacist.**

Before Using This Medicine

In order to decide on the best treatment for your medical problem, your doctor should be told:

—if you have ever had any unusual or allergic reaction to barbiturates, acetaminophen, codeine, or hydrocodone.

—if you are on a low-salt, low-sugar, or any other special diet, or if you are allergic to any substance, such as foods, sulfites or other preservatives, or dyes. Most medicines contain more than their active ingredient. Your doctor, nurse, or pharmacist can help you avoid products that may cause a problem.

—if you are **pregnant** or if you may become pregnant.

For butalbital

Barbiturates such as butalbital have been shown to increase the chance of birth defects in humans. Also, one study in humans has suggested that barbiturates taken during pregnancy may increase the chance of brain tumors in the baby.

For acetaminophen

Although acetaminophen has not been shown to cause birth defects or other problems in humans, studies on birth defects with acetaminophen have not been done in humans.

For codeine

Codeine has not been shown to cause birth defects in humans; however, studies on birth defects have not been done in humans. Studies in animals have not shown that codeine causes birth defects. However, it slowed development of bones and caused other toxic or harmful effects in the fetus.

For hydrocodone

Hydrocodone has not been shown to cause birth defects in humans; however, studies on birth defects have not been done in humans. Studies in animals have shown that hydrocodone causes birth defects when given in very large doses.

For butalbital, codeine, and hydrocodone
Taking a barbiturate such as butalbital regularly during the last 3 months of pregnancy or taking too much codeine or hydrocodone during pregnancy may cause the fetus to become dependent on the medicine. This may lead to withdrawal side effects in the newborn baby. Also, butalbital, codeine, or hydrocodone may cause breathing problems in the newborn baby if taken just before or during delivery.

For caffeine
Studies in humans have not shown that caffeine (contained in some of these combination medicines) causes birth defects. However, studies in animals have shown that caffeine causes birth defects when given in very large doses (amounts equal to the amount of caffeine present in 12 to 24 cups of coffee a day).

—if you are **breast-feeding**. Barbiturates such as butalbital pass into the breast milk and may cause drowsiness, unusually slow heartbeat, shortness of breath, or troubled breathing in nursing babies. Also, acetaminophen, caffeine, and codeine have been shown to pass into the breast milk. It is not known whether hydrocodone passes into the breast milk.

—if you have any of the following medical problems:
   Anemia (severe)
   Asthma (or history of), emphysema, or other chronic lung disease
   Brain disease or head injury
   Colitis
   Diabetes mellitus (sugar diabetes)
   Enlarged prostate or problems with urination
   Gallbladder disease or gallstones
   Heart disease
   Kidney disease
   Hepatitis or other liver disease
   Mental depression
   Overactive thyroid
   Porphyria (or history of)
   Underactive adrenal gland
   Underactive thyroid

—if you are taking **any** other prescription or nonprescription (OTC) medicine, especially:
   Central nervous system (CNS) depressants
   Naltrexone

Proper Use of This Medicine

Take this medicine only as directed by your doctor. Do not take more of it, do not take it more often, and do not take it for a longer period of time than your doctor ordered. If too much butalbital or too much of a narcotic analgesic is taken, it may become habit-forming (causing mental or physical dependence) or lead to medical problems because of an overdose. Also, too much acetaminophen may cause liver damage.

If you have been taking this medicine regularly for a few weeks and you think it is not working as well as before, **do not increase the dose.** To do so may increase the chance of your becoming dependent on the butalbital or the narcotic analgesic. Instead, check with your doctor.

If your doctor has ordered you to take this medicine according to a regular schedule and you miss a dose, take it as soon as you remember. However, if it is almost time for your next dose, skip the missed dose and go back to your regular dosing schedule. **Do not double doses.**

How to store this medicine:

• **Keep out of the reach of children** because overdose is especially dangerous in young children.

• Store away from heat and direct light.

• Do not store in the bathroom, near the kitchen sink, or in other damp places. Heat or moisture may cause the medicine to break down.

• Do not keep outdated medicine or medicine no longer needed. Be sure that any discarded medicine is out of the reach of children.

Precautions While Using This Medicine

If you will be taking this medicine in high doses or for a long period of time (for example, for several months at a time), your doctor should check your progress at regular visits.

Check the labels of all over-the-counter (OTC) or prescription medicines you now take. If any contain a barbiturate, acetaminophen, or a narcotic analgesic be especially careful, since taking them while taking this medicine may lead to overdose. If you have any questions about this, check with your doctor or pharmacist.

The butalbital and the narcotic analgesic in this medicine will add to the effects of alcohol and other CNS depressants (medicines that slow down the nervous system, possibly causing drowsiness). Some examples of CNS depressants are antihistamines or medicine for hay fever, other allergies, or colds; sedatives, tranquilizers, or sleeping medicine; other prescription pain medicine or narcotics; other barbiturates; medicine for convulsions (seizures); muscle relaxants; or anesthetics, including some dental anesthetics. Also, drinking large amounts of alcoholic beverages regularly while taking this medicine may increase the chance of liver damage, especially if you take more of this medicine than your doctor ordered or if you take it regularly for a long period of time. **Therefore, do not drink alcoholic beverages, and check with your doctor before taking any of the medicines listed above, while you are using this medicine.**

Too much use of the acetaminophen in this medicine together with certain other medicines may increase the chance of kidney problems. Therefore, do not regularly take this medicine with any of the following, unless directed to do so by your doctor:

   Aspirin or other salicylates
   Diclofenac (e.g., Voltaren)
   Diflunisal (e.g., Dolobid)
   Fenoprofen (e.g., Nalfon)
   Flurbiprofen, oral (e.g., Ansaid)
   Ibuprofen (e.g., Advil; Motrin; Nuprin)
   Indomethacin (e.g., Indocid; Indocin)

Ketoprofen (e.g., Orudis)
Meclofenamate (e.g., Meclomen)
Mefenamic acid (e.g., Ponstel)
Naproxen (e.g., Naprosyn)
Phenylbutazone (e.g., Butazolidin)
Piroxicam (e.g., Feldene)
Sulindac (e.g., Clinoril)
Tiaprofenic acid (e.g., Surgam)
Tolmetin (e.g., Tolectin)

This medicine may cause some people to become drowsy, dizzy, or lightheaded, or to feel a false sense of well-being. **Make sure you know how you react to this medicine before you drive, use machines, or do other jobs that require you to be alert and clearheaded.**

Dizziness, lightheadedness, or fainting may be especially likely to occur when you get up slowly from a lying or sitting position. Getting up slowly may lessen this problem.

Nausea or vomiting may occur, especially after the first couple of doses. This effect may go away if you lie down for a while. However, if nausea or vomiting continues, check with your doctor. Lying down for a while may also lessen some other side effects that may occur, such as dizziness or lightheadedness.

Before having any kind of surgery (including dental surgery or other dental treatment) or emergency treatment, tell the physician or dentist in charge that you are taking this medicine.

The narcotic analgesic in this combination medicine may cause dryness of the mouth. For temporary relief, use sugarless candy or gum, melt bits of ice in your mouth, or use a saliva substitute. However, if dry mouth continues for more than 2 weeks, check with your dentist. Continuing dryness of the mouth may increase the chance of dental disease, including tooth decay, gum disease, and fungal infections.

If you have been taking large amounts of this medicine, or if you have been taking it regularly for several weeks or more, **do not suddenly stop taking it without first checking with your doctor.** Your doctor may want you to reduce gradually the amount you are taking before stopping completely to lessen the chance of withdrawal side effects.

If you think you or anyone else may have taken an overdose of this medicine, get emergency help at once. Taking an overdose of this medicine or taking alcohol or CNS depressants with this medicine may lead to unconsciousness or possibly death. Signs of overdose of butalbital, codeine, or hydrocodone include convulsions (seizures), severe nervousness or restlessness, severe dizziness or drowsiness, confusion, severe weakness, shortness of breath or unusually slow or troubled breathing, slurred speech, staggering, and unusually slow heartbeat. Signs of severe acetaminophen poisoning may not occur until 2 to 4 days after the overdose is taken, but treatment to prevent liver damage or death must be started within 24 hours or less after the overdose is taken.

Side Effects of This Medicine

Along with its needed effects, a medicine may cause some unwanted effects. Although not all of these side effects may occur, if they do occur they may need medical attention.

Check with your doctor immediately if any of the following side effects occur:

Rare
Bleeding sores on lips
Chest pain
Muscle or joint pain
Red, thickened, or scaly skin
Skin rash or hives
Sores, ulcers, or white spots in mouth (painful)
Sore throat and/or fever
Swelling of eyelids, face, or lips
Wheezing or tightness in chest
Yellow eyes or skin

Signs of overdose
Cold, clammy skin
Confusion (severe)
Convulsions (seizures)
Decreased blood pressure
Diarrhea
Dizziness (severe)
Drowsiness (severe)
Increased sweating
Loss of appetite
Nausea or vomiting
Nervousness, restlessness, or irritability (severe)
Pinpoint pupils of eyes
Poor judgment
Shortness of breath or unusually slow, irregular, or troubled breathing
Slow heartbeat
Slurred speech
Staggering
Stomach cramps or pain
Swelling or tenderness in the upper abdomen or stomach area
Trouble in sleeping
Unusual movements of the eyes
Weakness (severe)

Also, check with your doctor as soon as possible if any of the following side effects occur:

Less common or rare
Bloody or cloudy urine
Confusion, feelings of unreality, or mental depression
Difficult or painful urination
Fast or pounding heartbeat
Hallucinations (seeing, hearing, or feeling things that are not there)
Itching of skin
Ringing or buzzing in the ears
Sudden decrease in amount of urine
Trembling or uncontrolled muscle movements
Unusual bleeding or bruising
Unusual excitement
Unusual tiredness or weakness

With long-term or chronic use
Bone pain, tenderness, or aching
Muscle weakness
Unusual weight loss

© 1988   The United States Pharmacopeial Convention, Inc.

Other side effects may occur that usually do not require medical attention. These side effects may go away during treatment as your body adjusts to the medicine. However, check with your doctor if any of the following side effects continue or are bothersome:

More common

    Clumsiness or unsteadiness
    Dizziness, lightheadedness, or feeling faint (mild)
    Drowsiness (mild)
    "Hangover" effect

Less common or rare

    Anxiety, irritability, nervousness, or restlessness (mild)
    Blurred or double vision or any change in vision
    Constipation
    Dry mouth
    False sense of well-being
    Frequent urge to urinate
    General feeling of discomfort or illness
    Headache
    Nightmares or unusual dreams
    Redness or flushing of face (more common with hydrocodone)

For children and elderly patients: Unusual excitement, confusion, mental depression, and/or breathing problems may be more likely to occur in children or elderly or very ill patients, who are usually more sensitive to the effects of the butalbital and the narcotic analgesic in this combination medicine.

After you stop using this medicine, your body may need time to adjust. The length of time this takes depends on which of these medicines you were taking, the amount of medicine you were using, and how long you used it. During this period of time check with your doctor if any of the following side effects occur:

    Anxiety, irritability, nervousness, or restlessness
    Body aches
    Convulsions (seizures)
    Diarrhea
    Dizziness, lightheadedness, or feeling faint
    Fast heartbeat
    Fever
    Gooseflesh
    Hallucinations (seeing, hearing, or feeling things that are not there)
    Increased dreaming, nightmares, or trouble in sleeping
    Increased sweating
    Increased yawning
    Loss of appetite
    Muscle twitching, shivering, or trembling
    Nausea or vomiting
    Runny nose or sneezing
    Stomach cramps
    Unusually large pupils of eyes
    Unusual weakness
    Vision problems

Other side effects not listed above may also occur in some patients. If you notice any other effects, check with your doctor.

December 1987

BUTALBITAL AND ASPIRIN (Systemic)

Some commonly used brand names and other names are:	Generic names:
Axotal	Butalbital and Aspirin
B-A-C Butalbital A-C Butalbital Compound Butal Compound Fiorgen PF Fiorinal Isollyl (Improved) Lanorinal Marnal Protension Tenstan	Butalbital, Aspirin, and Caffeine†

†Generic name product may also be available in the U.S.

To the Reader: If you do not recognize the names of medical conditions or medicines referred to in this information, check with your doctor, nurse, or pharmacist. Definitions for selected medical terms may be found in the Glossary. Brand names for the generic drug names listed can be found in the Index. In addition, selected brand names commonly associated with the generic name have been included in the text to help you recognize medicine you may be taking. The fact that a brand name product is not mentioned does not mean the information does not apply. It is a good idea for you to learn both the generic and brand names of your medicines and to write them down for future use.

Butalbital (byoo-TAL-bi-tal) and aspirin (AS-pir-in) combination is a pain reliever and relaxant. It is used to treat tension headaches. Butalbital belongs to the group of medicines called barbiturates. Barbiturates act in the central nervous system (CNS) to produce their effects. When butalbital is used for a long time, your body may get used to it so that larger amounts are needed to produce its effects. This is called tolerance to the medicine. Also, butalbital may become habit-forming (causing mental or physical dependence) when it is used for a long time or in large doses. Physical dependence may lead to withdrawal side effects when you stop taking the medicine.

Some of these medicines also contain caffeine (kaf-EEN).

Butalbital and aspirin combination is available only with your doctor's prescription.

Remember:

• **This medicine has been prescribed for your current medical problem only.** It must not be given to other people or used for other problems unless you are directed to do so by your doctor.

• **Keep all medicines out of the reach of children.**

• In order for this medicine to work, it must be used as directed.

• **It is very important that you read and understand the following information.** If any of the information causes you special concern, do not decide against using this medicine without first checking with your doctor.

• Before you begin using any new medicine (prescription or nonprescription) or if you develop any new medical problem while you are using this medicine, check with your doctor, nurse, or pharmacist.

• **If you have any questions** about the following information or if you want more information about this medicine or your medical problem, **ask your doctor, nurse, or pharmacist.**

Before Using This Medicine

In order to decide on the best treatment for your medical problem, your doctor should be told:

—if you have ever had any unusual or allergic reaction to barbiturates, caffeine, or aspirin or other salicylates including methyl salicylate (oil of wintergreen), or to any of the following medicines:

Diclofenac (e.g., Voltaren)
Diflunisal (e.g., Dolobid)
Fenoprofen (e.g., Nalfon)
Flurbiprofen, oral (e.g., Ansaid)
Ibuprofen (e.g., Motrin)
Indomethacin (e.g., Indocin)
Ketoprofen (e.g., Orudis)
Meclofenamate (e.g., Meclomen)
Mefenamic acid (e.g., Ponstel)
Naproxen (e.g., Naprosyn)
Oxyphenbutazone (e.g., Tandearil)
Phenylbutazone (e.g., Butazolidin)
Piroxicam (e.g., Feldene)
Sulindac (e.g., Clinoril)
Suprofen (e.g., Suprol)
Tiaprofenic acid (e.g., Surgam)
Tolmetin (e.g., Tolectin)
Zomepirac (e.g., Zomax)

—if you are on a low-salt, low-sugar, or any other special diet, or if you are allergic to any substance, such as foods, sulfites or other preservatives, or dyes. Most medicines contain more than their active ingredient. Your doctor, nurse, or pharmacist can help you avoid products that may cause a problem.

—if you are **pregnant** or if you may become pregnant.

For butalbital
Barbiturates such as butalbital have been shown to increase the chance of birth defects in humans. Also, one study in humans has suggested that barbiturates taken during pregnancy may increase the chance of brain tumors in the baby.

Taking a barbiturate regularly during the last 3 months of pregnancy may cause the fetus to become dependent on the medicine. This may lead to withdrawal side effects in the newborn baby. In addition, butalbital may cause breathing problems in the newborn baby if taken just before or during delivery.

For aspirin
Although studies in humans have not shown that aspirin causes birth defects, it has caused birth defects in animal studies.

Some reports have suggested that too much use of aspirin late in pregnancy may cause a decrease in the newborn's weight and possible death of the fetus or newborn baby. However, the mothers in these reports had been taking much larger amounts of aspirin than are usually recommended. Studies of mothers taking aspirin in the doses that are usually recommended did not show these unwanted effects.

There is a chance that regular use of aspirin late in pregnancy may cause unwanted effects on the heart or blood flow in the fetus or in the newborn baby. Also, use of aspirin during the last 2 weeks of pregnancy may cause bleeding problems in the fetus before or during delivery or in the newborn baby. In addition, too much use of aspirin during the last 3 months of pregnancy may increase the length of pregnancy, prolong labor, cause other problems during delivery, or cause severe bleeding in the mother before, during, or after delivery.

For caffeine

Studies in humans have not shown that caffeine causes birth defects. However, studies in animals have shown that caffeine causes birth defects when given in very large doses (amounts equal to the amount in 12 to 24 cups of coffee a day).

—if you are **breast-feeding**. Although this combination medicine has not been shown to cause problems, the chance always exists, especially if the medicine is taken for a long time or in large amounts. Barbiturates (such as butalbital) pass into the breast milk and may cause drowsiness, unusually slow heartbeat, shortness of breath, or troubled breathing in nursing babies. Aspirin and caffeine also pass into the breast milk.

—if you have any of the following medical problems:
   Anemia
   Asthma, allergies, and nasal polyps (history of)
   Emphysema, asthma, or chronic lung disease
   Gout
   Heart disease (severe)
   Hemophilia or other bleeding problems
   Hyperactivity (in children)
   Kidney disease
   Liver disease
   Mental depression
   Overactive thyroid
   Porphyria (or history of)
   Stomach ulcer or other stomach problems
   Vitamin K deficiency
—if you regularly take large amounts of antacids, especially calcium- and/or magnesium-containing antacids or sodium bicarbonate (baking soda).
—if you are taking **any** other prescription or nonprescription (OTC) medicine, especially:
   Anticoagulants (blood thinners)
   Antidiabetics, oral (diabetes medicine you take by mouth)
   Central nervous system (CNS) depressants
   Dipyridamole (e.g., Persantine)
   Divalproex (e.g., Depakote)
   Heparin
   Medicine for pain and/or inflammation
   Methotrexate (e.g., Folex; Mexate)
   Probenecid (e.g., Benemid)
   Sulfinpyrazone (e.g., Anturane)
   Urinary alkalizers (medicine that makes the urine less acid, such as acetazolamide [e.g., Diamox], dichlorphenamide [e.g., Daranide], methazolamide [e.g., Neptazane], potassium or sodium citrate and/or citric acid)
   Valproic acid (e.g., Depakene)
   Vancomycin (e.g., Vancocin)

Proper Use of This Medicine

Take this medicine with food or a full glass (8 ounces) of water to lessen stomach irritation.

There have been reports suggesting that use of aspirin in children or teenagers with fever due to a viral infection (especially flu or chickenpox) may cause a serious illness called Reye's syndrome. This medicine contains aspirin. Therefore, **do not give this medicine to a child or a teenager with symptoms of flu or chickenpox without first discussing this with your child's doctor.**

Take this medicine only as directed by your doctor. Do not take more of it, do not take it more often, and do not take it for a longer period of time than your doctor ordered. If too much butalbital is taken, it may become habit-forming (causing mental or physical dependence) or lead to medical problems because of an overdose. Also, taking too much aspirin may cause stomach problems or lead to medical problems because of an overdose.

Do not take this medicine if it has a strong vinegar-like odor, since this means the aspirin in it is breaking down. If you have any questions about this, check with your doctor or pharmacist.

If your doctor has ordered you to take this medicine according to a regular schedule and you miss a dose, take it as soon as you remember. However, if it is almost time for your next dose, skip the missed dose and go back to your regular dosing schedule. Do not double doses.

How to store this medicine:

• **Keep out of the reach of children** because overdose is especially dangerous in young children.

• Store away from heat and direct light.

• Do not store this medicine in the bathroom, near the kitchen sink, or in other damp places. Heat or moisture may cause the medicine to break down.

• Do not keep outdated medicine or medicine no longer needed. Be sure that any discarded medicine is out of the reach of children.

Precautions While Using This Medicine

If you will be taking this medicine for a long period of time (for example, for several months at a time), or in high doses, your doctor should check your progress at regular visits.

Check the labels of all over-the-counter (OTC), nonprescription, and prescription medicines you now take. If any contain a barbiturate, aspirin, or other salicylates, including diflunisal, be especially careful, since taking them while taking this medicine may lead to overdose. If you have any questions about this, check with your doctor or pharmacist.

The butalbital in this medicine will add to the effects of alcohol and other CNS depressants (medicines that slow down the nervous system, possibly causing drowsiness). Some examples of CNS depressants are antihistamines or medicine for hay fever, other allergies, or colds; sedatives, tranquilizers, or sleeping medicine; other prescription pain medicine or narcotics; other barbiturates; medicine for convulsions (seizures); tricyclic antidepressants (medicine for depression); muscle relaxants; or anesthetics, including some dental anesthetics. Also, stomach problems may be more likely to occur if you drink alcoholic beverages while you are taking aspirin. Therefore, **do not drink alcoholic beverages, and check with your doctor before taking any of the medicines listed above, while you are using this medicine.**

Too much use of acetaminophen together with this combination medicine may increase the chance of kidney or liver problems. Therefore, do not regularly take acetaminophen together with this medicine, unless directed to do so by your doctor.

Too much use of the aspirin in this medicine together with certain other medicines may increase the chance of side effects. Therefore, do not regularly take this medicine with any of the following, unless directed to do so by your doctor:

    Diclofenac (e.g., Voltaren)
    Diflunisal (e.g., Dolobid)
    Fenoprofen (e.g., Nalfon)
    Flurbiprofen, oral (e.g., Ansaid)
    Ibuprofen (e.g., Motrin)
    Indomethacin (e.g., Indocin)
    Ketoprofen (e.g., Orudis)
    Meclofenamate (e.g., Meclomen)
    Mefenamic acid (e.g., Ponstel)
    Naproxen (e.g., Naprosyn)
    Phenylbutazone (e.g., Butazolidin)
    Piroxicam (e.g., Feldene)
    Sulindac (e.g., Clinoril)
    Tiaprofenic acid (e.g., Surgam)
    Tolmetin (e.g., Tolectin)

This medicine may cause some people to become drowsy, dizzy, or lightheaded. **Make sure you know how you react to this medicine before you drive, use machines, or do other jobs that require you to be alert and clearheaded.**

Before having any kind of surgery (including dental surgery) or emergency treatment, tell the physician or dentist in charge that you are taking this medicine.

Do not take this medicine for 5 days before any surgery, including dental surgery, unless otherwise directed by your doctor. Taking aspirin during this time may cause bleeding problems.

For diabetics—The aspirin in this medicine may cause false urine sugar test results when it is taken regularly. Occasional use of aspirin usually will not affect urine sugar tests. If you have any questions about this, check with your doctor, nurse, or pharmacist, especially if your diabetes is not well controlled.

If you have been taking large amounts of this medicine, or if you have been taking it regularly for several weeks or more, **do not suddenly stop using it without first checking with your doctor.** Your doctor may want you to reduce gradually the amount you are taking before stopping completely, to lessen the chance of withdrawal side effects.

If you think you or anyone else may have taken an overdose of this medicine, get emergency help at once. Taking an overdose of this medicine or taking alcohol or CNS depressants with this medicine may lead to unconsciousness or death. Signs of overdose of this medicine include convulsions (seizures); hearing loss; confusion; ringing or buzzing in the ears; severe excitement, nervousness, or restlessness; severe dizziness; severe drowsiness; shortness of breath or troubled breathing; and severe weakness.

Side Effects of This Medicine

Along with its needed effects, a medicine may cause some unwanted effects. Although not all of these side effects may occur, if they do occur they may need medical attention.

Check with your doctor immediately if any of the following side effects occur:
Less common or rare
    Shortness of breath, troubled breathing, tightness in chest, or wheezing
Signs of overdose
    Any loss of hearing
    Bloody urine
    Convulsions (seizures)
    Diarrhea
    Dizziness, lightheadedness, or drowsiness (severe)
    Hallucinations (seeing, hearing, or feeling things that are not there)
    Headache (severe or continuing)
    Increased sweating
    Nausea or vomiting (continuing)
    Nervousness, excitement, or confusion (severe)
    Poor judgment
    Ringing or buzzing in ears (continuing)
    Slow heartbeat
    Slow or irregular breathing
    Slurred speech
    Staggering
    Trouble in sleeping
    Uncontrollable flapping movements of the hands, especially in elderly patients
    Unexplained fever
    Unusual irritability (continuing)
    Unusual movements of the eyes
    Unusual thirst
    Vision problems
    Weakness (severe)

Also, check with your doctor as soon as possible if any of the following side effects occur:
More common
    Nausea or vomiting
    Stomach pain
Less common or rare
    Bloody or black tarry stools
    Confusion or mental depression
    Skin rash, hives, or itching
    Sore throat and fever

Swelling of eyelids, face, or lips
Unusual bleeding or bruising
Unusual excitement
Unusual tiredness or weakness
Vomiting of blood or material that looks like coffee grounds
Yellow eyes or skin

Other side effects may occur that usually do not require medical attention. These side effects may go away during treatment as your body adjusts to the medicine. However, check with your doctor if any of the following side effects continue or are bothersome:

More common

Clumsiness or unsteadiness
Dizziness or lightheadedness
Drowsiness
"Hangover" effect
Heartburn or indigestion

Less common or rare

Anxiety or nervousness
Constipation
Feeling faint
Headache
Nightmares
Unusual irritability

For children and elderly patients: Some of the above side effects are more likely to occur in children, especially those with a fever or who have lost large amounts of body fluid because of vomiting, diarrhea, or sweating, and in elderly patients (60 years of age or older) or very ill patients. These patients are usually more sensitive to the effects of butalbital and aspirin.

After you stop using this medicine, your body may need time to adjust. The length of time this takes depends on the amount of medicine you were using and how long you used it. During this period of time check with your doctor if you notice any of the following side effects:

Convulsions (seizures)
Dizziness or lightheadedness
Feeling faint
Hallucinations (seeing, hearing, or feeling things that are not there)
Muscle twitching
Nausea or vomiting
Trembling of hands
Trouble in sleeping, increased dreaming, or nightmares
Unusual anxiety, nervousness, or restlessness
Unusual weakness
Vision problems

Other side effects not listed above may also occur in some patients. If you notice any other effects, check with your doctor.

_____

December 1987

_____

BUTALBITAL, ASPIRIN, AND CODEINE
(Systemic)

Some commonly used brand names are:

ABC Compound with Codeine	Fiorgen with Codeine
	Fiorinal with Codeine
B-A-C with Codeine	Isollyl with Codeine

To the Reader: If you do not recognize the names of medical conditions or medicines referred to in this information, check with your doctor, nurse, or pharmacist. Definitions for selected medical terms may be found in the Glossary. Brand names for the generic drug names listed can be found in the Index. In addition, selected brand names commonly associated with the generic name have been included in the text to help you recognize medicine you may be taking. The fact that a brand name product is not mentioned does not mean the information does not apply. It is a good idea for you to learn both the generic and brand names of your medicines and to write them down for future use.

Butalbital (byoo-TAL-bi-tal), aspirin (AS-pir-in), and codeine (KOE-deen) is a combination medicine used to relieve pain. This combination medicine may provide better pain relief than either aspirin or codeine used alone. In some cases, relief of pain may come at lower doses of each medicine. This combination medicine also contains caffeine (kaf-EEN).

Codeine is a narcotic analgesic (nar-KOT-ik an-al-JEE-zik) that acts in the central nervous system (CNS) to relieve pain. Many of its side effects are also caused by actions in the CNS. Butalbital belongs to the group of medicines called barbiturates. Barbiturates also act in the CNS to produce their effects. When you use butalbital or codeine for a long time, your body may get used to these medicines so that larger amounts are needed to produce their effects. This is called tolerance to the medicine. Also, butalbital and codeine may become habit-forming (causing mental or physical dependence) when they are used for a long time or in large doses. Physical dependence may lead to withdrawal symptoms when you stop taking the medicine.

Aspirin is not a narcotic and does not cause physical dependence. However, it may cause other unwanted effects if too much is taken.

This combination medicine is available only with your doctor's prescription.

Remember:
- **This medicine has been prescribed for your current medical problem only.** It must not be given to other people or used for other problems unless you are directed to do so by your doctor.
- **Keep all medicines out of the reach of children.**
- In order for this medicine to work, it must be used as directed.
- **It is very important that you read and understand the following information.** If any of the information causes you special concern, do not decide against using this medicine without first checking with your doctor.
- Before you begin using any new medicine (prescription or nonprescription) or if you develop any new medical problem while you are using this medicine, check with your doctor, nurse, or pharmacist.

- **If you have any questions** about the following information or if you want more information about this medicine or your medical problem, **ask your doctor, nurse, or pharmacist.**

Before Using This Medicine

In order to decide on the best treatment for your medical problem, your doctor should be told:

—if you have ever had any unusual or allergic reaction to a barbiturate, codeine, aspirin or other salicylates including methyl salicylate (oil of wintergreen), caffeine, or any of the following medicines:

Diclofenac (e.g., Voltaren)
Diflunisal (e.g., Dolobid)
Fenoprofen (e.g., Nalfon)
Flurbiprofen, oral (e.g., Ansaid)
Ibuprofen (e.g., Advil; Motrin; Nuprin)
Indomethacin (e.g., Indocid; Indocin)
Ketoprofen (e.g., Orudis)
Meclofenamate (e.g., Meclomen)
Mefenamic acid (e.g., Ponstan; Ponstel)
Naproxen (e.g., Anaprox; Naprosyn)
Oxyphenbutazone (e.g., Oxalid; Tandearil)
Phenylbutazone (e.g., Azolid; Butazolidin)
Piroxicam (e.g., Feldene)
Sulindac (e.g., Clinoril)
Suprofen (e.g., Suprol)
Tiaprofenic acid (e.g., Surgam)
Tolmetin (e.g., Tolectin)
Zomepirac (e.g., Zomax)

—if you are on a low-salt, low-sugar, or any other special diet, or if you are allergic to any substance, such as foods, sulfites or other preservatives, or dyes. Most medicines contain more than their active ingredient. Your doctor, nurse, or pharmacist can help you avoid products that may cause a problem.

—if you are **pregnant** or if you may become pregnant.

For aspirin
Although studies in humans have not shown that aspirin causes birth defects, aspirin has caused birth defects in animal studies.

Some reports have suggested that too much use of aspirin late in pregnancy may cause a decrease in the newborn's weight and possible death of the fetus or newborn baby. However, the mothers in these reports had been taking much larger amounts of aspirin than are usually recommended. Studies of mothers taking aspirin in the doses that are usually recommended did not show these unwanted effects.

There is a chance that regular use of aspirin late in pregnancy may cause unwanted effects on the heart or blood flow in the fetus or in the newborn baby. Also, use of aspirin during the last 2 weeks of pregnancy may cause bleeding problems in the fetus before or during delivery or in the newborn baby. In addition, too much use of aspirin during the last 3 months of pregnancy may increase the length of pregnancy, prolong labor, cause other problems during delivery, or cause severe bleeding in the mother before, during, or after delivery.

For butalbital
Barbiturates such as butalbital have been shown to increase the chance of birth defects in humans. Also, one study in humans has suggested that barbiturates taken during pregnancy may increase the chance of brain tumors in the baby.

For codeine
Codeine has not been shown to cause birth defects in humans; however, studies on birth defects have not been done in humans. Studies in animals have not shown that codeine causes birth defects. However, it caused slower development of bones and other toxic or harmful effects in the fetus.

For butalbital and codeine
Taking a barbiturate such as butalbital regularly during the last 3 months of pregnancy or taking too much codeine during pregnancy may cause the fetus to become dependent on these medicines. This may lead to withdrawal side effects in the newborn baby. Also, butalbital and codeine may cause breathing problems in the newborn baby if taken just before or during delivery.

For caffeine
Studies in humans have not shown that caffeine causes birth defects. However, studies in animals have shown that caffeine causes birth defects when given in very large doses (amounts equal to those in 12 to 24 cups of coffee a day).

—if you are **breast-feeding**. Although this combination medicine has not been shown to cause problems, the chance always exists, especially if the medicine is taken for a long time or in large amounts. Barbiturates (such as butalbital) pass into the breast milk and may cause drowsiness, unusually slow heartbeat, shortness of breath, or troubled breathing in nursing babies. Aspirin, caffeine, and codeine also pass into the breast milk.

—if you have any of the following medical problems:
Anemia
Asthma, allergies, and nasal polyps (history of)
Brain disease or head injury
Colitis
Convulsions (seizures) (history of)
Emphysema, asthma, or chronic lung disease
Enlarged prostate or problems with urination
Gallbladder disease or gallstones
Gout
Heart disease
Hemophilia or other bleeding problems
Hyperactivity (in children)
Kidney disease
Liver disease
Mental depression
Overactive thyroid
Porphyria (or history of)
Stomach ulcer or other stomach problems
Underactive thyroid
Vitamin K deficiency

—if you regularly take large amounts of antacids, especially calcium- and/or magnesium-containing antacids or sodium bicarbonate (baking soda).

—if you are taking **any** other prescription or nonprescription (OTC) medicine, especially:
Anticoagulants (blood thinners)
Antidiabetic agents, oral (diabetes medicine you take by mouth)
Central nervous system (CNS) depressants
Dipyridamole (e.g., Persantine)
Divalproex (e.g., Depakote)
Heparin
Medicine for pain and/or inflammation
Methotrexate (e.g., Mexate)
Naltrexone (e.g., Trexan)
Probenecid (e.g., Benemid)
Sulfinpyrazone (e.g., Anturane; Anturan)
Urinary alkalizers (medicine that makes the urine less acid, such as acetazolamide [e.g., Diamox], dichlorphenamide [e.g., Daranide], methazolamide [e.g., Neptazane], potassium or sodium citrate and/or citric acid)
Valproic acid (e.g., Depakene)
Vancomycin (e.g., Vancocin)

Proper Use of This Medicine

Take this medicine with food or a full glass (8 ounces) of water to lessen stomach irritation.

There have been reports suggesting that use of aspirin in children or teenagers with fever due to a viral infection (especially flu or chickenpox) may cause a serious illness called Reye's syndrome. This medicine contains aspirin. Therefore, **do not give this medicine to a child or a teenager with symptoms of flu or chickenpox without first discussing this with your child's doctor.**

Take this medicine only as directed by your doctor. Do not take more of it, do not take it more often, and do not take it for a longer period of time than your doctor ordered. If too much butalbital or codeine is taken, it may become habit-forming (causing mental or physical dependence) or lead to medical problems because of an overdose. Also, taking too much aspirin may cause stomach problems or lead to medical problems because of an overdose.

Do not take this medicine if it has a strong vinegar-like odor, since this means the aspirin in it is breaking down. If you have any questions about this, check with your doctor or pharmacist.

If your doctor has ordered you to take this medicine according to a regular schedule and you miss a dose, take it as soon as you remember. However, if it is almost time for your next dose, skip the missed dose and go back to your regular dosing schedule. Do not double doses.

How to store this medicine:

• **Keep out of the reach of children** because overdose is especially dangerous in young children.

• Store away from heat and direct light.

• Do not store this medicine in the bathroom, near the kitchen sink, or in other damp places. Heat or moisture may cause the medicine to break down.

• Do not keep outdated medicine or medicine no longer needed. Be sure that any discarded medicine is out of the reach of children.

Precautions While Using This Medicine

If you will be taking this medicine for a long period of time (for example, for several months at a time) or in high doses, your doctor should check your progress at regular visits.

Check the labels of all over-the-counter (OTC), nonprescription, and prescription medicines you now take. If any contain a narcotic, a barbiturate, aspirin, or other salicylates including diflunisal, be especially careful, since taking them while taking this medicine may lead to overdose. If you have any questions about this, check with your doctor or pharmacist.

The butalbital and the codeine in this medicine will add to the effects of alcohol and other CNS depressants (medicines that slow down the nervous system, possibly causing drowsiness). Some examples of CNS depressants are antihistamines or medicine for hay fever, other allergies, or colds; sedatives, tranquilizers, or sleeping medicine; other prescription pain medicine or narcotics; other barbiturates; medicine for convulsions (seizures); tricyclic antidepressants (medicine for depression); muscle relaxants; or anesthetics, including some dental anesthetics. Also, stomach problems may be more likely to occur if you drink alcoholic beverages while you are taking aspirin. Therefore, **do not drink alcoholic beverages, and check with your doctor before taking any of the medicines listed above, while you are using this medicine.**

Too much use of acetaminophen together with this combination medicine may increase the chance of kidney or liver problems. Therefore, do not regularly take acetaminophen together with this medicine, unless directed to do so by your doctor.

Too much use of aspirin in this medicine together with certain other medicines may increase the chance of unwanted effects. Therefore, do not regularly take this medicine with any of the following, unless directed to do so by your doctor.

Diclofenac (e.g., Voltaren)
Diflunisal (e.g., Dolobid)
Fenoprofen (e.g., Nalfon)
Flurbiprofen, oral (e.g., Ansaid)
Ibuprofen (e.g., Motrin)
Indomethacin (e.g., Indocin)
Ketoprofen (e.g., Orudis)
Meclofenamate (e.g., Meclomen)
Mefenamic acid (e.g., Ponstel)
Naproxen (e.g., Naprosyn)
Phenylbutazone (e.g., Butazolidin)
Piroxicam (e.g., Feldene)
Sulindac (e.g., Clinoril)
Tiaprofenic acid (e.g., Surgam)
Tolmetin (e.g., Tolectin)

This medicine may cause some people to become drowsy, dizzy, or lightheaded, or to feel a false sense of well-being. **Make sure you know how you react to this medicine before you drive, use machines, or do other jobs that require you to be alert and clearheaded.**

Dizziness, lightheadedness, or fainting may be especially likely to occur when you get up suddenly from a lying or sitting position. Getting up slowly may help lessen this problem.

Nausea or vomiting may occur, especially after the first couple of doses. This effect may go away if you lie down for a while. However, if nausea or vomiting continues, check with your doctor. Lying down for a while may also help some other side effects, such as dizziness or lightheadedness.

Before having any kind of surgery (including dental surgery) or emergency treatment, tell the physician or dentist in charge that you are taking this medicine.

Do not take this medicine for 5 days before any surgery, including dental surgery, unless otherwise directed by your physician or dentist. Taking aspirin during this time may cause bleeding problems.

For diabetics—The aspirin in this medicine may cause false urine sugar test results if you regularly take 8 tablets or capsules a day. Occasional use or lower doses of aspirin usually will not affect urine sugar tests. If you have any questions about this, check with your doctor, nurse, or pharmacist, especially if your diabetes is not well controlled.

If you have been taking large amounts of this medicine, or if you have been taking it regularly for several weeks or more, **do not suddenly stop using it without first checking with your doctor.** Your doctor may want you to reduce gradually the amount you are taking before stopping completely, to lessen the chance of withdrawal side effects.

If you think you or anyone else may have taken an overdose of this medicine, get emergency help at once. Taking an overdose of this medicine or taking alcohol or CNS depressants with this medicine may lead to unconsciousness or death. Signs of overdose of this medicine include convulsions (seizures); hearing loss; confusion; ringing or buzzing in the ears; severe excitement, nervousness, or restlessness; severe dizziness; severe drowsiness; unusually slow or troubled breathing; and severe weakness.

Side Effects of This Medicine

Along with its needed effects, a medicine may cause some unwanted effects. Although not all of these side effects may occur, if they do occur they may need medical attention.

Get emergency help immediately if any of the following side effects occur:
Less common or rare
   Shortness of breath, troubled breathing, tightness in chest, or wheezing

Signs of overdose
  Any loss of hearing
  Bloody urine
  Cold, clammy skin
  Convulsions (seizures)
  Diarrhea (severe or continuing)
  Dizziness, lightheadedness, or drowsiness (severe)
  Hallucinations (seeing, hearing, or feeling things that are not there)
  Headache (severe or continuing)
  Low blood pressure
  Nausea or vomiting (severe or continuing)
  Nervousness, excitement, or confusion (severe)
  Pinpoint pupils of eyes
  Poor judgment
  Ringing or buzzing in ears (continuing)
  Slow heartbeat
  Slow or irregular breathing
  Slurred speech
  Staggering
  Trouble in sleeping
  Uncontrollable flapping movements of the hands (especially in elderly patients)
  Unexplained fever
  Unusual irritability (continuing)
  Unusual movements of the eyes
  Unusual thirst
  Vision problems
  Weakness (severe)

Also, check with your doctor as soon as possible if any of the following side effects occur:

More common
  Nausea or vomiting
  Stomach pain

Less common or rare
  Bloody or black tarry stools
  Confusion or mental depression
  Fast or pounding heartbeat
  Skin rash, hives, or itching
  Sore throat and fever
  Stomach pain (severe)
  Swelling of eyelids, face or lips
  Trembling or uncontrolled muscle movements
  Unusual bleeding or bruising
  Unusual excitement
  Unusual tiredness or weakness
  Vomiting of blood or material that looks like coffee grounds
  Yellow eyes or skin

Other side effects may occur that usually do not require medical attention. These side effects may go away during treatment as your body adjusts to the medicine. However, check with your doctor if any of the following side effects continue or are bothersome:

More common
  Clumsiness or unsteadiness
  Constipation
  Dizziness, lightheadedness, or drowsiness
  "Hangover" effect
  Heartburn or indigestion

Less common or rare
  Blurred or double vision or other changes in vision
  Decrease in amount of urine
  Difficult or painful urination
  Dry mouth
  False sense of well-being
  Feeling faint
  Frequent urge to urinate
  General feeling of discomfort or illness
  Headache
  Increased sweating
  Loss of appetite
  Nightmares or unusual dreams
  Redness or flushing of face
  Trouble in sleeping
  Unusual anxiety, nervousness, restlessness, or irritability

For children or elderly patients: Some of the above side effects are more likely to occur in children, especially those with a fever or those who have lost large amounts of body fluid because of vomiting, diarrhea, or sweating, and in elderly patients (60 years of age or older) or very ill patients. These patients are usually more sensitive to the effects of butalbital, codeine (especially the breathing problems it can cause), and aspirin.

After you stop using this medicine, your body may need time to adjust. The length of time this takes depends on the amount of medicine you were using and how long you used it. During this period of time check with your doctor if you notice any of the following side effects:
  Body aches
  Convulsions (seizures)
  Diarrhea
  Dizziness, lightheadedness, or feeling faint
  Gooseflesh
  Hallucinations (seeing, hearing, or feeling things that are not there)
  Increased sweating
  Increased yawning
  Loss of appetite
  Nausea or vomiting
  Shivering, trembling, or muscle twitching
  Stomach cramps
  Trouble in sleeping, increased dreaming, or nightmares
  Unexplained fever or continuing runny nose or sneezing
  Unusual anxiety, nervousness, restlessness, or irritability
  Vision problems
  Weakness

Other side effects not listed above may also occur in some patients. If you notice any other effects, check with your doctor.

December 1987

CAFFEINE (Systemic)

Some commonly used brand names and other names are:

Caffedrine	Quick Pep
Citrated Caffeine	Tirend
Dexitac	Vivarin
NoDoz	

Generic name product may also be available in the U.S.

To the Reader: If you do not recognize the names of medical conditions or medicines referred to in this information, check with your doctor, nurse, or pharmacist. Definitions for selected medical terms may be found in the Glossary. Brand names for the generic drug names listed can be found in the Index. In addition, selected brand names commonly associated with the generic name have been included in the text to help you recognize medicine you may be taking. The fact that a brand name product is not mentioned does not mean the information does not apply. It is a good idea for you to learn both the generic and brand names of your medicines and to write them down for future use.

Caffeine (kaf-FEEN) belongs to the group of medicines called central nervous system (CNS) stimulants. It is taken by mouth to help restore mental alertness when fatigue or drowsiness occurs. It is not intended to replace sleep and should not be used routinely for this purpose.

Caffeine is also used in combination with ergotamine or with certain pain relievers such as aspirin or acetaminophen, for relief of headaches or menstrual tension. When used in this way, caffeine may increase the effectiveness of the other medicines. Caffeine is also used in combination with some antihistamines to overcome the drowsiness caused by them.

Caffeine may be given by mouth or injection to premature babies who have breathing problems. It may also be used for other conditions as determined by your doctor.

Caffeine is present in coffee, tea, cola drinks, cocoa, and chocolate.

As a medicine, it is available without a prescription; however, your doctor or pharmacist may have special instructions on its proper use.

Remember:

• **Keep all medicines out of the reach of children.**

• In order for this medicine to work, it must be used as directed. **If you are using this medicine without a prescription, it is very important that you follow the directions on the label.**

• **It is also very important that you read and understand the following information.** If any of the information causes you special concern, check with your doctor before using this medicine without a prescription.

• Before you begin using any new medicine (prescription or nonprescription) or if you develop any new medical problem while you are using this medicine, check with your doctor, nurse, or pharmacist.

• **If you have any questions** about the following information or if you want more information about this medicine or your medical problem, **ask your doctor, nurse, or pharmacist.**

Before Using This Medicine

Before you use caffeine, check with your doctor or pharmacist:

—if you have ever had any unusual or allergic reaction to aminophylline, caffeine, dyphylline, oxtriphylline, theobromine (also found in cocoa or chocolate), or theophylline.

—if you are on a low-salt, low-sugar, or any other special diet, or if you are allergic to any substance, such as foods, sulfites or other preservatives, or dyes. Most medicines contain more than their active ingredient.

—if you are **pregnant** or if you may become pregnant. Studies in humans have not shown that caffeine causes birth defects. However, studies in animals have shown that caffeine causes birth defects when given in very large doses (amounts equal to 12 to 24 cups of coffee a day) and problems with bone growth when given in smaller doses.

—if you are **breast-feeding**. Caffeine passes into breast milk in small amounts and may build up in the nursing baby. Studies have shown that babies may appear jittery and have trouble in sleeping when their mothers drink large amounts of caffeine-containing beverages.

—if you have any of the following medical problems:
Agoraphobia
Heart disease
High blood pressure
Liver disease
Panic attacks
Peptic ulcer
Trouble in sleeping

—if you are taking **any** prescription or nonprescription (OTC) medicine, especially:
Amantadine (e.g., Symmetrel)
Amphetamines (e.g., Desoxyn; Dexedrine)
Appetite suppressants (diet pills), except fenfluramine
Chlophedianol
Medicine for asthma or other breathing problems
Medicine for colds, sinus problems, hay fever or other allergies (including nose drops or sprays)
Methylphenidate (e.g., Ritalin)
Other medicines containing caffeine
Pemoline (e.g., Cylert)

—if you are now taking or have taken within the past 2 weeks monoamine oxidase (MAO) inhibitors, such as:

Furazolidone (e.g., Furoxone)
Isocarboxazid (e.g., Marplan)
Pargyline (e.g., Eutonyl)
Phenelzine (e.g., Nardil)
Procarbazine (e.g., Matulane)
Tranylcypromine (e.g., Parnate)

Proper Use of This Medicine

For patients taking the extended-release form of this medicine:

• Swallow the capsule whole.

• Do not break, crush, or chew the capsule before swallowing.

Take caffeine only as directed. Do not take more of it, do not take it more often, and do not take it for a longer period of time than directed. Taking too much may increase the chance of side effects. It may also become habit-forming.

If you think this medicine is not working as well after you have taken it for a long time, **do not increase the dose.** To do so may increase the chance of side effects.

How to store this medicine:

- **Keep out of the reach of children.** Young children are especially sensitive to caffeine's side effects.

- Store away from heat and direct light.

- Do not store in the bathroom, near the kitchen sink, or in other damp places. Heat or moisture may cause the medicine to break down.

- Do not keep outdated medicine or medicine no longer needed. Be sure that any discarded medicine is out of the reach of children.

Precautions While Using This Medicine

If fatigue or drowsiness continues for more than 2 weeks, or returns often, check with your doctor.

Do not drink large amounts of caffeine-containing coffee, tea, or colas while you are taking this medicine. To do so may cause unwanted effects.

The amount of caffeine in some common foods and beverages is as follows:
Coffee, brewed—100 to 150 mg per cup.
Coffee, instant—86 to 99 mg per cup.
Coffee, decaffeinated—2 to 4 mg per cup.
Tea—60 to 75 mg per cup.
Cola drinks—40 to 72 mg per 12 ounces.
Cocoa—6 to 42 mg per cup.
Chocolate, milk—3 to 6 mg per ounce.
Chocolate, bittersweet—25 mg per ounce.

Caffeine may cause dizziness or a fast or strong heartbeat. If this occurs, discontinue the use of caffeine-containing beverages or medicines.

Do not take caffeine-containing beverages or medicines too close to bedtime, to prevent trouble in sleeping.

Side Effects of This Medicine

Along with its needed effects, a medicine may cause some unwanted effects. Although not all of these side effects may occur, they may be more likely to occur if caffeine is taken in large doses or more often than recommended. If they do occur, they may need medical attention.

Check with your doctor as soon as possible if any of the following side effects occur:

More common
Diarrhea
Dizziness
Fast heartbeat
Nervousness
Trouble in sleeping

In newborn babies
Abdominal pain
Nervousness, severe jitters, or whole-body tremors
Vomiting

Signs of overdose
Abdominal or stomach pain
Agitation, anxiety, excitement, or restlessness
Confusion or delirium
Convulsions (seizures)—in acute overdose
Fever
Flashes of "zig-zag" lights in eyes
Frequent urination
Headache
Increased sensitivity to touch or pain
Irritability
Muscle trembling or twitching
Nausea and vomiting, sometimes with blood
Rapid or irregular heartbeat
Ringing or other sounds in ears
Trouble in sleeping

Other side effects may occur that usually do not require medical attention. These side effects may go away during treatment as your body adjusts to the medicine. However, check with your doctor if any of the following side effects continue or are bothersome:

More common
Nausea (mild)
Nervousness or jitters (mild)

After you stop using this medicine, your body may need time to adjust. The length of time this takes depends on the amount of medicine you were using and how long you used it. During this period of time check with your doctor if you notice any of the following side effects:

More common
Anxiety
Dizziness
Headache
Irritability
Muscle tension
Nausea
Nervousness
Stuffy nose

Side effects are more likely to occur in children, who usually are more sensitive to the effects of caffeine.

For elderly patients: Many medicines have not been tested in older people. Therefore, it is not known whether the medicine acts the same way it does in younger adults. Check with your doctor or pharmacist if you notice any unusual effects while taking this medicine or if you think it is not working as it should.

Other side effects not listed above may also occur in some patients. If you notice any other effects, check with your doctor.

December 1987

CALCIFEDIOL (Systemic)

A commonly used brand name is Calderol.

To the Reader: If you do not recognize the names of medical conditions or medicines referred to in this information, check with your doctor, nurse, or pharmacist. Definitions for selected medical terms may be found in the Glossary. Brand names for the generic drug names listed can be found in the Index. In addition, selected brand names commonly associated with the generic name have been included in the text to help you recognize medicine you may be taking. The fact that a brand name product is not mentioned does not mean the information does not apply. It is a good idea for you to learn both the generic and brand names of your medicines and to write them down for future use.

Calcifediol (kal-si-fe-DYE-ole) is a form of vitamin D which is taken by mouth to treat hypocalcemia (not enough calcium in the blood). It is also used to treat certain types of bone disease that may occur with kidney disease in patients who are undergoing renal dialysis. It may also be used for other conditions as determined by your doctor.

Calcifediol is available only with your doctor's prescription.

Remember:

• **This medicine has been prescribed for your current medical problem only.** It must not be given to other people or used for other problems unless you are directed to do so by your doctor.

• **Keep all medicines out of the reach of children.**

• In order for this medicine to work, it must be used as directed.

• **It is very important that you read and understand the following information.** If any of the information causes you special concern, do not decide against using this medicine without first checking with your doctor.

• Before you begin using any new medicine (prescription or nonprescription) or if you develop any new medical problem while you are using this medicine, check with your doctor, nurse, or pharmacist.

• **If you have any questions** about the following information or if you want more information about this medicine or your medical problem, **ask your doctor, nurse, or pharmacist.**

Before Using This Medicine

In order to decide on the best treatment for your medical problem, your doctor should be told:

—if you have ever had any unusual or allergic reaction to any form of vitamin D, including calcitriol or dihydrotachysterol.

—if you are on a low-salt, low-sugar, or any other special diet, or if you are allergic to any substance, such as foods, sulfites or other preservatives, or dyes. Most medicines contain more than their active ingredient. Your doctor, nurse, or pharmacist can help you avoid products that may cause a problem.

—if you are **pregnant** or if you may become pregnant. Normal amounts of vitamin D have not been shown to cause birth defects or other problems in humans.

However, studies in humans have not been done. In animal studies, calcifediol has been shown to cause birth defects when given in doses several times the human dose.

—if you are **breast-feeding**. Only small amounts of calcifediol pass into breast milk and it has not been shown to cause problems in nursing babies.

—if you have any of the following medical problems:
  Heart or blood vessel disease
  Kidney disease
  Sarcoidosis

—if you are taking **any** other prescription or nonprescription (OTC) medicine, especially:
  Antacids containing magnesium
  Vitamin D (other forms, including calcitriol or dihydrotachysterol)

Proper Use of This Medicine

Take this medicine only as directed. Do not take more of it and do not take it more often than your doctor ordered. To do so may increase the chance of overdose.

While you are taking this medicine, your doctor may want you to follow a special diet or take a calcium supplement. Be sure to follow instructions carefully. If you are already taking a calcium supplement or any medicine containing calcium, make sure your doctor knows.

If you miss a dose of this medicine and your dosing schedule is one dose to be taken:

Every other day—Take the missed dose as soon as possible if you remember it on the day it should be taken. However, if you do not remember the missed dose until the next day, take it at that time. Then skip a day and start your dosing schedule again. Do not double doses.

Once a day—Take the missed dose as soon as possible. However, if you do not remember the missed dose until the next day, skip the missed dose and go back to your regular dosing schedule. Do not double doses.

More than once a day—Take the missed dose as soon as possible. However, if it is almost time for your next dose, skip the missed dose and go back to your regular dosing schedule. Do not double doses.

If you have any questions about this, check with your doctor.

How to store this medicine:

• **Keep out of the reach of children.**

• Store away from heat and direct light.

• Do not store in the bathroom, near the kitchen sink, or in other damp places. Heat or moisture may cause the medicine to break down.

• Do not keep outdated medicine or medicine no longer needed. Be sure that any discarded medicine is out of the reach of children.

Precautions While Using This Medicine

Your doctor should check your progress at regular visits to make sure that this medicine does not cause unwanted effects.

Do not take any nonprescription or over-the-counter (OTC) medicine while you are taking this medicine, unless you have been told to do so by your doctor. The calcium, phosphorus, or vitamin D that these medicines may contain may increase the chance of side effects.

Do not take antacids containing magnesium while you are taking this medicine. Taking these medicines together may cause unwanted effects.

Side Effects of This Medicine

Along with its needed effects, a medicine may cause some unwanted effects. Vitamin D does not usually cause any side effects. However, **taking large amounts of vitamin D over a period of time may cause some unwanted effects that can be serious.**

Check with your doctor immediately if any of the following effects occur:

Late signs of severe overdose
   Convulsions (seizures)
   High blood pressure
   Irregular heartbeat
   Stomach pain (severe)

Check with your doctor as soon as possible if any of the following effects occur:

Early signs of overdose
   Constipation (especially in children or adolescents)
   Diarrhea
   Dry mouth
   Headache (continuing)
   Increase in thirst
   Loss of appetite
   Metallic taste
   Nausea or vomiting (especially in children or adolescents)
   Unusual tiredness or weakness

Late signs of overdose
   Bone pain
   Cloudy urine
   Increased sensitivity of eyes to light or irritation of eyes
   Increase in frequency of urination, especially at night, or in amount of urine
   Itching of skin
   Mood or mental changes
   Muscle pain
   Nausea or vomiting (severe)
   Weight loss

For children: Some of the above early signs of overdose, such as constipation and nausea or vomiting, are more likely to occur in children and adolescents. Also, children may show slowed growth when receiving vitamin D for a long time.

Other side effects not listed above may also occur in some patients. If you notice any other effects, check with your doctor.

December 1987

CALCITONIN (Systemic)

Some commonly used brand names are Calcimar, Cibacalcin, and Miacalcin.

To the Reader: If you do not recognize the names of medical conditions or medicines referred to in this information, check with your doctor, nurse, or pharmacist. Definitions for selected medical terms may be found in the Glossary. Brand names for the generic drug names listed can be found in the Index. In addition, selected brand names commonly associated with the generic name have been included in the text to help you recognize medicine you may be taking. The fact that a brand name product is not mentioned does not mean the information does not apply. It is a good idea for you to learn both the generic and brand names of your medicines and to write them down for future use.

Calcitonin (kal-si-TOE-nin) is given by injection to treat Paget's disease of bone. It also may be used to prevent continuing bone loss in women with postmenopausal osteoporosis and in the treatment of too much calcium in the blood.

Calcitonin is available only with your doctor's prescription.

Remember:

• **This medicine has been prescribed for your current medical problem only.** It must not be given to other people or used for other problems unless you are directed to do so by your doctor.

• **Keep all medicines out of the reach of children.**

• In order for this medicine to work, it must be used as directed.

• **It is very important that you read and understand the following information.** If any of the information causes you special concern, do not decide against using this medicine without first checking with your doctor.

• Before you begin using any new medicine (prescription or nonprescription) or if you develop any new medical problem while you are using this medicine, check with your doctor, nurse, or pharmacist.

• **If you have any questions** about the following information or if you want more information about this medicine or your medical problem, **ask your doctor, nurse, or pharmacist.**

Before Using This Medicine

In order to decide on the best treatment for your medical problem, your doctor should be told:

—if you have any allergies, especially to proteins. Calcitonin is a protein and some patients may be allergic to it.

—if you are on a low-salt, low-sugar, or any other special diet, or if you are allergic to any substance, such as foods or sulfites or other preservatives. Most medicines contain more than their active ingredient. Your doctor, nurse, or pharmacist can help you avoid products that may cause a problem.

—if you are **pregnant** or if you may become pregnant. Although studies have not been done in humans, calcitonin has not been shown to cause birth defects or

other problems in humans. However, studies in animals have shown that this medicine lowers the birth weight of the baby when the mother is given doses many times the human dose.

—if you are **breast-feeding.** Calcitonin has not been shown to cause problems in nursing babies. However, studies in animals have shown that calcitonin may decrease the flow of breast milk.

—if you are using this medicine for hypercalcemia (too much calcium in the blood) and are taking **any** other prescription or nonprescription (OTC) medicine, especially:

Medicine containing calcium
Vitamin D (including calcifediol and calcitriol)

Proper Use of This Medicine

This medicine is for injection only. If you will be giving yourself the injections, make sure you understand exactly how to give them. If you have any questions about this, check with your doctor.

Use the calcitonin only when the contents of the syringe are clear and colorless. Do not use it if it looks grainy or discolored.

Take this medicine only as directed by your doctor. Do not take more of it and do not take it more often than your doctor ordered.

If you miss a dose of this medicine and your dosing schedule is:

Every other day—Give the missed dose as soon as possible if you remember it on the day it should be given. Then go back to your regular dosing schedule. But if you do not remember the missed dose until the next day, give it at that time. Then skip a day and start your dosing schedule again.

Once a day—Give the missed dose as soon as possible. Then go back to your regular dosing schedule. But if you do not remember the missed dose until the next day, skip it and go back to your regular dosing schedule. Do not double doses.

Twice a day—If you remember within 2 hours of the missed dose, give it right away. Then go back to your regular dosing schedule. But if you do not remember the missed dose until later, skip it and go back to your regular dosing schedule. Do not double doses.

Three times a week—Give the missed dose the next day. Then set each injection back a day for the rest of the week. Go back to your regular Monday-Wednesday-Friday schedule the following week. Do not double doses.

How to store this medicine:

• **Keep out of the reach of children.**

• Store away from heat and direct light.

• Store the calcitonin-human at a temperature below 77 °F. Do not refrigerate. Use prepared solution within 6 hours.

© 1988   The United States Pharmacopeial Convention, Inc.

• Store calcitonin-salmon in the refrigerator. However, keep the medicine from freezing.

• Do not keep outdated medicine or medicine no longer needed. Be sure that any discarded medicine is out of the reach of children.

Precautions While Using This Medicine

Your doctor should check your progress at regular visits to make sure that this medicine does not cause unwanted effects.

If you are using this medicine for hypercalcemia (too much calcium in the blood), your doctor may want you to follow a low-calcium diet. If you have any questions about this, check with your doctor.

Side Effects of This Medicine

Along with its needed effects, a medicine may cause some unwanted effects. Although not all of these side effects may occur, if they do occur they may need medical attention.

Check with your doctor as soon as possible if either of the following side effects occurs:

Rare
   Skin rash or hives

Other side effects may occur that usually do not require medical attention. These side effects may go away during treatment as your body adjusts to the medicine.

However, check with your doctor if any of the following side effects continue or are bothersome:

More common
   Diarrhea
   Flushing or redness of face, ears, hands, or feet
   Loss of appetite
   Nausea or vomiting
   Pain, redness, soreness, or swelling at place of injection
   Stomach pain
Less common
   Increased frequency of urination
Rare
   Chills
   Dizziness
   Headache
   Pressure in chest
   Stuffy nose
   Tenderness or tingling of hands or feet
   Trouble in breathing
   Weakness

For elderly patients: Many medicines have not been tested in older people. Therefore, it is not known whether the medicine acts the same way it does in younger adults. Check with your doctor or pharmacist if you notice any unusual effects while taking this medicine or if you think it is not working as it should.

Other side effects not listed above may also occur in some patients. If you notice any other effects, check with your doctor.

December 1987

CALCITRIOL (Systemic)

Some commonly used brand names are Calcijex and Rocaltrol.

To the Reader: If you do not recognize the names of medical conditions or medicines referred to in this information, check with your doctor, nurse, or pharmacist. Definitions for selected medical terms may be found in the Glossary. Brand names for the generic drug names listed can be found in the Index. In addition, selected brand names commonly associated with the generic name have been included in the text to help you recognize medicine you may be taking. The fact that a brand name product is not mentioned does not mean the information does not apply. It is a good idea for you to learn both the generic and brand names of your medicines and to write them down for future use.

Calcitriol (kal-si-TRYE-ole) is a form of vitamin D taken by mouth to treat hypocalcemia (not enough calcium in the blood). It is also used to treat certain types of bone disease that may occur with kidney disease in patients who are undergoing renal dialysis. It may also be used for other conditions as determined by your doctor.

Calcitriol is available only with your doctor's prescription.

Remember:
• **This medicine has been prescribed for your current medical problem only.** It must not be given to other people or used for other problems unless you are directed to do so by your doctor.

• **Keep all medicines out of the reach of children.**

• If you are receiving this medicine by injection, some of the information about this medicine may not apply.

• In order for this medicine to work, it must be used as directed.

• **It is very important that you read and understand the following information.** If any of the information causes you special concern, do not decide against using this medicine without first checking with your doctor.

• Before you begin using any new medicine (prescription or nonprescription) or if you develop any new medical problem while you are using this medicine, check with your doctor, nurse, or pharmacist.

• **If you have any questions** about the following information or if you want more information about this medicine or your medical problem, **ask your doctor, nurse, or pharmacist.**

Before Using This Medicine

In order to decide on the best treatment for your medical problem, your doctor should be told:

—if you have ever had any unusual or allergic reaction to any form of vitamin D, including calcifediol or dihydrotachysterol.

—if you are on a low-salt, low-sugar, or any other special diet, or if you are allergic to any substance, such as foods, sulfites or other preservatives, or dyes. Most medicines contain more than their active ingredient. Your doctor, nurse, or pharmacist can help you avoid products that may cause a problem.

—if you are **pregnant** or if you may become pregnant. Normal amounts of vitamin D have not been shown to cause birth defects or other problems in humans. However, studies in humans have not been done. In animal studies, calcitriol has been shown to cause birth defects when given in doses several times the human dose.

—if you are **breast-feeding.** Only small amounts of calcitriol pass into breast milk and it has not been shown to cause problems in nursing babies.

—if you have any of the following medical problems:
Heart or blood vessel disease
Kidney disease
Sarcoidosis

—if you are taking **any** other prescription or nonprescription (OTC) medicine, especially:
Antacids containing magnesium
Vitamin D (other forms, including calcifediol or dihydrotachysterol)

Proper Use of This Medicine

Take this medicine only as directed. Do not take more of it and do not take it more often than your doctor ordered. To do so may increase the chance of overdose.

While you are taking this medicine, your doctor may want you to follow a special diet or take a calcium supplement. Be sure to follow instructions carefully. If you are already taking a calcium supplement or any medicine containing calcium, make sure your doctor knows.

If you miss a dose of this medicine and your dosing schedule is one dose to be taken:

Every other day—Take the missed dose as soon as possible if you remember it on the day it should be taken. However, if you do not remember the missed dose until the next day, take it at that time. Then skip a day and start your dosing schedule again. Do not double doses.

Once a day—Take the missed dose as soon as possible. Then go back to your regular dosing schedule. However, if you do not remember the missed dose until the next day, skip the missed dose and go back to your regular dosing schedule. Do not double doses.

More than once a day—Take the missed dose as soon as possible. Then go back to your regular dosing schedule. However, if it is almost time for your next dose, skip the missed dose and go back to your regular dosing schedule. Do not double doses.

If you have any questions about this, check with your doctor.

How to store this medicine:

• **Keep out of the reach of children.**

• Store away from heat and direct light.

• Do not store the capsule form of this medicine in the bathroom, near the kitchen sink, or in other damp places. Heat or moisture may cause the medicine to break down.

• Keep the injection form of this medicine from freezing.

• Do not keep outdated medicine or medicine no longer needed. Be sure that any discarded medicine is out of the reach of children.

Precautions While Using This Medicine

Your doctor should check your progress at regular visits to make sure that this medicine does not cause unwanted effects.

Do not take any nonprescription or over-the-counter (OTC) medicine while you are taking this medicine, unless you have been told to do so by your doctor. The calcium, phosphorus, or vitamin D that these medicines may contain may increase the chance of side effects.

Do not take antacids containing magnesium while you are taking this medicine. Taking these medicines together may cause unwanted effects.

Side Effects of This Medicine

Along with its needed effects, a medicine may cause some unwanted effects. Calcitriol does not usually cause any side effects. However, **taking large amounts of vitamin D over a period of time may cause some unwanted effects that can be serious.**

Check with your doctor immediately if any of the following effects occur:
Late signs of severe overdose
  Convulsions (seizures)
  High blood pressure
  Irregular heartbeat
  Stomach pain (severe)

Check with your doctor as soon as possible if any of the following effects occur:
Early signs of overdose
  Constipation (especially in children or adolescents)
  Diarrhea
  Dry mouth
  Headache (continuing)
  Increase in thirst
  Loss of appetite
  Metallic taste
  Nausea or vomiting (especially in children or adolescents)
  Unusual tiredness or weakness
Late signs of overdose
  Bone pain
  Cloudy urine
  Increased sensitivity of eyes to light or irritation of eyes
  Increase in frequency of urination, especially at night, or in amount of urine
  Itching of skin
  Mood or mental changes
  Muscle pain
  Nausea or vomiting (severe)
  Weight loss

For children: Some of the above early signs of overdose, such as constipation and nausea or vomiting, are more likely to occur in children and adolescents. Also, some children may show slowed growth when receiving vitamin D for a long time.

Other side effects not listed above may also occur in some patients. If you notice any other effects, check with your doctor.

December 1987

CALCIUM CHANNEL BLOCKING AGENTS (Systemic)

This information applies to the following medicines:

Diltiazem (dil-TYE-a-zem)
Nifedipine (nye-FED-i-peen)
Verapamil (ver-AP-a-mil)

Some commonly used brand names are:	Generic names:
Cardizem	Diltiazem
Adalat
Procardia	Nifedipine
Calan
Calan SR
Isoptin
Isoptin SR	Verapamil†

†Generic name product may also be available in the U.S.

To the Reader: If you do not recognize the names of medical conditions or medicines referred to in this information, check with your doctor, nurse, or pharmacist. Definitions for selected medical terms may be found in the Glossary. Brand names for the generic drug names listed can be found in the Index. In addition, selected brand names commonly associated with the generic name have been included in the text to help you recognize medicine you may be taking. The fact that a brand name product is not mentioned does not mean the information does not apply. It is a good idea for you to learn both the generic and brand names of your medicines and to write them down for future use.

Diltiazem, nifedipine, and verapamil belong to the group of medicines called calcium channel blockers. They are taken by mouth or given by injection to relieve and control angina (chest pain).

Calcium channel blocking agents affect the movement of calcium into the cells of the heart and blood vessels. As a result, they relax blood vessels and increase the supply of blood and oxygen to the heart while reducing its work load.

Some of these medicines are also used to treat high blood pressure. High blood pressure adds to the workload of the heart and arteries. If it continues for a long time, the heart and arteries may not function properly. This can damage the blood vessels of the brain, heart, and kidneys, resulting in a stroke, heart failure, or kidney failure. High blood pressure may also increase the risk of heart attacks. These problems may be less likely to occur if blood pressure is controlled.

Calcium channel blocking agents may also be used for other conditions as determined by your doctor.

These medicines are available only with your doctor's prescription.

Remember:

• **This medicine has been prescribed for your current medical problem only.** It must not be given to other people or used for other problems unless you are directed to do so by your doctor.

• **Keep all medicines out of the reach of children.**

• In order for this medicine to work, it must be used as directed.

• If you are receiving this medicine by injection, some of the information about this medicine may not apply.

• **It is very important that you read and understand the following information.** If any of the information causes you special concern, do not decide against using this medicine without first checking with your doctor.

• Before you begin using any new medicine (prescription or nonprescription) or if you develop any new medical problem while you are using this medicine, check with your doctor, nurse, or pharmacist.

• **If you have any questions** about the following information or if you want more information about this medicine or your medical problem, **ask your doctor, nurse, or pharmacist**.

Before Using This Medicine

In order to decide on the best treatment for your medical problem, your doctor should be told:

—if you have ever had any unusual or allergic reaction to diltiazem, nifedipine, or verapamil.

—if you are on a low-salt, low-sugar, or any other special diet, or if you are allergic to any substance, such as foods, sulfites or other preservatives, or dyes. Most medicines contain more than their active ingredient. Your doctor, nurse, or pharmacist can help you avoid products that may cause a problem.

—if you are **pregnant** or if you may become pregnant. Studies have not been done in humans. However, studies in animals have shown that large doses of calcium channel blockers cause birth defects, prolonged pregnancy, poor bone development, and stillbirth.

—if you are **breast-feeding**. Although these medicines may pass into breast milk, they have not been shown to cause problems in nursing babies.

—if you have any of the following medical problems:
Kidney disease
Liver disease
Other heart or blood vessel disorders

—if you are taking **any** other prescription or nonprescription (OTC) medicine, especially:
Beta-blockers (acebutolol, atenolol, labetalol, metoprolol, nadolol, oxprenolol, pindolol, propranolol, sotalol, timolol)
Carbamazepine (e.g., Tegretol)
Cyclosporine (e.g., Sandimmune)
Digitalis glycosides (heart medicine)
Disopyramide (e.g., Norpace)
Quinidine (e.g., Quinidex)

Proper Use of This Medicine

Take this medicine exactly as directed even if you feel well and do not notice any signs of chest pain. Do not take more of this medicine and do not take it more often than your doctor ordered. Do not miss any doses.

For patients taking extended-release verapamil tablets:

• Swallow the tablet whole, without breaking, crushing, or chewing it.

• Take the medicine with food or milk.

For patients taking this medicine for high blood pressure:

• **Importance of diet**—When prescribing medicine for your condition, your doctor may also prescribe a personal diet for you. Such a diet may be low in sodium (salt). **Most people eat much more sodium than they need and too much sodium in the diet may increase blood pressure.** Some foods that contain large amounts of sodium are canned soup, pickles, ketchup, green and ripe olives, relish, frankfurters, soy sauce, and carbonated beverages. Your doctor may want you to limit the amounts of these and other high-sodium foods in your diet. **High blood pressure medicine is usually more effective when such a diet is properly followed.**

Also, it may be very important for you to go on a reducing diet. However, check with your doctor before changing your diet.

• Many patients who have high blood pressure will not notice any signs of the problem. In fact, many may feel normal. It is very important that you **take your medicine exactly as directed** and that you keep your appointments with your doctor even if you feel well.

• Remember that this medicine will not cure your high blood pressure but it does help control it. Therefore, you must continue to take it as directed if you expect to lower your blood pressure and keep it down. **You may have to take high blood pressure medicine for the rest of your life.** If high blood pressure is not treated, it can cause serious problems such as heart failure, blood vessel disease, stroke, or kidney disease.

If you do miss a dose of this medicine, take it as soon as possible. However, if it is almost time for your next dose, skip the missed dose and go back to your regular dosing schedule. Do not double doses.

How to store this medicine:

• **Keep out of the reach of children.**

• Store away from heat and direct light.

• Do not store in the bathroom, near the kitchen sink, or in other damp places. Heat or moisture may cause the medicine to break down.

• Do not keep outdated medicine or medicine no longer needed. Be sure that any discarded medicine is out of the reach of children.

Precautions While Using This Medicine

It is important that your doctor check your progress at regular visits. This will allow your doctor to make sure the medicine is working properly and to change the dosage if needed.

If you have been using this medicine regularly for several weeks, do not suddenly stop using it. Stopping suddenly may bring on attacks of angina. Check with your doctor for the best way to reduce gradually the amount you are taking before stopping completely.

Dizziness, lightheadedness, or a fainting feeling may occur, especially when you get up quickly from a lying or sitting position. Getting up slowly may help. **Also, drinking alcohol may make these effects worse and may cause a serious drop in blood pressure.** Check with your doctor before drinking alcoholic beverages while you are taking this medicine.

Chest pain resulting from exercise or physical exertion is usually reduced or prevented by this medicine. This may tempt you to be overly active. **Make sure you discuss with your doctor a safe amount of exercise for your medical problem.**

After taking a dose of this medicine you may get a headache that lasts for a short time. This effect is more common if you are taking nifedipine. This should become less noticeable after you have taken this medicine for a while. If this effect continues or if the headaches are severe, check with your doctor.

In some patients, tenderness, swelling, or bleeding of the gums may appear soon after this treatment with this medicine is started. Brushing and flossing your teeth carefully and regularly and massaging your gums may help prevent this. **See your dentist regularly to have your teeth cleaned. Check with your physician or dentist if you have any questions about how to take care of your teeth and gums, or if you notice any tenderness, swelling, or bleeding of your gums.**

If you are taking diltiazem or verapamil:

• **Ask your doctor how to count your pulse rate. Then, while you are taking this medicine, check your pulse regularly.** If it is much slower than your usual rate, or less than 50 beats per minute, check with your doctor. A pulse rate that is too slow may cause circulation problems.

For patients taking this medicine for high blood pressure:

• **Do not take other medicines unless they have been discussed with your doctor.** This especially includes over-the-counter (nonprescription) medicines for appetite control, asthma, colds, cough, hay fever, or sinus problems, since they may tend to increase your blood pressure.

Side Effects of This Medicine

Along with its needed effects, a medicine may cause some unwanted effects. Although not all of these side effects may occur, if they do occur they may need medical attention.

Check with your doctor as soon as possible if any of the following side effects occur:

Less common
   Breathing difficulty, coughing, or wheezing
   Irregular or fast, pounding heartbeat
   Skin rash
   Slow heartbeat (less than 50 beats per minute—diltiazem and verapamil only)
   Swelling of ankles, feet, or lower legs (more common with nifedipine)

Rare
   Bleeding, tender, or swollen gums
   Chest pain (may appear about 30 minutes after nifedipine is taken)
   Fainting

Other side effects may occur that usually do not require medical attention. These side effects may go away during treatment as your body adjusts to the medicine. However, check with your doctor if any of the following side effects continue or are bothersome:

Less common or rare

Constipation
Dizziness or lightheadedness (more common with nifedipine)
Flushing and feeling of warmth (more common with nifedipine)
Headache (more common with nifedipine)
Nausea (more common with nifedipine)
Nervousness or mood changes
Shakiness or weakness
Stomach cramps
Stuffy nose
Unusual tiredness

Although not all of the side effects listed above have been reported for all of these medicines, they have been reported for at least one of them. Since some of the effects of calcium channel blockers are similar, some of the above side effects may occur with any of these medicines. However, they may be more common with some of these medicines than with others.

For elderly patients: The above side effects may be more likely to occur in the elderly, who are usually more sensitive to this medicine.

Other side effects not listed above may also occur in some patients. If you notice any other effects, check with your doctor.

December 1987

CALCIUM SUPPLEMENTS (Systemic)

This information applies to the following medicines:

Calcium Carbonate (KAL-see-um KAR-boh-nate)
Calcium Citrate (SIH-trayt)
Calcium Glubionate (gloo-BY-oh-nate)
Calcium Gluconate (GLOO-coh-nate)
Calcium Lactate (LAK-tate)
Dibasic (dy-BAY-sic) Calcium Phosphate (FOS-fate)
Tribasic (try-BAY-sic) Calcium Phosphate

This information does not apply to calcium carbonate used as an antacid.

Some commonly used brand names are:	Generic names:
BioCal Cal-Sup Caltrate Os-Cal 500 Suplical Tums‡ Tums E-X‡	Calcium Carbonate†
Citracal	Calcium Citrate
Neo-Calglucon	Calcium Glubionate
	Calcium Gluconate†
	Calcium Lactate†
	Dibasic Calcium Phosphate†
Posture	Tribasic Calcium Phosphate

†Generic name product may also be available in the U.S..
‡Antacid product being used as calcium supplement.

To the Reader: If you do not recognize the names of medical conditions or medicines referred to in this information, check with your doctor, nurse, or pharmacist. Definitions for selected medical terms may be found in the Glossary. Brand names for the generic drug names listed can be found in the Index. In addition, selected brand names commonly associated with the generic name have been included in the text to help you recognize medicine you may be taking. The fact that a brand name product is not mentioned does not mean the information does not apply. It is a good idea for you to learn both the generic and brand names of your medicines and to write them down for future use.

Calcium supplements are taken by mouth and sometimes by injection by patients who are unable to get enough calcium in their regular diet or who have a need for more calcium. They are used to prevent or treat several conditions that may cause hypocalcemia (not enough calcium in the blood). The body needs calcium to make strong bones. Calcium is also needed for the heart, muscles, and nervous system to work properly.

The bones serve as a storage site for the body's calcium. They are continuously giving up calcium to the bloodstream and then replacing it as the body's need for calcium changes from day to day. When there is not enough calcium in the blood to be used by the heart and other organs, your body will take the needed calcium from the bones. When you eat foods rich in calcium, the calcium balance between your blood and bones will be maintained.

Pregnant women and nursing mothers may need more calcium than they normally get from eating calcium-rich foods. Adult women may take calcium supplements to help prevent a bone disease called osteoporosis. Osteoporosis, which causes thin, porous, easily broken bones, appears most often in elderly women, but may sometimes occur in elderly men also. Although the exact cause of osteoporosis is not

known, a diet low in calcium for many years may add to the risk of developing it. Other bone diseases in children and adults are also treated with calcium supplements.

These medicines may also be used for other conditions as determined by your doctor.

Some of these preparations are available only with your doctor's prescription. Others are available without a prescription; however, your doctor may have special instructions on the proper use and dose for your medical problem.

Some calcium salts have more calcium (elemental calcium) than others. For example, the amount of calcium in calcium carbonate is greater than that in calcium gluconate. To give you an idea of how different calcium supplements vary in calcium content, the following chart explains how many tablets of each type of supplement will provide 1000 milligrams of elemental calcium. When you look for a calcium supplement, be sure the number of milligrams on the label refers to the amount of elemental calcium, and not to the amount of the salt.

Calcium supplement	Amount of "salt" in tablet (in milligrams)	Amount of calcium per tablet (in milligrams)	Number of tablets to provide 1000 milligrams of calcium
Calcium carbonate	625	250	4
	650	260	4
	750	300	4
	835	334	3
	1250	500	2
	1500	600	2
Calcium citrate	950	200	5
Calcium gluconate	500	45	22
	650	58	17
	1000	90	11
Calcium lactate	325	42	24
	650	84	12
Calcium phosphate, dibasic	500	115	9
Calcium phosphate, tribasic	800	304	4
	1600	608	2

Remember:

• **Keep all medicines out of the reach of children.**

• In order for this medicine to work, it must be used as directed. **If you are using this medicine without a prescription, it is very important that you follow the directions on the label.**

• **It is also very important that you read and understand the following information.** If any of the information causes you special concern, check with your doctor before using this medicine without a prescription.

• Before you begin using any new medicine (prescription or nonprescription) or if you develop any new medical problem while you are using this medicine, check with your doctor, nurse, or pharmacist.

• **If you have any questions** about the following information or if you want more information about this medicine or your medical problem, **ask your doctor, nurse, or pharmacist.**

Importance of Diet

Nutritionists recommend that, if possible, people should get all the calcium they need from foods. However, some people do not get enough calcium from food. For example, people on weight-loss diets may consume too little food. Others may not be able to tolerate milk products because their bodies lack an enzyme called lactase, which helps the body digest milk. Still others may need more calcium than normal. For such people, a calcium supplement is important. The body absorbs calcium in supplements in much the same way that it absorbs calcium in foods.

Experts have developed a list of Recommended Dietary Allowances (RDAs) of calcium. The RDA is not an exact number but a general idea of how much you need every day. The RDAs do not cover amounts needed for problems caused by a serious lack of calcium.

The daily RDAs for calcium are as follows:
 Infants up to 6 months of age—360 mg (milligrams)
 Children 6 months to 1 year of age—540 mg
 Children 1 to 10 years of age—800 mg
 Adolescents 11 to 18 years of age—1200 mg
 Adults—800 mg
 Pregnant and breastfeeding women—1200 mg

Some doctors and nutritionists believe that most adult women and some men generally need more calcium than is stated in the RDA. They recommend the following:
 Premenopausal women—1000 mg of calcium a day
 Women past menopause and elderly men—1500 mg
  of calcium a day

Getting the proper amount of calcium in the diet every day and participating in weight-bearing exercise (walking, dancing, bike riding, aerobics, jogging) during the early years of life (up to about 35 years of age) may be important in helping to prevent the development of osteoporosis in later life.

The following table includes some calcium-rich foods. The calcium content of these foods can supply the daily RDA for calcium if the foods are eaten regularly.

Food (amount)	Milligrams of calcium
Nonfat dry milk (1 cup)	375
Lowfat, skim, or whole milk (1 cup)	290 to 300
Yogurt (1 cup)	275 to 400
Sardines with bones (3 ounces)	370
Ricotta cheese, part skim (½ cup)	340
Salmon, canned, with bones (3 ounces)	285
Cheese, Swiss (1 ounce)	272
Turnip greens, cooked (1 cup)	267
Cheese, cheddar (1 ounce)	204
Broccoli, cooked (1 cup)	178
Cheese, American (1 ounce)	174
Collard greens (1 cup)	158
Cottage cheese, lowfat (1 cup)	154
Tofu (4 ounces)	154
Shrimp (1 cup)	147
Ice milk (¾ cup)	132

Vitamin D helps prevent calcium loss from your bones. It is sometimes called "the sunshine vitamin" because it is made in your skin when you are exposed to sunlight. If you get outside in the sunlight every day, you should get all the vitamin D you need.

Do not use bonemeal or dolomite as a source of calcium. The Food and Drug Administration has issued warnings that bonemeal and dolomite could be dangerous because they may contain lead.

Remember:
 • The total amount of calcium that you get every day includes what you get from the foods that you eat *and* what you may take as a supplement. Read the labels of processed foods that you eat. Many foods now have added calcium.

 • This total amount should not be greater than the RDA, unless ordered by your doctor.

Before Using This Medicine

Before you use calcium supplements, check with your doctor, nurse, or pharmacist:

—if you are on a low-salt, low-sugar, or any other special diet, or if you are allergic to any substance, such as foods, sulfites or other preservatives, or dyes. Most medicines contain more than their active ingredient, and many liquid medicines contain alcohol. Your doctor, nurse, or pharmacist can help you avoid products that may cause a problem.

—if you are **pregnant** or if you may become pregnant. Your doctor will help you decide whether you need to take a calcium supplement.

—if you are **breast-feeding**. Calcium supplements have not been shown to cause problems in either humans or animals. Although some extra calcium may pass into breast milk, there is not enough to have an effect on the baby.

—if you have any of the following medical problems:
 Diarrhea
 Heart disease
 Kidney disease or stones
 Sarcoidosis

—if your doctor has told you that you do not have enough stomach acid. Products containing calcium carbonate or calcium phosphate will be absorbed better if taken with meals. However, taking calcium supplements with meals may decrease the amount of iron your body uses from foods. Since another form of calcium may work better, your doctor, nurse, or pharmacist can help you choose the calcium salt that is best for you when stomach acid is low.

—if you are taking **any** other prescription or nonprescription (OTC) medicines, especially:
 Cellulose sodium phosphate (e.g., Calcibind)
 Digitalis glycosides (heart medicine)
 Etidronate (e.g., Didronel)
 Other calcium-containing medicines
 Tetracyclines taken by mouth

Proper Use of This Medicine

Take this medicine 1 to 1½ hours after meals and at bedtime, unless otherwise directed by your doctor.

For patients taking the chewable tablet form of this medicine:

- Chew the tablets completely before swallowing. Then
  drink a glass of water. This will allow the medicine to
  be more effective.

For patients taking the syrup form of this medicine:

- Take the syrup before meals. This will allow the
  medicine to work faster.
- Mix in water or fruit juice for infants or children.

Take this medicine only as directed. Do not take more
of it and do not take it more often than recommended
on the label. To do so may increase the chance of side
effects.

If you are taking this medicine on a regular schedule and
you miss a dose, take it as soon as possible, then go
back to your regular dosing schedule.

How to store this medicine:

- **Keep out of the reach of children.**
- Store away from heat and direct light.
- Do not store in the bathroom, near the kitchen sink,
  or in other damp places. Heat or moisture may cause
  the medicine to break down.
- Keep the liquid form of this medicine from freezing.
- Do not keep outdated medicine or medicine no longer
  needed. Be sure that any discarded medicine is out of
  the reach of children.

Precautions While Using This Medicine

If this medicine has been ordered by your doctor and you
will be taking it in large doses or for a long period of
time, your doctor should check your progress at regular visits. This is to make sure the medicine is working
properly and does not cause unwanted effects.

**Do not take calcium supplements within 1 to 2 hours of
taking other medicine by mouth.** To do so may keep
the other medicine from working as well.

Unless you are otherwise directed by your doctor, to make
sure that calcium is used properly by your body:

- **Do not take other medicines containing calcium, phosphates, magnesium, or vitamin D unless told to do so
  by your doctor.**

- **Do not take calcium supplements within 1 to 2 hours
  of eating spinach, rhubarb, bran or whole-grain cereals
  or breads, or fresh fruits and vegetables.**
- **Do not drink large amounts of alcohol or caffeine-
  containing beverages (usually more than 8 cups of coffee a day), or use tobacco.**

Side Effects of This Medicine

Along with its needed effects, a medicine may cause some
unwanted effects. Although the following side effects
occur very rarely when the calcium supplement is taken
as recommended, they may be more likely to occur if:

—it is taken in large doses.
—it is taken for a long period of time.
—it is taken by patients with kidney disease.

Check with your doctor as soon as possible if any of the
following side effects occur:

Rare
  Difficult or painful urination
Early signs of overdose
  Constipation (severe)
  Drowsiness
  Headache (continuing)
  Loss of appetite
  Metallic taste
  Unusually dry mouth
  Unusual tiredness or weakness

Late signs of overdose
  Confusion
  High blood pressure
  Increased sensitivity of eyes or skin to light
  Increased thirst
  Irregular or slow heartbeat
  Irritability
  Mental depression
  Muscle or bone pain
  Nausea and vomiting
  Skin rash or itching
  Unusually large amount of urine or increased frequency
    of urination

Other side effects not listed above may also occur in some
patients. If you notice any other effects, check with
your doctor.

December 1987

CAPREOMYCIN (Systemic)

A commonly used brand name is Capastat.

To the Reader: If you do not recognize the names of medical conditions or medicines referred to in this information, check with your doctor, nurse, or pharmacist. Definitions for selected medical terms may be found in the Glossary. Brand names for the generic drug names listed can be found in the Index. In addition, selected brand names commonly associated with the generic name have been included in the text to help you recognize medicine you may be taking. The fact that a brand name product is not mentioned does not mean the information does not apply. It is a good idea for you to learn both the generic and brand names of your medicines and to write them down for future use.

Capreomycin (kap-ree-oh-MYE-sin) belongs to the general family of medicines called antibiotics. It is used to help the body overcome tuberculosis (TB). It is given by injection with one or more other medicines for TB.

Capreomycin is available only with your doctor's prescription.

Remember:

• **It is very important that you read and understand the following information.** If any of the information causes you special concern, do not decide against using this medicine without first checking with your doctor.

• Before you begin using any new medicine (prescription or nonprescription) or if you develop any new medical problem while you are using this medicine, check with your doctor, nurse, or pharmacist.

• **If you have any questions** about the following information or if you want more information about this medicine or your medical problem, **ask your doctor, nurse, or pharmacist.**

Before Using This Medicine

In order to decide on the best treatment for your medical problem, your doctor should be told:

—if you have ever had any unusual or allergic reaction to capreomycin.

—if you are on a low-salt, low-sugar, or any other special diet, or if you are allergic to any substance, such as foods or sulfites or other preservatives. Most medicines contain more than their active ingredient. Your doctor, nurse, or pharmacist can help you avoid products that may cause a problem.

—if you are **pregnant** or if you may become pregnant. Capreomycin has not been shown to cause problems in humans. However, studies in rats given several times the human dose have shown that capreomycin may cause "wavy ribs."

—if you are **breast-feeding**. However, capreomycin has not been shown to cause problems in nursing babies.

—if you have any of the following medical problems:

Eighth-cranial-nerve disease (loss of hearing and/or balance)
Kidney disease
Myasthenia gravis
Parkinson's disease

—if you are taking **any** other prescription or nonprescription (OTC) medicine, especially:

Aminoglycosides by injection or topical application (amikacin, gentamicin, kanamycin, neomycin, netilmicin, streptomycin, tobramycin)
Amphotericin B by injection (e.g., Fungizone)
Bacitracin by injection
Bumetanide by injection (e.g., Bumex)
Cisplatin (e.g., Platinol)
Colistimethate (e.g., Coly-Mycin)
Cyclosporine (e.g., Sandimmune)
Ethacrynic acid by injection (e.g., Edecrin)
Furosemide by injection (e.g., Lasix)
Paromomycin (e.g., Humatin)
Polymyxin B by injection (e.g., Aerosporin)
Streptozocin (e.g., Zanosar)
Vancomycin (e.g., Vancocin)

—if you have ever had any problems with this medicine.

Side Effects of This Medicine

Along with its needed effects, a medicine may cause some unwanted effects. Although not all of these side effects may occur, if they do occur they may need medical attention.

Check with your doctor as soon as possible if any of the following side effects occur:

More common

Blood in urine
Greatly increased or decreased frequency of urination or amount of urine
Increased thirst
Loss of appetite

Less common

Any loss of hearing
Clumsiness or unsteadiness
Difficulty in breathing
Dizziness
Drowsiness
Irregular heartbeat
Mood or other mental changes
Muscle cramps or pain
Nausea or vomiting
Ringing or buzzing sound or a feeling of fullness in the ears
Stomach pain or bloating
Unusual tiredness or weakness
Weak pulse

Other side effects may occur that usually do not require medical attention. These side effects may go away during treatment as your body adjusts to the medicine.

However, check with your doctor if any of the following side effects continue or are bothersome:

Less common
    Fever
    Itching
    Pain, hardness, unusual bleeding, or a sore at the place
        of injection
    Redness
    Skin rash
    Swelling

Other side effects not listed above may also occur in some patients. If you notice any other effects, check with your doctor.

December 1987

CARBACHOL (Ophthalmic)

Some commonly used brand names are Isopto Carbachol and Miostat.

Generic name product may also be available in the U.S.

To the Reader: If you do not recognize the names of medical conditions or medicines referred to in this information, check with your doctor, nurse, or pharmacist. Definitions for selected medical terms may be found in the Glossary. Brand names for the generic drug names listed can be found in the Index. In addition, selected brand names commonly associated with the generic name have been included in the text to help you recognize medicine you may be taking. The fact that a brand name product is not mentioned does not mean the information does not apply. It is a good idea for you to learn both the generic and brand names of your medicines and to write them down for future use.

Carbachol (KAR-ba-kole) is used in the eye to treat glaucoma. Sometimes it is also used in eye surgery.

This medicine is available only with your doctor's prescription.

Remember:

• **This medicine has been prescribed for your current medical problem only.** It must not be given to other people or used for other problems unless you are directed to do so by your doctor.

• **Keep all medicines out of the reach of children.**

• In order for this medicine to work, it must be used as directed.

• **It is very important that you read and understand the following information.** If any of the information causes you special concern, do not decide against using this medicine without first checking with your doctor.

• Before you begin using any new medicine (prescription or nonprescription) or if you develop any new medical problem while you are using this medicine, check with your doctor, nurse, or pharmacist.

• **If you have any questions** about the following information or if you want more information about this medicine or your medical problem, **ask your doctor, nurse, or pharmacist.**

Before Using This Medicine

In order to decide on the best treatment for your medical problem, your doctor should be told:

—if you have ever had any unusual or allergic reaction to carbachol.

—if you are allergic to any substance, such as preservatives. Most medicines contain more than their active ingredient. Your doctor, nurse, or pharmacist can help you avoid products that may cause a problem.

—if you are **pregnant** or if you may become pregnant, since carbachol may be absorbed into the body. However, carbachol has not been shown to cause birth defects or other problems in humans.

—if you are **breast-feeding**, since carbachol may be absorbed into the body. However, carbachol has not been shown to cause problems in nursing babies.

—if you have any of the following medical problems:
  Asthma
  Eye problems (other)
  Heart disease
  Overactive thyroid
  Parkinson's disease
  Stomach ulcer or other stomach problems
  Urinary tract blockage

—if you are taking **any** other prescription or nonprescription (OTC) medicine.

Proper Use of This Medicine

Use this medicine only as directed. Do not use more of it and do not use it more often than your doctor ordered. To do so may increase the chance of too much medicine being absorbed into the body and the chance of side effects.

How to apply this medicine: First, wash your hands. With the middle finger, apply pressure to the inside corner of the eye (and continue to apply pressure for 1 or 2 minutes after the medicine has been placed in the eye). Tilt the head back and with the index finger of the same hand, pull the lower eyelid away from the eye to form a pouch. Drop the medicine into the pouch and gently close the eyes. Do not blink. Keep the eyes closed for 1 or 2 minutes to allow the medicine to be absorbed.

Immediately after applying the eye drops, wash your hands to remove any medicine that may be on them.

To prevent contamination of the eye drops, do not touch the applicator tip to any surface (including the eye) and keep the container tightly closed.

If you miss a dose of this medicine, apply it as soon as possible. However, if it is almost time for your next dose, skip the missed dose and apply your next dose at the regularly scheduled time. Then continue with your regular dosing schedule.

How to store this medicine:

• **Keep out of the reach of children.**

• Store away from heat and direct light.

• Keep the medicine from freezing.

• Do not keep outdated medicine or medicine no longer needed. Be sure that any discarded medicine is out of the reach of children.

Precautions While Using This Medicine

Your doctor should check your eye pressure at regular visits.

After you apply this medicine to your eyes, your pupils may become unusually small. This may cause you to see less well at night or in dim light. **Be especially careful if you drive or do other jobs at night or in dim light that require you to see well.**

Also, for a short time after you apply this medicine, your vision may be blurred or there may be a change in your near or distant vision. **Make sure your vision is clear before you drive or do other jobs that require you to see well.**

Side Effects of This Medicine

Along with its needed effects, a medicine may cause some unwanted effects. Although not all of these side effects may occur, if they do occur they may need medical attention.

Check with your doctor as soon as possible if any of the following side effects occur:

Signs of too much medicine being absorbed into the body
> Diarrhea, stomach cramps or pain, or vomiting
> Flushing or redness of face
> Frequent urge to urinate
> Shortness of breath, wheezing, or tightness in chest
> Unusual increase in sweating
> Unusual watering of mouth

Other side effects may occur that usually do not require medical attention. These side effects may go away during treatment as your body adjusts to the medicine. However, check with your doctor if any of the following side effects continue or are bothersome:

> Blurred vision or change in near or distant vision
> Eye pain
> Headache
> Irritation of eyes
> Twitching of eyelids

For elderly patients: Many medicines have not been tested in older people. Therefore, it is not known whether the medicine acts the same way it does in younger adults. Check with your doctor or pharmacist if you notice any unusual effects while using this medicine or if you think it is not working as it should.

Other side effects not listed above may also occur in some patients. If you notice any other effects, check with your doctor.

_____

December 1987

CARBAMAZEPINE (Systemic)

Some commonly used brand names are:

Apo-Carbamazepine*	Mazepine*
Epitol	Tegretol

Generic name product may also be available in the U.S.

*Not available in the U.S.

To the Reader: If you do not recognize the names of medical conditions or medicines referred to in this information, check with your doctor, nurse, or pharmacist. Definitions for selected medical terms may be found in the Glossary. Brand names for the generic drug names listed can be found in the Index. In addition, selected brand names commonly associated with the generic name have been included in the text to help you recognize medicine you may be taking. The fact that a brand name product is not mentioned does not mean the information does not apply. It is a good idea for you to learn both the generic and brand names of your medicines and to write them down for future use.

Carbamazepine (kar-ba-MAZ-e-peen) is taken by mouth to control some types of seizures in epilepsy. It is also used to relieve pain due to trigeminal neuralgia (tic douloureux) and other specific kinds of pain. It should not be used for other aches or pains.

This medicine may also be used for other conditions as determined by your doctor.

Carbamazepine is available only with your doctor's prescription.

Remember:

• **This medicine has been prescribed for your current medical problem only.** It must not be given to other people or used for other problems unless you are directed to do so by your doctor.

• **Keep all medicines out of the reach of children.**

• In order for this medicine to work, it must be used as directed.

• **It is very important that you read and understand the following information.** If any of the information causes you special concern, do not decide against using this medicine without first checking with your doctor.

• Before you begin using any new medicine (prescription or nonprescription) or if you develop any new medical problem while you are using this medicine, check with your doctor, nurse, or pharmacist.

• **If you have any questions** about the following information or if you want more information about this medicine or your medical problem, **ask your doctor, nurse, or pharmacist.**

Before Using This Medicine

In order to decide on the best treatment for your medical problem, your doctor should be told:

—if you have ever had any unusual or allergic reaction to carbamazepine or to any of the tricyclic antidepressants, such as amitriptyline, amoxapine, clomipramine, desipramine, doxepin, imipramine, nortriptyline, protriptyline, or trimipramine.

—if you are on a low-salt, low-sugar, or any other special diet, or if you are allergic to any substance, such as foods, sulfites or other preservatives, or dyes. Most medicines contain more than their active ingredient. Your doctor, nurse, or pharmacist can help you avoid products that may cause a problem.

—if any medicine you have taken has ever caused an allergy or reaction that affected your blood.

—if you are **pregnant** or if you may become pregnant. Studies on birth defects with carbamazepine have not been done in humans. However, there have been reports of babies having low birth weight and small head size when their mothers had taken carbamazepine during pregnancy. In addition, birth defects have been reported in some babies when the mothers took other medicines for epilepsy during pregnancy. Also, studies in animals have shown that carbamazepine causes birth defects when given in large doses. Therefore, the use of carbamazepine during pregnancy should be discussed with your doctor.

—if you are **breast-feeding**. Carbamazepine passes into the breast milk and in some cases the baby may receive enough of it to cause unwanted effects. In animal studies, carbamazepine has affected the growth and appearance of the nursing babies.

—if you have any of the following medical problems:

Anemia or other blood problems
Diabetes mellitus (sugar diabetes)
Glaucoma
Heart or blood vessel disease
Kidney disease
Liver disease
Problems with urination

—if you are taking **any** other prescription or nonprescription (OTC) medicine, especially:

Adrenocorticoids (cortisone-like medicine)
Anticoagulants (blood thinners)
Cimetidine (e.g., Tagamet)
Contraceptives, oral (birth control pills), containing estrogens
Diltiazem (e.g., Cardizem)
Erythromycin (e.g., E-Mycin; Erythrocin; Ilosone)
Estrogens (female hormones)
Isoniazid (e.g., INH)
Loxapine (e.g., Loxitane)
Maprotiline (e.g., Ludiomil)
Quinidine (e.g., Quinaglute)
Tricyclic antidepressants (amitriptyline, amoxapine, clomipramine, desipramine, doxepin, imipramine, nortriptyline, protriptyline, trimipramine)
Verapamil (e.g., Calan; Isoptin)

—if you are now taking or have taken within the past 2 weeks monoamine oxidase (MAO) inhibitors such as:

Furazolidone (e.g., Furoxone)
Isocarboxazid (e.g., Marplan)
Pargyline (e.g., Eutonyl)
Phenelzine (e.g., Nardil)
Procarbazine (e.g., Matulane)
Tranylcypromine (e.g., Parnate)

Proper Use of This Medicine

Carbamazepine may be taken with meals to lessen the chance of stomach upset (nausea and vomiting).

Carbamazepine is **not** an ordinary pain reliever. It should be used only when a doctor prescribes it for certain kinds of pain. **Do not take carbamazepine for any other aches or pains.**

It is very important that you take this medicine exactly as directed by your doctor to obtain the best results and lessen the chance of serious side effects. Do not take more of it, do not take it more often, and do not take it for a longer period of time than your doctor ordered.

If you are taking this medicine for epilepsy:

• **Do not suddenly stop taking this medicine without first checking with your doctor.** It is usually best to gradually reduce the amount of carbamazepine you are taking before stopping completely, to keep your seizures under control.

If you miss a dose of this medicine, take it as soon as possible. However, if it is almost time for your next dose, skip the missed dose and go back to your regular dosing schedule. Do not double doses. However, if you miss more than one dose a day, check with your doctor.

How to store this medicine:

• **Keep out of the reach of children.**

• Store away from heat and direct light.

• Do not store in the bathroom, near the kitchen sink, or in other damp places. Heat or moisture may cause the medicine to break down.

• Do not keep outdated medicine or medicine no longer needed. Be sure that any discarded medicine is out of the reach of children.

Precautions While Using This Medicine

It is very important that your doctor check your progress at regular visits. Your doctor may want to have certain tests done to see if you are receiving the right amount of medicine or if certain side effects may be occurring without your knowing it. Also, the amount of medicine you are taking may have to be changed often.

This medicine may cause some people to become drowsy, dizzy, lightheaded, or less alert than they are normally. It may also cause blurred vision, weakness, or loss of muscle control in some people. **Be sure you know how you react to this medicine before you drive, use machines, or do other jobs that require you to be alert and well-coordinated.**

Some people who take carbamazepine may become more sensitive to sunlight than they are normally. When you first begin taking this medicine, avoid too much sun or use of a sunlamp, and use a sunscreen and sunglasses until you know how you react, especially if you tend to burn easily. If you have a severe reaction, check with your doctor.

Carbamazepine may cause dryness of the mouth. For temporary relief, use sugarless gum or candy, melt bits of ice in your mouth, or use a saliva substitute. However, if dry mouth continues for more than 2 weeks, check with your physician or dentist. Continuing dryness of the mouth may increase the chance of dental disease, including tooth decay, gum disease, and fungal infections.

Diabetic patients—Carbamazepine may affect urine sugar levels. While you are using this medicine, be especially careful in testing for sugar in your urine. If you have any questions about this, check with your doctor.

Before having any kind of surgery, dental treatment, or emergency treatment, tell the physician or dentist in charge that you are taking this medicine.

Your doctor may want you to carry a medical identification card or bracelet stating that you are taking this medicine.

Side Effects of This Medicine

Along with its needed effects, a medicine may cause some unwanted effects. Although not all of these side effects may occur, if they do occur they may need medical attention.

Check with your doctor immediately if any of the following side effects occur:

Rare

 Bleeding or bruising
 Darkening of urine
 Pain, tenderness, swelling, or bluish color in leg or foot
 Pale stools
 Sores or ulcers in the mouth
 Sore throat and fever
 Unusual tiredness or weakness
 Yellow eyes and skin

Signs of overdose

 Convulsions (seizures)
 Dizziness (severe)
 Drowsiness (severe)
 Fast heartbeat
 Irregular, slow, or shallow breathing
 Trembling or twitching

In addition, check with your doctor as soon as possible if any of the following side effects occur:

More common

 Blurred vision or double vision
 Confusion, agitation, or hostility (especially in the elderly)
 Headache (continuing)
 Increase in seizures
 Nausea and vomiting (severe)
 Unusual drowsiness
 Weakness

Less common

 Hives, itching, or skin rash
 Behavioral changes (especially in children)

Rare

Chest pain
Continuous back-and-forth eye movements
Difficulty in speaking or slurred speech
Fainting
Frequent urination
Irregular, pounding, or unusually slow heartbeat
Mental depression with restlessness and nervousness or
  other mood or mental changes
Numbness, tingling, pain, or weakness in hands and feet
Rigidity
Ringing, buzzing, or other unexplained sounds in the ears
Sudden decrease in amount of urine
Swelling of feet or lower legs
Swollen glands
Trembling
Troubled breathing
Uncontrolled body movements
Visual hallucinations (seeing things that are not there)

Other side effects may occur that usually do not require
  medical attention. These side effects may go away
  during treatment as your body adjusts to the medicine.
  However, check with your doctor if any of the following side effects continue or are bothersome:

More common

Clumsiness or unsteadiness
Dizziness (mild)
Drowsiness (mild)
Lightheadedness
Nausea or vomiting (mild)

Less common or rare

Aching joints or muscles
Constipation
Diarrhea
Dryness of mouth
Headache
Increased sensitivity of skin and eyes to sunlight
Increased sweating
Irritation of tongue
Loss of appetite
Loss of hair
Sexual problems in males
Stomach pain or discomfort

For elderly patients: Confusion; restlessness and nervousness; irregular, pounding, or unusually slow heartbeat; and chest pain are more likely to occur in elderly
  patients, who may be more sensitive to some of the
  effects of carbamazepine.

Other side effects not listed above may also occur in some
  patients. If you notice any other effects, check with
  your doctor.

December 1987

CARBOL-FUCHSIN (Topical)

Some commonly used brand names or other names are Castel Plus and Castellani Paint.

To the Reader: If you do not recognize the names of medical conditions or medicines referred to in this information, check with your doctor, nurse, or pharmacist. Definitions for selected medical terms may be found in the Glossary. Brand names for the generic drug names listed can be found in the Index. In addition, selected brand names commonly associated with the generic name have been included in the text to help you recognize medicine you may be taking. The fact that a brand name product is not mentioned does not mean the information does not apply. It is a good idea for you to learn both the generic and brand names of your medicines and to write them down for future use.

Carbol-fuchsin (kar-bol-FOOK-sin) belongs to the general family of medicines called antifungals. Carbol-fuchsin is used on the skin and nails to help the body overcome fungal infections, including athlete's foot and ringworm of the nails. It may also be used as a drying agent in skin conditions where there is too much moisture.

Carbol-fuchsin is available only with your doctor's prescription.

Remember:

• **This medicine has been prescribed for your present infection only.** Another infection later on may require a different medicine. Also, even though other people may have the same symptoms as you, they may have a different kind of infection. Your medicine may not work for them and may even cause them harm. Therefore, **your medicine must not be given to other people or used for other infections** unless you are otherwise directed by your doctor.

• **Keep all medicines out of the reach of children.**

• In order for this medicine to work, it must be used as directed.

• **It is very important that you read and understand the following information.** If any of the information causes you special concern, do not decide against using this medicine without first checking with your doctor.

• Before you begin using any new medicine (prescription or nonprescription) or if you develop any new medical problem while you are using this medicine, check with your doctor, nurse, or pharmacist.

• **If you have any questions** about the following information or if you want more information about this medicine or your medical problem, **ask your doctor, nurse, or pharmacist.**

Before Using This Medicine

In order to decide on the best treatment for your medical problem, your doctor should be told:

—if you have ever had any unusual or allergic reaction to carbol-fuchsin.

—if you are allergic to any substance, such as certain foods or preservatives or dyes. Most medicines contain more than their active ingredient. Your doctor, nurse, or pharmacist can help you avoid products that may cause a problem.

—if you are **pregnant** or if you may become pregnant. However, carbol-fuchsin has not been shown to cause birth defects or other problems in humans.

—if you are **breast-feeding**. However, carbol-fuchsin has not been shown to cause problems in nursing babies.

Proper Use of This Medicine

Before applying this medicine, wash the affected areas with soap and water, and dry thoroughly.

Carbol-fuchsin is a poison. Use only on the affected areas as directed.

Using an applicator or swab, apply this medicine only to the affected areas. Do not apply to large areas of the body, unless otherwise directed by your doctor.

When this medicine is applied to the fingers or toes, do not bandage them.

To help clear up your infection completely, **it is very important that you keep using this medicine for the full time of treatment** even if your symptoms begin to clear up after a few days. Since fungal infections may be very slow to clear up, you may have to continue using this medicine every day for as long as several months or more. If you stop using this medicine too soon, your symptoms may return. **Do not miss any doses.**

If you do miss a dose of this medicine, apply it as soon as possible. However, if it is almost time for your next dose, skip the missed dose and go back to your regular dosing schedule.

How to store this medicine:

• **Keep out of the reach of children.**

• Store away from heat and direct light.

• Keep the medicine from freezing.

• Do not keep outdated medicine or medicine no longer needed. Be sure that any discarded medicine is out of the reach of children.

Precautions While Using This Medicine

If your skin problem does not improve within 1 week, or if it becomes worse, check with your doctor.

This medicine will stain clothing. Avoid getting it on your clothes.

Side Effects of This Medicine

Along with its needed effects, a medicine may cause some unwanted effects. Although not all of these side effects may occur, if they do occur they may need medical attention.

Check with your doctor as soon as possible if the following side effect occurs:

Skin irritation not present before using this medicine

Other side effects may occur that usually do not require medical attention. These side effects may go away during treatment as your body adjusts to the medicine. However, check with your doctor if the following side effect continues or is bothersome:

Mild, temporary stinging

Other side effects not listed above may also occur in some patients. If you notice any other effects, check with your doctor.

December 1987

CARBONIC ANHYDRASE INHIBITORS
(Systemic)

This information applies to the following medicines:

Acetazolamide (a-set-a-ZOLE-a-mide)
Dichlorphenamide (dye-klor-FEN-a-mide)
Methazolamide (meth-a-ZOLE-a-mide)

Some commonly used brand names are:	Generic names:
Acetazolam*	
Ak-Zol	
Apo-Acetazolamide*	
Dazamide	Acetazolamide†
Diamox	
Diamox Sequels	
Daranide	Dichlorphenamide
Neptazane	Methazolamide

*Not available in the U.S.
†Generic name product may also be available in the U.S.

To the Reader: If you do not recognize the names of medical conditions or medicines referred to in this information, check with your doctor, nurse, or pharmacist. Definitions for selected medical terms may be found in the Glossary. Brand names for the generic drug names listed can be found in the Index. In addition, selected brand names commonly associated with the generic name have been included in the text to help you recognize medicine you may be taking. The fact that a brand name product is not mentioned does not mean the information does not apply. It is a good idea for you to learn both the generic and brand names of your medicines and to write them down for future use.

Carbonic anhydrase inhibitors are taken by mouth to treat glaucoma. Acetazolamide is also sometimes given by injection.

Acetazolamide is also used as an anticonvulsant to control certain seizures in the treatment of epilepsy. It is also sometimes used to prevent or lessen some effects in mountain climbers who climb to high altitudes, and to treat other conditions as determined by your doctor.

These medicines are available only with your doctor's prescription.

Remember:
• **This medicine has been prescribed for your current medical problem only.** It must not be given to other people or used for other problems unless you are directed to do so by your doctor.

• **Keep all medicines out of the reach of children.**

• In order for this medicine to work, it must be used as directed.

• If you are receiving this medicine by injection, some of the information about this medicine may not apply.

• **It is very important that you read and understand the following information.** If any of the information causes you special concern, do not decide against using this medicine without first checking with your doctor.

• Before you begin using any new medicine (prescription or nonprescription) or if you develop any new medical problem while you are using this medicine, check with your doctor, nurse, or pharmacist.

• **If you have any questions** about the following information or if you want more information about this medicine or your medical problem, **ask your doctor, nurse, or pharmacist**.

Before Using This Medicine

In order to decide on the best treatment for your medical problem, your doctor should be told:

—if you have ever had any unusual or allergic reaction to this medicine or to sulfonamides (sulfa drugs) or thiazide diuretics (some kinds of water pills).

—if you are on a low-salt, low-sugar, or any other special diet, or if you are allergic to any substance, such as foods, sulfites or other preservatives, or dyes. Most medicines contain more than their active ingredient. Your doctor, nurse, or pharmacist can help you avoid products that may cause a problem.

—if you are **pregnant** or if you may become pregnant, although carbonic anhydrase inhibitors have not been shown to cause birth defects or other problems in humans. Studies in animals have shown that carbonic anhydrase inhibitors cause birth defects when given in very high doses. The studies with acetazolamide used doses greater than 10 times the human dose.

—if you are **breast-feeding**. Although these medicines may pass into the breast milk, they have not been shown to cause problems in nursing babies.

—if you have any of the following medical problems:
Diabetes mellitus (sugar diabetes)
Emphysema or other chronic lung disease
Gout
Kidney disease or stones
Liver disease
Low blood levels of potassium or sodium
Underactive adrenal gland (Addison's disease)

—if you are taking **any** other prescription or nonprescription (OTC) medicine, especially:
Amphetamines
Mecamylamine (e.g., Inversine)
Methenamine (e.g., Mandelamine)
Quinidine (e.g., Quinidex)

Proper Use of This Medicine

Take this medicine only as directed. Do not take more of it and do not take it more often than your doctor ordered. To do so may increase the chance of side effects without increasing the effectiveness of this medicine.

This medicine may be taken with meals to lessen the chance of stomach upset. However, if stomach upset (nausea or vomiting) continues, check with your doctor.

This medicine may cause an increase in the amount of urine or in your frequency of urination. If you continue to take the medicine every day, these effects should lessen or stop. In order to keep the increase in urine from affecting your sleep at night:

—if you are to take one dose a day, take it in the morning after breakfast, unless otherwise directed by your doctor.

—if you are to take more than one dose a day, take the last dose no later than 6 p.m., unless otherwise directed by your doctor.

However, it is best to plan your dose or doses according to a schedule that will least affect your personal activities and sleep. Ask your doctor, nurse, or pharmacist to help you plan the best time to take this medicine.

If you miss a dose of this medicine, take it as soon as possible. However, if it is almost time for your next dose, skip the missed dose and go back to your regular dosing schedule. Do not double doses.

How to store this medicine:

• **Keep out of the reach of children.**

• Store away from heat and direct light.

• Do not store the capsule or tablet form of this medicine in the bathroom, near the kitchen sink, or in other damp places. Heat or moisture may cause the medicine to break down.

• Do not keep outdated medicine or medicine no longer needed. Be sure that any discarded medicine is out of the reach of children.

Precautions While Using This Medicine

This medicine may cause some people to feel drowsy, dizzy, lightheaded, or more tired than they are normally. **Make sure you know how you react to this medicine before you drive, use machines, or do other jobs that require you to be alert.**

It is important that your doctor check your progress at regular visits. Your doctor may want to do certain tests to see if the medicine is working properly or if certain side effects may be occurring without your knowing it.

This medicine may cause a loss of potassium from your body. To help prevent this, your doctor may want you to eat or drink foods that have a high potassium content (for example, orange or other citrus fruit juices) or take a potassium supplement. It is very important to follow these directions. Also, it is important not to change your diet on your own. This is more important if you are already on a special diet (as for diabetes) or if you are taking a potassium supplement. Extra potassium may not be necessary and, in some cases, too much potassium could be harmful.

For diabetics—This medicine may raise blood and urine sugar levels. While you are using this medicine, be especially careful in testing for sugar in your blood or urine. If you have any questions about this, check with your doctor.

Your doctor may want you to increase the amount of fluids you drink while you are taking this medicine in order to prevent kidney stones. However, do not increase the amount of fluids you drink without first checking with your doctor.

For patients taking acetazolamide as an anticonvulsant:

• **If you have been taking acetazolamide regularly for several weeks or more, do not suddenly stop taking it.** Your doctor may want you to reduce gradually the amount you are taking before stopping completely.

Side Effects of This Medicine

Along with its needed effects, a medicine may cause some unwanted effects. Although not all of these side effects may occur, if they do occur they may need medical attention.

Check with your doctor immediately if either of the following side effects occurs:
   Rare
      Shortness of breath or trouble in breathing

Also, check with your doctor as soon as possible if any of the following side effects occur:
   More common
      Unusual tiredness or weakness
   Less common
      Blood in urine
      Difficult urination
      Mental depression
      Pain in lower back
      Pain or burning while urinating
      Sudden decrease in amount of urine
   Rare
      Bloody or black tarry stools
      Clumsiness or unsteadiness
      Confusion
      Convulsions (seizures)
      Darkening of urine
      Fever
      Hives, itching of skin, skin rash, or sores
      Muscle weakness (severe)
      Pale stools
      Ringing or buzzing in the ears
      Sore throat
      Trembling
      Unusual bruising or bleeding
      Yellow eyes and skin
   Signs of too much potassium loss
      Dryness of mouth
      Increased thirst
      Irregular heartbeats
      Mood or mental changes
      Muscle cramps or pain
      Nausea or vomiting
      Unusual tiredness or weakness
      Weak pulse

Also, check with your doctor if you have any changes in your vision (especially problems with seeing faraway objects) when you first begin taking this medicine.

Other side effects may occur that usually do not require medical attention. These side effects may go away during treatment as your body adjusts to the medicine.

However, check with your doctor if any of the following side effects continue or are bothersome:

More common

Diarrhea
General feeling of discomfort or illness
Increase in frequency of urination or amount of urine (rare with methazolamide)
Loss of appetite
Metallic taste in mouth
Nausea or vomiting
Numbness, tingling, or burning in hands or fingers, feet or toes, mouth, lips, tongue, or anus
Weight loss

Less common or rare

Constipation
Dizziness or lightheadedness
Drowsiness
Feeling of choking or lump in the throat

Headache
Loss of taste and smell
Nervousness or irritability

For elderly patients: Many medicines have not been tested in older people. Therefore, it is not known whether the medicine acts the same way it does in younger adults. Check with your doctor or pharmacist if you notice any unusual effects while taking this medicine or if you think it is not working as it should.

Other side effects not listed above may also occur in some patients. If you notice any other effects, check with your doctor.

December 1987

CARBOPROST (Systemic)

A commonly used brand name is Prostin/15M.

To the Reader: If you do not recognize the names of medical conditions or medicines referred to in this information, check with your doctor, nurse, or pharmacist. Definitions for selected medical terms may be found in the Glossary. Brand names for the generic drug names listed can be found in the Index. In addition, selected brand names commonly associated with the generic name have been included in the text to help you recognize medicine you may be taking. The fact that a brand name product is not mentioned does not mean the information does not apply. It is a good idea for you to learn both the generic and brand names of your medicines and to write them down for future use.

Carboprost (KAR-boe-prost) is given by injection to cause abortion. It acts by causing the uterus to contract the way it does during labor and also helps the cervix to dilate.

Carboprost may also be used for other purposes as determined by your doctor.

Carboprost is to be administered only by or under the immediate care of your doctor.

Remember:

• **It is very important that you read and understand the following information.** If any of the following information causes you special concern, do not decide against receiving this medicine without first checking with your doctor.

• **If you have any questions** about the following information or if you want more information about this medicine or your medical problem, ask your doctor, nurse, or pharmacist.

Before Using This Medicine

In order to decide on the best treatment for your medical problem, your doctor should be told:

—if you have ever had any unusual or allergic reaction to carboprost.

—if you have any of the following medical problems:
Adrenal gland disease (history of)
Anemia (history of)
Asthma (or history of)
Diabetes mellitus (sugar diabetes) (history of)
Epilepsy (history of)
Fibroid tumors of the uterus
Glaucoma

Heart or blood vessel disease (or history of)
High or low blood pressure (or history of)
Jaundice (history of)
Kidney disease (or history of)
Liver disease (or history of)
Lung disease
Pelvic inflammatory disease
Uterus surgery (history of)

Side Effects of This Medicine

Along with its needed effects, a medicine may cause some unwanted effects. Although not all of these side effects may occur, if they do occur they may need medical attention.

Tell the doctor or nurse immediately if any of the following side effects occur:
Less common or rare
Wheezing, troubled breathing, or tightness in chest

Other side effects may occur that usually do not require medical attention. These side effects usually go away after the medicine is stopped. However, let the doctor or nurse know if any of the following side effects continue or are bothersome:
More common
Diarrhea
Nausea
Vomiting
Less common
Chills or shivering
Fever
Flushing or redness of face
Headache
Stomach cramps or pain

After the procedure, this medicine may still produce some side effects that need attention. Check with your doctor if you notice any of the following:
Chills or shivering
Fever
Foul-smelling vaginal discharge
Pain in lower abdomen
Unusual increase in uterine bleeding

Other side effects not listed above may also occur in some patients. If you notice any other effects, check with your doctor or nurse.

December 1987

CARMUSTINE (Systemic)

Some commonly used brand names or other names are BCNU and BiCNU.

To the Reader: If you do not recognize the names of medical conditions or medicines referred to in this information, check with your doctor, nurse, or pharmacist. Definitions for selected medical terms may be found in the Glossary. Brand names for the generic drug names listed can be found in the Index. In addition, selected brand names commonly associated with the generic name have been included in the text to help you recognize medicine you may be taking. The fact that a brand name product is not mentioned does not mean the information does not apply. It is a good idea for you to learn both the generic and brand names of your medicines and to write them down for future use.

Carmustine (kar-MUS-teen) belongs to the group of medicines known as alkylating agents. It is given by injection to treat some kinds of cancer.

Carmustine interferes with the growth of cancer cells, which are eventually destroyed. Since the growth of normal body cells may also be affected by carmustine, other effects will also occur. Some of these may be serious and must be reported to your doctor. Other effects, like hair loss, may not be serious but may cause concern. Some effects may not occur for months or years after the medicine is used.

Before you begin treatment with carmustine, you and your doctor should talk about the good this medicine will do as well as the risks of using it.

Carmustine is to be administered only by or under the immediate supervision of your doctor.

Remember:

• **It is very important that you read and understand the following information.** If any of the information causes you special concern, do not decide against using this medicine without first checking with your doctor.

• Before you begin using any new medicine (prescription or nonprescription) or if you develop any new medical problem while you are using this medicine, check with your doctor, nurse, or pharmacist.

• **If you have any questions** about the following information or if you want more information about this medicine or your medical problem, **ask your doctor, nurse, or pharmacist.**

Before Using This Medicine

In order to decide on the best treatment for your medical problem, your doctor should be told:

—if you have ever had any unusual or allergic reaction to carmustine.

—if you are **pregnant** or if you intend to have children. There is a chance that this medicine may cause birth defects if either the male or female is taking it at the time of conception or if it is taken during pregnancy. Carmustine causes toxic or harmful effects in the fetus of rats and rabbits and causes birth defects in rats at doses about the same as the human dose. In addition, many cancer medicines may cause sterility which could be permanent. Although this has only been reported in animals with this medicine, the possibility should be kept in mind. Be sure that you have discussed this with your doctor before receiving this medicine.

—if you intend to **breast-feed.** Because this medicine may cause serious side effects, breast-feeding is generally not recommended while you are receiving it.

—if you have any of the following medical problems:
Chickenpox (including recent exposure)
Herpes zoster (shingles)
Infection
Kidney disease
Liver disease
Lung disease

—if you are using **any** other prescription or nonprescription (OTC) medicine, especially:
Amphotericin B by injection (e.g., Fungizone)
Antithyroid agents (medicine for overactive thyroid)
Azathioprine (e.g., Imuran)
Chloramphenicol (e.g., Chloromycetin)
Colchicine
Flucytosine (e.g., Ancobon)
Interferon (e.g., Intron A, Roferon-A)

—if you have ever been treated with x-rays or cancer medicines.

—if you smoke.

Proper Use of This Medicine

Carmustine is sometimes given together with certain other medicines. If you are using a combination of medicines, it is important that you receive each one at the proper time. If you are taking some of these medicines by mouth, ask your doctor, nurse, or pharmacist to help you plan a way to take them at the right time.

This medicine often causes nausea and vomiting, which usually last no longer than 4 to 6 hours. It is very important that you continue to receive the medicine, even if you begin to feel ill. Ask your doctor, nurse, or pharmacist for ways to lessen these effects.

Precautions While Using This Medicine

It is very important that your doctor check your progress at regular visits to make sure that this medicine is working properly and to check for unwanted effects.

While you are being treated with carmustine, and after you stop treatment with it, **do not have any immunizations without your doctor's approval.** Carmustine lowers your body's resistance and there is a chance you might get the infection the immunization is meant to prevent. In addition, other persons living in your household should not take oral polio vaccine since there is a chance they could pass the polio virus on to you. Also, you should avoid close contact with other persons (for example, at school or work) who have taken oral polio vaccine.

Carmustine can lower the number of white blood cells in your body. This may increase the chance of getting an infection. If you can, avoid people with colds or other infections. If you think you are getting a cold or other infection, check with your doctor.

If carmustine accidentally seeps out of the vein into which it is injected, it may damage some tissues and cause scarring. **Tell the doctor or nurse right away if you notice redness, pain, or swelling at the place of injection.**

Side Effects of This Medicine

Along with their needed effects, medicines like carmustine can sometimes cause unwanted effects such as blood problems, loss of hair, and other side effects; these are described below. Also, because of the way these medicines act on the body, there is a chance that they might cause other unwanted effects that may not occur until months or years after the medicine is used. These delayed effects may include certain types of cancer, such as leukemia. Discuss these possible effects with your doctor.

Although not all of these side effects may occur, if they do occur they may need medical attention.

Check with your doctor or nurse immediately if any of the following side effects occur:

More common
   Fever, chills, or sore throat
   Pain or redness at the place of injection
   Unusual bleeding or bruising

Check with your doctor or nurse as soon as possible if any of the following side effects occur:

More common
   Cough
   Shortness of breath
Less common
   Flushing of the face
   Sores in the mouth and on the lips
   Unusual tiredness or weakness
Rare
   Decrease in urination
   Swelling of feet or lower legs

Other side effects may occur that usually do not require medical attention. These side effects may go away during treatment as your body adjusts to the medicine.

Also, your doctor or nurse may be able to tell you about ways to prevent or reduce some of these side effects. Check with your doctor if any of the following side effects continue or are bothersome or if you have any questions about them:

More common
   Nausea and vomiting (usually lasting no longer than 4 to 6 hours)
Less common
   Diarrhea
   Difficulty in swallowing
   Difficulty in walking
   Discoloration of the skin along the vein of injection
   Dizziness
   Loss of appetite
   Skin rash and itching

This medicine may cause a temporary loss of hair in some people. After treatment with carmustine has ended, normal hair growth should return.

Side effects that affect your lungs (for example, cough and shortness of breath) may be more likely to occur if you smoke.

For elderly patients: Many medicines have not been tested in older people. Therefore, it is not known whether the medicine acts the same way it does in younger adults. Check with your doctor or pharmacist if you notice any unusual effects while taking this medicine or if you think it is not working as it should.

After you stop receiving carmustine, it may still produce some side effects that need attention. During this period of time check with your doctor or nurse if you notice any of the following:
   Cough
   Fever, chills, or sore throat
   Shortness of breath
   Unusual bleeding or bruising

Other side effects not listed above may also occur in some patients. If you notice any other effects, check with your doctor or nurse.

December 1987

CELLULOSE SODIUM PHOSPHATE
(Systemic)

A commonly used brand name is Calcibind.

To the Reader: If you do not recognize the names of medical conditions or medicines referred to in this information, check with your doctor, nurse, or pharmacist. Definitions for selected medical terms may be found in the Glossary. Brand names for the generic drug names listed can be found in the Index. In addition, selected brand names commonly associated with the generic name have been included in the text to help you recognize medicine you may be taking. The fact that a brand name product is not mentioned does not mean the information does not apply. It is a good idea for you to learn both the generic and brand names of your medicines and to write them down for future use.

Cellulose sodium phosphate (SELL-u-lose SO-dee-um FOS-fate) is taken by mouth to prevent the formation of calcium-containing kidney stones. It is used in patients whose bodies absorb too much calcium from their food.

Cellulose sodium phosphate works by combining with the calcium and some other minerals in food. This prevents the calcium from reaching the kidneys where the stones are formed.

Cellulose sodium phosphate is available only with your doctor's prescription.

Remember:
- **This medicine has been prescribed for your current medical problem only.** It must not be given to other people or used for other problems unless you are directed to do so by your doctor.

- **Keep all medicines out of the reach of children.**

- In order for this medicine to work, it must be used as directed.

- **It is very important that you read and understand the following information.** If any of the information causes you special concern, do not decide against using this medicine without first checking with your doctor.

- Before you begin using any new medicine (prescription or nonprescription) or if you develop any new medical problem while you are using this medicine, check with your doctor, nurse, or pharmacist.

- **If you have any questions** about the following information or if you want more information about this medicine or your medical problem, **ask your doctor, nurse, or pharmacist.**

Before Using This Medicine

In order to decide on the best treatment for your medical problem, your doctor should be told:
—if you have ever had any unusual or allergic reaction to cellulose sodium phosphate.

—if you are on a low-salt, low-sugar, or any other special diet, or if you are allergic to any substance, such as foods, sulfites or other preservatives, or dyes. Most medicines contain more than their active ingredient. Your doctor or pharmacist can help you avoid products that may cause a problem.

—if you are **pregnant** or if you may become pregnant. Studies have not been done in either humans or animals. However, pregnant women usually need more calcium in their diet, and should not take cellulose sodium phosphate unless it is clearly needed. Be sure you have discussed the risks and benefits with your doctor.

—if you are **breast-feeding**. It is not known whether cellulose sodium phosphate passes into breast milk. However, this medicine has not been shown to cause problems in nursing babies.

—if you have any of the following medical problems:
  Bone disease
  Edema or swelling
  Heart disease
  Intestinal problems
  Parathyroid disease or problems

—if you are taking **any** other prescription or nonprescription (OTC) medicine, especially:
  Antacids or laxatives containing calcium or magnesium
  Calcium supplements
  Magnesium supplements
  Vitamin C

Proper Use of This Medicine

Take this medicine mixed in a full glass (8 ounces) of water, soft drink, or fruit juice. After drinking all the liquid containing the medicine, rinse the glass with a little more liquid. Drink that also to make sure you get all the medicine.

It is very important that you take cellulose sodium phosphate with meals. If this medicine is taken an hour or more after a meal, it will not work as well.

Take cellulose sodium phosphate only as directed. Do not take more of it, do not take it more often, and do not take it for a longer period of time than your doctor ordered. To do so may increase the chance of side effects.

Drink at least a full glass (8 ounces) of water or other liquid every hour while you are awake, unless otherwise directed by your doctor. This also will help prevent kidney stones while you are taking cellulose sodium phosphate.

If you miss a dose of this medicine, skip the missed dose and go back to your regular dosing schedule. Do not double doses.

How to store this medicine:
- **Keep out of the reach of children.**

- Store away from heat and direct light.

- Do not store in the bathroom, near the kitchen sink, or in other damp places. Heat or moisture may cause the medicine to break down.

- Do not keep outdated medicine or medicine no longer needed. Be sure that any discarded medicine is out of the reach of children.

© 1988 The United States Pharmacopeial Convention, Inc.

Precautions While Using This Medicine

It is important that your doctor check your progress at regular visits. This is to make sure cellulose sodium phosphate is working properly and does not cause unwanted effects.

If you are taking a magnesium supplement, take it at least one hour before or after you take cellulose sodium phosphate. Otherwise, the magnesium may combine with this medicine and keep it from working as well.

Do not take vitamin C, or eat spinach (or other dark green leafy vegetables), chocolate, brewed tea, or rhubarb while you are taking cellulose sodium phosphate. They may increase the chance of kidney stones.

Do not drink milk or eat milk products (for example, cheese, ice cream, and yogurt) while you are taking this medicine, because dairy products are high in calcium. Eating or drinking milk or milk products may keep cellulose sodium phosphate from working as well.

While you are taking cellulose sodium phosphate, do not eat salty foods or use extra salt on foods. To do so may increase the chance of unwanted effects.

For patients on a sodium-restricted diet—This medicine contains sodium. If you have any questions about this, check with your doctor, nurse, or pharmacist.

Side Effects of This Medicine

Along with its needed effects, a medicine may cause some unwanted effects. Although not all of these side effects may occur, if they do occur they may need medical attention.

Check with your doctor as soon as possible if any of the following side effects occur:

With long-term use
    Drowsiness
    Loss of appetite
    Mood or mental changes
    Muscle spasms or twitching
    Nausea or vomiting
    Seizures
    Trembling
    Unusual tiredness or weakness

Other side effects may occur that usually do not require medical attention. These side effects may go away during treatment as your body adjusts to the medicine. However, check with your doctor if any of the following side effects continue or are bothersome:

More common
    Abdominal or stomach discomfort
    Loose bowel movements or diarrhea

For elderly patients: Many medicines have not been tested in older people. Therefore, it is not known whether the medicine acts the same way it does in younger adults. Check with your doctor or pharmacist if you notice any unusual effects while taking this medicine or if you think it is not working as it should.

Other side effects not listed above may also occur in some patients. If you notice any other effects, check with your doctor.

December 1987

CEPHALOSPORINS (Systemic)

This information applies to the following medicines:

Cefaclor (SEF-a-klor)
Cefadroxil (sef-a-DROX-ill)
Cefamandole (sef-a-MAN-dole)
Cefazolin (sef-A-zoe-lin)
Cefonicid (sef-FON-i-sid)
Cefoperazone (sef-oh-PER-a-zone)
Ceforanide (se-FOR-a-nide)
Cefotaxime (sef-oh-TAKS-eem)
Cefotetan (sef-oh-TEE-tan)
Cefoxitin (se-FOX-i-tin)
Ceftazidime (sef-TAY-zi-deem)
Ceftizoxime (sef-ti-ZOX-eem)
Ceftriaxone (sef-try-AX-one)
Cefuroxime (se-fyoor-OX-eem)
Cephalexin (sef-a-LEX-in)
Cephalothin (sef-A-loe-thin)
Cephapirin (sef-a-PYE-rin)
Cephradine (SEF-ra-deen)
Moxalactam (MOX-a-lak-tam)

Some commonly used brand names or other names are:	Generic names:
Ceclor	Cefaclor
Duricef Ultracef	Cefadroxil
Mandol	Cefamandole
Ancef Kefzol	Cefazolin†
Monocid	Cefonicid
Cefobid Cefobine*	Cefoperazone
Precef	Ceforanide
Claforan	Cefotaxime
Cefotan	Cefotetan
Mefoxin	Cefoxitin
Fortaz Magnacef* Tazicef Tazidime	Ceftazidime
Cefizox	Ceftizoxime
Rocephin	Ceftriaxone
Kefurox Zinacef	Cefuroxime
Ceporex* Keflet Keflex Novolexin*	Cephalexin†
Ceporacin* Keflin* Keflin Neutral Seffin Neutral	Cephalothin†
Cefadyl	Cephapirin†
Anspor Velosef	Cephradine†

Lamoxactam Latamoxef Moxam Oxalactam*	Moxalactam

*Not available in the U.S.
†Generic name product may also be available in the U.S.

To the Reader: If you do not recognize the names of medical conditions or medicines referred to in this information, check with your doctor, nurse, or pharmacist. Definitions for selected medical terms may be found in the Glossary. Brand names for the generic drug names listed can be found in the Index. In addition, selected brand names commonly associated with the generic name have been included in the text to help you recognize medicine you may be taking. The fact that a brand name product is not mentioned does not mean the information does not apply. It is a good idea for you to learn both the generic and brand names of your medicines and to write them down for future use.

Cephalosporins (sef-a-loe-SPOR-ins) belong to the family of medicines called antibiotics. Antibiotics are used in the treatment of infections caused by bacteria. They work by killing bacteria or preventing their growth.

Cephalosporins are taken by mouth or given by injection to treat bacterial infections in many different parts of the body. They are sometimes given with other antibiotics. Some cephalosporins are also given by injection to prevent infections before, during, and after surgery. However, cephalosporins will not work for colds, flu, or other viral infections.

Cephalosporins are available only with your doctor's prescription.

Remember:
• **This medicine has been prescribed for your present infection only.** Another infection later on may require a different medicine. Also, even though other people may have the same symptoms as you, they may have a different kind of infection. Your medicine may not work for them and may even cause them harm. Therefore, **your medicine must not be given to other people or used for other infections** unless you are otherwise directed by your doctor.

• **Keep all medicines out of the reach of children.**

• In order for this medicine to work, it must be used as directed.

• If you are receiving this medicine by injection, some of the information about this medicine may not apply.

• **It is very important that you read and understand the following information.** If any of the information causes you special concern, do not decide against using this medicine without first checking with your doctor.

• Before you begin using any new medicine (prescription or nonprescription) or if you develop any new medical problem while you are using this medicine, check with your doctor, nurse, or pharmacist.

• **If you have any questions** about the following information or if you want more information about this medicine or your medical problem, **ask your doctor, nurse, or pharmacist**.

Before Using This Medicine

In order to decide on the best treatment for your medical problem, your doctor should be told:

—if you have ever had any unusual or severe allergic reaction to any of the cephalosporins, penicillins, penicillin-like medicines, or penicillamine.

—if you are on a low-salt, low-sugar, or any other special diet, or if you are allergic to any substance, such as foods, sulfites or other preservatives, or dyes. Most medicines contain more than their active ingredient, and many liquid medicines contain alcohol. Your doctor, nurse, or pharmacist can help you avoid products that may cause a problem.

—if you are **pregnant** or if you may become pregnant. Studies have not been done in humans. However, most cephalosporins have not been shown to cause birth defects or other problems in animal studies. Studies in rats and mice have shown that moxalactam causes a decrease in the animal's ability to live after birth. Moxalactam has not been shown to cause birth defects or other problems in rats and mice given up to 20 times the usual human dose.

—if you are **breast-feeding**. Most cephalosporins pass into human breast milk, usually in small amounts. However, cephalosporins have not been shown to cause problems in nursing babies.

—if you have any of the following medical problems:
Bleeding problems, history of (cefamandole, cefoperazone, cefotetan, and moxalactam only)
Kidney disease
Liver disease (cefoperazone only)
Stomach or intestinal disease, history of (especially colitis, including colitis caused by antibiotics, or enteritis)

—if you are taking probenecid (e.g., Benemid), except with ceforanide, ceftazidime, or ceftriaxone.

—if you are receiving cefamandole, cefoperazone, cefotetan, or moxalactam and are also taking **any** other prescription or nonprescription (OTC) medicine, especially:
Alcohol-containing medicine
Anticoagulants (blood thinners)
Azlocillin (e.g., Azlin)
Carbenicillin by injection (e.g., Geopen)
Dipyridamole (e.g., Persantine)
Divalproex (e.g., Depakote)
Heparin (e.g., Panheprin)
Medicine for inflammation or pain (aspirin or other salicylates, diclofenac, diflunisal, fenoprofen, flurbiprofen [oral], ibuprofen, indomethacin, ketoprofen, meclofenamate, mefenamic acid, naproxen, oxyphenbutazone, phenylbutazone, piroxicam, sulindac, suprofen, tolmetin)
Mezlocillin (e.g., Mezlin)
Pentoxifylline (e.g., Trental)
Piperacillin (e.g., Pipracil)
Plicamycin (e.g., Mithracin)
Sulfinpyrazone (e.g., Anturane)
Ticarcillin (e.g., Ticar)
Valproic acid (e.g., Depakene)

—if you are receiving cephalothin and are also receiving **any** other prescription or nonprescription (OTC) medicine.

Proper Use of This Medicine

Cephalosporins may be taken on a full or empty stomach. If this medicine upsets your stomach, it may help to take it with food.

For patients taking the oral liquid form of this medicine:

• This medicine is to be taken by mouth even though it may come in a dropper bottle. If this medicine does not come in a dropper bottle, use a specially marked measuring spoon or other device to measure each dose accurately since the average household teaspoon may not hold the right amount of liquid.

• Do not use after the expiration date on the label since the medicine may not work as well. Check with your pharmacist if you have any questions about this.

To help clear up your infection completely, **keep taking this medicine for the full time of treatment,** even if you begin to feel better after a few days. **If you have a "strep" infection, you should keep taking this medicine for at least 10 days. This is especially important in "strep" infections since serious heart problems could develop later** if your infection is not cleared up completely. Also, if you stop taking this medicine too soon, your symptoms may return.

This medicine works best when there is a constant amount in the blood or urine. **To help keep the amount constant, do not miss any doses. Also, it is best to take the doses at evenly spaced times, day and night.** For example, if you are to take 4 doses a day, the doses should be spaced about 6 hours apart. If this interferes with your sleep or other daily activities, or if you need help in planning the best times to take your medicine, check with your doctor, nurse, or pharmacist.

If you do miss a dose of this medicine, take it as soon as possible. This will help to keep a constant amount of medicine in the blood or urine. However, if it is almost time for your next dose and your dosing schedule is:

• 1 dose a day—Space the missed dose and the next dose 10 to 12 hours apart.

• 2 doses a day—Space the missed dose and the next dose 5 to 6 hours apart.

• 3 or more doses a day—Space the missed dose and the next dose 2 to 4 hours apart or double your next dose.

Then go back to your regular dosing schedule.

How to store this medicine:

• **Keep out of the reach of children.**

• Store away from heat and direct light.

• Do not store the capsule or tablet form of this medicine in the bathroom, near the kitchen sink, or in other damp places. Heat or moisture may cause the medicine to break down.

• Store the oral liquid form of most cephalosporins in the refrigerator because heat will cause this medicine to break down. However, keep the medicine from freezing. Follow the directions on the label.

• Do not keep outdated medicine or medicine no longer needed. Be sure that any discarded medicine is out of the reach of children.

Precautions While Using This Medicine

If your symptoms do not improve within a few days, or if they become worse, check with your doctor.

Diabetics—This medicine may cause false test results with some urine sugar tests. Check with your doctor before changing your diet or the dosage of your diabetes medicine.

If diarrhea occurs, do not take any diarrhea medicine without first checking with your doctor or pharmacist. These medicines may make your diarrhea worse or make it last longer.

For patients receiving cefamandole, cefoperazone, cefotetan, or moxalactam by injection:
• Drinking alcoholic beverages or taking other alcohol-containing preparations (for example, elixirs, cough syrups, tonics, or injections of alcohol) while receiving these medicines may cause problems. The problems may last for several days after you stop taking these medicines. Drinking alcoholic beverages may result in increased side effects such as abdominal or stomach cramps, nausea, vomiting, headache, fainting, fast or irregular heartbeat, difficult breathing, sweating, or redness of the face or skin. These effects usually start within 15 to 30 minutes after you drink alcohol and may not go away for up to several hours. Therefore, **you should not drink alcoholic beverages or take other alcohol-containing preparations while you are receiving these medicines and for several days after stopping them.**

Side Effects of This Medicine

Along with its needed effects, a medicine may cause some unwanted effects. Although not all of these side effects may occur, if they do occur they may need medical attention.

Check with your doctor immediately if any of the following side effects occur:
Less common or rare
  Unusual bleeding or bruising (cefamandole, cefoperazone, cefotetan, and moxalactam only)
Rare
  Abdominal or stomach cramps, pain, and bloating (severe)
  Diarrhea (watery and severe), which may also be bloody
  Fever
  Increased thirst
  Nausea or vomiting
  Unusual tiredness or weakness
  Unusual weight loss
    (the above side effects may also occur up to several weeks after you stop taking this medicine)
  Convulsions (seizures)—moxalactam only

Other side effects may occur that usually do not require medical attention. These side effects may go away during treatment as your body adjusts to the medicine. However, check with your doctor if any of the following side effects continue or are bothersome:
More common (less common with some cephalosporins)
  Diarrhea (mild)
  Skin rash, itching, redness, or swelling
  Sore mouth or tongue
  Stomach cramps or upset (mild)
Less common or rare
  Itching of the rectal or genital (sex organ) areas

Other side effects not listed above may also occur in some patients. If you notice any other effects, check with your doctor.

December 1987

CHARCOAL, ACTIVATED (Oral)

Some commonly used brand names are:

Acta-Char	Charcocaps
Acta-Char Liquid	Aqueous Charcodote*
Actidose-Aqua	Insta-Char
Arm-a-char	Liquid-Antidose
CharcoalantiDote	

Generic name product available in the U.S.

---

*Not available in the U.S.

To the Reader: If you do not recognize the names of medical conditions or medicines referred to in this information, check with your doctor, nurse, or pharmacist. Definitions for selected medical terms may be found in the Glossary. Brand names for the generic drug names listed can be found in the Index. In addition, selected brand names commonly associated with the generic name have been included in the text to help you recognize medicine you may be taking. The fact that a brand name product is not mentioned does not mean the information does not apply. It is a good idea for you to learn both the generic and brand names of your medicines and to write them down for future use.

Activated charcoal (AK-ti-vay-ted CHAR-kole) is taken by mouth in the emergency treatment of certain kinds of poisoning. It helps prevent the poison from being absorbed by the body. Ordinarily, this medicine should not be used in poisoning if corrosive agents such as alkalis (lye) and strong acids, cyanide, iron, ethyl alcohol, or methyl alcohol have been swallowed, since it will not prevent these poisons from being absorbed into the body.

This medicine may also be used to relieve diarrhea and intestinal gas or stomach discomfort.

In babies and children under 3 years of age, activated charcoal should not be used for a long period of time to relieve diarrhea and gas, because it may affect the child's nutrition.

Activated charcoal is available without a doctor's prescription; however, before using this medicine for poisoning, call your doctor, a poison control center, or an emergency room for advice. Also, your doctor may have special instructions on the proper use of this medicine for diarrhea or intestinal gas.

Remember:

• **Keep all medicines out of the reach of children.**

• In order for this medicine to work, it must be used as directed. **If you are using this medicine without a prescription, it is very important to follow the directions on the label.**

• **It is also very important that you read and understand the following information.** If any of the information causes you special concern, check with your doctor before using this medicine without a prescription.

• Before you begin using any new medicine (prescription or nonprescription) or if you develop any new medical problem while you are using this medicine, check with your doctor, nurse, or pharmacist.

• **If you have any questions** about the following information or if you want more information about this medicine or your medical problem, **ask your doctor, nurse, or pharmacist.**

Before Using This Medicine

Before you use activated charcoal **for stomach or intestinal problems**, check with your doctor or pharmacist:

—if you have ever had any unusual or allergic reaction to activated charcoal.

—if you are on a low-salt, low-sugar, or any other special diet, or if you are allergic to any substance, such as foods, sulfites or other preservatives, or dyes. Most medicines contain more than their active ingredient. Your doctor, nurse, or pharmacist can help you avoid products that may cause a problem.

—if you are **pregnant** or if you may become pregnant while taking this medicine. Activated charcoal has not been shown to cause birth defects or other problems in humans.

—if you are **breast-feeding**. Activated charcoal has not been shown to cause problems in nursing babies.

—if you are taking **any** other prescription or nonprescription (OTC) medicine.

Proper Use of This Medicine

Do not take this medicine mixed with ice cream or sherbet, since it may prevent the medicine from working properly.

For patients taking this medicine for poisoning:

• **Before taking this medicine in the treatment of poisoning, call your doctor, a poison control center, or an emergency room for advice.** It is a good idea to have these telephone numbers readily available.

• If you have been told to take both this medicine and ipecac syrup to treat the poisoning, **do not take this medicine until after you have taken the ipecac syrup to cause vomiting and the vomiting has stopped. This is usually about 30 minutes.** Taking them together may prevent the ipecac syrup from causing vomiting of the poison.

How to store this medicine:

• **Keep out of the reach of children.**

• Store away from heat and direct light.

• Do not store the capsule, tablet, or powder form of this medicine in the bathroom, near the kitchen sink, or in other damp places. Heat or moisture may cause the medicine to break down.

• Keep the liquid form of this medicine from freezing.

• Do not keep outdated medicine or medicine no longer needed. Be sure that any discarded medicine is out of the reach of children.

Precautions While Using This Medicine

For patients taking this medicine for stomach or intestinal problems:

• If you are taking this medicine for intestinal gas or stomach discomfort and your condition has not improved after 7 days, check with your doctor.

• If you are taking this medicine for diarrhea and your condition has not improved after 2 days or if you have fever with the diarrhea, check with your doctor.

• **If you are taking any other medicine, do not take it within 2 hours of the activated charcoal.** Taking them together may prevent the other medicine from being absorbed by your body. If you have any questions about this, check with your doctor, nurse, or pharmacist.

Side Effects of This Medicine

This medicine will cause your stools to turn black. This is to be expected while you are taking this medicine.

There have not been any other side effects reported with this medicine. However, if you notice any other effects, check with your doctor.

December 1987

CHENODIOL (Systemic)

A commonly used brand name is Chenix.

To the Reader: If you do not recognize the names of medical conditions or medicines referred to in this information, check with your doctor, nurse, or pharmacist. Definitions for selected medical terms may be found in the Glossary. Brand names for the generic drug names listed can be found in the Index. In addition, selected brand names commonly associated with the generic name have been included in the text to help you recognize medicine you may be taking. The fact that a brand name product is not mentioned does not mean the information does not apply. It is a good idea for you to learn both the generic and brand names of your medicines and to write them down for future use.

Chenodiol (kee-noe-DYE-ole) is used in the treatment of gallstone disease. It is taken by mouth to dissolve the gallstones.

Chenodiol is used in patients who do not need to have their gallbladder removed or in those in whom surgery is best avoided because of other medical problems. However, chenodiol works only in those patients who have a working gallbladder and whose gallstones are made of cholesterol. Chenodiol works best when these stones are small and of the "floating" type.

Chenodiol is available only with your doctor's prescription.

Remember:

• **This medicine has been prescribed for your current medical problem only.** It must not be given to other people or used for other problems unless you are directed to do so by your doctor.

• **Keep all medicines out of the reach of children.**

• In order for this medicine to work, it must be used as directed.

• **It is very important that you read and understand the following information.** If any of the information causes you special concern, do not decide against using this medicine without first checking with your doctor.

• Before you begin using any new medicine (prescription or nonprescription) or if you develop any new medical problem while you are using this medicine, check with your doctor, nurse, or pharmacist.

• **If you have any questions** about the following information or if you want more information about this medicine or your medical problem, **ask your doctor, nurse, or pharmacist**.

Before Using This Medicine

Importance of diet—If you have gallstones, your doctor may prescribe chenodiol and a personal high-fiber diet for you. Some foods that are high in fiber are whole grain breads and cereals, bran, fruit, and green, leafy vegetables. It has been found that such a diet may help dissolve the stones faster and may keep new stones from forming.

It may also be important for you to go on a reducing diet. However, check with your doctor before going on any diet.

In order to decide on the best treatment for your medical problem, your doctor should be told:

—if you have ever had any unusual or allergic reaction to chenodiol.

—if you are **pregnant** or if you may become pregnant. Chenodiol is not recommended during pregnancy. It has been shown to cause liver and kidney problems in animals when given in doses many times the human dose. Be sure you have discussed this with your doctor.

—if you are **breast-feeding**. It is not known whether chenodiol passes into the breast milk. However, this medicine has not been shown to cause problems in nursing babies.

—if you have any of the following medical problems:
　Biliary tract problems
　Blood vessel disease
　Bowel inflammation disease
　Liver disease
　Pancreas disease

—if you are taking **any** other prescription or nonprescription (OTC) medicine.

Proper Use of This Medicine

Take chenodiol with food or milk for best results, unless otherwise directed by your doctor.

Take chenodiol for the full time of treatment, even if you begin to feel better. If you stop taking this medicine too soon, the gallstones may not dissolve as fast or may not dissolve at all.

If you miss a dose of this medicine, take it as soon as possible. However, if it is almost time for your next dose, skip the missed dose and go back to your regular dosing schedule. Do not double doses.

How to store this medicine:

• **Keep out of the reach of children.**

• Store away from heat and direct light.

• Do not store the tablet form of this medicine in the bathroom, near the kitchen sink, or in other damp places. Heat or moisture may cause the medicine to break down.

• Do not keep outdated medicine or medicine no longer needed. Be sure that any discarded medicine is out of the reach of children.

Precautions While Using This Medicine

It is important that your doctor check your progress at regular visits. Laboratory tests will have to be done every few months while you are taking this medicine in order to make sure the gallstones are dissolving and your liver is working properly.

Check with your doctor immediately if severe abdominal or stomach pain, especially toward the upper right side, and severe nausea and vomiting occur. These symptoms may mean that you have other medical problems or that your gallstone condition needs your doctor's attention.

Side Effects of This Medicine

Along with its needed effects, a medicine may cause some unwanted effects. Although not all of these side effects may occur, if they do occur they may need medical attention.

Check with your doctor as soon as possible if the following side effect occurs:

Less common or rare
    Diarrhea (severe)

Other side effects may occur that usually do not require medical attention. These side effects may go away during treatment as your body adjusts to the medicine. However, check with your doctor if any of the following side effects continue or are bothersome:

More common
    Diarrhea (mild)

Less common or rare
    Constipation
    Frequent urge for bowel movement
    Gas or indigestion (usually disappears within 2 to 4 weeks from the beginning of treatment)
    Loss of appetite
    Nausea or vomiting
    Stomach cramps or pain

For elderly patients: Many medicines have not been tested in older people. Therefore, it is not known whether the medicine acts the same way it does in younger adults. Check with your doctor or pharmacist if you notice any unusual effects while taking this medicine or if you think it is not working as it should.

Other side effects not listed above may also occur in some patients. If you notice any other effects, check with your doctor.

December 1987

© 1988   The United States Pharmacopeial Convention, Inc.

CHLOPHEDIANOL (Systemic)*

A commonly used brand name is Ulone*.

---

*Not commercially available in the U.S.

To the Reader: If you do not recognize the names of medical conditions or medicines referred to in this information, check with your doctor, nurse, or pharmacist. Definitions for selected medical terms may be found in the Glossary. Brand names for the generic drug names listed can be found in the Index. In addition, selected brand names commonly associated with the generic name have been included in the text to help you recognize medicine you may be taking. The fact that a brand name product is not mentioned does not mean the information does not apply. It is a good idea for you to learn both the generic and brand names of your medicines and to write them down for future use.

Chlophedianol (kloe-fe-DYE-a-nole) is used to relieve dry, irritating coughs. This medicine is not used when there is mucus or phlegm (pronounced flem) with the cough.

Chlophedianol is available only with your doctor's prescription.

Remember:

• **This medicine has been prescribed for your current medical problem only.** It must not be given to other people or used for other problems unless you are directed to do so by your doctor.

• **Keep all medicines out of the reach of children.**

• In order for this medicine to work, it must be used as directed.

• **It is very important that you read and understand the following information.** If any of the information causes you special concern, do not decide against using this medicine without first checking with your doctor.

• Before you begin using any new medicine (prescription or nonprescription) or if you develop any new medical problem while you are using this medicine, check with your doctor, nurse, or pharmacist.

• **If you have any questions** about the following information or if you want more information about this medicine or your medical problem, **ask your doctor, nurse, or pharmacist.**

Before Using This Medicine

In order to decide on the best treatment for your medical problem, your doctor should be told:

—if you have ever had any unusual or allergic reaction to chlophedianol.

—if you are on a low-salt, low-sugar, or any other special diet, or if you are allergic to any substance, such as foods, sulfites or other preservatives, or dyes. Most medicines contain more than their active ingredient. Your doctor, nurse, or pharmacist can help you avoid products that may cause a problem.

—if you are **pregnant** or if you may become pregnant. Chlophedianol has not been shown to cause birth defects or other problems in humans.

—if you are **breast-feeding**. Chlophedianol has not been shown to cause problems in nursing babies.

—if you have a productive cough (with phlegm).

—if you are now taking any of the following medicines or types of medicine:

    Amantadine
    Amphetamines
    Appetite suppressants (diet pills), except fenfluramine
    Caffeine
    Central nervous system (CNS) depressants
    Medicine for asthma or other breathing problems
    Medicine for colds, sinus problems, or hay fever or other allergies (including nose drops or sprays)
    Methylphenidate
    Pemoline

Proper Use of This Medicine

Do not take liquids immediately after taking this medicine. To do so may decrease the soothing effect of the syrup.

Take this medicine only as directed. Do not take more of it and do not take it more often than your doctor ordered. To do so may increase the chance of side effects.

If you are taking this medicine on a regular schedule and you miss a dose, take it as soon as possible. However, if it is almost time for your next dose, skip the missed dose and go back to your regular dosing schedule. Do not double doses.

How to store this medicine:

• **Keep out of the reach of children.**

• Store away from heat and direct light.

• Keep the syrup from freezing.

• Do not keep outdated medicine or medicine no longer needed. Be sure that any discarded medicine is out of the reach of children.

Precautions While Using This Medicine

If your cough has not improved after 7 days, or if you have a high fever, skin rash, or continuing headache with the cough, check with your doctor. These signs may mean that you have other medical problems.

This medicine will add to the effects of alcohol and other CNS depressants (medicines that slow down the nervous system, possibly causing drowsiness). Some examples of CNS depressants are antihistamines or medicine for hay fever, other allergies, or colds; sedatives, tranquilizers, or sleeping medicine; prescription pain medicine or narcotics; barbiturates; medicine for seizures; muscle relaxants; or anesthetics, including some dental anesthetics. **Check with your doctor before taking any of the above while you are taking this medicine.**

This medicine may also add to the effects of CNS stimulants, such as appetite suppressants and caffeine-containing beverages like tea, coffee, cocoa, and cola drinks. **Avoid drinking large amounts of these beverages while taking this medicine.** If you have any questions about this, check with your doctor.

This medicine may cause some people to become drowsy or less alert than they are normally. **Make sure you know how you react to this medicine before you drive, use machines, or do other jobs that require you to be alert.**

Side Effects of This Medicine

Along with its needed effects, a medicine may cause some unwanted effects. Although not all of these side effects may occur, if they do occur they may need medical attention.

Check with your doctor as soon as possible if any of the following side effects occur:

Rare
  Hallucinations (seeing, hearing, or feeling things that are not there)
  Nightmares
  Skin rash or hives
  Unusual excitement or irritability

With large doses
  Blurred vision
  Drowsiness or dizziness
  Dryness of the mouth
  Nausea or vomiting

For elderly patients: Many medicines have not been tested in older people. Therefore, it is not known whether the medicine acts the same way it does in younger adults. Check with your doctor or pharmacist if you notice any unusual effects while taking this medicine or if you think it is not working as it should.

Other side effects not listed above may also occur in some patients. If you notice any other effects, check with your doctor.

December 1987

CHLORAL HYDRATE (Systemic)

Some commonly used brand names are:

Aquachloral Supprettes   Novochlorhydrate*
Noctec

Generic name product may also be available in the U.S.

*Not available in the U.S.

To the Reader: If you do not recognize the names of medical conditions or medicines referred to in this information, check with your doctor, nurse, or pharmacist. Definitions for selected medical terms may be found in the Glossary. Brand names for the generic drug names listed can be found in the Index. In addition, selected brand names commonly associated with the generic name have been included in the text to help you recognize medicine you may be taking. The fact that a brand name product is not mentioned does not mean the information does not apply. It is a good idea for you to learn both the generic and brand names of your medicines and to write them down for future use.

Chloral hydrate (klor-al HYE-drate) belongs to the group of medicines called sedatives and hypnotics. It is used in the treatment of insomnia (sleeplessness) to help patients fall asleep and stay asleep through the night. Also, chloral hydrate may used to help calm or relax patients who are nervous or tense. It is sometimes used before surgery or certain procedures to relieve anxiety or tension or to produce sleep. In addition, chloral hydrate may be used with analgesics (pain medicine) for control of pain following surgery.

Chloral hydrate should not be used for nervousness or tension caused by the stress of everyday life.

This medicine is available only with your doctor's prescription.

Remember:

• **This medicine has been prescribed for your current medical problem only.** It must not be given to other people or used for other problems unless you are directed to do so by your doctor.

• **Keep all medicines out of the reach of children.**

• In order for this medicine to work, it must be used as directed.

• **It is very important that you read and understand the following information.** If any of the information causes you special concern, do not decide against using this medicine without first checking with your doctor.

• Before you begin using any new medicine (prescription or nonprescription) or if you develop any new medical problem while you are using this medicine, check with your doctor, nurse, or pharmacist.

• **If you have any questions** about the following information or if you want more information about this medicine or your medical problem, **ask your doctor, nurse, or pharmacist.**

Before Using This Medicine

In order to decide on the best treatment for your medical problem, your doctor should be told:

—if you have ever had any unusual or allergic reaction to chloral hydrate.

—if you are on a low-salt, low-sugar, or any other special diet, or if you are allergic to any substance, such as foods, sulfites or other preservatives, or dyes. Most medicines contain more than their active ingredient, and many liquid medicines contain alcohol. Your doctor, nurse, or pharmacist can help you avoid products that may cause a problem.

—if you are **pregnant** or if you may become pregnant. Studies on birth defects have not been done in either humans or animals. Too much use of chloral hydrate during pregnancy may cause the baby to become dependent on the medicine. This may lead to withdrawal side effects after birth.

—if you are **breast-feeding**. Chloral hydrate passes into the breast milk and may cause drowsiness in babies of mothers using this medicine.

—if you are taking this medicine by mouth or using the rectal suppository form of chloral hydrate and have any of the following medical problems:

Heart disease
Kidney disease
Liver disease
Porphyria

—if you are taking this medicine by mouth and have gastritis or inflammation of the stomach.

—if you are using the rectal suppository form of chloral hydrate and have either of the following medical problems:

Colitis
Proctitis or inflammation of the rectum

—if you are taking **any** other prescription or nonprescription (OTC) medicine, especially:

Anticoagulants (blood thinners)
Central nervous system (CNS) depressants

Proper Use of This Medicine

For patients taking the capsule form of chloral hydrate:

• Swallow the capsule whole. Do not chew since the medicine may cause an unpleasant taste.

• Take this medicine with a full glass (8 ounces) of water, fruit juice, or ginger ale to lessen stomach upset.

For patients taking the syrup form of chloral hydrate:

• Take each dose of medicine mixed with ½ glass (4 ounces) of water, fruit juice, or ginger ale to improve flavor and lessen stomach upset.

For patients using the rectal suppository form of chloral hydrate:

• How to insert suppository: First remove the foil wrapper and moisten the suppository with water. Lie down on your side and push the suppository well up into the rectum with the finger. If the suppository is too soft to insert because of storage in a warm place, before removing the foil wrapper chill the suppository in the refrigerator for 30 minutes or run cold water over it.

Use this medicine only as directed by your doctor. Do not use more of it, do not use it more often, and do not use it for a longer period of time than your doctor ordered. If too much is used, it may become habit-forming.

If you miss a dose of this medicine, skip the missed dose and go back to your regular dosing schedule. Do not double doses.

How to store this medicine:

• **Keep out of the reach of children** since overdose is especially dangerous in children.

• Store away from heat and direct light.

• Do not store the capsule form of this medicine in the bathroom, near the kitchen sink, or in other damp places. Heat or moisture may cause the medicine to break down.

• Keep the syrup form of this medicine from freezing.

• Do not keep outdated medicine or medicine no longer needed. Be sure that any discarded medicine is out of the reach of children.

Precautions While Using This Medicine

If you will be using this medicine regularly for a long period of time:

• Your doctor should check your progress at regular visits in order to make sure that this medicine does not cause unwanted effects.

• Do not stop using it without first checking with your doctor. Your doctor may want you to reduce gradually the amount you are using before stopping completely.

This medicine will add to the effects of alcohol and other CNS depressants (medicines that slow down the nervous system, possibly causing drowsiness). Some examples of CNS depressants are antihistamines or medicine for hay fever, other allergies, or colds; sedatives, tranquilizers, or sleeping medicine; prescription pain medicine or narcotics; barbiturates; medicine for convulsions (seizures); muscle relaxants; or anesthetics, including some dental anesthetics. **Check with your doctor before taking any of the above while you are using this medicine.**

If you think you or someone else may have taken an overdose, get emergency help at once. Taking an overdose of chloral hydrate or taking alcohol or other CNS depressants with chloral hydrate may lead to unconsciousness and possibly death. Some signs of an overdose are continuing confusion, difficulty in swallowing, convulsions (seizures), severe drowsiness, severe weakness, shortness of breath or troubled breathing, staggering, and slow or irregular heartbeat.

This medicine may cause some people to become dizzy, lightheaded, drowsy, or less alert than they are normally. Even if taken at bedtime, it may cause some people to feel drowsy or less alert on arising. **Make sure you know how you react to this medicine before you drive, use machines, or do other jobs that require you to be alert.**

Side Effects of This Medicine

Along with its needed effects, a medicine may cause some unwanted effects. Although not all of these side effects may occur, if they do occur they may need medical attention.

Check with your doctor as soon as possible if any of the following side effects occur:

Less common
  Skin rash or hives

Rare
  Confusion
  Hallucinations (seeing, hearing, or feeling things that are not there)
  Unusual excitement

Signs of overdose
  Confusion (continuing)
  Convulsions (seizures)
  Difficulty in swallowing
  Drowsiness (severe)
  Low body temperature
  Nausea, vomiting, or stomach pain (severe)
  Shortness of breath or troubled breathing
  Slow or irregular heartbeat
  Staggering
  Weakness (severe)

Other side effects may occur that do not require medical attention. These side effects may go away during treatment as your body adjusts to the medicine. However, check with your doctor if any of the following side effects continue or are bothersome:

More common
  Nausea
  Stomach pain
  Vomiting

Less common
  Clumsiness or unsteadiness
  Dizziness or lightheadedness
  Drowsiness
  "Hangover" effect

For elderly patients: Many medicines have not been tested in older people. Therefore, it is not known whether the medicine acts the same way it does in younger adults. Check with your doctor or pharmacist if you notice any unusual effects while taking this medicine or if you think it is not working as it should.

After you stop using this medicine, your body may need time to adjust. The length of time this takes depends on the amount of medicine you were using and how long you used it. During this period of time check with your doctor if you notice any of the following side effects:

    Confusion
    Hallucinations (seeing, hearing, or feeling things that are
        not there)
    Nausea or vomiting
    Nervousness
    Restlessness

    Stomach pain
    Trembling
    Unusual excitement

Other side effects not listed above may also occur in some patients. If you notice any other effects, check with your doctor.

December 1987

CHLORAMBUCIL (Systemic)

A commonly used brand name is Leukeran.

To the Reader: If you do not recognize the names of medical conditions or medicines referred to in this information, check with your doctor, nurse, or pharmacist. Definitions for selected medical terms may be found in the Glossary. Brand names for the generic drug names listed can be found in the Index. In addition, selected brand names commonly associated with the generic name have been included in the text to help you recognize medicine you may be taking. The fact that a brand name product is not mentioned does not mean the information does not apply. It is a good idea for you to learn both the generic and brand names of your medicines and to write them down for future use.

Chlorambucil (klor-AM-byoo-sill) belongs to the group of medicines called alkylating agents. It is used to treat some kinds of cancer.

Chlorambucil interferes with the growth of cancer cells, which are eventually destroyed. Since the growth of normal body cells may also be affected by chlorambucil, other effects will also occur. Some of these may be serious and must be reported to your doctor. Other effects may not be serious but may cause concern. Some effects may not occur for months or years after the medicine is used.

Before you begin treatment with chlorambucil, you and your doctor should talk about the good this medicine will do as well as the risks of using it.

Chlorambucil may also be used for other conditions as determined by your doctor.

Chlorambucil is available only with your doctor's prescription.

Remember:
* **This medicine has been prescribed for your current medical problem only.** It must not be given to other people or used for other problems unless you are directed to do so by your doctor.

* **Keep all medicines out of the reach of children.**

* In order for this medicine to work, it must be used as directed.

* **It is very important that you read and understand the following information.** If any of the information causes you special concern, do not decide against using this medicine without first checking with your doctor.

* Before you begin using any new medicine (prescription or nonprescription) or if you develop any new medical problem while you are using this medicine, check with your doctor, nurse, or pharmacist.

* **If you have any questions** about the following information or if you want more information about this medicine or your medical problem, **ask your doctor, nurse, or pharmacist.**

Before Using This Medicine

In order to decide on the best treatment for your medical problem, your doctor should be told:
—if you have ever had any unusual or allergic reaction to chlorambucil or melphalan.
—if you are **pregnant** or if you intend to have children. This medicine may cause birth defects if either the male or female is taking it at the time of conception

or if it is taken during pregnancy. In addition, many cancer medicines may cause sterility which could be permanent. This has been reported with this medicine and the possibility should be kept in mind. Be sure that you have discussed this with your doctor before taking this medicine.

—if you intend to **breast-feed**. Because of the serious side effects caused by this medicine, breast-feeding is generally not recommended while you are taking it.

—if you have any of the following medical problems:
Chickenpox (including recent exposure)
Gout
Herpes zoster (shingles)
Infection
Kidney stones (history of)

—if you are using **any** other prescription or nonprescription (OTC) medicine, especially:
Adrenocorticoids (cortisone-like medicine)
Amphotericin B by injection (e.g., Fungizone)
Antithyroid agents (medicine for overactive thyroid)
Azathioprine (e.g., Imuran)
Chloramphenicol (e.g., Chloromycetin)
Colchicine
Cyclophosphamide (e.g., Cytoxan)
Cyclosporine (e.g., Sandimmune)
Flucytosine (e.g., Ancobon)
Interferon (e.g., Intron A, Roferon-A)
Mercaptopurine (e.g., Purinethol)
Muromonab-CD3 (monoclonal antibody) (e.g., Orthoclone OKT3)

—if you have ever been treated with x-rays or cancer medicines.

Proper Use of This Medicine

Take this medicine only as directed by your doctor. Do not take more or less of it, and do not take it more often than your doctor ordered. The exact amount of medicine you need has been carefully worked out. Taking too much may increase the chance of side effects, while taking too little may not improve your condition.

Chlorambucil is sometimes given together with certain other medicines. If you are using a combination of medicines, make sure that you take each one at the proper time and do not mix them. Ask your doctor, nurse, or pharmacist to help you plan a way to remember to take your medicines at the right times.

While you are using chlorambucil, your doctor may want you to drink extra fluids so that you will pass more urine. This will help prevent kidney problems and keep your kidneys working well.

This medicine sometimes causes nausea and vomiting. However, it is very important that you continue to use the medicine, even if you begin to feel ill. **Do not stop using this medicine without first checking with your doctor.** Ask your doctor, nurse, or pharmacist for ways to lessen these effects.

If you vomit shortly after taking a dose of chlorambucil, check with your doctor. You will be told whether to take the dose again or wait until the next scheduled dose.

If you miss a dose of this medicine and your dosing schedule is:

Once a day—Take the missed dose as soon as possible. Then go back to your regular dosing schedule. However, if you do not remember the missed dose until the next day, do not take it at all. Instead, take your regularly scheduled dose. Do not double doses.

Several times a day—Take the missed dose as soon as possible. Then go back to your regular dosing schedule. However, if it is almost time for your next dose, skip the missed dose and go back to your regular dosing schedule. Do not double doses.

How to store this medicine:

• **Keep out of the reach of children.**

• Store away from heat and direct light.

• Do not store in the bathroom, near the kitchen sink, or in other damp places. Heat or moisture may cause the medicine to break down.

• Do not keep outdated medicine or medicine no longer needed. Be sure that any discarded medicine is out of the reach of children.

Precautions While Using This Medicine

It is very important that your doctor check your progress at regular visits to make sure this medicine is working properly and to check for unwanted effects.

While you are being treated with chlorambucil, and after you stop treatment with it, **do not have any immunizations without your doctor's approval**. Chlorambucil lowers your body's resistance and there is a chance you might get the infection the immunization is meant to prevent. In addition, other persons living in your household should not take oral polio vaccine since there is a chance they could pass the polio virus on to you. Also, you should avoid close contact with other persons (for example, at school or work) who have taken oral polio vaccine.

Chlorambucil can lower the number of white blood cells in your body. This may increase the chance of getting an infection. If you can, avoid people with colds or other infections. If you think you are getting a cold or other infection, check with your doctor.

Side Effects of This Medicine

Along with their needed effects, medicines like chlorambucil can sometimes cause unwanted effects such as blood problems and other side effects; these are described below. Also, because of the way these medicines act on the body, there is a chance that they might cause other unwanted effects that may not occur until months or years after the medicine is used. These delayed effects may include certain types of cancer, such as leukemia. Discuss these possible effects with your doctor.

Although not all of these side effects may occur, if they do occur they may need medical attention.

Check with your doctor immediately if any of the following side effects occur:

More common
Fever, chills, or sore throat
Sores in the mouth and on the lips
Unusual bleeding or bruising

Check with your doctor as soon as possible if any of the following side effects occur:

Less common
Joint pain
Lower back, side, or stomach pain
Skin rash
Swelling of feet or lower legs

Rare
Convulsions (seizures)
Cough
Shortness of breath
Yellow eyes and skin

Signs of overdose (in the order in which they may occur)
Difficulty in walking
Muscle twitching
Stomach pain
Vomiting
Unusual excitement
Convulsions (seizures)

Other side effects may occur that usually do not require medical attention. These side effects may go away during treatment as your body adjusts to the medicine. Also, your doctor or nurse may be able to tell you about ways to prevent or reduce some of these side effects. Check with your doctor if any of the following side effects continue or are bothersome or if you have any questions about them:

Less common
Changes in menstrual period
Itching of skin
Nausea and vomiting

For elderly patients: Many medicines have not been tested in older people. Therefore, it is not known whether the medicine acts the same way it does in younger adults. Check with your doctor or pharmacist if you notice any unusual effects while taking this medicine or if you think it is not working as it should.

After you stop using chlorambucil, it may still produce some side effects that need attention. During this period of time, check with your doctor if you notice any of the following side effects:
Cough
Fever, chills, or sore throat
Shortness of breath
Unusual bleeding or bruising

Other side effects not listed above may also occur in some patients. If you notice any other effects, check with your doctor.

December 1987

CHLORAMPHENICOL (Ophthalmic)

Some commonly used brand names are:

Chloromycetin	Isopto Fenicol*
Chloroptic	Ophthochlor
Fenicol*	Pentamycetin*

Generic name product may also be available in the U.S.

*Not available in the U.S.

To the Reader: If you do not recognize the names of medical conditions or medicines referred to in this information, check with your doctor, nurse, or pharmacist. Definitions for selected medical terms may be found in the Glossary. Brand names for the generic drug names listed can be found in the Index. In addition, selected brand names commonly associated with the generic name have been included in the text to help you recognize medicine you may be taking. The fact that a brand name product is not mentioned does not mean the information does not apply. It is a good idea for you to learn both the generic and brand names of your medicines and to write them down for future use.

Chloramphenicol (klor-am-FEN-i-kole) belongs to the general family of medicines called antibiotics. Chloramphenicol ophthalmic preparations are used in the eye to help the body overcome infections of the eye.

Chloramphenicol is available only with your doctor's prescription.

Remember:

• **This medicine has been prescribed for your present infection only.** Another infection later on may require a different medicine. Also, even though other people may have the same symptoms as you, they may have a different kind of infection. Your medicine may not work for them and may even cause them harm. Therefore, **your medicine must not be given to other people or used for other infections** unless you are otherwise directed by your doctor.

• **Keep all medicines out of the reach of children.**

• In order for this medicine to work, it must be used as directed.

• **It is very important that you read and understand the following information.** If any of the information causes you special concern, do not decide against using this medicine without first checking with your doctor.

• Before you begin using any new medicine (prescription or nonprescription) or if you develop any new medical problem while you are using this medicine, check with your doctor, nurse, or pharmacist.

• **If you have any questions** about the following information or if you want more information about this medicine or your medical problem, **ask your doctor, nurse, or pharmacist.**

Before Using This Medicine

In order to decide on the best treatment for your medical problem, your doctor should be told:

—if you have ever had any unusual or allergic reaction to chloramphenicol.

—if you are allergic to any substance, such as certain foods or preservatives or dyes. Most medicines contain more than their active ingredient. Your doctor, nurse, or pharmacist can help you avoid products that may cause a problem.

—if you are **pregnant** or if you may become pregnant. However, chloramphenicol ophthalmic preparations have not been shown to cause birth defects or other problems in humans.

—if you are **breast-feeding**. However, chloramphenicol ophthalmic preparations have not been shown to cause problems in nursing babies.

Proper Use of This Medicine

For patients using the eye drop form of chloramphenicol:

• Although the bottle may not be full, it contains exactly the amount of medicine your doctor ordered.

• How to apply this medicine: First, wash your hands. Then tilt the head back and pull the lower eyelid away from the eye to form a pouch. Drop the medicine into the pouch and gently close the eyes. Do not blink. Keep the eyes closed for 1 or 2 minutes to allow the medicine to come into contact with the infection.

• If you think you did not get the drop of medicine into your eye properly, use another drop.

• To prevent contamination of the eye drops, do not touch the applicator tip or dropper to any surface (including the eye). Also, keep the container tightly closed.

For patients using the eye ointment form of chloramphenicol:

• How to apply this medicine: First, wash your hands. Then pull the lower eyelid away from the eye to form a pouch. Squeeze a thin strip of ointment into the pouch. A 1-cm (approximately ⅓-inch) strip of ointment is usually enough unless otherwise directed by your doctor. Gently close the eyes and keep them closed for 1 or 2 minutes to allow the medicine to come into contact with the infection.

• To prevent contamination of the eye ointment, do not touch the applicator tip to any surface (including the eye). After using chloramphenicol eye ointment, wipe the tip of the ointment tube with a clean tissue and keep the tube tightly closed.

To help clear up your infection completely, **keep using this medicine for the full time of treatment**, even if your symptoms begin to clear up after a few days. If you stop using this medicine too soon, your symptoms may return. **Do not miss any doses.**

If you do miss a dose of this medicine, apply it as soon as possible. However, if it is almost time for your next dose, skip the missed dose and go back to your regular dosing schedule.

How to store this medicine:

• **Keep out of the reach of children.**

• Store away from heat and direct light.

• Keep the medicine from freezing.

• Do not keep outdated medicine or medicine no longer needed. Be sure that any discarded medicine is out of the reach of children.

Precautions While Using This Medicine

If your symptoms do not improve within a few days, or if they become worse, check with your doctor.

Side Effects of This Medicine

Along with its needed effects, a medicine may cause some unwanted effects. Although not all of these side effects may occur, if they do occur they may need medical attention.

Check with your doctor immediately if any of the following side effects occur:

Rare
    Pale skin
    Sore throat and fever
    Unusual bleeding or bruising
    Unusual tiredness or weakness
       (the above side effects may also occur weeks or months after you stop using this medicine)

Other side effects may occur that usually do not require medical attention. These side effects may go away during treatment as your body adjusts to the medicine. However, check with your doctor if either of the following side effects continues or is bothersome:

Less common
    Burning or stinging

After application, eye ointments may be expected to cause your vision to blur for a few minutes.

Other side effects not listed above may also occur in some patients. If you notice any other effects, check with your doctor.

_____

December 1987

_____

CHLORAMPHENICOL (Otic)

Some commonly used brand names are Chloromycetin and Pentamycetin*.

*Not available in the U.S.

To the Reader: If you do not recognize the names of medical conditions or medicines referred to in this information, check with your doctor, nurse, or pharmacist. Definitions for selected medical terms may be found in the Glossary. Brand names for the generic drug names listed can be found in the Index. In addition, selected brand names commonly associated with the generic name have been included in the text to help you recognize medicine you may be taking. The fact that a brand name product is not mentioned does not mean the information does not apply. It is a good idea for you to learn both the generic and brand names of your medicines and to write them down for future use.

Chloramphenicol (klor-am-FEN-i-kole) belongs to the general family of medicines called antibiotics. Chloramphenicol otic drops are used in the ear to treat infections of the ear canal.

Chloramphenicol is available only with your doctor's prescription.

Remember:

• **This medicine has been prescribed for your present infection only.** Another infection later on may require a different medicine. Also, even though other people may have the same symptoms as you, they may have a different kind of infection. Your medicine may not work for them and may even cause them harm. Therefore, **your medicine must not be given to other people or used for other infections** unless you are otherwise directed by your doctor.

• **Keep all medicines out of the reach of children.**

• In order for this medicine to work, it must be used as directed.

• **It is very important that you read and understand the following information.** If any of the information causes you special concern, do not decide against using this medicine without first checking with your doctor.

• Before you begin using any new medicine (prescription or nonprescription) or if you develop any new medical problem while you are using this medicine, check with your doctor, nurse, or pharmacist.

• **If you have any questions** about the following information or if you want more information about this medicine or your medical problem, **ask your doctor, nurse, or pharmacist.**

Before Using This Medicine

In order to decide on the best treatment for your medical problem, your doctor should be told:

—if you have ever had any unusual or allergic reaction to chloramphenicol.

—if you are allergic to any substance, such as certain foods or preservatives or dyes. Most medicines contain more than their active ingredient. Your doctor, nurse, or pharmacist can help you avoid products that may cause a problem.

—if you are **pregnant** or if you may become pregnant. However, chloramphenicol otic drops have not been shown to cause birth defects or other problems in humans.

—if you are **breast-feeding**. However, chloramphenicol otic drops have not been shown to cause problems in nursing babies.

Proper Use of This Medicine

How to apply this medicine: Lie down or tilt the head so that the infected ear faces up. Gently pull the earlobe up and back for adults (down and back for children) to straighten the ear canal. Drop the medicine into the ear canal. Keep the ear facing up for about 1 or 2 minutes to allow the medicine to come into contact with the infection. A sterile cotton plug may be gently inserted into the ear opening to prevent the medicine from leaking out.

To prevent contamination of the ear drops, do not touch the dropper to any surface (including the ear). Also, keep the container tightly closed.

To help clear up your infection completely, **keep using this medicine for the full time of treatment**, even if your symptoms begin to clear up after a few days. If you stop using this medicine too soon, your symptoms may return. **Do not miss any doses.**

If you do miss a dose of this medicine, apply it as soon as possible. However, if it is almost time for your next dose, skip the missed dose and go back to your regular dosing schedule.

How to store this medicine:

• **Keep out of the reach of children.**

• Store away from heat and direct light.

• Keep the medicine from freezing.

• Do not keep outdated medicine or medicine no longer needed. Be sure that any discarded medicine is out of the reach of children.

Precautions While Using This Medicine

If your symptoms do not improve within a few days, or if they become worse, check with your doctor.

Side Effects of This Medicine

Along with its needed effects, a medicine may cause some unwanted effects. Although not all of these side effects may occur, if they do occur they may need medical attention.

Check with your doctor as soon as possible if any of the following side effects occur:

Burning, itching, redness, skin rash, swelling, or other sign of irritation not present before using this medicine

Other side effects not listed above may also occur in some patients. If you notice any other effects, check with your doctor.

December 1987

CHLORAMPHENICOL (Systemic)

Some commonly used brand names are:

Chloromycetin	Novochlorocap*
Mychel	Pentamycetin*
Mychel-S	

Generic name product may also be available in the U.S.

*Not available in the U.S.

To the Reader: If you do not recognize the names of medical conditions or medicines referred to in this information, check with your doctor, nurse, or pharmacist. Definitions for selected medical terms may be found in the Glossary. Brand names for the generic drug names listed can be found in the Index. In addition, selected brand names commonly associated with the generic name have been included in the text to help you recognize medicine you may be taking. The fact that a brand name product is not mentioned does not mean the information does not apply. It is a good idea for you to learn both the generic and brand names of your medicines and to write them down for future use.

Chloramphenicol (klor-am-FEN-i-kole) belongs to the general family of medicines called antibiotics. Antibiotics are medicines used in the treatment of infections caused by bacteria. They work by killing bacteria or preventing their growth.

Chloramphenicol is taken by mouth or given by injection to treat serious infections in different parts of the body. It is sometimes given with other antibiotics. However, chloramphenicol should not be used for colds, flu, other virus infections, sore throats or other minor infections, or to prevent infections.

Chloramphenicol is usually used for serious infections in which other medicines may not work. However, this medicine may also cause some serious side effects, including blood problems and eye problems. Symptoms of the blood problems include pale skin, sore throat and fever, unusual bleeding or bruising, and unusual tiredness or weakness. **You and your doctor should talk about the good this medicine will do as well as the risks of taking it.**

Chloramphenicol is available only with your doctor's prescription.

Remember:

• **This medicine has been prescribed for your present infection only.** Another infection later on may require a different medicine. Also, even though other people may have the same symptoms as you, they may have a different kind of infection. Your medicine may not work for them and may even cause them harm. Therefore, **your medicine must not be given to other people or used for other infections** unless you are otherwise directed by your doctor.

• **Keep all medicines out of the reach of children.**

• In order for this medicine to work, it must be used as directed.

• If you are receiving this medicine by injection, some of the information about this medicine may not apply.

• **It is very important that you read and understand the following information.** If any of the information causes you special concern, do not decide against using this medicine without first checking with your doctor.

• Before you begin using any new medicine (prescription or nonprescription) or if you develop any new medical problem while you are using this medicine, check with your doctor, nurse, or pharmacist.

• **If you have any questions** about the following information or if you want more information about this medicine or your medical problem, **ask your doctor, nurse, or pharmacist**.

Before Using This Medicine

In order to decide on the best treatment for your medical problem, your doctor should be told:

—if you have ever had any unusual or allergic reaction to chloramphenicol.

—if you are on a low-salt, low-sugar, or any other special diet, or if you are allergic to any substance, such as foods, sulfites or other preservatives, or dyes. Most medicines contain more than their active ingredient, and many liquid medicines contain alcohol. Your doctor, nurse, or pharmacist can help you avoid products that may cause a problem.

—if you are **pregnant** and within a week or two of your delivery date. Chloramphenicol has not been shown to cause birth defects in humans. However, use is not recommended during this time. Chloramphenicol may cause gray skin color, low body temperature, bloated stomach, uneven breathing, drowsiness, pale skin, sore throat and fever, unusual bleeding or bruising, unusual tiredness or weakness, or other problems in the infant.

—if you are **breast-feeding**. Chloramphenicol passes into the breast milk and has been shown to cause unwanted effects, such as pale skin, sore throat and fever, unusual bleeding or bruising, unusual tiredness or weakness, or other problems, in nursing babies. It may be necessary for you to take another medicine or to stop breast-feeding during treatment. Be sure you have discussed the risks and benefits of the medicine with your doctor.

—if you have either of the following medical problems:

Kidney disease
Liver disease

—if you are taking **any** other prescription or nonprescription (OTC) medicine, especially:

Amphotericin B by injection (e.g., Fungizone)
Antidiabetic agents, oral (diabetes medicine you take by mouth)
Antineoplastics (cancer medicine)
Antithyroid agents (medicine for overactive thyroid)
Azathioprine (e.g., Imuran)
Chlorambucil (e.g., Leukeran)
Clindamycin (e.g., Cleocin)
Colchicine
Cyclophosphamide (e.g., Cytoxan)

Erythromycins
Ethotoin (e.g., Peganone)
Flucytosine (e.g., Ancobon)
Interferon (e.g., Intron A, Roferon-A)
Lincomycin (e.g., Lincocin)
Mephenytoin (e.g., Mesantoin)
Mercaptopurine (e.g., Purinethol)
Methotrexate (e.g., Mexate)
Phenytoin (e.g., Dilantin)
Zidovudine (e.g., Retrovir)

—if you have ever been treated with x-rays.

—if you have ever taken this medicine or if you have had any problems with it.

Proper Use of This Medicine

Chloramphenicol is best taken with a full glass (8 ounces) of water on an empty stomach (either 1 hour before or 2 hours after meals), unless otherwise directed by your doctor.

For patients taking the oral liquid form of this medicine:

• Use a specially marked measuring spoon or other device to measure each dose accurately since the average household teaspoon may not hold the right amount of liquid.

To help clear up your infection completely, **keep taking this medicine for the full time of treatment** even if you begin to feel better after a few days; **do not miss any doses.**

If you do miss a dose of this medicine, take it as soon as possible. However, if it is almost time for your next dose and your dosing schedule is:

• 2 doses a day—Space the missed dose and the next dose 5 to 6 hours apart.

• 3 or more doses a day—Space the missed dose and the next dose 2 to 4 hours apart or double your next dose.

Then go back to your regular dosing schedule.

How to store this medicine:

• **Keep out of the reach of children.**

• Store away from heat and direct light.

• Do not store the capsule form of this medicine in the bathroom, near the kitchen sink, or in other damp places. Heat or moisture may cause the medicine to break down.

• Keep the oral liquid form of this medicine from freezing.

• Do not keep outdated medicine or medicine no longer needed. Be sure that any discarded medicine is out of the reach of children.

Precautions While Using This Medicine

If your symptoms do not improve within a few days, or if they become worse, check with your doctor.

It is very important that your doctor check you at regular visits for any blood problems that may be caused by this medicine.

Chloramphenicol may cause blood problems. These problems may result in a greater chance of infection, slow healing, and bleeding of the gums. Therefore, you should be careful when using toothbrushes, dental floss, and toothpicks. Dental work, whenever possible, should be done before you begin taking this medicine or delayed until your blood counts have returned to normal. Check with your physician or dentist if you have any questions about proper oral hygiene (mouth care) during treatment.

This medicine may cause blurred vision or loss of vision. If either of these occurs, **do not drive, use machines, or do other jobs that require you to see clearly.**

Diabetics—This medicine may cause false test results with urine sugar tests. Check with your doctor before changing your diet or the dosage of your diabetes medicine.

Side Effects of This Medicine

Along with its needed effects, a medicine may cause some unwanted effects. Although not all of these side effects may occur, if they do occur they may need medical attention.

Stop taking this medicine and get emergency help immediately if any of the following side effects occur:

Rare

Bloated stomach
Drowsiness
Gray skin color
Low body temperature
Uneven breathing

Also, **check with your doctor immediately** if any of the following side effects occur:

Less common

Pale skin
Sore throat and fever
Unusual bleeding or bruising
Unusual tiredness or weakness
(the above side effects may also occur up to weeks or months after you stop taking this medicine)

Rare

Eye pain, blurred vision, or any loss of vision
Numbness, tingling, burning pain, or weakness in the hands or feet

Other side effects may occur that usually do not require medical attention. These side effects may go away during treatment as your body adjusts to the medicine. However, check with your doctor if any of the following side effects continue or are bothersome:

Less common

Diarrhea
Nausea or vomiting

For elderly patients: Many medicines have not been tested in older people. Therefore, it is not known whether the medicine acts the same way it does in younger adults. Check with your doctor or pharmacist if you notice any unusual effects while taking this medicine or if you think it is not working as it should.

Other side effects not listed above may also occur in some patients. If you notice any other effects, check with your doctor.

_____

December 1987

CHLORAMPHENICOL (Topical)

A commonly used brand name is Chloromycetin.

To the Reader: If you do not recognize the names of medical conditions or medicines referred to in this information, check with your doctor, nurse, or pharmacist. Definitions for selected medical terms may be found in the Glossary. Brand names for the generic drug names listed can be found in the Index. In addition, selected brand names commonly associated with the generic name have been included in the text to help you recognize medicine you may be taking. The fact that a brand name product is not mentioned does not mean the information does not apply. It is a good idea for you to learn both the generic and brand names of your medicines and to write them down for future use.

Chloramphenicol (klor-am-FEN-i-kole) belongs to the general family of medicines called antibiotics. Chloramphenicol cream is used on the skin to help the body overcome infections of the skin. It may be used alone or with other medicines that are taken by mouth for infections.

Chloramphenicol is available only with your doctor's prescription.

Remember:

• **This medicine has been prescribed for your present infection only.** Another infection later on may require a different medicine. Also, even though other people may have the same symptoms as you, they may have a different kind of infection. Your medicine may not work for them and may even cause them harm. Therefore, **your medicine must not be given to other people or used for other infections** unless you are otherwise directed by your doctor.

• **Keep all medicines out of the reach of children.**

• In order for this medicine to work, it must be used as directed.

• **It is very important that you read and understand the following information.** If any of the information causes you special concern, do not decide against using this medicine without first checking with your doctor.

• Before you begin using any new medicine (prescription or nonprescription) or if you develop any new medical problem while you are using this medicine, check with your doctor, nurse, or pharmacist.

• **If you have any questions** about the following information or if you want more information about this medicine or your medical problem, **ask your doctor, nurse, or pharmacist.**

Before Using This Medicine

In order to decide on the best treatment for your medical problem, your doctor should be told:

—if you have ever had any unusual or allergic reaction to chloramphenicol.

—if you are allergic to any substance, such as certain foods or preservatives or dyes. Most medicines contain more than their active ingredient. Your doctor, nurse, or pharmacist can help you avoid products that may cause a problem.

—if you are **pregnant** or if you may become pregnant. However, chloramphenicol cream has not been shown to cause birth defects or other problems in humans.

—if you are **breast-feeding.** However, chloramphenicol cream has not been shown to cause problems in nursing babies.

Proper Use of This Medicine

Before applying this medicine, wash the affected area with soap and water, and dry thoroughly.

To help clear up your infection completely, **keep using this medicine for the full time of treatment,** even if your symptoms begin to clear up after a few days. If you stop using this medicine too soon, your symptoms may return. **Do not miss any doses.** However, **do not use this medicine more often or for a longer period of time than your doctor ordered.**

If you do miss a dose of this medicine, apply it as soon as possible. However, if it is almost time for your next dose, skip the missed dose and go back to your regular dosing schedule.

How to store this medicine:

• **Keep out of the reach of children.**

• Store away from heat and direct light.

• Keep the medicine from freezing.

• Do not keep outdated medicine or medicine no longer needed. Be sure that any discarded medicine is out of the reach of children.

Precautions While Using This Medicine

If your skin problem does not improve within 1 week, or if it becomes worse, check with your doctor.

Side Effects of This Medicine

Along with its needed effects, a medicine may cause some unwanted effects. Although not all of these side effects may occur, if they do occur they may need medical attention.

Check with your doctor as soon as possible if any of the following side effects occur:

More common
　Burning, itching, redness, skin rash, swelling, or other sign of irritation not present before using this medicine

Other side effects not listed above may also occur in some patients. If you notice any other effects, check with your doctor.

December 1987

CHLORDIAZEPOXIDE AND AMITRIPTYLINE (Systemic)

Some commonly used brand names are Limbitrol and Limbitrol DS.

To the Reader: If you do not recognize the names of medical conditions or medicines referred to in this information, check with your doctor, nurse, or pharmacist. Definitions for selected medical terms may be found in the Glossary. Brand names for the generic drug names listed can be found in the Index. In addition, selected brand names commonly associated with the generic name have been included in the text to help you recognize medicine you may be taking. The fact that a brand name product is not mentioned does not mean the information does not apply. It is a good idea for you to learn both the generic and brand names of your medicines and to write them down for future use.

Chlordiazepoxide (klor-dye-az-e-POX-ide) and amitriptyline (a-mee-TRIP-ti-leen) combination is used to treat mental depression that occurs with anxiety or nervous tension.

This medicine is available only with your doctor's prescription.

Remember:

• **This medicine has been prescribed for your current medical problem only.** It must not be given to other people or used for other problems unless you are directed to do so by your doctor.

• **Keep all medicines out of the reach of children.**

• In order for this medicine to work, it must be used as directed.

• **It is very important that you read and understand the following information.** If any of the information causes you special concern, do not decide against using this medicine without first checking with your doctor.

• Before you begin using any new medicine (prescription or nonprescription) or if you develop any new medical problem while you are using this medicine, check with your doctor, nurse, or pharmacist.

• **If you have any questions** about the following information or if you want more information about this medicine or your medical problem, **ask your doctor, nurse, or pharmacist.**

Before Using This Medicine

In order to decide on the best treatment for your medical problem, your doctor should be told:

—if you have ever had any unusual or allergic reaction to benzodiazepines (such as alprazolam, chlordiazepoxide, clonazepam, clorazepate, diazepam, flurazepam, halazepam, lorazepam, oxazepam, prazepam, or temazepam) or to tricyclic antidepressants (such as amitriptyline, amoxapine, clomipramine, desipramine, doxepin, imipramine, nortriptyline, protriptyline, or trimipramine).

—if you are on a low-salt, low-sugar, or any other special diet, or if you are allergic to any substance, such as foods, sulfites or other preservatives, or dyes.

Most medicines contain more than their active ingredient. Your doctor, nurse, or pharmacist can help you avoid products that may cause a problem.

—if you are **pregnant** or if you may become pregnant. Chlordiazepoxide has been reported to increase the chance of birth defects when used during the first 3 months of pregnancy.

In addition, overuse of chlordiazepoxide during pregnancy may cause the baby to become dependent on the medicine. This may lead to withdrawal side effects after birth.

Use of chlordiazepoxide during pregnancy, especially during the last weeks, may cause drowsiness, unusually slow heartbeat, shortness of breath, or troubled breathing in the newborn baby. Chlordiazepoxide given just before or during labor may cause weakness in the newborn baby.

Studies with amitriptyline have not been done in humans. This medicine has not been shown to cause problems.

—if you are **breast-feeding.** Chlordiazepoxide may pass into the breast milk and cause drowsiness, unusually slow heartbeat, shortness of breath, or troubled breathing in babies of mothers taking this medicine.

Although amitriptyline has also been found in breast milk, it has not been shown to cause problems in nursing babies.

—if you have any of the following medical problems:

Alcoholism, active or treated
Blood disorders
Difficulty in urinating
Emphysema, asthma, bronchitis, or other chronic lung disease
Enlarged prostate
Epilepsy or history of seizures
Glaucoma or increased eye pressure
Heart disease
Hyperactivity
Kidney disease
Liver disease
Manic-depressive illness
Mental depression (severe)
Mental illness (severe)
Myasthenia gravis
Overactive thyroid
Porphyria
Stomach or intestinal problems

—if you are now taking **any** other prescription or nonprescription (OTC) medicine, especially:

Amphetamines
Antacids
Antihypertensives (high blood pressure medicine)
Antithyroid agents (medicine for overactive thyroid)
Appetite suppressants (diet pills)
Central nervous system (CNS) depressants
Cimetidine (e.g., Tagamet)
Medicine for asthma or other breathing problems
Medicine for colds, sinus problems, or hay fever or other allergies (including nose drops or sprays)
Oral contraceptives (birth control pills) containing estrogen

—if you are now taking or have taken within the past 2 weeks monoamine oxidase (MAO) inhibitors, such as:

Furazolidone (e.g., Furoxone)
Isocarboxazid (e.g., Marplan)
Pargyline (e.g., Eutonyl)
Phenelzine (e.g., Nardil)
Procarbazine (e.g., Matulane)
Tranylcypromine (e.g., Parnate)

Proper Use of This Medicine

To reduce stomach upset, take this medicine immediately after meals or with food unless your doctor has told you to take it on an empty stomach.

Sometimes this medicine must be taken for several weeks before you begin to feel better. Your doctor should check your progress at regular visits.

Take this medicine only as directed by your doctor. Do not take more of it, do not take it more often, and do not take it for a longer period of time than your doctor ordered. If too much is taken, it may increase unwanted effects or become habit-forming (causing mental or physical dependence).

If you think this medicine is not working as well after you have taken it for a few weeks, **do not increase the dose**. Instead, check with your doctor.

If you miss a dose of this medicine, skip the missed dose and go back to your regular dosing schedule. Do not double doses.

How to store this medicine:

• **Keep out of the reach of children.**

• Store away from heat and direct light.

• Do not store in the bathroom, near the kitchen sink, or in other damp places. Heat or moisture may cause the medicine to break down.

• Do not keep outdated medicine or medicine no longer needed. Be sure that any discarded medicine is out of the reach of children.

Precautions While Using This Medicine

It is very important that your doctor check your progress at regular visits to allow dose adjustments and help reduce side effects.

This medicine will add to the effects of alcohol and other CNS depressants (medicines that slow down the nervous system, possibly causing drowsiness). Some examples of CNS depressants are antihistamines or medicine for hay fever, other allergies, or colds; sedatives, tranquilizers, or sleeping medicine; prescription pain medicine or narcotics; barbiturates; medicine for seizures; muscle relaxants; or anesthetics, including some dental anesthetics. This effect may last for a few days after you stop taking this medicine. **Check with your doctor before taking any of the above while you are using this medicine.**

This medicine may cause some people to become dizzy, lightheaded, drowsy, or less alert than they are normally. Even if taken at bedtime, it may cause some people to feel drowsy or less alert on arising. **Make sure you know how you react to this medicine before you drive, use machines, or do other jobs that require you to be alert.**

Dizziness, lightheadedness, or fainting may occur when you get up from a lying or sitting position. Getting up slowly may help. If this problem continues or gets worse, check with your doctor.

Chlordiazepoxide and amitriptyline combination may cause dryness of the mouth. For temporary relief, use sugarless candy or gum, melt bits of ice in your mouth, or use a saliva substitute. However, if dry mouth continues for more than 2 weeks, check with your physician or dentist. Continuing dryness of the mouth may increase the chance of dental disease, including tooth decay, gum disease, and fungal infections.

Before having any surgery, any dental treatment, or emergency treatment, tell the physician or dentist in charge that you are using this medicine.

Do not stop taking this medicine without first checking with your doctor. Your doctor may want you to reduce gradually the amount you are using before stopping completely. This may help prevent a possible worsening of your condition and reduce the possibility of withdrawal symptoms such as headache, nausea, and/or an overall feeling of discomfort.

Side Effects of This Medicine

Along with its needed effects, a medicine may cause some unwanted effects. Although not all of these side effects may occur, if they do occur they may need medical attention.

Check with your doctor as soon as possible if any of the following side effects occur:

Less common

Blurred vision or other changes in vision
Confusion or hallucinations (seeing, hearing, or feeling things that are not there)
Constipation
Difficulty in urinating
Eye pain
Fainting
Irregular heartbeat
Mental depression
Shakiness
Trouble in sleeping
Unusual excitement, nervousness, or irritability

Rare

   Convulsions (seizures)
   Increased sensitivity to sunlight
   Skin rash and itching
   Sore throat and fever
   Yellow eyes or skin

Other side effects may occur that usually do not require medical attention. These side effects may go away during treatment as your body adjusts to the medicine. However, check with your doctor if any of the following side effects continue or are bothersome:

More common

   Bloating
   Clumsiness or unsteadiness
   Dizziness or lightheadedness
   Drowsiness
   Dry mouth or unpleasant taste
   Headache
   Weight gain

Less common

   Diarrhea
   Nausea or vomiting
   Unusual tiredness or weakness

After you stop using this medicine, your body may need time to adjust. If you took this medicine in high doses or for a long time, this may take up to 2 weeks. **During this period of time check with your doctor if you notice any of the following side effects:**

   Convulsions (seizures)
   Increased sweating
   Irritability or restlessness
   Muscle cramps
   Nausea or vomiting
   Stomach cramps
   Trembling
   Trouble in sleeping, with vivid dreams

The above side effects are more likely to occur in adolescent or elderly patients, who are usually more sensitive to the effects of chlordiazepoxide and amitriptyline combination.

Other side effects not listed above may also occur in some patients. If you notice any other effects, check with your doctor.

_____

December 1987

_____

CHLORDIAZEPOXIDE AND CLIDINIUM
(Systemic)

Some commonly used brand names are:

Apo-Chlorax*	Corium*
Clindex	Librax
Clinoxide	Lidox
Clipoxide	

*Not available in the U.S.

To the Reader: If you do not recognize the names of medical conditions or medicines referred to in this information, check with your doctor, nurse, or pharmacist. Definitions for selected medical terms may be found in the Glossary. Brand names for the generic drug names listed can be found in the Index. In addition, selected brand names commonly associated with the generic name have been included in the text to help you recognize medicine you may be taking. The fact that a brand name product is not mentioned does not mean the information does not apply. It is a good idea for you to learn both the generic and brand names of your medicines and to write them down for future use.

Chlordiazepoxide (klor-dye-az-e-POX-ide) and clidinium (kli-DI-nee-um) is a combination of medicines used to relax the digestive system and to reduce stomach acid. It is used to treat stomach and intestinal problems such as ulcers and colitis.

Chlordiazepoxide belongs to the group of medicines known as benzodiazepines. It is a central nervous system (CNS) depressant (a medicine that slows down the nervous system).

Clidinium belongs to the group of medicines known as antimuscarinics. It helps lessen the amount of acid formed in the stomach. Clidinium also helps relieve abdominal or stomach spasms or cramps.

This combination is available only with your doctor's prescription.

Remember:

• **This medicine has been prescribed for your current medical problem only.** It must not be given to other people or used for other problems unless you are directed to do so by your doctor.

• **Keep all medicines out of the reach of children.**

• In order for this medicine to work, it must be used as directed.

• **It is very important that you read and understand the following information.** If any of the information causes you special concern, do not decide against using this medicine without first checking with your doctor.

• Before you begin using any new medicine (prescription or nonprescription) or if you develop any new medical problem while you are using this medicine, check with your doctor, nurse, or pharmacist.

• **If you have any questions** about the following information or if you want more information about this medicine or your medical problem, **ask your doctor, nurse, or pharmacist.**

Before Using This Medicine

In order to decide on the best treatment for your medical problem, your doctor should be told:

—if you have ever had any unusual or allergic reaction to benzodiazepines such as alprazolam, chlordiazepoxide, clonazepam, clorazepate, diazepam, flurazepam, halazepam, lorazepam, oxazepam, prazepam, or temazepam, or to clidinium or any of the belladonna alkaloids (atropine, belladonna, hyoscyamine, and scopolamine).

—if you are on a low-salt, low-sugar, or any other special diet, or if you are allergic to any substance, such as foods, sulfites or other preservatives, or dyes. Most medicines contain more than their active ingredient. Your doctor, nurse, or pharmacist can help you avoid products that may cause a problem.

—if you are **pregnant** or if you may become pregnant while using this medicine. Studies with clidinium (contained in this combination) have not been done in humans. However, clidinium has not been shown to cause birth defects or other problems in animal studies. Chlordiazepoxide (contained also in this combination) may cause birth defects if taken during the first 3 months of pregnancy. In addition, too much use of this medicine during pregnancy may cause the baby to become dependent on the medicine. This may lead to withdrawal side effects after birth. Be sure that you have discussed this with your doctor before taking this medicine.

—if you are **breast-feeding**. Chlordiazepoxide may pass into the breast milk and cause unwanted effects, such as excessive drowsiness, in babies. Also, because clidinium tends to decrease the secretions of the body, it is possible that the flow of breast milk may be reduced in some patients.

—if you have any of the following medical problems:
Difficult urination
Dry mouth (severe and continuing)
Emphysema, asthma, bronchitis, or other chronic lung disease
Enlarged prostate
Glaucoma
Hiatal hernia
Hypertension (high blood pressure)
Intestinal blockage
Kidney disease
Liver disease
Mental depression
Mental illness (severe)
Myasthenia gravis
Overactive thyroid
Ulcerative colitis (severe)

—if you are taking **any** other prescription or nonprescription (OTC) medicine, especially:
Antacids
Central nervous system (CNS) depressants
Diarrhea medicine containing kaolin or attapulgite
Ketoconazole (e.g., Nizoral)
Other antimuscarinics (medicines for abdominal or stomach spasms or cramps)
Potassium chloride (e.g., Kay Ciel)

—if you are now taking or have taken within the past 2 weeks monoamine oxidase (MAO) inhibitors, such as:

> Furazolidone (e.g., Furoxone)
> Isocarboxazid (e.g., Marplan)
> Pargyline (e.g., Eutonyl)
> Phenelzine (e.g., Nardil)
> Procarbazine (e.g., Matulane)
> Tranylcypromine (e.g., Parnate)

Proper Use of This Medicine

Take this medicine about ½ to 1 hour before meals unless otherwise directed by your doctor.

Take this medicine only as directed by your doctor. Do not take more of it, do not take it more often, and do not take it for a longer period of time than your doctor ordered. If too much is taken, it may become habit-forming.

If you miss a dose of this medicine, take it as soon as possible. However, if it is almost time for your next dose, skip the missed dose and go back to your regular dosing schedule. Do not double doses.

How to store this medicine:

- **Keep out of the reach of children.**

- Store away from heat and direct light.

- Do not store the capsule form of this medicine in the bathroom, near the kitchen sink, or in other damp places. Heat or moisture may cause the medicine to break down.

- Do not keep outdated medicine or medicine no longer needed. Be sure that any discarded medicine is out of the reach of children.

Precautions While Using This Medicine

If you will be taking this medicine regularly for a long period of time your doctor should check your progress at regular visits.

Do not take this medicine within an hour of taking medicine for diarrhea. Taking them too close together will make this medicine less effective.

This medicine may cause some people to become dizzy, lightheaded, drowsy, or less alert than they are normally. **Make sure you know how you react to this medicine before you drive, use machines, or do other jobs that require you to be alert.**

This medicine will add to the effects of alcohol and other CNS depressants (medicines that slow down the nervous system, possibly causing drowsiness). Some examples of CNS depressants are sedatives, tranquilizers, or sleeping medicine; prescription pain medicine or narcotics; barbiturates; medicine for seizures; muscle relaxants; or anesthetics, including some dental anesthetics. **Check with your doctor before taking any of the above while you are using this medicine and also for a few days after you stop taking it.**

This medicine will often make you sweat less, causing your body temperature to increase. **Use extra care not to become overheated during exercise or hot weather while you are taking this medicine** as this could possibly result in heat stroke.

Your mouth, nose, and throat may feel very dry while you are taking this medicine. For temporary relief of mouth dryness, use sugarless candy or gum, melt bits of ice in your mouth, or use a saliva substitute. However, if dry mouth continues for more than 2 weeks, check with your dentist. Continuing dryness of the mouth may increase the chance of dental disease, including tooth decay, gum disease, and fungal infections.

Check with your doctor if you develop intestinal problems such as constipation. This is especially important if you are taking other medicine while you are taking chlordiazepoxide and clidinium. If these problems are not corrected, serious complications may result.

If you will be taking this medicine in large doses or for a long period of time, do not stop taking it without first checking with your doctor. Your doctor may want you to reduce gradually the amount you are taking before stopping completely.

Side Effects of This Medicine

Along with its needed effects, a medicine may cause some unwanted effects. Although not all of these side effects may occur, if they do occur they may need medical attention.

Check with your doctor as soon as possible if any of the following side effects occur:

Less common or rare

> Constipation
> Eye pain
> Mental depression
> Skin rash or hives
> Sore throat and fever
> Trouble in sleeping
> Unusual excitement, nervousness, or irritability
> Unusually slow heartbeat, shortness of breath, or troubled breathing
> Yellow eyes or skin

Signs of overdose

> Confusion
> Difficult urination
> Drowsiness (severe)
> Dryness of mouth, nose, or throat (severe)
> Fast heartbeat
> Unusual warmth, dryness, and flushing of skin

Other side effects may occur that usually do not require medical attention. These side effects may go away during treatment as your body adjusts to the medicine.

However, check with your doctor if any of the following side effects continue or are bothersome:

More common

Bloated feeling
Decreased sweating
Dizziness
Drowsiness
Dry mouth
Headache

Less common

Blurred vision
Decreased sexual ability
Loss of memory
Nausea
Unusual tiredness or weakness

After you stop using this medicine, your body may need time to adjust. The length of time this takes depends on the amount of medicine you were using and how long you used it. During this period of time check with your doctor if you notice any of the following side effects:

Convulsions (seizures)
Muscle cramps
Nausea or vomiting
Stomach cramps
Trembling

For children or elderly patients: Children and elderly patients are usually more sensitive to the effects of this medicine. Agitation, confusion, constipation, difficult urination, drowsiness, dryness of mouth, excitement, and memory loss may be more likely to occur in elderly patients.

Other side effects not listed above may also occur in some patients. If you notice any other effects, check with your doctor.

December 1987

CHLORHEXIDINE (Dental)

A commonly used brand name is Peridex.

To the Reader: If you do not recognize the names of medical conditions or medicines referred to in this information, check with your doctor, nurse, or pharmacist. Definitions for selected medical terms may be found in the Glossary. Brand names for the generic drug names listed can be found in the Index. In addition, selected brand names commonly associated with the generic name have been included in the text to help you recognize medicine you may be taking. The fact that a brand name product is not mentioned does not mean the information does not apply. It is a good idea for you to learn both the generic and brand names of your medicines and to write them down for future use.

Chlorhexidine (klor-HEX-i-deen) is used to treat gingivitis. It helps to reduce the inflammation (redness) and swelling of your gums and to control gum bleeding.

Gingivitis is caused by the bacteria that grow in the coating (plaque) that forms on your teeth between tooth brushings. Chlorhexidine destroys the bacteria, thereby preventing the gingivitis from occurring.

Chlorhexidine is available only with your doctor's prescription.

Remember:

• **This medicine has been prescribed for your current medical problem only.** It must not be given to other people or used for other problems unless you are directed to do so by your doctor.

• **Keep all medicines out of the reach of children.**

• In order for this medicine to work, it must be used as directed.

• **It is very important that you read and understand the following information.** If any of the information causes you special concern, do not decide against using this medicine without first checking with your doctor.

• Before you begin using any new medicine (prescription or nonprescription) or if you develop any new medical problem while you are using this medicine, check with your doctor, nurse, or pharmacist.

• **If you have any questions** about the following information or if you want more information about this medicine or your medical problem, **ask your doctor, nurse, or pharmacist.**

Before Using This Medicine

In order to decide on the best treatment for your medical problem, your doctor should be told:

—if you have ever had any unusual or allergic reaction to skin disinfectants containing chlorhexidine.

—if you are on a low-salt, low-sugar, or any other special diet, or if you are allergic to any substance, such as foods, sulfites or other preservatives, or dyes. Most medicines contain more than their active ingredient, and many liquid medicines contain alcohol. Your doctor, nurse, or pharmacist can help you avoid products that may cause a problem.

—if you are **pregnant** or if you may become pregnant. Studies have not been done in humans. However, chlorhexidine has not been shown to cause birth defects or other problems in animal studies.

—if you are **breast-feeding**. It is not known whether chlorhexidine passes into the breast milk. This medicine has not been shown to cause problems in nursing babies.

—if you have any other gum problems.

—if you have any front-tooth fillings, especially those having rough surfaces. Chlorhexidine may cause staining that, in some cases, may be impossible to remove and may require replacing the filling.

—if you are taking **any** other prescription or nonprescription (OTC) medicine.

Proper Use of This Medicine

Chlorhexidine oral rinse should be used after you have brushed and flossed your teeth. Rinse the toothpaste completely from your mouth with water before using the oral rinse. Do not eat or drink for several hours after using the oral rinse.

The cap on the original container of chlorhexidine can be used to measure the 15 mL (½ fluid ounce) dose of this medicine. Fill the cap to the 'fill line.' If you do not receive the dental rinse in its original container, make sure you have a measuring device to measure out the correct dose. Your pharmacist can help you with this.

Swish chlorhexidine around in the mouth for 30 seconds. Then spit out. **Use the medicine full strength.** Do not mix with water before using. **Do not swallow the medicine.**

If you miss a dose of this medicine, use it as soon as possible. However, if it is almost time for your next dose, skip the missed dose and go back to your regular dosing schedule. Do not double doses.

How to store this medicine:

• **Keep out of the reach of children.**

• Store away from heat and direct light.

• Keep the medicine from freezing.

• Do not keep outdated medicine or medicine that is no longer needed. Be sure any discarded medicine is out of the reach of children.

Precautions While Using This Medicine

Chlorhexidine may have a bitter aftertaste. Do not rinse your mouth with water immediately after using chlorhexidine, since this will increase the bitterness.

Chlorhexidine may change the way foods taste to you. Sometimes this effect may last up to 4 hours after you use the oral rinse. In most cases, this effect will become less noticeable as you continue to use the medicine. When you stop using chlorhexidine, your taste should return to normal.

Chlorhexidine may cause staining and an increase in tartar (calculus) on your teeth. Brushing with a tartar-control toothpaste and flossing your teeth daily may help reduce this tartar build-up and stain . In addition, you should visit your dentist at least every 6 months to have your teeth cleaned and your gums examined.

If you think that a child weighing 22 pounds (10 kg) or less has swallowed more than 4 ounces of the dental rinse, get emergency help at once. In addition, if a child of any age drinks the dental rinse, get emergency help at once if the child has symptoms of alcohol intoxication, such as slurred speech, sleepiness, or staggering or stumbling walk.

Side Effects of This Medicine

Along with its needed effects, a medicine may cause some unwanted effects. Although no serious side effects have been reported for chlorhexidine, the following side effects may be noticed by some patients.

Check with your doctor if any of the following side effects continue or are bothersome:

More common
- Change in taste
- Increase in tartar (calculus) on teeth
- Staining of teeth, mouth, tooth fillings, and dentures or other mouth appliances

Less common or rare
- Mouth irritation
- Tongue tip irritation

For elderly patients: Many medicines have not been tested in older people. Therefore, it is not known whether the medicine acts the same way it does in younger adults. Check with your doctor or pharmacist if you notice any unusual effects while using this medicine or if you do not think it is working as it should.

Other side effects not listed above may also occur in some patients. If you notice any other effects, check with your doctor.

December 1987

CHLOROXINE (Topical)

A commonly used brand name is Capitrol.

To the Reader: If you do not recognize the names of medical conditions or medicines referred to in this information, check with your doctor, nurse, or pharmacist. Definitions for selected medical terms may be found in the Glossary. Brand names for the generic drug names listed can be found in the Index. In addition, selected brand names commonly associated with the generic name have been included in the text to help you recognize medicine you may be taking. The fact that a brand name product is not mentioned does not mean the information does not apply. It is a good idea for you to learn both the generic and brand names of your medicines and to write them down for future use.

Chloroxine (klor-OX-een) is used in the treatment of dandruff and seborrheic dermatitis of the scalp.

This medicine is available only with your doctor's prescription.

Remember:

• **This medicine has been prescribed for your current medical problem only.** It must not be given to other people or used for other problems unless you are directed to do so by your doctor.

• **Keep all medicines out of the reach of children.**

• In order for this medicine to work, it must be used as directed.

• **It is very important that you read and understand the following information.** If any of the information causes you special concern, do not decide against using this medicine without first checking with your doctor.

• Before you begin using any new medicine (prescription or nonprescription) or if you develop any new medical problem while you are using this medicine, check with your doctor, nurse, or pharmacist.

• **If you have any questions** about the following information or if you want more information about this medicine or your medical problem, **ask your doctor, nurse, or pharmacist.**

Before Using This Medicine

In order to decide on the best treatment for your medical problem, your doctor should be told:

—if you have ever had any unusual or allergic reaction to clioquinol (iodochlorhydroxyquin), iodoquinol (diiodohydroxyquin), or edetate disodium.

—if you are **pregnant** or if you may become pregnant. Studies have not been done in either humans or animals.

—if you are **breast-feeding**. However, it is not known whether chloroxine passes into the breast milk and this medicine has not been shown to cause problems in nursing babies.

Proper Use of This Medicine

Do not use this medicine if blistered, raw, or oozing areas are present on your scalp, unless otherwise directed by your doctor.

Keep this medicine away from the eyes. If you should accidentally get some in your eyes, flush them thoroughly with cool water. Check with your doctor if eye irritation continues or is bothersome.

To apply this medicine: Wet the hair and scalp with lukewarm water. Apply enough chloroxine to the scalp to work up a lather, and rub in well. Allow the lather to remain on the scalp for about 3 minutes, then rinse. Apply the medicine again and rinse thoroughly.

How to store this medicine:

• **Keep out of the reach of children.**

• Store away from heat and direct light.

• Keep the medicine from freezing.

• Do not keep outdated medicine or medicine no longer needed. Be sure that any discarded medicine is out of the reach of children.

Precautions While Using This Medicine

This medicine may slightly discolor light-colored hair (for example, bleached, blond, or gray).

Side Effects of This Medicine

Along with its needed effects, a medicine may cause some unwanted effects. Although not all of these side effects may occur, if they do occur they may need medical attention.

Check with your doctor as soon as possible if any of the following side effects occur:

Irritation or burning of scalp not present before using this medicine
Skin rash

Other side effects may occur that usually do not require medical attention. However, check with your doctor if either of the following side effects continues or is bothersome:

Dryness or increased itching of scalp

For elderly patients: Many medicines have not been tested in older people. Therefore, it is not known whether the medicine acts the same way it does in younger adults. Check with your doctor or pharmacist if you notice any unusual effects while using this medicine or if you think it is not working as it should.

Other side effects not listed above may also occur in some patients. If you notice any other effects, check with your doctor.

December 1987

CHLORZOXAZONE AND ACETAMINOPHEN (Systemic)

Some commonly used brand names and other names are:

Algicin	Lobac
Blanex	Mus-Lax
Chlorofon-F	Paracet Forte
Chlorzone Forte	Parafon Forte
Chlorzoxazone with APAP	Polyflex
Flexaphen	Zoxaphen

Generic name product may also be available in the U.S.

To the Reader: If you do not recognize the names of medical conditions or medicines referred to in this information, check with your doctor, nurse, or pharmacist. Definitions for selected medical terms may be found in the Glossary. Brand names for the generic drug names listed can be found in the Index. In addition, selected brand names commonly associated with the generic name have been included in the text to help you recognize medicine you may be taking. The fact that a brand name product is not mentioned does not mean the information does not apply. It is a good idea for you to learn both the generic and brand names of your medicines and to write them down for future use.

Chlorzoxazone (klor-ZOX-a-zone) and acetaminophen (a-seat-a-MIN-oh-fen) combination medicine is taken by mouth to help relax certain muscles in your body and relieve the pain and discomfort caused by strains, sprains, or other injury to your muscles. However, this medicine does not take the place of rest, exercise or physical therapy, or other treatment that your doctor may recommend for your medical problem.

Chlorzoxazone acts in the central nervous system (CNS) to produce its muscle relaxant effects. Its actions in the CNS may also produce some of its side effects.

In the United States, this medicine is available only with your doctor's prescription. In Canada, this medicine is available without a prescripton.

Remember:

• **This medicine has been prescribed for your current medical problem only.** It must not be given to other people or used for other problems unless you are directed to do so by your doctor.

• **Keep all medicines out of the reach of children.**

• In order for this medicine to work, it must be used as directed.

• **It is very important that you read and understand the following information.** If any of the information causes you special concern, do not decide against using this medicine without first checking with your doctor.

• Before you begin using any new medicine (prescription or nonprescription) or if you develop any new medical problem while you are using this medicine, check with your doctor, nurse, or pharmacist.

• **If you have any questions** about the following information or if you want more information about this medicine or your medical problem, **ask your doctor, nurse, or pharmacist.**

Before Using This Medicine

In order to decide on the best treatment for your medical problem, your doctor should be told:

—if you have ever had any unusual reaction to acetaminophen or chlorzoxazone, or to other medicines.

—if you are on a low-salt, low-sugar, or any other special diet, or if you are allergic to any substance, such as foods, sulfites or other preservatives, or dyes. Most medicines contain more than their active ingredient. Your doctor, nurse, or pharmacist can help you avoid products that may cause a problem.

—if you are **pregnant** or if you may become pregnant. Although chlorzoxazone and acetaminophen have not been shown to cause birth defects or other problems, studies on birth defects with chlorzoxazone or acetaminophen have not been done in humans.

—if you are **breast-feeding**. Chlorzoxazone and acetaminophen have not been shown to cause problems in nursing babies. However, acetaminophen passes into the breast milk in small amounts.

—if you have any of the following medical problems:
Allergies (asthma, eczema, hay fever, hives)
Hepatitis or other liver disease
Kidney disease

—if you regularly drink large amounts of alcoholic beverages.

—if you are now taking **any** other prescription or nonprescription (OTC) medicine, especially central nervous system (CNS) depressants.

Proper Use of This Medicine

Take this medicine only as directed. Do not take more of it, do not take it more often, and do not take it for a longer time than your doctor ordered. To do so may increase the chance of side effects. Acetaminophen may cause liver damage if too much is taken.

If you miss a dose of this medicine, take it as soon as you remember. However, if it is almost time for your next dose, skip the missed dose and go back to your regular dosing schedule. Do not double doses.

How to store this medicine:

• **Keep out of the reach of children.**

• Store away from heat and direct light.

• Do not store this medicine in the bathroom, near the kitchen sink, or in other damp places. Heat or moisture may cause the medicine to break down.

• Do not keep outdated medicine or medicine no longer needed. Be sure that any discarded medicine is out of the reach of children.

Precautions While Using This Medicine

If you will be taking this medicine for a long period of time (for example, for several months at a time), your doctor should check your progress at regular visits.

Check the labels of all over-the-counter (OTC), nonprescription, and prescription medicines you now take. If any contain acetaminophen be especially careful, since taking them while taking this medicine may lead to overdose. If you have any questions about this, check with your doctor, nurse, or pharmacist.

This medicine will add to the effects of alcohol and other CNS depressants (medicines that slow down the nervous system, possibly causing drowsiness). Some examples of CNS depressants are antihistamines or medicine for hay fever, other allergies, or colds; sedatives, tranquilizers, or sleeping medicine; prescription pain medicine or narcotics; barbiturates; medicine for convulsions (seizures); or anesthetics, including some dental anesthetics. Also, the risk of liver damage from acetaminophen may be greater if you use large amounts of alcoholic beverages with acetaminophen. Therefore, **do not drink alcoholic beverages, and check with your doctor before taking any of the medicines listed above, while you are taking this medicine.**

Too much use of acetaminophen (contained in this combination medicine) together with certain other medicines may increase the chance of kidney problems. Therefore, do not regularly take this medicine together with any of the following, unless directed to do so by your doctor:

     Aspirin or other salicylates
     Diclofenac (e.g., Voltaren)
     Diflunisal (e.g., Dolobid)
     Fenoprofen (e.g., Nalfon)
     Flurbiprofen, oral (e.g., Ansaid)
     Ibuprofen (e.g., Motrin)
     Indomethacin (e.g., Indocin)
     Ketoprofen (e.g., Orudis)
     Meclofenamate (e.g., Meclomen)
     Mefenamic acid (e.g., Ponstel)
     Naproxen (e.g., Naprosyn)
     Phenylbutazone (e.g., Butazolidin)
     Piroxicam (e.g., Feldene)
     Sulindac (e.g., Clinoril)
     Tiaprofenic acid (e.g., Surgam)
     Tolmetin (e.g., Tolectin)

This medicine may cause some people to become drowsy, dizzy, or less alert than they are normally. **Make sure you know how you react to this medicine before you drive, use machines, or do other jobs that require you to be alert.**

If you think that you or anyone else may have taken an overdose of this medicine, get emergency help at once. Signs of overdose of this medicine include rapid or irregular breathing and severe muscle weakness. Signs of severe acetaminophen poisoning may not appear for 2 to 4 days after the overdose is taken, but treatment to prevent liver damage or death must be started within 24 hours or less after the overdose is taken.

Side Effects of This Medicine

Along with its needed effects, a medicine may cause some unwanted effects. Although not all of these side effects may occur, if they do occur they may need medical attention.

Check with your doctor immediately if any of the following side effects occur:

Rare

     Sudden decrease in amount of urine
     Swelling of lips, face, or tongue

Signs of overdose

     Diarrhea
     Increased sweating
     Loss of appetite
     Muscle weakness (severe)
     Nausea or vomiting
     Rapid or irregular breathing
     Stomach cramps or pain

Also, check with your doctor as soon as possible if any of the following side effects occur:

Rare

     Bloody or black tarry stools
     Bloody or cloudy urine
     Difficult or painful urination
     Frequent urge to urinate
     Skin rash, hives, itching, or redness
     Sore throat and fever
     Unusual bleeding or bruising
     Unusual tiredness or weakness
     Yellow eyes or skin

Other side effects may occur that usually do not require medical attention. These side effects may go away during treatment as your body adjusts to the medicine. However, check with your doctor if any of the following side effects continue or are bothersome:

More common

     Dizziness or lightheadedness
     Drowsiness

Less common

     Constipation
     Headache
     Heartburn
     Unusual excitement, nervousness, restlessness, or irritability

This medicine sometimes causes the urine to turn orange or reddish purple. This is not harmful and will go away when you stop taking the medicine. If you have any questions about this, check with your doctor.

For elderly patients: Many medicines have not been tested in older people. Therefore, it is not known whether the medicine acts the same way it does in younger adults. Check with your doctor or pharmacist if you notice any ususual effects while taking this medicine or if you think it is not working as it should.

Other side effects not listed above may also occur in some patients. If you notice any other effects, check with your doctor.

December 1987

CHOLECYSTOGRAPHIC AGENTS, ORAL
(Systemic)

This information applies to the following medicines:

Iocetamic Acid (eye-oh-se-TAM-ik)
Iopanoic Acid (eye-oh-pa-NOE-ik)
Ipodate (EYE-poe-date)
Tyropanoate (tye-roe-pa-NOE-ate)

Some commonly used brand names:	Generic names:
Cholebrine	Iocetamic Acid
Telepaque	Iopanoic Acid
Bilivist Oragrafin Calcium Oragrafin Sodium	Ipodate
Bilopaque	Tyropanoate

To the Reader: If you do not recognize the names of medical conditions or medicines referred to in this information, check with your doctor, nurse, or pharmacist. Definitions for selected medical terms may be found in the Glossary. Brand names for the generic drug names listed can be found in the Index. In addition, selected brand names commonly associated with the generic name have been included in the text to help you recognize medicine you may be taking. The fact that a brand name product is not mentioned does not mean the information does not apply. It is a good idea for you to learn both the generic and brand names of your medicines and to write them down for future use.

Oral cholecystographic (ko-le-sis-to-GRAF-ik) agents are radiopaque agents. These agents contain iodine, which absorbs x-rays. Depending on how the radiopaque agent is given, it builds up in certain areas of the body. The resulting high level of iodine allows the x-rays to make a "picture" of the area.

The oral cholecystographic agents are taken by mouth before x-ray tests to help check for problems of the gallbladder and the biliary tract. Ipodate may also be used for other conditions as determined by your doctor.

These radiopaque agents are to be given only by or under the direct supervision of a doctor.

Remember:
• **Keep all medicines out of the reach of children.**

• In order for this radiopaque agent to work, it must be used as directed.

• **It is very important that you read and understand the following information.** If any of the information causes you special concern, do not decide against using this radiopaque agent without first checking with your doctor.

• **If you have any questions** about the following information or if you want more information about this radiopaque agent or your medical problem, **ask your doctor, nurse, or pharmacist.**

Before Having This Test

Before this test is given, your doctor should be told:

—if you have ever had any unusual or allergic reaction to iodine, to products containing iodine (for example, iodine-containing foods, such as seafoods, cabbage, kale, rape, turnips, or iodized salt), or to other radiopaque agents.

—if you are on a low-salt, low-sugar, or any other special diet, or if you are allergic to any substance, such as foods, sulfites or other preservatives, or dyes. Most medicines contain more than their active ingredient. Your doctor can help you avoid products that may cause a problem.

—if you are **pregnant** or if you suspect that you may be pregnant when you are to receive a cholecystographic agent. Studies have not been done in humans; however, iocetamic acid has not been shown to cause birth defects or other problems in animal studies. Studies with ipodate, iopanoic acid, and tyropanoate have not been done in either humans or animals. However, x-rays of the abdomen are usually not recommended during pregnancy. This is to avoid exposing the fetus to radiation. Be sure you have discussed this with your doctor.

—if you are **breast-feeding**. Although these radiopaque agents have not been shown to cause problems in nursing babies, the chance always exists since iopanoic acid passes into the breast milk and the other agents may pass into the breast milk also.

—if you have any of the following medical problems:
Asthma, hay fever, or food allergies
Heart disease
Kidney disease
Liver disease (severe)

—if you are now taking cholestyramine or will be receiving any other radiopaque agent for another test.

Preparation For This Test

Unless otherwise directed by your doctor:

• Take this radiopaque agent with water after dinner the evening before the examination.

• Do not eat or drink anything, except water, after taking this radiopaque agent.

Your doctor may order a special diet or use of a laxative or enema in preparation for your test, depending on the type of test. If you have not received such instructions or if you do not understand them, check with your doctor in advance.

Precautions After Having This Test

Make sure your doctor knows if you are planning to have any future thyroid tests. The results of the thyroid test may be affected, even weeks or months later, by the iodine in this agent.

Side Effects of This Medicine

Along with its needed effects, a medicine may cause some unwanted effects. Although not all of these side effects may occur, if they do occur they may need medical attention.

Check with your doctor or nurse immediately if any of the following side effects occur:

Rare

    Itching
    Skin rash or hives
    Swelling of skin
    Unusual bleeding or bruising (with iopanoic acid)

Signs of overdose

    Diarrhea (severe)
    Nausea and vomiting (severe)
    Problems with urination

Other side effects may occur that usually do not require medical attention. These side effects should go away as the effects of the radiopaque agent wear off. However, check with your doctor if any of the following side effects continue or are bothersome:

Less common

    Abdominal or stomach spasms or cramps
    Diarrhea
    Difficult or painful urination
    Dizziness
    Frequent urge to urinate

    Headache
    Heartburn
    Nausea and vomiting

For elderly patients: The above side effects are more likely to occur in the elderly, who are usually more sensitive to the effects of cholecystographic agents.

Other side effects not listed above may also occur in some patients. If you notice any other effects, check with your doctor.

December 1987

Additional Information

In addition to the above information, for patients with Graves' disease taking ipodate:

• Ipodate is used in patients with Graves' disease, who have an overactive thyroid, to reduce the amount of thyroid hormone produced by the thyroid gland.

• **Use this medicine only as directed by your doctor.** Do not take more of it, do not take it more often, and do not take it for a longer period of time than your doctor ordered. To do so may increase the chance of side effects.

• In order for it to work properly, **ipodate must be taken every day, as ordered by your doctor**.

• The information given above in the section *Preparation For This Test* will not apply to you.

CHOLESTYRAMINE (Systemic)

A commonly used brand name is Questran.

To the Reader: If you do not recognize the names of medical conditions or medicines referred to in this information, check with your doctor, nurse, or pharmacist. Definitions for selected medical terms may be found in the Glossary. Brand names for the generic drug names listed can be found in the Index. In addition, selected brand names commonly associated with the generic name have been included in the text to help you recognize medicine you may be taking. The fact that a brand name product is not mentioned does not mean the information does not apply. It is a good idea for you to learn both the generic and brand names of your medicines and to write them down for future use.

Cholestyramine (koe-less-TEAR-a-meen) is used to remove substances called bile acids from your body. With some liver problems, there is too much bile acid in your body and this can cause severe itching. Cholestyramine is also used to lower high cholesterol levels in the blood. This may help prevent medical problems caused by cholesterol clogging the blood vessels.

Cholestyramine works by attaching to certain substances in the intestine. Since cholestyramine is not absorbed into the body, these substances also pass out of the body without being absorbed.

Cholestyramine may also be used for other conditions as determined by your doctor.

Cholestyramine is available only with your doctor's prescription.

Remember:

• **This medicine has been prescribed for your current medical problem only.** It must not be given to other people or used for other problems unless you are directed to do so by your doctor.

• **Keep all medicines out of the reach of children.**

• In order for this medicine to work, it must be used as directed.

• **It is very important that you read and understand the following information.** If any of the information causes you special concern, do not decide against using this medicine without first checking with your doctor.

• Before you begin using any new medicine (prescription or nonprescription) or if you develop any new medical problem while you are using this medicine, check with your doctor, nurse, or pharmacist.

• **If you have any questions** about the following information or if you want more information about this medicine or your medical problem, **ask your doctor, nurse, or pharmacist.**

Before Using This Medicine

In order to decide on the best treatment for your medical problem, your doctor should be told:

—if you have ever had any unusual or allergic reaction to cholestyramine.

—if you are on a low-salt, low-sugar, or any other special diet, or if you are allergic to any substance, such as foods, sulfites or other preservatives, or dyes.

Most medicines contain more than their active ingredient. Your doctor, nurse, or pharmacist can help you avoid products that may cause a problem.

—if you are **pregnant** or if you may become pregnant. Cholestyramine is not absorbed into the body and is not likely to cause problems. However, it may reduce absorption of vitamins into the body. Ask your doctor whether you need to take extra vitamins.

—if you are **breast-feeding**, although cholestyramine is not absorbed into the body and is not likely to cause problems.

—if you have any of the following medical problems:
Bleeding problems
Constipation
Gallstones
Heart or blood vessel disease
Hemorrhoids
Kidney disease
Stomach ulcer or other stomach problems

—if you are taking **any** other prescription or nonprescription (OTC) medicine, especially:
Anticoagulants (blood thinners)
Digitalis glycosides (heart medicine)
Penicillin G, taken by mouth
Tetracyclines, taken by mouth
Thyroid medicine
Vancomycin, taken by mouth

Proper Use of This Medicine

Take this medicine exactly as directed by your doctor. Try not to miss any doses and do not take more medicine than your doctor ordered.

This medicine should never be taken in its dry form, since it could cause you to choke. Instead, always mix as follows:

• Place the medicine on the surface of a glassful (4 to 6 ounces or more) of water, milk, flavored drink, or your favorite juice or carbonated drink. If you use a carbonated drink, use a large glass to prevent too much foaming. Allow it to sit, without stirring, for 1 or 2 minutes to keep it from becoming lumpy when mixed. Then stir until it is completely mixed (it will **not** dissolve) before drinking. After drinking all the liquid containing the medicine, rinse the glass with a little more liquid and drink that also, to make sure you get all the medicine.

• You may also mix this medicine with milk in hot or regular breakfast cereals, or in thin soups such as tomato or chicken noodle soup. Or you may add it to some pulpy fruits such as crushed pineapple, pears, peaches, or fruit cocktail.

For patients taking this medicine for high cholesterol:

• Importance of diet—Before prescribing medicine for your condition, your doctor will probably try to control your condition by prescribing a personal diet for you. Such a diet may be low in fats, sugars, and/or cholesterol. Many people are able to control their condition by carefully following their doctor's orders for proper diet and exercise. Medicine is prescribed only when additional help is needed. **Follow carefully the special diet your doctor gave you,** since the medicine is effective only when a schedule of diet and exercise is properly followed.

• Also, this medicine is less effective if you are greatly overweight. It may be very important for you to go on a reducing diet. However, check with your doctor before going on any diet.

• Remember that this medicine will not cure your cholesterol problem but it will help control it. Therefore, you must continue to take it as directed if you expect to lower your cholesterol level.

If you miss a dose of this medicine, take it as soon as possible. Then go back to your regular dosing schedule. However, if it is almost time for your next dose, skip the missed dose and go back to your regular dosing schedule. Do not double doses.

How to store this medicine:

• **Keep out of the reach of children.**

• Store away from heat and direct light.

• Do not store in the bathroom, near the kitchen sink, or in other damp places. Heat or moisture may cause the medicine to break down.

• Do not keep outdated medicine or medicine no longer needed. Be sure that any discarded medicine is out of the reach of children.

Precautions While Using This Medicine

It is very important that your doctor check your progress at regular visits. This will allow your doctor to see if the medicine is working properly and to decide if you should continue to take it.

Do not take any other medicine unless prescribed by your doctor since cholestyramine may change the effect of other medicines.

Side Effects of This Medicine

In some animal studies, cholestyramine was found to cause tumors. It is not known whether cholestyramine causes tumors in humans.

Along with its needed effects, a medicine may cause some unwanted effects. Although not all of these side effects may occur, if they do occur they may need medical attention.

Check with your doctor immediately if either of the following side effects occurs:
Rare
  Black tarry stools
  Stomach pain (severe) with nausea and vomiting

Check with your doctor as soon as possible if either of the following side effects occurs:
More common
  Constipation
Rare
  Loss of weight (sudden)

Other side effects may occur that usually do not require medical attention. These side effects may go away during treatment as your body adjusts to the medicine. However, check with your doctor if any of the following side effects continue or are bothersome:
More common
  Heartburn or indigestion
  Nausea or vomiting
  Stomach pain
Less common
  Belching
  Bloating
  Diarrhea

For elderly patients: The above side effects may be more likely to occur in the elderly (over 60 years of age), who are usually more sensitive to the effects of cholestyramine.

Other side effects not listed above may also occur in some patients. If you notice any other effects, check with your doctor.

December 1987

CHROMIC PHOSPHATE P 32 (Therapeutic)

A commonly used brand name is Phosphocol P 32.

To the Reader: If you do not recognize the names of medical conditions or medicines referred to in this information, check with your doctor, nurse, or pharmacist. Definitions for selected medical terms may be found in the Glossary. Brand names for the generic drug names listed can be found in the Index. In addition, selected brand names commonly associated with the generic name have been included in the text to help you recognize medicine you may be taking. The fact that a brand name product is not mentioned does not mean the information does not apply. It is a good idea for you to learn both the generic and brand names of your medicines and to write them down for future use.

Chromic phosphate (KROME-ik FOS-fate) P 32 is a radiopharmaceutical (ray-dee-oh-far-ma-SOO-ti-kal). Radiopharmaceuticals are agents used to diagnose certain medical problems or treat certain diseases.

A catheter is used to put the chromic phosphate P 32 into the pleura (sac that contains the lungs) or into the peritoneum (sac that contains the liver, stomach, and intestines). It is used to treat the leaking of fluid inside these areas that is caused by cancer. It may also be given by injection to treat cancer in certain organs such as the ovaries and prostate.

Chromic phosphate P 32 is to be given only by or under the direct supervision of a doctor with specialized training in nuclear medicine.

Remember:
• **It is very important that you read and understand the following information.** If any of the information causes you special concern, do not decide against using this medicine without first checking with your doctor.

• **If you have any questions** about the following information or if you want more information about this medicine or your medical problem, **ask your doctor, nuclear medicine physician and/or technician, nuclear pharmacist, or nurse.**

Before Using This Medicine

In order to decide on the best treatment for your medical problem, your doctor should be told:

—if you are **pregnant** or if you may become pregnant. Radiopharmaceuticals are usually not recommended for use during pregnancy to avoid exposing the fetus to radiation. However, some treatment using radiopharmaceuticals may be required even during pregnancy. Be sure you have discussed this with your doctor.

—if you are **breast-feeding**. Chromic phosphate P 32 passes into the breast milk. If you must receive this radiopharmaceutical, it may be necessary for you to stop breast-feeding during treatment. Be sure you have discussed this with your doctor.

Preparation for This Treatment

Your doctor may have special instructions for you in preparation for your treatment. If you have not received such instructions or if you do not understand them, check with your doctor in advance.

Side Effects of This Medicine

Along with its needed effects, a medicine may cause some unwanted effects. Although not all of these side effects may occur, if they do occur they may need medical attention.

Check with your doctor or nurse immediately if any of the following side effects occur:

Less common or rare
Abdominal or stomach pain (severe)
Chest pain
Chills and/or fever
Dry cough
Nausea and vomiting (severe)
Sore throat and fever
Troubled breathing
Unusual bleeding or bruising
Unusual tiredness or weakness

Other side effects may occur that usually do not require medical attention. These side effects may go away during treatment as your body adjusts to the medicine. However, check with your doctor if any of the following side effects continue or are bothersome:

More common
Abdominal or stomach cramps
Diarrhea
Feeling of discomfort
Loss of appetite
Nausea and vomiting
Weakness

Other side effects not listed above may also occur in some patients. If you notice any other effects, check with your doctor.

December 1987

CHYMOPAPAIN (Parenteral-Local)

Some commonly used brand names are Chymodiactin and Discase*.

---

*Not available in the U.S.

To the Reader: If you do not recognize the names of medical conditions or medicines referred to in this information, check with your doctor, nurse, or pharmacist. Definitions for selected medical terms may be found in the Glossary. Brand names for the generic drug names listed can be found in the Index. In addition, selected brand names commonly associated with the generic name have been included in the text to help you recognize medicine you may be taking. The fact that a brand name product is not mentioned does not mean the information does not apply. It is a good idea for you to learn both the generic and brand names of your medicines and to write them down for future use.

Chymopapain (kye-moe-PAP-ane) is injected directly into a herniated ("slipped") disk in the spine to dissolve part of the disk and relieve the pain and other problems caused by the disk pressing on a nerve. Before you receive chymopapain, you will be given an anesthetic (either a general anesthetic to put you to sleep or a local anesthetic).

Very rarely, use of chymopapain may cause serious side effects, including paralysis of the legs or death. Another dangerous side effect of chymopapain injection is a severe allergic reaction called anaphylaxis. This side effect occurs in less than 1% of the patients receiving the medicine, but it occurs more often in women than in men. Before receiving chymopapain, you should discuss the use of it, and the possibility of anaphylaxis or other serious side effects, with your doctor.

Chymopapain injections are given only in a hospital, usually in an operating room, by your surgeon.

Remember:

• **It is very important that you read and understand the following information.**

• **If you have any questions** about the following information or if you want more information about this medicine or your medical problem, **ask your doctor, nurse, or pharmacist**.

Before Receiving This Medicine

In order to decide on the best treatment for your medical problem, your doctor should be told:

—if you have ever had any unusual or allergic reaction to chymopapain, papaya, meat tenderizer, contact lens cleaning solutions, beer, or iodine.

—if you are **pregnant** or if you may become pregnant. Studies on birth defects or other problems with chymopapain have not been done in either humans or animals.

—if you are **breast-feeding**. Chymopapain has not been shown to cause problems in nursing babies.

—if you have ever received an injection of chymopapain or if you have had back surgery.

—if you have a history of allergies.

—if you or any member of your family has ever had a stroke or bleeding in the brain.

—if you have high blood pressure.

—if you are now using any of the following medicines in the eye:

Betaxolol (e.g., Betoptic)
Levobunolol (e.g., Betagan)
Timolol (e.g., Timoptic)

—if you are taking **any** other prescription or nonprescription (OTC) medicine, especially beta-blockers (acebutolol [e.g., Sectral], atenolol [e.g., Tenormin], esmolol [e.g., Brevibloc], labetalol [e.g., Normodyne], metoprolol [e.g., Lopressor], nadolol [e.g., Corgard], oxprenolol [e.g., Trasicor], pindolol [e.g., Visken], propranolol [e.g., Inderal], sotalol [e.g., Sotacor], timolol [e.g., Blocadren]).

Side Effects of This Medicine

Along with its needed effects, a medicine may cause some unwanted effects. Very rarely, use of chymopapain has caused serious side effects, including paralysis of the legs or death. Also, this medicine may cause dangerous allergic reactions, especially in women.

Although not all of the following side effects may occur, if they do occur they may need medical attention. Tell your doctor or nurse if any of the following side effects occur:

Rare

Abdominal or stomach cramps or pain
Constipation (severe)
Decreased or uncontrolled urination
Headache (sudden, severe, and continuing)
Pain, tenderness, blue color, or swelling of leg or foot
Runny nose
Shortness of breath, troubled breathing, tightness in chest, or wheezing
Skin rash, redness, hives, or itching
Swelling of abdomen or stomach
Uncontrolled bowel movements
Vomiting
Weakness in legs (severe) or problems with moving legs

Other side effects may occur that usually do not require medical attention. Pain and muscle spasms in the lower back may last for several days after you have received this medicine. Stiffness or soreness in the back may last for several months. Other side effects may go away after a short time. However, check with your doctor if any of the following side effects continue or are bothersome:

More common

Back pain, stiffness, or soreness
Muscle spasms in lower back

Less common or rare

Cramps or pain in legs
Dizziness
Feeling of burning in lower back
Headache
Nausea
Numbness or tingling in legs or toes

Some side effects may not appear until several days or weeks after you have received chymopapain. Check with your doctor as soon as possible if any of the following side effects occur within one month after you have received this medicine:

Back pain and muscle weakness (sudden and severe)
Skin rash, hives, or itching

Other side effects not listed above may also occur in some patients. If you notice any other effects, check with your doctor.

December 1987

CICLOPIROX (Topical)

A commonly used brand name is Loprox.

To the Reader: If you do not recognize the names of medical conditions or medicines referred to in this information, check with your doctor, nurse, or pharmacist. Definitions for selected medical terms may be found in the Glossary. Brand names for the generic drug names listed can be found in the Index. In addition, selected brand names commonly associated with the generic name have been included in the text to help you recognize medicine you may be taking. The fact that a brand name product is not mentioned does not mean the information does not apply. It is a good idea for you to learn both the generic and brand names of your medicines and to write them down for future use.

Ciclopirox (sye-kloe-PEER-ox) belongs to the general family of medicines called antifungals. Antifungals are used to treat infections caused by a fungus. They work by killing the fungus or preventing its growth.

Ciclopirox cream is applied to the skin to treat:

—ringworm of the body (tinea corporis);
—ringworm of the foot (tinea pedis; athlete's foot);
—ringworm of the groin (tinea cruris; jock itch);
—"sun fungus" (tinea versicolor; pityriasis versicolor); and
—certain other fungal infections, such as Candida or Monilia infections.

Ciclopirox is available only with your doctor's prescription.

Remember:
• **This medicine has been prescribed for your present infection only.** Another infection later on may require a different medicine. Also, even though other people may have the same symptoms as you, they may have a different kind of infection. Your medicine may not work for them and may even cause them harm. Therefore, **your medicine must not be given to other people or used for other infections** unless you are otherwise directed by your doctor.

• **Keep all medicines out of the reach of children.**

• In order for this medicine to work, it must be used as directed.

• **It is very important that you read and understand the following information.** If any of the information causes you special concern, do not decide against using this medicine without first checking with your doctor.

• Before you begin using any new medicine (prescription or nonprescription) or if you develop any new medical problem while you are using this medicine, check with your doctor, nurse, or pharmacist.

• **If you have any questions** about the following information or if you want more information about this medicine or your medical problem, **ask your doctor, nurse, or pharmacist.**

Before Using This Medicine

In order to decide on the best treatment for your medical problem, your doctor should be told:

—if you have ever had any unusual or allergic reaction to ciclopirox.

—if you are allergic to any substance, such as certain foods or preservatives or dyes. Most medicines contain more than their active ingredient. Your doctor, nurse, or pharmacist can help you avoid products that may cause a problem.

—if you are **pregnant** or if you may become pregnant. Studies have not been done in humans. However, ciclopirox has not been shown to cause birth defects or other problems in studies in mice, rats, rabbits, or monkeys given 10 or more times the usual human dose.

—if you are **breast-feeding**. It is not known whether ciclopirox passes into the breast milk. However, this medicine has not been shown to cause problems in nursing babies.

Proper Use of This Medicine

Apply enough ciclopirox to cover the affected and surrounding skin areas and rub in gently.

Keep this medicine away from the eyes.

When ciclopirox is used to treat certain types of fungal infections of the skin, an airtight covering or occlusive dressing (for example, kitchen plastic wrap) should *not* be applied over the medicine. To do so may irritate the skin. **Do not apply an airtight covering over this medicine unless you have been directed to do so by your doctor.**

To help clear up your infection completely, **it is very important that you keep using ciclopirox for the full time of treatment** even if your symptoms begin to clear up after a few days. Since fungal infections may be very slow to clear up, you may have to continue using this medicine every day for several weeks or more. If you stop using this medicine too soon, your symptoms may return. **Do not miss any doses.**

If you do miss a dose of this medicine, apply it as soon as possible. However, if it is almost time for your next dose, skip the missed dose and go back to your regular dosing schedule.

How to store this medicine:

• **Keep out of the reach of children.**
• Store away from heat and direct light.
• Keep the medicine from freezing.
• Do not keep outdated medicine or medicine no longer needed. Be sure that any discarded medicine is out of the reach of children.

Precautions While Using This Medicine

If your skin problem does not improve within 2 to 4 weeks, or if it becomes worse, check with your doctor.

To help clear up your infection completely and to help make sure it does not return, good health habits are

also required. The following measures will help reduce chafing and irritation and will also help keep the area cool and dry.

- For patients using ciclopirox for ringworm of the groin:

  —Avoid wearing underwear that is tight-fitting or made from synthetic materials (for example, rayon or nylon). Instead, wear loose-fitting, cotton underwear.

  —Use a bland, absorbent powder (for example, talcum powder) or an antifungal powder (for example, tolnaftate) on the skin. However, it is best to use the powder between the times you use ciclopirox cream or other antifungal cream.

- For patients using ciclopirox for ringworm of the foot:

  —Carefully dry the feet, especially between the toes, after bathing.

  —Avoid wearing socks made from wool or synthetic materials (for example, rayon or nylon). Instead, wear clean, cotton socks and change them daily or more often if the feet sweat freely.

  —Wear sandals or well-ventilated shoes (for example, shoes with holes).

—Use a bland, absorbent powder (for example, talcum powder) or an antifungal powder (for example, tolnaftate) between the toes, on the feet, and in socks and shoes freely once or twice a day. However, it is best to use the powder between the times you use ciclopirox cream or other antifungal cream.

If you have any questions about these instructions, check with your doctor, nurse, or pharmacist.

Side Effects of This Medicine

Along with its needed effects, a medicine may cause some unwanted effects. Although not all of these side effects may occur, if they do occur they may need medical attention.

Check with your doctor as soon as possible if any of the following side effects occur:

Rare

Burning, itching, redness, swelling, blistering, oozing, or other signs of irritation not present before therapy

Other side effects not listed above may also occur in some patients. If you notice any other effects, check with your doctor.

December 1987

CIMETIDINE (Systemic)

Some commonly used brand names are:

Apo-Cimetidine*	Peptol*
Novocimetine*	Tagamet

*Not available in the U.S.

To the Reader: If you do not recognize the names of medical conditions or medicines referred to in this information, check with your doctor, nurse, or pharmacist. Definitions for selected medical terms may be found in the Glossary. Brand names for the generic drug names listed can be found in the Index. In addition, selected brand names commonly associated with the generic name have been included in the text to help you recognize medicine you may be taking. The fact that a brand name product is not mentioned does not mean the information does not apply. It is a good idea for you to learn both the generic and brand names of your medicines and to write them down for future use.

Cimetidine (sye-MET-i-deen) is used to treat duodenal ulcers and prevent their return. It is also used to treat gastric ulcers and in some conditions, such as Zollinger-Ellison disease, in which the stomach produces too much acid. Cimetidine may also be used for other conditions as determined by your doctor.

Cimetidine works by decreasing the amount of acid produced by the stomach.

Cimetidine is available only with your doctor's prescription.

Remember:

• **This medicine has been prescribed for your current medical problem only.** It must not be given to other people or used for other problems unless you are directed to do so by your doctor.

• **Keep all medicines out of the reach of children.**

• In order for this medicine to work, it must be used as directed.

• If you are receiving this medicine by injection, some of the information about this medicine may not apply.

• **It is very important that you read and understand the following information.** If any of the information causes you special concern, do not decide against using this medicine without first checking with your doctor.

• Before you begin using any new medicine (prescription or nonprescription) or if you develop any new medical problem while you are using this medicine, check with your doctor, nurse, or pharmacist.

• **If you have any questions** about the following information or if you want more information about this medicine or your medical problem, **ask your doctor, nurse, or pharmacist.**

Before Using This Medicine

In order to decide on the best treatment for your medical problem, your doctor should be told:

—if you have ever had any unusual or allergic reaction to cimetidine, famotidine, or ranitidine.

—if you are on a low-salt, low-sugar, or any other special diet, or if you are allergic to any substance, such as foods, sulfites or other preservatives, or dyes.

Most medicines contain more than their active ingredient, and many liquid medicines contain alcohol. Your doctor, nurse, or pharmacist can help you avoid products that may cause a problem.

—if you are **pregnant** or if you may become pregnant. Studies have not been done in humans. However, one study in rats suggested that cimetidine may affect male sexual development. More studies are needed to confirm this.

—if you are **breast-feeding**. Cimetidine passes into the breast milk and may increase the chance of side effects, such as decreased amount of stomach acid and increased excitement, in the nursing baby.

—if you have any of the following medical problems:
  Kidney disease
  Liver disease

—if you are taking **any** other prescription or nonprescription (OTC) medicine, especially:
  Aminophylline (e.g., Somophyllin)
  Anticoagulants (blood thinners)
  Caffeine (e.g., No-Doz)
  Ketoconazole (e.g., Nizoral)
  Metoprolol (e.g., Lopressor)
  Oxtriphylline (e.g., Choledyl)
  Phenytoin (e.g., Dilantin)
  Propranolol (e.g., Inderal)
  Theophylline (e.g., Somophyllin-T)
  Tricyclic antidepressants (amitriptyline, amoxapine, clomipramine, desipramine, doxepin, imipramine, nortriptyline, protriptyline, trimipramine)

Proper Use of This Medicine

For patients taking:

• A single dose a day—Take it at bedtime, unless otherwise directed.

• Two doses a day—Take one in the morning and one at bedtime.

• Several doses a day—Take them with meals and at bedtime for best results.

It may take several days for cimetidine to begin to relieve stomach pain. To help relieve this pain, antacids may be taken with cimetidine, unless your doctor has told you not to use them. However, one hour should pass between taking the antacid and the cimetidine. For example, if you are taking cimetidine with meals, wait an hour after the meal before taking the antacid.

Take this medicine for the full time of treatment, even if you begin to feel better. Also, it is important that you keep your doctor's appointments for check-ups so that your doctor will be better able to tell you when to stop taking this medicine.

If you miss a dose of this medicine, take it as soon as possible. However, if it is almost time for your next dose, skip the missed dose and go back to your regular dosing schedule. Do not double doses.

How to store this medicine:

- **Keep out of the reach of children.**

- Store away from heat and direct light.

- Do not store the tablet form of this medicine in the bathroom, near the kitchen sink, or in other damp places. Heat or moisture may cause the medicine to break down.

- Keep the oral solution form of this medicine from freezing.

- Do not keep outdated medicine or medicine no longer needed. Be sure that any discarded medicine is out of the reach of children.

Precautions While Using This Medicine

Before you have any skin tests for allergies, tell the doctor in charge that you are taking this medicine. The results of the test may be affected by this medicine.

Remember that certain medicines, such as aspirin, and certain foods and drinks irritate the stomach and may make your problem worse.

Cigarette smoking tends to decrease the effect of cimetidine by increasing the amount of acid produced by the stomach. This is more likely to affect the stomach's nighttime production of acid. While taking cimetidine, stop smoking completely, or at least do not smoke after taking the last dose of the day.

Check with your doctor if your ulcer pain continues or gets worse.

Side Effects of This Medicine

Along with its needed effects, a medicine may cause some unwanted effects. Although not all of these side effects may occur, if they do occur they may need medical attention.

Check with your doctor as soon as possible if any of the following side effects occur:
Rare
 Confusion
 Sore throat and fever
 Unusual bleeding or bruising
 Unusual tiredness or weakness

Other side effects may occur that usually do not require medical attention. These side effects may go away during treatment as your body adjusts to the medicine. However, check with your doctor if any of the following side effects continue or are bothersome:
Less common or rare
 Decreased sexual ability (especially in patients with Zollinger-Ellison disease who have received high doses for at least 1 year)
 Diarrhea
 Dizziness or headache
 Muscle cramps or pain
 Skin rash
 Swelling of breasts or breast soreness in females and males

For elderly patients: Dizziness and confusion are more likely to occur in elderly patients with kidney or liver disease, who are usually more sensitive to the effects of cimetidine.

Other side effects not listed above may also occur in some patients. If you notice any other effects, check with your doctor.

December 1987

CINOXACIN (Systemic)

Some commonly used brand names or other names are Azolinic Acid, Cinobac, and Cinobactin*.

---

*Not available in the U.S.

To the Reader: If you do not recognize the names of medical conditions or medicines referred to in this information, check with your doctor, nurse, or pharmacist. Definitions for selected medical terms may be found in the Glossary. Brand names for the generic drug names listed can be found in the Index. In addition, selected brand names commonly associated with the generic name have been included in the text to help you recognize medicine you may be taking. The fact that a brand name product is not mentioned does not mean the information does not apply. It is a good idea for you to learn both the generic and brand names of your medicines and to write them down for future use.

Cinoxacin (sin-OX-a-sin) belongs to the general family of medicines called anti-infectives. It is taken by mouth to help the body overcome infections of the urinary tract. It will not work for other infections or for colds, flu, or other virus infections.

Cinoxacin is available only with your doctor's prescription.

Remember:

• **This medicine has been prescribed for your present infection only.** Another infection later on may require a different medicine. Also, even though other people may have the same symptoms as you, they may have a different kind of infection. Your medicine may not work for them and may even cause them harm. Therefore, **your medicine must not be given to other people or used for other infections** unless you are otherwise directed by your doctor.

• **Keep all medicines out of the reach of children.**

• In order for this medicine to work, it must be used as directed.

• **It is very important that you read and understand the following information.** If any of the information causes you special concern, do not decide against using this medicine without first checking with your doctor.

• Before you begin using any new medicine (prescription or nonprescription) or if you develop any new medical problem while you are using this medicine, check with your doctor, nurse, or pharmacist.

• **If you have any questions** about the following information or if you want more information about this medicine or your medical problem, **ask your doctor, nurse, or pharmacist.**

Before Using This Medicine

In order to decide on the best treatment for your medical problem, your doctor should be told:

—if you have ever had any unusual or allergic reaction to cinoxacin or to nalidixic acid, norfloxacin, or oxolinic acid.

—if you are on a low-salt, low-sugar, or any other special diet, or if you are allergic to any substance, such as foods, sulfites or other preservatives, or dyes.

Most medicines contain more than their active ingredient. Your doctor, nurse, or pharmacist can help you avoid products that may cause a problem.

—if you are **pregnant** or if you may become pregnant. Studies have not been done in humans. Cinoxacin has not been shown to cause birth defects in rat and rabbit fetuses when the adults were given doses up to 10 times the human dose. However, use is not recommended during pregnancy since cinoxacin given in single, very high doses has been shown to cause lameness in young dogs.

—if you are **breast-feeding**. It is not known whether cinoxacin passes into the breast milk. However, it may be necessary for you to take another medicine or to stop breast-feeding during treatment since nalidixic acid, a medicine similar to cinoxacin, does pass into the breast milk. Therefore, cinoxacin may also pass into the breast milk and may cause diarrhea, loss of appetite, vomiting, skin rash, or other problems in nursing babies. In addition, cinoxacin has been shown to cause lameness in some young animals. Be sure you have discussed the risks and benefits of the medicine with your doctor.

—if you have either of the following medical problems:
  Kidney disease
  Liver disease

—if you are taking **any** other prescription or nonprescription (OTC) medicine.

Proper Use of This Medicine

Cinoxacin may be taken with food, unless you are otherwise directed by your doctor.

Do not give this medicine to infants or children under 12 years of age, unless otherwise directed by your doctor.

To help clear up your infection completely, **keep taking this medicine for the full time of treatment** even if you begin to feel better after a few days. If you stop taking this medicine too soon, your symptoms may return.

This medicine works best when there is a constant amount in the urine. **To help keep this amount constant, do not miss any doses. Also, it is best to take the doses at evenly spaced times day and night.** For example, if you are to take 4 doses a day, the doses should be spaced about 6 hours apart. If this interferes with your sleep or other daily activities, or if you need help in planning the best times to take your medicine, check with your doctor, nurse, or pharmacist.

If you do miss a dose of this medicine, take it as soon as possible. This will help to keep a constant amount of medicine in the urine. However, if it is almost time for your next dose and your dosing schedule is:

• 2 doses a day—Space the missed dose and the next dose 5 to 6 hours apart.

• 3 or more doses a day—Space the missed dose and the next dose 2 to 4 hours apart or double your next dose.

Then go back to your regular dosing schedule.

How to store this medicine:

- **Keep out of the reach of children.**
- Store away from heat and direct light.
- Do not store in the bathroom, near the kitchen sink, or in other damp places. Heat or moisture may cause the medicine to break down.
- Do not keep outdated medicine or medicine no longer needed. Be sure that any discarded medicine is out of the reach of children.

Precautions While Using This Medicine

If your symptoms do not improve within a few days, or if they become worse, check with your doctor.

This medicine may cause your eyes to become more sensitive to light than they are normally. Wearing sunglasses and avoiding too much exposure to bright light may help lessen the discomfort.

This medicine may also cause some people to become dizzy. **Make sure you know how you react to this medicine before you drive, use machines, or do other jobs that require you to be alert.** If these reactions are especially bothersome, check with your doctor.

Side Effects of This Medicine

Along with its needed effects, a medicine may cause some unwanted effects. Although not all of these side effects may occur, if they do occur they may need medical attention.

Check with your doctor as soon as possible if any of the following side effects occur:

Less common
   Burning or tingling feeling
   Dizziness
   Headache

Increased sensitivity of the eyes to light
Ringing or buzzing sound in the ears
Trouble in sleeping

Other side effects may occur that usually do not require medical attention. These side effects may go away during treatment as your body adjusts to the medicine. However, check with your doctor if any of the following side effects continue or are bothersome:

More common
   Nausea
   Skin rash, itching, redness, or swelling

Less common
   Diarrhea
   Loss of appetite
   Stomach cramps
   Vomiting

For elderly patients: Many medicines have not been tested in older people. Therefore, it is not known whether the medicine acts the same way it does in younger adults. Check with your doctor or pharmacist if you notice any unusual effects while taking this medicine or if you think it is not working as it should.

Other side effects not listed above may also occur in some patients. If you notice any other effects, check with your doctor.

December 1987

CISPLATIN (Systemic)

Some commonly used brand names are Platinol and Platinol-AQ*.

Generic name product may also be available in Canada.

---

*Not available in the U.S.

To the Reader: If you do not recognize the names of medical conditions or medicines referred to in this information, check with your doctor, nurse, or pharmacist. Definitions for selected medical terms may be found in the Glossary. Brand names for the generic drug names listed can be found in the Index. In addition, selected brand names commonly associated with the generic name have been included in the text to help you recognize medicine you may be taking. The fact that a brand name product is not mentioned does not mean the information does not apply. It is a good idea for you to learn both the generic and brand names of your medicines and to write them down for future use.

Cisplatin (sis-PLA-tin) belongs to the group of medicines known as alkylating agents. It is given by injection to treat some kinds of cancer.

Cisplatin interferes with the growth of cancer cells, which are eventually destroyed. Since the growth of normal body cells may also be affected by cisplatin, other effects will also occur. Some of these may be serious and must be reported to your doctor. Other effects may not be serious but may cause concern. Some effects may not occur for months or years after the medicine is used.

Before you begin treatment with cisplatin, you and your doctor should talk about the good this medicine will do as well as the risks of using it.

Cisplatin is to be administered only by or under the immediate supervision of your doctor.

Remember:

• **It is very important that you read and understand the following information.** If any of the information causes you special concern, do not decide against using this medicine without first checking with your doctor.

• Before you begin using any new medicine (prescription or nonprescription) or if you develop any new medical problem while you are using this medicine, check with your doctor, nurse, or pharmacist.

• **If you have any questions** about the following information or if you want more information about this medicine or your medical problem, **ask your doctor, nurse, or pharmacist.**

Before Using This Medicine

In order to decide on the best treatment for your medical problem, your doctor should be told:

—if you have ever had any unusual or allergic reaction to cisplatin.

—if you are **pregnant** or if you intend to have children. There is a chance that this medicine may cause birth defects if either the male or female is taking it at the time of conception or if it is taken during pregnancy. Cisplatin causes toxic or harmful effects in the fetus in humans and birth defects in mice. In addition, many cancer medicines may cause sterility which could be

permanent. Although this has not been reported with this medicine, the possibility should be kept in mind. Be sure that you have discussed this with your doctor before receiving this medicine.

—if you intend to **breast-feed.** Because this medicine may cause serious side effects, breast-feeding is generally not recommended while you are receiving it.

—if you have any of the following medical problems:
   Chickenpox (including recent exposure)
   Gout (history of)
   Hearing problems
   Herpes zoster (shingles)
   Infection
   Kidney disease
   Kidney stones (history of)

—if you are taking **any** other prescription or nonprescription (OTC) medicine, especially:
   Aminoglycosides by injection or topical application (amikacin, gentamicin, kanamycin, neomycin, netilmicin, streptomycin, tobramycin)
   Amphotericin B by injection (e.g., Fungizone)
   Antithyroid agents (medicine for overactive thyroid)
   Azathioprine (e.g., Imuran)
   Capreomycin (e.g., Capastat)
   Captopril (e.g., Capoten)
   Chloramphenicol (e.g., Chloromycetin)
   Chloroquine (e.g., Aralen)
   Colchicine
   Cyclosporine (e.g., Sandimmune)
   Enalapril (e.g., Vasotec)
   Erythromycins
   Flucytosine (e.g., Ancobon)
   Gold salts
   Hydroxychloroquine (e.g., Plaquenil)
   Interferon (e.g., Intron A, Roferon-A)
   Lithium (e.g., Lithane)
   Medicine for inflammation or pain (diclofenac, diflunisal, fenoprofen, flurbiprofen [oral], ibuprofen, indomethacin, ketoprofen, meclofenamate, mefenamic acid, naproxen, phenylbutazone, piroxicam, sulindac, tiaprofenic acid, tolmetin)
   Neomycin by mouth
   Penicillamine (e.g., Cuprimine)
   Plicamycin (e.g., Mithracin)
   Probenecid (e.g., Benemid)
   Quinine (e.g., Quinamm)
   Rifampin (e.g., Rifadin)
   Sulfinpyrazone (e.g., Anturane)
   Sulfonamides (sulfa medicine)
   Tetracyclines, except doxycycline
   Vancomycin by injection (e.g., Vancocin)

—if you regularly take large amounts of combination pain medicine containing acetaminophen or aspirin or other salicylates.

—if you have ever been treated with x-rays or cancer medicines.

Proper Use of This Medicine

This medicine is sometimes given together with certain other medicines. If you are using a combination of medicines, it is important that you receive each one at the proper time. If you are taking some of these medicines by mouth, ask your doctor, nurse, or pharmacist to help you plan a way to take them at the right times.

While you are receiving this medicine, your doctor may want you to drink extra fluids so that you will pass more urine. This will help prevent kidney problems and keep your kidneys working well.

This medicine usually causes nausea and vomiting that may be severe. However, it is very important that you continue to receive the medicine, even if you begin to feel ill. Ask your doctor, nurse, or pharmacist for ways to lessen these effects, especially if they are severe.

Precautions While Using This Medicine

It is very important that your doctor check your progress at regular visits to make sure that this medicine is working properly and to check for unwanted effects.

While you are being treated with cisplatin, and after you stop treatment with it, **do not have any immunizations without your doctor's approval.** Cisplatin lowers your body's resistance and there is a chance you might get the infection the immunization is meant to prevent. In addition, other persons living in your household should not take oral polio vaccine since there is a chance they could pass the polio virus on to you. Also, you should avoid close contact with other persons (for example, at school or work) who have taken oral polio vaccine.

Cisplatin can lower the number of white blood cells in your body. This may increase the chance of getting an infection. If you can, avoid people with colds or other infections. If you think you are getting a cold or other infection, check with your doctor.

If cisplatin accidentally seeps out of the vein into which it is injected, it may damage some tissues and cause scarring. **Tell the doctor or nurse right away if you notice redness, pain, or swelling at the place of injection.**

Side Effects of This Medicine

Along with their needed effects, medicines like cisplatin can sometimes cause unwanted effects such as blood problems, ear and kidney problems, and other side effects; these are described below. Also, because of the way these medicines act on the body, there is a chance that they might cause other unwanted effects that may not occur until months or years after the medicine is used. These delayed effects may include certain types of cancer, such as leukemia. Discuss these possible effects with your doctor.

Although not all of these side effects may occur, if they do occur they may need medical attention.

Check with your doctor or nurse immediately if any of the following side effects occur:

More common
    Fever, chills, or sore throat
    Unusual bleeding or bruising

Less common
    Fast heartbeat
    Pain or redness at the place of injection
    Swelling of face
    Wheezing

Check with your doctor as soon as possible if any of the following side effects occur:

More common
    Difficulty in hearing
    Joint pain
    Lower back, side, or stomach pain
    Ringing in the ears
    Swelling of feet or lower legs
    Unusual tiredness or weakness

Less common
    Loss of taste
    Numbness or tingling in the fingers, toes, or face

Rare
    Blurred vision
    Change in ability to see colors
    Sores in the mouth and on the lips

Other side effects may occur that usually do not require medical attention. These side effects may go away during treatment as your body adjusts to the medicine. Also, your doctor or nurse may be able to tell you about ways to prevent or reduce some of these side effects. Check with your doctor if any of the following side effects continue or are bothersome or if you have any questions about them:

More common
    Nausea and vomiting (severe)

Less common
    Loss of appetite

For children: Hearing problems are more likely to occur in children, who are usually more sensitive to the effects of cisplatin.

For elderly patients: Many medicines have not been tested in older people. Therefore, it is not known whether the medicine acts the same way it does in younger adults. Check with your doctor if you notice any unusual effects while taking this medicine or if you think it is not working as it should.

After you stop receiving cisplatin, it may still produce some side effects that need attention. During this period of time check with your doctor if you notice any of the following side effects:

    Decrease in urination
    Difficulty in hearing
    Fever, chills, or sore throat
    Ringing in the ears
    Swelling of feet or lower legs
    Unusual bleeding or bruising

Other side effects not listed above may also occur in some patients. If you notice any other effects, check with your doctor.

December 1987

CITRATES (Systemic)

This information applies to the following medicines:
Potassium Citrate (poe-TASS-ee-um SIH-trayt)
Potassium Citrate and Citric Acid (SIH-trik A-sid)
Potassium Citrate and Sodium (SOE-dee-um) Citrate
Sodium Citrate and Citric Acid
Tricitrates (Try-SIH-trayts)

Some commonly used brand names and other names are:	Generic names:
Urocit-K	Potassium Citrate
Polycitra-K	Potassium Citrate and Citric Acid
Citrolith	Potassium Citrate and Sodium Citrate
Albright's solution Bicitra Modified Shohl's solution Oracit	Sodium Citrate and Citric Acid
Polycitra Polycitra-LC–Sugar-Free	Tricitrates

To the Reader: If you do not recognize the names of medical conditions or medicines referred to in this information, check with your doctor, nurse, or pharmacist. Definitions for selected medical terms may be found in the Glossary. Brand names for the generic drug names listed can be found in the Index. In addition, selected brand names commonly associated with the generic name have been included in the text to help you recognize medicine you may be taking. The fact that a brand name product is not mentioned does not mean the information does not apply. It is a good idea for you to learn both the generic and brand names of your medicines and to write them down for future use.

Citrates (SIH-trayts) are medicines taken by mouth to make the urine more alkaline (less acid). This helps prevent certain kinds of kidney stones. Citrates are sometimes used with other medicines to help treat kidney stones that may occur with gout. They are also used to make the blood more alkaline in certain conditions.

This medicine may also be used for other conditions as determined by your doctor.

Citrates are available only with your doctor's prescription.

Remember:
• **This medicine has been prescribed for your current medical problem only.** It must not be given to other people or used for other problems unless you are directed to do so by your doctor.

• **Keep all medicines out of the reach of children.**

• In order for this medicine to work, it must be used as directed.

• **It is very important that you read and understand the following information.** If any of the information causes you special concern, do not decide against using this medicine without first checking with your doctor.

• Before you begin using any new medicine (prescription or nonprescription) or if you develop any new medical problem while you are using this medicine, check with your doctor, nurse, or pharmacist.

• **If you have any questions** about the following information or if you want more information about this medicine or your medical problem, **ask your doctor, nurse, or pharmacist.**

Before Using This Medicine

In order to decide on the best treatment for your medical problem, your doctor should be told:

—if you are taking a potassium citrate-containing medicine and you have ever had any unusual reaction to other medicines containing potassium.

—if you are on a low-salt, low-sugar, or any other special diet, or if you are allergic to any substance, such as foods, sulfites or other preservatives, or dyes. Most medicines contain more than their active ingredient and some liquid medicines contain alcohol. Your doctor, nurse, or pharmacist can help you avoid products that may cause a problem.

—if you are **pregnant** or if you may become pregnant. Studies have not been done in either humans or animals.

—if you are **breast-feeding**. Although it is not known whether citrates pass into the breast milk, this medicine has not been shown to cause problems in nursing babies.

—if you have any of the following medical problems:
Addison's disease (underactive adrenal glands)
Diabetes mellitus (sugar diabetes)
Diarrhea (chronic)
Edema (swelling of the feet or lower legs)
Heart disease
High blood pressure
Intestinal or esophageal blockage
Kidney disease
Stomach ulcer or other stomach problems
Toxemia of pregnancy
Urinary tract infection

—if you are taking **any** other prescription or nonprescription (OTC) medicine, especially:
Amiloride (e.g., Midamor)
Antacids, especially calcium carbonate or sodium bicarbonate
Calcium-containing medicines, including calcium supplements
Digitalis glycosides (heart medicine)
Methenamine (e.g., Mandelamine)
Potassium-containing medicines (other)
Quinidine (e.g., Quinidex)
Sodium-containing medicines (other)
Spironolactone (e.g., Aldactone)
Triamterene (e.g., Dyrenium)

—if you are taking a potassium citrate–containing medicine and:

• you are using salt substitutes or drinking low-salt milk.

• you plan to start strenuous physical exercise but you are out of condition.

Proper Use of This Medicine

For patients taking the tablet forms of this medicine:
• Swallow the tablets whole. Do not crush, chew, or suck the tablet.

• Take with a full glass (8 ounces) of water.

• **If you have trouble swallowing the tablets or they seem to stick in your throat, check with your doctor at once.** If this medicine is not completely swallowed and not properly dissolved, it can cause severe irritation.

For patients taking the liquid form of this medicine:

• Dilute with a full glass (8 ounces) of water, followed by additional water, if desired.

• Chill, but do *not* freeze, this medicine before taking it, for a better taste.

Take each dose immediately after a meal or within 30 minutes after a meal or bedtime snack. This helps to prevent the medicine from causing stomach pain or a laxative effect.

Drink at least a full glass (8 ounces) of water or other liquid (except milk) every hour during the day (about 3 quarts a day), unless otherwise directed by your doctor. This will increase the flow of urine and help prevent kidney stones.

Take this medicine only as directed by your doctor. Do not take more of it, do not take it more often, and do not take it for a longer period of time than your doctor ordered. **This is especially important if you are also taking a diuretic (water pill) or digitalis medicine for your heart.**

If you miss a dose of this medicine, take it as soon as possible if remembered within 2 hours. However, if it is almost time for your next dose, skip the missed dose and go back to your regular dosing schedule. Do not double doses.

How to store this medicine:

• **Keep out of the reach of children.**

• Store away from heat and direct light.

• Do not store in the bathroom, near the kitchen sink, or in other damp places. Heat or moisture may cause the medicine to break down.

• Keep the medicine from freezing.

• Do not keep outdated medicine or medicine no longer needed. Be sure that any discarded medicine is out of the reach of children.

Precautions While Using This Medicine

It is important that your doctor check your progress at regular visits. This is to make sure the medicine is working properly and to check for unwanted effects.

Do not drink milk or eat other dairy products (for example, cheese, ice cream, or yogurt) while you are taking this medicine. To do so may increase the chance of kidney stones.

Do not eat salty foods or use extra table salt on your food while you are taking citrates. This will help prevent kidney stones and unwanted effects.

For patients taking potassium citrate–containing medicines:

• Do not use salt substitutes and low-salt milk unless told to do so by your doctor. They may contain potassium.

• **Check with your doctor at once if you notice black, tar-like stools or other signs of stomach or intestinal bleeding.**

For patients on a potassium-rich or potassium-restricted diet:

• Potassium citrate–containing medicines contain a large amount of potassium. If you have any questions about this, check with your doctor, nurse, or pharmacist.

For patients on a sodium-restricted diet:

• Sodium citrate–containing medicines contain a large amount of sodium. If you have any questions about this, check with your doctor, nurse, or pharmacist.

Side Effects of This Medicine

Along with its needed effects, a medicine may cause some unwanted effects. Although not all of these side effects may occur, if they do occur they may need medical attention.

Stop taking this medicine and check with your doctor immediately if any of the following side effects occur:

Rare

Abdominal or stomach pain or cramping (severe)
Black, tar-like stools
Vomiting (severe), sometimes with blood

Also, check with your doctor as soon as possible if any of the following side effects occur:

Bad taste
Confusion
Convulsions (seizures)
Dizziness
High blood pressure
Irregular or fast heartbeat
Irritability
Mood or mental changes
Muscle pain or twitching
Nervousness or restlessness
Numbness or tingling in hands, feet, or lips
Shortness of breath, difficult breathing, or slow breathing
Swelling of feet or lower legs
Unexplained anxiety
Unusual tiredness or weakness
Weakness or heaviness of legs

Other side effects may occur that usually do not require medical attention. These side effects may go away during treatment as your body adjusts to the medicine. However, check with your doctor if any of the following side effects continue or are bothersome:

Less common

Abdominal or stomach soreness or pain, mild
Diarrhea or loose bowel movements
Nausea or vomiting

For elderly patients: Many medicines have not been tested in older people. Therefore, it is not known whether the medicine acts the same way it does in younger adults. Check with your doctor or pharmacist if you notice any unusual effects while taking this medicine or if you do not think it is working as it should.

Other side effects not listed above may also occur in some patients. If you notice any other effects, check with your doctor.

December 1987

CLINDAMYCIN (Topical)

A commonly used brand name is Cleocin T.

To the Reader: If you do not recognize the names of medical conditions or medicines referred to in this information, check with your doctor, nurse, or pharmacist. Definitions for selected medical terms may be found in the Glossary. Brand names for the generic drug names listed can be found in the Index. In addition, selected brand names commonly associated with the generic name have been included in the text to help you recognize medicine you may be taking. The fact that a brand name product is not mentioned does not mean the information does not apply. It is a good idea for you to learn both the generic and brand names of your medicines and to write them down for future use.

Clindamycin (klin-da-MYE-sin) belongs to the general family of medicines called antibiotics. Topical clindamycin is used on the skin to help control acne. It may be used alone or with one or more other medicines that are used on the skin or taken by mouth for acne. Topical clindamycin may also be used for other problems as determined by your doctor.

Clindamycin is available only with your doctor's prescription.

Remember:

• **This medicine has been prescribed for your acne only.** Even though other people may also have acne, they may have a different kind. Your medicine may not work for them and may even cause them harm. Therefore, **your medicine must not be given to other people or used for other problems** unless you are otherwise directed by your doctor.

• **Keep all medicines out of the reach of children.**

• In order for this medicine to work, it must be used as directed.

• **It is very important that you read and understand the following information.** If any of the information causes you special concern, do not decide against using this medicine without first checking with your doctor.

• Before you begin using any new medicine (prescription or nonprescription) or if you develop any new medical problem while you are using this medicine, check with your doctor, nurse, or pharmacist.

• **If you have any questions** about the following information or if you want more information about this medicine or your medical problem, **ask your doctor, nurse, or pharmacist.**

Before Using This Medicine

In order to decide on the best treatment for your medical problem, your doctor should be told:

—if you have ever had any unusual or allergic reaction to any of the other clindamycins (by mouth or by injection) or lincomycin.

—if you are allergic to any substance, such as certain foods or preservatives or dyes. Most medicines contain more than their active ingredient. Your doctor, nurse, or pharmacist can help you avoid products that may cause a problem.

—if you are **pregnant** or if you may become pregnant. Studies have not been done in humans. However, clindamycin has not been shown to cause birth defects or other problems in studies in rats and mice receiving high doses of clindamycin by injection or by mouth.

—if you are **breast-feeding**. It is not known whether clindamycin used on the skin passes into the breast milk. Clindamycin taken by mouth or given by injection does pass into the breast milk. However, clindamycin used on the skin has not been shown to cause problems in nursing babies, even though small amounts are absorbed through the skin.

—if you have a history of stomach or intestinal disease (especially colitis, including colitis caused by antibiotics, or enteritis).

—if you are using **any** other prescription or nonprescription (OTC) medicine.

Proper Use of This Medicine

Before applying this medicine, thoroughly wash the affected areas with warm water and soap, rinse well, and pat dry.

You should avoid washing the acne-affected areas too often since this may dry your skin and make your acne worse. Washing with a mild, bland soap 2 or 3 times a day should be enough, unless you have oily skin. If you have any questions about this, check with your doctor.

Clindamycin will not cure your acne. However, to help keep your acne under control, **keep using this medicine for the full time of treatment,** even if your symptoms begin to clear up after a few days. You may have to continue using this medicine every day for months or even longer in some cases. If you stop using this medicine too soon, your symptoms may return. **It is important that you do not miss any doses.**

If you do miss a dose of this medicine, apply it as soon as possible. However, if it is almost time for your next dose, skip the missed dose and go back to your regular dosing schedule.

For patients using the topical solution form of clindamycin:

• After washing or shaving, it is best to wait 30 minutes before applying this medicine since the alcohol in it may irritate freshly washed or shaved skin.

• This medicine contains alcohol and is flammable. **Do not use near heat, near open flame, or while smoking.**

• How to apply this medicine:

—This medicine comes in a bottle with an applicator tip, which may be used to apply the medicine directly to the skin. Use the applicator with a dabbing motion instead of a rolling motion (not like a roll-on deodorant, for example). Tilt the bottle and press the tip firmly against your skin. If needed, you can make the medicine flow faster from the applicator tip by slightly increasing the pressure against the skin. If the medicine flows too fast, use less pressure. If the applicator tip becomes dry, turn the bottle upside down and press the tip several times to moisten it.

—Apply a thin film of medicine, using enough to cover the affected area lightly. **You should apply the medicine to the whole area usually affected by acne, not just to the pimples themselves.** This will help keep new pimples from breaking out.

—Since this medicine contains alcohol, it will sting or burn. In addition, it has a bad taste if it gets on the mouth or lips. Therefore, **do not get this medicine in the eyes, nose, mouth, or on other mucous membranes.** Spread the medicine away from these areas when applying. If this medicine does get in the eyes, wash them out immediately, but carefully, with large amounts of cool tap water. If your eyes still burn or are painful, check with your doctor.

• It is important that you do not use this medicine more often than your doctor ordered since it may cause your skin to become too dry or irritated.

• The bottle contains about a 4-week supply (30-mL size) or an 8-week supply (60-mL size) of medicine. Refills may be available at reduced cost.

How to store this medicine:

• **Keep out of the reach of children.**

• Store away from heat and direct light.

• Keep the medicine from freezing.

• Do not keep outdated medicine or medicine no longer needed. Be sure that any discarded medicine is out of the reach of children.

Precautions While Using This Medicine

If your acne does not improve within about 6 weeks, or if it becomes worse, check with your doctor or pharmacist. However, treatment of acne may take up to 8 to 12 weeks before full improvement is seen.

If your doctor has ordered another medicine to be applied to the skin along with this medicine, it is best to apply them at different times (for example, morning and evening). This may help keep your skin from becoming too irritated. Also, if the medicines are used too close together, they may not work as well.

For patients using the topical solution form of clindamycin:

• This medicine may cause the skin to become unusually dry, even with normal use. If this occurs, check with your doctor.

If diarrhea occurs, do not take any diarrhea medicine without first checking with your doctor or pharmacist. These medicines may make your diarrhea worse or make it last longer.

You may continue to use cosmetics (make-up) while you are using this medicine for acne. However, it is best to use only "water-base" cosmetics. Also, it is best not to use cosmetics too heavily or too often since they may make your acne worse. If you have any questions about this, check with your doctor.

Side Effects of This Medicine

Along with its needed effects, a medicine may cause some unwanted effects. Although not all of these side effects may occur, if they do occur they may need medical attention.

Check with your doctor immediately if any of the following side effects occur:
Very rare
   Abdominal or stomach cramps, pain, and bloating (severe)
   Diarrhea (watery and severe), which may also be bloody
   Fever
   Increased thirst
   Increased weight loss
   Nausea or vomiting
   Unusual tiredness or weakness
      (the above side effects may also occur up to several weeks after you stop using this medicine)

Also, check with your doctor as soon as possible if any of the following side effects occur:
Less common
   Skin rash, itching, redness, swelling, or other sign of irritation not present before using this medicine

Other side effects may occur that usually do not require medical attention. These side effects may go away during treatment as your body adjusts to the medicine. However, check with your doctor if any of the following side effects continue or are bothersome:
Less common—For topical gel and topical solution forms
   Diarrhea (mild)
Less common—For topical solution form only
   Dry or scaly skin
   Peeling of skin
   Stinging or burning feeling

For elderly patients: Many medicines have not been tested in older people. Therefore, it is not known whether the medicine acts the same way it does in younger adults. Check with your doctor or pharmacist if you notice any unusual effects while using this medicine or if you think it is not working as it should.

Other side effects not listed above may also occur in some patients. If you notice any other effects, check with your doctor.

December 1987

CLIOQUINOL (Topical)

Some commonly used brand names or other names are:

Iodo	Torofor
Iodochlorhydroxyquin	Vioform

Generic name product may also be available in the U.S.

To the Reader: If you do not recognize the names of medical conditions or medicines referred to in this information, check with your doctor, nurse, or pharmacist. Definitions for selected medical terms may be found in the Glossary. Brand names for the generic drug names listed can be found in the Index. In addition, selected brand names commonly associated with the generic name have been included in the text to help you recognize medicine you may be taking. The fact that a brand name product is not mentioned does not mean the information does not apply. It is a good idea for you to learn both the generic and brand names of your medicines and to write them down for future use.

Clioquinol (klye-oh-KWIN-ole) belongs to the general family of medicines called anti-infectives. Clioquinol topical preparations are used on the skin to treat skin infections.

Clioquinol is available without a prescription; however, your doctor may have special instructions on the proper use of this medicine for your medical problem.

Remember:

• **Keep all medicines out of the reach of children.**

• In order for this medicine to work, it must be used as directed. **If you are using this medicine without a prescription, it is very important to follow the directions on the label.**

• **It is also very important that you read and understand the following information.** If any of the information causes you special concern, check with your doctor or pharmacist.

• Before you begin using any new medicine (prescription or nonprescription) or if you develop any new medical problem while you are using this medicine, check with your doctor, nurse, or pharmacist.

• **If you have any questions** about the following information or if you want more information about this medicine or your medical problem, **ask your doctor, nurse, or pharmacist.**

Before Using This Medicine

Before you use clioquinol, check with your doctor or pharmacist:

—if you have ever had any unusual or allergic reaction to chloroxine, iodine, or iodine-containing preparations.

—if you are allergic to any substance, such as certain foods or preservatives or dyes. Most medicines contain more than their active ingredient. Your doctor, nurse, or pharmacist can help you avoid products that may cause a problem.

—if you are **pregnant** or if you may become pregnant. However, clioquinol topical preparations have not been shown to cause birth defects or other problems in humans.

—if you are **breast-feeding**. However, clioquinol topical preparations have not been shown to cause problems in nursing babies.

Proper Use of This Medicine

Before applying this medicine, wash the affected area with soap and water, and dry thoroughly.

Do not use this medicine in or around the eyes.

For patients using the cream form of this medicine:
• Apply a thin layer of cream to the affected area and rub in gently until the cream disappears.

For patients using the ointment form of this medicine:
• Apply a thin layer of ointment to the affected area and rub in gently.

To help clear up your infection completely, **keep using this medicine for the full time of treatment,** even though your symptoms may have disappeared; **do not miss any doses.**

If you do miss a dose of this medicine, apply it as soon as possible. However, if it is almost time for your next dose, skip the missed dose and go back to your regular dosing schedule.

How to store this medicine:

• **Keep out of the reach of children.**
• Store away from heat and direct light.
• Keep the medicine from freezing.
• Do not keep outdated medicine or medicine no longer needed. Be sure that any discarded medicine is out of the reach of children.

Precautions While Using This Medicine

If your skin problem does not improve within 1 to 2 weeks, or if it becomes worse, check with your doctor.

This medicine may stain clothing, skin, hair, and nails yellow. Avoid getting this medicine on your clothing since bleaching may not remove the stain.

Side Effects of This Medicine

Along with its needed effects, a medicine may cause some unwanted effects. Although not all of these side effects may occur, if they do occur they may need medical attention.

Check with your doctor immediately if any of the following side effects occur:
Rare
Itching, skin rash, redness, swelling, or other sign of irritation not present before using this medicine

Other side effects not listed above may also occur in some patients. If you notice any other effects, check with your doctor.

December 1987

CLIOQUINOL AND HYDROCORTISONE
(Topical)

Some commonly used brand names or other names are:

Clioquinol and Cortisol	Iodochlorhydroxyquin
Dek-Quin	and Hydrocortisone
HCV	Mity-Quin
Iodochlorhydroxyquin	Racet
and Cortisol	Vioform-Hydrocortisone

Generic name product may also be available in the U.S.

To the Reader: If you do not recognize the names of medical conditions or medicines referred to in this information, check with your doctor, nurse, or pharmacist. Definitions for selected medical terms may be found in the Glossary. Brand names for the generic drug names listed can be found in the Index. In addition, selected brand names commonly associated with the generic name have been included in the text to help you recognize medicine you may be taking. The fact that a brand name product is not mentioned does not mean the information does not apply. It is a good idea for you to learn both the generic and brand names of your medicines and to write them down for future use.

Clioquinol (klye-oh-KWIN-ole) and hydrocortisone (hye-droe-KOR-ti-sone) is a combined anti-infective and cortisone-like medicine. Clioquinol and hydrocortisone topical preparations are used on the skin to help the body overcome infections of the skin and to help provide relief from the redness, itching, and discomfort of many skin problems.

Clioquinol and hydrocortisone combination is available only with your doctor's prescription.

Remember:

• **This medicine has been prescribed for your present medical problem only.** Even though other people may have the same symptoms as you, they may have a different kind of problem. Your medicine may not work for them and may even cause them harm. Therefore, **your medicine must not be given to other people or used for other problems** unless you are otherwise directed by your doctor.

• **Keep all medicines out of the reach of children.**

• In order for this medicine to work, it must be used as directed.

• **It is very important that you read and understand the following information.** If any of the information causes you special concern, do not decide against using this medicine without first checking with your doctor.

• Before you begin using any new medicine (prescription or nonprescription) or if you develop any new medical problem while you are using this medicine, check with your doctor, nurse, or pharmacist.

• **If you have any questions** about the following information or if you want more information about this medicine or your medical problem, **ask your doctor, nurse, or pharmacist.**

Before Using This Medicine

In order to decide on the best treatment for your medical problem, your doctor should be told:

—if you have ever had any unusual or allergic reaction to chloroxine, iodine, or iodine-containing preparations.

—if you are allergic to any substance, such as certain foods or preservatives or dyes. Most medicines contain more than their active ingredient. Your doctor, nurse, or pharmacist can help you avoid products that may cause a problem.

—if you are **pregnant** or if you may become pregnant. Clioquinol and hydrocortisone topical preparations have not been shown to cause birth defects or other problems in humans. However, use of large amounts on the skin or use for a long time is not recommended during pregnancy.

—if you are **breast-feeding**. However, clioquinol and hydrocortisone topical preparations have not been shown to cause problems in nursing babies.

—if you have any other skin infection.

Proper Use of This Medicine

Before applying this medicine, wash the affected area with soap and water, and dry thoroughly.

Do not use this medicine in or around the eyes.

For patients using the cream form of this medicine:

• Apply a thin layer of cream to the affected area and rub in gently until cream disappears.

For patients using the lotion form of this medicine:

• Gently squeeze bottle and apply a few drops of lotion to the affected area. Rub in gently until lotion disappears.

For patients using the ointment form of this medicine:

• Apply a thin layer of ointment to the affected area and rub in gently.

Do not bandage or otherwise wrap the area of the skin being treated unless directed to do so by your doctor.

Check with your doctor before using this medicine on any other skin problems since it should not be used on certain kinds of bacterial, viral, or fungal skin infections.

To help clear up your infection completely, **keep using this medicine for the full time of treatment**, even though your symptoms may have disappeared; **do not miss any doses**. However, **do not use this medicine more often or for a longer period of time than your doctor ordered**. To do so may increase the chance of absorption through the skin and the chance of side effects. In addition, too much use, especially on thin skin areas (for example, face, armpits, groin), may result in thinning of the skin and stretch marks.

If you do miss a dose of this medicine, apply it as soon as possible. However, if it is almost time for your next dose, skip the missed dose and go back to your regular dosing schedule.

How to store this medicine:

- **Keep out of the reach of children.**

- Store away from heat and direct light.

- Keep the medicine from freezing.

- Do not keep outdated medicine or medicine no longer needed. Be sure that any discarded medicine is out of the reach of children.

Precautions While Using This Medicine

If your skin problem does not improve within 1 to 2 weeks, or if it becomes worse, check with your doctor.

This medicine may be absorbed through the skin, and too much use can affect growth. **Children who must use this medicine should be followed closely by their doctor.**

This medicine may stain clothing, skin, hair, and nails yellow. Avoid getting this medicine on your clothing since bleaching may not remove the stain.

Side Effects of This Medicine

Along with its needed effects, a medicine may cause some unwanted effects. Although not all of these side effects may occur, if they do occur they may need medical attention.

Check with your doctor immediately if any of the following side effects occur:
Rare
Blistering, burning, itching, peeling, skin rash, redness, swelling, or other sign of irritation not present before using this medicine
With prolonged use
Thinning of skin with easy bruising

For elderly patients: Many medicines have not been tested in older people. Therefore, it is not known whether the medicine acts the same way it does in younger adults. Check with your doctor or pharmacist if you notice any unusual effects while using this medicine or if you think it is not working as it should.

Other side effects not listed above may also occur in some patients. If you notice any other effects, check with your doctor.

December 1987

CLOFAZIMINE (Systemic)

A commonly used brand name is Lamprene.

To the Reader: If you do not recognize the names of medical conditions or medicines referred to in this information, check with your doctor, nurse, or pharmacist. Definitions for selected medical terms may be found in the Glossary. Brand names for the generic drug names listed can be found in the Index. In addition, selected brand names commonly associated with the generic name have been included in the text to help you recognize medicine you may be taking. The fact that a brand name product is not mentioned does not mean the information does not apply. It is a good idea for you to learn both the generic and brand names of your medicines and to write them down for future use.

Clofazimine (kloe-FA-zi-meen) belongs to the family of medicines called anti-infectives. Anti-infectives are used in the treatment of infections caused by bacteria. They work by killing bacteria or preventing their growth. This medicine will not work for colds, flu, or other virus infections.

Clofazimine is taken by mouth to treat leprosy (Hansen's disease). It is sometimes given with other medicines for leprosy. When this medicine is used to treat "flare-ups" of leprosy, it may be given with a cortisone-like medicine. Clofazimine may also be used for other problems as determined by your doctor.

This medicine is available only with your doctor's prescription.

Remember:

• **This medicine has been prescribed for your present infection only.** Another infection later on may require a different medicine. Also, even though other people may have the same symptoms as you, they may have a different kind of infection. Your medicine may not work for them and may even cause them harm. Therefore, **your medicine must not be given to other people or used for other infections** unless you are otherwise directed by your doctor.

• **Keep all medicines out of the reach of children.**

• In order for this medicine to work, it must be used as directed.

• **It is very important that you read and understand the following information.** If any of the information causes you special concern, do not decide against using this medicine without first checking with your doctor.

• Before you begin using any new medicine (prescription or nonprescription) or if you develop any new medical problem while you are using this medicine, check with your doctor, nurse, or pharmacist.

• **If you have any questions** about the following information or if you want more information about this medicine or your medical problem, **ask your doctor, nurse, or pharmacist.**

Before Using This Medicine

In order to decide on the best treatment for your medical problem, your doctor should be told:

—if you have ever had any unusual or allergic reaction to clofazimine.

—if you are on a low-salt, low-sugar, or any other special diet, or if you are allergic to any substance, such as foods, sulfites or other preservatives, or dyes. Most medicines contain more than their active ingredient. Your doctor, nurse, or pharmacist can help you avoid products that may cause a problem.

—if you are **pregnant** or if you may become pregnant. Studies have not been done in humans. Although the skin of babies born to mothers who took clofazimine during pregnancy was deeply discolored, this medicine has not been shown to cause birth defects or other problems in humans. Studies in rabbits and rats, given doses of up to 25 times the usual human dose, have not shown that clofazimine causes birth defects. However, studies in mice have shown that clofazimine may cause slow bone formation of the skull and a decrease in successful pregnancies.

—if you are **breast-feeding**. Clofazimine passes into the breast milk. Use is not recommended in nursing mothers.

—if you have any of the following medical problems:
  Liver disease
  Stomach or intestinal problems, history of

Proper Use of This Medicine

Clofazimine should be taken with meals or milk.

To help clear up your leprosy completely, **it is very important that you keep taking clofazimine for the full time of treatment,** even if you begin to feel better after a few months. You may have to take it every day for as long as 2 years to life. If you stop taking this medicine too soon, your symptoms may return.

This medicine works best when there is a constant amount in the blood. **To help keep the amount constant, do not miss any doses. Also, it is best to take each dose at the same time every day.** If you need help in planning the best time to take your medicine, check with your doctor, nurse, or pharmacist.

If you do miss a dose of this medicine, take it as soon as possible. However, if it is almost time for your next dose, skip the missed dose and go back to your regular dosing schedule. Do not double doses.

How to store this medicine:

• **Keep out of the reach of children.**

• Store away from heat and direct light.

• Do not store in the bathroom, near the kitchen sink, or in other damp places. Heat or moisture may cause the medicine to break down.

• Do not keep outdated medicine or medicine no longer needed. Be sure that any discarded medicine is out of the reach of children.

Precautions While Using This Medicine

If your symptoms do not improve within 1 to 3 months, or if they become worse, check with your doctor. It may take up to 6 months before the full benefit of this medicine is seen.

Diabetics—This medicine may cause false test results with some blood sugar tests. Check with your doctor before changing your diet or the dosage of your diabetes medicine.

Clofazimine may cause pink or red to brownish-black discoloration of the skin within a few weeks after you start taking it. Because of the skin discoloration, some patients may become depressed. The discoloration will go away when you stop taking this medicine. However, it may take several months or years for the skin to clear up completely. **If skin discoloration causes you to feel very depressed or to have thoughts of suicide, check with your doctor immediately.**

This medicine may also cause some loss of vision, or it may cause some people to become dizzy, drowsy, or less alert than they are normally. **Make sure you know how you react to this medicine before you drive, use machines, or do other jobs that require you to be alert or to see clearly.** If these reactions are especially bothersome, check with your doctor.

Some people who take clofazimine may become more sensitive to sunlight than they are normally. **When you first begin taking this medicine, avoid too much sun and do not use a sunlamp until you see how you react to the sun,** especially if you tend to burn easily. **If you have a severe reaction, check with your doctor.**

Clofazimine may also cause dry, rough, or scaly skin. A skin cream, lotion, or oil may help to treat this problem.

Side Effects of This Medicine

Along with its needed effects, a medicine may cause some unwanted effects. Although not all of these side effects may occur, if they do occur they may need medical attention.

Check with your doctor immediately if any of the following side effects occur:

More common
   Colicky or burning abdominal or stomach pain
   Diarrhea
   Nausea or vomiting
   Pink or red to brownish-black discoloration of skin

Rare
   Any loss of vision
   Bloody or black tarry stools
   Mental depression
   Yellow eyes or skin

Other side effects may occur that usually do not require medical attention. These side effects may go away during treatment as your body adjusts to the medicine. However, check with your doctor if any of the following side effects continue or are bothersome:

More common
   Dry, rough, or scaly skin

Less common or rare
   Changes in taste
   Dizziness
   Drowsiness
   Dryness, burning, itching, or irritation of the eyes
   Increased sensitivity of skin to sunlight
   Loss of appetite
   Skin rash and itching

This medicine commonly causes discoloration of the feces, lining of the eyelids, sputum, sweat, tears, and urine. This side effect does not require medical attention.

For elderly patients: Many medicines have not been tested in older people. Therefore, it is not known whether the medicine acts the same way it does in younger adults. Check with your doctor or pharmacist if you notice any unusual effects while taking this medicine or if you think it is not working as it should.

Other side effects not listed above may also occur in some patients. If you notice any other effects, check with your doctor.

December 1987

CLOFIBRATE (Systemic)

Some commonly used brand names are Atromid-S, Claripex*, and Novofibrate*.

Generic name product may also be available in the U.S.

*Not available in the U.S.

To the Reader: If you do not recognize the names of medical conditions or medicines referred to in this information, check with your doctor, nurse, or pharmacist. Definitions for selected medical terms may be found in the Glossary. Brand names for the generic drug names listed can be found in the Index. In addition, selected brand names commonly associated with the generic name have been included in the text to help you recognize medicine you may be taking. The fact that a brand name product is not mentioned does not mean the information does not apply. It is a good idea for you to learn both the generic and brand names of your medicines and to write them down for future use.

Clofibrate (kloe-FYE-brate) is used to lower cholesterol and triglyceride (fat-like substances) levels in the blood. This may help prevent medical problems caused by such substances clogging the blood vessels.

Clofibrate may also be used for other conditions as determined by your doctor.

Clofibrate is available only with your doctor's prescription.

Remember:

• **This medicine has been prescribed for your current medical problem only.** It must not be given to other people or used for other problems unless you are directed to do so by your doctor.

• **Keep all medicines out of the reach of children.**

• In order for this medicine to work, it must be used as directed.

• **It is very important that you read and understand the following information.** If any of the information causes you special concern, do not decide against using this medicine without first checking with your doctor.

• Before you begin using any new medicine (prescription or nonprescription) or if you develop any new medical problem while you are using this medicine, check with your doctor, nurse, or pharmacist.

• **If you have any questions** about the following information or if you want more information about this medicine or your medical problem, **ask your doctor, nurse, or pharmacist.**

Before Using This Medicine

In addition to its helpful effects in treating your medical problem, this medicine may have some harmful effects.

You may have read or heard about a study called the World Health Organization (WHO) Study. This study compared the effects in patients who used clofibrate with effects in those who used a placebo (sugar pill). The results of this study suggested that clofibrate might increase the patient's risk of cancer, liver disease, and

pancreatitis (inflammation of the pancreas), although it might also decrease the risk of heart attack. It may also increase the risk of gallstones and problems from gallbladder surgery. Other studies have not found all of these effects. Be sure you have discussed this with your doctor before taking this medicine.

Importance of diet—Before prescribing medicine for your condition, your doctor will probably try to control your condition by prescribing a personal diet for you. Such a diet may be low in fats, sugars, and/or cholesterol. Many people are able to control their condition by carefully following their doctors' orders for proper diet and exercise. **Medicine is prescribed only when additional help is needed** and is effective only when a schedule of diet and exercise is properly followed.

Also, this medicine is less effective if you are greatly overweight. It may be very important for you to go on a reducing diet. However, check with your doctor before going on any diet.

In order to decide on the best treatment for your medical problem, your doctor should be told:

—if you have ever had any unusual or allergic reaction to clofibrate.

—if you are on a low-salt, low-sugar, or any other special diet, or if you are allergic to any substance, such as foods, sulfites or other preservatives, or dyes. Most medicines contain more than their active ingredient. Your doctor, nurse, or pharmacist can help you avoid products that may cause a problem.

—if you are **pregnant** or if you may become pregnant. Use of clofibrate is not recommended during pregnancy. Although studies have not been done in humans, studies in rabbits have shown that the fetus may not be able to break down and get rid of this medicine as well as the mother. Because of this, it is possible that clofibrate may be harmful to your baby if you take it while you are pregnant or for up to several months before you become pregnant. Be sure that you have discussed this with your doctor before taking this medicine.

—if you are **breast-feeding**. It is not known whether clofibrate passes into breast milk. This medicine has not been shown to cause problems in nursing babies.

—if you have any of the following medical problems:
Gallstones
Heart disease
Kidney disease
Liver disease
Stomach or intestinal ulcer
Underactive thyroid

—if you are taking **any** other prescription or nonprescription (OTC) medicine, especially anticoagulants (blood thinners).

Proper Use of This Medicine

Use this medicine only as directed by your doctor. Do not use more or less of it, and do not use it more often or for a longer period of time than your doctor ordered.

Follow carefully the special diet your doctor gave you. This is the most important part of controlling your condition, and is necessary if the medicine is to work properly.

Stomach upset may occur but usually lessens after a few doses. Take this medicine with food or immediately after meals to lessen possible stomach upset.

If you miss a dose of this medicine, take it as soon as possible. However, if it is almost time for your next dose, skip the missed dose and go back to your regular dosing schedule. Do not double doses.

How to store this medicine:

- **Keep out of the reach of children.**
- Store away from heat and direct light.
- Do not store in the bathroom, near the kitchen sink, or in other damp places. Heat or moisture may cause the medicine to break down.
- Do not keep outdated medicine or medicine no longer needed. Be sure that any discarded medicine is out of the reach of children.

Precautions While Using This Medicine

It is very important that your doctor check your progress at regular visits. This will allow your doctor to see if the medicine is working properly to lower your cholesterol and triglyceride levels and to decide if you should continue to take it.

Do not stop taking this medicine without first checking with your doctor. When you stop taking this medicine, your blood fat levels may increase again. Your doctor may want you to follow a special diet to help prevent that.

Side Effects of This Medicine

Along with its needed effects, a medicine may cause some unwanted effects. Although not all of these side effects may occur, if they do occur they may need medical attention.

Check with your doctor immediately if you think you have taken an overdose or if any of the following side effects occur:

Rare

    Chest pain
    Irregular heartbeat
    Shortness of breath
    Stomach pain (severe) with nausea and vomiting

Check with your doctor as soon as possible if any of the following side effects occur:

Rare

    Blood in urine
    Decrease in urination
    Fever and chills or sore throat
    Swelling of feet or lower legs

Other side effects may occur that usually do not require medical attention. These side effects may go away during treatment as your body adjusts to the medicine. However, check with your doctor if any of the following side effects continue or are bothersome:

More common

    Diarrhea
    Nausea

Less common or rare

    Aching muscles
    Decreased sexual ability
    Headache
    Increased appetite or weight gain (slight)
    Muscle cramping
    Painful or difficult urination
    Sores in the mouth and on the lips
    Stomach pain, gas, or heartburn
    Tiredness
    Vomiting
    Weakness

For elderly patients: Many medicines have not been tested in older people. Therefore, it is not known whether the medicine acts the same way it does in younger adults. Check with your doctor or pharmacist if you notice any unusual effects while taking this medicine or if you think it is not working as it should.

Other side effects not listed above may also occur in some patients. If you notice any other effects, check with your doctor.

December 1987

CLOMIPHENE (Systemic)

Some commonly used brand names are Clomid and Serophene.

To the Reader: If you do not recognize the names of medical conditions or medicines referred to in this information, check with your doctor, nurse, or pharmacist. Definitions for selected medical terms may be found in the Glossary. Brand names for the generic drug names listed can be found in the Index. In addition, selected brand names commonly associated with the generic name have been included in the text to help you recognize medicine you may be taking. The fact that a brand name product is not mentioned does not mean the information does not apply. It is a good idea for you to learn both the generic and brand names of your medicines and to write them down for future use.

Clomiphene (KLOE-mi-feen) is used as a fertility medicine in some women who are unable to become pregnant.

Clomiphene probably changes the hormone balance of the body. In women, this causes ovulation to occur and prepares the body for pregnancy.

Clomiphene may also be used for other conditions in both females and males as determined by your doctor.

The following information is meant only for female patients taking clomiphene. Check with your doctor if you are a male and have any questions about the use of clomiphene.

Clomiphene is available only with your doctor's prescription.

Remember:

• **This medicine has been prescribed for your current medical problem only.** It must not be given to other people or used for other problems unless you are directed to do so by your doctor.

• **Keep all medicines out of the reach of children.**

• In order for this medicine to work, it must be used as directed.

• **It is very important that you read and understand the following information.** If any of the information causes you special concern, do not decide against using this medicine without first checking with your doctor.

• Before you begin using any new medicine (prescription or nonprescription) or if you develop any new medical problem while you are using this medicine, check with your doctor, nurse, or pharmacist.

• **If you have any questions** about the following information or if you want more information about this medicine or your medical problem, **ask your doctor, nurse, or pharmacist.**

Before Using This Medicine

If you become pregnant as a result of using this medicine, there is a chance of a multiple birth (for example, twins, triplets) occurring. If you have any questions about this, check with your doctor.

In order to decide on the best treatment for your medical problem, your doctor should be told:

—if you have ever had any unusual or allergic reaction to clomiphene.

—if you are on a low-salt, low-sugar, or any other special diet, or if you are allergic to any substance, such as foods, sulfites or other preservatives, or dyes. Most medicines contain more than their active ingredient. Your doctor, nurse, or pharmacist can help you avoid products that may cause a problem.

—if you have any of the following medical problems:
  Cyst on ovary
  Fibroid tumors of the womb
  Inflamed veins due to blood clots
  Liver disease
  Mental depression
  Unusual vaginal bleeding

Proper Use of This Medicine

Take this medicine only as directed by your doctor. If you are to begin on Day 5, count the first day of your menstrual period as Day 1. Beginning on Day 5, take the correct dose every day for as many days as your doctor ordered. To help you to remember to take your dose of medicine, take it at the same time every day.

If you miss a dose of this medicine, take it as soon as possible. If you do not remember until it is time for the next dose, take both doses together, then go back to your regular dosing schedule. If you miss more than one dose, check with your doctor.

How to store this medicine:

• **Keep out of the reach of children.**

• Store away from heat and direct light.

• Do not store in the bathroom, near the kitchen sink, or in other damp places. Heat or moisture may cause the medicine to break down.

• Do not keep outdated medicine or medicine no longer needed. Be sure that any discarded medicine is out of the reach of children.

Precautions While Using This Medicine

It is very important that your doctor check your progress at regular visits to make sure this medicine is working and to check for unwanted effects.

If your doctor has asked you to record your temperature daily, make sure that you do this every day as soon as you awaken and before getting up. This will help you know if you have begun to ovulate. It is important that intercourse take place at the correct time to give you the best chance of becoming pregnant. **Follow your doctor's instructions carefully.**

There is a chance that clomiphene may cause birth defects if it is taken after you become pregnant. **Stop taking this medicine and tell your doctor immediately if you think you have become pregnant** while still taking clomiphene.

This medicine may cause vision problems, dizziness, or lightheadedness. **Make sure you know how you react to this medicine before you drive, use machines, or do other jobs that require you to see well or be clearheaded.**

Side Effects of This Medicine

Along with its needed effects, a medicine may cause some unwanted effects. Although not all of these side effects may occur, if they do occur they may need medical attention.

When this medicine is used for short periods of time at low doses, side effects usually are rare. **However, check with your doctor immediately** if any of the following side effects occur:

More common
    Bloating
    Blurred vision
    Stomach or pelvic pain
Rare
    Shortness of breath (sudden)

Check with your doctor as soon as possible if any of the following side effects occur:

Rare
    Decreased or double vision
    Seeing flashes of light
    Sensitivity of eyes to light
    Yellow eyes and skin

Other side effects may occur that usually do not require medical attention. These side effects may go away during treatment as your body adjusts to the medicine. However, check with your doctor if any of the following side effects continue or are bothersome:

More common
    Hot flashes
Less common or rare
    Breast discomfort
    Dizziness or lightheadedness
    Headache
    Heavy menstrual periods or bleeding between periods
    Mental depression
    Nausea or vomiting
    Nervousness
    Restlessness or trouble in sleeping
    Tiredness

Other side effects not listed above may also occur in some patients. If you notice any other effects, check with your doctor.

December 1987

Additional Information

For men taking this medicine for infertility:
• Clomiphene is also used to treat infertility in men who are not producing enough sperm.

• In order to decide on the best treatment for your medical problem, your doctor should be told:

    —if you have ever had any unusual or allergic reaction to clomiphene.

    —if you have either of the following medical problems:

        Liver disease
        Mental depression

• If you miss a dose of this medicine, take it as soon as possible. If you do not remember until it is time for the next dose, take both doses together, then go back to your regular dosing schedule. If you miss more than one dose, check with your doctor.

• It is important that your doctor check your progress at regular visits to find out if clomiphene is working and to check for unwanted effects.

• This medicine may cause vision problems, dizziness, or lightheadedness. **Make sure you know how you react to this medicine before you drive, use machines, or do other jobs that require you to see well or be clearheaded.**

• Along with its needed effects, a medicine may cause some unwanted effects. Although not all of these side effects may occur, if they do occur they may need medical attention. When this medicine is used for short periods of time at low doses, side effects usually are rare. However, check with your doctor if any of the following side effects occur:

More common
    Blurred vision

Rare
    Decreased or double vision
    Seeing flashes of light
    Sensitivity of eyes to light
    Yellow eyes and skin

• Other side effects may occur that usually do not require medical attention. These side effects may go away during treatment as your body adjusts to the medicine. However, check with your doctor if any of the following side effects continue or are bothersome:

Less common or rare
    Breast enlargement
    Dizziness or lightheadedness
    Headache
    Mental depression, nervousness, restlessness, trouble in sleeping, or tiredness
    Nausea or vomiting

CLONIDINE (Systemic)

Some commonly used brand names are Catapres, Catapres-TTS, and Dixarit*.

Generic name product may also be available in the U.S.

*Not available in the U.S.

To the Reader: If you do not recognize the names of medical conditions or medicines referred to in this information, check with your doctor, nurse, or pharmacist. Definitions for selected medical terms may be found in the Glossary. Brand names for the generic drug names listed can be found in the Index. In addition, selected brand names commonly associated with the generic name have been included in the text to help you recognize medicine you may be taking. The fact that a brand name product is not mentioned does not mean the information does not apply. It is a good idea for you to learn both the generic and brand names of your medicines and to write them down for future use.

Clonidine (KLOE-ni-deen) belongs to the general class of medicines called antihypertensives. It is used to treat high blood pressure. High blood pressure adds to the workload of the heart and arteries. If it continues for a long time, the heart and arteries may not function properly. This can damage the blood vessels of the brain, heart, and kidneys, resulting in a stroke, heart failure, or kidney failure. Hypertension may also increase the risk of heart attacks. These problems may be less likely to occur if blood pressure is controlled.

Clonidine works by controlling nerve impulses along certain nerve pathways. As a result, it relaxes blood vessels so that blood passes through them more easily. This helps to lower blood pressure.

Clonidine may also be used for other conditions as determined by your doctor.

Clonidine is available only with your doctor's prescription.

Remember:

• **This medicine has been prescribed for your current medical problem only.** It must not be given to other people or used for other problems unless you are directed to do so by your doctor.

• **Keep all medicines out of the reach of children.**

• In order for this medicine to work, it must be used as directed.

• **It is very important that you read and understand the following information.** If any of the information causes you special concern, do not decide against using this medicine without first checking with your doctor.

• Before you begin using any new medicine (prescription or nonprescription) or if you develop any new medical problem while you are using this medicine, check with your doctor, nurse, or pharmacist.

• **If you have any questions** about the following information or if you want more information about this medicine or your medical problem, **ask your doctor, nurse, or pharmacist.**

Before Using This Medicine

In order to decide on the best treatment for your medical problem, your doctor should be told:

—if you have ever had any unusual or allergic reaction to clonidine.

—if you are on a low-salt, low-sugar, or any other special diet, or if you are allergic to any substance, such as food, sulfites or other preservatives, or dyes. Most medicines contain more than their active ingredient. Your doctor, nurse, or pharmacist can help you avoid products that may cause a problem.

—if you are **pregnant** or if you may become pregnant. Studies have not been done in humans. Although clonidine has not been shown to cause birth defects in animals, it has been shown to cause toxic or harmful effects in the animal fetus, even at doses of only one-third the maximum human dose.

—if you are **breast-feeding.** Although clonidine passes into breast milk, it has not been shown to cause problems in nursing babies.

—if you have any of the following medical problems:
Heart or blood vessel disease
Irritated or abraded skin—with transdermal system only
Kidney disease
Mental depression (history of)
Raynaud's syndrome
Systemic lupus erythematosus (SLE)—with transdermal (skin patch) system only

—if you are taking **any** other prescription or nonprescription (OTC) medicine, especially:
Beta-blockers (acebutolol, atenolol, labetalol, metoprolol, nadolol, oxprenolol, pindolol, propranolol, sotalol, timolol)
Tricyclic antidepressants (amitriptyline, amoxapine, clomipramine, desipramine, doxepin, imipramine, nortriptyline, protriptyline, trimipramine)

Proper Use of This Medicine

Importance of diet—When prescribing medicine for your condition, your doctor may also prescribe a personal diet for you. Such a diet may be low in sodium (salt). Most people eat much more sodium than they need and too much sodium in the diet may increase blood pressure. Some foods that contain large amounts of sodium are canned soup, pickles, ketchup, green and ripe olives, relish, frankfurters, soy sauce, and carbonated beverages. Your doctor may want you to limit the amounts of these and other high-sodium foods in your diet. High blood pressure medicine is usually more effective when such a diet is properly followed.

Also, it may be very important for you to go on a reducing diet. However, check with your doctor before changing your diet.

Many patients who have high blood pressure will not notice any signs of the problem. In fact, many may feel normal. It is very important that you **take your medicine exactly as directed** and that you keep your appointments with your doctor even if you feel well.

Remember that this medicine will not cure your high blood pressure but it does help control it. Therefore, you must continue to use it as directed if you expect to lower your blood pressure and keep it down. **You may have to take high blood pressure medicine for the rest of your life.** If high blood pressure is not treated, it can cause serious problems such as heart failure, blood vessel disease, stroke, or kidney disease.

For patients using the transdermal (stick-on patch) system:

- **Use this medicine exactly as directed by your doctor.** It will work only if applied correctly. **This medicine usually comes with patient instructions. Read them carefully before using.**

- Do not try to trim or cut the adhesive patch to adjust the dosage. Check with your doctor if you think the medicine is not working as it should.

- Apply the patch to a clean, dry skin area on your upper arm or chest with little or no hair and free of scars, cuts, or irritation.

- The system should stay in place even during showering, bathing, or swimming. If the patch becomes loose, cover it with the extra adhesive overlay. Apply a new patch if the first one becomes too loose or falls off.

- Each dose is best applied to a different area of skin to prevent skin problems or other irritation.

In order to help remember to use your medicine, try to get into the habit of using it at regular times. If you are taking the tablets, take them at the same time each day. If you are using the transdermal system, try to change it at the same time of day each week.

If you do miss a dose of this medicine, take it or use it as soon as possible. Then go back to your regular dosing schedule. **If you miss two or more doses of the tablets in a row or if you miss changing the transdermal patch for three or more days, check with your doctor right away.** If your body goes without this medicine for too long, your blood pressure may go up to a dangerously high level and some unpleasant effects may occur.

How to store this medicine:

- **Keep out of the reach of children.**

- Store away from heat and direct light.

- Do not store in the bathroom, near the kitchen sink, or in other damp places. Heat or moisture may cause the medicine to break down.

- Do not keep outdated medicine or medicine no longer needed. Be sure that any discarded medicine is out of the reach of children.

Precautions While Using This Medicine

It is important that your doctor check your progress at regular visits to make sure that this medicine is working properly.

Check with your doctor before you stop using this medicine. Your doctor may want you to reduce gradually the amount you are using before stopping completely.

Make sure that you have enough clonidine on hand to last through weekends, holidays, or vacations. You should not miss any doses. You may want to ask your doctor for another written prescription for clonidine to carry in your wallet or purse. You can then have it filled if you run out of medicine when you are away from home.

Do not take other medicines unless they have been discussed with your doctor. This especially includes over-the-counter (nonprescription) medicines for appetite control, asthma, colds, cough, hay fever, or sinus problems, since they may tend to increase your blood pressure.

Clonidine will add to the effects of alcohol and other CNS depressants (medicines that slow down the nervous system, possibly causing drowsiness). Some examples of CNS depressants are antihistamines or medicine for hay fever, other allergies, or colds; sedatives, tranquilizers, or sleeping medicine; prescription pain medicine or narcotics; barbiturates; medicine for seizures; muscle relaxants; or anesthetics, including some dental anesthetics. **Check with your doctor before taking any of the above while you are using this medicine.**

Clonidine may cause some people to become drowsy or less alert than they are normally. This is more likely to happen when you begin to take it or when you increase the amount of medicine you are taking. **Make sure you know how you react to this medicine before you drive, use machines, or do other jobs that require you to be alert.**

Before having any kind of surgery (including dental surgery) or emergency treatment, **tell the physician or dentist in charge that you are using this medicine.**

Dizziness, lightheadedness, or fainting may occur, especially when you get up from a lying or sitting position. Getting up slowly may help but if the problem continues or gets worse, check with your doctor.

The dizziness, lightheadedness, or fainting is also more likely to occur if you drink alcohol, stand for long periods of time, exercise, or if the weather is hot. While you are taking clonidine, be careful in the amount of alcohol you drink. Also, use extra care during exercise or hot weather or if you must stand for long periods of time.

Clonidine may cause dryness of the mouth. For temporary relief, use sugarless candy or gum, melt bits of ice in your mouth, or use a saliva substitute. However, if dry mouth continues for more than 2 weeks, check with your physician or dentist. Continuing dryness of the mouth may increase the chance of dental disease, including tooth decay, gum disease, and fungal infections.

Side Effects of This Medicine

Along with its needed effects, a medicine may cause some unwanted effects. Although not all of these side effects may occur, if they do occur they may need medical attention.

Check with your doctor immediately if any of the following side effects occur:

Signs of overdose
> Difficulty in breathing
> Dizziness (extreme) or faintness
> Slow heartbeat
> Unusual tiredness or weakness

Check with your doctor as soon as possible if any of the following side effects occur:

More common—with transdermal system only
> Itching or redness of skin

Less common
> Darkening of skin—with transdermal system only
> Mental depression
> Swelling of feet and lower legs

Rare
> Paleness or cold feeling in fingertips and toes
> Vivid dreams or nightmares

Other side effects may occur that usually do not require medical attention. These side effects may go away during treatment as your body adjusts to the medicine. However, check with your doctor if any of the following side effects continue or are bothersome:

More common
> Dizziness
> Drowsiness
> Dry mouth

Less common
> Constipation
> Decreased sexual ability
> Dizziness, lightheadedness, or fainting, especially when getting up from a lying or sitting position
> Dry, itching, or burning eyes
> Loss of appetite
> Nausea or vomiting
> Painful salivary glands
> Trouble in sleeping

After you have been using this medicine for a while, it may cause unpleasant or even harmful effects if you stop taking it too suddenly. After you stop taking this medicine, **check with your doctor immediately** if any of the following occur:

> Anxiety or tenseness
> Chest pain
> Fast or irregular heartbeat
> Headache
> Increased salivation
> Nausea
> Nervousness
> Restlessness
> Shaking or trembling of hands and fingers
> Stomach cramps
> Sweating
> Trouble in sleeping
> Vomiting

For elderly patients: Dizziness or faintness may be more likely to occur in the elderly, who are more sensitive to the effects of clonidine.

Other side effects not listed above may also occur in some patients. If you notice any other effects, check with your doctor.

_____

December 1987

CLONIDINE AND CHLORTHALIDONE
(Systemic)

A commonly used brand name is Combipres.

To the Reader: If you do not recognize the names of medical conditions or medicines referred to in this information, check with your doctor, nurse, or pharmacist. Definitions for selected medical terms may be found in the Glossary. Brand names for the generic drug names listed can be found in the Index. In addition, selected brand names commonly associated with the generic name have been included in the text to help you recognize medicine you may be taking. The fact that a brand name product is not mentioned does not mean the information does not apply. It is a good idea for you to learn both the generic and brand names of your medicines and to write them down for future use.

Clonidine (KLOE-ni-deen) and chlorthalidone (klor-THAL-i-done) combinations are used in the treatment of high blood pressure. High blood pressure adds to the workload of the heart and arteries. If it continues for a long time, the heart and arteries may not function properly. This can damage the blood vessels of the brain, heart, and kidneys resulting in a stroke, heart failure, or kidney failure. Hypertension may also increase the risk of heart attacks. These problems may be less likely to occur if blood pressure is controlled.

Clonidine works by controlling nerve impulses along certain body nerve pathways. As a result, it relaxes blood vessels so that blood passes through them more easily. The chlorthalidone in this combination helps reduce the amount of water in the body by increasing the flow of urine.

Clonidine and chlorthalidone combination is available only with your doctor's prescription.

Remember:

• **This medicine has been prescribed for your current medical problem only.** It must not be given to other people or used for other problems unless you are directed to do so by your doctor.

• **Keep all medicines out of the reach of children.**

• In order for this medicine to work, it must be used as directed.

• **It is very important that you read and understand the following information.** If any of the information causes you special concern, do not decide against using this medicine without first checking with your doctor.

• Before you begin using any new medicine (prescription or nonprescription) or if you develop any new medical problem while you are using this medicine, check with your doctor, nurse, or pharmacist.

• **If you have any questions** about the following information or if you want more information about this medicine or your medical problem, **ask your doctor, nurse, or pharmacist.**

Before Using This Medicine

In order to decide on the best treatment for your medical problem, your doctor should be told:

—if you have ever had any unusual or allergic reaction to clonidine, sulfonamides (sulfa drugs), or other thiazide diuretics (water pills).

—if you are on a low-salt, low-sugar, or any other special diet, or if you are allergic to any substance, such as foods, sulfites or other preservatives, or dyes. Most medicines contain more than their active ingredient. Your doctor, nurse, or pharmacist can help you avoid products that may cause a problem.

—if you are **pregnant** or if you may become pregnant. Studies with clonidine have not been done in humans. Although clonidine has not been shown to cause birth defects in animals, it has been shown to cause toxic or harmful effects in the fetus in animals even at doses of only one-third the maximum human dose. When chlorthalidone is used during pregnancy, it may cause side effects including jaundice, blood problems, and low potassium in the newborn infant.

—if you are **breast-feeding.** Although both clonidine and chlorthalidone pass into breast milk, they have not been shown to cause problems in nursing babies.

—if you have any of the following medical problems:
Diabetes mellitus (sugar diabetes)
Gout
Heart or blood vessel disease
Kidney disease
Liver disease
Lupus erythematosus (history of)
Mental depression (history of)
Pancreatitis (inflammation of the pancreas)
Problems with veins

—if you are now taking **any** prescription or nonprescription (OTC) medicine, especially:
Adrenocorticoids (cortisone-like medicines)
Beta-blockers (acebutolol, atenolol, labetalol, metoprolol, nadolol, oxprenolol, pindolol, propranolol, sotalol, timolol)
Digitalis glycosides (heart medicine)
Lithium (e.g., Lithane)
Methenamine (e.g., Mandelamine)
Tricyclic antidepressants (amitriptyline, amoxapine, clomipramine, desipramine, doxepin, imipramine, nortriptyline, protriptyline, trimipramine)

Proper Use of This Medicine

This medicine may cause you to have an unusual feeling of tiredness when you begin to take it. You may also notice an increase in the amount of urine or in your frequency of urination. After taking the medicine for a while, these effects should lessen. In general, in order to keep the increase in urine from affecting your sleep:

• If you are to take a single dose a day, take it in the morning after breakfast.

• If you are to take more than one dose a day, take the last dose no later than 6 p.m., unless otherwise directed by your doctor.

However, it is best to plan your dose or doses according to a schedule that will least affect your personal activities and sleep. Ask your doctor, nurse, or pharmacist to help you plan the best time to take this medicine.

Importance of diet—When prescribing medicine for your condition, your doctor may also prescribe a personal diet for you. Such a diet may be low in sodium (salt).

Most people eat much more sodium than they need and too much sodium in the diet may increase blood pressure. Some foods that contain large amounts of sodium are canned soup, pickles, ketchup, green and ripe olives, relish, frankfurters, soy sauce, and carbonated beverages. Your doctor may want you to limit the amounts of these and other high-sodium foods in your diet. High blood pressure medicine is usually more effective when such a diet is properly followed.

Also, it may be very important for you to go on a reducing diet. However, check with your doctor before changing your diet.

Many patients who have high blood pressure will not notice any signs of the problem. In fact, many may feel normal. It is very important that you **take your medicine exactly as directed** and that you keep your appointments with your doctor even if you feel well.

Remember that this medicine will not cure your high blood pressure but it does help control it. Therefore, you must continue to take it as directed if you expect to lower your blood pressure and keep it down. **You may have to take high blood pressure medicine for the rest of your life.** If high blood pressure is not treated, it can cause serious problems such as heart failure, blood vessel disease, stroke, or kidney disease.

In order to help remember to take your medicine, try to get into the habit of taking it at the same time each day.

If you do miss a dose of this medicine, take it as soon as possible. Then go back to your regular dosing schedule. **If you miss two or more doses in a row, check with your doctor right away.** If your body goes without this medicine for too long, your blood pressure may go up to a dangerously high level.

How to store this medicine:

• **Keep out of the reach of children.**

• Store away from heat and direct light.

• Do not store in the bathroom, near the kitchen sink, or in other damp places. Heat or moisture may cause the medicine to break down.

• Do not keep outdated medicine or medicine no longer needed. Be sure that any discarded medicine is out of the reach of children.

Precautions While Using This Medicine

It is important that your doctor check your progress at regular visits to make sure that this medicine is working properly.

Check with your doctor before you stop taking this medicine. Your doctor may want you to reduce gradually the amount you are taking before stopping completely.

Make sure that you have enough medicine on hand to last through weekends, holidays, or vacations. You should not miss taking any doses. You may want to ask your doctor for another written prescription to carry in your wallet or purse. You can then have it filled if you run out of medicine when you are away from home.

Before having any kind of surgery (including dental surgery) or emergency treatment, **make sure the physician or dentist in charge knows that you are taking this medicine.**

Do not take other medicines unless they have been discussed with your doctor. This especially includes over-the-counter (nonprescription) medicines for appetite control, asthma, colds, cough, hay fever, or sinus problems, since they may tend to increase your blood pressure.

This medicine will add to the effects of alcohol and other CNS depressants (medicines that slow down the nervous system, possibly causing drowsiness). Some examples of CNS depressants are antihistamines or medicine for hay fever, other allergies, or colds; sedatives, tranquilizers, or sleeping medicine; prescription pain medicine or narcotics; barbiturates; medicine for seizures; muscle relaxants; or anesthetics, including some dental anesthetics. **Check with your doctor before taking any of the above while you are using this medicine.**

This medicine may cause some people to become drowsy or less alert than they are normally. This is more likely to happen when you begin to take it or when you increase the amount of medicine you are taking. **Make sure you know how you react to this medicine before you drive, use machines, or do other jobs that require you to be alert.**

Dizziness, lightheadedness, or fainting may occur, especially when you get up from a lying or sitting position. Getting up slowly may help but if the problem continues or gets worse, check with your doctor.

The dizziness, lightheadedness, or fainting is also more likely to occur if you drink alcohol, stand for long periods of time, exercise, or if the weather is hot. Drinking alcoholic beverages may also make the drowsiness worse. While you are taking this medicine, be careful in the amount of alcohol you drink. Also, use extra care during exercise or hot weather or if you must stand for long periods of time.

This medicine may cause a loss of potassium from your body.

• To help prevent this, your doctor may want you to:
  —eat or drink foods that have a high potassium content (for example, orange or other citrus fruit juices), or
  —take a potassium supplement, or
  —take another medicine to help prevent the loss of the potassium in the first place.

• It is very important to follow these directions. Also, it is important not to change your diet on your own. This is more important if you are already on a special diet (as for diabetes), or if you are taking a potassium supplement or a medicine to reduce potassium loss. Extra potassium may not be necessary and, in some cases, too much potassium could be harmful.

Check with your doctor if you become sick and have severe or continuing vomiting or diarrhea. These problems may cause you to lose additional water and potassium.

Diabetics—Thiazide diuretics like chlorthalidone may raise blood sugar levels. While you are using this medicine, be especially careful in testing for sugar in your urine.

A few people who take this medicine may become more sensitive to sunlight than they are normally. When you first begin taking this medicine, avoid too much sun and do not use a sunlamp until you see how you react to the sun, especially if you tend to burn easily. If you have a severe reaction, check with your doctor.

This medicine may cause dryness of the mouth. For temporary relief, use sugarless candy or gum, melt bits of ice in your mouth, or use a saliva substitute. However, if dry mouth continues for more than 2 weeks, check with your physician or dentist. Continuing dryness of the mouth may increase the chance of dental disease, including tooth decay, gum disease, and fungal infections.

Side Effects of This Medicine

Along with its needed effects, a medicine may cause some unwanted effects. Although not all of these side effects may occur, if they do occur they may need medical attention.

Check with your doctor immediately if any of the following side effects occur:

Signs of overdose
　Difficulty in breathing
　Dizziness (extreme) or faintness
　Slow heartbeat
　Unusual tiredness or weakness

Check with your doctor as soon as possible if any of the following side effects occur, especially since some of them may mean that your body is losing too much potassium:

Signs of too much potassium loss
　Dryness of mouth
　Increased thirst
　Irregular heartbeats
　Mood or mental changes
　Muscle cramps or pain
　Nausea or vomiting
　Weak pulse

Rare
　Joint, flank, or stomach pain
　Paleness or cold feeling in fingertips and toes
　Skin rash or hives
　Sore throat and fever
　Stomach pain (severe) with nausea and vomiting
　Unusual bleeding or bruising
　Vivid dreams or nightmares
　Yellow eyes or skin

Other side effects may occur that usually do not require medical attention. These side effects may go away during treatment as your body adjusts to the medicine. However, check with your doctor if any of the following side effects continue or are bothersome:

More common
　Drowsiness

Less common
　Constipation
　Decreased sexual ability
　Diarrhea
　Dizziness or lightheadedness when getting up from a lying or sitting position
　Dry, itching, or burning eyes
　Increased sensitivity of skin to sunlight
　Loss of appetite
　Painful salivary glands
　Trouble in sleeping
　Upset stomach

After you have been using this medicine for a while, it may cause unpleasant or even harmful effects if you stop taking it too suddenly. After you stop taking this medicine, check with your doctor if any of the following occur:
　Anxiety or tenseness
　Chest pain
　Fast or irregular heartbeat
　Headache
　Increased salivation
　Nausea
　Nervousness
　Restlessness
　Shaking or trembling of hands and fingers
　Stomach cramps
　Sweating
　Trouble in sleeping
　Vomiting

For elderly patients: Dizziness or faintness may be more likely to occur in the elderly, who are more sensitive to the effects of clonidine and chlorthalidone.

Other side effects not listed above may also occur in some patients. If you notice any other effects, check with your doctor.

December 1987

CLOTRIMAZOLE (Oral)
A commonly used brand name is Mycelex.

To the Reader: If you do not recognize the names of medical conditions or medicines referred to in this information, check with your doctor, nurse, or pharmacist. Definitions for selected medical terms may be found in the Glossary. Brand names for the generic drug names listed can be found in the Index. In addition, selected brand names commonly associated with the generic name have been included in the text to help you recognize medicine you may be taking. The fact that a brand name product is not mentioned does not mean the information does not apply. It is a good idea for you to learn both the generic and brand names of your medicines and to write them down for future use.

Clotrimazole (kloe-TRIM-a-zole) belongs to the general family of medicines called antifungals. Antifungals are used to treat infections caused by a fungus. They work by killing the fungus or preventing its growth.

Clotrimazole lozenges are dissolved slowly in the mouth to treat thrush. Thrush, also called white mouth, is a fungal infection of the mouth and throat. This medicine may also be used for other problems as determined by your doctor.

Clotrimazole is available only with your doctor's prescription.

Remember:

• **This medicine has been prescribed for your present infection only.** Another infection later on may require a different medicine. Also, even though other people may have the same symptoms as you, they may have a different kind of infection. Your medicine may not work for them and may even cause them harm. Therefore, **your medicine must not be given to other people or used for other infections** unless you are otherwise directed by your doctor.

• **Keep all medicines out of the reach of children.**

• In order for this medicine to work, it must be used as directed.

• **It is very important that you read and understand the following information.** If any of the information causes you special concern, do not decide against using this medicine without first checking with your doctor.

• Before you begin using any new medicine (prescription or nonprescription) or if you develop any new medical problem while you are using this medicine, check with your doctor, nurse, or pharmacist.

• **If you have any questions** about the following information or if you want more information about this medicine or your medical problem, **ask your doctor, nurse, or pharmacist.**

Before Using This Medicine
In order to decide on the best treatment for your medical problem, your doctor should be told:

—if you have ever had any unusual or allergic reaction to clotrimazole.

—if you are on a low-salt, low-sugar, or any other special diet, or if you are allergic to any substance, such as foods, sulfites or other preservatives, or dyes.

Most medicines contain more than their active ingredient. Your doctor, nurse, or pharmacist can help you avoid products that may cause a problem.

—if you are **pregnant** or if you may become pregnant. Studies have not been done in humans. Studies in mice, rats, and rabbits given very high doses have not shown that clotrimazole causes birth defects. However, studies in rats and mice given high doses have shown that clotrimazole lozenges may cause other harmful effects in the fetus.

—if you are **breast-feeding**. Clotrimazole has not been shown to cause problems in nursing babies. In addition, only small amounts of clotrimazole are absorbed into the mother's body. Therefore, it is unlikely to pass into the breast milk in large amounts or to cause problems in nursing babies.

—if you have a history of liver disease.

Proper Use of This Medicine
Clotrimazole lozenges should be held in the mouth and allowed to dissolve slowly and completely. This may take 15 to 30 minutes. Also, the saliva should be swallowed during this time. **Do not chew or swallow the lozenges whole.**

Do not give clotrimazole lozenges to infants or children under 4 to 5 years of age since they may be too young to use the lozenges safely.

To help clear up your infection completely, **it is very important that you keep using clotrimazole for the full time of treatment** even if your symptoms begin to clear up after a few days. Since fungal infections may be very slow to clear up, you may have to continue using this medicine every day for two weeks or more. If you stop using this medicine too soon, your symptoms may return. **Do not miss any doses.**

If you do miss a dose of this medicine, use it as soon as possible. However, if it is almost time for your next dose, skip the missed dose and go back to your regular dosing schedule.

How to store this medicine:

• **Keep out of the reach of children.**

• Store away from heat and direct light.

• Do not store in the bathroom, near the kitchen sink, or in other damp places. Heat or moisture may cause the medicine to break down.

• Do not keep outdated medicine or medicine no longer needed. Be sure that any discarded medicine is out of the reach of children.

Precautions While Using This Medicine
If your symptoms do not improve within 1 week, or if they become worse, check with your doctor.

Side Effects of This Medicine

Along with its needed effects, a medicine may cause some unwanted effects. The following side effects may go away during treatment as your body adjusts to the medicine. However, check with your doctor if any of these effects continue or are bothersome:

More common—when swallowed
    Abdominal or stomach cramping or pain
    Diarrhea
    Nausea or vomiting

For elderly patients: Many medicines have not been tested in older people. Therefore, it is not known whether the medicine acts the same way it does in younger adults.

Check with your doctor or pharmacist if you notice any unusual effects while using this medicine or if you think it is not working as it should.

Other side effects not listed above may also occur in some patients. If you notice any other effects, check with your doctor.

December 1987

CLOTRIMAZOLE (Topical)

Some commonly used brand names are:

Canesten*	Mycelex
Lotrimin	Myclo*

*Not available in the U.S.

To the Reader: If you do not recognize the names of medical conditions or medicines referred to in this information, check with your doctor, nurse, or pharmacist. Definitions for selected medical terms may be found in the Glossary. Brand names for the generic drug names listed can be found in the Index. In addition, selected brand names commonly associated with the generic name have been included in the text to help you recognize medicine you may be taking. The fact that a brand name product is not mentioned does not mean the information does not apply. It is a good idea for you to learn both the generic and brand names of your medicines and to write them down for future use.

Clotrimazole (kloe-TRIM-a-zole) belongs to the general family of medicines called antifungals. Clotrimazole topical preparations are used on the skin to help the body overcome fungal infections.

Clotrimazole is available only with your doctor's prescription.

Remember:

• **This medicine has been prescribed for your present infection only.** Another infection later on may require a different medicine. Also, even though other people may have the same symptoms as you, they may have a different kind of infection. Your medicine may not work for them and may even cause them harm. Therefore, **your medicine must not be given to other people or used for other infections** unless you are otherwise directed by your doctor.

• **Keep all medicines out of the reach of children.**

• In order for this medicine to work, it must be used as directed.

• **It is very important that you read and understand the following information.** If any of the information causes you special concern, do not decide against using this medicine without first checking with your doctor.

• Before you begin using any new medicine (prescription or nonprescription) or if you develop any new medical problem while you are using this medicine, check with your doctor, nurse, or pharmacist.

• **If you have any questions** about the following information or if you want more information about this medicine or your medical problem, **ask your doctor, nurse, or pharmacist.**

Before Using This Medicine

In order to decide on the best treatment for your medical problem, your doctor should be told:

—if you have ever had any unusual or allergic reaction to clotrimazole.

—if you are allergic to any substance, such as certain foods or preservatives or dyes. Most medicines contain more than their active ingredient. Your doctor, nurse, or pharmacist can help you avoid products that may cause a problem.

—if you are **pregnant** or if you may become pregnant. Clotrimazole topical preparations have not been shown to cause birth defects or other problems in humans, even though small amounts of clotrimazole are absorbed through the skin.

—if you are **breast-feeding**. Clotrimazole topical preparations have not been shown to cause problems in nursing babies, even though small amounts of clotrimazole are absorbed through the skin.

Proper Use of This Medicine

Apply enough clotrimazole to cover the affected and surrounding skin areas, and rub in gently.

Keep this medicine away from the eyes.

When clotrimazole is used to treat certain types of fungal infections of the skin, an occlusive dressing or airtight covering (for example, kitchen plastic wrap) should *not* be applied over the medicine. To do so may cause irritation of the skin. **Do not apply an occlusive dressing over this medicine unless you have been directed to do so by your doctor.**

To help clear up your infection completely, **it is very important that you keep using this medicine for the full time of treatment** even if your symptoms begin to clear up after a few days. Since fungal infections may be very slow to clear up, you may have to continue using this medicine every day for several weeks or more. If you stop using this medicine too soon, your symptoms may return. **Do not miss any doses.**

If you do miss a dose of this medicine, apply it as soon as possible. However, if it is almost time for your next dose, skip the missed dose and go back to your regular dosing schedule.

How to store this medicine:

• **Keep out of the reach of children.**

• Store away from heat and direct light.

• Keep the medicine from freezing.

• Do not keep outdated medicine or medicine no longer needed. Be sure that any discarded medicine is out of the reach of children.

Precautions While Using This Medicine

If your skin problem does not improve within 4 weeks, or if it becomes worse, check with your doctor.

Side Effects of This Medicine

Along with its needed effects, a medicine may cause some unwanted effects. Although not all of these side effects may occur, if they do occur they may need medical attention.

© 1988   The United States Pharmacopeial Convention, Inc.

Check with your doctor as soon as possible if any of the following side effects occur:

> Skin rash, hives, blistering, burning, itching, peeling, redness, stinging, swelling, or other sign of skin irritation not present before using this medicine

Other side effects not listed above may also occur in some patients. If you notice any other effects, check with your doctor.

December 1987

CLOTRIMAZOLE (Vaginal)

Some commonly used brand names are:

Canesten*	Gyne-Lotrimin
Canesten 1*	Mycelex-G
Canesten 3*	Myclo*

*Not available in the U.S.

To the Reader: If you do not recognize the names of medical conditions or medicines referred to in this information, check with your doctor, nurse, or pharmacist. Definitions for selected medical terms may be found in the Glossary. Brand names for the generic drug names listed can be found in the Index. In addition, selected brand names commonly associated with the generic name have been included in the text to help you recognize medicine you may be taking. The fact that a brand name product is not mentioned does not mean the information does not apply. It is a good idea for you to learn both the generic and brand names of your medicines and to write them down for future use.

Clotrimazole (kloe-TRIM-a-zole) belongs to the general family of medicines called antifungals. Clotrimazole vaginal preparations are used in the vagina to help the body overcome fungal infections of the vagina.

Clotrimazole is available only with your doctor's prescription.

Remember:

• **This medicine has been prescribed for your present infection only.** Another infection later on may require a different medicine. Also, even though other people may have the same symptoms as you, they may have a different kind of infection. Your medicine may not work for them and may even cause them harm. Therefore, **your medicine must not be given to other people or used for other infections** unless you are otherwise directed by your doctor.

• **Keep all medicines out of the reach of children.**

• In order for this medicine to work, it must be used as directed.

• **It is very important that you read and understand the following information.** If any of the information causes you special concern, do not decide against using this medicine without first checking with your doctor.

• Before you begin using any new medicine (prescription or nonprescription) or if you develop any new medical problem while you are using this medicine, check with your doctor, nurse, or pharmacist.

• **If you have any questions** about the following information or if you want more information about this medicine or your medical problem, **ask your doctor, nurse, or pharmacist.**

Before Using This Medicine

In order to decide on the best treatment for your medical problem, your doctor should be told:

—if you have ever had any unusual or allergic reaction to clotrimazole.

—if you are allergic to any substance, such as certain foods or preservatives or dyes. Most medicines contain more than their active ingredient. Your doctor, nurse, or pharmacist can help you avoid products that may cause a problem.

—if you are **pregnant** or if you may become pregnant. However, clotrimazole vaginal preparations have not been shown to cause birth defects or other problems in humans, even though small amounts of clotrimazole are absorbed through the vagina.

—if you are **breast-feeding**. However, clotrimazole vaginal preparations have not been shown to cause problems in nursing babies, even though small amounts of clotrimazole are absorbed through the vagina.

Proper Use of This Medicine

Clotrimazole usually comes with patient directions. Read them carefully before using this medicine.

Use this medicine at bedtime, unless otherwise directed by your doctor.

Clotrimazole is usually inserted into the vagina with an applicator. However, if you are pregnant, check with your doctor before using the applicator to insert the vaginal cream or tablet.

For patients using clotrimazole vaginal cream or the 3-day or 7-day treatment with clotrimazole vaginal tablets:

• To help clear up your infection completely, **it is very important that you keep using this medicine for the full time of treatment** even if your symptoms begin to clear up after a few days. Also, keep using this medicine even if you begin to menstruate during the time of treatment. If you stop using this medicine too soon, your symptoms may return. **Do not miss any doses.**

• If you do miss a dose of this medicine, insert it as soon as possible. However, if it is almost time for your next dose, skip the missed dose and go back to your regular dosing schedule.

How to store this medicine:

• **Keep out of the reach of children.**

• Store away from heat and direct light.

• Do not store the vaginal tablet form of this medicine in the bathroom, near the kitchen sink, or in other damp places. Heat or moisture may cause the medicine to break down.

• Keep the vaginal cream form of this medicine from freezing.

• Do not keep outdated medicine or medicine no longer needed. Be sure that any discarded medicine is out of the reach of children.

Precautions While Using This Medicine

To help cure the infection and to help prevent reinfection, good health habits are required.

• Wear cotton panties (or panties or pantyhose with cotton crotches) instead of synthetic (for example, nylon, rayon) underclothes.

• Wear freshly laundered underclothes.

If you have any questions about this, check with your doctor, nurse, or pharmacist.

If you have any questions about douching and intercourse during the time of treatment with clotrimazole, check with your doctor.

Since there may be some vaginal drainage while you are using this medicine, a sanitary napkin may be worn to protect your clothing.

Side Effects of This Medicine

Along with its needed effects, a medicine may cause some unwanted effects. Although not all of these side effects may occur, if they do occur they may need medical attention.

Check with your doctor as soon as possible if any of the following side effects occur:

Less common
>   Vaginal burning or other irritation not present before using this medicine

Rare
>   Skin rash

Other side effects may occur that usually do not require medical attention. These side effects may go away during treatment as your body adjusts to the medicine. However, check with your doctor if any of the following side effects continue or are bothersome:

Less common or rare
>   Burning or irritation of penis of sexual partner
>   Increased frequency of urination
>   Lower stomach cramps or pain

Other side effects not listed above may also occur in some patients. If you notice any other effects, check with your doctor.

December 1987

COAL TAR (Topical)

Some commonly used brand names are:

Alphosyl	Doak Tar	Taraphilic
Aquatar	Duplex T	Tarbonis
Balnetar	Estar	Tar Doak*
Cutar Bath Oil	Fototar	Tarpaste Doak
Emulsion	Iocon	T/Derm
Denorex	Ionil-T Plus	Tegrin Medicated
Dermatologic	Lavatar	Tersa-Tar
Shower System	Medotar	T/Gel
DHS Tar	Pentrax	Zetar
Doak Oil	Psorex Medicated	Zetar Emulsion
Doak Oil Forte	psoriGel	

Generic name product may also be available in the U.S.

---

*Not available in the U.S.

To the Reader: If you do not recognize the names of medical conditions or medicines referred to in this information, check with your doctor, nurse, or pharmacist. Definitions for selected medical terms may be found in the Glossary. Brand names for the generic drug names listed can be found in the Index. In addition, selected brand names commonly associated with the generic name have been included in the text to help you recognize medicine you may be taking. The fact that a brand name product is not mentioned does not mean the information does not apply. It is a good idea for you to learn both the generic and brand names of your medicines and to write them down for future use.

Coal tar is applied to the skin to treat eczema, psoriasis, seborrheic dermatitis, and other skin disorders.

Some of these preparations are available only with your doctor's prescription. Others are available without a prescription; however, your doctor may have special instructions on the proper use of coal tar for your medical condition.

Remember:
• **Keep all medicines out of the reach of children.**

• In order for this medicine to work, it must be used as directed. **If you are using this medicine without a prescription, it is very important to follow the directions on the label.**

• **It is also very important that you read and understand the following information.** If any of the information causes you special concern, check with your doctor or pharmacist.

• Before you begin using any new medicine (prescription or nonprescription) or if you develop any new medical problem while you are using this medicine, check with your doctor, nurse, or pharmacist.

• **If you have any questions** about the following information or if you want more information about this medicine or your medical problem, **ask your doctor, nurse, or pharmacist.**

Before Using This Medicine

Before you use coal tar, check with your doctor or pharmacist:

—if you have ever had any unusual or allergic reaction to coal tar.

—if you are **pregnant** or if you may become pregnant. Studies on birth defects have not been done in either humans or animals.

—if you are **breast-feeding**, although it is not known whether coal tar passes into the breast milk and this medicine has not been shown to cause problems in nursing babies.

—if you are taking **any** other prescription or nonprescription (OTC) medicine.

Proper Use of This Medicine

Use this medicine only as directed. Do not use more of it and do not use it more often than recommended on the label, unless otherwise directed by your doctor. To do so may increase the chance of side effects.

After applying coal tar, **protect the treated area from direct sunlight for at least 24 hours**, unless otherwise directed by your doctor, since it may cause a severe reaction.

Do not apply this medicine to infected, blistered, raw, or oozing areas of the skin.

Keep this medicine away from the eyes. If you should accidentally get some in your eyes, flush them thoroughly with water at once.

For patients using the cream or ointment form of this medicine:

• Apply enough medicine to cover the affected area, and rub in gently.

For patients using the gel form of this medicine:

• Apply enough gel to cover the affected area, and rub in gently. Allow the gel to remain on the affected area for 5 minutes, then remove excess gel by patting with a clean tissue.

For patients using the shampoo form of this medicine:

• Wet the scalp and hair with lukewarm water. Apply a generous amount of shampoo and rub into the scalp, then rinse. Apply the shampoo again, working up a rich lather, and allow to remain on the scalp for 5 minutes. Then rinse thoroughly.

For patients using the nonshampoo liquid form of this medicine:

• Some of these preparations are to be applied directly to dry or wet skin, some are to be added to lukewarm bath water, and some may be applied directly to dry or wet skin or added to lukewarm bath water. Make sure you know exactly how you should use this medicine. If you have any questions about this, check with your doctor or pharmacist.

• If this medicine is to be applied directly to the skin, apply enough to cover the affected area, and rub in gently.

• Some of these preparations contain alcohol and are flammable. Do not use near heat, near open flame, or while smoking.

If you miss a dose of this medicine, apply it as soon as possible. However, if it is almost time for your next dose, skip the missed dose and go back to your regular dosing schedule.

How to store this medicine:

- **Keep out of the reach of children.**
- Store away from heat and direct light.
- Keep the medicine from freezing.
- Do not keep outdated medicine or medicine no longer needed. Be sure that any discarded medicine is out of the reach of children.

Precautions While Using This Medicine

If this medicine is used on the scalp, it may temporarily discolor blond, bleached, or tinted hair.

Coal tar may stain the skin or clothing. Avoid getting it on your clothing. The stain on the skin will wear off after you stop using the medicine.

Side Effects of This Medicine

In animal studies, coal tar has been shown to increase the chance of skin cancer.

Along with its needed effects, a medicine may cause some unwanted effects. Although not all of these side effects may occur, if they do occur they may need medical attention.

Check with your doctor as soon as possible if either of the following side effects occurs:

Rare

Skin irritation not present before using this medicine
Skin rash

Other side effects may occur that usually do not require medical attention. These side effects may go away during treatment as your body adjusts to the medicine. However, check with your doctor or pharmacist if the following side effect continues or is bothersome:

More common

Stinging (mild)—especially for gel and solution dosage forms

For elderly patients: Many medicines have not been tested in older people. Therefore, it is not known whether the medicine acts the same way it does in younger adults. Check with your doctor or pharmacist if you notice any unusual effects while using this medicine or if you think it is not working as it should.

Other side effects not listed above may also occur in some patients. If you notice any other effects, check with your doctor or pharmacist.

December 1987

COLCHICINE (Systemic)

To the Reader: If you do not recognize the names of medical conditions or medicines referred to in this information, check with your doctor, nurse, or pharmacist. Definitions for selected medical terms may be found in the Glossary. Brand names for the generic drug names listed can be found in the Index. In addition, selected brand names commonly associated with the generic name have been included in the text to help you recognize medicine you may be taking. The fact that a brand name product is not mentioned does not mean the information does not apply. It is a good idea for you to learn both the generic and brand names of your medicines and to write them down for future use.

Colchicine (KOL-chi-seen) is taken by mouth or given by injection to prevent or treat attacks of gout or gouty arthritis. Some patients take it only when an attack occurs, to relieve inflammation, pain, and swelling. Other patients take small amounts of it regularly every day to prevent an attack from occurring.

Colchicine may also be used for other conditions as determined by your doctor. For some of these conditions, colchicine is taken only when an attack occurs. For other conditions, the medicine is taken regularly every day. If you are taking colchicine for one of these other conditions, the information about gout will not apply to you. However, your doctor may have other instructions for you to follow.

In addition to its helpful effects in treating your medical problem, colchicine has side effects that can be very serious. Before you take colchicine, you should discuss with your doctor the good that this medicine will do as well as the risks of using it. Make sure that you understand exactly how you are to use this medicine, and follow the instructions very carefully, to lessen the chance of unwanted effects.

This medicine is available only with your doctor's prescription.

Remember:

• **This medicine has been prescribed for your current medical problem only.** It must not be given to other people or used for other problems unless you are directed to do so by your doctor.

• **Keep all medicines out of the reach of children.**

• In order for this medicine to work, it must be used as directed.

• If you are receiving this medicine by injection, some of the information about this medicine may not apply.

• **It is very important that you read and understand the following information.** If any of the information causes you special concern, do not decide against using this medicine without first checking with your doctor.

• Before you begin using any new medicine (prescription or nonprescription) or if you develop any new medical problem while you are using this medicine, check with your doctor, nurse, or pharmacist.

• **If you have any questions** about the following information or if you want more information about this medicine or your medical problem, **ask your doctor, nurse, or pharmacist.**

Before Using This Medicine

In order to decide on the best treatment for your medical problem, your doctor should be told:

—if you have ever had any unusual or allergic reaction to colchicine.

—if you are on a low-salt, low-sugar, or any other special diet, or if you are allergic to any substance, such as foods, sulfites or other preservatives, or dyes. Most medicines contain more than their active ingredient. Your doctor, nurse, or pharmacist can help you avoid products that may cause a problem.

—if you are **pregnant** or if you may become pregnant. Although studies in humans have not been done, some reports have suggested that use of colchicine during pregnancy can cause harm to the fetus. Also, this medicine has been shown to cause birth defects in animal studies. Therefore, do not begin taking colchicine during pregnancy, and do not become pregnant while taking this medicine, unless you have first discussed this problem with your doctor. Also, check with your doctor at once if you suspect that you have become pregnant while taking colchicine.

—if you are **breast-feeding**. Although it is not known whether colchicine passes into the breast milk and this medicine has not been shown to cause problems in humans, the chance always exists.

—if you have any of the following medical problems:
Blood disease
Heart disease
Intestinal disease (severe)
Kidney disease (severe)
Liver disease
Stomach ulcer or other stomach problems

—if you are taking **any** other prescription or nonprescription (OTC) medicine, especially:
Antineoplastics (cancer medicine)
Antithyroid agents (medicine for overactive thyroid)
Azathioprine (e.g., Imuran)
Chlorambucil (e.g., Leukeran)
Chloramphenicol (e.g., Chloromycetin)
Cyclophosphamide (e.g., Cytoxan)
Flucytosine (e.g., Ancobon)
Interferon (e.g., Intron-A; Roferon-A)
Mercaptopurine (e.g., Purinethol)
Methotrexate (e.g., Mexate)

Proper Use of This Medicine

For patients taking colchicine only when an attack occurs:

• Start taking it at the first sign of the attack for best results.

• **Stop taking this medicine as soon as the pain is relieved or at the first sign of nausea, vomiting, stomach pain, or diarrhea.** Also, stop taking colchicine when you have taken the largest amount that your doctor ordered for each attack, even if the pain is not relieved or none of these side effects occurs.

• Unless otherwise directed by your doctor, **do not take colchicine more often than every three days.**

• If you are taking colchicine for an attack of gout, and you are also taking other medicine for gout, **do not stop taking the other medicine.** Continue taking the other medicine as directed by your doctor.

For patients taking colchicine regularly to prevent gout attacks:

• You should increase the dose you normally take at the first sign of an attack as advised by your doctor.

• **Stop taking the larger dose of medicine as soon as the gout pain is relieved or at the first sign of nausea, vomiting, stomach pain, or diarrhea.**

• After the gout attack is over, start taking the lower dose of colchicine again as ordered by your doctor.

Take this medicine only as directed by your doctor. Do not take more of it, do not take it more often, and do not take it for a longer period of time than your doctor ordered. To do so may cause serious side effects.

If you are taking colchicine regularly (for example, every day) and you miss a dose of this medicine, take it as soon as possible. However, if it is almost time for your next dose, skip the missed dose and go back to your regular dosing schedule. Do not double doses.

How to store this medicine:

• **Keep out of the reach of children.**

• Store away from heat and direct light.

• Do not store this medicine in the bathroom, near the kitchen sink, or in other damp places. Heat or moisture may cause the medicine to break down.

• Do not keep outdated medicine or medicine no longer needed. Be sure that any discarded medicine is out of the reach of children.

Precautions While Using This Medicine

If you will be taking colchicine for more than a few days at a time, your doctor should check your progress at regular visits.

Stomach problems may be more likely to occur if you drink large amounts of alcoholic beverages while taking colchicine. Also, drinking too much alcohol may increase the amount of uric acid in your blood. This may lessen the effects of colchicine when it is used to treat gout. Therefore, **do not drink alcoholic beverages while you are taking this medicine,** unless you have first checked with your doctor.

Side Effects of This Medicine

Along with its needed effects, a medicine may cause some unwanted effects. Although not all of these side effects may occur, if they do occur they may need medical attention.

Stop taking this medicine immediately if any of the following side effects occur:
More common
　　Diarrhea
　　Nausea or vomiting
　　Stomach pain

If any of these side effects continue for 3 hours or longer after you have stopped taking colchicine, check with your doctor.

Also, **check with your doctor immediately** if any of the following side effects occur:
Rare
　　Redness, swelling, or pain at place of injection
With long-term use
　　Numbness, tingling, pain, or weakness in hands or feet
　　Skin rash
　　Sore throat, fever, and chills
　　Unusual bleeding or bruising
　　Unusual tiredness or weakness
Signs of overdose
　　Bloody urine
　　Burning feeling in stomach, throat, or skin
　　Convulsions (seizures)
　　Diarrhea (severe or bloody)
　　Fever
　　Mood or mental changes
　　Muscle weakness (severe)
　　Sudden decrease in amount of urine
　　Troubled breathing
　　Vomiting (severe)

Other side effects may occur that usually do not require medical attention. However, check with your doctor if either of the following side effects continues or is bothersome:
Less common
　　Loss of appetite
With long-term use
　　Loss of hair

For elderly patients: The above side effects are more likely to occur in the elderly, who are usually more sensitive to the effects of colchicine.

Other side effects not listed above may also occur in some patients. If you notice any other effects, check with your doctor.

December 1987

COLESTIPOL (Systemic)

A commonly used brand name is Colestid.

To the Reader: If you do not recognize the names of medical conditions or medicines referred to in this information, check with your doctor, nurse, or pharmacist. Definitions for selected medical terms may be found in the Glossary. Brand names for the generic drug names listed can be found in the Index. In addition, selected brand names commonly associated with the generic name have been included in the text to help you recognize medicine you may be taking. The fact that a brand name product is not mentioned does not mean the information does not apply. It is a good idea for you to learn both the generic and brand names of your medicines and to write them down for future use.

Colestipol (koe-LES-ti-pole) is used to lower high cholesterol levels in the blood. This may help prevent medical problems caused by cholesterol clogging the blood vessels.

Colestipol works by attaching to certain substances in the intestine. Since colestipol is not absorbed into the body, these substances also pass out of the body without being absorbed.

Colestipol may also be used for other conditions as determined by your doctor.

Colestipol is available only with your doctor's prescription.

Remember:

• **This medicine has been prescribed for your current medical problem only.** It must not be given to other people or used for other problems unless you are directed to do so by your doctor.

• **Keep all medicines out of the reach of children.**

• In order for this medicine to work, it must be used as directed.

• **It is very important that you read and understand the following information.** If any of the information causes you special concern, do not decide against using this medicine without first checking with your doctor.

• Before you begin using any new medicine (prescription or nonprescription) or if you develop any new medical problem while you are using this medicine, check with your doctor, nurse, or pharmacist.

• **If you have any questions** about the following information or if you want more information about this medicine or your medical problem, **ask your doctor, nurse, or pharmacist.**

Before Using This Medicine

Importance of diet—Before prescribing medicine for your condition, your doctor will probably try to control your condition by prescribing a personal diet for you. Such a diet may be low in fats, sugars, and/or cholesterol. Many people are able to control their condition by carefully following their doctor's orders for proper diet and exercise. Medicine is prescribed only when additional help is needed and is effective only when a schedule of diet and exercise is properly followed.

Also, this medicine is less effective if you are greatly overweight. It may be very important for you to go on a reducing diet. However, check with your doctor before going on any diet.

Remember that this medicine will not cure your cholesterol problem but it does help control it. Therefore, you must continue to take it as directed if you expect to lower your cholesterol level.

In order to decide on the best treatment for your medical problem, your doctor should be told:

—if you have ever had any unusual or allergic reaction to colestipol.

—if you are on a low-salt, low-sugar, or any other special diet, or if you are allergic to any substance, such as foods, sulfites or other preservatives, or dyes. Most medicines contain more than their active ingredient. Your doctor, nurse, or pharmacist can help you avoid products that may cause a problem.

—if you are **pregnant** or if you may become pregnant. Colestipol is not absorbed into the body and is not likely to cause problems. However, it may reduce absorption of vitamins into the body. Ask your doctor whether you need to take extra vitamins.

—if you are **breast-feeding**, although colestipol is not absorbed into the body and is not likely to cause problems.

—if you have any of the following medical problems:
    Bleeding problems
    Constipation
    Gallstones
    Heart or blood vessel disease
    Hemorrhoids
    Liver disease
    Stomach ulcer or other stomach problems

—if you are taking **any** other prescription or nonprescription (OTC) medicine, especially:
    Anticoagulants (blood thinners)
    Digitalis glycosides (heart medicine)
    Penicillin G, taken by mouth
    Tetracyclines, taken by mouth
    Thyroid hormones
    Vancomycin, taken by mouth

Proper Use of This Medicine

Take this medicine exactly as directed by your doctor. Try not to miss any doses and do not take more medicine than your doctor ordered.

This medicine should never be taken in its dry form, since it could cause you to choke. Instead, always mix as follows:

• Add this medicine to 3 ounces or more of water, milk, flavored drink, or your favorite juice or carbonated drink. If you use a carbonated drink, slowly mix in the powder in a large glass to prevent too much foaming. Stir until it is completely mixed (it will **not** dissolve) before drinking. After drinking all the liquid containing the medicine, rinse the glass with a little more liquid and drink that also, to make sure you get all the medicine.

• You may also mix this medicine with milk in hot or regular breakfast cereals, or in thin soups such as tomato or chicken noodle soup. Or you may add it to some pulpy fruits such as crushed pineapple, pears, peaches, or fruit cocktail.

If you miss a dose of this medicine, take it as soon as possible. Then go back to your regular dosing schedule. However, if it is almost time for your next dose, skip the missed dose and go back to your regular dosing schedule. Do not double doses.

How to store this medicine:

• **Keep out of the reach of children.**

• Store away from heat and direct light.

• Do not store in the bathroom, near the kitchen sink or in other damp places. Heat or moisture may cause the medicine to break down.

• Do not keep outdated medicine or medicine no longer needed. Be sure that any discarded medicine is out of the reach of children.

Precautions While Using This Medicine

It is very important that your doctor check your progress at regular visits. This will allow your doctor to see if the medicine is working properly to lower your cholesterol levels and to decide if you should continue to take it.

Do not take any other medicine unless prescribed by your doctor since colestipol may interfere with other medicines.

Side Effects of This Medicine

Along with its needed effects, a medicine may cause some unwanted effects. Although not all of these side effects may occur, if they do occur they may need medical attention.

Check with your doctor immediately if either of the following side effects occurs:

Rare
Black, tarry stools
Stomach pain (severe) with nausea and vomiting

Check with your doctor as soon as possible if either of the following side effects occurs:

More common
Constipation

Rare
Loss of weight (sudden)

Other side effects may occur that usually do not require medical attention. These side effects may go away during treatment as your body adjusts to the medicine. However, check with your doctor if any of the following side effects continue or are bothersome:

Less common
Belching
Bloating
Diarrhea
Nausea or vomiting
Stomach pain

For elderly patients: The above side effects may be more likely to occur in the elderly (over 60 years of age), who are usually more sensitive to the effects of colestipol.

Other side effects not listed above may also occur in some patients. If you notice any other effects, check with your doctor.

December 1987

COLISTIN, NEOMYCIN, AND HYDROCORTISONE (Otic)

Some commonly used brand names are Coly-Mycin* and Coly-Mycin S.

*Not available in the U.S.

To the Reader: If you do not recognize the names of medical conditions or medicines referred to in this information, check with your doctor, nurse, or pharmacist. Definitions for selected medical terms may be found in the Glossary. Brand names for the generic drug names listed can be found in the Index. In addition, selected brand names commonly associated with the generic name have been included in the text to help you recognize medicine you may be taking. The fact that a brand name product is not mentioned does not mean the information does not apply. It is a good idea for you to learn both the generic and brand names of your medicines and to write them down for future use.

Colistin (koe-LIS-tin), neomycin (nee-oh-MYE-sin), and hydrocortisone (hye-droe-KOR-ti-sone) combination contains an antibiotic and a cortisone-like medicine. It is used in the ear to help the body overcome infections of the ear canal and to help provide relief from redness, irritation, and discomfort of certain ear problems.

Colistin, neomycin, and hydrocortisone combination is available only with your doctor's prescription.

Remember:

• **This medicine has been prescribed for your present infection only.** Another infection later on may require a different medicine. Also, even though other people may have the same symptoms as you, they may have a different kind of infection. Your medicine may not work for them and may even cause them harm. Therefore, **your medicine must not be given to other people or used for other infections** unless you are otherwise directed by your doctor.

• **Keep all medicines out of the reach of children.**

• In order for this medicine to work, it must be used as directed.

• **It is very important that you read and understand the following information.** If any of the information causes you special concern, do not decide against using this medicine without first checking with your doctor.

• Before you begin using any new medicine (prescription or nonprescription) or if you develop any new medical problem while you are using this medicine, check with your doctor, nurse, or pharmacist.

• **If you have any questions** about the following information or if you want more information about this medicine or your medical problem, **ask your doctor, nurse, or pharmacist.**

Before Using This Medicine

In order to decide on the best treatment for your medical problem, your doctor should be told:

—if you have ever had any unusual or allergic reaction to this medicine or to any related antibiotics such as amikacin, colistin (by mouth or by injection), gentamicin, kanamycin, neomycin (by mouth or by injection), netilmicin, paromomycin, polymyxin B, streptomycin, or tobramycin.

—if you are allergic to any substance, such as certain foods or preservatives or dyes. Most medicines contain more than their active ingredient. Your doctor, nurse, or pharmacist can help you avoid products that may cause a problem.

—if you are **pregnant** or if you may become pregnant. However, colistin, neomycin, and hydrocortisone otic drops have not been shown to cause birth defects or other problems in humans.

—if you are **breast-feeding.** However, colistin, neomycin, and hydrocortisone otic drops have not been shown to cause problems in nursing babies.

—if you have any other ear infection or problem (including punctured eardrum).

Proper Use of This Medicine

You may warm the ear drops to body temperature (37 °C or 98.6 °F), but no higher, by holding the bottle in your hand for a few minutes before applying. If this medicine gets too warm, it may break down and not work as well.

How to apply this medicine: Lie down or tilt the head so that the infected ear faces up. Gently pull the earlobe up and back for adults (down and back for children) to straighten the ear canal. Drop the medicine into the ear canal. Keep the ear facing up for about 5 minutes to allow the medicine to come into contact with the infection. A sterile cotton plug may be gently inserted into the ear opening to prevent the medicine from leaking out. However, your doctor may want you to keep a sterile cotton plug moistened with this medicine in your ear for the full time of treatment. If you have any questions about this, check with your doctor.

To prevent contamination of the ear drops, do not touch the dropper to any surface (including the ear). Also, keep the container tightly closed.

Do not use this medicine for more than 10 days unless otherwise directed by your doctor.

To help clear up your infection completely, **keep using this medicine for the full time of treatment,** even if your symptoms begin to clear up after a few days. If you stop using this medicine too soon, your symptoms may return. **Do not miss any doses.**

If you do miss a dose of this medicine, apply it as soon as possible. However, if it is almost time for your next dose, skip the missed dose and go back to your regular dosing schedule.

How to store this medicine:

• **Keep out of the reach of children.**

• Store away from heat and direct light.

• Keep the medicine from freezing

• Do not keep outdated medicine or medicine no longer needed. Be sure that any discarded medicine is out of the reach of children.

Precautions While Using This Medicine

If your symptoms do not improve within 1 week, or if they become worse, check with your doctor immediately.

Side Effects of This Medicine

Along with its needed effects, a medicine may cause some unwanted effects. Although not all of these side effects may occur, if they do occur they may need medical attention.

Check with your doctor immediately if any of the following side effects occur:

More common

Itching, skin rash, redness, swelling, or other sign of irritation not present before using this medicine

Other side effects not listed above may also occur in some patients. If you notice any other effects, check with your doctor.

December 1987

COUGH/COLD COMBINATIONS (Systemic)

Some commonly used brand names are:

Actifed with Codeine Cough[42]
Actifed DM*[43]
Adatuss D.C. Expectorant[103]
Alamine-C Liquid[28]
Alamine Expectorant[119]
Ambay Cough[1]
Ambenyl Cough[1]
Ambenyl-D Decongestant Cough Formula[120]
Ambophen Expectorant[9]
Anatuss[77]
Anatuss with Codeine[78]
Anti-Tuss DM Expectorant[100]
Banex[126]
Banex-LA[127]
Bayaminic Expectorant[127]
Bayaminicol[27]
Baycodan[92]
Baycomine[109]
Baycomine Pediatric[109]
BayCotussend Liquid[112]
Baydec DM Drops[20]
Bayer Cough Syrup for Children[108]
Bayhistine-DH[28]
Bayhistine Expectorant[119]
Baytussin AC[95]
Baytussin DM[100]
Benylin with Codeine*[11]
Benylin-DM*[12]
Benylin DME[100]
Biphetane DC Cough[19]
Brexin[84]
Broncholate[124]
Bronkotuss Expectorant[85]
Calcidrine[94]
Caldomine-DH Forte*[37]
Caldomine-DH Pediatric*[37]
Calmylin with Codeine*[11]
Carbodec DM Drops[20]
Cerose-DM[22]
Cheracol[95]
Cheracol D Cough[100]
Cheracol Plus[27]
Chexit[82]
Citra Forte[15 45]
CoActifed*[42]
CoActifed Expectorant*[76]
Co-Apap[51]
Codamine[109]
Codehist DH[28]
Codiclear DH[103]
Codimal DH[41]
Codimal DM[40]

Codimal Expectorant[127]
Codimal PH[39]
Codistan No.1[100]
Colrex Compound[46]
Colrex Cough[22]
Comtrex Multi-Symptom Cold Reliever[49]
Conar[106]
Conar-A[122]
Conar Expectorant[115]
Concentrin[120]
Conex[127]
Conex with Codeine Liquid[117]
Congess JR[128]
Congess SR[128]
Contac Jr. Children's Cold Medicine[113]
Contac Severe Cold Formula[51]
Contac Severe Cold Formula Night Strength[52]
Cophene-S[26]
Cophene-X[66]
Cophene-XP[66]
Coricidin with Codeine*[7]
Coricidin Cough[118]
Coristex-DH*[33]
Coristine-DH*[33]
Coryban-D Cough[122]
CoTylenol Cold Medication[51]
Cremacoat 3 Throat Coating Cough Medicine[118]
Cremacoat 4 Throat Coating Cough Medicine[34]
C-Tussin Expectorant[119]
DayCare[123]
Deproist Expectorant with Codeine[119]
De-Tuss[112]
Detussin Expectorant[121]
Detussin Liquid[112]
Dilaudid Cough[105]
Dimacol[120]
Dimetane-DC Cough[19]
Dimetane-DX Cough[19b]
Dimetane Expectorant*[83]
Dimetane Expectorant-C*[56]
Dimetane Expectorant-DC*[57]
Dimetapp with Codeine*[17]
Dimetapp-DM*[18]
Donatussin[64]
Donatussin DC[116]
Donatussin Drops[86]
Dondril[22]
Dorcol Children's Cough[120]

Dura-Vent[127]
Efficol Cough Whip (Cough Suppressant/Decongestant)[108]
Efficol Cough Whip (Cough Suppressant/Decongestant/Antihistamine)[27]
Efficol Cough Whip (Cough Suppressant/Expectorant)[100]
Efricon Expectorant Liquid[62]
Entex[126]
Entex LA[127]
Entex Liquid[126]
Entuss-D[112 121]
Entuss Expectorant[103 104]
Father John's Medicine Plus[65]
Fedahist Expectorant[89]
2/G-DM Cough[100]
Glycotuss-dM[100]
Glydeine Cough[95]
Glydm Cough[100]
Guaifed[128]
Guaifed-PD[128]
Guiamid D.M. Liquid[100]
Guiatuss A.C.[95]
Guiatuss-DM[100]
Guiatussin with Codeine Liquid[95]
Guistrey Fortis[86]
Halls Mentho-Lyptus Decongestant Cough Formula[108]
Halotussin-DM Expectorant[100]
Head & Chest[127]
Histadyl E.C.[58]
Histafed C[42]
Histalet-DM[29]
Histalet X[128]
Hold (Children's Formula)[108]
Hycodan[92]
Hycomine[109]
Hycomine*[75]
Hycomine Compound[48]
Hycomine Pediatric[109]
Hycomine-S Pediatric*[75]
Hycotuss Expectorant[103]
Hydropane[92]
Hydrophen[109]
Improved Sino-Tuss[47]
Iophen-C Liquid[96]
Isoclor Expectorant[119]
Kiddy Koff[118]
KIE[125]
Kolephrin/DM[50]
Kolephrin GG/DM[100]
Kolephrin NN Liquid[55]
Kophane[67]

Kwelcof Liquid[103]
Lanatuss Expectorant[88]
Mediquell Decongestant Formula[111]
Naldecon-CX[117]
Naldecon-DX[118]
Naldecon-EX[127]
Noratuss II Liquid[120]
Nortussin with Codeine[95]
Novahistex C*[31]
Novahistex DH*[33]
Novahistex DH Expectorant*[70]
Novahistex DM*[32]
Novahistine Cough & Cold Formula Liquid[29]
Novahistine DH*[33]
Novahistine DH Expectorant*[70]
Novahistine DH Liquid[28]
Novahistine DMX Liquid[120]
Novahistine Expectorant[119]
Nucofed[110]
Nucofed Expectorant[119]
Nucofed Pediatric Expectorant[119]
NyQuil Nighttime Colds Medicine[52]
Nytime Cold Medicine Liquid[52]
Omnicol[44]
Omni-Tuss*[69]
Ornade-DM 10*[27]
Ornade-DM 15*[27]
Ornade-DM 30*[27]
Ornade Expectorant*[87]
Orthoxicol Cough[93]
PediaCare 3 Children's Cold Relief[29]
Pediacof Cough[63]
Penntuss[2]
Pertussin AM[27]
Pertussin CS[100]
Pertussin PM[52]
Phenergan with Codeine[5]
Phenergan with Dextromethorphan[6]
Phenergan VC with Codeine[38]
Phenhist Expectorant[119]
Polaramine Expectorant[90]
Poly-Histine-CS[19]
Poly-Histine-DM[19a]
Poly-Histine Expectorant Plain[127]
Prominic Expectorant[127]
Prominicol Cough[72]
Promist HD Liquid[30]

Prunicodeine[98]
Pseudo-Bid[128]
Pseudo-Car DM[20]
Pseudodine C Cough[42]
Pseudo-Hist Expectorant[121]
P-V-Tussin[13 60]
Quelidrine Cough[59]
Queltuss[100]
Remcol-C[8]
Rescaps-D S.R.[107]
Respaire-60 SR[128]
Respaire-120 SR[128]
Respinol-G[126]
Respinol LA[126]
Rhinosyn-DM[29]
Rhinosyn-DMX Expectorant[100]
Rhinosyn-X[120]
Robitussin A-C[95]
Robitussin A-C*[14]
Robitussin-CF[118]
Robitussin with Codeine*[14]
Robitussin-DAC[119]
Robitussin-DM[100]
Robitussin-DM Cough Calmers[100]
Robitussin Night Relief Colds Formula Liquid[54]
Robitussin-PE[128]
Rondec-DM[20]
Rondec-DM Drops[20]
Ru-Tuss Expectorant[61]
Ru-Tuss with Hydrocodone Liquid[35]
Rymed[126]
Rymed-Jr[126]
Rymed Liquid[126]
Rymed-TR[126]
Ryna-C Liquid[28]
Ryna-CX Liquid[119]
Rynatuss[21]
Rynatuss Pediatric[21]
Saleto-CF[113]
Silexin Cough[100]
Sinufed Timecelles[128]
Spantuss[22]
SRC Expectorant[121]
Sudafed Cough[120]
Sudafed DM*[111]
Sudafed Expectorant*[128]
Syracol Liquid[108]
Terphan[102]
Terpin-Dex[102]
T-Koff[24]
T-Moist[128]
Tolu-Sed Cough[95]
Tolu-Sed DM Cough[100]
Triaminic-DM Cough Formula[108]
Triaminic-DM Expectorant*[73]
Triaminic Expectorant[127]

Triaminic Expectorant*[91]
Triaminic Expectorant with Codeine[117]
Triaminic Expectorant DH[74]
Triaminicin with Codeine*[53]
Triaminicol DM*[36]
Triaminicol Multi-Symptom Cold[27]
Tricodene #1[16]
Tricodene Forte[27]
Tricodene NN Cough and Cold Medication[68]
Tricodene Pediatric[108]
Trimedine Liquid[22]
Trind DM Liquid[27]
Trinex[89]
Triphenyl Expectorant[127]
Trocal[100]
Tusquelin[25]
Tuss-Ade[107]
Tussafed[20]
Tussagesic[82]
Tuss Allergine Modified T.D.[107]
Tussaminic DH Forte*[37]
Tussaminic DH Pediatric*[37]
Tussanil DH[23 79]
Tussar-2 Cough[10]
Tussar DM Cough[22]
Tussar SF[10]
Tussend[112]
Tussend Expectorant[121]
Tussend Liquid[112]
Tussigon[92]
Tussionex[4]
Tussi-Organidin DM Liquid[101]
Tussi-Organidin Liquid[96]
Tussirex with Codeine Liquid[81]
Tussogest[107]
Tuss-Ornade Liquid[107]
Tuss-Ornade Spansules[107]
Tuss-Ornade Spansules*[26a]
Unproco[100]
Vicks Children's Cough[100]
Vicks Formula 44 Cough Mixture[3]
Vicks Formula 44D Decongestant Cough Mixture[120]
Vicks Formula 44M Multi-symptom Cough Mixture[123]
Viro-Med[80]
Zephrex[128]
Zephrex-LA[128]

---

*Not available in the U.S.

Note: For quick reference the following cough/cold combinations are numbered to match the corresponding brand names.

Antihistamine and antitussive combinations—
1. Bromodiphenhydramine (broe-moe-dye-fen-HYE-dra-meen) and Codeine (KOE-deen)
2. Chlorpheniramine (klor-fen-EER-a-meen) and Codeine
3. Chlorpheniramine and Dextromethorphan (dex-troe-meth-OR-fan)
4. Phenyltoloxamine (fen-ill-tole-OX-a-meen) and Hydrocodone (hye-droe-KOE-done)
5. Promethazine (proe-METH-a-zeen) and Codeine†
6. Promethazine and Dextromethorphan

Antihistamine, antitussive, and analgesic combinations—
7. Chlorpheniramine (klor-fen-EER-a-meen), Codeine (KOE-deen), Aspirin, and Caffeine*
8. Chlorpheniramine, Dextromethorphan (dex-troe-meth-OR-fan), and Acetaminophen (a-seat-a-MEE-noe-fen)

Antihistamine, antitussive, and expectorant combinations—
9. Bromodiphenhydramine (broe-moe-dye-fen-HYE-dra-meen), Diphenhydramine (dye-fen-HYE-dra-meen), Codeine (KOE-deen), Ammonium Chloride (a-MOE-nee-um KLOR-ide), and Potassium Guaiacolsulfonate (poe-TAS-ee-um gwye-a-kol-SUL-fon-ate)
10. Chlorpheniramine (klor-fen-EER-a-meen), Codeine, Carbetapentane, Guaifenesin (gwye-FEN-e-sin), Sodium Citrate (SOE-dee-um SI-trate), and Citric (SI-trik) Acid
11. Diphenhydramine, Codeine, and Ammonium Chloride*
12. Diphenhydramine, Dextromethorphan, and Ammonium Chloride*
13. Phenindamine (fen-IN-da-meen), Hydrocodone (hye-droe-KOE-done), and Guaifenesin
14. Pheniramine (fen-EER-a-meen), Codeine, and Guaifenesin*
15. Pheniramine, Pyrilamine (peer-ILL-a-meen), Hydrocodone, and Potassium Citrate
16. Pyrilamine, Codeine, and Terpin Hydrate (TER-pin HYE-drate)

Antihistamine, decongestant, and antitussive combinations—
17. Brompheniramine (brome-fen-EER-a-meen), Phenylephrine (fen-ill-EF-rin), Phenylpropanolamine (fen-ill-proe-pa-NOLE-a-meen), and Codeine (KOE-deen)*
18. Brompheniramine, Phenylephrine, Phenylpropanolamine, and Dextromethorphan (dex-troe-meth-OR-fan)*
19. Brompheniramine, Phenylpropanolamine, and Codeine
19a. Brompheniramine, Phenylpropanolamine, and Dextromethorphan
19b. Brompheniramine, Pseudoephedrine (soo-doe-e-FED-rin), and Dextromethorphan
20. Carbinoxamine, Pseudoephedrine and Dextromethorphan
21. Chlorpheniramine (klor-fen-EER-a-meen), Ephedrine (e-FED-rin), Phenylephrine, and Carbetapentane
22. Chlorpheniramine, Phenylephrine, and Dextromethorphan
23. Chlorpheniramine, Phenylephrine, and Hydrocodone (hye-droe-KOE-done)
24. Chlorpheniramine, Phenylephrine, Phenylpropanolamine, and Codeine
25. Chlorpheniramine, Phenylephrine, Phenylpropanolamine, and Dextromethorphan
26. Chlorpheniramine, Phenylephrine, Phenylpropanolamine, and Dihydrocodeine
26a. Chlorpheniramine, Phenylpropanolamine, and Caramiphen*
27. Chlorpheniramine, Phenylpropanolamine, and Dextromethorphan
28. Chlorpheniramine, Pseudoephedrine, and Codeine
29. Chlorpheniramine, Pseudoephedrine, and Dextromethorphan
30. Chlorpheniramine, Pseudoephedrine, and Hydrocodone
31. Diphenylpyraline (dye-fen-il-PEER-a-leen), Phenylephrine, and Codeine*
32. Diphenylpyraline, Phenylephrine, and Dextromethorphan*
33. Diphenylpyraline, Phenylephrine, and Hydrocodone*
34. Doxylamine, Phenylpropanolamine, and Dextromethorphan
35. Pheniramine, Pyrilamine (peer-ILL-a-meen), Phenylephrine, Phenylpropanolamine, and Hydrocodone
36. Pheniramine, Pyrilamine, Phenylpropanolamine, and Dextromethorphan*
37. Pheniramine, Pyrilamine, Phenylpropanolamine, and Hydrocodone*
38. Promethazine, Phenylephrine, and Codeine
39. Pyrilamine, Phenylephrine, and Codeine
40. Pyrilamine, Phenylephrine, and Dextromethorphan
41. Pyrilamine, Phenylephrine, and Hydrocodone
42. Triprolidine (trye-PROE-li-deen), Pseudoephedrine, and Codeine
43. Triprolidine, Pseudoephedrine, and Dextromethorphan*

Antihistamine, decongestant, antitussive, and analgesic combinations—
44. Chlorpheniramine (klor-fen-EER-a-meen), Phenindamine (fen-IN-da-meen), Phenylephrine (fen-ill-EF-rin), Dextromethorphan (dex-troe-meth-OR-fan), Acetaminophen (a-seat-a-MEE-noe-fen), Salicylamide (sal-i-SILL-a-mide), Caffeine, and Ascorbic (a-SKOR-bik) Acid
45. Chlorpheniramine, Pheniramine, Pyrilamine, Phenylephrine, Hydrocodone, Salicylamide, Caffeine, and Ascorbic Acid
46. Chlorpheniramine, Phenylephrine, Codeine (KOE-deen), and Acetaminophen
47. Chlorpheniramine, Phenylephrine, Dextromethorphan, Acetaminophen, and Salicylamide
48. Chlorpheniramine, Phenylephrine, Hydrocodone (hye-droe-KOE-done), Acetaminophen, and Caffeine
49. Chlorpheniramine, Phenylpropanolamine (fen-ill-proe-pa-NOLE-a-meen), Dextromethorphan, and Acetaminophen
50. Chlorpheniramine, Phenylpropanolamine, Dextromethorphan, Acetaminophen, and Caffeine
51. Chlorpheniramine, Pseudoephedrine (soo-doe-e-FED-rin), Dextromethorphan, and Acetaminophen
52. Doxylamine (dox-ILL-a-meen), Pseudoephedrine, Dextromethorphan, and Acetaminophen
53. Pheniramine, Pyrilamine (peer-ILL-a-meen), Phenylpropanolamine, Codeine, Acetaminophen, and Caffeine*
54. Pyrilamine, Phenylephrine, Dextromethorphan, and Acetaminophen
55. Pyrilamine, Phenylpropanolamine, Dextromethorphan, and Sodium Salicylate

Antihistamine, decongestant, antitussive, and expectorant combinations—
56. Brompheniramine (brome-fen-EER-a-meen), Phenylephrine (fen-ill-EF-rin), Phenylpropanolamine (fen-ill-proe-pa-NOLE-a-meen), Codeine (KOE-deen), and Guaifenesin (gwye-FEN-e-sin)*

57. Brompheniramine, Phenylephrine, Phenylpropanolamine, Hydrocodone (hye-droe-KOE-done), and Guaifenesin*
58. Chlorpheniramine, Ephedrine, Codeine, and Ammonium Chloride
59. Chlorpheniramine, Ephedrine, Phenylephrine, Dextromethorphan (dex-troe-meth-OR-fan), Ammonium Chloride, and Ipecac
60. Chlorpheniramine (klor-fen-EER-a-meen), Phenindamine (fen-IN-da-meen), Pyrilamine (peer-ILL-a-meen), Phenylephrine, Hydrocodone, and Ammonium Chloride
61. Chlorpheniramine, Phenylephrine, Codeine, and Ammonium Chloride
62. Chlorpheniramine, Phenylephrine, Codeine, Ammonium Chloride, Potassium Guaiacolsulfonate, and Sodium Citrate
63. Chlorpheniramine, Phenylephrine, Codeine, and Potassium Iodide
64. Chlorpheniramine, Phenylephrine, Dextromethorphan, and Guaifenesin
65. Chlorpheniramine, Phenylephrine, Dextromethorphan, Guaifenesin, and Ammonium Chloride
66. Chlorpheniramine, Phenylephrine, Phenylpropanolamine, Carbetapentane, and Potassium Guaiacolsulfonate
67. Chlorpheniramine, Phenylpropanolamine, Dextromethorphan, and Ammonium Chloride
68. Chlorpheniramine, Phenylpropanolamine, Dextromethorphan, Ammonium Chloride, Terpin Hydrate (TER-pin HYE-drate), and Sodium Citrate
69. Chlorpheniramine, Phenyltoloxamine (fen-ill-tole-OX-a-meen), Ephedrine (e-FED-rin), Codeine, and Guaiacol Carbonate*
70. Diphenylpyraline (dye-fen-il-PEER-a-leen), Phenylephrine, Hydrocodone, and Guaifenesin*
71. Discontinued
72. Pheniramine (fen-EER-a-meen), Pyrilamine, Phenylpropanolamine, Dextromethorphan, and Ammonium Chloride
73. Pheniramine, Pyrilamine, Phenylpropanolamine, Dextromethorphan, and Guaifenesin*
74. Pheniramine, Pyrilamine, Phenylpropanolamine, Hydrocodone, and Guaifenesin
75. Pyrilamine, Phenylephrine, Hydrocodone, and Ammonium Chloride*
76. Triprolidine (trye-PROE-li-deen), Pseudoephedrine (soo-doe-e-FED-rin), Codeine, and Guaifenesin*

Antihistamine, decongestant, antitussive, expectorant, and analgesic combinations—
77. Chlorpheniramine (klor-fen-EER-a-meen), Phenylephrine (fen-ill-EF-rin), Phenylpropanolamine (fen-ill-proe-pa-NOLE-a-meen), Dextromethorphan (dex-troe-meth-OR-fan), Guaifenesin (gwye-FEN-e-sin), and Acetaminophen (a-seat-a-MEE-noe-fen)
78. Chlorpheniramine, Phenylpropanolamine, Codeine (KOE-deen), Guaifenesin, and Acetaminophen
79. Chlorpheniramine, Phenylpropanolamine, Hydrocodone (hye-droe-KOE-done), Guaifenesin, and Salicylamide (sal-i-SILL-a-mide)
80. Chlorpheniramine, Pseudoephedrine (soo-doe-e-FED-rin), Dextromethorphan, Guaifenesin, and Aspirin
81. Pheniramine, Phenylephrine, Codeine, Sodium Citrate (SOE-dee-um SI-trate), Sodium Salicylate (sa-LI-sill-ate), and Caffeine
82. Pheniramine (fen-EER-a-meen), Pyrilamine (peer-ILL-a-meen), Phenylpropanolamine, Dextromethorphan, Terpin Hydrate (TER-pin HYE-drate), and Acetaminophen

Antihistamine, decongestant, and expectorant combinations—
83. Brompheniramine (brome-fen-EER-a-meen), Phenylephrine (fen-ill-EF-rin), Phenylpropanolamine (fen-ill-proe-pa-NOLE-a-meen), and Guaifenesin (gwye-FEN-e-sin)*
84. Carbinoxamine (kar-bi-NOX-a-meen), Pseudoephedrine (soo-doe-e-FED-rin), and Guaifenesin
85. Chlorpheniramine (klor-fen-EER-a-meen), Ephedrine (e-FED-rin), and Guaifenesin
86. Chlorpheniramine, Phenylephrine, and Guaifenesin
87. Chlorpheniramine, Phenylpropanolamine, and Guaifenesin*
88. Chlorpheniramine, Phenylpropanolamine, Guaifenesin, Sodium Citrate (SOE-dee-um SI-trate), and Citric (SI-trik) Acid
89. Chlorpheniramine, Pseudoephedrine, and Guaifenesin
90. Dexchlorpheniramine (dex-klor-fen-EER-a-meen), Pseudoephedrine, and Guaifenesin
91. Pheniramine (fen-EER-a-meen), Pyrilamine (peer-ILL-a-meen), Phenylpropanolamine, and Guaifenesin*

Antitussive and antimuscarinic combinations—
92. Hydrocodone (hye-droe-KOE-done) and Homatropine (hoe-MA-troe-peen)†

Antitussive and bronchodilator combinations—
93. Dextromethorphan (dex-troe-meth-OR-fan) and Methoxyphenamine (meth-ox-ee-FEN-a-meen)

Antitussive and expectorant combinations—
94. Codeine (KOE-deen) and Calcium Iodide (KAL-see-um EYE-oh-dyed)
95. Codeine and Guaifenesin (gwye-FEN-e-sin)
96. Codeine and Iodinated Glycerol (EYE-oh-di-nay-ted GLI-ser-ole)
97. Discontinued
98. Codeine and Terpin Hydrate (TER-pin HYE-drate)†
99. Discontinued
100. Dextromethorphan and Guaifenesin
101. Dextromethorphan and Iodinated Glycerol
102. Dextromethorphan and Terpin Hydrate†
103. Hydrocodone (hye-droe-KOE-done) and Guaifenesin
104. Hydrocodone and Potassium Guaiacolsulfonate
105. Hydromorphone (hye-droe-MOR-fone) and Guaifenesin

Decongestant and antitussive combinations—
106. Phenylephrine (fen-ill-EF-rin) and Dextromethorphan (dex-troe-meth-OR-fan)
107. Phenylpropanolamine and Caramiphen (kar-AM-i-fen)
108. Phenylpropanolamine and Dextromethorphan
109. Phenylpropanolamine and Hydrocodone (hye-droe-KOE-done)
110. Pseudoephedrine (soo-doe-e-FED-rin) and Codeine
111. Pseudoephedrine and Dextromethorphan
112. Pseudoephedrine and Hydrocodone

Decongestant, antitussive, and analgesic combinations—
113. Phenylpropanolamine (fen-ill-proe-pa-NOLE-a-meen), Dextromethorphan (dex-troe-meth-OR-fan), and Acetaminophen (a-seat-a-MEE-noe-fen)
114. Discontinued

Decongestant, antitussive, and expectorant combinations—
115. Phenylephrine, Dextromethorphan (dex-troe-meth-OR-fan), and Guaifenesin
116. Phenylephrine (fen-ill-EF-rin), Hydrocodone (hye-droe-KOE-done), and Guaifenesin (gwye-FEN-e-sin)
117. Phenylpropanolamine, Codeine (KOE-deen), and Guaifenesin
118. Phenylpropanolamine (fen-ill-proe-pa-NOLE-a-meen), Dextromethorphan, and Guaifenesin

119. Pseudoephedrine (soo-doe-e-FED-rin), Codeine, and Guaifenesin
120. Pseudoephedrine, Dextromethorphan, and Guaifenesin
121. Pseudoephedrine, Hydrocodone, and Guaifenesin

Decongestant, antitussive, expectorant, and analgesic combinations—
122. Phenylephrine (fen-ill-EF-rin), Dextromethorphan (dex-troe-meth-OR-fan), Guaifenesin (gwye-FEN-e-sin), and Acetaminophen (a-seat-a-MEE-noe-fen)
123. Pseudoephedrine (soo-doe-e-FED-rin), Dextromethorphan, Guaifenesin, and Acetaminophen

Decongestant and expectorant combinations—
124. Ephedrine (e-FED-rin) and Guaifenesin (gwye-FEN-e-sin)
125. Ephedrine and Potassium Iodide (poe-TAS-ee-um EYE-oh-dyed)
126. Phenylephrine (fen-ill-EF-rin), Phenylpropanolamine (fen-ill-proe-pa-NOLE-a-meen), and Guaifenesin
127. Phenylpropanolamine and Guaifenesin
128. Pseudoephedrine (soo-doe-e-FED-rin) and Guaifenesin

---

*Not available in the U.S.
†Generic name product available in the U.S.

To the Reader: If you do not recognize the names of medical conditions or medicines referred to in this information, check with your doctor, nurse, or pharmacist. Definitions for selected medical terms may be found in the Glossary. Brand names for the generic drug names listed can be found in the Index. In addition, selected brand names commonly associated with the generic name have been included in the text to help you recognize medicine you may be taking. The fact that a brand name product is not mentioned does not mean the information does not apply. It is a good idea for you to learn both the generic and brand names of your medicines and to write them down for future use.

Cough/cold combinations are used mainly to relieve the cough due to colds, influenza, or hay fever. They are not to be used for the chronic cough that occurs with smoking, asthma, or emphysema or when there is an unusually large amount of mucus or phlegm (pronounced flem) with the cough.

Cough/cold combination products contain more than one ingredient. For example, some products may contain an antihistamine, a decongestant, and an analgesic, in addition to a medicine for coughing. If you are treating yourself, it is important to select a product that is best for your symptoms. Also, in general, it is best to buy a product that includes only those medicines you really need. If you have questions about which product to buy, check with your pharmacist.

Since different products contain ingredients that will have different precautions and side effects, it is important that you know the ingredients of the medicine you are taking. The different kind of ingredients that may be found in cough/cold combinations include:

—**Antihistamines**

Antihistamines are used to relieve or prevent the symptoms of hay fever and other types of allergy. They also help relieve some symptoms of the common cold, such as sneezing and runny nose. They work by preventing the effects of a substance called histamine, which is produced by the body. Some examples of antihistamines contained in these combinations are: chlorpheniramine, diphenhydramine, pheniramine, promethazine, and triprolidine.

—**Decongestants**

Decongestants, such as ephedrine, phenylephrine, phenylpropanolamine (also known as PPA), and pseudoephedrine, produce a narrowing of blood vessels. This leads to clearing of nasal congestion. However, this effect may also increase blood pressure in patients who have high blood pressure.

—**Antitussives**

To help relieve coughing these combinations contain either a narcotic (codeine, dihydrocodeine, hydrocodone or hydromorphone) or a non-narcotic (carbetapentane, dextromethorphan, or noscapine) antitussive. These antitussives act directly on the cough center in the brain. Narcotics may become habit-forming, causing mental or physical dependence, if used for a long time. Physical dependence may lead to withdrawal side effects when you stop taking the medicine.

—**Expectorants**

Guaifenesin works by loosening the mucus or phlegm in the lungs. Other expectorants (for example, ammonium chloride, calcium iodide, iodinated glycerol, ipecac, potassium guaiacolsulfonate, potassium iodide, and sodium citrate) may have a similar effect, although their effectiveness has not been proven. In general, the best thing you can do to loosen mucus or phlegm is to drink plenty of water.

—**Analgesics**

Analgesics, such as acetaminophen, aspirin, and other salicylates (such as salicylamide and sodium salicylate), are used in these combination medicines to help relieve the aches and pain that may occur with the common cold.

The use of too much acetaminophen and salicylates at the same time may cause kidney damage or cancer of the kidney or urinary bladder. This may occur if large amounts of both medicines are taken together for a long period of time. However, taking the recommended amounts of combination medicines that contain both acetaminophen and a salicylate for short periods of time has not been shown to cause these unwanted effects.

There have been reports suggesting that use of aspirin in children or teenagers with fever due to a viral infection (especially flu or chickenpox) may cause a serious illness called Reye's syndrome. **Do not give medicines containing aspirin or other salicylates to a child or a teenager with symptoms of flu or chickenpox** unless you have first discussed this with your child's doctor.

—**Antimuscarinics**

Antimuscarinics such as homatropine may help produce a drying effect in the nose and chest.

—**Bronchodilators**

The bronchodilator methoxyphenamine helps relieve cough probably by increasing the flow of air through the bronchial tubes.

Some of these combinations are available only with your doctor's prescription. Others are available without a prescription; however, your doctor or pharmacist may have special instructions on the proper dose of the medicine for your medical condition.

Remember:
• **Keep all medicines out of the reach of children.**

• In order for this medicine to work, it must be used as directed. **If you are using this medicine without a prescription, it is very important that you follow the directions on the label.**

• **It is also very important that you read and understand the following information.** If any of the information causes you special concern, check with your doctor before using this medicine without a prescription.

• Before you begin using any new medicine (prescription or nonprescription) or if you develop any new medical problem while you are using this medicine, check with your doctor, nurse, or pharmacist.

• **If you have any questions** about the following information or if you want more information about this medicine or your medical problem, **ask your doctor, nurse, or pharmacist.**

Before Using This Medicine

Before you use this medicine, check with your doctor or pharmacist:

—if you have ever had any unusual or allergic reaction to any of the ingredients contained in this medicine. Also, if this medicine contains *aspirin or other salicylate*, before taking it, check with your doctor if you have ever had any unusual or allergic reaction to any of the following medicines:

   Diflunisal
   Fenoprofen
   Flurbiprofen (Oral)
   Ibuprofen
   Indomethacin
   Meclofenamate
   Mefenamic acid
   Methyl salicylate (oil of wintergreen)
   Naproxen
   Phenylbutazone
   Piroxicam
   Sulindac
   Tiaprofenic acid
   Tolmetin
   Zomepirac

—if you are on a low-salt, low-sugar, or any other special diet, or if you are allergic to any substance, such as foods, sulfites or other preservatives, or dyes. Most medicines contain more than their active ingredient, and many liquid medicines contain alcohol. Check the label or ask your doctor, nurse, or pharmacist; they can help you avoid products that may cause a problem.

—if you are **pregnant** or if you may become pregnant and your medicine contains:

• *Alcohol*—Some of these combination medicines contain a large amount of alcohol. Too much use of alcohol during pregnancy may cause birth defects.

• *Caffeine*—Studies in humans have not shown that caffeine causes birth defects. However, studies in animals have shown that caffeine causes birth defects

when given in very large doses (amounts equal to the amount of caffeine contained in 12 to 24 cups of coffee a day).

• *Codeine*—Although studies on birth defects with codeine have not been done in humans, it has not been reported to cause birth defects in humans. Codeine has not been shown to cause birth defects in animal studies, but it caused other unwanted effects. Also, regular use of narcotics during pregnancy may cause the baby to become dependent on the medicine. This may lead to withdrawal side effects after birth. In addition, narcotics may cause breathing problems in the newborn baby if taken by the mother just before delivery.

• *Hydrocodone*—Although studies on birth defects with hydrocodone have not been done in humans, it has not been reported to cause birth defects in humans. However, hydrocodone has been shown to cause birth defects in animals when given in very large doses. Also, regular use of narcotics during pregnancy may cause the baby to become dependent on the medicine. This may lead to withdrawal side effects after birth. In addition, narcotics may cause breathing problems in the newborn baby if taken by the mother just before delivery.

• *Iodides (e.g., calcium iodide and iodinated glycerol)*– Not recommended during pregnancy. Iodides have caused enlargement of the thyroid gland in the fetus and resulted in breathing problems in newborn babies whose mothers took iodides in large doses for a long period of time.

• *Phenylephrine*—Studies on birth defects have not been done in either humans or animals with decongestants such as phenylephrine.

• *Phenylpropanolamine*—Studies on birth defects have not been done in either humans or animals with decongestants such as phenylpropanolamine.

• *Pseudoephedrine*—Studies on birth defects with pseudoephedrine have not been done in humans; however, in animal studies pseudoephedrine did not cause birth defects but did cause a reduction in average weight, length, and rate of bone formation in the animal fetus when administered in high doses.

• *Salicylates (e.g., aspirin)*—Have not been shown to cause birth defects in humans. Studies on birth defects in humans have been done with aspirin, but not with salicylamide or sodium salicylate. However, salicylates have been shown to cause birth defects in animals.

Regular use of salicylates late in pregnancy may cause unwanted effects on the heart or blood flow in the fetus or newborn baby. Use of salicylates during the last 2 weeks of pregnancy may cause bleeding problems in the fetus before or during delivery, or in the newborn baby. Also, too much use of salicylates during the last 3 months of pregnancy may increase the length of pregnancy, prolong labor, cause other problems during delivery, or cause severe bleeding in the mother before, during, or after delivery.

—if you are **breast-feeding** and your medicine contains:

• *Acetaminophen*—Passes into the breast milk. However, it has not been shown to cause problems in nursing babies.

• *Alcohol*—Passes into the breast milk. However, the amount of alcohol in recommended doses of this medicine does not usually cause problems in nursing babies.

• *Antihistamines*—Small amounts pass into the breast milk. Antihistamine-containing medicine is not recommended while breast-feeding since the chances are greater for most antihistamines to cause side effects, such as unusual excitement or irritability, in the baby. Also, since antihistamines tend to decrease the secretions of the body, it is possible that the flow of breast milk may be reduced in some patients.

• *Caffeine*—Small amounts pass into the breast milk and may build up in the breast-fed baby. However, the amount of caffeine in recommended doses of this medicine does not usually cause problems in nursing babies.

• *Decongestants (e.g., phenyleprhine, phenylpropanolamine, pseudoephedrine)*—Phenylephrine and phenylpropanolamine have not been shown to cause problems in nursing babies. Pseudoephedrine passes into the breast milk and may cause unwanted side effects in nursing babies (especially newborn and premature babies) of mothers taking this medicine.

• *Iodides (e.g., calcium iodide and iodinated glycerol)*—Pass into the breast milk and may cause unwanted effects, such as underactive thyroid, in the baby.

• *Narcotic antitussives (e.g., codeine, dihydrocodeine, hydrocodone, and hydromorphone)*—Small amounts of codeine have been shown to pass into the breast milk. However, the amount of codeine or other narcotic antitussives in recommended doses of this medicine have not been shown to cause problems in nursing babies.

• *Salicylates (e.g., aspirin)*—Pass into the breast milk. However, they have not been shown to cause problems in nursing babies.

—if you have any of the following medical problems:

    Diabetes mellitus (sugar diabetes)
    Emphysema, asthma, or chronic lung disease (especially in children)
    Enlarged prostate
    Glaucoma
    Heart or blood vessel disease
    High blood pressure
    Kidney disease
    Liver disease
    Overactive thyroid
    Urinary tract blockage or problems with urination

—if you are taking a combination medicine containing *codeine, dihydrocodeine, hydrocodone,* or *hydromorphone*, and have any of the following medical problems:

    Brain disease or injury
    Colitis
    Convulsions (seizures) (history of)
    Gallbladder disease or gallstones
    Underactive thyroid

—if you are taking a combination medicine containing *aspirin* or another *salicylate* and have any of the following medical problems:

    Anemia
    Gout
    Hemophilia or other bleeding problems
    Stomach ulcer or other stomach problems

—if you are taking **any** other prescription or nonprescription (OTC) medicine (for example, aspirin or other medicine for allergies). Some medicines may change the way this medicine affects your body. Also, the effect of other medicines may be increased or reduced by some of the ingredients in this medicine. Check with your doctor or pharmacist about what medicines you should not take together with this medicine.

Proper Use of This Medicine

To help loosen mucus or phlegm in the lungs, **drink a glass of water after each dose of this medicine**, unless otherwise directed by your doctor.

Take this medicine only as directed. Do not take more of it and do not take it more often than recommended on the label, unless otherwise directed by your doctor. To do so may increase the chance of side effects.

For patients taking the extended-release capsule or tablet form of this medicine:

• Swallow it whole.

• Do not crush, break, or chew before swallowing.

• If the capsule is too large to swallow, you may mix the contents of the capsule with applesauce, jelly, honey, or syrup and swallow without chewing.

For patients taking a combination medicine containing an antihistamine and/or aspirin or other salicylate:

• Take with food or a glass of water or milk to lessen stomach irritation, if necessary.

If a combination medicine containing aspirin has a strong vinegar-like odor, do not use it. This means the medicine is breaking down. If you have any questions about this, check with your pharmacist.

If you must take this medicine regularly and you miss a dose, take it as soon as possible. However, if it is almost time for your next dose, skip the missed dose and go back to your regular dosing schedule. Do not double doses.

How to store this medicine:

- **Keep this medicine out of the reach of children** since overdose is very dangerous in young children.

- Store away from heat and direct light.

- Do not store the capsule or tablet form of this medicine in the bathroom, near the kitchen sink, or in other damp places. Heat or moisture may cause the medicine to break down.

- Keep the liquid form of this medicine from freezing. Do not refrigerate the syrup.

- Do not keep outdated medicine or medicine no longer needed. Be sure that any discarded medicine is out of the reach of children.

Precautions While Using This Medicine

If your cough has not improved after 7 days or if you have a high fever, skin rash, continuing headache, or sore throat with the cough, check with your doctor. These signs may mean that you have other medical problems.

For patients taking antihistamine-containing medicine:

- Tell the doctor in charge that you are taking this medicine before you have any skin tests for allergies. The results of the test may be affected by the antihistamine in this medicine.

- This medicine will add to the effects of alcohol and other CNS depressants (medicines that slow down the nervous system, possibly causing drowsiness). Some examples of CNS depressants are antihistamines or medicine for hay fever, other allergies, or colds; sedatives, tranquilizers, or sleeping medicine; prescription pain medicine or narcotics; barbiturates; medicine for convulsions (seizures); muscle relaxants; or anesthetics, including some dental anesthetics. **Check with your doctor before taking any of the above while you are taking this medicine.**

- This medicine may cause some people to become drowsy, dizzy, or less alert than they are normally. **Make sure you know how you react to this medicine before you drive, use machines, or do other jobs that require you to be alert.**

- When taking antihistamines on a regular basis, make sure your doctor knows if you are taking large amounts of aspirin at the same time (as in arthritis or rheumatism). Effects of too much aspirin, such as ringing in the ears, may be covered up by the antihistamine.

For patients taking decongestant-containing medicine:

- This medicine may add to the central nervous system (CNS) stimulant and other effects of phenylpropanolamine (PPA)-containing diet aids. **Do not use medicines for diet or appetite control while taking this medicine unless you have checked with your doctor.**

- This medicine may cause some people to be nervous or restless or to have trouble in sleeping. If you have trouble in sleeping, **take the last dose of this medicine for each day a few hours before bedtime.** If you have any questions about this, check with your doctor.

- Before having any kind of surgery (including dental surgery) or emergency treatment, tell the physician or dentist in charge that you are taking this medicine.

For patients taking narcotic antitussive (codeine, dihydrocodeine, hydrocodone, or hydromorphone)–containing medicine:

- This medicine will add to the effects of alcohol and other CNS depressants (medicines that slow down the nervous system, possibly causing drowsiness). Some examples of CNS depressants are antihistamines or medicine for hay fever, other allergies, or colds; sedatives, tranquilizers, or sleeping medicine; prescription pain medicine or narcotics; barbiturates; medicine for convulsions (seizures); muscle relaxants; or anesthetics, including some dental anesthetics. **Check with your doctor before taking any of the above while you are taking this medicine.**

- This medicine may cause some people to become drowsy, dizzy, or less alert than they are normally. **Make sure you know how you react to this medicine before you drive, use machines, or do other jobs that require you to be alert.**

- Nausea or vomiting may occur after taking a narcotic antitussive. This effect may go away if you lie down for a while. However, if nausea or vomiting continues, check with your doctor.

- Dizziness, lightheadedness, or fainting may be especially likely to occur when you get up suddenly from a lying or sitting position. Getting up slowly may help lessen this problem.

- Before having any kind of surgery (including dental surgery) or emergency treatment, tell the physician or dentist in charge that you are taking this medicine.

For patients taking iodide (calcium iodide, iodinated glycerol, or potassium iodide)-containing medicine:

- Make sure your doctor knows if you are planning to have any future thyroid tests. The results of the thyroid test may be affected by the iodine in this medicine.

For patients taking analgesic-containing medicine:

- **Check the label of all over-the-counter (OTC), nonprescription, and prescription medicines you now take.** If any contain acetaminophen or aspirin or other salicylates, including diflunisal or bismuth subsalicylate, be especially careful. Taking them while taking a cough/cold combination medicine which already contains them may lead to overdose. If you have any questions about this, check with your doctor or pharmacist.

- Do not take aspirin-containing medicine for 5 days before any surgery, including dental surgery, unless otherwise directed by your physician or dentist. Taking aspirin during this time may cause bleeding problems.

For diabetic patients taking aspirin- or sodium salicylate–containing medicine:

- False urine sugar test results may occur if you take 8 or more 325-mg (5-grain) doses of aspirin or sodium salicylate every day for several days in a row. Smaller doses or occasional use of aspirin or sodium salicylate usually will not affect urine sugar tests. If you have any questions about this, check with your doctor, nurse, or pharmacist, especially if your diabetes is not well controlled.

For patients taking homatropine-containing medicine:

• This medicine may make you sweat less, causing your body temperature to increase. **Use extra care not to become overheated during exercise or hot weather while you are taking this medicine,** since overheating may result in heat stroke.

Side Effects of This Medicine

Along with its needed effects, a medicine may cause some unwanted effects. Although serious side effects occur rarely when this medicine is taken as recommended, they may be more likely to occur if:

—too much medicine is taken.
—it is taken in large doses.
—it is taken for a long period of time.

Get emergency help immediately if any of the following signs of overdose occur:

For narcotic antitussive (codeine, dihydrocodeine, hydrocodone, or hydromorphone)–containing

Cold, clammy skin
Confusion (severe)
Convulsions (seizures)
Drowsiness or dizziness (severe)
Nervousness or restlessness (severe)
Pinpoint pupils of eyes
Slow heartbeat
Slow or troubled breathing
Weakness (severe)

For acetaminophen-containing

Diarrhea
Increase in sweating
Loss of appetite
Nausea or vomiting
Stomach cramps or pain
Swelling or tenderness in the upper abdomen or stomach area

For salicylate-containing

Any loss of hearing
Bloody urine
Confusion
Convulsions (seizures)
Diarrhea (severe)
Dizziness or lightheadedness
Drowsiness (severe)
Excitement or nervousness (severe)
Fast or deep breathing
Fever
Hallucinations (seeing, hearing, or feeling things that are not there)
Increase in sweating
Nausea or vomiting (severe or continuing)
Shortness of breath or troubled breathing (for salicylamide only)
Stomach pain (severe or continuing)

Uncontrollable flapping movements of the hands, especially in elderly patients
Unusual thirst
Vision problems

For decongestant-containing

Fast, pounding, or irregular heartbeat
Headache (continuing and severe)
Nausea or vomiting (severe)
Nervousness or restlessness (severe)
Shortness of breath or troubled breathing (severe or continuing)

Also, check with your doctor as soon as possible if any of the following side effects occur:

For antihistamine- or antimuscarinic-containing

Clumsiness or unsteadiness
Convulsions (seizures)
Drowsiness (severe)
Dryness of mouth, nose, or throat (severe)
Flushing or redness of face
Hallucinations (seeing, hearing, or feeling things that are not there)
Restlessness (severe)
Shortness of breath or troubled breathing
Slow or fast heartbeat

For iodine-containing

Headache (continuing)
Increase in salivation
Loss of appetite
Metallic taste
Skin rash, hives, or redness
Sore throat
Swelling of face, lips, or eyelids

For bronchodilator-containing

Chest pain (severe)
Dizziness (severe)
Fast, pounding, or irregular heartbeat
Headache (continuing or severe)
Increase in blood pressure
Nausea or vomiting (severe)

Other side effects may occur that usually do not require medical attention. These side effects may go away during treatment as your body adjusts to the medicine. However, check with your doctor if any of the following side effects continue or are bothersome:

Constipation
Difficult or painful urination
Dizziness or lightheadedness
Drowsiness
Dryness of mouth, nose, or throat
False sense of well-being
Nausea or vomiting
Nightmares
Skin rash
Trouble in sleeping
Unusual excitement, nervousness, restlessness, or irritability

Although not all of the side effects listed above have been reported for all of these medicines, they have been reported for at least one of them. However, since there are some similarities among these combination medicines, many of the above side effects may occur with any of these medicines.

For children or elderly patients: Very young children and elderly patients are usually more sensitive to the effects of this medicine.

Other side effects not listed above may also occur in some patients. If you notice any other effects, check with your doctor.

December 1987

CROMOLYN (Inhalation)

Some commonly used brand names or other names are Fivent*, Intal, and Sodium Cromoglycate.

*Not available in the U.S.

To the Reader: If you do not recognize the names of medical conditions or medicines referred to in this information, check with your doctor, nurse, or pharmacist. Definitions for selected medical terms may be found in the Glossary. Brand names for the generic drug names listed can be found in the Index. In addition, selected brand names commonly associated with the generic name have been included in the text to help you recognize medicine you may be taking. The fact that a brand name product is not mentioned does not mean the information does not apply. It is a good idea for you to learn both the generic and brand names of your medicines and to write them down for future use.

Cromolyn (KROE-moe-lin) is taken by oral inhalation to prevent asthma attacks. It is also used before and during exposure to substances that cause allergic reactions to prevent bronchospasm (wheezing or difficulty in breathing). In addition, this medicine is used to prevent bronchospasm caused by exercise.

Cromolyn inhalation works by acting on certain cells in the body, called mast cells, to prevent them from releasing substances that cause the asthma or bronchospasm attack.

Cromolyn will not help an asthma attack that has already started. If this medicine is used during a severe attack, it may cause irritation and make the attack worse.

This medicine is available only with your doctor's prescription.

Remember:

• **This medicine has been prescribed for your current medical problem only.** It must not be given to other people or used for other problems unless you are directed to do so by your doctor.

• **Keep all medicines out of the reach of children.**

• In order for this medicine to work, it must be used as directed.

• **It is very important that you read and understand the following information.** If any of the information causes you special concern, do not decide against using this medicine without first checking with your doctor.

• Before you begin using any new medicine (prescription or nonprescription) or if you develop any new medical problem while you are using this medicine, check with your doctor, nurse, or pharmacist.

• **If you have any questions** about the following information or if you want more information about this medicine or your medical problem, **ask your doctor, nurse, or pharmacist.**

Before Using This Medicine

In order to decide on the best treatment for your medical problem, your doctor should be told:

—if you have ever had any unusual or allergic reaction to cromolyn.

—if you are using the aerosol form of cromolyn and you have ever had any unusual or allergic reaction to other inhalation aerosols.

—if you are using the capsule form of cromolyn for oral inhalation and you have ever had any unusual or allergic reaction to lactose, milk, or milk products.

—if you are **pregnant** or if you may become pregnant. Studies have not been done in humans. However, studies in animals have shown that cromolyn causes a decrease in successful pregnancies and a decrease in the weight of the animal fetus when given by injection in very large amounts.

—if you are **breast-feeding**. It is not known whether cromolyn passes into the breast milk. This medicine has not been shown to cause problems in nursing babies.

—if you have any of the following medical problems:
Heart disease (or history of) (for aerosol only)
Kidney disease
Liver disease

Proper Use of This Medicine

Cromolyn oral inhalation is used to prevent asthma or bronchospasm (wheezing or difficulty in breathing) attacks. It will not relieve an attack that has already started. If this medicine is used during a severe attack, it may cause irritation and make the attack worse.

For patients using cromolyn aerosol:

• This medicine usually comes with patient directions. Read them carefully before using this medicine.

• Keep the spray away from the eyes because it may cause irritation.

For patients using cromolyn capsules for inhalation:

• This medicine is used with a special inhaler and usually comes with patient directions. Read the directions carefully before using.

• **Do not swallow the capsules because the medicine will not work if you swallow it.**

For patients using cromolyn solution for inhalation:

• Use this medicine only in a power-operated nebulizer with an adequate flow rate and equipped with a face mask or mouthpiece. Make sure you understand exactly how to use it. Hand-operated nebulizers are not suitable for using this medicine. If you have any questions about this, check with your doctor.

Use cromolyn oral inhalation only as directed. Do not use more of it and do not use it more often than your doctor ordered. To do so may increase the chance of side effects.

For patients using cromolyn oral inhalation regularly (for example, every day):

- **In order for cromolyn to work properly, it must be inhaled every day in regularly spaced doses as ordered by your doctor.** Up to 4 weeks may pass before you feel the full effects of the medicine.

- If you miss a dose of this medicine, take it as soon as possible. Then take any remaining doses for that day at regularly spaced intervals. Do not double doses.

How to store this medicine:

- **Keep out of the reach of children.**

- Store away from heat.

- Store the capsule or solution form of this medicine away from direct light. Store the aerosol form of this medicine away from direct sunlight.

- Do not store the capsule form of this medicine in the bathroom, near the kitchen sink, or in other damp places. Heat or moisture may cause the medicine to break down.

- Keep the aerosol or solution form of this medicine from freezing.

- Do not puncture, break, or burn the aerosol container, even if it is empty.

- Do not keep outdated medicine or medicine no longer needed. Be sure that any discarded medicine is out of the reach of children.

Precautions While Using This Medicine

If your symptoms do not improve or if your condition gets worse, check with your doctor.

If you are also taking an adrenocorticoid (cortisone-like medicine, such as cortisone or prednisone) for your asthma along with this medicine, do not stop taking the adrenocorticoid even if your asthma seems better, unless you are told to do so by your doctor.

If you are also using a bronchodilator inhaler to help you breathe better, use the bronchodilator first. Then wait about 5 minutes before using cromolyn, unless otherwise directed by your doctor. In order to lessen the chance of unwanted effects, it is best not to use the two kinds of aerosols too close together. If your bronchodilator does not seem to be working or if you have any questions, check with your doctor.

Dryness of the mouth or throat, throat irritation, and hoarseness may occur after using this medicine. Gargling and rinsing the mouth after each dose may help prevent these effects.

Side Effects of This Medicine

Along with its needed effects, a medicine may cause some unwanted effects. Although not all of these side effects may occur, if they do occur they may need medical attention.

Check with your doctor as soon as possible if any of the following side effects occur:
Less common
    Difficult or painful urination
    Dizziness
    Frequent urge to urinate
    Headache (severe or continuing)
    Increased wheezing
    Joint pain or swelling
    Muscle pain or weakness
    Nausea or vomiting
    Skin rash, hives, or itching
    Swelling of the lips and eyes
    Tightness in chest
    Troubled breathing
    Trouble in swallowing
Rare
    Chest pain
    Chills
    Difficulty in breathing (severe)
    Sweating
    Wheezing (severe)

Other side effects may occur that usually do not require medical attention. These side effects may go away during treatment as your body adjusts to the medicine. However, check with your doctor if any of the following side effects continue or are bothersome:
More common
    Cough
    Hoarseness
Less common
    Dryness of the mouth or throat
    Sneezing
    Stuffy nose
    Throat irritation
    Watering of the eyes

If you are using cromolyn aerosol, you may notice an unpleasant taste. This may be expected and will go away when you stop using the medicine.

For elderly patients: Many medicines have not been tested in older people. Therefore, it is not known whether the medicine acts the same way it does in younger adults. Check with your doctor or pharmacist if you notice any unusual effects while using this medicine or if you think it is not working as it should.

Other side effects not listed above may also occur in some patients. If you notice any other effects, check with your doctor.

December 1987

CROMOLYN (Nasal)

Some commonly used brand names or other names are Nasalcrom, Rynacrom*, and Sodium Cromoglycate.

---

*Not commercially available in the U.S.

To the Reader: If you do not recognize the names of medical conditions or medicines referred to in this information, check with your doctor, nurse, or pharmacist. Definitions for selected medical terms may be found in the Glossary. Brand names for the generic drug names listed can be found in the Index. In addition, selected brand names commonly associated with the generic name have been included in the text to help you recognize medicine you may be taking. The fact that a brand name product is not mentioned does not mean the information does not apply. It is a good idea for you to learn both the generic and brand names of your medicines and to write them down for future use.

Cromolyn (KROE-moe-lin) nasal solution is used in the nose to prevent or treat the symptoms (sneezing, wheezing, runny nose, itching) of seasonal (short-term) or chronic (long-term) allergic rhinitis. Cromolyn powder for nasal inhalation is used in the nose to prevent seasonal (short-term) allergic rhinitis.

This medicine works by acting on certain cells in the body, called mast cells, to prevent them from releasing substances that cause the allergic reaction.

When cromolyn is used to treat chronic (long-term) allergic rhinitis, an antihistamine and/or a nasal decongestant may be used with this medicine, especially during the first few weeks of treatment.

Cromolyn nasal solution and cromolyn powder for nasal inhalation are available only with your doctor's prescription.

Remember:

• **This medicine has been prescribed for your current medical problem only.** It must not be given to other people or used for other problems unless you are directed to do so by your doctor.

• **Keep all medicines out of the reach of children.**

• In order for this medicine to work, it must be used as directed.

• **It is very important that you read and understand the following information.** If any of the information causes you special concern, do not decide against using this medicine without first checking with your doctor.

• Before you begin using any new medicine (prescription or nonprescription) or if you develop any new medical problem while you are using this medicine, check with your doctor, nurse, or pharmacist.

• **If you have any questions** about the following information or if you want more information about this medicine or your medical problem, **ask your doctor, nurse, or pharmacist.**

Before Using This Medicine

In order to decide on the best treatment for your medical problem, your doctor should be told:

—if you have ever had any unusual or allergic reaction to cromolyn.

—if you are **pregnant** or if you may become pregnant. Studies have not been done in humans. However, studies in animals have shown that cromolyn causes a decrease in successful pregnancies and a decrease in the weight of the animal fetus when given by injection in very large amounts.

—if you are **breast-feeding**. It is not known whether cromolyn passes into the breast milk. This medicine has not been shown to cause problems in nursing babies.

—if you have any of the following medical problems:
Kidney disease
Liver disease
Polyps or growths inside the nose

Proper Use of This Medicine

This medicine usually comes with patient directions. Read them carefully before using.

Before using this medicine, clear the nasal passages by blowing nose.

For patients using cromolyn nasal solution:

• Cromolyn nasal solution is used with a special spray device. Cleaning of this device is not recommended. The spray device should be replaced every 6 months.

For patients using cromolyn powder for nasal inhalation:

• This medicine is used with a special inhaler. Be sure you understand exactly how to use it.

Use this medicine only as directed. Do not use more of it and do not use it more often than your doctor ordered. To do so may increase the chance of side effects.

In order for this medicine to work properly, it must be used every day in regularly spaced doses as ordered by your doctor.

For patients using cromolyn for seasonal (short-term) allergic rhinitis:

• Up to 1 week may pass before you begin to feel better.

For patients using cromolyn for chronic (long-term) allergic rhinitis:

• Up to 4 weeks may pass before you feel the full effects of this medicine.

If you miss a dose of this medicine, use it as soon as possible. Then use any remaining doses for that day at regularly spaced intervals. Do not double doses.

How to store this medicine:

• **Keep out of the reach of children.**

• Store away from heat and direct light.

• Store the powder form of this medicine in a dry place. Do not store it in the bathroom, near the kitchen sink, or in other damp places. Heat or moisture may cause the medicine to break down.

• Keep the solution form of this medicine from freezing.

• Do not keep outdated medicine or medicine no longer needed. Be sure that any discarded medicine is out of the reach of children.

Precautions While Using This Medicine

If your symptoms do not improve or if your condition gets worse, check with your doctor.

Side Effects of This Medicine

Along with its needed effects, a medicine may cause some unwanted effects. Although not all of these side effects may occur, if they do occur they may need medical attention.

Check with your doctor as soon as possible if any of the following side effects occur:

Rare
   Coughing
   Difficulty in swallowing
   Nosebleed
   Skin rash, hives, or itching
   Swelling of face, lips, or eyelids
   Wheezing or difficulty in breathing

Other side effects may occur that usually do not require medical attention. These side effects may go away during treatment as your body adjusts to the medicine. However, check with your doctor if any of the following side effects continue or are bothersome:

More common
   Burning, stinging, or irritation inside of nose
   Increase in sneezing

Less common
   Headache
   Postnasal drip
   Unpleasant taste

For elderly patients: Many medicines have not been tested in older people. Therefore, it is not known whether the medicine acts the same way it does in younger adults. Check with your doctor or pharmacist if you notice any unusual effects while using this medicine or if you think it is not working as it should.

Other side effects not listed above may also occur in some patients. If you notice any other effects, check with your doctor.

December 1987

CROMOLYN (Ophthalmic)

Some commonly used brand names or other names are Opticrom and Sodium Cromoglycate.

To the Reader: If you do not recognize the names of medical conditions or medicines referred to in this information, check with your doctor, nurse, or pharmacist. Definitions for selected medical terms may be found in the Glossary. Brand names for the generic drug names listed can be found in the Index. In addition, selected brand names commonly associated with the generic name have been included in the text to help you recognize medicine you may be taking. The fact that a brand name product is not mentioned does not mean the information does not apply. It is a good idea for you to learn both the generic and brand names of your medicines and to write them down for future use.

Cromolyn (KROE-moe-lin) ophthalmic solution is used in the eye to treat certain disorders of the eye caused by allergies. It works by acting on certain cells, called mast cells, to prevent them from releasing substances that cause the allergic reaction.

Cromolyn is available only with your doctor's prescription.

Remember:

• **This medicine has been prescribed for your current medical problem only.** It must not be given to other people or used for other problems unless you are directed to do so by your doctor.

• **Keep all medicines out of the reach of children.**

• In order for this medicine to work, it must be used as directed.

• **It is very important that you read and understand the following information.** If any of the information causes you special concern, do not decide against using this medicine without first checking with your doctor.

• Before you begin using any new medicine (prescription or nonprescription) or if you develop any new medical problem while you are using this medicine, check with your doctor, nurse, or pharmacist.

• **If you have any questions** about the following information or if you want more information about this medicine or your medical problem, **ask your doctor, nurse, or pharmacist.**

Before Using This Medicine

In order to decide on the best treatment for your medical problem, your doctor should be told:

—if you have ever had any unusual or allergic reaction to cromolyn.

—if you are allergic to any substance, such as preservatives. Most medicines contain more than their active ingredient. Your doctor, nurse, or pharmacist can help you avoid products that may cause a problem.

—if you are **pregnant** or if you may become pregnant. Studies have not been done in humans. However, studies in animals have shown that cromolyn causes a decrease in successful pregnancies and a decrease in the

weight of the animal fetus when given by injection in very large amounts. It is unlikely that cromolyn will cause problems in humans when used in the eye as directed.

—if you are **breast-feeding**. It is not known whether cromolyn passes into the breast milk. This medicine has not been shown to cause problems in nursing babies.

Proper Use of This Medicine

How to apply this medicine: First, wash your hands. Then tilt the head back and pull the lower eyelid away from the eye to form a pouch. Drop the medicine into the pouch and gently close the eyes. Do not blink. Keep the eyes closed for 1 or 2 minutes to allow the medicine to be absorbed.

To prevent contamination of the eye drops, do not touch the applicator tip to any surface (including the eye) and keep the container tightly closed.

Use cromolyn eye drops only as directed. Do not use more of this medicine and do not use it more often than your doctor ordered. To do so may increase the chance of side effects.

In order for this medicine to work properly, it must be used every day in regularly spaced doses as ordered by your doctor. A few days may pass before you begin to feel better.

If you miss a dose of this medicine, apply it as soon as possible. Then go back to your regular dosing schedule.

How to store this medicine:

• **Keep out of the reach of children.**

• Store away from heat and direct light.

• Keep the medicine from freezing.

• Do not keep outdated medicine or medicine no longer needed. Be sure that any discarded medicine is out of the reach of children.

Precautions While Using This Medicine

If your symptoms do not improve or if your condition gets worse, check with your doctor.

Side Effects of This Medicine

Along with its needed effects, a medicine may cause some unwanted effects. Although not all of these side effects may occur, if they do occur they may need medical attention.

Check with your doctor as soon as possible if either of the following side effects occurs:

Rare

Eye irritation not present before using this medicine, including styes

Swelling of conjunctiva (in eye) (severe)

© 1988   The United States Pharmacopeial Convention, Inc.

Other side effects may occur that usually do not require medical attention. These side effects may go away during treatment as your body adjusts to the medicine. However, check with your doctor if any of the following side effects continue or are bothersome:

More common

Burning or stinging of eye (mild and temporary)

Less common or rare

Dryness or puffiness around the eye
Watering or itching of eye (increased)

For elderly patients: Many medicines have not been tested in older people. Therefore, it is not known whether the medicine acts the same way it does in younger adults. Check with your doctor or pharmacist if you notice any unusual effects while using this medicine or if you think it is not working as it should.

Other side effects not listed above may also occur in some patients. If you notice any other effects, check with your doctor.

December 1987

CROMOLYN (Oral)*

Some commonly used brand names or other names are Nalcrom* and Sodium Cromoglycate.

---

*Not commercially available in the U.S.

To the Reader: If you do not recognize the names of medical conditions or medicines referred to in this information, check with your doctor, nurse, or pharmacist. Definitions for selected medical terms may be found in the Glossary. Brand names for the generic drug names listed can be found in the Index. In addition, selected brand names commonly associated with the generic name have been included in the text to help you recognize medicine you may be taking. The fact that a brand name product is not mentioned does not mean the information does not apply. It is a good idea for you to learn both the generic and brand names of your medicines and to write them down for future use.

Cromolyn (KROE-moe-lin) is taken by mouth to treat the symptoms of mastocytosis. It may also be used to prevent the symptoms of food allergies. It works by acting on certain cells in the body, called mast cells, to prevent them from releasing substances that cause the symptoms of these conditions.

Cromolyn is available only with your doctor's prescription.

Remember:

• **This medicine has been prescribed for your current medical problem only.** It must not be given to other people or used for other problems unless you are directed to do so by your doctor.

• **Keep all medicines out of the reach of children.**

• In order for this medicine to work, it must be used as directed.

• **It is very important that you read and understand the following information.** If any of the information causes you special concern, do not decide against using this medicine without first checking with your doctor.

• Before you begin using any new medicine (prescription or nonprescription) or if you develop any new medical problem while you are using this medicine, check with your doctor, nurse, or pharmacist.

• **If you have any questions** about the following information or if you want more information about this medicine or your medical problem, **ask your doctor, nurse, or pharmacist.**

Before Using This Medicine

In order to decide on the best treatment for your medical problem, your doctor should be told:

—if you have ever had any unusual or allergic reaction to cromolyn, lactose, milk, or milk products.

—if you are on a low-salt, low-sugar, or any other special diet, or if you are allergic to any substance, such as foods, sulfites or other preservatives, or dyes. Most medicines contain more than their active ingredient, and many liquid medicines contain alcohol. Your doctor, nurse, or pharmacist can help you avoid products that may cause a problem.

—if you are **pregnant** or if you may become pregnant. Studies have not been done in humans. However, studies in animals have shown that cromolyn causes a decrease in successful pregnancies and a decrease in the weight of the animal fetus when given by injection in very large amounts.

—if you are **breast-feeding**. It is not known whether cromolyn passes into the breast milk. This medicine has not been shown to cause problems in nursing babies.

—if you have either of the following medical problems:
Kidney disease
Liver disease

Proper Use of This Medicine

Take cromolyn only as directed. Do not take more of it and do not take it more often than your doctor ordered. To do so may increase the chance of side effects.

If you miss a dose of this medicine, take it as soon as possible. Then take any remaining doses for that day at regularly spaced intervals. Do not double doses.

How to store this medicine:

• **Keep out of the reach of children.**

• Store away from heat and direct light.

• Do not store the capsule form of this medicine in the bathroom, near the kitchen sink, or in other damp places. Heat or moisture may cause the medicine to break down.

• Keep the liquid form of this medicine from freezing.

• Do not keep outdated medicine or medicine no longer needed. Be sure that any discarded medicine is out of the reach of children.

Precautions While Using This Medicine

If your symptoms do not improve or if your condition gets worse, check with your doctor.

Side Effects of This Medicine

Along with its needed effects, a medicine may cause some unwanted effects. Although not all of these side effects may occur, if they do occur they may need medical attention.

Check with your doctor as soon as possible if the following side effect occurs:

Less common
Skin rash

Other side effects may occur that usually do not require medical attention. These side effects may go away during treatment as your body adjusts to the medicine. However, check with your doctor if any of the following side effects continue or are bothersome:

Less common
Headache
Joint pain
Nausea
Trouble in sleeping

For elderly patients: Many medicines have not been tested in older people. Therefore, it is not known whether the medicine acts the same way it does in younger adults. Check with your doctor or pharmacist if you notice any unusual effects while taking this medicine or if you think it is not working as it should.

Other side effects not listed above may also occur in some patients. If you notice any other effects, check with your doctor.

December 1987

CROTAMITON (Topical)

A commonly used brand name is Eurax.

To the Reader: If you do not recognize the names of medical conditions or medicines referred to in this information, check with your doctor, nurse, or pharmacist. Definitions for selected medical terms may be found in the Glossary. Brand names for the generic drug names listed can be found in the Index. In addition, selected brand names commonly associated with the generic name have been included in the text to help you recognize medicine you may be taking. The fact that a brand name product is not mentioned does not mean the information does not apply. It is a good idea for you to learn both the generic and brand names of your medicines and to write them down for future use.

Crotamiton (kroe-TAM-i-tonn) is applied to the skin to treat scabies infection. It is also used to relieve the itching of certain skin conditions.

This medicine is available only with your doctor's prescription.

Remember:

• **This medicine has been prescribed for your current medical problem only.** It must not be given to other people or used for other problems unless you are directed to do so by your doctor.

• **Keep all medicines out of the reach of children.**

• In order for this medicine to work, it must be used as directed.

• **It is very important that you read and understand the following information.** If any of the information causes you special concern, do not decide against using this medicine without first checking with your doctor.

• Before you begin using any new medicine (prescription or nonprescription) or if you develop any new medical problem while you are using this medicine, check with your doctor, nurse, or pharmacist.

• **If you have any questions** about the following information or if you want more information about this medicine or your medical problem, **ask your doctor, nurse, or pharmacist.**

Before Using This Medicine

In order to decide on the best treatment for your medical problem, your doctor should be told:

—if you have ever had any unusual or allergic reaction to crotamiton.

—if you are **pregnant** or if you may become pregnant. Studies have not been done in either humans or animals.

—if you are **breast-feeding,** although topical crotamiton has not been shown to cause problems in nursing babies.

—if you have severely inflamed skin or raw oozing areas of the skin.

Proper Use of This Medicine

Keep crotamiton away from the mouth. It may be harmful if swallowed.

Use this medicine only as directed. Do not use more of it and do not use it more often than your doctor ordered. To do so may increase the chance of side effects.

Keep crotamiton away from the eyes and other mucous membranes, such as the inside of the nose. It may cause irritation. If you should accidentally get some in your eyes, flush them thoroughly with water at once.

This medicine usually comes with patient directions. Read them carefully before using.

If you take a bath or shower before using this medicine, dry the skin well before applying crotamiton.

For patients using this medicine for scabies:

• Apply enough medicine to cover the entire skin surface from the chin down, and rub in well. This applies especially to folds and creases in the skin and to the hands, feet (including the soles), between fingers and toes, and moist areas (such as underarms and groin).

• Do not wash off the first coat of this medicine.

• Apply a second coat of this medicine 24 hours after the first one.

• Then, 48 hours after the second application of this medicine, take a cleansing bath to remove the medicine.

• Put on freshly washed or dry-cleaned clothing and change bedding in order to prevent reinfection.

• Your sexual partner, especially, and all members of your household may need to be treated also, since the infection may spread to persons in close contact. If these persons are not being treated or if you have any questions about this, check with your doctor.

How to store this medicine:

• **Keep out of the reach of children.**

• Store away from heat and direct light.

• Keep the medicine from freezing.

• Do not keep outdated medicine or medicine no longer needed. Be sure that any discarded medicine is out of the reach of children.

Precautions While Using This Medicine

If your condition does not improve or if it becomes worse, check with your doctor.

For patients using this medicine for scabies:

• To prevent reinfection or spreading of the infection to other people, good health habits are also required. These include machine washing all underwear, pajamas, sheets, pillowcases, towels, and washcloths in very hot water and drying them using the hot cycle of a dryer. Clothing or bedding that cannot be washed in this way should be dry cleaned.

Side Effects of This Medicine

Along with its needed effects, a medicine may cause some unwanted effects. Although not all of these side effects may occur, if they do occur they may need medical attention.

Check with your doctor as soon as possible if either of the following side effects occur:

Rare
Skin irritation not present before using this medicine
Skin rash

For elderly patients: Many medicines have not been tested in older people. Therefore, it is not known whether the medicine acts the same way it does in younger adults. Check with your doctor or pharmacist if you notice any unusual effects while using this medicine or if you think it is not working as it should.

Other side effects not listed above may also occur in some patients. If you notice any other effects, check with your doctor.

December 1987

CYCLANDELATE (Systemic)

A commonly used brand name is Cyclospasmol.

Generic name product may also be available in the U.S.

To the Reader: If you do not recognize the names of medical conditions or medicines referred to in this information, check with your doctor, nurse, or pharmacist. Definitions for selected medical terms may be found in the Glossary. Brand names for the generic drug names listed can be found in the Index. In addition, selected brand names commonly associated with the generic name have been included in the text to help you recognize medicine you may be taking. The fact that a brand name product is not mentioned does not mean the information does not apply. It is a good idea for you to learn both the generic and brand names of your medicines and to write them down for future use.

Cyclandelate (sye-KLAN-de-late) belongs to the group of medicines commonly called vasodilators. These medicines increase the size of blood vessels. Cyclandelate is used to treat problems resulting from poor blood circulation.

Cyclandelate is available only with your doctor's prescription.

Remember:

• **This medicine has been prescribed for your current medical problem only.** It must not be given to other people or used for other problems unless you are directed to do so by your doctor.

• **Keep all medicines out of the reach of children.**

• In order for this medicine to work, it must be used as directed.

• **It is very important that you read and understand the following information.** If any of the information causes you special concern, do not decide against using this medicine without first checking with your doctor.

• Before you begin using any new medicine (prescription or nonprescription) or if you develop any new medical problem while you are using this medicine, check with your doctor, nurse, or pharmacist.

• **If you have any questions** about the following information or if you want more information about this medicine or your medical problem, **ask your doctor, nurse, or pharmacist.**

Before Using This Medicine

In order to decide on the best treatment for your medical problem, your doctor should be told:

—if you have ever had any unusual or allergic reaction to cyclandelate.

—if you are on a low-salt, low-sugar, or any other special diet, or if you are allergic to any substance, such as foods, sulfites or other preservatives, or dyes. Most medicines contain more than their active ingredient. Your doctor, nurse, or pharmacist can help you avoid products that may cause a problem.

—if you are **pregnant** or if you may become pregnant. Studies have not been done in either humans or animals.

—if you are **breast-feeding**. Cyclandelate has not been shown to cause problems in nursing babies.

—if you have any of the following medical problems:
Angina (chest pain)
Bleeding problems
Glaucoma
Hardening of the arteries

—if you have recently had a heart attack or stroke.

—if you are taking **any** other prescription or nonprescription (OTC) medicine.

—if you smoke.

Proper Use of This Medicine

If this medicine upsets your stomach, it may be taken with meals, milk, or antacids.

If you miss a dose of this medicine, take it as soon as you remember. Then go back to your regular dosing schedule. However, if it is almost time for your next dose, skip the missed dose and go back to your regular dosing schedule. Do not double doses.

How to store this medicine:

• **Keep out of the reach of children.**

• Store away from heat and direct light.

• Do not store in the bathroom, near the kitchen sink, or in other damp places. Heat or moisture may cause the medicine to break down.

• Do not keep outdated medicine or medicine no longer needed. Be sure that any discarded medicine is out of the reach of children.

Precautions While Using This Medicine

It may take some time for this medicine to work. If you feel that the medicine is not working, do not stop taking it on your own. Instead, check with your doctor.

The helpful effects of this medicine may be decreased if you smoke.

Dizziness may occur, especially when you get up from a lying or sitting position or climb stairs. Getting up slowly may help. If this problem continues or gets worse, check with your doctor.

Side Effects of This Medicine

Along with its needed effects, a medicine may cause some unwanted effects. The following side effects may go away during treatment as your body adjusts to the medicine. However, check with your doctor if any of these effects continue or are bothersome:

Less common
Belching, heartburn, nausea, or stomach pain
Dizziness
Fast heartbeat
Flushing of the face
Headache
Sweating
Tingling sensation in face, fingers, or toes
Weakness

For elderly patients: Many medicines have not been tested in older people. Therefore, it is not known whether the medicine acts the same way it does in younger adults. Check with your doctor or pharmacist if you notice any unusual effects while taking this medicine or if you think it is not working as it should.

Other side effects not listed above may also occur in some patients. If you notice any other effects, check with your doctor.

———————

December 1987

CYCLOBENZAPRINE (Systemic)

A commonly used brand name is Flexeril.

To the Reader: If you do not recognize the names of medical conditions or medicines referred to in this information, check with your doctor, nurse, or pharmacist. Definitions for selected medical terms may be found in the Glossary. Brand names for the generic drug names listed can be found in the Index. In addition, selected brand names commonly associated with the generic name have been included in the text to help you recognize medicine you may be taking. The fact that a brand name product is not mentioned does not mean the information does not apply. It is a good idea for you to learn both the generic and brand names of your medicines and to write them down for future use.

Cyclobenzaprine (sye-kloe-BEN-za-preen) is used to help relax certain muscles in your body. It helps relieve the pain and discomfort caused by strains, sprains, or other injury to your muscles. However, this medicine does not take the place of rest, exercise or physical therapy, or other treatment that your doctor may recommend for your medical problem. Cyclobenzaprine acts on the central nervous system (CNS) to produce its muscle relaxant effects. Its actions on the CNS may also cause some of this medicine's side effects.

Cyclobenzaprine is available only with your doctor's prescription.

Remember:

• **This medicine has been prescribed for your current medical problem only.** It must not be given to other people or used for other problems unless you are directed to do so by your doctor.

• **Keep all medicines out of the reach of children.**

• In order for this medicine to work, it must be used as directed.

• **It is very important that you read and understand the following information.** If any of the information causes you special concern, do not decide against using this medicine without first checking with your doctor.

• Before you begin using any new medicine (prescription or nonprescription) or if you develop any new medical problem while you are using this medicine, check with your doctor, nurse, or pharmacist.

• **If you have any questions** about the following information or if you want more information about this medicine or your medical problem, **ask your doctor, nurse, or pharmacist.**

Before Using This Medicine

In order to decide on the best treatment for your medical problem, your doctor should be told:

—if you have ever had any unusual or allergic reaction to cyclobenzaprine.

—if you are on a low-salt, low-sugar, or any other special diet, or if you are allergic to any substance, such as foods, sulfites or other preservatives, or dyes. Most medicines contain more than their active ingredient. Your doctor, nurse, or pharmacist can help you avoid products that may cause a problem.

—if you are **pregnant** or if you may become pregnant. Studies on birth defects with cyclobenzaprine have not been done in humans. However, cyclobenzaprine has not been shown to cause birth defects or other problems in animal studies.

—if you are **breast-feeding**. Although it is not known whether cyclobenzaprine passes into the breast milk, cyclobenzaprine has not been shown to cause problems in nursing babies.

—if you have any of the following medical problems:
   Glaucoma
   Heart or blood vessel disease
   Overactive thyroid
   Problems with urination

—if you are now taking or have taken within the past 2 weeks monoamine oxidase (MAO) inhibitors such as:

   Furazolidone (e.g., Furoxone)
   Isocarboxazid (e.g., Marplan)
   Pargyline (e.g., Eutonyl)
   Phenelzine (e.g., Nardil)
   Procarbazine (e.g., Matulane)
   Tranylcypromine (e.g., Parnate)

—if you are taking **any** other prescription or nonprescription (OTC) medicine, especially:

   Central nervous system (CNS) depressants
   Tricyclic antidepressants (amitriptyline [e.g., Elavil], amoxapine, [e.g., Asendin], clomipramine [e.g., Anafranil], desipramine [e.g., Pertofrane], doxepin [e.g., Sinequan], imipramine [e.g., Tofranil], nortriptyline [e.g., Aventyl], protriptyline [e.g., Vivactil], trimipramine [e.g., Surmontil])

Proper Use of This Medicine

Take this medicine only as directed by your doctor. Do not take more of it and do not take it more often than your doctor ordered. To do so may increase the chance of serious side effects.

If you miss a dose of this medicine and remember within an hour or so of the missed dose, take it right away. Then go back to your regular dosing schedule. But if you do not remember until later, skip the missed dose and go back to your regular dosing schedule. Do not double doses.

How to store this medicine:

• **Keep out of the reach of children.**

• Store away from heat and direct light.

• Do not store this medicine in the bathroom, near the kitchen sink, or in other damp places. Heat or moisture may cause the medicine to break down.

• Do not keep outdated medicine or medicine no longer needed. Be sure that any discarded medicine is out of the reach of children.

Precautions While Using This Medicine

This medicine will add to the effects of alcohol and other CNS depressants (medicines that slow down the nervous system, possibly causing drowsiness). Some examples of CNS depressants are antihistamines or medicine for hay fever, other allergies, or colds; sedatives,

tranquilizers, or sleeping medicine; prescription pain medicine or narcotics; barbiturates; medicine for seizures; other muscle relaxants; or anesthetics, including some dental anesthetics. Therefore, **do not drink alcoholic beverages, and check with your doctor before taking any of the medicines listed above, while you are using this medicine.**

This medicine may cause some people to have blurred vision or to become drowsy, dizzy, or less alert than they are normally. **Make sure you know how you react to this medicine before you drive, use machines, or do other jobs that require you to be alert and see well.**

Cyclobenzaprine may cause dryness of the mouth. For temporary relief, use sugarless candy or gum, melt bits of ice in your mouth, or use a saliva substitute. However, if dry mouth continues for more than 2 weeks, check with your dentist. Continuing dryness of the mouth may increase the chance of dental disease, including tooth decay, gum disease, and fungal infections.

Side Effects of This Medicine

Along with its needed effects, a medicine may cause some unwanted effects. Although not all of these side effects may occur, if they do occur they may need medical attention.

Check with your doctor immediately if any of the following side effects occur:

Rare
   Swelling of face, lips, or tongue

Signs of overdose
   Convulsions (seizures)
   Drowsiness (severe)
   Fainting
   Fast or irregular heartbeat
   Hallucinations (seeing, hearing, or feeling things that are
      not there)
   Increase or decrease in body temperature
   Troubled breathing
   Unexplained muscle stiffness
   Unusual nervousness or restlessness (severe)
   Vomiting

Also, check with your doctor as soon as possible if any of the following side effects occur:

Rare
   Clumsiness or unsteadiness
   Confusion
   Mental depression
   Problems in urinating
   Ringing or buzzing in the ears
   Skin rash, hives, or itching
   Yellow eyes or skin

Other side effects may occur that usually do not require medical attention. These side effects may go away during treatment as your body adjusts to the medicine. However, check with your doctor if any of the following side effects continue or are bothersome:

More common
   Dizziness or lightheadedness
   Drowsiness
   Dry mouth

Less common or rare
   Blurred vision
   Constipation
   Headache
   Indigestion
   Nausea
   Numbness, tingling, pain, or weakness in hands or feet
   Pounding heartbeat
   Problems in speaking
   Trembling
   Trouble in sleeping
   Unpleasant taste
   Unusual muscle weakness
   Unusual tiredness

For elderly patients: Many medicines have not been tested in older people. Therefore, it is not known whether the medicine acts the same way it does in younger adults. Check with your doctor or pharmacist if you notice any ususual effects while taking this medicine or if you think it is not working as it should.

Other side effects not listed above may also occur in some patients. If you notice any other effects, check with your doctor.

December 1987

CYCLOPENTOLATE (Ophthalmic)

Some commonly used brand names are:

Ak-Pentolate
Cyclogyl   Minims Cyclopentolate*
I-Pentolate   Pentolair

Generic name product may also be available in the U.S.

*Not available in the U.S.

To the Reader: If you do not recognize the names of medical conditions or medicines referred to in this information, check with your doctor, nurse, or pharmacist. Definitions for selected medical terms may be found in the Glossary. Brand names for the generic drug names listed can be found in the Index. In addition, selected brand names commonly associated with the generic name have been included in the text to help you recognize medicine you may be taking. The fact that a brand name product is not mentioned does not mean the information does not apply. It is a good idea for you to learn both the generic and brand names of your medicines and to write them down for future use.

Cyclopentolate (sye-kloe-PEN-toe-late) is used in the eye to dilate (enlarge) the pupil. It is used before eye examinations and to treat certain eye conditions.

This medicine is available only with your doctor's prescription.

Remember:

• **This medicine has been prescribed for your current medical problem only.** It must not be given to other people or used for other problems unless you are directed to do so by your doctor.

• **Keep all medicines out of the reach of children.**

• In order for this medicine to work, it must be used as directed.

• **It is very important that you read and understand the following information.** If any of the information causes you special concern, do not decide against using this medicine without first checking with your doctor.

• Before you begin using any new medicine (prescription or nonprescription) or if you develop any new medical problem while you are using this medicine, check with your doctor, nurse, or pharmacist.

• **If you have any questions** about the following information or if you want more information about this medicine or your medical problem, **ask your doctor, nurse, or pharmacist**.

Before Using This Medicine

In order to decide on the best treatment for your medical problem, your doctor should be told:

—if you have ever had any unusual or allergic reaction to cyclopentolate.

—if you are **pregnant** or if you may become pregnant, since cyclopentolate may be absorbed into the body. However, cyclopentolate has not been shown to cause birth defects or other problems in humans.

—if you are **breast-feeding**, since cyclopentolate may be absorbed into the body. However, cyclopentolate has not been shown to cause problems in nursing babies.

—if you have any of the following medical problems:
Brain damage (in children)
Down's syndrome (mongolism)
Spastic paralysis (in children)

—if you are taking **any** other prescription or nonprescription (OTC) medicine.

Proper Use of This Medicine

How to apply this medicine: First, wash your hands. With the middle finger, apply pressure to the inside corner of the eye (and continue to apply pressure for 1 or 2 minutes after the medicine has been placed in the eye). Tilt the head back and with the index finger of the same hand, pull the lower eyelid away from the eye to form a pouch. Drop the medicine into the pouch and gently close the eyes. Do not blink. Keep the eyes closed for 1 or 2 minutes to allow the medicine to be absorbed.

Immediately after applying the eye drops, wash your hands to remove any medicine that may be on them.

To prevent contamination of the eye drops, do not touch the applicator tip to any surface (including the eye) and keep the container tightly closed.

Use this medicine only as directed. Do not use more of it and do not use it more often than your doctor ordered. To do so may increase the chance of too much medicine being absorbed into the body and the chance of side effects.

If you miss a dose of this medicine, apply it as soon as possible. However, if it is almost time for your next dose, skip the missed dose and apply your next dose at the regularly scheduled time. Then continue with your regular dosing schedule.

How to store this medicine:

• **Keep out of the reach of children.**

• Store away from heat and direct light.

• Keep the medicine from freezing.

• Do not keep outdated medicine or medicine no longer needed. Be sure that any discarded medicine is out of the reach of children.

Precautions While Using This Medicine

After you apply this medicine to your eyes:

• Your pupils will become unusually large and you will have blurring of vision, especially for close objects. **Make sure your vision is clear before you drive, use machines, or do other jobs that require you to see well.**

• Your eyes will become more sensitive to light than they are normally. **Wear sunglasses to protect your eyes from sunlight and other bright lights.**

If these side effects continue for longer than 36 hours after you have stopped using this medicine, check with your doctor.

Side Effects of This Medicine

Along with its needed effects, a medicine may cause some unwanted effects. Although not all of these side effects may occur, if they do occur they may need medical attention.

Check with your doctor as soon as possible if any of the following side effects occur:

Signs of too much medicine being absorbed into the body

    Clumsiness or unsteadiness
    Confusion
    Fast heartbeat
    Fever
    Flushing or redness of face
    Hallucinations (seeing, hearing, or feeling things that are
      not there)
    Increased thirst or dryness of mouth
    Skin rash
    Slurred speech

    Swollen stomach in infants
    Unusual behavior, especially in children
    Unusual drowsiness, tiredness, or weakness

Other side effects may occur that usually do not require medical attention. These side effects may go away during treatment as your body adjusts to the medicine. However, check with your doctor if either of the following side effects continues or is bothersome:

    Burning of eye
    Increased sensitivity of eyes to light

For infants and for children with spastic paralysis or brain damage: The above side effects are more likely to occur in infants and in children with spastic paralysis or brain damage, who are usually more sensitive to the effects of cyclopentolate.

For elderly patients: Many medicines have not been tested in older people. Therefore, it is not known whether the medicine acts the same way it does in younger adults. Check with your doctor or pharmacist if you notice any unusual effects while using this medicine or if you think it is not working as it should.

Other side effects not listed above may also occur in some patients. If you notice any other effects, check with your doctor.

_____

December 1987

CYCLOPHOSPHAMIDE (Systemic)

Some commonly used brand names are Cytoxan, Neosar, and Procytox*.

---

*Not available in the U.S.

To the Reader: If you do not recognize the names of medical conditions or medicines referred to in this information, check with your doctor, nurse, or pharmacist. Definitions for selected medical terms may be found in the Glossary. Brand names for the generic drug names listed can be found in the Index. In addition, selected brand names commonly associated with the generic name have been included in the text to help you recognize medicine you may be taking. The fact that a brand name product is not mentioned does not mean the information does not apply. It is a good idea for you to learn both the generic and brand names of your medicines and to write them down for future use.

Cyclophosphamide (sye-kloe-FOSS-fa-mide) belongs to the group of medicines called alkylating agents. It is taken by mouth or given by injection to treat some kinds of cancer.

Cyclophosphamide interferes with the growth of cancer cells, which are eventually destroyed. Since the growth of normal body cells may also be affected by cyclophosphamide, other effects will also occur. Some of these may be serious and must be reported to your doctor. Other effects, like hair loss, may not be serious but may cause concern. Some effects may not occur for months or years after the medicine is used.

Cyclophosphamide is also used for treatment of some kinds of kidney disease.

Cyclophosphamide may also be used for other conditions as determined by your doctor.

Before you begin treatment with cyclophosphamide, you and your doctor should talk about the good this medicine will do as well as the risks of using it.

Cyclophosphamide is available only with your doctor's prescription.

Remember:

• **This medicine has been prescribed for your current medical problem only.** It must not be given to other people or used for other problems unless you are directed to do so by your doctor.

• **Keep all medicines out of the reach of children.**

• In order for this medicine to work, it must be used as directed.

• If you are receiving this medicine by injection, some of the information about this medicine may not apply.

• **It is very important that you read and understand the following information.** If any of the information causes you special concern, do not decide against using this medicine without first checking with your doctor.

• Before you begin using any new medicine (prescription or nonprescription) or if you develop any new medical problem while you are using this medicine, check with your doctor, nurse, or pharmacist.

• **If you have any questions** about the following information or if you want more information about this medicine or your medical problem, **ask your doctor, nurse, or pharmacist.**

Before Using This Medicine

In order to decide on the best treatment for your medical problem, your doctor should be told:

—if you have ever had any unusual or allergic reaction to cyclophosphamide.

—if you are **pregnant** or if you intend to have children. This medicine may cause several different birth defects if either the male or female is taking it at the time of conception or if it is taken during pregnancy. In addition, many cancer medicines may cause sterility. Although this occurs commonly with cyclophosphamide, it is usually only temporary. Be sure that you have discussed this with your doctor before taking this medicine.

—if you intend to **breast-feed**. Cyclophosphamide passes into the breast milk. Because this medicine may cause serious side effects, breast-feeding is generally not recommended while you are taking it.

—if you have any of the following medical problems:
  Chickenpox (including recent exposure)
  Gout
  Herpes zoster (shingles)
  Infection
  Kidney disease
  Kidney stones
  Liver disease

—if you are taking **any** other prescription or nonprescription (OTC) medicine, especially:
  Adrenocorticoids (cortisone-like medicine)
  Antithyroid agents (medicine for overactive thyroid)
  Azathioprine (e.g., Imuran)
  Chloramphenicol (e.g., Chloromycetin)
  Colchicine
  Cyclosporine (e.g., Sandimmune)
  Flucytosine (e.g., Ancobon)
  Interferon (e.g., Intron A; Roferon-A)
  Muromonab-CD3 (monoclonal antibody; e.g., Orthoclone OKT3)
  Probenecid (e.g., Benemid)
  Sulfinpyrazone (e.g., Anturane)

—if you have ever been treated with x-rays or cancer medicines.

Proper Use of This Medicine

Take this medicine only as directed by your doctor. Do not take more or less of it, and do not take it more often than your doctor ordered. The exact amount of medicine you need has been carefully worked out. Taking too much may increase the chance of side effects while taking too little may not improve your condition.

Cyclophosphamide is sometimes given together with certain other medicines. If you are using a combination of medicines, make sure that you take each one at the proper time and do not mix them. Ask your doctor, nurse, or pharmacist to help you plan a way to remember to take your medicines at the right times.

While you are using cyclophosphamide, it is important that you drink extra fluids so that you will pass more urine. Also, empty your bladder frequently, including at least once during the night. This will help prevent kidney and bladder problems and keep your kidneys working well. Cyclophosphamide passes from the body in the urine. If too much of it appears in the urine or if the urine stays in the bladder too long, it can cause dangerous irritation. **Follow your doctor's instructions carefully about how much fluid to drink every day.** Some patients may have to drink up to 7 to 12 cups (3 quarts) of fluid a day.

Usually it is best to take cyclophosphamide first thing in the morning, to reduce the risk of bladder problems. However, your doctor may want you to take it with food in smaller doses over the day, to lessen stomach upset or help the medicine work better. Follow your doctor's instructions carefully about when to take cyclophosphamide.

Cyclophosphamide often causes nausea, vomiting, and loss of appetite. However, it is very important that you continue to use the medicine even if you begin to feel ill. **Do not stop taking this medicine without first checking with your doctor.** Ask your doctor, nurse, or pharmacist for ways to lessen these effects.

If you vomit shortly after taking a dose of cyclophosphamide, check with your doctor. You will be told whether to take the dose again or wait until the next scheduled dose.

If you miss a dose of this medicine, do not take the missed dose at all and do not double the next one. Instead, go back to your regular dosing schedule and check with your doctor.

How to store this medicine:

• **Keep out of the reach of children.**

• Store away from heat and direct light.

• Do not store in the bathroom, near the kitchen sink, or in other damp places. Heat or moisture may cause the medicine to break down.

• Store the oral solution form of this medicine in the refrigerator. Keep it from freezing.

• Do not keep outdated medicine or medicine no longer needed. Be sure that any discarded medicine is out of the reach of children.

Precautions While Using This Medicine

It is very important that your doctor check your progress at regular visits to make sure that this medicine is working properly and to check for unwanted effects.

While you are being treated with cyclophosphamide, and after you stop treatment with it, **do not have any immunizations without your doctor's approval**. Cyclophosphamide lowers your body's resistance and there is a chance you might get the infection the immunization is meant to prevent. In addition, other persons living in your house should not take oral polio vaccine since there is a chance they could pass the polio virus on to you. Also, you should avoid close contact with other persons (for example, at school or work) who have taken oral polio vaccine.

Cyclophosphamide can lower the number of white blood cells in your body. This may increase the chance of getting an infection. If you can, avoid people with colds or other infections. If you think you are getting a cold or other infection, check with your doctor.

Before having any kind of surgery, including dental surgery, or emergency treatment, make sure the physician or dentist in charge knows that you are taking this medicine.

Side Effects of This Medicine

Along with their needed effects, medicines like cyclophosphamide can sometimes cause unwanted effects such as blood problems; loss of hair; problems with the lungs, heart, or bladder; and other side effects. These are described below. Also, because of the way these medicines act on the body, there is a chance that they might cause other unwanted effects that may not occur until months or years after the medicine is used. These may include certain types of cancer, such as leukemia or bladder cancer. Discuss these possible effects with your doctor.

Although not all of these side effects may occur, if they do occur they may need medical attention.

Stop taking this medicine and check with your doctor immediately if the following side effects occur:
With high doses and/or long-term treatment
    Blood in urine
    Painful urination

Check with your doctor immediately if any of the following side effects occur:
More common
    Fever, chills, or sore throat
Less common
    Unusual bleeding or bruising

Check with your doctor as soon as possible if any of the following side effects occur:
More common
    Dizziness, confusion, or agitation
    Missing menstrual periods
    Tiredness or weakness
Less common
    Cough
    Fast heartbeat
    Joint pain
    Lower back, side, or stomach pain
    Shortness of breath
    Swelling of feet or lower legs
Rare
    Black, tarry stools
    Frequent urination
    Redness, swelling, or pain at the place of injection
    Sores in the mouth and on the lips
    Unusual thirst
    Yellow eyes and skin

Other side effects may occur that usually do not require medical attention. These side effects may go away during treatment as your body adjusts to the medicine. Also, your doctor or nurse may be able to tell you about ways to prevent or reduce some of these side effects. Check with your doctor if any of the following side effects continue or are bothersome or if you have any questions about them:

More common

Darkening of skin and fingernails
Loss of appetite
Nausea or vomiting

Less common

Flushing or redness of the face
Headache
Increase in sweating
Skin rash, hives, or itching
Swollen lips

Cyclophosphamide may cause a temporary loss of hair in some people. After treatment has ended, normal hair growth should return, although the new hair may be a slightly different color or texture.

For elderly patients: Many medicines have not been tested in older people. Therefore, it is not known whether the medicine acts the same way it does in younger adults. Check with your doctor or pharmacist if you notice any unusual effects while taking this medicine or if you think it is not working as it should.

After you stop using cyclophosphamide, it may still produce some side effects that need attention. During this period of time, **check with your doctor immediately** if you notice the following side effect:

Blood in urine

Other side effects not listed above may also occur in some patients. If you notice any other effects, check with your doctor.

December 1987

CYCLOSERINE (Systemic)

A commonly used brand name is Seromycin.

To the Reader: If you do not recognize the names of medical conditions or medicines referred to in this information, check with your doctor, nurse, or pharmacist. Definitions for selected medical terms may be found in the Glossary. Brand names for the generic drug names listed can be found in the Index. In addition, selected brand names commonly associated with the generic name have been included in the text to help you recognize medicine you may be taking. The fact that a brand name product is not mentioned does not mean the information does not apply. It is a good idea for you to learn both the generic and brand names of your medicines and to write them down for future use.

Cycloserine (sye-kloe-SER-een) belongs to the general family of medicines called antibiotics. It is taken by mouth to help the body overcome tuberculosis (TB) and certain infections of the urinary tract. When cycloserine is used for TB, it is given with one or more other medicines for TB. Cycloserine may also be used for other conditions as determined by your doctor.

Cycloserine is available only with your doctor's prescription.

Remember:

• **This medicine has been prescribed for your present infection only.** Another infection later on may require a different medicine. Also, even though other people may have the same symptoms as you, they may have a different kind of infection. Your medicine may not work for them and may even cause them harm. Therefore, **your medicine must not be given to other people or used for other infections** unless you are otherwise directed by your doctor.

• **Keep all medicines out of the reach of children.**

• In order for this medicine to work, it must be used as directed.

• **It is very important that you read and understand the following information.** If any of the information causes you special concern, do not decide against using this medicine without first checking with your doctor.

• Before you begin using any new medicine (prescription or nonprescription) or if you develop any new medical problem while you are using this medicine, check with your doctor, nurse, or pharmacist.

• **If you have any questions** about the following information or if you want more information about this medicine or your medical problem, **ask your doctor, nurse, or pharmacist.**

Before Using This Medicine

In order to decide on the best treatment for your medical problem, your doctor should be told:

—if you have ever had any unusual or allergic reaction to cycloserine.

—if you are on a low-salt, low-sugar, or any other special diet, or if you are allergic to any substance, such as foods, sulfites or other preservatives, or dyes.

Most medicines contain more than their active ingredient. Your doctor, nurse, or pharmacist can help you avoid products that may cause a problem.

—if you are **pregnant** or if you may become pregnant. However, cycloserine has not been shown to cause birth defects or other problems in humans. In addition, it is not known whether this medicine causes problems when taken with other TB medicines during pregnancy.

—if you are **breast-feeding**. Cycloserine passes into the breast milk. However, cycloserine has not been shown to cause problems in nursing babies.

—if you have any of the following medical problems:
  Alcoholism (active or treated)
  Convulsive disorders such as seizures or epilepsy
  Kidney disease (severe)
  Mental disorders such as depression, psychosis, or severe anxiety

—if you are taking **any** other prescription or nonprescription (OTC) medicine, especially ethionamide (e.g., Trecator-SC).

Proper Use of This Medicine

Cycloserine may be taken after meals if it upsets your stomach.

Your doctor may also want you to take some other medicines (for example, seizure medicine, a sedative, or vitamin B_6) to help prevent or lessen some of the side effects of cycloserine. If so, **it is very important to take these medicines every day along with cycloserine.** If you have any questions about this, check with your doctor.

To help clear up your infection completely, **it is very important that you keep taking this medicine for the full time of treatment** even if you begin to feel better after a few weeks. If you are taking this medicine for TB, you may have to take it every day for as long as 1 to 2 years or more. If you stop taking this medicine too soon, your symptoms may return.

This medicine works best when there is a constant amount in the blood or urine. **To help keep this amount constant, do not miss any doses. Also, it is best to take the doses at evenly spaced times day and night.** For example, if you are to take 2 doses a day, each dose should be spaced about 12 hours apart. If this interferes with your sleep or other daily activities, or if you need help in planning the best times to take your medicine, check with your doctor, nurse, or pharmacist.

If you do miss a dose of this medicine, take it as soon as possible. This will help to keep a constant amount of medicine in the blood or urine. However, if it is almost time for your next dose, skip the missed dose and go back to your regular dosing schedule. Do not double doses.

How to store this medicine:

- **Keep out of the reach of children.**

- Store away from heat and direct light.

- Do not store in the bathroom, near the kitchen sink, or in other damp places. Heat or moisture may cause the medicine to break down.

- Do not keep outdated medicine or medicine no longer needed. Be sure that any discarded medicine is out of the reach of children.

Precautions While Using This Medicine

It is very important that your doctor check your progress at regular visits.

If your symptoms do not improve within 2 to 3 weeks, or if they become worse, check with your doctor.

If cycloserine causes you to feel very depressed or to have thoughts of suicide, check with your doctor immediately. Your doctor will probably want to change your medicine.

Some people who take cycloserine may become more sensitive to sunlight than they are normally. **When you first begin taking this medicine, avoid too much sun or overuse of sunlamps until you see how you react,** especially if you tend to burn easily. **If you have a severe reaction, check with your doctor.**

This medicine may also cause blurred vision or loss of vision, or it may cause some people to become dizzy, drowsy, or less alert than they are normally. **Make sure you know how you react to this medicine before you drive, use machines, or do other jobs that require you to be alert or to see clearly.** If these reactions are especially bothersome, check with your doctor.

Some of cycloserine's side effects (for example, seizures) may be more likely to occur if you drink alcoholic beverages regularly while you are taking this medicine. Therefore, **you should not drink alcoholic beverages while you are taking this medicine.**

Side Effects of This Medicine

Along with its needed effects, a medicine may cause some unwanted effects. Although not all of these side effects may occur, if they do occur they may need medical attention.

Check with your doctor immediately if any of the following side effects occur:

More common
    Anxiety
    Confusion
    Dizziness
    Drowsiness
    Increased irritable feeling
    Increased restlessness
    Mental depression
    Muscle twitching or trembling
    Nervousness
    Nightmares
    Other mood or mental changes
    Speech problems
    Thoughts of suicide

Less common
    Blurred vision or any loss of vision, with or without eye pain
    Increased sensitivity of the skin to sunlight
    Numbness, tingling, burning pain, or weakness in the hands or feet
    Skin rash
    Yellow eyes or skin

Rare
    Convulsions (seizures)

Other side effects may occur that usually do not require medical attention. These side effects may go away during treatment as your body adjusts to the medicine. However, check with your doctor if any of the following side effects continue or are bothersome:

More common
    Headache

Less common
    Pale skin
    Unusual bleeding or bruising
    Unusual tiredness or weakness

For elderly patients: Many medicines have not been tested in older people. Therefore, it is not known whether the medicine acts the same way it does in younger adults. Check with your doctor or pharmacist if you notice any unusual effects while taking this medicine or if you think it is not working as it should.

Other side effects not listed above may also occur in some patients. If you notice any other effects, check with your doctor.

December 1987

CYCLOSPORINE (Systemic)

A commonly used brand name is Sandimmune.

To the Reader: If you do not recognize the names of medical conditions or medicines referred to in this information, check with your doctor, nurse, or pharmacist. Definitions for selected medical terms may be found in the Glossary. Brand names for the generic drug names listed can be found in the Index. In addition, selected brand names commonly associated with the generic name have been included in the text to help you recognize medicine you may be taking. The fact that a brand name product is not mentioned does not mean the information does not apply. It is a good idea for you to learn both the generic and brand names of your medicines and to write them down for future use.

Cyclosporine (SYE-kloe-spor-een) belongs to the group of medicines known as immunosuppressive agents. It is used to reduce the body's natural immunity in patients who receive organ (for example, kidney, liver, and heart) transplants.

When a patient receives an organ transplant, the body's white blood cells will try to get rid of (reject) the transplanted organ. Cyclosporine works by preventing the white blood cells from doing this.

Cyclosporine is a very strong medicine. It may cause side effects that could be very serious, such as high blood pressure and kidney and liver problems. It may also reduce the body's ability to fight infections. You and your doctor should talk about the good this medicine will do as well as the risks of using it.

Cyclosporine is available only with your doctor's prescription.

Remember:

• **This medicine has been prescribed for your current medical problem only.** It must not be given to other people or used for other problems unless you are directed to do so by your doctor.

• **Keep all medicines out of the reach of children.**

• In order for this medicine to work, it must be used as directed.

• If you are receiving this medicine by injection, some of the information about this medicine may not apply.

• **It is very important that you read and understand the following information.** If any of the information causes you special concern, do not decide against using this medicine without first checking with your doctor.

• Before you begin using any new medicine (prescription or nonprescription) or if you develop any new medical problem while you are using this medicine, check with your doctor, nurse, or pharmacist.

• **If you have any questions** about the following information or if you want more information about this medicine or your medical problem, **ask your doctor, nurse, or pharmacist.**

Before Using This Medicine

In order to decide on the best treatment for your medical problem, your doctor should be told:

—if you have ever had any unusual or allergic reaction to cyclosporine.

—if you are **pregnant** or if you may become pregnant. Studies have not been done in humans. However, studies in rats and rabbits have shown that cyclosporine at toxic doses (2 to 5 times the human dose) causes birth defects or death of the fetus.

—if you are **breast-feeding**. Although cyclosporine passes into breast milk, it has not been shown to cause problems in nursing babies. However, there is a chance that it could cause the same side effects in the baby that it does in patients. It may be necessary for you to stop breast-feeding during treatment. Be sure you have discussed the risks and benefits of the medicine with your doctor.

—if you have any of the following medical problems:
Chickenpox (including recent exposure)
Herpes zoster (shingles)
Infection
Intestine problems
Kidney disease
Liver disease

—if you are taking **any** other prescription or non-prescription (OTC) medicine, especially:
Adrenocorticoids (cortisone-like medicine)
Azathioprine (e.g., Imuran)
Chlorambucil (e.g., Leukeran)
Cyclophosphamide (e.g., Cytoxan)
Ketoconazole (e.g., Nizoral)
Mercaptopurine (e.g., Purinethol)
Muromonab-CD3 (monoclonal antibody, e.g., Orthoclone OKT3)

Proper Use of This Medicine

Take this medicine only as directed by your doctor. Do not take more or less of it and do not take it more often than your doctor ordered. The exact amount of medicine you need has been carefully worked out. Taking too much may increase the chance of side effects, while taking too little may not improve your condition.

In order to help you remember to take your medicine, try to get into the habit of taking it at the same time each day. This will also help cyclosporine work better by keeping a constant amount in the blood.

This medicine is to be taken by mouth even though it may come in a dropper bottle. The amount you should take is to be measured only with the specially marked dropper.

To make cyclosporine taste better, mix it in a glass container with milk, chocolate milk, or orange juice (preferably at room temperature). Stir it well, then drink it immediately. After drinking all the liquid containing the medicine, rinse the glass with a little more liquid and drink that also, to make sure you get all the medicine.

If this medicine upsets your stomach, your doctor may recommend that you take it with meals. However, check with your doctor before you decide to do this on your own.

Do not stop taking this medicine without first checking with your doctor. You may have to take medicine for the rest of your life to prevent your body from rejecting the transplant.

If you miss a dose of cyclosporine and remember it within 12 hours, take the missed dose as soon as you remember. However, if it is almost time for the next dose, skip the missed dose, go back to your regular dosing schedule, and check with your doctor. Do not double doses.

How to store this medicine:

- **Keep out of the reach of children.**

- Store away from heat and direct light.

- Do not store in the bathroom, near the kitchen sink, or in other damp places. Heat or moisture may cause the medicine to break down.

- Do not store the oral solution in the refrigerator.

- Do not keep outdated medicine or medicine no longer needed. Be sure that any discarded medicine is out of the reach of children.

Precautions While Using This Medicine

It is very important that your doctor check your progress at regular visits. Your doctor will want to do laboratory tests to make sure that cyclosporine is working properly and to check for unwanted effects.

While you are being treated with cyclosporine, and after you stop treatment with it, **do not have any immunizations without your doctor's approval.** Cyclosporine lowers your body's resistance and there is a chance you might get the infection the immunization is meant to prevent. In addition, other persons living in your house should not take oral polio vaccine since there is a chance they could pass the polio virus on to you. Also, you should avoid close contact with other persons (for example, at school or work) who have taken oral polio vaccine.

In some patients (usually younger patients), tenderness, swelling, or bleeding of the gums may appear soon after starting treatment with cyclosporine. Brushing and flossing your teeth carefully and regularly and massaging your gums may help prevent this. **See your dentist regularly to have your teeth cleaned. Check with your physician or dentist if you have any questions about how to take care of your teeth and gums, or if you notice any tenderness, swelling, or bleeding of your gums.**

Side Effects of This Medicine

Along with its needed effects, a medicine may cause some unwanted effects. Because of the way that cyclosporine acts on the body, there is a chance that it may cause effects that may not occur until years after the medicine is used. These delayed effects may include certain types of cancer, such as lymphomas. Discuss these possible effects with your doctor.

Although not all of these side effects may occur, if they do occur they may need medical attention.

Check with your doctor immediately if any of the following side effects occur:
Less common
    Fever, chills, or sore throat
    Frequent urge to urinate
Rare
    Blood in urine

Check with your doctor as soon as possible if any of the following side effects occur:
More common
    Bleeding, tender, or enlarged gums
Less common
    Convulsions (seizures)
Rare
    Confusion
    Irregular heartbeat
    Numbness or tingling in hands, feet, or lips
    Shortness of breath or difficult breathing
    Stomach pain (severe) with nausea and vomiting
    Unexplained nervousness
    Unusual tiredness or weakness
    Weakness or heaviness of legs

Other side effects may occur that usually do not require medical attention. These side effects may go away during treatment as your body adjusts to the medicine. However, check with your doctor if any of the following side effects continue or are bothersome:
More common
    Increase in hair growth
    Trembling and shaking of hands
Less common
    Acne or oily skin
    Headache
    Leg cramps
    Nausea or vomiting

For elderly patients: Many medicines have not been tested in older people. Therefore, it is not known whether the medicine acts the same way it does in younger adults. Check with your doctor or pharmacist if you notice any unusual effects while taking this medicine or if you think it is not working as it should.

Other side effects not listed above may also occur in some patients. If you notice any other effects, check with your doctor.

December 1987

CYTARABINE (Systemic)

Some commonly used brand names or other names are Ara-C, Cytosar*, and Cytosar-U.

---

*Not available in the U.S.

To the Reader: If you do not recognize the names of medical conditions or medicines referred to in this information, check with your doctor, nurse, or pharmacist. Definitions for selected medical terms may be found in the Glossary. Brand names for the generic drug names listed can be found in the Index. In addition, selected brand names commonly associated with the generic name have been included in the text to help you recognize medicine you may be taking. The fact that a brand name product is not mentioned does not mean the information does not apply. It is a good idea for you to learn both the generic and brand names of your medicines and to write them down for future use.

Cytarabine (sye-TARE-a-been) belongs to the group of medicines called antimetabolites. It is given by injection to treat some kinds of cancer.

Cytarabine interferes with the growth of cancer cells, which are eventually destroyed. Since the growth of normal body cells may also be affected by cytarabine, other effects will also occur. Some of these may be serious and must be reported to your doctor. Other effects, like hair loss, may not be serious but may cause concern. Some effects may not occur for months or years after the medicine is used.

Before you begin treatment with cytarabine, you and your doctor should talk about the good this medicine will do as well as the risks of using it.

Cytarabine is to be administered only by or under the immediate supervision of your doctor.

Remember:

• **It is very important that you read and understand the following information.** If any of the information causes you special concern, do not decide against using this medicine without first checking with your doctor.

• Before you begin using any new medicine (prescription or nonprescription) or if you develop any new medical problem while you are using this medicine, check with your doctor, nurse, or pharmacist.

• **If you have any questions** about the following information or if you want more information about this medicine or your medical problem, **ask your doctor, nurse, or pharmacist.**

Before Using This Medicine

In order to decide on the best treatment for your medical problem, your doctor should be told:

—if you have ever had any unusual or allergic reaction to cytarabine.

—if you are **pregnant** or if you intend to have children. This medicine may cause birth defects (such as defects of the arms, legs, or ears, which occurred in two babies) if either the male or female is taking it at the time of conception or if it is taken during pregnancy.

In addition, many cancer medicines may cause sterility. Although this has been reported with this medicine, it is usually only temporary. Be sure that you have discussed this with your doctor before taking this medicine.

—if you intend to **breast-feed**. Because this medicine may cause serious side effects, breast-feeding is generally not recommended while you are receiving it.

—if you have any of the following medical problems:
Chickenpox (including recent exposure)
Gout (history of)
Herpes zoster (shingles)
Infection
Kidney disease
Kidney stones (history of)
Liver disease

—if you are taking **any** other prescription or nonprescription (OTC) medicine, especially:
Amphotericin B by injection (e.g., Fungizone)
Antithyroid agents (medicine for overactive thyroid)
Azathioprine (e.g., Imuran)
Chloramphenicol (e.g., Chloromycetin)
Colchicine
Flucytosine (e.g., Ancobon)
Interferon (e.g., Intron A; Roferon-A)
Probenecid (e.g., Benemid)
Sulfinpyrazone (e.g., Anturane)

—if you have ever been treated with x-rays or cancer medicines.

Proper Use of This Medicine

This medicine is sometimes given together with certain other medicines. If you are using a combination of medicines, it is important that you receive each one at the proper time. If you are taking some of these medicines by mouth, ask your doctor, nurse, or pharmacist to help you plan a way to take them at the right times.

While you are receiving this medicine, your doctor may want you to drink extra fluids so that you will pass more urine. This will help prevent kidney problems and keep your kidneys working well.

This medicine often causes nausea and vomiting. However, it is very important that you continue to receive the medicine even if you begin to feel ill. Ask your doctor, nurse, or pharmacist for ways to lessen these effects.

Precautions While Using This Medicine

It is very important that your doctor check your progress at regular visits to make sure that this medicine is working properly and to check for unwanted effects.

While you are being treated with cytarabine, and after you stop treatment with it, **do not have any immunizations without your doctor's approval.** Cytarabine lowers your body's resistance and there is a chance you might get the infection the immunization is meant to prevent. In addition, other persons living in your household should not take oral polio vaccine since there is a chance they could pass the polio virus on to you. Also, you should avoid close contact with other persons (for example, at school or work) who have taken oral polio vaccine.

Cytarabine can lower the number of white blood cells in your body. This may increase the chance of getting an infection. If you can, avoid people with colds or other infections. If you think you are getting a cold or other infection, check with your doctor.

Side Effects of This Medicine

Along with their needed effects, medicines like cytarabine can sometimes cause unwanted effects such as blood problems and other side effects; these are described below. Also, because of the way these medicines act on the body, there is a chance that they might cause other unwanted effects that may not occur until months or years after the medicine is used. These delayed effects may include certain types of cancer, such as leukemia. Discuss these possible effects with your doctor.

Although not all of these side effects may occur, if they do occur they may need medical attention.

Check with your doctor or nurse immediately if any of the following side effects occur:

More common
   Fever, chills, or sore throat
   Unusual bleeding or bruising

Check with your doctor or nurse as soon as possible if any of the following side effects occur:

More common
   Sores in the mouth and on the lips

Less common
   Joint pain
   Lower back, side, or stomach pain
   Numbness or tingling in fingers, toes, or face
   Swelling of feet or lower legs
   Tiredness

Rare
   Black tarry stools
   Bone or muscle pain
   Chest pain
   Cough
   Decrease in urination
   Difficulty in swallowing
   Fainting spells

   General feeling of body discomfort or weakness
   Heartburn
   Irregular heartbeat
   Pain at place of injection
   Reddened eyes
   Shortness of breath
   Skin rash
   Weakness
   Yellow eyes and skin

Other side effects may occur that usually do not require medical attention. These side effects may go away during treatment as your body adjusts to the medicine. Also, your doctor or nurse may be able to tell you about ways to prevent or reduce some of these side effects. Check with your doctor if any of the following side effects continue or are bothersome or if you have any questions about them:

More common
   Loss of appetite
   Nausea and vomiting

Less common or rare
   Diarrhea
   Dizziness
   Headache
   Itching of skin
   Skin freckling

This medicine may cause a temporary loss of hair in some people. After treatment with cytarabine has ended, normal hair growth should return.

After you stop receiving cytarabine, it may still produce some side effects that need attention. During this period of time check with your doctor if you notice any of the following:
   Fever, chills, or sore throat
   Unusual bleeding or bruising

For elderly patients: Many medicines have not been tested in older people. Therefore, it is not known whether the medicine acts the same way it does in younger adults. Check with your doctor or pharmacist if you notice any unusual effects while taking this medicine or if you think it is not working as it should.

Other side effects not listed above may also occur in some patients. If you notice any other effects, check with your doctor.

December 1987

DACARBAZINE (Systemic)

Some commonly used brand names are DTIC* and DTIC-Dome. Generic name product may also be available in the U.S.

*Not available in the U.S.

To the Reader: If you do not recognize the names of medical conditions or medicines referred to in this information, check with your doctor, nurse, or pharmacist. Definitions for selected medical terms may be found in the Glossary. Brand names for the generic drug names listed can be found in the Index. In addition, selected brand names commonly associated with the generic name have been included in the text to help you recognize medicine you may be taking. The fact that a brand name product is not mentioned does not mean the information does not apply. It is a good idea for you to learn both the generic and brand names of your medicines and to write them down for future use.

Dacarbazine (da-KAR-ba-zeen) belongs to the group of medicines called alkylating agents. It is given by injection to treat some kinds of cancer.

Dacarbazine interferes with the growth of cancer cells, which are eventually destroyed. Since the growth of normal body cells may also be affected by dacarbazine, other effects will also occur. Some of these may be serious and must be reported to your doctor. Other effects, like hair loss, may not be serious but may cause concern. Some effects may not occur for months or years after the medicine is used.

Before you begin treatment with dacarbazine, you and your doctor should talk about the good this medicine will do as well as the risks of using it.

Dacarbazine is to be administered only by or under the immediate supervision of your doctor.

Remember:

• **It is very important that you read and understand the following information.** If any of the information causes you special concern, do not decide against receiving this medicine without first checking with your doctor.

• Before you begin using any new medicine (prescription or nonprescription) or if you develop any new medical problem while you are receiving this medicine, check with your doctor, nurse, or pharmacist.

• **If you have any questions** about the following information or if you want more information about this medicine or your medical problem, **ask your doctor, nurse, or pharmacist.**

Before Using This Medicine

In order to decide on the best treatment for your medical problem, your doctor should be told:

—if you have ever had any unusual or allergic reaction to dacarbazine.

—if you are **pregnant** or if you intend to have children. There is a chance that this medicine may cause birth defects if either the male or female is taking it at the time of conception or if it is taken during pregnancy. In addition, many cancer medicines may cause sterility, which could be permanent. Although this has not been reported with this medicine, the possibility should

be kept in mind. Dacarbazine has caused birth defects and a decrease in successful pregnancies in animal studies involving rats and rabbits given doses several times the usual human adult dose. Be sure that you have discussed this with your doctor before taking this medicine.

—if you intend to **breast-feed**. It is not known whether dacarbazine passes into breast milk. However, because this medicine may cause serious side effects, breast-feeding is generally not recommended while you are receiving it.

—if you have any of the following medical problems:
Chickenpox (including recent exposure)
Herpes zoster (shingles)
Infection
Kidney disease
Liver disease

—if you are taking **any** other prescription or nonprescription (OTC) medicine, especially:
Amphotericin B by injection (e.g., Fungizone)
Antithyroid agents (medicine for overactive thyroid)
Azathioprine (e.g., Imuran)
Chloramphenicol (e.g., Chloromycetin)
Colchicine
Flucytosine (e.g., Ancobon)
Interferon (e.g., Intron A; Roferon-A)

—if you have ever been treated with x-rays or cancer medicines.

Proper Use of This Medicine

Dacarbazine is sometimes given together with certain other medicines. If you are using a combination of medicines, it is important that you receive each one at the proper time. If you are taking some of these medicines by mouth, ask your doctor, nurse, or pharmacist to help you plan a way to remember to take them at the right times.

This medicine often causes nausea, vomiting, and loss of appetite. The injection may also cause a feeling of burning or pain. However, it is very important that you continue to receive the medicine, even if you begin to feel ill. After 1 or 2 days, your stomach upset should lessen. Ask your doctor, nurse, or pharmacist for ways to lessen these effects.

Precautions While Using This Medicine

It is very important that your doctor check your progress at regular visits to make sure that this medicine is working properly and to check for unwanted effects.

While you are being treated with dacarbazine, and after you stop treatment with it, **do not have any immunizations without your doctor's approval**. Dacarbazine lowers your body's resistance and there is a chance you might get the infection the immunization is meant to prevent. In addition, other persons living in your household should not take oral polio vaccine since there is a chance they could pass the polio virus on to you. Also, you should avoid close contact with other persons (for example, at school or work) who have taken oral polio vaccine.

© 1988   The United States Pharmacopeial Convention, Inc.

Dacarbazine can lower the number of white blood cells in your body. This may increase the chance of getting an infection. If you can, avoid people with colds or other infections. If you think you are getting a cold or other infection, check with your doctor.

If dacarbazine accidentally seeps out of the vein into which it is injected, it may damage some tissues and cause scarring. **Tell the doctor or nurse right away if you notice redness, pain, or swelling at the place of injection.**

Side Effects of This Medicine

Along with their needed effects, medicines like dacarbazine can sometimes cause unwanted effects such as blood problems, loss of hair, and other side effects; these are described below. Also, because of the way these medicines act on the body, there is a chance that they might cause other unwanted effects that may not occur until months or years after the medicine is used. These delayed effects may include certain types of cancer, such as leukemia. Discuss these possible effects with your doctor.

Although not all of these side effects may occur, if they do occur they may need medical attention.

Check with your doctor or nurse immediately if any of the following side effects occur:

More common
    Redness, pain, or swelling at the place of injection
    Fever, chills, or sore throat
    Unusual bleeding or bruising

Check with your doctor or nurse as soon as possible if the following side effect occurs:

Rare
    Sores in the mouth and on the lips

Other side effects may occur that usually do not require medical attention. These side effects may go away during treatment as your body adjusts to the medicine. Also, your doctor or nurse may be able to tell you about ways to prevent or reduce some of these side effects. Check with your doctor if any of the following side effects continue or are bothersome or if you have any questions about them:

More common
    Loss of appetite
    Nausea or vomiting (should lessen after 1 or 2 days)

Less common
    Feelings of uneasiness
    Flushing of the face
    Joint or muscle pain
    Numbness of the face

This medicine may cause a temporary loss of hair in some people. After treatment with dacarbazine has ended, normal hair growth should return.

After you stop receiving dacarbazine, it may still produce some side effects that need attention. During this period of time check with your doctor if you notice any of the following:
    Fever, chills, or sore throat
    Unusual bleeding or bruising.

Other side effects not listed above may also occur in some patients. If you notice any other effects, check with your doctor.

December 1987

DACTINOMYCIN (Systemic)

Some commonly used brand names or other names are Actinomycin-D and Cosmegen.

To the Reader: If you do not recognize the names of medical conditions or medicines referred to in this information, check with your doctor, nurse, or pharmacist. Definitions for selected medical terms may be found in the Glossary. Brand names for the generic drug names listed can be found in the Index. In addition, selected brand names commonly associated with the generic name have been included in the text to help you recognize medicine you may be taking. The fact that a brand name product is not mentioned does not mean the information does not apply. It is a good idea for you to learn both the generic and brand names of your medicines and to write them down for future use.

Dactinomycin (dak-ti-noe-MYE-sin) belongs to the group of medicines known as antineoplastics. It is given by injection to treat some kinds of cancer.

Dactinomycin interferes with the growth of cancer cells, which are eventually destroyed. Since the growth of normal body cells may also be affected by dactinomycin, other effects will also occur. Some of these may be serious and must be reported to your doctor. Other effects, like hair loss, may not be serious but may cause concern. Some effects may not occur for months or years after the medicine is used.

Before you begin treatment with dactinomycin, you and your doctor should talk about the good this medicine will do as well as the risks of using it.

Dactinomycin is to be administered only by or under the immediate supervision of your doctor.

Remember:
- **It is very important that you read and understand the following information.** If any of the information causes you special concern, do not decide against receiving this medicine without first checking with your doctor.

- Before you begin using any new medicine (prescription or nonprescription) or if you develop any new medical problem while you are receiving this medicine, check with your doctor, nurse, or pharmacist.

- **If you have any questions** about the following information or if you want more information about this medicine or your medical problem, **ask your doctor, nurse, or pharmacist.**

Before Using This Medicine

In order to decide on the best treatment for your medical problem, your doctor should be told:

—if you have ever had any unusual or allergic reaction to dactinomycin.

—if you are **pregnant** or if you intend to have children. There is a chance that this medicine may cause birth defects if either the male or female is receiving it at the time of conception or if it is taken during pregnancy. Studies have shown that dactinomycin causes birth defects in animals. In addition, many cancer medicines may cause sterility which could be permanent. Although this has not been reported with this

medicine, the possibility should be kept in mind. Be sure that you have discussed this with your doctor before receiving this medicine.

—if you intend to **breast-feed**. It is not known whether dactinomycin passes into breast milk. However, because this medicine may cause serious side effects, breast-feeding is generally not recommended while you are receiving it.

—if you have any of the following medical problems:
Chickenpox (including recent exposure)
Gout (or history of)
Herpes zoster (shingles)
Infection
Kidney stones
Liver disease

—if you are taking **any** other prescription or nonprescription (OTC) medicine, especially:
Amphotericin B by injection (e.g., Fungizone)
Antithyroid agents (medicine for overactive thyroid)
Azathioprine (e.g., Imuran)
Chloramphenicol (e.g., Chloromycetin)
Flucytosine (e.g., Ancobon)
Interferon (e.g., Intron A; Roferon-A)
Probenecid (e.g., Benemid)
Sulfinpyrazone (e.g., Anturane)

—if you have ever been treated with x-rays or cancer medicines.

Proper Use of This Medicine

Dactinomycin is sometimes given together with certain other medicines. If you are receiving a combination of medicines, it is important that you receive each one at the proper time. If you are taking some of these medicines by mouth, ask your doctor, nurse, or pharmacist to help you plan a way to remember to take them at the right times.

This medicine often causes nausea and vomiting. However, it is very important that you continue to receive the medicine, even if you begin to feel ill. Ask your doctor, nurse, or pharmacist for ways to lessen these effects.

Precautions While Using This Medicine

It is very important that your doctor check your progress at regular visits to make sure that this medicine is working properly and to check for unwanted effects.

While you are being treated with dactinomycin, and after you stop treatment with it, **do not have any immunizations without your doctor's approval.** Dactinomycin lowers your body's resistance, and there is a chance you might get the infection the immunization is meant to prevent. In addition, other persons living in your household should not take oral polio vaccine since there is a chance they could pass the polio virus on to you. Also, you should avoid close contact with other persons (for example, at school or work) who have taken oral polio vaccine.

Dactinomycin can lower the number of white blood cells in your body. This may increase the chance of getting an infection. If you can, avoid people with colds or other infections. If you think you are getting a cold or other infection, check with your doctor.

If dactinomycin accidentally seeps out of the vein into which it is injected, it may severely damage some tissues and cause scarring. **Tell the doctor or nurse right away if you notice redness, pain, or swelling at the place of injection.**

Side Effects of This Medicine

Along with their needed effects, medicines like dactinomycin can sometimes cause unwanted effects such as blood problems, loss of hair, and other side effects; these are described below. Also, because of the way these medicines act on the body, there is a chance that they might cause other unwanted effects that may not occur until months or years after the medicine is used. These delayed effects may include certain types of cancer, such as leukemia. Discuss these possible effects with your doctor.

Although not all of these side effects may occur, if they do occur they may need medical attention.

Check with your doctor or nurse immediately if any of the following side effects occur:

More common
   Fever, chills, or sore throat
   Unusual bleeding or bruising

Rare
   Pain at the place of injection
   Wheezing

Check with your doctor or nurse as soon as possible if any of the following side effects occur:

More common
   Black tarry stools
   Diarrhea (continuing)
   Difficulty in swallowing
   Heartburn
   Sores in the mouth and on the lips
   Stomach pain (continuing)

Rare
   Joint pain
   Lower back, side, or stomach pain
   Swelling of feet or lower legs
   Yellow eyes and skin

Other side effects may occur that usually do not require medical attention. These side effects may go away during treatment as your body adjusts to the medicine. Also, your doctor or nurse may be able to tell you about ways to prevent or reduce some of these side effects. Check with your doctor if any of the following side effects continue or are bothersome or if you have any questions about them:

More common
   Darkening of the skin
   Nausea and vomiting
   Redness of skin
   Skin rash or acne
   Tiredness

This medicine often causes a temporary loss of hair, sometimes including the eyebrows. After treatment with dactinomycin has ended, normal hair growth should return.

For elderly patients: Many medicines have not been tested in older people. Therefore, it is not known whether the medicine acts the same way it does in younger adults. Check with your doctor if you notice any unusual effects while taking this medicine or if you think it is not working as it should.

After you stop receiving dactinomycin, it may still produce some side effects that need attention. During this period of time check with your doctor if you notice any of the following:
   Black tarry stools
   Diarrhea
   Fever, chills, or sore throat
   Sores in the mouth and on the lips
   Stomach pain
   Unusual bleeding or bruising
   Yellow eyes and skin

Other side effects not listed above may also occur in some patients. If you notice any other effects, check with your doctor.

December 1987

DANAZOL (Systemic)

Some commonly used brand names are Cyclomen* and Danocrine.

*Not available in the U.S.

To the Reader: If you do not recognize the names of medical conditions or medicines referred to in this information, check with your doctor, nurse, or pharmacist. Definitions for selected medical terms may be found in the Glossary. Brand names for the generic drug names listed can be found in the Index. In addition, selected brand names commonly associated with the generic name have been included in the text to help you recognize medicine you may be taking. The fact that a brand name product is not mentioned does not mean the information does not apply. It is a good idea for you to learn both the generic and brand names of your medicines and to write them down for future use.

Danazol (DA-na-zole) is taken by mouth and may be used for a number of different medical problems. These include treatment of:

—pain and/or infertility due to endometriosis;
—a tendency for females to develop cysts in the breasts (fibrocystic breast disease); or
—hereditary angioedema (a disease involving swellings of the skin) in both males and females.

Danazol may also be used for other conditions as determined by your doctor.

This medicine is available only with your doctor's prescription.

Remember:

• **This medicine has been prescribed for your current medical problem only.** It must not be given to other people or used for other problems unless you are directed to do so by your doctor.

• **Keep all medicines out of the reach of children.**

• **In order for this medicine to work, it must be used as directed.**

• **It is very important that you read and understand the following information.** If any of the information causes you special concern, do not decide against using this medicine without first checking with your doctor.

• Before you begin using any new medicine (prescription or nonprescription) or if you develop any new medical problem while you are using this medicine, check with your doctor, nurse, or pharmacist.

• **If you have any questions** about the following information or if you want more information about this medicine or your medical problem, **ask your doctor, nurse, or pharmacist.**

Before Using This Medicine

In order to decide on the best treatment for your medical problem, your doctor should be told:

—if you have ever had any unusual or allergic reaction to danazol.

—if you are on a low-salt, low-sugar, or any other special diet, or if you are allergic to any substance, such as foods, sulfites or other preservatives, or dyes.

Most medicines contain more than their active ingredient. Your doctor, nurse, or pharmacist can help you avoid products that may cause a problem.

—if you are **pregnant** or may become pregnant. Danazol is not recommended for use during pregnancy, since it may cause a female baby to develop certain male characteristics.

—if you are **breast-feeding**. Breast-feeding is usually not recommended while you are taking this medicine because it may cause unwanted effects in the baby. Be sure you have discussed this with your doctor before taking danazol.

—if you have any of the following medical problems:
  Diabetes mellitus (sugar diabetes)
  Epilepsy
  Heart disease
  Kidney disease
  Liver disease
  Migraine headaches

—if you are taking **any** other prescription or nonprescription (OTC) medicine, especially anticoagulants (blood thinners).

Proper Use of This Medicine

In order for danazol to help you, **it must be taken regularly for the full time of treatment** as ordered by your doctor.

If you miss a dose of this medicine, take it as soon as possible. However, if it is almost time for your next dose, skip the missed dose and go back to your regular dosing schedule. Do not double doses.

How to store this medicine:

• **Keep out of the reach of children.**

• Store away from heat and direct light.

• Do not store in the bathroom, near the kitchen sink, or in other damp places. Heat or moisture may cause the medicine to break down.

• Do not keep outdated medicine or medicine no longer needed. Be sure that any discarded medicine is out of the reach of children.

Precautions While Using This Medicine

Your doctor should check your progress at regular visits to make sure that this medicine does not cause unwanted effects.

Diabetics—This medicine may affect blood sugar levels. If you notice a change in the results of your urine sugar test or if you have any questions about this, check with your doctor.

If you are taking danazol for endometriosis or fibrocystic breast disease:

• During the time you are taking danazol, your menstrual period may not be regular or you may not have a menstrual period at all. This is to be expected when taking this medicine. If regular menstruation does not begin within 60 to 90 days after you stop taking this medicine, check with your doctor.

• During the time you are taking danazol, you should use birth control methods which do not contain hormones. If you have any questions about this, check with your doctor, nurse, or pharmacist.

• **If you suspect that you may have become pregnant, stop taking this medicine and check with your doctor.** Continued use of danazol during pregnancy may cause female babies to develop male characteristics.

Side Effects of This Medicine

Along with its needed effects, a medicine may cause some unwanted effects. Although not all of these side effects may occur, if they do occur they may need medical attention.

Check with your doctor as soon as possible if any of the following side effects occur:

For both females and males
  Less common
    Acne or increased oiliness of skin or hair
    Muscle cramps or spasms
    Swelling of feet or lower legs
    Unusual tiredness or weakness
    Weight gain
  Rare
    Blood in urine
    Yellow eyes or skin

For females only
  Less common
    Decrease in breast size
    Hoarseness or deepening of voice
    Unnatural hair growth
  Rare
    Enlarged clitoris

For males only
  Rare
    Decrease in size of testicles

Other side effects may occur that usually do not require medical attention. These side effects may go away during treatment as your body adjusts to the medicine. However, check with your doctor if any of the following side effects continue or are bothersome:

For both females and males
  Less common
    Flushing or redness of skin
    Mood or mental changes
    Nervousness
    Sweating

For females only
  Less common
    Burning, dryness, or itching of vagina or vaginal bleeding

For elderly patients: Many medicines have not been tested in older people. Therefore, it is not known whether the medicine acts the same way it does in younger adults. Check with your doctor or pharmacist if you notice any unusual effects while taking this medicine or if you think it is not working as it should.

Other side effects not listed above may also occur in some patients. If you notice any other effects, check with your doctor.

December 1987

DANTROLENE (Systemic)

A commonly used brand name is Dantrium.

To the Reader: If you do not recognize the names of medical conditions or medicines referred to in this information, check with your doctor, nurse, or pharmacist. Definitions for selected medical terms may be found in the Glossary. Brand names for the generic drug names listed can be found in the Index. In addition, selected brand names commonly associated with the generic name have been included in the text to help you recognize medicine you may be taking. The fact that a brand name product is not mentioned does not mean the information does not apply. It is a good idea for you to learn both the generic and brand names of your medicines and to write them down for future use.

Dantrolene (DAN-troe-leen) is used to help relax certain muscles in your body. It relieves the spasms, cramping, and tightness of muscles caused by certain medical problems such as multiple sclerosis (MS), cerebral palsy, stroke, or injury to the spine. Dantrolene does not cure these problems, but it may allow other treatment, such as physical therapy, to be more helpful in improving your condition. Dantrolene acts directly on the muscles to produce its relaxant effects.

Dantrolene is also used to prevent or treat a medical problem called malignant hyperthermia that may occur in some people during or following surgery or anesthesia. Malignant hyperthermia consists of a group of symptoms including very high fever, fast and irregular heartbeat, and breathing problems. It is believed that the tendency to develop malignant hyperthermia is inherited.

Dantrolene may also be used for other conditions as determined by your doctor.

Dantrolene has been shown to cause cancer and noncancerous tumors in some animals (but not in others) when given in large doses for a long period of time. It is not known whether long-term use of dantrolene causes cancer or tumors in humans. Before taking this medicine, be sure that you have discussed this with your doctor.

This medicine is available only with your doctor's prescription.

Remember:

• **This medicine has been prescribed for your current medical problem only.** It must not be given to other people or used for other problems unless you are directed to do so by your doctor.

• **Keep all medicines out of the reach of children.**

• In order for this medicine to work, it must be used as directed.

• If you are receiving this medicine by injection, some of the information about this medicine may not apply.

• **It is very important that you read and understand the following information.** If any of the information causes you special concern, do not decide against using this medicine without first checking with your doctor.

• Before you begin using any new medicine (prescription or nonprescription) or if you develop any new medical problem while you are using this medicine, check with your doctor, nurse, or pharmacist.

• **If you have any questions** about the following information or if you want more information about this medicine or your medical problem, **ask your doctor, nurse, or pharmacist**.

Before Using This Medicine

In order to decide on the best treatment for your medical problem, your doctor should be told:

—if you have ever had any unusual or allergic reaction to dantrolene.

—if you are on a low-salt, low-sugar, or any other special diet, or if you are allergic to any substance, such as foods, sulfites or other preservatives, or dyes. Most medicines contain more than their active ingredient.

—if you are **pregnant** or if you may become pregnant. Dantrolene has not been shown to cause birth defects or other problems in humans.

—if you are **breast-feeding**. Dantrolene has not been shown to cause problems in nursing babies.

—if you have any of the following medical problems:
  Emphysema, asthma, bronchitis, or other chronic lung disease
  Heart disease
  Liver disease, such as hepatitis or cirrhosis (or history of)

—if you are now taking **any** other medicine or type of medicine, especially:
  Acetaminophen (e.g., Tylenol) (with long-term, high-dose use)
  Amiodarone (e.g., Cordarone)
  Anabolic steroids (dromostanolone [e.g., Drolban], ethylestrenol [e.g., Maxibolin], nandrolone [e.g., Durabolin], oxandrolone [e.g., Anavar], oxymetholone [e.g., Anadrol], stanozolol [e.g., Winstrol])
  Androgens (male hormones)
  Antithyroid agents (medicine for overactive thyroid)
  Carbamazepine (e.g., Tegretol)
  Central nervous system (CNS) depressants
  Chloroquine (e.g., Aralen)
  Disulfiram (e.g., Antabuse)
  Divalproex (e.g., Depakote)
  Erythromycins
  Estrogens (female hormones)
  Etretinate (e.g., Tegison)
  Furazolidone (e.g., Furoxone)
  Gold salts (medicine for arthritis)
  Hydroxychloroquine (e.g., Plaquenil)
  Isoniazid (e.g., Nydrazid)
  Ketoconazole (e.g., Nizoral)
  Mercaptopurine (e.g., Purinethol)
  Methotrexate (e.g., Mexate)
  Methyldopa (e.g., Aldomet)
  Naltrexone (e.g., Trexan) (with long-term, high-dose use)
  Nitrofurantoin (e.g., Furadantin)
  Oral contraceptives (birth control pills) containing estrogen
  Phenothiazines (acetophenazine [e.g., Tindal], chlorpromazine [e.g., Thorazine], fluphenazine [e.g., Permitil; Prolixin], mesoridazine [e.g., Serentil], perphenazine [e.g., Trilafon], prochlorperazine [e.g., Compazine], promazine [e.g., Sparine], promethazine [e.g., Phenergan], thioridazine [e.g., Mellaril], trifluoperazine [e.g., Stelazine], triflupromazine [e.g., Vesprin], trimeprazine [e.g., Temaril])

Phenytoin (e.g., Dilantin)
Rifampin (e.g., Rimactane)
Sulfonamides (sulfa medicine)
Tricyclic antidepressants (amitriptyline [e.g., Elavil],
amoxapine, [e.g., Asendin], clomipramine [e.g., An-
afranil], desipramine [e.g., Pertofrane], doxepin [e.g.,
Sinequan], imipramine [e.g., Tofranil], nortriptyline
[e.g., Aventyl], protriptyline [e.g., Vivactil], trimipra-
mine [e.g., Surmontil])
Valproic acid (e.g., Depakene)

Proper Use of This Medicine

If you are unable to swallow the capsules, you may empty
the number of capsules needed for one dose into a
small amount of fruit juice or other liquid. Stir gently
to mix the powder with the liquid before drinking.
Drink the medicine right away. Rinse the glass with
a little more liquid and drink that also to make sure
that you have taken all of the medicine.

Take this medicine only as directed by your doctor. Do
not take more of it and do not take it more often than
your doctor ordered. Dantrolene may cause liver damage or other unwanted effects if too much is taken.

If you miss a dose of this medicine and remember within
an hour or so of the missed dose, take it right away.
Then go back to your regular dosing schedule. But if
you do not remember until later, skip the missed dose
and go back to your regular dosing schedule. Do not
double doses.

How to store this medicine:

• **Keep out of the reach of children.**

• Store away from heat and direct light.

• Do not store this medicine in the bathroom, near the
kitchen sink, or in other damp places. Heat or moisture
may cause the medicine to break down.

• Do not keep outdated medicine or medicine no longer
needed. Be sure that any discarded medicine is out of
the reach of children.

Precautions While Using This Medicine

If you will be taking dantrolene for a long period of time
(for example, for several months at a time), your doctor should check your progress at regular visits. It may
be necessary to have certain blood tests to check for
unwanted effects while you are taking dantrolene.

This medicine will add to the effects of alcohol and other
CNS depressants (medicines that slow down the nervous system, possibly causing drowsiness). Some examples of CNS depressants are antihistamines or medicine for hay fever, other allergies, or colds; sedatives,
tranquilizers, or sleeping medicine; prescription pain
medicine or narcotics; barbiturates; medicine for seizures; other muscle relaxants; or anesthetics, including
some dental anesthetics. Therefore, **do not drink alcoholic beverages, and check with your doctor before
taking any of the medicines listed above, while you are
using this medicine.**

This medicine may cause drowsiness, dizziness or lightheadedness, vision problems, or muscle weakness in
some people. **Make sure you know how you react to
this medicine before you drive, use machines, or do
other jobs that require you to be alert, well-coordinated,
and able to see well.**

Side Effects of This Medicine

Along with its needed effects, a medicine may cause some
unwanted effects. Although not all of these side effects
may occur, if they do occur they may need medical
attention. Serious side effects are very rare when dantrolene is taken for a short period of time (for example,
when it is used for a few days before, during, or after
surgery or anesthesia to prevent or treat malignant
hyperthermia). However, serious side effects may occur, especially when the medicine is taken for a long
period of time.

Check with your doctor immediately if any of the following side effects occur:

Less common

Convulsions (seizures)
Pain, tenderness, bluish color, or swelling of foot or leg
Shortness of breath or unusually slow or troubled breath-
ing

Also, check with your doctor as soon as possible if any
of the following side effects occur:

Less common

Bloody or dark urine
Chest pain
Constipation (severe)
Diarrhea (severe)
Difficult urination
Mental depression or confusion
Skin rash, hives, or itching
Yellow eyes or skin

Other side effects may occur that usually do not require
medical attention. These side effects may go away
during treatment as your body adjusts to the medicine.
However, check with your doctor if any of the following side effects continue or are bothersome:

More common

Diarrhea (mild)
Dizziness or lightheadedness
Drowsiness
General feeling of discomfort or illness
Muscle weakness
Nausea or vomiting
Unusual tiredness

Less common

Abdominal or stomach cramps or discomfort
Blurred or double vision or any change in vision
Chills and fever
Constipation (mild)
Difficulty in swallowing
Frequent urge to urinate or uncontrolled urination
Headache
Loss of appetite
Slurring of speech or other speech problems

Sudden decrease in amount of urine
Trouble in sleeping
Unusual nervousness

For elderly patients: Many medicines have not been tested in older people. Therefore, it is not known whether the medicine acts the same way it does in younger adults. Check with your doctor or pharmacist if you notice any unusual effects while taking this medicine or if you think it is not working as it should.

Other side effects not listed above may also occur in some patients. If you notice any other effects, check with your doctor.

December 1987

DAPSONE (Systemic)

Some commonly used brand names or other names are Avlosulfon* and DDS.

Generic name product may also be available in the U.S.

*Not available in the U.S.

To the Reader: If you do not recognize the names of medical conditions or medicines referred to in this information, check with your doctor, nurse, or pharmacist. Definitions for selected medical terms may be found in the Glossary. Brand names for the generic drug names listed can be found in the Index. In addition, selected brand names commonly associated with the generic name have been included in the text to help you recognize medicine you may be taking. The fact that a brand name product is not mentioned does not mean the information does not apply. It is a good idea for you to learn both the generic and brand names of your medicines and to write them down for future use.

Dapsone (DAP-sone), a sulfone, belongs to the general family of medicines called anti-infectives.

Dapsone is taken by mouth to help the body overcome leprosy (Hansen's disease) and to help control dermatitis herpetiformis, a skin problem. It may be given alone or with one or more other medicines for leprosy. Dapsone may also be used for other conditions as determined by your doctor.

Dapsone is available only with your doctor's prescription.

Remember:

• **This medicine has been prescribed for your present medical problem only.** Even though other people may have the same symptoms as you, they may have a different kind of problem. Your medicine may not work for them and may even cause them harm. Therefore, **your medicine must not be given to other people or used for other problems** unless you are otherwise directed by your doctor.

• **Keep all medicines out of the reach of children.**

• In order for this medicine to work, it must be used as directed.

• **It is very important that you read and understand the following information.** If any of the information causes you special concern, do not decide against using this medicine without first checking with your doctor.

• Before you begin using any new medicine (prescription or nonprescription) or if you develop any new medical problem while you are using this medicine, check with your doctor, nurse, or pharmacist.

• **If you have any questions** about the following information or if you want more information about this medicine or your medical problem, **ask your doctor, nurse, or pharmacist.**

Before Using This Medicine

In order to decide on the best treatment for your medical problem, your doctor should be told:

—if you have ever had any unusual or allergic reaction to dapsone, sulfoxone, furosemide or thiazide diuretics (water pills), oral antidiabetic agents (diabetes medicine you take by mouth), or glaucoma medicine you take by mouth (for example, acetazolamide, dichlorphenamide, methazolamide).

—if you are on a low-salt, low-sugar, or any other special diet, or if you are allergic to any substance, such as foods, sulfites or other preservatives, or dyes. Most medicines contain more than their active ingredient. Your doctor, nurse, or pharmacist can help you avoid products that may cause a problem.

—if you are **pregnant** or if you may become pregnant. Studies in humans have not shown that dapsone causes birth defects or other problems.

—if you are **breast-feeding.** Dapsone passes into the breast milk. It may cause blood problems in nursing babies with glucose-6-phosphate dehydrogenase (G6PD) deficiency.

—if you have any of the following medical problems:
Anemia (severe)
Glucose-6-phosphate dehydrogenase (G6PD) deficiency
Kidney disease
Liver disease
Methemoglobin reductase deficiency

—if you are taking dapsone for leprosy and are also taking aminobenzoic acid (PABA).

—if you are taking **any** other prescription or nonprescription (OTC) medicine, especially:
Antidiabetic agents, oral (diabetes medicine you take by mouth)
Furazolidone (e.g., Furoxone)
Methyldopa (e.g., Aldomet)
Nitrofurantoin (e.g., Furadantin)
Primaquine
Procainamide (e.g., Pronestyl)
Quinidine (e.g., Quinidex)
Quinine (e.g., Quinamm)
Sulfonamides (sulfa medicine)
Sulfoxone (e.g., Diasone)
Vitamin K (e.g., AquaMEPHYTON, Synkayvite)

—if you have ever had any problems with this medicine.

Proper Use of This Medicine

For patients taking dapsone for leprosy:

• To help clear up your leprosy completely or to keep it from coming back, **it is very important that you keep taking this medicine for the full time of treatment** even if you begin to feel better after a few weeks or months. You may have to take it every day for as long as 3 years or more, or for life. If you stop taking this medicine too soon, your symptoms may return.

• This medicine works best when there is a constant amount in the blood. **To help keep this amount constant, do not miss any doses. Also, it is best to take each dose at the same time every day.** If you need help in planning the best time to take your medicine, check with your doctor, nurse, or pharmacist.

• If you do miss a dose of this medicine, take it as soon as possible. This will help keep a constant amount of medicine in the blood. However, if it is almost time for your next dose, skip the missed dose and go back to your regular dosing schedule. Do not double doses.

For patients taking dapsone for dermatitis herpetiformis:

• Your doctor may want you to follow a gluten-free diet. If you have any questions about this, check with your doctor.

• You may skip a missed dose if it does not make your symptoms come back or get worse. If your symptoms do come back or get worse, take the missed dose as soon as possible. Then go back to your regular dosing schedule.

How to store this medicine:

• **Keep out of the reach of children**.

• Store away from heat and direct light.

• Do not store in the bathroom, near the kitchen sink, or in other damp places. Heat or moisture may cause the medicine to break down.

• Do not keep outdated medicine or medicine no longer needed. Be sure that any discarded medicine is out of the reach of children.

Precautions While Using This Medicine

It is very important that your doctor check your progress at regular visits.

If your symptoms do not improve within 2 to 3 months (for leprosy) or within a few days (for dermatitis herpetiformis), or if they become worse, check with your doctor.

Dapsone may cause blood problems. These problems may result in a greater chance of infection, slow healing, and bleeding of the gums. Therefore, you should be careful when using toothbrushes, dental floss, and toothpicks. Dental work should be delayed until your blood counts have returned to normal. Check with your physician or dentist if you have any questions about proper oral hygiene (mouth care) during treatment.

This medicine may also cause some people to become dizzy or lightheaded. **Make sure you know how you react to this medicine before you drive, use machines, or do other jobs that require you to be alert.** If these reactions are especially bothersome, check with your doctor.

Side Effects of This Medicine

Along with its needed effects, a medicine may cause some unwanted effects. Although not all of these side effects may occur, if they do occur they may need medical attention.

Check with your doctor immediately if any of the following side effects occur:
More common
  Back, leg, or stomach pains
  Fever
  Loss of appetite
  Pale skin
  Skin rash
  Unusual tiredness or weakness
Rare
  Bluish fingernails, lips, or skin
  Difficult breathing
  Itching, dryness, redness, scaling, or peeling of the skin, or loss of hair
  Mood or other mental changes
  Numbness, tingling, pain, burning, or weakness in hands or feet
  Sore throat
  Yellow eyes or skin

Other side effects may occur that usually do not require medical attention. These side effects may go away during treatment as your body adjusts to the medicine. However, check with your doctor if any of the following side effects continue or are bothersome:
Rare
  Dizziness
  Headache
  Lightheadedness
  Nausea or vomiting

For elderly patients: Many medicines have not been tested in older people. Therefore, it is not known whether the medicine acts the same way it does in younger adults. Check with your doctor or pharmacist if you notice any unusual effects while taking this medicine or if you think it is not working as it should.

Other side effects not listed above may also occur in some patients. If you notice any other effects, check with your doctor.

December 1987

DAUNORUBICIN (Systemic)

A commonly used brand name is Cerubidine.

To the Reader: If you do not recognize the names of medical conditions or medicines referred to in this information, check with your doctor, nurse, or pharmacist. Definitions for selected medical terms may be found in the Glossary. Brand names for the generic drug names listed can be found in the Index. In addition, selected brand names commonly associated with the generic name have been included in the text to help you recognize medicine you may be taking. The fact that a brand name product is not mentioned does not mean the information does not apply. It is a good idea for you to learn both the generic and brand names of your medicines and to write them down for future use.

Daunorubicin (daw-noe-ROO-bi-sin) belongs to the general group of medicines known as antineoplastics. It is given by injection to treat some kinds of cancer.

Daunorubicin seems to interfere with the growth of cancer cells, which are eventually destroyed. Since the growth of normal body cells may also be affected by daunorubicin, other effects will also occur. Some of these may be serious and must be reported to your doctor. Other effects, like hair loss, may not be serious but may cause concern. Some effects may not occur for months or years after the medicine is used.

Before you begin treatment with daunorubicin, you and your doctor should talk about the good this medicine will do as well as the risks of using it.

Daunorubicin is to be administered only by or under the immediate supervision of your doctor.

Remember:

• **It is very important that you read and understand the following information.** If any of the information causes you special concern, do not decide against receiving this medicine without first checking with your doctor.

• Before you begin using any new medicine (prescription or nonprescription) or if you develop any new medical problem while you are receiving this medicine, check with your doctor, nurse, or pharmacist.

• **If you have any questions** about the following information or if you want more information about this medicine or your medical problem, **ask your doctor, nurse, or pharmacist.**

Before Using This Medicine

In order to decide on the best treatment for your medical problem, your doctor should be told:

—if you have ever had any unusual or allergic reaction to daunorubicin.

—if you are **pregnant** or if you intend to have children. This medicine may cause birth defects if either the male or female is receiving it at the time of conception or if it is taken during pregnancy. In addition, many cancer medicines may cause sterility which could be permanent. Although this has been reported only in male dogs with this medicine, the possibility of an effect in human males should be kept in mind. Be sure that you have discussed this with your doctor before receiving this medicine.

—if you intend to **breast-feed**. Because this medicine may cause serious side effects, breast-feeding is generally not recommended while you are receiving it.

—if you have any of the following medical problems:
Chickenpox (including recent exposure)
Gout (history of)
Heart disease
Herpes zoster (shingles)
Infection
Kidney disease
Kidney stones
Liver disease

—if you are taking **any** other prescription or nonprescription (OTC) medicine, especially:
Amphotericin B by injection (e.g., Fungizone)
Antithyroid agents (medicine for overactive thyroid)
Azathioprine (e.g., Imuran)
Chloramphenicol (e.g., Chloromycetin)
Colchicine
Flucytosine (e.g., Ancobon)
Interferon (e.g., Intron A; Roferon-A)
Probenecid (e.g., Benemid)
Sulfinpyrazone (e.g., Anturane)

—if you have ever been treated with x-rays or cancer medicines.

Proper Use of This Medicine

Daunorubicin is sometimes given together with certain other medicines. If you are using a combination of medicines, it is important that you receive each one at the proper time. If you are taking some of these medicines by mouth, ask your doctor, nurse, or pharmacist to help you plan a way to take them at the right times.

While you are receiving daunorubicin, your doctor may want you to drink extra fluids so that you will pass more urine. This will help prevent kidney problems and keep your kidneys working well.

This medicine often causes nausea and vomiting. However, it is very important that you continue to receive it, even if you begin to feel ill. Ask your doctor, nurse, or pharmacist for ways to lessen these effects.

Precautions While Using This Medicine

It is very important that your doctor check your progress at regular visits to make sure that this medicine is working properly and to check for unwanted effects.

While you are being treated with daunorubicin, and after you stop treatment with it, **do not have any immunizations without your doctor's approval**. Daunorubicin lowers your body's resistance and there is a chance you might get the infection the immunization is meant to prevent. In addition, other persons living in your household should not take oral polio vaccine since there is a chance they could pass the polio virus on to you. Also, you should avoid close contact with other persons (for example, at school or work) who have taken oral polio vaccine.

Daunorubicin can lower the number of white blood cells in your body. This may increase the chance of getting an infection. If you can, avoid people with colds or other infections. If you think you are getting a cold or other infection, check with your doctor.

If daunorubicin accidentally seeps out of the vein into which it is injected, it may damage some tissues and cause scarring. **Tell the doctor or nurse right away if you notice redness, pain, or swelling at the place of injection.**

Side Effects of This Medicine

Along with their needed effects, medicines like daunorubicin can sometimes cause unwanted effects such as blood problems, loss of hair, heart problems, and other side effects; these are described below. Also, because of the way these medicines act on the body, there is a chance that they might cause other unwanted effects that may not occur until months or years after the medicine is used. These delayed effects may include certain types of cancer, such as leukemia. Discuss these possible effects with your doctor.

Although not all of these side effects may occur, if they do occur they may need medical attention.

Check with your doctor or nurse immediately if any of the following side effects occur:

More common
> Fever, chills, or sore throat

Less common
> Irregular heartbeat
> Pain at the place of injection
> Shortness of breath
> Swelling of feet and lower legs
> Unusual bleeding or bruising

Check with your doctor or nurse as soon as possible if any of the following side effects occur:

More common
> Sores in the mouth and on the lips

Less common
> Joint pain
> Lower back, side, or stomach pain

Rare
> Skin rash or itching

Other side effects may occur that usually do not require medical attention. These side effects may go away during treatment as your body adjusts to the medicine. Also, your doctor or nurse may be able to tell you about ways to prevent or reduce some of these side effects. Check with your doctor or nurse if any of the following side effects continue or are bothersome or if you have any questions about them:

More common
> Nausea and vomiting

Less common or rare
> Darkening or redness of the skin
> Diarrhea

Daunorubicin causes the urine to turn reddish in color, which may stain clothes. This is not blood. It is perfectly normal and lasts for only 1 or 2 days after each dose is given.

This medicine often causes a temporary and total loss of hair. After treatment with daunorubicin has ended, normal hair growth should return.

After you stop receiving daunorubicin, it may still produce some side effects that need attention. During this period of time **check with your doctor immediately** if you notice any of the following side effects:

> Irregular heartbeat
> Shortness of breath
> Swelling of feet and lower legs

For children and elderly patients: Heart problems are more likely to occur in children under 2 years of age and in the elderly, who are usually more sensitive to the effects of daunorubicin. The elderly may also be more likely to have blood problems.

Other side effects not listed above may also occur in some patients. If you notice any other effects, check with your doctor or nurse.

December 1987

DEFEROXAMINE (Systemic)

A commonly used brand name is Desferal.

To the Reader: If you do not recognize the names of medical conditions or medicines referred to in this information, check with your doctor, nurse, or pharmacist. Definitions for selected medical terms may be found in the Glossary. Brand names for the generic drug names listed can be found in the Index. In addition, selected brand names commonly associated with the generic name have been included in the text to help you recognize medicine you may be taking. The fact that a brand name product is not mentioned does not mean the information does not apply. It is a good idea for you to learn both the generic and brand names of your medicines and to write them down for future use.

Deferoxamine (dee-fer-OX-a-meen) is given by injection to remove excess iron from the body. This may be necessary in certain patients with anemia who must receive many blood transfusions. It is also used to treat acute iron poisoning, especially in small children.

Deferoxamine combines with iron in the bloodstream. The combination of iron and deferoxamine is then removed from the body by the kidneys. By removing the excess iron, the medicine lessens damage to various organs and tissues of the body.

Deferoxamine is available only with your doctor's prescription.

Remember:

• **It is very important that you read and understand the following information.** If any of the information causes you special concern, do not decide against using this medicine without first checking with your doctor.

• Before you begin using any new medicine (prescription or nonprescription) or if you develop any new medical problem while you are using this medicine, check with your doctor, nurse, or pharmacist.

• **If you have any questions** about the following information or if you want more information about this medicine or your medical problem, **ask your doctor, nurse, or pharmacist.**

Before Using This Medicine

In order to decide on the best treatment for your medical problem, your doctor should be told:

—if you have ever had any unusual or allergic reaction to deferoxamine.

—if you are on a low-salt, low-sugar, or any other special diet, or if you are allergic to any substance, such as foods or sulfites or other preservatives. Most medicines contain more than their active ingredient. Your doctor, nurse, or pharmacist can help you avoid products that may cause a problem.

—if you are **pregnant** or if you may become pregnant. Deferoxamine has not been shown to cause birth defects or other problems in humans. However, studies in animals have shown that this medicine given in doses just above the recommended human dose causes birth

defects. In general, deferoxamine is not recommended for women who may become pregnant or during early pregnancy, unless their life is in danger from too much iron.

—if you are **breast-feeding**. It is not known whether deferoxamine is excreted in breast milk. However, this medicine has not been shown to cause problems in nursing babies.

—if you have kidney disease.

—if you are now taking **any** other prescription or nonprescription (OTC) medicine, especially ascorbic acid (vitamin C).

Proper Use of This Medicine

Some medicines given by injection may sometimes be given at home to patients who do not need to be in the hospital. If you are using this medicine at home, **make sure you clearly understand and carefully follow your doctor's instructions.**

How to store this medicine:

• **Keep out of the reach of children.**

• Store away from heat and direct light.

• Store the mixed medicine at room temperature for no more than one week. Do not refrigerate.

• Do not keep outdated medicine or medicine that is no longer needed. Be sure any discarded medicine is out of the reach of children.

Precautions While Using This Medicine

It is important that your doctor check your progress at regular visits to make sure that this medicine is working properly and to prevent unwanted effects. Certain blood and urine tests must be done regularly to allow for dosage changes.

Deferoxamine may cause some people, especially younger patients, to have hearing and vision problems within a few weeks after they start taking it. **If you notice any problems with your vision, such as blurred vision, difficulty in seeing at night, or difficulty in seeing colors, or difficulty with your hearing, check with your doctor as soon as possible.** The dose of deferoxamine may need to be adjusted.

Do not take vitamin C unless your doctor has told you to do so.

Side Effects of This Medicine

Along with its needed effects, a medicine may cause some unwanted effects. Although not all of these side effects may occur, if they do occur they may need medical attention.

Check with your doctor as soon as possible if any of the following side effects occur:

More common

Blurred vision or other changes in vision
Difficulty in breathing (wheezing)
Hearing problems

Pain or swelling at place of injection
Skin rash
Less common
Abdominal (stomach) discomfort
Diarrhea
Difficult urination
Fast heartbeat
Fever
Leg cramps

Hearing and vision problems are more likely to occur in younger patients taking high doses and on long-term treatment.

Deferoxamine may cause the urine to turn orange-rose in color. This is to be expected while you are using this medicine.

For elderly patients: Many medicines have not been tested in older people. Therefore, it is not known whether the medicine acts the same way it does in younger adults. Check with your doctor or pharmacist if you notice any unusual effects while taking this medicine or if you do not think it is working as it should.

Other side effects not listed above may also occur in some patients. If you notice any other effects, check with your doctor.

December 1987

DESMOPRESSIN (Systemic)

Some commonly used brand names are DDAVP and Stimate.

To the Reader: If you do not recognize the names of medical conditions or medicines referred to in this information, check with your doctor, nurse, or pharmacist. Definitions for selected medical terms may be found in the Glossary. Brand names for the generic drug names listed can be found in the Index. In addition, selected brand names commonly associated with the generic name have been included in the text to help you recognize medicine you may be taking. The fact that a brand name product is not mentioned does not mean the information does not apply. It is a good idea for you to learn both the generic and brand names of your medicines and to write them down for future use.

Desmopressin (des-moe-PRESS-in) is a hormone taken through the nose or given by injection to prevent or control the frequent urination, increased thirst, and loss of water associated with diabetes insipidus (water diabetes). It is used also to control frequent urination and increased thirst associated with certain types of brain injuries or brain surgery. Desmopressin works by acting on the kidneys to reduce the flow of urine.

Desmopressin is also given by injection to treat some patients with certain bleeding problems such as hemophilia or von Willebrand's disease.

It may also be used for other conditions as determined by your doctor.

Desmopressin is available only with your doctor's prescription.

Remember:

• **This medicine has been prescribed for your current medical problem only.** It must not be given to other people or used for other problems unless you are directed to do so by your doctor.

• **Keep all medicines out of the reach of children.**

• In order for this medicine to work, it must be used as directed.

• If you are receiving this medicine by injection, some of the information about this medicine may not apply.

• **It is very important that you read and understand the following information.** If any of the information causes you special concern, do not decide against using this medicine without first checking with your doctor.

• Before you begin using any new medicine (prescription or nonprescription) or if you develop any new medical problem while you are using this medicine, check with your doctor, nurse, or pharmacist.

• **If you have any questions** about the following information or if you want more information about this medicine or your medical problem, **ask your doctor, nurse, or pharmacist.**

Before Using This Medicine

In order to decide on the best treatment for your medical problem, your doctor should be told:

—if you have ever had any unusual or allergic reaction to desmopressin.

—if you are allergic to any substance, such as certain preservatives or dyes. Most medicines contain more than their active ingredient. Your doctor, nurse, or pharmacist can help you avoid products that may cause a problem.

—if you are **pregnant** or if you may become pregnant. Studies have not been done in humans. However, desmopressin has not been shown to cause birth defects or other problems in rats or rabbits given up to 12.5 times the human dose.

—if you are **breast-feeding**. Desmopressin has not been shown to cause problems in nursing babies.

—if you have any of the following medical problems:
  Heart or blood vessel disease
  High blood pressure
  Stuffy nose caused by cold or allergy

—if you are taking **any** other prescription or nonprescription (OTC) medicine.

Proper Use of This Medicine

For patients using the nasal solution form of this medicine:

• **Use this medicine only as directed.** Do not use more of it and do not use it more often than your doctor ordered. To do so may increase the chance of side effects.

• This medicine usually comes with patient directions. Read them carefully before using this medicine.

• If you miss a dose of this medicine and your dosing schedule is one dose to be used:
  Once a day—
    Use the missed dose as soon as possible. Then go back to your regular dosing schedule. However, if you do not remember the missed dose until the next day, skip the missed dose and go back to your regular dosing schedule. Do not double doses.
  More than once a day—
    Use the missed dose as soon as possible. Then go back to your regular dosing schedule. However, if it is almost time for your next dose, skip the missed dose and go back to your regular dosing schedule. Do not double doses.

How to store this medicine:

• **Keep out of the reach of children.**

• Store away from heat and direct light.

• Do not keep outdated medicine or medicine no longer needed. Be sure that any discarded medicine is out of the reach of children.

Side Effects of This Medicine

Along with its needed effects, a medicine may cause some
unwanted effects. Although not all of these effects
may occur, if they do occur they may need medical
attention.

Check with your doctor immediately if any of the following side effects occur since they may be signs of an
overdose:

> Confusion
> Convulsions (seizures)
> Drowsiness
> Headache (continuing)
> Problem with urination
> Weight gain

Other side effects may occur that usually do not require
medical attention. These side effects may go away
during treatment as your body adjusts to the medicine.

However, check with your doctor if any of the following side effects continue or are bothersome:

Less common or rare
> Abdominal or stomach cramps
> Flushing or redness of skin
> Headache
> Nausea
> Pain in the vulva

With intranasal (through the nose) use
> Runny or stuffy nose

With intravenous use
> Pain, redness, or swelling at the place of injection

Other side effects not listed above may also occur in some
patients. If you notice any other effects, check with
your doctor.

December 1987

DEXTROMETHORPHAN (Systemic)

Some commonly used brand names are:

Balminil D.M.*	Koffex*
Benylin DM Cough	Mediquell
Broncho-Grippol-DM*	Neo-DM*
Congespirin	PediaCare 1
Cremacoat 1	Pertussin 8 Hour Cough
Delsym	Formula
Demo-Cineol*	Robidex*
DM Cough	Sedatuss*
DM Syrup*	St. Joseph for Children
Hold	Sucrets Cough Control

*Not available in the U.S.

To the Reader: If you do not recognize the names of medical conditions or medicines referred to in this information, check with your doctor, nurse, or pharmacist. Definitions for selected medical terms may be found in the Glossary. Brand names for the generic drug names listed can be found in the Index. In addition, selected brand names commonly associated with the generic name have been included in the text to help you recognize medicine you may be taking. The fact that a brand name product is not mentioned does not mean the information does not apply. It is a good idea for you to learn both the generic and brand names of your medicines and to write them down for future use.

Dextromethorphan (dex-troe-meth-OR-fan) is taken by mouth to relieve coughs due to colds or influenza (flu). It is not to be used for chronic cough that occurs with smoking, asthma, or emphysema or when there is an unusually large amount of mucus or phlegm with the cough.

Dextromethorphan relieves cough by acting directly on the cough center in the brain.

This medicine is available without a prescription; however, your doctor may have special instructions on the proper use of this medicine for your medical condition.

Remember:
- **Keep all medicines out of the reach of children.**
- In order for this medicine to work, it must be used as directed. **If you are using this medicine without a prescription, it is very important to follow the directions on the label.**
- **It is also very important that you read and understand the following information.** If any of the information causes you special concern, check with your doctor before using this medicine without a prescription.
- Before you begin using any new medicine (prescription or nonprescription) or if you develop any new medical problem while you are using this medicine, check with your doctor, nurse, or pharmacist.
- **If you have any questions** about the following information or if you want more information about this medicine or your medical problem, **ask your doctor, nurse, or pharmacist.**

Before Using This Medicine

Before you use dextromethorphan, check with your doctor or pharmacist:

—if you have ever had any unusual or allergic reaction to dextromethorphan.

—if you are on a low-salt, low-sugar, or any other special diet, or if you are allergic to any substance, such as foods, sulfites or other preservatives, or dyes.

Most medicines contain more than their active ingredient, and many liquid medicines contain alcohol. Your doctor, nurse, or pharmacist can help you avoid products that may cause a problem.

—if you are **pregnant** or if you may become pregnant. Dextromethorphan has not been shown to cause problems in humans.

—if you are **breast-feeding.** Dextromethorphan has not been shown to cause problems in nursing babies.

—if you have either of the following medical problems:
   Asthma
   Liver disease

—if you are taking **any** other prescription or nonprescription (OTC) medicine, especially central nervous system (CNS) depressants.

—if you are now taking or have taken within the past 2 weeks monoamine oxidase (MAO) inhibitors, such as:

   Furazolidone (e.g., Furoxone)
   Isocarboxazid (e.g., Marplan)
   Pargyline (e.g., Eutonyl)
   Phenelzine (e.g., Nardil)
   Procarbazine (e.g., Matulane)
   Tranylcypromine (e.g., Parnate)

Proper Use of This Medicine

If you must take this medicine regularly and you miss a dose, take it as soon as possible. However, if it is almost time for your next dose, skip the missed dose and go back to your regular dosing schedule. Do not double doses.

How to store this medicine:

- Store away from heat and direct light.

- **Keep out of the reach of children.**

- Do not store the tablet form of this medicine in the bathroom, near the kitchen sink, or in other damp places. Heat or moisture may cause the medicine to break down.

- Keep the liquid form of this medicine from freezing.

- Do not keep outdated medicine or medicine no longer needed. Be sure that any discarded medicine is out of the reach of children.

Precautions While Using This Medicine

If your cough has not improved after 7 days or if you have a high fever, skin rash, or continuing headache with the cough, check with your doctor. These signs may mean that you have other medical problems.

Side Effects of This Medicine

Along with its needed effects, a medicine may cause some unwanted effects. Although not all of these side effects may occur, if they do occur they may need medical attention.

Check with your doctor as soon as possible if any of the following side effects occur:

Signs of overdose
   Confusion
   Unusual excitement, nervousness, restlessness, or irritability (severe)

Other side effects may occur that usually do not require medical attention. These side effects may go away during treatment as your body adjusts to the medicine. However, check with your doctor or pharmacist if any of the following side effects continue or are bothersome:

Less common or rare
   Dizziness
   Drowsiness
   Nausea or vomiting
   Stomach pain

For elderly patients: Many medicines have not been tested in older people. Therefore, it is not known whether the medicine acts the same way it does in younger adults. Check with your doctor or pharmacist if you notice any unusual effects while taking this medicine or if you think it is not working as it should.

Other side effects not listed above may also occur in some patients. If you notice any other effects, check with your doctor.

December 1987

DEXTROTHYROXINE (Systemic)

A commonly used brand name is Choloxin.

To the Reader: If you do not recognize the names of medical conditions or medicines referred to in this information, check with your doctor, nurse, or pharmacist. Definitions for selected medical terms may be found in the Glossary. Brand names for the generic drug names listed can be found in the Index. In addition, selected brand names commonly associated with the generic name have been included in the text to help you recognize medicine you may be taking. The fact that a brand name product is not mentioned does not mean the information does not apply. It is a good idea for you to learn both the generic and brand names of your medicines and to write them down for future use.

Dextrothyroxine (dex-troe-thye-ROX-een) is used to lower high cholesterol levels in the blood. This may help prevent medical problems caused by cholesterol clogging the blood vessels.

Dextrothyroxine is available only with your doctor's prescription.

Remember:
- **This medicine has been prescribed for your current medical problem only.** It must not be given to other people or used for other problems unless you are directed to do so by your doctor.

- **Keep all medicines out of the reach of children.**

- In order for this medicine to work, it must be used as directed.

- **It is very important that you read and understand the following information.** If any of the information causes you special concern, do not decide against using this medicine without first checking with your doctor.

- Before you begin using any new medicine (prescription or nonprescription) or if you develop any new medical problem while you are using this medicine, check with your doctor, nurse, or pharmacist.

- **If you have any questions** about the following information or if you want more information about this medicine or your medical problem, **ask your doctor, nurse, or pharmacist.**

Before Using This Medicine

Importance of diet—Before prescribing medicine for your condition, your doctor will probably try to control your condition by prescribing a personal diet for you. Such a diet may be low in fats, sugars, and/or cholesterol. Many people are able to control their condition by carefully following their doctor's orders for proper diet and exercise. Medicine is prescribed only when additional help is needed and is effective only when a schedule of diet and exercise is properly followed.

Also, this medicine is less effective if you are greatly overweight. It may be very important for you to go on a reducing diet. However, check with your doctor before going on any diet.

In order to decide on the best treatment for your medical problem, your doctor should be told:
—if you have ever had any unusual or allergic reaction to dextrothyroxine or other thyroid medicines.

—if you are on a low-salt, low-sugar, or any other special diet, or if you are allergic to any substance, such as foods, sulfites or other preservatives, or dyes. Most medicines contain more than their active ingredient. Your doctor, nurse, or pharmacist can help you avoid products that may cause a problem.

—if you are **pregnant** or if you may become pregnant, although dextrothyroxine has not been shown to cause birth defects or other problems in humans. Your doctor should check your progress at regular visits while you are pregnant.

—if you are **breast-feeding**. Although dextrothyroxine passes into the breast milk, it has not been shown to cause problems in nursing babies.

—if you have any of the following medical problems:
  Diabetes mellitus (sugar diabetes)
  Heart or blood vessel disease
  High blood pressure
  Kidney disease
  Liver disease
  Overactive or underactive thyroid

—if you are taking **any** other prescription or nonprescription (OTC) medicine, especially:
  Anticoagulants (blood thinners)
  Cholestyramine (e.g., Questran)
  Colestipol (e.g., Colestid)

Proper Use of This Medicine

Take this medicine exactly as directed by your doctor. Try not to miss any doses and do not take more medicine than your doctor ordered.

Remember that this medicine will not cure your cholesterol problem but it does help control it. Therefore, you must continue to take it as directed if you expect to lower your cholesterol level.

If you miss a dose of this medicine, take it as soon as possible. However, if it is almost time for your next dose, skip the missed dose and go back to your regular dosing schedule. Do not double doses.

How to store this medicine:
- **Keep out of the reach of children.**
- Store away from heat and direct light.
- Do not store in the bathroom, near the kitchen sink, or in other damp places. Heat or moisture may cause the medicine to break down.
- Do not keep outdated medicine or medicine no longer needed. Be sure that any discarded medicine is out of the reach of children.

Precautions While Using This Medicine

It is very important that your doctor check your progress at regular visits. This will allow your doctor to see if the medicine is working properly to lower your cholesterol levels and if you should continue to take it.

Before having any kind of surgery (including dental surgery) or emergency treatment, **tell the physician or dentist in charge that you are taking this medicine.**

Side Effects of This Medicine

Along with its needed effects, a medicine may cause some unwanted effects. Although not all of these side effects may occur, if they do occur they may need medical attention.

Check with your doctor immediately if any of the following side effects occur:

Rare

   Chest pain
   Fast or irregular heartbeat
   Stomach pain (severe) with nausea and vomiting

Check with your doctor as soon as possible if the following side effects occur, since they may indicate too much medicine is being taken:

Rare

   Changes in menstrual periods
   Diarrhea
   Fever

   Hand tremors
   Headache
   Increase in urination
   Irritability, nervousness, or trouble in sleeping
   Leg cramps
   Shortness of breath
   Skin rash or itching
   Sweating, flushing, or increased sensitivity to heat
   Vomiting, weight loss, or changes in appetite

For elderly patients: The above side effects are more likely to occur in the elderly (over 60 years of age), who are usually more sensitive to the effects of dextrothyroxine.

Other side effects not listed above may also occur in some patients. If you notice any other effects, check with your doctor.

December 1987

DIATRIZOATE AND IODIPAMIDE
(Mucosal)

A commonly used brand name is Sinografin.

Generic name product may also be available in the U.S.

To the Reader: If you do not recognize the names of medical conditions or medicines referred to in this information, check with your doctor, nurse, or pharmacist. Definitions for selected medical terms may be found in the Glossary. Brand names for the generic drug names listed can be found in the Index. In addition, selected brand names commonly associated with the generic name have been included in the text to help you recognize medicine you may be taking. The fact that a brand name product is not mentioned does not mean the information does not apply. It is a good idea for you to learn both the generic and brand names of your medicines and to write them down for future use.

Diatrizoate (dye-a-tri-ZOE-ate) and iodipamide (eye-oh-DI-pa-mide) combination is a radiopaque agent. This agent contains iodine, which absorbs x-rays. Depending on how the radiopaque agent is given, it builds up in certain areas of the body. The resulting high level of iodine allows the x-rays to make a "picture" of the area.

The solution of diatrizoate and iodipamide is instilled into the uterus and fallopian tubes to help diagnose problems or disease of these organs.

Diatrizoate and iodipamide combination is to be used only by or under the supervision of a doctor.

Remember:

• **It is very important that you read and understand the following information.** If any of the information causes you special concern, do not decide against receiving this radiopaque agent without first checking with your doctor.

• **If you have any questions** about the following information or if you want more information about this radiopaque agent or your medical problem, **ask your doctor, nurse, or pharmacist.**

Before Having This Test

Before this test is given, your doctor should be told:

—if you have ever had any unusual or allergic reaction to iodine, to products containing iodine (for example, iodine-containing foods, such as seafoods, cabbage, kale, rape, turnips, or iodized salt), or to other radiopaque agents.

—if you are allergic to any substance, such as sulfites or other preservatives. Most medicines contain more than their active ingredient. Your doctor can help you avoid products that may cause a problem.

—if you are **pregnant** or if you suspect that you may be pregnant when you are to receive this radiopaque agent. Diatrizoate and iodipamide combination is not recommended during pregnancy or for at least 3 months after a pregnancy has ended. The test may cause other problems, such as infection in the uterus. Also, other radiopaque agents containing iodine have caused, on rare occasions, hypothyroidism (underactive thyroid) in the baby. In addition, x-rays of the abdomen during pregnancy may have harmful effects on the fetus.

—if you are **breast-feeding**. Although diatrizoate and iodipamide combination has not been shown to cause problems in nursing babies, the chance always exists since it passes into the breast milk.

—if you have any of the following medical problems:
   Asthma, hay fever, or other allergies
   Genital tract infection
   Pelvic inflammatory disease (severe)

Preparation for This Test

Your doctor may have special instructions for you in preparation for your test. If you have not received such instructions or if you do not understand them, check with your doctor in advance.

Precautions After Having This Test

Make sure your doctor knows if you are planning to have any future thyroid tests. Even after several weeks or months, the results of the thyroid test may be affected by the iodine in this agent.

Side Effects of This Medicine

Along with its needed effects, radiopaque agents like diatrizoate and iodipamide can cause serious side effects such as allergic reactions. These effects may occur almost immediately or a few minutes after the radiopaque agent is given. Although these serious side effects appear only rarely, your doctor or nurse will be prepared to give you immediate medical attention if needed. If you have any questions about this, check with your doctor.

Other side effects may occur that usually do not require medical attention. These side effects should go away as the effects of the radiopaque agent wear off. However, check with your doctor if any of the following side effects continue or are bothersome:

Less common
   Abdominal or stomach pain and discomfort
   Chills
   Fever
   Nausea and vomiting

For elderly patients: Many medicines have not been tested in older people. Therefore, it is not known whether the medicine acts the same way it does in younger adults. Check with your doctor if you notice any unusual effects after receiving this medicine.

Other side effects not listed above may also occur in some patients. If you notice any other effects, check with your doctor.

December 1987

DIATRIZOATES (Mucosal)

Some commonly used brand names are:

Cystografin	Hypaque-Cysto
Cystografin Dilute	Reno-M-30
Hypaque	Urovist Cysto

To the Reader: If you do not recognize the names of medical conditions or medicines referred to in this information, check with your doctor, nurse, or pharmacist. Definitions for selected medical terms may be found in the Glossary. Brand names for the generic drug names listed can be found in the Index. In addition, selected brand names commonly associated with the generic name have been included in the text to help you recognize medicine you may be taking. The fact that a brand name product is not mentioned does not mean the information does not apply. It is a good idea for you to learn both the generic and brand names of your medicines and to write them down for future use.

Diatrizoates (dye-a-tri-ZOE-ates) are radiopaque agents. These agents contain iodine, which absorbs x-rays. Depending on how the radiopaque agent is given, it builds up in certain areas of the body. The resulting high level of iodine allows the x-rays to make a "picture" of the area.

A catheter or syringe is used to put the solution of diatrizoate into the bladder or ureters to help diagnose problems or diseases of the kidneys or other areas of the urinary tract. After the test is done, the solution is expelled by urinating.

Diatrizoate is to be used only by or under the supervision of a doctor.

Remember:

• **It is very important that you read and understand the following information.** If any of the information causes you special concern, do not decide against receiving this radiopaque agent without first checking with your doctor.

• **If you have any questions** about the following information or if you want more information about this radiopaque agent or your medical problem, **ask your doctor, nurse, or pharmacist**.

Before Having This Test

Before this test is given, your doctor should be told:

—if you have ever had any unusual or allergic reaction to iodine, to products containing iodine (for example, iodine-containing foods, such as seafood, cabbage, kale, rape (turnip-like vegetable) or turnips, or iodized salt), or to other radiopaque agents.

—if you are allergic to any substance, such as sulfites or other preservatives. Most medicines contain more than their active ingredient. Your doctor can help you avoid products that may cause a problem.

—if you are **pregnant** or if you suspect that you may be pregnant when you are to receive this radiopaque agent. Studies have not been done in either humans or animals. However, other radiopaque agents containing iodine have caused, on rare occasions, hypothyroidism (underactive thyroid) in the baby. Also, x-rays of the abdomen are usually not recommended during pregnancy. This is to avoid exposing the fetus to radiation. Be sure you have discussed this with your doctor.

—if you are **breast-feeding**. Although diatrizoate has not been shown to cause problems in nursing babies, the chance always exists since it passes into the breast milk.

—if you have any of the following medical problems:
Asthma, hay fever, or other allergies
Enlarged prostate
Urinary tract infection

Preparation for This Test

Your doctor may have special instructions for you in preparation for your test. If you have not received such instructions or if you do not understand them, check with your doctor in advance.

Precautions After Having This Test

Make sure your doctor knows if you are planning to have any future thyroid tests. Even after several weeks the results of the thyroid test may be affected by the iodine in this agent.

Side Effects of This Medicine

Along with its needed effects, a medicine may cause some unwanted effects. Although not all of these side effects may occur, if they do occur they may need medical attention.

Check with your doctor or nurse immediately if any of the following side effects occur:
Less common
Abdominal or stomach pain and discomfort
Backache

For elderly patients: Many medicines have not been tested in older people. Therefore, it is not known whether the medicine acts the same way it does in younger adults. Check with your doctor if you notice any unusual effects after receiving this medicine.

Other side effects not listed above may also occur in some patients. If you notice any other effects, check with your doctor.

December 1987

DIATRIZOATES (Systemic)

Some commonly used brand names are:

Gastrografin	Reno-M
Hypaque	Reno-M Dip
Hypaque Meglumine	Renovist
Hypaque Sodium	Urovist Meglumine DIU/CT
MD-Gastroview	Urovist Sodium
Renografin	

To the Reader: If you do not recognize the names of medical conditions or medicines referred to in this information, check with your doctor, nurse, or pharmacist. Definitions for selected medical terms may be found in the Glossary. Brand names for the generic drug names listed can be found in the Index. In addition, selected brand names commonly associated with the generic name have been included in the text to help you recognize medicine you may be taking. The fact that a brand name product is not mentioned does not mean the information does not apply. It is a good idea for you to learn both the generic and brand names of your medicines and to write them down for future use.

Diatrizoates (dye-a-tri-ZOE-ates) are radiopaque agents. Radiopaque agents contain iodine, which absorbs x-rays. Depending on how they are given, radiopaque agents build up in a particular area of the body. The resulting high level of iodine allows the x-rays to make a "picture" of the area.

Diatrizoates are taken by mouth or given by enema or injection. X-rays are then used to check if there are any problems with the stomach, intestines, kidneys, or other parts of the body.

Radiopaque agents are to be used only by or under the direct supervision of a doctor.

Remember:

• **It is very important that you read and understand the following information.** If any of the information causes you special concern, do not decide against taking or receiving this radiopaque agent without first checking with your doctor.

• **If you have any questions** about the following information or if you want more information about this radiopaque agent or your medical problem, **ask your doctor, nurse, or pharmacist**.

Before Having This Test

Before this test is given, your doctor should be told:

—if you have ever had any unusual or allergic reaction to iodine, to products containing iodine (for example, iodine-containing foods, such as seafoods, cabbage, kale, rape, turnips, or iodized salt), or to other radiopaque agents.

—if you are allergic to any substance, such as sulfites or other preservatives. Most medicines contain more than their active ingredient. Your doctor can help you avoid products that may cause a problem.

—if you are **pregnant** or if you suspect that you may be pregnant when you are to receive this radiopaque agent. Studies on birth defects have not been done in either humans or animals. However, other radiopaque agents containing iodine have, on rare occasions, caused

hypothyroidism (underactive thyroid) in the infant. Also, x-rays of the abdomen are usually not recommended during pregnancy. This is to avoid exposing the fetus to radiation. Be sure you have discussed this with your doctor.

—if you are **breast-feeding**. Although diatrizoates have not been shown to cause problems in nursing babies, the chance always exists since these agents pass into the breast milk.

—if you have or have had **any** medical problems, especially:

    Asthma, hay fever, or food allergies
    Bleeding problems
    Diabetes mellitus (sugar diabetes)
    Heart or blood vessel disease
    High blood pressure
    Infection
    Kidney disease
    Liver disease (severe)
    Migraine
    Multiple myeloma (bone cancer)
    Overactive thyroid
    Pheochromocytoma (PCC)
    Sickle cell disease

—if you are taking **any** other prescription or nonprescription (OTC) medicine.

Preparation For This Test

Your doctor may have special instructions for you in preparation for your test. He or she might prescribe a special diet or use of a laxative, depending on the type of test. If you have not received such instructions or if you do not understand them, check with your doctor in advance.

Do not have any food for several hours before having the test, unless otherwise directed by your doctor. This is to prevent any food from coming back up and entering your lungs during the test. You may be allowed to drink small amounts of clear liquids; however, check first with your doctor.

Precautions After Having This Test

Make sure your doctor knows if you are planning to have any future thyroid tests. Even after several weeks or months the results of the thyroid test may be affected by the iodine in this agent.

Side Effects of This Medicine

Along with their needed effects, radiopaque agents like diatrizoates can sometimes cause serious effects such as severe allergic reactions or heart problems. These effects may occur almost immediately or a few minutes after the radiopaque agent is given. Although these serious side effects appear only rarely, your doctor or nurse will be prepared to give you immediate medical attention if needed. If you have any questions about this, check with your doctor.

Other side effects may occur that usually do not require medical attention. These side effects may go away as your body adjusts to this agent. However, check with your doctor if any of the following side effects continue or are bothersome:

More common

Unusual warmth and flushing of skin

Less common

Chills
Diarrhea or laxative effect
Dizziness or lightheadedness
Headache

Nausea or vomiting
Sweating
Unusual thirst

For children or elderly patients: The above side effects are more likely to occur in children and the elderly, who are usually more sensitive to the effects of diatrizoates.

Other side effects not listed above may also occur in some patients. If you notice any other effects, check with your doctor.

December 1987

DIAZOXIDE (Oral)

A commonly used brand name is Proglycem.

To the Reader: If you do not recognize the names of medical conditions or medicines referred to in this information, check with your doctor, nurse, or pharmacist. Definitions for selected medical terms may be found in the Glossary. Brand names for the generic drug names listed can be found in the Index. In addition, selected brand names commonly associated with the generic name have been included in the text to help you recognize medicine you may be taking. The fact that a brand name product is not mentioned does not mean the information does not apply. It is a good idea for you to learn both the generic and brand names of your medicines and to write them down for future use.

Diazoxide (dye-az-OX-ide) when taken by mouth is used in the treatment of hypoglycemia (low blood sugar). It works by preventing release of insulin from the pancreas.

Diazoxide is available only with your doctor's prescription.

Remember:

• **This medicine has been prescribed for your current medical problem only.** It must not be given to other people or used for other problems unless you are directed to do so by your doctor.

• **Keep all medicines out of the reach of children.**

• In order for this medicine to work, it must be used as directed.

• **It is very important that you read and understand the following information.** If any of the information causes you special concern, do not decide against using this medicine without first checking with your doctor.

• Before you begin using any new medicine (prescription or nonprescription) or if you develop any new medical problem while you are using this medicine, check with your doctor, nurse, or pharmacist.

• **If you have any questions** about the following information or if you want more information about this medicine or your medical problem, **ask your doctor, nurse, or pharmacist.**

Before Using This Medicine

In order to decide on the best treatment for your medical problem, your doctor should be told:

—if you have ever had any unusual or allergic reaction to diazoxide, sulfonamides (sulfa drugs), or thiazide diuretics (water pills).

—if you are on a low-salt, low-sugar, or any other special diet, or if you are allergic to any substance, such as foods, sulfites or other preservatives, or dyes. Most medicines contain more than their active ingredient, and many liquid medicines contain alcohol. Your doctor, nurse, or pharmacist can help you avoid products that may cause a problem.

—if you are **pregnant** or if you may become pregnant. Studies have not been done in humans. However, too much use of diazoxide during pregnancy may cause unwanted effects (high blood sugar, loss of hair or increased hair growth, blood problems) in the baby. Studies in animals have shown that diazoxide causes some birth defects (in the skeleton, heart, and pancreas) and other problems (delayed birth, decrease in successful pregnancies).

—if you are **breast-feeding**. It is not known whether diazoxide passes into breast milk. This medicine has not been shown to cause problems in nursing babies.

—if you have any of the following medical problems:

Angina (chest pain)
Gout
Heart or blood vessel disease
Kidney disease
Liver disease

—if you have had a recent heart attack or stroke.

—if you are taking **any** other prescription or nonprescription (OTC) medicine, especially:

Amantadine (e.g., Symmetrel)
Amyl nitrite
Antidepressants (medicine for depression)
Antihypertensives (high blood pressure medicine)
Beta-blockers (acebutolol, atenolol, esmolol, labetalol, metoprolol, nadolol, oxprenolol, pindolol, propranolol, sotalol, timolol)
Bromocriptine (e.g., Parlodel)
Captopril (e.g., Capoten)
Chlorprothixene (e.g., Taractan)
Cyclandelate (e.g., Cyclospasmol)
Diltiazem (e.g., Cardizem)
Diuretics (water pills)
Enalapril (e.g., Vasotec)
Ethotoin (e.g., Peganone)
Haloperidol (e.g., Haldol)
Hydralazine (e.g., Apresoline)
Isoxsuprine (e.g., Vasodilan)
Levodopa (e.g., Dopar)
Loxapine (e.g., Loxitane)
Mephenytoin (e.g., Mesantoin)
Molindone (e.g., Moban)
Narcotic pain medicine
Nicotinyl alcohol (e.g., Roniacol)
Nifedipine (e.g., Procardia)
Nitrates (medicine for angina)
Nylidrin (e.g., Arlidin)
Papaverine (e.g., Pavabid)
Phenothiazines (acetophenazine, chlorpromazine, fluphenazine, mesoridazine, perphenazine, prochlorperazine, promazine, promethazine, thioridazine, trifluoperazine, triflupromazine, trimeprazine)
Phenytoin (e.g., Dilantin)
Pimozide (e.g., Orap)
Prazosin (e.g., Minipress)
Procainamide (e.g., Pronestyl)
Quinidine (e.g., Quinidex)
Thiothixene (e.g., Navane)
Verapamil (e.g., Calan)

—if you are now taking or have taken within the past 2 weeks monoamine oxidase (MAO) inhibitors, such as:

Furazolidone (e.g., Furoxone)
Isocarboxazid (e.g., Marplan)
Pargyline (e.g., Eutonyl)

Phenelzine (e.g., Nardil)
Procarbazine (e.g., Matulane)
Tranylcypromine (e.g., Parnate)

—if you are now using any of the following medicines in the eye:

Levobunolol (e.g., Betagan)
Timolol (e.g., Timoptic)

Proper Use of This Medicine

Take this medicine only as directed by your doctor. Do not take more or less of it than your doctor ordered, and take it at the same time each day.

Follow carefully the special diet your doctor gave you. This is an important part of controlling your condition, and is necessary if the medicine is to work properly.

Test for sugar in your urine as directed by your doctor. This is a convenient way to make sure your condition is being controlled, and it provides an early warning when it is not. Two urine tests for sugar are widely used: the tablet urine test and the paper-strip urine test. The results of these two tests are read differently. For example, a 3-plus reading of a tablet urine test is not equal to a 3-plus reading of a paper-strip urine test. Do not change from one test to the other unless told to do so by your doctor. In addition, your doctor may instruct you to test your urine for acetone.

If you miss a dose of this medicine, take it as soon as possible. However, if it is almost time for your next dose, skip the missed dose and go back to your regular dosing schedule. Do not double doses.

How to store this medicine:

• **Keep out of the reach of children.**

• Store away from heat and direct light.

• Do not store in the bathroom, near the kitchen sink, or in other damp places. Heat or moisture may cause the medicine to break down.

• Keep the oral liquid form of this medicine from freezing.

• Do not keep outdated medicine or medicine no longer needed. Be sure that any discarded medicine is out of the reach of children.

Precautions While Using This Medicine

It is very important that your doctor check your progress at regular visits, especially during the first few weeks of treatment, to make sure that this medicine is working properly.

Do not take any other medicine, unless prescribed or approved by your doctor, since some may interfere with this medicine's effects. This especially includes over-the-counter (OTC) or nonprescription medicine such as that for colds, cough, asthma, hay fever, or appetite control.

Check with your doctor right away if signs of high blood sugar (hyperglycemia) occur. These signs usually include:

Drowsiness
Flushed, dry skin
Fruit-like breath odor
Increased urination
Loss of appetite
Unusual thirst

These signs may occur if the dose of the medicine is too high, or if you have a fever or infection or are experiencing unusual stress.

Check with your doctor as soon as possible also if these signs of low blood sugar (hypoglycemia) occur:

Anxiety
Chills
Cold sweats
Cool pale skin
Drowsiness
Excessive hunger
Fast pulse
Headache
Nausea
Nervousness
Shakiness
Unusual tiredness or weakness

Signs of both low blood sugar and high blood sugar must be corrected before they progress to a more serious condition. In either situation, you should check with your doctor immediately.

Side Effects of This Medicine

Along with its needed effects, a medicine may cause some unwanted effects. Although not all of these side effects may occur, if they do occur they may need medical attention.

Check with your doctor as soon as possible if any of the following side effects occur:
More common
Decrease in urination
Swelling of hands, feet, or lower legs
Weight gain
Less common
Fast or irregular heartbeat
Rare
Chest pain
Confusion
Fever
Numbness of the hands
Skin rash
Unusual bleeding or bruising

Other side effects may occur that usually do not require medical attention. These side effects may go away during treatment as your body adjusts to the medicine. However, check with your doctor if any of the following side effects continue or are bothersome:
Less common
Changes in ability to taste
Constipation
Increased hair growth on forehead, back, arms, and legs

Loss of appetite
Nausea and vomiting
Stiffness
Stomach pain
Trembling and shaking of hands and fingers

This medicine may cause a temporary increase in hair growth in some people. After treatment with diazoxide has ended, normal hair growth should return.

For elderly patients: Many medicines have not been tested in older people. Therefore, it is not known whether the medicine acts the same way it does in younger adults.

Check with your doctor or pharmacist if you notice any unusual effects while taking this medicine or if you think it is not working as it should.

Other side effects not listed above may also occur in some patients. If you notice any other effects, check with your doctor.

December 1987

DIFENOXIN AND ATROPINE (Systemic)

A commonly used brand name is Motofen.

To the Reader: If you do not recognize the names of medical conditions or medicines referred to in this information, check with your doctor, nurse, or pharmacist. Definitions for selected medical terms may be found in the Glossary. Brand names for the generic drug names listed can be found in the Index. In addition, selected brand names commonly associated with the generic name have been included in the text to help you recognize medicine you may be taking. The fact that a brand name product is not mentioned does not mean the information does not apply. It is a good idea for you to learn both the generic and brand names of your medicines and to write them down for future use.

Difenoxin (dye-fen-OX-in) and atropine (A-troe-peen) combination medicine is used along with other measures to treat severe diarrhea. Difenoxin helps stop diarrhea by slowing down the movements of the intestines. The atropine is included to prevent possible abuse, since difenoxin is chemically related to some narcotics.

This medicine is available only with your doctor's prescription.

Remember:

• **This medicine has been prescribed for your current medical problem only.** It must not be given to other people or used for other problems unless you are directed to do so by your doctor.

• **Keep all medicines out of the reach of children.**

• In order for this medicine to work, it must be used as directed.

• **It is very important that you read and understand the following information.** If any of the information causes you special concern, do not decide against using this medicine without first checking with your doctor.

• Before you begin using any new medicine (prescription or nonprescription) or if you develop any new medical problem while you are using this medicine, check with your doctor, nurse, or pharmacist.

• **If you have any questions** about the following information or if you want more information about this medicine or your medical problem, **ask your doctor, nurse, or pharmacist.**

Before Using This Medicine

In order to decide on the best treatment for your medical problem, your doctor should be told:

—if you have ever had any unusual or allergic reaction to difenoxin or atropine.

—if you are on a low-salt, low-sugar, or any other special diet, or if you are allergic to any substance, such as foods, sulfites or other preservatives, or dyes. Most medicines contain more than their active ingredient. Your doctor, nurse, or pharmacist can help you avoid products that may cause a problem.

—if you are **pregnant** or if you may become pregnant. Studies have not been done in humans. Studies in rats have shown that difenoxin and atropine when given in doses many times the human dose increases the delivery time and the chance of death in the newborn.

—if you are **breast-feeding**. Both difenoxin and atropine pass into the breast milk. However, this medicine has not been shown to cause problems in nursing babies.

—if you have any of the following medical problems:
Colitis (severe)
Difficult urination
Down's syndrome (mongolism) in children
Emphysema, asthma, bronchitis, or other chronic lung disease
Enlarged prostate
Gallbladder disease or gallstones
Glaucoma
Heart disease
Hiatal hernia
High blood pressure
Kidney disease
Liver disease
Myasthenia gravis
Overactive or underactive thyroid
Urinary tract blockage

—if you are taking **any** other prescription or nonprescription (OTC) medicine, especially:
Antimuscarinics, other (medicine for abdominal or stomach spasms or cramps)
Central nervous system (CNS) depressants

—if you are now taking an antibiotic. Some antibiotics may cause diarrhea. This medicine may make the diarrhea caused by antibiotics worse or make it last longer.

Proper Use of This Medicine

If this medicine upsets your stomach, your doctor may want you to take it with food.

Take this medicine only as directed by your doctor. Do not take more of it, do not take it more often, and do not take it for a longer period of time than your doctor ordered. If too much is taken, it may become habit-forming.

If you are taking this medicine on a regular schedule and you miss a dose, take it as soon as possible. However, if it is almost time for your next dose, skip the missed dose and go back to your regular dosing schedule. Do not double doses.

How to store this medicine:

• **Keep out of the reach of children** since overdose is especially dangerous in children.

• Store away from heat and direct light.

• Do not store in the bathroom, near the kitchen sink, or in other damp places. Heat or moisture may cause the medicine to break down.

• Do not keep outdated medicine or medicine no longer needed. Be sure that any discarded medicine is out of the reach of children.

Precautions While Using This Medicine

Your doctor should check your progress at regular visits if you will be taking this medicine regularly for a long period of time.

Check with your doctor if your diarrhea does not stop after a few days or if you develop a fever.

This medicine will add to the effects of alcohol and other CNS depressants (medicines that slow down the nervous system, possibly causing drowsiness). Some examples of CNS depressants are antihistamines or medicine for hay fever, other allergies, or colds; sedatives, tranquilizers, or sleeping medicine; prescription pain medicine or narcotics; barbiturates; medicine for convulsions (seizures); muscle relaxants; or anesthetics, including some dental anesthetics. **Check with your doctor before taking any of the above while you are taking this medicine.**

If you think you or someone else in your home may have taken an overdose of this medicine, get emergency help at once. Taking an overdose of this medicine may lead to unconsciousness and possibly death. Signs of overdose include severe drowsiness; fast heartbeat; shortness of breath or troubled breathing; and unusual warmth, dryness, and flushing of skin.

Before having any kind of surgery (including dental surgery) or emergency treatment, tell the doctor or dentist in charge that you are using this medicine.

This medicine may cause some people to become dizzy, drowsy, or less alert than they are normally. Even if taken at bedtime, it may cause some people to feel drowsy or less alert on arising. **Make sure you know how you react to this medicine before you drive, use machines, or do other jobs that require you to be alert.**

Side Effects of This Medicine

Along with its needed effects, a medicine may cause some unwanted effects. Although not all of these side effects may occur, if they do occur they may need medical attention. **When this medicine is used for short periods of time at low doses, side effects usually are rare.**

Check with your doctor immediately if any of the following side effects are severe and occur suddenly, since they may indicate a more severe and dangerous problem with your bowels:

    Bloating
    Constipation
    Loss of appetite
    Nausea and vomiting
    Stomach pain

Check with your doctor also if the following effects occur, since they may indicate an overdose:

    Blurred vision (continuing) or changes in near vision
    Drowsiness (severe)
    Dryness of mouth, nose, and throat (severe)
    Fast heartbeat
    Shortness of breath or troubled breathing (severe)
    Unusual excitement, nervousness, restlessness, or irritability (especially in children)
    Unusual warmth, dryness, and flushing of skin

Other side effects may occur that usually do not require medical attention. These side effects may go away during treatment as your body adjusts to the medicine. However, check with your doctor if any of the following side effects continue, worsen, or are bothersome:

Less common or rare
    Blurred vision
    Confusion
    Difficult urination
    Dizziness or lightheadedness
    Drowsiness
    Dryness of skin and mouth
    Fever
    Headache
    Trouble in sleeping
    Unusual tiredness or weakness

After you stop using this medicine, your body may need time to adjust. The length of time this takes depends on the amount of medicine you were using and how long you used it. During this period of time check with your doctor if you notice any of the following side effects:

    Increased sweating
    Muscle cramps
    Nausea or vomiting
    Shivering or trembling
    Stomach cramps

For children: The above side effects are more likely to occur in infants, young children, and in children with Down's syndrome.

For elderly patients: Shortness of breath or troubled breathing are more likely to occur in elderly patients.

Other side effects not listed above may also occur in some patients. If you notice any other effects, check with your doctor.

December 1987

DIGITALIS MEDICINES (Systemic)

This information applies to the following medicines:
Deslanoside (des-LAN-oh-side)
Digitalis (di-ji-TAL-iss)
Digitoxin (di-ji-TOX-in)
Digoxin (di-JOX-in)

Some commonly used brand names are:	Generic names:
Cedilanid* Cedilanid-D	Deslanoside
	Digitalist
Crystodigin	Digitoxint
Lanoxin Lanoxicaps Novodigoxin*	Digoxint‡

*Not available in the United States.
†Generic name product may also be available in the U.S.
‡Generic name product may also be available in Canada.

To the Reader: If you do not recognize the names of medical conditions or medicines referred to in this information, check with your doctor, nurse, or pharmacist. Definitions for selected medical terms may be found in the Glossary. Brand names for the generic drug names listed can be found in the Index. In addition, selected brand names commonly associated with the generic name have been included in the text to help you recognize medicine you may be taking. The fact that a brand name product is not mentioned does not mean the information does not apply. It is a good idea for you to learn both the generic and brand names of your medicines and to write them down for future use.

Digitalis medicines are taken by mouth or given by injection to improve the strength and efficiency of the heart, or to control the rate and rhythm of the heartbeat. This leads to better blood circulation and reduced swelling of hands and ankles in patients with heart problems.

Although digitalis has been prescribed to help some patients lose weight, it should **never** be used in this way. When used improperly, digitalis can cause serious problems.

Digitalis medicines are available only with your doctor's prescription.

Remember:

• **This medicine has been prescribed for your current medical problem only.** It must not be given to other people or used for other problems unless you are directed to do so by your doctor.

• **Keep all medicines out of the reach of children.**

• In order for this medicine to work, it must be used as directed.

• If you are receiving this medicine by injection, some of the information about this medicine may not apply.

• **It is very important that you read and understand the following information.** If any of the information causes you special concern, do not decide against using this medicine without first checking with your doctor.

• Before you begin using any new medicine (prescription or nonprescription) or if you develop any new medical problem while you are using this medicine, check with your doctor, nurse, or pharmacist.

• **If you have any questions** about the following information or if you want more information about this medicine or your medical problem, **ask your doctor, nurse, or pharmacist**.

Before Using This Medicine

In order to decide on the best treatment for your medical problem, your doctor should be told:

—if you have ever had any unusual or allergic reaction to digitalis medicine.

—if you are on a low-salt, low-sugar, or any other special diet, or if you are allergic to any substance, such as foods, sulfites or other preservatives, or dyes. Most medicines contain more than their active ingredient, and many liquid medicines contain alcohol. Your doctor, nurse, or pharmacist can help you avoid products that may cause a problem.

—if you are **pregnant** or if you may become pregnant. Studies have not been done in either humans or animals. However, these medicines pass from the mother to the fetus.

—if you are **breast-feeding**. Although small amounts of digitalis medicines pass into the breast milk, they have not been shown to cause problems in nursing babies.

—if you have any of the following medical problems:
  Kidney disease
  Liver disease
  Lung disease (severe)

—if you have recently had a heart attack.

—if you have ever had rheumatic fever.

—if you are now taking **any** prescription or nonprescription (OTC) medicine, especially:
  Adrenocorticoids (cortisone-like medicine)
  Amphetamines
  Amphotericin B by injection (e.g., Fungizone)
  Any other digitalis medicines or other heart medicine
  Appetite suppressants (diet pills)
  Cholestyramine (e.g., Questran)
  Colestipol (e.g., Colestid)
  Diarrhea medicine
  Diltiazem (e.g., Cardizem)
  Diuretics (water pills)
  Medicine for asthma or other breathing problems
  Medicine for colds, sinus problems, or hay fever or other allergies (including nose drops or sprays)
  Potassium-containing medicines or supplements
  Quinidine (e.g., Quinidex)
  Verapamil (e.g., Calan)

—if your diet contains large amounts of fiber, such as bran.

Proper Use of This Medicine

To keep your heart working properly, **take this medicine exactly as directed even though you may feel well.** Do not take more of it than your doctor ordered and do not miss any doses.

For patients taking the liquid form of digoxin:
- This medicine is to be taken by mouth even though it may come in a dropper bottle. The amount you should take is to be measured only with the specially marked dropper.

To help you remember to take your dose of medicine, try to take it at the same time every day.

Ask your doctor about checking your pulse rate. Then, while you are taking this medicine, check your pulse regularly. If it is much slower, or faster, than your usual rate (or less than 60 beats per minute), or if it changes in rhythm or force, check with your doctor. Such changes may mean that side effects are developing.

If you do miss a dose of this medicine, and you remember it within 12 hours, take it as soon as you remember. However, if you do not remember until later, do not take the missed dose at all and do not double the next one. Instead, go back to your regular dosing schedule. If you have any questions about this or if you miss doses for 2 or more days in a row, check with your doctor.

How to store this medicine:
- **Keep out of the reach of children.**
- Store away from heat and direct light.
- Do not store in the bathroom, near the kitchen sink, or in other damp places. Heat or moisture may cause the medicine to break down.
- Keep the oral liquid form of this medicine from freezing.
- Do not keep outdated medicine or medicine no longer needed. Be sure that any discarded medicine is out of the reach of children.

Precautions While Using This Medicine

It is important that your doctor check your progress at regular visits to make sure the medicine is working properly. This will allow your doctor to make any changes in directions for taking it, if necessary.

Do not stop taking this medicine without first checking with your doctor. Stopping suddenly may cause a serious change in heart function.

Keep this medicine out of the reach of children. Digitalis medicines are a major cause of accidental poisoning in children.

Watch for signs of overdose while you are taking digitalis medicine. Follow your doctor's directions carefully. The amount of this medicine needed to help most people is very close to the amount that could cause serious problems from overdose. Some early warning signs of overdose are loss of appetite, nausea, vomiting, diarrhea, or extremely slow heartbeat. In infants and small children, the earliest signs of overdose are changes in the rate and rhythm of the heartbeat. Children may not show the other signs as soon as adults.

Before having any kind of surgery (including dental surgery) or emergency treatment, tell the physician or dentist in charge that you are using this medicine.

Your doctor may want you to carry a medical identification card or bracelet stating that you are taking this medicine.

Do not take any other medicine unless ordered by your doctor. Many over-the-counter (OTC) or nonprescription medicines contain ingredients that interfere with digitalis medicines or that may make your condition worse. These medicines include antacids; laxatives; asthma remedies; cold, cough, or sinus preparations; medicine for diarrhea; and reducing or diet medicines.

For patients taking the tablet or capsule form of this medicine:
- This medicine may look like other tablets or capsules you now take. It is very important that you do not get the medicines mixed up since this may have serious results. Ask your pharmacist for ways to avoid mix-ups with medicines that look alike.

Side Effects of This Medicine

Along with its needed effects, a medicine may cause some unwanted effects. Although not all of these side effects may occur, if they do occur they may need medical attention.

Check with your doctor as soon as possible if any of the following side effects or signs of overdose occur:
Rare
  Skin rash or hives
Signs of overdose (in the order in which they may occur)
  Loss of appetite
  Nausea or vomiting
  Lower stomach pain
  Diarrhea
  Unusual tiredness or weakness (extreme)
  Slow or irregular heartbeat (may be fast heartbeat in children)
  Blurred vision or "yellow, green, or white vision" (yellow, green, or white halo seen around objects)
  Drowsiness
  Confusion or mental depression
  Headache
  Fainting
Note: Overdose symptoms in infants and small children may occur at first only as changes in the heartbeat rate or rhythm, while in adults and older children the first symptoms may be mostly stomach upset, stomach pain, loss of appetite, or unusually slow heartbeat.

For elderly patients: The above signs of overdose may be more likely to occur in the elderly, who are usually more sensitive to the effects of digitalis medicines.

Other side effects not listed above may also occur in some patients. If you notice any other effects, check with your doctor.

December 1987

DIHYDROERGOTAMINE (Systemic)

A commonly used brand name is D.H.E. 45.
Generic name product may also be available in Canada.

To the Reader: If you do not recognize the names of medical conditions or medicines referred to in this information, check with your doctor, nurse, or pharmacist. Definitions for selected medical terms may be found in the Glossary. Brand names for the generic drug names listed can be found in the Index. In addition, selected brand names commonly associated with the generic name have been included in the text to help you recognize medicine you may be taking. The fact that a brand name product is not mentioned does not mean the information does not apply. It is a good idea for you to learn both the generic and brand names of your medicines and to write them down for future use.

Dihydroergotamine (dye-hye-droe-er-GOT-a-meen) belongs to the group of medicines known as ergot alkaloids. It is given by injection to treat migraine headaches and some kinds of throbbing headaches. Dihydroergotamine is not used to prevent headaches, but is used by injection to treat an attack once it has started. It works by causing the blood vessels to constrict or narrow.

Dihydroergotamine may also be used for other conditions as determined by your doctor.

This medicine is available only with your doctor's prescription.

Remember:

• **This medicine has been prescribed for your current medical problem only.** It must not be given to other people or used for other problems unless you are directed to do so by your doctor.

• **Keep all medicines out of the reach of children.**

• In order for this medicine to work, it must be used as directed.

• **It is very important that you read and understand the following information.** If any of the information causes you special concern, do not decide against using this medicine without first checking with your doctor.

• Before you begin using any new medicine (prescription or nonprescription) or if you develop any new medical problem while you are using this medicine, check with your doctor, nurse, or pharmacist.

• **If you have any questions** about the following information or if you want more information about this medicine or your medical problem, **ask your doctor, nurse, or pharmacist.**

Before Using This Medicine

In order to decide on the best treatment for your medical problem, your doctor should be told:

—if you have ever had any unusual or allergic reaction to dihydroergotamine or other ergot medicines.

—if you are on a low-salt, low-sugar, or any other special diet, or if you are allergic to any substance, such as foods, sulfites or other preservatives. Most medicines contain more than their active ingredient. Your doctor, nurse, or pharmacist can help you avoid products that may cause a problem.

—if you are **pregnant** or if you may become pregnant. Dihydroergotamine is not recommended during pregnancy since ergot alkaloids have been shown to stimulate labor, which could result in a miscarriage.

—if you are **breast-feeding**. Dihydroergotamine passes into the breast milk and may cause unwanted effects (vomiting, diarrhea, weak pulse, unstable blood pressure, seizures) in babies of mothers receiving large doses of it.

—if you have any of the following medical problems:
  Heart or blood vessel disease
  High blood pressure
  Infection
  Itching (severe)
  Kidney disease
  Liver disease

—if you are taking **any** other prescription or nonprescription (OTC) medicine.

—if you smoke.

Proper Use of This Medicine

Use this medicine only as directed by your doctor. If the amount you are to use does not relieve your headache, do not use more than your doctor ordered. Instead, check with your doctor. Using too much of this medicine or using it too frequently may cause serious effects such as nausea and vomiting; cold, painful hands or feet; or even gangrene.

This medicine works best if you:

• **Use it at the first sign of headache or migraine attack.**

• **Lie down in a quiet, dark room for at least 2 hours after using it.**

How to store this medicine:

• **Keep out of the reach of children.**

• Store away from heat and direct light.

• Keep the medicine from freezing.

• Do not keep outdated medicine or medicine no longer needed. Be sure that any discarded medicine is out of the reach of children.

Precautions While Using This Medicine

Since drinking alcoholic beverages may make headaches worse, it is best to avoid alcohol while you are suffering from them.

Since smoking may increase some of the harmful effects of this medicine, it is best to avoid smoking while you are using it.

Avoid prolonged exposure to very cold temperatures while you are using this medicine, since cold may increase the harmful effects of the medicine.

If you have an infection or illness of any kind, check with your doctor before using this medicine, since you may be more sensitive to the effects of it.

Side Effects of This Medicine

Along with its needed effects, a medicine may cause some unwanted effects. Although not all of these side effects may occur, if they do occur they may need medical attention.

Check with your doctor immediately if any of the following side effects occur:

Less common

    Numbness and tingling of fingers, toes, or face

Rare

    Red or violet blisters on skin of hands or feet

Check with your doctor as soon as possible if the following side effects occur:

Less common

    Itching
    Pain in arms, legs, or lower back
    Pale or cold hands or feet
    Swelling of feet or lower legs
    Weakness in legs

Rare

    Fast or slow heartbeat

Other side effects may occur that usually do not require medical attention. These side effects may go away during treatment as your body adjusts to the medicine. However, check with your doctor if any of the following side effects continue or are bothersome:

Less common

    Dizziness
    Headache
    Nausea or vomiting

For elderly patients: The above side effects may be more likely to occur in the elderly, who are more likely to already have problems with blood vessels. In addition, dihydroergotamine may reduce tolerance to cold temperatures in elderly patients.

After you stop using this medicine, your body may need time to adjust. The length of time this takes depends on the amount of medicine you were using and how long you used it. During this period of time check with your doctor if your headaches begin again or get worse.

Other side effects not listed above may also occur in some patients. If you notice any other effects, check with your doctor.

December 1987

DIHYDROTACHYSTEROL (Systemic)

Some commonly used brand names are DHT, DHT Intensol, and Hytakerol.

Generic name product may also be available in the U.S.

To the Reader: If you do not recognize the names of medical conditions or medicines referred to in this information, check with your doctor, nurse, or pharmacist. Definitions for selected medical terms may be found in the Glossary. Brand names for the generic drug names listed can be found in the Index. In addition, selected brand names commonly associated with the generic name have been included in the text to help you recognize medicine you may be taking. The fact that a brand name product is not mentioned does not mean the information does not apply. It is a good idea for you to learn both the generic and brand names of your medicines and to write them down for future use.

Dihydrotachysterol (dye-hye-droe-tak-ISS-ter-ole) is a form of vitamin D taken by mouth to treat hypocalcemia (not enough calcium in the blood) or other conditions in which calcium is not used properly by the body. It may also be used for other conditions as determined by your doctor.

This medicine is available only with your doctor's prescription.

Remember:

• **This medicine has been prescribed for your current medical problem only.** It must not be given to other people or used for other problems unless you are directed to do so by your doctor.

• **Keep all medicines out of the reach of children.**

• In order for this medicine to work, it must be used as directed.

• **It is very important that you read and understand the following information.** If any of the information causes you special concern, do not decide against using this medicine without first checking with your doctor.

• Before you begin using any new medicine (prescription or nonprescription) or if you develop any new medical problem while you are using this medicine, check with your doctor, nurse, or pharmacist.

• **If you have any questions** about the following information or if you want more information about this medicine or your medical problem, **ask your doctor, nurse, or pharmacist.**

Before Using This Medicine

In order to decide on the best treatment for your medical problem, your doctor should be told:

—if you have ever had any unusual or allergic reaction to any form of vitamin D (including calcifediol or calcitriol).

—if you are on a low-salt, low-sugar, or any other special diet, or if you are allergic to any substance, such as foods, sulfites or other preservatives, or dyes. Most medicines contain more than their active ingredient, and many liquid medicines contain alcohol. Your doctor, nurse, or pharmacist can help you avoid products that may cause a problem.

—if you are **pregnant** or if you may become pregnant. Studies in humans have not been done. Although normal amounts of vitamin D have not been shown to cause birth defects or other problems in humans, very high doses of dihydrotachysterol have been shown to cause birth defects in animals.

—if you are **breast-feeding**. Only small amounts of dihydrotachysterol pass into breast milk and it has not been shown to cause problems in nursing babies.

—if you have any of the following medical problems:
Heart or blood vessel disease
Kidney disease
Sarcoidosis

—if you are taking **any** other prescription or nonprescription (OTC) medicine, especially other forms of vitamin D.

Proper Use of This Medicine

Take this medicine only as directed. Do not take more of it and do not take it more often than your doctor ordered. To do so may increase the chance of overdose.

For patients taking the oral liquid form:

• This preparation is to be taken by mouth even though it comes in a dropper bottle.

• This medicine may be dropped directly into the mouth or mixed with cereal, fruit juice, or other food.

While you are taking this medicine, your doctor may want you to follow a special diet or take a calcium supplement. Be sure to follow instructions carefully. If you are already taking a calcium supplement or any medicine containing calcium, make sure your doctor knows.

If you miss a dose of this medicine and your dosing schedule is one dose to be taken:

Every other day—Take the missed dose as soon as possible if you remember it on the day it should be taken. However, if you do not remember the missed dose until the next day, take it at that time. Then skip a day and start your dosing schedule again. Do not double doses.

Once a day—Take the missed dose as soon as possible. Then go back to your regular dosing schedule. However, if you do not remember the missed dose until the next day, skip the missed dose and back to your regular dosing schedule. Do not double doses.

More than once a day—Take the missed dose as soon as possible. Then go back to your regular dosing schedule. However, if it is almost time for your next dose, skip the missed dose and go back to your regular dosing schedule. Do not double doses.

If you have any questions about this, check with your doctor.

How to store this medicine:

• **Keep out of the reach of children.**

• Store away from heat and direct light.

• Do not store in the bathroom, near the kitchen sink, or in other damp places. Heat or moisture may cause the medicine to break down.

• Keep the oral liquid form of this medicine from freezing.

• Do not keep outdated medicine or medicine no longer needed. Be sure that any discarded medicine is out of the reach of children.

Precautions While Using This Medicine

Your doctor should check your progress at regular visits to make sure that this medicine does not cause unwanted effects.

Do not take any nonprescription or over-the-counter (OTC) medicine while you are taking this medicine, unless you have been told to do so by your doctor. The calcium, phosphorus, or vitamin D that these medicines may contain may increase the chance of side effects.

Side Effects of This Medicine

Along with its needed effects, a medicine may cause some unwanted effects. Vitamin D does not usually cause any side effects. However, **taking large amounts of vitamin D over a period of time may cause some unwanted effects that can be serious.**

Check with your doctor immediately if any of the following effects occur:
 Late signs of severe overdose
   Convulsions (seizures)
   High blood pressure
   Irregular heartbeat
   Stomach pain (severe)

Check with your doctor as soon as possible if any of the following effects occur:
 Early signs of overdose
   Constipation (especially in children or adolescents)
   Diarrhea
   Dry mouth
   Headache (continuing)
   Increase in thirst
   Loss of appetite
   Metallic taste
   Nausea or vomiting (especially in children or adolescents)
   Unusual tiredness or weakness
 Late signs of overdose
   Bone pain
   Cloudy urine
   Increased sensitivity of eyes to light or irritation of eyes
   Increase in frequency of urination, especially at night, or in amount of urine
   Itching of skin
   Mood or mental changes
   Muscle pain
   Nausea or vomiting (severe)
   Weight loss

For children: Some of the above early signs of overdose, such as constipation and nausea or vomiting, are more likely to occur in children and adolescents. Also, children may show slowed growth when receiving vitamin D for a long time.

Other side effects not listed above may also occur in some patients. If you notice any other effects, check with your doctor.

December 1987

DIMETHYL SULFOXIDE (Mucosal)

Some commonly used brand names or other names are DMSO and Rimso-50.

Generic name product may also be available in the U.S.

To the Reader: If you do not recognize the names of medical conditions or medicines referred to in this information, check with your doctor, nurse, or pharmacist. Definitions for selected medical terms may be found in the Glossary. Brand names for the generic drug names listed can be found in the Index. In addition, selected brand names commonly associated with the generic name have been included in the text to help you recognize medicine you may be taking. The fact that a brand name product is not mentioned does not mean the information does not apply. It is a good idea for you to learn both the generic and brand names of your medicines and to write them down for future use.

Dimethyl sulfoxide (dye-METH-il sul-FOX-ide) is a purified preparation used in the bladder to relieve the symptoms of the bladder condition called interstitial cystitis. A catheter or syringe is used to put the solution into the bladder where it is allowed to remain for about 15 minutes. Then, the solution is expelled by urinating.

Interstitial cystitis is the only human use for dimethyl sulfoxide that is approved by the Food and Drug Administration (FDA). Although other preparations of dimethyl sulfoxide are available for industrial and veterinary (animal) use, they must not be used by humans because of their unknown purity. Impurities in these preparations may cause serious unwanted effects in humans. Even if dimethyl sulfoxide is applied to the skin, it is absorbed into the body through the skin and mucous membranes.

Claims that dimethyl sulfoxide is effective for treating various types of arthritis, ulcers in scleroderma, muscle sprains and strains, bruises, infections of the skin, burns, wounds, and mental conditions have not been proven.

This medicine is available only with your doctor's prescription.

Remember:

• **It is very important that you read and understand the following information.** If any of the information causes you special concern, do not decide against receiving this medicine without first checking with your doctor.

• Before you begin using any new medicine (prescription or nonprescription) or if you develop any new medical problem while you are receiving this medicine, check with your doctor, nurse, or pharmacist.

• **If you have any questions** about the following information or if you want more information about this medicine or your medical problem, **ask your doctor, nurse, or pharmacist.**

Before Using This Medicine

In order to decide on the best treatment for your medical problem, your doctor should be told:

—if you have ever had any unusual or allergic reaction to dimethyl sulfoxide.

—if you are **pregnant** or if you may become pregnant. Studies in humans have not been done. However, some studies in animals have shown that dimethyl sulfoxide causes birth defects when used on the skin and when given in high doses by injection.

—if you are **breast-feeding**, since dimethyl sulfoxide is absorbed into the body. It is not known whether dimethyl sulfoxide passes into the breast milk and this medicine has not been shown to cause problems in nursing babies.

Side Effects of This Medicine

Along with its needed effects, a medicine may cause some unwanted effects. Although not all of these side effects may occur, if they do occur they may need medical attention.

Check with your doctor immediately if any of the following side effects occur:
Nasal congestion
Shortness of breath or troubled breathing
Skin rash, hives, or itching
Swelling of face

Some patients may have some discomfort during the time this medicine is being put into the bladder. However, the discomfort usually becomes less each time the medicine is used.

Dimethyl sulfoxide may cause you to have a garlic-like taste within a few minutes after the medicine is put into the bladder. This effect may last for several hours. It may also cause your breath and skin to have a garlic-like odor, which may last up to 72 hours.

For elderly patients: Many medicines have not been tested in older people. Therefore, it is not known whether the medicine acts the same way it does in younger adults. Check with your doctor or pharmacist if you notice any unusual effects while using this medicine or if you think it is not working as it should.

Other side effects not listed above may also occur in some patients. If you notice any other effects, check with your doctor.

December 1987

DINOPROST (Intra-amniotic)

A commonly used brand name is Prostin F$_2$ Alpha.

To the Reader: If you do not recognize the names of medical conditions or medicines referred to in this information, check with your doctor, nurse, or pharmacist. Definitions for selected medical terms may be found in the Glossary. Brand names for the generic drug names listed can be found in the Index. In addition, selected brand names commonly associated with the generic name have been included in the text to help you recognize medicine you may be taking. The fact that a brand name product is not mentioned does not mean the information does not apply. It is a good idea for you to learn both the generic and brand names of your medicines and to write them down for future use.

Dinoprost (DYE-noe-prost) is given by injection to cause abortion. It may also be used for other purposes as determined by your doctor.

Dinoprost is to be administered only by or under the immediate care of your doctor.

Remember:

• **It is very important that you read and understand the following information.** If any of the information causes you special concern, do not decide against using this medicine without first checking with your doctor.

• **If you have any questions** about the following information or if you want more information about this medicine or your medical problem, **ask your doctor, nurse, or pharmacist**.

Before Using This Medicine

In order to decide on the best treatment for your medical problem, your doctor should be told:

—if you have ever had any unusual or allergic reaction to dinoprost.

—if you have any of the following medical problems:
Anemia (history of)
Asthma (history of)
Diabetes mellitus (sugar diabetes) (history of)
Epilepsy
Fibroid tumors of the uterus
Glaucoma
Heart or blood vessel disease (or history of)
High blood pressure (history of)
Jaundice (history of)
Kidney disease (or history of)
Liver disease (or history of)
Low blood pressure (history of)
Lung disease
Uterus surgery (history of)

—if you are using **any** other prescription or nonprescription (OTC) medicine.

Side Effects of This Medicine

Along with its needed effects, a medicine may cause some unwanted effects. Although not all of these side effects may occur, if they do occur they may need medical attention.

Tell the doctor or nurse immediately if any of the following side effects occur:

Less common or rare
Wheezing, troubled breathing, or tightness in chest

Other side effects may occur that usually do not require medical attention. These side effects usually go away after the medicine is stopped. However, let the doctor or nurse know if any of the following side effects continue or are bothersome:

More common
Diarrhea
Nausea and vomiting
Stomach cramps or pain

Less common
Breast tenderness
Chills or shivering
Dizziness
Fever
Flushing or redness of face
Headache

After the procedure, this medicine may still produce some side effects that need attention. Check with your doctor if you notice any of the following side effects:
Chills or shivering
Fever
Foul-smelling vaginal discharge
Increase in uterine bleeding
Pain in lower abdomen

Other side effects not listed above may also occur in some patients. If you notice any other effects, check with your doctor or nurse.

December 1987

DINOPROSTONE (Vaginal)

A commonly used brand name is Prostin E$_2$.

To the Reader: If you do not recognize the names of medical conditions or medicines referred to in this information, check with your doctor, nurse, or pharmacist. Definitions for selected medical terms may be found in the Glossary. Brand names for the generic drug names listed can be found in the Index. In addition, selected brand names commonly associated with the generic name have been included in the text to help you recognize medicine you may be taking. The fact that a brand name product is not mentioned does not mean the information does not apply. It is a good idea for you to learn both the generic and brand names of your medicines and to write them down for future use.

Dinoprostone (dye-noe-PROST-one) suppositories are inserted into the vagina to cause abortion. They may also be used for other purposes as determined by your doctor.

Dinoprostone is to be administered only by or under the immediate care of your doctor.

Remember:

• **It is very important that you read and understand the following information.** If any of the information causes you special concern, do not decide against using this medicine without first checking with your doctor.

• **If you have any questions** about the following information or if you want more information about this medicine or your medical problem, **ask your doctor, nurse, or pharmacist.**

Before Using This Medicine

In order to decide on the best treatment for your medical problem, your doctor should be told:

—if you have ever had any unusual or allergic reaction to dinoprostone.

—if you have any of the following medical problems:

Anemia (history of)
Asthma (history of)
Diabetes mellitus (sugar diabetes) (history of)
Epilepsy (history of)
Fibroid tumors of the uterus
Glaucoma
Heart or blood vessel disease (or history of)
High blood pressure (history of)
Inflammation or infection of cervix or vagina
Jaundice (history of)
Kidney disease (or history of)
Liver disease (or history of)
Low blood pressure (history of)
Lung disease
Uterus surgery (history of)

—if you are using **any** other prescription or nonprescription (OTC) medicine.

Proper Use of This Medicine

After the suppository is inserted into the vagina, remain lying down for at least 10 minutes so that the medicine can be absorbed.

Side Effects of This Medicine

Along with its needed effects, a medicine may cause some unwanted effects. Although not all of these side effects may occur, if they do occur they may need medical attention.

Tell the doctor or nurse immediately if any of the following side effects occur:

Less common or rare
Wheezing, troubled breathing, or tightness in chest

Other side effects may occur that usually do not require medical attention. These side effects usually go away after the medicine is stopped. However, let the doctor or nurse know if any of the following side effects continue or are bothersome:

More common
Diarrhea
Fever
Nausea
Vomiting

Less common
Chills or shivering
Headache

After the procedure, this medicine may still produce some side effects that need attention. Check with your doctor if any of the following side effects occur:
Chills or shivering
Fever
Foul-smelling vaginal discharge
Increase in uterine bleeding
Pain in lower abdomen

Other side effects not listed above may also occur in some patients. If you notice any other effects, check with your doctor or nurse.

December 1987

DIPHENIDOL (Systemic)

A commonly used brand name is Vontrol.

To the Reader: If you do not recognize the names of medical conditions or medicines referred to in this information, check with your doctor, nurse, or pharmacist. Definitions for selected medical terms may be found in the Glossary. Brand names for the generic drug names listed can be found in the Index. In addition, selected brand names commonly associated with the generic name have been included in the text to help you recognize medicine you may be taking. The fact that a brand name product is not mentioned does not mean the information does not apply. It is a good idea for you to learn both the generic and brand names of your medicines and to write them down for future use.

Diphenidol (dye-FEN-i-dole) is taken by mouth to relieve or prevent nausea, vomiting, and dizziness caused by certain medical problems.

Diphenidol is available only with your doctor's prescription.

Remember:

• **This medicine has been prescribed for your current medical problem only.** It must not be given to other people or used for other problems unless you are directed to do so by your doctor.

• **Keep all medicines out of the reach of children.**

• In order for this medicine to work, it must be used as directed.

• **It is very important that you read and understand the following information.** If any of the information causes you special concern, do not decide against using this medicine without first checking with your doctor.

• Before you begin using any new medicine (prescription or nonprescription) or if you develop any new medical problem while you are using this medicine, check with your doctor, nurse, or pharmacist.

• **If you have any questions** about the following information or if you want more information about this medicine or your medical problem, **ask your doctor, nurse, or pharmacist.**

Before Using This Medicine

In order to decide on the best treatment for your medical problem, your doctor should be told:

—if you have ever had any unusual or allergic reaction to diphenidol.

—if you are on a low-salt, low-sugar, or any other special diet, or if you are allergic to any substance, such as foods, sulfites or other preservatives, or dyes. Most medicines contain more than their active ingredient. Your doctor, nurse, or pharmacist can help you avoid products that may cause a problem.

—if you are **pregnant** or if you may become pregnant. Diphenidol has not been shown to cause birth defects or other problems in human or animal studies.

—if you are **breast-feeding**. Diphenidol has not been shown to cause problems in nursing babies.

—if you have any of the following medical problems:
Enlarged prostate
Glaucoma
Intestinal blockage
Kidney disease
Low blood pressure
Stomach ulcer
Urinary tract blockage

—if you are taking **any** other prescription or nonprescription (OTC) medicine, especially central nervous system (CNS) depressants.

Proper Use of This Medicine

If you are taking diphenidol to prevent nausea and vomiting, it may be taken with food or a glass of water or milk to lessen stomach irritation, unless otherwise directed by your doctor. However, if you are already suffering from nausea and vomiting it is best to keep the stomach empty, and this medicine should be taken only with a small amount of water.

Take this medicine only as directed. Do not take more of it and do not take it more often than directed by your doctor. To do so may increase the chance of side effects.

If this medicine has been ordered by your doctor to be taken on a regular schedule and you miss a dose, take it as soon as possible. However, if it is almost time for your next dose, skip the missed dose and go back to your regular dosing schedule. Do not double doses.

How to store this medicine:

• **Keep out of the reach of children.**

• Store away from heat and direct light.

• Do not store the tablet form of this medicine in the bathroom, near the kitchen sink, or in other damp places. Heat or moisture may cause the medicine to break down.

• Do not keep outdated medicine or medicine no longer needed. Be sure that any discarded medicine is out of the reach of children.

Precautions While Using This Medicine

This medicine will add to the effects of alcohol and other CNS depressants (medicines that slow down the nervous system, possibly causing drowsiness). Some examples of CNS depressants are antihistamines or medicine for hay fever, other allergies, or colds; sedatives, tranquilizers, or sleeping medicine; prescription pain medicine or narcotics; barbiturates; medicine for seizures; muscle relaxants; or anesthetics, including some dental anesthetics. **Check with your doctor before taking any of the above while you are using this medicine.**

This medicine may cause some people to have blurred vision or to become drowsy or less alert than they are normally. **Make sure you know how you react to this medicine before you drive, use machines, or do other jobs that require you to be alert.**

© 1988   The United States Pharmacopeial Convention, Inc.

Side Effects of This Medicine

Along with its needed effects, a medicine may cause some unwanted effects. Although not all of these side effects may occur, if they do occur they may need medical attention.

Check with your doctor as soon as possible if any of the following side effects occur:

Rare
> Confusion
> Hallucinations (seeing, hearing, or feeling things that are not there)

Signs of overdose
> Drowsiness (severe)
> Shortness of breath or troubled breathing
> Unusual tiredness or weakness (severe)

Other side effects may occur that usually do not require medical attention. These side effects may go away during treatment as your body adjusts to the medicine. However, check with your doctor if any of the following side effects continue or are bothersome:

More common
> Drowsiness

Less common or rare
> Blurred vision
> Dizziness
> Dryness of mouth
> Headache
> Heartburn
> Nervousness, restlessness, or trouble in sleeping
> Skin rash
> Stomach upset or pain
> Unusual tiredness or weakness

For elderly patients: Many medicines have not been tested in older people. Therefore, it is not known whether the medicine acts the same way it does in younger adults. Check with your doctor or pharmacist if you notice any unusual effects while taking this medicine or if you think it is not working as it should.

Other side effects not listed above may also occur in some patients. If you notice any other effects, check with your doctor.

December 1987

DIPHENOXYLATE AND ATROPINE
(Systemic)

Some commonly used brand names are:

Diphenatol	Lonox
Latropine	Lo-Trol
Lofene	Low-Quel
Lomanate	Nor-Mil
Lomotil	

Generic name product may also be available.

To the Reader: If you do not recognize the names of medical conditions or medicines referred to in this information, check with your doctor, nurse, or pharmacist. Definitions for selected medical terms may be found in the Glossary. Brand names for the generic drug names listed can be found in the Index. In addition, selected brand names commonly associated with the generic name have been included in the text to help you recognize medicine you may be taking. The fact that a brand name product is not mentioned does not mean the information does not apply. It is a good idea for you to learn both the generic and brand names of your medicines and to write them down for future use.

Diphenoxylate (dye-fen-OX-i-late) and atropine (A-troe-peen) is a combination medicine used along with other measures to treat severe diarrhea. Diphenoxylate helps stop diarrhea by slowing down the movements of the intestines. The atropine is included to prevent possible abuse, since diphenoxylate is chemically related to some narcotics.

This medicine is available only with your doctor's prescription.

Remember:

• **This medicine has been prescribed for your current medical problem only.** It must not be given to other people or used for other problems unless you are directed to do so by your doctor.

• **Keep all medicines out of the reach of children.**

• In order for this medicine to work, it must be used as directed.

• **It is very important that you read and understand the following information.** If any of the information causes you special concern, do not decide against using this medicine without first checking with your doctor.

• Before you begin using any new medicine (prescription or nonprescription) or if you develop any new medical problem while you are using this medicine, check with your doctor, nurse, or pharmacist.

• **If you have any questions** about the following information or if you want more information about this medicine or your medical problem, **ask your doctor, nurse, or pharmacist.**

Before Using This Medicine

In order to decide on the best treatment for your medical problem, your doctor should be told:

—if you have ever had any unusual or allergic reaction to diphenoxylate or atropine.

—if you are on a low-salt, low-sugar, or any other special diet, or if you are allergic to any substance, such as foods, sulfites or other preservatives, or dyes. Most medicines contain more than their active ingredient, and many liquid medicines contain alcohol. Your doctor, nurse, or pharmacist can help you avoid products that may cause a problem.

—if you are **pregnant** or if you may become pregnant. Studies have not been done in humans. In animal studies this medicine given in larger doses than the usual human dose has not been shown to cause birth defects. However, some studies in animals have shown that this medicine may retard growth and lessen the chance of conceiving or becoming pregnant.

—if you are **breast-feeding**. Although this medicine has not been shown to cause problems in nursing babies, the chance always exists since both diphenoxylate and atropine pass into the breast milk.

—if you have any of the following medical problems:
Colitis (severe)
Down's syndrome (mongolism) in children
Emphysema, asthma, bronchitis, or other chronic lung disease
Enlarged prostate
Gallbladder disease or gallstones
Heart disease
Hiatal hernia
High blood pressure
Kidney disease
Liver disease
Myasthenia gravis
Overactive or underactive thyroid
Urinary tract blockage or difficult urination

—if you are taking **any** other prescription or nonprescription (OTC) medicine, especially:
Central nervous system (CNS) depressants
Other antimuscarinics (medicine for abdominal or stomach spasms or cramps)

—if you are now taking an antibiotic. Some antibiotics may cause diarrhea. This medicine may make the diarrhea caused by antibiotics worse or make it last longer.

Proper Use of This Medicine

If this medicine upsets your stomach, your doctor may want you to take it with food.

Take this medicine only as directed by your doctor. Do not take more of it, do not take it more often, and do not take it for a longer period of time than your doctor ordered. If too much is taken, it may become habit-forming, or may cause overdose in a child.

For patients taking the liquid form of this medicine:

• This medicine is to be taken by mouth even though it may come in a dropper bottle. The amount to be taken is to be measured with the specially marked dropper.

If you are taking this medicine on a regular schedule and you miss a dose, take it as soon as possible. However, if it is almost time for your next dose, skip the missed dose and go back to your regular dosing schedule. Do not double doses.

How to store this medicine:

- **Keep out of the reach of children** since overdose is especially dangerous in children.

- Store away from heat and direct light.

- Do not store the tablet form of this medicine in the bathroom, near the kitchen sink, or in other damp places. Heat or moisture may cause the medicine to break down.

- Keep the liquid form of this medicine from freezing.

- Do not keep outdated medicine or medicine no longer needed. Be sure that any discarded medicine is out of the reach of children.

Precautions While Using This Medicine

Your doctor should check your progress at regular visits if you will be taking this medicine regularly for a long period of time.

Check with your doctor if your diarrhea does not stop after a few days or if you develop a fever.

This medicine will add to the effects of alcohol and other central nervous system (CNS) depressants (medicines that slow down the nervous system, possibly causing drowsiness). Some examples of CNS depressants are antihistamines or medicine for hay fever, other allergies, or colds; sedatives, tranquilizers, or sleeping medicine; prescription pain medicine or narcotics; barbiturates; medicine for seizures; muscle relaxants; or anesthetics, including some dental anesthetics. **Check with your doctor before taking any of the above while you are taking this medicine.**

If you think you or anyone else may have taken an overdose, get emergency help at once. Taking an overdose of this medicine may lead to unconsciousness and possibly death. Signs of overdose include severe drowsiness; shortness of breath or troubled breathing; fast heartbeat; and unusual warmth, dryness, and flushing of skin.

Before having any kind of surgery (including dental surgery) or emergency treatment, tell the physician or dentist in charge that you are taking this medicine.

This medicine may cause some people to become dizzy, drowsy, or less alert than they are normally. Even if taken at bedtime, it may cause some people to feel drowsy or less alert on arising. **Make sure you know how you react to this medicine before you drive, use machines, or do other jobs that require you to be alert.**

Side Effects of This Medicine

Along with its needed effects, a medicine may cause some unwanted effects. Although not all of these side effects may occur, if they do occur they may need medical attention.

When this medicine is used for short periods of time at low doses, side effects usually are rare. However, check with your doctor immediately if any of the following side effects are severe and occur suddenly since they may indicate a more severe and dangerous problem with your bowels:

Bloating
Constipation
Loss of appetite
Nausea or vomiting
Stomach pain

Check with your doctor immediately also if the following effects occur, since they may indicate an overdose:

Blurred vision (continuing) or changes in near vision
Drowsiness (severe)
Dryness of mouth, nose, and throat (severe)
Fast heartbeat
Shortness of breath or troubled breathing (severe)
Unusual excitement, nervousness, restlessness, or irritability (especially in children)
Unusual warmth, dryness, and flushing of skin

Other side effects may occur that usually do not require medical attention. These side effects may go away during treatment as your body adjusts to the medicine. However, check with your doctor if any of the following side effects continue, worsen, or are bothersome:

Less common or rare
Blurred vision
Difficult urination
Dizziness or lightheadedness
Drowsiness
Dryness of skin and mouth
Fever
Headache
Mental depression
Numbness of hands or feet
Skin rash or itching
Swelling of the gums

After you stop using this medicine, your body may need time to adjust. The length of time this takes depends on the amount of medicine you were using and how long you used it. During this period of time check with your doctor if you notice any of the following side effects:

Rare
Increased sweating
Muscle cramps
Nausea or vomiting
Shivering or trembling
Stomach cramps

For children: The above side effects may be more likely to occur in infants, young children, and children with Down's syndrome.

For elderly patients: Shortness of breath or troubled breathing may be more likely to occur in elderly patients.

Other side effects not listed above may also occur in some patients. If you notice any other effects, check with your doctor.

December 1987

DIPHTHERIA AND TETANUS TOXOIDS AND PERTUSSIS VACCINE ADSORBED
(Systemic)

A commonly used brand name is Tri-Immunol.

Generic name product may also be available in the U.S. and Canada.

To the Reader: If you do not recognize the names of medical conditions or medicines referred to in this information, check with your doctor, nurse, or pharmacist. Definitions for selected medical terms may be found in the Glossary. Brand names for the generic drug names listed can be found in the Index. In addition, selected brand names commonly associated with the generic name have been included in the text to help you recognize medicine you may be taking. The fact that a brand name product is not mentioned does not mean the information does not apply. It is a good idea for you to learn both the generic and brand names of your medicines and to write them down for future use.

Diphtheria (dif-THEER-ee-a) and Tetanus (TET-n-us) Toxoids and Pertussis (per-TUSS-iss) Vaccine is a combination immunizing agent given by injection to prevent diphtheria, tetanus, and pertussis. Diphtheria and Tetanus Toxoids and Pertussis Vaccine is also known as DTP.

Diphtheria is a serious illness that can cause heart problems, nerve damage, pneumonia, and possibly death. The risk of serious complications and death is greater in very young children and in the elderly.

Tetanus (also known as lockjaw) is a serious illness that causes seizures and severe spasms of the muscles that can be strong enough to cause bone fractures of the spine. In addition, tetanus causes death in 30 to 40 percent of cases.

Pertussis (also known as whooping cough) is a serious disease that causes severe spells of coughing that can interfere with breathing. Pertussis can also cause pneumonia, long-lasting bronchitis, seizures, brain damage, and death.

Immunization against diphtheria, tetanus, and pertussis is recommended for all infants and children from 6 or 8 weeks of age up until their 7th birthday. Children 7 years of age and older and adults should receive immunizing agents that contain only diphtheria and tetanus toxoids and not pertussis vaccine. The diphtheria and tetanus injections should be taken every 10 years for the rest of their lives.

Diphtheria, tetanus, and pertussis are serious diseases that can cause life-threatening illnesses. Although some serious side effects can occur after a dose of DTP (usually from the pertussis vaccine in DTP), this rarely happens. The chance of your child catching one of these diseases and being permanently injured or possibly dying as a result is much greater than the chance of your child getting a serious side effect from the DTP vaccine.

Remember:

• **It is very important that you read and understand the following information.** If any of the information causes you special concern, do not decide against your child receiving this vaccine without first checking with your doctor.

• If your child develops any new medical problem while he or she is receiving this vaccine, check with your doctor, nurse, or pharmacist.

• **If you have any questions** about the following information or if you want more information about this vaccine, **ask your doctor, nurse, or pharmacist.**

Before Receiving This Vaccine

In order to decide on the best treatment for your child, your doctor should be told:

—if your child has ever had any unusual or allergic reaction to thimerosal or any other mercury-type product. The DTP products available in the U.S. contain thimerosal; products available in other countries may contain other preservatives.

—if your child has any of the following medical problems:

  Brain disease
  Central nervous system (CNS) disease
  Epilepsy
  Fever
  Seizures
  Spasms

—if your child is taking **any** other prescription or nonprescription (OTC) medicine.

—if your child has ever been treated with x-rays or cancer medicines.

Side Effects of This Vaccine

Along with its needed effects, a vaccine may cause some unwanted effects. Although not all of these side effects may occur, if they do occur they may need medical attention.

Get emergency help immediately if any of the following side effects occur:

Rare

  Collapse
  Confusion
  Convulsions (seizures)
  Crying or screaming for three or more hours or an unusual high-pitched cry
  Difficulty in breathing or swallowing
  Fever of 40.5 °C (105 °F) or more
  Headache (severe or continuing)
  Hives
  Irritability (unusual)
  Itching, especially of feet or hands
  Periods of unconsciousness or lack of awareness
  Reddening of skin, especially around ears

Sleepiness (unusual and continuing)
Swelling of eyes, face, or inside of nose
Unusual tiredness, weakness, or limpness (sudden and severe)
Vomiting (severe or continuing)

Other side effects may occur that usually do not require medical attention. These side effects may go away as your child's body adjusts to the vaccine. However, check with your doctor if any of the following side effects continue or are bothersome:

More common

Fever between 38 and 39 °C (100.4 and 102.2 °F) (may be accompanied by fretfulness, drowsiness, vomiting, and loss of appetite)
Lump at place of injection (may be present for a few weeks after injection)
Redness, swelling, tenderness, or pain at site of injection

Less common

Fever between 39 and 40 °C (102.2 and 104 °F) (may be accompanied by fretfulness, drowsiness, vomiting, and loss of appetite)

Rare

Fever between 40 and 40.5 °C (104 and 105 °F) (may be accompanied by fretfulness, drowsiness, vomiting, and loss of appetite)
Swollen glands on side of neck (following DTP injection into arm)

It is very important that you tell your doctor about any side effect that occurs after a dose of DTP, even though the side effect may have gone away without treatment. Some types of side effects may mean that your child should not receive any more doses of DTP.

Other side effects not listed above may also occur in some patients. If you notice any other effects, check with your doctor.

_____

December 1987

DIPIVEFRIN (Ophthalmic)

A commonly used brand name is Propine.

To the Reader: If you do not recognize the names of medical conditions or medicines referred to in this information, check with your doctor, nurse, or pharmacist. Definitions for selected medical terms may be found in the Glossary. Brand names for the generic drug names listed can be found in the Index. In addition, selected brand names commonly associated with the generic name have been included in the text to help you recognize medicine you may be taking. The fact that a brand name product is not mentioned does not mean the information does not apply. It is a good idea for you to learn both the generic and brand names of your medicines and to write them down for future use.

Dipivefrin (dye-PI-ve-frin) is used in the eye to treat certain types of glaucoma.

This medicine is available only with your doctor's prescription.

Remember:

• **This medicine has been prescribed for your current medical problem only.** It must not be given to other people or used for other problems unless you are directed to do so by your doctor.

• **Keep all medicines out of the reach of children.**

• In order for this medicine to work, it must be used as directed.

• **It is very important that you read and understand the following information.** If any of the information causes you special concern, do not decide against using this medicine without first checking with your doctor.

• Before you begin using any new medicine (prescription or nonprescription) or if you develop any new medical problem while you are using this medicine, check with your doctor, nurse, or pharmacist.

• **If you have any questions** about the following information or if you want more information about this medicine or your medical problem, **ask your doctor, nurse, or pharmacist.**

Before Using This Medicine

In order to decide on the best treatment for your medical problem, your doctor should be told:

—if you have ever had any unusual or allergic reaction to dipivefrin or epinephrine.

—if you are **pregnant** or if you may become pregnant. Studies have not been done in humans. However, dipivefrin has not been shown to cause birth defects or other problems in animal studies.

—if you are **breast-feeding**, since dipivefrin may be absorbed into the body. It is not known whether dipivefrin passes into the breast milk and this medicine has not been shown to cause problems in humans.

—if you are taking **any** other prescription or nonprescription (OTC) medicine.

Proper Use of This Medicine

Use this medicine only as directed. Do not use more of it and do not use it more often than your doctor ordered. To do so may increase the chance of too much medicine being absorbed into the body and the chance of side effects.

How to apply this medicine: First, wash your hands. With the middle finger, apply pressure to the inside corner of the eye (and continue to apply pressure for 1 or 2 minutes after the medicine has been placed in the eye). Tilt the head back and with the index finger of the same hand, pull the lower eyelid away from the eye to form a pouch. Drop the medicine into the pouch and gently close the eyes. Do not blink. Keep the eyes closed for 1 or 2 minutes to allow the medicine to be absorbed.

Immediately after applying the eye drops, wash your hands to remove any medicine that may be on them.

To prevent contamination of the eye drops, do not touch the applicator tip to any surface (including the eye). Also, keep the container tightly closed.

If you miss a dose of this medicine, apply the missed dose as soon as possible. However, if it is almost time for your next dose, skip the missed dose and apply your next dose at the regularly scheduled time. Then continue with your regular dosing schedule.

How to store this medicine:

• **Keep out of the reach of children.**

• Store away from heat and direct light.

• Keep the medicine from freezing.

• Do not keep outdated medicine or medicine no longer needed. Be sure that any discarded medicine is out of the reach of children.

Precautions While Using This Medicine

Your doctor should check your eye pressure at regular visits.

Side Effects of This Medicine

Along with its needed effects, a medicine may cause some unwanted effects. Although not all of these side effects may occur, if they do occur they may need medical attention.

Check with your doctor as soon as possible if either of the following side effects occurs:
Rare—Signs of too much medicine being absorbed into the body

Fast or irregular heartbeat
Increase in blood pressure

© 1988   The United States Pharmacopeial Convention, Inc.

Other side effects may occur that usually do not require medical attention. These side effects may go away during treatment as your body adjusts to the medicine. However, check with your doctor if any of the following side effects continue or are bothersome:

More common
    Burning, stinging, or other eye irritation

For elderly patients: Many medicines have not been tested in older people. Therefore, it is not known whether the medicine acts the same way it does in younger adults.

Check with your doctor or pharmacist if you notice any unusual effects while using this medicine or if you think it is not working as it should.

Other side effects not listed above may also occur in some patients. If you notice any other effects, check with your doctor.

_____

December 1987

DIPYRIDAMOLE (Systemic)

Some commonly used brand names are Apo-Dipyridamole* and Persantine.

Generic name product may also be available in the U.S.

---

*Not available in the U.S.

To the Reader: If you do not recognize the names of medical conditions or medicines referred to in this information, check with your doctor, nurse, or pharmacist. Definitions for selected medical terms may be found in the Glossary. Brand names for the generic drug names listed can be found in the Index. In addition, selected brand names commonly associated with the generic name have been included in the text to help you recognize medicine you may be taking. The fact that a brand name product is not mentioned does not mean the information does not apply. It is a good idea for you to learn both the generic and brand names of your medicines and to write them down for future use.

Dipyridamole (dye-peer-ID-a-mole) is used to reduce blood-clot formation in patients who have had surgery to replace heart valves. It works by affecting the blood so that clots are less likely to form. Although dipyridamole reduces clot formation, this medicine is **not** an anticoagulant (blood thinner) since it does not change the blood's bleeding time.

Dipyridamole may also be used for other heart and blood conditions as determined by your doctor.

Dipyridamole is available only with your doctor's prescription.

Remember:

• **This medicine has been prescribed for your current medical problem only.** It must not be given to other people or used for other problems unless you are directed to do so by your doctor.

• **Keep all medicines out of the reach of children.**

• In order for this medicine to work, it must be used as directed.

• If you are receiving this medicine by injection, some of the information about this medicine may not apply.

• **It is very important that you read and understand the following information.** If any of the information causes you special concern, do not decide against using this medicine without first checking with your doctor.

• Before you begin using any new medicine (prescription or nonprescription) or if you develop any new medical problem while you are using this medicine, check with your doctor, nurse, or pharmacist.

• **If you have any questions** about the following information or if you want more information about this medicine or your medical problem, **ask your doctor, nurse, or pharmacist.**

Before Using This Medicine

In order to decide on the best treatment for your medical problem, your doctor should be told:

—if you have ever had any unusual or allergic reaction to dipyridamole.

—if you are on a low-salt, low-sugar, or any other special diet, or if you are allergic to any substance, such as foods, sulfites or other preservatives, or dyes.

Most medicines contain more than their active ingredient. Your doctor, nurse, or pharmacist can help you avoid products that may cause a problem.

—if you are **pregnant** or if you may become pregnant. Studies have not been done in humans. However, dipyridamole has not been shown to cause birth defects or other problems in mice, rats, or rabbits given over 15 times the maximum human dose.

—if you are **breast-feeding**. Although dipyridamole passes into breast milk, it has not been shown to cause problems in nursing babies.

—if you are taking **any** other prescription or nonprescription (OTC) medicine, especially:

    Anticoagulants (blood thinners)
    Azlocillin (e.g., Azlin)
    Carbenicillin by injection (e.g., Geopen)
    Cefamandole (e.g., Mandol)
    Cefoperazone (e.g., Cefobid)
    Divalproex (e.g., Depakote)
    Mezlocillin (e.g., Mezlin)
    Moxalactam (e.g., Moxam)
    Pentoxifylline (e.g., Trental)
    Piperacillin (e.g., Pipracil)
    Plicamycin (e.g., Mithracin)
    Sulfinpyrazone (e.g., Anturane)
    Ticarcillin (e.g., Ticar)
    Valproic acid (e.g., Depakene)

Proper Use of This Medicine

This medicine works best when there is a constant amount in the blood. To help keep this amount constant, **dipyridamole must be taken in regularly spaced doses,** as ordered by your doctor.

This medicine works best when taken with a full glass (8 ounces) of water at least 1 hour before or 2 hours after meals. However, to lessen stomach upset, your doctor may want you to take the medicine with food or milk.

If you miss a dose of this medicine, take it as soon as possible. However, if it is within 4 hours of your next scheduled dose, skip the missed dose and go back to your regular dosing schedule. Do not double doses.

How to store this medicine:

• **Keep out of the reach of children.**

• Store away from heat and direct light.

• Do not store in the bathroom, near the kitchen sink, or in other damp places. Heat or moisture may cause the medicine to break down.

• Do not keep outdated medicine or medicine no longer needed. Be sure that any discarded medicine is out of the reach of children.

Precautions While Using This Medicine

Dizziness, lightheadedness, or fainting may occur, especially when you get up from a lying or sitting position. Getting up slowly may help. If this problem continues or gets worse, check with your doctor.

Side Effects of This Medicine

Along with its needed effects, a medicine may cause some unwanted effects. Although not all of these side effects may occur, if they do occur they may need medical attention.

Check with your doctor as soon as possible if the following side effect occurs shortly after you start taking this medicine:

Rare

Chest pain or tightness in chest

Other side effects may occur that usually do not require medical attention. These side effects may go away during treatment as your body adjusts to the medicine.

However, check with your doctor if they continue or are bothersome:

More common
Dizziness

Less common
Flushing
Headache
Nausea or vomiting
Skin rash
Stomach cramping
Weakness

Other side effects not listed above may also occur in some patients. If you notice any other effects, check with your doctor.

December 1987

DISOPYRAMIDE (Systemic)

Some commonly used brand names are Norpace, Norpace CR, Rythmodan*, and Rythmodan-LA*.

Generic name product may also be available in the U.S.

*Not commercially available in the U.S.

To the Reader: If you do not recognize the names of medical conditions or medicines referred to in this information, check with your doctor, nurse, or pharmacist. Definitions for selected medical terms may be found in the Glossary. Brand names for the generic drug names listed can be found in the Index. In addition, selected brand names commonly associated with the generic name have been included in the text to help you recognize medicine you may be taking. The fact that a brand name product is not mentioned does not mean the information does not apply. It is a good idea for you to learn both the generic and brand names of your medicines and to write them down for future use.

Disopyramide (dye-soe-PEER-a-mide) is used to correct irregular heartbeats to a normal rhythm and to slow an overactive heart. This allows the heart to work more efficiently.

Disopyramide is available only with your doctor's prescription.

Remember:

• **This medicine has been prescribed for your current medical problem only.** It must not be given to other people or used for other problems unless you are directed to do so by your doctor.

• **Keep all medicines out of the reach of children.**

• In order for this medicine to work, it must be used as directed.

• **It is very important that you read and understand the following information.** If any of the information causes you special concern, do not decide against using this medicine without first checking with your doctor.

• Before you begin using any new medicine (prescription or nonprescription) or if you develop any new medical problem while you are using this medicine, check with your doctor, nurse, or pharmacist.

• **If you have any questions** about the following information or if you want more information about this medicine or your medical problem, **ask your doctor, nurse, or pharmacist.**

Before Using This Medicine

In order to decide on the best treatment for your medical problem, your doctor should be told:

—if you have ever had any unusual or allergic reaction to disopyramide.

—if you are on a low-salt, low-sugar, or any other special diet, or if you are allergic to any substance, such as foods, sulfites or other preservatives, or dyes. Most medicines contain more than their active ingredient. Your doctor, nurse, or pharmacist can help you avoid products that may cause a problem.

—if you are **pregnant** or if you may become pregnant. Studies have not been done in humans. Use in pregnant patients is limited. However, there are some reports that disopyramide caused contractions of the uterus when taken during pregnancy. Studies in animals have not shown disopyramide to cause birth defects.

—if you are **breast-feeding.** Although disopyramide passes into breast milk, this medicine has not been shown to cause problems in nursing babies.

—if you have any of the following medical problems:
Diabetes mellitus (sugar diabetes)
Difficult urination
Enlarged prostate
Glaucoma (history of)
Kidney disease
Liver disease
Myasthenia gravis

—if you are taking **any** other prescription or nonprescription (OTC) medicine, especially:
Other heart medicine
Pimozide (e.g., Orap)

Proper Use of This Medicine

Take disopyramide exactly as directed by your doctor even though you may feel well. Do not take more medicine than ordered and do not miss any doses.

Take disopyramide on an empty stomach, either 1 hour before or 2 hours after meals, unless otherwise directed by your doctor. This will allow it to work better.

For patients taking the extended-release capsules or tablets:

• Swallow the capsule whole without breaking, crushing, or chewing.

If you do miss a dose of this medicine, take it as soon as possible unless the next scheduled dose is in less than 4 hours. If you do not remember until later, skip the missed dose and go back to your regular dosing schedule. Do not double doses.

How to store this medicine:

• **Keep out of the reach of children.**

• Store away from heat and direct light.

• Do not store in the bathroom, near the kitchen sink, or in other damp places. Heat or moisture may cause the medicine to break down.

• Do not keep outdated medicine or medicine no longer needed. Be sure that any discarded medicine is out of the reach of children.

Precautions While Using This Medicine

Your doctor should check your progress at regular visits to make sure the medicine is working properly.

Do not stop taking this medicine without first checking with your doctor. Stopping suddenly may cause a serious change in heart function.

Dizziness, lightheadedness, or fainting may occur, especially when you get up from a lying or sitting position. This is due to lowered blood pressure. Getting up slowly may help. This effect does not occur often at doses of disopyramide usually used; however, **make sure you know how you react to this medicine before you drive, use machines, or do other jobs that require you to be alert.** If the problem continues or gets worse, check with your doctor.

Avoid alcoholic beverages until you have discussed their use with your doctor. Alcohol may make the low blood sugar effect worse and/or increase the possibility of dizziness or fainting.

Disopyramide may cause hypoglycemia (low blood sugar) in some people. Patients with congestive heart disease or diabetes especially should be aware of the signs of hypoglycemia. (See *Side Effects of This Medicine*.) If these signs appear, eat or drink a food containing sugar and call your doctor right away.

This medicine may cause blurred vision or other vision problems. If any of these occur, **do not drive, use machines, or do other jobs that require you to see well.**

Disopyramide may cause dryness of the mouth, nose, and throat. For temporary relief of mouth dryness, use sugarless candy or gum, melt bits of ice in your mouth, or use a saliva substitute. However, if dry mouth continues for more than 2 weeks, check with your physician or dentist. Continuing dryness of the mouth may increase the chance of dental disease, including tooth decay, gum disease, and fungal infections.

This medicine will often make you sweat less, allowing your body temperature to increase. **Use extra care not to become overheated during exercise or hot weather while you are taking this medicine** since overheating could possibly result in heat stroke.

Side Effects of This Medicine

Along with its needed effects, a medicine may cause some unwanted effects. Although not all of these side effects may occur, if they do occur they may need medical attention.

Check with your doctor as soon as possible if any of the following side effects occur:

More common
    Difficult urination

Less common
    Chest pains
    Dizziness, lightheadedness, or fainting
    Fast or slow heartbeat
    Muscle weakness
    Shortness of breath (unexplained)
    Swelling of feet or lower legs
    Weight gain (rapid)

Rare
    Eye pain
    Mental depression
    Sore throat and fever
    Yellow eyes and skin

Signs of hypoglycemia (low blood sugar)
    Anxious feeling
    Chills
    Cold sweats
    Confusion
    Cool, pale skin
    Drowsiness
    Fast heartbeat
    Headache
    Hunger (excessive)
    Nausea
    Nervousness
    Shakiness
    Unsteady walk
    Unusual tiredness or weakness

Other side effects may occur that usually do not require medical attention. These side effects may go away during treatment as your body adjusts to the medicine. However, check with your doctor if any of the following side effects continue or are bothersome:

More common
    Dry mouth and throat

Less common
    Bloating or stomach pain
    Blurred vision
    Constipation
    Decreased sexual ability
    Dry eyes and nose
    Frequent urge to urinate
    Loss of appetite

For elderly patients: Some of the above side effects may be more likely to occur in the elderly, who are usually more sensitive to the effects of disopyramide.

Other side effects not listed above may also occur in some patients. If you notice any other effects, check with your doctor.

December 1987

DISULFIRAM (Systemic)

A commonly used brand name is Antabuse.

Generic name product may also be available in the U.S.

To the Reader: If you do not recognize the names of medical conditions or medicines referred to in this information, check with your doctor, nurse, or pharmacist. Definitions for selected medical terms may be found in the Glossary. Brand names for the generic drug names listed can be found in the Index. In addition, selected brand names commonly associated with the generic name have been included in the text to help you recognize medicine you may be taking. The fact that a brand name product is not mentioned does not mean the information does not apply. It is a good idea for you to learn both the generic and brand names of your medicines and to write them down for future use.

Disulfiram (dye-SUL-fi-ram) is used to help overcome your drinking problem. It is not a cure for alcoholism, but rather will discourage you from drinking.

Disulfiram is available only with your doctor's prescription.

Remember:

• **This medicine has been prescribed for your current medical problem only.** It must not be given to other people or used for other problems unless you are directed to do so by your doctor.

• **Keep all medicines out of the reach of children.**

• In order for this medicine to work, it must be used as directed.

• **It is very important that you read and understand the following information.** If any of the information causes you special concern, do not decide against using this medicine without first checking with your doctor.

• Before you begin using any new medicine (prescription or nonprescription) or if you develop any new medical problem while you are using this medicine, check with your doctor, nurse, or pharmacist.

• **If you have any questions** about the following information or if you want more information about this medicine or your medical problem, **ask your doctor, nurse, or pharmacist**.

Before Using This Medicine

In order to decide on the best treatment for your medical problem, your doctor should be told:

—if you have had any unusual or allergic reactions to disulfiram, rubber, pesticides, or fungicides.

—if you are on a low-salt, low-sugar, or any other special diet, or if you are allergic to any substance, such as foods, sulfites or other preservatives, or dyes. Most medicines contain more than their active ingredient. Your doctor, nurse, or pharmacist can help you avoid products that may cause a problem.

—if you are **pregnant** or if you may become pregnant. However, disulfiram has not been shown to cause problems in humans.

—if you are **breast-feeding**, although disulfiram has not been shown to cause problems in nursing babies.

—if you have any of the following medical problems:
   Brain damage
   Diabetes mellitus (sugar diabetes)
   Epilepsy
   Heart or blood vessel disease
   Kidney disease
   Liver disease or cirrhosis of the liver
   Severe mental illness
   Skin allergy
   Underactive thyroid

—if you are taking **any** other prescription or nonprescription (OTC) medicine, especially:
   Anticoagulants (blood thinners)
   Ethotoin (e.g., Peganone)
   Isoniazid (e.g., INH; Nydrazid)
   Mephenytoin (e.g., Mesantoin)
   Phenytoin (e.g., Dilantin)

—if you are now taking or have taken within the past several days either of the following medicines:
   Metronidazole (e.g., Flagyl)
   Paraldehyde (e.g., Paral)

Proper Use of This Medicine

Before you take the first dose of this medicine, **make sure you have not taken any alcoholic beverage or alcohol-containing product or medicine** (for example, tonics, elixirs, and cough syrups) **during the past 12 hours.** If you are not sure about the alcohol content of medicines you may have taken, check with your doctor or pharmacist.

Take this medicine every day as directed by your doctor. The medicine is usually taken each morning. However, if it makes you drowsy, ask your doctor if you may take it at bedtime instead.

How to store this medicine:

• **Keep out of the reach of children.**

• Store away from heat and direct light.

• Do not store in the bathroom, near the kitchen sink, or in other damp places. Heat or moisture may cause the medicine to break down.

• Do not keep outdated medicine or medicine no longer needed. Be sure that any discarded medicine is out of the reach of children.

Precautions While Using This Medicine

Do not drink any alcohol, even small amounts, while you are taking this medicine and for 14 days after stopping this medicine because it may make you very sick. This includes alcohol-containing foods, products, or medicines, such as elixirs, tonics, sauces, vinegars, cough syrups, mouth washes, or gargles. **In addition, do not apply to your skin any alcohol-containing liniments or lotions,** such as rubbing alcohol, back rubs, after-shave lotions, cologne, toilet waters, or after-bath preparations because the alcohol they contain may be absorbed into your body. Reading the list of ingredients on foods or other products before using them will help you to avoid alcohol.

Some of the symptoms you may experience if you use any alcohol while taking this medicine are:

> Blurred vision
> Chest pain
> Confusion
> Dizziness or fainting
> Fast or pounding heartbeat
> Flushing or redness of face
> Nausea and vomiting
> Sweating
> Throbbing headache
> Troubled breathing
> Weakness

These symptoms will last as long as there is any alcohol left in your system, from 30 minutes to several hours. On rare occasions, if you have a severe reaction or have taken a large enough amount of alcohol, a heart attack, unconsciousness, convulsions (seizures), and death may occur.

Your doctor may want you to carry an identification card stating that you are using this medicine. This card should list the symptoms most likely to occur if alcohol is taken, and the doctor, clinic, or hospital to be contacted in case of an emergency. These cards may be available from the manufacturer. Ask your doctor or pharmacist if you have any questions about this.

If you will be taking this medicine for a long period of time (for example, for several months at a time), your doctor should check your progress at regular visits.

Before buying or using any liquid prescription or nonprescription medicine, check with your pharmacist to see if it contains any alcohol.

This medicine may cause some people to become drowsy or less alert than they are normally. If this occurs, **do not drive, use machines, or do other jobs that require you to be alert** while you are taking disulfiram.

Disulfiram will add to the effects of other CNS depressants (medicines that slow down the nervous system, possibly causing drowsiness). Some examples of CNS depressants are antihistamines or medicine for hay fever, other allergies, or colds; sedatives, tranquilizers, or sleeping medicine; prescription pain medicine or narcotics; barbiturates; medicine for seizures; muscle relaxants; or anesthetics, including some dental anesthetics. **Check with your doctor before taking any of the above while you are using this medicine.**

Side Effects of This Medicine

Along with its needed effects, a medicine may cause some unwanted effects. Although not all of these side effects may occur, if they do occur they may need medical attention.

Check with your doctor as soon as possible if any of the following side effects occur:

Less common
> Eye pain or tenderness or any change in vision
> Mood or mental changes
> Numbness, tingling, pain, or weakness in hands or feet

Rare
> Yellow eyes or skin

Other side effects may occur that usually do not require medical attention. These side effects may go away during treatment as your body adjusts to the medicine. However, check with your doctor if any of the following side effects continue or are bothersome:

More common
> Drowsiness

Less common or rare
> Decreased sexual ability in males
> Headache
> Metallic or garlic-like taste in mouth
> Skin rash
> Stomach discomfort
> Unusual tiredness

For elderly patients: Many medicines have not been tested in older people. Therefore, it is not known whether the medicine acts the same way it does in younger adults. Check with your doctor or pharmacist if you notice any unusual effects while taking this medicine or if you think it is not working as it should.

Other side effects not listed above may also occur in some patients. If you notice any other effects, check with your doctor.

December 1987

DIURETICS, LOOP (Systemic)

This information applies to the following medicines:

Bumetanide (byoo-MET-a-nide)
Ethacrynic acid (eth-a-KRIN-ik AS-id)
Furosemide (fur-OH-se-mide)

Some commonly used brand names are:	Generic names:
Bumex	Bumetanide
Edecrin	Ethacrynic acid
Apo-Furosemide* Furoside* Lasix Lasix Special* Novosemide* Uritol*	Furosemide†‡

*Not available in the U.S.
†Generic name product may also be available in the U.S.
‡Generic name product may also be available in Canada.

To the Reader: If you do not recognize the names of medical conditions or medicines referred to in this information, check with your doctor, nurse, or pharmacist. Definitions for selected medical terms may be found in the Glossary. Brand names for the generic drug names listed can be found in the Index. In addition, selected brand names commonly associated with the generic name have been included in the text to help you recognize medicine you may be taking. The fact that a brand name product is not mentioned does not mean the information does not apply. It is a good idea for you to learn both the generic and brand names of your medicines and to write them down for future use.

Loop diuretics are given to help reduce the amount of water in the body. They work by acting on the kidneys to increase the flow of urine.

Furosemide is also used to treat high blood pressure in those patients who are not helped by other medicines or in those patients who have kidney problems. High blood pressure adds to the workload of the heart and arteries. If it continues for a long time, the heart and arteries may not function properly. This can damage the blood vessels of the brain, heart, and kidneys, resulting in a stroke, heart failure, or kidney failure. High blood pressure may also increase the risk of heart attacks. These problems may be less likely to occur if blood pressure is controlled.

Loop diuretics may also be used for other conditions as determined by your doctor.

This medicine is available only with your doctor's prescription.

Remember:

• **This medicine has been prescribed for your current medical problem only.** It must not be given to other people or used for other problems unless you are directed to do so by your doctor.

• **Keep all medicines out of the reach of children.**

• In order for this medicine to work, it must be used as directed.

• If you are receiving this medicine by injection, some of the information about this medicine may not apply.

• **It is very important that you read and understand the following information.** If any of the information causes you special concern, do not decide against using this medicine without first checking with your doctor.

• Before you begin using any new medicine (prescription or nonprescription) or if you develop any new medical problem while you are using this medicine, check with your doctor, nurse, or pharmacist.

• **If you have any questions** about the following information or if you want more information about this medicine or your medical problem, **ask your doctor, nurse, or pharmacist.**

Before Using This Medicine

In order to decide on the best treatment for your medical problem, your doctor should be told:

—if you have ever had any unusual or allergic reaction to bumetanide, ethacrynic acid, furosemide, sulfonamides (sulfa drugs), or thiazide diuretics (water pills).

—if you are on a low-salt, low-sugar, or any other special diet, or if you are allergic to any substance, such as foods, sulfites or other preservatives, or dyes. Most medicines contain more than their active ingredient, and many liquid medicines contain alcohol. Your doctor, nurse, or pharmacist can help you avoid products that may cause a problem.

—if you are **pregnant** or if you may become pregnant. Although studies have not been done in humans, studies in animals have shown this medicine to cause harmful effects on the fetus. Also, ethacrynic acid causes birth defects in animals.

In general, diuretics are not useful for normal swelling of feet and hands that occurs during pregnancy. Diuretics should not be taken during pregnancy unless recommended by your doctor.

—if you are **breast-feeding**. This medicine has not been shown to cause problems in nursing babies. Furosemide passes into breast milk; it is not known whether bumetanide or ethacrynic acid passes into breast milk.

—if you have any of the following medical problems:
  Diabetes mellitus (sugar diabetes)
  Diarrhea
  Gout
  Hearing problems
  Kidney disease (severe)
  Liver disease
  Lupus erythematosus (history of)
  Pancreas disease

—if you have recently had a heart attack.

—if you are taking **any** other prescription or nonprescription (OTC) medicine, especially:
  Adrenocorticoids (cortisone-like medicines)
  Aminoglycosides by injection or topical application (amikacin, gentamicin, kanamycin, neomycin, netilmicin, streptomycin, tobramycin)
  Amphotericin B by injection (e.g., Fungizone)
  Anticoagulants (blood thinners)
  Capreomycin (e.g., Capastat)
  Captopril (e.g., Capoten)
  Carmustine (e.g., BiCNU)

Cisplatin (e.g., Platinol)
Cyclosporine (e.g., Sandimmune)
Enalapril (e.g., Vasotec)
Gold salts
Lithium (e.g., Lithane)
Medicine for inflammation or pain (diclofenac, diflunisal, fenoprofen, flurbiprofen [oral], ibuprofen, indomethacin, ketoprofen, meclofenamate, mefenamic acid, naproxen, phenylbutazone, piroxicam, sulindac, tiaprofenic acid, tolmetin)
Methotrexate (e.g., Mexate)
Neomycin by mouth (e.g., Mycifradin)
Penicillamine (e.g., Cuprimine)
Plicamycin (e.g., Mithracin)
Rifampin (e.g., Rifadin)
Streptozocin (e.g., Zanosar)
Sulfonamides (sulfa medicine)
Tetracyclines, except doxycycline and minocycline
Vancomycin by injection (e.g., Vancocin)

—if you regularly take large amounts of combination pain medicine containing acetaminophen and aspirin or other salicylates.

Proper Use of This Medicine

This medicine may cause you to have an unusual feeling of tiredness when you begin to take it. You may also notice an increase in the amount of urine or in your frequency of urination. After taking the medicine for a while, these effects should lessen. In order to keep the increase in urine from affecting your nighttime sleep:

• If you are to take a single dose a day, take it in the morning after breakfast.

• If you are to take more than one dose a day, take the last dose no later than 6 p.m., unless otherwise directed by your doctor.

However, it is best to plan your dose or doses according to a schedule that will least affect your personal activities and sleep. Ask your doctor, nurse, or pharmacist to help you plan the best time to take this medicine.

In order to help remember to take your medicine, try to get into the habit of taking it at the same time each day.

For patients taking the oral liquid form of furosemide:

• This medicine is to be taken by mouth even though it may come in a dropper bottle. If this medicine does not come in a dropper bottle, use a specially marked measuring spoon or other device to measure each dose accurately, since the average household teaspoon may not hold the right amount of liquid.

For patients taking this medicine for high blood pressure:

• Importance of diet—When prescribing medicine for your condition, your doctor may prescribe a personal diet for you. Such a diet may be low in sodium (salt). Most people eat much more sodium than they need and too much sodium in the diet may increase blood pressure. Some foods that contain large amounts of sodium are canned soup, pickles, ketchup, green and

ripe olives, relish, frankfurters, soy sauce, and carbonated beverages. Your doctor may want you to limit the amounts of these and other high-sodium foods in your diet. High blood pressure medicine is usually more effective when such a diet is properly followed.

Also, it may be very important for you to go on a reducing diet. However, check with your doctor before changing your diet.

• Many patients who have high blood pressure will not notice any signs of the problem. In fact, many may feel normal. It is very important that you **take your medicine exactly as directed** and that you keep your appointments with your doctor even if you feel well.

• Remember that this medicine will not cure your high blood pressure but it does help control it. Therefore, you must continue to take it as directed if you expect to lower your blood pressure and keep it down. **You may have to take high blood pressure medicine for the rest of your life.** If high blood pressure is not treated, it can cause serious problems such as heart failure, blood vessel disease, stroke, or kidney disease.

If this medicine upsets your stomach, it may be taken with meals or milk. If stomach upset (nausea, vomiting, or stomach pain) continues or gets worse, or if you suddenly get severe diarrhea, check with your doctor.

If you miss a dose of this medicine, take it as soon as possible. However, if it is almost time for your next dose, skip the missed dose and go back to your regular dosing schedule. Do not double doses.

How to store this medicine:

• **Keep out of the reach of children.**

• Store away from heat and direct light.

• Do not store in the bathroom, near the kitchen sink, or in other damp places. Heat or moisture may cause the medicine to break down.

• Keep the oral liquid form of this medicine from freezing.

• Do not keep outdated medicine or medicine no longer needed. Be sure that any discarded medicine is out of the reach of children.

Precautions While Using This Medicine

It is important that your doctor check your progress at regular visits to make sure that this medicine is working properly.

This medicine may cause a loss of potassium from your body.

• To help prevent this, your doctor may want you to:

    —eat or drink foods that have a high potassium content (for example, orange or other citrus fruit juices), or

    —take a potassium supplement, or

    —take another medicine to help prevent the loss of the potassium in the first place.

• It is very important to follow these directions. Also, it is important not to change your diet on your own. This is more important if you are already on a special diet (as for diabetes), or if you are taking a potassium supplement or a medicine to reduce potassium loss. Extra potassium may not be necessary and, in some cases, too much potassium could be harmful.

To prevent the loss of too much water and potassium, tell your doctor if you become sick, especially with severe or continuing nausea and vomiting or diarrhea.

Before having any kind of surgery (including dental surgery) or emergency treatment, make sure the physician or dentist in charge knows that you are taking this medicine.

Dizziness, lightheadedness, or fainting may occur, especially when you get up from a lying or sitting position. This is more likely to occur in the morning. **Getting up slowly may help**, but if the problem continues or gets worse, check with your doctor.

The dizziness, lightheadedness, or fainting is also more likely to occur if you drink alcohol, stand for long periods of time, or exercise, or if the weather is hot. **While you are taking this medicine, be careful of the amount of alcohol you drink. Also, use extra care during exercise or hot weather or if you must stand for long periods of time.**

Diabetics—This medicine may affect blood sugar levels. While you are using this medicine, be especially careful in testing for sugar in your urine.

For patients taking this medicine for high blood pressure:

• **Do not take other medicines unless they have been discussed with your doctor.** This especially includes over-the-counter (nonprescription) medicines for appetite control, asthma, colds, cough, hay fever, or sinus problems, since they may tend to increase your blood pressure.

For patients taking furosemide:

• Some people who take this medicine may become more sensitive to sunlight than they are normally. When you first begin taking this medicine, avoid too much sun and do not use a sunlamp until you see how you react to the sun, especially if you tend to burn easily. If you have a severe reaction, check with your doctor.

Side Effects of This Medicine

Along with its needed effects, a medicine may cause some unwanted effects. Although not all of these side effects may occur, if they do occur they may need medical attention.

Check with your doctor as soon as possible if any of the following side effects occur:

Rare

Black tarry stools—for ethacrynic acid injection only
Blood in urine—for ethacrynic acid injection only
Joint, lower back or side, or stomach pain
Ringing or buzzing sound in ears or any loss of hearing—more common with ethacrynic acid
Skin rash or hives
Sore throat and fever
Stomach pain (severe) with nausea and vomiting
Unusual bleeding or bruising
Yellow eyes or skin
Yellow vision—for furosemide only

Signs of loss of too much potassium

Dryness of mouth
Increased thirst
Irregular heartbeats
Mood or mental changes
Muscle cramps or pain
Nausea or vomiting
Unusual tiredness or weakness
Weak pulse

Other side effects may occur that usually do not require medical attention. These side effects may go away during treatment as your body adjusts to the medicine. However, check with your doctor if any of the following side effects continue or are bothersome:

More common

Dizziness or lightheadedness when getting up from a lying or sitting position

Less common or rare

Blurred vision
Chest pain—with bumetanide only
Confusion—with ethacrynic acid only
Diarrhea—more common with ethacrynic acid
Headache
Increased sensitivity of skin to sunlight—with furosemide only
Loss of appetite—more common with ethacrynic acid
Nervousness—with ethacrynic acid only
Premature ejaculation or difficulty in keeping an erection—with bumetanide only
Redness or pain at the place of injection
Stomach cramps or pain

For elderly patients: Dizziness, lightheadedness, or signs of too much potassium loss may be more likely to occur in the elderly, who are more sensitive to the effects of this medicine.

Other side effects not listed above may also occur in some patients. If you notice any other effects, check with your doctor.

December 1987

DIURETICS, POTASSIUM-SPARING
(Systemic)

This information applies to the following medicines:

Amiloride (a-MILL-oh-ride)
Spironolactone (speer-on-oh-LAK-tone)
Triamterene (trye-AM-ter-een)

Some commonly used brand names are:	Generic names
Midamor	Amiloride†
Aldactone Novospiroton* Sincomen*	Spironolactone†
Dyrenium	Triamterene

*Not available in the U.S.
†Generic name product may also be available in the U.S.

To the Reader: If you do not recognize the names of medical conditions or medicines referred to in this information, check with your doctor, nurse, or pharmacist. Definitions for selected medical terms may be found in the Glossary. Brand names for the generic drug names listed can be found in the Index. In addition, selected brand names commonly associated with the generic name have been included in the text to help you recognize medicine you may be taking. The fact that a brand name product is not mentioned does not mean the information does not apply. It is a good idea for you to learn both the generic and brand names of your medicines and to write them down for future use.

Potassium-sparing diuretics are commonly taken by mouth to help reduce the amount of water in the body. Unlike some other diuretics, these medicines do not cause your body to lose potassium.

Amiloride and spironolactone are also used to treat high blood pressure. High blood pressure adds to the workload of the heart and arteries. If it continues for a long time, the heart and arteries may not function properly. This can damage the blood vessels of the brain, heart, and kidneys resulting in a stroke, heart failure, or kidney failure. High blood pressure may also increase the risk of heart attacks. These problems may be less likely to occur if blood pressure is controlled.

Spironolactone is also used to help increase the amount of potassium in the body when it is getting too low.

Potassium-sparing diuretics help to reduce the amount of water in the body by acting on the kidneys to increase the flow of urine. This also helps to lower blood pressure.

These medicines can also be used for other conditions as determined by your doctor.

Potassium-sparing diuretics are available only with your doctor's prescription.

Remember:

• **This medicine has been prescribed for your current medical problem only.** It must not be given to other people or used for other problems unless you are directed to do so by your doctor.

• **Keep all medicines out of the reach of children.**

• In order for this medicine to work, it must be used as directed.

• It is very important that you read and understand the following information. If any of the information causes you special concern, do not decide against using this medicine without first checking with your doctor.

• Before you begin using any new medicine (prescription or nonprescription) or if you develop any new medical problem while you are using this medicine, check with your doctor, nurse, or pharmacist.

• **If you have any questions** about the following information or if you want more information about this medicine or your medical problem, **ask your doctor, nurse, or pharmacist.**

Before Using This Medicine

In order to decide on the best treatment for your medical problem, your doctor should be told:

—if you have ever had any unusual or allergic reaction to amiloride, spironolactone, or triamterene.

—if you are on a low-salt, low-sugar, or any other special diet, or if you are allergic to any substance, such as foods, sulfites or other preservatives, or dyes. Most medicines contain more than their active ingredient. Your doctor, nurse, or pharmacist can help you avoid products that may cause a problem.

—if you are **pregnant** or if you may become pregnant. Studies have not been done in humans. However, this medicine has not been shown to cause birth defects or other problems in animals.

In general, diuretics are not useful for normal swelling of feet and hands that occurs during pregnancy. Diuretics should not be taken during pregnancy unless recommended by your doctor.

—if you are **breast-feeding**. Although spironolactone and triamterene may pass into breast milk, these medicines have not been shown to cause problems in nursing babies. It is not known whether amiloride passes into breast milk.

—if you have any of the following medical problems:
Diabetes mellitus (sugar diabetes)
Gout (triamterene only)
Kidney disease
Kidney stones (history of; triamterene only)
Liver disease
Menstrual problems or breast enlargement (spironolactone only)

—if you are taking **any** other prescription or nonprescription (OTC) medicine, especially:
Captopril (e.g., Capoten)
Cyclosporine (e.g., Sandimmune)
Enalapril (e.g., Vasotec)
Lithium (e.g., Lithane)
Potassium-containing medicines or supplements

Proper Use of This Medicine

This medicine may cause you to have an unusual feeling of tiredness when you begin to take it. You may also notice an increase in the amount of urine or in your frequency of urination. After taking the medicine for a while, these effects should lessen. In general, in order to keep the increase in urine from affecting your night-time sleep:

• If you are to take a single dose a day, take it in the morning after breakfast.

• If you are to take more than one dose a day, take the last dose no later than 6 p.m., unless otherwise directed by your doctor.

However, it is best to plan your dose or doses according to a schedule that will least affect your personal activities and sleep. Ask your doctor, nurse, or pharmacist to help you plan the best time to take this medicine.

In order to help you remember to take your medicine, try to get into the habit of taking it at the same time each day.

If this medicine upsets your stomach, it may be taken with meals or milk. If stomach upset (nausea, vomiting, stomach pain or cramps) continues, check with your doctor.

For patients taking this medicine for high blood pressure:

• Importance of diet—When prescribing medicine for your condition, your doctor may also prescribe a personal diet for you. Such a diet may be low in sodium (salt). Most people eat much more sodium than they need and too much sodium in the diet may increase blood pressure. Some foods that contain large amounts of sodium are canned soup, pickles, ketchup, green and ripe olives, relish, frankfurters, soy sauce, and carbonated beverages. Your doctor may want you to limit the amounts of these and other high-sodium foods in your diet. High blood pressure medicine is usually more effective when such a diet is properly followed.

Also, it may be very important for you to go on a reducing diet. However, check with your doctor before changing your diet.

• Many patients who have high blood pressure will not notice any signs of the problem. In fact, many may feel normal. It is very important that you **take your medicine exactly as directed** and that you keep your appointments with your doctor even if you feel well.

• Remember that this medicine will not cure your high blood pressure but it does help control it. Therefore, you must continue to take it as directed if you expect to lower your blood pressure and keep it down. **You may have to take high blood pressure medicine for the rest of your life.** If high blood pressure is not treated, it can cause serious problems such as heart failure, blood vessel disease, stroke, or kidney disease.

If you miss a dose of this medicine, take it as soon as possible. However, if it is almost time for your next dose, skip the missed dose and go back to your regular dosing schedule. Do not double doses.

How to store this medicine:

• **Keep out of the reach of children.**

• Store away from heat and direct light.

• Do not store in the bathroom, near the kitchen sink, or in other damp places. Heat or moisture may cause the medicine to break down.

• Do not keep outdated medicine or medicine no longer needed. Be sure that any discarded medicine is out of the reach of children.

Precautions While Using This Medicine

It is important that your doctor check your progress at regular visits to make sure that this medicine is working properly.

This medicine does not cause a loss of potassium from your body as some other diuretics (water pills) do. Therefore, it is not necessary for you to get extra potassium in your diet, and too much potassium could even be harmful. Since salt substitutes and low-salt milk may contain potassium, do not use them unless told to do so by your doctor.

Check with your doctor if you become sick and have severe or continuing nausea, vomiting, or diarrhea. These problems may cause you to lose additional water, which could be harmful, or to lose potassium, which could lessen the medicine's helpful effects.

Before having any kind of surgery (including dental surgery) or emergency treatment, tell the physician or dentist in charge that you are taking this medicine.

For patients taking this medicine for high blood pressure:

• **Do not take other medicines unless they have been discussed with your doctor.** This especially includes over-the-counter (nonprescription) medicines for appetite control, asthma, colds, cough, hay fever, or sinus problems, since they may tend to increase your blood pressure.

For patients taking triamterene:

• Diabetics—This medicine may raise blood sugar levels. While you are using triamterene, be especially careful in testing for sugar in your urine. If you have any questions about this, check with your doctor.

• A few people who take this medicine may become more sensitive to sunlight than they are normally. When you first begin taking triamterene, avoid too much sun and do not use a sunlamp until you see how you react to the sun, especially if you tend to burn easily. If you have a severe reaction, check with your doctor.

Side Effects of This Medicine

In rats, spironolactone has been found to increase the risk of tumors. It is not known if spironolactone increases the chance of tumors in humans.

Along with its needed effects, a medicine may cause some unwanted effects. Although not all of these side effects may occur, if they do occur they may need medical attention.

Check with your doctor as soon as possible if any of the following side effects occur:

Rare

Shortness of breath
Skin rash or itching

Signs of too much potassium

Confusion
Irregular heartbeat
Nervousness
Numbness or tingling in hands, feet, or lips
Shortness of breath or difficult breathing
Unusual tiredness or weakness
Weakness or heaviness of legs

Reported for triamterene only (rare)

Bright red tongue
Burning, inflamed feeling in tongue
Cracked corners of mouth
Lower back or side pain (severe)
Sore throat and fever
Unusual bleeding or bruising
Weakness

For elderly patients: Signs of too much potassium are more likely to occur in the elderly, who are more sensitive to the effects of this medicine.

Other side effects may occur that usually do not require medical attention. These side effects may go away during treatment as your body adjusts to the medicine. However, check with your doctor if any of the following side effects continue or are bothersome:

More common (less common with amiloride and triamterene)

Nausea and vomiting
Stomach cramps and diarrhea

Less common

Dizziness
Headache

Signs of too little sodium

Drowsiness
Dryness of mouth
Increased thirst
Lack of energy

Reported for amiloride and spironolactone only (less common)

Constipation
Decreased sexual ability
Muscle cramps

Reported for spironolactone only (less common)

Breast tenderness in females
Clumsiness
Deepening of voice in females
Enlargement of breasts in males
Inability to have or keep an erection
Increased hair growth in females
Irregular menstrual periods
Sweating

Reported for triamterene only (less common)

Increased sensitivity of skin to sunlight

For male patients: Spironolactone sometimes causes enlarged breasts in males, especially when they take large doses of it for a long time. Breasts usually decrease in size gradually over several months after this medicine is stopped. If you have any questions about this, check with your doctor.

Other side effects not listed above may also occur in some patients. If you notice any other effects, check with your doctor.

December 1987

DIURETICS, POTASSIUM-SPARING, AND HYDROCHLOROTHIAZIDE (Systemic)

This information applies to the following medicines:

Amiloride (a-MILL-oh-ride) and Hydrochlorothiazide (hye-droe-klor-oh-THYE-a-zide)

Spironolactone (speer-on-oh-LAK-tone) and Hydrochlorothiazide

Triamterene (trye-AM-ter-een) and Hydrochlorothiazide

Some commonly used brand names are:	Generic names:
Moduret* Moduretic	Amiloride and Hydrochlorothiazide†
Aldactazide Novospirozine*	Spironolactone and Hydrochlorothiazide†
Apo-Triazide* Dyazide Maxzide Novotriamzide*	Triamterene and Hydrochlorothiazide†

*Not available in the U.S.

†Generic name product may also be available in the U.S.

To the Reader: If you do not recognize the names of medical conditions or medicines referred to in this information, check with your doctor, nurse, or pharmacist. Definitions for selected medical terms may be found in the Glossary. Brand names for the generic drug names listed can be found in the Index. In addition, selected brand names commonly associated with the generic name have been included in the text to help you recognize medicine you may be taking. The fact that a brand name product is not mentioned does not mean the information does not apply. It is a good idea for you to learn both the generic and brand names of your medicines and to write them down for future use.

This medicine is a combination of two diuretics (water pills). It is commonly taken by mouth to help reduce the amount of water in the body.

This combination is also used to treat high blood pressure. High blood pressure adds to the workload of the heart and arteries. If it continues for a long time, the heart and arteries may not function properly. This can damage the blood vessels of the brain, heart, and kidneys, resulting in a stroke, heart failure, or kidney failure. High blood pressure may also increase the risk of heart attacks. These problems may be less likely to occur if blood pressure is controlled.

Diuretics help to reduce the amount of water in the body by acting on the kidneys to increase the flow of urine. This also helps to lower blood pressure.

This combination is also used to treat problems caused by too little potassium in the body.

This medicine is available only with your doctor's prescription.

Remember:

• **This medicine has been prescribed for your current medical problem only.** It must not be given to other people or used for other problems unless you are directed to do so by your doctor.

• **Keep all medicines out of the reach of children.**

• In order for this medicine to work, it must be used as directed.

• **It is very important that you read and understand the following information.** If any of the information causes you special concern, do not decide against using this medicine without first checking with your doctor.

• Before you begin using any new medicine (prescription or nonprescription) or if you develop any new medical problem while you are using this medicine, check with your doctor, nurse, or pharmacist.

• **If you have any questions** about the following information or if you want more information about this medicine or your medical problem, **ask your doctor, nurse, or pharmacist.**

Before Using This Medicine

In order to decide on the best treatment for your medical problem, your doctor should be told:

—if you have ever had any unusual or allergic reaction to amiloride, spironolactone, triamterene, sulfonamides (sulfa drugs), bumetanide, furosemide, acetazolamide, dichlorphenamide, methazolamide, or to hydrochlorothiazide or any of the other thiazide diuretics.

—if you are on a low-salt, low-sugar, or any other special diet, or if you are allergic to any substance, such as foods, sulfites or other preservatives, or dyes. Most medicines contain more than their active ingredient. Your doctor, nurse, or pharmacist can help you avoid products that may cause a problem.

—if you are **pregnant** or if you may become pregnant. When hydrochlorothiazide is used during pregnancy, it may cause side effects including jaundice, blood problems, and low potassium in the newborn infant. In addition, although this medicine has not been shown to cause birth defects, the chance always exists.

In general, diuretics are not useful for normal swelling of feet and hands that occurs during pregnancy. They should not be taken during pregnancy unless recommended by your doctor.

—if you are **breast-feeding**. Although spironolactone, triamterene, and hydrochlorothiazide may pass into breast milk, they have not been shown to cause problems in nursing babies. It is not known whether amiloride passes into breast milk.

—if you have any of the following medical problems:

Diabetes mellitus (sugar diabetes)

Gout (history of)

Kidney disease

Kidney stones (history of—triamterene only)

Liver disease

Lupus erythematosus (history of)

Menstrual problems or breast enlargement (spironolactone only)

Pancreatitis (inflammation of pancreas)

—if you are taking **any** other prescription or nonprescription (OTC) medicine, especially:

Adrenocorticoids (cortisone-like medicine)

Captopril (e.g., Capoten)

Cyclosporine (e.g., Sandimmune)

Digitalis glycosides (heart medicine)

Enalapril (e.g., Vasotec)

Lithium (e.g., Lithane)
Methenamine (e.g., Mandelamine)
Other diuretics (water pills) or antihypertensives (high
  blood pressure medicine)
Potassium-containing medicines or supplements

Proper Use of This Medicine

This medicine may cause you to have an unusual feeling
of tiredness when you begin to take it. You may also
notice an increase in the amount of urine or in your
frequency of urination. After you have taken the medicine for a while, these effects should lessen. In general, in order to keep the increase in urine from affecting your nighttime sleep:

• If you are to take a single dose a day, take it in the
morning after breakfast.

• If you are to take more than one dose a day, take
the last dose no later than 6 p.m., unless otherwise
directed by your doctor.

However, it is best to plan your dose or doses according
to a schedule that will least affect your personal activities and sleep. Ask your doctor, nurse, or pharmacist to help you plan the best time to take this
medicine.

In order to help you remember to take your medicine,
try to get into the habit of taking it at the same time
each day.

If this medicine upsets your stomach, it may be taken
with meals or milk. If stomach upset (nausea, vomiting, stomach pain, or cramps) continues, check with
your doctor.

For patients taking this medicine for high blood pressure:
• Importance of diet—When prescribing medicine for
your condition, your doctor may also prescribe a personal diet for you. Such a diet may be low in sodium
(salt). Most people eat much more sodium than they
need and too much sodium in the diet may increase
blood pressure. Some foods that contain large amounts
of sodium are canned soup, pickles, ketchup, green
and ripe olives, relish, frankfurters, soy sauce, and carbonated beverages. Your doctor may want you to limit
the amounts of these and other high-sodium foods in
your diet. High blood pressure medicine is usually more
effective when such a diet is properly followed.

However, some foods low in sodium, and some salt
substitutes, are high in potassium. If they are used
together with this medicine, they may lead to too much
potassium in the body. Discuss with your doctor what
low-sodium foods you may use.

Also, it may be very important for you to go on a
reducing diet. However, check with your doctor before
changing your diet.

• Many patients who have high blood pressure will not
notice any signs of the problem. In fact, many may
feel normal. It is very important that you **take your
medicine exactly as directed** and that you keep your
appointments with your doctor even if you feel well.

• Remember that this medicine will not cure your high
blood pressure but it does help control it. Therefore,
you must continue to take it as directed if you expect
to lower your blood pressure and keep it down. **You
may have to take high blood pressure medicine for the
rest of your life.** If high blood pressure is not treated,
it can cause serious problems such as heart failure,
blood vessel disease, stroke, or kidney disease.

If you miss a dose of this medicine, take it as soon as
possible. However, if it is almost time for your next
dose, skip the missed dose and go back to your regular
dosing schedule. Do not double doses.

How to store this medicine:

• **Keep out of the reach of children.**

• Store away from heat and direct light.

• Do not store in the bathroom, near the kitchen sink,
or in other damp places. Heat or moisture may cause
the medicine to break down.

• Do not keep outdated medicine or medicine no longer
needed. Be sure that any discarded medicine is out of
the reach of children.

Precautions While Using This Medicine

It is important that your doctor check your progress at
regular visits to make sure that this medicine is working properly.

**This medicine may cause a loss or increase of potassium
in your body. Your doctor may have special instructions
about whether or not you need to eat or drink foods or
beverages that have a high potassium content (for example, orange or other citrus fruit juices), taking a
potassium supplement, or using salt substitutes.** Since
too much potassium can be harmful, it is important
not to change your diet on your own. Tell your doctor
if you are already on a special diet (as for diabetes).
Since salt substitutes and low-salt milk may contain
potassium, do not use them unless told to do so by
your doctor. Check with your doctor, nurse, or pharmacist if you need a list of foods that are high in
potassium or if you have any questions.

Check with your doctor if you become sick and have
severe or continuing vomiting or diarrhea. These problems may cause you to lose additional water and potassium and lead to low blood pressure.

Diabetics—Hydrochlorothiazide (contained in this combination medicine) may raise blood sugar levels. While
you are taking this medicine, be especially careful in
testing for sugar in your urine.

A few people who take this medicine may become more
sensitive to sunlight than they are normally. When you
first begin taking this medicine, avoid too much sun
and do not use a sunlamp until you see how you react
to the sun, especially if you tend to burn easily. If you
have a severe reaction, check with your doctor.

Before having any kind of surgery (including dental surgery) or emergency treatment, tell the physician or dentist in charge that you are taking this medicine.

For patients taking triamterene and hydrochlorothiazide combination:
• Do not change brands of triamterene and hydrochlorothiazide without first checking with your doctor. Different products may not work the same way. If you refill your medicine and it looks different, check with your pharmacist.

For patients taking this medicine for high blood pressure:
• **Do not take other medicines unless they have been discussed with your doctor.** This especially includes over-the-counter (nonprescription) medicines for appetite control, asthma, colds, cough, hay fever, or sinus problems, since they may tend to increase your blood pressure.

Side Effects of This Medicine

In rats, spironolactone has been found to increase the risk of development of tumors. However, the doses given were many times the dose of spironolactone given to humans. It is not known whether spironolactone causes tumors in humans.

Along with its needed effects, a medicine may cause some unwanted effects. Although not all of these side effects may occur, if they do occur they may need medical attention.

Check with your doctor as soon as possible if any of the following side effects occur:
Rare
  Joint, lower back or side, or stomach pain
  Skin rash or hives
  Sore throat and fever
  Stomach pain (severe) with nausea and vomiting
  Unusual bleeding or bruising
  Yellow eyes or skin
Signs of changes in potassium
  Dryness of mouth
  Increased thirst
  Irregular heartbeats
  Mood or mental changes
  Muscle cramps or pain
  Numbness or tingling in hands, feet, or lips
  Shortness of breath or difficulty breathing
  Unusual tiredness or weakness
  Weak pulse

Reported for triamterene only (rare)
  Bright red tongue
  Burning, inflamed feeling in tongue
  Cracked corners of mouth

Other side effects may occur that usually do not require medical attention. These side effects may go away during treatment as your body adjusts to the medicine. However, check with your doctor if any of the following side effects continue or are bothersome:
More common (less common with triamterene)
  Loss of appetite
  Nausea and vomiting
  Stomach cramps and diarrhea
  Upset stomach
Less common
  Decreased sexual ability
  Dizziness or lightheadedness when getting up from a lying or sitting position
  Headache (more common with amiloride)
  Increased sensitivity of skin to sunlight
Reported for amiloride and triamterene only (less common)
  Constipation
Reported for spironolactone only (less common)
  Breast tenderness in females
  Clumsiness
  Deepening of voice in females
  Enlargement of breasts in males
  Increased hair growth in females
  Irregular menstrual periods
  Sweating

For elderly patients: Dizziness or lightheadedness and signs of too much potassium loss may be more likely to occur in the elderly, who are more sensitive to the effects of this medicine.

Spironolactone sometimes causes enlarged breasts in males, especially when they take large doses of it for a long time. Breasts usually decrease in size gradually over several months after this medicine is stopped. If you have any questions about this, check with your doctor.

Other side effects not listed above may also occur in some patients. If you notice any other effects, check with your doctor.

December 1987

DIURETICS, THIAZIDE (Systemic)

This information applies to the following medicines:

Bendroflumethiazide (ben-droe-floo-meth-EYE-a-zide)
Benzthiazide (benz-THYE-a-zide)
Chlorothiazide (klor-oh-THYE-a-zide)
Chlorthalidone (klor-THAL-i-doan)
Cyclothiazide (sye-kloe-THYE-a-zide)
Hydrochlorothiazide (hye-droe-klor-oh-THYE-a-zide)
Hydroflumethiazide (hye-droe-floo-meth-EYE-a-zide)
Methyclothiazide (meth-ee-kloe-THYE-a-zide)
Metolazone (me-TOLE-a-zone)
Polythiazide (pol-i-THYE-a-zide)
Quinethazone (kwin-ETH-a-zone)
Trichlormethiazide (trye-klor-meth-EYE-a-zide)

Some commonly used brand names are:	Generic names:
Naturetin	Bendroflumethiazide
Aquatag Exna Hydrex	Benzthiazide†
Diuril	Chlorothiazide†
Apo-Chlorthalidone* Hygroton Novothalidone* Thalitone Uridon*	Chlorthalidone†‡
Anhydron Fluidil	Cyclothiazide
Apo-Hydro* Diuchlor H* Esidrix Hydrochlorothiazide Intensol HydroDIURIL Mictrin Natrimax* Neo-Codema* Novohydrazide* Oretic Thiuretic Urozide*	Hydrochlorothiazide†‡
Diucardin Saluron	Hydroflumethiazide†
Aquatensen Duretic* Enduron	Methyclothiazide†
Diulo Zaroxolyn	Metolazone
Renese	Polythiazide
Aquamox* Hydromox	Quinethazone
Metahydrin Naqua	Trichlormethiazide†

*Not available in the U.S.
†Generic name product may also be available in the U.S.
‡Generic name product may also be available in Canada.

To the Reader: If you do not recognize the names of medical conditions or medicines referred to in this information, check with your doctor, nurse, or pharmacist. Definitions for selected medical terms may be found in the Glossary. Brand names for the generic drug names listed can be found in the Index. In addition, selected brand names commonly associated with the generic name have been included in the text to help you recognize medicine you may be taking. The fact that a brand name product is not mentioned does not mean the information does not apply. It is a good idea for you to learn both the generic and brand names of your medicines and to write them down for future use.

Thiazide or thiazide-like diuretics are commonly used to treat high blood pressure. High blood pressure adds to the workload of the heart and arteries. If it continues for a long time, the heart and arteries may not function properly. This can damage the blood vessels of the brain, heart, and kidneys, resulting in a stroke, heart failure, or kidney failure. High blood pressure may also increase the risk of heart attacks. These problems may be less likely to occur if blood pressure is controlled.

Thiazide diuretics are also used to help reduce the amount of water in the body by increasing the flow of urine. They may also be used for other conditions as determined by your doctor.

Thiazide diuretics are available only with your doctor's prescription.

Remember:

• **This medicine has been prescribed for your current medical problem only.** It must not be given to other people or used for other problems unless you are directed to do so by your doctor.

• **Keep all medicines out of the reach of children.**

• In order for this medicine to work, it must be used as directed.

• If you are receiving this medicine by injection, some of the information about this medicine may not apply.

• **It is very important that you read and understand the following information.** If any of the information causes you special concern, do not decide against using this medicine without first checking with your doctor.

• Before you begin using any new medicine (prescription or nonprescription) or if you develop any new medical problem while you are using this medicine, check with your doctor, nurse, or pharmacist.

• **If you have any questions** about the following information or if you want more information about this medicine or your medical problem, **ask your doctor, nurse, or pharmacist.**

Before Using This Medicine

In order to decide on the best treatment for your medical problem, your doctor should be told:

—if you have ever had any unusual or allergic reaction to sulfonamides (sulfa drugs) or any of the thiazide diuretics.

—if you are on a low-salt, low-sugar, or any other special diet, or if you are allergic to any substance, such as foods, sulfites or other preservatives, or dyes. Most medicines contain more than their active ingredient, and many liquid medicines contain alcohol. Your doctor, nurse, or pharmacist can help you avoid products that may cause a problem.

—if you are **pregnant** or if you may become pregnant. When this medicine is used during pregnancy, it may cause side effects including jaundice, blood problems, and low potassium in the newborn infant. In addition, although this medicine has not been shown to cause birth defects or other problems in animals, studies have not been done in humans.

In general, diuretics are not useful for normal swelling of feet and hands that occurs during pregnancy. They should not be taken during pregnancy unless recommended by your doctor.

—if you are **breast-feeding**. Although thiazide diuretics pass into breast milk, they have not been shown to cause problems in nursing babies.

—if you have any of the following medical problems:

Diabetes mellitus (sugar diabetes)
Gout (history of)
Kidney disease (severe)
Liver disease
Lupus erythematosus (history of)
Pancreas disease

—if you are taking or using **any** other prescription or nonprescription (OTC) medicine, especially:

Adrenocorticoids (cortisone-like medicines)
Digitalis glycosides (heart medicine)
Lithium (e.g., Lithane)
Methenamine (e.g., Mandelamine)

Proper Use of This Medicine

This medicine may cause you to have an unusual feeling of tiredness when you begin to take it. You may also notice an increase in the amount of urine or in your frequency of urination. After you have taken the medicine for a while, these effects should lessen. In order to keep the increase in urine from affecting your nighttime sleep:

• If you are to take a single dose a day, take it in the morning after breakfast.

• If you are to take more than one dose a day, take the last dose no later than 6 p.m., unless otherwise directed by your doctor.

However, it is best to plan your dose or doses according to a schedule that will least affect your personal activities and sleep. Ask your doctor, nurse, or pharmacist to help you plan the best time to take this medicine.

In order to help remember to take your medicine, try to get into the habit of taking it at the same time each day.

For patients taking this medicine for high blood pressure:

• Importance of diet—When prescribing medicine for your condition, your doctor may also prescribe a personal diet for you. Such a diet may be low in sodium (salt). Most people eat much more sodium than they need and too much sodium in the diet may increase blood pressure. Some foods that contain large amounts of sodium are canned soup, pickles, ketchup, green and ripe olives, relish, frankfurters, soy sauce, and carbonated beverages. Your doctor may want you to limit the amounts of these and other high-sodium foods in your diet. High blood pressure medicine is usually more effective when such a diet is properly followed.

Also, it may be very important for you to go on a reducing diet. However, check with your doctor before changing your diet.

• Many patients who have high blood pressure will not notice any signs of the problem. In fact, many may feel normal. It is very important that you **take your medicine exactly as directed** and that you keep your appointments with your doctor even if you feel well.

• Remember that this medicine will not cure your high blood pressure but it does control it. Therefore, you must continue to take it as directed if you expect to lower your blood pressure and keep it down. **You may have to take high blood pressure medicine for the rest of your life.** If high blood pressure is not treated, it can cause serious problems such as heart failure, blood vessel disease, stroke, or kidney disease.

For patients taking the oral liquid form of hydrochlorothiazide, which comes in a dropper bottle:

• This medicine is to be taken by mouth. The amount you should take is to be measured only with the specially marked dropper.

If you miss a dose of this medicine, take it as soon as possible. However, if it is almost time for your next dose, skip the missed dose and go back to your regular dosing schedule. Do not double doses.

How to store this medicine:

• **Keep out of the reach of children.**

• Store away from heat and direct light.

• Do not store in the bathroom, near the kitchen sink, or in other damp places. Heat or moisture may cause the medicine to break down.

• Keep the oral liquid form of this medicine from freezing.

• Do not keep outdated medicine or medicine no longer needed. Be sure that any discarded medicine is out of the reach of children.

Precautions While Using This Medicine

It is important that your doctor check your progress at regular visits to make sure that this medicine is working properly.

This medicine may cause a loss of potassium from your body.

• To help prevent this, your doctor may want you to:
   —eat or drink foods that have a high potassium content (for example, orange or other citrus fruit juices), or
   —take a potassium supplement, or
   —take another medicine to help prevent the loss of the potassium in the first place.

• It is very important to follow these directions. Also, it is important not to change your diet on your own. This is more important if you are already on a special diet (as for diabetes), or if you are taking a potassium supplement or a medicine to reduce potassium loss. Extra potassium may not be necessary and, in some cases, too much potassium could be harmful.

Check with your doctor if you become sick and have severe or continuing vomiting or diarrhea. These problems may cause you to lose additional water and potassium.

Diabetics—Thiazide diuretics may raise blood sugar levels. While you are using this medicine, be especially careful in testing for sugar in your urine.

A few people who take this medicine may become more sensitive to sunlight than they are normally. When you first begin taking this medicine, avoid too much sun and do not use a sunlamp until you see how you react to the sun, especially if you tend to burn easily. If you have a severe reaction, check with your doctor.

For patients taking this medicine for high blood pressure:
• **Do not take other medicines unless they have been discussed with your doctor.** This especially includes over-the-counter (nonprescription) medicines for appetite control, asthma, colds, cough, hay fever, or sinus problems, since they may tend to increase your blood pressure.

Side Effects of This Medicine

Along with its needed effects, a medicine may cause some unwanted effects. Although not all of these side effects may occur, if they do occur they may need medical attention.

Check with your doctor as soon as possible if any of the following side effects occur:
Rare
　Joint, lower back or side, or stomach pain
　Skin rash or hives
　Sore throat and fever
　Stomach pain (severe) with nausea and vomiting
　Unusual bleeding or bruising
　Yellow eyes or skin
Signs of too much potassium loss
　Dryness of mouth
　Increased thirst
　Irregular heartbeats

　Mood or mental changes
　Muscle cramps or pain
　Nausea or vomiting
　Unusual tiredness or weakness
　Weak pulse

Other side effects may occur that usually do not require medical attention. These side effects may go away during treatment as your body adjusts to the medicine. However, check with your doctor if any of the following side effects continue or are bothersome:
Less common
　Decreased sexual ability
　Diarrhea
　Dizziness or lightheadedness when getting up from a lying or sitting position
　Increased sensitivity of skin to sunlight
　Loss of appetite
　Upset stomach

For elderly patients: Dizziness or lightheadedness and signs of too much potassium loss may be more likely to occur in the elderly, who are more sensitive to the effects of thiazide diuretics.

Other side effects not listed above may also occur in some patients. If you notice any other effects, check with your doctor.

December 1987

Additional Information

In addition to the above information, for patients taking this medicine for diabetes insipidus (water diabetes):
• Some thiazide diuretics are used in the treatment of diabetes insipidus (water diabetes). In patients with water diabetes, this medicine causes a decrease in the flow of urine and helps the body hold water. Thus, the information given above about increased urine flow will not apply to you.

DOXORUBICIN (Systemic)

A commonly used brand name is Adriamycin RDF.

To the Reader: If you do not recognize the names of medical conditions or medicines referred to in this information, check with your doctor, nurse, or pharmacist. Definitions for selected medical terms may be found in the Glossary. Brand names for the generic drug names listed can be found in the Index. In addition, selected brand names commonly associated with the generic name have been included in the text to help you recognize medicine you may be taking. The fact that a brand name product is not mentioned does not mean the information does not apply. It is a good idea for you to learn both the generic and brand names of your medicines and to write them down for future use.

Doxorubicin (dox-oh-ROO-bi-sin) belongs to the general group of medicines known as antineoplastics. It is given by injection to treat some kinds of cancer.

Doxorubicin seems to interfere with the growth of cancer cells, which are eventually destroyed. Since the growth of normal body cells may also be affected by doxorubicin, other effects will also occur. Some of these may be serious and must be reported to your doctor. Other effects, like hair loss, may not be serious but may cause concern. Some effects may not occur for months or years after the medicine is used.

Before you begin treatment with doxorubicin, you and your doctor should talk about the good this medicine will do as well as the risks of using it.

Doxorubicin is to be administered only by or under the immediate supervision of your doctor.

Remember:

• **It is very important that you read and understand the following information.** If any of the information causes you special concern, do not decide against receiving this medicine without first checking with your doctor.

• Before you begin using any new medicine (prescription or nonprescription) or if you develop any new medical problem while you are receiving this medicine, check with your doctor, nurse, or pharmacist.

• **If you have any questions** about the following information or if you want more information about this medicine or your medical problem, **ask your doctor, nurse, or pharmacist.**

Before Using This Medicine

In order to decide on the best treatment for your medical problem, your doctor should be told:

—if you have ever had any unusual or allergic reaction to doxorubicin, lincomycin, or clindamycin.

—if you are **pregnant** or if you intend to have children. There is a chance that this medicine may cause birth defects if either the male or female is receiving it at the time of conception or if it is taken during pregnancy. Studies in rats and rabbits have shown that doxorubicin causes birth defects in the fetus and other problems (including miscarriage). In addition, many cancer medicines may cause sterility which could be permanent. Although sterility has been reported in animals and humans with this medicine, the effect is weaker in humans than in animals. Be sure that you have discussed these possible effects with your doctor before receiving this medicine.

—if you intend to **breast-feed**. Because this medicine may cause serious side effects, breast-feeding is generally not recommended while you are receiving it.

—if you have any of the following medical problems:
Chickenpox (including recent exposure)
Gout
Heart disease
Herpes zoster (shingles)
Kidney stones
Liver disease

—if you are taking **any** other prescription or nonprescription (OTC) medicine, especially:
Amphotericin B by injection (e.g., Fungizone)
Antithyroid agents (medicine for overactive thyroid)
Azathioprine (e.g., Imuran)
Chloramphenicol (e.g., Chloromycetin)
Colchicine
Flucytosine (e.g., Ancobon)
Interferon (e.g., Intron A; Roferon-A)
Probenecid (e.g., Benemid)
Sulfinpyrazone (e.g., Anturane)

—if you have ever been treated with x-rays or cancer medicines.

Proper Use of This Medicine

Doxorubicin is sometimes given together with certain other medicines. If you are receiving a combination of medicines, it is important that you receive each one at the proper time. If you are taking some of these medicines by mouth, ask your doctor, nurse, or pharmacist to help you plan a way to take them at the right times.

While you are using this medicine, your doctor may want you to drink extra fluids so that you will pass more urine. This will help prevent kidney problems and keep your kidneys working well.

Doxorubicin often causes nausea and vomiting. However, it is very important that you continue to receive it, even if you begin to feel ill. Ask your doctor, nurse, or pharmacist for ways to lessen these effects.

Precautions While Using This Medicine

It is very important that your doctor check your progress at regular visits to make sure that this medicine is working properly and to check for unwanted effects.

While you are being treated with doxorubicin, and after you stop treatment with it, **do not have any immunizations without your doctor's approval.** Doxorubicin lowers your body's resistance, and there is a chance you might get the infection the immunization is meant to prevent. In addition, other persons living in your household should not take oral polio vaccine since there is a chance they could pass the polio virus on to you. Also, you should avoid close contact with other persons (for example, at school or work) who have taken oral polio vaccine.

Doxorubicin can lower the number of white blood cells in your body. This may increase the chance of getting an infection. If you can, avoid people with colds or other infections. If you think you are getting a cold or other infection, check with your doctor.

If doxorubicin accidentally seeps out of the vein into which it is injected, it may damage some tissues and cause scarring. **Tell the doctor or nurse right away if you notice redness, pain, or swelling at the place of injection**.

Side Effects of This Medicine

Along with their needed effects, medicines like doxorubicin can sometimes cause unwanted effects such as heart problems, blood problems, loss of hair, and other side effects; these are described below. Also, because of the way these medicines act on the body, there is a chance that they might cause other unwanted effects that may not occur until months or years after the medicine is used. These delayed effects may include certain types of cancer, such as leukemia. Discuss these possible effects with your doctor.

Although not all of these side effects may occur, if they do occur they may need medical attention.

Check with your doctor or nurse immediately if any of the following side effects occur:

More common
    Fever, chills, or sore throat
Less common
    Fast or irregular heartbeat
    Pain at the place of injection
    Shortness of breath
    Swelling of feet and lower legs
    Unusual bleeding or bruising
Rare
    Wheezing

Check with your doctor or nurse as soon as possible if any of the following side effects occur:

More common
    Sores in the mouth and on the lips
Less common
    Darkening or redness of the skin (after x-ray treatment)
    Joint pain
    Lower back, side, or stomach pain
Rare
    Skin rash or itching

Other side effects may occur that usually do not require medical attention. These side effects may go away during treatment as your body adjusts to the medicine. Also, your doctor or nurse may be able to tell you about ways to prevent or reduce some of these side effects. Check with your doctor or nurse if any of the following side effects continue or are bothersome or if you have any questions about them:

More common
    Nausea and vomiting
Less common
    Darkening of the soles, palms, or nails
    Diarrhea

Doxorubicin causes the urine to turn reddish in color, which may stain clothes. This is not blood. It is to be expected and only lasts for 1 or 2 days after each dose is given.

This medicine often causes a temporary and total loss of hair. After treatment with doxorubicin has ended, normal hair growth should return.

After you stop receiving doxorubicin, it may still produce some side effects that need attention. During this period of time, **check with your doctor or nurse immediately** if you notice any of the following side effects:

    Fast or irregular heartbeat
    Shortness of breath
    Swelling of feet and lower legs

For children and elderly patients: Heart problems are more likely to occur in children under 2 years of age and in the elderly, who are usually more sensitive to the effects of doxorubicin. The elderly may also be more likely to have blood problems.

Other side effects not listed above may also occur in some patients. If you notice any other effects, check with your doctor or nurse.

December 1987

DRONABINOL (Systemic)

A commonly used brand name is Marinol.

To the Reader: If you do not recognize the names of medical conditions or medicines referred to in this information, check with your doctor, nurse, or pharmacist. Definitions for selected medical terms may be found in the Glossary. Brand names for the generic drug names listed can be found in the Index. In addition, selected brand names commonly associated with the generic name have been included in the text to help you recognize medicine you may be taking. The fact that a brand name product is not mentioned does not mean the information does not apply. It is a good idea for you to learn both the generic and brand names of your medicines and to write them down for future use.

Dronabinol (droe-NAB-i-nol) is taken by mouth to prevent the nausea and vomiting that may occur after treatment with anti-cancer medicines. It is used only when other kinds of medicine for nausea and vomiting do not work.

Dronabinol is available only with your doctor's prescription. Prescriptions cannot be refilled and you must obtain a new prescription from your doctor each time you need this medicine.

Remember:

• **This medicine has been prescribed for your current medical problem only.** It must not be given to other people or used for other problems unless you are directed to do so by your doctor.

• **Keep all medicines out of the reach of children.**

• In order for this medicine to work, it must be used as directed.

• **It is very important that you read and understand the following information.** If any of the information causes you special concern, do not decide against using this medicine without first checking with your doctor.

• Before you begin using any new medicine (prescription or nonprescription) or if you develop any new medical problem while you are using this medicine, check with your doctor, nurse, or pharmacist.

• **If you have any questions** about the following information or if you want more information about this medicine or your medical problem, **ask your doctor, nurse, or pharmacist.**

Before Using This Medicine

In order to decide on the best treatment for your medical problem, your doctor should be told:

—if you have ever had any unusual or allergic reaction to marijuana products.

—if you are on a low-salt, low sugar, or any other special diet, or if you are allergic to any substance, such as sesame oil or other foods, sulfites or other preservatives, or dyes. Most medicines contain more than their active ingredient. Your doctor, nurse, or pharmacist can help you avoid products that may cause a problem.

—if you are **pregnant** or if you may become pregnant. Studies have not been done in humans. However, studies in animals have shown that dronabinol given in doses many times the usual human dose increases the risk of death in the fetus and decreases the number of live babies born.

—if you are **breast-feeding**. Dronabinol passes into the breast milk. There is the possibility the baby may become dependent on it.

—if you have any of the following medical problems:

> Alcoholism
> Heart disease
> High blood pressure
> Manic depression
> Schizophrenia

—if you are taking **any** other prescription or nonprescription (OTC) medicine, especially central nervous system (CNS) depressants.

Proper Use of This Medicine

Take this medicine only as directed by your physician. Do not take more of it, do not take it more often, and do not take it for a longer period of time than your doctor ordered. If too much is taken, it may lead to medical problems because of an overdose.

If you miss a dose of this medicine, take it as soon as you remember. However, if it is almost time for your next dose, skip the missed dose and go back to your regular dosing schedule. **Do not double doses.**

How to store this medicine:

• **Keep out of the reach of children** since overdose is very dangerous in young children.

• Store away from heat and direct light.

• Do not store the capsule form of this medicine in the bathroom, near the kitchen sink, or in other damp places. Heat or moisture may cause the medicine to break down.

• Keep the capsule form of this medicine in the refrigerator but keep it from freezing.

• Do not keep outdated medicine or medicine no longer needed. Be sure that any discarded medicine is out of the reach of children.

Precautions While Using This Medicine

Dronabinol will add to the effects of alcohol and other central nervous system (CNS) depressants (medicines that slow down the nervous system, possibly causing drowsiness). Some examples of CNS depressants are antihistamines or medicine for hay fever, other allergies, or colds; sedatives, tranquilizers, or sleeping medicine; prescription pain medicines including other narcotics; barbiturates; medicine for seizures; muscle relaxants; or anesthetics, including some dental anesthetics. **Check with your doctor before taking any of the above while you are taking this medicine.**

This medicine may cause some people to become drowsy, dizzy, or lightheaded, or to feel a false sense of well-being. **Make sure you know how you react to this medicine before you drive, use machines, or do other jobs that require you to be alert and clearheaded.**

Dizziness, lightheadedness, or fainting may occur, especially when you get up suddenly from a lying or sitting position. Getting up slowly may help lessen this problem.

If you think you or someone else may have taken an overdose, get emergency help at once. Taking an overdose of this medicine or taking alcohol or CNS depressants with this medicine may lead to severe mental effects. Signs of overdose include changes in mood, confusion, hallucinations, mental depression, nervousness or anxiety, and fast or pounding heartbeat.

Side Effects of This Medicine

Along with its needed effects, a medicine may cause some unwanted effects. Although not all of these side effects may occur, if they do occur they may need medical attention.

Check with your doctor or nurse immediately if any of the following side effects occur:

Less common (may also be signs of overdose)
  Changes in mood
  Confusion
  Fast or pounding heartbeat

  Hallucinations (seeing, hearing, or feeling things that are not there)
  Mental depression
  Nervousness or anxiety

Other side effects may occur that usually do not require medical attention. These side effects may go away during treatment as your body adjusts to the medicine. However, check with your doctor if any of the following side effects continue or are bothersome:

More common
  Dizziness
  Drowsiness
  Inability to think
  Loss of coordination

Less common or rare
  Blurred vision or any changes in vision
  Dry mouth
  Feeling faint or lightheaded
  Restlessness
  Unusual tiredness or weakness

For elderly patients: The above side effects may be more likely to occur in the elderly.

Other side effects not listed above may also occur in some patients. If you notice any other effects, check with your doctor.

December 1987

ECONAZOLE (Topical)

Some commonly used brand names are Ecostatin*, Pevaryl*, and Spectazole.

---

*Not available in the U.S.

To the Reader: If you do not recognize the names of medical conditions or medicines referred to in this information, check with your doctor, nurse, or pharmacist. Definitions for selected medical terms may be found in the Glossary. Brand names for the generic drug names listed can be found in the Index. In addition, selected brand names commonly associated with the generic name have been included in the text to help you recognize medicine you may be taking. The fact that a brand name product is not mentioned does not mean the information does not apply. It is a good idea for you to learn both the generic and brand names of your medicines and to write them down for future use.

Econazole (e-KONE-a-zole) belongs to the general family of medicines called antifungals. Antifungals are used to treat infections caused by a fungus. They work by killing the fungus or preventing its growth.

Econazole cream is applied to the skin to treat fungal infections. These include:

—ringworm of the body (tinea corporis);
—ringworm of the foot (tinea pedis; athlete's foot);
—ringworm of the groin (tinea cruris; jock itch);
—tinea versicolor (sometimes called "sun fungus"); and
—certain other fungal infections, such as Candida (Monilia) infections.

Econazole is available only with your doctor's prescription.

Remember:

• **This medicine has been prescribed for your present infection only.** Another infection later on may require a different medicine. Also, even though other people may have the same symptoms as you, they may have a different kind of infection. Your medicine may not work for them and may even cause them harm. Therefore, **your medicine must not be given to other people or used for other infections** unless you are otherwise directed by your doctor.

• **Keep all medicines out of the reach of children.**

• In order for this medicine to work, it must be used as directed.

• **It is very important that you read and understand the following information.** If any of the information causes you special concern, do not decide against using this medicine without first checking with your doctor.

• Before you begin using any new medicine (prescription or nonprescription) or if you develop any new medical problem while you are using this medicine, check with your doctor, nurse, or pharmacist.

• **If you have any questions** about the following information or if you want more information about this medicine or your medical problem, **ask your doctor, nurse, or pharmacist.**

Before Using This Medicine

In order to decide on the best treatment for your medical problem, your doctor should be told:

—if you have ever had any unusual or allergic reaction to econazole.

—if you are allergic to any substance, such as certain foods or preservatives or dyes. Most medicines contain more than their active ingredient. Your doctor, nurse, or pharmacist can help you avoid products that may cause a problem.

—if you are **pregnant** or if you may become pregnant. Studies have not been done in humans. Econazole, when given by mouth, has not been shown to cause birth defects in studies in mice, rabbits, or rats. However, studies in these animals have shown that econazole, when given by mouth in high doses, causes other problems in the fetus.

—if you are **breast-feeding**. It is not known whether econazole passes into human breast milk. This medicine has not been shown to cause problems in nursing babies. However, econazole, when given by mouth, does pass into the milk of rats and has caused problems in the young.

Proper Use of This Medicine

Apply enough econazole to cover the affected and surrounding skin areas, and rub in gently.

Keep this medicine away from the eyes.

When econazole is used to treat certain types of fungal infections of the skin, an airtight covering or occlusive dressing (for example, kitchen plastic wrap) should *not* be applied over the medicine. To do so may cause irritation of the skin. **Do not apply an airtight covering over this medicine unless you have been directed to do so by your doctor.**

To help clear up your infection completely, **it is very important that you keep using econazole for the full time of treatment** even if your symptoms begin to clear up after a few days. Since fungal infections may be very slow to clear up, you may have to continue using this medicine every day for several weeks or more. If you stop using this medicine too soon, your symptoms may return. **Do not miss any doses.**

If you do miss a dose of this medicine, apply it as soon as possible. However, if it is almost time for your next dose, skip the missed dose and go back to your regular dosing schedule.

How to store this medicine:

• **Keep out of the reach of children.**

• Store away from heat and direct light.

• Keep the medicine from freezing.

• Do not keep outdated medicine or medicine no longer needed. Be sure that any discarded medicine is out of the reach of children.

© 1988   The United States Pharmacopeial Convention, Inc.

Precautions While Using This Medicine

If your skin problem does not improve within 2 weeks or more, or if it becomes worse, check with your doctor.

To help clear up your infection completely and to help make sure it does not return, good health habits are also required.

• For patients using econazole for ringworm of the groin (tinea cruris; jock itch):

—Avoid wearing underwear that is tight-fitting or made from synthetic materials (for example, rayon or nylon). Instead, wear loose-fitting, cotton underwear.

—Use a bland, absorbent powder (for example, talcum powder) or an antifungal powder (for example, tolnaftate) on the skin. It is best not to use econazole cream or other antifungal cream at the same time that you use the powder.

These measures will help reduce chafing and irritation and will also help keep the groin area cool and dry.

• For patients using econazole for ringworm of the foot (tinea pedis; athlete's foot):

—Carefully dry the feet, especially between the toes, after bathing.

—Avoid wearing socks made from wool or synthetic materials (for example, rayon or nylon). Instead, wear clean, cotton socks and change them daily or more often if the feet sweat freely.

—Wear well-ventilated shoes (for example, shoes with holes) or sandals.

—Use a bland, absorbent powder (for example, talcum powder) or an antifungal powder (for example, tolnaftate) between the toes, on the feet, and in socks and shoes freely once or twice a day. It is best not to use econazole cream or other antifungal cream at the same time that you use the powder.

These measures will help keep the feet cool and dry.

If you have any questions about this, check with your doctor, nurse, or pharmacist.

Side Effects of This Medicine

Along with its needed effects, a medicine may cause some unwanted effects. Although not all of these side effects may occur, if they do occur they may need medical attention.

Check with your doctor as soon as possible if any of the following side effects occur:

More common

Burning, itching, stinging, redness, or other sign of irritation not present before using this medicine

Other side effects not listed above may also occur in some patients. If you notice any other effects, check with your doctor.

December 1987

ENCAINIDE (Systemic)

A commonly used brand name is Enkaid.

To the Reader: If you do not recognize the names of medical conditions or medicines referred to in this information, check with your doctor, nurse, or pharmacist. Definitions for selected medical terms may be found in the Glossary. Brand names for the generic drug names listed can be found in the Index. In addition, selected brand names commonly associated with the generic name have been included in the text to help you recognize medicine you may be taking. The fact that a brand name product is not mentioned does not mean the information does not apply. It is a good idea for you to learn both the generic and brand names of your medicines and to write them down for future use.

Encainide (en-KAY-nide) belongs to the group of medicines known as antiarrhythmics. It is taken by mouth to convert irregular heartbeats to a normal rhythm.

Encainide produces its helpful effects by slowing nerve impulses in the heart and making the heart tissue less sensitive.

This medicine is available only with your doctor's prescription.

Remember:

• **This medicine has been prescribed for your current medical problem only.** It must not be given to other people or used for other problems unless you are directed to do so by your doctor.

• **Keep all medicines out of the reach of children.**

• In order for this medicine to work, it must be used as directed.

• **It is very important that you read and understand the following information.** If any of the information causes you special concern, do not decide against using this medicine without first checking with your doctor.

• Before you begin using any new medicine (prescription or nonprescription) or if you develop any new medical problem while you are using this medicine, check with your doctor, nurse, or pharmacist.

• **If you have any questions** about the following information or if you want more information about this medicine or your medical problem, **ask your doctor, nurse, or pharmacist.**

Before Using This Medicine

In order to decide on the best treatment for your medical problem, your doctor should be told:

—if you have ever had any unusual or allergic reaction to encainide.

—if you are on a low-salt, low-sugar, or any other special diet, or if you are allergic to any substance, such as foods, sulfites or other preservatives, or dyes. Most medicines contain more than their active ingredient. Your doctor, nurse, or pharmacist can help you avoid products that may cause a problem.

—if you are **pregnant** or if you may become pregnant. Studies have not been done in humans. Encainide has not been shown to cause birth defects or other problems in animal studies, but has been shown to reduce fertility in rats.

—if you are **breast-feeding**. Encainide passes into the milk of some animals and may also pass into the milk of humans. However, this medicine has not been shown to cause problems in nursing babies.

—if you have either of the following medical problems:
  Kidney disease
  Liver disease

—if you have recently had a heart attack.

—if you have a pacemaker.

—if you are taking **any** other prescription or nonprescription (OTC) medicine.

Proper Use of This Medicine

Take encainide exactly as directed by your doctor, even though you may feel well. Do not take more or less of it than your doctor ordered.

This medicine works best when there is a constant amount in the blood. **To help keep the amount constant, do not miss any doses. Also, it is best to take each dose at evenly spaced times day and night.** For example, if you are to take 3 doses a day, doses should be spaced about 8 hours apart. If you need help in planning the best times to take your medicine, check with your doctor or pharmacist.

If you do miss a dose of encainide and remember within 4 hours, take it as soon as possible. However, if you do not remember until later, skip the missed dose and go back to your regular dosing schedule. Do not double doses.

How to store this medicine:

• **Keep out of the reach of children.**

• Store away from heat and direct light.

• Do not store in the bathroom, near the kitchen sink, or in other damp places. Heat or moisture may cause the medicine to break down.

• Do not keep outdated medicine or medicine no longer needed. Be sure that any discarded medicine is out of the reach of children.

Precautions While Using This Medicine

It is important that your doctor check your progress at regular visits to make sure the medicine is working properly. This will allow changes to be made in the amount of medicine you are taking, if necessary.

Your doctor may want you to carry a medical identification card or bracelet stating that you are using this medicine.

Before having any kind of surgery (including dental surgery) or emergency treatment, tell the physician or dentist in charge that you are taking this medicine.

Encainide may cause some people to become dizzy, light-headed, or less alert than they are normally. **Make sure you know how you react to this medicine before you drive, use machines, or do other jobs that require you to be alert.**

Side Effects of This Medicine

Along with its needed effects, a medicine may cause some unwanted effects. Although not all of these side effects may occur, if they do occur they may need medical attention.

Check with your doctor as soon as possible if any of the following side effects occur:

Less common
>   Chest pain
>   Fast or irregular heartbeat

Rare
>   Shortness of breath
>   Swelling of feet or lower legs
>   Trembling or shaking

Other side effects may occur that usually do not require medical attention. These side effects may go away during treatment as your body adjusts to the medicine.

However, check with your doctor if any of the following side effects continue or are bothersome:

Less common
>   Blurred or double vision
>   Dizziness
>   Headache
>   Nausea
>   Pain in arms or legs
>   Skin rash
>   Unusual tiredness or weakness

For elderly patients: Many medicines have not been tested in older people. Therefore, it is not known whether the medicine acts the same way it does in younger adults. Check with your doctor or pharmacist if you notice any unusual effects while taking this medicine or if you do not think it is working as it should.

Other side effects not listed above may also occur in some patients. If you notice any other effects, check with your doctor.

December 1987

EPINEPHRINE (Ophthalmic)

This information applies to the following medicines:
Epinephrine (ep-i-NEF-rin)
Epinephryl Borate (ep-i-NEF-rill BOR-ate)

Some commonly used brand names are:	Generic names:
Epifrin	
Epitrate	Epinephrine†
Glaucon	
Epinal	
Eppy/N	Epinephryl Borate

†Generic name product may also be available in the U.S.

To the Reader: If you do not recognize the names of medical conditions or medicines referred to in this information, check with your doctor, nurse, or pharmacist. Definitions for selected medical terms may be found in the Glossary. Brand names for the generic drug names listed can be found in the Index. In addition, selected brand names commonly associated with the generic name have been included in the text to help you recognize medicine you may be taking. The fact that a brand name product is not mentioned does not mean the information does not apply. It is a good idea for you to learn both the generic and brand names of your medicines and to write them down for future use.

Ophthalmic epinephrine is used in the eye to treat certain types of glaucoma. It may also be used in eye surgery.

This medicine is available only with your doctor's prescription.

Remember:

• **This medicine has been prescribed for your current medical problem only.** It must not be given to other people or used for other problems unless you are directed to do so by your doctor.

• **Keep all medicines out of the reach of children.**

• In order for this medicine to work, it must be used as directed.

• **It is very important that you read and understand the following information.** If any of the information causes you special concern, do not decide against using this medicine without first checking with your doctor.

• Before you begin using any new medicine (prescription or nonprescription) or if you develop any new medical problem while you are using this medicine, check with your doctor, nurse, or pharmacist.

• **If you have any questions** about the following information or if you want more information about this medicine or your medical problem, **ask your doctor, nurse, or pharmacist.**

Before Using This Medicine

In order to decide on the best treatment for your medical problem, your doctor should be told:

—if you have ever had any unusual or allergic reaction to epinephrine.

—if you are **pregnant** or if you may become pregnant, since ophthalmic epinephrine may be absorbed into the body. Studies on birth defects have not been done in either humans or animals.

—if you are **breast-feeding**, since ophthalmic epinephrine may be absorbed into the body. However, it is not known whether epinephrine passes into the breast milk and this medicine has not been shown to cause problems in nursing babies.

—if you are having dental surgery on your gums.

—if you have any of the following medical problems:
Diabetes mellitus (sugar diabetes)
Eye disease (other)
Heart or blood vessel disease
High blood pressure
Overactive thyroid

—if you are taking **any** other prescription or nonprescription (OTC) medicine.

Proper Use of This Medicine

Use this medicine only as directed. Do not use more of it and do not use it more often than your doctor ordered. To do so may increase the chance of too much medicine being absorbed into the body and the chance of side effects.

How to apply this medicine: First, wash your hands. With the middle finger, apply pressure to the inside corner of the eye (and continue to apply pressure for 1 or 2 minutes after the medicine has been placed in the eye). Tilt the head back and with the index finger of the same hand, pull the lower eyelid away from eye to form a pouch. Drop the medicine into the pouch and gently close the eyes. Do not blink. Keep the eyes closed for 1 or 2 minutes to allow the medicine to be absorbed.

Immediately after applying the eye drops, wash your hands to remove any medicine that may be on them.

To prevent contamination of the eye drops, do not touch the applicator tip to any surface (including the eye) and keep the container tightly closed.

For patients using epinephrine ophthalmic solution:

• Do not use if the solution turns pinkish or brownish in color, or if it becomes cloudy.

For patients using epinephryl borate ophthalmic solution:

• The color of this solution may vary from colorless to amber yellow. Do not use if the solution turns dark brown or becomes cloudy.

If you miss a dose of this medicine, apply the missed dose as soon as possible. However, if it is almost time for your next dose, skip the missed dose and apply your next dose at the regularly scheduled time. Then continue with your regular dosing schedule.

How to store this medicine:

• **Keep out of the reach of children.**

• Store away from heat and direct light.

• Keep the medicine from freezing.

• Do not keep outdated medicine or medicine no longer needed. Be sure that any discarded medicine is out of the reach of children.

Precautions While Using This Medicine

Your doctor should check your eye pressure at regular visits.

Side Effects of This Medicine

Along with its needed effects, a medicine may cause some unwanted effects. Although not all of these side effects may occur, if they do occur they may need medical attention.

Check with your doctor as soon as possible if any of the following side effects occur:

Less common
    Blurred or decreased vision

Signs of too much medicine being absorbed into the body
    Fast, irregular, or pounding heartbeat
    Feeling faint
    Increase in sweating
    Paleness
    Trembling

Other side effects may occur that usually do not require medical attention. These side effects may go away during treatment as your body adjusts to the medicine. However, check with your doctor if any of the following side effects continue or are bothersome:

More common
    Headache or browache
    Stinging, burning or other eye irritation
    Watering of eyes

Less common
    Eye pain

For elderly patients: Many medicines have not been tested in older people. Therefore, it is not known whether the medicine acts the same way it does in younger adults. Check with your doctor or pharmacist if you notice any unusual effects while using this medicine or if you think it is not working as it should.

Other side effects not listed above may also occur in some patients. If you notice any other effects, check with your doctor.

December 1987

ERGOLOID MESYLATES (Systemic)

Some commonly used brand names or other names are:

Deapril-ST   Hydergine
Dihydrogenated   Hydergine LC
  Ergot Alkaloids

Generic name product may also be available in the U.S.

To the Reader: If you do not recognize the names of medical conditions or medicines referred to in this information, check with your doctor, nurse, or pharmacist. Definitions for selected medical terms may be found in the Glossary. Brand names for the generic drug names listed can be found in the Index. In addition, selected brand names commonly associated with the generic name have been included in the text to help you recognize medicine you may be taking. The fact that a brand name product is not mentioned does not mean the information does not apply. It is a good idea for you to learn both the generic and brand names of your medicines and to write them down for future use.

Ergoloid mesylates (ER-goe-loid MESS-i-lates) belongs to the group of medicines known as ergot alkaloids. It is used to treat some changes in mood, memory, or behavior, or dizziness, and other problems that may be due to poor blood circulation to the brain. This medicine is different from other ergot alkaloids such as ergotamine and methysergide. It is not useful for treating migraine headache. The exact way ergoloid mesylates acts on the body is not known.

This medicine is available only with your doctor's prescription.

Remember:

• **This medicine has been prescribed for your current medical problem only.** It must not be given to other people or used for other problems unless you are directed to do so by your doctor.

• **Keep all medicines out of the reach of children.**

• In order for this medicine to work, it must be used as directed.

• **It is very important that you read and understand the following information.** If any of the information causes you special concern, do not decide against using this medicine without first checking with your doctor.

• Before you begin using any new medicine (prescription or nonprescription) or if you develop any new medical problem while you are using this medicine, check with your doctor, nurse, or pharmacist.

• **If you have any questions** about the following information or if you want more information about this medicine or your medical problem, **ask your doctor, nurse, or pharmacist.**

Before Using This Medicine

In order to decide on the best treatment for your medical problem, your doctor should be told:

—if you have ever had any unusual or allergic reaction to ergot alkaloids.

—if you are on a low-salt, low-sugar, or any other special diet, or if you are allergic to any substance, such as foods, sulfites or other preservatives, or dyes.

Most medicines contain more than their active ingredient, and many liquid medicines contain alcohol. Your doctor, nurse, or pharmacist can help you avoid products that may cause a problem.

—if you have any of the following medical problems:
  Liver disease
  Low blood pressure
  Other mental problems
  Slow pulse

—if you are taking **any** other prescription or nonprescription (OTC) medicine, especially medicines containing other ergot alkaloids (such as dihydroergotamine, ergonovine, ergotamine, methylergonovine, methysergide).

—if you smoke.

Proper Use of This Medicine

Take this medicine only as directed by your doctor. Do not take more or less of it, and do not take it more often or for a longer period of time than your doctor ordered. To do so may increase the chance of unwanted effects.

For patients taking the sublingual (under-the-tongue) tablets:

• Dissolve the tablet under your tongue. The sublingual tablet should not be chewed or swallowed, since it works much faster when absorbed through the lining of the mouth. Do not eat, drink, or smoke while a tablet is dissolving.

If you miss a dose of this medicine, skip the missed dose and go back to your regular dosing schedule. Do not double doses. If you have any questions about this, or if you miss two or more doses in a row, check with your doctor.

How to store this medicine:

• **Keep out of the reach of children.**

• Store away from heat and direct light.

• Do not store in the bathroom, near the kitchen sink, or in other damp places. Heat or moisture may cause the medicine to break down.

• Keep the oral solution from freezing.

• Do not keep outdated medicine or medicine no longer needed. Be sure that any discarded medicine is out of the reach of children.

Precautions While Using This Medicine

It is important that your doctor check your progress at regular visits to make sure this medicine is working and to check for unwanted effects.

While you are taking this medicine, do not expose your body to very cold temperatures for long periods of time. The medicine may lessen your body's ability to adjust to the cold.

© 1988   The United States Pharmacopeial Convention, Inc.

It may take several weeks for this medicine to work. **However, do not stop taking this medicine without first checking with your doctor.**

Side Effects of This Medicine

Along with its needed effects, a medicine may cause some unwanted effects. The following side effects may go away as your body adjusts to the medicine. However, check with your doctor if any of these effects continue or are bothersome, especially since some may indicate that you are taking too much medicine:

Rare

Dizziness or lightheadedness when getting up from a lying or sitting position
Drowsiness
Skin rash
Slow pulse
Soreness under the tongue (with sublingual use)

Signs of overdose

Blurred vision
Dizziness
Fainting
Flushing
Headache
Loss of appetite
Nausea or vomiting
Stomach cramps
Stuffy nose

For elderly patients: This medicine may reduce tolerance to cold temperatures in elderly patients.

Other side effects not listed above may also occur in some patients. If you notice any other effects, check with your doctor.

December 1987

ERGONOVINE (Systemic)

This information applies to the following medicines:

Ergonovine (er-goe-NOE-veen)
Methylergonovine (meth-ill-er-goe-NOE-veen)

Some commonly used brand names or other names are:	Generic names:
Ergometrine Ergotrate	Ergonovine‡
Methergine Methylergobasine-Sandoz* Methylergometrine	Methylergonovine

*Not available in the U.S.
‡Generic name product may also be available in Canada.

To the Reader: If you do not recognize the names of medical conditions or medicines referred to in this information, check with your doctor, nurse, or pharmacist. Definitions for selected medical terms may be found in the Glossary. Brand names for the generic drug names listed can be found in the Index. In addition, selected brand names commonly associated with the generic name have been included in the text to help you recognize medicine you may be taking. The fact that a brand name product is not mentioned does not mean the information does not apply. It is a good idea for you to learn both the generic and brand names of your medicines and to write them down for future use.

Ergonovine and methylergonovine belong to the group of medicines known as ergot alkaloids. These medicines are usually given to stop excessive bleeding that sometimes occurs after a baby is delivered. They work by causing the muscle of the uterus to contract. Ergonovine and methylergonovine may also be used for other conditions as determined by your doctor.

These medicines are available only on prescription and are to be administered only by or under the supervision of your doctor.

Remember:

• **This medicine has been prescribed for your current medical problem only.** It must not be given to other people or used for other problems unless you are directed to do so by your doctor.

• **Keep all medicines out of the reach of children.**

• In order for this medicine to work, it must be used as directed.

• If you are receiving this medicine by injection, some of the information about this medicine may not apply.

• **It is very important that you read and understand the following information.** If any of the information causes you special concern, do not decide against using this medicine without first checking with your doctor.

• Before you begin using any new medicine (prescription or nonprescription) or if you develop any new medical problem while you are using this medicine, check with your doctor, nurse, or pharmacist.

• **If you have any questions** about the following information or if you want more information about this medicine or your medical problem, **ask your doctor, nurse, or pharmacist.**

Before Using This Medicine

In order to decide on the best treatment for your medical problem, your doctor should be told:

—if you have ever had any unusual or allergic reaction to ergonovine, methylergonovine, or other ergot medicines.

—if you are on a low-salt, low-sugar, or any other special diet, or if you are allergic to any substance, such as foods, sulfites or other preservatives, or dyes. Most medicines contain more than their active ingredient. Your doctor, nurse, or pharmacist can help you avoid products that may cause a problem.

—if you are **breast-feeding**. This medicine passes into the breast milk and may cause unwanted effects, such as vomiting, diarrhea, weak pulse, unstable blood pressure, or convulsions (seizures) in infants of mothers taking large doses of it. Be sure you have discussed this with your doctor before taking this medicine.

—if you have any of the following medical problems:

Angina (chest pain)
Blood vessel disease
High blood pressure
Infection
Kidney disease
Liver disease

—if you are taking **any** other prescription or nonprescription (OTC) medicine.

Proper Use of This Medicine

Take this medicine only as directed by your doctor. Do not take more of it, do not take it more often, and do not take it for a longer period of time than your doctor ordered. If too much is taken, it may cause serious effects such as nausea and vomiting; cold, painful hands or feet; or even gangrene.

If you miss a dose of this medicine, do not take the missed dose at all and do not double the next one. Instead, go back to your regular dosing schedule. If you have any questions about this, check with your doctor.

How to store this medicine:

• **Keep out of the reach of children.**

• Store away from heat and direct light.

• Do not store in the bathroom, near the kitchen sink, or in other damp places. Heat or moisture may cause the medicine to break down.

• Do not keep outdated medicine or medicine no longer needed. Be sure that any discarded medicine is out of the reach of children.

Precautions While Using This Medicine

Since smoking may increase some of the harmful effects of this medicine, it is best to avoid smoking while you are being treated with it. If you have any questions about this, check with your doctor.

If you have an infection or illness of any kind, check with your doctor before taking this medicine, since you may be more sensitive to its effects.

Side Effects of This Medicine

Along with its needed effects, a medicine may cause some unwanted effects. Although not all of these side effects may occur, if they do occur they may need medical attention.

Check with your doctor as soon as possible if any of the following side effects occur:

Less common
   Chest pain

Rare
   Headache (sudden severe)
   Itching of skin
   Pain in arms, legs, or lower back
   Pale or cold hands or feet
   Shortness of breath
   Weakness in legs

Other side effects may occur that usually do not require medical attention. These side effects may go away during treatment as your body adjusts to the medicine. However, check with your doctor if any of the following side effects continue or are bothersome:

More common
   Nausea or vomiting

Less common
   Confusion
   Cramping
   Diarrhea
   Dizziness
   Ringing in the ears
   Sweating

Other side effects not listed above may also occur in some patients. If you notice any other effects, check with your doctor.

December 1987

ERGOTAMINE (Systemic)

Some commonly used brand names are:

Ergomar	Medihaler Ergotamine
Ergostat	Wigrettes
Gynergen*	

*Not available in the U.S.

To the Reader: If you do not recognize the names of medical conditions or medicines referred to in this information, check with your doctor, nurse, or pharmacist. Definitions for selected medical terms may be found in the Glossary. Brand names for the generic drug names listed can be found in the Index. In addition, selected brand names commonly associated with the generic name have been included in the text to help you recognize medicine you may be taking. The fact that a brand name product is not mentioned does not mean the information does not apply. It is a good idea for you to learn both the generic and brand names of your medicines and to write them down for future use.

Ergotamine (er-GOT-a-meen) belongs to the group of medicines known as ergot alkaloids. It is used to treat migraine headaches and some kinds of throbbing headaches. It is not used to prevent headaches, but is used to treat an attack once it has started. Ergotamine works by causing the blood vessels to constrict or narrow.

This medicine is available only with your doctor's prescription.

Remember:

• **This medicine has been prescribed for your current medical problem only.** It must not be given to other people or used for other problems unless you are directed to do so by your doctor.

• **Keep all medicines out of the reach of children.**

• In order for this medicine to work, it must be used as directed.

• **It is very important that you read and understand the following information.** If any of the information causes you special concern, do not decide against using this medicine without first checking with your doctor.

• Before you begin using any new medicine (prescription or nonprescription) or if you develop any new medical problem while you are using this medicine, check with your doctor, nurse, or pharmacist.

• **If you have any questions** about the following information or if you want more information about this medicine or your medical problem, **ask your doctor, nurse, or pharmacist.**

Before Using This Medicine

In order to decide on the best treatment for your medical problem, your doctor should be told:

—if you have ever had any unusual or allergic reaction to ergotamine or other ergot medicines.

—if you are on a low-salt, low-sugar, or any other special diet, or if you are allergic to any substance, such as foods, sulfites or other preservatives, or dyes. Most medicines contain more than their active ingredient. Your doctor, nurse, or pharmacist can help you avoid products that may cause a problem.

—if you are **pregnant** or if you may become pregnant. Ergotamine is not recommended during pregnancy since it has been shown to stimulate labor, which could result in a miscarriage.

—if you are **breast-feeding**. Ergotamine passes into the breast milk and may cause unwanted effects, such as vomiting, diarrhea, weak pulse, unstable blood pressure, or convulsions (seizures), in infants of mothers taking large doses of it.

—if you have any of the following medical problems:
Heart or blood vessel disease
High blood pressure
Infection
Itching (severe)
Kidney disease
Liver disease
Overactive thyroid

—if you are taking **any** other prescription or nonprescription (OTC) medicine, especially other medicines containing ergotamine for treatment of migraine headaches or medicine containing other ergot alkaloids (such as dihydroergotamine, ergoloid mesylates, ergonovine, methylergonovine, methysergide).

—if you smoke.

Proper Use of This Medicine

Take this medicine only as directed by your doctor. If the amount you are to take does not relieve your headache, do not take more than your doctor ordered. Instead, check with your doctor. Taking too much of this medicine or taking it too frequently may cause serious effects such as nausea and vomiting; cold, painful hands or feet; or even gangrene.

This medicine works best if you:

• **Take it at the first sign of headache or migraine attack.**

• **Lie down in a quiet, dark room for at least 2 hours after taking it.**

For patients taking the sublingual (under-the-tongue) tablets:

• Dissolve the tablet under your tongue. The sublingual tablet should not be chewed or swallowed since it works much faster when absorbed through the lining of the mouth. Do not eat, drink, or smoke while a tablet is dissolving.

For patients using the inhalation form of this medicine:

• This medicine comes with patient directions. Read them carefully before using this medicine.

• This medicine is used with a special inhaler. Save your inhaler. Refill units of the medicine may be available at lower cost.

• Container provides about 300 measured sprays.

How to store this medicine:

• **Keep out of the reach of children.**

• Store away from heat and direct light.

• Do not store in the bathroom, near the kitchen sink, or in other damp places. Heat and moisture may cause the medicine to break down.

• If you are using the inhalation form of this medicine, do not puncture, break, or burn the container.

• Do not keep outdated medicine or medicine no longer needed. Be sure that any discarded medicine is out of the reach of children.

Precautions While Using This Medicine

If you have been taking this medicine regularly, **do not stop taking it without first checking with your doctor.** Your doctor may want you to reduce gradually the amount you are using before stopping completely. If you stop taking it suddenly, your headaches may return or worsen.

Since drinking alcoholic beverages may make headaches worse, it is best to avoid alcohol while you are suffering from them. If you have any questions about this, check with your doctor.

Since smoking may increase some of the harmful effects of this medicine, it is best to avoid smoking while you are using it. If you have any questions about this, check with your doctor.

Avoid prolonged exposure to very cold temperatures while you are using this medicine, since cold may increase the harmful effects of the medicine.

If you have an infection or illness of any kind, check with your doctor before taking this medicine, since you may be more sensitive to the effects of it.

For patients using the inhalation form of this medicine:

• If signs of a mouth, throat, or lung infection occur, if your condition gets worse, or if your symptoms do not improve, check with your doctor.

• Cough, hoarseness, or throat irritation may occur. Gargling and rinsing your mouth after each dose may help prevent the hoarseness and irritation; however, check with your doctor if these or any other side effects continue or are bothersome.

Side Effects of This Medicine

Along with its needed effects, a medicine may cause some unwanted effects. Although not all of these side effects may occur, if they do occur they may need medical attention.

Check with your doctor immediately if any of the following side effects occur since they may be signs of an overdose:

    Confusion
    Fast or slow heartbeat
    Numbness and tingling of fingers, toes, or face
    Red or violet blisters on skin of hands or feet
    Shortness of breath
    Stomach pain or bloating
    Weakness

Check with your doctor as soon as possible if the following side effects occur:

More common

    Headache
    Swelling of feet and lower legs

Less common or rare

    Anxiety
    Changes in vision
    Chest pain
    Itching of skin
    Mental depression
    Nausea or vomiting (continuing or severe)
    Pain in arms, legs, or lower back
    Pale or cold hands or feet
    Tiredness
    Weakness in legs

Other side effects may occur that usually do not require medical attention. These side effects may go away during treatment as your body adjusts to the medicine. However, check with your doctor if any of the following side effects continue or are bothersome:

More common

    Diarrhea
    Dizziness
    Nausea or vomiting

After you stop using this medicine, your body may need time to adjust. The length of time this takes depends on the amount of medicine you were using and how long you used it. During this period of time check with your doctor if your headaches begin again or worsen.

For elderly patients: The above side effects are more likely to occur in the elderly, who are more likely to already have problems with blood vessels. In addition, this medicine may reduce tolerance to cold temperatures in elderly patients.

Other side effects not listed above may also occur in some patients. If you notice any other effects, check with your doctor.

December 1987

ERGOTAMINE, BELLADONNA ALKALOIDS, AND PHENOBARBITAL
(Systemic)

Some commonly used brand names are Bellergal*, Bellergal-S, and Bellergal Spacetabs*.

*Not available in the U.S.

To the Reader: If you do not recognize the names of medical conditions or medicines referred to in this information, check with your doctor, nurse, or pharmacist. Definitions for selected medical terms may be found in the Glossary. Brand names for the generic drug names listed can be found in the Index. In addition, selected brand names commonly associated with the generic name have been included in the text to help you recognize medicine you may be taking. The fact that a brand name product is not mentioned does not mean the information does not apply. It is a good idea for you to learn both the generic and brand names of your medicines and to write them down for future use.

Ergotamine (er-GOT-a-meen), belladonna alkaloids (bell-a-DON-a AL-ka-loids), and phenobarbital (feen-oh-BAR-bi-tal) combination is taken by mouth for a variety of problems including menstrual and stomach problems and some kinds of throbbing headaches.

This medicine is available only with your doctor's prescription.

Remember:

• **This medicine has been prescribed for your current medical problem only.** It must not be given to other people or used for other problems unless you are directed to do so by your doctor.

• **Keep all medicines out of the reach of children.**

• In order for this medicine to work, it must be used as directed.

• **It is very important that you read and understand the following information.** If any of the information causes you special concern, do not decide against using this medicine without first checking with your doctor.

• Before you begin using any new medicine (prescription or nonprescription) or if you develop any new medical problem while you are using this medicine, check with your doctor, nurse, or pharmacist.

• **If you have any questions** about the following information or if you want more information about this medicine or your medical problem, **ask your doctor, nurse, or pharmacist.**

Before Using This Medicine

In order to decide on the best treatment for your medical problem, your doctor should be told:

—if you have ever had any unusual or allergic reaction to ergotamine or other ergot medicines, atropine, belladonna, or barbiturates.

—if you are on a low-salt, low-sugar, or any other special diet, or if you are allergic to any substance, such as foods, sulfites or other preservatives, or dyes. Most medicines contain more than their active ingredient. Your doctor, nurse, or pharmacist can help you avoid products that may cause a problem.

—if you are **pregnant** or if you may become pregnant. Ergotamine is not recommended during pregnancy since it has been shown to stimulate labor, which could result in a miscarriage. The amount of belladonna alkaloids contained in this medicine should not cause any problems. Barbiturates have been shown to increase the chance of birth defects and may increase the chance of some tumors in the baby.

—if you are **breast-feeding**. Ergotamine passes into the breast milk and may cause unwanted effects, such as vomiting, diarrhea, weak pulse, unstable blood pressure, or convulsions (seizures) in infants of mothers taking large doses of it. Although belladonna alkaloids or barbiturates have not been shown to cause problems in humans, traces of belladonna alkaloids and barbiturates pass into the breast milk. Also, because the belladonna alkaloids tend to decrease the secretions of the body, it is possible that the flow of breast milk may be reduced in some patients. Be sure you have discussed this with your doctor before taking this medicine.

—if you have any of the following medical problems:
  Anemia (severe)
  Asthma (or history of), emphysema, or chronic lung disease
  Brain damage (in children)
  Diabetes
  Difficult urination
  Enlarged prostate
  Glaucoma
  Heart or blood vessel disease
  High blood pressure (severe)
  Infection
  Intestinal disease
  Itching (severe)
  Kidney disease
  Liver disease
  Mental depression
  Overactive thyroid
  Porphyria
  Spastic paralysis (in children)
  Underactive adrenal gland

—if you are now taking **any** other prescription or nonprescription (OTC) medicine, especially:
  Antacids
  Anticoagulants (blood thinners)
  Antimuscarinics (medicine for abdominal or stomach spasms or cramps)
  Central nervous system (CNS) depressants
  Diarrhea medicine
  Digitalis glycosides (heart medicine)
  Ketoconazole (e.g., Nizoral)
  Potassium chloride

—if you are now taking or have taken within the past 2 weeks monoamine oxidase (MAO) inhibitors, such as:
  Furazolidone (e.g., Furoxone)
  Isocarboxazid (e.g., Marplan)
  Pargyline (e.g., Eutonyl)
  Phenelzine (e.g., Nardil)
  Procarbazine (e.g., Matulane)
  Tranylcypromine (e.g., Parnate)

—if you are taking other medicines containing ergotamine for treatment of migraine headaches or medicines containing other ergot alkaloids (such as dihydroergotamine, ergoloid mesylates, ergonovine, methylergonovine, methysergide).

—if you smoke.

Proper Use of This Medicine

Take this medicine only as directed by your doctor. If the amount you are to take does not seem to work, do not take more than your doctor ordered. Instead, check with your doctor. Taking too much of this medicine or taking it too frequently may cause serious effects such as nausea and vomiting; cold, painful hands or feet; or even gangrene. Also, if too much is used, it may become habit-forming.

For patients taking the extended-release tablet form of this medicine:

• Swallow the tablet whole.

• Do not crush, break, or chew before swallowing.

If you miss a dose of this medicine, skip the missed dose and go back to your regular dosing schedule. Do not double doses.

How to store this medicine:

• **Keep out of the reach of children** since overdose is especially dangerous in children.

• Store away from heat and direct light.

• Do not store in the bathroom, near the kitchen sink, or in other damp places. Heat and moisture may cause the medicine to break down.

• Do not keep outdated medicine or medicine no longer needed. Be sure that any discarded medicine is out of the reach of children.

Precautions While Using This Medicine

If you have been taking this medicine regularly, **do not stop taking it without first checking with your doctor.** Your doctor may want you to reduce gradually the amount you are using before stopping completely.

Do not take antacids or medicine for diarrhea within 1 hour of taking this medicine. Taking them too close together will make the belladonna less effective.

This medicine will add to the effects of alcohol and other CNS depressants (medicines that slow down the nervous system, possibly causing drowsiness). Some examples of CNS depressants are antihistamines or medicine for hay fever, other allergies, or colds; sedatives, tranquilizers, or sleeping medicine; prescription pain medicine or narcotics; barbiturates; medicine for convulsions (seizures); tricyclic antidepressants (medicine for depression); muscle relaxants; or anesthetics, including some dental anesthetics. **Check with your doctor before taking any of the above while you are taking this medicine.**

This medicine may cause some people to become drowsy, dizzy, lightheaded, or less alert than they are normally. **Make sure you know how you react to this medicine before you drive, use machines, or do other jobs that require you to be alert.**

Since smoking may increase some of the harmful effects of this medicine, it is best to avoid smoking while you are using it. If you have any questions about this, check with your doctor.

Avoid prolonged exposure to very cold temperatures while you are using this medicine, since cold may increase the harmful effects of the medicine.

If you have an infection or illness of any kind, check with your doctor before taking this medicine, since you may be more sensitive to the effects of it.

This medicine may cause dryness of the mouth, nose and throat. For temporary relief of mouth dryness, use sugarless candy or gum, melt bits of ice in your mouth, or use a saliva substitute. However, if dry mouth continues for more than 2 weeks, check with your physician or dentist. Continuing dryness of the mouth may increase the chance of dental disease, including tooth decay, gum disease, and fungal infections.

Side Effects of This Medicine

Along with its needed effects, a medicine may cause some unwanted effects. Although not all of these side effects may occur, if they do occur they may need medical attention.

Check with your doctor immediately if any of the following side effects occur since they may be signs of an overdose:

    Blurred vision
    Clumsiness or unsteadiness
    Confusion, especially in the elderly
    Extreme drowsiness or irritability
    Fast heartbeat
    Fever
    Flushing of skin
    Hallucinations (seeing, hearing, or feeling things that are not there)
    Mental depression
    Numbness and tingling of fingers, toes, or face
    Red or violet blisters on skin of hands or feet
    Shortness of breath or troubled breathing
    Stomach pain or bloating
    Unusual excitement

Check with your doctor as soon as possible if any of the following side effects occur:

More common
    Swelling of feet and lower legs

Less common or rare
    Chest pain
    Pain in arms, legs, or lower back
    Pale or cold hands or feet
    Skin rash or itching
    Weakness in legs
    Yellow eyes or skin

Other side effects may occur that usually do not require medical attention. These side effects may go away during treatment as your body adjusts to the medicine. However, check with your doctor if any of the following side effects continue or are bothersome:

More common

> Constipation
> Dizziness or lightheadedness
> Drowsiness
> "Hangover" effect

Less common or rare

> Difficult urination (especially in older men)
> Difficulty in swallowing
> Dryness of mouth or skin
> Increased sensitivity of eyes to sunlight
> Nausea or vomiting
> Reduced sweating

After you stop taking this medicine, your body may need time to adjust. The length of time this takes depends on the amount of medicine you were taking and how long you took it. During this period of time check with your doctor if your headaches begin again or worsen.

For children and elderly patients: The above side effects may be more likely to occur in children and elderly patients, who are usually more sensitive to the effects of this medicine. In addition, this medicine may decrease tolerance to cold temperatures in elderly patients.

Other side effects not listed above may also occur in some patients. If you notice any other effects, check with your doctor.

_____

December 1987

ERGOTAMINE AND CAFFEINE (Systemic)

Some commonly used brand names are:

Cafatine	Ercaf
Cafergot	Ergo-Caff
Cafetrate	Wigraine

To the Reader: If you do not recognize the names of medical conditions or medicines referred to in this information, check with your doctor, nurse, or pharmacist. Definitions for selected medical terms may be found in the Glossary. Brand names for the generic drug names listed can be found in the Index. In addition, selected brand names commonly associated with the generic name have been included in the text to help you recognize medicine you may be taking. The fact that a brand name product is not mentioned does not mean the information does not apply. It is a good idea for you to learn both the generic and brand names of your medicines and to write them down for future use.

Ergotamine (er-GOT-a-meen) and caffeine (KAF-een) combination medicine is used to treat migraine headaches and some kinds of throbbing headaches. It is not used to prevent headaches, but is used to treat an attack once it has started. Ergotamine belongs to the group of medicines known as ergot alkaloids. It works by causing the blood vessels to constrict or narrow. Caffeine helps ergotamine to be absorbed into the body.

This medicine is available only with your doctor's prescription.

Remember:

• **This medicine has been prescribed for your current medical problem only.** It must not be given to other people or used for other problems unless you are directed to do so by your doctor.

• **Keep all medicines out of the reach of children.**

• In order for this medicine to work, it must be used as directed.

• **It is very important that you read and understand the following information.** If any of the information causes you special concern, do not decide against using this medicine without first checking with your doctor.

• Before you begin using any new medicine (prescription or nonprescription) or if you develop any new medical problem while you are using this medicine, check with your doctor, nurse, or pharmacist.

• **If you have any questions** about the following information or if you want more information about this medicine or your medical problem, **ask your doctor, nurse, or pharmacist.**

Before Using This Medicine

In order to decide on the best treatment for your medical problem, your doctor should be told:

—if you have ever had any unusual or allergic reaction to ergotamine or other ergot medicines.

—if you are on a low-salt, low-sugar, or any other special diet, or if you are allergic to any substance, such as foods, sulfites or other preservatives, or dyes.

Most medicines contain more than their active ingredient. Your doctor, nurse, or pharmacist can help you avoid products that may cause a problem.

—if you are **pregnant** or if you may become pregnant. Ergotamine is not recommended during pregnancy since it has been shown to stimulate labor, which could result in a miscarriage. Studies in animals have shown that caffeine causes birth defects when given in very large doses (amounts equal to the amount of caffeine contained in 12 to 24 cups of coffee). However, studies in humans have not shown that caffeine causes birth defects.

—if you are **breast-feeding**. This medicine passes into the breast milk and may cause unwanted effects, such as vomiting, diarrhea, weak pulse, unstable blood pressure, or convulsions (seizures), in infants of mothers using large doses of it.

—if you have any of the following medical problems:

Agoraphobia
Fibrocystic breast disease
Heart or blood vessel disease
High blood pressure
Infection
Itching (severe)
Kidney disease
Liver disease
Overactive thyroid
Panic attacks
Stomach ulcer
Trouble in sleeping

—if you are taking **any** other prescription or nonprescription (OTC) medicine, especially:

Amantadine (e.g., Symmetrel)
Amphetamines
Appetite suppressants (diet pills), except fenfluramine (e.g., Pondimin)
Chlophedianol (e.g., Ulo)
Medicine for asthma or other breathing problems
Medicine for colds, sinus problems, or hay fever or other allergies (including nose drops or sprays)
Methylphenidate (e.g., Ritalin)
Other medicines containing caffeine
Pemoline (e.g., Cylert)

—if you are now taking or have taken within the past 2 weeks monoamine oxidase (MAO) inhibitors, such as:

Furazolidone (e.g., Furoxone)
Isocarboxazid (e.g., Marplan)
Pargyline (e.g., Eutonyl)
Phenelzine (e.g., Nardil)
Procarbazine (e.g., Matulane)
Tranylcypromine (e.g., Parnate)

—if you are taking other medicines containing ergotamine for treatment of migraine headaches or medicine containing other ergot alkaloids (such as dihydroergotamine, ergoloid mesylates, ergonovine, methylergonovine, methysergide).

—if you smoke.

Proper Use of This Medicine

Use this medicine only as directed by your doctor. If the amount you are to use does not relieve your headache, do not use more than your doctor ordered. Instead, check with your doctor. Using too much of this medicine or taking it too often may cause serious effects such as nausea and vomiting; cold, painful hands or feet; or even gangrene.

This medicine works best if you:

• **Use it at the first sign of headache or migraine attack.**

• **Lie down in a quiet, dark room for at least 2 hours after using it.**

For patients using the rectal suppository form of this medicine:

• If suppository is too soft to insert because of storage in a warm place, before removing the foil wrapper chill the suppository in the refrigerator for 30 minutes or run cold water over it.

• How to insert suppository—First remove the foil wrapper and moisten the suppository with water. Lie down on side and push the suppository well up into rectum with finger.

How to store this medicine:

• **Keep out of the reach of children.**

• Store away from heat and direct light.

• Do not store in the bathroom, near the kitchen sink, or in other damp places. Heat and moisture may cause the medicine to break down.

• Do not keep outdated medicine or medicine no longer needed. Be sure that any discarded medicine is out of the reach of children.

Precautions While Using This Medicine

If you have been using this medicine regularly, **do not stop using it without first checking with your doctor.** Your doctor may want you to reduce gradually the amount you are using before stopping completely. If you stop using it suddenly, your headaches may return or worsen.

Since drinking alcoholic beverages may make headaches worse, it is best to avoid alcohol while you are suffering from them. If you have any questions about this, check with your doctor.

Since smoking may increase some of the harmful effects of this medicine, it is best to avoid smoking while you are using it. If you have any questions about this, check with your doctor.

Avoid prolonged exposure to very cold temperatures while you are using this medicine, since cold may increase the harmful effects of the medicine.

If you have an infection or illness of any kind, check with your doctor before using this medicine, since you may be more sensitive to its effects.

Side Effects of This Medicine

Along with its needed effects, a medicine may cause some unwanted effects. Although not all of these side effects may occur, if they do occur they may need medical attention.

Check with your doctor immediately if any of the following side effects occur, since they may be signs of an overdose:

    Confusion
    Fast or slow heartbeat
    Numbness and tingling of fingers, toes, or face
    Red or violet blisters on skin of hands or feet
    Shortness of breath
    Stomach pain or bloating
    Weakness

Check with your doctor as soon as possible if the following side effects occur:

More common

    Headache
    Swelling of feet and lower legs

Less common or rare

    Anxiety
    Changes in vision
    Chest pain
    Itching of skin
    Mental depression
    Nausea or vomiting (continuing or severe)
    Pain in arms, legs, or lower back
    Pale or cold hands or feet
    Tiredness
    Weakness in legs

Other side effects may occur that usually do not require medical attention. These side effects may go away during treatment as your body adjusts to the medicine. However, check with your doctor if any of the following side effects continue or are bothersome:

More common

    Diarrhea
    Dizziness
    Nausea or vomiting
    Nervousness or jitters

After you stop using this medicine, your body may need time to adjust. The length of time this takes depends on the amount of medicine you were using and how long you used it. During this period of time check with your doctor if your headaches begin again or worsen.

For elderly patients: The above side effects are more likely to occur in the elderly, who are more likely to have problems with blood vessels. In addition, this medicine may reduce tolerance to cold temperatures in elderly patients.

Other side effects not listed above may also occur in some patients. If you notice any other effects, check with your doctor.

———————————

December 1987

———————————

ERGOTAMINE, CAFFEINE, BELLADONNA ALKALOIDS, AND PENTOBARBITAL (Systemic)

Some commonly used brand names are Cafatine PB, Cafergot-PB, Cafermine PB, Cafetrate-PB, and Migergot-PB.

To the Reader: If you do not recognize the names of medical conditions or medicines referred to in this information, check with your doctor, nurse, or pharmacist. Definitions for selected medical terms may be found in the Glossary. Brand names for the generic drug names listed can be found in the Index. In addition, selected brand names commonly associated with the generic name have been included in the text to help you recognize medicine you may be taking. The fact that a brand name product is not mentioned does not mean the information does not apply. It is a good idea for you to learn both the generic and brand names of your medicines and to write them down for future use.

Ergotamine (er-GOT-a-meen), caffeine (KAF-een), belladonna alkaloids (bell-a-DON-a AL-ka-loids), and pentobarbital (pen-toe-BAR-bi-tal) combination medicine is used as needed to treat migraine headaches and some kinds of throbbing headaches. It is not used to prevent headaches, but is used to treat an attack once it has started.

This medicine is available only with your doctor's prescription.

Remember:
• **This medicine has been prescribed for your current medical problem only.** It must not be given to other people or used for other problems unless you are directed to do so by your doctor.

• **Keep all medicines out of the reach of children.**

• In order for this medicine to work, it must be used as directed.

• **It is very important that you read and understand the following information.** If any of the information causes you special concern, do not decide against using this medicine without first checking with your doctor.

• Before you begin using any new medicine (prescription or nonprescription) or if you develop any new medical problem while you are using this medicine, check with your doctor, nurse, or pharmacist.

• **If you have any questions** about the following information or if you want more information about this medicine or your medical problem, **ask your doctor, nurse, or pharmacist.**

Before Using This Medicine

In order to decide on the best treatment for your medical problem, your doctor should be told:

—if you have ever had any unusual or allergic reaction to atropine, belladonna, barbiturates, or ergot medicines.

—if you are on a low-salt, low-sugar, or any other special diet, or if you are allergic to any substance, such as foods, sulfites or other preservatives, or dyes.

Most medicines contain more than their active ingredient. Your doctor, nurse, or pharmacist can help you avoid products that may cause a problem.

—if you are **pregnant** or if you may become pregnant. Ergotamine is not recommended during pregnancy since it has been shown to stimulate labor, which could result in a miscarriage. Studies in animals have shown that caffeine causes birth defects when given in very large doses (amounts equal to the amount of caffeine contained in 12 to 24 cups of coffee). However, studies in humans have not shown that caffeine causes birth defects. The amount of belladonna alkaloids contained in this medicine should not cause any problems. Barbiturates have been shown to increase the chance of birth defects and may increase the chance of some tumors in the baby.

—if you are **breast-feeding**. Ergotamine passes into the breast milk and may cause unwanted effects, such as vomiting, diarrhea, weak pulse, unstable blood pressure, or convulsions (seizures) in infants of mothers taking large doses of it. Although belladonna alkaloids or barbiturates have not been shown to cause problems in humans, traces of belladonna alkaloids and barbiturates pass into the breast milk. Also, because the belladonna alkaloids tend to decrease the secretions of the body, it is possible that the flow of breast milk may be reduced in some patients. Be sure you have discussed this with your doctor before taking this medicine.

—if you have any of the following medical problems:
Agoraphobia (fear of open or public places)
Anemia (severe)
Asthma (or history of), emphysema, or chronic lung disease
Brain damage (in children)
Diabetes
Difficult urination
Enlarged prostate
Fibrocystic breast disease
Glaucoma
Heart or blood vessel disease
High blood pressure
Infection
Intestinal disease
Itching (severe)
Kidney disease
Liver disease
Mental depression
Overactive thyroid
Panic attacks
Spastic paralysis (in children)
Stomach ulcer
Trouble in sleeping
Underactive adrenal gland

—if you are taking **any** other prescription or nonprescription (OTC) medicine, especially:
Amantadine (e.g., Symmetrel)
Amphetamines
Antacids
Anticoagulants (blood thinners)
Antimuscarinics (medicine for abdominal or stomach spasms or cramps)
Appetite suppressants (diet pills), except fenfluramine
Central nervous system (CNS) depressants

Diarrhea medicine
Digitalis glycosides (heart medicine)
Ketoconazole (e.g., Nizoral)
Medicine for asthma or other breathing problems
Medicine for colds, sinus problems, or hay fever or other allergies (including nose drops or sprays)
Methylphenidate (e.g., Ritalin)
Other medicines containing caffeine
Pemoline (e.g., Cylert)
Potassium chloride

—if you are now taking or have taken within the past 2 weeks monoamine oxidase (MAO) inhibitors such as:

Furazolidone (e.g., Furoxone)
Isocarboxazid (e.g., Marplan)
Pargyline (e.g., Eutonyl)
Phenelzine (e.g., Nardil)
Procarbazine (e.g., Matulane)
Tranylcypromine (e.g., Parnate)

—if you are taking other medicines containing ergotamine for treatment of migraine headaches or medicine containing other ergot alkaloids (such as dihydroergotamine, ergoloid mesylates, ergonovine, methylergonovine, methysergide).

—if you smoke.

Proper Use of This Medicine

Use this medicine only as directed by your doctor. If the amount you are to use does not relieve your headache, do not use more than your doctor ordered. Instead, check with your doctor. Using too much of this medicine or taking it too often may cause serious effects such as nausea and vomiting; cold, painful hands or feet; or even gangrene. Also, if too much is used, it may become habit-forming.

This medicine works best if you:

• **Use it at the first sign of headache or migraine attack.**

• **Lie down in a quiet, dark room for at least 2 hours after using it.**

For patients using the rectal suppository form of this medicine:

• If suppository is too soft to insert because of storage in a warm place, before removing the foil wrapper chill the suppository in the refrigerator for 30 minutes or run cold water over it.

• How to insert suppository—First remove the foil wrapper and moisten the suppository with water. Lie down on side and push the suppository well up into rectum with finger.

How to store this medicine:

• **Keep out of the reach of children** since overdose is especially dangerous in children.

• Store away from heat and direct light.

• Do not store in the bathroom, near the kitchen sink, or in other damp places. Heat or moisture may cause the medicine to break down.

• Do not keep outdated medicine or medicine no longer needed. Be sure that any discarded medicine is out of the reach of children.

Precautions While Using This Medicine

If you have been using this medicine regularly, **do not stop taking it without first checking with your doctor.** Your doctor may want you to reduce gradually the amount you are using before stopping completely. If you stop using it suddenly, your headaches may return or worsen.

Do not take antacids or medicine for diarrhea within 1 hour of using this medicine. Using them too close together will make the belladonna less effective.

This medicine will add to the effects of alcohol and other CNS depressants (medicines that slow down the nervous system, possibly causing drowsiness). Some examples of CNS depressants are antihistamines or medicine for hay fever, other allergies, or colds; sedatives, tranquilizers, or sleeping medicine; prescription pain medicine or narcotics; barbiturates; medicine for convulsions (seizures); tricyclic antidepressants (medicine for depression); muscle relaxants; or anesthetics, including dental anesthetics. **Check with your doctor before taking any of the above while you are using this medicine.**

This medicine may cause some people to become drowsy, dizzy, lightheaded, or less alert than they are normally. **Make sure you know how you react to this medicine before you drive, use machines, or do other jobs that require you to be alert.**

Since smoking may increase some of the harmful effects of this medicine, it is best to avoid smoking while you are using it. If you have any questions about this, check with your doctor.

Avoid prolonged exposure to very cold temperatures while you are using this medicine, since cold may increase the harmful effects of the medicine.

If you have an infection or illness of any kind, check with your doctor before using this medicine, since you may be more sensitive to the effects of it.

This medicine may cause dryness of the mouth, nose, and throat. For temporary relief of mouth dryness, use sugarless candy or gum, melt bits of ice in your mouth, or use a saliva substitute. However, if dry mouth continues for more than 2 weeks, check with your physician or dentist. Continuing dryness of the mouth may increase the chance of dental disease, including tooth decay, gum disease, and fungal infections.

Side Effects of This Medicine

Along with its needed effects, a medicine may cause some unwanted effects. Although not all of these side effects may occur, if they do occur they may need medical attention.

Check with your doctor immediately if any of the following side effects occur since they may be signs of an overdose:

Blurred vision
Clumsiness or unsteadiness
Confusion, especially in the elderly

Extreme drowsiness or irritability
Fast heartbeat
Fever
Flushing of skin
Hallucinations (seeing, hearing, or feeling things that are not there)
Mental depression
Numbness and tingling of fingers, toes, or face
Red or violet blisters on skin of hands or feet
Shortness of breath or troubled breathing
Stomach pain or bloating

Check with your doctor as soon as possible if any of the following side effects occur:

More common

Swelling of feet and lower legs
Unusual excitement

Less common or rare

Chest pain
Pain in arms, legs, or lower back
Pale or cold hands or feet
Skin rash or itching
Weakness in legs
Yellow eyes or skin

Other side effects may occur that usually do not require medical attention. These side effects may go away during treatment as your body adjusts to the medicine.

However, check with your doctor if any of the following side effects continue or are bothersome:

More common

Constipation
Dizziness or lightheadedness
Drowsiness
Dryness of mouth or skin
"Hangover" effect
Nervousness or jitters
Reduced sweating

Less common or rare

Difficult urination (especially in older men)
Difficulty in swallowing
Increased sensitivity of eyes to sunlight
Nausea or vomiting

After you stop taking this medicine, your body may need time to adjust. The length of time this takes depends on the amount of medicine you were taking and how long you took it. During this period of time check with your doctor if your headaches begin again or worsen.

For children and elderly patients: The above side effects may be more likely to occur in children and elderly patients, who are usually more sensitive to the effects of this medicine. In addition, this medicine may reduce tolerance to cold temperatures in elderly patients.

Other side effects not listed above may also occur in some patients. If you notice any other effects, check with your doctor.

December 1987

ERYTHROMYCIN (Ophthalmic)

A commonly used brand name is Ilotycin.

Generic name product may also be available in the U.S.

To the Reader: If you do not recognize the names of medical conditions or medicines referred to in this information, check with your doctor, nurse, or pharmacist. Definitions for selected medical terms may be found in the Glossary. Brand names for the generic drug names listed can be found in the Index. In addition, selected brand names commonly associated with the generic name have been included in the text to help you recognize medicine you may be taking. The fact that a brand name product is not mentioned does not mean the information does not apply. It is a good idea for you to learn both the generic and brand names of your medicines and to write them down for future use.

Erythromycin (eh-rith-roe-MYE-sin) belongs to the general family of medicines called antibiotics. Erythromycin ophthalmic preparations are used in the eye to help the body overcome infections of the eye.

Erythromycin is available only with your doctor's prescription.

Remember:

• **This medicine has been prescribed for your present infection only.** Another infection later on may require a different medicine. Also, even though other people may have the same symptoms as you, they may have a different kind of infection. Your medicine may not work for them and may even cause them harm. Therefore, **your medicine must not be given to other people or used for other infections** unless you are otherwise directed by your doctor.

• **Keep all medicines out of the reach of children.**

• In order for this medicine to work, it must be used as directed.

• **It is very important that you read and understand the following information.** If any of the information causes you special concern, do not decide against using this medicine without first checking with your doctor.

• Before you begin using any new medicine (prescription or nonprescription) or if you develop any new medical problem while you are using this medicine, check with your doctor, nurse, or pharmacist.

• **If you have any questions** about the following information or if you want more information about this medicine or your medical problem, **ask your doctor, nurse, or pharmacist.**

Before Using This Medicine

In order to decide on the best treatment for your medical problem, your doctor should be told:

—if you have ever had any unusual or allergic reaction to this or any of the other erythromycins.

—if you are allergic to any substance, such as certain foods or preservatives or dyes. Most medicines contain more than their active ingredient. Your doctor, nurse, or pharmacist can help you avoid products that may cause a problem.

—if you are **pregnant** or if you may become pregnant. However, erythromycin ophthalmic ointment has not been shown to cause birth defects or other problems in humans.

—if you are **breast-feeding**. However, erythromycin ophthalmic ointment has not been shown to cause problems in nursing babies.

Proper Use of This Medicine

How to apply this medicine: First, wash your hands. Then pull the lower eyelid away from the eye to form a pouch. Squeeze a thin strip of ointment into the pouch. A 1-cm (approximately ⅓-inch) strip of ointment is usually enough unless otherwise directed by your doctor. Gently close the eyes and keep them closed for 1 or 2 minutes to allow the medicine to come into contact with the infection.

To prevent contamination of the eye ointment, do not touch the applicator tip to any surface (including the eye). After using erythromycin eye ointment, wipe the tip of the ointment tube with a clean tissue and keep the tube tightly closed.

To help clear up your infection completely, **keep using this medicine for the full time of treatment,** even if your symptoms begin to clear up after a few days. If you stop using this medicine too soon, your symptoms may return. **Do not miss any doses.**

If you do miss a dose of this medicine, apply it as soon as possible. However, if it is almost time for your next dose, skip the missed dose and go back to your regular dosing schedule.

How to store this medicine:

• **Keep out of the reach of children.**

• Store away from heat and direct light.

• Keep the medicine from freezing.

• Do not keep outdated medicine or medicine no longer needed. Be sure that any discarded medicine is out of the reach of children.

Precautions While Using This Medicine

If your symptoms do not improve within a few days, or if they become worse, check with your doctor.

After application, eye ointments usually cause your vision to blur for a few minutes.

Side Effects of This Medicine

There have not been any common or important side effects reported with this medicine. However, if you notice any side effects, check with your doctor.

December 1987

ERYTHROMYCIN (Topical)

Some commonly used brand names are:

Akne-mycin	Erymax
A/T/S	Sansac*
Erycette	Staticin
EryDerm	T-Stat

Generic name product may also be available in the U.S.

---

*Not available in the U.S.

To the Reader: If you do not recognize the names of medical conditions or medicines referred to in this information, check with your doctor, nurse, or pharmacist. Definitions for selected medical terms may be found in the Glossary. Brand names for the generic drug names listed can be found in the Index. In addition, selected brand names commonly associated with the generic name have been included in the text to help you recognize medicine you may be taking. The fact that a brand name product is not mentioned does not mean the information does not apply. It is a good idea for you to learn both the generic and brand names of your medicines and to write them down for future use.

Erythromycin (eh-rith-roe-MYE-sin) belongs to the general family of medicines called antibiotics. Erythromycin topical preparations are used on the skin to help control acne. They may be used alone or with one or more other medicines that are applied to the skin or taken by mouth for acne. They may also be used for other problems as determined by your doctor.

Erythromycin is available only with your doctor's prescription.

Remember:
• **This medicine has been prescribed for your acne only.** Even though other people may also have acne, they may have a different kind. Your medicine may not work for them and may even cause them harm. Therefore, **your medicine must not be given to other people or used for other problems** unless you are otherwise directed by your doctor.

• **Keep all medicines out of the reach of children.**

• In order for this medicine to work, it must be used as directed.

• **It is very important that you read and understand the following information.** If any of the information causes you special concern, do not decide against using this medicine without first checking with your doctor.

• Before you begin using any new medicine (prescription or nonprescription) or if you develop any new medical problem while you are using this medicine, check with your doctor, nurse, or pharmacist.

• **If you have any questions** about the following information or if you want more information about this medicine or your medical problem, **ask your doctor, nurse, or pharmacist.**

Before Using This Medicine

In order to decide on the best treatment for your medical problem, your doctor should be told:

—if you have ever had any unusual or allergic reaction to this or any of the other erythromycins.

—if you are allergic to any substance, such as certain foods or preservatives or dyes. Most medicines contain more than their active ingredient. Your doctor, nurse, or pharmacist can help you avoid products that may cause a problem.

—if you are **pregnant** or if you may become pregnant. However, erythromycin topical preparations have not been shown to cause birth defects or other problems in humans.

—if you are **breast-feeding**. However, erythromycin topical preparations have not been shown to cause problems in nursing babies.

—if you are using **any** other prescription or nonprescription (OTC) preparation.

Proper Use of This Medicine

Before applying this medicine, thoroughly wash the affected area with warm water and soap, rinse well, and pat dry. After washing or shaving, it is best to wait 30 minutes before applying the pledget or topical liquid form since the alcohol in them may irritate freshly washed or shaved skin.

This medicine will not cure your acne. However, to help keep your acne under control, **keep using this medicine for the full time of treatment,** even if your symptoms begin to clear up after a few days. You may have to continue using this medicine every day for months or even longer in some cases. If you stop using this medicine too soon, your symptoms may return. **It is important that you do not miss any doses.**

If you do miss a dose of this medicine, apply it as soon as possible. However, if it is almost time for your next dose, skip the missed dose and go back to your regular dosing schedule.

For patients using the pledget (swab) or topical liquid form of erythromycin:

• These forms contain alcohol and are flammable. **Do not use near heat, near open flame, or while smoking.**

• It is important that you do not use this medicine more often than your doctor ordered since it may cause your skin to become too dry or irritated.

• Also, you should avoid washing the acne-affected areas too often since this may dry your skin and make your acne worse. Washing with a mild, bland soap 2 or 3 times a day should be enough, unless you have oily skin. If you have any questions about this, check with your doctor.

• How to apply these medicines:
—The topical liquid form of this medicine may come in a bottle with an applicator tip, which may be used to apply the medicine directly to the skin. Use

the applicator with a dabbing motion instead of a rolling motion (not like a roll-on deodorant, for example). If the medicine does not come in an applicator bottle, you may moisten a pad with the medicine and then rub the pad over the whole affected area. Or you may also apply this medicine with your fingertips. Be sure to wash the medicine off your hands afterward.

—Apply a thin film of medicine, using enough to cover the affected area lightly. **You should apply the medicine to the whole area usually affected by acne, not just to the pimples themselves.** This will help keep new pimples from breaking out.

—The pledget form should be rubbed over the whole affected area. You may use extra pledgets, if needed, to cover larger areas.

—Since these medicines contain alcohol, they may sting or burn. Therefore, **do not get these medicines in the eyes, nose, mouth, or on other mucous membranes.** Spread the medicine away from these areas when applying. If these medicines do get in the eyes, wash them out immediately, but carefully, with large amounts of cool tap water. If your eyes still burn or are painful, check with your doctor.

How to store this medicine:

• **Keep out of the reach of children.**

• Store away from heat and direct light.

• Keep the medicine from freezing.

• Do not keep outdated medicine or medicine no longer needed. Be sure that any discarded medicine is out of the reach of children.

Precautions While Using This Medicine

If your acne does not improve within 3 to 4 weeks, or if it becomes worse, check with your doctor or pharmacist. However, treatment of acne may take up to 8 to 12 weeks before you see full improvement.

For patients using the pledget (swab) or topical liquid form of erythromycin:

• If your doctor has ordered another medicine to be applied to the skin along with this medicine, it is best to wait at least 1 hour before you apply the second medicine. This may help keep your skin from becoming too irritated. Also, if the medicines are used too close together, they may not work as well.

• After application of this medicine to the skin, mild stinging or burning may be expected and may last up to a few minutes or more.

• This medicine may also cause the skin to become unusually dry, even with normal use. If this occurs, check with your doctor.

• You may continue to use cosmetics (make-up) while you are using this medicine for acne. However, it is best to use only "water-base" cosmetics. Also, it is best not to use cosmetics too heavily or too often since they may make your acne worse. If you have any questions about this, check with your doctor.

Side Effects of This Medicine

Along with its needed effects, a medicine may cause some unwanted effects. The following side effects may go away during treatment as your body adjusts to the medicine. However, check with your doctor if any of the following side effects continue or are bothersome:

For erythromycin ointment

Less common
    Peeling
    Redness

For erythromycin pledget (swab) or topical liquid form

More common
    Dry or scaly skin
    Irritation
    Itching
    Peeling
    Redness
    Stinging or burning feeling

Other side effects not listed above may also occur in some patients. If you notice any other effects, check with your doctor.

December 1987

ERYTHROMYCINS (Systemic)

Some commonly used brand names are:	Generic names:
E-Mycin Eryc Eryc Sprinkle* Ery-Tab Erythromid* Ilotycin Novorythro* PCE Dispersatabs Robimycin RP-Mycin	Erythromycin†
Ilosone Novorythro*	Erythromycin Estolate†
E.E.S. E-Mycin E EryPed Pediamycin Wyamycin E	Erythromycin Ethylsuccinate†
Ilotycin	Erythromycin Gluceptate
Erythrocin	Erythromycin Lactobionate†
Apo-Erythro-S* Erypar Erythrocin Ethril Novorythro* SK-Erythromycin Wyamycin S	Erythromycin Stearate†

*Not available in the U.S.
†Generic name product may also be available in the U.S.

To the Reader: If you do not recognize the names of medical conditions or medicines referred to in this information, check with your doctor, nurse, or pharmacist. Definitions for selected medical terms may be found in the Glossary. Brand names for the generic drug names listed can be found in the Index. In addition, selected brand names commonly associated with the generic name have been included in the text to help you recognize medicine you may be taking. The fact that a brand name product is not mentioned does not mean the information does not apply. It is a good idea for you to learn both the generic and brand names of your medicines and to write them down for future use.

Erythromycins (eh-rith-roe-MYE-sins) belong to the general family of medicines called antibiotics. They are taken by mouth or given by injection to treat infections. Erythromycins are also used to prevent "strep" infections in patients with a history of rheumatic heart disease who may be allergic to penicillin.

These medicines may also be used to treat Legionnaires' disease and for other problems as determined by your doctor. They will not work for colds, flu, or other virus infections.

Erythromycins are available only with your doctor's prescription.

Remember:

• **This medicine has been prescribed for your present infection only.** Another infection later on may require a different medicine. Also, even though other people may have the same symptoms as you, they may have a different kind of infection. Your medicine may not work for them and may even cause them harm. Therefore, **your medicine must not be given to other people or used for other infections** unless you are otherwise directed by your doctor.

• **Keep all medicines out of the reach of children.**

• In order for this medicine to work, it must be used as directed.

• If you are receiving this medicine by injection, some of the information about this medicine may not apply.

• **It is very important that you read and understand the following information.** If any of the information causes you special concern, do not decide against using this medicine without first checking with your doctor.

• Before you begin using any new medicine (prescription or nonprescription) or if you develop any new medical problem while you are using this medicine, check with your doctor, nurse, or pharmacist.

• **If you have any questions** about the following information or if you want more information about this medicine or your medical problem, **ask your doctor, nurse, or pharmacist.**

Before Using This Medicine

In order to decide on the best treatment for your medical problem, your doctor should be told:

—if you have ever had any unusual or allergic reaction to any of the erythromycins.

—if you are on a low-salt, low-sugar, or any other special diet, or if you are allergic to any substance, such as foods, sulfites or other preservatives, or dyes. Most medicines contain more than their active ingredient, and many liquid medicines contain alcohol. Your doctor, nurse, or pharmacist can help you avoid products that may cause a problem.

—if you are **pregnant** or if you may become pregnant. However, erythromycins have not been shown to cause birth defects or other problems in humans.

—if you are **breast-feeding.** Erythromycins pass into the breast milk. However, erythromycins have not been shown to cause problems in nursing babies.

—if you have either of the following medical problems:
　　Liver disease
　　Loss of hearing

—if you are taking **any** other prescription or nonprescription (OTC) medicine, especially:
　　Acetaminophen (with long-term, high-dose use) (e.g., Tylenol)
　　Aminophylline (e.g., Somophyllin)
　　Amiodarone (e.g., Cordarone)
　　Anabolic steroids (dromostanolone, ethylestrenol, nandrolone, oxandrolone, oxymetholone, stanozolol)
　　Androgens (male hormones)
　　Antithyroid agents (medicine for overactive thyroid)
　　Azlocillin (e.g., Azlin)
　　Caffeine (e.g., NoDoz)
　　Carbamazepine (e.g., Tegretol)
　　Carmustine (e.g., BiCNU)
　　Chloramphenicol (e.g., Chloromycetin)
　　Chloroquine (e.g., Aralen)

Clindamycin (e.g., Cleocin)
Dantrolene (e.g., Dantrium)
Daunorubicin (e.g., Cerubidine)
Disulfiram (e.g., Antabuse)
Divalproex (e.g., Depakote)
Doxorubicin (e.g., Adriamycin)
Estrogens (female hormones)
Etretinate (e.g., Tegison)
Furazolidone (e.g., Furoxone)
Gold salts
Hydroxychloroquine (e.g., Plaquenil)
Isoniazid (e.g., INH, Nydrazid)
Ketoconazole by mouth (e.g., Nizoral)
Lincomycin (e.g., Lincocin)
Mercaptopurine (e.g., Purinethol)
Methotrexate (e.g., Mexate)
Methyldopa (e.g., Aldomet)
Mezlocillin (e.g., Mezlin)
Naltrexone (with long-term, high-dose use) (e.g., Trexan)
Nitrofurantoin (e.g., Furadantin)
Oral contraceptives (birth control pills) containing estrogen
Oxtriphylline (e.g., Choledyl)
Phenothiazines (acetophenazine, chlorpromazine, fluphenazine, mesoridazine, perphenazine, prochlorperazine, promazine, promethazine, thioridazine, trifluoperazine, triflupromazine, trimeprazine)
Phenytoin (e.g., Dilantin)
Piperacillin (e.g., Pipracil)
Plicamycin (e.g., Mithracin)
Rifampin (e.g., Rifadin)
Sulfonamides (sulfa medicine)
Theophylline (e.g., Somophyllin-T)
Valproic acid (e.g., Depakene)
Warfarin (e.g., Coumadin)

—if you have ever had any problems with erythromycin estolate.

Proper Use of This Medicine

Generally, erythromycins are best taken with a full glass (8 ounces) of water on an empty stomach (for example, 1 hour before or 3 to 4 hours after meals), unless otherwise directed by your doctor. However, certain brands of erythromycin delayed-release tablets, as well as erythromycin estolate and erythromycin ethylsuccinate, may be taken on a full or empty stomach. In addition, certain brands of erythromycin stearate tablets may be taken on an empty stomach or immediately before meals. If you have any questions about this, check with your doctor or pharmacist.

For patients taking the oral liquid form of this medicine:

• This medicine is to be taken by mouth even though it may come in a dropper bottle. If this medicine does not come in a dropper bottle, use a specially marked measuring spoon or other device to measure each dose accurately since the average household teaspoon may not hold the right amount of liquid.

• Do not use after the expiration date on the label since the medicine may not work as well. Check with your pharmacist if you have any questions about this.

For patients taking the chewable tablet form of this medicine:

• Tablets must be chewed or crushed before they are swallowed.

For patients taking the delayed-release capsule form (with enteric-coated pellets) or the delayed-release tablet form of this medicine:

• Swallow capsules or tablets whole. Do not break or crush. If you are not sure about which type of capsule or tablet you are taking, check with your pharmacist.

To help clear up your infection completely, **keep taking this medicine for the full time of treatment** even if you begin to feel better after a few days. **If you have a "strep" infection, you should keep taking this medicine for at least 10 days. This is especially important in "strep" infections since serious heart problems could develop later** if your infection is not cleared up completely. Also, if you stop taking this medicine too soon, your symptoms may return.

This medicine works best when there is a constant amount in the blood. **To help keep this amount constant, do not miss any doses. Also, it is best to take each dose at evenly spaced times day and night.** For example, if you are to take 4 doses a day, each dose should be spaced about 6 hours apart. If this interferes with your sleep or other daily activities, or if you need help in planning the best times to take your medicine, check with your doctor, nurse, or pharmacist.

If you do miss a dose of this medicine, take it as soon as possible. This will help to keep a constant amount of medicine in the blood. However, if it is almost time for your next dose and your dosing schedule is:

• 2 doses a day—Space the missed dose and the next dose 5 to 6 hours apart.

• 3 or more doses a day—Space the missed dose and the next dose 2 to 4 hours apart or double your next dose.

Then go back to your regular dosing schedule.

How to store this medicine:

• **Keep out of the reach of children.**

• Store away from heat and direct light.

• Do not store the capsule or tablet form of erythromycins in the bathroom, near the kitchen sink, or in other damp places. Heat or moisture may cause the medicine to break down.

• Store the oral liquid form of some erythromycins in the refrigerator because heat will cause this medicine to break down. However, keep the medicine from freezing. Follow the directions on the label.

• Do not keep outdated medicine or medicine no longer needed. Be sure that any discarded medicine is out of the reach of children.

Precautions While Using This Medicine

If your symptoms do not improve within a few days, or if they become worse, check with your doctor.

Side Effects of This Medicine

Along with its needed effects, a medicine may cause some unwanted effects. Although not all of these side effects may occur, if they do occur they may need medical attention.

Check with your doctor immediately if any of the following side effects occur:

Rare (more common with erythromycin estolate)

 Dark or amber urine
 Pale stools
 Stomach pain (severe)
 Unusual tiredness or weakness
 Yellow eyes or skin

Rare (with kidney disease and high doses)

 Loss of hearing (temporary)

Other side effects may occur that usually do not require medical attention. These side effects may go away during treatment as your body adjusts to the medicine.

However, check with your doctor if any of the following side effects continue or are bothersome:

Less common

 Diarrhea
 Nausea or vomiting
 Sore mouth or tongue
 Stomach cramping and discomfort

For elderly patients: Many medicines have not been tested in older people. Therefore, it is not known whether the medicine acts the same way it does in younger adults. Check with your doctor or pharmacist if you notice any unusual effects while taking this medicine or if you think it is not working as it should.

Other side effects not listed above may also occur in some patients. If you notice any other effects, check with your doctor.

December 1987

ERYTHROMYCIN AND SULFISOXAZOLE
(Systemic)

A commonly used brand name is Pediazole.

To the Reader: If you do not recognize the names of medical conditions or medicines referred to in this information, check with your doctor, nurse, or pharmacist. Definitions for selected medical terms may be found in the Glossary. Brand names for the generic drug names listed can be found in the Index. In addition, selected brand names commonly associated with the generic name have been included in the text to help you recognize medicine you may be taking. The fact that a brand name product is not mentioned does not mean the information does not apply. It is a good idea for you to learn both the generic and brand names of your medicines and to write them down for future use.

Erythromycin (eh-rith-roe-MYE-sin) and sulfisoxazole (sul-fi-SOX-a-zole) is a combination antibiotic and sulfa medicine. Antibiotics and sulfas are used in the treatment of infections caused by bacteria. They work by killing bacteria or preventing their growth.

Erythromycin and sulfisoxazole combination is taken by mouth to treat ear infections. It may also be used for other problems as determined by your doctor. It will not work for colds, flu, or other virus infections.

Erythromycin and sulfisoxazole combination is available only with your doctor's prescription.

Remember:

• **This medicine has been prescribed for your present infection only.** Another infection later on may require a different medicine. Also, even though other people may have the same symptoms as you, they may have a different kind of infection. Your medicine may not work for them and may even cause them harm. Therefore, **your medicine must not be given to other people or used for other infections** unless you are otherwise directed by your doctor.

• **Keep all medicines out of the reach of children.**

• In order for this medicine to work, it must be used as directed.

• **It is very important that you read and understand the following information.** If any of the information causes you special concern, do not decide against using this medicine without first checking with your doctor.

• Before you begin using any new medicine (prescription or nonprescription) or if you develop any new medical problem while you are using this medicine, check with your doctor, nurse, or pharmacist.

• **If you have any questions** about the following information or if you want more information about this medicine or your medical problem, **ask your doctor, nurse, or pharmacist.**

Before Using This Medicine

In order to decide on the best treatment for your medical problem, your doctor should be told:

—if you have ever had any unusual or allergic reaction to any of the erythromycins or sulfas, furosemide or thiazide diuretics (water pills), oral antidiabetic agents (diabetes medicine you take by mouth), or glaucoma medicine you take by mouth (for example, acetazolamide, dichlorphenamide, methazolamide).

—if you are on a low-salt, low-sugar, or any other special diet, or if you are allergic to any substance, such as foods, sulfites or other preservatives, or dyes. Most medicines contain more than their active ingredient, and many liquid medicines contain alcohol. Your doctor, nurse, or pharmacist can help you avoid products that may cause a problem.

—if you are **pregnant** or if you may become pregnant. However, erythromycins and sulfas have not been shown to cause birth defects in humans. Liver problems, although possible, do not usually occur.

—if you are **breast-feeding**. Erythromycins and sulfas pass into the breast milk. Although only small amounts of sulfas appear in breast milk, they may cause unwanted effects in nursing babies with glucose-6-phosphate dehydrogenase (G6PD) deficiency.

—if you have any of the following medical problems:
Glucose-6-phosphate dehydrogenase (G6PD) deficiency
Kidney disease
Liver disease
Porphyria

—if you are taking **any** other prescription or nonprescription (OTC) medicine, especially:
Acetaminophen (with long-term, high-dose use) (e.g., Tylenol)
Aminobenzoic acid (PABA)
Aminophylline (e.g., Somophyllin)
Amiodarone (e.g., Cordarone)
Anabolic steroids (dromostanolone, ethylestrenol, nandrolone, oxandrolone, oxymetholone, stanozolol)
Androgens (male hormones)
Anticoagulants (blood thinners)
Antidiabetic agents, oral (diabetes medicine you take by mouth)
Antithyroid agents (medicine for overactive thyroid)
Azlocillin (e.g., Azlin)
Caffeine (e.g., NoDoz)
Carbamazepine (e.g., Tegretol)
Carmustine (e.g., BiCNU)
Chloramphenicol (e.g., Chloromycetin)
Chloroquine (e.g., Aralen)
Clindamycin (e.g., Cleocin)
Dantrolene (e.g., Dantrium)
Dapsone
Daunorubicin (e.g., Cerubidine)
Disulfiram (e.g., Antabuse)
Divalproex (e.g., Depakote)
Doxorubicin (e.g., Adriamycin)
Estrogens (female hormones)
Ethotoin (e.g., Peganone)
Etretinate (e.g., Tegison)
Furazolidone (e.g., Furoxone)
Gold salts
Hydroxychloroquine (e.g., Plaquenil)
Isoniazid (e.g., INH, Nydrazid)
Ketoconazole by mouth (e.g., Nizoral)
Lincomycin (e.g., Lincocin)
Mephenytoin (e.g., Mesantoin)
Mercaptopurine (e.g., Purinethol)
Methenamine (e.g., Mandelamine)
Methotrexate (e.g., Mexate)
Methyldopa (e.g., Aldomet)

Mezlocillin (e.g., Mezlin)
Naltrexone (with long-term, high-dose use) (e.g., Trexan)
Nitrofurantoin (e.g., Furadantin)
Oral contraceptives (birth control pills) containing estrogen
Oxtriphylline (e.g., Choledyl)
Phenothiazines (acetophenazine, chlorpromazine, fluphenazine, mesoridazine, perphenazine, prochlorperazine, promazine, promethazine, thioridazine, trifluoperazine, triflupromazine, trimeprazine)
Phenytoin (e.g., Dilantin)
Piperacillin (e.g., Pipracil)
Plicamycin (e.g., Mithracin)
Primaquine
Procainamide (e.g., Pronestyl)
Quinidine (e.g., Quinidex)
Quinine (e.g., Quinamm)
Rifampin (e.g., Rifadin)
Sulfoxone (e.g., Diasone)
Theophylline (e.g., Somophyllin-T)
Valproic acid (e.g., Depakene)
Vitamin K (e.g., AquaMEPHYTON, Synkayvite)

Proper Use of This Medicine

Erythromycin and sulfisoxazole combination may be taken on a full or empty stomach.

Do not give this medicine to infants under 1 month of age unless otherwise directed by your doctor. Sulfas may cause liver problems in these infants.

Use a specially marked measuring spoon or other device to measure each dose accurately since the average household teaspoon may not hold the right amount of liquid.

Do not use after the expiration date on the label since the medicine may not work as well. Check with your pharmacist if you have any questions about this.

To help clear up your infection completely, **keep taking this medicine for the full time of treatment** even if you begin to feel better after a few days. If you stop taking this medicine too soon, your symptoms may return.

This medicine works best when there is a constant amount in the blood. **To help keep the amount constant, do not miss any doses. Also, it is best to take the doses at evenly spaced times day and night.** For example, if you are to take 4 doses a day, the doses should be spaced about 6 hours apart. If this interferes with your sleep or other daily activities, or if you need help in planning the best times to take your medicine, check with your doctor, nurse, or pharmacist.

If you do miss a dose of this medicine, take it as soon as possible. This will help to keep a constant amount of medicine in the blood. However, if it is almost time for your next dose and your dosing schedule is:

• 3 or more doses a day—Space the missed dose and the next dose 2 to 4 hours apart or double your next dose.

Then go back to your regular dosing schedule.

How to store this medicine:

• **Keep out of the reach of children.**

• Store away from heat and direct light.

• Store in the refrigerator because heat will cause this medicine to break down. However, keep the medicine from freezing. Follow the directions on the label.

• Do not keep outdated medicine or medicine no longer needed. Be sure that any discarded medicine is out of the reach of children.

Precautions While Using This Medicine

It is important that your doctor check your progress at regular visits if you will be taking this medicine for a long time.

If your symptoms do not improve within a few days, or if they become worse, check with your doctor.

Some people who take medicines containing a sulfonamide may become more sensitive to sunlight than they are normally. **When you first begin taking this medicine, avoid too much sun and do not use a sunlamp until you see how you react to the sun,** especially if you tend to burn easily. You may still be more sensitive to sunlight or sunlamps for many months after you stop taking this medicine. **If you have a severe reaction, check with your doctor.**

Erythromycin and sulfisoxazole combination may cause blood problems. These problems may result in a greater chance of infection, slow healing, and bleeding of the gums. Therefore, you should be careful when using toothbrushes, dental floss, and toothpicks. Dental work should be delayed until your blood counts have returned to normal. Check with your physician or dentist if you have any questions about proper oral hygiene (mouth care) during treatment.

This medicine may also cause some people to become dizzy. **Make sure you know how you react to this medicine before you drive, use machines, or do other jobs that require you to be alert.** If this reaction is especially bothersome, check with your doctor.

Side Effects of This Medicine

Along with its needed effects, a medicine may cause some unwanted effects. Although not all of these side effects may occur, if they do occur they may need medical attention.

Check with your doctor immediately if any of the following side effects occur:
More common
  Itching
  Skin rash
Less common
  Aching of joints and muscles
  Difficulty in swallowing
  Pale skin
  Redness, blistering, peeling, or loosening of skin
  Sore throat and fever

Unusual bleeding or bruising
Unusual tiredness or weakness
Yellow eyes or skin
Rare
Blood in urine
Dark or amber urine
Lower back pain
Pain or burning while urinating
Pale stools
Stomach pain (severe)
Swelling of front part of neck

In addition to the side effects listed above, check with your doctor as soon as possible if the following side effect occurs:

More common
Increased sensitivity of the skin to sunlight

Other side effects may occur that usually do not require medical attention. These side effects may go away during treatment as your body adjusts to the medicine.

However, check with your doctor if any of the following side effects continue or are bothersome:

More common
Diarrhea
Dizziness
Headache
Loss of appetite
Nausea or vomiting
Less common
Sore mouth or tongue
Stomach cramping and discomfort

Other side effects not listed above may also occur in some patients. If you notice any other effects, check with your doctor.

_____

December 1987

_____

ESTRAMUSTINE (Systemic)

A commonly used brand name is Emcyt.

To the Reader: If you do not recognize the names of medical conditions or medicines referred to in this information, check with your doctor, nurse, or pharmacist. Definitions for selected medical terms may be found in the Glossary. Brand names for the generic drug names listed can be found in the Index. In addition, selected brand names commonly associated with the generic name have been included in the text to help you recognize medicine you may be taking. The fact that a brand name product is not mentioned does not mean the information does not apply. It is a good idea for you to learn both the generic and brand names of your medicines and to write them down for future use.

Estramustine (ess-tra-MUSS-teen) belongs to the general group of medicines called antineoplastics. It is taken by mouth to treat some cases of prostate cancer.

Estramustine is a combination of two medicines, an estrogen and mechlorethamine. The way that estramustine works against cancer is not completely understood. However, it seems to interfere with the growth of cancer cells, which are eventually destroyed.

Estramustine is available only with your doctor's prescription.

Remember:

• **This medicine has been prescribed for your current medical problem only.** It must not be given to other people or used for other problems unless you are directed to do so by your doctor.

• **Keep all medicines out of the reach of children.**

• In order for this medicine to work, it must be used as directed.

• **It is very important that you read and understand the following information.** If any of the information causes you special concern, do not decide against using this medicine without first checking with your doctor.

• Before you begin using any new medicine (prescription or nonprescription) or if you develop any new medical problem while you are using this medicine, check with your doctor, nurse, or pharmacist.

• **If you have any questions** about the following information or if you want more information about this medicine or your medical problem, **ask your doctor, nurse, or pharmacist.**

Before Using This Medicine

In order to decide on the best treatment for your medical problem, your doctor should be told:

—if you have ever had any unusual or allergic reaction to estramustine, estrogens, or mechlorethamine.

—if you intend to have children. There is a chance that this medicine may cause birth defects if the male is taking it at the time of conception. It may also cause permanent sterility after it has been taken for a while. Be sure that you have discussed this with your doctor before taking this medicine.

—if you have any of the following medical problems:
  Asthma
  Blood clots (or history of)
  Chickenpox (including recent exposure)
  Diabetes mellitus (sugar diabetes)
  Epilepsy
  Gallbladder disease (or history of)
  Heart or blood vessel disease
  Herpes zoster (shingles)
  Jaundice or hepatitis (or history of) or other liver disease
  Kidney disease
  Mental depression (or history of)
  Migraine headaches
  Stomach ulcer
  Stroke (or history of)

—if you are now taking/using **any** prescription or non-prescription (OTC) medicine, especially:
  Acetaminophen (with long-term, high-dose use) (e.g., Tylenol)
  Amiodarone (e.g., Cordarone)
  Anabolic steroids (dromostanolone, ethylestrenol, nandrolone, oxandrolone, oxymetholone, stanozolol)
  Androgens (male hormones)
  Antithyroid agents (medicine for overactive thyroid)
  Azlocillin (e.g., Azlin)
  Carbamazepine (e.g., Tegretol)
  Carmustine (e.g., BiCNU)
  Chloroquine (e.g., Aralen)
  Dantrolene (e.g., Dantrium)
  Daunorubicin (e.g., Cerubidine)
  Disulfiram (e.g., Antabuse)
  Divalproex (e.g., Depakote)
  Doxorubicin (e.g., Adriamycin)
  Erythromycins
  Etretinate (e.g., Tegison)
  Furazolidone (e.g., Furoxone)
  Gold salts
  Hydroxychloroquine (e.g., Plaquenil)
  Isoniazid (e.g., Nydrazid)
  Ketoconazole (e.g., Nizoral)
  Mercaptopurine (e.g., Purinethol)
  Methotrexate (e.g., Mexate)
  Methyldopa (e.g., Aldomet)
  Mezlocillin (e.g., Mezlin)
  Naltrexone (with long-term, high-dose use) (e.g., Trexan)
  Nitrofurantoin (e.g., Furadantin)
  Phenothiazines (acetophenazine, chlorpromazine, fluphenazine, mesoridazine, perphenazine, prochlorperazine, promazine, promethazine, thioridazine, trifluoperazine, triflupromazine, trimeprazine)
  Phenytoin (e.g., Dilantin)
  Piperacillin (e.g., Pipracil)
  Plicamycin (e.g., Mithracin)
  Rifampin (e.g., Rifadin)
  Sulfonamides (sulfa medicine)
  Valproic acid (e.g., Depakene)

—if you smoke.

Proper Use of This Medicine

Use this medicine only as directed by your doctor. Do not use more or less of it, and do not use it more often than your doctor ordered. The exact amount of medicine you need has been carefully worked out. Taking too much may increase the chance of side effects, while taking too little may not improve your condition.

Do not take estramustine within 1 hour before or 2 hours after the time you take milk, milk formulas, or other dairy products, since they may keep the medicine from working as well.

This medicine commonly causes nausea and sometimes causes vomiting. However, it may have to be taken for several weeks to months to be effective. Even if you begin to feel ill, **do not stop using this medicine without first checking with your doctor.** Ask your doctor, nurse, or pharmacist for ways to lessen these effects.

If you vomit shortly after taking a dose of estramustine, check with your doctor. You will be told whether to take the dose again or wait until the next scheduled dose.

If you miss a dose of this medicine, skip the missed dose and go back to your regular dosing schedule. Do not double doses.

How to store this medicine:

• **Keep out of the reach of children.**

• Store in the refrigerator, away from direct light.

• Do not store in the bathroom, near the kitchen sink, or in other damp places. Heat or moisture may cause the medicine to break down.

• Do not keep outdated medicine or medicine no longer needed. Be sure that any discarded medicine is out of the reach of children.

Precautions While Using This Medicine

It is very important that your doctor check your progress at regular visits to make sure that the medicine is working properly and does not cause unwanted effects.

While you are being treated with estramustine, and after you stop treatment with it, **do not have any immunizations without your doctor's approval.** Estramustine lowers your body's resistance and there is a chance you might get the infection the immunization is meant to prevent. In addition, other persons living in your household should not take oral polio vaccine since there is a chance they could pass the polio virus on to you. Also, you should avoid close contact with other persons (for example, at school or work) who have taken oral polio vaccine.

Side Effects of This Medicine

Along with its needed effects, a medicine may cause some unwanted effects. Although not all of these side effects may occur, if they do occur they may need medical attention.

Check with your doctor immediately if any of the following side effects occur. If your doctor is not available, go to the nearest hospital emergency room.

Rare

  Fever, chills, or sore throat
  Headaches (severe or sudden)
  Loss of coordination (sudden)
  Pains in chest, groin, or leg (especially calf of leg)
  Shortness of breath (sudden, for no apparent reason)
  Slurred speech (sudden)
  Unusual bleeding or bruising
  Vision changes (sudden)
  Weakness or numbness in arm or leg

Check with your doctor as soon as possible if any of the following side effects occur:

More common

  Swelling of feet or lower legs

Rare

  Skin rash or fever
  Unusual tiredness or weakness

Other side effects may occur that usually do not require medical attention. These side effects may go away during treatment as your body adjusts to the medicine. However, check with your doctor if any of the following side effects continue or are bothersome or if you have any questions about them:

More common

  Breast tenderness or enlargement
  Diarrhea
  Nausea

Less common

  Trouble in sleeping
  Vomiting

Other side effects not listed above may also occur in some patients. If you notice any other effects, check with your doctor.

December 1987

ESTROGENS (Systemic)

This information applies to the following medicines:

Chlorotrianisene (klor-oh-trye-AN-i-seen)
Diethylstilbestrol (dye-eth-il-stil-BESS-trole)
Estradiol (ess-tra-DYE-ole)
Conjugated Estrogens (ESS-troe-jenz)
Esterified Estrogens
Estrone (ESS-trone)
Estropipate (ess-troe-PI-pate)
Ethinyl Estradiol (ETH-in-il ess-tra-DYE-ole)
Quinestrol (quin-ESS-trole)

Some commonly used brand names and other names are:	Generic names:
TACE	Chlorotrianisene
DES Honvol* Stilphostrol	Diethylstilbestrol†
Delestrogen Depanate Depestro depGynogen Depo-Estradiol Depogen Dioval Dura-Estrin Duragen E-Cypionate E-Ionate P.A. Estrace Estra-D Estraderm Estradiol L.A. Estra-L Estraval Estraval P.A. Estro-Cyp Estrofem Estroject-LA Estronol-LA Feminate Femogex* Gynogen L.A. Hormogen Depot L.A.E. Menaval Valergen	Estradiol†
C.E.S.* Conjugated Estrogens C.S.D.* Premarin Premarin Intravenous Progens	Conjugated Estrogens†
Estratab Estromed* Menest Neo-Estrone*	Esterified Estrogens
Bestrone Estaqua Estrofol Estroject Estrone-A Estronol Femogen* Foygen Aqueous	Estrone†
Gynogen Hormogen-A Kestrin Aqueous Kestrone Theelin Aqueous Theogen Unigen Wehgen	Estrone†
Ogen Piperazine estrone sulfate	Estropipate
Estinyl Feminone	Ethinyl Estradiol
Estrovis	Quinestrol

*Not available in the U.S.
†Generic name product may also be available in the U.S.

To the Reader: If you do not recognize the names of medical conditions or medicines referred to in this information, check with your doctor, nurse, or pharmacist. Definitions for selected medical terms may be found in the Glossary. Brand names for the generic drug names listed can be found in the Index. In addition, selected brand names commonly associated with the generic name have been included in the text to help you recognize medicine you may be taking. The fact that a brand name product is not mentioned does not mean the information does not apply. It is a good idea for you to learn both the generic and brand names of your medicines and to write them down for future use.

Estrogens (ESS-troe-jenz) are often called female hormones. They are produced by the body and are necessary for the normal sexual development of the female and for the regulation of the menstrual cycle during the childbearing years.

Estrogens are prescribed for several reasons:

—to provide additional hormone when the body does not produce enough of its own, as during the menopause or following certain kinds of surgery.
—in the treatment of selected cases of breast cancer in men and women.
—in the treatment of men with certain kinds of cancer of the prostate.
—to help treat weakening of bones (osteoporosis) in women past menopause.

Estrogens may also be used for other conditions as determined by your doctor.

Estrogens are very useful medicines. However, in addition to their helpful effects in treating your medical problem, they sometimes have side effects that could be very serious. **A paper called "Information for the Patient" is given to you with your prescription. Read this carefully.** Also, before you use an estrogen, you and your doctor should discuss the good that it will do as well as the risks of using it.

Estrogens are usually taken by mouth as tablets or capsules because this method is easier and less costly than injection. However, to suit the individual needs of the patient, they are sometimes given by injection into a vein to produce a rapid effect, or injected into a muscle for a more lasting effect. Estradiol is used also by transdermal disk (a transparent patch the size of a silver dollar that is applied to the skin).

There is no medical evidence to support the belief that the use of estrogens will keep the patient feeling young, keep the skin soft, or delay the appearance of wrinkles. Nor has it been proven that the use of estrogens during the menopause will relieve emotional and nervous symptoms, unless these symptoms are associated with other menopausal symptoms, such as hot flashes or hot flushes.

Estrogens are available only with your doctor's prescription.

Remember:

• **This medicine has been prescribed for your current medical problem only.** It must not be given to other people or used for other problems unless you are directed to do so by your doctor.

• **Keep all medicines out of the reach of children.**

• In order for this medicine to work, it must be used as directed.

• If you are receiving this medicine by injection, some of the information about this medicine may not apply.

• **It is very important that you read and understand the following information.** If any of the information causes you special concern, do not decide against using this medicine without first checking with your doctor.

• Before you begin using any new medicine (prescription or nonprescription) or if you develop any new medical problem while you are using this medicine, check with your doctor, nurse, or pharmacist.

• **If you have any questions** about the following information or if you want more information about this medicine or your medical problem, **ask your doctor, nurse, or pharmacist.**

Before Using This Medicine

In order to decide on the best treatment for your medical problem, your doctor should be told:

—if you have ever had any unusual or allergic reaction to estrogens.

—if you are on a low-salt, low-sugar, or any other special diet, or if you are allergic to any substance, such as foods, sulfites or other preservatives, or dyes. Most medicines contain more than their active ingredient. Your doctor, nurse, or pharmacist can help you avoid products that may cause a problem.

—if you are **pregnant** or if you may become pregnant. Estrogens are not recommended for use during pregnancy, since they have been shown to cause serious birth defects in humans and animals. Daughters of women who took diethylstilbestrol (DES) during pregnancy have developed reproductive tract problems and, rarely, cancer of the vagina and/or uterine cervix when they reached childbearing age. Sons of women who took DES during pregnancy have developed urinary-genital tract problems.

—if you are **breast-feeding.** Use is not recommended in nursing mothers, since estrogens pass into the breast milk and may reduce the flow of the milk and lower its nutritional value.

—if you have any of the following medical problems:

Asthma
Blood clots (or history of)
Bone disease
Cancer (or history of)
Changes in vaginal bleeding
Endometriosis
Epilepsy
Gallbladder disease or gallstones (or history of)
Heart or circulation disease
High blood pressure
Jaundice (or history of during pregnancy)
Kidney disease
Liver disease (such as jaundice or porphyria)
Migraine headaches
Stroke (or history of)
Too much calcium in the blood
Tumors or growths in uterus (not cancerous, such as fibroids)

—if you smoke.

—if you are taking **any** other prescription or nonprescription (OTC) medicine, especially:

Acetaminophen (with long-term, high-dose use)
Amiodarone
Anabolic steroids (dromostanolone, ethylstrenol, nandrolone, oxandrolone, oxymetholone, stanozolol)
Androgens (male hormones)
Antithyroid agents (medicine for overactive thyroid)
Azlocillin
Bromocriptine
Carbamazepine
Carmustine
Chloroquine
Dantrolene
Daunorubicin
Disulfiram
Divalproex
Doxorubicin
Erythromycins
Etretinate
Furazolidone
Gold salts
Hydroxychloroquine
Isoniazid
Ketoconazole
Mercaptopurine
Methotrexate
Methyldopa
Mezlocillin
Naltrexone (with long-term, high-dose use)
Nitrofurantoin
Oral contraceptives (birth control pills) containing estrogen
Phenothiazines (acetophenazine, chlorpromazine, fluphenazine, mesoridazine, perphenazine, prochlorperazine, promazine, promethazine, thioridazine, trifluoperazine, triflupromazine, trimeprazine)
Phenytoin
Piperacillin
Plicamycin
Rifampin
Sulfonamides (sulfa medicine)
Valproic acid

Proper Use of This Medicine

For patients taking any of the estrogens by mouth:

• **Take this medicine only as directed by your doctor. Do not take more of it and do not take it for a longer period of time than your doctor ordered.** Try to take the medicine at the same time each day to reduce the possibility of side effects and to allow it to work better.

• Nausea may occur during the first few weeks after you start taking estrogens. This effect usually disappears with continued use. If the nausea is bothersome, it can usually be prevented or reduced by taking each dose with food or immediately after food.

• If you miss a dose of this medicine, take it as soon as possible. However, if it is almost time for your next dose, skip the missed dose and go back to your regular dosing schedule. Do not double doses.

For patients using the transdermal (stick-on patch) form of estradiol:

• This medicine comes with patient directions. Read them carefully before using this medicine.

• Wash and dry your hands thoroughly before and after handling.

• Apply the patch to a clean, dry, non-oily skin area of your abdomen (stomach) that has little or no hair and is free of cuts or irritation.

• **Do not apply to the breasts.** Also, do not apply to the waistline or anywhere else where tight clothes may rub the patch loose.

• Press the patch firmly in place with the palm of your hand for about 10 seconds. Make sure there is good contact, especially around the edges.

• If a patch becomes loose or falls off, you may reapply it or discard it and apply a new patch.

• Each dose is best applied to a different area of skin on your abdomen so that at least 1 week goes by before the same area is used again. This will help prevent skin irritation.

• If you forget to apply a new patch when you are supposed to, apply it as soon as possible. However, if it is almost time for the next patch, skip the missed one and go back to your regular schedule. Do not apply more than one patch at a time.

How to store this medicine:

• **Keep out of the reach of children.**

• Store away from heat and direct light.

• Do not store in the bathroom medicine cabinet because the heat or moisture may cause the medicine to break down.

• Keep the injectable form of this medicine from freezing.

• Do not keep outdated medicine or medicine no longer needed. Be sure that any discarded medicine is out of the reach of children.

Precautions While Using This Medicine

It is very important that your doctor check your progress at regular visits to make sure this medicine does not cause unwanted effects. These visits will usually be every 6 to 12 months, but many doctors require them more often.

In some patients using estrogens, tenderness, swelling, or bleeding of the gums may occur. Brushing and flossing your teeth carefully and regularly and massaging your gums may help prevent this. See your dentist regularly to have your teeth cleaned. Check with your physician or dentist if you have any questions about how to take care of your teeth and gums, or if you notice any tenderness, swelling, or bleeding of your gums.

While taking this medicine, use caution during exposure to the sun or sunlamps. Some people may develop brown, blotchy spots on exposed areas of their skin. These spots usually disappear gradually when the medicine is stopped.

If you suspect that you may have become pregnant, stop using the medicine immediately and check with your doctor. Continued use of this medicine during pregnancy may cause birth defects in the child. It may also increase the risk of vaginal cancer developing in daughters when they reach childbearing age.

Do not give this medicine to anyone else. Your doctor has prescribed it only for you after studying your health record and the results of your physical examination. Estrogens may be dangerous for other people because of differences in their health and body make-up.

Side Effects of This Medicine

Discuss these possible effects with your doctor:

• The prolonged use of estrogens has been reported to increase the risk of endometrial cancer (cancer of the uterus lining) in women after the menopause. This risk seems to increase as the dose and the length of use increase. When estrogens are used in low doses for less than 1 year, there is less risk. The risk is also reduced if a progestin is added to, or replaces part of, your estrogen dose. If the uterus has been removed by surgery (total hysterectomy), there is no risk of endometrial cancer.

• Cigarette smoking during treatment with estrogens may cause increased risk of serious side effects affecting the heart and/or blood circulation, such as dangerous blood clots, heart attack, or stroke. The risk increases as the amount of smoking and the age of the smoker increase.

The following side effects may be caused by blood clots, which could lead to stroke, heart attack, or death. These side effects rarely occur, and, when they do occur, they usually occur in men treated for cancer using high doses of estrogens. These side effects may need immediate medical attention. **Get emergency help immediately** if any of the following side effects occur:
        Headache (sudden or severe)
        Loss of coordination (sudden)
        Loss of vision or change of vision (sudden)

Pains in chest, groin, or leg, especially in calf of leg
Shortness of breath (sudden and unexplained)
Slurring of speech (sudden)
Weakness or numbness in arm or leg

Also, check with your doctor as soon as possible if any of the following side effects occur:

More common

Swelling of ankles and feet

Less common or rare

Changes in vaginal bleeding (spotting, breakthrough bleeding, prolonged bleeding, or complete stoppage of bleeding)
Dribbling or sudden loss of urine (usually with high doses)
Increased blood pressure
Lumps in, or discharge from, breast
Pains in stomach, side, or abdomen
Skin rash
Uncontrolled jerky movements
Yellow eyes or skin

Other side effects may occur that usually do not require medical attention. These side effects may go away during treatment as your body adjusts to the medicine.

However, check with your doctor if any of the following side effects continue or are bothersome:

More common

Bloating of stomach
Cramps of lower stomach
Loss of appetite
Nausea
Skin irritation or redness (with the estradiol skin patch)
Swelling and increased tenderness of breasts in males or females

Less common

Brown, blotchy spots on exposed skin
Diarrhea (mild)
Dizziness
Headaches or migraine headaches
Increased sensitivity to contact lenses
Unusual decrease in sexual desire (in males)
Unusual increase in sexual desire (in females)
Vomiting (usually with high doses)

Other side effects not listed above may also occur in some patients. If you notice any other effects, check with your doctor.

December 1987

ESTROGENS (Vaginal)

This information applies to the following medicines:

Dienestrol (dye-en-ESS-trole)
Conjugated Estrogens (ESS-troe-jenz)
Estradiol (ess-tra-DYE-ole)
Estrone (ESS-trone)
Estropipate (ess-troe-PI-pate)

Some commonly used brand names or other names are:	Generic names:
DV Estraguard Ortho Dienestrol	Dienestrol†
Estrace	Estradiol
Premarin	Conjugated Estrogens
Oestrilin*	Estrone
Ogen Piperazine Estrone Sulfate	Estropipate

*Not commercially available in the U.S.
†Generic name product may also be available in the U.S.

To the Reader: If you do not recognize the names of medical conditions or medicines referred to in this information, check with your doctor, nurse, or pharmacist. Definitions for selected medical terms may be found in the Glossary. Brand names for the generic drug names listed can be found in the Index. In addition, selected brand names commonly associated with the generic name have been included in the text to help you recognize medicine you may be taking. The fact that a brand name product is not mentioned does not mean the information does not apply. It is a good idea for you to learn both the generic and brand names of your medicines and to write them down for future use.

Estrogens (ESS-troe-jenz) are often called female hormones. They are produced by the body and are necessary for the normal sexual development of the female and for the regulation of the menstrual cycle during the childbearing years.

Uncomfortable changes may occur in vaginal tissues when the body does not produce enough estrogens, as during the menopause or following certain kinds of surgery. In order to relieve such uncomfortable conditions, estrogens are sometimes prescribed for vaginal use in the form of special creams or suppositories.

When used vaginally or on the skin, most estrogens are absorbed into the blood stream and produce many of the same effects in the body as when they are taken by mouth or given by injection.

Estrogens are very useful medicines. However, in addition to their helpful effects in treating your medical problem, they sometimes have side effects that could be very serious. **A paper called "Information for the Patient" is given to you with your prescription. Read this carefully.** Also, you should discuss with your doctor the good that this medicine will do as well as the risks of using it.

Estrogens for vaginal use are available only with your doctor's prescription.

Remember:
• **This medicine has been prescribed for your current medical problem only.** It must not be given to other people or used for other problems unless you are directed to do so by your doctor.

• **Keep all medicines out of the reach of children.**

• In order for this medicine to work, it must be used as directed.

• **It is very important that you read and understand the following information.** If any of the information causes you special concern, do not decide against using this medicine without first checking with your doctor.

• Before you begin using any new medicine (prescription or nonprescription) or if you develop any new medical problem while you are using this medicine, check with your doctor, nurse, or pharmacist.

• **If you have any questions** about the following information or if you want more information about this medicine or your medical problem, **ask your doctor, nurse, or pharmacist**.

Before Using This Medicine

In order to decide on the best treatment for your medical problem, your doctor should be told:

—if you have ever had any unusual or allergic reaction to estrogens.

—if you are allergic to any substance, such as sulfites or other preservatives or dyes. Most medicines contain more than their active ingredient. Your doctor, nurse, or pharmacist can help you avoid products that may cause a problem.

—if you are **pregnant** or if you may become pregnant. Estrogens are not recommended during pregnancy, since they have been shown to cause serious birth defects in humans and animals.

—if you are **breast-feeding**. Use is not recommended in nursing mothers, since estrogens pass into the breast milk and may stop the flow of the milk.

—if you have any of the following medical problems:
  Asthma
  Blood clots (or history of)
  Bone disease
  Cancer (or history of)
  Changes in vaginal bleeding
  Endometriosis
  Epilepsy
  Gallbladder disease or gallstones (or history of)
  Heart or circulation disease
  High blood pressure
  Jaundice (or history of during pregnancy)
  Kidney disease
  Liver disease (such as jaundice or porphyria)
  Migraine headaches
  Stroke (or history of)
  Too much calcium in the blood
  Tumors or growths in uterus (not cancerous, such as fibroids)

—if you smoke.

—if you are now taking **any** other medicine, nonprescription (over-the-counter) or prescription, especially:

Acetaminophen (with long-term, high-dose use)
Amiodarone
Anabolic steroids (dromostanolone, ethylestrenol, nandrolone, oxandrolone, oxymetholone, stanozolol)
Androgens (male hormones)
Antithyroid agents (medicine for overactive thyroid)
Azlocillin
Bromocriptine
Carbamazepine
Carmustine
Chloroquine
Dantrolene
Daunorubicin
Disulfiram
Divalproex
Doxorubicin
Erythromycins
Etretinate
Furazolidone
Gold salts
Hydroxychloroquine
Isoniazid
Ketoconazole
Mercaptopurine
Methotrexate
Methyldopa
Mezlocillin
Naltrexone (with long-term, high-dose use)
Nitrofurantoin
Oral contraceptives (birth control pills) containing estrogen
Phenothiazines (acetophenazine, chlorpromazine, fluphenazine, mesoridazine, perphenazine, prochlorperazine, promazine, promethazine, thioridazine, trifluoperazine, triflupromazine, trimeprazine)
Phenytoin
Piperacillin
Plicamycin
Rifampin
Sulfonamides (sulfa medicine)
Valproic acid

Proper Use of This Medicine

Use this medicine only as directed. Do not use more of it and do not use it for a longer period of time than your doctor ordered.

This medicine is often used at bedtime to increase effectiveness through better absorption. To protect your clothing while using this medicine, you may find sanitary napkins helpful.

Nausea may occur during the first few weeks after you start using estrogens. This effect usually disappears with continued use. If the nausea is bothersome, it can usually be prevented or reduced if you eat a solid breakfast or a mid-morning snack.

Vaginal creams and some vaginal suppositories are inserted with a plastic dose applicator. Directions for using the applicator are included with your medicine. If you do not receive the directions or do not understand them, ask your doctor, pharmacist, or nurse for information or additional explanation.

If you miss a dose of this medicine and do not remember it until the next day, do not use the missed dose at all. Instead, go back to your regular dosing schedule.

How to store this medicine:

• **Keep out of the reach of children.**

• Store away from heat and direct light.

• Keep the medicine from freezing.

• Do not keep outdated medicine or medicine no longer needed. Be sure that any discarded medicine is out of the reach of children.

Precautions While Using This Medicine

It is very important that your doctor check your progress at regular visits to make sure this medicine does not cause unwanted effects. These visits will usually be every 6 to 12 months, but some doctors require them more often.

In some patients using estrogens, tenderness, swelling, or bleeding of the gums may occur. Brushing and flossing your teeth carefully and regularly and massaging your gums may help prevent this. See your dentist regularly to have your teeth cleaned. Check with your physician or dentist if you have any questions about how to take care of your teeth and gums, or if you notice any tenderness, swelling, or bleeding of your gums.

While using this medicine, use caution during exposure to the sun or sunlamps. Some people may develop brown, blotchy spots on exposed areas of their skin. These spots usually disappear gradually when the medicine is stopped.

If you suspect that you may have become pregnant, stop using the medicine immediately and check with your doctor. Continued use of estrogens during pregnancy may cause birth defects in the child.

Do not give this medicine to anyone else. Your doctor has prescribed it only for you after studying your health record and the results of your physical examination. Estrogens may be dangerous for other people because of differences in their health and body make-up.

Side Effects of This Medicine

Discuss these possible effects with your doctor:

• The prolonged use of estrogens has been reported to increase the risk of endometrial cancer (cancer of the uterus lining) in women after the menopause. This risk seems to increase as the dose and the length of use increase. When estrogens are used in low doses for less than 1 year, there is less risk. The risk is also reduced if a progestin is added to, or replaces part of, your estrogen dose. If the uterus has been removed by surgery (total hysterectomy), there is no risk of endometrial cancer.

• Cigarette smoking during treatment with estrogens may cause increased risk of serious side effects affecting the heart and/or blood circulation, such as dangerous blood clots, heart attack, or stroke. The risk increases as the amount of smoking and the age of the smoker increase.

Check with your doctor as soon as possible if any of the following side effects occur:

More common
> Swelling of ankles and feet

Less common or rare
> Changes in vaginal bleeding (spotting, breakthrough bleeding, prolonged bleeding, or complete stoppage of bleeding)
> Increased blood pressure
> Lumps in, or discharge from, breast
> Pains in stomach, side, or abdomen
> Skin rash
> Swelling, redness, or itching around vaginal area
> Uncontrolled jerky movements
> Yellow eyes or skin

Other side effects may occur that usually do not require medical attention. These side effects may go away during treatment as your body adjusts to the medicine. However, check with your doctor if any of the following side effects continue or are bothersome:

More common
> Bloating of stomach
> Cramps of lower stomach
> Loss of appetite
> Nausea
> Swelling and increased tenderness of breasts

Less common
> Brown, blotchy spots on exposed skin
> Diarrhea (mild)
> Dizziness
> Headaches or migraine headaches
> Increased sensitivity to contact lenses
> Unusual increase in sexual desire

Other side effects not listed above may also occur in some patients. If you notice any other effects, check with your doctor.

_____

December 1987

ESTROGENS AND PROGESTINS
(Systemic)
Oral Contraceptives

This information applies to the following medicines:

Ethynodiol (e-thye-noe-DYE-ole) Diacetate and Ethinyl Estradiol (ETH-in-il ess-tra-DYE-ole)

Ethynodiol Diacetate and Mestranol (MES-tra-nole)

Levonorgestrel (LEE-voe-nor-jess-trel) and Ethinyl Estradiol

Norethindrone (nor-eth-IN-drone) Acetate and Ethinyl Estradiol

Norethindrone and Ethinyl Estradiol

Norethindrone and Mestranol

Norethynodrel (nor-e-THYE-noe-drel) and Mestranol

Norgestrel (nor-JESS-trel) and Ethinyl Estradiol

For information about Norethindrone or Norgestrel when used as single-ingredient oral contraceptives, see *Progestins (Systemic)*.

Some commonly used brand names are:	Generic names:
Demulen	Ethynodiol Diacetate and Ethinyl Estradiol
Ovulen	Ethynodiol Diacetate and Mestranol
Levlen Nordette Tri-Levlen Triphasil	Levonorgestrel and Ethinyl Estradiol
Loestrin Minestrin* Norlestrin	Norethindrone Acetate and Ethinyl Estradiol
Brevicon Genora 1/35 ModiCon Norinyl 1+35 Norquest Ortho* Ortho-Novum 1/35 Ortho-Novum 7/7/7 Ortho-Novum 10/11 Ovcon Synphasic* Tri-Norinyl	Norethindrone and Ethinyl Estradiol
Genora 1/50 Norinyl 1+50 Norinyl 1+80 Norinyl 2 Ortho-Novum 0.5* Ortho-Novum 1/50 Ortho-Novum 1/80 Ortho-Novum 2 Program*	Norethindrone and Mestranol
Enovid Enovid-E	Norethynodrel and Mestranol
Lo/Ovral Min-Ovral* Ovral	Norgestrel and Ethinyl Estradiol

To the Reader: If you do not recognize the names of medical conditions or medicines referred to in this information, check with your doctor, nurse, or pharmacist. Definitions for selected medical terms may be found in the Glossary. Brand names for the generic drug names listed can be found in the Index. In addition, selected brand names commonly associated with the generic name have been included in the text to help you recognize medicine you may be taking. The fact that a brand name

product is not mentioned does not mean the information does not apply. It is a good idea for you to learn both the generic and brand names of your medicines and to write them down for future use.

Oral contraceptives are known also as the Pill, OC's, BC's, BC tablets, or birth control pills. They usually contain two types of female hormones, estrogens (ESS-troe-jenz) and progestins (proe-JESS-tins). When taken by mouth on a regular schedule, they change the hormone balance of the body, which prevents pregnancy.

Sometimes these preparations can be used in the treatment of conditions that are helped by added hormones. Oral contraceptives (birth control pills) do not prevent or cure venereal diseases (VD), however.

Before you take an oral contraceptive, you and your doctor should discuss the benefits and risks of using these medicines. These medicines are the most effective method of preventing pregnancy although they sometimes have side effects that could be very serious.

In order to make the use of oral contraceptives (birth control tablets) as safe and reliable as possible, you should understand how and when to take them and what effects may be expected. **A paper with information for the patient will be given to you with your filled prescription, and will provide many details concerning the use of oral contraceptives. Read this paper carefully** and ask your doctor, nurse, or pharmacist if you need additional information or explanation.

Oral contraceptives are available only with your doctor's prescription.

Remember:

• **This medicine has been prescribed for your use only.** It must not be given to other people or used for other purposes unless you are directed to do so by your doctor.

• **Keep all medicines out of the reach of children.**

• In order for this medicine to work, it must be used as directed.

• **It is very important that you read and understand the following information.** If any of the information causes you special concern, do not decide against using this medicine without first checking with your doctor.

• Before you begin using any new medicine (prescription or nonprescription) or if you develop any new medical problem while you are using this medicine, check with your doctor, nurse, or pharmacist.

• **If you have any questions** about the following information or if you want more information about this medicine or your medical problem, **ask your doctor, nurse, or pharmacist.**

Before Using This Medicine

In order to decide on the best treatment for your medical problem, your doctor should be told:

—if you have ever had any unusual or allergic reaction to estrogens or progestins.

—if you are on a low-salt, low-sugar, or any other special diet, or if you are allergic to any substance, such as foods, sulfites or other preservatives, or dyes. Most medicines contain more than their active ingredient. Your doctor, nurse, or pharmacist can help you avoid products that may cause a problem.

—if you suspect that you are **pregnant**. Oral contraceptives are not recommended during pregnancy, since they have been shown to cause birth defects in humans and animals. Daughters of women who took one kind of estrogen, diethylstilbestrol (DES), during pregnancy have developed reproductive tract problems and, rarely, cancer of the vagina and/or uterine cervix when they reached childbearing age. Sons of women who took DES during pregnancy have developed urinary-genital tract problems. It is not yet known if the estrogens in oral contraceptives also cause this effect, but the chance does exist.

—if you are **breast-feeding**. The estrogens in oral contraceptives pass into the breast milk and may reduce the quantity and quality of milk. Studies have shown oral contraceptives to cause tumors in humans and animals. Use of "high-dose" birth control medicines is not recommended during breast-feeding. It may be necessary for you to use another method of birth control or to stop breast-feeding while taking oral contraceptives. However, your doctor may allow you to begin using one of the "low-dose" oral contraceptives after you have been breast-feeding for a while. Be sure you have discussed the risks and benefits with your doctor.

—if your mother took diethylstilbestrol (DES) while she was pregnant with you.

—if you have any of the following medical problems:
 Angina pectoris (chest pains on exertion)
 Asthma
 Blood clots (or history of)
 Bone disease
 Breast disease (not cancerous, such as fibrocystic disease [breast cysts], breast lumps, or abnormal mammograms [x-ray pictures of the breast])
 Cancer (or history of)
 Changes in vaginal bleeding
 Diabetes mellitus (sugar diabetes)
 Endometriosis
 Epilepsy
 Gallbladder disease or gallstones (or history of)
 Heart or circulation disease
 High blood pressure
 Jaundice (or history of during pregnancy)
 Kidney disease
 Liver disease (such as jaundice or porphyria)
 Lumps in breasts
 Mental depression (or history of)
 Migraine headaches
 Scanty or irregular menstrual periods
 Stroke (or history of)
 Too much calcium in the blood
 Tuberculosis
 Tumors or growths in uterus (not cancerous, such as fibroids)
 Varicose veins

—if you are bedridden or if you expect to have surgery in the near future.

—if you smoke cigarettes. Smoking increases the risk of serious adverse effects.

—if you are taking **any** other prescription or nonprescription (OTC) medicine, especially:
 Acetaminophen (with long-term, high-dose use)
 Adrenocorticoids (cortisone-like medicine)
 Amiodarone
 Anabolic steroids (dromostanolone, ethylestrenol, nandrolone, oxandrolone, oxymetholone, stanozolol)
 Androgens (male hormones)
 Anticoagulants (blood thinners)
 Antithyroid agents (medicine for overactive thyroid)
 Azlocillin
 Barbiturates
 Bromocriptine
 Carbamazepine
 Carmustine
 Chloroquine
 Dantrolene
 Daunorubicin
 Disulfiram
 Divalproex
 Doxorubicin
 Erythromycins
 Estrogens (female hormones)
 Etretinate
 Furazolidone
 Gold salts
 Griseofulvin
 Hydroxychloroquine
 Isoniazid
 Ketoconazole
 Mercaptopurine
 Methotrexate
 Methyldopa
 Mezlocillin
 Naltrexone (with long-term, high-dose use)
 Nitrofurantoin
 Phenothiazines (acetophenazine, chlorpromazine, fluphenazine, mesoridazine, perphenazine, prochlorperazine, promazine, promethazine, thioridazine, trifluoperazine, triflupromazine, trimeprazine)
 Phenylbutazone
 Phenytoin
 Piperacillin
 Plicamycin
 Primidone
 Rifampin
 Sulfonamides (sulfa medicine)
 Tricyclic antidepressants (amitriptyline, amoxapine, clomipramine, desipramine, doxepin, imipramine, nortriptyline, protriptyline, trimipramine)
 Valproic acid

Proper Use of This Medicine

Take this medicine only as directed by your doctor. This medicine must be taken exactly on schedule to prevent pregnancy. Try to take the medicine at the same time each day, not more than 24 hours apart, to reduce the possibility of side effects and to provide the best protection.

Nausea may occur during the first few weeks after you start taking this medicine. This effect usually disappears with continued use. If the nausea is bothersome, it can usually be prevented or reduced by taking each dose with food or immediately after food.

Since one of the most important factors in the proper use of oral contraceptives is taking every dose exactly on schedule, you should never let your tablet supply run out. Always keep 1 extra month's supply of tablets on hand. To keep the extra month's supply from becoming too old, use it next, after the pills now being used, and replace the extra supply each month on a regular schedule. The tablets will keep well when kept dry and at room temperature (light will fade some tablet colors but will not change the medicine's effect).

Keep the tablets in the container in which you received them. Most containers aid you in keeping track of your dosage schedule.

Monophasic, biphasic, and triphasic dosing schedules—

• Monophasic cycle dosing schedule: Most available dosing schedules are of the monophasic type. If you are taking tablets of one strength (color) for 20 or 21 days, you are using a monophasic schedule. For the 28-day monophasic cycle you will also take an additional 7 inactive tablets, which are of another color.

• Biphasic cycle dosing schedule:
—If you are using a biphasic 21-day schedule, you are taking tablets of one strength (color) for 10 days (the 1st phase). You then take tablets of a second strength (color) for the next 11 days (the 2nd phase). For the 28-day biphasic cycle you will also take an additional 7 inactive tablets, which are of a third color.
—If you are using a biphasic 24-day schedule, you are taking tablets of one strength (color) for 17 days (the 1st phase). You then take tablets of a second strength (color) for the next 7 days (the 2nd phase).

• Triphasic cycle dosing schedule: If you are using a triphasic 21-day schedule, you are taking tablets of one strength (color) for 6 or 7 days depending on the medicine prescribed (the 1st phase). You then take tablets of a second strength (color) for the next 5 to 9 days depending on the medicine prescribed (the 2nd phase). After that, you take tablets of a third strength (color) for the next 5 to 10 days depending on the medicine prescribed (the 3rd phase). At this point, you will have taken a total of 21 tablets. For the 28-day triphasic cycle you will also take an additional 7 inactive tablets, which are of a fourth color.

It is very important that you take the tablets in the same order that they appear in the container. Tablets of different colors in the same package are also different in strength. Taking the tablets out of order may reduce the effectiveness of the medicine.

If you miss a dose of this medicine:

• For monophasic or biphasic cycles—
If you are using a 20-, 21-, or a 24-day schedule and you miss a dose of this medicine for one day, take the missed tablet as soon as you remember. If it is not remembered until the next day, take the missed tablet plus the tablet that is regularly scheduled for that day. This means that you will take 2 tablets on the same day. Then continue on your regular dosing schedule.

If you are using a 20-, 21-, or a 24-day schedule and you miss a dose for 2 days in a row, take 2 tablets a day for each of the next 2 days, then continue on your regular dosing schedule. In addition, you should use a second method of birth control to make sure that you are fully protected for the rest of the cycle. Report to your doctor.

If you are using a 20-, 21-, or a 24-day schedule and you miss a dose for 3 days or more in a row, stop taking the medicine completely and use another method of birth control until your period begins or until your doctor determines that you are not pregnant. Then restart protection with a new cycle of tablets.

If you are using a 28-day schedule and you miss any of the first 21 (active) tablets, follow the instructions for the 21-day schedule depending on how many doses you have missed. If you miss any of the last 7 (inactive) tablets, there is no danger of pregnancy. However, the first tablet (active) of the next month's cycle must be taken on the regularly scheduled day, in spite of any missed doses, if pregnancy is to be avoided. The active and inactive tablets are colored differently for your convenience.

• For triphasic cycles—
If you are using a 21-day schedule and you miss a dose of this medicine for one day, take the missed tablet as soon as you remember. If it is not remembered until the next day, take the missed tablet plus the tablet that is regularly scheduled for that day. This means that you will take 2 tablets on the same day. Then continue on your regular dosing schedule. In addition, you should use a second method of birth control to make sure that you are fully protected for the rest of the cycle. Report to your doctor.

If you are using a 21-day schedule and you miss a dose for 2 days in a row, take 2 tablets a day for each of the next 2 days, then continue on your regular dosing schedule. In addition, you should use a second method of birth control to make sure that you are fully protected for the rest of the cycle. Report to your doctor.

If you are using a 21-day schedule and you miss a dose for 3 days or more in a row, stop taking the medicine completely and use another method of birth control until your period begins or until your doctor determines that you are not pregnant. Then restart protection with a new cycle of tablets.

If you are using a 28-day schedule and you miss any of the first 21 (active) tablets, follow the instructions for the 21-day schedule depending on how many doses you have missed. If you miss any of the last 7 (inactive) tablets, there is no danger of pregnancy. However, the first tablet (active) of the next month's cycle must be taken on the regularly scheduled day, in spite of any missed doses, if pregnancy is to be avoided. The active and inactive tablets are colored differently for your convenience.

How to store this medicine:

- **Keep out of the reach of children.**

- Store away from heat and direct light.

- Do not store in the bathroom, near the kitchen sink, or in other damp places. Heat and moisture may cause the medicine to break down.

- Do not keep outdated medicine or medicine no longer needed. Be sure that any discarded medicine is out of the reach of children.

Precautions While Using This Medicine

It is very important that your doctor check your progress at regular visits to make sure this medicine does not cause unwanted effects. These visits will usually be every 6 to 12 months, but some doctors require them more often.

When you begin to use oral contraceptives, your body will require at least 7 days to adjust before pregnancy will be prevented; therefore, you should **use a second method of birth control for the first cycle (or 3 weeks)** to ensure full protection.

Tell the physician or dentist in charge that you are taking this medicine before any kind of surgery (including dental surgery) or emergency treatment, since this medicine may cause serious blood clots, heart attack, or stroke.

The following medicines may reduce the effectiveness of oral contraceptives. **You should use a second method of birth control during each cycle in which any of the following medicines are used:**

    Ampicillin
    Adrenocorticoids (cortisone-like medicine)
    Bacampicillin
    Barbiturates
    Carbamazepine
    Chloramphenicol
    Dihydroergotamine
    Griseofulvin
    Mineral oil
    Neomycin, oral
    Penicillin V
    Phenylbutazone
    Phenytoin
    Primidone
    Rifampin
    Sulfonamides (sulfa medicine)
    Tetracyclines
    Tranquilizers
    Valproic acid

Check with your doctor if you have any questions about this.

Vaginal bleeding of various amounts may occur between your regular menstrual periods during the first 2 months of use. This is sometimes called spotting when slight, or breakthrough bleeding when heavier. If this should occur:

- Continue on your regular dosing schedule.

- The bleeding usually stops within 1 week.

- Check with your doctor if the bleeding continues for more than 1 week.

- After you have been taking oral contraceptives on schedule and for more than 2 months, check with your doctor.

Missed menstrual periods may occur:

—if you have not taken the medicine exactly as scheduled. Pregnancy must be considered a possibility.

—if the medicine is not properly adjusted for your needs.

—if you have taken oral contraceptives for a long time, usually 2 or more years, and stop their use.

Check with your doctor if you miss any menstrual periods so that the cause may be determined.

In some patients using estrogen-containing oral contraceptives, tenderness, swelling, or bleeding of the gums may occur. Brushing and flossing your teeth carefully and regularly and massaging your gums may help prevent this. See your dentist regularly to have your teeth cleaned. Check with your physician or dentist if you have any questions about how to take care of your teeth and gums, or if you notice any tenderness, swelling, or bleeding of your gums.

A few people who take this medicine may become more sensitive to sunlight than they are normally. When you begin to take this medicine, avoid too much sun or use of a sunlamp until you see how you react. Some people may develop brown, blotchy spots on exposed areas. These spots usually disappear gradually when the medicine is stopped.

If you wear contact lenses and notice a change in vision or an inability to wear them, check with your doctor.

If you suspect that you may have become pregnant, stop taking this medicine immediately and check with your doctor. Continued use of this medicine during pregnancy may cause birth defects in the child. It may also increase the risk of vaginal cancer developing in daughters when they reach childbearing age.

If you are scheduled for any laboratory tests, tell your doctor that you are taking birth control pills.

The hormones in oral contraceptives may cause birth defects. Since it takes a while for the effects of this medicine to wear off, birth defects may occur even though the tablets are no longer being used. Therefore, **when you stop using oral contraceptives, it is very important that you wait at least 3 months before becoming pregnant. Be sure to use another method of birth control during that time.**

Do not give this medicine to anyone else. Your doctor has prescribed it only for you after studying your health record and the results of your physical examination. Oral contraceptives may be dangerous for other people because of differences in their health and body make-up.

Check with your doctor before taking any leftover oral contraceptives from an old prescription, especially after a pregnancy. Your old prescription may be dangerous to you now or may allow you to become pregnant if your health has changed since your last physical examination.

Side Effects of This Medicine

Discuss these possible effects with your doctor:

• Along with their needed effects, birth control tablets sometimes cause some unwanted effects such as benign (not cancerous) liver tumors, liver cancer, blood clots, heart attack, and stroke, and problems of the gallbladder, liver, and uterus. Although these effects are rare, they can be very serious and may cause death.

• **Cigarette smoking** during the use of oral contraceptives has been found to increase the risk of serious side effects affecting the heart and/or blood circulation, such as dangerous blood clots, heart attack, or stroke. The risk increases as the age of the patient and the amount of smoking increase. This risk is greater in women of age 35 to the age of menopause. **To reduce the risk of serious side effects, do not smoke cigarettes while using oral contraceptives.**

The following side effects may be caused by blood clots, which could lead to stroke, heart attack, or death. Although these side effects rarely occur, they require immediate medical attention. **Get emergency help immediately** if any of the following side effects occur:

 Coughing up blood
 Headache (severe or sudden)
 Loss of coordination (sudden)
 Loss of vision or change in vision (sudden)
 Pains in chest, groin, or leg (especially in calf of leg)
 Shortness of breath (sudden)
 Slurring of speech (sudden)
 Weakness, numbness, or pain in arm or leg (unexplained)

Check with your doctor as soon as possible if any of the following side effects occur:

Less common or rare
 Bulging eyes
 Changes in vaginal bleeding (spotting, breakthrough bleeding, prolonged bleeding, or complete stoppage of bleeding)
 Double vision

Fainting
Frequent urge to urinate or painful urination
Increased blood pressure
Loss of vision (gradual, partial, or complete)
Lumps in, or discharge from, breast
Mental depression
Pain, numbness, and coldness of fingers or toes (continuing)
Pains in stomach, side, or abdomen
Skin rash
Swelling, pain, or tenderness in upper abdomen (stomach) area
Uncontrolled jerky movements
Unusual or dark-colored mole
Vaginal discharge (thick, white, and curd-like)
Yellow eyes or skin

Other side effects may occur that usually do not require medical attention. These side effects may go away during treatment as your body adjusts to the medicine. However, check with your doctor if any of the following side effects continue or are bothersome:

More common
 Acne (usually less common after first 3 months)
 Bloating of stomach
 Cramps of lower stomach
 Loss of appetite
 Nausea
 Swelling of ankles and feet
 Swelling and increased tenderness of breasts
 Unusual tiredness or weakness
 Unusual weight gain

Less common or rare
 Brown, blotchy spots on exposed skin
 Diarrhea (mild)
 Dizziness
 Headaches or migraine headaches
 Increased body and facial hair
 Increased sensitivity to contact lenses
 Increased skin sensitivity to sun
 Irritability
 Some loss of scalp hair
 Unusual decrease or increase in sexual desire
 Vomiting

Other side effects not listed above may also occur in some patients. If you notice any other effects, check with your doctor.

December 1987

ETHAMBUTOL (Systemic)

Some commonly used brand names are Etibi* and Myambutol.

---

*Not available in the U.S.

To the Reader: If you do not recognize the names of medical conditions or medicines referred to in this information, check with your doctor, nurse, or pharmacist. Definitions for selected medical terms may be found in the Glossary. Brand names for the generic drug names listed can be found in the Index. In addition, selected brand names commonly associated with the generic name have been included in the text to help you recognize medicine you may be taking. The fact that a brand name product is not mentioned does not mean the information does not apply. It is a good idea for you to learn both the generic and brand names of your medicines and to write them down for future use.

Ethambutol (e-THAM-byoo-tole) belongs to the general family of medicines called anti-infectives. It is used to help the body overcome tuberculosis (TB) and is taken by mouth with one or more other medicines for TB. This medicine may also be used for other problems as determined by your doctor.

Ethambutol is available only with your doctor's prescription.

Remember:

• **This medicine has been prescribed for your present TB infection only.** Another TB infection later on may require a different medicine. Also, even though other people may have the same symptoms as you, they may have a different kind of TB. Your medicine may not work for them and may even cause them harm. Therefore, **your medicine must not be given to other people or used for other infections** unless you are otherwise directed by your doctor.

• **Keep all medicines out of the reach of children.**

• In order for this medicine to work, it must be used as directed.

• **It is very important that you read and understand the following information.** If any of the information causes you special concern, do not decide against using this medicine without first checking with your doctor.

• Before you begin using any new medicine (prescription or nonprescription) or if you develop any new medical problem while you are using this medicine, check with your doctor, nurse, or pharmacist.

• **If you have any questions** about the following information or if you want more information about this medicine or your medical problem, **ask your doctor, nurse, or pharmacist.**

Before Using This Medicine

In order to decide on the best treatment for your medical problem, your doctor should be told:

—if you have ever had any unusual or allergic reaction to ethambutol.

—if you are on a low-salt, low-sugar, or any other special diet, or if you are allergic to any substance, such as foods, sulfites or other preservatives, or dyes.

Most medicines contain more than their active ingredient. Your doctor, nurse, or pharmacist can help you avoid products that may cause a problem.

—if you are **pregnant** or if you may become pregnant. Ethambutol has not been shown to cause birth defects or other problems in humans. However, studies in animals have shown that ethambutol causes cleft palate, skull and spine defects, absence of one eye, and hare lip. In addition, it is not known whether this medicine causes problems when taken with other TB medicines.

—if you are **breast-feeding**. Ethambutol passes into the breast milk. However, ethambutol has not been shown to cause problems in nursing babies.

—if you have any of the following medical problems:
   Gout
   Kidney disease
   Optic neuritis (eye nerve damage)

—if you are taking **any** other prescription or nonprescription (OTC) medicine.

Proper Use of This Medicine

Ethambutol may be taken with food if it upsets your stomach.

To help clear up your tuberculosis (TB) completely, **it is very important that you keep taking this medicine for the full time of treatment** even if you begin to feel better after a few weeks. You may have to take it every day for as long as 1 to 2 years or more. **It is important that you do not miss any doses.**

If you do miss a dose of this medicine, take it as soon as possible. However, if it is almost time for your next dose, skip the missed dose and go back to your regular dosing schedule. Do not double doses.

How to store this medicine:

• **Keep out of the reach of children.**

• Store away from heat and direct light.

• Do not store in the bathroom, near the kitchen sink, or in other damp places. Heat or moisture may cause the medicine to break down.

• Do not keep outdated medicine or medicine no longer needed. Be sure that any discarded medicine is out of the reach of children.

Precautions While Using This Medicine

If your symptoms do not improve within 2 to 3 weeks, or if they become worse, check with your doctor.

It is very important that your doctor check your progress at regular visits. In addition, you should **check with your doctor immediately if blurred vision, eye pain, red-green color blindness, or loss of vision occurs during treatment.** Your doctor may want you to have your eyes checked by an ophthalmologist (eye doctor).

In addition to this medicine causing blurred vision or any loss of vision, it may also cause some people to become dizzy. **Make sure you know how you react to this medicine before you drive, use machines, or do other jobs that require you to be alert or to see clearly.** If these reactions are especially bothersome, check with your doctor.

Side Effects of This Medicine

Along with its needed effects, a medicine may cause some unwanted effects. Although not all of these side effects may occur, if they do occur they may need medical attention.

Check with your doctor immediately if any of the following side effects occur:

Less common

Chills

Pain and swelling of joints, especially big toe, ankle, or knee

Tense, hot skin over affected joints

Rare

Blurred vision, eye pain, red-green color blindness, or any loss of vision (more common with high doses)

Numbness, tingling, burning pain, or weakness in hands or feet

Other side effects may occur that usually do not require medical attention. These side effects may go away during treatment as your body adjusts to the medicine. However, check with your doctor if any of the following side effects continue or are bothersome:

Less common

Dizziness

Skin rash or itching

Stomach upset

For elderly patients: Many medicines have not been tested in older people. Therefore, it is not known whether the medicine acts the same way it does in younger adults. Check with your doctor or pharmacist if you notice any unusual effects while taking this medicine or if you think it is not working as it should.

Other side effects not listed above may also occur in some patients. If you notice any other effects, check with your doctor.

December 1987

ETHCHLORVYNOL (Systemic)

A commonly used brand name is Placidyl.

To the Reader: If you do not recognize the names of medical conditions or medicines referred to in this information, check with your doctor, nurse, or pharmacist. Definitions for selected medical terms may be found in the Glossary. Brand names for the generic drug names listed can be found in the Index. In addition, selected brand names commonly associated with the generic name have been included in the text to help you recognize medicine you may be taking. The fact that a brand name product is not mentioned does not mean the information does not apply. It is a good idea for you to learn both the generic and brand names of your medicines and to write them down for future use.

Ethchlorvynol (eth-klor-VI-nole) is taken by mouth to treat insomnia (sleeplessness). It helps patients to sleep. However, if used regularly (for example, every day) for insomnia, it is usually not effective for more than 1 week.

This medicine is available only with your doctor's prescription.

Remember:

• **This medicine has been prescribed for your current medical problem only.** It must not be given to other people or used for other problems unless you are directed to do so by your doctor.

• **Keep all medicines out of the reach of children.**

• In order for this medicine to work, it must be used as directed.

• **It is very important that you read and understand the following information.** If any of the information causes you special concern, do not decide against using this medicine without first checking with your doctor.

• Before you begin using any new medicine (prescription or nonprescription) or if you develop any new medical problem while you are using this medicine, check with your doctor, nurse, or pharmacist.

• **If you have any questions** about the following information or if you want more information about this medicine or your medical problem, **ask your doctor, nurse, or pharmacist.**

Before Using This Medicine

In order to decide on the best treatment for your medical problem, your doctor should be told:

—if you have ever had any unusual or allergic reaction to ethchlorvynol.

—if you are on a low-salt, low-sugar, or any other special diet, or if you are allergic to any substance, such as foods, sulfites or other preservatives, or dyes. Most medicines contain more than their active ingredient. Your doctor, nurse, or pharmacist can help you avoid products that may cause a problem.

—if you are **pregnant** or if you may become pregnant. Studies have not been done in humans. However, use of ethchlorvynol during the first 6 months of pregnancy is not recommended because studies in animals have shown that high doses of ethchlorvynol increase the chance of stillbirths and decrease the chance of the newborn surviving. Taking ethchlorvynol during the last 3 months of pregnancy may cause slow heartbeat, shortness of breath, troubled breathing, or withdrawal side effects in the newborn baby.

—if you are **breast-feeding.** It is not known whether ethchlorvynol passes into the breast milk. This medicine has not been shown to cause problems in nursing babies.

—if you have any of the following medical problems:

    Kidney disease
    Liver disease
    Mental depression
    Porphyria

—if you are taking **any** other prescription or nonprescription (OTC) medicine, especially:

    Anticoagulants (blood thinners)
    Central nervous system (CNS) depressants

Proper Use of This Medicine

Ethchlorvynol is best taken with food or a glass of milk to lessen the possibility of dizziness, clumsiness, or unsteadiness, which may occur shortly after you take this medicine.

Take this medicine only as directed by your doctor. Do not take more of it, do not take it more often, and do not take it for a longer period of time than your doctor ordered. If too much is taken, it may become habit-forming.

How to store this medicine:

• **Keep out of the reach of children** since overdose is especially dangerous in children.

• Store away from heat and direct light.

• Do not store in the bathroom, near the kitchen sink, or in other damp places. Heat or moisture may cause the medicine to break down.

• Do not keep outdated medicine or medicine no longer needed. Be sure that any discarded medicine is out of the reach of children.

Precautions While Using This Medicine

If you will be taking this medicine regularly for a long period of time:

• Your doctor should check your progress at regular visits.

• Do not stop taking it without first checking with your doctor. Your doctor may want you to reduce gradually the amount you are taking before stopping completely.

This medicine will add to the effects of alcohol and other CNS depressants (medicines that slow down the nervous system, possibly causing drowsiness). Some examples of CNS depressants are antihistamines or medicine for hay fever, other allergies, or colds; sedatives, tranquilizers, or sleeping medicine; prescription pain

medicine or narcotics; barbiturates; medicine for convulsions (seizures); muscle relaxants; or anesthetics, including some dental anesthetics. **Check with your doctor before taking any of the above while you are taking this medicine.**

If you think you or someone else may have taken an overdose of this medicine, get emergency help at once. Taking an overdose of ethchlorvynol or taking alcohol or other CNS depressants with ethchlorvynol may lead to unconsciousness and possibly death. Some signs of an overdose are continuing confusion, severe weakness, shortness of breath or slow or troubled breathing, slurred speech, staggering, and slow heartbeat.

This medicine may cause some people to become dizzy, lightheaded, drowsy, or less alert than they are normally. Even if taken at bedtime, it may cause some people to feel drowsy or less alert on arising. **Make sure you know how you react to this medicine before you drive, use machines, or do other jobs that require you to be alert.**

Side Effects of This Medicine

Along with its needed effects, a medicine may cause some unwanted effects. Although not all of these side effects may occur, if they do occur they may need medical attention.

Check with your doctor as soon as possible if any of the following side effects occur:

Less common
 Skin rash or hives
 Unusual bleeding or bruising
 Unusual excitement, nervousness, or restlessness

Rare
 Darkening of urine
 Itching
 Pale stools
 Yellow eyes or skin

Signs of overdose
 Confusion (continuing)
 Double vision
 Low body temperature
 Numbness, tingling, pain, or weakness in hands or feet
 Shortness of breath or slow or troubled breathing
 Slow heartbeat
 Slurred speech

 Staggering
 Trembling
 Unusual movements of the eyes
 Weakness (severe)

Other side effects may occur that usually do not require medical attention. These side effects may go away during treatment as your body adjusts to the medicine. However, check with your doctor if any of the following side effects continue or are bothersome:

More common
 Blurred vision
 Dizziness or lightheadedness
 Indigestion
 Nausea or vomiting
 Numbness of face
 Stomach pain
 Unpleasant aftertaste
 Unusual tiredness or weakness

Less common
 Clumsiness or unsteadiness
 Confusion
 Drowsiness (daytime)

For elderly patients: The above side effects are more likely to occur in the elderly, who are usually more sensitive to the effects of ethchlorvynol.

After you stop using this medicine, your body may need time to adjust. If you took this medicine in high doses or for a long time, this may take up to 2 weeks. During this period of time check with your doctor if you notice any of the following side effects:

 Convulsions (seizures)
 Hallucinations (seeing, hearing, or feeling things that are not there)
 Muscle twitching
 Nausea or vomiting
 Restlessness, nervousness, or irritability
 Sweating
 Trembling
 Trouble in sleeping
 Weakness

Other side effects not listed above may also occur in some patients. If you notice any other effects, check with your doctor.

December 1987

ETHINAMATE (Systemic)

A commonly used brand name is Valmid.

To the Reader: If you do not recognize the names of medical conditions or medicines referred to in this information, check with your doctor, nurse, or pharmacist. Definitions for selected medical terms may be found in the Glossary. Brand names for the generic drug names listed can be found in the Index. In addition, selected brand names commonly associated with the generic name have been included in the text to help you recognize medicine you may be taking. The fact that a brand name product is not mentioned does not mean the information does not apply. It is a good idea for you to learn both the generic and brand names of your medicines and to write them down for future use.

Ethinamate (e-THIN-a-mate) is taken by mouth to treat insomnia (sleeplessness). It helps patients to sleep. However, if used regularly (for example, every day) for insomnia, it is usually not effective for more than 7 days.

This medicine is available only with your doctor's prescription.

Remember:
- **This medicine has been prescribed for your current medical problem only.** It must not be given to other people or used for other problems unless you are directed to do so by your doctor.

- **Keep all medicines out of the reach of children.**

- In order for this medicine to work, it must be used as directed.

- **It is very important that you read and understand the following information.** If any of the information causes you special concern, do not decide against using this medicine without first checking with your doctor.

- Before you begin using any new medicine (prescription or nonprescription) or if you develop any new medical problem while you are using this medicine, check with your doctor, nurse, or pharmacist.

- **If you have any questions** about the following information or if you want more information about this medicine or your medical problem, **ask your doctor, nurse, or pharmacist.**

Before Using This Medicine

In order to decide on the best treatment for your medical problem, your doctor should be told:

—if you have ever had any unusual or allergic reaction to ethinamate.

—if you are on a low-salt, low-sugar, or any other special diet, or if you are allergic to any substance, such as foods, sulfites or other preservatives, or dyes. Most medicines contain more than their active ingredient. Your doctor, nurse, or pharmacist can help you avoid products that may cause a problem.

—if you are **pregnant** or if you may become pregnant. Studies on birth defects have not been done in either humans or animals.

—if you are **breast-feeding**. It is not known whether ethinamate passes into the breast milk. This medicine has not been shown to cause problems in nursing babies.

—if you have mental depression.

—if you are taking **any** other prescription or nonprescription (OTC) medicine, especially central nervous system (CNS) depressants.

Proper Use of This Medicine

Take this medicine only as directed by your doctor. Do not take more of it, do not take it more often, and do not take it for a longer period of time than your doctor ordered. If too much is taken, it may become habit-forming.

How to store this medicine:

- **Keep out of the reach of children** since overdose is especially dangerous in children.

- Store away from heat and direct light.

- Do not store in the bathroom, near the kitchen sink, or in other damp places. Heat or moisture may cause the medicine to break down.

- Do not keep outdated medicine or medicine no longer needed. Be sure that any discarded medicine is out of the reach of children.

Precautions While Using This Medicine

If you will be taking this medicine regularly for a long period of time:

—your doctor should check your progress at regular visits.

—do not stop taking it without first checking with your doctor. Your doctor may want you to reduce gradually the amount you are taking before stopping completely.

This medicine will add to the effects of alcohol and other CNS depressants (medicines that slow down the nervous system, possibly causing drowsiness.) Some examples of CNS depressants are antihistamines or medicine for hay fever, other allergies, or colds; sedatives, tranquilizers, or sleeping medicine; prescription pain medicine or narcotics; barbiturates; medicine for convulsions (seizures); muscle relaxants; or anesthetics, including some dental anesthetics. **Check with your doctor before taking any of the above while you are taking this medicine.**

If you think you or someone else may have taken an overdose of this medicine, get emergency help at once. Taking an overdose of ethinamate or taking alcohol or other CNS depressants with ethinamate may lead to unconsciousness and possibly death. Some signs of an overdose are confusion, severe weakness, shortness of breath or slow or troubled breathing, slurred speech, staggering, and slow heartbeat.

This medicine may cause some people to become drowsy or less alert than they are normally. Even if taken at bedtime, it may cause some people to feel drowsy or less alert on arising. **Make sure you know how you react to this medicine before you drive, use machines, or do other jobs that require you to be alert.**

Side Effects of This Medicine

Along with its needed effects, a medicine may cause some unwanted effects. Although not all of these side effects may occur, if they do occur they may need medical attention.

Check with your doctor as soon as possible if any of the following side effects occur:

Less common
   Skin rash
   Unusual excitement (especially in children)

Rare
   Unusual bleeding or bruising

Signs of overdose
   Confusion
   Shortness of breath or slow or troubled breathing
   Slow heartbeat
   Slurred speech
   Staggering
   Weakness (severe)

Other side effects may occur that usually do not require medical attention. These side effects may go away during treatment as your body adjusts to the medicine.

However, check with your doctor if any of the following side effects continue or are bothersome:

Less common
   Indigestion
   Nausea
   Stomach pain
   Vomiting

Rare
   Drowsiness (daytime)

For elderly patients: The above side effects are more likely to occur in the elderly, who are usually more sensitive to the effects of ethinamate.

After you stop using this medicine, your body may need time to adjust. The length of time this takes depends on the amount of medicine you were using and how long you used it. During this period of time check with your doctor if you notice any of the following side effects:
   Confusion
   Convulsions (seizures)
   Hallucinations (seeing, hearing, or feeling things that are not there)
   Restlessness, nervousness, or irritability
   Trembling
   Trouble in sleeping

Other side effects not listed above may also occur in some patients. If you notice any other effects, check with your doctor.

December 1987

ETHIONAMIDE (Systemic)

A commonly used brand name is Trecator-SC.

To the Reader: If you do not recognize the names of medical conditions or medicines referred to in this information, check with your doctor, nurse, or pharmacist. Definitions for selected medical terms may be found in the Glossary. Brand names for the generic drug names listed can be found in the Index. In addition, selected brand names commonly associated with the generic name have been included in the text to help you recognize medicine you may be taking. The fact that a brand name product is not mentioned does not mean the information does not apply. It is a good idea for you to learn both the generic and brand names of your medicines and to write them down for future use.

Ethionamide (e-thye-on-AM-ide) belongs to the general family of medicines called anti-infectives. It is used to help the body overcome tuberculosis (TB). It is taken by mouth with one or more other medicines for TB. Ethionamide may also be used for other problems as determined by your doctor.

Ethionamide is available only with your doctor's prescription.

Remember:

• **This medicine has been prescribed for your present TB infection only.** Another TB infection later on may require a different medicine. Also, even though other people may have the same symptoms as you, they may have a different kind of TB. Your medicine may not work for them and may even cause them harm. Therefore, **your medicine must not be given to other people or used for other infections** unless you are otherwise directed by your doctor.

• **Keep all medicines out of the reach of children.**

• In order for this medicine to work, it must be used as directed.

• **It is very important that you read and understand the following information.** If any of the information causes you special concern, do not decide against using this medicine without first checking with your doctor.

• Before you begin using any new medicine (prescription or nonprescription) or if you develop any new medical problem while you are using this medicine, check with your doctor, nurse, or pharmacist.

• **If you have any questions** about the following information or if you want more information about this medicine or your medical problem, **ask your doctor, nurse, or pharmacist.**

Before Using This Medicine

In order to decide on the best treatment for your medical problem, your doctor should be told:

—if you have ever had any unusual or allergic reaction to isoniazid, pyrazinamide, or niacin (nicotinic acid).

—if you are on a low-salt, low-sugar, or any other special diet, or if you are allergic to any substance, such as foods, sulfites or other preservatives, or dyes.

Most medicines contain more than their active ingredient. Your doctor, nurse, or pharmacist can help you avoid products that may cause a problem.

—if you are **pregnant** or if you may become pregnant. Use is not recommended during pregnancy since ethionamide causes birth defects in rats and rabbits given doses greater than the usual human dose. In addition, it is not known whether this medicine causes problems when taken with other TB medicines.

—if you are **breast-feeding**. However, ethionamide has not been shown to cause problems in nursing babies.

—if you have either of the following medical problems:
   Diabetes mellitus (sugar diabetes)
   Liver disease (severe)

—if you are taking **any** other prescription or nonprescription (OTC) medicine, especially cycloserine (e.g., Seromycin).

Proper Use of This Medicine

Ethionamide may be taken with or after meals if it upsets your stomach.

To help clear up your tuberculosis (TB) completely, **it is very important that you keep taking this medicine for the full time of treatment** even if you begin to feel better after a few weeks. You may have to take it every day for 1 to 2 years or more. **It is important that you do not miss any doses.**

Your doctor may also want you to take pyridoxine (vitamin B_6) every day to help prevent or lessen some of the side effects of ethionamide. If so, **it is very important to take pyridoxine every day along with this medicine. Do not miss any doses.**

If you do miss a dose of either of these medicines, take it as soon as possible. However, if it is almost time for your next dose, skip the missed dose and go back to your regular dosing schedule. Do not double doses.

How to store this medicine:

• **Keep out of the reach of children.**

• Store away from heat and direct light.

• Do not store in the bathroom, near the kitchen sink, or in other damp places. Heat or moisture may cause the medicine to break down.

• Do not keep outdated medicine or medicine no longer needed. Be sure that any discarded medicine is out of the reach of children.

Precautions While Using This Medicine

If your symptoms do not improve within 2 to 3 weeks, or if they become worse, check with your doctor.

It is very important that your doctor check your progress at regular visits. Also, **check with your doctor immediately if blurred vision or any loss of vision, with or without eye pain, occurs during treatment.** Your doctor may want you to have your eyes checked by an ophthalmologist (eye doctor).

Some people who take ethionamide may become more sensitive to sunlight than they are normally. **When you first begin taking this medicine, avoid too much sun and do not use a sunlamp until you see how you react to the sun,** especially if you tend to burn easily. **If you have a severe reaction, check with your doctor.**

This medicine may also cause blurred vision or loss of vision, or it may cause some people to become dizzy, drowsy, or less alert than they are normally. **Make sure you know how you react to this medicine before you drive, use machines, or do other jobs that require you to be alert or to see clearly.** If these reactions are especially bothersome, check with your doctor.

If this medicine causes clumsiness; unsteadiness; or numbness, tingling, burning, or pain in the hands and feet, check with your doctor immediately. These may be early warning signs of more serious nerve problems that could develop later.

Side Effects of This Medicine

Along with its needed effects, a medicine may cause some unwanted effects. Although not all of these side effects may occur, if they do occur they may need medical attention.

Check with your doctor immediately if any of the following side effects occur:

More common

Mental depression

Less common

Clumsiness or unsteadiness
Confusion
Mood or other mental changes
Numbness, tingling, burning, or pain in hands and feet
Yellow eyes or skin

Rare

Blurred vision or any loss of vision, with or without eye pain
Changes in menstrual periods
Coldness

Decreased sexual ability (in males)
Dry, puffy skin
Pain, stiffness, or swelling of joints
Swelling of front part of neck
Weight gain

Other side effects may occur that usually do not require medical attention. These side effects may go away during treatment as your body adjusts to the medicine. However, check with your doctor if any of the following side effects continue or are bothersome:

More common

Diarrhea
Dizziness (especially when getting up from a lying or sitting position)
Drowsiness
Increased amount of saliva or drooling
Loss of appetite
Metallic taste
Nausea or vomiting
Sore mouth
Stomach pain or upset
Weakness

Less common or rare

Acne
Enlargement of the breasts (in males)
Hair loss
Increased sensitivity of skin to sunlight
Skin rash

For elderly patients: Many medicines have not been tested in older people. Therefore, it is not known whether the medicine acts the same way it does in younger adults. Check with your doctor or pharmacist if you notice any unusual effects while taking this medicine or if you think it is not working as it should.

Other side effects not listed above may also occur in some patients. If you notice any other effects, check with your doctor.

December 1987

ETIDRONATE (Systemic)

A commonly used brand name is Didronel.

To the Reader: If you do not recognize the names of medical conditions or medicines referred to in this information, check with your doctor, nurse, or pharmacist. Definitions for selected medical terms may be found in the Glossary. Brand names for the generic drug names listed can be found in the Index. In addition, selected brand names commonly associated with the generic name have been included in the text to help you recognize medicine you may be taking. The fact that a brand name product is not mentioned does not mean the information does not apply. It is a good idea for you to learn both the generic and brand names of your medicines and to write them down for future use.

Etidronate (eh-tih-DROE-nate) is taken by mouth to treat Paget's disease of bone. It may also be used to treat or prevent a certain type of bone problem that may occur after hip replacement surgery or spinal injury.

Etidronate is given by injection and sometimes taken by mouth to treat hypercalcemia (too much calcium in the blood) that may occur with some types of cancer.

This medicine is available only with your doctor's prescription.

Remember:

• **This medicine has been prescribed for your current medical problem only.** It must not be given to other people or used for other problems unless you are directed to do so by your doctor.

• **Keep all medicines out of the reach of children.**

• In order for this medicine to work, it must be used as directed.

• If you are receiving this medicine by injection, some of the information about this medicine may not apply.

• **It is very important that you read and understand the following information.** If any of the information causes you special concern, do not decide against using this medicine without first checking with your doctor.

• Before you begin using any new medicine (prescription or nonprescription) or if you develop any new medical problem while you are using this medicine, check with your doctor, nurse, or pharmacist.

• **If you have any questions** about the following information or if you want more information about this medicine or your medical problem, **ask your doctor, nurse, or pharmacist.**

Before Using This Medicine

In order to decide on the best treatment for your medical problem, your doctor should be told:

—if you have ever had any unusual or allergic reaction to etidronate.

—if you are on a low-salt, low-sugar, or any other special diet, or if you are allergic to any substance, such as foods, sulfites or other preservatives, or dyes. Most medicines contain more than their active ingredient. Your doctor, nurse, or pharmacist can help you avoid products that may cause a problem.

—if you are **pregnant** or if you may become pregnant. Studies have not been done in humans. However, studies in rats injected with large doses of etidronate have shown that etidronate causes deformed bones in the fetus.

—if you are **breast-feeding**. It is not known if etidronate passes into breast milk. However, this medicine has not been shown to cause problems in nursing babies.

—if you have any of the following medical problems:
  Bone fracture, especially of arm or leg
  Intestinal or bowel disease
  Kidney disease

—if you are taking **any** other prescription or nonprescription (OTC) medicine, especially:
  Antacids containing calcium, magnesium, or aluminum
  Mineral supplements or other medicines containing calcium, iron, magnesium, or aluminum

—if your diet now includes foods containing large amounts of calcium, such as milk or other dairy products.

Proper Use of This Medicine

Take etidronate with black coffee, tea, fruit juice, or water on an empty stomach at least 2 hours before or after food (midmorning is best) or at bedtime. Food may decrease the amount of etidronate absorbed by your body.

Take etidronate only as directed. Do not take more of it, do not take it more often, and do not take it for a longer period of time than your doctor ordered. To do so may increase the chance of side effects.

In some patients, etidronate takes up to three months to work. If you feel that the medicine is not working, do not stop taking it on your own. Instead, check with your doctor.

It is important that you eat a well-balanced diet with an adequate amount of calcium and vitamin D (found in milk or other dairy products). Too much or too little of either may increase the chance of side effects while you are taking etidronate. Your doctor can help you choose the meal plan that is best for you. **However, do not take milk, milk formulas, or other dairy products, antacids, mineral supplements, or other medicines that are high in calcium or iron (high amounts of these minerals may also be in some vitamin preparations), magnesium, or aluminum** within 2 hours of taking etidronate. To do so may keep this medicine from working as well.

If you miss a dose of this medicine, take it as soon as possible. However, if it is almost time for your next dose, skip the missed dose and go back to your regular dosing schedule. Do not double doses.

How to store this medicine:

• **Keep out of the reach of children.**

• Store away from heat and direct light.

• Do not store in the bathroom, near the kitchen sink, or in other damp places. Heat or moisture may cause the medicine to break down.

• Do not keep outdated medicine or medicine no longer needed. Be sure that any discarded medicine is out of the reach of children.

Precautions While Using This Medicine

It is important that your doctor check your progress at regular visits even if you are between treatments and are not taking this medicine. If your condition has improved and your doctor has told you to stop taking etidronate, your progress must still be checked. The results of laboratory tests or the occurrence of certain symptoms will tell your doctor if more medicine must be taken. Your doctor may want you to begin another course of treatment after you have been off the medicine for at least 3 months.

If this medicine causes you to have nausea or diarrhea and it continues, check with your doctor. The dose may need to be changed.

Side Effects of This Medicine

Along with its needed effects, a medicine may cause some unwanted effects. Although not all of these side effects may occur, if they do occur they may need medical attention.

Check with your doctor as soon as possible if any of the following side effects occur:

More common

Bone pain or tenderness (increased, continuing, or returning—in patients with Paget's disease)

Less common

Bone fractures, especially of the thigh bone

Rare

Skin rash (red, raised, and itchy)

Other side effects may occur that usually do not require medical attention. These side effects may go away during treatment as your body adjusts to the medicine. However, check with your doctor if any of the following side effects continue or are bothersome:

More common—at higher doses

Diarrhea
Nausea

Less common—with injection

Loss of taste or metallic or altered taste

Other side effects not listed above may also occur in some patients. If you notice any other effects, check with your doctor.

December 1987

ETOPOSIDE (Systemic)

Some commonly used brand names or other names are VePesid and
VP-16.

To the Reader: If you do not recognize the names of medical
conditions or medicines referred to in this information, check
with your doctor, nurse, or pharmacist. Definitions for selected
medical terms may be found in the Glossary. Brand names for
the generic drug names listed can be found in the Index. In
addition, selected brand names commonly associated with the
generic name have been included in the text to help you recognize medicine you may be taking. The fact that a brand name
product is not mentioned does not mean the information does
not apply. It is a good idea for you to learn both the generic
and brand names of your medicines and to write them down
for future use.

Etoposide (e-TOE-poe-side) belongs to the group of
medicines known as antineoplastic agents. It is used to
treat cancer of the testicles and certain types of lung
cancer. It is also sometimes given to treat some other
kinds of cancer in both males and females.

The exact way that etoposide acts against cancer is
not known. However, it seems to interfere with the growth
of the cancer cells, which are eventually destroyed. Since
the growth of normal body cells may also be affected by
etoposide, other effects will also occur. Some of these
may be serious and must be reported to your doctor.
Other effects, like hair loss, may not be serious but may
cause concern. Some effects may not occur for months
or years after the medicine is used.

Before you begin treatment with etoposide, you and
your doctor should talk about the good this medicine will
do as well as the risks of using it.

This medicine is available only with your doctor's prescription.

Remember:

• **This medicine has been prescribed for your current
medical problem only.** It must not be given to other
people or used for other problems unless you are directed to do so by your doctor.

• **Keep all medicines out of the reach of children.**

• In order for this medicine to work, it must be used
as directed.

• If you are receiving this medicine by injection, some
of the information about this medicine may not apply.

• **It is very important that you read and understand the
following information.** If any of the information causes
you special concern, do not decide against using this
medicine without first checking with your doctor.

• Before you begin using any new medicine (prescription or nonprescription) or if you develop any new
medical problem while you are using this medicine,
check with your doctor, nurse, or pharmacist.

• **If you have any questions** about the following information or if you want more information about this
medicine or your medical problem, **ask your doctor,
nurse, or pharmacist.**

Before Using This Medicine

In order to decide on the best treatment for your medical
problem, your doctor should be told:

—if you have ever had any unusual or allergic reaction
to etoposide.

—if you are **pregnant** or if you intend to have children.
There is a good chance that this medicine will cause
birth defects if it is being used at the time of conception or during pregnancy. In addition, many cancer
medicines may cause sterility which could be permanent. Although this has not been reported with etoposide, the possibility should be kept in mind. Be sure
that you have discussed this with your doctor before
receiving this medicine.

—if you intend to **breast-feed**. Because etoposide may
cause serious side effects, breast-feeding is generally
not recommended while you are receiving it.

—if you have any of the following medical problems:
  Chickenpox (including recent exposure)
  Herpes zoster (shingles)
  Infection
  Kidney disease
  Liver disease

—if you are taking **any** other prescription or nonpre-
cription (OTC) medicine, especially:
  Amphotericin B by injection (e.g., Fungizone)
  Antithyroid agents (medicine for overactive thyroid)
  Azathioprine (e.g., Imuran)
  Chloramphenicol (e.g., Chloromycetin)
  Colchicine
  Flucytosine (e.g., Ancobon)
  Interferon (e.g., Intron A; Roferon-A)

—if you have ever been treated with x-rays or cancer
medicines.

Proper Use of This Medicine

Take etoposide only as directed by your doctor. Do not
use more or less of it, and do not use it more often
than your doctor ordered. The exact amount of medicine you need has been carefully worked out. Taking
too much may increase the chance of side effects,
while taking too little may not improve your condition.

Etoposide is sometimes given together with certain other
medicines. If you are using a combination of medicines, make sure that you take each one at the proper
time and do not mix them. If you are taking some of
these medicines by mouth, ask your doctor, nurse, or
pharmacist to help you plan a way to remember to
take your medicines at the right times.

Etoposide often causes nausea, vomiting, and loss of appetite, which may be severe. However, it is very important that you continue to receive the medicine, even
if you begin to feel ill. Ask your doctor, nurse, or
pharmacist for ways to lessen these effects.

If you vomit shortly after taking a dose of etoposide,
check with your doctor. You will be told whether to
take the dose again or to wait until the next dose.

© 1988   The United States Pharmacopeial Convention, Inc.

If you miss a dose of this medicine, do not take the missed dose at all and do not double the next one. Instead, go back to your regular dosing schedule and check with your doctor.

How to store this medicine:

• **Keep out of the reach of children.**

• Store away from heat and direct light.

• Do not store in the bathroom, near the kitchen sink, or in other damp places. Heat or moisture may cause the medicine to break down.

• Do not keep outdated medicine or medicine no longer needed. Be sure that any discarded medicine is out of the reach of children.

Precautions While Using This Medicine

It is very important that your doctor check your progress at regular visits to make sure that etoposide is working properly and to check for unwanted effects.

While you are being treated with etoposide, and after you stop treatment with it, **do not have any immunizations without your doctor's approval**. Etoposide lowers your body's resistance and there is a chance you might get the infection the immunization is meant to prevent. In addition, other persons living in your household should not take oral polio vaccine since there is a chance they could pass the polio virus on to you. Also, you should avoid close contact with other persons (for example, at school or work) who have taken oral polio vaccine.

Etoposide can lower the number of white blood cells in your body. This may increase the chance of getting an infection. If you can, avoid people with colds or other infections. If you think you are getting a cold or other infection, check with your doctor.

Side Effects of This Medicine

Along with their needed effects, medicines like etoposide can sometimes cause unwanted effects such as blood problems, loss of hair, and other side effects; these are described below. Also, because of the way these medicines act on the body, there is a chance that they might cause other unwanted effects that may not occur until months or years after the medicine is used. These delayed effects may include certain types of cancer, such as leukemia. Discuss these possible effects with your doctor.

Although not all of these side effects may occur, if they do occur they may need medical attention.

Check with your doctor or nurse immediately if any of the following side effects occur:
More common
    Fever, chills, or sore throat
    Unusual bleeding or bruising

Check with your doctor or nurse as soon as possible if any of the following side effects occur:
Less common
    Sores in the mouth or on the lips
Rare
    Difficulty in walking
    Fast heartbeat
    Numbness or tingling in fingers and toes
    Pain at the place of injection
    Shortness of breath or wheezing
    Weakness

Other side effects may occur that usually do not require medical attention. These side effects may go away during treatment as your body adjusts to the medicine. Also, your doctor or nurse may be able to tell you about ways to prevent or reduce some of these side effects. Check with your doctor or nurse if any of the following side effects continue or are bothersome or if you have any questions about them:
More common
    Loss of appetite
    Nausea and vomiting
Less common
    Diarrhea
    Unusual tiredness

This medicine often causes a temporary loss of hair. After treatment with etoposide has ended, normal hair growth should return.

For elderly patients: Many medicines have not been tested in older people. Therefore, it is not known whether the medicine acts the same way it does in younger adults. Check with your doctor or pharmacist if you notice any unusual effects while taking this medicine or if you think it is not working as it should.

Other side effects not listed above may also occur in some patients. If you notice any other effects, check with your doctor or nurse.

December 1987

ETRETINATE (Systemic)

A commonly used brand name is Tegison.

To the Reader: If you do not recognize the names of medical conditions or medicines referred to in this information, check with your doctor, nurse, or pharmacist. Definitions for selected medical terms may be found in the Glossary. Brand names for the generic drug names listed can be found in the Index. In addition, selected brand names commonly associated with the generic name have been included in the text to help you recognize medicine you may be taking. The fact that a brand name product is not mentioned does not mean the information does not apply. It is a good idea for you to learn both the generic and brand names of your medicines and to write them down for future use.

Etretinate (e-TRET-i-nate) is taken by mouth to treat severe psoriasis. It is usually used only after other medicines have been used and have failed to help the psoriasis.

It is recommended that etretinate not be used to treat children unless all other forms of therapy have been tried first and have failed. Etretinate may interfere with bone growth. In addition, children may be more sensitive to the side effects of the medicine.

This medicine is available only with your doctor's prescription.

Remember:

• **This medicine has been prescribed for your current medical problem only.** It must not be given to other people or used for other problems unless you are directed to do so by your doctor.

• **Keep all medicines out of the reach of children.**

• In order for this medicine to work, it must be used as directed.

• **It is very important that you read and understand the following information.** If any of the information causes you special concern, do not decide against using this medicine without first checking with your doctor.

• Before you begin using any new medicine (prescription or nonprescription) or if you develop any new medical problem while you are using this medicine, check with your doctor, nurse, or pharmacist.

• **If you have any questions** about the following information or if you want more information about this medicine or your medical problem, **ask your doctor, nurse, or pharmacist.**

Before Using This Medicine

In order to decide on the best treatment for your medical problem, your doctor should be told:

—if you have ever had any unusual or allergic reaction to etretinate, isotretinoin, or tretinoin or to vitamin A–like preparations.

—if you are on a low-salt, low-sugar, or any other special diet, or if you are allergic to any substance, such as foods, sulfites or other preservatives, or dyes. Most medicines contain more than their active ingredient. Your doctor or pharmacist can help you avoid products that may cause a problem.

—if you are **pregnant** or if you may become pregnant. Etretinate must not be taken during pregnancy because it has been shown to cause birth defects in humans. In addition, since it is not known how long pregnancy should be avoided after treatment stops, you should plan on not having children during or after you are treated with etretinate. If you are able to bear children, you should have a pregnancy test within 2 weeks before beginning treatment with etretinate to make sure you are not pregnant. Therapy with etretinate should then be started on the second or third day of your next normal menstrual period. Also, etretinate should not be taken unless an effective form of contraception (birth control) is used for at least 1 month before beginning treatment. Contraception should be continued during treatment and for as long as you are able to become pregnant after etretinate is stopped. Be sure you have discussed this with your doctor.

—if you are **breast-feeding**. It is not known whether etretinate passes into the breast milk. However, etretinate is not recommended during breast-feeding or if you plan to breast-feed in the future because it may cause unwanted effects in nursing babies.

—if you have any of the following medical problems:
    Diabetes mellitus (sugar diabetes) (or a family history of)
    Heart or blood vessel disease (or history of increased risk of or family history of)
    Liver disease (or history of or family history of)
    Overweight (severe)

—if you or any member of your family has a history of high triglyceride (fat-like substance) levels in the blood.

—if you drink or have a history of drinking a lot of alcoholic beverages.

—if you are taking **any** other prescription or nonprescription (OTC) medicine, especially:
    Isotretinoin (e.g., Accutane)
    Methotrexate
    Tetracyclines
    Tretinoin (vitamin A acid) (e.g., Retin A)
    Vitamin A or any preparation containing vitamin A

—if you are now using any other topical acne preparation or preparation containing a peeling agent, such as benzoyl peroxide, resorcinol, salicylic acid, sulfur, or tretinoin (vitamin A acid).

—if you are now using any topical alcohol-containing preparation such as after-shave lotion, astringent, cologne, perfume, or shaving cream or lotion.

—if you are now using any of the following preparations:
    Abrasive or medicated soaps or cleansers
    Cosmetics or soaps that dry the skin
    Medicated cosmetics or "cover-ups"
    Other topical medicine for the skin

Proper Use of This Medicine

Take each dose of etretinate with milk or a fatty food. This is important because fats taken with etretinate help the medicine to be absorbed better. However, the rest of the time, you should follow a low-fat diet.

It is very important that you take etretinate only as directed. Do not take more of it, do not take it more often, and do not take it for a longer period of time than your doctor ordered. To do so may increase the chance of side effects.

If you miss a dose of this medicine, take it as soon as possible with milk or a fatty food. However, if it is almost time for your next dose, skip the missed dose and go back to your regular dosing schedule. Do not double doses.

How to store this medicine:

- **Keep out of the reach of children.**

- Store away from heat and direct light.

- Do not store in the bathroom, near the kitchen sink, or in other damp places. Heat or moisture may cause the medicine to break down.

- Do not keep outdated medicine or medicine no longer needed. Be sure that any discarded medicine is out of the reach of children.

Precautions While Using This Medicine

Your doctor should check your progress at regular visits to make sure this medicine does not cause unwanted effects.

Etretinate has been shown to cause birth defects in humans if taken during pregnancy. In addition, it is not known how long pregnancy should be avoided after treatment stops in order to prevent birth defects. Therefore, you should plan on not having children during treatment or in the future after being treated with etretinate. For as long as you are able to become pregnant, you should use a reliable form of birth control. In addition, you should not change your birth control method unless you have checked with your doctor first. If you suspect that you may have become pregnant while taking etretinate, stop taking the medicine immediately and check with your doctor. Also, if you become pregnant at any time after you have stopped taking this medicine, check with your doctor as soon as possible. In either case, you should talk to your doctor about the risks of continuing the pregnancy.

Do not donate blood to a blood bank while you are taking etretinate and for several years or longer after you stop taking it. This is to prevent the possibility of a pregnant patient receiving your blood. Check with your doctor to see how long you should wait before donating blood.

Do not take vitamin A or any vitamin supplement containing vitamin A while you are taking this medicine. To do so may increase the chance of side effects.

Drinking too much alcohol or eating a high-fat diet while you are taking this medicine may cause high triglyceride (fat-like substance) levels in the blood. This may possibly increase the chance of heart and blood vessel disease. Therefore, **while taking this medicine, do not drink alcoholic beverages or, at least, reduce the amount**

you usually drink. In addition, you should reduce the amount of high-fat foods that you eat. If you have any questions about this, check with your doctor.

Diabetics—Etretinate may cause a change in your blood sugar levels. If you notice a change in the results of your blood or urine sugar test or if you have any questions, check with your doctor.

Etretinate may cause dryness of the eyes. Therefore, if you wear contact lenses, your eyes may be more sensitive to them during the time you are taking etretinate and for several weeks or longer after you stop taking it. To help relieve dryness of the eyes, check with your doctor about using an eye lubricating solution, such as artificial tears. If your eyes become inflamed, check with your doctor.

Some people who take this medicine may become more sensitive to sunlight than they are normally. When you first begin taking this medicine, avoid too much sun and do not use a sunlamp until you see how you react to the sun, especially if you tend to burn easily. If you have a severe reaction, check with your doctor.

Your mouth and nose may feel very dry while you are taking this medicine. For temporary relief of mouth dryness, use sugarless candy or gum, melt bits of ice in your mouth, or use a saliva substitute. However, if dry mouth continues for more than 2 weeks, check with your dentist. Continuing dryness of the mouth may increase the chance of dental disease, including tooth decay, gum disease, and fungal infections.

During the first month of treatment with etretinate, your psoriasis may seem to get worse before it gets better. There may be more redness or itching, but this usually goes away during treatment. It may take 2 or 3 months before the full effects of etretinate are seen. If irritation or other symptoms of your condition become severe, check with your doctor.

Side Effects of This Medicine

Along with its needed effects, a medicine may cause some unwanted effects. Although not all of these side effects may occur, if they do occur they may need medical attention.

Stop taking this medicine and check with your doctor immediately if any of the following side effects occur:

Less common

    Blurred or double vision or other changes in vision
    Dark-colored urine
    Flu-like symptoms
    Yellow eyes or skin

Rare

    Headache (severe or continuing)
    Nausea and vomiting

Check with your doctor as soon as possible if any of the following side effects occur:

More common

Bone or joint pain, tenderness, or stiffness; muscle cramps

Burning, redness, itching, feeling of dryness, pain, tenderness, excessive tearing (continuing), or other sign of inflammation or irritation of eyes

Cramps or pain in upper abdomen or stomach area

Unusual bruising

Less common

Change in hearing, earache or pain in ear, or drainage from ear

Rare

Bleeding or inflammation of gums

Confusion, mental depression, or mood or mental changes

Other side effects may occur that usually do not require medical attention. These side effects may go away during treatment as your body adjusts to the medicine. However, check with your doctor if any of the following side effects continue or are bothersome:

More common

Changes in appetite

Chapped lips

Dryness of nose or nosebleeds

Dryness, redness, scaling, itching, rash, or other sign of inflammation or irritation of the skin; increased sensitivity of skin to sunlight

Headache (mild)

Increased sensitivity to contact lenses (may occur during and after therapy)

Peeling of skin on fingertips, palms of hands, or soles of feet

Thinning of hair

Unusual thirst

Unusual tiredness

Less common

Dizziness

Dryness of mouth; soreness of tongue; or soreness, cracking, swelling, or unusual redness of lips

Fever

Nausea (mild)

Redness or soreness around fingernails; loosening of the fingernails

For elderly patients: Many medicines have not been tested in older people. Therefore, it is not known whether the medicine acts the same way it does in younger adults. Check with your doctor or pharmacist if you notice any unusual effects while taking this medicine or if you do not think it is working as it should.

Other side effects not listed above may also occur in some patients. If you notice any other effects, check with your doctor.

_____

December 1987

FAMOTIDINE (Systemic)

A commonly used brand name is Pepcid.

To the Reader: If you do not recognize the names of medical conditions or medicines referred to in this information, check with your doctor, nurse, or pharmacist. Definitions for selected medical terms may be found in the Glossary. Brand names for the generic drug names listed can be found in the Index. In addition, selected brand names commonly associated with the generic name have been included in the text to help you recognize medicine you may be taking. The fact that a brand name product is not mentioned does not mean the information does not apply. It is a good idea for you to learn both the generic and brand names of your medicines and to write them down for future use.

Famotidine (fa-MOE-ti-deen) is used to treat duodenal ulcers and prevent their return. It is also used to treat some conditions in which the stomach produces too much acid, such as in Zollinger-Ellison disease.

Famotidine works by decreasing the amount of acid produced by the stomach.

Famotidine is available only with your doctor's prescription.

Remember:

• **This medicine has been prescribed for your current medical problem only.** It must not be given to other people or used for other problems unless you are directed to do so by your doctor.

• **Keep all medicines out of the reach of children.**

• In order for this medicine to work, it must be used as directed.

• If you are receiving this medicine by injection, some of the information about this medicine may not apply.

• **It is very important that you read and understand the following information.** If any of the information causes you special concern, do not decide against using this medicine without first checking with your doctor.

• Before you begin using any new medicine (prescription or nonprescription) or if you develop any new medical problem while you are using this medicine, check with your doctor, nurse, or pharmacist.

• **If you have any questions** about the following information or if you want more information about this medicine or your medical problem, **ask your doctor, nurse, or pharmacist.**

Before Using This Medicine

In order to decide on the best treatment for your medical problem, your doctor should be told:

—if you have ever had any unusual or allergic reaction to cimetidine, famotidine, or ranitidine.

—if you are on a low-salt, low-sugar, or any other special diet, or if you are allergic to any substance, such as foods, sulfites or other preservatives, or dyes. Most medicines contain more than their active ingredient. Your doctor, nurse, or pharmacist can help you avoid products that may cause a problem.

—if you are **pregnant** or if you may become pregnant. Studies have not been done in humans. However, famotidine has not been shown to cause birth defects or other problems in animal studies.

—if you are **breast-feeding**. It is not known whether famotidine passes into the breast milk. However, this medicine has not been shown to cause problems in nursing babies.

—if you have any of the following medical problems:
Kidney disease
Liver disease

—if you are taking **any** other prescription or nonprescription (OTC) medicine, especially ketoconazole (e.g., Nizoral).

Proper Use of This Medicine

For patients taking:

• A single dose a day—Take it at bedtime.

• Two doses a day—Take one dose in the morning and one at bedtime.

It may take several days for famotidine to begin to relieve stomach pain. Antacids may be taken with famotidine to help relieve pain, unless your doctor has told you not to use them.

Take this medicine for the full time of treatment, even if you begin to feel better. Also, it is important that you keep your doctor's appointments for check-ups so that your doctor will be better able to tell you when to stop taking this medicine.

If you miss a dose of this medicine, take it as soon as possible. However, if it is almost time for your next dose, skip the missed dose and go back to your regular dosing schedule. Do not double doses.

How to store this medicine:

• **Keep out of the reach of children.**

• Store away from heat and direct light.

• Do not store the tablet form of this medicine in the bathroom, near the kitchen sink, or in other damp places. Heat or moisture may cause the medicine to break down.

• Protect the liquid form of this medicine from freezing.

• Do not keep outdated medicine or medicine no longer needed. Be sure that any discarded medicine is out of the reach of children.

Precautions While Using This Medicine

Before you have any skin tests for allergies, tell the doctor in charge that you are taking this medicine. The results of the test may be affected by this medicine.

Remember that certain medicines, such as aspirin, and certain foods and drinks irritate the stomach and may make your problem worse.

Cigarette smoking tends to decrease the effect of famotidine by increasing the amount of acid produced by the stomach. This is more likely to affect the stomach's night-time production of acid. While taking famotidine, stop smoking completely, or at least do not smoke after taking the last dose of the day.

Follow your doctor's orders and check with him or her if your ulcer pain continues or gets worse.

Side Effects of This Medicine

Along with its needed effects, a medicine may cause some unwanted effects. Although not all of these side effects may occur, if they do occur they may need medical attention.

Check with your doctor as soon as possible if any of the following side effects occur:

Rare
   Fast or pounding heartbeat
   Fever
   Swelling of eyelids
   Tightness in chest
   Unusual bleeding or bruising
   Unusual tiredness or weakness (severe)

Other side effects may occur that usually do not require medical attention. These side effects may go away during treatment as your body adjusts to the medicine.

However, check with your doctor if any of the following side effects continue or are bothersome:

Less common or rare
   Anxiety
   Constipation
   Decrease in sexual desire
   Diarrhea
   Dizziness or headache
   Drowsiness
   Dryness of mouth or skin
   Joint or muscle pain
   Loss of appetite
   Mental depression
   Nausea or vomiting
   Ringing or buzzing in ears
   Skin rash or itching
   Stomach pain
   Temporary loss of hair
   Unusual taste

For elderly patients: Many medicines have not been tested in older people. Therefore, it is not known whether the medicine acts the same way it does in younger adults. Check with your doctor or pharmacist if you notice any unusual effects while taking this medicine or if you think it is not working as it should.

Other side effects not listed above may also occur in some patients. If you notice any other effects, check with your doctor.

_____

December 1987

_____

FENFLURAMINE (Systemic)

Some commonly used brand names are:

Ponderal*	Pondimin
Ponderal Pacaps*	Pondimin Extentabs*

*Not available in the United States.

To the Reader: If you do not recognize the names of medical conditions or medicines referred to in this information, check with your doctor, nurse, or pharmacist. Definitions for selected medical terms may be found in the Glossary. Brand names for the generic drug names listed can be found in the Index. In addition, selected brand names commonly associated with the generic name have been included in the text to help you recognize medicine you may be taking. The fact that a brand name product is not mentioned does not mean the information does not apply. It is a good idea for you to learn both the generic and brand names of your medicines and to write them down for future use.

Fenfluramine (fen-FLURE-a-meen) belongs to the group of medicines called appetite suppressants. It is used in the short-term (a few weeks) treatment of obesity to help patients lose weight.

For a few weeks (6 to 12), fenfluramine in combination with dieting, exercise, and changes in eating habits can help patients lose weight. However, since its appetite-reducing effect is only temporary, it is useful only for the first few weeks of dieting until new eating habits are established. It is not effective for continuous use in diet control.

Fenfluramine may also be used for other conditions as determined by your doctor.

This medicine is available only with your doctor's prescription.

Remember:

• **This medicine has been prescribed for your current medical problem only.** It must not be given to other people or used for other problems unless you are directed to do so by your doctor.

• **Keep all medicines out of the reach of children.**

• In order for this medicine to work, it must be used as directed.

• **It is very important that you read and understand the following information.** If any of the information causes you special concern, do not decide against using this medicine without first checking with your doctor.

• Before you begin using any new medicine (prescription or nonprescription) or if you develop any new medical problem while you are using this medicine, check with your doctor, nurse, or pharmacist.

• **If you have any questions** about the following information or if you want more information about this medicine or your medical problem, **ask your doctor, nurse, or pharmacist.**

Before Using This Medicine

In order to decide on the best treatment for your medical problem, your doctor should be told:

—if you have ever had any unusual or allergic reaction to amphetamine, dextroamphetamine, ephedrine, epinephrine, isoproterenol, metaproterenol, methamphetamine, norepinephrine, phenylephrine, phenylpropanolamine, pseudoephedrine, or terbutaline.

—if you are on a low-salt, low-sugar, or any other special diet, or if you are allergic to any substance, such as foods, sulfites or other preservatives, or dyes. Most medicines contain more than their active ingredient. Your doctor, nurse, or pharmacist can help you avoid products that may cause a problem.

—if you are **pregnant** or if you may become pregnant. Studies have not been done in humans. However, animal studies have shown that fenfluramine, when given at many times the human dose, reduces fertility and causes toxic or harmful effects on the fetus.

—if you are **breast-feeding.** It is not known if fenfluramine is excreted in breast milk. This medicine has not been shown to cause problems in nursing babies.

—if you have any of the following medical problems:
Diabetes mellitus (sugar diabetes)
Glaucoma
Heart or blood vessel disease
High blood pressure
Mental depression (or history of)
Mental illness (severe)
Migraine headache
Overactive thyroid

—if you are taking **any** other prescription or nonprescription (OTC) medicine, especially central nervous system (CNS) depressants.

—if you are now taking or have taken within the past 2 weeks monoamine oxidase (MAO) inhibitors such as:
Furazolidone (e.g., Furoxone)
Isocarboxazid (e.g., Marplan)
Pargyline (e.g., Eutonyl)
Phenelzine (e.g., Nardil)
Procarbazine (e.g., Matulane)
Tranylcypromine (e.g., Parnate)

Proper Use of This Medicine

Take fenfluramine only as directed by your doctor. Do not take more of it, do not take it more often, and do not take it for a longer period of time than your doctor ordered. If too much is taken, it may beome habit-forming.

If you think this medicine is not working as well after you have taken it for a few weeks, **do not increase the dose.** Instead, check with your doctor.

For patients taking the long-acting form of this medicine:

• These capsules or tablets are to be swallowed whole. Do not break, crush, or chew before swallowing.

How to store this medicine:

- **Keep out of the reach of children.**

- Store away from heat and direct light.

- Do not store in the bathroom, near the kitchen sink, or in other damp places. Heat or moisture may cause the medicine to break down.

- Do not keep outdated medicine or medicine no longer needed. Be sure that any discarded medicine is out of the reach of children.

Precautions While Using This Medicine

Your doctor should check your progress at regular visits in order to make sure that this medicine does not cause unwanted effects.

Fenfluramine will add to the effects of alcohol and other CNS depressants (medicines that slow down the nervous system, possibly causing drowsiness). Some examples of CNS depressants are antihistamines or medicine for hay fever, other allergies, or colds; sedatives, tranquilizers, or sleeping medicine; prescription pain medicine or narcotics; barbiturates; medicine for seizures; muscle relaxants; or anesthetics, including some dental anesthetics. **Check with your doctor before taking any such depressants while you are using this medicine.**

Fenfluramine may cause dryness of the mouth. For temporary relief, use sugarless candy or gum, melt bits of ice in your mouth, or use a saliva substitute. However, if dry mouth continues for more than 2 weeks, check with your physician or dentist. Continuing dryness of the mouth may increase the chance of dental disease, including tooth decay, gum disease, and fungal infections.

This medicine may cause some people to have a false sense of well-being or to become dizzy, lightheaded, drowsy, or less alert than they are normally. If this occurs, **do not drive, use machines, or do other jobs that require you to be alert** while you are taking fenfluramine.

Before having any kind of surgery, dental treatment, or emergency treatment, tell the physician or dentist in charge that you are using this medicine.

If you have been taking fenfluramine for a long time or in large doses and **you think you may have become mentally or physically dependent on it, check with your doctor.**

Some signs of dependence on fenfluramine are:

—a strong desire or need to continue taking the medicine

—a need to increase the dose to receive the effects of the medicine

—withdrawal side effects (for example, mental depression, trouble in sleeping, or nightmares when you stop taking the medicine)

Diabetic patients—This medicine may affect blood sugar levels. If you notice a change in the results of your urine or blood sugar test or if you have any questions, check with your doctor.

If you will be taking fenfluramine in large doses for a long period of time, **do not stop taking it without first checking with your doctor.** Your doctor may want you to reduce gradually the amount you are taking before stopping completely.

Side Effects of This Medicine

Along with its needed effects, a medicine may cause some unwanted effects. Although not all of these side effects may occur, if they do occur they may need medical attention.

Check with your doctor as soon as possible if any of the following side effects occur:

Less common

Confusion
Mental depression
Skin rash or hives
Sore throat and fever

Other side effects may occur that usually do not require medical attention. These side effects may go away during treatment as your body adjusts to the medicine. However, check with your doctor if any of the following side effects continue or are bothersome:

More common

Diarrhea
Drowsiness
Dryness of mouth

Less common

Blurred vision
Changes in sexual desire
Clumsiness or unsteadiness
Constipation
Difficult or painful urination
Difficulty in talking
Dizziness or lightheadedness
False sense of well-being
Frequent urge to urinate or increased urination
Headache
Increased sweating
Irritability
Nausea or vomiting
Nervousness or restlessness
Pounding heartbeat
Stomach cramps or pain
Trouble in sleeping or nightmares
Unpleasant taste
Unusual tiredness or weakness

After you stop using this medicine, your body may need time to adjust. The length of time this takes depends on the amount of medicine you were using and how long you used it. During this period of time check with your doctor if you notice any of the following side effects:

Mental depression
Trouble in sleeping or nightmares

For elderly patients: Many medicines have not been tested in older people. Therefore, it is not known whether the medicine acts the same way it does in younger adults. Check with your doctor or pharmacist if you notice any unusual effects while taking this medicine or if you think it is not working as it should.

For children: Fenfluramine should not be used as an appetite suppressant by children under 12 years of age.

Other side effects not listed above may also occur in some patients. If you notice any other effects, check with your doctor.

December 1987

FLAVOXATE (Systemic)

A commonly used brand name is Urispas.

To the Reader: If you do not recognize the names of medical conditions or medicines referred to in this information, check with your doctor, nurse, or pharmacist. Definitions for selected medical terms may be found in the Glossary. Brand names for the generic drug names listed can be found in the Index. In addition, selected brand names commonly associated with the generic name have been included in the text to help you recognize medicine you may be taking. The fact that a brand name product is not mentioned does not mean the information does not apply. It is a good idea for you to learn both the generic and brand names of your medicines and to write them down for future use.

Flavoxate (fla-VOX-ate) belongs to the general group of medicines called antispasmodics. It is taken by mouth to help decrease muscle spasms of the bladder and relieve difficult urination.

Flavoxate is available only with your doctor's prescription.

Remember:

• **This medicine has been prescribed for your current medical problem only.** It must not be given to other people or used for other problems unless you are directed to do so by your doctor.

• **Keep all medicines out of the reach of children.**

• In order for this medicine to work, it must be used as directed.

• **It is very important that you read and understand the following information.** If any of the information causes you special concern, do not decide against using this medicine without first checking with your doctor.

• Before you begin using any new medicine (prescription or nonprescription) or if you develop any new medical problem while you are using this medicine, check with your doctor, nurse, or pharmacist.

• **If you have any questions** about the following information or if you want more information about this medicine or your medical problem, **ask your doctor, nurse, or pharmacist.**

Before Using This Medicine

In order to decide on the best treatment for your medical problem, your doctor should be told:

—if you have ever had any unusual or allergic reaction to flavoxate.

—if you are on a low-salt, low-sugar, or any other special diet, or if you are allergic to any substance, such as foods, sulfites or other preservatives, or dyes. Most medicines contain more than their active ingredient. Your doctor, nurse, or pharmacist can help you avoid products that may cause a problem.

—if you are **pregnant** or if you may become pregnant. Studies have not been done in humans. However, flavoxate has not been shown to cause birth defects or other problems in animal studies.

—if you are **breast-feeding**. Flavoxate has not been shown to cause problems in nursing babies.

—if you have any of the following medical problems:
Bleeding (severe)
Enlarged prostate
Intestinal blockage or other intestinal or stomach problems
Urinary tract blockage

—if you are taking **any** other prescription or nonprescription (OTC) medicine, especially antimuscarinics (medicines for abdominal or stomach spasms or cramps).

Proper Use of This Medicine

Take this medicine on an empty stomach with water, or with food or milk to lessen stomach upset unless otherwise directed by your doctor.

Take this medicine only as directed. Do not take more of it, do not take it more often, and do not take it for a longer period of time than your doctor ordered. To do so may increase the chance of side effects.

If you miss a dose of this medicine, take it as soon as possible. However, if it is almost time for your next dose, skip the missed dose and go back to your regular dosing schedule. Do not double doses.

How to store this medicine:

• **Keep out of the reach of children.**

• Store away from heat and direct light.

• Do not store in the bathroom, near the kitchen sink, or in other damp places. Heat or moisture may cause the medicine to break down.

• Do not keep outdated medicine or medicine no longer needed. Be sure that any discarded medicine is out of the reach of children.

Precautions While Using This Medicine

This medicine may cause your eyes to become more sensitive to light than they are normally. Wearing sunglasses may help lessen the discomfort from bright light.

This medicine may cause some people to become drowsy or have blurred vision. **Make sure you know how you react to this medicine before you drive, use machines, or do other jobs that require you to be alert.**

Flavoxate may make you sweat less, causing your body temperature to increase. **Use extra care not to become overheated during exercise or hot weather while you are taking this medicine,** since overheating may result in heat stroke.

Your mouth and throat may feel very dry while you are taking this medicine. For temporary relief of mouth dryness, use sugarless candy or gum, melt bits of ice in your mouth, or use a saliva substitute. However, if

---

dry mouth continues for more than 2 weeks, check with your physician or dentist. Continuing dryness of the mouth may increase the chance of dental disease, including tooth decay, gum disease, and fungal infections.

Side Effects of This Medicine

Along with its needed effects, a medicine may cause some unwanted effects. Although not all of these side effects may occur, if they do occur they may need medical attention.

Check with your doctor as soon as possible if any of the following side effects occur:

Rare

    Confusion
    Eye pain
    Skin rash or hives
    Sore throat and fever

Signs of overdose

    Clumsiness or unsteadiness
    Dizziness (severe)
    Drowsiness (severe)
    Fever
    Flushing or redness of face
    Hallucinations (seeing, hearing, or feeling things that are not there)
    Shortness of breath or troubled breathing
    Unusual excitement, nervousness, restlessness, or irritability

Other side effects may occur that usually do not require medical attention. These side effects may go away during treatment as your body adjusts to the medicine. However, check with your doctor if any of the following side effects continue or are bothersome:

More common

    Drowsiness
    Dryness of mouth and throat

Less common or rare

    Blurred vision
    Constipation
    Difficult urination
    Difficulty concentrating
    Dizziness
    Fast heartbeat
    Headache
    Increased sensitivity of eyes to light
    Increased sweating
    Nausea or vomiting
    Nervousness
    Stomach pain

For elderly patients: Confusion is more likely to occur in the elderly, who are usually more sensitive to the effects of flavoxate.

Other side effects not listed above may also occur in some patients. If you notice any other effects, check with your doctor.

December 1987

FLECAINIDE (Systemic)

A commonly used brand name is Tambocor.

To the Reader: If you do not recognize the names of medical conditions or medicines referred to in this information, check with your doctor, nurse, or pharmacist. Definitions for selected medical terms may be found in the Glossary. Brand names for the generic drug names listed can be found in the Index. In addition, selected brand names commonly associated with the generic name have been included in the text to help you recognize medicine you may be taking. The fact that a brand name product is not mentioned does not mean the information does not apply. It is a good idea for you to learn both the generic and brand names of your medicines and to write them down for future use.

Flecainide (FLEK-a-nide) belongs to the group of medicines known as antiarrhythmics. It is taken by mouth to convert irregular heartbeats to a normal rhythm.

Flecainide produces its helpful effects by slowing nerve impulses in the heart and making the heart tissue less sensitive.

This medicine is available only with your doctor's prescription.

Remember:

• **This medicine has been prescribed for your current medical problem only.** It must not be given to other people or used for other problems unless you are directed to do so by your doctor.

• **Keep all medicines out of the reach of children.**

• In order for this medicine to work, it must be used as directed.

• **It is very important that you read and understand the following information.** If any of the information causes you special concern, do not decide against using this medicine without first checking with your doctor.

• Before you begin using any new medicine (prescription or nonprescription) or if you develop any new medical problem while you are using this medicine, check with your doctor, nurse, or pharmacist.

• **If you have any questions** about the following information or if you want more information about this medicine or your medical problem, **ask your doctor, nurse, or pharmacist.**

Before Using This Medicine

In order to decide on the best treatment for your medical problem, your doctor should be told:

—if you have ever had any unusual or allergic reaction to flecainide, lidocaine, tocainide, or anesthetics.

—if you are on a low-salt, low-sugar, or any other special diet, or if you are allergic to any substance, such as foods, sulfites or other preservatives, or dyes. Most medicines contain more than their active ingredient. Your doctor, nurse, or pharmacist can help you avoid products that may cause a problem.

—if you are **pregnant** or if you may become pregnant. Studies have not been done in humans. However, studies in one kind of rabbit given about 4 times the usual human dose have shown that flecainide causes birth defects.

—if you are **breast-feeding**. It is not known whether flecainide passes into breast milk. This medicine has not been shown to cause problems in nursing babies.

—if you have either of the following medical problems:
Kidney disease
Liver disease

—if you have a pacemaker.

—if you have recently had a heart attack.

—if you are taking **any** other prescription or nonprescription (OTC) medicine, especially other heart medicine.

Proper Use of This Medicine

Take flecainide exactly as directed by your doctor, even though you may feel well. Do not take more medicine than ordered.

This medicine works best when there is a constant amount in the blood. **To help keep this amount constant, do not miss any doses. Also, it is best to take the doses 12 hours apart, in the morning and at night**, unless otherwise directed by your doctor. If you need help in planning the best times to take your medicine, check with your doctor or pharmacist.

If you do miss a dose of flecainide and remember within 6 hours, take it as soon as possible. However, if you do not remember until later, skip the missed dose and go back to your regular dosing schedule. Do not double doses.

How to store this medicine:

• **Keep out of the reach of children.**

• Store away from heat and direct light.

• Do not store in the bathroom, near the kitchen sink, or in other damp places. Heat or moisture may cause the medicine to break down.

• Do not keep outdated medicine or medicine no longer needed. Be sure that any discarded medicine is out of the reach of children.

Precautions While Using This Medicine

It is important that your doctor check your progress at regular visits to make sure the medicine is working properly. This will allow for changes to be made in the amount of medicine you are taking, if necessary.

Your doctor may want you to carry a medical identification card or bracelet stating that you are using this medicine.

Before having any kind of surgery (including dental surgery) or emergency treatment, tell the physician or dentist in charge that you are taking this medicine.

Flecainide may cause some people to become dizzy, lightheaded, or less alert than they are normally. **Make sure you know how you react to this medicine before you drive, use machines, or do other jobs that require you to be alert.**

If you have been using this medicine regularly for several weeks, do not suddenly stop using it. Check with your doctor for the best way to reduce gradually the amount you are taking before stopping completely.

Side Effects of This Medicine

Along with its needed effects, a medicine may cause some unwanted effects. Although not all of these side effects may occur, if they do occur they may need medical attention.

Check with your doctor as soon as possible if any of the following side effects occur:

Less common
> Chest pain
> Irregular heartbeat
> Shortness of breath
> Swelling of feet or lower legs
> Trembling or shaking

Rare
> Fever, chills, or sore throat
> Unusual bleeding or bruising
> Yellow eyes and skin

Other side effects may occur that usually do not require medical attention. These side effects may go away during treatment as your body adjusts to the medicine.

However, check with your doctor if any of the following side effects continue or are bothersome:

More common
> Blurred vision
> Dizziness or lightheadedness

Less common
> Anxiety or mental depression
> Constipation
> Headache
> Nausea or vomiting
> Skin rash
> Stomach pain or loss of appetite
> Tiredness or weakness

For elderly patients: Many medicines have not been tested in older people. Therefore, it is not known whether the medicine acts the same way it does in younger adults. Check with your doctor or pharmacist if you notice any unusual effects while taking this medicine or if you think it is not working as it should.

Other side effects not listed above may also occur in some patients. If you notice any other effects, check with your doctor.

December 1987

FLOXURIDINE (Systemic)

A commonly used brand name is FUDR.

To the Reader: If you do not recognize the names of medical conditions or medicines referred to in this information, check with your doctor, nurse, or pharmacist. Definitions for selected medical terms may be found in the Glossary. Brand names for the generic drug names listed can be found in the Index. In addition, selected brand names commonly associated with the generic name have been included in the text to help you recognize medicine you may be taking. The fact that a brand name product is not mentioned does not mean the information does not apply. It is a good idea for you to learn both the generic and brand names of your medicines and to write them down for future use.

Floxuridine (flox-YOOR-i-deen) belongs to the group of medicines known as antimetabolites. It is given by injection to treat some kinds of cancer.

Floxuridine interferes with the growth of cancer cells, which are eventually destroyed. Since the growth of normal body cells may also be affected by floxuridine, other effects will also occur. Some of these may be serious and must be reported to your doctor. Other effects, like hair loss, may not be serious but may cause concern. Some effects may not occur for months or years after the medicine is used.

Before you begin treatment with floxuridine, you and your doctor should talk about the good this medicine will do as well as the risks of using it.

Floxuridine is to be administered only by or under the immediate supervision of your doctor.

Remember:
• **It is very important that you read and understand the following information.** If any of the information causes you special concern, do not decide against receiving this medicine without first checking with your doctor.

• Before you begin using any new medicine (prescription or nonprescription) or if you develop any new medical problem while you are receiving this medicine, check with your doctor, nurse, or pharmacist.

• **If you have any questions** about the following information or if you want more information about this medicine or your medical problem, **ask your doctor, nurse, or pharmacist.**

Before Using This Medicine

In order to decide on the best treatment for your medical problem, your doctor should be told:

—if you have ever had any unusual or allergic reaction to floxuridine.

—if you are **pregnant** or if you intend to have children. There is a chance that this medicine may cause birth defects if either the male or female is receiving it at the time of conception or if it is taken during pregnancy. Floxuridine has been shown to cause birth defects in mice and rats. In addition, many cancer medicines may cause sterility which could be permanent. Although this has not been reported with this medicine, the possibility should be kept in mind. Be sure that you have discussed this with your doctor before receiving this medicine.

—if you intend to **breast-feed.** Because this medicine may cause serious side effects, breast-feeding is generally not recommended while you are receiving it.

—if you have any of the following medical problems:
Chickenpox (including recent exposure)
Hepatitis (history of) or other liver disease
Herpes zoster (shingles)
Infection
Kidney disease

—if you are now taking/using **any** prescription or non-prescription (OTC) medicine, especially:
Amphotericin B by injection (e.g., Fungizone)
Antithyroid agents (medicine for overactive thyroid)
Azathioprine (e.g., Imuran)
Chloramphenicol (e.g., Chloromycetin)
Colchicine
Flucytosine (e.g., Ancobon)

—if you have ever been treated with x-rays or cancer medicines.

Proper Use of This Medicine

Floxuridine sometimes causes nausea and vomiting. **Tell your doctor if this occurs, especially if you have stomach pain.**

Precautions While Using This Medicine

It is very important that your doctor check your progress at regular visits to make sure that this medicine is working properly and to check for unwanted effects.

While you are being treated with floxuridine, and after you stop treatment with it, **do not have any immunizations without your doctor's approval.** Floxuridine lowers your body's resistance and there is a chance you might get the infection the immunization is meant to prevent. In addition, other persons living in your household should not take oral polio vaccine since there is a chance they could pass the polio virus on to you. Also, you should avoid close contact with other persons (for example, at school or work) who have taken oral polio vaccine.

Side Effects of This Medicine

Along with their needed effects, medicines like floxuridine can sometimes cause unwanted effects such as blood problems, inflammation of the digestive tract, liver problems, and other side effects; these are described below. Also, because of the way these medicines act on the body, there is a chance that they might cause other unwanted effects that may not occur until months or years after the medicine is used. These delayed effects may include certain types of cancer, such as leukemia. Discuss these possible effects with your doctor.

Although some side effects may appear only rarely, if they do occur they may need medical attention.

Check with your doctor or nurse immediately if any of the following side effects occur:

More common
    Diarrhea
    Sores in the mouth and on the lips
    Stomach pain or cramps

Less common
    Black tarry stools
    Heartburn
    Nausea and vomiting
    Scaling or redness of hands or feet
    Swelling or soreness of the tongue

Rare
    Difficulty in walking
    Fever, chills, or sore throat
    Unusual bleeding or bruising
    Yellow eyes and skin

Other side effects may occur that usually do not require medical attention. These side effects may go away during treatment as your body adjusts to the medicine.

Also, your doctor or nurse may be able to tell you about ways to prevent or reduce some of these side effects. Check with your doctor or nurse if any of the following side effects continue or are bothersome or if you have any questions about them:

Less common or rare
    Loss of appetite
    Skin rash or itching

This medicine sometimes causes temporary thinning of hair. After treatment with floxuridine has ended, normal hair growth should return.

Other side effects not listed above may also occur in some patients. If you notice any other effects, check with your doctor or nurse.

_____

December 1987
_____

FLUCYTOSINE (Systemic)

Some commonly used brand names or other names are:

Ancobon	5-FC
Ancotil*	5-Fluorocytosine

*Not available in the U.S.

To the Reader: If you do not recognize the names of medical conditions or medicines referred to in this information, check with your doctor, nurse, or pharmacist. Definitions for selected medical terms may be found in the Glossary. Brand names for the generic drug names listed can be found in the Index. In addition, selected brand names commonly associated with the generic name have been included in the text to help you recognize medicine you may be taking. The fact that a brand name product is not mentioned does not mean the information does not apply. It is a good idea for you to learn both the generic and brand names of your medicines and to write them down for future use.

Flucytosine (floo-SYE-toe-seen) belongs to the group of medicines called antifungals. It is taken by mouth to treat certain fungus infections.

Flucytosine is available only with your doctor's prescription.

Remember:

• **This medicine has been prescribed for your present infection only.** Another infection later on may require a different medicine. Also, even though other people may have the same symptoms as you, they may have a different kind of infection. Your medicine may not work for them and may even cause them harm. Therefore, **your medicine must not be given to other people or used for other infections** unless you are otherwise directed by your doctor.

• **Keep all medicines out of the reach of children.**

• In order for this medicine to work, it must be used as directed.

• **It is very important that you read and understand the following information.** If any of the information causes you special concern, do not decide against using this medicine without first checking with your doctor.

• Before you begin using any new medicine (prescription of nonprescription) or if you develop any new medical problem while you are using this medicine, check with your doctor, nurse, or pharmacist.

• **If you have any questions** about the following information or if you want more information about this medicine or your medical problem, **ask your doctor, nurse, or pharmacist.**

Before Using This Medicine

In order to decide on the best treatment for your medical problem, your doctor should be told:

—if you have ever had any unusual or allergic reaction to flucytosine.

—if you are on a low-salt, low-sugar, or any other special diet, or if you are allergic to any substance, such as foods, sulfites or other preservatives, or dyes.

Most medicines contain more than their active ingredient. Your doctor, nurse, or pharmacist can help you avoid products that may cause a problem.

—if you are **pregnant** or if you may become pregnant. Flucytosine has not been shown to cause birth defects or other problems in humans. However, studies in rats have shown that flucytosine causes birth defects.

—if you are **breast-feeding.** However, flucytosine has not been shown to cause problems in nursing babies.

—if you have any of the following medical problems:
  Blood disease
  Kidney disease
  Liver disease

—if you are taking **any** other prescription or nonprescription (OTC) medicine, especially:
  Amphotericin B by injection (e.g., Fungizone)
  Antineoplastics (cancer medicine)
  Antithyroid agents (medicine for overactive thyroid)
  Azathioprine (e.g., Imuran)
  Chlorambucil (e.g., Leukeran)
  Chloramphenicol (e.g., Chloromycetin)
  Colchicine
  Cyclophosphamide (e.g., Cytoxan)
  Interferon (e.g., Intron A, Roferon-A)
  Mercaptopurine (e.g., Purinethol)
  Methotrexate (e.g., Mexate)
  Zidovudine (e.g., Retrovir)

—if you have ever been treated with x-rays.

Proper Use of This Medicine

In some patients this medicine may cause nausea or vomiting. If you are taking more than 1 capsule for each dose, you may space them out over a period of 15 minutes to help lessen the nausea or vomiting. If this does not help or if you have any questions, check with your doctor.

To help clear up your infection completely, **keep taking this medicine for the full time of treatment** even if you begin to feel better after a few days; **do not miss any doses.**

If you do miss a dose of this medicine, take it as soon as possible. However, if it is almost time for your next dose, skip the missed dose and go back to your regular dosing schedule. Do not double doses.

How to store this medicine:

• **Keep out of the reach of children.**

• Store away from heat and direct light.

• Do not store in the bathroom, near the kitchen sink, or in other damp places. Heat or moisture may cause the medicine to break down.

• Do not keep outdated medicine or medicine no longer needed. Be sure that any discarded medicine is out of the reach of children.

Precautions While Using This Medicine

Your doctor should check your progress at regular visits to make sure that this medicine does not cause unwanted effects.

Flucytosine may cause blood problems. These problems may result in a greater chance of infection, slow healing, and bleeding of the gums. Therefore, you should be careful when using toothbrushes, dental floss, and toothpicks. Dental work, whenever possible, should be done before you begin taking this medicine or delayed until your blood counts have returned to normal. Check with your physician or dentist if you have any questions about proper oral hygiene (mouth care) during treatment.

This medicine may also cause some people to become dizzy, lightheaded, drowsy, or less alert than they are normally. **Make sure you know how you react to this medicine before you drive, use machines, or do other jobs that require you to be alert.** If these reactions are especially bothersome, check with your doctor.

Side Effects of This Medicine

Along with its needed effects, a medicine may cause some unwanted effects. Although not all of these side effects may occur, if they do occur they may need medical attention.

Check with your doctor immediately if any of the following side effects occur:

More common

Skin rash
Sore throat and fever
Unusual bleeding or bruising
Unusual tiredness or weakness

Less common

Confusion
Hallucinations (seeing, hearing, or feeling things that are not there)

Other side effects may occur that usually do not require medical attention. These side effects may go away during treatment as your body adjusts to the medicine. However, check with your doctor if any of the following side effects continue or are bothersome:

More common

Diarrhea
Nausea or vomiting

Less common

Dizziness or lightheadedness
Drowsiness
Headache

For elderly patients: Many medicines have not been tested in older people. Therefore, it is not known whether the medicine acts the same way it does in younger adults. Check with your doctor or pharmacist if you notice any unusual effects while taking this medicine or if you think it is not working as it should.

Other side effects not listed above may also occur in some patients. If you notice any other effects, check with your doctor.

————————

December 1987

———————————————————————————————————

FLUOROURACIL (Systemic)

Some commonly used brand names or other names are Adrucil and 5-FU.

Generic name product may also be available in the U.S. and Canada.

To the Reader: If you do not recognize the names of medical conditions or medicines referred to in this information, check with your doctor, nurse, or pharmacist. Definitions for selected medical terms may be found in the Glossary. Brand names for the generic drug names listed can be found in the Index. In addition, selected brand names commonly associated with the generic name have been included in the text to help you recognize medicine you may be taking. The fact that a brand name product is not mentioned does not mean the information does not apply. It is a good idea for you to learn both the generic and brand names of your medicines and to write them down for future use.

Fluorouracil (flure-oh-YOOR-a-sill) belongs to the group of medicines known as antimetabolites. It is given by injection to treat some kinds of cancer.

Fluorouracil interferes with the growth of cancer cells, which are eventually destroyed. Since the growth of normal body cells may also be affected by fluorouracil, other effects will also occur. Some of these may be serious and must be reported to your doctor. Other effects, like hair loss, may not be serious but may cause concern. Some effects may not occur for months or years after the medicine is used.

Before you begin treatment with fluorouracil, you and your doctor should talk about the good this medicine will do as well as the risks of using it.

Fluorouracil is to be administered only by or under the immediate supervision of your doctor.

Remember:
- **It is very important that you read and understand the following information.** If any of the information causes you special concern, do not decide against receiving this medicine without first checking with your doctor.

- Before you begin using any new medicine (prescription or nonprescription) or if you develop any new medical problem while you are receiving this medicine, check with your doctor, nurse, or pharmacist.

- **If you have any questions** about the following information or if you want more information about this medicine or your medical problem, **ask your doctor, nurse, or pharmacist.**

Before Using This Medicine

In order to decide on the best treatment for your medical problem, your doctor should be told:

—if you have ever had any unusual or allergic reaction to fluorouracil.

—if you are **pregnant** or if you intend to have children. There is a chance that this medicine may cause birth defects if either the male or female is receiving it at the time of conception or if it is taken during pregnancy. Fluorouracil has been reported to cause birth defects in mice given doses slightly higher than the human dose. Also, there has been one case of a baby born with several birth defects after the mother received fluorouracil. In addition, many cancer medicines may cause sterility. Although this has been reported with this medicine, it is usually only temporary; the possibility should be kept in mind. Be sure that you have discussed this with your doctor before receiving this medicine.

—if you intend to **breast-feed**. Because this medicine may cause serious side effects, breast-feeding is generally not recommended while you are receiving it.

—if you have any of the following medical problems:
Chickenpox (including recent exposure)
Herpes zoster (shingles)
Infection
Kidney disease
Liver disease

—if you are taking **any** other prescription or nonprescription (OTC) medicine, especially:
Amphotericin B by injection (e.g., Fungizone)
Antithyroid agents (medicine for overactive thyroid)
Azathioprine (e.g., Imuran)
Chloramphenicol (e.g., Chloromycetin)
Colchicine
Flucytosine (e.g., Ancobon)
Interferon (e.g., Intron A; Roferon-A)

—if you have ever been treated with x-rays or cancer medicines.

Proper Use of This Medicine

This medicine is sometimes given together with certain other medicines. If you are using a combination of medicines, it is important that you receive each one at the proper time. If you are taking some of these medicines by mouth, ask your doctor, nurse, or pharmacist to help you plan a way to remember to take them at the right times.

Fluorouracil often causes nausea and vomiting. However, it is very important that you continue to receive the medicine, even if your stomach is upset. Ask your doctor, nurse, or pharmacist for ways to lessen these effects.

Precautions While Using This Medicine

It is very important that your doctor check your progress at regular visits to make sure that this medicine is working properly and to check for unwanted effects.

While you are being treated with fluorouracil, and after you stop treatment with it, **do not have any immunizations without your doctor's approval.** Fluorouracil lowers your body's resistance and there is a chance you might get the infection the immunization is meant to prevent. In addition, other persons living in your household should not take oral polio vaccine since there is a chance they could pass the polio virus on to you. Also, you should avoid close contact with other persons (for example, at school or work) who have taken oral polio vaccine.

Fluorouracil can lower the number of white blood cells in your body. This may increase the chance of getting an infection. If you can, avoid people with colds or other infections. If you think you are getting a cold or other infection, check with your doctor.

Side Effects of This Medicine

Along with their needed effects, medicines like fluorouracil can sometimes cause unwanted effects such as blood problems, loss of hair, and other side effects; these are described below. Also, because of the way these medicines act on the body, there is a chance that they might cause other unwanted effects that may not occur until months or years after the medicine is used. These delayed effects may include certain types of cancer, such as leukemia. Discuss these possible effects with your doctor.

Although not all of these side effects may occur, if they do occur they may need medical attention.

Check with your doctor or nurse immediately if any of the following side effects occur:

More common
    Diarrhea
    Fever, chills, or sore throat
    Heartburn
    Sores in the mouth and on the lips

Less common
    Black, tarry stools
    Nausea and vomiting (severe)
    Stomach cramps
    Unusual bleeding or bruising

Check with your doctor or nurse as soon as possible if any of the following side effects occur:

Rare
    Chest pain
    Cough
    Difficulty with balance
    Shortness of breath

Other side effects may occur that usually do not require medical attention. These side effects may go away during treatment as your body adjusts to the medicine. Also, your doctor or nurse may be able to tell you about ways to prevent or reduce some of these side effects. Check with your doctor or nurse if any of the following side effects continue or are bothersome or if you have any questions about them:

More common
    Loss of appetite
    Nausea and vomiting
    Skin rash and itching
    Weakness

This medicine often causes a temporary loss of hair. After treatment with fluorouracil has ended, normal hair growth should return.

For elderly patients: Many medicines have not been tested in older people. Therefore, it is not known whether the medicine acts the same way it does in younger adults. Check with your doctor if you notice any unusual effects while taking this medicine or if you think it is not working as it should.

After you stop receiving fluorouracil, it may still produce some side effects that need attention. During this period of time, **check with your doctor or nurse immediately** if you notice any of the following:
    Fever, chills, or sore throat
    Unusual bleeding or bruising

Other side effects not listed above may also occur in some patients. If you notice any other effects, check with your doctor or nurse.

December 1987

FLUOROURACIL (Topical)

Some commonly used brand names or other names are Efudex, Fluoroplex, and 5-FU.

To the Reader: If you do not recognize the names of medical conditions or medicines referred to in this information, check with your doctor, nurse, or pharmacist. Definitions for selected medical terms may be found in the Glossary. Brand names for the generic drug names listed can be found in the Index. In addition, selected brand names commonly associated with the generic name have been included in the text to help you recognize medicine you may be taking. The fact that a brand name product is not mentioned does not mean the information does not apply. It is a good idea for you to learn both the generic and brand names of your medicines and to write them down for future use.

Fluorouracil (flure-oh-YOOR-a-sill) belongs to the group of medicines known as antimetabolites. When applied to the skin, it is used to treat certain skin problems, including cancer or conditions that could become cancerous if not treated.

Fluorouracil interferes with the growth of abnormal cells, which are eventually destroyed.

Fluorouracil is available only with your doctor's prescription.

Remember:

• **This medicine has been prescribed for your current medical problem only.** It must not be given to other people or used for other problems unless you are directed to do so by your doctor.

• **Keep all medicines out of the reach of children.**

• In order for this medicine to work, it must be used as directed.

• **It is very important that you read and understand the following information.** If any of the information causes you special concern, do not decide against using this medicine without first checking with your doctor.

• Before you begin using any new medicine (prescription or nonprescription) or if you develop any new medical problem while you are using this medicine, check with your doctor, nurse, or pharmacist.

• **If you have any questions** about the following information or if you want more information about this medicine or your medical problem, **ask your doctor, nurse, or pharmacist**.

Before Using This Medicine

In order to decide on the best treatment for your medical problem, your doctor should be told:

—if you have ever had any unusual or allergic reaction to fluorouracil.

—if you are **pregnant** or if you intend to become pregnant. Although fluorouracil applied to the skin has not been shown to cause problems in humans, some of it is absorbed through the skin.

—if you are **breast-feeding**. Although fluorouracil applied to the skin has not been shown to cause problems in nursing babies, some of it is absorbed through the skin.

—if you have any other skin problems.

—if you are using **any** other prescription or nonprescription (OTC) medicine.

Proper Use of This Medicine

Keep using this medicine for the full time of treatment. However, **do not use this medicine more often or for a longer period of time than your doctor ordered.** Apply enough medicine each time to cover the entire affected area with a thin layer.

After washing the area with soap and water and drying carefully, use a cotton-tipped applicator or your fingertips to apply the medicine in a thin layer to your skin.

If you apply this medicine with your fingertips, make sure you **wash your hands immediately afterwards,** to prevent any of the medicine from accidentally getting in your eyes or mouth.

Fluorouracil may cause redness, soreness, scaling, and peeling of affected skin after 1 or 2 weeks of use. This effect may last for several weeks after you stop using the medicine and is to be expected. Sometimes a pink, smooth area is left when the skin treated with this medicine heals. This area will usually fade after 1 to 2 months. Do not stop using this medicine without first checking with your doctor. If the reaction is very uncomfortable, check with your doctor.

If you miss a dose of this medicine, apply it as soon as you remember. However, if more than a few hours have passed, skip the missed dose and go back to your regular dosing schedule. If you miss more than one dose, check with your doctor.

How to store this medicine:

• **Keep out of the reach of children.**

• Store away from heat and direct light.

• Do not store in the bathroom, near the kitchen sink, or in other damp places. Heat or moisture may cause the medicine to break down.

• Protect the solution from freezing.

• Do not keep outdated medicine or medicine no longer needed. Be sure that any discarded medicine is out of the reach of children.

Precautions While Using This Medicine

It is very important that your doctor check your progress at regular visits to make sure that this medicine is working properly and to check for unwanted effects.

Apply this medicine very carefully when using it on your face. Avoid getting any in your eyes, nose, or mouth.

While using this medicine, and for 1 or 2 months after you stop using it, your skin may become more sensitive to sunlight than usual and too much sunlight may increase the effect of the drug. During this period of time, avoid too much sun and do not use a sunlamp. In case of a severe burn, check with your doctor.

Side Effects of This Medicine

Along with its needed effects, a medicine may cause some unwanted effects. Although not all of these side effects may occur, if they do occur they may need medical attention.

Check with your doctor immediately if the following side effects occur:

    Redness and swelling of normal skin

Other side effects may occur that usually do not require medical attention. These side effects may go away during treatment as your body adjusts to the medicine. However, check with your doctor if any of the following side effects continue, worsen, or are bothersome:

More common

    Burning sensation where medicine is applied
    Increased sensitivity of skin to sunlight
    Itching
    Oozing
    Skin rash
    Soreness or tenderness

Less common or rare

    Darkening of skin
    Scaling
    Watery eyes

For elderly patients: Many medicines have not been tested in older people. Therefore, it is not known whether the medicine acts the same way it does in younger adults. Check with your doctor if you notice any unusual effects while taking this medicine or if you think it is not working as it should.

Other side effects not listed above may also occur in some patients. If you notice any other effects, check with your doctor.

December 1987

FLURBIPROFEN (Ophthalmic)

A commonly used brand name is Ocufen.

To the Reader: If you do not recognize the names of medical conditions or medicines referred to in this information, check with your doctor, nurse, or pharmacist. Definitions for selected medical terms may be found in the Glossary. Brand names for the generic drug names listed can be found in the Index. In addition, selected brand names commonly associated with the generic name have been included in the text to help you recognize medicine you may be taking. The fact that a brand name product is not mentioned does not mean the information does not apply. It is a good idea for you to learn both the generic and brand names of your medicines and to write them down for future use.

Flurbiprofen (flur-bi-PROE-fen) is used in the eye before some kinds of eye surgery. Sometimes, the pupil of the eye gets smaller during an operation. This makes it more difficult for the surgeon to reach some areas of the eye. Flurbiprofen helps to prevent this. When this medicine is used before surgery, it will be placed in the eye by your doctor or your doctor's assistant shortly before the operation begins.

Flurbiprofen may also be used for other conditions as determined by your doctor.

Flurbiprofen is available only with your doctor's prescription.

Remember:
• **This medicine has been prescribed for your current medical problem only.** It must not be given to other people or used for other problems unless you are directed to do so by your doctor.

• **Keep all medicines out of the reach of children.**

• In order for this medicine to work, it must be used as directed.

• **It is very important that you read and understand the following information.** If any of the information causes you special concern, do not decide against using this medicine without first checking with your doctor.

• Before you begin using any new medicine (prescription or nonprescription) or if you develop any new medical problem while you are using this medicine, check with your doctor, nurse, or pharmacist.

• **If you have any questions** about the following information or if you want more information about this medicine or your medical problem, **ask your doctor, nurse, or pharmacist.**

Before Receiving This Medicine

In order to decide whether or not you should receive flurbiprofen, your doctor should be told:
—if you have ever had any unusual or allergic reaction, especially asthma or wheezing, runny nose, or hives, to any of the following medicines:

Aspirin or other salicylates
Diclofenac (e.g., Voltaren)
Diflunisal (e.g., Dolobid)
Fenoprofen (e.g., Nalfon)
Flurbiprofen, oral (e.g., Ansaid)
Ibuprofen (e.g., Motrin)

Indomethacin (e.g., Indocin)
Ketoprofen (e.g., Orudis)
Meclofenamate (e.g., Meclomen)
Mefenamic acid (e.g., Ponstel)
Naproxen (e.g., Naprosyn)
Oxyphenbutazone (e.g., Tandearil)
Phenylbutazone (e.g., Butazolidin)
Piroxicam (e.g., Feldene)
Sulindac (e.g., Clinoril)
Suprofen (e.g., Suprol)
Tiaprofenic acid (e.g., Surgam)
Tolmetin (e.g., Tolectin)
Zomepirac (e.g., Zomax)

—if you are allergic to any substance, such as certain preservatives. Most medicines contain more than their active ingredient. Your doctor can help you avoid products that may cause a problem.

—if you are **pregnant** or if you may become pregnant. Flurbiprofen has not been shown to cause birth defects or other problems in humans. However, studies on birth defects have not been done in humans. Studies have been done in animals receiving flurbiprofen by mouth in amounts that are much greater than the amounts used in the eye. Flurbiprofen did not cause birth defects in these studies. However, it decreased the weight or slowed the growth of the fetus and caused other, more serious, harmful effects. Also, when flurbiprofen was given to animals late in pregnancy, it increased the length of pregnancy or prolonged labor.

—if you are **breast-feeding**. Although it is not known whether flurbiprofen passes into the breast milk, this medicine has not been shown to cause problems in nursing babies.

—if you have hemophilia or other bleeding problems.

—if you are taking or using medicine for glaucoma.

Proper Use of This Medicine

How to apply this medicine: First, wash your hands. With the middle finger, apply pressure to the inside corner of the eye (and continue to apply pressure for 1 or 2 minutes after the medicine has been placed in the eye). Tilt the head back and with the index finger of the same hand, pull the lower eyelid away from the eye to form a pouch. Drop the medicine into the pouch and gently close your eyes. Do not blink. Keep your eyes closed for 1 or 2 minutes to allow the medicine to come into contact with the irritation. If you think you did not get the drop of medicine into your eye properly, use another drop.

Remove any excess solution around the eye with a clean tissue, being careful not to touch the eye.

Immediately after applying the eye drops, wash your hands to remove any medicine that may be on them.

To prevent contamination of the eye drops, do not touch the dropper or the applicator tip to any surface (including the eye). Also, always keep the container tightly closed.

Do not use this medicine more often or for a longer period of time than your doctor ordered. To do so may increase the chance of side effects.

Do not use any leftover medicine for future eye problems without first checking with your doctor. If certain kinds of infection are present, using this medicine may make the infection worse and possibly lead to eye damage.

If you miss a dose of this medicine, apply it as soon as possible. But if it is almost time for your next dose, skip the missed dose and go back to your regular dosing schedule.

How to store this medicine:

- **Keep out of the reach of children.**

- Store away from heat and direct light.

- Keep the medicine from freezing.

- Do not keep outdated medicine or medicine no longer needed. Be sure that any discarded medicine is out of the reach of children.

Side Effects of This Medicine

Along with its needed effects, a medicine may cause some unwanted effects. Flurbiprofen may cause temporary burning, itching, or stinging in the eye when it is applied. These side effects usually do not need medical attention. However, check with your doctor if they continue or are bothersome.

There have not been any other common or important side effects reported with this medicine. However, if you notice any unusual effects, check with your doctor.

December 1987

Additional Information

For patients who are using flurbiprofen eye drops at home:
- Check with your doctor as soon as possible if you notice any bleeding or redness in the eye that was not present before you started using this medicine, or if any bleeding or redness caused by eye surgery becomes worse while you are using this medicine.

FOLIC ACID (Vitamin B₉) (Systemic)

Some commonly used brand names are Apo-Folic*, Folvite, and Novo-folacid*.

Generic name product may also be available in the U.S. and Canada.

* Not available in the U.S.

To the Reader: If you do not recognize the names of medical conditions or medicines referred to in this information, check with your doctor, nurse, or pharmacist. Definitions for selected medical terms may be found in the Glossary. Brand names for the generic drug names listed can be found in the Index. In addition, selected brand names commonly associated with the generic name have been included in the text to help you recognize medicine you may be taking. The fact that a brand name product is not mentioned does not mean the information does not apply. It is a good idea for you to learn both the generic and brand names of your medicines and to write them down for future use.

Vitamins (VYE-ta-mins) are compounds that you *must* have for growth and health. They are needed in small amounts only and are usually available in the foods that you eat. Folic acid (FOE-lik) or vitamin B₉ is necessary for strong blood.

Lack of folic acid may lead to anemia (weak blood). Your doctor may treat this by prescribing folic acid for you.

Claims that folic acid and other B vitamins are effective for preventing mental problems have not been proven. Many of these treatments involve large and expensive amounts of vitamins.

Some strengths of folic acid are available only with your doctor's prescription. Others are available without a prescription. However, it may be a good idea to check with your doctor before taking folic acid on your own.

Remember:
• **Keep all medicines out of the reach of children.**

• In order for this medicine to work, it must be used as directed. **If you are using this medicine without a prescription, it is very important that you follow the directions on the label.**

• **It is also very important that you read and understand the following information.** If any of the information causes you special concern, check with your doctor before using this medicine without a prescription.

• Before you begin using any new medicine (prescription or nonprescription) or if you develop any new medical problem while you are using this medicine, check with your doctor, nurse, or pharmacist.

• **If you have any questions** about the following information or if you want more information about this medicine or your medical problem, **ask your doctor, nurse, or pharmacist.**

Importance of Diet

Vitamin supplements should be taken only if you cannot get enough vitamins in your diet. A balanced diet should provide all the vitamins you normally need.

Nutritionists recommend that you eat:
• Cereal or bread—4 or more servings per day and
• Dairy products (milk, cheese, ice cream, cottage cheese)—3 or more servings per day and
• Meat, fish, or eggs—2 or more servings per day and
• Vegetables and fruits—4 or more servings per day.

If you are not getting all of these foods every day, you may not be getting enough vitamins in your diet. The best way to correct this is to start eating the foods that contain what you need.

Folic acid is found in various foods, including vegetables, fruits, and organ meats (for example, liver or kidney). It is best to eat fresh fruits and vegetables whenever possible since they contain the most vitamins. Food processing may destroy some of the vitamins. For example, heat may reduce the amount of folic acid in foods.

Vitamins alone will not take the place of a good diet and will not provide energy. Your body also needs other substances found in food such as protein, minerals, carbohydrates, and fat. Vitamins themselves often cannot work without the presence of other foods.

In some cases, it may not be possible for you to get enough food to supply you with the proper vitamins. In other cases, the amount of vitamins you need may be increased above normal. Therefore, a vitamin supplement may be needed.

Experts have developed a list of recommended dietary allowances (RDA) for most of the vitamins. The RDA are not an exact number but a general idea of how much you need. They do not cover amounts needed for problems caused by a serious lack of vitamins.

The RDA for folic acid are:
    Children 4 to 6 years of age—200 mcg (micrograms) per day
    Adult males—400 mcg per day
    Adult females—400 mcg per day
    Pregnant females—800 mcg per day
    Breast-feeding females—500 mcg per day.

Remember:
• The total amount of each vitamin that you get every day includes what you get from the foods that you eat *and* what you may take as a supplement.

• This total amount should not be greater than the RDA, unless ordered by your doctor.

Before Using This Medicine

In deciding whether you need additional folic acid, the following should be kept in mind and/or your doctor should be told:

—if you have ever had any unusual or allergic reaction to folic acid.

—if you are on a low-salt, low-sugar, or any other special diet, or if you are allergic to any substance, such as foods, sulfites or other preservatives, or dyes.

Most medicines contain more than their active ingredient. Your doctor, nurse, or pharmacist can help you avoid products that may cause a problem.

—if you are **pregnant** or if you may become pregnant. It is especially important that you are receiving enough vitamins when you become pregnant and that you continue to receive the right amount of vitamins, especially folic acid, throughout your pregnancy. The healthy growth and development of the fetus depend on a steady supply of nutrients from the mother.

—if you are **breast-feeding**. It is especially important that you receive the right amounts of vitamins so that your baby will also get the vitamins needed to grow properly. You should also check with your doctor if you are giving your baby an unfortified formula. In that case, the baby must get the vitamins needed some other way.

—if you are not able to get a diet that contains all of the vitamins you need. This may occur with rapid weight loss, unusual diets (such as some reducing diets in which choice of foods is very limited), prolonged intravenous feeding, or malnutrition.

—if you have had a large part of your stomach removed.

—if you have been under a lot of stress for a long time, or if you have had a long illness or serious injury.

—if you have any of the following medical problems:

Alcoholism
Diarrhea (prolonged)
Hemolytic anemia
Intestinal problems
Liver disease
Pernicious anemia (a special blood problem)

—if you are taking **any** other prescription or nonprescription (OTC) medicine.

Proper Use of This Medicine

Some people believe that taking very large doses of vitamins (called megadoses or megavitamin therapy) is useful for treating certain medical problems. Studies have not proven this. Large doses should be taken only under the direction of your doctor after need has been identified.

If you miss taking a vitamin for one or more days there is no cause for concern, since it takes some time for your body to become seriously low in vitamins. However, if your doctor has recommended that you take this vitamin, try to remember to take it as directed every day.

How to store this medicine:

• **Keep out of the reach of children.**

• Store away from heat and direct light.

• Do not store in the bathroom, near the kitchen sink, or in other damp places. Heat or moisture may cause the medicine to break down.

• Do not keep outdated medicine or medicine no longer needed. Be sure that any discarded medicine is out of the reach of children.

Side Effects of This Medicine

Along with its needed effects, a medicine may cause some unwanted effects. Although folic acid does not usually cause any side effects, check with your doctor as soon as possible if either of the following side effects occurs:
Rare

Fever
Skin rash

This medicine may cause urine to have a more yellow color than normal. This is to be expected and is no cause for alarm.

Other side effects not listed above may also occur in some patients. If you notice any other effects, check with your doctor.

December 1987

GEMFIBROZIL (Systemic)

A commonly used brand name is Lopid.

To the Reader: If you do not recognize the names of medical conditions or medicines referred to in this information, check with your doctor, nurse, or pharmacist. Definitions for selected medical terms may be found in the Glossary. Brand names for the generic drug names listed can be found in the Index. In addition, selected brand names commonly associated with the generic name have been included in the text to help you recognize medicine you may be taking. The fact that a brand name product is not mentioned does not mean the information does not apply. It is a good idea for you to learn both the generic and brand names of your medicines and to write them down for future use.

Gemfibrozil (gem-FI-broe-zil) is taken by mouth to lower cholesterol and triglyceride (fat-like substances) levels in the blood. This may help prevent medical problems caused by such substances clogging the blood vessels.

Gemfibrozil is available only with your doctor's prescription.

Remember:

• **This medicine has been prescribed for your current medical problem only.** It must not be given to other people or used for other problems unless you are directed to do so by your doctor.

• **Keep all medicines out of the reach of children.**

• In order for this medicine to work, it must be used as directed.

• **It is very important that you read and understand the following information.** If any of the information causes you special concern, do not decide against using this medicine without first checking with your doctor.

• Before you begin using any new medicine (prescription or nonprescription) or if you develop any new medical problem while you are using this medicine, check with your doctor, nurse, or pharmacist.

• **If you have any questions** about the following information or if you want more information about this medicine or your medical problem, **ask your doctor, nurse, or pharmacist.**

Before Using This Medicine

In addition to its helpful effects in treating your medical problem, this type of medicine may have some harmful effects.

Although problems have not been found with gemfibrozil, it is similar in action to another medicine called clofibrate. Studies with clofibrate have suggested that it may increase the risk of gallstones and problems from gallbladder surgery, although it may also decrease the risk of heart attack. Other studies have not found all of these effects.

Studies with gemfibrozil in male rats found an increased risk of noncancerous tumors when doses up to 10 times the human dose were given for long periods. Be sure you have discussed this with your doctor before taking this medicine.

Importance of diet—Before prescribing medicine for your condition, your doctor will probably try to control your condition by prescribing a personal diet for you. Such a diet may be low in fats, sugars, and/or cholesterol. Many people are able to control their condition by carefully following their doctor's orders for proper diet and exercise. **Medicine is prescribed only when additional help is needed** and is effective only when a schedule of diet and exercise is properly followed.

Also, this medicine is less effective if you are greatly overweight. It may be very important for you to go on a reducing diet. However, check with your doctor before going on any diet.

In order to decide on the best treatment for your medical problem, your doctor should be told:

—if you have ever had any unusual or allergic reaction to gemfibrozil.

—if you are on a low-salt, low-sugar, or any other special diet, or if you are allergic to any substance, such as foods, sulfites or other preservatives, or dyes. Most medicines contain more than their active ingredient. Your doctor, nurse, or pharmacist can help you avoid products that may cause a problem.

—if you are **pregnant** or if you may become pregnant. Studies have not been done in humans. However, studies in animals have shown that high doses of gemfibrozil may increase the number of fetal deaths, although it does not cause birth defects.

—if you are **breast-feeding**. Studies in male animals have shown that high doses of gemfibrozil may increase the incidence of some kinds of tumors. You should consider this when deciding whether to breast-feed your baby while taking this medicine.

—if you have any of the following medical problems:
   Gallbladder disease
   Gallstones
   Kidney disease
   Liver disease

—if you are taking **any** other prescription or nonprescription (OTC) medicine, especially anticoagulants (blood thinners).

Proper Use of This Medicine

Use this medicine only as directed by your doctor. Do not use more or less of it, and do not use it more often or for a longer period of time than your doctor ordered.

Follow carefully the special diet your doctor gave you. This is the most important part of controlling your condition, and is necessary if the medicine is to work properly.

If you miss a dose of this medicine, take it as soon as possible. However, if it is almost time for your next dose, skip the missed dose and go back to your regular dosing schedule. Do not double doses.

How to store this medicine:

• **Keep out of the reach of children.**

• **Store away from heat and direct light.**

• Do not store in the bathroom, near the kitchen sink, or in other damp places. Heat or moisture may cause the medicine to break down.

• Do not keep outdated medicine or medicine no longer needed. Be sure that any discarded medicine is out of the reach of children.

Precautions While Using This Medicine

It is very important that your doctor check your progress at regular visits. This will allow your doctor to see if the medicine is working properly to lower your cholesterol and triglyceride levels and to decide if you should continue to take it.

Side Effects of This Medicine

Along with its needed effects, a medicine may cause some unwanted effects. Although not all of these side effects may occur, if they do occur they may need medical attention.

Check with your doctor immediately if any of the following side effects occur:
Rare
    Fever and chills or sore throat
    Stomach pain (severe) with nausea and vomiting

Other side effects may occur that usually do not require medical attention. These side effects may go away during treatment as your body adjusts to the medicine. However, check with your doctor if any of the following side effects continue or are bothersome:
Less common
    Aching muscles
    Diarrhea
    Muscle cramping
    Nausea or vomiting
    Skin rash
    Stomach pain, gas, or heartburn

For elderly patients: Many medicines have not been tested in older people. Therefore, it is not known whether the medicine acts the same way it does in younger adults. Check with your doctor or pharmacist if you notice any unusual effects while taking this medicine or if you think it is not working as it should.

Other side effects not listed above may also occur in some patients. If you notice any other effects, check with your doctor.

December 1987

GENTAMICIN (Ophthalmic)

Some commonly used brand names are:

Alcomicin*	Genoptic
Garamycin	Gentacidin

Generic name product may also be available in the U.S.

*Not available in the U.S.

To the Reader: If you do not recognize the names of medical conditions or medicines referred to in this information, check with your doctor, nurse, or pharmacist. Definitions for selected medical terms may be found in the Glossary. Brand names for the generic drug names listed can be found in the Index. In addition, selected brand names commonly associated with the generic name have been included in the text to help you recognize medicine you may be taking. The fact that a brand name product is not mentioned does not mean the information does not apply. It is a good idea for you to learn both the generic and brand names of your medicines and to write them down for future use.

Gentamicin (jen-ta-MYE-sin) belongs to the family of medicines called antibiotics. Gentamicin ophthalmic preparations are used in the eye to treat infections of the eye.

Gentamicin is available only with your doctor's prescription.

Remember:

• **This medicine has been prescribed for your present infection only.** Another infection later on may require a different medicine. Also, even though other people may have the same symptoms as you, they may have a different kind of infection. Your medicine may not work for them and may even cause them harm. Therefore, **your medicine must not be given to other people or used for other infections** unless you are otherwise directed by your doctor.

• **Keep all medicines out of the reach of children.**

• In order for this medicine to work, it must be used as directed.

• **It is very important that you read and understand the following information.** If any of the information causes you special concern, do not decide against using this medicine without first checking with your doctor.

• Before you begin using any new medicine (prescription or nonprescription) or if you develop any new medical problem while you are using this medicine, check with your doctor, nurse, or pharmacist.

• **If you have any questions** about the following information or if you want more information about this medicine or your medical problem, **ask your doctor, nurse, or pharmacist.**

Before Using This Medicine

In order to decide on the best treatment for your medical problem, your doctor should be told:

—if you have ever had any unusual or allergic reaction to this medicine or to any related antibiotics such as amikacin, gentamicin (by injection), kanamycin, neomycin, netilmicin, streptomycin, or tobramycin.

—if you are allergic to any substance, such as certain foods or preservative or dyes. Most medicines contain more than their active ingredient. Your doctor, nurse, or pharmacist can help you avoid products that may cause a problem.

—if you are **pregnant** or if you may become pregnant. However, gentamicin ophthalmic preparations have not been shown to cause birth defects or other problems in humans.

—if you are **breast-feeding**. However, gentamicin ophthalmic preparations have not been shown to cause problems in nursing babies.

Proper Use of This Medicine

For patients using the eye drop form of this medicine:

• The bottle is only partially full to provide proper drop control.

• How to apply this medicine: First, wash your hands. Then tilt the head back and pull the lower eyelid away from the eye to form a pouch. Drop the medicine into the pouch and gently close the eyes. Do not blink. Keep the eyes closed for 1 or 2 minutes to allow the medicine to come into contact with the infection.

• If you think you did not get the drop of medicine into your eye properly, use another drop.

• To prevent contamination of the eye drops, do not touch the applicator tip to any surface (including the eye). Also, keep the container tightly closed.

For patients using the eye ointment form of this medicine:

• How to apply this medicine: First, wash your hands. Then pull the lower eyelid away from the eye to form a pouch. Squeeze a thin strip of ointment into the pouch. A 1-cm (approximately ⅓-inch) strip of ointment is usually enough unless otherwise directed by your doctor. Gently close the eyes and keep them closed for 1 or 2 minutes to allow the medicine to come into contact with the infection.

• To prevent contamination of the eye ointment, do not touch the applicator tip to any surface (including the eye). After using gentamicin eye ointment, wipe the tip of the ointment tube with a clean tissue and keep the tube tightly closed.

To help clear up your infection completely, **keep using this medicine for the full time of treatment,** even though your symptoms may have disappeared; **do not miss any doses.**

If you do miss a dose of this medicine, apply it as soon as possible. However, if it is almost time for your next dose, skip the missed dose and go back to your regular dosing schedule.

How to store this medicine:

• **Keep out of the reach of children.**

• Store away from heat and direct light.

• Keep the medicine from freezing.

• Do not keep outdated medicine or medicine no longer needed. Be sure that any discarded medicine is out of the reach of children.

Precautions While Using This Medicine

If your symptoms do not improve within a few days, or if they become worse, check with your doctor.

Side Effects of This Medicine

Along with its needed effects, a medicine may cause some unwanted effects. Although not all of these side effects may occur, if they do occur they may need medical attention.

Check with your doctor immediately if any of the following side effects occur:

Less common

    Itching, redness, swelling, or other sign of irritation not present before using this medicine

Other side effects may occur that usually do not require medical attention. These side effects may go away during treatment as your body adjusts to the medicine. However, check with your doctor if either of the following side effects continues or is bothersome:

Less common

    Burning or stinging

After application, eye ointments usually cause your vision to blur for a few minutes.

Other side effects not listed above may also occur in some patients. If you notice any other effects, check with your doctor.

_____

December 1987

GENTAMICIN (Otic)*

A commonly used brand name is Garamycin*.

*Not commercially available in the U.S.

To the Reader: If you do not recognize the names of medical conditions or medicines referred to in this information, check with your doctor, nurse, or pharmacist. Definitions for selected medical terms may be found in the Glossary. Brand names for the generic drug names listed can be found in the Index. In addition, selected brand names commonly associated with the generic name have been included in the text to help you recognize medicine you may be taking. The fact that a brand name product is not mentioned does not mean the information does not apply. It is a good idea for you to learn both the generic and brand names of your medicines and to write them down for future use.

Gentamicin (jen-ta-MYE-sin) belongs to the family of medicines called antibiotics. Gentamicin otic preparations are used in the ear to treat infections of the ear canal.

Gentamicin is available only with your doctor's prescription.

Remember:
• **This medicine has been prescribed for your present infection only.** Another infection later on may require a different medicine. Also, even though other people may have the same symptoms as you, they may have a different kind of infection. Your medicine may not work for them and may even cause them harm. Therefore, **your medicine must not be given to other people or used for other infections** unless you are otherwise directed by your doctor.

• **Keep all medicines out of the reach of children.**

• In order for this medicine to work, it must be used as directed.

• **It is very important that you read and understand the following information.** If any of the information causes you special concern, do not decide against using this medicine without first checking with your doctor.

• Before you begin using any new medicine (prescription or nonprescription) or if you develop any new medical problem while you are using this medicine, check with your doctor, nurse, or pharmacist.

• **If you have any questions** about the following information or if you want more information about this medicine or your medical problem, **ask your doctor, nurse, or pharmacist.**

Before Using This Medicine

In order to decide on the best treatment for your medical problem, your doctor should be told:

—if you have ever had any unusual or allergic reaction to this medicine or to any related antibiotics such as amikacin, gentamicin (by injection), kanamycin, neomycin, netilmicin, streptomycin, or tobramycin.

—if you are allergic to any substance, such as certain foods or preservative or dyes. Most medicines contain more than their active ingredient. Your doctor, nurse, or pharmacist can help you avoid products that may cause a problem.

—if you are **pregnant** or if you may become pregnant. However, gentamicin otic preparations have not been shown to cause birth defects or other problems in humans.

—if you are **breast-feeding**. However, gentamicin otic preparations have not been shown to cause problems in nursing babies.

—if you have any other ear infection or problem (including punctured eardrum).

Proper Use of This Medicine

How to apply this medicine: Lie down or tilt the head so that the infected ear faces up. Gently pull the earlobe up and back for adults (down and back for children) to straighten the ear canal. Drop the medicine into the ear canal. Keep the ear facing up for about 1 or 2 minutes to allow the medicine to come into contact with the infection. A sterile cotton plug may be gently inserted into the ear opening to prevent the medicine from leaking out.

To prevent contamination of the ear drops, do not touch the applicator tip to any surface (including the ear). Also, keep the container tightly closed.

To help clear up your infection completely, **keep using this medicine for the full time of treatment,** even though your symptoms may have disappeared; **do not miss any doses.**

If you do miss a dose of this medicine, apply it as soon as possible. However, if it is almost time for your next dose, skip the missed dose and go back to your regular dosing schedule.

How to store this medicine:

• **Keep out of the reach of children.**

• Store away from heat and direct light.

• Keep the medicine from freezing.

• Do not keep outdated medicine or medicine no longer needed. Be sure that any discarded medicine is out of the reach of children.

Precautions While Using This Medicine

If your symptoms do not improve within a few days, or if they become worse, check with your doctor.

Side Effects of This Medicine

Along with its needed effects, a medicine may cause some unwanted effects. Although not all of these side effects may occur, if they do occur they may need medical attention.

Check with your doctor immediately if any of the following side effects occur:

Less common
　Itching, redness, swelling, or other sign of irritation not present before using this medicine

Other side effects may occur that usually do not require medical attention. These side effects may go away during treatment as your body adjusts to the medicine.

However, check with your doctor if either of the following side effects continues or is bothersome:

Less common
　Burning or stinging

Other side effects not listed above may also occur in some patients. If you notice any other effects, check with your doctor.

_____

December 1987

GENTAMICIN (Topical)

A commonly used brand name is Garamycin.

Generic name product may also be available in the U.S.

To the Reader: If you do not recognize the names of medical conditions or medicines referred to in this information, check with your doctor, nurse, or pharmacist. Definitions for selected medical terms may be found in the Glossary. Brand names for the generic drug names listed can be found in the Index. In addition, selected brand names commonly associated with the generic name have been included in the text to help you recognize medicine you may be taking. The fact that a brand name product is not mentioned does not mean the information does not apply. It is a good idea for you to learn both the generic and brand names of your medicines and to write them down for future use.

Gentamicin (jen-ta-MYE-sin) belongs to the general family of medicines called antibiotics. Gentamicin topical preparations are used on the skin to help the body overcome infections of the skin.

Gentamicin is available only with your doctor's prescription.

Remember:

• **This medicine has been prescribed for your present infection only.** Another infection later on may require a different medicine. Also, even though other people may have the same symptoms as you, they may have a different kind of infection. Your medicine may not work for them and may even cause them harm. Therefore, **your medicine must not be given to other people or used for other infections** unless you are otherwise directed by your doctor.

• **Keep all medicines out of the reach of children.**

• In order for this medicine to work, it must be used as directed.

• **It is very important that you read and understand the following information.** If any of the information causes you special concern, do not decide against using this medicine without first checking with your doctor.

• Before you begin using any new medicine (prescription or nonprescription) or if you develop any new medical problem while you are using this medicine, check with your doctor, nurse, or pharmacist.

• **If you have any questions** about the following information or if you want more information about this medicine or your medical problem, **ask your doctor, nurse, or pharmacist.**

Before Using This Medicine

In order to decide on the best treatment for your medical problem, your doctor should be told:

—if you have ever had any unusual or allergic reaction to this medicine or any related antibiotics such as amikacin, gentamicin (by injection), kanamycin, neomycin, netilmicin, streptomycin, or tobramycin.

—if you are allergic to any substance, such as certain foods or preservatives or dyes. Most medicines contain more than their active ingredient. Your doctor, nurse, or pharmacist can help you avoid products that may cause a problem.

—if you are **pregnant** or if you may become pregnant. However, gentamicin topical preparations have not been shown to cause birth defects or other problems in humans.

—if you are **breast-feeding**. However, gentamicin topical preparations have not been shown to cause problems in nursing babies.

—if you are taking **any** other prescription or nonprescription (OTC) medicine.

Proper Use of This Medicine

Before applying this medicine, wash the affected area with soap and water, and dry thoroughly. Apply a small amount to the affected area and rub in gently.

After this medicine is applied, the treated area may be covered with a gauze dressing if desired.

To help clear up your infection completely, **keep using this medicine for the full time of treatment,** even though your symptoms may have disappeared; **do not miss any doses.**

If you do miss a dose of this medicine, apply it as soon as possible. However, if it is almost time for your next dose, skip the missed dose and go back to your regular dosing schedule.

How to store this medicine:

• **Keep out of the reach of children.**

• Store away from heat and direct light.

• Keep the medicine from freezing.

• Do not keep outdated medicine or medicine no longer needed. Be sure that any discarded medicine is out of the reach of children.

Precautions While Using This Medicine

If your skin problem does not improve within 1 week, or if it becomes worse, check with your doctor.

Side Effects of This Medicine

Along with its needed effects, a medicine may cause some unwanted effects. Although not all of these side effects may occur, if they do occur they may need medical attention.

Check with your doctor immediately if any of the following side effects occur:
Less common

Itching, redness, swelling, or other sign of irritation not present before using this medicine

Other side effects not listed above may also occur in some patients. If you notice any other effects, check with your doctor.

December 1987

GENTIAN VIOLET (Topical)

To the Reader: If you do not recognize the names of medical conditions or medicines referred to in this information, check with your doctor, nurse, or pharmacist. Definitions for selected medical terms may be found in the Glossary. Brand names for the generic drug names listed can be found in the Index. In addition, selected brand names commonly associated with the generic name have been included in the text to help you recognize medicine you may be taking. The fact that a brand name product is not mentioned does not mean the information does not apply. It is a good idea for you to learn both the generic and brand names of your medicines and to write them down for future use.

Gentian violet (JEN-shun VYE-oh-let) belongs to the group of medicines called antifungals. Topical gentian violet is used on the skin or mucous membranes to treat some types of fungal infections inside the mouth (thrush) and of the skin.

Gentian violet is available without a prescription; however, your doctor may have special instructions on the proper use of gentian violet for your medical condition.

Remember:

• **Keep all medicines out of the reach of children.**

• In order for this medicine to work, it must be used as directed. **If you are using this medicine without a prescription, it is very important to follow the directions on the label.**

• **It is also very important that you read and understand the following information.** If any of the information causes you special concern, check with your doctor or pharmacist.

• Before you begin using any new medicine (prescription or nonprescription) or if you develop any new medical problem while you are using this medicine, check with your doctor, nurse, or pharmacist.

• **If you have any questions** about the following information or if you want more information about this medicine or your medical problem, **ask your doctor, nurse, or pharmacist.**

Before Using This Medicine

Before you use gentian violet, check with your doctor or pharmacist:

—if you have ever had any unusual or allergic reaction to gentian violet.

—if you are allergic to any substance, such as certain foods or preservatives or dyes. Most medicines contain more than their active ingredient. Your doctor, nurse, or pharmacist can help you avoid products that may cause a problem.

—if you are **pregnant** or if you may become pregnant. However, gentian violet topical solution has not been shown to cause birth defects or other problems in humans.

—if you are **breast-feeding**. However, gentian violet topical solution has not been shown to cause problems in nursing babies.

Proper Use of This Medicine

Using a cotton swab, apply enough gentian violet to cover only the affected area.

If you are applying this medicine to affected areas in the mouth, avoid swallowing any of the medicine.

If you are using this medicine in a child's mouth, make sure you understand exactly how to apply it so that it is not swallowed. If you have any questions about this, check with your doctor, nurse, or pharmacist.

Do not apply an occlusive dressing or airtight covering (for example, kitchen plastic wrap) over this medicine, since it may cause irritation of the skin.

To help clear up your infection completely, **keep using this medicine for the full time of treatment** even though your condition may have improved. **Do not miss any doses.**

If you do miss a dose of this medicine, apply it as soon as possible. However, if it is almost time for your next dose, skip the missed dose and go back to your regular dosing schedule.

How to store this medicine:

• **Keep out of the reach of children.**

• Store away from heat and direct light.

• Keep the medicine from freezing.

• Do not keep outdated medicine or medicine no longer needed. Be sure that any discarded medicine is out of the reach of children.

Precautions While Using This Medicine

Gentian violet will stain the skin and clothing. Avoid getting the medicine on your clothes.

Side Effects of This Medicine

Along with its needed effects, a medicine may cause some unwanted effects. Although not all of these side effects may occur, if they do occur they may need medical attention.

Check with your doctor as soon as possible if the following side effect occurs:

Skin irritation not present before using this medicine

Other side effects not listed above may also occur in some patients. If you notice any other effects, check with your doctor.

December 1987

GENTIAN VIOLET (Vaginal)

A commonly used brand name is Genapax.

To the Reader: If you do not recognize the names of medical conditions or medicines referred to in this information, check with your doctor, nurse, or pharmacist. Definitions for selected medical terms may be found in the Glossary. Brand names for the generic drug names listed can be found in the Index. In addition, selected brand names commonly associated with the generic name have been included in the text to help you recognize medicine you may be taking. The fact that a brand name product is not mentioned does not mean the information does not apply. It is a good idea for you to learn both the generic and brand names of your medicines and to write them down for future use.

Gentian violet (JEN-shun VYE-oh-let) belongs to the group of medicines called antifungals. Vaginal gentian violet is used in the vagina to treat fungal infections of the vagina.

Gentian violet is available only with your doctor's prescription.

Remember:

• **This medicine has been prescribed for your present infection only.** Another infection later on may require a different medicine. Also, even though other people may have the same symptoms as you, they may have a different kind of infection. Your medicine may not work for them and may even cause them harm. Therefore, **your medicine must not be given to other people or used for other infections** unless you are otherwise directed by your doctor.

• **Keep all medicines out of the reach of children.**

• In order for this medicine to work, it must be used as directed.

• **It is very important that you read and understand the following information.** If any of the information causes you special concern, do not decide against using this medicine without first checking with your doctor.

• Before you begin using any new medicine (prescription or nonprescription) or if you develop any new medical problem while you are using this medicine, check with your doctor, nurse, or pharmacist.

• **If you have any questions** about the following information or if you want more information about this medicine or your medical problem, **ask your doctor, nurse, or pharmacist.**

Before Using This Medicine

In order to decide on the best treatment for your medical problem, your doctor should be told:

—if you have ever had any unusual or allergic reaction to gentian violet.

—if you are allergic to any substance, such as certain foods or preservatives or dyes. Most medicines contain more than their active ingredient. Your doctor, nurse, or pharmacist can help you avoid products that may cause a problem.

—if you are **pregnant** or if you may become pregnant. However, gentian violet tampons have not been shown to cause birth defects or other problems in humans.

—if you are **breast-feeding**. However, gentian violet tampons have not been shown to cause problems in nursing babies.

Proper Use of This Medicine

Gentian violet usually comes with patient directions. Read them carefully before using this medicine.

After insertion, remove the tampon from the vagina after 3 to 4 hours unless otherwise directed by your doctor.

To help clear up your infection completely, **keep using this medicine for the full time of treatment** even though your condition may have improved. Also, keep using this medicine even if you begin to menstruate during the time of treatment. **Do not miss any doses.**

If you do miss a dose of this medicine, insert it as soon as possible. However, if it is almost time for your next dose, skip the missed dose and go back to your regular dosing schedule.

How to store this medicine:

• **Keep out of the reach of children.**

• Store away from heat and direct light.

• Do not keep outdated medicine or medicine no longer needed. Be sure that any discarded medicine is out of the reach of children.

Precautions While Using This Medicine

To help cure the infection and to help prevent reinfection, good health habits are required.

• Wear cotton panties (or panties or pantyhose with cotton crotches) instead of synthetic (for example, nylon, rayon) underclothes.

• Wear freshly laundered underclothes.

If you have any questions about this, check with your doctor, nurse, or pharmacist.

If you have intercourse during the time of treatment with this medicine, make sure your partner wears a condom (prophylactic). If you have any questions about this, check with your doctor or pharmacist.

If you have any questions about douching during the time of treatment with this medicine, check with your doctor.

Gentian violet will stain the skin and clothing. Avoid getting the medicine on your clothes.

Since there may be some vaginal drainage while you are using this medicine, a sanitary napkin may be worn to protect your clothing.

Side Effects of This Medicine

Along with its needed effects, a medicine may cause some
unwanted effects. Although not all of these side effects
may occur, if they do occur they may need medical
attention.

Check with your doctor as soon as possible if any of the
following side effects occur:
  Vaginal burning, itching, pain, or other sign of irritation
  not present before using this medicine

Other side effects not listed above may also occur in some
patients. If you notice any other effects, check with
your doctor.

_____

December 1987

_____

GLUCAGON (Systemic)

To the Reader: If you do not recognize the names of medical conditions or medicines referred to in this information, check with your doctor, nurse, or pharmacist. Definitions for selected medical terms may be found in the Glossary. Brand names for the generic drug names listed can be found in the Index. In addition, selected brand names commonly associated with the generic name have been included in the text to help you recognize medicine you may be taking. The fact that a brand name product is not mentioned does not mean the information does not apply. It is a good idea for you to learn both the generic and brand names of your medicines and to write them down for future use.

Glucagon (GLOO-ka-gon) belongs to the group of medicines called hormones. It is an emergency medicine given by injection to treat severe hypoglycemia (low blood sugar) reactions in diabetic patients who are unconscious or unable to take some form of sugar by mouth. Discuss with your doctor the importance of its use.

Glucagon is also used during certain examination procedures to improve patient comfort and examination results. It may also be used for other conditions as determined by your doctor.

Glucagon is available only with your doctor's prescription.

Remember:

• **This medicine has been prescribed for your current medical problem only.** It must not be given to other people or used for other problems unless you are directed to do so by your doctor.

• **Keep all medicines out of the reach of children.**

• In order for this medicine to work, it must be used as directed.

• **It is very important that you read and understand the following information.** If any of the information causes you special concern, do not decide against using this medicine without first checking with your doctor.

• **If you have any questions** about the following information or if you want more information about this medicine or your medical problem, **ask your doctor, nurse, or pharmacist.**

Before Using This Medicine

Before glucagon is prescribed for you, make sure that your doctor knows if you have any allergies, especially to proteins. Glucagon is a protein and some patients may be allergic to it.

Proper Use of This Medicine

Glucagon is an emergency medicine and must be used only as directed by your doctor. **Make sure that you and your family or a friend understand exactly when and how to use this medicine before it must be used.**

Glucagon is packaged in a kit containing two vials (one powder and one liquid) whose contents must be mixed before use. **Directions for mixing and injecting are in the package. Read them carefully** and ask your doctor, nurse, or pharmacist for additional explanation, if necessary.

Your doctor may want you to inject glucagon with the type of syringe you normally use to inject your insulin. Other patients may be told to use a different type of syringe that will allow a deeper injection. If you have any questions about the type of syringe you should be using, check with your doctor. Also, you should **regularly check to see if you have a sterile syringe and needles always available** to be used for the glucagon.

Glucagon may be mixed when an emergency occurs. However, if glucagon is needed often, it may be mixed ahead of time and kept in the refrigerator, ready for use. The date of mixing should then be written on the package. Mixed glucagon kept more than 1 month should be discarded and replaced by a fresh preparation.

Glucagon should not be mixed after the expiration date printed on the kit and on one vial. **Check the date regularly and replace the medicine before it expires.** The printed expiration date does not apply after mixing.

How to store this medicine.

• **Keep out of the reach of children.**

• Store away from heat and direct light.

• **Store the unmixed medication at room temperature.**

• Do not store the unmixed or mixed medication in the bathroom, near the kitchen sink, or in other damp places. Heat or moisture may cause the medicine to break down.

• **Store the mixed solution in the refrigerator for no longer than 1 month and keep it from freezing.**

• Do not keep outdated medicine or medicine no longer needed. Be sure that any discarded medicine is out of the reach of children.

Precautions While Using This Medicine

Diabetic patients should be aware of the symptoms of hypoglycemia (low blood sugar). These symptoms may develop in a very short time and may result from:

—using too much insulin ("insulin reaction").

—delaying or missing a scheduled snack or meal.

—sickness (especially with vomiting).

—exercising more than usual.

Unless corrected, hypoglycemia will lead to unconsciousness and possibly death. Early symptoms of hypoglycemia include:

Anxious feeling
Chills
Cool pale skin
Difficulty in concentrating
Headache
Hunger
Nausea
Nervousness
Shakiness
Sweating
Unusual tiredness
Weakness

Eating some form of sugar when symptoms of hypoglycemia first appear will usually prevent them from getting worse, and will probably make the use of glucagon unnecessary. Good sources of sugar include orange juice, corn syrup, and honey. Sugar cubes or table sugar dissolved in water will also work well.

If it becomes necessary to inject glucagon in an unconscious patient, a family member or friend should know the following:

• **After injection, turn the unconscious patient on one side.** Glucagon may cause some patients to vomit and this position will reduce the possibility of choking.

• **Call the patient's doctor at once.**

• The patient will usually become conscious in 5 to 20 minutes, but if not, a second dose may be given. **Get the patient to a doctor or to hospital emergency care as soon as possible,** since being unconscious too long may be harmful.

• **When the patient is conscious and can swallow, give some form of sugar to eat.** Glucagon is not effective for much longer than 1½ hours and is **used only until the patient is able to swallow.** Orange juice, corn syrup, honey, and sugar cubes or table sugar (dissolved in water) all work quickly. Then, if a snack or meal is not scheduled for an hour or more, the patient should also eat some crackers and cheese or half a sandwich, or drink a glass of milk. This will prevent hypoglycemia from occurring again before the next meal or snack.

• **If nausea prevents a patient from swallowing some form of sugar for an hour after glucagon is given, medical help should be obtained.**

Keep your doctor informed of any hypoglycemic attacks or use of glucagon even if the symptoms are successfully controlled and there seem to be no continuing problems. Complete information is necessary to provide the best possible treatment of any condition.

Replace your supply of glucagon as soon as possible, in case of another hypoglycemic episode.

Side Effects of This Medicine

Along with its needed effects, a medicine may cause some unwanted effects. Although not all of these side effects may occur, if they do occur they may need medical attention.

Check with your doctor as soon as possible if any of the following side effects occur:

Less common
   Dizziness
   Nausea or vomiting
   Skin rash
   Trouble in breathing

Other side effects not listed above may also occur in some patients. If you notice any other effects, check with your doctor.

December 1987

GLUTETHIMIDE (Systemic)

A commonly used brand name is Doriden.

Generic name product may also be available in the U.S.

To the Reader: If you do not recognize the names of medical conditions or medicines referred to in this information, check with your doctor, nurse, or pharmacist. Definitions for selected medical terms may be found in the Glossary. Brand names for the generic drug names listed can be found in the Index. In addition, selected brand names commonly associated with the generic name have been included in the text to help you recognize medicine you may be taking. The fact that a brand name product is not mentioned does not mean the information does not apply. It is a good idea for you to learn both the generic and brand names of your medicines and to write them down for future use.

Glutethimide (gloo-TETH-i-mide) is taken by mouth and may be used in the treatment of insomnia (sleeplessness). It helps patients to sleep. However, if used regularly (for example, every day) for insomnia, it is usually not effective for more than 7 days.

This medicine is available only with your doctor's prescription.

Remember:
- **This medicine has been prescribed for your current medical problem only.** It must not be given to other people or used for other problems unless you are directed to do so by your doctor.

- **Keep all medicines out of the reach of children.**

- In order for this medicine to work, it must be used as directed.

- **It is very important that you read and understand the following information.** If any of the information causes you special concern, do not decide against using this medicine without first checking with your doctor.

- Before you begin using any new medicine (prescription or nonprescription) or if you develop any new medical problem while you are using this medicine, check with your doctor, nurse, or pharmacist.

- **If you have any questions** about the following information or if you want more information about this medicine or your medical problem, **ask your doctor, nurse, or pharmacist**.

Before Using This Medicine

In order to decide on the best treatment for your medical problem, your doctor should be told:
- —if you have ever had any unusual or allergic reaction to glutethimide.

- —if you are on a low-salt, low-sugar, or any other special diet, or if you are allergic to any substance, such as foods, sulfites or other preservatives, or dyes. Most medicines contain more than their active ingredient. Your doctor, nurse, or pharmacist can help you avoid products that may cause a problem.

—if you are **pregnant** or if you may become pregnant. Studies on birth defects have not been done in either humans or animals. Too much use of glutethimide during pregnancy may cause the baby to become dependent on the medicine. This may lead to withdrawal side effects after birth.

—if you are **breast-feeding**. Glutethimide passes into the breast milk and may cause drowsiness in babies of mothers taking this medicine.

—if you have any of the following medical problems:
Enlarged prostate
Intestinal blockage
Irregular heartbeat
Kidney disease
Porphyria
Stomach ulcer
Urinary tract blockage

—if you are taking **any** other prescription or nonprescription (OTC) medicine, especially:
Anticoagulants (blood thinners)
Central nervous system (CNS) depressants

Proper Use of This Medicine

Take this medicine only as directed by your doctor. Do not take more of it, do not take it more often, and do not take it for a longer period of time than your doctor ordered. If too much is taken, it may become habit-forming.

How to store this medicine:
- **Keep out of the reach of children** since overdose is especially dangerous in children.

- Store away from heat and direct light.

- Do not store in the bathroom, near the kitchen sink, or in other damp places. Heat or moisture may cause the medicine to break down.

- Do not keep outdated medicine or medicine no longer needed. Be sure that any discarded medicine is out of the reach of children.

Precautions While Using This Medicine

If you will be taking this medicine regularly for a long period of time:
- —your doctor should check your progress at regular visits.

- —do not stop taking it without first checking with your doctor. Your doctor may want you to reduce gradually the amount you are taking before stopping completely.

This medicine will add to the effects of alcohol and other CNS depressants (medicines that slow down the nervous system, possibly causing drowsiness). Some examples of CNS depressants are antihistamines or medicine for hay fever, other allergies, or colds; sedatives, tranquilizers, or sleeping medicine; prescription pain medicine or narcotics; barbiturates; medicine for convulsions (seizures); muscle relaxants; or anesthetics, including some dental anesthetics. **Check with your doctor before taking any of the above while you are using this medicine.**

If you think you or someone else may have taken an overdose of this medicine, get emergency help at once. Taking an overdose of glutethimide or taking alcohol or other CNS depressants with glutethimide may lead to unconsciousness and possibly death. Some signs of an overdose are continuing confusion, severe weakness, shortness of breath or slow or troubled breathing, convulsions (seizures), slurred speech, staggering, and slow heartbeat.

This medicine may cause some people to become dizzy, drowsy, or less alert than they are normally. Even if taken at bedtime, it may cause some people to feel drowsy or less alert on arising. **Make sure you know how you react to this medicine before you drive, use machines, or do other jobs that require you to be alert.**

Side Effects of This Medicine

Along with its needed effects, a medicine may cause some unwanted effects. Although not all of these side effects may occur, if they do occur they may need medical attention.

Check with your doctor as soon as possible if any of the following side effects occur:

Less common
   Skin rash

Rare
   Sore throat and fever
   Unusual bleeding or bruising
   Unusual excitement
   Unusual tiredness or weakness

Signs of overdose
   Bluish coloration of skin
   Confusion (continuing)
   Convulsions (seizures)
   Fever
   Low body temperature
   Memory problems
   Muscle spasms or twitching
   Shortness of breath or slow or troubled breathing
   Slow heartbeat
   Slowness or loss of reflexes
   Slurred speech
   Staggering
   Trembling
   Trouble in concentrating
   Weakness (severe)

Other side effects may occur that usually do not require medical attention. These side effects may go away during treatment as your body adjusts to the medicine. However, check with your doctor if any of the following side effects continue or are bothersome:

More common
   Drowsiness (daytime)

Less common
   Blurred vision
   Clumsiness or unsteadiness
   Confusion
   Dizziness
   "Hangover" effect
   Headache
   Nausea
   Vomiting

For elderly patients: The above side effects are more likely to occur in the elderly, who are usually more sensitive to the effects of glutethimide.

After you stop using this medicine, your body may need time to adjust. The length of time this takes depends on the amount of medicine you were using and how long you used it. During this period of time check with your doctor if you notice any of the following side effects:

   Convulsions (seizures)
   Fast heartbeat
   Hallucinations (seeing, hearing, or feeling things that are not there)
   Increased dreaming
   Muscle cramps or spasms
   Nausea or vomiting
   Nightmares
   Stomach cramps or pain
   Trembling
   Trouble in sleeping

Other side effects not listed above may also occur in some patients. If you notice any other effects, check with your doctor.

December 1987

GLYCERIN (Systemic)

Some commonly used brand names are Glyrol and Osmoglyn.

Generic name product may also be available in the U.S.

To the Reader: If you do not recognize the names of medical conditions or medicines referred to in this information, check with your doctor, nurse, or pharmacist. Definitions for selected medical terms may be found in the Glossary. Brand names for the generic drug names listed can be found in the Index. In addition, selected brand names commonly associated with the generic name have been included in the text to help you recognize medicine you may be taking. The fact that a brand name product is not mentioned does not mean the information does not apply. It is a good idea for you to learn both the generic and brand names of your medicines and to write them down for future use.

Glycerin (GLI-ser-in), when taken by mouth, is used to treat certain conditions in which there is increased eye pressure, such as glaucoma. It may also be used before eye surgery to reduce pressure in the eye.

Glycerin may also be used for other conditions as determined by your doctor.

This medicine is available only with your doctor's prescription.

Remember:

• **This medicine has been prescribed for your current medical problem only.** It must not be given to other people or used for other problems unless you are directed to do so by your doctor.

• **Keep all medicines out of the reach of children.**

• In order for this medicine to work, it must be used as directed.

• **It is very important that you read and understand the following information.** If any of the information causes you special concern, do not decide against using this medicine without first checking with your doctor.

• Before you begin using any new medicine (prescription or nonprescription) or if you develop any new medical problem while you are using this medicine, check with your doctor, nurse, or pharmacist.

• **If you have any questions** about the following information or if you want more information about this medicine or your medical problem, **ask your doctor, nurse, or pharmacist.**

Before Using This Medicine

In order to decide on the best treatment for your medical problem, your doctor should be told:

—if you have ever had any unusual or allergic reaction to glycerin.

—if you are on a low-salt, low-sugar, or any other special diet, or if you are allergic to any substance, such as foods, sulfites or other preservatives, or dyes. Most medicines contain more than their active ingredient, and many liquid medicines contain alcohol. Your doctor, nurse, or pharmacist can help you avoid products that may cause a problem.

—if you are **pregnant** or if you may become pregnant. Studies have not been done in either humans or animals.

—if you are **breast-feeding**. It is not known whether glycerin passes into breast milk. This medicine has not been shown to cause problems in nursing babies.

—if you have any of the following medical problems:
Diabetes mellitus (sugar diabetes)
Heart disease
Kidney disease

—if you are taking **any** other prescription or nonprescription (OTC) medicine.

Proper Use of This Medicine

It is very important that you take this medicine only as directed. Do not take more of it and do not take it more often than your doctor ordered.

To improve the taste of this medicine, mix it with a small amount of unsweetened lemon, lime, or orange juice, pour over cracked ice, and sip through a straw.

If you miss a dose of this medicine, take it as soon as possible. However, if it is almost time for your next dose, skip the missed dose and go back to your regular dosing schedule. Do not double doses.

How to store this medicine:

• **Keep out of the reach of children.**

• Store away from heat and direct light.

• Do not store in the bathroom, near the kitchen sink, or in other damp places. Heat or moisture may cause the medicine to break down.

• Keep the medicine from freezing.

• Do not keep outdated medicine or medicine no longer needed. Be sure that any discarded medicine is out of the reach of children.

Precautions While Using This Medicine

Your doctor should check your progress at regular visits to make sure that this medicine is working properly.

In some patients, headaches may occur when this medicine is taken. To help prevent or relieve the headache, lie down while you are taking this medicine and for a short time after taking it. If headaches become severe or continue, check with your doctor.

Side Effects of This Medicine

Along with its needed effects, a medicine may cause some unwanted effects. Although not all of these side effects may occur, if they do occur they may need medical attention.

Check with your doctor as soon as possible if either of the following side effects occurs:

Less common
    Confusion

Rare
    Irregular heartbeat

Other side effects may occur that usually do not require medical attention. These side effects may go away during treatment as your body adjusts to the medicine. However, check with your doctor if any of the following side effects continue or are bothersome:

More common
    Headache
    Nausea or vomiting

Less common
    Diarrhea
    Dizziness
    Dryness of mouth or increased thirst

Other side effects not listed above may also occur in some patients. If you notice any other effects, check with your doctor.

December 1987

GOLD COMPOUNDS (Systemic)

This information applies to the following medicines:

Auranofin (au-RANE-oh-fin)
Aurothioglucose (aur-oh-thye-oh-GLOO-kose)
Gold Sodium Thiomalate (gold SO-dee-um thye-oh-MAH-late)

Some commonly used brand names or other names are:	Generic names:
Ridaura	Auranofin
Solganal	Aurothioglucose
Myochrysine Myocrisin* Sodium Aurothiomalate	Gold Sodium Thiomalate

*Not available in the U.S.

To the Reader: If you do not recognize the names of medical conditions or medicines referred to in this information, check with your doctor, nurse, or pharmacist. Definitions for selected medical terms may be found in the Glossary. Brand names for the generic drug names listed can be found in the Index. In addition, selected brand names commonly associated with the generic name have been included in the text to help you recognize medicine you may be taking. The fact that a brand name product is not mentioned does not mean the information does not apply. It is a good idea for you to learn both the generic and brand names of your medicines and to write them down for future use.

The gold compounds are used in the treatment of rheumatoid arthritis. They may also be used for other conditions as determined by your doctor.

In addition to the helpful effects of this medicine in treating your medical problem, it has side effects that can be very serious. Before you take this medicine, you should discuss with your doctor the good that this medicine will do as well as the risks of using it.

Auranofin is taken by mouth and is available only with your doctor's prescription. The other gold compounds are given by injection.

Remember:
• **This medicine has been prescribed for your current medical problem only.** It must not be given to other people or used for other problems unless you are directed to do so by your doctor.

• **Keep all medicines out of the reach of children.**

• In order for this medicine to work, it must be used as directed.

• If you are receiving this medicine by injection, some of the information about this medicine may not apply.

• **It is very important that you read and understand the following information.** If any of the information causes you special concern, do not decide against using this medicine without first checking with your doctor.

• Before you begin using any new medicine (prescription or nonprescription) or if you develop any new medical problem while you are using this medicine, check with your doctor, nurse, or pharmacist.

• **If you have any questions** about the following information or if you want more information about this medicine or your medical problem, **ask your doctor, nurse, or pharmacist**.

Before Using This Medicine

In order to decide on the best treatment for your medical problem, your doctor should be told:

—if you have ever had any unusual or allergic reaction to gold or other metals.

—if you are on a low-salt, low-sugar, or any other special diet, if you are allergic to sesame seeds or sesame oil, or if you are allergic to any other substance, such as foods, sulfites or other preservatives, or dyes. Most medicines contain more than their active ingredient. Your doctor, nurse, or pharmacist can help you avoid products that may cause a problem.

—if you have received a gold compound before and developed serious side effects from it.

—if any medicine you have taken has ever caused an allergy or reaction that affected your blood or lungs.

—if you are **pregnant** or if you may become pregnant. Studies on birth defects with gold compounds have not been done in humans. However, studies in animals have shown that gold compounds may cause birth defects.

—if you are **breast-feeding**. Aurothioglucose and gold sodium thiomalate pass into the breast milk and may cause unwanted effects in nursing babies. It is not known whether auranofin passes into the breast milk.

—if you have any of the following medical problems:
   Blood or blood vessel disease
   Colitis
   Kidney disease (or history of)
   Lupus erythematosus
   Sjögren's syndrome
   Skin disease

—if you are taking **any** other prescription or nonprescription (OTC) medicine, especially penicillamine (e.g., Cuprimine).

Proper Use of This Medicine

In order for this medicine to work, it must be taken regularly as ordered by your doctor. Continue receiving the injections or taking auranofin even if you think the medicine is not working. You may not notice the effects of this medicine until after three to six months of regular use.

For patients taking auranofin:

• **Do not take more of this medicine than ordered by your doctor.** Taking too much auranofin may increase the chance of serious unwanted effects.

• If you miss a dose of this medicine, and your dosing schedule is one dose to be taken:

Once a day—Take the missed dose as soon as possible. However, if you do not remember until the next day, skip the missed dose and go back to your regular dosing schedule. Do not double doses.

© 1988   The United States Pharmacopeial Convention, Inc.

More than once a day—Take the missed dose as soon as possible. However, if it is almost time for your next dose, skip the missed dose and go back to your regular dosing schedule. Do not double doses.

How to store this medicine:

- **Keep out of the reach of children.**
- Store away from heat and direct light.
- Do not store this medicine in the bathroom, near the kitchen sink, or in other damp places. Heat or moisture may cause the medicine to break down.
- Do not keep outdated medicine or medicine no longer needed. Be sure that any discarded medicine is out of the reach of children.

Precautions While Using This Medicine

Gold compounds may cause some people to become more sensitive to sunlight than they are normally. These people may break out in a rash after being in the sun, or a skin rash that is already present may become worse. It is best to avoid too much sun or use of a sunlamp while being treated with a gold compound. You may protect yourself against sunlight with clothing, or ask your doctor if you may use a factor-15 (or higher) sunscreen. If you have a severe reaction, check with your doctor.

For patients taking auranofin:

- Your doctor should check your progress at regular visits. Blood and urine tests may be needed to make certain that this medicine is not causing unwanted effects.

For patients receiving gold injections:

- Immediately following an injection of this medicine, side effects such as dizziness, feeling faint, flushing or redness of the face, nausea or vomiting, unusual sweating, or unusual weakness may occur. These will usually go away after you lie down for a few minutes. If any of these effects continue or become worse, check with your doctor.
- Joint pain may occur for 1 or 2 days after you receive an injection of this medicine. This effect usually disappears after the first few injections. However, if this continues or is bothersome, check with your doctor.

Side Effects of This Medicine

Gold compounds have been shown to cause tumors and cancer of the kidney when given to animals in large amounts for a long period of time. However, these effects have not been reported in humans receiving gold compounds for arthritis. If you have any questions about this, check with your doctor.

Along with its needed effects, a medicine may cause some unwanted effects. Although not all of these side effects may occur, side effects may occur at any time during treatment with this medicine **and up to many months after treatment has ended,** and they may need medical attention.

Check with your doctor as soon as possible if any of the following side effects occur:

More common
Irritation or soreness of tongue or gums—less common with auranofin
Metallic taste—less common with auranofin
Skin rash or itching
Ulcers, sores, or white spots in mouth or throat

Less common
Bloody or cloudy urine
Hives
Sore throat and fever
Unusual bleeding or bruising
Unusual tiredness or weakness

Rare
Abdominal or stomach pain (severe)
Bloody or black tarry stools
Coughing or shortness of breath
Red, thickened, or scaly skin
Yellow eyes or skin

With long-term use
Numbness, tingling, pain, or weakness in hands or feet
Red or irritated eyes

Other side effects may occur that usually do not require medical attention. These side effects may go away during treatment as your body adjusts to the medicine. However, check with your doctor if the following side effects continue or are bothersome:

More common with auranofin; rare with injections
Abdominal or stomach cramps or pain (mild or moderate)
Bloated feeling, gas, or indigestion
Decrease or loss of appetite
Diarrhea
Nausea or vomiting

Less common
Constipation—with auranofin
Joint pain—with injections

Some patients receiving auranofin have noticed changes in the taste of certain foods. If you notice a metallic taste while receiving any gold compound, check with your doctor as soon as possible. If you notice any other taste changes while you are taking auranofin, it is not necessary to check with your doctor unless you find this effect especially bothersome.

For elderly patients: Many medicines have not been tested in older people. Therefore, it is not known whether the medicine acts the same way it does in younger adults. Check with your doctor or pharmacist if you notice any unusual effects while taking this medicine.

Other side effects not listed above may also occur in some patients. If you notice any other effects, check with your doctor.

December 1987

GONADORELIN (Systemic)

Some commonly used brand names or other names are Factrel and LHRH.

To the Reader: If you do not recognize the names of medical conditions or medicines referred to in this information, check with your doctor, nurse, or pharmacist. Definitions for selected medical terms may be found in the Glossary. Brand names for the generic drug names listed can be found in the Index. In addition, selected brand names commonly associated with the generic name have been included in the text to help you recognize medicine you may be taking. The fact that a brand name product is not mentioned does not mean the information does not apply. It is a good idea for you to learn both the generic and brand names of your medicines and to write them down for future use.

Gonadorelin (goe-nad-oh-RELL-in) is a man-made chemical identical to a hormone normally released from the hypothalamus gland. This hormone causes the release of other hormones from the anterior pituitary gland. These hormones are necessary for normal development in children and fertility in adults. Gonadorelin is used to test how well the hypothalamus and the anterior pituitary are working.

It may also be used for other conditions as determined by your doctor.

How test is done: First, one or more samples of your blood are taken. Then gonadorelin is given by intravenous (into a vein) or subcutaneous (under the skin) injection. At regular times after it is given, more blood samples are taken. Then the results of the test are studied.

Gonadorelin is to be used only under the supervision of a doctor.

Remember:
• **If you have any questions** about the following information or if you want more information about this test or your medical problem, **ask your doctor, nurse, or pharmacist**.

Before Having This Test
Before this test is given, your doctor should be told:
— if you have ever had any unusual or allergic reaction to gonadorelin.

— if you are on a low-salt, low-sugar, or any other special diet, or if you are allergic to any substance, such as foods or sulfites or other preservatives. Most medicines contain more than their active ingredient. Your doctor, nurse, or pharmacist can help you avoid products that may cause a problem.

— if you are taking **any** other prescription or nonprescription (OTC) medicine.

Side Effects of This Medicine
Along with its needed effects, a medicine may cause some unwanted effects. No serious side effects have been reported with gonadorelin. However, pain or itching may occur at the place of injection. If this continues or is bothersome or if you notice any other effects, check with your doctor.

December 1987

GONADOTROPIN, CHORIONIC
(Systemic)

Some commonly used brand or other names are:

Antuitrin*	HCG
A.P.L.	Pregnyl
Follutein	Profasi HP

Generic name product may also be available in Canada.

*Not available in the U.S.

To the Reader: If you do not recognize the names of medical conditions or medicines referred to in this information, check with your doctor, nurse, or pharmacist. Definitions for selected medical terms may be found in the Glossary. Brand names for the generic drug names listed can be found in the Index. In addition, selected brand names commonly associated with the generic name have been included in the text to help you recognize medicine you may be taking. The fact that a brand name product is not mentioned does not mean the information does not apply. It is a good idea for you to learn both the generic and brand names of your medicines and to write them down for future use.

Chorionic gonadotropin (kor-ee-ON-ik goe-NAD-oh-troe-pin) has different uses for males and females.

In women who are unable to become pregnant, it is used with another medicine as a fertility drug.

In men or boys, it is used to treat some sexual problems that are caused by a lack of hormones.

Although chorionic gonadotropin has been prescribed to help some patients lose weight, it should **never** be used this way. When used improperly, chorionic gonadotropin can cause serious problems.

Chorionic gonadotropin is to be administered only by or under the immediate supervision of your doctor.

Remember:

• **It is very important that you read and understand the following information.** If any of the information causes you special concern, do not decide against receiving this medicine without first checking with your doctor.

• Before you begin using any new medicine (prescription or nonprescription) or if you develop any new medical problem while you are receiving this medicine, check with your doctor, nurse, or pharmacist.

• **If you have any questions** about the following information or if you want more information about this medicine or your medical problem, **ask your doctor, nurse, or pharmacist.**

Before Using This Medicine

If you become pregnant as a result of using this medicine, you have an increased chance of a multiple birth (for example, twins, triplets) occurring. If you have any questions about this, check with your doctor.

In order to decide on the best treatment for your medical problem, your doctor should be told:

—if you have ever had any unusual or allergic reaction to chorionic gonadotropin.

—if you are on a low-salt, low-sugar, or any other special diet, or if you are allergic to any substance, such as foods or sulfites or other preservatives. Most medicines contain more than their active ingredient. Your doctor, nurse, or pharmacist can help you avoid products that may cause a problem.

—if you have any of the following medical problems:

For males

Cancer of the prostate

For females

Cyst on ovary
Fibroid tumors of the uterus
Problems with veins
Unusual vaginal bleeding

For males and females

Asthma
Epilepsy
Heart disease
Kidney disease
Migraine headaches
Pituitary disease

Precautions While Using This Medicine

It is very important that your doctor check your progress at regular visits to make sure that the medicine is working and to check for unwanted effects.

It may take some time for this medicine to work. **It is very important that you continue to receive the medicine.** If you are concerned that it is not working, discuss it with your doctor.

For women taking this medicine to become pregnant:

• Record your temperature every day if told to do so by your doctor, so that you will know if you have begun to ovulate. It is important that intercourse take place at the correct time to give you the best chance of becoming pregnant. **Follow your doctor's instructions carefully.**

Side Effects of This Medicine

Along with its needed effects, a medicine may cause some other effects. Although not all of these side effects may occur, if they do occur they may need medical attention.

Check with your doctor as soon as possible if any of the following side effects occur:

For females only
More common

Bloating
Stomach or pelvic pain

For boys only
  Less common

    Acne
    Enlargement of penis and testes
    Growth of pubic hair
    Rapid increase in height

Other side effects may occur that usually do not require medical attention. These side effects may go away during treatment as your body adjusts to the medicine. However, check with your doctor if any of the following side effects continue or are bothersome:

Less common

    Enlargement of breasts
    Headache
    Irritability
    Mental depression

    Pain at place of injection
    Swelling of feet or lower legs
    Tiredness

After you stop receiving this medicine, it may continue to cause some side effects which require medical attention. During this period of time check with your doctor if you notice either of the following side effects:

For females only
    Bloating
    Stomach or pelvic pain

Other side effects not listed above may also occur in some patients. If you notice any other effects, check with your doctor.

_____

December 1987

_____

GRISEOFULVIN (Systemic)

Some commonly used brand names are:

Fulvicin P/G	Grisactin Ultra
Fulvicin-U/F	Gris-PEG
Grifulvin V	Grisovin-FP*
Grisactin	

Generic name product may also be available in the U.S.

*Not available in the U.S.

To the Reader: If you do not recognize the names of medical conditions or medicines referred to in this information, check with your doctor, nurse, or pharmacist. Definitions for selected medical terms may be found in the Glossary. Brand names for the generic drug names listed can be found in the Index. In addition, selected brand names commonly associated with the generic name have been included in the text to help you recognize medicine you may be taking. The fact that a brand name product is not mentioned does not mean the information does not apply. It is a good idea for you to learn both the generic and brand names of your medicines and to write them down for future use.

Griseofulvin (gri-see-oh-FUL-vin) belongs to the group of medicines called antifungals. It is taken by mouth to treat fungus infections of the skin, hair, fingernails, and toenails.

Griseofulvin is available only with your doctor's prescription.

Remember:

• **This medicine has been prescribed for your present infection only.** Another infection later on may require a different medicine. Also, even though other people may have the same symptoms as you, they may have a different kind of infection. Your medicine may not work for them and may even cause them harm. Therefore, **your medicine must not be given to other people or used for other infections** unless you are otherwise directed by your doctor.

• **Keep all medicines out of the reach of children.**

• In order for this medicine to work, it must be used as directed.

• **It is very important that you read and understand the following information.** If any of the information causes you special concern, do not decide against using this medicine without first checking with your doctor.

• Before you begin using any new medicine (prescription or nonprescription) or if you develop any new medical problem while you are using this medicine, check with your doctor, nurse, or pharmacist.

• **If you have any questions** about the following information or if you want more information about this medicine or your medical problem, **ask your doctor, nurse, or pharmacist.**

Before Using This Medicine

In order to decide on the best treatment for your medical problem, your doctor should be told:

—if you have ever had any unusual or allergic reaction to penicillin, penicillamine, or griseofulvin.

—if you are on a low-salt, low-sugar, or any other special diet, or if you are allergic to any substance, such as foods, sulfites or other preservatives, or dyes.

Most medicines contain more than their active ingredient, and many liquid medicines contain alcohol. Your doctor, nurse, or pharmacist can help you avoid products that may cause a problem.

—if you are **pregnant** or if you may become pregnant. Griseofulvin has not been shown to cause birth defects or other problems in humans. However, studies in rats have shown that griseofulvin causes birth defects and other problems.

—if you are **breast-feeding**. However, griseofulvin has not been shown to cause problems in nursing babies.

—if you have any of the following medical problems:
Liver disease
Lupus erythematosus
Porphyria

—if you are taking **any** other prescription or nonprescription (OTC) medicine, especially:
Aminobenzoic acid (PABA)
Amiodarone (e.g., Cordarone)
Anthralin (e.g., Anthra-Derm)
Anticoagulants (blood thinners)
Antidiabetic agents, oral (diabetes medicine you take by mouth)
Antihistamines
Chlorprothixene (e.g., Taractan)
Coal tar (e.g., Estar)
Estrogens (female hormones)
Ethionamide (e.g., Trecator-SC)
Etretinate (e.g., Tegison)
Fluorouracil (topical) (e.g., Efudex)
Furosemide (e.g., Lasix)
Isotretinoin (e.g., Accutane)
Methoxsalen (e.g., Oxsoralen)
Nalidixic acid (e.g., NegGram)
Oral contraceptives (birth control pills) containing estrogen
Phenothiazines (acetophenazine, chlorpromazine, fluphenazine, mesoridazine, perphenazine, prochlorperazine, promazine, promethazine, thioridazine, trifluoperazine, triflupromazine, trimeprazine)
Pyrazinamide
Sulfonamides (sulfa medicine)
Tetracyclines
Thiazide diuretics (water pills)
Thiothixene (e.g., Navane)
Tretinoin (e.g., Retin-A)
Trioxsalen (e.g., Trisoralen)

Proper Use of This Medicine

Griseofulvin is best taken with or after meals, especially fatty ones (for example, whole milk or ice cream). This lessens possible stomach upset and helps to clear up the infection by helping your body absorb the medicine better. **However, if you are on a low-fat diet, check with your doctor.**

For patients taking the oral liquid form of griseofulvin:

• Use a specially marked measuring spoon or other device to measure each dose accurately since the average household teaspoon may not hold the right amount of liquid.

To help clear up your infection completely, **keep taking this medicine for the full time of treatment** even if you begin to feel better after a few days; do not miss any doses.

If you do miss a dose of this medicine, take it as soon as possible. However, if it is almost time for your next dose, skip the missed dose and go back to your regular dosing schedule. Do not double doses.

How to store this medicine:

- **Keep out of the reach of children.**

- Store away from heat and direct light.

- Do not store the capsule or tablet form of this medicine in the bathroom, near the kitchen sink, or in other damp places. Heat or moisture may cause the medicine to break down.

- Keep the oral liquid form of this medicine from freezing.

- Do not keep outdated medicine or medicine no longer needed. Be sure that any discarded medicine is out of the reach of children.

Precautions While Using This Medicine

Your doctor should check your progress at regular visits to make sure that griseofulvin does not cause unwanted effects.

Oral contraceptives (birth control pills) containing estrogen may not work as well if you take them while you are taking griseofulvin. Unplanned pregnancies may occur. You should use a different or additional means of birth control while you are taking griseofulvin. If you have any questions about this, check with your doctor or pharmacist.

Griseofulvin may increase the effects of alcohol. If taken with alcohol it may also cause unusually fast heartbeat, flushing, increased sweating, or redness of the face. Therefore, **do not drink alcoholic beverages while you are taking this medicine,** unless you have first checked with your doctor.

This medicine may cause some people to become dizzy or less alert than they are normally. **Make sure you know how you react to this medicine before you drive, use machines, or do other jobs that require you to be alert.** If these reactions are especially bothersome, check with your doctor.

Some people who take griseofulvin may become more sensitive to sunlight than they are normally. **When you first begin taking this medicine, avoid too much sun and do not use a sunlamp until you see how you react to the sun,** especially if you tend to burn easily. **If you have a severe reaction, check with your doctor.**

Side Effects of This Medicine

Along with its needed effects, a medicine may cause some unwanted effects. Although not all of these side effects may occur, if they do occur they may need medical attention.

Check with your doctor as soon as possible if any of the following side effects occur:

Less common
    Confusion
    Increased sensitivity of skin to sunlight
    Skin rash, hives, or itching
    Soreness or irritation of mouth or tongue
Rare
    Numbness, tingling, pain, or weakness in hands or feet
    Sore throat and fever

Other side effects may occur that usually do not require medical attention. These side effects may go away during treatment as your body adjusts to the medicine. However, check with your doctor if any of the following side effects continue or are bothersome:

More common
    Headache

Less common
    Diarrhea
    Dizziness
    Nausea or vomiting
    Stomach pain
    Trouble in sleeping
    Unusual tiredness

For elderly patients: Many medicines have not been tested in older people. Therefore, it is not known whether the medicine acts the same way it does in younger adults. Check with your doctor or pharmacist if you notice any unusual effects while taking this medicine or if you think it is not working as it should.

Other side effects not listed above may also occur in some patients. If you notice any other effects, check with your doctor.

December 1987

GUAIFENESIN (Systemic)

Some commonly used brand names and other names are:

Anti-Tuss	Guiatuss
Balminil Expectorant*	Halotussin
Baytussin	Humibid L.A.
Breonesin	Hytuss
Colrex Expectorant	Hytuss-2X
Cremacoat 2	Malotuss
Gee-Gee	Neo-Spec*
GG-CEN	Nortussin
Glyate	Resyl*
Glyceryl guaiacolate	Robafen
Glycotuss	Robitussin
Glytuss	S-T Expectorant

Generic name product may also be available.

*Not available in the U.S.

To the Reader: If you do not recognize the names of medical conditions or medicines referred to in this information, check with your doctor, nurse, or pharmacist. Definitions for selected medical terms may be found in the Glossary. Brand names for the generic drug names listed can be found in the Index. In addition, selected brand names commonly associated with the generic name have been included in the text to help you recognize medicine you may be taking. The fact that a brand name product is not mentioned does not mean the information does not apply. It is a good idea for you to learn both the generic and brand names of your medicines and to write them down for future use.

Guaifenesin (gwye-FEN-e-sin) is taken by mouth to relieve coughs due to colds or influenza. Guaifenesin works by loosening the mucus or phlegm (pronounced flem) in the lungs.

This medicine is not to be used for the chronic cough that occurs with smoking, asthma, or emphysema or when there is an unusually large amount of mucus or phlegm with the cough.

Guaifenesin is available without a prescription; however, your doctor may have special instructions on the proper dose of this medicine for your medical condition.

Remember:
• **Keep all medicines out of the reach of children.**

• In order for this medicine to work, it must be used as directed. **If you are using this medicine without a prescription, it is very important to follow the directions on the label.**

• **It is also very important that you read and understand the following information.** If any of the information causes you special concern, check with your doctor before using this medicine without a prescription.

• Before you begin using any new medicine (prescription or nonprescription) or if you develop any new medical problem while you are using this medicine, check with your doctor, nurse, or pharmacist.

• **If you have any questions** about the following information or if you want more information about this medicine or your medical problem, **ask your doctor, nurse, or pharmacist.**

Before Using This Medicine

Before you use this medicine, check with your doctor, nurse, or pharmacist:

—if you have ever had any unusual or allergic reaction to guaifenesin.

—if you are on a low-salt, low-sugar, or any other special diet, or if you are allergic to any substance, such as foods, sulfites or other preservatives, or dyes. Most medicines contain more than their active ingredient, and many liquid medicines contain alcohol. Your doctor, nurse, or pharmacist can help you avoid products that may cause a problem.

—if you are **pregnant** or if you may become pregnant. Studies have not been done in either humans or animals.

—if you are **breast-feeding**. Guaifenesin has not been shown to cause problems in nursing babies.

Proper Use of This Medicine

To help loosen mucus or phlegm in the lungs, **drink a glass of water after each dose of this medicine,** unless otherwise directed by your doctor.

If you must take this medicine regularly and you miss a dose, take it as soon as possible. However, if it is almost time for your next dose, skip the missed dose and go back to your regular dosing schedule. Do not double doses.

How to store this medicine:

• **Keep out of the reach of children.**

• Store away from heat and direct light.

• Do not store the capsule or tablet form of this medicine in the bathroom, near the kitchen sink, or in other damp places. Heat or moisture may cause the medicine to break down.

• Do not refrigerate the syrup form of this medicine.

• Do not keep outdated medicine or medicine no longer needed. Be sure that any discarded medicine is out of the reach of children.

Precautions While Using This Medicine

If your cough has not improved after 7 days or if you have a high fever, skin rash, continuing headache, or sore throat with the cough, check with your doctor. These signs may mean that you have other medical problems.

Side Effects of This Medicine

Along with its needed effects, a medicine may cause some unwanted effects. Although not all of these side effects may occur, if they do occur they may need medical attention.

Check with your doctor as soon as possible if any of the following side effects occur:

Less common or rare

Diarrhea
Drowsiness
Nausea or vomiting
Stomach pain

For elderly patients: Many medicines have not been tested in older people. Therefore, it is not known whether the medicine acts the same way it does in younger adults.

Check with your doctor or pharmacist if you notice any unusual effects while taking this medicine or if you think it is not working as it should.

Other side effects not listed above may also occur in some patients. If you notice any other effects, check with your doctor.

December 1987

GUANABENZ (Systemic)

A commonly used brand name is Wytensin.

To the Reader: If you do not recognize the names of medical conditions or medicines referred to in this information, check with your doctor, nurse, or pharmacist. Definitions for selected medical terms may be found in the Glossary. Brand names for the generic drug names listed can be found in the Index. In addition, selected brand names commonly associated with the generic name have been included in the text to help you recognize medicine you may be taking. The fact that a brand name product is not mentioned does not mean the information does not apply. It is a good idea for you to learn both the generic and brand names of your medicines and to write them down for future use.

Guanabenz (GWAHN-a-benz) belongs to the general class of medicines called antihypertensives. It is taken by mouth to treat high blood pressure. High blood pressure adds to the workload of the heart and arteries. If it continues for a long time, the heart and arteries may not function properly. This can damage the blood vessels of the brain, heart, and kidneys, resulting in a stroke, heart failure, or kidney failure. High blood pressure may also increase the risk of heart attacks. These problems may be less likely to occur if blood pressure is controlled.

Guanabenz works by controlling nerve impulses along certain nerve pathways. As a result, it relaxes blood vessels so that blood passes through them more easily. This helps to lower blood pressure.

Guanabenz is available only with your doctor's prescription.

Remember:

• **This medicine has been prescribed for your current medical problem only.** It must not be given to other people or used for other problems unless you are directed to do so by your doctor.

• **Keep all medicines out of the reach of children.**

• In order for this medicine to work, it must be used as directed.

• **It is very important that you read and understand the following information.** If any of the information causes you special concern, do not decide against using this medicine without first checking with your doctor.

• Before you begin using any new medicine (prescription or nonprescription) or if you develop any new medical problem while you are using this medicine, check with your doctor, nurse, or pharmacist.

• **If you have any questions** about the following information or if you want more information about this medicine or your medical problem, **ask your doctor, nurse, or pharmacist.**

Before Using This Medicine

In order to decide on the best treatment for your medical problem, your doctor should be told:

—if you have ever had any unusual or allergic reaction to guanabenz.

—if you are on a low-salt, low-sugar, or any other special diet, or if you are allergic to any substance, such as foods, sulfites or other preservatives, or dyes.

Most medicines contain more than their active ingredient. Your doctor, nurse, or pharmacist can help you avoid products that may cause a problem.

—if you are **pregnant** or if you may become pregnant. Studies have not been done in humans. However, studies in rats have shown that guanabenz given in doses 9 to 10 times the maximum human dose caused a decrease in fertility. In addition, 3 to 6 times the maximum human dose caused birth defects (in the skeleton) in mice, and 6 to 9 times the maximum human dose caused death of the fetus in rats.

—if you are **breast-feeding**. It is not known whether guanabenz passes into the breast milk. This medicine has not been shown to cause problems in nursing babies.

—if you have any of the following medical problems:
   Heart or blood vessel disease
   Kidney disease
   Liver disease

—if you are taking **any** other prescription or nonprescription (OTC) medicine.

Proper Use of This Medicine

Importance of diet—When prescribing medicine for your condition, your doctor may also prescribe a personal diet for you. Such a diet may be low in sodium (salt). Most people eat much more sodium than they need and too much sodium in the diet may increase blood pressure. Some foods that contain large amounts of sodium are canned soup, pickles, ketchup, green and ripe olives, relish, frankfurters, soy sauce, and carbonated beverages. Your doctor may want you to limit the amounts of these and other high-sodium foods in your diet. High blood pressure medicine is usually more effective when such a diet is properly followed.

Also, it may be very important for you to go on a reducing diet. However, check with your doctor before changing your diet.

Many patients who have high blood pressure will not notice any signs of the problem. In fact, many may feel normal. It is very important that you **take your medicine exactly as directed** and that you keep your appointments with your doctor even if you feel well.

Remember that this medicine will not cure your high blood pressure but it does control it. Therefore, you must continue to take it as directed if you expect to lower your blood pressure and keep it down. **You may have to take high blood pressure medicine for the rest of your life.** If high blood pressure is not treated, it can cause serious problems such as heart failure, blood vessel disease, stroke, or kidney disease.

In order to help remember to take your medicine, try to get into the habit of taking it at the same time each day.

If you miss a dose of this medicine, take it as soon as possible. However, if it is almost time for your next dose, skip the missed dose and go back to your regular dosing schedule. Do not double doses. If you miss two or more doses in a row, check with your doctor. If your body suddenly goes without this medicine, some unpleasant effects may occur. If you have any questions about this, check with your doctor.

How to store this medicine:

- **Keep out of the reach of children.**

- Store away from heat and direct light.

- Do not store in the bathroom, near the kitchen sink, or in other damp places. Heat or moisture may cause the medicine to break down.

- Do not keep outdated medicine or medicine no longer needed. Be sure that any discarded medicine is out of the reach of children.

Precautions While Using This Medicine

It is important that your doctor check your progress at regular visits to make sure that this medicine is working properly.

Check with your doctor before you stop taking guanabenz. Your doctor may want you to reduce gradually the amount you are taking before stopping completely.

Before having any kind of surgery (including dental surgery) or emergency treatment, tell the physician or dentist in charge that you are using this medicine.

Do not take other medicines unless they have been discussed with your doctor. This especially includes over-the-counter (nonprescription) medicines for appetite control, asthma, colds, cough, hay fever, or sinus problems, since they may tend to increase your blood pressure.

Guanabenz will add to the effects of alcohol and other CNS depressants (medicines that slow down the nervous system, possibly causing drowsiness). Some examples of CNS depressants are antihistamines or medicine for hay fever, other allergies, or colds; sedatives, tranquilizers, or sleeping medicine; prescription pain medicine or narcotics; barbiturates; medicine for seizures; muscle relaxants; or anesthetics, including some dental anesthetics. **Check with your doctor before taking any of the above while you are using this medicine.**

Guanabenz may cause some people to become dizzy, drowsy, or less alert than they are normally. **Make sure you know how you react to this medicine before you drive, use machines, or do other jobs that require you to be alert.**

Guanabenz may cause dryness of the mouth, nose, and throat. For temporary relief of mouth dryness, use sugarless candy or gum, melt bits of ice in your mouth, or use a saliva substitute. However, if dry mouth continues for more than 2 weeks, check with your physician or dentist. Continuing dryness of the mouth may increase the chance of dental disease, including tooth decay, gum disease, and fungal infections.

Side Effects of This Medicine

Along with its needed effects, a medicine may cause some unwanted effects. Although not all of these side effects may occur, if they do occur they may need medical attention.

Check with your doctor as soon as possible if any of the following side effects occur:
Signs of overdose
    Dizziness (severe)
    Faintness
    Irritability
    Nervousness
    Pinpoint pupils
    Slow heartbeat
    Unusual tiredness or weakness

Other side effects may occur that usually do not require medical attention. These side effects may go away during treatment as your body adjusts to the medicine. However, check with your doctor if any of the following side effects continue or are bothersome:
More common
    Dizziness
    Drowsiness
    Dry mouth
    Weakness
Less common or rare
    Decreased sexual ability
    Headache
    Nausea

After you have been using this medicine for a while, unpleasant effects may occur if you stop taking it too suddenly. After you stop taking this medicine, check with your doctor if any of the following effects occur:
    Anxiety or tenseness
    Chest pain
    Fast or irregular heartbeat
    Headache
    Increased salivation
    Increase in sweating
    Nausea or vomiting
    Nervousness or restlessness
    Shaking or trembling of hands or fingers
    Stomach cramps
    Trouble in sleeping

For elderly patients: Dizziness, faintness, or drowsiness may be more likely to occur in the elderly, who are usually more sensitive to the effects of guanabenz.

Other side effects not listed above may also occur in some patients. If you notice any other effects, check with your doctor.

December 1987

GUANADREL (Systemic)

A commonly used brand name is Hylorel.

To the Reader: If you do not recognize the names of medical conditions or medicines referred to in this information, check with your doctor, nurse, or pharmacist. Definitions for selected medical terms may be found in the Glossary. Brand names for the generic drug names listed can be found in the Index. In addition, selected brand names commonly associated with the generic name have been included in the text to help you recognize medicine you may be taking. The fact that a brand name product is not mentioned does not mean the information does not apply. It is a good idea for you to learn both the generic and brand names of your medicines and to write them down for future use.

Guanadrel (GWAHN-a-drel) belongs to the general class of medicines called antihypertensives. It is used to treat high blood pressure.

High blood pressure adds to the workload of the heart and arteries. If it continues for a long time, the heart and arteries may not function properly. This can damage the blood vessels of the brain, heart, and kidneys resulting in a stroke, heart failure, or kidney failure. High blood pressure may also increase the risk of heart attacks. These problems may be less likely to occur if blood pressure is controlled.

Guanadrel works by controlling nerve impulses along certain nerve pathways. As a result, it relaxes the blood vessels so that blood passes through them more easily. This helps to lower blood pressure.

Guanadrel is available only with your doctor's prescription.

Remember:

• **This medicine has been prescribed for your current medical problem only.** It must not be given to other people or used for other problems unless you are directed to do so by your doctor.

• **Keep all medicines out of the reach of children.**

• In order for this medicine to work, it must be used as directed.

• **It is very important that you read and understand the following information.** If any of the information causes you special concern, do not decide against using this medicine without first checking with your doctor.

• Before you begin using any new medicine (prescription or nonprescription) or if you develop any new medical problem while you are using this medicine, check with your doctor, nurse, or pharmacist.

• **If you have any questions** about the following information or if you want more information about this medicine or your medical problem, **ask your doctor, nurse, or pharmacist.**

Before Using This Medicine

In order to decide on the best treatment for your medical problem, your doctor should be told:

—if you have ever had any unusual or allergic reaction to guanadrel.

—if you are on a low-salt, low-sugar, or any other special diet, or if you are allergic to any substance, such as foods, sulfites or other preservatives, or dyes.

Most medicines contain more than their active ingredient. Your doctor, nurse, or pharmacist can help you avoid products that may cause a problem.

—if you are **pregnant** or if you may become pregnant. Studies have not been done in humans. However, guanadrel has not been shown to cause birth defects or other problems in rats and rabbits given up to 12 times the highest human dose.

—if you are **breast-feeding**. It is not known whether guanadrel passes into breast milk. However, it has not been shown to cause problems in nursing babies.

—if you have any of the following medical problems:

    Asthma (history of)
    Diarrhea
    Fever
    Heart or blood vessel disease
    Pheochromocytoma
    Stomach ulcer (history of)

—if you have recently had a heart attack or stroke.

—if you are taking **any** other prescription or nonprescription (OTC) medicine, especially:

    Chlorprothixene (e.g., Taractan)
    Loxapine (e.g., Loxitane)
    Thiothixene (e.g., Navane)
    Tricyclic antidepressants (amitriptyline, amoxapine, clomipramine, desipramine, doxepin, imipramine, nortriptyline, protriptyline, trimipramine)

—if you are now taking or have taken within the past 2 weeks monoamine oxidase (MAO) inhibitors such as:

    Furazolidone (e.g., Furoxone)
    Isocarboxazid (e.g., Marplan)
    Pargyline (e.g., Eutonyl)
    Phenelzine (e.g., Nardil)
    Procarbazine (e.g., Matulane)
    Tranylcypromine (e.g., Parnate)

Proper Use of This Medicine

Importance of diet—When prescribing medicine for your condition, your doctor may also prescribe a personal diet for you. Such a diet may be low in sodium (salt). Most people eat much more sodium than they need and too much sodium in the diet may increase blood pressure. Some foods that contain large amounts of sodium are canned soup, pickles, ketchup, green and ripe olives, relish, frankfurters, soy sauce, and carbonated beverages. Your doctor may want you to limit the amounts of these and other high-sodium foods in your diet. High blood pressure medicine is usually more effective when such a diet is properly followed.

Also, it may be very important for you to go on a reducing diet. However, check with your doctor before changing your diet.

Many patients who have high blood pressure will not notice any signs of the problem. In fact, many may feel normal. It is very important that you **take your medicine exactly as directed** and that you keep your appointments with your doctor even if you feel well.

© 1988   The United States Pharmacopeial Convention, Inc.

Remember that guanadrel will not cure your high blood pressure but it does help control it. Therefore, you must continue to take it as directed if you expect to lower your blood pressure and keep it down. **You may have to take high blood pressure medicine for the rest of your life.** If high blood pressure is not treated, it can cause serious problems such as heart failure, blood vessel disease, stroke, or kidney disease.

In order to help remember to take your medicine, try to get into the habit of taking it at the same time each day.

If you miss a dose of guanadrel, take it as soon as possible. However, if it is almost time for your next dose, skip the missed dose and go back to your regular dosing schedule. Do not double doses.

How to store this medicine:

- **Keep out of the reach of children.**

- Store away from heat and direct light.

- Do not store in the bathroom, near the kitchen sink, or in other damp places. Heat or moisture may cause the medicine to break down.

- Do not keep outdated medicine or medicine no longer needed. Be sure that any discarded medicine is out of the reach of children.

Precautions While Using This Medicine

It is important that your doctor check your progress at regular visits to make sure that this medicine is working properly.

Dizziness, lightheadedness, or fainting may occur, especially when you get up from a lying or sitting position. This may be more likely to occur in the morning. **Getting up slowly may help.** If you feel dizzy, sit or lie down. When you get up from lying down, sit on the edge of the bed with your feet dangling for 1 or 2 minutes. Then stand up slowly. If the problem continues or gets worse, check with your doctor.

The dizziness, lightheadedness, or fainting is also more likely to occur if you drink alcohol, stand for long periods of time, exercise, or if the weather is hot. **While you are taking guanadrel, be careful in the amount of alcohol you drink. Also, use extra care during exercise or hot weather or if you must stand for long periods of time.**

Do not take other medicines unless they have been discussed with your doctor. This especially includes over-the-counter (nonprescription) medicines for appetite control, asthma, colds, cough, hay fever, or sinus problems, since they may tend to increase your blood pressure.

Before having any kind of surgery (including dental surgery) or emergency treatment, tell the physician or dentist in charge that you are taking guanadrel.

Tell your doctor if you get a fever since that may change the amount of medicine you have to take.

Side Effects of This Medicine

Along with its needed effects, a medicine may cause some unwanted effects. Although not all of these side effects may occur, if they do occur they may need medical attention.

Check with your doctor immediately if either of the following side effects occurs since they may be signs of an overdose:
Rare
    Blurred vision
    Dizziness or faintness (severe)

Check with your doctor as soon as possible if any of the following side effects occur:
More common
    Swelling of feet or lower legs
Less common or rare
    Chest pain
    Shortness of breath

Other side effects may occur that usually do not require medical attention. These side effects may go away during treatment as your body adjusts to the medicine. However, check with your doctor if any of the following side effects continue or are bothersome:
More common
    Difficulty in ejaculating
    Dizziness, lightheadedness, or fainting, especially when getting up from a lying or sitting position
    Drowsiness or tiredness
Less common or rare
    Diarrhea or increase in bowel movements
    Dry mouth
    Headache
    Muscle pain or tremors
    Nighttime urination

For elderly patients: Dizziness or faintness may be more likely to occur in the elderly, who are usually more sensitive to the effects of guanadrel.

Other side effects not listed above may also occur in some patients. If you notice any other effects, check with your doctor.

December 1987

GUANETHIDINE (Systemic)

Some commonly used brand names are Apo-Guanethidine* and Ismelin.

Generic name product may also be available in the U.S.

*Not available in the U.S.

To the Reader: If you do not recognize the names of medical conditions or medicines referred to in this information, check with your doctor, nurse, or pharmacist. Definitions for selected medical terms may be found in the Glossary. Brand names for the generic drug names listed can be found in the Index. In addition, selected brand names commonly associated with the generic name have been included in the text to help you recognize medicine you may be taking. The fact that a brand name product is not mentioned does not mean the information does not apply. It is a good idea for you to learn both the generic and brand names of your medicines and to write them down for future use.

Guanethidine (gwahn-ETH-i-deen) belongs to the general class of medicines called antihypertensives. It is taken by mouth to treat high blood pressure. High blood pressure adds to the workload of the heart and arteries. If it continues for a long time, the heart and arteries may not function properly. This can damage the blood vessels of the brain, heart, and kidneys, resulting in a stroke, heart failure, or kidney failure. High blood pressure may also increase the risk of heart attacks. These problems may be less likely to occur if blood pressure is controlled.

Guanethidine works by controlling nerve impulses along certain nerve pathways. As a result, it relaxes the blood vessels so that blood passes through them more easily. This helps to lower blood pressure.

Guanethidine is available only with your doctor's prescription.

Remember:
• **This medicine has been prescribed for your current medical problem only.** It must not be given to other people or used for other problems unless you are directed to do so by your doctor.

• **Keep all medicines out of the reach of children.**

• In order for this medicine to work, it must be used as directed.

• **It is very important that you read and understand the following information.** If any of the information causes you special concern, do not decide against using this medicine without first checking with your doctor.

• Before you begin using any new medicine (prescription or nonprescription) or if you develop any new medical problem while you are using this medicine, check with your doctor, nurse, or pharmacist.

• **If you have any questions** about the following information or if you want more information about this medicine or your medical problem, **ask your doctor, nurse, or pharmacist.**

Before Using This Medicine

In order to decide on the best treatment for your medical problem, your doctor should be told:

—if you have ever had any unusual or allergic reaction to guanethidine.

—if you are on a low-salt, low-sugar, or any other special diet, or if you are allergic to any substance, such as foods, sulfites or other preservatives, or dyes. Most medicines contain more than their active ingredient. Your doctor, nurse, or pharmacist can help you avoid products that may cause a problem.

—if you are **pregnant** or if you may become pregnant. Studies have not been done in either humans or animals.

—if you are **breast-feeding**. Guanethidine has not been shown to cause problems in nursing babies.

—if you have any of the following medical problems:
Asthma (history of)
Diabetes mellitus (sugar diabetes)
Diarrhea
Fever
Heart or blood vessel disease
Kidney disease
Liver disease
Pheochromocytoma
Stomach ulcer (history of)

—if you hve recently had a heart attack or stroke.

—if you are taking **any** other prescription or nonprescription (OTC) medicine, especially:
Antidiabetic agents, oral (diabetes medicine you take by mouth)
Chlorprothixene (e.g., Taractan)
Loxapine (e.g., Loxitane)
Minoxidil (e.g., Loniten)
Thiothixene (e.g., Navane)
Tricyclic antidepressants (amitriptyline, amoxapine, clomipramine, desipramine, doxepin, imipramine, nortriptyline, protriptyline, trimipramine)

—if you are now taking or have taken within the past 2 weeks monoamine oxidase (MAO) inhibitors such as:
Furazolidone (e.g., Furoxone)
Isocarboxazid (e.g., Marplan)
Pargyline (e.g., Eutonyl)
Phenelzine (e.g., Nardil)
Procarbazine (e.g., Matulane)
Tranylcypromine (e.g., Parnate)

Proper Use of This Medicine

Importance of diet—When prescribing medicine for your condition, your doctor may also prescribe a personal diet for you. Such a diet may be low in sodium (salt). Most people eat much more sodium than they need and too much sodium in the diet may increase blood pressure. Some foods that contain large amounts of sodium are canned soup, pickles, ketchup, green and ripe olives, relish, frankfurters, soy sauce, and carbonated beverages. Your doctor may want you to limit the amounts of these and other high-sodium foods in your diet. High blood pressure medicine is usually more effective when such a diet is properly followed.

Also, it may be very important for you to go on a reducing diet. However, check with your doctor before changing your diet.

Many patients who have high blood pressure will not notice any signs of the problem. In fact, many may feel normal. It is very important that you **take your medicine exactly as directed** and that you keep your appointments with your doctor even if you feel well.

Remember that guanethidine will not cure your high blood pressure but it does help control it. Therefore, you must continue to take it as directed if you expect to lower your blood pressure and keep it down. **You may have to take high blood pressure medicine for the rest of your life.** If high blood pressure is not treated, it can cause serious problems such as heart failure, blood vessel disease, stroke, or kidney disease.

In order to help remember to take your medicine, try to get into the habit of taking it at the same time each day.

If you miss a dose of guanethidine, take it as soon as possible. However, if it is almost time for your next dose, skip the missed dose and go back to your regular dosing schedule. Do not double doses.

How to store this medicine:

• **Keep out of the reach of children.**

• Store away from heat and direct light.

• Do not store in the bathroom, near the kitchen sink, or in other damp places. Heat or moisture may cause the medicine to break down.

• Do not keep outdated medicine or medicine no longer needed. Be sure that any discarded medicine is out of the reach of children.

Precautions While Using This Medicine

It is important that your doctor check your progress at regular visits to make sure that this medicine is working properly.

Dizziness, lightheadedness, or fainting may occur, especially when you get up from a lying or sitting position. This is more likely to occur in the morning. **Getting up slowly may help.** When you get up from lying down, sit on the edge of the bed with your feet dangling for 1 or 2 minutes. Then stand up slowly. If the problem continues or gets worse, check with your doctor.

The dizziness, lightheadedness, or fainting is also more likely to occur if you drink alcohol, stand for long periods of time, exercise, or if the weather is hot. **While you are taking this medicine, be careful in the amount of alcohol you drink. Also, use extra care during exercise or hot weather or if you must stand for long periods of time.**

Do not take other medicines unless they have been discussed with your doctor. This especially includes over-the-counter (nonprescription) medicines for appetite control, asthma, colds, cough, hay fever, or sinus problems, since they may tend to increase your blood pressure.

Before having any kind of surgery (including dental surgery) or emergency treatment, tell the physician or dentist in charge that you are taking this medicine.

Tell your doctor if you get a fever since that may change the amount of medicine you have to take.

Side Effects of This Medicine

Along with its needed effects, a medicine may cause some unwanted effects. Although not all of these side effects may occur, if they do occur they may need medical attention.

Check with your doctor as soon as possible if any of the following side effects occur:
More common
    Swelling of feet or lower legs
Less common or rare
    Chest pain
    Shortness of breath

Other side effects may occur that usually do not require medical attention. These side effects may go away during treatment as your body adjusts to the medicine. However, check with your doctor if any of the following side effects continue or are bothersome:
More common
    Diarrhea or increase in bowel movements
    Dizziness, lightheadedness, or fainting, especially when getting up from a lying or sitting position
    Sexual problems in males
    Slow heartbeat
    Stuffy nose
    Tiredness or weakness
Less common or rare
    Blurred vision
    Drooping eyelids
    Dry mouth
    Headache
    Loss of hair on scalp
    Muscle pain or tremors
    Nausea or vomiting
    Nighttime urination
    Skin rash

For elderly patients: Dizziness, lightheadedness, or fainting may be more likely to occur in the elderly, who are more sensitive to the effects of guanethidine.

Other side effects not listed above may also occur in some patients. If you notice any other effects, check with your doctor.

December 1987

GUANETHIDINE AND HYDROCHLOROTHIAZIDE (Systemic)

A commonly used brand name is Esimil.

To the Reader: If you do not recognize the names of medical conditions or medicines referred to in this information, check with your doctor, nurse, or pharmacist. Definitions for selected medical terms may be found in the Glossary. Brand names for the generic drug names listed can be found in the Index. In addition, selected brand names commonly associated with the generic name have been included in the text to help you recognize medicine you may be taking. The fact that a brand name product is not mentioned does not mean the information does not apply. It is a good idea for you to learn both the generic and brand names of your medicines and to write them down for future use.

Guanethidine (gwahn-ETH-i-deen) and hydrochlorothiazide (hye-droe-klor-oh-THYE-a-zide) combination is taken by mouth to treat high blood pressure.

High blood pressure adds to the workload of the heart and arteries. If it continues for a long time, the heart and arteries may not function properly. This can damage the blood vessels of the brain, heart, and kidneys, resulting in a stroke, heart failure, or kidney failure. High blood pressure may also increase the risk of heart attacks. These problems may be less likely to occur if blood pressure is controlled.

Guanethidine works by controlling nerve impulses along certain nerve pathways. As a result, it relaxes the blood vessels so that blood passes through them more easily. The hydrochlorothiazide in this combination is a thiazide diuretic (water pill) that helps reduce the amount of water in the body by increasing the flow of urine.

Guanethidine and hydrochlorothiazide combination is available only with your doctor's prescription.

Remember:
- **This medicine has been prescribed for your current medical problem only.** It must not be given to other people or used for other problems unless you are directed to do so by your doctor.

- **Keep all medicines out of the reach of children.**

- In order for this medicine to work, it must be used as directed.

- **It is very important that you read and understand the following information.** If any of the information causes you special concern, do not decide against using this medicine without first checking with your doctor.

- Before you begin using any new medicine (prescription or nonprescription) or if you develop any new medical problem while you are using this medicine, check with your doctor, nurse, or pharmacist.

- **If you have any questions** about the following information or if you want more information about this medicine or your medical problem, **ask your doctor, nurse, or pharmacist.**

Before Using This Medicine

In order to decide on the best treatment for your medical problem, your doctor should be told:

—if you have ever had any unusual or allergic reaction to guanethidine, sulfonamides (sulfa drugs), hydrochlorothiazide, or other thiazide diuretics (water pills).

—if you are on a low-salt, low-sugar, or any other special diet, or if you are allergic to any substance, such as foods, sulfites or other preservatives, or dyes. Most medicines contain more than their active ingredient. Your doctor, nurse, or pharmacist can help you avoid products that may cause a problem.

—if you are **pregnant** or if you may become pregnant. When hydrochlorothiazide is used during pregnancy, it may cause side effects including jaundice, blood problems, and low potassium in the newborn infant. However, this medicine has not been shown to cause birth defects.

—if you are **breast-feeding**. Although hydrochlorothiazide passes into breast milk, this medicine has not been shown to cause problems in nursing babies.

—if you have any of the following medical problems:
  Asthma (history of)
  Diabetes mellitus (sugar diabetes)
  Diarrhea
  Fever
  Gout
  Heart or blood vessel disease
  Kidney disease
  Liver disease
  Lupus erythematosus (history of)
  Pancreas disease
  Pheochromocytoma (PCC)
  Stomach ulcer (history of)

—if you have recently had a heart attack or stroke.

—if you are taking **any** other prescription or nonprescription (OTC) medicine, especially:
  Adrenocorticoids (cortisone-like medicines)
  Antidiabetic agents, oral (diabetes medicine you take by mouth)
  Chlorprothixene (e.g., Taractan)
  Lithium (e.g., Lithane)
  Loxapine (e.g., Loxitane)
  Methenamine (e.g., Mandelamine)
  Thiothixene (e.g., Navane)
  Tricyclic antidepressants (amitriptyline, amoxapine, clomipramine, desipramine, doxepin, imipramine, nortriptyline, protriptyline, trimipramine)

—if you are now taking or have taken within the past 2 weeks monoamine oxidase (MAO) inhibitors such as:
  Furazolidone (e.g., Furoxone)
  Isocarboxazid (e.g., Marplan)
  Pargyline (e.g., Eutonyl)
  Phenelzine (e.g., Nardil)
  Procarbazine (e.g., Matulane)
  Tranylcypromine (e.g., Parnate)

Proper Use of This Medicine

This medicine may cause you to have an unusual feeling of tiredness when you begin to take it. You may also notice an increase in the amount of urine or in your frequency of urination. After taking the medicine for a while, these effects should lessen. In general, in order to keep the increase in urine from affecting your sleep:

• If you are to take a single dose a day, take it in the morning after breakfast.

• If you are to take more than one dose a day, take the last dose no later than 6 p.m., unless otherwise directed by your doctor.

However, it is best to plan your dose or doses according to a schedule that will least affect your personal activities and sleep. Ask your doctor, nurse, or pharmacist to help you plan the best time to take this medicine.

Importance of diet—When prescribing medicine for your condition, your doctor may also prescribe a personal diet for you. Such a diet may be low in sodium (salt). Most people eat much more sodium than they need and too much sodium in the diet may increase blood pressure. Some foods that contain large amounts of sodium are canned soup, pickles, ketchup, green and ripe olives, relish, frankfurters, soy sauce, and carbonated beverages. Your doctor may want you to limit the amounts of these and other high-sodium foods in your diet. High blood pressure medicine is usually more effective when such a diet is properly followed.

Also, it may be very important for you to go on a reducing diet. However, check with your doctor before changing your diet.

Many patients who have high blood pressure will not notice any signs of the problem. In fact, many may feel normal. It is very important that you **take your medicine exactly as directed** and that you keep your appointments with your doctor even if you feel well.

Remember that this medicine will not cure your high blood pressure but it does help control it. Therefore, you must continue to take it as directed if you expect to lower your blood pressure and keep it down. **You may have to take high blood pressure medicine for the rest of your life.** If high blood pressure is not treated, it can cause serious problems such as heart failure, blood vessel disease, stroke, or kidney disease.

In order to help remember to take your medicine, try to get into the habit of taking it at the same time each day.

If you miss a dose of this medicine, take it as soon as possible. However, if it is almost time for your next dose, skip the missed dose and go back to your regular dosing schedule. Do not double doses.

How to store this medicine:

• **Keep out of the reach of children.**

• Store away from heat and direct light.

• Do not store in the bathroom, near the kitchen sink, or in other damp places. Heat or moisture may cause the medicine to break down.

• Do not keep outdated medicine or medicine no longer needed. Be sure that any discarded medicine is out of the reach of children.

Precautions While Using This Medicine

It is important that your doctor check your progress at regular visits to make sure that this medicine is working properly.

Do not take other medicines unless they have been discussed with your doctor. This especially includes over-the-counter (nonprescription) medicines for appetite control, asthma, colds, cough, hay fever, or sinus problems, since they may tend to increase your blood pressure.

This medicine may cause a loss of potassium from your body.

• To help prevent this, your doctor may want you to:

—eat or drink foods that have a high potassium content (for example, orange or other citrus fruit juices), or

—take a potassium supplement, or

—take another medicine to help prevent the loss of the potassium in the first place.

• It is very important to follow these directions. Also, it is important not to change your diet on your own. This is more important if you are already on a special diet (as for diabetes), or if you are taking a potassium supplement or a medicine to reduce potassium loss. Extra potassium may not be necessary and, in some cases, too much potassium could be harmful.

Check with your doctor if you become sick and have severe or continuing vomiting or diarrhea. These problems may cause you to lose additional water and potassium.

Dizziness, lightheadedness, or fainting may occur, especially when you get up from a lying or sitting position. This is more likely to occur in the morning. **Getting up slowly** may help. When you get up from lying down, sit on the edge of the bed with your feet dangling for 1 or 2 minutes. Then stand up slowly. If the problem continues or gets worse, check with your doctor.

The dizziness, lightheadedness, or fainting is also more likely to occur if you drink alcohol, stand for long periods of time or exercise, or if the weather is hot. **While you are taking this medicine, be careful in the amount of alcohol you drink. Also, use extra care during exercise or hot weather or if you must stand for long periods of time.**

Diabetics—This medicine may raise blood sugar levels. While you are using this medicine, be especially careful in testing for sugar in your urine. If you have any questions about this, check with your doctor.

Some people who take this medicine may become more sensitive to sunlight than they are normally. When you first begin taking this medicine, avoid too much sun and do not use a sunlamp until you see how you react to the sun, especially if you tend to burn easily. If you have a severe reaction, check with your doctor.

Tell your doctor if you get a fever since that may change the amount of medicine you have to take.

Before having any kind of surgery (including dental surgery) or emergency treatment, tell the physician or dentist in charge that you are taking this medicine.

Side Effects of This Medicine

Along with its needed effects, a medicine may cause some unwanted effects. Although not all of these side effects may occur, if they do occur they may need medical attention.

Check with your doctor as soon as possible if any of the following side effects occur, especially since some of them may mean that your body is losing too much potassium:

Signs of too much potassium loss

    Dryness of mouth
    Increased thirst
    Irregular heartbeats
    Mood or mental changes
    Muscle cramps or pain
    Nausea or vomiting
    Unusual tiredness or weakness
    Weak pulse

Less common

    Chest pain

Rare

    Joint, lower back or side, or stomach pain
    Skin rash or hives
    Sore throat and fever

    Stomach pain (severe) with nausea and vomiting
    Unusual bleeding or bruising
    Yellow eyes or skin

Other side effects may occur that usually do not require medical attention. These side effects may go away during treatment as your body adjusts to the medicine. However, check with your doctor if any of the following side effects continue or are bothersome:

More common

    Diarrhea or increase in bowel movements
    Dizziness, lightheadedness, or fainting, especially when getting up from a lying or sitting position
    Sexual problems in males
    Slow heartbeat
    Stuffy nose

Less common or rare

    Blurred vision
    Drooping eyelids
    Headache
    Increased sensitivity to sunlight
    Loss of appetite
    Loss of hair
    Nighttime urination

For elderly patients: Dizziness, lightheadedness, fainting, or signs of too much potassium loss may be more likely to occur in the elderly, who are more sensitive to the effects of guanethidine and hydrochlorothiazide.

Other side effects not listed above may also occur in some patients. If you notice any other effects, check with your doctor.

December 1987

GUANFACINE (Systemic)

A commonly used brand name is Tenex.

To the Reader: If you do not recognize the names of medical conditions or medicines referred to in this information, check with your doctor, nurse, or pharmacist. Definitions for selected medical terms may be found in the Glossary. Brand names for the generic drug names listed can be found in the Index. In addition, selected brand names commonly associated with the generic name have been included in the text to help you recognize medicine you may be taking. The fact that a brand name product is not mentioned does not mean the information does not apply. It is a good idea for you to learn both the generic and brand names of your medicines and to write them down for future use.

Guanfacine (GWAHN-fa-seen) belongs to the general class of medicines called antihypertensives. It is used to treat high blood pressure. High blood pressure adds to the workload of the heart and arteries. If it continues for a long time, the heart and arteries may not function properly. This can damage the blood vessels of the brain, heart, and kidneys, resulting in a stroke, heart failure, or kidney failure. High blood pressure may also increase the risk of heart attacks. These problems may be less likely to occur if blood pressure is controlled.

Guanfacine works by controlling nerve impulses along certain nerve pathways. As a result, it relaxes blood vessels so that blood passes through them more easily. This helps to lower blood pressure.

Guanfacine is available only with your doctor's prescription.

Remember:
• **This medicine has been prescribed for your current medical problem only.** It must not be given to other people or used for other problems unless you are directed to do so by your doctor.

• **Keep all medicines out of the reach of children.**

• In order for this medicine to work, it must be used as directed.

• **It is very important that you read and understand the following information.** If any of the information causes you special concern, do not decide against using this medicine without first checking with your doctor.

• Before you begin using any new medicine (prescription or nonprescription) or if you develop any new medical problem while you are using this medicine, check with your doctor, nurse, or pharmacist.

• **If you have any questions** about the following information or if you want more information about this medicine or your medical problem, **ask your doctor, nurse, or pharmacist.**

Before Using This Medicine

In order to decide on the best treatment for your medical problem, your doctor should be told:
—if you have ever had any unusual or allergic reaction to guanfacine.

—if you are on a low-salt, low-sugar, or any other special diet, or if you are allergic to any substance, such as foods, sulfites or other preservatives, or dyes.

Most medicines contain more than their active ingredient. Your doctor, nurse, or pharmacist can help you avoid products that may cause a problem.

—if you are **pregnant** or if you may become pregnant. Studies have not been done in humans. However, guanfacine has not been shown to cause birth defects or other problems in rats or rabbits given many times the human dose. In rats and rabbits given extremely high doses (up to 200 times the human dose), there was an increase in deaths of the animal fetus.

—if you are **breast-feeding.** It is not known whether guanfacine passes into the breast milk. It has not been shown to cause problems in nursing babies.

—if you have any of the following medical problems:
Heart disease
Liver disease
Mental depression

—if you have recently had a heart attack or stroke.

—if you are taking **any** other prescription or nonprescription (OTC) medicine.

Proper Use of This Medicine

Importance of diet—When prescribing medicine for your condition, your doctor may also prescribe a personal diet for you. Such a diet may be low in sodium (salt). Most people eat much more sodium than they need and too much sodium in the diet may increase blood pressure. Some foods that contain large amounts of sodium are canned soup, pickles, ketchup, green and ripe olives, relish, frankfurters, soy sauce, and carbonated beverages. Your doctor may want you to limit the amounts of these and other high-sodium foods in your diet. High blood pressure medicine is usually more effective when such a diet is properly followed.

Also, it may be very important for you to go on a reducing diet. However, check with your doctor before changing your diet.

Many patients who have high blood pressure will not notice any signs of the problem. In fact, many may feel normal. It is very important that you **take your medicine exactly as directed** and that you keep your appointments with your doctor even if you feel well.

Remember that this medicine will not cure your high blood pressure but it does help control it. Therefore, you must continue to use it as directed if you expect to lower your blood pressure and keep it down. **You may have to take high blood pressure medicine for the rest of your life.** If high blood pressure is not treated, it can cause serious problems such as heart failure, blood vessel disease, stroke, or kidney disease.

Take your daily dose of guanfacine at bedtime. (If you are taking more than one dose a day, take your last dose at bedtime). Taking it this way will help lessen daytime drowsiness.

If you miss a dose of this medicine, take it as soon as possible. However, if it is almost time for your next dose, skip the missed dose and go back to your regular dosing schedule. Do not double doses. **If you miss taking guanfacine for two or more days in a row, check with your doctor.** If your body suddenly goes without this medicine, some unwanted effects may occur. If you have any questions about this, check with your doctor.

How to store this medicine:

- **Keep out of the reach of children.**
- Store away from heat and direct light.
- Do not store in the bathroom, near the kitchen sink, or in other damp places. Heat or moisture may cause the medicine to break down.
- Do not keep outdated medicine or medicine no longer needed. Be sure any discarded medicine is out of the reach of children.

Precautions While Using This Medicine

It is important that your doctor check your progress at regular visits to make sure this medicine is working properly.

Check with your doctor before you stop taking guanfacine. Your doctor may want you to reduce gradually the amount you are taking before stopping completely.

Make sure that you have enough guanfacine on hand to last through weekends, holidays, and vacations. You should not miss any doses. You may want to ask your doctor for another written prescription for guanfacine to carry in your wallet or purse. You can then have it filled if you run out when you are away from home.

Before having any kind of surgery (including dental surgery) or emergency treatment, tell the physician or dentist in charge that you are using this medicine.

Do not take other medicines unless they have been discussed with your doctor. This especially includes over-the-counter (nonprescription) medicines for appetite control, asthma, colds, cough, hay fever, or sinus problems, since they may tend to increase your blood pressure.

Guanfacine will add to the effects of alcohol and other CNS depressants (medicines that slow down the nervous system, possibly causing drowsiness). Some examples of CNS depressants are antihistamines or medicine for hay fever, other allergies, or colds; sedatives, tranquilizers, or sleeping medicine; prescription pain medicine or narcotics; barbiturates; medicine for convulsions (seizures); muscle relaxants; or anesthetics, including some dental anesthetics. **Check with your doctor before taking any of the above while you are using this medicine.**

Guanfacine may cause some people to become dizzy, drowsy, or less alert than they are normally. **Make sure you know how you react to this medicine before you drive, use machines, or do other jobs that require you to be alert.**

Guanfacine may cause dryness of the mouth, nose, and throat. For temporary relief of mouth dryness, use sugarless candy or gum, melt bits of ice in your mouth, or use a saliva substitute. However, if dry mouth continues for more than 2 weeks, check with your physician or dentist. Continuing dryness of the mouth may increase the chance of dental disease, including tooth decay, gum disease, and fungal infections.

Side Effects of This Medicine

Along with its needed effects, a medicine may cause some unwanted effects. Although not all of these side effects may occur, if they do occur they may need medical attention.

Check with your doctor as soon as possible if any of the following side effects occur:

Less common

Confusion
Mental depression

Signs of overdose

Difficulty in breathing
Dizziness (extreme) or faintness
Slow heartbeat
Unusual tiredness or weakness (severe)

Other side effects may occur that usually do not require medical attention. These side effects may go away during treatment as your body adjusts to the medicine. However, check with your doctor if any of the following side effects continue or are bothersome:

More common

Constipation
Dizziness
Drowsiness
Dry mouth

Less common

Decreased sexual ability
Dry, itching, or burning eyes
Headache
Nausea or vomiting
Trouble in sleeping
Unusual tiredness or weakness

After you have been using this medicine for a while, unwanted effects may occur if you stop taking it too suddenly. After you stop taking this medicine, check with your doctor if any of the following side effects occur:

Anxiety or tenseness
Chest pain
Fast or irregular heartbeat
Headache
Increased salivation
Nausea or vomiting
Nervousness or restlessness

Shaking or trembling of hands and fingers
Stomach cramps
Sweating
Trouble in sleeping

For elderly patients: Dizziness, drowsiness, or faintness may be more likely to occur in the elderly, who are more sensitive to the effects of guanfacine.

Other side effects not listed above may also occur in some patients. If you notice any other effects, check with your doctor.

December 1987

HALOPERIDOL (Systemic)

Some commonly used brand names are:

Apo-Haloperidol*	Haldol LA*
Haldol	Novoperidol*
Haldol Decanoate	Peridol*

Generic name product may also be available in the U.S.

---

*Not available in the U.S.

To the Reader: If you do not recognize the names of medical conditions or medicines referred to in this information, check with your doctor, nurse, or pharmacist. Definitions for selected medical terms may be found in the Glossary. Brand names for the generic drug names listed can be found in the Index. In addition, selected brand names commonly associated with the generic name have been included in the text to help you recognize medicine you may be taking. The fact that a brand name product is not mentioned does not mean the information does not apply. It is a good idea for you to learn both the generic and brand names of your medicines and to write them down for future use.

Haloperidol (ha-loe-PER-i-dole) is used to treat nervous, mental, and emotional conditions. It is also used to control the symptoms of Tourette's disorder. Haloperidol may also be used for other conditions as determined by your doctor.

Haloperidol is available only with your doctor's prescription.

Remember:

• **This medicine has been prescribed for your current medical problem only.** It must not be given to other people or used for other problems unless you are directed to do so by your doctor.

• **Keep all medicines out of the reach of children.**

• In order for this medicine to work, it must be used as directed.

• If you are receiving this medicine by injection, some of the information about this medicine may not apply.

• **It is very important that you read and understand the following information.** If any of the information causes you special concern, do not decide against using this medicine without first checking with your doctor.

• Before you begin using any new medicine (prescription or nonprescription) or if you develop any new medical problem while you are using this medicine, check with your doctor, nurse, or pharmacist.

• **If you have any questions** about the following information or if you want more information about this medicine or your medical problem, **ask your doctor, nurse, or pharmacist.**

Before Using This Medicine

In order to decide on the best treatment for your medical problem, your doctor should be told:

—if you have any allergies or have ever had any unusual or allergic reaction to haloperidol or any other medicine.

—if you are on a low-salt, low-sugar, or any other special diet, or if you are allergic to any substance, such as foods, sulfites or other preservatives, or dyes.

Most medicines contain more than their active ingredient, and many liquid medicines contain alcohol. Your doctor, nurse, or pharmacist can help you avoid products that may cause a problem.

—if you are **pregnant** or if you may become pregnant. Adequate studies have not been done in humans. However, studies in animals given 2 to 20 times the usual maximum human dose of haloperidol have shown reduced fertility, delayed delivery, cleft palate, and an increase in the number of stillbirths and newborn deaths.

—if you are **breast-feeding**. Haloperidol passes into breast milk. Animal studies have shown that haloperidol in breast milk causes drowsiness and difficulty with body movements in the nursing offspring. Breast-feeding is not recommended during treatment with haloperidol.

—if you have any of the following medical problems:

Alcoholism, active
Difficult urination
Epilepsy
Glaucoma
Heart or blood vessel disease
Kidney disease
Liver disease
Lung disease
Overactive thyroid
Parkinson's disease

—if you are taking **any** other prescription or nonprescription (OTC) medicine, especially:

Amoxapine (e.g., Asendin)
Central nervous system (CNS) depressants
Chlorprothixene (e.g., Taractan)
Epinephrine (e.g., Adrenalin)
Levodopa (e.g., Dopar; Larodopa)
Lithium (e.g., Eskalith; Lithane)
Loxapine (e.g., Loxitane)
Methyldopa (e.g., Aldomet)
Metoclopramide (e.g., Reglan)
Metyrosine (e.g., Demser)
Molindone (e.g., Moban)
Phenothiazines (acetophenazine, chlorpromazine, fluphenazine, mesoridazine, perphenazine, prochlorperazine, promazine, promethazine, thioridazine, trifluoperazine, triflupromazine, trimeprazine)
Pemoline (e.g., Cylert)
Pimozide (e.g., Orap)
Rauwolfia alkaloids (alseroxylon, deserpidine, rauwolfia serpentina, reserpine)
Thiothixene (e.g., Navane)

Proper Use of This Medicine

If this medicine upsets your stomach, it may be taken with food or milk to lessen stomach irritation.

For patients taking the liquid form of this medicine:

• This medicine is to be taken by mouth even though it may come in a dropper bottle. Each dose is to be measured with the included, specially marked dropper. Do not use other droppers since they may not deliver the correct amount of medicine.

© 1988   The United States Pharmacopeial Convention, Inc.

• This medicine is best taken alone. However, if necessary, it may be mixed with water. If this is done, the mixture should be taken immediately after mixing. Haloperidol should not be taken in tea or coffee, since they cause the medicine to separate out of solution.

Take this medicine only as directed by your doctor. Do not take more of it, do not take it more often, and do not take it for a longer period of time than your doctor ordered.

Continue taking this medicine for the full time of treatment. **Sometimes haloperidol must be taken for several days to several weeks before its full effect is reached.**

If you miss a dose of this medicine, take it as soon as possible. Then take any remaining doses for that day at regularly spaced intervals. Do not double doses.

How to store this medicine:

• **Keep out of the reach of children.**

• Store away from heat and direct light.

• Do not store in the bathroom, near the kitchen sink, or in other damp places. Heat or moisture may cause the medicine to break down.

• Keep the liquid form of this medicine from freezing.

• Do not keep outdated medicine or medicine no longer needed. Be sure that any discarded medicine is out of the reach of children.

Precautions While Using This Medicine

Your doctor should check your progress at regular visits, especially for the first few months you take this medicine. The amount of haloperidol you take may be changed often to meet the needs of your condition. This also helps avoid side effects.

Do not suddenly stop taking this medicine without first checking with your doctor. Your doctor may want you to reduce gradually the amount you are taking before stopping completely. This will allow your body time to adjust and help avoid a worsening of your medical condition.

This medicine will add to the effects of alcohol and other CNS depressants (medicines that slow down the nervous system, possibly causing drowsiness). Some examples of CNS depressants are antihistamines or medicine for hay fever, other allergies, or colds; sedatives, tranquilizers, or sleeping medicine; prescription pain medicine or narcotics; barbiturates; medicine for convulsions (seizures); muscle relaxants; or anesthetics, including some dental anesthetics. **Check with your doctor before taking any of the above while you are taking this medicine.**

This medicine may cause some people to become drowsy or less alert than they are normally, especially as the amount of medicine is increased. Even if you take this medicine at bedtime, you may feel drowsy or less alert

on arising. **Make sure you know how you react to this medicine before you drive, use machines, or do other jobs that require you to be alert.**

Although not a problem for many patients, dizziness, lightheadedness, or fainting may occur, especially when you get up from a lying or sitting position. Getting up slowly may help. However, if the problem continues or gets worse, check with your doctor.

This medicine will often make you sweat less, allowing your body temperature to rise. **Use extra care not to become overheated during exercise or hot weather, or during hot baths, while you are taking this medicine.** Overheating could possibly result in heat stroke. Also, hot baths may make you feel dizzy or faint while you are taking haloperidol.

Before having any kind of surgery, dental treatment, or emergency treatment, tell the physician or dentist in charge that you are using this medicine.

Some people who take haloperidol may become more sensitive to sunlight than they are normally. When you first begin taking this medicine, use sunscreen lotions, avoid too much sun, and do not use a sunlamp until you see how you react to the sun, especially if you tend to burn easily. If you have a severe reaction, check with your doctor.

Haloperidol may cause dryness of the mouth. For temporary relief, use sugarless candy or gum, melt bits of ice in your mouth, or use a saliva substitute. However, if dry mouth continues for more than 2 weeks, check with your physician or dentist. Continuing dryness of the mouth may increase the chance of dental disease, including tooth decay, gum disease, and fungal infections.

Side Effects of This Medicine

Along with its needed effects, a medicine may cause some unwanted effects. Although not all of these side effects may occur, if they do occur they may need medical attention.

Stop taking haloperidol and get emergency help immediately if any of the following side effects occur:

Rare
    Convulsions (seizures)
    Difficult or unusually fast breathing
    Fast heartbeat or irregular pulse
    Fever (high)
    Increased sweating
    Loss of bladder control
    Muscle stiffness (severe)
    Unusual feeling of tiredness or weakness
    Unusually pale skin

Check with your doctor as soon as possible if any of the following side effects occur:

More common
    Difficulty in speaking or swallowing
    Fixation of eyes
    Loss of balance control

Mask-like face
Muscle spasms, especially of the neck and back
Restlessness or need to keep moving (severe)
Shuffling walk
Stiffness of arms and legs
Trembling and shaking of fingers and hands
Twisting movements of body

Less common

Chewing movements
Decreased feeling of thirst
Difficulty in urination
Dizziness, lightheadedness, or fainting
Hallucinations (seeing or hearing things that are not there)
Lip smacking or puckering
Puffing of cheeks
Rapid or worm-like movements of tongue
Skin rash
Uncontrolled movements of arms and legs

Rare

Sore throat and fever
Yellow eyes or skin

Signs of overdose

Difficulty in breathing (severe)
Dizziness or lightheadedness (severe)
Drowsiness (severe)
Muscle trembling, jerking, stiffness, or uncontrolled movements (severe)
Unusual tiredness or weakness

Other side effects may occur that usually do not require medical attention. These side effects may go away during treatment as your body adjusts to the medicine.

However, check with your doctor if any of the following side effects continue or are bothersome:

More common

Blurred vision
Changes in menstrual period
Constipation
Dry mouth
Swelling or pain in breasts (in females)
Unusual secretion of milk
Weight gain

Less common

Decreased sexual ability
Drowsiness
Increased sensitivity of skin to sun
Nausea or vomiting

Some side effects, such as dizziness, stomach pain, nausea or vomiting, trembling of fingers and hands, or uncontrolled movements of the mouth, tongue, and jaw, may occur after you have stopped taking this medicine. If you notice any of these effects, check with your doctor as soon as possible.

For children and elderly patients: Side effects are more likely to occur in children and the elderly, who usually are more sensitive to the effects of haloperidol.

Other side effects not listed above may also occur in some patients. If you notice any other effects, check with your doctor.

December 1987

HALOPROGIN (Topical)

A commonly used brand name is Halotex.

To the Reader: If you do not recognize the names of medical conditions or medicines referred to in this information, check with your doctor, nurse, or pharmacist. Definitions for selected medical terms may be found in the Glossary. Brand names for the generic drug names listed can be found in the Index. In addition, selected brand names commonly associated with the generic name have been included in the text to help you recognize medicine you may be taking. The fact that a brand name product is not mentioned does not mean the information does not apply. It is a good idea for you to learn both the generic and brand names of your medicines and to write them down for future use.

Haloprogin (ha-loe-PROE-jin) belongs to the group of medicines called antifungals. It is used on the skin to treat some types of fungal infections.

Haloprogin is available only with your doctor's prescription.

Remember:

• **This medicine has been prescribed for your present infection only.** Another infection later on may require a different medicine. Also, even though other people may have the same symptoms as you, they may have a different kind of infection. Your medicine may not work for them and may even cause them harm. Therefore, **your medicine must not be given to other people or used for other infections** unless you are otherwise directed by your doctor.

• **Keep all medicines out of the reach of children.**

• In order for this medicine to work, it must be used as directed.

• **It is very important that you read and understand the following information.** If any of the information causes you special concern, do not decide against using this medicine without first checking with your doctor.

• Before you begin using any new medicine (prescription or nonprescription) or if you develop any new medical problem while you are using this medicine, check with your doctor, nurse, or pharmacist.

• **If you have any questions** about the following information or if you want more information about this medicine or your medical problem, **ask your doctor, nurse, or pharmacist.**

Before Using This Medicine

In order to decide on the best treatment for your medical problem, your doctor should be told:

—if you have ever had any unusual or allergic reaction to haloprogin.

—if you are allergic to any substance, such as certain foods or preservatives or dyes. Most medicines contain more than their active ingredient. Your doctor, nurse, or pharmacist can help you avoid products that may cause a problem.

—if you are **pregnant** or if you may become pregnant. Studies have not been done in humans. However, haloprogin has not been shown to cause birth defects or other problems in studies in rats and rabbits. These animals were given topical doses equivalent to up to 3 times the human dose for a 30-day course of treatment.

—if you are **breast-feeding**. It is not known whether haloprogin passes into the breast milk. However, this medicine has not been shown to cause problems in nursing babies.

Proper Use of This Medicine

Apply enough haloprogin to cover the affected area, and rub in gently.

Keep this medicine away from the eyes.

To help clear up your infection completely, **keep using this medicine for the full time of treatment** even though your condition may have improved. **Do not miss any doses.**

If you do miss a dose of this medicine, apply it as soon as possible. However, if it is almost time for your next dose, skip the missed dose and go back to your regular dosing schedule.

How to store this medicine:

• **Keep out of the reach of children.**

• Store away from heat and direct light.

• Keep the medicine from freezing.

• Do not keep outdated medicine or medicine no longer needed. Be sure that any discarded medicine is out of the reach of children.

Precautions While Using This Medicine

If your skin problem does not improve within 4 weeks, or if it becomes worse, check with your doctor.

Side Effects of This Medicine

Along with its needed effects, a medicine may cause some unwanted effects. Although not all of these side effects may occur, if they do occur they may need medical attention.

Check with your doctor as soon as possible if any of the following side effects occur:

Blistering, burning, itching, or other sign of skin irritation not present before using this medicine

When you apply the solution form of this medicine, a mild temporary stinging may be expected.

Other side effects not listed above may also occur in some patients. If you notice any other effects, check with your doctor.

December 1987

HEPARIN (Systemic)

Some commonly used brand names are:

Calcilean*	Monoparin*
Calciparine	Multiparin*
Hepalean*	Pump-Hep*
Hepsal*	Unihep*
Liquaemin	Uniparin*
Minihep*	

Generic name product may also be available in the U.S.

---

* Not available in the U.S.

To the Reader: If you do not recognize the names of medical conditions or medicines referred to in this information, check with your doctor, nurse, or pharmacist. Definitions for selected medical terms may be found in the Glossary. Brand names for the generic drug names listed can be found in the Index. In addition, selected brand names commonly associated with the generic name have been included in the text to help you recognize medicine you may be taking. The fact that a brand name product is not mentioned does not mean the information does not apply. It is a good idea for you to learn both the generic and brand names of your medicines and to write them down for future use.

Heparin (HEP-a-rin) is an anticoagulant. It is given by injection to decrease the clotting ability of the blood and help prevent harmful clots from forming in the blood vessels. This medicine is sometimes called a blood thinner, although it does not actually thin the blood. Heparin will not dissolve blood clots that have already formed, but it may prevent the clots from becoming larger and causing more serious problems.

Heparin is often used as a treatment for certain blood vessel, heart, and lung conditions. Heparin is also used to prevent blood clotting during open-heart surgery, bypass surgery, and dialysis. It is also used in low doses to prevent the formation of blood clots in certain patients, especially those who must have certain types of surgery or who must remain in bed for a long time.

Heparin is available only with your doctor's prescription.

Remember:

• **This medicine has been prescribed for your current medical problem only.** It must not be given to other people or used for other problems unless you are directed to do so by your doctor.

• **Keep all medicines out of the reach of children.**

• In order for this medicine to work, it must be used as directed.

• **It is very important that you read and understand the following information.** If any of the information causes you special concern, do not decide against using this medicine without first checking with your doctor.

• Before you begin using any new medicine (prescription or nonprescription) or if you develop any new medical problem while you are using this medicine, check with your doctor, nurse, or pharmacist.

• **If you have any questions** about the following information or if you want more information about this medicine or your medical problem, **ask your doctor, nurse, or pharmacist.**

Before Using This Medicine

In order to decide on the best treatment for your medical problem, your doctor should be told:

—if you have ever had any unusual or allergic reaction to heparin, to beef, or to pork.

—if you are on a low-salt, low-sugar, or any other special diet, or if you are allergic to any substance, such as sulfites or other preservatives. Most medicines contain more than their active ingredient. Your doctor, nurse, or pharmacist can help you avoid products that may cause a problem.

—if you are **pregnant** (especially if you are within 3 months of your delivery date), or if you have delivered a baby within the past month. Heparin has not been shown to cause birth defects or bleeding problems in the baby. However, use during the last 3 months of pregnancy or during the month following the baby's delivery may cause bleeding problems in the mother.

—if you are **breast-feeding**. Heparin does not pass into the breast milk. However, heparin can rarely cause bone problems in the nursing mother. This effect has been reported to occur when heparin is used for 2 weeks or more. Be sure to discuss this with your doctor.

—if you have any of the following medical problems:

  Allergies or asthma (history of)
  Blood disease or bleeding problems
  Colitis or stomach ulcer (or history of)
  Diabetes (severe)
  High blood pressure
  Kidney disease
  Liver disease
  Tuberculosis (active)

—if you have recently had any of the following conditions:

  Falls or blows to the body or head
  Heavy or unusual menstrual bleeding
  Insertion of intrauterine device (IUD)
  Medical or dental surgery
  Spinal anesthesia
  X-ray (radiation) treatment

—if you are taking **any** other prescription or nonprescription (OTC) medicine, especially:

  Dipyridamole (e.g., Persantine)
  Divalproex (e.g., Depakote)
  Medicine for pain and/or inflammation (aspirin or other salicylates, diclofenac [e.g., Voltaren], diflunisal [e.g., Dolobid], fenoprofen [e.g., Nalfon], flurbiprofen [oral] [e.g., Ansaid], ibuprofen [e.g., Motrin], indomethacin [e.g., Indocin], ketoprofen [e.g., Orudis], meclofenamate [e.g., Meclomen], mefenamic acid [e.g., Ponstel], naproxen [e.g., Naprosyn], phenylbutazone [e.g., Butazolidin], piroxicam [e.g., Feldene], sulindac [e.g., Clinoril], tiaprofenic acid [e.g., Surgam], tolmetin [e.g., Tolectin])
  Medicine for overactive thyroid
  Probenecid (e.g., Benemid)
  Sulfinpyrazone (e.g., Anturane)
  Valproic acid (e.g., Depakene)

—if you are now receiving any kind of medicine by intramuscular (IM) injection.

Proper Use of This Medicine

If you are using these injections at home, make sure your doctor has explained exactly how this medicine is to be given.

In order to obtain the best results without causing serious bleeding, **use this medicine exactly as directed by your doctor. Be certain that you are using the right amount of heparin, and that you use it according to schedule.** Be especially careful that you do not use more of it, do not use it more often, and do not use it for a longer period of time than your doctor ordered.

Your doctor should check your progress at regular visits. A blood test must be taken regularly to see how fast your blood is clotting so that your doctor can decide on the proper amount of heparin you should be receiving each day.

If you miss a dose of this medicine, use it as soon as possible. However, if it is almost time for your next dose, do not use the missed dose at all and do not double the next one. **Doubling the dose may cause bleeding.** Instead, go back to your regular dosing schedule. It is best to keep a record of each dose as you use it to avoid mistakes. Be sure to give your doctor a record of any doses you miss. If you have any questions about this, check with your doctor.

How to store this medicine:

• **Keep out of the reach of children.**

• Store away from heat and direct light.

• Keep the medicine from freezing.

• Do not keep outdated medicine or medicine no longer needed. Be sure that any discarded medicine is out of the reach of children.

Precautions While Using This Medicine

Do not take aspirin while using this medicine. Many over-the-counter (OTC) or nonprescription medicines and some prescription medicines contain aspirin. Check the labels of all medicines you take. Also, do not take ibuprofen unless it has been ordered by your doctor. In addition, there are many other medicines that may change the way heparin works or increase the chance of bleeding if they are used together with heparin. It is best to check with your doctor or pharmacist before taking any other medicine while you are using heparin.

Tell all physicians and dentists you visit that you are using this medicine.

It is recommended that you carry identification stating that you are using heparin. If you have any questions about what kind of identification to carry, check with your doctor, nurse, or pharmacist.

While you are using this medicine, it is very important that you avoid sports and other activities which may cause you to be injured. Report to your doctor any falls, blows to the body or head, or other injuries, since serious bleeding inside the body may occur without your knowing about it.

Take special care in brushing your teeth and in shaving. Use a soft toothbrush and floss gently. Also, it is best to use an electric shaver rather than a blade.

Side Effects of This Medicine

Since many things can affect the way your body reacts to this medicine, you should always watch for signs of unusual bleeding. Unusual bleeding may mean that your body is getting more heparin than it needs.

Along with its needed effects, a medicine may cause some unwanted effects. Although not all of these side effects may occur, if they do occur they may need medical attention.

Check with your doctor immediately if any of the following signs of bleeding inside the body occur:

  Abdominal or stomach pain or swelling
  Back pain or backaches
  Blood in urine
  Bloody or black tarry stools
  Constipation
  Coughing up blood
  Dizziness
  Headaches (severe or continuing)
  Joint pain, stiffness, or swelling
  Vomiting of blood or material that looks like coffee grounds

Also, check with your doctor as soon as possible if any of the following early signs of overdose occur:

  Bleeding from gums when brushing teeth
  Heavy bleeding or oozing from cuts or wounds
  Unexplained bruising or purplish areas on skin
  Unexplained nosebleeds
  Unusually heavy or unexpected menstrual bleeding

For elderly patients: Bleeding problems may be more likely to occur in elderly patients, especially women, who may be more sensitive to the effects of heparin.

Other side effects that may require medical attention may occur while you are using this medicine. Check with your doctor as soon as possible if any of the following side effects occur:

Less common or rare

  Back or rib pain (with long-term use only)
  Change in skin color, especially near the place of injection or in the fingers, toes, arms, or legs
  Chest pain
  Chills or fever
  Collection of blood under skin (blood blister) at place of injection
  Decrease in height (with long-term use only)
  Frequent or persistent erection
  Numbness or tingling in hands or feet

Pain or irritation at place of injection
Pains in arms or legs
Peeling of skin at place of injection
Runny nose
Shortness of breath, troubled breathing, wheezing, or
    tightness in chest
Skin rash, itching, or hives
Unusual hair loss (with long-term use only)

Other side effects not listed above may also occur in some
    patients. If you notice any other effects, check with
    your doctor.

_____

December 1987

HISTAMINE (Systemic)

To the Reader: If you do not recognize the names of medical conditions or medicines referred to in this information, check with your doctor, nurse, or pharmacist. Definitions for selected medical terms may be found in the Glossary. Brand names for the generic drug names listed can be found in the Index. In addition, selected brand names commonly associated with the generic name have been included in the text to help you recognize medicine you may be taking. The fact that a brand name product is not mentioned does not mean the information does not apply. It is a good idea for you to learn both the generic and brand names of your medicines and to write them down for future use.

Histamine (HISS-ta-meen) is used by injection as a test to help diagnose problems or disease of the stomach. This test determines how much acid your stomach produces.

How the stomach test is done: Before this medicine is given, the stomach contents are emptied through a tube. Then histamine is injected and, fifteen minutes later, the stomach contents are emptied and tested for acidity. This procedure may be repeated several times. An antihistamine medicine may be given before the histamine is injected.

Histamine is to be used only under the supervision of a doctor.

Remember:
• **It is very important that you read and understand the following information.** If any of the information causes you special concern, do not decide against having this test without first checking with your doctor.

• **If you have any questions** about the following information or if you want more information about this test or your medical problem, **ask your doctor, nurse, or pharmacist.**

Before Having This Test

Before this test is given, your doctor should be told:

—if you have ever had any unusual or allergic reaction to histamine.

—if you are allergic to any substance, such as sulfites or other preservatives or dyes. Most medicines contain more than their active ingredient. Your doctor can help you avoid products that may cause a problem.

—if you are **pregnant** or if you suspect that you may be pregnant. Histamine has not been shown to cause problems in humans.

—if you are **breast-feeding.** Histamine has not been shown to cause problems in nursing babies.

—if you have any of the following medical problems:
Heart disease
High blood pressure (severe)
Kidney disease (severe)
Low blood pressure
Lung disease (especially asthma)
Skin rash

—if you are taking **any** other prescription or nonprescription (OTC) medicine, especially:

Antacids
Antimuscarinics (medicine for abdominal or stomach spasms or cramps)
Cimetidine (e.g., Tagamet)
Famotidine (e.g., Pepcid)
Ranitidine (e.g., Zantac)

Preparation For This Test

Your doctor may ask you to avoid certain medicines before the histamine test is done. **Follow your doctor's instructions carefully.** Otherwise, this test may not work and may have to be done again.

Do not eat anything for twelve hours before the test, unless otherwise directed by your doctor. Having food in the stomach may affect the interpretation of the test results.

Precautions During This Test

Do not swallow saliva during the test. The saliva may affect the results of the test.

Side Effects of This Medicine

Along with its needed effects, histamine may cause some unwanted effects. Although not all of these side effects may occur, if they do occur they may need medical attention.

Check with your doctor or nurse immediately if any of the following side effects occur:

More common

Dizziness, lightheadedness, or fainting
Fast or pounding heartbeat
Headache (continuing or severe)
Nervousness
Unusually slow heartbeat

Less common or rare

Convulsions (seizures)
Difficulty in breathing
Flushing or redness of face
Skin rash or hives

With large doses

Bluish coloration of face
Blurred vision
Chest discomfort or pain
Decrease in blood pressure (sudden)
Diarrhea (severe)
Difficulty in breathing (severe)
Flushing or redness of face
Vomiting (severe)

© 1988   The United States Pharmacopeial Convention, Inc.

Other side effects may occur that usually do not require medical attention. These side effects should go away as the effects of the medicine wear off. However, check with your doctor if any of the following side effects continue or are bothersome:

More common

 Abdominal or stomach spasms or cramps
 Diarrhea
 Metallic taste

 Nausea or vomiting
 Stomach pain
 Swelling or redness at injection site

Other side effects not listed above may also occur in some patients. If you notice any other effects, check with your doctor.

   ———————

December 1987

HYDRALAZINE (Systemic)

Some commonly used brand names are Apresoline and Dralzine.

Generic name product may also be available in the U.S.

To the Reader: If you do not recognize the names of medical conditions or medicines referred to in this information, check with your doctor, nurse, or pharmacist. Definitions for selected medical terms may be found in the Glossary. Brand names for the generic drug names listed can be found in the Index. In addition, selected brand names commonly associated with the generic name have been included in the text to help you recognize medicine you may be taking. The fact that a brand name product is not mentioned does not mean the information does not apply. It is a good idea for you to learn both the generic and brand names of your medicines and to write them down for future use.

Hydralazine (hye-DRAL-a-zeen) belongs to the general class of medicines called antihypertensives. It is used to treat high blood pressure.

High blood pressure adds to the workload of the heart and arteries. If it continues for a long time, the heart and arteries may not function properly. This can damage the blood vessels of the brain, heart, and kidneys, resulting in a stroke, heart failure, or kidney failure. High blood pressure may also increase the risk of heart attacks. These problems may be less likely to occur if blood pressure is controlled.

Hydralazine works by relaxing blood vessels and increasing the supply of blood and oxygen to the heart while reducing its work load.

Hydralazine may also be used for other conditions as determined by your doctor.

Hydralazine is available only with your doctor's prescription.

Remember:

• **This medicine has been prescribed for your current medical problem only.** It must not be given to other people or used for other problems unless you are directed to do so by your doctor.

• **Keep all medicines out of the reach of children.**

• In order for this medicine to work, it must be used as directed.

• If you are receiving this medicine by injection, some of the information about this medicine may not apply.

• **It is very important that you read and understand the following information.** If any of the information causes you special concern, do not decide against using this medicine without first checking with your doctor.

• Before you begin using any new medicine (prescription or nonprescription) or if you develop any new medical problem while you are using this medicine, check with your doctor, nurse, or pharmacist.

• **If you have any questions** about the following information or if you want more information about this medicine or your medical problem, **ask your doctor, nurse, or pharmacist.**

Before Using This Medicine

In order to decide on the best treatment for your medical problem, your doctor should be told:

—if you have ever had any unusual or allergic reaction to hydralazine.

—if you are on a low-salt, low-sugar, or any other special diet, or if you are allergic to any substance, such as foods, sulfites or other preservatives, or dyes. Most medicines contain more than their active ingredient, and many liquid medicines contain alcohol. Your doctor, nurse, or pharmacist can help you avoid products that may cause a problem.

—if you are **pregnant** or if you may become pregnant. Studies have not been done in humans. However, studies in mice have shown that hydralazine causes birth defects (cleft palate, defects in head and face bones). These birth defects may also occur in rabbits, but do not occur in rats.

—if you are **breast-feeding**. Hydralazine has not been shown to cause problems in nursing babies.

—if you have either of the following medical problems:
Heart or blood vessel disease
Kidney disease

—if you have recently had a stroke.

—if you are taking **any** other prescription or nonprescription (OTC) medicine, especially diazoxide (e.g., Proglycem).

Proper Use of This Medicine

Importance of diet—When prescribing medicine for your condition, your doctor may also prescribe a personal diet for you. Such a diet may be low in sodium (salt). Most people eat much more sodium than they need and too much sodium in the diet may increase blood pressure. Some foods that contain large amounts of sodium are canned soup, pickles, ketchup, green and ripe olives, relish, frankfurters, soy sauce, and carbonated beverages. Your doctor may want you to limit the amounts of these and other high-sodium foods in your diet. High blood pressure medicine is usually more effective when such a diet is properly followed.

Also, it may be very important for you to go on a reducing diet. However, check with your doctor before changing your diet.

Many patients who have high blood pressure will not notice any signs of the problem. In fact, many may feel normal. It is very important that you **take your medicine exactly as directed** and that you keep your appointments with your doctor even if you feel well.

Remember that hydralazine will not cure your high blood pressure but it does help control it. Therefore, you must continue to take it as directed if you expect to lower your blood pressure and keep it down. **You may have to take high blood pressure medicine for the rest of your life.** If high blood pressure is not treated, it can cause serious problems such as heart failure, blood vessel disease, stroke, or kidney disease.

In order to help remember to take your medicine, try to get into the habit of taking it at the same time each day.

If you miss a dose of this medicine, take it as soon as possible. However, if it is almost time for your next dose, skip the missed dose and go back to your regular dosing schedule. Do not double doses.

How to store this medicine:

- **Keep out of the reach of children.**
- Store the tablets away from heat and direct light.
- Do not store in the bathroom, near the kitchen sink, or in other damp places. Heat or moisture may cause the medicine to break down.
- Store the oral solution in the refrigerator. Protect it from freezing.
- Do not keep outdated medicine or medicine no longer needed. Be sure that any discarded medicine is out of the reach of children.

Precautions While Using This Medicine

It is important that your doctor check your progress at regular visits to make sure that this medicine is working properly.

Do not take other medicines unless they have been discussed with your doctor. This especially includes over-the-counter (nonprescription) medicines for appetite control, asthma, colds, cough, hay fever, or sinus, since they may tend to increase your blood pressure.

Hydralazine may cause some people to have headaches or to feel dizzy. **Make sure you know how you react to this medicine before you drive, use machines, or do other jobs that require you to be alert.**

Side Effects of This Medicine

Along with its needed effects, a medicine may cause some unwanted effects. Although not all of these side effects may occur, if they do occur they may need medical attention.

In general, side effects with hydralazine are rare at lower doses. However, check with your doctor as soon as possible if any of the following occur:

Less common

Blisters on skin
Chest pain
General feeling of body discomfort or weakness
Joint pain
Numbness, tingling, pain, or weakness in hands or feet
Skin rash or itching
Sore throat and fever
Swelling of feet or lower legs
Swelling of the lymph glands

Other side effects may occur that usually do not require medical attention. These side effects may go away during treatment as your body adjusts to the medicine. However, check with your doctor if any of the following side effects continue or are bothersome:

More common

Diarrhea
Fast or irregular heartbeat
Headache
Loss of appetite
Nausea or vomiting

Less common

Constipation
Dizziness or lightheadedness
Redness or flushing of face
Shortness of breath with exercise or work
Stuffy nose
Watering or irritated eyes

For elderly patients: Dizziness or lightheadedness may be more likely to occur in the elderly, who are more sensitive to the effects of hydralazine.

Other side effects not listed above may also occur in some patients. If you notice any other effects, check with your doctor.

December 1987

HYDRALAZINE AND HYDROCHLOROTHIAZIDE
(Systemic)

Some commonly used brand names are:

Apresazide	Apresoline-Esidrix
Apresodex	Hydral

Generic name product may also be available in the U.S.

To the Reader: If you do not recognize the names of medical conditions or medicines referred to in this information, check with your doctor, nurse, or pharmacist. Definitions for selected medical terms may be found in the Glossary. Brand names for the generic drug names listed can be found in the Index. In addition, selected brand names commonly associated with the generic name have been included in the text to help you recognize medicine you may be taking. The fact that a brand name product is not mentioned does not mean the information does not apply. It is a good idea for you to learn both the generic and brand names of your medicines and to write them down for future use.

Hydralazine (hye-DRAL-a-zeen) and hydrochlorothiazide (hye-droe-klor-oh-THYE-a-zide) combination is taken by mouth to treat high blood pressure.

High blood pressure adds to the workload of the heart and arteries. If it continues for a long time, the heart and arteries may not function properly. This can damage the blood vessels of the brain, heart, and kidneys, resulting in a stroke, heart failure, or kidney failure. High blood pressure may also increase the risk of heart attacks. These problems may be less likely to occur if blood pressure is controlled.

Hydralazine works by relaxing blood vessels and increasing the supply of blood and oxygen to the heart while reducing its work load. The hydrochlorothiazide in this combination helps reduce the amount of water in the body by acting on the kidneys to increase the flow of urine.

This medicine is available only with your doctor's prescription.

Remember:

• **This medicine has been prescribed for your current medical problem only.** It must not be given to other people or used for other problems unless you are directed to do so by your doctor.

• **Keep all medicines out of the reach of children.**

• In order for this medicine to work, it must be used as directed.

• **It is very important that you read and understand the following information.** If any of the information causes you special concern, do not decide against using this medicine without first checking with your doctor.

• Before you begin using any new medicine (prescription or nonprescription) or if you develop any new medical problem while you are using this medicine, check with your doctor, nurse, or pharmacist.

• **If you have any questions** about the following information or if you want more information about this medicine or your medical problem, **ask your doctor, nurse, or pharmacist.**

Before Using This Medicine

In order to decide on the best treatment for your medical problem, your doctor should be told:

—if you have ever had any unusual or allergic reaction to hydralazine, sulfonamides (sulfa drugs), or any of the thiazide diuretics.

—if you are on a low-salt, low-sugar, or any other special diet, or if you are allergic to any substance, such as foods, sulfites or other preservatives, or dyes. Most medicines contain more than their active ingredient. Your doctor, nurse, or pharmacist can help you avoid products that may cause a problem.

—if you are **pregnant** or if you may become pregnant. When hydrochlorothiazide is used during pregnancy, it may cause side effects including jaundice, blood problems, and low potassium in the newborn infant. Studies with hydralazine have not been done in humans. However, studies in mice have shown that hydralazine causes birth defects (cleft palate, defects in head and face bones); these birth defects may also occur in rabbits, but do not occur in rats.

—if you are **breast-feeding**. Hydrochlorothiazide passes into breast milk. However, neither hydralazine nor hydrochlorothiazide has been shown to cause problems in nursing babies.

—if you have any of the following medical problems:
   Diabetes mellitus (sugar diabetes)
   Gout
   Heart or blood vessel disease
   Kidney disease
   Liver disease
   Lupus erythematosus (history of)
   Pancreas disease

—if you have recently had a stroke.

—if you are taking **any** other prescription or nonprescription (OTC) medicine, especially:
   Adrenocorticoids (cortisone-like medicine)
   Diazoxide (e.g., Proglycem)
   Digitalis glycosides (heart medicine)
   Lithium (e.g., Lithane)
   Methenamine (e.g., Mandelamine)

Proper Use of This Medicine

This medicine may cause you to have an unusual feeling of tiredness when you begin to take it. You may also notice an increase in the amount of urine or in your frequency of urination. After taking the medicine for a while, these effects should lessen. In order to keep the increase in urine from affecting your nighttime sleep:

• If you are to take a single dose a day, take it in the morning after breakfast.

• If you are to take more than one dose a day, take the last dose no later than 6 p.m., unless otherwise directed by your doctor.

However, it is best to plan your dose or doses according to a schedule that will least affect your personal activities and sleep. Ask your doctor, nurse, or pharmacist to help you plan the best time to take this medicine.

Importance of diet—When prescribing medicine for your condition, your doctor may also prescribe a personal diet for you. Such a diet may be low in sodium (salt). Most people eat much more sodium than they need and too much sodium in the diet may increase blood pressure. Some foods that contain large amounts of sodium are canned soup, pickles, ketchup, green and ripe olives, relish, frankfurters, soy sauce, and carbonated beverages. Your doctor may want you to limit the amounts of these and other high-sodium foods in your diet. High blood pressure medicine is usually more effective when such a diet is properly followed.

Also, it may be very important for you to go on a reducing diet. However, check with your doctor before changing your diet.

Many patients who have high blood pressure will not notice any signs of the problem. In fact, many may feel normal. It is very important that you **take your medicine exactly as directed** and that you keep your appointments with your doctor even if you feel well.

Remember that this medicine will not cure your high blood pressure but it does help control it. Therefore, you must continue to take it as directed if you expect to lower your blood pressure and keep it down. **You may have to take high blood pressure medicine for the rest of your life.** If high blood pressure is not treated, it can cause serious problems such as heart failure, blood vessel disease, stroke, or kidney disease.

In order to help remember to take your medicine, try to get into the habit of taking it at the same time each day.

If you miss a dose of this medicine, take it as soon as possible. However, if it is almost time for your next dose, skip the missed dose and go back to your regular dosing schedule. Do not double doses.

How to store this medicine:
- **Keep out of the reach of children.**
- Store away from heat and direct light.
- Do not store in the bathroom, near the kitchen sink, or in other damp places. Heat or moisture may cause the medicine to break down.
- Do not keep outdated medicine or medicine no longer needed. Be sure that any discarded medicine is out of the reach of children.

Precautions While Using This Medicine

It is important that your doctor check your progress at regular visits to make sure that this medicine is working properly.

Do not take other medicines unless they have been discussed with your doctor. This especially includes over-the-counter (nonprescription) medicines for appetite control, asthma, colds, cough, hay fever, or sinus problems, since they may tend to increase your blood pressure.

This medicine may cause some people to have headaches or to feel dizzy. **Make sure you know how you react to this medicine before you drive, use machines, or do other jobs that require you to be alert.**

Dizziness, lightheadedness, or fainting may occur, especially when you get up from a lying or sitting position. Getting up slowly may help, but if the problem continues or gets worse, check with your doctor.

The dizziness, lightheadedness, or fainting is also more likely to occur if you drink alcohol, stand for long periods of time, exercise, or if the weather is hot. **While you are taking this medicine, be careful in the amount of alcohol you drink. Also, use extra care during exercise or hot weather or if you must stand for long periods of time.**

This medicine may cause a loss of potassium from your body.
- To help prevent this, your doctor may want you to:
  —eat or drink foods that have a high potassium content (for example, orange or other citrus fruit juices), or
  —take a potassium supplement, or
  —take another medicine to help prevent the loss of the potassium in the first place.

- It is very important to follow these directions. Also, it is important not to change your diet on your own. This is more important if you are already on a special diet (as for diabetes), or if you are taking a potassium supplement or a medicine to reduce potassium loss. Extra potassium may not be necessary and, in some cases, too much potassium could be harmful.

Check with your doctor if you become sick and have severe or continuing nausea, vomiting, or diarrhea. These problems may cause you to lose additional water and potassium.

Diabetics—Thiazide diuretics may raise blood sugar levels. While you are using this medicine, be especially careful in testing for sugar in your urine. If you have any questions about this, check with your doctor.

Some people who take this medicine may become more sensitive to sunlight than they are normally. When you first begin taking this medicine, avoid too much sun and do not use a sunlamp until you see how you react to the sun, especially if you tend to burn easily. If you have a severe reaction, check with your doctor.

Side Effects of This Medicine

Along with its needed effects, a medicine may cause some unwanted effects. Although not all of these side effects may occur, if they do occur they may need medical attention.

Check with your doctor as soon as possible if any of the following side effects occur:
Less common
    Blisters on skin
    Chest pain
    General feeling of body discomfort or weakness

Joint pain
Numbness, tingling, pain, or weakness in hands or feet
Skin rash or itching
Sore throat and fever
Swelling of the lymph glands
Rare
Flank or stomach pain
Severe stomach pain with nausea and vomiting
Unusual bleeding or bruising
Yellow eyes or skin
Signs of too much potassium loss
Dryness of mouth
Increased thirst
Irregular heartbeats
Mood or mental changes
Muscle cramps or pain
Weak pulse

Other side effects may occur that usually do not require medical attention. These side effects may go away during treatment as your body adjusts to the medicine. However, check with your doctor if any of the following side effects continue or are bothersome:
More common
Decreased sexual ability
Diarrhea
Fast or irregular heartbeat

Headache
Loss of appetite
Nausea or vomiting
Less common
Dizziness or lightheadedness, especially when getting up from a lying or sitting position
Increased sensitivity of skin to sunlight
Redness or flushing of the face
Shortness of breath with exercise or work
Stuffy nose
Watering or irritated eyes

For elderly patients: Dizziness or lightheadedness or signs of too much potassium loss may be more likely to occur in the elderly, who are usually more sensitive to the effects of this medicine.

Other side effects not listed above may also occur in some patients. If you notice any other effects, check with your doctor.

_____

December 1987

HYDROCORTISONE (Rectal)

Some commonly used brand names are:

Cort-Dome	Dermolate
Corticaine	Rectocort*
Cortiment*	

*Not available in the U.S.

To the Reader: If you do not recognize the names of medical conditions or medicines referred to in this information, check with your doctor, nurse, or pharmacist. Definitions for selected medical terms may be found in the Glossary. Brand names for the generic drug names listed can be found in the Index. In addition, selected brand names commonly associated with the generic name have been included in the text to help you recognize medicine you may be taking. The fact that a brand name product is not mentioned does not mean the information does not apply. It is a good idea for you to learn both the generic and brand names of your medicines and to write them down for future use.

Hydrocortisone (hye-droe-KOR-ti-sone) is an adrenocorticoid (a-dree-noe-KOR-ti-koid) (cortisone-like medicine). It belongs to the general family of medicines called steroids. Cortisone-like medicines are used in the rectum to help relieve swelling, itching, and discomfort of some rectal problems. They may also be applied to the area around the anus or rectum to relieve itching and discomfort. Hydrocortisone is used in the form of a rectal cream, ointment, or suppository.

Rectal adrenocorticoids may be absorbed through the lining of the rectum and may rarely affect growth in children, especially if used in large amounts or for a long time. Before using this medicine in children, you should discuss the use of it with your doctor.

Some hydrocortisone products for rectal use are available without a prescription; however, your doctor may have special instructions on the proper dose for your medical condition. Other hydrocortisone products for rectal use are available only with your doctor's prescription.

Remember:
• If this medicine has been prescribed for you, **it is for your current medical problem only.** It must not be given to other people or used for other problems unless you are directed to do so by your doctor.

• **Keep all medicines out of the reach of children.**

• In order for this medicine to work, it must be used as directed by your doctor or on the package label.

• **It is very important that you read and understand the following information.** If this medicine has been prescribed for you and any of the information causes you special concern, do not decide against using this medicine without first checking with your doctor.

• Before you begin using any new medicine (prescription or nonprescription) or if you develop any new medical problem while you are using this medicine, check with your doctor, nurse, or pharmacist.

• **If you have any questions** about the following information or if you want more information about this medicine or your medical problem, **ask your doctor, nurse, or pharmacist.**

Before Using This Medicine

Before you use rectal hydrocortisone without a prescription, check with your doctor, nurse, or pharmacist:

—if you have ever had any unusual or allergic reaction to hydrocortisone.

—if you are allergic to any substance, such as certain preservatives or dyes. Most medicines contain more than their active ingredient. Your doctor, nurse, or pharmacist can help you avoid products that may cause a problem.

—if you are **pregnant** or if you may become pregnant. Studies on birth defects with rectal hydrocortisone have not been done in humans. However, studies in animals have shown that topical adrenocorticoids, such as hydrocortisone contained in this medicine, when used in large amounts or for prolonged periods of time, may be absorbed through the skin and cause birth defects.

—if you are **breast-feeding**. Although rectal adrenocorticoids have not been shown to cause problems in nursing babies, the chance always exists since they may be absorbed into the body.

—if you have any of the following medical problems:
Diabetes mellitus (sugar diabetes)
Infection at the place of treatment
Tuberculosis

Proper Use of This Medicine

For patients using hydrocortisone rectal cream or ointment:

• This medicine usually comes with patient directions. Read them carefully before using this medicine.

For patients using hydrocortisone suppositories:

• How to insert suppository: First remove the foil wrapper and moisten the suppository with water. Lie down on side and push the suppository well up into rectum with your finger. If the suppository is too soft to insert because of storage in a warm place, chill the suppository in the refrigerator for 30 minutes or run cold water over it before removing the foil wrapper.

Do not use rectal hydrocortisone in larger amounts, more often, or for a longer period of time than your doctor ordered or the package label directs. To do so may increase the chance of absorption through the lining of the rectum and the chance of side effects.

If this medicine was ordered by your doctor, do not use any leftover medicine for future rectal problems without first checking with your doctor. Also, if you are treating yourself, check with your doctor before using rectal hydrocortisone for problems other than those stated on the package, or if you suspect that an infection may be present. The medicine should not be used to treat many kinds of bacterial, viral, or fungal infections.

If your doctor has ordered you to use this medicine according to a regular schedule and you miss a dose, use it as soon as you remember. However, if it is almost time for your next dose, skip the missed dose and go back to your regular dosing schedule. Do not double doses.

How to store this medicine:

- **Keep out of the reach of children.**
- Store away from heat and direct light.
- Do not store hydrocortisone suppositories in the bathroom medicine cabinet because the heat or moisture may cause the medicine to break down.
- Keep the medicine from freezing.
- Do not keep outdated medicine or medicine no longer needed. Be sure that any discarded medicine is out of the reach of children.

Precautions While Using This Medicine

Children who must use this medicine should be checked by their doctor during frequent visits. Hydrocortisone may be absorbed through the lining of the rectum and can affect growth.

Side Effects of This Medicine

Along with its needed effects, a medicine may cause some unwanted effects. Although not all of these side effects may occur, if they do occur they may need medical attention.

Check with your doctor as soon as possible if any of the following side effects occur:

> Signs of irritation or infection such as rectal bleeding, pain, burning, itching, or blistering not present before using this medicine

Additional side effects may occur if you use this medicine for a long period of time. Check with your doctor as soon as possible if any of the following side effects occur:

> Acne or oily skin
> Filling or rounding out of the face
> Reddish-purple lines on arms, legs, trunk, or groin
> Thinning of skin with easy bruising
> Unusual increase in hair growth
> Unusual loss of hair

Other side effects not listed above may also occur in some patients. If you notice any other effects, check with your doctor.

December 1987

HYDROCORTISONE, BISMUTH, BENZYL BENZOATE, PERUVIAN BALSAM, AND ZINC OXIDE (Rectal)

A commonly used brand name is Anusol-HC (U.S. only).

To the Reader: If you do not recognize the names of medical conditions or medicines referred to in this information, check with your doctor, nurse, or pharmacist. Definitions for selected medical terms may be found in the Glossary. Brand names for the generic drug names listed can be found in the Index. In addition, selected brand names commonly associated with the generic name have been included in the text to help you recognize medicine you may be taking. The fact that a brand name product is not mentioned does not mean the information does not apply. It is a good idea for you to learn both the generic and brand names of your medicines and to write them down for future use.

Hydrocortisone (hye-droe-KOR-ti-sone), bismuth (BIZ-muth), benzyl benzoate (BEN-zill BENZ-oh-ate), Peruvian balsam (pe-ROO-vee-an BAL-sam), and zinc oxide (ZINK OX-ide) combination is used to relieve the swelling, itching, and discomfort of hemorrhoids and certain other rectal problems.

Since topical adrenocorticoids (such as the hydrocortisone present in this combination medicine) may be absorbed through the lining of the rectum, they may affect the growth of children. Before this medicine is used in children, you should discuss the use of it with your doctor.

This medicine is used as a rectal cream or suppository and is available only with your doctor's prescription.

Remember:
• **This medicine has been prescribed for your current medical problem only.** It must not be given to other people or used for other problems unless you are directed to do so by your doctor.

• **Keep all medicines out of the reach of children.**

• In order for this medicine to work, it must be used as directed.

• **It is very important that you read and understand the following information.** If any of the information causes you special concern, do not decide against using this medicine without first checking with your doctor.

• Before you begin using any new medicine (prescription or nonprescription) or if you develop any new medical problem while you are using this medicine, check with your doctor, nurse, or pharmacist.

• **If you have any questions** about the following information or if you want more information about this medicine or your medical problem, **ask your doctor, nurse, or pharmacist.**

Before Using This Medicine

In order to decide on the best treatment for your medical problem, your doctor should be told:

—if you have ever had any unusual or allergic reaction to hydrocortisone or to hemorrhoid or other rectal medicines.

—if you are allergic to any substance, such as certain preservatives or dyes. Most medicines contain more than their active ingredient. Your doctor, nurse, or pharmacist can help you avoid products that may cause a problem.

—if you are **pregnant** or if you may become pregnant. Studies on birth defects with this medicine have not been done in humans. However, hydrocortisone used in large amounts or for long periods of time may cause unwanted effects if it is absorbed into the body. Also, studies in animals have shown that hydrocortisone causes birth defects.

—if you are **breast-feeding**. This medicine has not been shown to cause problems in humans. However, the chance always exists.

—if you have an infection at the place of treatment.

Proper Use of This Medicine

For patients using the rectal cream form of this medicine:

• If you are applying this medicine to the rectal area, first bathe and dry the rectal area. Then apply a small amount of cream and rub it in gently.

• If you have been directed to insert the cream into the rectum, first attach the plastic applicator tip onto the opened tube. Insert the applicator tip into the rectum and gently squeeze the tube to deliver the cream. Remove the applicator tip from the tube and wash with hot, soapy water. Replace the cap of the tube after use.

For patients using the suppository form of this medicine:

• This medicine usually comes with patient directions. Read them carefully before using this medicine.

• How to insert the suppository: First remove the foil wrapper and moisten the suppository with water. Lie down on your side and push the suppository well up into the rectum with your finger. If the suppository is too soft to insert because of storage in a warm place, chill the suppository in the refrigerator for 30 minutes or run cold water over it before removing the foil wrapper.

Do not use more of this medicine, or use it for a longer period of time than your doctor ordered. To do so may increase the chance of absorption through the lining of the rectum and the chance of side effects.

Do not use any leftover medicine for future rectal problems without first checking with your doctor. The hydrocortisone in this medicine should not be used if many kinds of bacterial, viral, or fungal infections are present.

If you miss a dose of this medicine, use it as soon as you remember. However, if it is almost time for your next dose, skip the missed dose and go back to your regular dosing schedule. Do not double doses.

© 1988   The United States Pharmacopeial Convention, Inc.

How to store this medicine:

- **Keep out of the reach of children.**
- Store away from heat and direct light.
- Keep the medicine from freezing.
- Do not keep outdated medicine or medicine no longer needed. Be sure that any discarded medicine is out of the reach of children.

Precautions While Using This Medicine

Children who must use this medicine should be followed closely by their doctor since the hydrocortisone in this medicine may be absorbed through the lining of the rectum and can affect growth.

If this medicine stains your clothing, the stain may be removed by hand- or machine-washing with laundry detergent.

Side Effects of This Medicine

Along with its needed effects, a medicine may cause some unwanted effects. Although not all of these side effects may occur, if they do occur they may need medical attention.

Check with your doctor as soon as possible if any of the following side effects occur:

Rare

Signs of irritation or infection such as rectal bleeding, pain, burning, itching, or blistering not present before using this medicine

Other side effects not listed above may also occur in some patients. If you notice any other effects, check with your doctor.

_____

December 1987

HYDROXYPROPYL CELLULOSE
(Ophthalmic)

A commonly used brand name is Lacrisert.

To the Reader: If you do not recognize the names of medical conditions or medicines referred to in this information, check with your doctor, nurse, or pharmacist. Definitions for selected medical terms may be found in the Glossary. Brand names for the generic drug names listed can be found in the Index. In addition, selected brand names commonly associated with the generic name have been included in the text to help you recognize medicine you may be taking. The fact that a brand name product is not mentioned does not mean the information does not apply. It is a good idea for you to learn both the generic and brand names of your medicines and to write them down for future use.

Hydroxypropyl cellulose (hye-drox-ee-PROE-pil SELL-yoo-lose) belongs to the group of medicines known as artificial tears. It is inserted in the eye to relieve dryness and irritation caused by reduced tear flow that occurs in certain eye diseases.

This medicine is available only with your doctor's prescription.

Remember:

• **This medicine has been prescribed for your current medical problem only.** It must not be given to other people or used for other problems unless you are directed to do so by your doctor.

• **Keep all medicines out of the reach of children.**

• In order for this medicine to work, it must be used as directed.

• **It is very important that you read and understand the following information.** If any of the information causes you special concern, do not decide against using this medicine without first checking with your doctor.

• Before you begin using any new medicine (prescription or nonprescription) or if you develop any new medical problem while you are using this medicine, check with your doctor, nurse, or pharmacist.

• **If you have any questions** about the following information or if you want more information about this medicine or your medical problem, **ask your doctor, nurse, or pharmacist.**

Before Using This Medicine

In order to decide on the best treatment for your medical problem, your doctor should be told:

—if you have ever had any unusual or allergic reaction to hydroxypropyl cellulose.

—if you are **pregnant** or if you may become pregnant. However, hydroxypropyl cellulose has not been shown to cause birth defects or other problems in humans.

—if you are **breast-feeding**. However, hydroxypropyl cellulose has not been shown to cause problems in nursing babies.

Proper Use of This Medicine

This medicine usually comes with patient directions. Read them carefully before using this medicine. It is very important that you understand how to insert this eye system properly. If you have any questions about this, check with your doctor.

If the eye system accidentally comes out of your eye, as sometimes occurs when the eye is rubbed, do not put it back in the eye, since it may be contaminated. Instead, insert another eye system if needed.

If you miss a dose of this medicine, insert it as soon as possible. Then go back to your regular dosing schedule.

How to store this medicine:

• **Keep out of the reach of children.**

• Store away from heat and direct light.

• Do not keep outdated medicine or medicine no longer needed. Be sure that any discarded medicine is out of the reach of children.

Precautions While Using This Medicine

This medicine may cause blurred vision. **Make sure your vision is clear before you drive, use machines, or do other jobs that require you to see well.**

This medicine may also cause your eyes to become more sensitive to light than they are normally. Wearing sunglasses may help relieve the discomfort from bright light.

Side Effects of This Medicine

Along with its needed effects, a medicine may cause some unwanted effects. The following side effects may go away during treatment as your body adjusts to the medicine. However, check with your doctor if any of these effects continue or are bothersome:

Less common
  Blurred vision
  Eye discomfort or other irritation not present before using this medicine
  Increased sensitivity of eyes to light
  Matting or stickiness of eyelids
  Swelling of eyelids

For elderly patients: Many medicines have not been tested in older people. Therefore, it is not known whether the medicine acts the same way it does in younger adults. Check with your doctor or pharmacist if you notice any unusual effects while using this medicine or if you think it is not working as it should.

Other side effects not listed above may also occur in some patients. If you notice any other effects, check with your doctor.

December 1987

HYDROXYPROPYL METHYLCELLULOSE
(Ophthalmic)

Some commonly used brand names are:

Gonak	Moisture Drops
Goniosol	Muro Tears
Isopto Alkaline	Tearisol
Isopto Plain	Tears Naturale
Isopto Tears	Ultra Tears
Lacril	

To the Reader: If you do not recognize the names of medical conditions or medicines referred to in this information, check with your doctor, nurse, or pharmacist. Definitions for selected medical terms may be found in the Glossary. Brand names for the generic drug names listed can be found in the Index. In addition, selected brand names commonly associated with the generic name have been included in the text to help you recognize medicine you may be taking. The fact that a brand name product is not mentioned does not mean the information does not apply. It is a good idea for you to learn both the generic and brand names of your medicines and to write them down for future use.

Hydroxypropyl methylcellulose (hye-drox-ee-PROE-pil meth-ill-SELL-yoo-lose) belongs to the group of medicines known as artificial tears. It is used in the eye to relieve dryness and irritation caused by reduced tear flow. It helps prevent damage to the eye in certain eye diseases. Hydroxypropyl methylcellulose may also be used to moisten hard contact lenses and artificial eyes. In addition, it may be used in certain eye examinations.

Some of these preparations are available only with your doctor's prescription. Others are available without a prescription; however, your doctor may have special instructions on the proper use of this medicine for your medical problem.

Remember:
• **Keep all medicines out of the reach of children.**

• In order for this medicine to work, it must be used as directed. **If you are using this medicine without a prescription, it is very important to follow the directions on the label.**

• **It is also very important that you read and understand the following information.** If any of the information causes you special concern, check with your doctor or pharmacist.

• Before you begin using any new medicine (prescription or nonprescription) or if you develop any new medical problem while you are using this medicine, check with your doctor, nurse, or pharmacist.

• **If you have any questions** about the following information or if you want more information about this medicine or your medical problem, **ask your doctor, nurse, or pharmacist.**

Before Using This Medicine

Before you use hydroxypropyl methylcellulose, check with your doctor or pharmacist:

—if you have ever had any unusual or allergic reaction to hydroxypropyl methylcellulose.

—if you are allergic to any substance, such as certain preservatives. Most medicines contain more than their active ingredient. Your doctor or pharmacist can help you avoid products that may cause a problem.

—if you are **pregnant** or if you may become pregnant, although hydroxypropyl methylcellulose has not been shown to cause birth defects or other problems in humans.

—if you are **breast-feeding**, although hydroxypropyl methylcellulose has not been shown to cause problems in nursing babies.

Proper Use of This Medicine

How to apply this medicine: First, wash your hands. Then tilt the head back and pull the lower eyelid away from the eye to form a pouch. Drop the medicine into the pouch and gently close the eyes. Do not blink. Keep the eyes closed for 1 or 2 minutes to allow the medicine to be absorbed.

To prevent contamination of the eye drops, do not touch the applicator tip to any surface (including the eye) and keep the container tightly closed.

Do not use this medicine for more than 3 days, unless otherwise directed by your doctor. To do so may increase the chance of side effects.

For patients wearing hard contact lenses:
• Take care not to float the lens from your eye when applying this medicine. If you have any questions about this, check with your doctor, nurse, or pharmacist.

How to store this medicine:
• **Keep out of the reach of children.**
• Store away from heat and direct light.
• Keep the medicine from freezing.
• Do not keep outdated medicine or medicine no longer needed. Be sure that any discarded medicine is out of the reach of children.

Precautions While Using This Medicine

If your symptoms continue or become worse, check with your doctor.

Side Effects of This Medicine

Along with its needed effects, a medicine may cause some unwanted effects. Although not all of these side effects may occur, if they do occur they may need medical attention.

Check with your doctor as soon as possible if the following side effect occurs:

> Eye irritation not present before using this medicine

Other side effects may occur that usually do not require medical attention. These side effects may go away during treatment as your body adjusts to the medicine. However, check with your doctor or pharmacist if either of the following side effects continues or is bothersome:

Less common—more common with 1% solution

> Blurred vision
> Matting or stickiness of eyelids

For elderly patients: Many medicines have not been tested in older people. Therefore, it is not known whether the medicine acts the same way it does in younger adults. Check with your doctor or pharmacist if you notice any unusual effects while using this medicine or if you think it is not working as it should.

Other side effects not listed above may also occur in some patients. If you notice any other effects, check with your doctor or pharmacist.

December 1987

HYDROXYSTILBAMIDINE (Systemic)*

*Not commercially available in the U.S.

To the Reader: If you do not recognize the names of medical conditions or medicines referred to in this information, check with your doctor, nurse, or pharmacist. Definitions for selected medical terms may be found in the Glossary. Brand names for the generic drug names listed can be found in the Index. In addition, selected brand names commonly associated with the generic name have been included in the text to help you recognize medicine you may be taking. The fact that a brand name product is not mentioned does not mean the information does not apply. It is a good idea for you to learn both the generic and brand names of your medicines and to write them down for future use.

Hydroxystilbamidine (hye-drox-ee-stil-BAM-i-deen) belongs to the group of medicines called antifungals. It is given by injection to treat certain fungal infections.

Hydroxystilbamidine is available only with your doctor's prescription.

Remember:
• **It is very important that you read and understand the following information.** If any of the information causes you special concern, do not decide against using this medicine without first checking with your doctor.

• Before you begin using any new medicine (prescription or nonprescription) or if you develop any new medical problem while you are using this medicine, check with your doctor, nurse, or pharmacist.

• **If you have any questions** about the following information or if you want more information about this medicine or your medical problem, **ask your doctor, nurse, or pharmacist.**

Before Using This Medicine

In order to decide on the best treatment for your medical problem, your doctor should be told:

—if you have ever had any unusual or allergic reaction to hydroxystilbamidine.

—if you are on a low-salt, low-sugar, or any other special diet, or if you are allergic to any substance, such as foods or sulfites or other preservatives. Most medicines contain more than their active ingredient. Your doctor, nurse, or pharmacist can help you avoid products that may cause a problem.

—if you are **pregnant** or if you may become pregnant. However, hydroxystilbamidine has not been shown to cause birth defects or other problems in humans.

—if you are **breast-feeding**. However, hydroxystilbamidine has not been shown to cause problems in nursing babies.

—if you have either of the following medical problems:
  Kidney disease
  Liver disease

Side Effects of This Medicine

Along with its needed effects, a medicine may cause some unwanted effects. Although not all of these side effects may occur, if they do occur they may need medical attention.

Check with your doctor as soon as possible if any of the following side effects occur:
Less common
  Chills and fever
  Fast heartbeat
  Redness, swelling, or pain at place of injection
  Skin rash or itching
  Sore throat and fever
  Swelling of face or eyelids
  Troubled breathing
  Unusual tiredness or weakness
Rare
  Numbness, tingling, pain, or weakness in hands or feet
  Yellow eyes or skin

Other side effects may occur that usually do not require medical attention. These side effects may go away during treatment as your body adjusts to the medicine. However, check with your doctor if any of the following side effects continue or are bothersome:
More common
  Diarrhea
  Loss of appetite
  Nausea or vomiting
Less common
  Dizziness or lightheadedness
  Drowsiness
  Headache
  Joint pain

For elderly patients: Many medicines have not been tested in older people. Therefore, it is not known whether the medicine acts the same way it does in younger adults. Check with your doctor or pharmacist if you notice any unusual effects while receiving this medicine or if you think it is not working as it should.

Other side effects not listed above may also occur in some patients. If you notice any other effects, check with your doctor.

December 1987

HYDROXYUREA (Systemic)
A commonly used brand name is Hydrea.

To the Reader: If you do not recognize the names of medical conditions or medicines referred to in this information, check with your doctor, nurse, or pharmacist. Definitions for selected medical terms may be found in the Glossary. Brand names for the generic drug names listed can be found in the Index. In addition, selected brand names commonly associated with the generic name have been included in the text to help you recognize medicine you may be taking. The fact that a brand name product is not mentioned does not mean the information does not apply. It is a good idea for you to learn both the generic and brand names of your medicines and to write them down for future use.

Hydroxyurea (hye-DROX-ee-yoo-REE-ah) belongs to the group of medicines called antimetabolites. It is taken by mouth to treat some kinds of cancer.

Hydroxyurea seems to interfere with the growth of cancer cells, which are eventually destroyed. Since the growth of normal body cells may also be affected by hydroxyurea, other effects will also occur. Some of these may be serious and must be reported to your doctor. Other effects may not be serious but may cause concern. Some effects may not occur for months or years after the medicine is used.

Before you begin treatment with hydroxyurea, you and your doctor should talk about the good this medicine will do as well as the risks of using it.

Hydroxyurea is available only with your doctor's prescription.

Remember:

• **This medicine has been prescribed for your current medical problem only.** It must not be given to other people or used for other problems unless you are directed to do so by your doctor.

• **Keep all medicines out of the reach of children.**

• In order for this medicine to work, it must be used as directed.

• **It is very important that you read and understand the following information.** If any of the information causes you special concern, do not decide against using this medicine without first checking with your doctor.

• Before you begin using any new medicine (prescription or nonprescription) or if you develop any new medical problem while you are using this medicine, check with your doctor, nurse, or pharmacist.

• **If you have any questions** about the following information or if you want more information about this medicine or your medical problem, **ask your doctor, nurse, or pharmacist.**

Before Using This Medicine
In order to decide on the best treatment for your medical problem, your doctor should be told:

—if you have ever had any unusual or allergic reaction to hydroxyurea.

—if you are **pregnant** or if you intend to have children. There is a chance that this medicine may cause birth defects if either the male or female is taking it at the time of conception or if it is taken during pregnancy. Studies have shown that hydroxyurea causes birth defects in animals. In addition, many cancer medicines may cause sterility. Although this seems to be only temporary with this medicine, the possibility should be kept in mind. Be sure that you have discussed this with your doctor before taking this medicine.

—if you intend to **breast-feed**. Because this medicine may cause serious side effects, breast-feeding is generally not recommended while you are taking it.

—if you have any of the following medical problems:
Anemia
Chickenpox (including recent exposure)
Gout
Herpes zoster (shingles)
Infection
Kidney disease
Kidney stones

—if you are taking **any** other prescription or nonprescription (OTC) medicine, especially:
Amphotericin B by injection (e.g., Fungizone)
Antithyroid agents (medicine for overactive thyroid)
Azathioprine (e.g., Imuran)
Chloramphenicol (e.g., Chloromycetin)
Colchicine
Flucytosine (e.g., Ancobon)
Inteferon (e.g., Intron A; Roferon-A)
Probenecid (e.g., Benemid)
Sulfinpyrazone (e.g., Anturane)

—if you have ever been treated with x-rays or cancer medicines.

Proper Use of This Medicine
Take hydroxyurea only as directed by your doctor. Do not use more or less of it, and do not use it more often than your doctor ordered. The exact amount of medicine you need has been carefully worked out. Taking too much may increase the chance of side effects, while taking too little may not improve your condition.

This medicine is sometimes given together with certain other medicines. If you are using a combination of medicines, make sure that you take each one at the right time and do not mix them. Ask your doctor, nurse, or pharmacist to help you plan a way to take your medicine at the right times.

While you are using this medicine, your doctor may want you to drink extra fluids so that you will pass more urine. This will help prevent kidney problems and keep your kidneys working well.

This medicine commonly causes nausea, vomiting, and diarrhea. However, it is very important that you continue to use the medicine, even if you begin to feel ill. Ask your doctor, nurse, or pharmacist for ways to lessen these effects.

If you vomit shortly after taking a dose of hydroxyurea, check with your doctor. You will be told whether to take the dose again or to wait until the next scheduled dose.

If you miss a dose of this medicine, do not take the missed dose at all and do not double the next one. Instead, go back to your regular dosing schedule and check with your doctor.

How to store this medicine:

• **Keep out of the reach of children.**

• Store away from heat and direct light.

• Do not store in the bathroom, near the kitchen sink, or in other damp places. Heat or moisture may cause the medicine to break down.

• Do not keep outdated medicine or medicine no longer needed. Be sure that any discarded medicine is out of the reach of children.

Precautions While Using This Medicine

It is very important that your doctor check your progress at regular visits to make sure that this medicine is working properly and to check for unwanted effects.

While you are being treated with hydroxyurea, and after you stop treatment with it, **do not have any immunizations without your doctor's approval.** Hydroxyurea lowers your body's resistance and there is a chance you might get the infection the immunization is meant to prevent. In addition, other persons in your household should not take oral polio vaccine since there is a chance they could pass the polio virus on to you. Also, you should avoid close contact with other persons (for example, at school or work) who have taken oral polio vaccine.

Hydroxyurea can lower the number of white blood cells in your body. This may increase the chance of getting an infection. If you can, avoid people with colds or other infections. If you think you are getting a cold or other infection, check with your doctor.

Side Effects of This Medicine

Along with their needed effects, medicines like hydroxyurea can sometimes cause unwanted effects such as blood problems and other side effects. These are described below. Also, because of the way these medicines act on the body, there is a chance that they might cause other unwanted effects that may not occur until months or years after the medicine is used. These delayed effects may include certain types of cancer, such as leukemia. Ask your doctor, nurse, or pharmacist for ways to lessen these effects.

Although not all of these side effects may occur, if they do occur they may need medical attention.

Check with your doctor immediately if any of the following side effects occur:
More common
  Fever, chills, or sore throat
Less common
  Unusual bleeding or bruising

Check with your doctor as soon as possible if any of the following side effects occur:
Less common
  Sores in the mouth and on the lips
Rare
  Confusion
  Convulsions (seizures)
  Dizziness
  Hallucinations (seeing, hearing, or feeling things that are not there)
  Headache
  Joint pain
  Lower back, side, or stomach pain
  Swelling of feet or lower legs

Other side effects may occur that usually do not require medical attention. These side effects may go away during treatment as your body adjusts to the medicine. Also, your doctor or nurse may be able to tell you about ways to prevent or reduce some of these side effects. Check with your doctor if any of the following side effects continue or are bothersome or if you have any questions about them:
More common
  Diarrhea
  Drowsiness
  Loss of appetite
  Nausea or vomiting
Less common
  Constipation
  Redness of the face
  Skin rash and itching

After you stop taking hydroxyurea, your body may need time to adjust. The length of time this takes depends on the amount of medicine you were using and how long you used it. During this period of time check with your doctor if you notice any of the following side effects:
  Fever, chills, or sore throat
  Unusual bleeding or bruising

For children and elderly patients: The above side effects are more likely to occur in children and in elderly patients, who are usually more sensitive to the effects of hydroxyurea.

Other side effects not listed above may also occur in some patients. If you notice any other effects, check with your doctor.

December 1987

HYDROXYZINE (Systemic)

Some commonly used brand names are:

Anxanil	Orgatrax
Atarax	Quiess
Atozine	Vamate
Durrax	Vistacon
E-Vista	Vistaject
Hydroxacen	Vistaquel
Hy-Pam	Vistaril
Hyzine	Vistazine
Multipax*	

Generic name product may also be available in the U.S.

---

*Not available in the U.S.

To the Reader: If you do not recognize the names of medical conditions or medicines referred to in this information, check with your doctor, nurse, or pharmacist. Definitions for selected medical terms may be found in the Glossary. Brand names for the generic drug names listed can be found in the Index. In addition, selected brand names commonly associated with the generic name have been included in the text to help you recognize medicine you may be taking. The fact that a brand name product is not mentioned does not mean the information does not apply. It is a good idea for you to learn both the generic and brand names of your medicines and to write them down for future use.

Hydroxyzine (hye-DROX-i-zeen) is used in the treatment of nervous and emotional conditions to help control anxiety. It can also be used to help control anxiety and induce sleep before surgery.

Because hydroxyzine has antihistamine action, it is used to relieve the itching caused by allergic conditions. In addition, hydroxyzine when given by injection can be used to prevent nausea and vomiting.

Hydroxyzine is available only with your doctor's prescription.

Remember:

• **This medicine has been prescribed for your current medical problem only.** It must not be given to other people or used for other problems unless you are directed to do so by your doctor.

• **Keep all medicines out of the reach of children.**

• In order for this medicine to work, it must be used as directed.

• If you are receiving this medicine by injection, some of the information about this medicine may not apply.

• **It is very important that you read and understand the following information.** If any of the information causes you special concern, do not decide against using this medicine without first checking with your doctor.

• Before you begin using any new medicine (prescription or nonprescription) or if you develop any new medical problem while you are using this medicine, check with your doctor, nurse, or pharmacist.

• **If you have any questions** about the following information or if you want more information about this medicine or your medical problem, **ask your doctor, nurse, or pharmacist.**

Before Using This Medicine

In order to decide on the best treatment for your medical problem, your doctor should be told:

—if you have ever had any unusual or allergic reaction to hydroxyzine.

—if you are on a low-salt, low-sugar, or any other special diet, or if you are allergic to any substance, such as foods, sulfites or other preservatives, or dyes. Most medicines contain more than their active ingredient, and many liquid medicines contain alcohol. Your doctor, nurse, or pharmacist can help you avoid products that may cause a problem.

—if you are **pregnant** or if you may become pregnant. Hydroxyzine is not recommended in the first months of pregnancy since it has been shown to cause birth defects in rats when given in doses up to many times the usual human dose. Be sure you have discussed this with your doctor.

—if you are **breast-feeding**. Hydroxyzine has not been shown to cause problems in nursing babies.

—if you are taking **any** other prescription or nonprescription (OTC) medicine, especially central nervous system (CNS) depressants.

Proper Use of This Medicine

Take hydroxyzine only as directed by your doctor. Do not take more of it and do not take it more often than your doctor ordered. To do so may increase the chance of side effects.

If you miss a dose of this medicine, take it as soon as possible. However, if it is almost time for your next dose, skip the missed dose and go back to your regular dosing schedule. Do not double doses.

How to store this medicine:

• **Keep out of the reach of children.**

• Store away from heat and direct light.

• Do not store the capsule or tablet form of this medicine in the bathroom, near the kitchen sink, or in other damp places. Heat or moisture may cause the medicine to break down.

• Keep the liquid form of this medicine from freezing.

• Do not keep outdated medicine or medicine no longer needed. Be sure that any discarded medicine is out of the reach of children.

Precautions While Using This Medicine

Tell the doctor in charge that you are taking this medicine before you have any skin tests for allergies. The results of the test may be affected by this medicine.

Hydroxyzine will add to the effects of alcohol and other central nervous system (CNS) depressants (medicines that slow down the nervous system, possibly causing drowsiness). Some examples of CNS depressants are antihistamines or medicine for hay fever, other allergies, or colds; sedatives, tranquilizers, or sleeping medicine; prescription pain medicine or narcotics; barbiturates; medicine for convulsions (seizures); muscle relaxants; or anesthetics, including some dental anesthetics. **Check with your doctor before taking any of the above while you are using this medicine.**

This medicine may cause some people to become drowsy or less alert than they are normally. Even if taken at bedtime, it may cause some people to feel drowsy or less alert on arising. **Make sure you know how you react to this medicine before you drive, use machines, or do other jobs that require you to be alert.**

Hydroxyzine may cause dryness of the mouth. For temporary relief of mouth dryness, use sugarless candy or gum, melt bits of ice in your mouth, or use a saliva substitute. However, if dry mouth continues for more than 2 weeks, check with your physician or dentist. Continuing dryness of the mouth may increase the chance of dental disease, including tooth decay, gum disease, and fungal infections.

Side Effects of This Medicine

Along with its needed effects, a medicine may cause some unwanted effects. Although not all of these side effects may occur, if they do occur they may need medical attention.

Check with your doctor as soon as possible if any of the following side effects occur:

Rare
   Seizures
   Skin rash
   Trembling or shakiness
Signs of overdose
   Drowsiness (severe)
   Feeling faint

Other side effects may occur that usually do not require medical attention. These side effects may go away during treatment as your body adjusts to the medicine. However, check with your doctor if either of the following side effects continues or is bothersome:

More common
   Drowsiness
Less common
   Dryness of the mouth

For elderly patients: The above side effects are more likely to occur in elderly patients, who are usually more sensitive to the effects of hydroxyzine.

Other side effects not listed above may also occur in some patients. If you notice any other effects, check with your doctor.

December 1987

IDOXURIDINE (Ophthalmic)

Some commonly used brand names are Herplex and Stoxil.

To the Reader: If you do not recognize the names of medical conditions or medicines referred to in this information, check with your doctor, nurse, or pharmacist. Definitions for selected medical terms may be found in the Glossary. Brand names for the generic drug names listed can be found in the Index. In addition, selected brand names commonly associated with the generic name have been included in the text to help you recognize medicine you may be taking. The fact that a brand name product is not mentioned does not mean the information does not apply. It is a good idea for you to learn both the generic and brand names of your medicines and to write them down for future use.

Idoxuridine (eye-dox-YOOR-i-deen) belongs to the general family of medicines called antivirals. Idoxuridine ophthalmic preparations are used in the eye to help the body overcome virus infections of the eye.

Idoxuridine is available only with your doctor's prescription.

Remember:

• **This medicine has been prescribed for your present infection only.** Another infection later on may require a different medicine. Also, even though other people may have the same symptoms as you, they may have a different kind of infection. Your medicine may not work for them and may even cause them harm. Therefore, **your medicine must not be given to other people or used for other infections** unless you are otherwise directed by your doctor.

• **Keep all medicines out of the reach of children.**

• In order for this medicine to work, it must be used as directed.

• **It is also very important that you read and understand the following information.** If any of the information causes you special concern, do not decide against using this medicine without first checking with your doctor.

• Before you begin using any new medicine (prescription or nonprescription) or if you develop any new medical problem while you are using this medicine, check with your doctor, nurse, or pharmacist.

• **If you have any questions** about the following information or if you want more information about this medicine or your medical problem, **ask your doctor, nurse, or pharmacist.**

Before Using This Medicine

In order to decide on the best treatment for your medical problem, your doctor should be told:

—if you have ever had any unusual or allergic reaction to iodine or iodine-containing preparations.

—if you are allergic to any substance, such as certain foods or preservatives or dyes. Most medicines contain more than their active ingredient. Your doctor, nurse, or pharmacist can help you avoid products that may cause a problem.

—if you are **pregnant** or if you may become pregnant. Idoxuridine ophthalmic preparations have not been shown to cause birth defects or other problems in humans. However, idoxuridine has been shown to cause protruding eyes (eyes that stick out too far) and deformed forelegs in rabbits.

—if you are **breast-feeding**. It is not known whether idoxuridine passes into the breast milk. However, this medicine has not been shown to cause problems in nursing babies.

—if you are using **any** other prescription or nonprescription (OTC) medicine, especially boric acid in the eyes.

Proper Use of This Medicine

For patients using the eye drop form of idoxuridine:

• The bottle is only partially full to provide proper drop control.

• How to apply this medicine: First, wash your hands. Then tilt the head back and pull the lower eyelid away from the eye to form a pouch. Drop the medicine into the pouch and gently close the eyes. Do not blink. Keep the eyes closed for 1 or 2 minutes to allow the medicine to come into contact with the infection.

• If you think you did not get the drop of medicine into your eye properly, use another drop.

• To prevent contamination of the eye drops, do not touch the applicator tip to any surface (including the eye). Also, keep the container tightly closed.

For patients using the eye ointment form of idoxuridine:

• How to apply this medicine: First, wash your hands. Then pull the lower eyelid away from the eye to form a pouch. Squeeze a thin strip of ointment into the pouch. A 1-cm (approximately ⅓-inch) strip of ointment is usually enough unless otherwise directed by your doctor. Gently close the eyes and keep them closed for 1 or 2 minutes to allow the medicine to come into contact with the infection.

• To prevent contamination of the eye ointment, do not touch the applicator tip to any surface (including the eye). After using idoxuridine eye ointment, wipe the tip of the ointment tube with a clean tissue and keep the tube tightly closed.

Do not use this medicine more often or for a longer time than your doctor ordered. To do so may cause problems in the eyes. If you have any questions about this, check with your doctor.

To help clear up your infection completely, **keep using this medicine for the full time of treatment,** even though your symptoms may have disappeared; **do not miss any doses.**

If you do miss a dose of this medicine, apply it as soon as possible. However, if it is almost time for your next dose, skip the missed dose and go back to your regular dosing schedule.

How to store this medicine:

- **Keep out of the reach of children.**

- Store in the refrigerator or in a cool place because heat will cause this medicine to break down. However, keep the medicine from freezing. Follow the directions on the label.

- Do not keep outdated medicine or medicine no longer needed. Be sure that any discarded medicine is out of the reach of children.

Precautions While Using This Medicine

It is very important that your doctor check your progress at regular visits.

If your symptoms do not improve within a week, or if they become worse, check with your doctor.

This medicine may cause your eyes to become more sensitive to light than they are normally. Wearing sunglasses and avoiding too much exposure to bright light may help lessen the discomfort.

Side Effects of This Medicine

Along with its needed effects, a medicine may cause some unwanted effects. Although not all of these side effects may occur, if they do occur they may need medical attention.

Check with your doctor as soon as possible if any of the following side effects occur:

Less common
 Increased sensitivity of eyes to light
 Itching, redness, swelling, pain, or other sign of irritation not present before using this medicine

Rare
 Blurring, dimming, or haziness of vision

Other side effects may occur that usually do not require medical attention. These side effects may go away during treatment as your body adjusts to the medicine. However, check with your doctor if the following side effect continues or is bothersome:

Less common
 Excess flow of tears

After application, eye ointments usually cause your vision to blur for a few minutes.

Other side effects not listed above may also occur in some patients. If you notice any other effects, check with your doctor.

December 1987

IMIPENEM AND CILASTATIN (Systemic)

Some commonly used brand names or other names are Imipemide and cilastatin, Primaxin, and Zienam*.

*Not available in the U.S.

To the Reader: If you do not recognize the names of medical conditions or medicines referred to in this information, check with your doctor, nurse, or pharmacist. Definitions for selected medical terms may be found in the Glossary. Brand names for the generic drug names listed can be found in the Index. In addition, selected brand names commonly associated with the generic name have been included in the text to help you recognize medicine you may be taking. The fact that a brand name product is not mentioned does not mean the information does not apply. It is a good idea for you to learn both the generic and brand names of your medicines and to write them down for future use.

Imipenem (i-mi-PEN-em) and cilastatin (sye-la-STAT-in) combination belongs to the family of medicines called antibiotics. Antibiotics are medicines used in the treatment of infections caused by bacteria. They work by killing bacteria or preventing their growth. This medicine will not work for colds, flu, or other virus infections.

Imipenem and cilastatin combination is given by injection into a vein to treat infections in many different parts of the body. It is sometimes given with other antibiotics.

This medicine is available only with your doctor's prescription.

Remember:

• **It is very important that you read and understand the following information.** If any of the information causes you special concern, do not decide against using this medicine without first checking with your doctor.

• Before you begin using any new medicine (prescription or nonprescription) or if you develop any new medical problem while you are using this medicine, check with your doctor, nurse, or pharmacist.

• **If you have any questions** about the following information or if you want more information about this medicine or your medical problem, **ask your doctor, nurse, or pharmacist.**

Before Using This Medicine

In order to decide on the best treatment for your medical problem, your doctor should be told:

—if you have ever had any unusual or allergic reaction to any of the penicillins or cephalosporins.

—if you are on a low-salt, low-sugar, or any other special diet, or if you are allergic to any substance, such as foods or sulfites or other preservatives. Most medicines contain more than their active ingredient. Your doctor, nurse, or pharmacist can help you avoid products that may cause a problem.

—if you are **pregnant** or if you may become pregnant. Studies have not been done in humans. However, imipenem and cilastatin combination has not been shown to cause birth defects or other problems in animal studies.

—if you are **breast-feeding**. It is not known whether imipenem or cilastatin passes into the breast milk. However, this medicine has not been shown to cause problems in nursing babies.

—if you have any of the following medical problems:
Central nervous system disorders (for example, brain disease or history of seizures)
Kidney disease

—if you are taking **any** other prescription or nonprescription (OTC) medicine.

Proper Use of This Medicine

To help clear up your infection completely, **imipenem and cilastatin combination must be given for the full time of treatment** even if you begin to feel better after a few days. Also, this medicine works best when there is a constant amount in the blood or urine. To help keep this amount constant, it must be given on a regular schedule.

Precautions While Using This Medicine

Some patients may develop tremors or seizures while receiving this medicine. If either of these occurs, your doctor may want you to take anticonvulsants (seizure medicine) along with this medicine. **If you already have a history of seizures and you are taking anticonvulsants, you should continue to take them** unless otherwise directed by your doctor.

If diarrhea occurs, do not take any diarrhea medicine without first checking with your doctor or pharmacist. These medicines may make your diarrhea worse or make it last longer.

Side Effects of This Medicine

Along with its needed effects, a medicine may cause some unwanted effects. Although not all of these side effects may occur, if they do occur they may need medical attention.

Check with your doctor or nurse immediately if any of the following side effects occur:

More common
Skin rash, hives, itching, or wheezing

Less common
Confusion
Convulsions (seizures)
Dizziness
Increased sweating
Nausea or vomiting
Tremors

Rare
Abdominal or stomach cramps, pain, and bloating (severe)
Diarrhea (watery and severe), which may also be bloody
Fever
Increased thirst
Increased weight loss
Unusual tiredness or weakness
(the above side effects may also occur up to several weeks after you stop receiving this medicine)

Other side effects may occur that usually do not require medical attention. These side effects may go away during treatment as your body adjusts to the medicine. However, check with your doctor if the following side effect continues or is bothersome:

More common
    Diarrhea (mild)

For elderly patients: Many medicines have not been tested in older people. Therefore, it is not known whether the medicine acts the same way it does in younger adults.

Check with your doctor or pharmacist if you notice any unusual effects while receiving this medicine or if you think it is not working as it should.

Other side effects not listed above may also occur in some patients. If you notice any other effects, check with your doctor.

December 1987

INDAPAMIDE (Systemic)

Some commonly used brand names are Lozide* and Lozol.

*Not available in the U.S.

To the Reader: If you do not recognize the names of medical conditions or medicines referred to in this information, check with your doctor, nurse, or pharmacist. Definitions for selected medical terms may be found in the Glossary. Brand names for the generic drug names listed can be found in the Index. In addition, selected brand names commonly associated with the generic name have been included in the text to help you recognize medicine you may be taking. The fact that a brand name product is not mentioned does not mean the information does not apply. It is a good idea for you to learn both the generic and brand names of your medicines and to write them down for future use.

Indapamide (in-DAP-a-mide) belongs to the group of medicines known as diuretics. It is commonly used to treat high blood pressure.

High blood pressure adds to the workload of the heart and arteries. If it continues for a long time, the heart and arteries may not function properly. This can damage the blood vessels of the brain, heart, and kidneys resulting in a stroke, heart failure, or kidney failure. High blood pressure may also increase the risk of heart attacks. These problems may be less likely to occur if blood pressure is controlled.

Indapamide is also used to help reduce the amount of water in the body by increasing the flow of urine.

Indapamide is available only with your doctor's prescription.

Remember:

• **This medicine has been prescribed for your current medical problem only.** It must not be given to other people or used for other problems unless you are directed to do so by your doctor.

• **Keep all medicines out of the reach of children.**

• In order for this medicine to work, it must be used as directed.

• **It is very important that you read and understand the following information.** If any of the information causes you special concern, do not decide against using this medicine without first checking with your doctor.

• Before you begin using any new medicine (prescription or nonprescription) or if you develop any new medical problem while you are using this medicine, check with your doctor, nurse, or pharmacist.

• **If you have any questions** about the following information or if you want more information about this medicine or your medical problem, **ask your doctor, nurse, or pharmacist.**

Before Using This Medicine

In order to decide on the best treatment for your medical problem, your doctor should be told:

—if you have ever had any unusual or allergic reaction to indapamide, sulfonamides (sulfa drugs), or thiazide diuretics (other water pills).

—if you are on a low-salt, low-sugar, or any other special diet, or if you are allergic to any substance, such as foods, sulfites or other preservatives, or dyes. Most medicines contain more than their active ingredient. Your doctor, nurse, or pharmacist can help you avoid products that may cause a problem.

—if you are **pregnant** or if you may become pregnant. Studies have not been done in humans. However, indapamide has not been shown to cause birth defects or other problems in animal studies.

In general, diuretics are not useful for normal swelling of feet and hands that occurs during pregnancy. Diuretics should not be taken during pregnancy unless recommended by your doctor.

—if you are **breast-feeding**. It is not known whether indapamide passes into the breast milk. This medicine has not been shown to cause problems in nursing babies.

—if you have any of the following medical problems:
   Diabetes mellitus (sugar diabetes)
   Gout (history of)
   Kidney disease
   Liver disease

—if you are taking **any** other prescription or nonprescription (OTC) medicine, especially:
   Adrenocorticoids (cortisone-like medicine)
   Digitalis glycosides (heart medicine)
   Lithium (e.g., Lithane)

Proper Use of This Medicine

Indapamide may cause you to have an unusual feeling of tiredness when you begin to take it. You may also notice an increase in the amount of urine or in your frequency of urination. After taking the medicine for a while, these effects should lessen. In order to keep the increase in urine from affecting your nighttime sleep:

   —if you are to take a single dose a day, take it in the morning after breakfast.

   —if you are to take more than one dose a day, take the last dose no later than 6 p.m., unless otherwise directed by your doctor.

However, it is best to plan your dose or doses according to a schedule that will least affect your personal activities and sleep. Ask your doctor, nurse, or pharmacist to help you plan the best time to take this medicine.

In order to help remember to take indapamide, try to get into the habit of taking it at the same time each day.

For patients taking indapamide for high blood pressure:

• Importance of diet—When prescribing medicine for your condition your doctor may also prescribe a personal diet for you. Such a diet may be low in sodium (salt). Most people eat much more sodium than they need. Too much sodium in the diet may increase blood pressure. Some foods that contain large amounts of sodium are canned soup, pickles, ketchup, green and ripe olives, relish, frankfurters, soy sauce, and carbonated beverages. Your doctor may want you to limit the amounts of these and other high-sodium foods in your diet. High blood pressure medicine is usually more effective when such a diet is properly followed.

Also, it may be very important for you to go on a reducing diet. However, check with your doctor before changing your diet.

• Many patients who have high blood pressure will not notice any signs of the problem. In fact, many may feel normal. It is very important that you **take your medicine exactly as directed** and that you keep your appointments with your doctor even if you feel well.

• Remember that this medicine will not cure your high blood pressure but it does control it. Therefore, you must continue to take it as directed if you expect to lower your blood pressure and keep it down. **You may have to take high blood pressure medicine for the rest of your life.** If high blood pressure is not treated, it can cause serious problems such as heart failure, blood vessel disease, stroke, or kidney disease.

If you miss a dose of this medicine, take it as soon as possible. However, if it is almost time for your next dose, skip the missed dose and go back to your regular dosing schedule. Do not double doses.

How to store this medicine:

• **Keep out of the reach of children.**

• Store away from heat and direct light.

• Do not store in the bathroom, near the kitchen sink, or in other damp places. Heat or moisture may cause the medicine to break down.

• Do not keep outdated medicine or medicine no longer needed. Be sure that any discarded medicine is out of the reach of children.

Precautions While Using This Medicine

It is important that your doctor check your progress at regular visits to make sure that indapamide is working properly.

This medicine may cause a loss of potassium from your body:

• To help prevent this, your doctor may want you to:
  —eat or drink foods that have a high potassium content (for example, orange or other citrus fruit juices), or
  —take a potassium supplement, or
  —take another medication to help prevent the loss of the potassium in the first place.

• It is very important to follow these directions. Also, it is important not to change your diet on your own. This is more important if you are already on a special diet (as for diabetes), or if you are taking a potassium supplement or a medicine to reduce potassium loss. Extra potassium may not be necessary and, in some cases, too much potassium could be harmful.

Check with your doctor if you become sick and have severe or continuing vomiting or diarrhea. These problems may cause you to lose additional water and potassium.

For patients taking this medicine for high blood pressure:

• **Do not take other medicines unless they have been discussed with your doctor.** This especially includes over-the-counter (nonprescription) medicines for appetite control, asthma, colds, hay fever, or sinus problems, since they may tend to increase your blood pressure.

Side Effects of This Medicine

Along with its needed effects, a medicine may cause some unwanted effects. Although not all of these side effects may occur, if they do occur they may need medical attention.

Check with your doctor as soon as possible if any of the following side effects occur:
Signs of too much potassium loss
   Dryness of mouth
   Increased thirst
   Irregular heartbeat
   Mood or mental changes
   Muscle cramps or pain
   Nausea or vomiting
   Unusual tiredness or weakness
   Weak pulse
Rare
   Skin rash, itching, or hives

Other side effects may occur that usually do not require medical attention. These side effects may go away during treatment as your body adjusts to the medicine. However, check with your doctor if any of the following side effects continue or are bothersome:
Less common or rare
   Diarrhea
   Dizziness or lightheadedness, especially when getting up from a lying or sitting position
   Headache
   Loss of appetite
   Trouble in sleeping
   Upset stomach

For elderly patients: Dizziness or lightheadedness and signs of too much potassium loss are more likely to occur in the elderly, who are usually more sensitive to the effects of indapamide.

Other side effects not listed above may also occur in some patients. If you notice any other effects, check with your doctor.

December 1987

INDOMETHACIN
(Systemic—Anti-inflammatory)

Some commonly used brand names and other names are:

Apo-Indomethacin*	Indocin SR
Imbrilon*	Indolar SR*
Indocid*	Indo-Lemmon
Indocid R*	Indometacin
Indocid SR*	Novomethacin*
Indocin	Zendole

Generic name product may also be available in the U.S.

*Not available in the U.S.

To the Reader: If you do not recognize the names of medical conditions or medicines referred to in this information, check with your doctor, nurse, or pharmacist. Definitions for selected medical terms may be found in the Glossary. Brand names for the generic drug names listed can be found in the Index. In addition, selected brand names commonly associated with the generic name have been included in the text to help you recognize medicine you may be taking. The fact that a brand name product is not mentioned does not mean the information does not apply. It is a good idea for you to learn both the generic and brand names of your medicines and to write them down for future use.

Indomethacin (in-doe-METH-a-sin) is used to treat the symptoms of many painful conditions, including certain types of arthritis and gout. It may be taken by mouth or used rectally as a suppository to help relieve inflammation, swelling, stiffness, joint pain, and fever.

When used to treat arthritis, indomethacin only relieves the symptoms of the disease. It does not cure arthritis and will help you only as long as you continue to take it.

Indomethacin is also used by injection to treat patent ductus arteriosus (PDA) in premature babies. PDA is a condition that causes heart and breathing problems in some premature babies. Indomethacin helps to correct this condition. However, some premature babies with PDA may need heart surgery if indomethacin does not correct the condition completely or permanently. Because this use of indomethacin by injection is so different from the medicine's other uses, the information that follows applies only to the oral and rectal uses of indomethacin. If you have any questions about the use of indomethacin to treat PDA, check with your doctor, nurse, or pharmacist.

Indomethacin may also be used for other conditions as determined by your doctor.

This medicine is available only with your doctor's prescription.

Remember:
- **This medicine has been prescribed for your current medical problem only.** It must not be given to other people or used for other problems unless you are directed to do so by your doctor.
- **Keep all medicines out of the reach of children.**
- In order for this medicine to work, it must be used as directed.
- **It is very important that you read and understand the following information.** If any of the information causes you special concern, do not decide against using this medicine without first checking with your doctor.

- Before you begin using any new medicine (prescription or nonprescription) or if you develop any new medical problem while you are using this medicine, check with your doctor, nurse, or pharmacist.

- **If you have any questions** about the following information or if you want more information about this medicine or your medical problem, **ask your doctor, nurse, or pharmacist.**

Before Using This Medicine

In order to decide on the best treatment for your medical problem, your doctor should be told:

—if you have ever had any unusual or allergic reaction, especially asthma or wheezing, runny nose, or hives, to indomethacin or to any of the following medicines:

Aspirin or other salicylates
Diclofenac (e.g., Voltaren)
Diflunisal (e.g., Dolobid)
Fenoprofen (e.g., Nalfon)
Flurbiprofen, oral (e.g., Ansaid)
Ibuprofen (e.g., Motrin)
Ketoprofen (e.g., Orudis)
Meclofenamate (e.g., Meclomen)
Mefenamic acid (e.g., Ponstel)
Naproxen (e.g., Naprosyn)
Oxyphenbutazone (e.g., Tandearil)
Phenylbutazone (e.g., Butazolidin)
Piroxicam (e.g., Feldene)
Sulindac (e.g., Clinoril)
Suprofen (e.g., Suprol)
Tiaprofenic acid (e.g., Surgam)
Tolmetin (e.g., Tolectin)
Zomepirac (e.g., Zomax)

—if you are on a low-sugar or any other special diet, or if you are allergic to any substance, such as foods, sulfites or other preservatives, or dyes. Most medicines contain more than their active ingredient, and many liquid medicines contain alcohol. Your doctor, nurse, or pharmacist can help you avoid products that may cause a problem.

—if you are **pregnant** or if you may become pregnant. Studies on birth defects with indomethacin have not been done in humans. However, if indomethacin is used late in pregnancy, it may cause unwanted effects on the heart or blood flow in the fetus or in the newborn baby. Studies in animals have shown that indomethacin causes several unwanted effects such as a lowering of the newborn's weight, slower development of bones, and damage to nerves. Also, studies in animals have shown that indomethacin, if taken late in pregnancy, may increase the length of pregnancy and prolong labor.

—if you are **breast-feeding**. Indomethacin passes into the breast milk and has been reported to cause unwanted effects in a nursing baby. It may be necessary for you to take another medicine or to stop breast-feeding during treatment. Be sure you have discussed the risks and benefits of the medicine with your doctor.

—if you have any of the following medical problems:
Bleeding problems
Colitis, stomach ulcer, or other stomach problems
Epilepsy

Heart disease
High blood pressure
Infection
Kidney disease
Liver disease
Mental illness
Parkinson's disease
Rectal irritation or bleeding, recent (for the suppository only)
Systemic lupus erythematosus (SLE)

—if you regularly take acetaminophen or aspirin or other salicylates.

—if you are taking **any** other prescription or nonprescription (OTC) medicine, especially:

Anticoagulants (blood thinners)
Diflunisal (e.g., Dolobid)
Lithium (e.g., Lithane)
Methotrexate (e.g., Mexate)
Probenecid (e.g., Benemid)
Triamterene (e.g., Dyrenium)

Proper Use of This Medicine

For patients taking the capsule or liquid form of indomethacin:

• **Take indomethacin capsules or liquid immediately after meals or with food or antacids to lessen stomach upset.** However, do not mix the liquid form of indomethacin together with an antacid or with other liquids before taking it. To do so may cause the indomethacin to break down. If stomach upset (indigestion, heartburn, nausea, vomiting, stomach pain, or diarrhea) continues, check with your doctor.

• **Take indomethacin capsules with a full glass (8 ounces) of water.** Also, do not lie down for about 15 to 30 minutes after taking the medicine. This helps to prevent irritation that may lead to trouble in swallowing.

For patients using the rectal suppository form of indomethacin:

• If the suppository is too soft to insert because of storage in a warm place, chill the suppository in the refrigerator for 30 minutes or run cold water over it before removing the foil wrapper.

• How to insert the suppository: First, remove the foil wrapper and moisten the suppository with water. Lie down on your side and push the suppository well up into the rectum with the finger.

• Keep the suppository inside the rectum for at least one hour so that all of the medicine can be absorbed by your body. This helps the medicine work better.

Use this medicine only as directed by your doctor. Do not use more of it, do not use it more often, and do not use it for a longer period of time than your doctor ordered. To do so may increase the chance of serious side effects.

If you are using this medicine to relieve arthritis, you must use it regularly as ordered by your doctor. In some types of arthritis, up to 2 weeks may pass before you begin to feel better and up to 1 month may pass before you feel the full effects of this medicine.

If you miss a dose of this medicine and remember within an hour or so of the missed dose, take it right away. But if you do not remember until later, skip the missed dose and go back to your regular dosing schedule. Do not double doses.

How to store this medicine:

• **Keep out of the reach of children.**

• Store away from heat and direct light.

• Do not store capsule forms of this medicine in the bathroom, near the kitchen sink, or in other damp places. Heat or moisture may cause the medicine to break down.

• Keep the liquid and suppository forms of this medicine from freezing.

• Do not keep outdated medicine or medicine no longer needed. Be sure that any discarded medicine is out of the reach of children.

Precautions While Using This Medicine

If you will be using this medicine for a long period of time, your doctor should check your progress at regular visits.

Before having any kind of surgery (including dental surgery), tell the physician or dentist in charge that you are using indomethacin.

Stomach problems may be more likely to occur if you take aspirin or other salicylates, ibuprofen, or other anti-inflammatory analgesics (medicines used to relieve pain and/or inflammation) regularly (for example, every day) or drink alcoholic beverages while being treated with indomethacin. Therefore, **do not take aspirin, ibuprofen, or other anti-inflammatory analgesics regularly or drink alcoholic beverages while taking indomethacin,** unless otherwise directed by your doctor.

Too much use of acetaminophen together with indomethacin may increase the chance of kidney problems. Therefore, do not regularly take acetaminophen together with indomethacin, unless your doctor has directed you to do so.

This medicine may cause some people to become dizzy, lightheaded, drowsy, or less alert than they are normally. **Make sure you know how you react to this medicine before you drive, use machines, or do other jobs that require you to be alert.**

Check with your doctor immediately if chills, fever, muscle aches or pains, or other influenza-like symptoms occur shortly before, or together with, a skin rash. Very rarely, these effects may be the first signs of a serious reaction to this medicine.

Side Effects of This Medicine

Along with its needed effects, a medicine may cause some unwanted effects. Although not all of these side effects may occur, if they do occur they may need medical attention.

Check with your doctor immediately if any of the following side effects occur:

Rare

Convulsions (seizures)

Shortness of breath, troubled breathing, wheezing, or tightness in chest

Also, check with your doctor as soon as possible if any of the following side effects occur:

More common

Headache, especially in the morning

Less common

Bloody or black tarry stools

Confusion or forgetfulness

Mental depression or other mood or mental changes

Rectal irritation, pain, or bleeding, especially with the suppository

Ringing or buzzing in ears

Swelling of face, feet, or lower legs

Weight gain

Rare

Abdominal or stomach pain, cramping, or burning (severe)

Bleeding sores on lips

Bloody urine

Blurred vision, other vision problems, or eye pain (with prolonged use)

Chest pain

Decreased hearing, loss of hearing, or any other change in hearing

Diarrhea (severe and/or bloody)

Fainting

Fast, irregular, or pounding heartbeat

Hallucinations (seeing, hearing, or feeling things that are not there)

Increased blood pressure

Muscle weakness or uncontrollable muscle movements

Numbness, tingling, pain, or weakness in hands or feet

Redness, tenderness, itching, burning, or peeling of skin

Red, thickened, or scaly skin

Skin rash, hives, or itching

Sores, ulcers, or white spots in mouth (painful)

Sore throat, fever, and chills

Sudden decrease in amount of urine

Unexplained nosebleeds

Unexplained or unusual vaginal bleeding

Unusual bleeding or bruising

Unusual tiredness or weakness

Vomiting blood or material that looks like coffee grounds

Yellow eyes or skin

Other side effects may occur that usually do not require medical attention. These side effects may go away during treatment as your body adjusts to the medicine. However, check with your doctor if any of the following side effects continue or are bothersome:

More common

Abdominal or stomach pain (mild to moderate)

Dizziness or lightheadedness

Heartburn or indigestion

Nausea or vomiting

Less common

Constipation

Diarrhea

Drowsiness

General feeling of discomfort or illness

For elderly patients: Some of the above side effects, especially stomach problems or confusion, may be more likely to occur in elderly patients, who are usually more sensitive to the effects of indomethacin.

Other side effects not listed above may also occur in some patients. If you notice any other effects, check with your doctor.

_____

December 1987

_____

INSULIN (Systemic)

This information applies to the following medicines:

Insulin (IN-su-lin)
Insulin Human (HYOO-man)
Buffered Insulin Human
Isophane (EYE-so-fayn) Insulin
Isophane Insulin, Human
Isophane Insulin and Insulin
Isophane Insulin, Human and Insulin Human
Insulin Zinc
Insulin Zinc, Human
Extended Insulin Zinc
Prompt Insulin Zinc
Protamine (PRO-tah-meen) Zinc Insulin

Some commonly used brand names and other names are:	Generic names:
Regular Regular (Concentrated) Iletin II, U-500 Regular Iletin I Regular Iletin II Regular insulin Velosulin	Insulin
Humulin R Novolin R Velosulin Human	Insulin Human
Humulin BR	Buffered Insulin Human
Insulatard NPH NPH NPH Iletin I NPH Iletin II NPH insulin	Isophane Insulin
Humulin N Insulatard NPH Human Novolin N	Isophane Insulin, Human
Mixtard	Isophane Insulin and Insulin
Novolin 70/30	Isophane Insulin, Human and Insulin Human
Lente Lente Iletin I Lente Iletin II Lente insulin	Insulin Zinc
Humulin L Novolin L	Insulin Zinc, Human
Ultralente Ultralente Iletin I Ultralente insulin	Extended Insulin Zinc
Semilente Semilente Iletin I Semilente insulin	Prompt Insulin Zinc
Protamine Zinc & Iletin I Protamine Zinc & Iletin II PZI insulin	Protamine Zinc Insulin

To the Reader: If you do not recognize the names of medical conditions or medicines referred to in this information, check

with your doctor, nurse, or pharmacist. Definitions for selected medical terms may be found in the Glossary. Brand names for the generic drug names listed can be found in the Index. In addition, selected brand names commonly associated with the generic name have been included in the text to help you recognize medicine you may be taking. The fact that a brand name product is not mentioned does not mean the information does not apply. It is a good idea for you to learn both the generic and brand names of your medicines and to write them down for future use.

Insulin (IN-su-lin) belongs to the group of medicines called hormones. It is made naturally by the body to help produce energy from the carbohydrates and sugars in food.

If the body does not make enough insulin to meet its needs or does not properly use the insulin it makes, a condition known as diabetes mellitus (sugar diabetes) may develop. Proper diet and exercise may control this condition. However, if they do not, your doctor may prescribe insulin along with a special meal plan and exercise to help keep your health in balance.

Insulin is obtained from beef or pork, or from new processes resulting in products that are the same as human insulin. Insulin must be injected under the skin because when taken by mouth, it is destroyed by stomach acids.

A prescription is not necessary to purchase most insulin. However, your doctor must first determine your personal insulin needs and provide you with special instructions for control of your diabetic condition.

Remember:
• In order for this medicine to work, it must be used as directed.

• **It is very important that you read and understand the following information.** If any of the information causes you special concern, do not decide against using this medicine without first checking with your doctor.

• Before you begin using any new medicine (prescription or nonprescription) or if you develop any new medical problem while you are using this medicine, check with your doctor, nurse, or pharmacist.

• **If you have any questions** about the following information or if you want more information about this medicine or your medical problem, **ask your doctor, nurse, or pharmacist**.

Before Using This Medicine

Importance of diet—If you have insulin-dependent diabetes (IDDM, type I), your doctor will prescribe both insulin and a personal diabetic meal plan for you. If you have non–insulin-dependent diabetes (NIDDM, type II), your doctor will probably try to control your condition by changing your diet to promote weight loss before prescribing medicine for your diabetes. A diabetic meal plan is low in refined carbohydrates (foods, such as sugar and candy, used for quick energy). The daily number of calories in this meal plan should be adjusted to help you reach and maintain your ideal body weight. In addition, meals and snacks are arranged to meet the energy needs of your body at different times of the day. **It is very important that you carefully follow the meal plan that is prescribed for you.**

Many diabetic patients are able to control their condition by carefully following their doctor's orders for proper diet and exercise. **Medicine is prescribed only when additional help is needed.**

In order to decide on the best treatment for your medical problem, your doctor should be told:

—if you are allergic to beef or pork insulins.

—if you are pregnant.

—if you have any of the following medical problems:

Infection
Kidney disease
Liver disease
Thyroid disease

—if you are taking **any** other prescription or nonprescription (OTC) medicine, especially:

Adrenocorticoids (cortisone-like medicine)
Antidiabetic agents, oral (diabetes medicine you take by mouth)
Beta-blockers (acebutolol, atenolol, labetalol, metoprolol, nadolol, oxprenolol, pindolol, propranolol, sotalol, timolol)

Proper Use of This Medicine

Make sure you have the correct type and strength of insulin as ordered for you by your doctor. You may find that keeping an insulin label with you is helpful when buying insulin supplies. The strength (concentration) of insulin is measured by Units and is sometimes expressed in terms such as U-100 insulin instead of insulin 100 Units.

Insulin doses are measured and given with specially marked insulin syringes. For patients using only 50 units or less of U-100 insulin per dose, a special low-dose syringe is available to make dose measurement easier and more accurate. The syringes are marked with a scale in Units that match the Unit strength of insulin being used. For example, a U-100 syringe is used to give U-100 insulin.

A prescription from your doctor may be required to purchase insulin syringes in some states.

How to draw insulin into the syringe:

• First wash your hands.

• Be sure insulin is completely mixed. However, do not shake the insulin bottle hard before using. Frothing or bubbles can cause an incorrect dose. Mix contents well by rolling the bottle slowly between the palms of the hands or by gently tipping the bottle over a few times.

Do not use if contents look lumpy or grainy or stick to the bottle. Do not use regular insulin if it becomes discolored or cloudy. Use regular insulin only when it is clear and colorless.

• Remove the colored protective cap on the bottle. Do *not* remove the rubber stopper.

• Wipe the top of the bottle with an alcohol swab.

• Draw air into the syringe by pulling back on the plunger. The amount of air should be equal to your insulin dose.

• Remove the needle cover. Put the needle through rubber top of bottle.

• Push plunger in all the way.

• Turn bottle with syringe upside down in one hand. Be sure tip of needle is in insulin. With other hand, draw plunger back slowly to draw the correct dose of insulin into the syringe.

• Check for air bubbles. To remove air bubbles, push insulin slowly back into bottle and measure again your correct dose.

• Double check your dose. Remove needle from the bottle. Cover needle carefully with needle cover or lay syringe down so the needle does not touch anything.

For patients mixing more than one type of insulin in the same syringe:

• Your doctor may want you to mix two types of insulin in the same syringe to match your needs more closely with one injection.

• When mixing regular insulin with another type of insulin, always draw the regular insulin (the clear one) into the syringe first. When mixing other insulins, it does not matter which type is drawn into the syringe first. However, once you have established an order of mixing, always mix them in that same order.

• Some mixtures of insulins have to be injected immediately after they are mixed. Other mixtures may be stable (that is, the two kinds of insulin will not interact chemically) for a longer period of time. If you have any questions about the stability of the mixture you are using, check with your doctor or pharmacist.

• If your mixture of insulins is stable and mixed for you ahead of time, gently turn the filled syringe back-and-forth to remix the insulins before you inject them. Do not shake the syringe hard.

How to inject the insulin:

• Clean the skin where the injection is to be made (on thighs, upper arms, buttocks, or abdomen) with an alcohol swab and let the area dry.

• Pinch up a large area of skin and hold it firmly. With the other hand hold the syringe like a pencil. Push the needle straight into the pinched-up skin. Be sure the needle is in all the way.

• To inject the insulin, push the plunger all the way down, using less than 5 seconds to inject the dose.

• Hold an alcohol swab near the needle and pull the needle straight out of the skin. Press the swab against the injection site for several seconds. Do not rub.

In addition, each package of insulin contains a patient instruction sheet. Read this sheet carefully for information concerning your syringe and needle and steps to follow when injecting a dose of insulin.

For patients using disposable syringes:

• Disposable insulin syringes and needles are presterilized and designed to be used one time only and then discarded. If you have any questions about the use of disposable syringes, check with your doctor, nurse, or pharmacist.

For patients using a glass syringe and metal needle:

• A glass insulin syringe with a metal needle may be used repeatedly if it is sterilized each time. The patient instruction sheet included in each insulin package will explain how to sterilize the syringe and needle. For more information or for explanation of instructions you do not understand, ask your doctor, nurse, or pharmacist.

For patients using an insulin-infusion pump:

• Regular insulin is the only insulin product that should be used with insulin infusion pumps.

• Do not use the insulin injection if it looks lumpy, cloudy, unusually thick, or even slightly discolored, or if it contains crystals. Use the insulin only if it is clear and colorless.

• Do not mix the buffered regular insulin injection with any other insulin. If you do, crystals may form that will block the pump catheter. Also, the activity of the insulin may change.

• It is important to follow the pump manufacturer's directions on how to load the syringe and/or pump reservoir. You will receive too much or too little insulin if loading is not done correctly. This may lead to serious problems of high or low blood sugar.

• Check the infusion tubing and infusion-site dressing often for improper insulin infusion, as your physician or nurse recommends.

It is very important to use insulin only as directed. Do not change the strength, brand, or type of insulin unless told to do so by your doctor.

Storage and expiration date:

• When buying insulin, always check the package expiration date to make sure the insulin will be used before it expires. This expiration date applies only when the insulin has been stored under refrigeration.

• Do not use insulin after the expiration date stated on the label even if the bottle has never been opened. Check with your pharmacist about the possibility of exchanging an outdated bottle not yet opened.

• Insulin should be refrigerated until it is to be used. It should never be frozen. Remove the insulin from the refrigerator and allow it to reach room temperature before injection. Insulin you are now using regularly may be kept at room temperature if it will be used up within a month. Insulin that has been opened and stored at room temperature and has not been used for a month or more should be discarded. Insulin that is used only occasionally should be kept refrigerated.

• Do not expose insulin to extremely hot temperatures or sunlight. Do not leave insulin in the hot summer sun or in a hot, closed automobile. Extreme heat will cause insulin to spoil more quickly.

Precautions While Using This Medicine

It is very important that your doctor check your progress at regular visits, especially during the first few weeks of insulin treatment.

It is very important to follow carefully any instructions from your doctor about:

• Alcohol. Drinking alcohol may cause severe hypoglycemia (low blood sugar). Discuss the use of alcoholic beverages with your doctor.

• Tobacco. If you have been smoking for a long time and suddenly stop, your dosage of insulin may need to be reduced. If you decide to quit smoking, first check with your doctor.

• Diabetic meal plan. The success of your treatment depends on your closely following the diet your doctor or dietitian prescribed for you.

• Exercise. Your doctor will tell you what kind of exercise to do, the best time of day to do it, and how much you should do daily.

• Foot care. Special care of your feet will help to prevent possible future trouble.

• Urine tests. These tests are used to guide you in the control of your condition and must be done properly. Two urine tests for sugar are widely used: the tablet urine test and the paper-strip urine test. Your doctor may also instruct you to test your urine for acetone.

• Blood tests. Many patients have learned to measure their own blood sugar levels and make changes in their insulin dosage as needed. If you are taking blood tests, follow directions carefully.

• Injection sites. Careful selection and rotation of the injection sites on your body, following your doctor's recommendations, may prevent skin problems and difficulties in injecting. The insulin may also be absorbed better.

Do not take other medicines unless they have been discussed with your doctor. This especially includes over-the-counter (nonprescription) medicines such as aspirin, and those for appetite control, asthma, colds, cough, hay fever, or sinus.

In case of emergency:

- A medical I.D. bracelet or chain should be worn at all times. In addition, you should carry a diabetic identification card.

- Keep handy an extra supply of insulin and a syringe with needles.

- Keep handy a glucagon kit if your doctor has prescribed one for you, with syringe and needle, and know how it is used; also, members of your household should know how it is used and when to use it. Check the date on the glucagon bottle often to make sure you will not mix it after that date.

- Make sure a source of sugar such as orange juice, non-diet soft drinks, honey, table sugar, corn syrup, sugar cubes, sugar tablets, or some candy is always available to correct an insulin reaction (hypoglycemia).

- Have on hand several phone numbers that you can call for help, such as those of your doctor, the emergency room, your pharmacy, friends, and neighbors.

Check with your doctor immediately if these symptoms of low blood sugar (hypoglycemia or insulin reaction) appear:

Anxious feeling
Chills
Cold sweats
Confusion
Cool pale skin
Difficulty in concentration
Drowsiness
Excessive hunger
Headache
Nausea
Nervousness
Rapid pulse
Shakiness
Unusual tiredness or weakness
Vision changes

These symptoms of hypoglycemia (low blood sugar) may develop suddenly and may result from:

—using too much insulin.

—delaying or missing a scheduled snack or meal.

—sickness (especially with vomiting or diarrhea).

—exercising more than usual just before a meal.

—drinking alcohol

—taking certain medicines

Eating some form of sugar when symptoms of hypoglycemia first appear will usually prevent them from getting worse. Good sources of sugar include orange juice, corn syrup, honey, sugar cubes or table sugar (dissolved in water), and sugar tablets. Also, you should eat some crackers or half a sandwich or drink a glass of milk if you will not be having a snack or a meal for an hour or more.

If you become sick, especially with nausea, vomiting, diarrhea, or fever, you still need insulin. Call your doctor for instructions. Continue taking your insulin and try to stay on your regular diet. However, if you have trouble eating solid food, drink fruit juices, soft drinks, or clear soups, or eat small amounts of bland foods. Test your glucose level regularly and check your urine for acetone. If acetone is present, call your doctor at once. If you have severe or prolonged vomiting, check with your doctor. Even if you control the symptoms of low blood sugar and have no continuing problems, you should let your doctor know how you are feeling. In addition, before you become sick, check with your doctor for instructions regarding days when you are ill.

Check with your doctor right away if the symptoms of high blood sugar (hyperglycemia) occur. These symptoms appear more slowly than those of hypoglycemia, and usually include:

Dry mouth
Drowsiness
Flushed, dry skin
Fruit-like breath odor
Increased urination
Loss of appetite
Stomach ache, nausea, or vomiting
Tiredness
Troubled breathing (rapid and deep)
Unusual thirst
Weight loss (rapid)

These symptoms may occur if you do not take enough insulin, if you skip a dose, if you overeat or do not follow a proper diet, or if you have a fever or infection.

Symptoms of both low blood sugar and high blood sugar must be corrected before they progress to more serious conditions. In either situation, you should check with your doctor immediately.

When traveling:

- Carry a recent prescription from your doctor for your diabetes medicine and also for the correct syringe and needles, since some state and city laws and regulations may require a prescription for syringes and needles.

- Do not change your diet or medicine schedule. Before you leave, discuss your trip with your doctor.

- Consider the use of disposable syringes, since they are presterilized.

- Carry your diabetic supplies on your person or in a purse or briefcase to reduce the possibility of loss.

- Remember time zone changes and changes in meal times. Such changes may affect your diabetic schedule unless you allow for them.

- In hot climates, consider the use of an insulated container to help maintain the temperature of your insulin. These containers can be obtained at most pharmacies.

• In foreign countries, it is advisable to carry enough diabetic supplies to last until you return home, although most countries have some form of insulin available. Carry a letter from your doctor stating that you are diabetic, the type of insulin that you are taking, and that you need to carry syringes and needles. This will help to avoid customs problems. It may also help you to get new insulin supplies, if needed.

• When carrying a large quantity of diabetic supplies, divide the supplies equally throughout your pieces of luggage or have a companion carry some for you. This will reduce the amount of loss if any of your luggage is lost or delayed.

December 1987

INTERFERONS (Systemic)

This information applies to the following medicines:
Interferon Alfa-2a, Recombinant
Interferon Alfa-2b, Recombinant

Some commonly used brand names are:	Generic names:
Roferon-A	Interferon Alfa-2a, Recombinant
Intron A	Interferon Alfa-2b, Recombinant

To the Reader: If you do not recognize the names of medical conditions or medicines referred to in this information, check with your doctor, nurse, or pharmacist. Definitions for selected medical terms may be found in the Glossary. Brand names for the generic drug names listed can be found in the Index. In addition, selected brand names commonly associated with the generic name have been included in the text to help you recognize medicine you may be taking. The fact that a brand name product is not mentioned does not mean the information does not apply. It is a good idea for you to learn both the generic and brand names of your medicines and to write them down for future use.

Interferons (in-ter-FEER-ons) are synthetic (man-made) versions of substances naturally produced by cells in the body to help fight infections and tumors. They are given by injection to treat hairy cell leukemia.

Interferons may also be used for other conditions as determined by your doctor.

Interferons are available only with your doctor's prescription.

Remember:

• **This medicine has been prescribed for your current medical problem only.** It must not be given to other people or used for other problems unless you are directed to do so by your doctor.

• **Keep all medicines out of the reach of children.**

• In order for this medicine to work, it must be used as directed.

• **It is very important that you read and understand the following information.** If any of the information causes you special concern, do not decide against using this medicine without first checking with your doctor.

• Before you begin using any new medicine (prescription or nonprescription) or if you develop any new medical problem while you are using this medicine, check with your doctor, nurse, or pharmacist.

• **If you have any questions** about the following information or if you want more information about this medicine or your medical problem, **ask your doctor, nurse, or pharmacist.**

Before Using This Medicine

In order to decide on the best treatment for your medical problem, your doctor should be told:

—if you have ever had any unusual or allergic reaction to interferon.

—if you are **pregnant** or if you may become pregnant. Interferons have not been shown to cause birth defects or other problems in humans. However, in monkeys given 20 to 500 times the human dose of interferon alfa-2a, recombinant, there was an increase in deaths of the fetus.

—if you are **breast-feeding**. It is not known whether interferons pass into the breast milk and they have not been shown to cause problems in nursing babies. However, because this medicine may cause serious side effects, breast-feeding is generally not recommended while you are receiving it.

—if you have any of the following medical problems:
  Bleeding problems
  Convulsions (seizures)
  Diabetes mellitus (sugar diabetes)
  Heart disease
  Kidney disease
  Liver disease
  Lung disease

—if you have recently had a heart attack.

—if you are taking **any** other prescription or nonprescription (OTC) medicine.

Proper Use of This Medicine

If you are injecting this medicine yourself, **use it exactly as directed by your doctor.** Do not use more or less of it, and do not use it more often than your doctor ordered. The exact amount of medicine you need has been carefully worked out. Using too much will increase the risk of side effects, while using too little may not improve your condition.

Each package of interferon contains a patient instruction sheet. Read this sheet carefully and make sure you understand:

—How to prepare the injection.

—Proper use of disposable syringes.

—How to give the injection.

—How long the injection is stable.

If you have any questions about any of this, check with your doctor, nurse, or pharmacist.

While you are using interferon, your doctor may want you to drink extra fluids. This will help prevent low blood pressure due to loss of too much water.

Interferons often cause unusual tiredness, which can be severe. This effect is less likely to cause problems if you inject your interferon at bedtime.

If you miss a dose of this medicine, do not give the missed dose at all and do not double the next one. Check with your doctor for further instructions.

How to store this medicine:

• **Keep out of the reach of children.**

• Store in the refrigerator.

- Keep the medicine from freezing.
- Do not keep outdated medicine or medicine no longer needed. Ask your doctor or pharmacist how you should dispose of any medicine you do not use. Be sure that any discarded medicine is out of the reach of children.

Precautions While Using This Medicine

It is very important that your doctor check your progress at regular visits to make sure that this medicine is working properly and to check for unwanted effects.

Do not change to another brand of interferon without checking with your physician. Different kinds of interferon have different doses. If you refill your medicine and it looks different, check with your pharmacist.

Interferon may cause some people to become unusually tired or dizzy, or less alert than they are normally. **Make sure you know how you react to this medicine before you drive, use machines, or do other jobs that require you to be alert.**

This medicine will add to the effects of alcohol and other CNS depressants (medicines that slow down the nervous system, possibly causing drowsiness). Some examples of CNS depressants are antihistamines or medicine for hay fever, other allergies, or colds; sedatives, tranquilizers, or sleeping medicine; prescription pain medicine or narcotics; barbiturates; medicine for convulsions (seizures); muscle relaxants; or anesthetics, including some dental anesthetics. **Check with your doctor before taking any of the above while you are using this medicine.**

This medicine commonly causes a flu-like reaction, with aching muscles, fever and chills, and headache. To prevent problems from your temperature going too high, your doctor may ask you to take acetaminophen before each dose of interferon. You may also need to take it after a dose to bring your temperature down. **Follow your doctor's instructions carefully about taking your temperature, and how much and when to take the acetaminophen.**

While you are being treated with interferon, and after you stop treatment with it, **do not have any immunizations without your doctor's approval.** Interferon lowers your body's resistance and there is a chance you might get the infection the immunization is meant to prevent. In addition, other persons living in your house should not take oral polio vaccine since they could pass the polio virus on to you. Also, you should avoid close contact with other persons (for example, at school or work) who have taken oral polio vaccine.

Side Effects of This Medicine

Along with its needed effects, a medicine may cause some unwanted effects. Although not all of these side effects may occur, if they do occur they may need medical attention.

Check with your doctor as soon as possible if any of the following side effects occur:

Less common

Chest pain
Confusion
Difficulty in thinking or concentrating
Irregular heartbeat
Mental depression
Nervousness
Numbness or tingling of fingers, toes, and face
Trouble in sleeping

Rare

Fever, chills, or sore throat (beginning after 3 weeks of treatment)
Unusual bleeding or bruising

Other side effects may occur that usually do not require medical attention. These side effects may go away during treatment as your body adjusts to the medicine. However, check with your doctor if any of the following side effects continue or are bothersome:

More common

Aching muscles
Change in taste
Diarrhea
Fever and chills (should lessen after the first 1 or 2 weeks of treatment)
Headache
Loss of appetite
Nausea and vomiting
Unusual tiredness
Weight loss

Less common

Dizziness
Dry mouth
Dry skin or itching
Inability to have or keep an erection
Joint pain
Skin rash
Sores in the mouth and on the lips

Interferons may cause a temporary loss of some hair. After treatment has ended, normal hair growth should return.

For elderly patients: Some side effects of interferons (chest pain, irregular heartbeat, unusual tiredness, confusion, mental depression, difficulty in thinking or concentrating) may be more likely to occur in the elderly, who are usually more sensitive to the effects of interferons.

Other side effects not listed above may also occur in some patients. If you notice any other effects, check with your doctor.

December 1987

INULIN (Systemic)

To the Reader: If you do not recognize the names of medical conditions or medicines referred to in this information, check with your doctor, nurse, or pharmacist. Definitions for selected medical terms may be found in the Glossary. Brand names for the generic drug names listed can be found in the Index. In addition, selected brand names commonly associated with the generic name have been included in the text to help you recognize medicine you may be taking. The fact that a brand name product is not mentioned does not mean the information does not apply. It is a good idea for you to learn both the generic and brand names of your medicines and to write them down for future use.

Inulin (IN-yoo-lin) is used as a test to help diagnose problems or disease of the kidneys. This test determines how well your kidneys are working.

Inulin passes out of the body entirely in the urine. Measuring the amount of inulin in the blood after it has been given can help the doctor determine if the kidneys are working properly.

How test is done: Inulin is given through an intravenous infusion (run into a vein). Several times during the test, blood and sometimes urine samples are taken. A tube called a catheter may be placed in your bladder to help take the urine samples. The amount of inulin in your blood or urine is measured. Then the results of the test are studied.

Inulin is to be used only under the supervision of a doctor.

Remember:

• **It is very important that you read and understand the following information.** If any of the information causes you special concern, check with your doctor or pharmacist.

• Before you begin using any new medicine (prescription or nonprescription) or if you develop any new medical problem while you are using this medicine, check with your doctor, nurse, or pharmacist.

• **If you have any questions** about the following information or if you want more information about this test or your medical problem, **ask your doctor, nurse, or pharmacist**.

Before Having This Test

Before this test is given, your doctor should be told:

—if you have ever had any unusual or allergic reaction to inulin.

—if you are **pregnant** or if you suspect that you may be pregnant. Inulin has not been shown to cause birth defects or other problems in humans.

—if you are **breast-feeding**. Inulin has not been shown to cause problems in nursing babies.

—if you have any of the following medical problems:
Heart disease
Liver disease
Underactive adrenal gland
Underactive thyroid

Side Effects of This Medicine

Along with its needed effects, a medicine may cause some unwanted effects. Although inulin does not usually cause any side effects, check with your doctor if you notice any unusual effects.

December 1987

IODINATED GLYCEROL (Systemic)

A commonly used brand name is Organidin.

To the Reader: If you do not recognize the names of medical conditions or medicines referred to in this information, check with your doctor, nurse, or pharmacist. Definitions for selected medical terms may be found in the Glossary. Brand names for the generic drug names listed can be found in the Index. In addition, selected brand names commonly associated with the generic name have been included in the text to help you recognize medicine you may be taking. The fact that a brand name product is not mentioned does not mean the information does not apply. It is a good idea for you to learn both the generic and brand names of your medicines and to write them down for future use.

Iodinated glycerol (EYE-oh-di-nay-ted GLI-ser-ole) is taken by mouth to thin and loosen mucus secretions. It is used in the treatment of respiratory tract conditions such as asthma, bronchitis, emphysema, sinusitis, and cystic fibrosis.

Iodinated glycerol is available only with your doctor's prescription.

Remember:

• **This medicine has been prescribed for your current medical problem only.** It must not be given to other people or used for other problems unless you are directed to do so by your doctor.

• **Keep all medicines out of the reach of children.**

• In order for this medicine to work, it must be used as directed.

• **It is very important that you read and understand the following information.** If any of the information causes you special concern, do not decide against using this medicine without first checking with your doctor.

• Before you begin using any new medicine (prescription or nonprescription) or if you develop any new medical problem while you are using this medicine, check with your doctor, nurse, or pharmacist.

• **If you have any questions** about the following information or if you want more information about this medicine or your medical problem, **ask your doctor, nurse, or pharmacist.**

Before Using This Medicine

In order to decide on the best treatment for your medical problem, your doctor should be told:

—if you have ever had any unusual or allergic reaction to iodinated glycerol, iodine, or iodine-containing preparations or foods.

—if you are on a low-salt, low-sugar, or any other special diet, or if you are allergic to any substance, such as foods, sulfites or other preservatives, or dyes. Most medicines contain more than their active ingredient, and many liquid medicines contain alcohol. Your doctor, nurse, or pharmacist can help you avoid products that may cause a problem.

—if you are **pregnant** or if you may become pregnant. Iodinated glycerol is not recommended during pregnancy because it may cause enlargement of the thyroid gland in the fetus and result in breathing problems.

—if you are **breast-feeding**. Iodinated glycerol is not recommended in nursing mothers because it may cause skin rash and thyroid problems in the baby.

—if you have any of the following medical problems:
   Acne (teenage)
   Cystic fibrosis (in children)
   Thyroid disease (or history of)

—if you are taking **any** other prescription or nonprescription (OTC) medicine, especially:
   Antithyroid agents (medicine for overactive thyroid)
   Lithium (e.g., Lithane)

Proper Use of This Medicine

For patients taking the oral solution form of iodinated glycerol:

• This medicine is to be taken by mouth even though it may come in a dropper bottle.

• Take this medicine mixed in water or other liquid. Be sure to drink all of the liquid in order to get the full dose of medicine.

To help thin and loosen mucus in the lungs, **drink a glass of water after each dose of this medicine** unless otherwise directed by your doctor.

Take iodinated glycerol only as directed. Do not take more of it, do not take it more often, and do not take it for a longer period of time than your doctor ordered. To do so may increase the chance of side effects.

If you miss a dose of this medicine, take it as soon as possible. However, if it is almost time for your next dose, skip the missed dose and go back to your regular dosing schedule. Do not double doses.

How to store this medicine:

• **Keep out of the reach of children.**

• Store away from heat and direct light.

• Do not store the tablet form of this medicine in the bathroom, near the kitchen sink, or in other damp places. Heat or moisture may cause the medicine to break down.

• Keep the liquid form of this medicine from freezing.

• Do not keep outdated medicine or medicine no longer needed. Be sure that any discarded medicine is out of the reach of children.

Precautions While Using This Medicine

Your doctor should check your progress at regular visits to make sure this medicine is working properly and does not cause unwanted effects.

Side Effects of This Medicine

Along with its needed effects, a medicine may cause some unwanted effects. Although not all of these side effects may occur, if they do occur they may need medical attention.

Check with your doctor as soon as possible if any of the following side effects occur:

Rare

Chills or fever
Headache (continuing)
Joint pain
Loss of appetite
Pain on chewing or swallowing
Skin rash, hives, or redness
Sore throat
Swelling of face, lips, or eyelids
Tenderness or swelling below or in front of ear

With long-term use

Burning of mouth and throat
Dry skin
Headache (severe)
Increase in salivation
Irritation of eyes or swelling of eyelids
Metallic taste
Runny nose, sneezing, and other symptoms of head cold
Soreness of teeth and gums
Swelling around the eyes
Swelling of neck

Unusual sensitivity to cold
Unusual tiredness or weakness
Unusual weight gain

Other side effects may occur that usually do not require medical attention. These side effects may go away during treatment as your body adjusts to the medicine. However, check with your doctor if any of the following side effects continue or are bothersome:

More common

Diarrhea
Nausea or vomiting
Stomach pain

For children: Swelling of the neck (goiter or enlarged thyroid gland) is more likely to occur in children with cystic fibrosis. These patients are usually more sensitive to this effect of iodinated glycerol.

For elderly patients: Many medicines have not been tested in older people. Therefore, it is not known whether the medicine acts the same way it does in younger adults. Check with your doctor or pharmacist if you notice any unusual effects while taking this medicine or if you think it is not working as it should.

Other side effects not listed above may also occur in some patients. If you notice any other effects, check with your doctor.

December 1987

IODIPAMIDE (Systemic)
A commonly used brand name is Cholografin.

To the Reader: If you do not recognize the names of medical conditions or medicines referred to in this information, check with your doctor, nurse, or pharmacist. Definitions for selected medical terms may be found in the Glossary. Brand names for the generic drug names listed can be found in the Index. In addition, selected brand names commonly associated with the generic name have been included in the text to help you recognize medicine you may be taking. The fact that a brand name product is not mentioned does not mean the information does not apply. It is a good idea for you to learn both the generic and brand names of your medicines and to write them down for future use.

Iodipamide (eye-oh-DI-pa-mide) is a radiopaque agent. This agent contains iodine, which absorbs x-rays. Depending on how the radiopaque agent is given, it builds up in certain areas of the body. The resulting high level of iodine allows the x-rays to make a "picture" of the area.

Iodipamide is given by injection before x-ray tests to help check for problems with the gallbladder and biliary tract.

Iodipamide is to be used only by or under the supervision of a doctor.

Remember:
- **It is very important that you read and understand the following information.** If any of the information causes you special concern, do not decide against receiving this radiopaque agent without first checking with your doctor.

- **If you have any questions** about the following information or if you want more information about this radiopaque agent or your medical problem, **ask your doctor, nurse, or pharmacist.**

Before Having This Test
Before this test is given, your doctor should be told:

—if you have ever had any unusual or allergic reaction to iodine, to products containing iodine (for example, iodine-containing foods, such as seafood, cabbage, kale, rape, turnips, or iodized salt), or to other radiopaque agents.

—if you are allergic to any substance, such as sulfites or other preservatives. Most medicines contain more than their active ingredient. Your doctor can help you avoid products that may cause a problem.

—if you are **pregnant** or if you suspect that you may be pregnant while using this radiopaque agent. Studies have not been done in either humans or animals. However, other radiopaque agents containing iodine have, on rare occasions, caused hypothyroidism (underactive thyroid) in the infant. Also, x-rays of the abdomen during pregnancy may cause harmful effects in the fetus.

—if you are **breast-feeding**. Although iodipamide has not been shown to cause problems in nursing babies, the chance always exists since it passes into the breast milk.

—if you have any of the following medical problems:
   Asthma, hay fever, or other allergies (history of)
   Diabetes mellitus (sugar diabetes)
   Heart or blood vessel disease
   High blood pressure (severe)
   Kidney disease (severe)
   Liver disease (severe)
   Overactive thyroid
   Pheochromocytoma (PCC)
   Sickle cell disease

—if you are taking **any** other prescription or nonprescription (OTC) medicine.

—if you have been given or will be receiving radiopaque agents for other tests.

Preparation for This Test
Your doctor may order a special diet and/or use of a laxative or enema in preparation for your test, depending on the type of test. If you have not received such instructions or if you do not understand them, check with your doctor in advance.

Precautions After Having This Test
Make sure your doctor knows if you are planning to have any future thyroid tests. Even after several weeks or months the results of the thyroid test may be affected by the iodine in this agent.

Side Effects of This Medicine
Along with its needed effects, radiopaque agents like iodipamide can sometimes cause serious effects such as severe allergic reactions or heart problems. These effects may occur almost immediately or a few minutes after the radiopaque agent is given. Although these serious side effects appear only rarely, your doctor or nurse will be prepared to give you immediate medical attention if needed. If you have any questions about this, check with your doctor.

Other side effects may occur that usually do not require medical attention. These side effects should go away as the effects of the radiopaque agent wear off. However, check with your doctor if any of the following side effects continue or are bothersome:
More common
   Unusual warmth and flushing of skin
Less common
   Chills
   Dizziness or lightheadedness
   Headache
   Nausea or vomiting
   Unusual sweating
   Unusual watering of mouth

For children and elderly patients: The above side effects are more likely to occur in children and elderly patients, who are usually more sensitive to the effects of iodipamide.

Other side effects not listed above may also occur in some patients. If you notice any other effects, check with your doctor.

December 1987

IODOQUINOL (Oral)

Some commonly used brand names or other names are:

Diiodohydroxyquin	Diquinol
Diodoquin*	Yodoxin

Generic name product may also be available in the U.S.

*Not available in the U.S.

To the Reader: If you do not recognize the names of medical conditions or medicines referred to in this information, check with your doctor, nurse, or pharmacist. Definitions for selected medical terms may be found in the Glossary. Brand names for the generic drug names listed can be found in the Index. In addition, selected brand names commonly associated with the generic name have been included in the text to help you recognize medicine you may be taking. The fact that a brand name product is not mentioned does not mean the information does not apply. It is a good idea for you to learn both the generic and brand names of your medicines and to write them down for future use.

Iodoquinol (eye-oh-doe-KWIN-ole) belongs to the group of medicines called antiprotozoals. Although sometimes used to treat other types of infection, it is taken by mouth most often in the treatment of intestinal infections.

Iodoquinol is available only with your doctor's prescription.

Remember:

• **This medicine has been prescribed for your present infection only.** Another infection later on may require a different medicine. Also, even though other people may have the same symptoms as you, they may have a different kind of infection. Your medicine may not work for them and may even cause them harm. Therefore, **your medicine must not be given to other people or used for other infections** unless you are otherwise directed by your doctor.

• **Keep all medicines out of the reach of children.**

• In order for this medicine to work, it must be used as directed.

• **It is also very important that you read and understand the following information.** If any of the information causes you special concern, do not decide against using this medicine without first checking with your doctor.

• Before you begin using any new medicine (prescription or nonprescription) or if you develop any new medical problem while you are using this medicine, check with your doctor, nurse, or pharmacist.

• **If you have any questions** about the following information or if you want more information about this medicine or your medical problem, **ask your doctor, nurse, or pharmacist.**

Before Using This Medicine

In order to decide on the best treatment for your medical problem, your doctor should be told:

—if you have ever had any unusual or allergic reaction to chloroxine, clioquinol (iodochlorhydroxyquin), iodine, pamaquine, pentaquine, primaquine, seafood, or shellfish.

—if you are on a low-salt, low-sugar, or any other special diet, or if you are allergic to any substance, such as foods, sulfites or other preservatives, or dyes. Most medicines contain more than their active ingredient. Your doctor, nurse, or pharmacist can help you avoid products that may cause a problem.

—if you are **pregnant** or if you may become pregnant. However, iodoquinol has not been shown to cause birth defects or other problems in humans.

—if you are **breast-feeding**. However, iodoquinol has not been shown to cause problems in nursing babies.

—if you have any of the following medical problems:
Eye disease
Kidney disease
Liver disease
Thyroid disease

Proper Use of This Medicine

Take this medicine after meals to lessen possible stomach upset, unless otherwise directed by your doctor.

If these tablets are too large to swallow whole, they may be crushed and mixed with a small amount of applesauce or chocolate syrup.

To help clear up your infection completely, **keep taking this medicine for the full time of treatment** even if you begin to feel better after a few days; **do not miss any doses.**

If you do miss a dose of this medicine, take it as soon as possible. However, if it is almost time for your next dose, skip the missed dose and go back to your regular dosing schedule. Do not double doses.

How to store this medicine:

• **Keep out of the reach of children.**

• Store away from heat and direct light.

• Do not store in the bathroom, near the kitchen sink, or in other damp places. Heat or moisture may cause the medicine to break down.

• Do not keep outdated medicine or medicine no longer needed. Be sure that any discarded medicine is out of the reach of children.

Precautions While Using This Medicine

This medicine may cause blurred vision or loss of vision, or it may cause some people to become dizzy or lightheaded. **Make sure you know how you react to this medicine before you drive, use machines, or do other jobs that require you to be alert or to see clearly.** If these reactions are especially bothersome, check with your doctor.

If you must have thyroid function tests, make sure the doctor knows that you are taking this medicine or have taken it within the past 6 months.

Side Effects of This Medicine

Along with its needed effects, a medicine may cause some unwanted effects. Although not all of these side effects may occur, if they do occur they may need medical attention.

Check with your doctor immediately if any of the following side effects occur:

Less common

   Fever or chills
   Skin rash, hives, or itching
   Swelling of neck

With long-term use of high doses

   Blurred vision or any change in vision (especially in children)
   Clumsiness or unsteadiness
   Decreased vision or eye pain (especially in children)
   Increased weakness
   Muscle pain
   Numbness, tingling, pain, or weakness in hands or feet (especially in children)

Other side effects may occur that usually do not require medical attention. These side effects may go away during treatment as your body adjusts to the medicine.

However, check with your doctor if any of the following side effects continue or are bothersome:

More common

   Diarrhea
   Nausea or vomiting
   Stomach pain

Less common

   Dizziness or lightheadedness
   Headache
   Itching of the rectal area

Blurred vision or any change in vision; decreased vision; eye pain; or numbness, tingling, pain, or weakness in hands or feet may be more likely to occur in children, especially with long-term use of high doses.

For elderly patients: Many medicines have not been tested in older people. Therefore, it is not known whether the medicine acts the same way it does in younger adults. Check with your doctor or pharmacist if you notice any unusual effects while taking this medicine or if you think it is not working as it should.

Other side effects not listed above may also occur in some patients. If you notice any other effects, check with your doctor.

December 1987

IOHEXOL (Systemic)

A commonly used brand name is Omnipaque.

To the Reader: If you do not recognize the names of medical conditions or medicines referred to in this information, check with your doctor, nurse, or pharmacist. Definitions for selected medical terms may be found in the Glossary. Brand names for the generic drug names listed can be found in the Index. In addition, selected brand names commonly associated with the generic name have been included in the text to help you recognize medicine you may be taking. The fact that a brand name product is not mentioned does not mean the information does not apply. It is a good idea for you to learn both the generic and brand names of your medicines and to write them down for future use.

Iohexol (eye-oh-HEX-ole) is a radiopaque agent. This agent contains iodine, which absorbs x-rays. Depending on how the radiopaque agent is given, it builds up in certain areas of the body. The resulting high level of iodine allows the x-rays to make a "picture" of the area.

Iohexol is given by injection into the spinal canal before x-ray tests to help diagnose problems or diseases in different areas of the head, spinal canal, and nervous system. It may be injected into a specific vein or artery to help check for problems with the heart, blood vessels, and kidneys.

Iohexol is to be used only by or under the supervision of a doctor.

Remember:

• **It is very important that you read and understand the following information.** If any of the information causes you special concern, do not decide against receiving this radiopaque agent without first checking with your doctor.

• **If you have any questions** about the following information or if you want more information about this radiopaque agent or your medical problem, **ask your doctor, nurse, or pharmacist.**

Before Having This Test

Before this test is given, your doctor should be told:

—if you have ever had any unusual or allergic reaction to iodine, to products containing iodine (for example, iodine-containing foods such as seafood, cabbage, kale, rape, turnips, or iodized salt), or to other radiopaque agents.

—if you are allergic to any substance, such as sulfites or other preservatives. Most medicines contain more than their active ingredient. Your doctor can help you avoid products that may cause a problem.

—if you are **pregnant** or if you suspect that you may be pregnant while receiving this radiopaque agent. Studies have not been done in humans; however, iohexol has not been shown to cause birth defects or other problems in animal studies when given in doses many times the usual human dose. Other radiopaque

agents containing iodine have caused, on rare occasions, hypothyroidism (underactive thyroid) in the infant. Also, x-rays of the abdomen are usually not recommended during pregnancy. This is to avoid exposing the fetus to radiation. Be sure you have discussed this with your doctor.

—if you are **breast-feeding**. Although it is not known how much iohexol passes into the breast milk, it may be necessary for you to stop breast-feeding after receiving it. Be sure you have discussed this with your doctor.

—if you have or have had **any** other medical problems, especially:
  Alcoholism (chronic)
  Asthma, hay fever, or other allergies (history of)
  Diabetes mellitus (sugar diabetes)
  Epilepsy (history of)
  Heart or blood vessel disease
  High blood pressure (severe)
  Infection
  Kidney disease (severe)
  Liver disease
  Multiple myeloma (bone disease)
  Multiple sclerosis
  Overactive thyroid
  Pheochromocytoma
  Sickle cell disease

—if you are taking **any** of the following medicines or types of medicine:
  Amantadine
  Aminoglycosides by injection (amikacin, gentamicin, kanamycin, neomycin, netilmicin, streptomycin, tobramycin)
  Amphetamines
  Amphotericin B by injection
  Appetite suppressants (diet pills), except fenfluramine
  Caffeine
  Capreomycin
  Captopril
  Carmustine
  Chlophedianol
  Cisplatin
  Cyclosporine
  Gold salts
  Lithium
  Medicine for asthma or other breathing problems
  Medicine for hay fever or other allergies (including nose drops or sprays)
  Medicine for inflammation or pain (aspirin or other salicylates, diclofenac, diflunisal, fenoprofen, ibuprofen, indomethacin, ketoprofen, meclofenamate, mefenamic acid, naproxen, phenylbutazone, piroxicam, sulindac, suprofen, tolmetin)
  Methicillin
  Methotrexate
  Methylphenidate
  Metoprolol
  Nafcillin
  Oxacillin
  Oxprenolol
  Pemoline
  Penicillamine
  Penicillin G
  Phenothiazines (acetophenazine, chlorpromazine, fluphenazine, mesoridazine, perphenazine, prochlorperazine, promazine, promethazine, thioridazine, trifluoperazine, triflupromazine, trimeprazine)

Pindolol
Plicamycin
Propranolol
Rifampin
Streptozocin
Sulfonamides (sulfa medicine)
Tetracyclines, except doxycycline and minocycline
Tricyclic antidepressants (amitriptyline, amoxapine, clomipramine, desipramine, doxepin, imipramine, nortriptyline, protriptyline, trimipramine)
Vancomycin by injection

—if you regularly take large amounts of combination pain medicine containing acetaminophen and aspirin or other salicylates.

—if you are now taking or have taken within the past 2 weeks monoamine oxidase (MAO) inhibitors such as:

Furazolidone
Isocarboxazid
Pargyline
Phenelzine
Procarbazine
Tranylcypromine

Preparation for This Test

Your doctor may have special instructions for you in preparation for your test. If you have not received such instructions or if you do not understand them, check with your doctor in advance.

For patients having this radiopaque agent injected into the spinal canal, unless otherwise directed by your doctor:

• You may eat and drink your usual diet up to 2 hours before the test, and you may drink clear liquids up to the time of the test.

Precautions After Having This Test

Make sure your doctor knows if you are planning to have any future thyroid tests. Even after several weeks the results of the thyroid test may be affected by the iodine in this agent.

For patients having this radiopaque agent injected into the spinal canal, unless otherwise directed by your doctor or radiologist:

• Remain still during and for several hours after the test.

• Keep head high as instructed during and after test.

Side Effects of This Medicine

Along with its needed effects, radiopaque agents like iohexol can sometimes cause serious effects such as severe allergic reactions or heart problems. These effects may occur almost immediately or a few minutes after the radiopaque agent is given. Although these serious side effects appear only rarely, your doctor or nurse will be prepared to give you immediate medical attention if needed. If you have any questions about this, check with your doctor.

Other side effects may occur that usually do not require medical attention. These side effects should go away as the effects of the radiopaque agent wear off. However, check with your doctor if any of the following side effects continue or are bothersome:

With injection into the spinal canal, a vein, or an artery
More common
Headache (mild to moderate)
Nausea and vomiting
Less common or rare
Unusual feeling of warmth
With injection into the spinal canal
More common
Backache
Dizziness
Stiffness of neck
Less common or rare
Difficult urination
Drowsiness
Headache (severe)
Increased sensitivity of eyes to light
Loss of appetite
Ringing or buzzing sound in ears
Unusual sweating
Unusual tiredness or weakness
With injection into a vein or an artery
Less common or rare
Blurred vision or other changes in vision
Drowsiness or lightheadedness
Metallic taste
Pain or burning at injection site

For elderly patients: The above side effects are more likely to occur in the elderly, who are usually more sensitive to the effects of iohexol.

Other side effects not listed above may also occur in some patients. If you notice any other effects, check with your doctor.

December 1987

IOPAMIDOL (Systemic)

Some commonly used brand names are Isovue and Isovue-M.

Read the bold information first. Then go back and read the rest. If you do not recognize the names of medical conditions or medicines included in this information, check with your doctor, nurse, or pharmacist. Brand names for the generic drug names listed can also be found in the index. It is a good idea for you to learn both the generic and brand names of your medicines and to write them down for future use.

Iopamidol (eye-oh-PA-mi-dole) is a radiopaque agent. This agent contains iodine, which absorbs x-rays. Depending on how the radiopaque agent is given, it builds up in certain areas of the body. The resulting high level of iodine allows the x-rays to make a "picture" of the area.

Iopamidol is given by injection into the spinal canal before x-ray tests to help diagnose problems or diseases in different areas of the head, spinal canal, and nervous system. It may be injected into a specific vein or artery to help check for problems with the heart and blood vessels, brain, or other organs.

Iopamidol is to be used only by or under the supervision of a doctor.

Remember:

• **It is very important that you read and understand the following information.** If any of the information causes you special concern, do not decide against receiving this radiopaque agent without first checking with your doctor.

• **If you have any questions** about the following information or if you want more information about this radiopaque agent or your medical problem, **ask your doctor, nurse, or pharmacist.**

Before Having This Test

Before this test is given, your doctor should be told:

—if you have ever had any unusual or allergic reaction to iodine, to products containing iodine (for example, iodine-containing foods such as seafoods, cabbage, kale, rape, turnips, or iodized salt), or to other radiopaque agents.

—if you are allergic to any substance, such as sulfites or other preservatives. Most medicines contain more than their active ingredient. Your doctor can help you avoid products that may cause a problem.

—if you are pregnant or if you suspect that you may be pregnant while receiving this radiopaque agent. Studies have not been done in humans; however, iopamidol has not been shown to cause birth defects or other problems in animal studies. Other radiopaque agents containing iodine have caused, on rare occasions, hypothyroidism (underactive thyroid) in the baby. Also, x-rays of the abdomen are usually not recommended during pregnancy. This is to avoid exposing the fetus to radiation. Be sure you have discussed this with your doctor.

—if you are breast-feeding. Although it is not known whether iopamidol passes into the breast milk, the chance always exists.

—if you have any of the following medical problems:

Alcoholism (chronic)
Asthma, hay fever, or other allergies (history of)
Epilepsy (history of)
Heart or blood vessel disease
High blood pressure (severe)
Kidney disease (severe)
Liver disease
Multiple myeloma (bone cancer)
Multiple sclerosis
Overactive thyroid
Pheochromocytoma (PCC)
Sickle cell disease

—if you now have or have had any other medical problems or diseases.

—if you are taking any of the following medicines or types of medicines:

Amantadine
Amphetamines
Appetite suppressants (diet pills), except fenfluramine
Caffeine
Chlophedianol
Medicine for asthma or other breathing problems
Medicine for hay fever or other allergies (including nose drops or sprays)
Methylphenidate
Metoprolol
Oxprenolol
Pemoline
Phenothiazines (acetophenazine, chlorpromazine, fluphenazine, mesoridazine, perphenazine, prochlorperazine, promazine, promethazine, thioridazine, trifluoperazine, triflupromazine, trimeprazine)
Pindolol
Propranolol
Tricyclic antidepressants (amitriptyline, amoxapine, clomipramine, desipramine, doxepin, imipramine, nortriptyline, protriptyline, trimipramine)

—if you are now taking or have taken within the past 2 weeks monoamine oxidase (MAO) inhibitors such as:

Furazolidone
Isocarboxazid
Pargyline
Phenelzine
Procarbazine
Tranylcypromine

Preparation for This Test

Your doctor may have special instructions for you in preparation for your test. If you have not received such instructions or if you do not understand them, check with your doctor in advance.

For patients having this radiopaque agent injected into the spinal canal, unless otherwise directed by your doctor:

• You may eat and drink your usual diet up to 2 hours before the test, and you may drink clear liquids up to the time of the test.

Precautions After Having This Test

Make sure your doctor knows if you are planning to have any future thyroid tests. Even after several weeks, the results of the thyroid test may be affected by the iodine in this agent.

For patients having this radiopaque agent injected into the spinal canal, unless otherwise directed by your doctor or radiologist:

• Remain still during and for several hours after the test.

• Keep head high as instructed during and after the test.

Side Effects of This Medicine

Along with their needed effects, radiopaque agents like iopamidol can sometimes cause serious effects such as severe allergic reactions or heart problems. These effects may occur almost immediately or a few minutes after the radiopaque agent is given. Although these serious side effects appear only rarely, your doctor or nurse will be prepared to give you immediate medical attention if needed. If you have any questions about this, check with your doctor.

Other side effects may occur which usually do not require medical attention. These side effects should go away as the effects of the radiopaque agent wear off. However, check with your doctor if any of the following side effects continue or are bothersome:

With injection into the spinal canal, a vein, or an artery
More common
  Headache (mild to moderate)
  Nausea and vomiting

With injection into the spinal canal
More common
  Backache
  Dizziness
  Stiffness of neck
Less common or rare
  Difficult urination
  Drowsiness
  Headache (severe)
  Increased sensitivity of eyes to light
  Loss of appetite
  Ringing or buzzing in ears
  Unusual sweating
  Unusual tiredness or weakness

With injection into a vein or an artery
More common
  Hot flashes or sudden feeling of warmth
  Pain or burning sensation at injection site
Less common or rare
  Blurred vision or other changes in vision
  Lightheadedness
  Unusual taste

The above side effects are more likely to occur in the elderly, who are usually more sensitive to the effects of iopamidol.

Other side effects not listed above may also occur in some patients. If you notice any other effects, check with your doctor.

_____

December 1987

IOPHENDYLATE (Systemic)

A commonly used brand name is Pantopaque.

To the Reader: If you do not recognize the names of medical conditions or medicines referred to in this information, check with your doctor, nurse, or pharmacist. Definitions for selected medical terms may be found in the Glossary. Brand names for the generic drug names listed can be found in the Index. In addition, selected brand names commonly associated with the generic name have been included in the text to help you recognize medicine you may be taking. The fact that a brand name product is not mentioned does not mean the information does not apply. It is a good idea for you to learn both the generic and brand names of your medicines and to write them down for future use.

Iophendylate (eye-oh-FEN-di-late) is a radiopaque agent. This agent contains iodine, which absorbs x-rays. Depending on how the radiopaque agent is given, it builds up in certain areas of the body. The resulting high level of iodine allows the x-rays to make a "picture" of the area.

Iophendylate is given by injection into the spinal canal. X-rays are then used to help diagnose problems or diseases in the head, spinal canal, and nervous system. After the test is completed, iophendylate is removed with a special needle and syringe, to help lessen the chance of side effects.

Iophendylate is to be used only by or under the supervision of a doctor.

Remember:
• **It is very important that you read and understand the following information.** If any of the information causes you special concern, do not decide against taking or receiving this radiopaque agent without first checking with your doctor.

• **If you have any questions** about the following information or if you want more information about this radiopaque agent or your medical problem, **ask your doctor, nurse, or pharmacist.**

Before Having This Test

Before this test is given, your doctor should be told:

—if you have ever had any unusual or allergic reaction to iodine, to products containing iodine (for example iodine-containing foods, such as seafoods, cabbage, kale, rape, turnips, or iodized salt), or to other radiopaque agents.

—if you are allergic to any substance, such as sulfites or other preservatives. Most medicines contain more than their active ingredient. Your doctor can help you avoid products that may cause a problem.

—if you are **pregnant** or if you suspect that you may be pregnant while receiving this radiopaque agent. Studies have not been done in either humans or animals with iophendylate. However, x-rays of the abdomen are usually not recommended during pregnancy. This is to avoid exposing the fetus to radiation. Be sure you have discussed this with your doctor.

—if you are **breast-feeding**. Although it is not known whether iophendylate passes into breast milk, it has not been shown to cause problems in nursing babies.

—if you have any of the following medical problems:
Asthma, hay fever, or other allergies (history of)
Multiple sclerosis (MS)

Preparation for This Test

Your doctor may have special instructions for you in preparation for your test. If you have not received such instructions or if you do not understand them, check with your doctor in advance.

You may eat and drink your usual diet up to 4 to 6 hours before the test, unless otherwise directed by your doctor.

Precautions After Having This Test

Make sure your doctor knows if you are planning to have any future thyroid tests. The results of the thyroid test may be affected by the iodine in this agent.

It is important to remain still during and for 6 to 24 hours after the test. Follow your doctor's instructions.

Side Effects of This Medicine

Along with its needed effects, a medicine may cause some unwanted effects. Although not all of these side effects may occur, if they do occur they may need medical attention.

Check with your doctor as soon as possible if any of the following side effects occur:
Rare
Nausea and/or vomiting (severe)
Paralysis of one side of body or of arm(s) or leg(s)
Skin rash or hives
Stuffy nose
Swelling of face or skin
Wheezing, tightness in chest, or troubled breathing

Other side effects may occur that usually do not require medical attention. These side effects should go away as the effects of the radiopaque agent wear off. However, check with your doctor if any of the following side effects continue or are bothersome:
More common
Backache
Fever
Headache
Stiffness of neck
Less common or rare
Blurred or double vision or other changes in vision
Chest pain
Decrease in amount of urine
Dizziness
Unusual tiredness or weakness

Other side effects not listed above may also occur in some patients. If you notice any other effects, check with your doctor.

December 1987

IOTHALAMATE (Mucosal)

A commonly used brand name is Cysto-Conray.

To the Reader: If you do not recognize the names of medical conditions or medicines referred to in this information, check with your doctor, nurse, or pharmacist. Definitions for selected medical terms may be found in the Glossary. Brand names for the generic drug names listed can be found in the Index. In addition, selected brand names commonly associated with the generic name have been included in the text to help you recognize medicine you may be taking. The fact that a brand name product is not mentioned does not mean the information does not apply. It is a good idea for you to learn both the generic and brand names of your medicines and to write them down for future use.

Iothalamate (eye-oh-thal-A-mate) is a radiopaque agent. This agent contains iodine, which absorbs x-rays. Depending on how the radiopaque agent is given, it builds up in certain areas of the body. The resulting high level of iodine allows the x-rays to make a "picture" of the area.

The solution of iothalamate is instilled into the bladder or ureters to help diagnose problems or diseases of the kidneys or other areas of the urinary tract. After the test is done, the solution is expelled by urinating.

Iothalamate is to be used only by or under the supervision of a doctor.

Remember:

• **It is very important that you read and understand the following information.** If any of the information causes you special concern, do not decide against receiving this radiopaque agent without first checking with your doctor.

• **If you have any questions** about the following information or if you want more information about this radiopaque agent or your medical problem, **ask your doctor, nurse, or pharmacist.**

Before Having This Test

Before this test is given, your doctor should be told:

—if you have ever had any unusual or allergic reaction to iodine, to products containing iodine (for example, iodine-containing foods, such as seafoods, cabbage, kale, rape, turnips, or iodized salt), or to other radiopaque agents.

—if you are allergic to any substance, such as sulfites or other preservatives. Most medicines contain more than their active ingredient. Your doctor can help you avoid products that may cause a problem.

—if you are **pregnant** or if you suspect that you may be pregnant when you are to receive this radiopaque agent. Studies have not been done in humans; however, iothalamate has not been shown to cause birth defects or other problems in animal studies. Other radiopaque agents containing iodine have caused, on rare occasions, hypothyroidism (underactive thyroid) in the baby. Also, x-rays of the abdomen are usually not recommended during pregnancy. This is to avoid exposing the fetus to radiation. Be sure you have discussed this with your doctor.

—if you are **breast-feeding**. Although iothalamate passes into the breast milk, it has not been shown to cause problems in nursing babies.

—if you have any of the following medical problems:

Asthma, hay fever, or other allergies
Enlarged prostate
Kidney disease
Urinary tract infection

Preparation for This Test

Your doctor may have special instructions for you in preparation for your test. He or she may order a special diet and/or use of a laxative in preparation for your test depending on the type of test. If you have not received such instructions or if you do not understand them, check with your doctor in advance.

Side Effects of This Medicine

Along with its needed effects, a medicine may cause some unwanted effects. Although iothalamate does not usually cause any side effects when used for instillation into the bladder or ureters, side effects have occurred when iothalamate was not given properly.

December 1987

IOTHALAMATE (Systemic)

Some commonly used brand names are:

Angio-Conray	Conray-400
Conray	Vascoray

To the Reader: If you do not recognize the names of medical conditions or medicines referred to in this information, check with your doctor, nurse, or pharmacist. Definitions for selected medical terms may be found in the Glossary. Brand names for the generic drug names listed can be found in the Index. In addition, selected brand names commonly associated with the generic name have been included in the text to help you recognize medicine you may be taking. The fact that a brand name product is not mentioned does not mean the information does not apply. It is a good idea for you to learn both the generic and brand names of your medicines and to write them down for future use.

Iothalamate (eye-oh-thal-A-mate) is a radiopaque agent. This agent contains iodine, which absorbs x-rays. Depending on how the radiopaque agent is given, it builds up in certain areas of the body. The resulting high level of iodine allows the x-rays to make a "picture" of the area.

Iothalamate is given by injection before x-ray tests to help diagnose problems or diseases of the heart and blood vessels, gallbladder and biliary tract, pancreas, kidneys, or other parts of the body.

Iothalamate is to be used only by or under the supervision of a doctor.

Remember:

• **It is very important that you read and understand the following information.** If any of the information causes you special concern, do not decide against receiving this radiopaque agent without first checking with your doctor.

• **If you have any questions** about the following information or if you want more information about this radiopaque agent or your medical problem, **ask your doctor, nurse, or pharmacist.**

Before Having This Test

Before this test is given, your doctor should be told:

—if you have ever had any unusual or allergic reaction to iodine, to products containing iodine (for example, iodine-containing foods, such as seafood, cabbage, kale, rape, turnips, or iodized salt), or to other radiopaque agents.

—if you are allergic to any substance, such as sulfites or other preservatives. Most medicines contain more than their active ingredient. Your doctor can help you avoid products that may cause a problem.

—if you are **pregnant** or if you suspect that you may be pregnant. Studies have not been done in humans. However, iothalamate has not been shown to cause birth defects or other problems in animal studies. Other radiopaque agents containing iodine have caused, on rare occasions, hypothyroidism (underactive thyroid)

in the baby. Also, x-rays of the abdomen are usually not recommended during pregnancy. This is to avoid exposing the fetus to radiation. Be sure you have discussed this with your doctor.

—if you are **breast-feeding.** Although iothalamate passes into the breast milk, it has not been shown to cause problems in nursing babies.

—if you now have or have had **any** medical problems, especially:

> Asthma, hay fever, or other allergies (history of)
> Bleeding problems
> Diabetes mellitus (sugar diabetes)
> Heart or blood vessel disease
> Kidney disease
> Liver disease (severe)
> Multiple myeloma (bone cancer)
> Overactive thyroid
> Pheochromocytoma (PCC)
> Sickle cell disease

—if you are now taking any of the following medicines or types of medicine:

> Aminoglycosides by injection (amikacin, gentamicin, kanamycin, neomycin, netilmicin, streptomycin, tobramycin)
> Amphotericin B by injection
> Capreomycin
> Captopril
> Carmustine
> Cisplatin
> Cyclosporine
> Gold salts
> Lithium
> Medicine for inflammation or pain (aspirin or other salicylates, diclofenac, diflunisal, fenoprofen, ibuprofen, indomethacin, ketoprofen, meclofenamate, mefenamic acid, naproxen, phenylbutazone, piroxicam, sulindac, suprofen, tolmetin)
> Methicillin
> Methotrexate
> Nafcillin
> Oxacillin
> Penicillamine
> Penicillin G
> Plicamycin
> Rifampin
> Streptozocin
> Sulfonamides (sulfa medicine)
> Tetracyclines, except doxycycline and minocycline
> Vancomycin by injection

—if you regularly take large amounts of combination pain medicine containing acetaminophen and aspirin or other salicylates.

Preparation for This Test

Your doctor may order a special diet and/or use of a laxative for you in preparation for your test, depending on the type of test. If you have not received such instructions or if you do not understand them, check with your doctor in advance.

Do not have any food for several hours before having the test, unless otherwise directed by your doctor. This is to prevent any food from coming back up and entering your lungs during the test. You may be allowed to drink clear liquids; however, check first with your doctor.

Precautions After Having This Test

Make sure your doctor knows if you are planning to have any future thyroid tests. Even after several weeks, the results of the thyroid test may be affected by the iodine in this agent.

Side Effects of This Medicine

Along with their needed effects, radiopaque agents like iothalamate can sometimes cause serious side effects such as severe allergic reactions or heart problems. These effects may occur almost immediately or a few minutes after the radiopaque agent is given. Although these serious side effects appear only rarely, your doctor or nurse will be prepared to give you immediate medical attention if needed. If you have any questions about this, check with your doctor.

Other side effects may occur that usually do not require medical attention. These side effects should go away as the effects of the radiopaque agent wear off. However, check with your doctor if any of the following side effects continue or are bothersome:

More common
Unusual warmth and flushing of skin

Less common
Changes in vision
Chills
Confusion
Dizziness or lightheadedness
Headache
Nausea or vomiting
Numbness, tingling, pain, or weakness in hands or feet
Unusual sweating
Unusual tiredness or weakness
Unusual watering of the mouth

For children and elderly patients: The above side effects are more likely to occur in children and the elderly, who are usually more sensitive to the effects of iothalamate.

Other side effects not listed above may also occur in some patients. If you notice any other effects, check with your doctor.

December 1987

IOXAGLATE (Systemic)

A commonly used brand name is Hexabrix.

To the Reader: If you do not recognize the names of medical conditions or medicines referred to in this information, check with your doctor, nurse, or pharmacist. Definitions for selected medical terms may be found in the Glossary. Brand names for the generic drug names listed can be found in the Index. In addition, selected brand names commonly associated with the generic name have been included in the text to help you recognize medicine you may be taking. The fact that a brand name product is not mentioned does not mean the information does not apply. It is a good idea for you to learn both the generic and brand names of your medicines and to write them down for future use.

Ioxaglate (eye-OX-a-glate) is a radiopaque agent. This agent contains iodine, which absorbs x-rays. Depending on how the radiopaque agent is given, it builds up in certain areas of the body. The resulting high level of iodine allows the x-rays to make a "picture" of the area.

Ioxaglate is given by injection before x-rays to help diagnose problems or diseases of the heart and blood vessels, kidneys, or other parts of the body.

Ioxaglate is to be used only by or under the supervision of a doctor.

Remember:

• **It is very important that you read and understand the following information.** If any of the information causes you special concern, do not decide against receiving this radiopaque agent without first discussing this with your doctor.

• **If you have any questions** about the following information or if you want more information about this radiopaque agent or your medical problem, **ask your doctor, nurse, or pharmacist.**

Before Having This Test

Before this test is given, your doctor should be told:

—if you have ever had any unusual or allergic reaction to iodine, to other products containing iodine (for example iodine-containing foods, such as seafoods, cabbage, kale, rape, turnips, or iodized salt), or to other radiopaque agents.

—if you are allergic to any substance, such as sulfites or other preservatives. Most medicines contain more than their active ingredient. Your doctor can help you avoid products that may cause a problem.

—if you are **pregnant** or if you suspect that you may be pregnant when you are to receive ioxaglate. Studies have not been done in humans. However, ioxaglate has not been shown to cause birth defects or other problems in animal studies. Other radiopaque agents containing iodine have caused, on rare occasions, hypothyroidism (underactive thyroid) in the baby. Also, x-rays of the abdomen are usually not recommended during pregnancy. This is to avoid exposing the fetus to radiation. Be sure you have discussed this with your doctor.

—if you are **breast-feeding**. Ioxaglate passes into the breast milk. If you must receive ioxaglate, it may be necessary for you to stop breast-feeding for 24 hours after receiving it. Be sure you have discussed this with your doctor.

—if you have or have had **any** medical problems, especially:

　　Asthma, hay fever, or other allergies (history of)
　　Bleeding problems
　　Diabetes mellitus (sugar diabetes)
　　Heart or blood vessel disease
　　High blood pressure (severe)
　　Kidney disease
　　Liver disease (severe)
　　Migraine
　　Multiple myeloma (bone cancer)
　　Overactive thyroid
　　Pheochromocytoma (PCC)
　　Sickle cell disease

—if you are taking **any** other prescription or nonprescription (OTC) medicine.

Preparation for This Test

Your doctor may have special instructions for you in preparation for your test, depending on the type of test. If you have not received such instructions or if you do not understand them, check with your doctor in advance.

Do not eat any food for several hours before having the test, unless otherwise directed by your doctor. This is to prevent any food from coming back up and entering your lungs during the test. You may be allowed to drink clear liquids; however, check first with your doctor.

Precautions After Having This Test

Make sure your doctor knows if you are planning to have any future thyroid tests. Even after several weeks, the results of the thyroid test may be affected by the iodine in this agent.

Side Effects of This Medicine

Along with their needed effects, radiopaque agents like ioxaglate can sometimes cause serious effects such as severe allergic reactions or heart problems. These effects may occur almost immediately or a few minutes after the radiopaque agent is given. Although these serious side effects appear only rarely, your doctor or nurse will be prepared to give you immediate medical attention if needed. If you have any questions about this, ask your doctor.

Other side effects may occur which usually do not require medical attention. These side effects should go away as the effects of the radiopaque agent wear off. However, check with your doctor if any of the following side effects continue or are bothersome:

More common

　　Nausea or vomiting
　　Unusual warmth and flushing of skin

Less common or rare
    Changes in vision
    Chills
    Dizziness or lightheadedness
    Headache
    Numbness, tingling, pain, or weakness in hands or feet
    Trembling
    Unusual sweating
    Unusual tiredness or weakness

Other side effects not listed above may also occur in some patients. If you notice any other effects, check with your doctor.

_____

December 1987

IPECAC (Oral)

To the Reader: If you do not recognize the names of medical conditions or medicines referred to in this information, check with your doctor, nurse, or pharmacist. Definitions for selected medical terms may be found in the Glossary. Brand names for the generic drug names listed can be found in the Index. In addition, selected brand names commonly associated with the generic name have been included in the text to help you recognize medicine you may be taking. The fact that a brand name product is not mentioned does not mean the information does not apply. It is a good idea for you to learn both the generic and brand names of your medicines and to write them down for future use.

Ipecac (IP-e-kak) is used in the emergency treatment of certain kinds of poisoning. Only the syrup form of ipecac should be used. It is taken by mouth to cause vomiting of the poison.

A bottle of ipecac labeled as being Ipecac Fluidextract or Ipecac Tincture should not be used. These dosage forms are too strong and may cause serious side effects or death. Only ipecac syrup contains the proper strength of ipecac for treating poisonings.

Ordinarily, this medicine should not be used if strychnine, corrosives such as alkalies (lye) and strong acids, or petroleum distillates such as kerosene, gasoline, coal oil, fuel oil, paint thinner, or cleaning fluid have been swallowed, since it may cause seizures, additional injury to the throat, or pneumonia.

Ipecac should not be used to cause vomiting as a means of losing weight. If used regularly for this purpose, serious heart problems or even death may occur.

This medicine in amounts of more than 1 ounce is available only with your doctor's prescription. It is available in 1-ounce bottles without a prescription. However, before using ipecac syrup, call your doctor, a poison control center, or an emergency room for advice.

Remember:

• **Keep all medicines out of the reach of children.**

• In order for this medicine to work, it must be used as directed. **If you are using this medicine without a prescription, it is very important to follow the directions on the label.**

• **If you have any questions** about the following information or if you want more information about this medicine or your medical problem, **ask your doctor, nurse, or pharmacist.**

Before Using This Medicine

Before using this medicine to cause vomiting in poisoning, call your doctor, a poison control center, or an emergency room for advice. It is a good idea to have these telephone numbers readily available. Be sure to tell them:

—if you are **pregnant**. Studies with ipecac have not been done in either humans or animals.

—if you have heart disease. There is an increased risk of heart problems such as unusually fast heartbeat if the ipecac is not vomited.

Proper Use of This Medicine

It is very important that you take this medicine only as directed. Do not take more of it and do not take it more often than recommended on the label, unless otherwise directed. When too much ipecac is used, it can cause damage to the heart and other muscles, and may even cause death.

Do not give this medicine to unconscious or very drowsy persons, since the vomited material may enter the lungs and cause pneumonia.

To help this medicine cause vomiting of the poison, adults should drink 1 full glass (8 ounces) of water and children should drink ½ to 1 full glass (4 to 8 ounces) of water immediately after taking this medicine. Water may be given first in the case of a small or scared child.

Do not take this medicine with milk, milk products, or with carbonated beverages. Milk or milk products may prevent this medicine from working properly, and carbonated beverages may cause swelling of the stomach.

If vomiting does not occur within 20 minutes after you have taken the first dose of this medicine, take a second dose. If vomiting does not occur after you have taken the second dose, you must immediately see your doctor or go to an emergency room.

If you have been told to take both this medicine and activated charcoal to treat the poisoning, **do not take the activated charcoal until after you have taken this medicine to cause vomiting and the vomiting has stopped. This is usually about 30 minutes.** Taking the activated charcoal before or with this medicine may prevent this medicine from causing vomiting of the poison.

How to store this medicine:

• **Keep out of the reach of children** since overdose is very dangerous in children.

• Store away from heat and direct light.

• Keep the syrup from freezing.

• Do not keep outdated medicine or medicine no longer needed. Be sure that any discarded medicine is out of the reach of children.

• Do not keep a bottle of ipecac that has been opened. Ipecac may evaporate over a period of time. It is best to replace it with a new one.

Side Effects of This Medicine

Along with its needed effects, a medicine may cause some unwanted effects. Although side effects usually do not occur with recommended doses of ipecac, if they do occur they may need medical attention.

Check with your doctor as soon as possible if any of the following side effects occur:

Signs of overdose (may also occur if ipecac is taken regularly)

　　Diarrhea
　　Nausea or vomiting (continuing more than 30 minutes)
　　Stomach cramps or pain
　　Troubled breathing

Unusual tiredness or weakness
Unusually fast or irregular heartbeat
Weakness, aching, and stiffness of muscles, especially those of the neck, arms, and legs

Other side effects not listed above may also occur in some patients. If you notice any other effects, check with your doctor.

December 1987

IPRATROPIUM (Inhalation)

A commonly used brand name is Atrovent.

To the Reader: If you do not recognize the names of medical conditions or medicines referred to in this information, check with your doctor, nurse, or pharmacist. Definitions for selected medical terms may be found in the Glossary. Brand names for the generic drug names listed can be found in the Index. In addition, selected brand names commonly associated with the generic name have been included in the text to help you recognize medicine you may be taking. The fact that a brand name product is not mentioned does not mean the information does not apply. It is a good idea for you to learn both the generic and brand names of your medicines and to write them down for future use.

Ipratropium (i-pra-TROE-pee-um) belongs to the group of medicines called bronchodilators (medicines that open up the bronchial tubes [air passages] of the lungs). It is taken by oral inhalation to control the symptoms of lung diseases, such as chronic bronchitis and emphysema.

Ipratropium may also be used for other conditions as determined by your doctor.

Ipratropium is available only with your doctor's prescription.

Remember:

• **This medicine has been prescribed for your current medical problem only.** It must not be given to other people or used for other problems unless you are directed to do so by your doctor.

• **Keep all medicines out of the reach of children.**

• In order for this medicine to work, it must be used as directed.

• **It is very important that you read and understand the following information.** If any of the information causes you special concern, do not decide against using this medicine without first checking with your doctor.

• Before you begin using any new medicine (prescription or nonprescription) or if you develop any new medical problem while you are using this medicine, check with your doctor, nurse, or pharmacist.

• **If you have any questions** about the following information or if you want more information about this medicine or your medical problem, **ask your doctor, nurse, or pharmacist.**

Before Using This Medicine

In order to decide on the best treatment for your medical problem, your doctor should be told:

—if you have ever had any unusual or allergic reaction to ipratropium, atropine, belladonna, hyoscyamine, or scopolamine or to other inhalation aerosol medicines.

—if you are **pregnant** or if you may become pregnant. Studies have not been done in humans. Although ipratropium has not been shown to cause birth defects in animals, it has been shown to cause fetal death and a slight decrease in successful pregnancies when the medicine was given to rats in very high doses.

—if you are **breast-feeding**. It is not known whether ipratropium passes into the breast milk. However, this medicine has not been shown to cause problems in nursing babies.

—if you have any of the following medical problems:
  Difficult urination
  Enlarged prostate

—if you are taking **any** other prescription or nonprescription (OTC) medicine.

Proper Use of This Medicine

Ipratropium usually comes with patient directions. Read them carefully before using this medicine.

If you are directed to use more than 1 inhalation of this medicine for each dose, allow 1 minute between the inhalations in order to receive the full effect of the medicine.

It is very important that you use ipratropium only as directed. Do not use more of it and do not use it more often than your doctor ordered. To do so may increase the chance of serious side effects.

Keep the spray away from the eyes because it may cause irritation. Also, if the spray gets in the eyes, the medicine may cause blurred vision for a short period of time.

If you miss a dose of this medicine, use it as soon as possible. However, if it is almost time for your next dose, skip the missed dose and go back to your regular dosing schedule. Do not double doses.

How to store this medicine:

• **Keep out of the reach of children.**

• Store away from heat and direct sunlight.

• Keep the medicine from freezing.

• Do not puncture, break, or burn the container, even if it is empty.

• Do not keep outdated medicine or medicine no longer needed. Be sure that any discarded medicine is out of the reach of children.

Precautions While Using This Medicine

Check with your doctor at once if your symptoms do not improve within 30 minutes after using a dose of this medicine or if your condition gets worse.

For patients who are also using another bronchodilator inhalation aerosol:

• Unless otherwise directed by your doctor, use the other bronchodilator inhalation aerosol first, then wait about 5 minutes before using this medicine. It is best not to use the 2 kinds of aerosols too close together, to lessen the chance of unwanted effects.

© 1988   The United States Pharmacopeial Convention, Inc.

For patients who are also using an adrenocorticoid inhalation aerosol or cromolyn inhalation aerosol:

- Unless otherwise directed by your doctor, use the ipratropium inhalation aerosol first, then wait about 5 minutes before using the adrenocorticoid aerosol or cromolyn aerosol. It is best not to use the ipratropium aerosol and the adrenocorticoid or cromolyn aerosol too close together, to lessen the chance of unwanted effects.

Ipratropium may cause dryness of the mouth or throat. For temporary relief of mouth dryness, use sugarless candy or gum, melt bits of ice in your mouth, or use a saliva substitute. However, if dry mouth continues for more than 2 weeks, check with your physician or dentist. Continuing dryness of the mouth may increase the chance of dental disease, including tooth decay, gum disease, and fungal infections.

Side Effects of This Medicine

Along with its needed effects, a medicine may cause some unwanted effects. Although not all of these side effects may occur, if they do occur they may require medical attention.

Check with your doctor as soon as possible if any of the following side effects occur:

Rare

Skin rash or hives
Ulcers or sores in mouth and on lips

Other side effects may occur that usually do not require medical attention. These side effects may go away during treatment as your body adjusts to the medicine. However, check with your doctor if any of the following side effects continue or are bothersome:

More common

Cough or dryness of mouth or throat
Headache or dizziness
Nervousness
Stomach upset or nausea

Less common or rare

Blurred vision or other changes in vision
Difficult urination
Metallic or unpleasant taste
Pounding heartbeat
Stuffy nose
Trembling
Trouble in sleeping
Unusual tiredness or weakness

Other side effects not listed above may also occur in some patients. If you notice any other effects, check with your doctor.

December 1987

IRON SUPPLEMENTS (Systemic)

This information applies to the following medicines:

Ferrous Fumarate (FER-us FYOO-ma-rate)
Ferrous Gluconate (FER-us GLOO-koe-nate)
Ferrous Sulfate (FER-us SUL-fate)
Iron Dextran (DEX-tran)
Iron-Polysaccharide (pol-i-SAK-a-ride)

Some commonly used brand names are:	Generic names:
Femiron Feostat Fumasorb Fumerin Hemocyte Ircon Neo-Fer* Novofumar* Palafer* Palmiron Span-FF	Ferrous Fumarate†
Apo-Ferrous Gluconate* Fergon Ferralet Fertinic* Novoferrogluc* Simron	Ferrous Gluconate†
Apo-Ferrous Sulfate* Feosol Fer-In-Sol Fer-Iron Fero-Grad* Fero-Gradumet Ferralyn Ferra-TD Fesofor* Mol-Iron Novoferrosulfa* PMS Ferrous Sulfate* Slow-Fe	Ferrous Sulfate†
Feostat Feronim Hematran Hydextran Imfergen Imferon Irodex K-Feron Nor-Feron Proferdex	Iron Dextran†
Hytinic Niferex Nu-Iron	Iron-Polysaccharide

*Not available in the U.S.
†Generic name product also available in the U.S.

To the Reader: If you do not recognize the names of medical conditions or medicines referred to in this information, check with your doctor, nurse, or pharmacist. Definitions for selected medical terms may be found in the Glossary. Brand names for the generic drug names listed can be found in the Index. In addition, selected brand names commonly associated with the generic name have been included in the text to help you recognize medicine you may be taking. The fact that a brand name

product is not mentioned does not mean the information does not apply. It is a good idea for you to learn both the generic and brand names of your medicines and to write them down for future use.

Iron is a mineral that the body needs to produce red blood cells. When the body does not get enough iron, it cannot produce the number of normal red blood cells needed to keep you in good health. This condition is called iron deficiency (iron shortage) or iron deficiency anemia. Although most people get enough iron from their diet, some must take additional amounts to meet their needs. For example, iron is sometimes lost with slow or small amounts of bleeding in the body that you would not be aware of and which can only be detected by your doctor. Your doctor can determine if you have an iron deficiency, what is causing the deficiency, and if an iron supplement is necessary.

After you start using this medicine, continue to return to your doctor to see if you are benefiting from the iron. Some blood tests may be necessary for this.

Some iron preparations are available only with your doctor's prescription. Others are available without a prescription; however, your doctor may have special instructions on the proper use and dose for your condition.

Remember:
- **This medicine has been prescribed for your current medical problem only.** It must not be given to other people or used for other problems unless you are directed to do so by your doctor.

- **Keep all medicines out of the reach of children.**

- In order for this medicine to work, it must be used as directed.

- If you are receiving this medicine by injection, some of the information about this medicine may not apply.

- **It is very important that you read and understand the following information.** If any of the information causes you special concern, do not decide against using this medicine without first checking with your doctor.

- Before you begin using any new medicine (prescription or nonprescription) or if you develop any new medical problem while you are using this medicine, check with your doctor, nurse, or pharmacist.

- **If you have any questions** about the following information or if you want more information about this medicine or your medical problem, **ask your doctor, nurse, or pharmacist.**

Before Using This Medicine

In order to decide on the best treatment for your medical problem, your doctor should be told:

—if you have ever had any unusual or allergic reaction to iron medicine.

—if you are on a low-salt, low-sugar, or any other special diet, or if you are allergic to any substance, such as foods, sulfites or other preservatives, or dyes. Most medicines contain more than their active ingredient, and many liquid medicines contain alcohol. Your doctor, nurse, or pharmacist can help you avoid products that may cause a problem.

—if you are **pregnant** or if you may become pregnant. During the first 3 months of pregnancy, a proper diet usually provides enough iron. However, during the last 6 months, in order to meet the increased needs of the developing baby, an iron supplement may be recommended by your doctor.

—if you are **breast-feeding**. Iron normally is present in breast milk in small amounts. When prescribed by a doctor, iron preparations are not known to cause problems during breast-feeding. However, nursing mothers are advised to check with their doctor before taking iron supplements or any other medication.

—if you have any of the following medical problems:
   Arthritis (rheumatoid)
   Asthma or allergies
   Blood disease (other than iron-deficiency anemia)
   Kidney infection
   Pancreatitis (inflammation of the pancreas)
   Colitis or other intestinal problems
   Liver disease
   Stomach ulcer

—if you are taking **any** other prescription or nonprescription (OTC) medicine, especially:
   Calcium supplements or other medicines containing calcium
   Tetracyclines
   Vitamin E

Proper Use of This Medicine

Iron is best taken on an empty stomach, with water or fruit juice (adults: full glass or 8 ounces; children: ½ glass or 4 ounces), about 1 hour before or 2 hours after meals. However, to lessen the possibility of stomach upset, iron may be taken with food or immediately after meals.

For safe and effective use of iron supplements:

• Follow your doctor's instructions if this medicine was prescribed.

• Follow the manufacturer's package directions if you are treating yourself. If you think you still need iron after taking it for 1 or 2 months, check with your doctor.

Liquid forms of iron medicine tend to stain the teeth. To prevent, reduce, or remove these stains:

• Mix each dose in water, fruit juice, or tomato juice. You may use a drinking tube or straw to help keep the medicine from getting on the teeth.

• When doses of liquid iron medicine are to be given by dropper, the dose may be placed well back on the tongue and followed with water or juice.

• Iron stains on teeth can usually be removed by brushing with baking soda (sodium bicarbonate) or medicinal peroxide (hydrogen peroxide 3%).

If you miss a dose of this medicine, skip the missed dose and go back to your regular dosing schedule. Do not double doses.

How to store this medicine:

• **Keep out of the reach of children because iron overdose is especially dangerous in children.** As few as 3 or 4 adult iron tablets can cause serious poisoning in small children. Vitamin-iron products for use during pregnancy and flavored vitamins with iron often cause iron overdose in small children..

• Store away from heat and direct light.

• Do not store in the bathroom, near the kitchen sink, or in other damp places. Heat or moisture may cause the medicine to break down.

• Keep the liquid form of this medicine from freezing.

• Do not keep outdated medicine or medicine no longer needed. Be sure that any discarded medicine is out of the reach of children.

Precautions While Using This Medicine

When iron combines with certain foods it loses much of its value. If you are taking iron, the following foods should be avoided or only taken in very small amounts for at least 1 hour before or 2 hours after taking iron:
   Cheese and yogurt
   Eggs
   Milk
   Tea or coffee
   Whole-grain breads and cereals

Do not take iron supplements at the same time as taking calcium supplements. It is best to space them 1 to 2 hours apart, to get the full benefit from each medicine.

If you are taking iron medicine without a doctor's prescription:

• Do not take iron medicine by mouth if you are receiving iron injections. To do so may result in iron poisoning.

• Do not regularly take large amounts of iron for longer than 6 months without checking with your doctor. People differ in their need for iron, and those with certain medical conditions can gradually become poisoned by taking too much iron over a period of time. Also, unabsorbed iron can mask the presence of blood in the stool, which may delay discovery of a serious condition.

• Your total daily intake of iron must be considered, not just the amount contained in iron medicine. Iron-fortified bread, cereals, and other foods must be added for the total amount.

If you have been taking a long-acting or coated iron tablet and your stools have *not* become black, check with your doctor. The tablets may not be breaking down properly in your stomach, and you may not be receiving enough iron.

Keep a 1-ounce bottle of *syrup* of ipecac available at home to be taken in case of an emergency when a doctor, poison control center, or emergency room orders its use.

If you think you or anyone else has taken an overdose of iron medicine:

- **Immediate medical attention is very important.**

- **Call your doctor, a poison control center, or the nearest hospital emergency room at once.** Always keep these phone numbers readily available.

- **Follow any instructions given to you.** If syrup of ipecac has been ordered and given, do not delay going to the emergency room while waiting for the ipecac syrup to empty the stomach, since it may require 20 to 30 minutes to show results.

- **Go to the emergency room without delay.**

- **Take the container of iron medicine with you.**

Early signs of iron overdose may not appear for up to 60 minutes or more. Do not delay going to the emergency room while waiting for signs to appear.

Side Effects of This Medicine

Along with its needed effects, a medicine may cause some unwanted effects. Although not all of these effects may occur, if they do occur they may need medical attention.

Check with your doctor if any of the following side effects occur:

More common—with the injection only
    Backache or muscle pain
    Chills
    Dizziness
    Fever with increased sweating
    Headache
    Nausea or vomiting
    Numbness, pain, or tingling of hands or feet
    Pain or redness at injection site
    Skin rash or hives
    Troubled breathing

More common—when taken by mouth only
    Abdominal or stomach pain, cramping, or soreness (continuing)

Less common or rare—when taken by mouth only
    Chest or throat pain, especially when swallowing
    Stools with signs of blood (red or black color)

Early signs of iron overdose
    Diarrhea (may contain blood)
    Nausea
    Stomach pain or cramping (sharp)
    Vomiting (severe; may contain blood)

Note: May not be noticed for up to 60 minutes or more. By this time you should have had emergency room treatment. Do not delay going to emergency room while waiting for signs to appear.

Late signs of iron overdose
    Bluish-colored lips, fingernails, and palms of hands
    Drowsiness
    Pale, clammy skin
    Unusual tiredness and/or weakness
    Weak and unusually fast heartbeat

Other side effects may occur that usually do not require medical attention. These side effects may go away during treatment as your body adjusts to the medicine. However, check with your doctor if any of the following side effects continue or are bothersome:

More common
    Nausea
    Vomiting

Less common
    Constipation
    Darkened urine
    Diarrhea
    Heartburn

Stools commonly become black when iron preparations are taken by mouth. This is caused by unabsorbed iron and is harmless. However, in rare cases, black stools of a sticky consistency may occur along with other side effects such as red streaks in the stool, cramping, soreness, or sharp pains in the stomach or abdominal area. Check with your doctor immediately if these side effects appear.

If you have been receiving injections of iron, you may notice a brown discoloration of your skin. This color usually fades within several weeks or months.

For the elderly: Elderly patients sometimes do not absorb iron as easily and may need a larger dose. Your doctor will decide if you need iron supplements and how much you should take.

Other side effects not listed above may also occur in some patients. If you notice any other effects, check with your doctor.

December 1987

ISOMETHEPTENE, DICHLORALPHENAZONE, AND ACETAMINOPHEN (Systemic)

Some commonly used brand names are Isocom and Midrin.

To the Reader: If you do not recognize the names of medical conditions or medicines referred to in this information, check with your doctor, nurse, or pharmacist. Definitions for selected medical terms may be found in the Glossary. Brand names for the generic drug names listed can be found in the Index. In addition, selected brand names commonly associated with the generic name have been included in the text to help you recognize medicine you may be taking. The fact that a brand name product is not mentioned does not mean the information does not apply. It is a good idea for you to learn both the generic and brand names of your medicines and to write them down for future use.

Isometheptene (eye-soe-meth-EP-teen), dichloralphenazone (dye-klor-al-FEN-a-zone), and acetaminophen (a-set-a-MEE-noe-fen) combination is taken by mouth to treat migraine headaches and some kinds of throbbing headaches. It is not used to prevent headaches, but is used to treat an attack once it has started. Isometheptene probably works by causing the blood vessels to constrict or narrow. Dichloralphenazone is a mild sedative and acetaminophen relieves pain.

This medicine is available only with your doctor's prescription.

Remember:

• **This medicine has been prescribed for your current medical problem only.** It must not be given to other people or used for other problems unless you are directed to do so by your doctor.

• **Keep all medicines out of the reach of children.**

• In order for this medicine to work, it must be used as directed.

• **It is very important that you read and understand the following information.** If any of the information causes you special concern, do not decide against using this medicine without first checking with your doctor.

• Before you begin using any new medicine (prescription or nonprescription) or if you develop any new medical problem while you are using this medicine, check with your doctor, nurse, or pharmacist.

• **If you have any questions** about the following information or if you want more information about this medicine or your medical problem, **ask your doctor, nurse, or pharmacist**.

Before Using This Medicine

In order to decide on the best treatment for your medical problem, your doctor should be told:

—if you have ever had any unusual or allergic reaction to isometheptene, dichloralphenazone, or acetaminophen.

—if you are on a low-salt, low-sugar, or any other special diet, or if you are allergic to any substance, such as foods, sulfites or other preservatives, or dyes.

Most medicines contain more than their active ingredient. Your doctor, nurse, or pharmacist can help you avoid products that may cause a problem.

—if you are **pregnant** or if you may become pregnant. Studies have not been done in either humans or animals.

—if you are **breast-feeding**. Although acetaminophen passes into breast milk in small amounts, this medicine has not been shown to cause problems in nursing babies.

—if you have any of the following medical problems:
Glaucoma
Heart or blood vessel disease
High blood pressure
Kidney disease
Liver disease
Virus infection of the liver

—if you have recently had a heart attack or stroke.

—if you are now taking or have taken within the past 2 weeks monoamine oxidase (MAO) inhibitors, such as:

Furazolidone (e.g., Furoxone)
Isocarboxazid (e.g., Marplan)
Pargyline (e.g., Eutonyl)
Phenelzine (e.g., Nardil)
Procarbazine (e.g., Matulane)
Tranylcypromine (e.g., Parnate)

—if you are taking **any** other prescription or nonprescription (OTC) medicine.

Proper Use of This Medicine

Take this medicine only as directed by your doctor. Do not take more of it, do not take it more often, and do not take it for a longer period of time than your doctor ordered. If too much acetaminophen (contained in this combination) is taken, liver damage may occur.

This medicine works best if you:

• **Take it at the first sign of headache.**

• **Lie down in a quiet, dark room for at least 2 hours** after taking it.

How to store this medicine:

• **Keep out of the reach of children.**

• Store away from heat and direct light.

• Do not store in the bathroom, near the kitchen sink, or in other damp places. Heat and moisture may cause the medicine to break down.

• Do not keep outdated medicine or medicine no longer needed. Be sure that any discarded medicine is out of the reach of children.

Precautions While Using This Medicine

If you will be taking this medicine regularly for a long period of time, your doctor should check your progress at regular visits to make sure that it is not causing any unwanted effects.

Check the labels of all over-the-counter (OTC), nonprescription, and prescription medicines you now take. If any contain acetaminophen be especially careful, since taking them while taking this medicine may lead to overdose. If you have any questions about this, check with your doctor or pharmacist.

Side Effects of This Medicine

Along with its needed effects, a medicine may cause some unwanted effects. Although not all of these side effects may occur, if they do occur they may need medical attention.

Check with your doctor as soon as possible if any of the following side effects occur:

Less common
> Unusual tiredness or weakness

Rare
> Skin rash or itching
> Sore throat and fever
> Unusual bleeding or bruising
> Yellow eyes or skin

Signs of acetaminophen overdose
> Diarrhea
> Nausea or vomiting
> Stomach cramps or pain

Other side effects may occur that usually do not require medical attention. These side effects may go away during treatment as your body adjusts to the medicine. However, check with your doctor if any of the following side effects continue or are bothersome:

Rare
> Dizziness
> Drowsiness
> Fast or irregular heartbeat

For elderly patients: Many medicines have not been tested in older people. Therefore, it is not known whether the medicine acts the same way it does in younger adults. Check with your doctor or pharmacist if you notice any unusual effects while taking this medicine or if you think it is not working as it should.

Other side effects not listed above may also occur in some patients. If you notice any other effects, check with your doctor.

December 1987

ISONIAZID (Systemic)

Some commonly used brand names or other names are:

DOW-Isoniazid	Nydrazid
INH	PMS Isoniazid*
Isotamine*	Rimifon*
Laniazid	

Generic name product may also be available in the U.S.

---

*Not available in the U.S.

To the Reader: If you do not recognize the names of medical conditions or medicines referred to in this information, check with your doctor, nurse, or pharmacist. Definitions for selected medical terms may be found in the Glossary. Brand names for the generic drug names listed can be found in the Index. In addition, selected brand names commonly associated with the generic name have been included in the text to help you recognize medicine you may be taking. The fact that a brand name product is not mentioned does not mean the information does not apply. It is a good idea for you to learn both the generic and brand names of your medicines and to write them down for future use.

Isoniazid (eye-soe-NYE-a-zid) belongs to the family of medicines called anti-infectives. It is used to prevent or help the body overcome tuberculosis (TB). It is taken by mouth or given by injection and may be given alone or with one or more other medicines for TB. This medicine may also be used for other problems as determined by your doctor.

Isoniazid is available only with your doctor's prescription.

Remember:

• **This medicine has been prescribed for your present TB infection only.** Another TB infection later on may require a different medicine. Also, even though other people may have the same symptoms as you, they may have a different kind of TB. Your medicine may not work for them and may even cause them harm. Therefore, **your medicine must not be given to other people or used for other infections** unless you are otherwise directed by your doctor.

• **Keep all medicines out of the reach of children.**

• In order for this medicine to work, it must be used as directed.

• If you are receiving this medicine by injection, some of the information about this medicine may not apply.

• **It is also very important that you read and understand the following information.** If any of the information causes you special concern, do not decide against using this medicine without first checking with your doctor.

• Before you begin using any new medicine (prescription or nonprescription) or if you develop any new medical problem while you are using this medicine, check with your doctor, nurse, or pharmacist.

• **If you have any questions** about the following information or if you want more information about this medicine or your medical problem, **ask your doctor, nurse, or pharmacist.**

Before Using This Medicine

In order to decide on the best treatment for your medical problem, your doctor should be told:

—if you have ever had any unusual or allergic reaction to ethionamide, isoniazid, pyrazinamide, or niacin (nicotinic acid).

—if you are on a low-salt, low-sugar, or any other special diet, or if you are allergic to any substance, such as foods, sulfites or other preservatives, or dyes. Most medicines contain more than their active ingredient, and many liquid medicines contain alcohol. Your doctor, nurse, or pharmacist can help you avoid products that may cause a problem.

—if you are **pregnant** or if you may become pregnant. Isoniazid has not been shown to cause birth defects or other problems in humans or animals. However, studies in rats and rabbits have shown that isoniazid may kill the fetus. In addition, it is not known whether this medicine causes problems when taken with other TB medicines.

—if you are **breast-feeding**. Isoniazid passes into the breast milk. However, isoniazid has not been shown to cause problems in nursing babies.

—if you have any of the following medical problems:
Alcoholism (active or treated)
Convulsive disorders such as seizures or epilepsy
Kidney disease (severe)
Liver disease

—if you are taking **any** other prescription or nonprescription (OTC) medicine, especially:
Acetaminophen (with long-term, high-dose use) (e.g., Tylenol)
Amiodarone (e.g., Cordarone)
Anabolic steroids (dromostanolone, ethylestrenol, nandrolone, oxandrolone, oxymetholone, stanozolol)
Androgens (male hormones)
Antithyroid agents (medicine for overactive thyroid)
Azlocillin (e.g., Azlin)
Carbamazepine (e.g., Tegretol)
Carmustine (e.g., BiCNU)
Chloroquine (e.g., Aralen)
Dantrolene (e.g., Dantrium)
Daunorubicin (e.g., Cerubidine)
Disulfiram (e.g., Antabuse)
Divalproex (e.g., Depakote)
Doxorubicin (e.g., Adriamycin)
Erythromycins
Estrogens (female hormones)
Etretinate (e.g., Tegison)
Furazolidone (e.g., Furoxone)
Gold salts
Hydroxychloroquine (e.g., Plaquenil)
Ketoconazole by mouth (e.g., Nizoral)
Mercaptopurine (e.g., Purinethol)
Methotrexate (e.g., Mexate)
Methyldopa (e.g., Aldomet)
Mezlocillin (e.g., Mezlin)
Miconazole by injection (e.g., Monistat)
Naltrexone (with long-term, high-dose use) (e.g., Trexan)
Nitrofurantoin (e.g., Furadantin)
Oral contraceptives (birth control pills) containing estrogen

Phenothiazines (acetophenazine, chlorpromazine, flu-
phenazine, mesoridazine, perphenazine, prochlorper-
azine, promazine, promethazine, thioridazine, trifluo-
perazine, triflupromazine, trimeprazine)
Phenytoin (e.g., Dilantin)
Piperacillin (e.g., Pipracil)
Plicamycin (e.g., Mithracin)
Rifampin (e.g., Rifadin)
Sulfonamides (sulfa medicine)
Valproic acid (e.g., Depakene)

—if you have ever had any problems with this medicine.

Proper Use of This Medicine

If you are taking isoniazid by mouth and it upsets your
stomach, you may take it with food. Antacids may also
help. However, do not take aluminum-containing antacids within 1 hour of the time you take isoniazid since
they may keep this medicine from working as well.

For patients taking the oral liquid form of isoniazid:

• Use a specially marked measuring spoon or other
device to measure each dose accurately since the average household teaspoon may not hold the right
amount of liquid.

To help clear up your tuberculosis (TB) completely, **it is
very important that you keep taking this medicine for
the full time of treatment** even if you begin to feel
better after a few weeks. You may have to take it
every day for as long as 6 months to 2 years. **It is
important that you do not miss any doses.**

Your doctor may also want you to take pyridoxine (vitamin B_6) every day to help prevent or lessen some of
the side effects of isoniazid. This is not usually needed
in children who receive enough pyridoxine in their diet.
If it is needed, **it is very important to take pyridoxine
every day along with this medicine. Do not miss any
doses.**

If you do miss a dose of either of these medicines, take
it as soon as possible. However, if it is almost time for
your next dose, skip the missed dose and go back to
your regular dosing schedule. Do not double doses.

How to store this medicine:

• **Keep out of the reach of children.**

• Store away from heat and direct light.

• Do not store the tablet form of this medicine in the
bathroom, near the kitchen sink, or in other damp
places. Heat or moisture may cause the medicine to
break down.

• Keep the oral liquid form of this medicine from freezing.

• Do not keep outdated medicine or medicine no longer
needed. Be sure that any discarded medicine is out of
the reach of children.

Precautions While Using This Medicine

It is very important that your doctor check your progress
at regular visits. Also, **check with your doctor immediately if blurred vision or any loss of vision, with or
without eye pain, occurs in either adults or children
during treatment.** Your doctor may want you to have
your eyes checked by an ophthalmologist (eye doctor).

If your symptoms do not improve within 2 to 3 weeks,
or if they become worse, check with your doctor.

Certain foods such as cheese (Swiss or Cheshire) or fish
(tuna, skipjack, or Sardinella) may rarely cause reactions in some patients taking isoniazid. Check with
your doctor if redness or itching of the skin, hot feeling,
rapid or pounding heartbeat, sweating, chills or clammy
feeling, headache, or lightheadedness occurs while you
are taking this medicine.

Liver problems may be more likely to occur if you drink
alcoholic beverages regularly while you are taking this
medicine. Also, the regular use of alcohol may keep
this medicine from working as well. Therefore, **you
should not drink alcoholic beverages while you are taking this medicine.**

**If this medicine causes you to feel very tired or very weak;
or causes clumsiness; unsteadiness; a loss of appetite;
nausea; numbness, tingling, burning, or pain in the hands
and feet; or vomiting, check with your doctor immediately.** These may be early warning signs of more
serious liver or nerve problems that could develop later.

This medicine may also cause blurred vision or loss of
vision, or it may cause some people to become dizzy.
**Make sure you know how you react to this medicine
before you drive, use machines, or do other jobs that
require you to be alert or to see clearly.** If these reactions are especially bothersome, check with your
doctor.

**Diabetics—This medicine may cause false test results with
some urine sugar tests.** Check with your doctor before
changing your diet or the dosage of your diabetes medicine.

Side Effects of This Medicine

In some types of mice, isoniazid was shown to cause lung
tumors.

Along with its needed effects, a medicine may cause some
unwanted effects. Although not all of these side effects
may occur, if they do occur they may need medical
attention.

Check with your doctor immediately if any of the follow-
ing side effects occur:
More common
Clumsiness or unsteadiness
Dark urine
Loss of appetite

Nausea or vomiting
Numbness, tingling, burning, or pain in hands and feet
Unusual tiredness or weakness
Yellow eyes or skin

Rare

Blurred vision or any loss of vision, with or without eye pain

Other side effects may occur that usually do not require medical attention. These side effects may go away during treatment as your body adjusts to the medicine. However, check with your doctor if any of the following side effects continue or are bothersome:

More common

Dizziness
Stomach upset

Less common

Enlargement of the breasts—males

For injection form

Irritation at the place of injection

Dark urine and yellowing of the eyes or skin are more likely to occur in patients over 35 years of age.

Other side effects not listed above may also occur in some patients. If you notice any other effects, check with your doctor.

December 1987

ISOPROTERENOL AND PHENYLEPHRINE (Systemic)

A commonly used brand name is Duo-Medihaler.

To the Reader: If you do not recognize the names of medical conditions or medicines referred to in this information, check with your doctor, nurse, or pharmacist. Definitions for selected medical terms may be found in the Glossary. Brand names for the generic drug names listed can be found in the Index. In addition, selected brand names commonly associated with the generic name have been included in the text to help you recognize medicine you may be taking. The fact that a brand name product is not mentioned does not mean the information does not apply. It is a good idea for you to learn both the generic and brand names of your medicines and to write them down for future use.

Isoproterenol (eye-soe-proe-TER-e-nole) and phenylephrine (fen-ill-EF-rin) combination medicine is taken by oral inhalation to treat bronchial asthma, bronchitis, emphysema, and other lung diseases. It relieves wheezing, shortness of breath, and troubled breathing.

This medicine is available only with your doctor's prescription.

Remember:

• **This medicine has been prescribed for your current medical problem only.** It must not be given to other people or used for other problems unless you are directed to do so by your doctor.

• **Keep all medicines out of the reach of children.**

• In order for this medicine to work, it must be used as directed.

• **It is very important that you read and understand the following information.** If any of the information causes you special concern, do not decide against using this medicine without first checking with your doctor.

• Before you begin using any new medicine (prescription or nonprescription) or if you develop any new medical problem while you are using this medicine, check with your doctor, nurse, or pharmacist.

• **If you have any questions** about the following information or if you want more information about this medicine or your medical problem, **ask your doctor, nurse, or pharmacist.**

Before Using This Medicine

In order to decide on the best treatment for your medical problem, your doctor should be told:

—if you have ever had any unusual or allergic reaction to medicines like isoproterenol and phenylephrine, such as amphetamines, ephedrine, epinephrine, metaproterenol, norepinephrine, phenylpropanolamine, pseudoephedrine, or terbutaline, or to other inhalation aerosol medicines.

—if you are **pregnant** or if you may become pregnant. Studies on birth defects with isoproterenol and phenylephrine have not been done in either humans or animals. However, use of phenylephrine during late pregnancy or during labor may cause a lack of oxygen and slow heartbeat in the fetus.

—if you are **breast-feeding**. It is not known whether isoproterenol and phenylephrine pass into the breast milk. This combination medicine has not been shown to cause problems in nursing babies.

—if you have any of the following medical problems:
Diabetes mellitus (sugar diabetes)
Heart or blood vessel disease
High blood pressure
Overactive thyroid

—if you are taking **any** other prescription or nonprescription (OTC) medicine, especially:
Beta-blockers (acebutolol [e.g., Sectral], atenolol [e.g., Tenormin], esmolol [e.g., Brevibloc], labetalol [e.g., Normodyne], metoprolol [e.g., Lopressor], nadolol [e.g., Corgard], oxprenolol [e.g., Trasicor], pindolol [e.g., Visken], propranolol [e.g., Inderal], sotalol [e.g., Sotacor], timolol [e.g., Blocadren])
Digitalis glycosides (heart medicine)
Maprotiline (e.g., Ludiomil)
Tricyclic antidepressants (amitriptyline [e.g., Elavil], amoxapine [e.g., Asendin], clomipramine, desipramine [e.g., Pertofrane], doxepin [e.g., Sinequan], imipramine [e.g., Tofranil], nortriptyline [e.g., Aventyl], protriptyline [e.g., Vivactil], trimipramine [e.g., Surmontil])

Proper Use of This Medicine

This medicine usually comes with patient directions. Read them carefully before using this medicine.

Keep spray away from the eyes.

Do not take more than 2 inhalations of this medicine at any one time, unless otherwise directed by your doctor. Allow 2 to 5 minutes after the first inhalation to make certain that a second inhalation is necessary.

Save your applicator. Refill units of this medicine may be available.

Use this medicine only as directed. Do not use more of it and do not use it more often than your doctor ordered. To do so may increase the chance of serious side effects. Isoproterenol inhalation preparations have been reported to cause death when too much of the medicine was used.

How to store this medicine:

• **Keep out of the reach of children.**

• Store away from heat and direct sunlight.

• Keep the medicine from freezing.

• Do not puncture, break, or burn container, even if it is empty.

• Do not keep outdated medicine or medicine no longer needed. Be sure that any discarded medicine is out of the reach of children.

Precautions While Using This Medicine

If you still have trouble breathing after using this medicine, or if your condition gets worse, check with your doctor at once.

If you are also using the inhalation aerosol form of an adrenocorticoid (cortisone-like medicine, such as beclomethasone, dexamethasone, flunisolide, or triamcinolone) or ipratropium, **allow 5 minutes between using the isoproterenol and phenylephrine combination and an adrenocorticoid or ipratropium,** unless otherwise directed by your doctor. This will help to reduce the possibility of side effects.

Side Effects of This Medicine

Along with its needed effects, a medicine may cause some unwanted effects. Although not all of these side effects may occur, if they do occur they may need medical attention.

Check with your doctor as soon as possible if any of the following side effects occur:

Rare
   Chest pain
   Irregular heartbeat

Signs of overdose
   Chest pain (continuing or severe)
   Dizziness or lightheadedness (continuing or severe)
   Fast, slow, or pounding heartbeat (continuing)
   Headache (continuing or severe)
   Increase in blood pressure
   Irregular heartbeat (continuing or severe)
   Nausea or vomiting (continuing or severe)
   Sensation of fullness in head
   Tingling in hands or feet
   Trembling (severe)
   Unusual anxiety, nervousness, or restlessness
   Weakness (severe)

Other side effects may occur that usually do not require medical attention. These side effects may go away during treatment as your body adjusts to the medicine.

However, check with your doctor if any of the following side effects continue or are bothersome:

More common
   Nervousness
   Restlessness
   Trouble in sleeping

Less common
   Dizziness or lightheadedness
   Fast or pounding heartbeat
   Flushing or redness of face or skin
   Headache
   Increase in sweating
   Nausea or vomiting
   Trembling
   Weakness

This medicine may cause the saliva to turn pinkish to red in color. This is to be expected while you are using this medicine.

For elderly patients: Many medicines have not been tested in older people. Therefore, it is not known whether the medicine acts the same way it does in younger adults. Check with your doctor or pharmacist if you notice any unusual effects while using this medicine or if you think it is not working as it should.

Other side effects not listed above may also occur in some patients. If you notice any other effects, check with your doctor.

December 1987

ISOTRETINOIN (Systemic)

A commonly used brand name is Accutane.

To the Reader: If you do not recognize the names of medical conditions or medicines referred to in this information, check with your doctor, nurse, or pharmacist. Definitions for selected medical terms may be found in the Glossary. Brand names for the generic drug names listed can be found in the Index. In addition, selected brand names commonly associated with the generic name have been included in the text to help you recognize medicine you may be taking. The fact that a brand name product is not mentioned does not mean the information does not apply. It is a good idea for you to learn both the generic and brand names of your medicines and to write them down for future use.

Isotretinoin (eye-soe-TRET-i-noyn) is taken by mouth and is used in the treatment of severe cystic acne. It is usually used only after other acne medicines have been used and have failed to help the acne. Isotretinoin may also be used to treat other skin diseases as determined by your doctor.

This medicine is available only with your doctor's prescription.

Remember:
• **This medicine has been prescribed for your current medical problem only.** It must not be given to other people or used for other problems unless you are directed to do so by your doctor.

• **Keep all medicines out of the reach of children.**

• In order for this medicine to work, it must be used as directed.

• **It is very important that you read and understand the following information.** If any of the information causes you special concern, do not decide against using this medicine without first checking with your doctor.

• Before you begin using any new medicine (prescription or nonprescription) or if you develop any new medical problem while you are using this medicine, check with your doctor, nurse, or pharmacist.

• **If you have any questions** about the following information or if you want more information about this medicine or your medical problem, **ask your doctor, nurse, or pharmacist.**

Before Using This Medicine

In order to decide on the best treatment for your medical problem, your doctor should be told:

—if you have ever had any unusual or allergic reaction to isotretinoin.

—if you are on a low-salt, low-sugar, or any other special diet, or if you are allergic to any substance, such as foods, sulfites or other preservatives, or dyes. Most medicines contain more than their active ingredient. Your doctor, nurse, or pharmacist can help you avoid products that may cause a problem.

—if you are **pregnant** or if you may become pregnant. Isotretinoin must not be taken during pregnancy because it has been shown to cause birth defects in humans. Women of childbearing potential should have a pregnancy test within 2 weeks before beginning treatment with isotretinoin to make sure they are not pregnant. Therapy with isotretinoin should then be started on the second or third day of your next normal menstrual period. Also, isotretinoin should not be taken unless an effective form of contraception (birth control) is used for at least 1 month before beginning treatment. Contraception should be continued during the period of treatment and for 1 month after isotretinoin is stopped. Be sure you have discussed this with your doctor.

—if you are **breast-feeding**. It is not known whether isotretinoin passes into the breast milk. However, isotretinoin is not recommended during breast-feeding because it may cause unwanted effects in nursing babies.

—if you have either of the following medical problems:
Diabetes mellitus (sugar diabetes) (or a family history of)
Overweight (severe)

—if any member of your family has a history of high triglyceride (fat-like substance) levels in the blood.

—if you drink a lot of alcoholic beverages.

—if you are taking **any** other prescription or nonprescription (OTC) medicine, especially:
Tetracyclines
Vitamin A or any preparation containing vitamin A

Proper Use of This Medicine

It is very important that you take isotretinoin only as directed. Do not take more of it, do not take it more often, and do not take it for a longer period of time than your doctor ordered. To do so may increase the chance of side effects.

If you miss a dose of this medicine, take it as soon as possible. However, if it is almost time for your next dose, skip the missed dose and go back to your regular dosing schedule. Do not double doses.

How to store this medicine:
• **Keep out of the reach of children.**
• Store away from heat and direct light.
• Do not store in the bathroom, near the kitchen sink, or in other damp places. Heat or moisture may cause the medicine to break down.
• Do not keep outdated medicine or medicine no longer needed. Be sure that any discarded medicine is out of the reach of children.

Precautions While Using This Medicine

Your doctor should check your progress at regular visits to make sure this medicine does not cause unwanted effects.

Isotretinoin has been shown to cause birth defects in humans if taken during pregnancy. Therefore, if you suspect that you may have become pregnant, stop taking this medicine immediately and check with your doctor.

Do not donate blood to a blood bank while you are taking isotretinoin or for 30 days after you stop taking it. This is to prevent the possibility of a pregnant patient receiving the blood.

Do not take vitamin A or any vitamin supplement containing vitamin A while taking this medicine, unless otherwise directed by your doctor. To do so may increase the chance of side effects.

Drinking too much alcohol while taking this medicine may cause high triglyceride (fat-like substance) levels in the blood and possibly increase the chance of unwanted effects on the heart and blood vessels. Therefore, **while taking this medicine, it is best that you do not drink alcoholic beverages or at least reduce the amount you usually drink.** If you have any questions about this, check with your doctor.

Diabetics—Isotretinoin may cause a change in your blood sugar levels. If you notice a change in the results of your urine sugar test or if you have any questions, check with your doctor.

In some patients, isotretinoin may cause a decrease in night vision. This decrease may occur suddenly. Also, for a short time after you apply this medicine, your vision may be blurred or there may be a change in your near or distant vision, especially at night. **Make sure your vision is clear before you drive or do other jobs that require you to see well.**

Isotretinoin may cause dryness of the eyes. Therefore, if you wear contact lenses, your eyes may be more sensitive to them during the time you are taking isotretinoin and for up to about 2 weeks after you stop taking it. To help relieve dryness of the eyes, check with your doctor about using an eye lubricating solution, such as artificial tears. If inflammation of the eyes occurs, check with your doctor.

Some people who take this medicine may become more sensitive to sunlight than they are normally. When you first begin taking this medicine, avoid too much sun and do not use a sunlamp until you see how you react to the sun, especially if you tend to burn easily. If you have a severe reaction, check with your doctor.

Isotretinoin may cause dryness of the mouth and nose. For temporary relief of mouth dryness, use sugarless candy or gum, melt bits of ice in your mouth, or use a saliva substitute. However, if dry mouth continues for more than 2 weeks, check with your physician or dentist. Continuing dryness of the mouth may increase the chance of dental disease, including tooth decay, gum disease, and fungal infections.

For patients taking isotretinoin for acne:

• When you begin taking isotretinoin, your acne may seem to get worse before it gets better. If irritation or other symptoms of your condition become severe, check with your doctor.

Side Effects of This Medicine

Along with its needed effects, a medicine may cause some unwanted effects. Although not all of these side effects may occur, if they do occur they may need medical attention.

Check with your doctor as soon as possible if any of the following side effects occur:
More common
   Burning, redness, itching, or other sign of inflammation of eyes
   Nosebleeds
   Scaling, redness, burning, pain, or other sign of inflammation of lips
Less common
   Mental depression
   Skin infection or rash
Rare
   Abdominal or stomach pain (severe)
   Bleeding or inflammation of gums
   Blurred vision or other changes in vision
   Diarrhea (severe)
   Headache (severe or continuing)
   Mood changes
   Nausea and vomiting
   Pain or tenderness of eyes
   Rectal bleeding
   Yellow eyes or skin

Other side effects may occur that usually do not require medical attention. These side effects may go away during treatment as your body adjusts to the medicine. However, check with your doctor if any of the following side effects continue or are bothersome:
More common
   Dryness or itching of skin
   Dryness of mouth or nose
Less common
   Dryness of eyes
   Headache (mild)
   Increased sensitivity of skin to sunlight
   Pain, tenderness, or stiffness in muscles, bones, or joints
   Peeling of skin on palms of hands or soles of feet
   Stomach upset
   Thinning of hair
   Unusual tiredness

For elderly patients: Many medicines have not been tested in older people. Therefore, it is not known whether the medicine acts the same way it does in younger adults. Check with your doctor or pharmacist if you notice any unusual effects while taking this medicine or if you think it is not working as it should.

Other side effects not listed above may also occur in some patients. If you notice any other effects, check with your doctor.

December 1987

ISOXSUPRINE (Systemic)

Some commonly used brand names are Vasodilan and Vasoprine.

Generic name product may also be available in the U.S.

To the Reader: If you do not recognize the names of medical conditions or medicines referred to in this information, check with your doctor, nurse, or pharmacist. Definitions for selected medical terms may be found in the Glossary. Brand names for the generic drug names listed can be found in the Index. In addition, selected brand names commonly associated with the generic name have been included in the text to help you recognize medicine you may be taking. The fact that a brand name product is not mentioned does not mean the information does not apply. It is a good idea for you to learn both the generic and brand names of your medicines and to write them down for future use.

Isoxsuprine (eye-SOX-syoo-preen) belongs to the group of medicines called vasodilators. Vasodilators increase the size of blood vessels. Isoxsuprine is used to treat problems resulting from poor blood circulation.

It may also be used for other conditions as determined by your doctor.

Isoxsuprine is available only with your doctor's prescription.

Remember:

• **This medicine has been prescribed for your current medical problem only.** It must not be given to other people or used for other problems unless you are directed to do so by your doctor.

• **Keep all medicines out of the reach of children.**

• In order for this medicine to work, it must be used as directed.

• If you are receiving this medicine by injection, some of the information about this medicine may not apply.

• **It is very important that you read and understand the following information.** If any of the information causes you special concern, do not decide against using this medicine without first checking with your doctor.

• Before you begin using any new medicine (prescription or nonprescription) or if you develop any new medical problem while you are using this medicine, check with your doctor, nurse, or pharmacist.

• **If you have any questions** about the following information or if you want more information about this medicine or your medical problem, **ask your doctor, nurse, or pharmacist.**

Before Using This Medicine

In order to decide on the best treatment for your medical problem, your doctor should be told:

—if you have ever had any unusual or allergic reaction to isoxsuprine.

—if you are on a low-salt, low-sugar, or any other special diet, or if you are allergic to any substance, such as foods, sulfites or other preservatives, or dyes. Most medicines contain more than their active ingredient. Your doctor, nurse, or pharmacist can help you avoid products that may cause a problem.

—if you are **pregnant** or if you may become pregnant. Isoxsuprine has not been shown to cause birth defects in humans. However, isoxsuprine given shortly before delivery may cause fast heartbeat and other problems (low blood sugar, bowel problems, low blood pressure) in the newborn.

—if you are **breast-feeding**. Isoxsuprine has not been shown to cause problems in nursing babies.

—if you have any of the following medical problems:
Angina (chest pain)
Bleeding problems
Glaucoma
Hardening of the arteries

—if you have recently had a heart attack or stroke.

—if you are taking **any** other prescription or nonprescription (OTC) medicine.

—if you smoke.

Proper Use of This Medicine

If this medicine upsets your stomach, it may be taken with meals, milk, or antacids.

If you miss a dose of this medicine, take it as soon as possible. However, if it is almost time for your next dose, skip the missed dose and go back to your regular dosing schedule. Do not double doses.

How to store this medicine:

• **Keep out of the reach of children.**

• Store away from heat and direct light.

• Do not store in the bathroom, near the kitchen sink, or in other damp places. Heat or moisture may cause the medicine to break down.

• Do not keep outdated medicine or medicine no longer needed. Be sure that any discarded medicine is out of the reach of children.

Precautions While Using This Medicine

It may take some time for this medicine to work. If you feel that the medicine is not working, do not stop taking it on your own. Instead, check with your doctor.

The helpful effects of this medicine may be decreased if you smoke. If you have any questions about this, check with your doctor.

Dizziness may occur, especially when you get up from a lying or sitting position or climb stairs. Getting up slowly may help. If this problem continues or gets worse, check with your doctor.

Side Effects of This Medicine

Along with its needed effects, a medicine may cause some unwanted effects. Although not all of these side effects may occur, if they do occur they may need medical attention.

Check with your doctor as soon as possible if any of the following side effects occur:

Rare

Chest pain
Dizziness or faintness (more common for injection)
Fast or irregular heartbeat (more common for injection)
Shortness of breath
Skin rash

Other side effects may occur that usually do not require medical attention. These side effects may go away during treatment as your body adjusts to the medicine. However, check with your doctor if the following side effects continue or are bothersome:

Rare

Nausea or vomiting (more common for injection)

For elderly patients: Many medicines have not been tested in older people. Therefore, it is not known whether the medicine acts the same way it does in younger adults. Isoxsuprine may reduce tolerance to cold temperatures in elderly patients. Check with your doctor or pharmacist if you notice any unusual effects while taking this medicine or if you think it is not working as it should.

Other side effects not listed above may also occur in some patients. If you notice any other effects, check with your doctor.

December 1987

Additional Information

In addition to the above information, for women taking isoxsuprine to prevent labor:

• Isoxsuprine is also used to stop premature labor.

• In order to decide on the best treatment for your medical problem, your doctor should be told:

—if you have any of the following medical problems:

Asthma
Diabetes mellitus (sugar diabetes)
Heart disease
High blood pressure
Overactive thyroid

• **Check with your doctor immediately:**

—if your contractions begin again or your water breaks.

—if you notice chest pain or shortness of breath while taking isoxsuprine.

KANAMYCIN (Oral)

A commonly used brand name is Kantrex.

To the Reader: If you do not recognize the names of medical conditions or medicines referred to in this information, check with your doctor, nurse, or pharmacist. Definitions for selected medical terms may be found in the Glossary. Brand names for the generic drug names listed can be found in the Index. In addition, selected brand names commonly associated with the generic name have been included in the text to help you recognize medicine you may be taking. The fact that a brand name product is not mentioned does not mean the information does not apply. It is a good idea for you to learn both the generic and brand names of your medicines and to write them down for future use.

Oral kanamycin (kan-a-MYE-sin) belongs to the family of medicines called antibiotics. Oral kanamycin is taken by mouth to help lessen the symptoms of hepatic coma, a complication of liver disease. This medicine may also be used before any surgery affecting the bowels to help prevent infection during surgery.

Kanamycin is available only with your doctor's prescription.

Remember:

• **This medicine has been prescribed for your present medical problem only.** Even though other people may have the same symptoms as you, they may have a different kind of problem. Your medicine may not work for them and may even cause them harm. Therefore, **your medicine must not be given to other people or used for other problems** unless you are otherwise directed by your doctor.

• **Keep all medicines out of the reach of children.**

• In order for this medicine to work, it must be used as directed.

• **It is very important that you read and understand the following information.** If any of the information causes you special concern, do not decide against using this medicine without first checking with your doctor.

• Before you begin using any new medicine (prescription or nonprescription) or if you develop any new medical problem while you are using this medicine, check with your doctor, nurse, or pharmacist.

• **If you have any questions** about the following information or if you want more information about this medicine or your medical problem, **ask your doctor, nurse, or pharmacist.**

Before Using This Medicine

In order to decide on the best treatment for your medical problem, your doctor should be told:

—if you have ever had any unusual or allergic reaction to this medicine or to any related antibiotics such as amikacin, gentamicin, kanamycin (by injection), neomycin, netilmicin, streptomycin, or tobramycin.

—if you are on a low-salt, low-sugar, or any other special diet, or if you are allergic to any substance, such as foods, sulfites or other preservatives, or dyes.

Most medicines contain more than their active ingredient. Your doctor, nurse, or pharmacist can help you avoid products that may cause a problem.

—if you are **pregnant** or if you may become pregnant. However, oral kanamycin has not been shown to cause birth defects or other problems in humans.

—if you are **breast-feeding**. However, oral kanamycin has not been shown to cause problems in nursing babies.

—if you have any of the following medical problems:
   Blockage of the bowel
   Eighth-cranial-nerve disease (loss of hearing and/or balance)
   Kidney disease
   Ulcers of the bowel

Proper Use of This Medicine

This medicine may be taken on a full or empty stomach.

Keep taking this medicine for the full time of treatment; do not miss any doses.

For patients taking oral kanamycin for hepatic coma:

• If you do miss a dose of this medicine, take it as soon as possible. However, if it is almost time for your next dose, skip the missed dose and go back to your regular dosing schedule. Do not double doses.

For patients taking oral kanamycin before any surgery affecting the bowels:

• If you do miss a dose of this medicine, take it as soon as possible. However, if it is almost time for your next dose and your dosing schedule is:

   —1 dose every hour (for 4 hours): Space the missed dose and the next dose ½ hour apart.

   —3 or more doses a day: Space the missed dose and the next dose 2 to 4 hours apart or double your next dose. Then go back to your regular dosing schedule.

How to store this medicine:

• **Keep out of the reach of children.**

• Store away from heat and direct light.

• Do not store in the bathroom, near the kitchen sink, or in other damp places. Heat and moisture may cause the medicine to break down.

• Do not keep outdated medicine or medicine no longer needed. Be sure that any discarded medicine is out of the reach of children.

Precautions While Using This Medicine

This medicine may cause some people to become dizzy or less alert than they are normally. **Make sure you know how you react to this medicine before you drive, use machines, or do other jobs that require you to be alert.** If these reactions are especially bothersome, check with your doctor.

Side Effects of This Medicine

Along with its needed effects, a medicine may cause some unwanted effects. Although not all of these side effects may occur, if they do occur they may need medical attention.

Check with your doctor immediately if any of the following side effects occur:

Rare
- Any loss of hearing
- Clumsiness
- Dizziness
- Greatly decreased frequency of urination or amount of urine
- Increased thirst
- Ringing or buzzing or a feeling of fullness in the ears
- Unsteadiness

Other side effects may occur that usually do not require medical attention. These side effects may go away during treatment as your body adjusts to the medicine. However, check with your doctor if any of the following side effects continue or are bothersome:

More common
- Irritation or soreness of the mouth or rectal area
- Nausea or vomiting

Rare
- Diarrhea
- Increased amount of gas
- Light-colored, frothy, fatty-appearing stools
- Skin rash

For elderly patients: Many medicines have not been tested in older people. Therefore, it is not known whether the medicine acts the same way it does in younger adults. Check with your doctor or pharmacist if you notice any unusual effects while taking this medicine or if you think it is not working as it should.

Other side effects not listed above may also occur in some patients. If you notice any other effects, check with your doctor.

December 1987

KAOLIN AND PECTIN (Oral)

Some commonly used brand names are:

Donnagel-MB*	K-C
Kao-Con*	K-P
Kaopectate	K-Pek
Kapectolin	Pecto Kay
Kaypectol	

*Not available in the United States.

Read the bold information first. Then go back and read the rest. If you do not recognize the names of medical conditions or medicines included in this information, check with your doctor, nurse, or pharmacist. Brand names for the generic drug names listed can also be found in the index. It is a good idea for you to learn both the generic and brand names of your medicines and to write them down for future use.

Kaolin (KAY-oh-lin) and pectin (PEK-tin) combination medicine is taken by mouth to treat diarrhea.

In babies and children, the fluid loss caused by diarrhea may result in a severe condition. Do not give any antidiarrhea medicine to children without first checking with your doctor.

In persons over 60 years of age, the fluid loss caused by diarrhea may result in a severe condition. These persons also should check with their doctor before taking any antidiarrhea medicine.

This medicine is available without a prescription; however, the product's directions and warnings should be carefully followed. In addition, your doctor may have special instructions on the proper dose or use of kaolin and pectin combination medicine for your medical condition.

Remember:

• **Keep all medicines out of the reach of children.**

• In order for this medicine to work, it must be used as directed. **If you are using this medicine without a prescription, it is very important to follow the directions on the label.**

• **It is also very important that you read and understand the following information.** If any of the information causes you special concern, check with your doctor before using this medicine without a prescription.

• Before you begin using any new medicine (prescription or nonprescription) or if you develop any new medical problem while you are using this medicine, check with your doctor, nurse, or pharmacist.

• **If you have any questions** about the following information or if you want more information about this medicine or your medical problem, **ask your doctor, nurse, or pharmacist.**

Before Using This Medicine

Before you use this medicine, check with your doctor or pharmacist:

—if you are on a low-salt, low-sugar, or any other special diet, or if you are allergic to any substance, such as foods, sulfites or other preservatives, or dyes. Most medicines contain more than their active ingredient. Your doctor, nurse, or pharmacist can help you avoid products that may cause a problem.

—if you are pregnant or if you intend to become pregnant while taking this medicine. Although this medicine is not absorbed into the body and is not likely to cause problems, the chance always exists.

—if you are breast-feeding. Although this medicine is not absorbed into the body and is not likely to cause problems, the chance always exists.

—if you have a chronic medical problem, including such problems as asthma, heart disease, or stomach ulcer.

—if you are now taking any of the following medicines or types of medicine:

Aminophylline
Antimuscarinics (medicine for abdominal or stomach spasms or cramps)
Caffeine
Chlorprothixene
Clindamycin
Dicyclomine
Digitalis glycosides (heart medicine)
Dyphylline
Lincomycin
Loxapine
Medicine for Parkinson's disease or other conditions affecting control of muscles
Oxtriphylline
Phenothiazines (acetophenazine, chlorpromazine, fluphenazine, mesoridazine, perphenazine, prochlorperazine, promazine, promethazine, thioridazine, trifluoperazine, triflupromazine, trimeprazine)
Theophylline
Thiothixene

—if you are now taking any other medicines by mouth.

Proper Use of This Medicine

Take this medicine after each loose bowel movement until the diarrhea is controlled, unless otherwise directed by your doctor.

How to store this medicine:

• Store away from heat and direct light.

• **Keep out of the reach of children.**

• Keep this medicine from freezing.

• Do not keep outdated medicine or medicine no longer needed. Flush the contents of the container down the toilet, unless otherwise directed.

Precautions While Using This Medicine

Check with your doctor if your diarrhea does not stop after 1 or 2 days or if you develop a fever.

© 1988   The United States Pharmacopeial Convention, Inc.

Side Effects of This Medicine

Along with its needed effects, a medicine may cause some unwanted effects. No serious side effects have been reported for this medicine. However, constipation may occur in some patients, especially if they take a lot of it. This is particularly true of elderly patients and children. Check with your doctor as soon as possible if constipation continues or is bothersome.

Other side effects not listed above may also occur in some patients. If you notice any other effects, check with your doctor.

December 1987

KAOLIN, PECTIN, BELLADONNA ALKALOIDS, AND OPIUM (Systemic)

Some commonly used brand names are:

Amogel PG	Kaodonna-PG
Donnagel-PG	Kapectolin PG
Kaodene with Paregoric	Quiagel PG

Read the bold information first. Then go back and read the rest. If you do not recognize the names of medical conditions or medicines included in this information, check with your doctor, nurse, or pharmacist. Brand names for the generic drug names listed can also be found in the index. It is a good idea for you to learn both the generic and brand names of your medicines and to write them down for future use.

Kaolin (KAY-oh-lin), pectin (PEK-tin), belladonna alkaloids (bell-a-DON-a AL-ka-loyds), and opium (OH-pee-um) combination medicine is taken by mouth to treat diarrhea.

In babies and children, the fluid loss caused by diarrhea may result in a severe condition. Do not give any antidiarrhea medicine to children without first checking with your doctor.

In persons over 60 years of age, the fluid loss caused by diarrhea may result in a severe condition. These persons also should check with their doctor before taking any antidiarrhea medicine.

In some states, this medicine is available without a prescription. However, the product's directions and warnings should be carefully followed. In addition, your doctor may have special instructions on the proper dose or use of this medicine for your medical condition.

Remember:

• **Keep all medicines out of the reach of children.**

• In order for this medicine to work, it must be used as directed. **If you are using this medicine without a prescription, it is very important to follow the directions on the label.**

• **It is also very important that you read and understand the following information.** If any of the information causes you special concern, check with your doctor before using this medicine without a prescription.

• Before you begin using any new medicine (prescription or nonprescription) or if you develop any new medical problem while you are using this medicine, check with your doctor, nurse, or pharmacist.

• **If you have any questions** about the following information or if you want more information about this medicine or your medical problem, **ask your doctor, nurse, or pharmacist.**

Before Using This Medicine

Before you use this medicine, check with your doctor, nurse, or pharmacist:

—if you have ever had any unusual or allergic reaction to any of the belladonna alkaloids (atropine, hyoscyamine, scopolamine) or medicines like morphine, codeine, or papaverine.

—if you are on a low-salt, low-sugar, or any other special diet, or if you are allergic to any substance, such as foods, sulfites or other preservatives, or dyes. Most medicines contain more than their active ingredient, and many liquid medicines contain alcohol. Your doctor, nurse, or pharmacist can help you avoid products that may cause a problem.

—if you are pregnant or if you intend to become pregnant. Although this medicine has not been shown to cause problems in humans, the chance always exists. Too much use of opium (contained in this combination medicine) during pregnancy may cause the baby to become dependent on the medicine. This may lead to withdrawal side effects after birth. Also, opium may cause breathing problems in the newborn baby if taken by the mother just before delivery.

—if you are breast-feeding. Although this medicine has not been shown to cause problems in humans, the chance always exists.

—if you have any of the following medical problems:
  Alcoholism
  Brain damage (children)
  Colitis or other intestinal disease
  Difficult urination
  Down's syndrome (mongolism)
  Dry mouth (severe and continuing)
  Emphysema, asthma, bronchitis, or other chronic lung disease
  Enlarged prostate
  Gallbladder disease or gallstones
  Glaucoma
  Heart disease
  Hiatal hernia
  Irregular heartbeat
  Kidney disease
  Liver disease
  Spastic paralysis (children)
  Underactive thyroid

—if you are now taking **any** of the following medicines or types of medicine:
  Antimuscarinics (medicine for abdominal or stomach spasms or cramps)
  Ketoconazole
  Lincomycin
  Potassium chloride

—if you are now taking other central nervous system (CNS) depressants, such as:
  Anticonvulsants (seizure medicine)
  Antihistamines or medicine for hay fever, other allergies, or colds
  Barbiturates
  Other narcotics
  Prescription pain medicine
  Sedatives, tranquilizers, or sleeping medicine

—if you are now taking or have taken within the past 2 weeks monoamine oxidase (MAO) inhibitors, such as:
  Furazolidone
  Isocarboxazid
  Pargyline
  Phenelzine
  Procarbazine
  Tranylcypromine

—if you are also taking **any** other medicines, including over-the-counter (OTC) or nonprescription medicines (for example, antacids). Many medicines change the way belladonna alkaloids (contained in this combination medicine) affect your body. Also, the effect of other medicines may be reduced by belladonna alkaloids.

Proper Use of This Medicine

If this medicine upsets your stomach, you may take it with food.

Take this medicine only as directed on the label or as ordered by your doctor. Do not take more of it, do not take it more often, and do not take it for a long period of time. If too much is taken, it may become habit-forming.

How to store this medicine:

• Store away from heat and direct light.

• **Keep out of the reach of children** since overdose is especially dangerous in children.

• Keep this medicine from freezing.

• Do not keep outdated medicine or medicine no longer needed. Flush the contents of the container down the toilet, unless otherwise directed.

Precautions While Using This Medicine

Check with your doctor if your diarrhea does not stop after 1 or 2 days or if you develop a fever.

This medicine will add to the effects of alcohol and other CNS depressants (medicines that slow down the nervous system, possibly causing drowsiness). Some examples of CNS depressants are antihistamines or medicine for hay fever, other allergies, or colds; sedatives, tranquilizers, or sleeping medicine; prescription pain medicine or narcotics; barbiturates; medicine for seizures; muscle relaxants; or anesthetics, including some dental anesthetics. **Check with your doctor before taking any of the above while you are taking this medicine.**

This medicine may cause some people to become dizzy, drowsy, or less alert than they are normally. Even if taken at bedtime, it may cause some people to feel drowsy or less alert on arising. **Make sure you know how you react to this medicine before you drive, use machines, or do other jobs that require you to be alert.**

This medicine may cause your eyes to become more sensitive to light than they are normally. Wearing sunglasses may help lessen the discomfort from bright light.

This medicine may make you sweat less, causing your body temperature to increase. **Use extra care not to become overheated during exercise or hot weather while you are taking this medicine,** as overheating could possibly result in heat stroke.

Your mouth, nose, and throat may feel very dry while you are taking this medicine. For temporary relief of mouth dryness, use sugarless candy or gum, melt bits of ice in your mouth, or use a saliva substitute. However, if dry mouth continues for more than 2 weeks, check with your dentist. Continuing dryness of the mouth may increase the chance of dental disease, including tooth decay, gum disease, and fungal infections.

Side Effects of This Medicine

Along with its needed effects, a medicine may cause some unwanted effects. Although not all of these side effects appear very often, when they do occur they may require medical attention. **Check with your doctor immediately** if any of the following side effects are severe and occur suddenly since they may indicate a more severe and dangerous problem with your bowels:

Rare

   Bloating
   Stomach pain (severe) with nausea and vomiting

Also, check with your doctor as soon as possible if the following effects occur:

Rare

   Eye pain
   Hallucinations (seeing, hearing, or feeling things that are
      not there)
   Shortness of breath
   Skin rash or itching
   Troubled breathing
   Unusually slow heartbeat

Other side effects may occur which usually do not require medical attention. These side effects may go away during treatment as your body adjusts to the medicine. However, check with your doctor if any of the following side effects continue or are bothersome:

More common with large doses

   Confusion
   Constipation
   Decrease in sweating
   Difficult urination
   Dizziness
   Drowsiness
   Dryness of mouth, nose, throat, or skin
   Faintness
   Headache
   Lightheadedness
   Rapid heartbeat
   Redness or flushing of face
   Unusual increase in sweating
   Unusual tiredness or weakness

Less common

   Blurred vision
   Decreased sexual ability
   Increased sensitivity of eyes to sunlight

Loss of memory (especially in the elderly)
Nervousness
Reduced sense of taste

The above side effects are more likely to occur in children and elderly patients, who are usually more sensitive to the effects of belladonna alkaloids and opium.

Other side effects not listed above may also occur in some patients. If you notice any other effects, check with your doctor.

December 1987

KAOLIN, PECTIN, AND PAREGORIC
(Systemic)

Some commonly used brand names are Donnagel-PG*, Kapectolin with Paregoric, and Parepectolin.

*Not available in the United States.

Read the bold information first. Then go back and read the rest. If you do not recognize the names of medical conditions or medicines included in this information, check with your doctor, nurse, or pharmacist. Brand names for the generic drug names listed can also be found in the index. It is a good idea for you to learn both the generic and brand names of your medicines and to write them down for future use.

Kaolin (KAY-oh-lin), pectin (PEK-tin), and paregoric (par-e-GOR-ik) combination medicine is taken by mouth to treat diarrhea.

In babies and children, the fluid loss caused by diarrhea may result in a severe condition. Do not give any antidiarrhea medicine to children without first checking with your doctor.

In persons over 60 years of age, the fluid loss caused by diarrhea may result in a severe condition. These persons also should check with their doctor before taking any antidiarrhea medicine.

In some states, this medicine is available without a prescription; however, the product's directions and warnings should be carefully followed. In addition, your doctor may have special instructions on the proper dose or use of this medicine for your medical condition.

Remember:
• **Keep all medicines out of the reach of children.**

• In order for this medicine to work, it must be used as directed. **If you are using this medicine without a prescription, it is very important to follow the directions on the label.**

• **It is also very important that you read and understand the following information.** If any of the information causes you special concern, check with your doctor before using this medicine without a prescription.

• Before you begin using any new medicine (prescription or nonprescription) or if you develop any new medical problem while you are using this medicine, check with your doctor, nurse, or pharmacist.

• **If you have any questions** about the following information or if you want more information about this medicine or your medical problem, **ask your doctor, nurse, or pharmacist.**

Before Using This Medicine

Before you use this medicine, check with your doctor, nurse, or pharmacist:

—if you have ever had an unusual or allergic reaction to morphine, codeine, or papaverine.

—if you are on a low-salt, low-sugar, or any other special diet, or if you are allergic to any substance, such as foods, sulfites or other preservatives, or dyes.

Most medicines contain more than their active ingredient, and many liquid medicines contain alcohol. Your doctor, nurse, or pharmacist can help you avoid products that may cause a problem.

—if you are pregnant or if you intend to become pregnant while taking this medicine. Although this medicine has not been shown to cause problems in humans, the chance always exists. Too much use of opium preparations (such as paregoric contained in this combination medicine) during pregnancy may cause the baby to become dependent on the medicine. This may lead to withdrawal side effects after birth. Also, opium preparations may cause breathing problems in the newborn baby if taken by the mother just before delivery.

—if you are breast-feeding. Although this medicine has not been shown to cause problems in humans, the chance always exists.

—if you have any of the following medical problems:
  Alcoholism
  Colitis or other intestinal disease
  Difficult urination
  Emphysema, asthma, bronchitis, or other chronic lung disease
  Enlarged prostate
  Gallbladder disease or gallstones
  Heart disease
  Irregular heartbeat
  Kidney disease
  Liver disease
  Underactive thyroid

—if you are now taking any of the following medicines or types of medicine:
  Aminophylline
  Antimuscarinics (medicine for abdominal or stomach spasms or cramps)
  Caffeine
  Chlorprothixene
  Clindamycin
  Dicyclomine
  Digitalis glycosides (heart medicine)
  Dyphylline
  Lincomycins
  Loxapine
  Medicine for Parkinson's disease or other conditions affecting control of muscles
  Oxtriphylline
  Phenothiazines (acetophenazine, chlorpromazine, fluphenazine, mesoridazine, perphenazine, prochlorperazine, promazine, promethazine, thioridazine, trifluoperazine, triflupromazine, trimeprazine)
  Theophylline
  Thiothixene
  Tricyclic antidepressants (amitriptyline, amoxapine, clomipramine, desipramine, doxepin, imipramine, nortriptyline, protriptyline, trimipramine)

—if you are now taking other central nervous system (CNS) depressants, such as:
  Anticonvulsants (seizure medicine)
  Antihistamines or medicine for hay fever, other allergies, or colds
  Barbiturates
  Other narcotics
  Prescription pain medicine
  Sedatives, tranquilizers, or sleeping medicine

© 1988   The United States Pharmacopeial Convention, Inc.

—if you are now taking or have taken within the past 2 weeks monoamine oxidase (MAO) inhibitors, such as:

Furazolidone
Isocarboxazid
Pargyline
Phenelzine
Procarbazine
Tranylcypromine

Proper Use of This Medicine

If this medicine upsets your stomach, you may take it with food.

Take this medicine only as directed on the label or as ordered by your doctor. Do not take more of it, do not take it more often, and do not take it for a long period of time. If too much is taken, it may become habit-forming.

How to store this medicine:

• Store away from heat and direct light.

• **Keep out of the reach of children** since overdose is especially dangerous in children.

• Do not store this medicine in the refrigerator. If it does get cold and you notice any solid particles in it, throw it away.

• Keep this medicine from freezing.

• Keep the container for this medicine tightly closed to prevent the alcohol from evaporating and the medicine from becoming stronger.

• Do not keep outdated medicine or medicine no longer needed. Flush the contents of the container down the toilet, unless otherwise directed.

Precautions While Using This Medicine

Check with your doctor if your diarrhea does not stop after 1 or 2 days or if you develop a fever.

This medicine will add to the effects of alcohol and other CNS depressants (medicines that slow down the nervous system, possibly causing drowsiness). Some examples of CNS depressants are antihistamines or medicine for hay fever, other allergies, or colds; sedatives, tranquilizers, or sleeping medicine; prescription pain medicine or narcotics; barbiturates; medicine for seizures; muscle relaxants; or anesthetics, including some dental anesthetics. **Check with your doctor before taking any of the above while you are taking this medicine.**

This medicine may cause some people to become dizzy, drowsy, or less alert than they are normally. Even if taken at bedtime, it may cause some people to feel drowsy or less alert on arising. **Make sure you know how you react to this medicine before you drive, use machines, or do other jobs that require you to be alert.**

Side Effects of This Medicine

Along with its needed effects, a medicine may cause some unwanted effects. Although not all of these side effects appear very often, when they do occur they may require medical attention. **Check with your doctor immediately** if any of the following side effects are severe and occur suddenly since they may indicate a more severe and dangerous problem with your bowels:

Rare
Bloating
Stomach pain (severe) with nausea and vomiting

Also, check with your doctor as soon as possible if the following effects occur:

Rare
Shortness of breath
Skin rash or itching
Troubled breathing
Unusually slow heartbeat

Other side effects may occur which usually do not require medical attention. These side effects may go away during treatment as your body adjusts to the medicine. However, check with your doctor if any of the following side effects continue or are bothersome:

More common with large doses
Constipation
Difficult urination or frequent urge to urinate
Dizziness
Drowsiness
Faintness
Lightheadedness
Redness or flushing of face
Unusual increase in sweating
Unusual tiredness or weakness

The above side effects are more likely to occur in children and elderly patients, who are usually more sensitive to the effects of paregoric.

Other side effects not listed above may also occur in some patients. If you notice any other effects, check with your doctor.

December 1987

KETOCONAZOLE (Systemic)

A commonly used brand name is Nizoral.

To the Reader: If you do not recognize the names of medical conditions or medicines referred to in this information, check with your doctor, nurse, or pharmacist. Definitions for selected medical terms may be found in the Glossary. Brand names for the generic drug names listed can be found in the Index. In addition, selected brand names commonly associated with the generic name have been included in the text to help you recognize medicine you may be taking. The fact that a brand name product is not mentioned does not mean the information does not apply. It is a good idea for you to learn both the generic and brand names of your medicines and to write them down for future use.

Ketoconazole (kee-toe-KOE-na-zole) belongs to the general family of medicines called antifungals. It is taken by mouth to help the body overcome fungal infections. It may be given alone or with other medicines that are used on the skin for fungal infections. This medicine may also be used for other problems as determined by your doctor.

Ketoconazole is available only with your doctor's prescription.

Remember:
• **This medicine has been prescribed for your present medical problem only.** Even though other people may have the same symptoms as you, they may have a different kind of problem. Your medicine may not work for them and may even cause them harm. Therefore, **your medicine must not be given to other people or used for other problems** unless you are otherwise directed by your doctor.

• **Keep all medicines out of the reach of children.**

• In order for this medicine to work, it must be used as directed.

• **It is very important that you read and understand the following information.** If any of the information causes you special concern, do not decide against using this medicine without first checking with your doctor.

• Before you begin using any new medicine (prescription or nonprescription) or if you develop any new medical problem while you are using this medicine, check with your doctor, nurse, or pharmacist.

• **If you have any questions** about the following information or if you want more information about this medicine or your medical problem, **ask your doctor, nurse, or pharmacist.**

Before Using This Medicine

In order to decide on the best treatment for your medical problem, your doctor should be told:

—if you have ever had any unusual or allergic reaction to ketoconazole.

—if you are on a low-salt, low-sugar, or any other special diet, or if you are allergic to any substance, such as foods, sulfites or other preservatives, or dyes.

Most medicines contain more than their active ingredient. Your doctor, nurse, or pharmacist can help you avoid products that may cause a problem.

—if you are **pregnant** or if you may become pregnant. Studies have not been done in humans. However, studies in rats given doses 10 times the highest recommended human dose have shown that ketoconazole causes webbed toes or fewer toes than normal. When given in higher doses, ketoconazole may also cause other problems in the fetus. Ketoconazole has also been shown to cause difficult labor in rats given doses slightly higher than the highest recommended human dose.

—if you are **breast-feeding**. Ketoconazole passes into the breast milk and may increase the chance of liver problems in nursing babies. Therefore, you should stop breast-feeding when you begin taking ketoconazole, during treatment, and for 48 to 72 hours thereafter. During this time the breast milk should be squeezed out or sucked out with a breast pump and thrown away. Then you may go back to breast-feeding.

—if you have any of the following medical problems:
  Achlorhydria (absence of stomach acid)
  Alcoholism (active or treated)
  Liver disease

—if you are taking **any** other prescription or nonprescription (OTC) medicine, especially:
  Acetaminophen (with long-term, high-dose use) (e.g., Tylenol)
  Amiodarone (e.g., Cordarone)
  Anabolic steroids (dromostanolone, ethylestrenol, nandrolone, oxandrolone, oxymetholone, stanozolol)
  Androgens (male hormones)
  Antithyroid agents (medicine for overactive thyroid)
  Azlocillin (e.g., Azlin)
  Carbamazepine (e.g., Tegretol)
  Carmustine (e.g., BiCNU)
  Chloroquine (e.g., Aralen)
  Cimetidine (e.g., Tagamet)
  Cyclosporine (e.g., Sandimmune)
  Dantrolene (e.g., Dantrium)
  Daunorubicin (e.g., Cerubidine)
  Disulfiram (e.g., Antabuse)
  Divalproex (e.g., Depakote)
  Doxorubicin (e.g., Adriamycin)
  Erythromycins
  Estrogens (female hormones)
  Etretinate (e.g., Tegison)
  Famotidine (e.g., Pepcid)
  Furazolidone (e.g., Furoxone)
  Gold salts
  Hydroxychloroquine (e.g., Plaquenil)
  Isoniazid (e.g., INH; Nydrazid)
  Mercaptopurine (e.g., Purinethol)
  Methotrexate (e.g., Mexate)
  Methyldopa (e.g., Aldomet)
  Mezlocillin (e.g., Mezlin)
  Naltrexone (with long-term, high-dose use) (e.g., Trexan)
  Nitrofurantoin (e.g., Furadantin)
  Oral contraceptives (birth control pills) containing estrogen
  Phenothiazines (acetophenazine, chlorpromazine, fluphenazine, mesoridazine, perphenazine, prochlorperazine, promazine, promethazine, thioridazine, trifluoperazine, triflupromazine, trimeprazine)
  Phenytoin (e.g., Dilantin)

Piperacillin (e.g., Pipracil)
Plicamycin (e.g., Mithracin)
Ranitidine (e.g., Zantac)
Rifampin (e.g., Rifadin)
Sulfonamides (sulfa medicine)
Valproic acid (e.g., Depakene)

Proper Use of This Medicine

If this medicine causes nausea or vomiting, it may be taken with a meal or snack.

For patients taking the oral liquid form of ketoconazole:

• Use a specially marked measuring spoon or other device to measure each dose accurately since the average household teaspoon may not hold the right amount of liquid.

If you have achlorhydria (absence of stomach acid), your doctor may want you to dissolve each tablet in a teaspoonful of weak hydrochloric acid solution to help you absorb the medicine better. Your doctor or pharmacist can prepare the solution for you. After you dissolve the tablet in the acid solution, add this mixture to a small amount (1 or 2 teaspoonfuls) of water in a glass. Drink the mixture through a plastic or glass drinking straw. Place the straw behind your teeth, as far back in your mouth as you can. This will keep the acid from harming your teeth. Be sure to drink all the liquid in order to get the full dose of medicine. Then drink about ½ glass of water, swish it around in your mouth, and swallow it.

To help clear up your infection completely, **it is very important that you keep taking this medicine for the full time of treatment** even if your symptoms begin to clear up or you begin to feel better after a few days. Since fungal infections may be very slow to clear up, you may have to continue taking this medicine every day for as long as 6 months to a year or more. Some fungal infections never clear up completely and require continuous treatment. If you stop taking this medicine too soon, your symptoms may return.

This medicine works best when there is a constant amount in the blood or urine. **To help keep the amount constant, do not miss any doses. Also, it is best to take each dose at the same time every day.** If you need help in planning the best time to take your medicine, check with your doctor, nurse, or pharmacist.

If you do miss a dose of this medicine, take it as soon as possible. This will help to keep a constant amount of medicine in the blood or urine. However, if it is almost time for your next dose, space the missed dose and the next dose 10 to 12 hours apart. Then go back to your regular dosing schedule.

How to store this medicine:

• **Keep out of the reach of children.**

• Store away from heat and direct light.

• Do not store the tablet form of this medicine in the bathroom, near the kitchen sink, or in other damp places. Heat or moisture may cause the medicine to break down.

• Keep the oral liquid form of this medicine from freezing.

• Do not keep outdated medicine or medicine no longer needed. Be sure that any discarded medicine is out of the reach of children.

Precautions While Using This Medicine

It is important that your doctor check your progress at regular visits. This will allow your doctor to check for any unwanted effects.

If your symptoms do not improve within a few weeks (or months for some infections), or if they become worse, check with your doctor.

If you are taking cimetidine, famotidine, or ranitidine while you are taking ketoconazole, take them at least 2 hours after you take ketoconazole. If you take them at the same time, they will keep ketoconazole from working as well.

Liver problems may be more likely to occur if you drink alcoholic beverages while you are taking this medicine. Therefore, **you should not drink alcoholic beverages while you are taking this medicine.**

This medicine may cause your eyes to become more sensitive to light than they are normally. Wearing sunglasses and avoiding too much exposure to bright light may help lessen the discomfort.

This medicine may also cause some people to become dizzy, drowsy, or less alert than they are normally. **Make sure you know how you react to this medicine before you drive, use machines, or do other jobs that require you to be alert.** If these reactions are especially bothersome, check with your doctor.

Side Effects of This Medicine

Along with its needed effects, a medicine may cause some unwanted effects. Although not all of these effects may occur, if they do occur they may need medical attention.

Check with your doctor immediately if any of the following side effects occur:
Rare
Dark or amber urine
Enlargement of the breasts—in males
Pale stools
Stomach pain
Unusual tiredness or weakness
Yellow eyes or skin

Other side effects may occur that usually do not require medical attention. These side effects may go away during treatment as your body adjusts to the medicine. However, check with your doctor if any of the following side effects continue or are bothersome:
More common
Nausea or vomiting

Less common
  Decreased sexual ability in males
  Diarrhea
  Dizziness
  Drowsiness
  Increased sensitivity of the eyes to light
  Skin rash or itching
  Trouble in sleeping

For elderly patients: Many medicines have not been tested in older people. Therefore, it is not known whether the medicine acts the same way it does in younger adults.

Check with your doctor or pharmacist if you notice any unusual effects while taking this medicine or if you think it is not working as it should.

Other side effects not listed above may also occur in some patients. If you notice any other effects, check with your doctor.

December 1987

KETOCONAZOLE (Topical)

A commonly used brand name is Nizoral.

To the Reader: If you do not recognize the names of medical conditions or medicines referred to in this information, check with your doctor, nurse, or pharmacist. Definitions for selected medical terms may be found in the Glossary. Brand names for the generic drug names listed can be found in the Index. In addition, selected brand names commonly associated with the generic name have been included in the text to help you recognize medicine you may be taking. The fact that a brand name product is not mentioned does not mean the information does not apply. It is a good idea for you to learn both the generic and brand names of your medicines and to write them down for future use.

Ketoconazole (kee-toe-KOE-na-zole) belongs to the family of medicines called antifungals. Antifungals are used to treat infections caused by a fungus. They work by killing the fungus or preventing its growth.

Ketoconazole cream is applied to the skin to treat:

—ringworm of the body (tinea corporis);
—ringworm of the groin (tinea cruris; jock itch); and
—"sun fungus" (tinea versicolor; pityriasis versicolor).

This medicine may also be used for other fungal infections of the skin as determined by your doctor.

Ketoconazole is available only with your doctor's prescription.

Remember:

• **This medicine has been prescribed for your present infection only.** Another infection later on may require a different medicine. Also, even though other people may have the same symptoms as you, they may have a different kind of infection. Your medicine may not work for them and may even cause them harm. Therefore, **your medicine must not be given to other people or used for other infections** unless you are otherwise directed by your doctor.

• **Keep all medicines out of the reach of children.**

• In order for this medicine to work, it must be used as directed.

• **It is very important that you read and understand the following information.** If any of the information causes you special concern, do not decide against using this medicine without first checking with your doctor.

• Before you begin using any new medicine (prescription or nonprescription) or if you develop any new medical problem while you are using this medicine, check with your doctor, nurse, or pharmacist.

• **If you have any questions** about the following information or if you want more information about this medicine or your medical problem, **ask your doctor, nurse, or pharmacist.**

Before Using This Medicine

In order to decide on the best treatment for your medical problem, your doctor should be told:

—if you have ever had any unusual or allergic reaction to ketoconazole.

—if you are allergic to any substance, such as certain foods or preservatives or dyes. Most medicines contain more than their active ingredient. Your doctor, nurse, or pharmacist can help you avoid products that may cause a problem.

—if you are **pregnant** or if you may become pregnant. Studies have not been done in humans. However, studies in rats, given doses 10 times the highest recommended human dose by mouth, have shown that ketoconazole causes webbed toes or fewer toes than normal in offspring.

—if you are **breast-feeding**. It is not known whether ketoconazole, applied to the skin on a regular basis, is absorbed into the body enough to pass into the breast milk. However, this medicine was not absorbed through the skin after a single dose. Therefore, it is unlikely to cause problems in nursing babies.

Proper Use of This Medicine

Keep this medicine away from the eyes.

Apply enough ketoconazole to cover the affected and surrounding skin areas, and rub in gently.

To help clear up your infection completely, **it is very important that you keep using ketoconazole for the full time of treatment,** even if your symptoms begin to clear up after a few days. Since fungal infections may be very slow to clear up, you may have to continue using this medicine every day for up to several weeks. If you stop using this medicine too soon, your symptoms may return. **Do not miss any doses.**

If you do miss a dose of this medicine, apply it as soon as possible. However, if it is almost time for your next dose, skip the missed dose and go back to your regular dosing schedule.

How to store this medicine:

• **Keep out of the reach of children.**

• Store away from heat and direct light.

• Keep the medicine from freezing.

• Do not keep outdated medicine or medicine no longer needed. Be sure that any discarded medicine is out of the reach of children.

Precautions While Using This Medicine

If your skin problem does not improve within 2 to 4 weeks, or if it becomes worse, check with your doctor.

To help clear up your infection completely and to help make sure it does not return, good health habits are also required.

• For patients using ketoconazole for ringworm of the groin (tinea cruris; jock itch):

—Avoid wearing underwear that is tight-fitting or made from synthetic materials (for example, rayon or nylon). Instead, wear loose-fitting, cotton underwear.

—Use a bland, absorbent powder (for example, talcum powder) or an antifungal powder (for example, tolnaftate) on the skin. It is best to use the powder between the times you use ketoconazole cream or other antifungal cream.

These measures will help reduce chafing and irritation and will also help keep the groin area cool and dry.

If you have any questions about these instructions, check with your doctor, nurse or pharmacist.

Side Effects of This Medicine

Along with its needed effects, a medicine may cause some unwanted effects. Although not all of these side effects may occur, if they do occur they may need medical attention.

Check with your doctor as soon as possible if any of the following side effects occur:

More common
   Itching, stinging, or irritation

Other side effects not listed above may also occur in some patients. If you notice any other effects, check with your doctor.

December 1987

Additional Information

In addition to the above information, for patients using ketoconazole for ringworm of the foot (tinea pedis; athlete's foot):

—Carefully dry the feet, especially between the toes, after bathing.

—Avoid wearing socks made from wool or synthetic materials (for example, rayon or nylon). Instead, wear clean, cotton socks and change them daily or more often if your feet sweat freely.

—Wear sandals or well-ventilated shoes (for example, shoes with holes).

—Use a bland, absorbent powder (for example, talcum powder) or an antifungal powder (for example, tolnaftate) between the toes, on the feet, and in socks and shoes freely once or twice a day. It is best to use the powder between the times you use ketoconazole cream or other antifungal cream.

These measures will help keep the feet cool and dry.

If you have any questions about these instructions, check with your doctor, nurse, or pharmacist.

KETOPROFEN (Systemic)

Some commonly used brand names are:

Alrheumat* Orudis-E*
Orudis Profenid*

*Not available in the U.S.

To the Reader: If you do not recognize the names of medical conditions or medicines referred to in this information, check with your doctor, nurse, or pharmacist. Definitions for selected medical terms may be found in the Glossary. Brand names for the generic drug names listed can be found in the Index. In addition, selected brand names commonly associated with the generic name have been included in the text to help you recognize medicine you may be taking. The fact that a brand name product is not mentioned does not mean the information does not apply. It is a good idea for you to learn both the generic and brand names of your medicines and to write them down for future use.

Ketoprofen (kee-toe-PROE-fen) belongs to the family of medicines known as anti-inflammatory analgesics. It is used to relieve some symptoms caused by arthritis or rheumatism, such as inflammation, swelling, stiffness, and joint pain. However, ketoprofen does not cure arthritis and will help you only as long as you continue to take it.

Ketoprofen may also be used for treating other kinds of pain, including menstrual cramps, or other conditions as determined by your doctor.

Ketoprofen is available only with your doctor's prescription.

Remember:

• **This medicine has been prescribed for your current medical problem only.** It must not be given to other people or used for other problems unless you are directed to do so by your doctor.

• **Keep all medicines out of the reach of children.**

• In order for this medicine to work, it must be used as directed.

• **It is very important that you read and understand the following information.** If any of the information causes you special concern, do not decide against using this medicine without first checking with your doctor.

• Before you begin using any new medicine (prescription or nonprescription) or if you develop any new medical problem while you are using this medicine, check with your doctor, nurse, or pharmacist.

• **If you have any questions** about the following information or if you want more information about this medicine or your medical problem, **ask your doctor, nurse, or pharmacist.**

Before Using This Medicine

In order to decide on the best treatment for your medical problem, your doctor should be told:

—if you have ever had any unusual or allergic reaction to ketoprofen or to any of the following medicines:

Aspirin or other salicylates
Diclofenac (e.g., Voltaren)
Diflunisal (e.g., Dolobid)
Fenoprofen (e.g., Nalfon)
Flurbiprofen, oral (e.g., Ansaid)
Ibuprofen (e.g., Motrin)
Indomethacin (e.g., Indocin)
Meclofenamate (e.g., Meclomen)
Mefenamic acid (e.g., Ponstel)
Naproxen (e.g., Naprosyn)
Oxyphenbutazone (e.g., Tandearil)
Phenylbutazone (e.g., Butazolidin)
Piroxicam (e.g., Feldene)
Sulindac (e.g., Clinoril)
Suprofen (e.g., Suprol)
Tiaprofenic acid (e.g., Surgam)
Tolmetin (e.g., Tolectin)
Zomepirac (e.g., Zomax)

—if you are on a low-salt, low-sugar, or any other special diet, or if you are allergic to any substance, such as foods, sulfites or other preservatives, or dyes. Most medicines contain more than their active ingredient. Your doctor, nurse, or pharmacist can help you avoid products that may cause a problem.

—if you are **pregnant** or if you may become pregnant. Studies on birth defects with ketoprofen have not been done in humans. However, if taken regularly during the last few months of pregnancy, there is a chance that ketoprofen may cause unwanted effects on the heart or blood flow in the newborn infant. Studies in animals have not shown that ketoprofen causes birth defects. However, studies in animals have shown that ketoprofen, if taken late in pregnancy, may increase the length of pregnancy, prolong labor, or cause other problems during delivery.

—if you are **breast-feeding**. It is not known whether ketoprofen passes into human breast milk. However, this medicine has not been shown to cause problems in nursing babies.

—if you have any of the following medical problems:

Anemia
Asthma
Bleeding problems
Colitis, stomach ulcer, or other stomach problems
Heart disease
High blood pressure
Kidney disease
Liver disease

—if you regularly take acetaminophen or aspirin or other salicylates.

—if you are taking the enteric-coated tablet form of ketoprofen and are also taking antacids.

—if you are taking **any** other prescription or nonprescription (OTC) medicine, especially:

Methotrexate (e.g., Mexate)
Probenecid (e.g., Benemid)

Proper Use of This Medicine

For patients taking ketoprofen by mouth:

• Ketoprofen will get into the blood more quickly if it is taken 30 minutes before meals or at least 2 hours after meals. This may help the medicine work a little faster when you first begin to take it. However, if you will be taking ketoprofen capsules (but not the enteric-coated tablets) for more than a few days, your doctor may want you to take them with food or with antacids to lessen stomach upset. An antacid containing aluminum hydroxide and magnesium hydroxide will not interfere with the way this medicine works and may be the best kind of antacid to use. If stomach upset (indigestion, nausea, vomiting, stomach pain, or diarrhea) continues or if you have any questions about how you should be taking this medicine, check with your doctor, nurse, or pharmacist.

• **Take this medicine with a full glass (8 ounces) of water.** Also, do not lie down for about 15 to 30 minutes after taking it. This helps to prevent irritation that may lead to trouble in swallowing.

For patients using the rectal suppository form of ketoprofen:

• If the suppository is too soft to insert because of storage in a warm place, before removing the foil wrapper chill the suppository in the refrigerator for 30 minutes or run cold water over it.

• How to insert the suppository: First, remove the foil wrapper and moisten the suppository with water. Lie down on your side and push the suppository well up into the rectum with a finger.

Do not take more of this medicine, do not take it more often, and do not take it for a longer period of time than ordered by your doctor. To do so may increase the chance of unwanted effects.

When used for severe or continuing arthritis, ketoprofen must be taken regularly as ordered by your doctor in order for it to help you. Ketoprofen usually begins to work in about one week, but several weeks may pass before you feel the full effects of the medicine.

If you miss a dose of this medicine, take it as soon as possible. However, if it is almost time for your next dose, skip the missed dose and go back to your regular dosing schedule. Do not double doses.

How to store this medicine:

• **Keep out of the reach of children.**

• Store away from heat and direct light.

• Do not store the tablet or capsule forms of this medicine in the bathroom, near the kitchen sink, or in other damp places. Heat or moisture may cause the medicine to break down.

• Keep the suppository form of this medicine from freezing.

• Do not keep outdated medicine or medicine no longer needed. Be sure that any discarded medicine is out of the reach of children.

Precautions While Using This Medicine

If you will be using this medicine for a long period of time, your doctor should check your progress at regular visits.

Stomach problems may be more likely to occur if you drink alcoholic beverages or if you are also regularly

taking certain other medicines while being treated with ketoprofen. Therefore, **do not drink alcoholic beverages or take any of the following medicines while being treated with this medicine,** unless otherwise directed by your doctor:

> Aspirin or other salicylates
> Diclofenac (e.g., Voltaren)
> Diflunisal (e.g., Dolobid)
> Fenoprofen (e.g., Nalfon)
> Flurbiprofen, oral (e.g., Ansaid)
> Ibuprofen (e.g., Motrin)
> Indomethacin (e.g., Indocin)
> Meclofenamate (e.g., Meclomen)
> Mefenamic acid (e.g., Ponstel)
> Naproxen (e.g., Naprosyn)
> Phenylbutazone (e.g., Butazolidin)
> Piroxicam (e.g., Feldene)
> Sulindac (e.g., Clinoril)
> Tiaprofenic acid (e.g., Surgam)
> Tolmetin (e.g., Tolectin)

Too much use of acetaminophen with ketoprofen may increase the chance of kidney problems. Therefore, do not regularly take acetaminophen together with this medicine, unless your doctor has directed you to do so.

Before having any kind of surgery (including dental surgery), tell the physician or dentist in charge that you are taking ketoprofen.

Ketoprofen may cause some people to become drowsy or dizzy, or to have blurred vision or other vision problems. **Make sure you know how you react to this medicine before you drive, use machines, or do other jobs that require you to be alert and able to see well.**

Some people who take ketoprofen may become more sensitive to sunlight than they are normally. These people may become sunburned more easily or break out in a rash after being in the sun. When you first begin taking this medicine, avoid too much sun or too much use of a sunlamp. You may protect yourself against sunlight with clothing or by using a factor-15 (or higher) sunscreen until you see how you react, especially if you tend to burn easily. **If you have a severe reaction, check with your doctor.**

Ketoprofen may cause a serious type of allergic reaction called anaphylaxis. Although this is very rare, it may occur more often in people who are allergic to aspirin or to other anti-inflammatory analgesics. **Anaphylaxis requires immediate medical attention.** The most serious signs of this reaction are very fast or irregular breathing, gasping for breath, wheezing, or fainting. Other signs may include very pale, gray, or blue color of the skin of the face; very fast but irregular heartbeat or pulse; hive-like swellings on the skin; and puffiness or swellings of the eyelids or around the eyes. If these effects occur, get emergency help at once. Ask someone to drive you to the nearest hospital emergency room. Do not try to drive yourself. If this is not possible, call an ambulance, lie down, cover yourself to keep warm, and prop your feet higher than your head. Stay in that position until help arrives.

Side Effects of This Medicine

Along with its needed effects, a medicine may cause some unwanted effects. Although not all of these side effects may occur, if they do occur they may need medical attention.

Stop taking this medicine and get emergency help immediately if any of the following side effects occur:

Shortness of breath, troubled breathing, wheezing, or pain or tightness in chest

Also, check with your doctor as soon as possible if any of the following side effects occur:

More common

Bleeding from rectum (with suppository dosage form)
Swelling of feet or lower legs
Weight gain

Less common

Abdominal or stomach pain (severe)
Blurred vision or any change in vision
Difficult or painful urination
Frequent urge to urinate
Mental depression
Ringing or buzzing sound in ears
Skin rash
Sores, ulcers, or white spots in mouth

Rare

Bloody or black, tarry stools
Bloody or cloudy urine
Chills
Confusion
Coughing or spitting up blood
Decreased hearing
Eye pain or redness
Fever
Headache (severe and throbbing)
Hives or itching of skin
Loosening of fingernails
Loss of memory
Red, thickened, or scaly skin
Sore throat and fever
Sudden decrease in amount of urine
Swelling of face
Unexplained nosebleeds
Unusual bruising or bleeding
Unusual or unexplained runny nose

Unusual tiredness or weakness
Vomiting blood or material that looks like coffee grounds
Yellow eyes or skin

Other side effects may occur that usually do not require medical attention. These side effects may go away during treatment as your body adjusts to the medicine. However, check with your doctor if any of the following side effects continue or are bothersome:

More common

Bloated feeling, gas, or indigestion
Burning, itching, or pain in rectum (with suppository dosage form)
Constipation
Diarrhea
Headache
Nausea
Nervousness
Stomach pain or discomfort
Trouble in sleeping

Less common or rare

Decreased sexual ability in men
Dizziness or lightheadedness
Drowsiness
Dryness or irritation of nose or throat
Fast or pounding heartbeat
General feeling of discomfort or illness
Increased sensitivity of skin to sunlight
Irritation or soreness of tongue, mouth, or gums
Loss of appetite
Numbness, tingling, pain, or weakness in hands or feet
Unusual hair loss
Unusual thirst
Vomiting

For elderly patients: Swelling of the face, feet, or lower legs; a sudden decrease in the amount of urine; or stomach problems may be more likely to occur in the elderly, who are usually more sensitive to the effects of ketoprofen.

Other side effects not listed above may also occur in some patients. If you notice any other effects, check with your doctor.

December 1987

LAXATIVES (Oral)

Some commonly used brand names and other names are:

Afko-Lube[16]	DSMC Plus[20]	Modane Soft[16]
Afko-Lube Lax[20]	D-S-S[16]	Molatoc[16]
Agarol*[34]	D-S-S plus[20]	Molatoc-CST[20]
Agoral[37]	Dulcodos*[19]	M.O.M.[29]
Agoral Marshmallow[37]	Dulcolax[38]	Naturacil[6]
Agoral Plain[35]	Duosol[16]	Nature's Remedy[41]
Agoral Raspberry[37]	Effer-syllium[7]	Neo-Cultol[35]
Alaxin[17]	Emulsoil[43]	Neolax[23]
Alophen[46]	Epsom salts[31]	Neoloid[43]
Alphamul[43]	Espotabs[46]	Nujol[35]
Bilagog[31]	Evac-U-Gen[46]	Nytilax[48]
Bilax[23]	Evac-U-Lax[46]	Perdiem[13]
Black-Draught[39]	Ex-Lax[46]	Perdiem Plain[6]
Black-Draught	Ex-Lax Pills[46]	Peri-Colace[20]
Lax-Senna[47]	Extra Gentle Ex-Lax[25]	Petrogalar Plain[35]
Carter's Little	Feen-a-Mint[25]	Phenolphthalein
Pills[38]	Feen-a-Mint Gum[46]	Petrogalar[37]
Caroid Laxative[42]	Feen-a-Mint Pills[25]	Phenolax[46]
Cholan-HMB[45]	FiberCon[5]	Phillips' LaxCaps[25]
Chronulac[27]	Fiberall[7]	Phillips' Milk of
Cillium[6]	Fleet Bisacodyl[38]	Magnesia[29]
Citrate of magnesia[28]	Fleet Flavored Castor	Poloxalkol[17]
Citroma[28]	Oil[43]	Pro-Cal-Sof[16]
Citro-Mag*[28]	Fleet Phospho-Soda[32]	Prodiem*[14]
Citro-Nesia[28]	Fletcher's Castoria[47]	Prodiem Plain*[7]
Citrucel[4]	Gentlax S[26]	Pro-Lax[7]
Colace[16]	Gentle Nature[48]	Prompt[15]
Colax[25]	Glysennid*[48]	Pro-Sof[16]
Cologel[4]	Haley's M-O[33]	Pro-Sof Liquid
Correctol[25 46]	Hepahydrin[45]	Concentrate[16]
Dacodyl[38]	Hydrocil Instant[7]	Pro-Sof Plus[20]
D-C-S[16]	Kasof[16]	Purge[43]
Decholin[45]	Kellogg's Castor Oil[43]	Regulace[20]
Deficol[38]	Kondremul*[35]	Regulax SS[16]
Dialose[16]	Kondremul Plain[35]	Regulex*[16]
Dialose Plus[20]	Kondremul with	Regulex-D*[21]
Dioctyl sodium	Cascara[36]	Reguloid Natural[7]
sulfosuccinate[16]	Kondremul with	Reguloid Orange[7]
Diocto[16]	Phenolphthalein[37]	Regutol[16]
Diocto-C[20]	Konsyl[6]	Roydan*[44]
Diocto-K[16]	Konsyl-D[7]	Roydan Mild*[44]
Diocto-K Plus[20]	Lansoÿl*[35]	Sal hepatica[32]
Diocto Plus[11]	Laxinate 100[16]	Senexon[47]
Dioeze[16]	Liqui-Doss[18]	Senokap DSS[26]
Diolax[20]	Liquid petrolatum[35]	Senokot[47]
Diosuccin[16]	Mag-Ox 400[30]	Senokot-S[26]
Dio-Sul[16]	Maltsupex[2]	Senolax[47]
Diothron[20]	Maox[30]	Serutan[7]
Disanthrol[20]	Metamucil[7]	Serutan Toasted
Disolan[25]	Metamucil Instant	Granules[8]
Disolan Forte[9a]	Mix[7]	Siblin[6]
Disonate[16]	Metamucil Instant	Sterculia gum[1]
Disoplex[9]	Mix, Orange Flavor[7]	Stulex[16]
Di-Sosul[16]	Metamucil Orange	Surfak[16]
Di-Sosul Forte[20]	Flavor[7]	Syllact[6]
Docu-K Plus[20]	Metamucil Strawberry	Syllamalt[3]
Dorbane[44]	Flavor[7]	Trilax[24]
Dorbanex*[22]	Metamucil Sugar Free[7]	Versabran[7]
Doss[16]	Milkinol[35]	V-Lax[7]
Doss*[21]	Mitrolan[5]	X-Prep Liquid[47]
Doxidan[25]	Modane[46]	Zymenol[35]
Doxinate[16]	Modane Bulk[7]	

*Not available in the U.S.

Note: For quick reference the following laxatives are numbered
   to match the corresponding brand names.

Bulk-forming laxatives—
   1. Karaya Gum*
   2. Malt Soup Extract
   3. Malt Soup Extract and Psyllium (SILL-i-yum)
   4. Methylcellulose (meth-ill-SELL-yoo-lose)†
   5. Polycarbophil (pol-i-KAR-boe-fil)
   6. Psyllium
   7. Psyllium Hydrophilic Mucilloid
   8. Psyllium Hydrophilic Mucilloid and Carboxymethylcellulose
Bulk-forming and emollient (stool softener) combinations—
   9. Carboxymethylcellulose (kar-box-ee-meth-ill-SELL-yoo-
lose) and Docusate (DOK-yoo-sate)
Bulk-forming, emollient (stool softener), and stimulant combinations—
   9a. Carboxymethylcellulose, Casanthranol (ka-SAN-thra-
nole), and Docusate
   10. Carboxymethylcellulose, Danthron (DAN-thron), and
Docusate*
   11. Docusate, Carboxymethylcellulose, and Casanthranol
   12. Docusate, Danthron, and Guar Gum*
Bulk-forming and stimulant combinations—
   13. Psyllium and Senna
   14. Psyllium Hydrophilic Mucilloid and Senna
   15. Psyllium Hydrophilic Mucilloid and Sennosides
Emollient (stool softener) laxatives—
   16. Docusate†
   17. Poloxamer 188 (pol-OX-a-mer)
Emollient (stool softener) and lubricant combinations—
   18. Docusate and Mineral Oil
Emollient (stool softener) and stimulant combinations—
   19. Bisacodyl (bis-a-KOE-dill) and Docusate
   20. Casanthranol and Docusate†
   21. Danthron and Docusate*
   22. Danthron and Poloxamer 188*
   23. Dehydrocholic (dee-hye-droe-KOE-lik) Acid and Docusate
   24. Dehydrocholic Acid, Docusate, and Phenolphthalein (fee-
nole-THAY-leen)
   25. Docusate and Phenolphthalein
   26. Senna and Docusate
Hyperosmotic laxatives—Lactulose:
   27. Lactulose
Hyperosmotic laxatives—Saline:
   28. Magnesium Citrate (mag-NEE-zhum SI-trate)†
   29. Magnesium Hydroxide†
   30. Magnesium Oxide
   31. Magnesium Sulfate (SUL-fate)†
   32. Sodium Phosphate† (SOE-dee-um FOS-fate)
Hyperosmotic and lubricant combinations—
   33. Milk of Magnesia and Mineral Oil
Hyperosmotic, lubricant, and stimulant combinations—
   34. Mineral Oil, Glycerin, and Phenolphthalein
Lubricant laxatives—
   35. Mineral Oil†
Lubricant and stimulant combinations—
   36. Mineral Oil and Cascara Sagrada
   37. Mineral Oil and Phenolphthalein
Stimulant laxatives—
   38. Bisacodyl†
   39. Casanthranol
   40. Cascara (kas-KAR-a) Sagrada†
   41. Cascara Sagrada and Aloe
   42. Cascara Sagrada and Phenolphthalein
   43. Castor (KAS-tor) Oil†
   44. Danthron*
   45. Dehydrocholic Acid†
   46. Phenolphthalein
   47. Senna
   48. Sennosides

*Not commercially available in the U.S.
†Generic name product may also be available.

Oral laxatives are medicines taken by mouth to encourage bowel movements to relieve constipation.

There are several different types of oral laxatives and they work in different ways. Since directions for use are different for each type, it is important to know which one you are taking. The different types of oral laxatives include:

—Bulk-formers

Bulk-forming laxatives are not digested but absorb liquid in the intestines and swell to form a soft, bulky stool. The bowel is then stimulated normally by the presence of the bulky mass. Some bulk-forming laxatives, like psyllium and polycarbophil, may be prescribed by your doctor to treat diarrhea.

—Emollients (stool softeners)

Emollient laxatives encourage bowel movements by helping liquids mix into the stool and prevent dry, hard stool masses. This type of laxative has been said not to *cause* a bowel movement but instead *allows* the patient to have a bowel movement without straining.

—Hyperosmotics

Hyperosmotic laxatives encourage bowel movements by drawing water into the bowel from surrounding body tissues. This provides a soft stool mass and increased bowel action.

There are two types of hyperosmotic laxatives taken by mouth—the saline and the lactulose types. The *saline type* is often called "salts." They are used for rapid emptying of the lower intestine and bowel. They are not used for long-term or repeated correction of constipation. With smaller doses than those used for the laxative effect, some saline laxatives are used as antacids. The information that follows applies only to their use as laxatives. Sodium phosphate may also be prescribed for other conditions as determined by your doctor.

The *lactulose type* is a special sugar-like laxative that works the same way as the saline type. However, it produces results much more slowly and is often used for long-term treatment of chronic constipation. Lactulose may sometimes be used in the treatment of certain medical conditions to reduce the amount of ammonia in the blood. It is available only with your doctor's prescription.

—Lubricants

Lubricant laxatives, such as mineral oil, taken by mouth encourage bowel movements by coating the bowel and the stool mass with a waterproof film. This keeps moisture in the stool. The stool remains soft and its passage is made easier.

—Stimulants

Stimulant laxatives, also known as contact laxatives, encourage bowel movements by acting on the intestinal wall. They increase the muscle contractions that move along the stool mass. Stimulant laxatives are a popular type of laxative for self-treatment. However, they also are more likely to cause side effects. One of the stimulant laxatives, dehydrocholic acid, may also be used for treating certain conditions of the biliary tract.

—Combinations

There are many products that you can buy for constipation that contain more than one type of laxative. For example, a product may contain both an emollient laxative and a stimulant laxative. In general, combination products may be more likely to cause side effects because of the multiple ingredients. In addition, they may not offer any advantage over products containing only one type of laxative. *If you are taking a combination laxative, make certain you know the proper use and precautions for each of the different ingredients.*

Laxatives should not be given to young children (up to 6 years of age) unless prescribed by their doctor. Since children cannot usually describe their symptoms very well, a doctor should check the child before giving this medicine. This is to prevent an unknown condition from getting worse and to avoid causing unwanted effects in the child.

Most laxatives are available without a prescription; however, your doctor may have special instructions for the proper use and dose for your medical condition.

Most laxatives (except saline laxatives) may be used to provide relief:

—during pregnancy.

—for a few days after giving birth.

—during preparation for examination or surgery.

—for constipation of bedfast patients.

—for constipation caused by other medicines.

—following surgery when straining should be avoided.

—following a period of poor eating habits or a lack of physical exercise in order to develop normal bowel function (bulk-forming laxatives only).

—for some medical conditions that may be made worse by straining, for example:

  Heart disease
  Hemorrhoids
  Hernia (rupture)
  High blood pressure
  History of stroke

Saline laxatives have more limited uses and may be used to provide rapid results:

—during preparation for examination or surgery.

—for elimination of food or drugs from the body in cases of poisoning or overdose.

—for simple constipation that happens on occasion (although another type of laxative may be preferred).

—in supplying a fresh stool sample for diagnosis.

Remember:
• **Keep all medicines out of the reach of children.**

• In order for this medicine to work, it must be used as directed. **If you are using this medicine without a prescription, it is very important to follow the directions on the label.**

• **It is also very important that you read and understand the following information.** If any of the information causes you special concern, check with your doctor before using this medicine without a prescription.

• Before you begin using any new medicine (prescription or nonprescription) or if you develop any new medical problem while you are using this medicine, check with your doctor, nurse, or pharmacist.

• **If you have any questions** about the following information or if you want more information about this medicine or your medical problem, **ask your doctor, nurse, or pharmacist.**

Before Using This Medicine

Importance of diet, fluids, and exercise to prevent constipation—Laxatives are to be used to provide short-term relief only, unless otherwise directed by a doctor. A proper diet containing roughage (whole grain breads and cereals, bran, fruit, and green, leafy vegetables), with 6 to 8 full glasses (8 ounces each) of liquids each day, and daily exercise are most important in maintaining a healthy bowel function. Also, for individuals who have problems with constipation, foods such as pastries, puddings, sugar, candy, cake, and cheese may make the constipation worse.

Before you use this medicine check with your doctor or pharmacist.

—if you have ever had any unusual or allergic reaction to laxatives.

—if you are on a low-salt, low-sugar, or any other special diet, or if you are allergic to any substance, such as foods, sulfites or other preservatives, or dyes. Most medicines contain more than their active ingredient, and many liquid medicines contain alcohol. Your doctor, nurse, or pharmacist can help you avoid products that may cause a problem.

—if you are **pregnant**. Although laxatives are often used during pregnancy, some types are better than others. Emollient (stool softeners) laxatives and bulk-forming laxatives are probably used most often. If you are using a laxative during pregnancy, remember that:

• Some laxatives (in particular, the bulk-formers) contain a large amount of sodium or sugars, which may have possible unwanted effects such as increasing blood pressure or causing water to be held in the tissues.

• Saline laxatives containing magnesium, potassium, or phosphates may have to be avoided if your kidney function is not normal.

• Mineral oil is usually not used during pregnancy because of possible unwanted effects on the mother or infant. Mineral oil may interfere with the absorption of nutrients and vitamins in the mother. Also, if taken for a long period of time during pregnancy, mineral oil may cause severe bleeding in the newborn infant.

• Stimulant laxatives may cause unwanted effects in the expectant mother if improperly used. Castor oil in particular should not be used as it may cause contractions of the womb.

—if you are **breast-feeding**. Laxatives containing cascara, danthron, and phenolphthalein may pass into the breast milk. Although the amount of laxative in the milk is generally thought to be too small to cause problems in the baby, your doctor should be told that you plan to use such laxatives. Some reports claim that diarrhea has been caused in the infant.

—if you have any of the following medical problems:
    Appendicitis (or signs of)
    Colostomy
    Diabetes mellitus (sugar diabetes)
    Heart disease
    High blood pressure
    Ileostomy
    Intestinal blockage
    Kidney disease
    Laxative habit
    Rectal bleeding of unknown cause
    Swallowing difficulty

—if you are now taking any of the following medicines or types of medicine:
    Amiloride
    Antacids
    Anticoagulants, coumarin- or indandione-type, oral (blood thinners you take by mouth)
    Aspirin or other salicylates
    Cimetidine
    Contraceptives, oral (birth control pills)
    Digitalis glycosides (heart medicine)
    Famotidine
    Laxatives (other)
    Medicine containing potassium
    Phenothiazines (acetophenazine, chlorpromazine, fluphenazine, mesoridazine, perphenazine, prochlorperazine, promazine, promethazine, thioridazine, trifluoperazine, triflupromazine, trimeprazine)
    Ranitidine
    Sodium polysterene sulfonate
    Spironolactone
    Tetracyclines
    Triamterene
    Vitamin A
    Vitamin D
    Vitamin E
    Vitamin K

Proper Use of This Medicine

For safe and effective use of your laxative:

• Follow your doctor's instructions if this laxative was prescribed.

• Follow the manufacturer's package directions if you are treating yourself.

With all kinds of laxatives, at least 6 to 8 glasses (8 ounces each) of liquids should be taken each day. This will help make the stool softer.

For patients taking laxatives containing a bulk-forming ingredient:

• Do not try to swallow in the dry form. Take with liquid.

• To allow bulk-forming laxatives to work properly and to prevent intestinal blockage, it is necessary to drink plenty of fluids during their use. Each dose should be taken in or with a full glass (8 ounces) or more of cold water or fruit juice. This will provide enough liquid for the laxative to work properly. A second glass of water or juice by itself is often recommended with each dose for best effect and to avoid side effects.

• When taking a product that contains only a bulk-forming ingredient, results often may be obtained in 12 hours. However, this may not occur for some individuals until after 2 or 3 days.

For patients taking laxatives containing an emollient (stool softener):

• Liquid forms may be taken in milk or fruit juice to improve flavor.

• When taking a product that contains only an emollient, results usually occur 1 to 2 days after the first dose. However, this may not occur for some individuals until after 3 to 5 days.

For patients taking laxatives containing a hyperosmotic ingredient:

• Each dose should be taken in or with a full glass (8 ounces) or more of cold water or fruit juice. This will provide enough liquid for the laxative to work properly. A second glass of water or juice by itself is often recommended with each dose for best effect and, in the case of saline laxatives, to prevent you from becoming dehydrated.

• The unpleasant taste produced by some hyperosmotic laxatives may be improved by following each dose with citrus fruit juice or citrus-flavored carbonated beverage.

• Lactulose may not produce laxative results for 24 to 48 hours.

• Saline laxatives usually produce results within ½ to 3 hours following a dose. When a larger dose is taken on an empty stomach, the results are quicker. When a smaller dose is taken with food, the results are delayed. Therefore, large doses of saline laxatives are usually not taken late in the day on an empty stomach.

For patients taking laxatives containing mineral oil:

• Mineral oil should not be taken within 2 hours of meals because of possible interference with food digestion and absorption of nutrients and vitamins.

• Mineral oil is usually taken at bedtime (but not while lying down) for convenience and because they require about 6 to 8 hours to produce results.

For patients taking laxatives containing a stimulant ingredient:

• Stimulant laxatives are usually taken on an empty stomach for rapid effect. Results are slowed if taken with food.

• Many stimulant laxatives (but not castor oil) are often taken at bedtime to produce results the next morning (although some may require 24 hours or more).

• **Castor oil** is not usually taken late in the day because its results occur within 2 to 6 hours.

• The unpleasant taste of **castor oil** may be improved by chilling in the refrigerator for at least an hour and then stirring the dose into a full glass of cold orange juice just before it is taken. Also, flavored preparations of castor oil are available.

• **Bisacodyl tablets** are specially coated to allow them to work properly without causing irritation and/or nausea. To protect this coating, do not chew, crush, or take the tablets within an hour of milk or antacids.

• Because of the way **phenolphthalein** works in the body, a single dose may cause a laxative effect in some people for up to 3 days.

How to store this medicine:

• **Keep out of the reach of children.**

• Store away from heat and direct light.

• Do not store the capsule, tablet, granules, or powder form of this medicine in the bathroom, near the kitchen sink, or in other damp places. Heat or moisture may cause the medicine to break down.

• Keep the liquid form of this medicine from freezing.

• Do not keep outdated medicine or medicine no longer needed. Be sure that any discarded medicine is out of the reach of children.

Precautions While Using This Medicine

Do not take any type of laxative:

—**if you have signs of appendicitis or inflamed bowel** (such as stomach or lower abdominal pain, cramping, bloating, soreness, nausea, or vomiting). Instead, check with your doctor as soon as possible.

—**for more than 1 week** unless your doctor has prescribed or ordered a special schedule for you. This is true even when you have had no results from the laxative.

—**within 2 hours of taking other medicine** because the desired effect of the other medicine may be reduced.

—**if you do not need it,** as for the common cold, "to clean out your system," or as a "tonic to make you feel better."

—**if you miss a bowel movement for a day or two.**

—**if you develop a skin rash** while taking a laxative or if you had a rash the last time you took it. Instead, check with your doctor.

If you notice a sudden change in bowel habits or function that lasts longer than 2 weeks, or that keeps returning off and on, check with your doctor before using a laxative. This will allow the cause of your problem to be determined before it may become more serious.

The "laxative habit"—Laxative products are overused by many people. Such a practice often leads to dependence on the laxative action to produce a bowel movement. In severe cases, overuse of some laxatives has caused damage to the nerves, muscles, and tissues of the intestines and bowel. If you have any questions about the use of laxatives, check with your doctor or pharmacist.

Many laxatives often contain large amounts of sugars, carbohydrates, and sodium. If you are on a low-sugar, low-caloric, or low-salt diet, check with your doctor or pharmacist before using a laxative.

For patients taking laxatives containing mineral oil:

• Mineral oil should not be taken often or for long periods of time because:

—gradual build-up in body tissues may create additional problems.

—the use of mineral oil may interfere with the body's ability to absorb certain food nutrients and vitamins A, D, E, and K.

• Large doses of mineral oil may cause some leakage from the rectum. The use of absorbent pads or a decrease in dose may be necessary to prevent the soiling of clothing.

• With the use of mineral oil, a form of pneumonia may be caused by the inhalation of oil droplets into the lungs. Young children (up to 6 years of age) and bedridden elderly patients seem more likely to suffer from this effect, and use by such patients is discouraged.

• Do not take mineral oil within 2 hours of an emollient (stool softener) laxative. The emollient laxative may increase the amount of mineral oil absorbed.

For patients taking laxatives containing a stimulant ingredient:

• Stimulant laxatives are most often associated with:

—overuse and the laxative habit.

—skin rashes.

—intestinal cramping after dosing (especially if taken on an empty stomach).

—potassium loss.

Side Effects of This Medicine

Along with its needed effects, a medicine may cause some unwanted effects. Although not all of these side effects may occur, if they do occur they may need medical attention.

Check with your doctor as soon as possible if any of the following side effects occur:

For bulk-forming–containing

Asthma
Intestinal blockage
Skin rash or itching
Swallowing difficulty (feeling of lump in throat)

For emollient (stool softener)-containing

Skin rash

For hyperosmotic-containing

Confusion
Dizziness or lightheadedness
Irregular heartbeat
Muscle cramps
Unusual tiredness or weakness

For stimulant-containing

Confusion
Irregular heartbeat
Muscle cramps
Pink to red coloration of alkaline urine and stools (for phenolphthalein only)
Pink to red, red to violet, or red to brown coloration of alkaline urine (for cascara, danthron, and/or senna only)
Skin rash
Unusual tiredness or weakness
Yellow to brown coloration of acid urine (for cascara, phenolphthalein, and/or senna only)

Other side effects may occur that usually do not require medical attention. These side effects are less common and may go away during treatment as your body adjusts to the medicine. However, check with your doctor if any of the following side effects continue or are bothersome:

For emollient (stool softener)-containing

Stomach and/or intestinal cramping
Throat irritation (liquid forms only)

For hyperosmotic-containing

Cramping
Diarrhea
Gas
Increased thirst

For lubricant-containing

Skin irritation—surrounding rectal area

For stimulant-containing

Belching
Cramping
Diarrhea
Nausea

Other side effects not listed above may also occur in some patients. If you notice any other effects, check with your doctor.

December 1987

LAXATIVES (Rectal)

This information applies to the following medicines:

Carbon dioxide–releasing laxatives—
  Potassium Bitartrate and Sodium Bicarbonate (SOE-dee-um bye-KAR-boe-nate)
Emollient (stool softener) laxatives—
  Docusate (DOK-yoo-sate)
Hyperosmotic laxatives—
  Glycerin (GLI-ser-in)
  Sodium Phosphates (soe-dee-um FOS-fates)
Lubricant laxatives—
  Mineral Oil
Stimulant laxatives—
  Bisacodyl (bis-a-KOE-dill)
  Senna

Some commonly used brand names are:	Generic names:
Bisco-Lax Clysodrast Dacodyl Deficol Dulcolax Fleet Bisacodyl Fleet Bisacodyl Prep Theralax	Bisacodyl†
Therevac Plus Therevac-SB	Docusate
Fleet Babylax Sani-Supp	Glycerin†
Fleet Mineral Oil	Mineral Oil
Ceo-Two	Potassium Bitartrate and Sodium Bicarbonate
Senokot	Senna
Fleet Enema	Sodium Phosphates

†Generic name product may also be available.

To the Reader: If you do not recognize the names of medical conditions or medicines referred to in this information, check with your doctor, nurse, or pharmacist. Definitions for selected medical terms may be found in the Glossary. Brand names for the generic drug names listed can be found in the Index. In addition, selected brand names commonly associated with the generic name have been included in the text to help you recognize medicine you may be taking. The fact that a brand name product is not mentioned does not mean the information does not apply. It is a good idea for you to learn both the generic and brand names of your medicines and to write them down for future use.

Rectal laxatives are used as enemas or suppositories to produce bowel movements in a short period of time.

There are several different types of rectal laxatives and they work in different ways. Since directions for use are different for each type, it is important to know which one you are taking. The different types of rectal laxatives include:

—Carbon dioxide–releasing
Carbon dioxide–releasing laxatives are suppositories that encourage bowel movements by forming carbon dioxide, a gas. This gas pushes against the intestinal wall, causing contractions that move along the stool mass.

—Emollients (stool softeners)
Emollient laxatives encourage bowel movements by helping liquids mix into the stool and prevent dry, hard stool masses. This type of laxative has been said not to *cause* a bowel movement but instead *allows* the patient to have a bowel movement without straining.

—Hyperosmotic
Hyperosmotic laxatives draw water into the bowel from surrounding body tissues. This provides a soft stool mass and increased bowel action.

—Mineral Oil
Mineral oil coats the bowel and the stool mass with a waterproof film. This keeps moisture in the stool. The stool remains soft and its passage is made easier.

—Stimulants
Stimulant laxatives, also known as contact laxatives, act on the intestinal wall. They increase the muscle contractions that move along the stool mass.

Rectal laxatives may provide relief in a number of situations such as:

—before giving birth.

—for a few days after giving birth.

—preparation for examination or surgery.

—to aid in developing normal bowel function following a period of poor eating habits or a lack of physical exercise (glycerin suppositories only).

—following surgery when straining should be avoided.

—constipation caused by other medicines.

Laxatives should not be given to young children (up to 6 years of age) unless prescribed by their doctor. Since children cannot usually describe their symptoms very well, a doctor should check the child before giving this medicine. This is to prevent an unknown condition from getting worse and to avoid causing unwanted effects in the child.

Some of these laxatives are available only with your doctor's prescription. Others are available without a prescription; however, your doctor may have special instructions for the proper use and dose for your medical condition.

Remember:
• **Keep all medicines out of the reach of children.**

• In order for this medicine to work, it must be used as directed. **If you are using this medicine without a prescription, it is very important to follow the directions on the label.**

• **It is also very important that you read and understand the following information.** If any of the information causes you special concern, check with your doctor before using this medicine without a prescription.

• Before you begin using any new medicine (prescription or nonprescription) or if you develop any new medical problem while you are using this medicine, check with your doctor, nurse, or pharmacist.

• **If you have any questions** about the following information or if you want more information about this medicine or your medical problem, **ask your doctor, nurse, or pharmacist.**

Before Using This Medicine

Importance of diet, fluids, and exercise to prevent constipation—Laxatives are to be used to provide short-term relief only, unless otherwise directed by your doctor. A proper diet containing roughage (whole grain breads and cereals, bran, fruit, and green, leafy vegetables), with 6 to 8 full glasses (8 ounces each) of liquids each day, and daily exercise are most important in maintaining a healthy bowel function. Also, for individuals who have problems with constipation, foods such as pastries, puddings, sugar, candy, cake, and cheese may make the constipation worse.

Before you use this medicine, check with your doctor or pharmacist:

—if you have ever had any unusual or allergic reaction to laxatives.

—if you are on a low-salt, low-sugar, or any other special diet, or if you are allergic to any substance, such as foods, sulfites or other preservatives, or dyes. Most medicines contain more than their active ingredient. Your doctor, nurse, or pharmacist can help you avoid products that may cause a problem.

—if you have any of the following medical problems:
  Appendicitis (or signs of)
  Intestinal blockage
  Laxative habit
  Rectal bleeding of unknown cause

—if you are now taking any of the following medicines or types of medicine:
  Amiloride
  Anticoagulants, coumarin- or indandione-type, oral (blood thinners you take by mouth)
  Contraceptives, oral (birth control pills)
  Digitalis glycosides (heart medicine)
  Laxatives (other)
  Medicine containing potassium
  Spironolactone
  Triamterene
  Vitamin A
  Vitamin D
  Vitamin E
  Vitamin K

Proper Use of This Medicine

For safe and effective use of laxatives:

• Follow your doctor's orders if this laxative was prescribed.

• Follow the manufacturer's package directions if you are treating yourself.

For patients using the enema form of this medicine:

• This medicine usually comes with patient directions. Read them carefully before using this medicine.

• Lubricate anus with petroleum jelly before inserting the enema applicator.

• Gently insert the rectal tip of the enema applicator to prevent damage to the rectal wall.

• Results often may be obtained with:
  —bisacodyl enema in 15 minutes to 1 hour.
  —docusate enema in 2 to 15 minutes.
  —glycerin enema in 15 minutes to 1 hour.
  —mineral oil enema in 2 to 15 minutes.
  —senna enema in 30 minutes, but may not occur for some individuals up to 2 hours.
  —sodium phosphates enema in 2 to 5 minutes.

For patients using the suppository form of this medicine:

• To insert suppository: First remove the foil wrapper and moisten the suppository with water (place under water tap for 30 seconds or in a cup of water for at least 10 seconds). Lie down on side and push the suppository well up into the rectum with finger.

• If the suppository is too soft to insert because of storage in a warm place, before removing the foil wrapper chill the suppository in the refrigerator for 30 minutes or run cold water over it.

• Results often may be obtained with:
  —bisacodyl suppositories in 15 minutes to 1 hour.
  —carbon dioxide–releasing suppositories in 5 to 30 minutes.
  —glycerin suppositories in 15 minutes to 1 hour.
  —senna suppositories in 30 minutes, but may not occur for some individuals up to 2 hours.

How to store this medicine:

• **Keep out of the reach of children.**

• Store away from heat and direct light.

• Do not store in the bathroom, near the kitchen sink, or in other damp places. Heat or moisture may cause the medicine to break down.

• Do not keep outdated medicine or medicine no longer needed. Be sure that any discarded medicine is out of the reach of children.

Precautions While Using This Medicine

Do not use any type of laxative:

—**if you have signs of appendicitis or inflamed bowel** (such as stomach or lower abdominal pain, cramping, bloating, soreness, nausea, or vomiting). Instead, check with your doctor as soon as possible.

—**more often than your doctor prescribed. This is true even when you have had no results from the laxative.**

—**if you do not need it,** as for the common cold, "to clean out your system," or as a "tonic to make you feel better."

—**if you miss a bowel movement for a day or two.**

If you notice a sudden change in bowel habits or function that lasts longer than 2 weeks, or that keeps returning off and on, check with your doctor before using a laxative. This will allow the cause of your problem to be determined before it becomes more serious.

The "laxative habit"—Laxative products are overused by many people. Such a practice often leads to dependence on the laxative action to produce a bowel movement. In severe cases, overuse of some laxatives has caused damage to the nerves, muscles, and tissues of the intestines and bowel. If you have any questions about the use of laxatives, check with your doctor or pharmacist.

For patients using the enema form of this medicine:
• **Check with your doctor if you notice rectal bleeding, blistering, pain, burning, itching, or other sign of irritation not present before you started using this medicine.**

For patients using the suppository form of this medicine:
• Do not lubricate the suppository with mineral oil or petroleum jelly before inserting into the rectum. To do so may affect the way the suppository works. Moisten only with water.

Side Effects of This Medicine

Along with its needed effects, a medicine may cause some unwanted effects. Although not all of these side effects may occur, if they do occur they may need medical attention.

Check with your doctor as soon as possible if any of the following side effects occur:
Less common
   Rectal bleeding, blistering, burning, itching, or pain (with enemas only)

Other side effects may occur that usually do not require medical attention. These side effects may go away during treatment as your body adjusts to the medicine. However, check with your doctor if the following side effect continues or is bothersome:
Less common
   Skin irritation—surrounding rectal area

For children and elderly persons: Weakness, increased sweating, and convulsions may be more likely to occur in children or elderly patients using enemas since these patients are more sensitive to the effects of enemas.

Other side effects not listed above may also occur in some patients. If you notice any other effects, check with your doctor.

_____
December 1987

LEUCOVORIN (Systemic)

A commonly used brand name is Wellcovorin.

Generic name product may also be available in the U.S. and Canada.

To the Reader: If you do not recognize the names of medical conditions or medicines referred to in this information, check with your doctor, nurse, or pharmacist. Definitions for selected medical terms may be found in the Glossary. Brand names for the generic drug names listed can be found in the Index. In addition, selected brand names commonly associated with the generic name have been included in the text to help you recognize medicine you may be taking. The fact that a brand name product is not mentioned does not mean the information does not apply. It is a good idea for you to learn both the generic and brand names of your medicines and to write them down for future use.

Leucovorin (loo-koe-VOR-in) is used as an antidote to the harmful effects of some cancer medicines that are given in high doses. It is used also to prevent or treat certain kinds of anemia. Leucovorin acts the same way in the body as folic acid, which may be low in these patients.

Leucovorin is available only with a prescription and is to be given only by or under the supervision of your doctor.

Remember:

• **This medicine has been prescribed for your current medical problem only.** It must not be given to other people or used for other problems unless you are directed to do so by your doctor.

• **Keep all medicines out of the reach of children.**

• In order for this medicine to work, it must be used as directed.

• If you are receiving this medicine by injection, some of the information about this medicine may not apply.

• **It is very important that you read and understand the following information.** If any of the information causes you special concern, do not decide against using this medicine without first checking with your doctor.

• Before you begin using any new medicine (prescription or nonprescription) or if you develop any new medical problem while you are using this medicine, check with your doctor, nurse, or pharmacist.

• **If you have any questions** about the following information or if you want more information about this medicine or your medical problem, **ask your doctor, nurse, or pharmacist.**

Before Using This Medicine

In order to decide on the best treatment for your medical problem, your doctor should be told:

—if you are on a low-salt, low-sugar, or any other special diet, or if you are allergic to any substance, such as foods, sulfites or other preservatives, or dyes. Most medicines contain more than their active ingredient, and many liquid medicines contain alcohol. Your doctor, nurse, or pharmacist can help you avoid products that may cause a problem.

—if you are **pregnant** or if you may become pregnant. Studies have not been done in either humans or animals.

—if you are **breast-feeding**. It is not known whether leucovorin passes into the breast milk. It has not been shown to cause problems in nursing babies.

—if you have either of the following medical problems:
   Kidney disease
   Nausea and vomiting

—if you are taking **any** other prescription or nonprescription (OTC) medicine.

Proper Use of This Medicine

Leucovorin works best when there is a constant amount in the blood. **To help keep this amount constant, do not miss any doses. Also, it is best to take each dose at evenly spaced times day and night.** For example, if you are to take 4 doses a day, the doses should be spaced about 6 hours apart. If this interferes with your sleep or other daily activities, or if you need help in planning the best times to take your medicine, check with your doctor, nurse, or pharmacist.

Do not stop taking leucovorin without checking with your doctor. It is very important that you get exactly the right amount.

If you miss a dose of leucovorin, **check with your doctor right away.** Your doctor may want you to take extra leucovorin to make up for what you missed. Do not take more medicine on your own, however, since it is very important that you receive just the right dose at the right time.

How to store this medicine:

• **Keep out of the reach of children.**

• Store away from heat and direct light.

• Do not store in the bathroom, near the kitchen sink, or in other damp places. Heat or moisture may cause the medicine to break down.

• Do not keep outdated medicine or medicine no longer needed. Be sure that any discarded medicine is out of the reach of children.

Side Effects of This Medicine

Along with its needed effects, a medicine may cause some unwanted effects. Leucovorin usually does not cause any side effects. However, **check with your doctor immediately** if any of the following side effects occur shortly after you receive this medicine:
   Skin rash, hives, or itching
   Wheezing

For elderly patients: Many medicines have not been tested in older people. Therefore, it is not known whether the medicine acts the same way it does in younger adults. Check with your doctor or pharmacist if you notice any unusual effects while taking this medicine or if you think it is not working as it should.

Other side effects not listed above may also occur in some patients. If you notice any other effects, check with your doctor.

December 1987

LEUPROLIDE (Systemic)

A commonly used brand name is Lupron.

To the Reader: If you do not recognize the names of medical conditions or medicines referred to in this information, check with your doctor, nurse, or pharmacist. Definitions for selected medical terms may be found in the Glossary. Brand names for the generic drug names listed can be found in the Index. In addition, selected brand names commonly associated with the generic name have been included in the text to help you recognize medicine you may be taking. The fact that a brand name product is not mentioned does not mean the information does not apply. It is a good idea for you to learn both the generic and brand names of your medicines and to write them down for future use.

Leuprolide (loo-PROE-lide) is given by injection to treat cancer of the prostate gland.

It is similar to a hormone normally released from the hypothalamus gland. When given regularly, leuprolide decreases testosterone levels. Reducing the amount of testosterone in the body is one way of treating cancer of the prostate.

Leuprolide is available only with your doctor's prescription.

Remember:

• **It is very important that you read and understand the following information.** If any of the information causes you special concern, do not decide against using this medicine without first checking with your doctor.

• Before you begin using any new medicine (prescription or nonprescription) or if you develop any new medical problem while you are using this medicine, check with your doctor, nurse, or pharmacist.

• **If you have any questions** about the following information or if you want more information about this medicine or your medical problem, **ask your doctor, nurse, or pharmacist.**

Before Using This Medicine

In order to decide on the best treatment for your medical problem, your doctor should be told:

—if you have ever had any unusual or allergic reaction to leuprolide.

—if you intend to have children. Leuprolide causes sterility which may be permanent. Be sure that you have discussed this with your doctor before receiving this medicine.

Proper Use of This Medicine

Leuprolide comes with patient directions. Read these instructions carefully.

Use the syringes provided in the kit. Other syringes may not provide the correct dose. These disposable syringes and needles are already sterilized and designed to be used one time only and then discarded. If you have any questions about the use of disposable syringes, check with your doctor, nurse, or pharmacist.

Use this medicine only as directed by your doctor. Do not use more or less of it, and do not use it more often than your doctor ordered. The exact amount of medicine you need has been carefully worked out. Using too much may increase the chance of side effects while using too little may not improve your condition.

Leuprolide sometimes causes unwanted effects such as hot flashes or decreased sexual ability. It may also cause an increase in pain or difficulty in urinating when you begin to use it. However, it is very important that you continue to use the medicine, even after you begin to feel better. **Do not stop using this medicine without first checking with your doctor.**

If you miss a dose of this medicine, give it as soon as possible. However, if you do not remember until the next day, skip the missed dose and go back to your regular dosing schedule. Do not double doses.

How to store this medicine:

• **Keep out of the reach of children.**

• Store away from heat and direct light.

• Keep the medicine from freezing.

• Do not keep outdated medicine or medicine no longer needed. Dispose of used syringes properly in the container provided. Be sure that any discarded medicine is out of the reach of children.

Precautions While Using This Medicine

It is very important that your doctor check your progress at regular visits to make sure that this medicine is working properly and to check for unwanted effects.

Side Effects of This Medicine

Along with its needed effects, a medicine may cause some unwanted effects. Although not all of these side effects may occur, if they do occur they may need medical attention.

The following side effects may be caused by blood clots but occur only rarely. However, they require immediate medical attention. **Get emergency help immediately** if any of the following side effects occur:

Pains in chest, groin, or legs (especially in calves of legs)
Shortness of breath (sudden)

Other side effects may occur that usually do not require medical attention. These side effects may go away during treatment as your body adjusts to the medicine. However, check with your doctor if any of the following side effects continue or are bothersome:

More common

Sudden sweating and feelings of warmth ("hot flashes")

Less common

Blurred vision
Bone pain
Burning, itching, redness, or swelling at place of injection
Constipation
Decrease in sexual desire or impotence
Dizziness

Headache
Loss of appetite
Nausea or vomiting
Numbness or tingling of hands or feet
Swelling and increased tenderness of breasts
Swelling of feet or lower legs

For elderly patients: Many medicines have not been tested in older people. Therefore, it is not known whether the medicine acts the same way it does in younger adults.

Check with your doctor or pharmacist if you notice any unusual effects while receiving this medicine or if you think it is not working as it should.

Other side effects not listed above may also occur in some patients. If you notice any other effects, check with your doctor.

December 1987

LEVOBUNOLOL (Ophthalmic)

A commonly used brand name is Betagan.

To the Reader: If you do not recognize the names of medical conditions or medicines referred to in this information, check with your doctor, nurse, or pharmacist. Definitions for selected medical terms may be found in the Glossary. Brand names for the generic drug names listed can be found in the Index. In addition, selected brand names commonly associated with the generic name have been included in the text to help you recognize medicine you may be taking. The fact that a brand name product is not mentioned does not mean the information does not apply. It is a good idea for you to learn both the generic and brand names of your medicines and to write them down for future use.

Levobunolol (lee-voe-BYOO-noe-lole) is used in the eye to treat certain types of glaucoma. It appears to work by reducing production of fluid in the eye to lower pressure in the eye.

This medicine is available only with your doctor's prescription.

Remember:

• **This medicine has been prescribed for your current medical problem only.** It must not be given to other people or used for other problems unless you are directed to do so by your doctor.

• **Keep all medicines out of the reach of children.**

• In order for this medicine to work, it must be used as directed.

• **It is very important that you read and understand the following information.** If any of the information causes you special concern, do not decide against using this medicine without first checking with your doctor.

• Before you begin using any new medicine (prescription or nonprescription) or if you develop any new medical problem while you are using this medicine, check with your doctor, nurse, or pharmacist.

• **If you have any questions** about the following information or if you want more information about this medicine or your medical problem, **ask your doctor, nurse, or pharmacist.**

Before Using This Medicine

In order to decide on the best treatment for your medical problem, your doctor should be told:

—if you have ever had any unusual or allergic reaction to levobunolol or other beta-blockers (such as acebutolol, atenolol, betaxolol, labetalol, metoprolol, nadolol, oxprenolol, pindolol, propranolol, sotalol, or timolol).

—if you are allergic to any substance, such as certain preservatives. Most medicines contain more than their active ingredient. Your doctor, nurse, or pharmacist can help you avoid products that may cause a problem.

—if you are **pregnant** or if you may become pregnant, since ophthalmic levobunolol may be absorbed into the body. Studies on birth defects have not been done in humans. However, studies in animals have not shown

that levobunolol causes birth defects. Some studies in animals have shown that levobunolol causes harm to the fetus when given in doses many times the recommended human dose for glaucoma.

—if you are **breast-feeding**, since this medicine may be absorbed into the body. However, ophthalmic levobunolol has not been shown to cause problems in nursing babies.

—if you have any of the following medical problems:
Asthma (or history of), chronic bronchitis, emphysema, or other lung disease
Diabetes mellitus (sugar diabetes)
Heart disease
Myasthenia gravis
Overactive thyroid

—if you are taking **any** other prescription or nonprescription (OTC) medicine.

Proper Use of This Medicine

How to apply levobunolol eye drops: First, wash your hands. With the middle finger, apply pressure to the inside corner of the eye (and continue to apply pressure for 1 or 2 minutes after the medicine has been placed in the eye). Tilt the head back and with the index finger of the same hand, pull the lower eyelid away from the eye to form a pouch. Drop the medicine into the pouch and gently close the eyes. Do not blink. Keep the eyes closed for 1 or 2 minutes to allow the medicine to be absorbed.

To prevent contamination of the eye drops, do not touch the applicator tip to any surface (including the eye) and keep the container tightly closed.

Use this medicine only as directed. Do not use more of it and do not use it more often than your doctor ordered. To do so may increase the chance of too much medicine being absorbed into the body and the chance of side effects.

If you miss a dose of this medicine and your dosing schedule is one dose to be applied:

Once a day—Apply the missed dose as soon as possible. However, if you do not remember the missed dose until the next day, skip it and apply your regularly scheduled dose.

More than once a day—Apply the missed dose as soon as possible. However, if it is almost time for your next dose, skip the missed dose and apply your next dose at the regularly scheduled time. Then continue with your regular dosing schedule.

How to store this medicine:

• **Keep out of the reach of children.**

• Store away from heat and direct light.

• Keep the medicine from freezing.

• Do not keep outdated medicine or medicine no longer needed. Be sure that any discarded medicine is out of the reach of children.

Precautions While Using This Medicine

Your doctor should check your eye pressure at regular visits in order to make certain that your glaucoma is being controlled.

Before having any kind of surgery (including dental surgery) or emergency treatment, tell the physician or dentist in charge that you are using this medicine.

Diabetics—**This medicine may cause a change in your blood sugar level. Also, this medicine may cover up signs of hypoglycemia (low blood sugar),** such as increase in pulse rate or increased blood pressure. However, other signs of low blood sugar, such as dizziness and sweating, are not affected. If you have any questions about this, check with your doctor.

Side Effects of This Medicine

In some animal studies, levobunolol has been shown to increase the chance of benign (not cancerous) tumors when taken by mouth in doses many times the recommended human dose for glaucoma. However, it is not known if levobunolol has the same effect in humans when used in the eye in much smaller doses. You should discuss this possible effect with your doctor.

Along with its needed effects, a medicine may cause some unwanted effects. Although not all of these side effects may occur, if they do occur they may need medical attention.

Check with your doctor as soon as possible if any of the following side effects occur:

Rare

    Irritation or inflammation of eye (severe)
    Skin rash, hives, or itching
    Vision disturbances

Signs of too much medicine being absorbed into the body

    Chest pain
    Clumsiness or unsteadiness
    Confusion or mental depression
    Dizziness or feeling faint
    Headache
    Irregular, slow, or pounding heartbeat
    Nausea or vomiting
    Swelling of feet, ankles, or lower legs
    Unusual tiredness or weakness
    Wheezing or troubled breathing

Other side effects may occur that usually do not require medical attention. These side effects may go away during treatment as your body adjusts to the medicine. However, check with your doctor if either of the following side effects continues or is bothersome:

Less common or rare

    Burning or stinging of eye

For elderly patients: Many medicines have not been tested in older people. Therefore, it is not known whether the medicine acts the same way it does in younger adults. Check with your doctor or pharmacist if you notice any unusual effects while using this medicine or if you think it is not working as it should.

Other side effects not listed above may also occur in some patients. If you notice any other effects, check with your doctor.

December 1987

LEVOCARNITINE (Systemic)

Some commonly used brand names are Carnitor and VitaCarn.

To the Reader: If you do not recognize the names of medical conditions or medicines referred to in this information, check with your doctor, nurse, or pharmacist. Definitions for selected medical terms may be found in the Glossary. Brand names for the generic drug names listed can be found in the Index. In addition, selected brand names commonly associated with the generic name have been included in the text to help you recognize medicine you may be taking. The fact that a brand name product is not mentioned does not mean the information does not apply. It is a good idea for you to learn both the generic and brand names of your medicines and to write them down for future use.

Levocarnitine (lee-voe-KAR-ni-teen) is a substance that helps the cells use fat to produce energy needed by the body. It is needed in small amounts only and is usually available in the foods that you eat. Lack of carnitine can lead to liver, heart, and muscle problems. Your doctor may treat lack of carnitine by prescribing levocarnitine for you.

Carnitine comes in two forms. Levocarnitine (L-Carnitine) should not be confused with D,L-carnitine (sold in some health food stores labeled as "vitamin B_T"). Only the L-form of carnitine is used by the body. The D,L-form does not help the body use fat and can actually interfere with and cause a lack of levocarnitine.

Levocarnitine is available only with your doctor's prescription.

Remember:

• **This medicine has been prescribed for your current medical problem only.** It must not be given to other people or used for other problems unless you are directed to do so by your doctor.

• **Keep all medicines out of the reach of children.**

• In order for this medicine to work, it must be used as directed.

• **It is very important that you read and understand the following information.** If any of the information causes you special concern, do not decide against using this medicine without first checking with your doctor.

• Before you begin using any new medicine (prescription or nonprescription) or if you develop any new medical problem while you are using this medicine, check with your doctor, nurse, or pharmacist.

• **If you have any questions** about the following information or if you want more information about this medicine or your medical problem, **ask your doctor, nurse, or pharmacist.**

Before Using This Medicine

In order to decide on the best treatment for your medical problem, your doctor should be told:

—if you have ever had any unusual or allergic reaction to carnitine.

—if you are on a low-salt, low-sugar, or any other special diet, or if you are allergic to any substance, such as foods, sulfites or other preservatives, or dyes. Most medicines contain more than their active ingredient, and many liquid medicines contain alcohol. Your doctor or pharmacist can help you avoid products that may cause a problem.

—if you are **pregnant** or if you may become pregnant. Studies have not been done in humans. However, levocarnitine has not been shown to cause birth defects or other problems in animal studies. Normal healthy fetal growth and development depend on a steady supply of nutrients such as levocarnitine from mother to fetus.

—if you are **breast-feeding**. Levocarnitine has not been shown to cause problems in nursing babies. It normally passes into breast milk, even in women not taking it, because it is obtained from the diet.

—if you are taking **any** other prescription or nonprescription (OTC) medicine, especially valproic acid.

Proper Use of This Medicine

Take levocarnitine with or just after meals. Also, if you are taking it in liquid form, drink it slowly. It will be less likely to upset your stomach if you take it this way.

This medicine is also less likely to cause unwanted effects when there is a constant amount in the blood. If you are taking more than one dose a day, take each dose at evenly spaced times throughout the day. Doses should be spaced at least 3 to 4 hours apart. If you need help in planning the best times to take your medicine, check with your doctor or pharmacist.

If you miss a dose of this medicine, skip the missed dose and go back to your regular dosing schedule. Do not double doses. Taking doses too close together may increase stomach upset.

How to store this medicine:

• **Keep out of the reach of children.**

• Store away from heat and direct light.

• Do not store in the bathroom, near the kitchen sink, or in other damp places. Heat or moisture may cause the medicine to break down.

• Keep the oral solution form of this medicine from freezing. Do not refrigerate.

• Do not keep outdated medicine or medicine that is no longer needed. Be sure any discarded medicine is out of the reach of children.

Side Effects of This Medicine

Along with its needed effects, a medicine may cause some unwanted effects. The following side effects may go away during treatment as your body adjusts to the medicine. However, check with your doctor if any of these effects continue or are bothersome:

More common
  Body odor
  Diarrhea or stomach cramps
  Nausea or vomiting

Other side effects not listed above may also occur in some patients. If you notice any other effects, check with your doctor.

December 1987

LEVODOPA (Systemic)

This information applies to the following medicines:
Carbidopa and Levodopa (KAR-bi-doe-pa and LEE-voe-doe-pa)
Levodopa

Some commonly used brand names are:	Generic names:
Sinemet	Carbidopa and Levodopa
Dopar Larodopa	Levodopa†

†Generic name product may also be available in the U.S.

To the Reader: If you do not recognize the names of medical conditions or medicines referred to in this information, check with your doctor, nurse, or pharmacist. Definitions for selected medical terms may be found in the Glossary. Brand names for the generic drug names listed can be found in the Index. In addition, selected brand names commonly associated with the generic name have been included in the text to help you recognize medicine you may be taking. The fact that a brand name product is not mentioned does not mean the information does not apply. It is a good idea for you to learn both the generic and brand names of your medicines and to write them down for future use.

Levodopa used alone or in combination with carbidopa is used to treat Parkinson's disease, sometimes referred to as shaking palsy or paralysis agitans. Some patients require the combination of medicine, while others benefit from levodopa alone. By improving muscle control, this medicine allows more normal movements of the body.

Levodopa alone or in combination is available only with your doctor's prescription.

Remember:

• **This medicine has been prescribed for your current medical problem only.** It must not be given to other people or used for other problems unless you are directed to do so by your doctor.

• **Keep all medicines out of the reach of children.**

• In order for this medicine to work, it must be used as directed.

• **It is very important that you read and understand the following information.** If any of the information causes you special concern, do not decide against using this medicine without first checking with your doctor.

• Before you begin using any new medicine (prescription or nonprescription) or if you develop any new medical problem while you are using this medicine, check with your doctor, nurse, or pharmacist.

• **If you have any questions** about the following information or if you want more information about this medicine or your medical problem, **ask your doctor, nurse, or pharmacist.**

Before Using This Medicine

In order to decide on the best treatment for your medical problem, your doctor should be told:

—if you have ever had any unusual or allergic reaction to levodopa alone or in combination with carbidopa.

—if you are on a low-salt, low-sugar, or any other special diet, or if you are allergic to any substance, such as foods, sulfites or other preservatives, or dyes.

Most medicines contain more than their active ingredient. Your doctor, nurse, or pharmacist can help you avoid products that may cause a problem.

—if you are **pregnant** or if you may become pregnant. Studies have not been done in humans. However, studies in animals have shown that levodopa affects the baby's growth both before and after birth if given during pregnancy in doses many times the human dose. Also, studies in rabbits have shown that levodopa alone or in combination with carbidopa causes birth defects.

—if you are **breast-feeding**. Levodopa and carbidopa pass into the breast milk and may cause unwanted side effects in the nursing baby. Also, levodopa may reduce the flow of breast milk.

—if you have any of the following medical problems:
Diabetes mellitus (sugar diabetes)
Emphysema, asthma, bronchitis, or other chronic lung disease
Heart or blood vessel disease
Hormone problems
Kidney disease
Liver disease
Mental illness
Seizure disorders, such as epilepsy (history of)
Skin cancer (or history of)
Stomach ulcer (history of)

—if you are now taking any of the following medicines or types of medicine:
Amantadine
Antacids
Antihypertensives (high blood pressure medicine)
Benzodiazepines (alprazolam, chlordiazepoxide, clonazepam, clorazepate, diazepam, flurazepam, halazepam, lorazepam, midazolam, oxazepam, prazepam, temazepam, triazolam)
Benztropine
Beta-blockers (acebutolol, atenolol, labetalol, metoprolol, nadolol, oxprenolol, pindolol, propranolol, sotalol, timolol)
Bromocriptine
Chlorprothixene
Diltiazem
Disopyramide
Diuretics (water pills)
Droperidol
Ethotoin
Haloperidol
Loxapine
Maprotiline
Medicine for asthma or breathing problems (for levodopa used alone)
Medicine for hay fever or other allergies (including nose drops or sprays) (for levodopa used alone)
Mephenytoin
Methyldopa
Metoclopramide
Metyrosine
Molindone
Narcotic pain medicine
Nifedipine
Nitrates (medicine for angina)
Papaverine
Phenothiazines (acetophenazine, chlorpromazine, fluphenazine, mesoridazine, perphenazine, prochlorperazine, promazine, promethazine, thioridazine, trifluoperazine, triflupromazine, trimeprazine)

Phenytoin
Pimozide
Procainamide
Procyclidine
Pyridoxine (vitamin B$_6$), present in some foods and vi-
tamin formulas (for levodopa used alone)
Rauwolfia alkaloids (alseroxylon, deserpidine, rauwolfia
serpentina, reserpine)
Thiothixene
Trazodone
Tricyclic antidepressants (amitriptyline, amoxapine,
clomipramine, desipramine, doxepin, imipramine, nor-
triptyline, protriptyline, trimipramine)
Trihexyphenidyl

—if you are now taking or have taken within the past
2 weeks monoamine oxidase (MAO) inhibitors, such
as:

Furazolidone
Isocarboxazid
Pargyline
Phenelzine
Procarbazine
Tranylcypromine

Proper Use of This Medicine

It is best not to take this medicine with or after food,
especially high-protein food, since food may decrease
levodopa's effect. However, **to lessen possible stomach
upset, take food shortly after taking this medicine (about
15 minutes after).** If stomach upset is severe or continues, check with your doctor.

Take this medicine only as directed. Do not take more or
less of it, and do not take it more often than ordered.

Some people must take this medicine for several weeks
or months before full benefit is received. **Do not stop
taking it even if you do not think it is working.** Instead,
check with your doctor.

If you miss a dose of this medicine, take it as soon as
possible. However, if your next scheduled dose is within
2 hours, skip the missed dose and go back to your
regular dosing schedule. Do not double doses.

How to store this medicine:

• Store away from heat and direct light.

• **Keep out of the reach of children.**

• Do not store the capsule or tablet form of this medicine in the bathroom medicine cabinet because the
heat or moisture may cause the medicine to break
down.

• Do not keep outdated medicine or medicine no longer
needed. Flush the contents of the container down the
toilet, unless otherwise directed.

Precautions While Using This Medicine

Before having any kind of surgery (including dental surgery) or emergency treatment, tell the physician or
dentist in charge that you are taking this medicine.

Diabetics—This medicine may cause test results for urine
sugar or ketones to be wrong. Check with your doctor
before depending on home tests using the paper-strip
or tablet method.

This medicine may cause some people to become drowsy
or less alert than they are normally. **Make sure you
know how you react to this medicine before you drive,
use machines, or do other jobs that require you to be
alert.**

**Dizziness, lightheadedness, or fainting may occur, espe-
cially when you get up from a lying or sitting position.**
Getting up slowly may help. If the problem continues
or gets worse, check with your doctor.

For patients taking levodopa by itself:

• Pyridoxine (vitamin B$_6$) has been found to reduce
the effects of levodopa when taken by itself. This does
not happen with the combination of carbidopa and
levodopa. **If you are taking levodopa by itself, do not
take vitamin products containing vitamin B$_6$ during
treatment, unless prescribed by your doctor.**

• Large amounts of pyridoxine are also contained in
some foods such as avocado, bacon, beans, beef liver,
dry skim milk, oatmeal, peas, pork, sweet potato, tuna,
and certain health foods. Check with your doctor about
how much of these foods you may have in your diet
while you are taking levodopa. Also, ask your doctor
or pharmacist for help when selecting vitamin products.

As your condition improves and your body movements
become easier, **be careful not to overdo physical activities. Injuries resulting from falls may occur.** Physical activities must be gradually increased to allow
your body to adjust to changing balance, circulation,
and coordination. **This is especially important in the
elderly.**

After taking this medicine for long periods of time, such
as a year or more, some patients suddenly lose the
ability to move. Their muscles do not seem to work.
This loss of movement may last from a few minutes
to several hours. The patient then is able to move as
before. This condition may unexpectedly occur again
and again. If you should have this problem, sometimes
called the "on-off" effect, check with your doctor.

Side Effects of This Medicine

Along with its needed effects, a medicine may cause some
unwanted effects. Although not all of these side effects
may occur, if they do occur they may need medical
attention.

Check with your doctor as soon as possible if any of the
following side effects occur:
More common
Mental depression
Mood or mental changes (such as aggressive behavior)
Unusual and uncontrolled movements of the body

Less common—more common when levodopa is used alone
>   Difficult urination
>   Dizziness or lightheadedness when getting up from a lying or sitting position
>   Irregular heartbeat
>   Nausea or vomiting (severe or continuing)
>   Spasm or closing of eyelid (not more common when levodopa is used alone)

Rare
>   High blood pressure
>   Stomach pain
>   Unusual tiredness or weakness

Other side effects may occur that usually do not require medical attention. These side effects may go away during treatment as your body adjusts to the medicine. However, check with your doctor if any of the following side effects continue or are bothersome:

More common
>   Anxiety, confusion, or nervousness (especially in elderly patients receiving other medicine for Parkinson's disease)

Less common
>   Constipation (more common when levodopa is used alone)
>   Diarrhea
>   Dry mouth
>   Flushing of skin

>   Headache
>   Loss of appetite
>   Muscle twitching
>   Nightmares (more common when levodopa is used alone)
>   Tiredness
>   Trouble in sleeping

This medicine may sometimes cause the urine and sweat to be darker in color than usual. The urine may at first be reddish, then turn to nearly black after being exposed to air. Some bathroom cleaning products will produce a similar effect when in contact with urine containing this medicine. This is to be expected during treatment with this medicine.

For elderly patients: The above side effects are more likely to occur in elderly patients, who are usually more sensitive to the effects of levodopa alone or in combination with carbidopa.

Other side effects not listed above may also occur in some patients. If you notice any other effects, check with your doctor.

December 1987

LIDOCAINE
(Systemic—For Self-Injection)

A commonly used brand name is LidoPen.

This information does *not* apply to any other dosage forms or brand names of lidocaine.

To the Reader: If you do not recognize the names of medical conditions or medicines referred to in this information, check with your doctor, nurse, or pharmacist. Definitions for selected medical terms may be found in the Glossary. Brand names for the generic drug names listed can be found in the Index. In addition, selected brand names commonly associated with the generic name have been included in the text to help you recognize medicine you may be taking. The fact that a brand name product is not mentioned does not mean the information does not apply. It is a good idea for you to learn both the generic and brand names of your medicines and to write them down for future use.

Lidocaine (LYE-doe-kane) belongs to the group of medicines called antiarrhythmics. It is given by injection to change an abnormal rhythm in the heart back to normal. Lidocaine produces its helpful effects by slowing abnormal nerve impulses in the heart and reducing irritability of heart tissues.

Lidocaine is usually given by a doctor or nurse when a rapid effect is needed. However, this dosage form has been prescribed by your doctor as part of the early management of a heart attack when certain abnormal heart rhythms occur. It is designed to be used by the patient under instructions from a doctor.

This form of lidocaine is available only with your doctor's prescription and **is to be administered only under direct orders from your doctor**.

Remember:

• **This medicine has been prescribed for your current medical problem only.** It must not be given to other people or used for other problems unless you are directed to do so by your doctor.

• **Keep all medicines out of the reach of children.**

• In order for this medicine to work, it must be used as directed.

• **It is very important that you read and understand the following information.** If any of the information causes you special concern, do not decide against using this medicine without first checking with your doctor.

• Before you begin using any new medicine (prescription or nonprescription) or if you develop any new medical problem while you are using this medicine, check with your doctor, nurse, or pharmacist.

• **If you have any questions** about the following information or if you want more information about this medicine or your medical problem, **ask your doctor, nurse, or pharmacist.**

Before Using This Medicine

In order to decide on the best treatment for your medical problem, your doctor should be told:

—if you have ever had any unusual or allergic reaction to lidocaine, flecainide, tocainide, or anesthetics.

—if you are **pregnant** or if you suspect that you may be pregnant. This medicine has not been shown to cause problems in humans.

—if you are **breast-feeding**. This medicine has not been shown to cause problems in nursing babies.

—if you have either of the following medical problems:
Kidney disease
Liver disease

—if you are taking **any** other prescription or nonprescription (OTC) medicine, especially:
Ethotoin (e.g., Peganone)
Mephenytoin (e.g., Mesantoin)
Phenytoin (e.g., Dilantin)

Proper Use of This Medicine

This medicine should be kept within easy reach, along with your doctor's telephone number. Check the expiration date on the lidocaine regularly. Replace the medicine before it expires.

Be familiar with possible symptoms of a heart attack and how to recognize them. If they occur, **telephone your doctor immediately**. The special device your doctor gave you will transmit your electrocardiogram (ECG or EKG) over the telephone. Your doctor will look at your ECG and tell you whether you need to use this medicine.

Lidocaine comes with patient directions. Read them carefully before you actually need to use this medicine. Then, when an emergency arises, you will know how to inject the lidocaine.

How to use the lidocaine self-injector:

• Remove the gray safety cap.

• Place the black end of the self-injector on the thickest part of your thigh and press hard until the injector functions. You should feel a needle prick.

• Hold the device firmly in place for 10 seconds, then remove it. Massage the injection area for 10 seconds.

Proper storage:

• **Keep out of the reach of children**.

• Store away from heat and direct light.

• Keep the medicine from freezing.

Precautions While Using This Medicine

Do not administer this injection unless instructed to do so by your doctor. Your doctor is trained to read the electrocardiogram and decide whether an arrhythmia is occurring.

© 1988   The United States Pharmacopeial Convention, Inc.

Unless it is absolutely necessary, **do not attempt to drive after using this medicine.** Follow your doctor's instructions about what to do next, including going to the doctor's office or hospital emergency room, if necessary.

Side Effects of This Medicine

Along with its needed effects, a medicine may cause some unwanted effects. Although not all of these side effects may occur, if they do occur they may need medical attention.

Check with your doctor immediately if any of the following side effects occur:

Rare
>   Convulsions (seizures)
>   Difficulty in breathing
>   Itching
>   Skin rash
>   Swelling of skin

Check with your doctor as soon as possible if any of the following side effects occur:

Signs of overdose
>   Blurred or double vision
>   Dizziness (severe) or fainting
>   Nausea or vomiting
>   Ringing in ears
>   Slow heartbeat
>   Tremors or twitching

Other side effects may occur that usually do not require medical attention. However, check with your doctor if the following side effects continue or are bothersome:

Less common or rare
>   Anxiety or nervousness
>   Dizziness
>   Drowsiness
>   Feelings of coldness, heat, or numbness
>   Pain at the place of injection

For elderly patients: The above side effects are more likely to occur in the elderly, who are usually more sensitive to the effects of this medicine.

Other side effects not listed above may also occur in some patients. If you notice any other effects, check with your doctor.

_____

December 1987

_____

LINCOMYCINS (Systemic)

This information applies to the following medicines:

Clindamycin (klin-da-MYE-sin)
Lincomycin (lin-koe-MYE-sin)

Some commonly used brand names are:	Generic names:
Cleocin Dalacin C*	Clindamycin
Lincocin	Lincomycin

*Not available in the U.S.

To the Reader: If you do not recognize the names of medical conditions or medicines referred to in this information, check with your doctor, nurse, or pharmacist. Definitions for selected medical terms may be found in the Glossary. Brand names for the generic drug names listed can be found in the Index. In addition, selected brand names commonly associated with the generic name have been included in the text to help you recognize medicine you may be taking. The fact that a brand name product is not mentioned does not mean the information does not apply. It is a good idea for you to learn both the generic and brand names of your medicines and to write them down for future use.

Lincomycins belong to the family of medicines called antibiotics. They are taken by mouth or given by injection to help the body overcome infections. They will not work for colds, flu, or other virus infections.

Lincomycins are available only with your doctor's prescription.

Remember:
- **This medicine has been prescribed for your present infection only.** Another infection later on may require a different medicine. Also, even though other people may have the same symptoms as you, they may have a different kind of infection. Your medicine may not work for them and may even cause them harm. Therefore, **your medicine must not be given to other people or used for other infections** unless you are otherwise directed by your doctor.

- **Keep all medicines out of the reach of children.**

- In order for this medicine to work, it must be used as directed.

- If you are receiving this medicine by injection, some of the information about this medicine may not apply.

- **It is very important that you read and understand the following information.** If any of the information causes you special concern, do not decide against using this medicine without first checking with your doctor.

- Before you begin using any new medicine (prescription or nonprescription) or if you develop any new medical problem while you are using this medicine, check with your doctor, nurse, or pharmacist.

- **If you have any questions** about the following information or if you want more information about this medicine or your medical problem, **ask your doctor, nurse, or pharmacist.**

Before Using This Medicine

In order to decide on the best treatment for your medical problem, your doctor should be told:
—if you have ever had any unusual or allergic reaction to any of the lincomycins.

—if you are on a low-salt, low-sugar, or any other special diet, or if you are allergic to any substance, such as foods, sulfites or other preservatives, or dyes. Most medicines contain more than their active ingredient, and many liquid medicines contain alcohol. Your doctor, nurse, or pharmacist can help you avoid products that may cause a problem.

—if you are **pregnant** or if you may become pregnant. However, lincomycins have not been shown to cause birth defects or other problems in humans.

—if you are **breast-feeding**. Lincomycins pass into the breast milk. However, lincomycins have not been shown to cause problems in nursing babies.

—if you have any of the following medical problems:
Kidney disease (severe)
Liver disease
Stomach or intestinal disease, history of (especially colitis, including colitis caused by antibiotics, or enteritis)

—if you are taking **any** other prescription or nonprescription (OTC) medicine, especially:
Chloramphenicol (e.g., Chloromycetin)
Diarrhea medicine containing kaolin or attapulgite
Erythromycins

—if you have ever had any problems with this medicine.

Proper Use of This Medicine

For patients taking the capsule form of clindamycin:

- **The capsule form of clindamycin should be taken with a full glass (8 ounces) of water or with meals** to prevent irritation of the esophagus (tube between the throat and stomach).

For patients taking the oral liquid form of clindamycin:

- Use a specially marked measuring spoon or other device to measure each dose accurately since the average household teaspoon may not hold the right amount of liquid.

- Do not use after the expiration date on the label since the medicine may not work as well. Check with your pharmacist if you have any questions about this.

For patients taking lincomycin:

- Lincomycin is best taken with a full glass (8 ounces) of water on an empty stomach (either 1 hour before or 2 hours after meals), unless otherwise directed by your doctor.

To help clear up your infection completely, **keep taking this medicine for the full time of treatment** even if you begin to feel better after a few days. **If you have a "strep" infection, you should keep taking this medicine for at least 10 days. This is especially important in "strep" infections since serious heart problems could**

develop later if your infection is not cleared up completely. Also, if you stop taking this medicine too soon, your symptoms may return.

This medicine works best when there is a constant amount in the blood. **To help keep the amount constant, do not miss any doses. Also, it is best to take each dose at evenly spaced times day and night.** For example, if you are to take 4 doses a day, each dose should be spaced about 6 hours apart. If this interferes with your sleep or other daily activities, or if you need help in planning the best times to take your medicine, check with your doctor, nurse, or pharmacist.

If you do miss a dose of this medicine, take it as soon as possible. This will help to keep a constant amount of medicine in the blood. However, if it is almost time for your next dose and your dosing schedule is:

• 3 or more doses a day—Space the missed dose and the next dose 2 to 4 hours apart or double your next dose.

Then go back to your regular dosing schedule.

How to store this medicine:

• **Keep out of the reach of children.**

• Store away from heat and direct light.

• Do not store the capsule form of this medicine in the bathroom, near the kitchen sink, or in other damp places. Heat or moisture may cause the medicine to break down.

• Do not refrigerate the oral liquid form of clindamycin. If chilled, the liquid may thicken and be difficult to pour. Follow the directions on the label.

• Do not keep outdated medicine or medicine no longer needed. Be sure that any discarded medicine is out of the reach of children.

Precautions While Using This Medicine

It is important that your doctor check your progress at regular visits.

If your symptoms do not improve within a few days, or if they become worse, check with your doctor.

In some patients, lincomycins may cause diarrhea.

• For severe diarrhea, check with your doctor as soon as possible since this could be a sign of a serious side effect. Do not take any diarrhea medicine without first checking with your doctor since these medicines could make your diarrhea worse or make it last longer.

• For mild diarrhea, diarrhea medicine containing kaolin or attapulgite may be taken. However, kaolin or attapulgite may keep lincomycins from being absorbed into the body. Therefore, these diarrhea medicines should be taken at least 2 hours before or 3 to 4 hours after you take lincomycins by mouth. Other types of diarrhea medicine should not be taken since they could make your diarrhea worse or make it last longer.

If you have any questions about this or if mild diarrhea continues or gets worse, check with your doctor or pharmacist.

Before having surgery (including dental surgery) with a general anesthetic, tell the physician or dentist in charge that you are taking a lincomycin.

Side Effects of This Medicine

Along with its needed effects, a medicine may cause some unwanted effects. Although not all of these side effects may occur, if they do occur they may need medical attention.

Check with your doctor immediately if any of the following side effects occur:

More common
    Abdominal or stomach cramps, pain, and bloating (severe)
    Diarrhea (watery and severe), which may also be bloody
    Fever
    Increased thirst
    Increased weight loss
    Nausea or vomiting
    Unusual tiredness or weakness
        (the above side effects may also occur up to several weeks after you stop taking this medicine)

Other side effects may occur which usually do not require medical attention. These side effects may go away during treatment as your body adjusts to the medicine. However, check with your doctor if any of the following side effects continue or are bothersome:

More common
    Diarrhea (mild)
    Skin rash
Less common
    Itching of skin, rectal, or genital (sex organ) areas

For elderly patients: Many medicines have not been tested in older people. Therefore, it is not known whether the medicine acts the same way it does in younger adults. Check with your doctor or pharmacist if you notice any unusual effects while taking this medicine or if you think it is not working as it should.

Other side effects not listed above may also occur in some patients. If you notice any other effects, check with your doctor.

December 1987

LINDANE (Topical)

Some commonly used brand names are:

gBh*	Kwellada*
G-well	Kwildane
Kwell	Scabene

Generic name product may also be available in the U.S.

*Not available in the U.S.

To the Reader: If you do not recognize the names of medical conditions or medicines referred to in this information, check with your doctor, nurse, or pharmacist. Definitions for selected medical terms may be found in the Glossary. Brand names for the generic drug names listed can be found in the Index. In addition, selected brand names commonly associated with the generic name have been included in the text to help you recognize medicine you may be taking. The fact that a brand name product is not mentioned does not mean the information does not apply. It is a good idea for you to learn both the generic and brand names of your medicines and to write them down for future use.

Lindane (LIN-dane), formerly known as gamma benzene hexachloride, is applied to the skin or scalp to treat scabies and lice infections.

Lindane cream and lotion are used to treat only scabies infection. Lindane shampoo is used to treat only lice infections.

This medicine is available only with your doctor's prescription.

Remember:

• **This medicine has been prescribed for your current medical problem only.** It must not be given to other people or used for other problems unless you are directed to do so by your doctor.

• **Keep all medicines out of the reach of children.**

• In order for this medicine to work, it must be used as directed.

• **It is very important that you read and understand the following information.** If any of the information causes you special concern, do not decide against using this medicine without first checking with your doctor.

• Before you begin using any new medicine (prescription or nonprescription) or if you develop any new medical problem while you are using this medicine, check with your doctor, nurse, or pharmacist.

• **If you have any questions** about the following information or if you want more information about this medicine or your medical problem, **ask your doctor, nurse, or pharmacist.**

Before Using This Medicine

In order to decide on the best treatment for your medical problem, your doctor should be told:

—if you have ever had any unusual or allergic reaction to lindane.

—if you are allergic to any substance, such as certain preservatives or dyes. Most medicines contain more than their active ingredient. Your doctor, nurse, or pharmacist can help you avoid products that may cause a problem.

—if you are **pregnant** or if you may become pregnant, since lindane is absorbed through the skin and may cause toxic effects on the central nervous system (CNS) of the unborn baby.

—if you are **breast-feeding**, since this medicine is absorbed through the skin and is present in small amounts in breast milk. Even though lindane has not been shown to cause problems in nursing babies, your doctor may want you to use another method of feeding your baby for 2 days after you use lindane.

—if you have any seizure disorder.

—if you have a skin rash or raw or broken skin.

—if you are taking **any** other prescription or nonprescription (OTC) medicine.

Proper Use of This Medicine

Lindane is a poisonous medicine. Keep it away from the mouth because it is harmful if swallowed.

Use this medicine only as directed by your doctor. Do not use more of it, do not use it more often, and do not use it for a longer period of time than your doctor ordered. To do so may increase the chance of absorption through the skin and the chance of lindane poisoning.

Keep this medicine away from the eyes. If you should accidentally get some in your eyes, flush them thoroughly with water at once.

Do not use this medicine on open wounds such as scratches, cuts, or sores on the skin or scalp. To do so may increase the chance of lindane poisoning.

When applying lindane to another person, you should wear plastic disposable or rubber gloves. This will prevent the medicine from being absorbed through your skin. If you have any questions about this, check with your doctor.

This medicine usually comes with patient directions. Read them carefully before using this medicine.

For patients using the cream or lotion form of this medicine for scabies:

• If your skin has any cream, lotion, ointment, or oil on it, wash, rinse, and dry your skin well before applying this medicine.

• If you take a warm bath or shower before using this medicine, dry and cool the skin well before applying this medicine.

• Apply enough medicine to your dry skin to cover the entire skin surface from the neck down, including the soles of your feet, and rub in well. Adults and older children do not need to treat their heads, since scabies does not affect this area. However, if this medicine is being applied to an infant, ask your doctor if the medicine should be applied to the infant's head also.

• Leave the medicine on for no more than 8 to 12 hours, then remove by washing thoroughly.

• Put on freshly washed or dry-cleaned clothing to prevent reinfection.

For patients using the shampoo form of this medicine for lice:

• If your hair has an oil-based hair dressing on it, shampoo, rinse, and dry your hair and scalp well before applying this medicine.

• If you apply this shampoo in the shower or in the bathtub, make sure the shampoo is not allowed to run down on other parts of your body. Also, do not apply this shampoo in a bathtub where the shampoo may run into the bath water in which you are sitting. To do so may increase the chance of absorption through the skin. When you rinse out the shampoo, be sure to thoroughly rinse your entire body also to remove any shampoo that may have gotten on it.

• Apply enough shampoo to your dry hair (1 ounce for short hair, 1½ ounces for medium length hair, and 2 ounces for long hair) to thoroughly wet the hair and skin or scalp of the affected and surrounding hairy areas.

• Thoroughly rub the shampoo into the hair and skin or scalp and allow to remain in place for 4 minutes. Then, use just enough water to work up a good lather.

• Rinse thoroughly and dry with a clean towel.

• When the hair is dry, comb with a fine-toothed comb to remove any remaining nits (eggs) or nit shells.

• This shampoo may also be used to wash combs and brushes to prevent spread of the infection.

• Do not use as a regular shampoo.

For patients using this medicine for pubic (crab) lice or scabies: Your sexual partner, especially, and all members of your household may need to be treated also, since the infection may spread to persons in close contact. If these persons are not being treated or if you have any questions about this, check with your doctor.

How to store this medicine:

• **Keep out of the reach of children.**

• Store away from heat and direct light.

• Keep the medicine from freezing.

• Do not keep outdated medicine or medicine no longer needed. Be sure that any discarded medicine is out of the reach of children.

Precautions While Using This Medicine

To prevent reinfection or spreading of the infection to other people, all recently worn clothing and used bed linens and towels should be washed in very hot water or dry-cleaned.

Side Effects of This Medicine

In infants and children, the risk of lindane being absorbed through the skin and causing unwanted side effects is greater than in adults. In premature newborn infants, use of lindane is not recommended because this medicine may be more likely to be absorbed through their skin than through the skin of older infants. You should discuss these possible effects with your doctor.

Along with its needed effects, a medicine may cause some unwanted effects. Although not all of these side effects may occur, if they do occur they may need medical attention.

Check with your doctor as soon as possible if any of the following side effects occur:

Rare

    Skin irritation not present before using this medicine

    Skin rash

Signs of lindane poisoning

    Convulsions (seizures)

    Dizziness, clumsiness, or unsteadiness

    Fast heartbeat

    Muscle cramps

    Nervousness, restlessness, or irritability

    Vomiting

After you stop using this medicine, itching may occur and continue for 1 to several weeks. If this continues longer or is bothersome, check with your doctor.

For elderly patients: Many medicines have not been tested in older people. Therefore, it is not known whether the medicine acts the same way it does in younger adults. Check with your doctor or pharmacist if you notice any unusual effects while using this medicine or if you think it is not working as it should.

Other side effects not listed above may also occur in some patients. If you notice any other effects, check with your doctor.

December 1987

LITHIUM (Systemic)

Some commonly used brand names are:

Carbolith*	Lithane
Cibalith-S	Lithizine*
Duralith*	Lithobid
Eskalith	Lithonate
Eskalith CR	Lithotabs

Generic name product may also be available.

---

*Not available in the U.S.

To the Reader: If you do not recognize the names of medical conditions or medicines referred to in this information, check with your doctor, nurse, or pharmacist. Definitions for selected medical terms may be found in the Glossary. Brand names for the generic drug names listed can be found in the Index. In addition, selected brand names commonly associated with the generic name have been included in the text to help you recognize medicine you may be taking. The fact that a brand name product is not mentioned does not mean the information does not apply. It is a good idea for you to learn both the generic and brand names of your medicines and to write them down for future use.

Lithium (LITH-ee-um) is taken by mouth to treat the manic stage of manic-depressive illness. Manic-depressive patients experience severe mood changes, ranging from an excited or manic state (for example, unusual anger or a false sense of well-being) to depression or sadness. Lithium is also used to reduce the frequency and severity of manic states. Lithium may also reduce the frequency and severity of depression in manic-depressive illness.

The way lithium works to affect a person's mood is not known. However, it does act on the central nervous system. It helps you to have more stable emotions and to be better able to cope with the problems of living.

It is important that you and your family understand all the effects of lithium. These effects depend on your individual condition and response and the amount of lithium you use. You also must know when to contact your doctor if there are problems with the medicine's use. Lithium may also be used for other conditions as determined by your doctor.

This medicine is available only with your doctor's prescription.

Remember:

• **This medicine has been prescribed for your current medical problem only.** It must not be given to other people or used for other problems unless you are directed to do so by your doctor.

• **Keep all medicines out of the reach of children.**

• In order for this medicine to work, it must be used as directed.

• **It is very important that you read and understand the following information.** If any of the information causes you special concern, do not decide against using this medicine without first checking with your doctor.

• Before you begin using any new medicine (prescription or nonprescription) or if you develop any new medical problem while you are using this medicine, check with your doctor, nurse, or pharmacist.

• **If you have any questions** about the following information or if you want more information about this medicine or your medical problem, **ask your doctor, nurse, or pharmacist**.

Before Using This Medicine

In order to decide on the best treatment for your medical problem, your doctor should be told:

—if you have ever had any unusual or allergic reaction to lithium.

—if you are on a low-salt, low-sugar, or any other special diet, or if you are allergic to any substance, such as foods, sulfites or other preservatives, or dyes. Most medicines contain more than their active ingredient. Your doctor, nurse, or pharmacist can help you avoid products that may cause a problem.

—if you are **pregnant** or if you may become pregnant. Lithium is not recommended for use during pregnancy, especially during the first three months. Studies have shown that lithium may cause thyroid problems and heart or blood vessel defects in the baby. It has also been shown to cause muscle weakness and severe drowsiness in newborn babies of mothers taking lithium near time of delivery.

—if you are **breast-feeding**. Lithium passes into the breast milk. It has been reported to cause unwanted effects such as muscle weakness, lowered body temperature, and heart problems in nursing babies. Before taking this medicine, be sure you have discussed with your doctor the risks and benefits of breast-feeding.

—if you have any of the following medical problems:
Brain disease
Diabetes mellitus (sugar diabetes)
Difficult urination
Epilepsy
Heart disease
Infection (severe)
Kidney disease
Parkinson's disease
Schizophrenia
Thyroid disease

—if you are taking **any** other prescription or nonprescription (OTC) medicine, especially:
Antithyroid agents (medicine for overactive thyroid)
Diuretics (water pills)
Haloperidol (e.g., Haldol)
Medicine for inflammation or pain (aspirin or other salicylates, diclofenac, diflunisal, fenoprofen, flurbiprofen, ibuprofen, indomethacin, ketoprofen, meclofenamate, mefenamic acid, naproxen, phenylbutazone, piroxicam, sulindac, suprofen, tolmetin)
Molindone (e.g., Moban)

—if you are now taking medicine for asthma, bronchitis, emphysema, sinusitis, or cystic fibrosis that contains the following:
Calcium iodide–containing preparations
Iodinated glycerol
Potassium iodide

—if you drink large amounts of caffeine-containing beverages, such as coffee, tea, or some colas.

—if you are on a low-salt diet.

Proper Use of This Medicine

For patients taking the long-acting form of lithium:

- Swallow the tablets whole.
- Do not break, crush, or chew the tablets before swallowing.

While taking this medicine, drink 2 or 3 quarts of water or other fluids each day, and use a normal amount of salt in your food, unless otherwise directed by your doctor.

Take this medicine exactly as directed. Do not take more of it, do not take it more often, and do not take it for a longer period of time than your doctor ordered. To do so may increase the chance of unwanted effects.

Sometimes lithium must be taken for 1 to several weeks before you begin to feel better.

In order for lithium to work properly, it must be taken every day in regularly spaced doses as ordered by your doctor. This is necessary to keep a constant amount of lithium in your blood. To help keep the amount constant, do not miss any doses and do not stop taking the medicine even if you feel better.

If you do miss a dose of this medicine, take it as soon as possible. However, if it is within 2 hours (6 hours for extended-release tablets) of your next dose, skip the missed dose and go back to your regular dosing schedule. Do not double doses.

How to store this medicine:

- **Keep out of the reach of children.**
- Store away from heat and direct light.
- Do not store in the bathroom, near the kitchen sink, or in other damp places. Heat or moisture may cause the medicine to break down.
- Keep the syrup form of this medicine from freezing.
- Do not keep outdated medicine or medicine no longer needed. Be sure that any discarded medicine is out of the reach of children.

Precautions While Using This Medicine

Your doctor should check your progress at regular visits to make sure that the medicine is working properly and that possible side effects are avoided. Laboratory tests may be necessary.

Lithium may not work as well as it should if you drink large amounts of caffeine-containing coffee, tea, or colas. Check with your doctor before drinking large amounts of these beverages.

This medicine may cause some people to become dizzy, drowsy, or less alert than they are normally. **Make sure you know how you react to this medicine before you drive, use machines, or do other jobs that require you to be alert.**

Use extra care in hot weather and during activities that cause you to sweat heavily, such as hot baths, saunas, or exercising. The loss of too much water and salt from your body may lead to serious side effects from this medicine.

If you have an infection or illness that causes heavy sweating, vomiting, or diarrhea, check with your doctor. The loss of too much water and salt from your body may lead to serious side effects from lithium.

Do not go on a diet to lose weight without first checking with your doctor. Improper dieting may cause the loss of too much water and salt from your body and may lead to serious side effects from this medicine.

It is important that you and your family know the early signs of lithium overdose and when to call the doctor.

Side Effects of This Medicine

Along with its needed effects, a medicine may cause some unwanted effects. Although not all of these side effects may occur, if they do occur they may need medical attention.

Check with your doctor immediately if any of the following side effects occur:

Early signs of overdose

  Diarrhea
  Drowsiness
  Loss of appetite
  Muscle weakness
  Nausea or vomiting
  Slurred speech
  Trembling

Late signs of overdose

  Blurred vision
  Clumsiness or unsteadiness
  Confusion
  Convulsions (seizures)
  Dizziness
  Increase in amount of urine
  Trembling (severe)

Check with your doctor as soon as possible if any of the following side effects occur:

Less common

  Fainting
  Fast heartbeat
  Irregular pulse
  Troubled breathing (especially during hard work or exercise)
  Unusual tiredness or weakness
  Weight gain

Rare

  Blue color and pain in fingers and toes
  Coldness of arms and legs
  Dizziness
  Eye pain
  Headache
  Noises in the ears
  Vision problems

Signs of low thyroid function
  Dry, rough skin
  Hair loss
  Hoarseness
  Sensitivity to cold
  Swelling of feet or lower legs
  Swelling of neck

Other side effects may occur that usually do not require medical attention. These side effects may go away during treatment as your body adjusts to the medicine. However, check with your doctor if any of the following side effects continue or are bothersome:

More common
  Increased frequency of urination
  Increased thirst
  Nausea (mild)
  Trembling of hands (slight)

Less common
  Acne or skin rash
  Bloated feeling or pressure in the stomach
  Muscle twitching (slight)

For elderly patients: The above side effects, especially the signs of overdose and low thyroid function, are more likely to occur in the elderly, who are usually more sensitive to the effects of lithium.

Other side effects not listed above may also occur in some patients. If you notice any other effects, check with your doctor.

_____

December 1987

LOMUSTINE (Systemic)

Some commonly used brand names and other names are CeeNU and CCNU.

To the Reader: If you do not recognize the names of medical conditions or medicines referred to in this information, check with your doctor, nurse, or pharmacist. Definitions for selected medical terms may be found in the Glossary. Brand names for the generic drug names listed can be found in the Index. In addition, selected brand names commonly associated with the generic name have been included in the text to help you recognize medicine you may be taking. The fact that a brand name product is not mentioned does not mean the information does not apply. It is a good idea for you to learn both the generic and brand names of your medicines and to write them down for future use.

Lomustine (loe-MUS-teen) belongs to the group of medicines known as alkylating agents. It is taken by mouth to treat some kinds of cancer.

Lomustine interferes with the growth of cancer cells, which are eventually destroyed. Since the growth of normal body cells may also be affected by lomustine, other effects will also occur. Some of these may be serious and must be reported to your doctor. Other effects, like hair loss, may not be serious but may cause concern. Some effects may not occur for months or years after the medicine is used.

Before you begin treatment with lomustine, you and your doctor should talk about the good this medicine will do as well as the risks of using it.

Lomustine is available only with your doctor's prescription.

Remember:

• **This medicine has been prescribed for your current medical problem only.** It must not be given to other people or used for other problems unless you are directed to do so by your doctor.

• **Keep all medicines out of the reach of children.**

• In order for this medicine to work, it must be used as directed.

• **It is very important that you read and understand the following information.** If any of the information causes you special concern, do not decide against using this medicine without first checking with your doctor.

• Before you begin using any new medicine (prescription or nonprescription) or if you develop any new medical problem while you are using this medicine, check with your doctor, nurse, or pharmacist.

• **If you have any questions** about the following information or if you want more information about this medicine or your medical problem, **ask your doctor, nurse, or pharmacist.**

Before Using This Medicine

In order to decide on the best treatment for your medical problem, your doctor should be told:

—if you have ever had any unusual or allergic reaction to lomustine.

—if you are **pregnant** or if you intend to have children. There is a chance that this medicine may cause birth defects if either the male or female is taking it at the time of conception or if it is taken during pregnancy. Lomustine causes birth defects in rats and causes toxic or harmful effects in the fetus of rats and rabbits at doses about the same as the human dose. In addition, many cancer medicines may cause sterility which could be permanent. This has been reported in animals and humans with this medicine, and the possibility should be kept in mind. Be sure that you have discussed this with your doctor before taking this medicine.

—if you intend to **breast-feed**. Because this medicine may cause serious side effects, breast-feeding is generally not recommended while you are receiving it.

—if you have any of the following medical problems:
Chickenpox (including recent exposure)
Herpes zoster (shingles)
Infection
Kidney disease

—if you are taking **any** other prescription or nonprescription (OTC) medicine, especially:
Amphotericin B by injection (e.g., Fungizone)
Antithyroid agents (medicine for overactive thyroid)
Azathioprine (e.g., Imuran)
Chloramphenicol (e.g., Chloromycetin)
Colchicine
Flucytosine (e.g., Ancobon)
Interferon (e.g., Intron A; Roferon-A)

—if you ever have been treated with x-rays or cancer medicines.

Proper Use of This Medicine

Take this medicine only as directed by your doctor. Do not take more or less of it than your doctor ordered. The exact amount of medicine you need has been carefully worked out. Taking too much may increase the chance of side effects, while taking too little may not improve your condition.

In order that you receive the proper dose of lomustine, there may be two or more different types of capsules in the container. This is not an error. It is important that you take all of the capsules in the container as one dose so that you receive the right dose of the medicine.

This medicine is sometimes given together with certain other medicines. If you are using a combination of medicines, make sure that you take each one at the right time and do not mix them. Ask your doctor, nurse, or pharmacist to help you plan a way to remember to take your medicines at the right times.

Nausea and vomiting occur often after lomustine is taken, but usually last less than 24 hours. Loss of appetite may last for several days. This medicine is best taken on an empty stomach at bedtime so that it will cause less stomach upset. Ask your doctor, nurse, or pharmacist for other ways to lessen these effects.

If you vomit shortly after taking a dose of lomustine, check with your doctor. You may be told to take the dose again.

Precautions While Using This Medicine

It is important that your doctor check your progress at regular visits to make sure that this medicine is working properly and to check for unwanted effects.

While you are being treated with lomustine, and after you stop treatment with it, **do not have any immunizations without your doctor's approval.** Lomustine lowers your body's resistance and there is a chance you might get the infection the immunization is meant to prevent. In addition, other persons living in your household should not take oral polio vaccine since there is a chance they could pass the polio virus on to you. Also, you should avoid close contact with other persons (for example, at school or work) who have taken oral polio vaccine.

Lomustine can lower the number of white blood cells in your body. This may increase the chance of getting an infection. If you can, avoid people with colds or other infections. If you think you are getting a cold or other infection, check with your doctor.

Side Effects of This Medicine

Along with their needed effects, medicines like lomustine can sometimes cause unwanted effects such as blood problems, loss of hair, and other side effects; these are described below. Also, because of the way these medicines act on the body, there is a chance that they might cause other unwanted effects that may not occur until months or years after the medicine is used. These delayed effects may include certain types of cancer, such as leukemia. Discuss these possible effects with your doctor.

Although not all of these side effects may occur, if they do occur they may need medical attention.

Check with your doctor immediately if any of the following side effects occur:

More common
   Fever, chills, or sore throat
   Unusual bleeding or bruising

Check with your doctor as soon as possible if any of the following side effects occur:

Less common
   Awkwardness
   Confusion
   Decrease in urination

   Slurred speech
   Sores in the mouth and on the lips
   Swelling of feet or lower legs
   Unusual tiredness or weakness

Rare
   Cough
   Shortness of breath
   Yellow eyes and skin

Other side effects may occur that usually do not require medical attention. These side effects may go away during treatment as your body adjusts to the medicine. Also, your doctor or nurse may be able to tell you about ways to prevent or reduce some of these side effects. Check with your doctor if any of the following side effects continue or are bothersome or if you have any questions about them:

More common
   Loss of appetite
   Nausea and vomiting (usually last less than 24 hours)

Less common
   Darkening of skin
   Diarrhea
   Skin rash and itching

This medicine may cause a temporary loss of hair in some people. After treatment with lomustine has ended, normal hair growth should return.

For elderly patients: Many medicines have not been tested in older people. Therefore, it is not known whether the medicine acts the same way it does in younger adults. Check with your doctor or pharmacist if you notice any unusual effects while taking this medicine or if you think it is not working as it should.

After you stop using this medicine, it may still produce some side effects that need attention. During this period of time, check with your doctor if you notice any of the following side effects:

   Fever, chills, or sore throat
   Unusual bleeding or bruising

Other side effects not listed above may also occur in some patients. If you notice any other effects, check with your doctor.

December 1987

LOPERAMIDE (Oral)

A commonly used brand name is Imodium.

To the Reader: If you do not recognize the names of medical conditions or medicines referred to in this information, check with your doctor, nurse, or pharmacist. Definitions for selected medical terms may be found in the Glossary. Brand names for the generic drug names listed can be found in the Index. In addition, selected brand names commonly associated with the generic name have been included in the text to help you recognize medicine you may be taking. The fact that a brand name product is not mentioned does not mean the information does not apply. It is a good idea for you to learn both the generic and brand names of your medicines and to write them down for future use.

Loperamide (loe-PER-a-mide) is a medicine used along with other measures to treat severe diarrhea.

In babies and children and in persons over 60 years of age, the fluid loss caused by diarrhea may result in a severe condition. These persons should not take any anti-diarrhea medicine unless prescribed by their doctor.

Loperamide is available only with your doctor's prescription.

Remember:
• **This medicine has been prescribed for your current medical problem only.** It must not be given to other people or used for other problems unless you are directed to do so by your doctor.

• **Keep all medicines out of the reach of children.**

• In order for this medicine to work, it must be used as directed.

• **It is very important that you read and understand the following information.** If any of the information causes you special concern, do not decide against using this medicine without first checking with your doctor.

• Before you begin using any new medicine (prescription or nonprescription) or if you develop any new medical problem while you are using this medicine, check with your doctor, nurse, or pharmacist.

• **If you have any questions** about the following information or if you want more information about this medicine or your medical problem, **ask your doctor, nurse, or pharmacist.**

Before Using This Medicine

In order to decide on the best treatment for your medical problem, your doctor should be told:

—if you have ever had any unusual or allergic reaction to loperamide.

—if you are on a low-salt, low-sugar, or any other special diet, or if you are allergic to any substance, such as foods, sulfites or other preservatives, or dyes. Most medicines contain more than their active ingredient. Your doctor, nurse, or pharmacist can help you avoid products that may cause a problem.

—if you are **pregnant** or if you may become pregnant. Studies have not been done in humans. However, studies in animals have not shown that loperamide causes cancer or birth defects or lessens the chances of becoming pregnant when given in doses many times the human dose.

—if you are **breast-feeding**. Loperamide has not been shown to cause problems in nursing babies.

—if you have either of the following medical problems:
Colitis (severe)
Liver disease

—if you are taking **any** other prescription or nonprescription (OTC) medicine, especially narcotic pain medicine.

—if you are now taking an antibiotic. Some antibiotics may cause diarrhea. This medicine may make the diarrhea caused by antibiotics worse or make it last longer.

Proper Use of This Medicine

Take this medicine only as directed by your doctor. Do not take more of it, do not take it more often, and do not take it for a longer period of time than your doctor ordered. To do so may increase the chance of side effects.

If you must take this medicine regularly and you miss a dose, skip the missed dose and go back to your regular dosing schedule. Do not double doses.

How to store this medicine:
• Store away from heat and direct light.
• **Keep out of the reach of children**
• Do not store the capsule form of this medicine in the bathroom medicine cabinet because the heat or moisture may cause the medicine to break down.
• Keep the liquid form of this medicine from freezing.
• Do not keep outdated medicine or medicine no longer needed. Flush the contents of the container down the toilet, unless otherwise directed.

Precautions While Using This Medicine

If you will be taking this medicine regularly for a long period of time, your doctor should check your progress at regular visits.

Check with your doctor if your diarrhea doesn't stop after a few days or if you develop a fever.

Side Effects of This Medicine

Along with its needed effects, a medicine may cause some unwanted effects. **When this medicine is used for short periods of time at low doses, side effects usually are rare,** and they may go away during treatment as your body adjusts to the medicine.

Check with your doctor as soon as possible if any of the following side effects continue, worsen, or are bothersome:

Rare
  Bloating
  Constipation
  Dizziness
  Drowsiness
  Dry mouth
  Fever
  Loss of appetite

  Nausea and vomiting
  Skin rash
  Stomach pain

Other side effects not listed above may also occur in some patients. If you notice any other effects, check with your doctor.

December 1987

LOXAPINE (Systemic)

Some commonly used brand names are:

Loxapac*	Loxitane C
Loxitane	Loxitane IM

*Not available in the U.S.

To the Reader: If you do not recognize the names of medical conditions or medicines referred to in this information, check with your doctor, nurse, or pharmacist. Definitions for selected medical terms may be found in the Glossary. Brand names for the generic drug names listed can be found in the Index. In addition, selected brand names commonly associated with the generic name have been included in the text to help you recognize medicine you may be taking. The fact that a brand name product is not mentioned does not mean the information does not apply. It is a good idea for you to learn both the generic and brand names of your medicines and to write them down for future use.

Loxapine (LOX-a-peen) is used to treat nervous, mental, and emotional conditions. It is taken by mouth as a tablet, capsule, or liquid and sometimes is given by injection.

Loxapine is available only with your doctor's prescription.

Remember:

• **This medicine has been prescribed for your current medical problem only.** It must not be given to other people or used for other problems unless you are directed to do so by your doctor.

• **Keep all medicines out of the reach of children.**

• In order for this medicine to work, it must be used as directed.

• If you are receiving this medicine by injection, some of the information about this medicine may not apply.

• **It is very important that you read and understand the following information.** If any of the information causes you special concern, do not decide against using this medicine without first checking with your doctor.

• Before you begin using any new medicine (prescription or nonprescription) or if you develop any new medical problem while you are using this medicine, check with your doctor, nurse, or pharmacist.

• **If you have any questions** about the following information or if you want more information about this medicine or your medical problem, **ask your doctor, nurse, or pharmacist.**

Before Using This Medicine

In order to decide on the best treatment for your medical problem, your doctor should be told:

—if you have ever had any unusual or allergic reaction to loxapine or amoxapine.

—if you are on a low-salt, low-sugar, or any other special diet, or if you are allergic to any substance, such as foods, sulfites or other preservatives, or dyes.

Most medicines contain more than their active ingredient, and many liquid medicines contain alcohol. Your doctor, nurse, or pharmacist can help you avoid products that may cause a problem.

—if you are **pregnant** or if you may become pregnant. Loxapine has not been shown to cause birth defects or other problems in humans. However, animal studies have shown unwanted effects in the fetus.

—if you are **breast-feeding**. It is not known if loxapine passes into breast milk. This medicine has not been shown to cause problems in nursing babies.

—if you have any of the following medical problems:
Enlarged prostate
Glaucoma (or predisposition to)
Heart or blood vessel disease
Liver disease
Parkinson's disease
Seizure disorders
Difficult urination

—if you are taking **any** other prescription or nonprescription (OTC) medicine, especially:
Amoxapine (e.g., Asendin)
Central nervous system (CNS) depressants
Chlorprothixene (e.g., Taractan)
Epinephrine (e.g., Adrenalin)
Guanadrel (e.g., Hylorel)
Guanethidine (e.g., Ismelin)
Haloperidol (e.g., Haldol)
Methyldopa (e.g., Aldomet)
Metoclopramide (e.g., Reglan)
Metyrosine (e.g., Demser)
Molindone (e.g., Moban)
Pemoline (e.g., Cylert)
Phenothiazines (acetophenazine, chlorpromazine, fluphenazine, mesoridazine, perphenazine, prochlorperazine, promazine, promethazine, thioridazine, trifluoperazine, triflupromazine, trimeprazine)
Pimozide (e.g., Orap)
Rauwolfia alkaloids (alseroxylon, deserpidine, rauwolfia serpentina, reserpine)
Thiothixene (e.g., Navane)

Proper Use of This Medicine

This medicine may be taken with food or a full glass (8 ounces) of water or milk to reduce stomach irritation.

For patients taking the oral solution:
• Measure the solution only with the dropper provided by the manufacturer. This will give a more accurate dose.

The liquid medicine must be mixed with orange juice or grapefruit juice just before you take it to make it easier to take.

Do not take more of this medicine, do not take it more often, and do not take it for a longer time than your doctor ordered. To do so may increase the chance of unwanted effects.

If you miss a dose of this medicine, take it as soon as possible. However, if it is within one hour of your next dose, skip the missed dose and go back to your regular dosing schedule. Do not double doses.

How to store this medicine:

- **Keep out of the reach of children.**

- Store away from heat and direct light.

- Do not store the capsule or tablet form of this medicine in the bathroom, near the kitchen sink, or in other damp places. Heat or moisture may cause the medicine to break down.

- Keep the liquid form of this medicine from freezing.

- Do not keep outdated medicine or medicine no longer needed. Be sure that any discarded medicine is out of the reach of children.

Precautions While Using This Medicine

Your doctor should check your progress at regular visits, especially for the first few months you take this medicine. The amount of loxapine you take may be changed often to meet the needs of your condition and to help avoid side effects.

This medicine will add to the effects of alcohol and other CNS depressants (medicines that slow down the nervous system, possibly causing drowsiness). Some examples of CNS depressants are antihistamines or medicine for hay fever, other allergies, or colds; sedatives, tranquilizers, or sleeping medicine; prescription pain medicine or narcotics; barbiturates; medicine for seizures; or anesthetics, including some dental anesthetics. **Check with your doctor before taking any of the above while you are taking this medicine.**

Do not take this medicine within an hour or two of taking antacids or medicine for diarrhea. Taking them too close together may make this medicine less effective.

This medicine may cause some people to become drowsy or less alert than they are normally, especially as the amount of medicine is increased. Even if you take this medicine at bedtime, you may feel drowsy or less alert on arising. **Make sure you know how you react to this medicine before you drive, use machines, or do other jobs that require you to be alert.**

Although not a problem for most patients, dizziness, lightheadedness, or fainting may occur, especially when you get up from a lying or sitting position. Getting up slowly may help. However, if the problem continues or gets worse, check with your doctor.

A few people who take this medicine may become more sensitive to sunlight than they are normally. When you first begin taking this medicine, use sunscreen lotions or avoid too much sun or too much use of a sunlamp until you see how you react. If you have a severe reaction, check with your doctor.

Loxapine may cause dryness of the mouth. For temporary relief, use sugarless candy or gum, melt bits of ice in your mouth, or use a saliva substitute. However, if dry mouth continues for more than 2 weeks, check with

your physician or dentist. Continuing dryness of the mouth may increase the chance of dental disease, including tooth decay, gum disease, and fungal infections.

Before having any kind of surgery, dental treatment, or emergency treatment, tell the physician or dentist in charge that you are taking this medicine.

Do not suddenly stop taking this medicine without first checking with your doctor. Your doctor may want you to reduce gradually the amount you are taking before stopping completely. This will allow your body time to adjust and helps to avoid a worsening of your medical condition.

Side Effects of This Medicine

Along with its needed effects, a medicine may cause some unwanted effects. Although not all of these side effects may occur, if they do occur they may need medical attention.

Stop taking loxapine and get emergency help immediately if any of the following side effects occur:

Rare

    Convulsions (seizures)
    Difficult or unusually fast breathing
    Fast heartbeat or irregular pulse
    Fever (high)
    Increased sweating
    Loss of bladder control
    Muscle stiffness (severe)
    Unusual feeling of tiredness or weakness
    Unusually pale skin

Check with your doctor as soon as possible if any of the following side effects occur:

More common (occurring with increase of dosage)

    Difficulty in speaking or swallowing
    Loss of balance control
    Mask-like face
    Restlessness or desire to keep moving
    Shuffling walk
    Slowed movements
    Stiffness of arms and legs
    Trembling and shaking of fingers and hands

Less common

    Chewing movements
    Constipation (severe)
    Difficult urination
    Fixation of the eyes
    Lip smacking or puckering
    Muscle spasms, especially of the neck and back
    Puffing of cheeks
    Rapid or worm-like movements of tongue
    Skin rash
    Twisting movements of the body
    Uncontrolled movements of the arms and legs

Rare

    Sore throat and fever
    Yellow eyes or skin

Signs of overdose
   Dizziness (severe)
   Drowsiness (severe)
   Muscle trembling, jerking, stiffness, or uncontrolled
      movements (severe)
   Troubled breathing (severe)
   Unusual tiredness or weakness (severe)

Other side effects may occur that usually do not require
   medical attention. These side effects may go away
   during treatment as your body adjusts to the medicine.
   However, check with your doctor if any of the following side effects continue or are bothersome:

More common
   Blurred vision
   Confusion
   Dizziness, lightheadedness, or fainting
   Drowsiness
   Dry mouth

Less common
   Constipation (mild)
   Decreased sexual ability
   Enlargement of breasts (males and females)
   Headache
   Increased sensitivity of skin to sun
   Missing menstrual periods
   Nausea or vomiting
   Trouble in sleeping
   Unusual secretion of milk
   Weight gain

Certain side effects of this medicine may occur after you
   have stopped taking it. Check with your doctor as soon
   as possible if you notice any of the following effects
   after you have stopped taking loxapine:

   Chewing movements
   Dizziness
   Nausea and vomiting
   Puffing of cheeks
   Rapid or worm-like movements of the tongue
   Stomach upset or pain
   Trembling of fingers and hands

For elderly patients: The above side effects are more
   likely to occur in elderly patients, who are usually more
   sensitive to the effects of loxapine.

Other side effects not listed above may also occur in some
   patients. If you notice any other effects, check with
   your doctor.

_____

December 1987

LYPRESSIN (Systemic)

A commonly used brand name is Diapid.

To the Reader: If you do not recognize the names of medical conditions or medicines referred to in this information, check with your doctor, nurse, or pharmacist. Definitions for selected medical terms may be found in the Glossary. Brand names for the generic drug names listed can be found in the Index. In addition, selected brand names commonly associated with the generic name have been included in the text to help you recognize medicine you may be taking. The fact that a brand name product is not mentioned does not mean the information does not apply. It is a good idea for you to learn both the generic and brand names of your medicines and to write them down for future use.

Lypressin (lye-PRESS-in) is a hormone used as a nose spray to prevent or control the frequent urination, increased thirst, and loss of water associated with diabetes insipidus (water diabetes).

Lypressin is available only with your doctor's prescription.

Remember:

• **This medicine has been prescribed for your current medical problem only.** It must not be given to other people or used for other problems unless you are directed to do so by your doctor.

• **Keep all medicines out of the reach of children.**

• In order for this medicine to work, it must be used as directed.

• **It is very important that you read and understand the following information.** If any of the information causes you special concern, do not decide against using this medicine without first checking with your doctor.

• Before you begin using any new medicine (prescription or nonprescription) or if you develop any new medical problem while you are using this medicine, check with your doctor, nurse, or pharmacist.

• **If you have any questions** about the following information or if you want more information about this medicine or your medical problem, **ask your doctor, nurse, or pharmacist.**

Before Using This Medicine

In order to decide on the best treatment for your medical problem, your doctor should be told:

—if you have ever had any unusual or allergic reaction to lypressin or vasopressin.

—if you are allergic to any substance, such as certain preservatives or dyes. Most medicines contain more than their active ingredient. Your doctor, nurse, or pharmacist can help you avoid products that may cause a problem.

—if you are **pregnant** or if you may become pregnant. Lypressin has not been shown to cause birth defects or other problems in humans.

—if you are **breast-feeding**. Lypressin has not been shown to cause problems in nursing babies.

—if you have any of the following medical problems:

Hay fever or other allergies
High blood pressure
Infection of ears, lungs, nose, or throat
Stuffy nose

—if you are taking **any** other prescription or nonprescription (OTC) medicine.

Proper Use of This Medicine

Use this medicine only as directed. Do not use more of it and do not use it more often than your doctor ordered. To do so may increase the chance of unwanted effects.

How to use: Blow nose gently. Hold the bottle in an upright position. With head upright, spray the medicine into each nostril by squeezing the bottle quickly and firmly. Do not lie down when spraying this medicine.

Rinse the tip of the bottle with hot water, taking care not to suck water into the bottle, and dry with a clean tissue. Replace the cap right after use.

If you miss a dose of this medicine, use it as soon as possible. However, if it is almost time for your next dose, skip the missed dose and go back to your regular dosing schedule. Do not double doses.

How to store this medicine:

• **Keep out of the reach of children.**

• Store away from heat and direct light.

• Do not store in the bathroom, near the kitchen sink, or in other damp places. Heat or moisture may cause the medicine to break down.

• Keep the medicine from freezing.

• Do not keep outdated medicine or medicine no longer needed. Be sure that any discarded medicine is out of the reach of children.

Side Effects of This Medicine

Along with its needed effects, a medicine may cause some unwanted effects. Although not all of these effects may occur, if they do occur they may need medical attention.

Check with your doctor as soon as possible if any of the following side effects occur:

Rare

Cough (continuing)
Feeling of tightness in chest
Shortness of breath or troubled breathing

Other side effects may occur that usually do not require medical attention. These side effects may go away during treatment as your body adjusts to the medicine.

However, check with your doctor if any of the following side effects continue or are bothersome:

Less common or rare

    Abdominal or stomach cramps
    Headache
    Heartburn
    Increased bowel movements
    Irritation or pain in the eye
    Itching, irritation, or sores inside the nose
    Runny or stuffy nose

For elderly patients: Many medicines have not been tested in older people. Therefore, it is not known whether the medicine acts the same way it does in younger adults. Check with your doctor or pharmacist if you notice any unusual effects while taking this medicine or if you think it is not working as it should.

Other side effects not listed above may also occur in some patients. If you notice any other effects, check with your doctor.

December 1987

MALATHION (Topical)*

Some commonly used brand names are Derbac* and Prioderm*.

*Not commercially available in the U.S. or Canada.

To the Reader: If you do not recognize the names of medical conditions or medicines referred to in this information, check with your doctor, nurse, or pharmacist. Definitions for selected medical terms may be found in the Glossary. Brand names for the generic drug names listed can be found in the Index. In addition, selected brand names commonly associated with the generic name have been included in the text to help you recognize medicine you may be taking. The fact that a brand name product is not mentioned does not mean the information does not apply. It is a good idea for you to learn both the generic and brand names of your medicines and to write them down for future use.

Malathion (mal-a-THYE-on) belongs to the group of medicines known as pediculicides (medicines that destroy lice).

Malathion is applied to the hair and scalp to treat head lice infections. It acts by destroying both the lice and their eggs.

This medicine is available only with your doctor's prescription.

Remember:

• **This medicine has been prescribed for your current medical problem only.** It must not be given to other people or used for other problems unless you are directed to do so by your doctor.

• **Keep all medicines out of the reach of children.**

• In order for this medicine to work, it must be used as directed.

• **It is very important that you read and understand the following information.** If any of the information causes you special concern, do not decide against using this medicine without first checking with your doctor.

• Before you begin using any new medicine (prescription or nonprescription) or if you develop any new medical problem while you are using this medicine, check with your doctor, nurse, or pharmacist.

• **If you have any questions** about the following information or if you want more information about this medicine or your medical problem, **ask your doctor, nurse, or pharmacist.**

Before Using This Medicine

In order to decide on the best treatment for your medical problem, your doctor should be told:

—if you have ever had any unusual or allergic reaction to malathion.

—if you are allergic to any substance, such as certain preservatives or dyes. Most medicines contain more than their active ingredient, and many liquid medicines contain alcohol. Your doctor, nurse, or pharmacist can help you avoid products that may cause a problem.

—if you are **pregnant** or if you may become pregnant, since malathion may be absorbed through the skin. Studies have not been done in humans. However, malathion has not been shown to cause birth defects or other problems in animal studies.

—if you are **breast-feeding**, since malathion may be absorbed through the skin. However, it is not known whether malathion passes into the breast milk and this medicine has not been shown to cause problems in nursing babies.

—if you have any of the following medical problems:
 Anemia (severe)
 Asthma
 Epilepsy or other seizure disorder
 Heart disease
 Liver disease
 Malnutrition
 Myasthenia gravis or other neuromuscular disease
 Parkinson's disease
 Stomach ulcer or other stomach or intestinal problems

—if you have recently had brain surgery.

—if you are taking **any** other prescription or nonprescription (OTC) medicine, especially antimyasthenics (ambenonium, neostigmine, pyridostigmine).

—if you are now using demecarium, echothiophate, or isoflurophate eye medicine.

Proper Use of This Medicine

Malathion is a poisonous medicine. Keep it away from the mouth because it is harmful if swallowed.

Use this medicine only as directed by your doctor. Do not use more of it, do not use it more often, and do not use it for a longer period of time than your doctor ordered. To do so may increase the chance of absorption through the skin and the chance of malathion poisoning.

Apply malathion by sprinkling on the hair and rubbing in until the hair and scalp are thoroughly moistened.

Allow the hair to dry naturally. Use no heat (as from a hair dryer) and leave the hair uncovered.

After the medicine has been allowed to remain on the hair and scalp for 8 to 12 hours, **wash the hair with a nonmedicated shampoo and then rinse thoroughly**.

After rinsing, use a fine-toothed comb to remove the dead lice and eggs from the hair.

Immediately after using this medicine, wash your hands to remove any medicine that may be on them.

Keep this medicine away from the eyes. If you should accidentally get some in your eyes, flush them thoroughly with water at once.

This medicine is flammable. Do not use near heat, near open flame, or while smoking.

Head lice can be easily transferred from one person to another by direct contact with clothing, hats, scarves, bedding, towels, washcloths, hairbrushes and combs, or hairs from infected persons. Therefore, **all household members of your family should be examined for head lice and receive treatment if they are found to be infected.** If you have any questions about this, check with your doctor.

How to store this medicine:

- **Keep out of the reach of children.**

- Store away from heat and direct light.

- Keep the medicine from freezing.

- Do not keep outdated medicine or medicine no longer needed. Be sure that any discarded medicine is out of the reach of children.

Precautions While Using This Medicine

To prevent reinfection or the spreading of the infection to other people, good health habits are also required. These include the following:

- Wash all clothing, bedding, towels, and washcloths in very hot water or dry clean them.
- Wash all hairbrushes and combs in very hot soapy water and do not share them with other people.
- Clean the house or room by thorough vacuuming.

If you have any questions about this, check with your doctor.

Breathing in even small amounts of carbamate- or organophosphate-type insecticides or pesticides (for example, carbaryl [Sevin], demeton [Systox], diazinon, malathion, parathion, ronnel [Trolene]) may add to the effects of this medicine. Farmers, gardeners, residents of communities undergoing insecticide or pesticide spraying or dusting, workers in plants manufacturing such products, or other persons exposed to such poisons should protect themselves by wearing a mask over the nose and mouth, changing clothes frequently, and washing hands often while using this medicine.

Side Effects of This Medicine

Along with its needed effects, a medicine may cause some unwanted effects. Although not all of these side effects may occur, if they do occur they may need medical attention.

Check with your doctor as soon as possible if any of the following side effects occur:

Rare

   Skin rash

When malathion is applied to the skin in recommended doses, signs of poisoning have not been reported. However, the chance may exist, especially if the skin is broken. *Signs of malathion poisoning* include:

   Abdominal or stomach cramps
   Anxiety or restlessness
   Clumsiness or unsteadiness
   Confusion or mental depression
   Convulsions (seizures)
   Diarrhea
   Difficult or labored breathing
   Dizziness
   Drowsiness
   Increase in sweating
   Increase in watering of mouth or eyes
   Loss of bowel or bladder control
   Muscle twitching of eyelids, face, and neck
   Pinpoint pupils
   Slow heartbeat
   Trembling
   Unusual weakness

Other side effects may occur that usually do not require medical attention. These side effects may go away during treatment as your body adjusts to the medicine. However, check with your doctor if the following side effect continues or is bothersome:

Less common or rare

   Stinging or irritation of scalp

For elderly patients: Many medicines have not been tested in older people. Therefore, it is not known whether the medicine acts the same way it does in younger adults. Check with your doctor or pharmacist if you notice any unusual effects while using this medicine or if you think it is not working as it should.

Other side effects not listed above may also occur in some patients. If you notice any other effects, check with your doctor.

_____

December 1987

MAPROTILINE (Systemic)

A commonly used brand name is Ludiomil.

To the Reader: If you do not recognize the names of medical conditions or medicines referred to in this information, check with your doctor, nurse, or pharmacist. Definitions for selected medical terms may be found in the Glossary. Brand names for the generic drug names listed can be found in the Index. In addition, selected brand names commonly associated with the generic name have been included in the text to help you recognize medicine you may be taking. The fact that a brand name product is not mentioned does not mean the information does not apply. It is a good idea for you to learn both the generic and brand names of your medicines and to write them down for future use.

Maprotiline (ma-PROE-ti-leen) belongs to the group of medicines known as tetracyclic antidepressants or "mood elevators." It is used to relieve mental depression, including anxiety that sometimes occurs with depression.

Maprotiline is available only with your doctor's prescription.

Remember:

• **This medicine has been prescribed for your current medical problem only.** It must not be given to other people or used for other problems unless you are directed to do so by your doctor.

• **Keep all medicines out of the reach of children.**

• In order for this medicine to work, it must be used as directed.

• **It is very important that you read and understand the following information.** If any of the information causes you special concern, do not decide against using this medicine without first checking with your doctor.

• Before you begin using any new medicine (prescription or nonprescription) or if you develop any new medical problem while you are using this medicine, check with your doctor, nurse, or pharmacist.

• **If you have any questions** about the following information or if you want more information about this medicine or your medical problem, **ask your doctor, nurse, or pharmacist.**

Before Using This Medicine

In order to decide on the best treatment for your medical problem, your doctor should be told:

—if you have ever had any unusual or allergic reaction to maprotiline or tricyclic antidepressants.

—if you are on a low-salt, low-sugar, or any other special diet, or if you are allergic to any substance, such as foods, sulfites or other preservatives, or dyes. Most medicines contain more than their active ingredient. Your doctor, nurse, or pharmacist can help you avoid products that may cause a problem.

—if you are **pregnant** or if you may become pregnant. Studies have not been done in humans. Maprotiline has not been shown to cause birth defects or other problems in animal studies.

—if you are **breast-feeding**. Maprotiline passes into the breast milk. However, this medicine has not been shown to cause problems in humans.

—if you have any of the following medical problems:

    Asthma
    Difficult urination
    Enlarged prostate
    Glaucoma
    Heart or blood vessel disease
    Liver disease
    Mental illness (severe)
    Overactive thyroid
    Seizure disorders (including epilepsy)
    Stomach or intestinal problems

—if you are taking **any** other prescription or nonprescription (OTC) medicine, especially:

    Amphetamines
    Appetite suppressants (diet pills)
    Central nervous system (CNS) depressants
    Medicine for asthma or other breathing problems
    Medicine for colds, sinus problems, or hay fever or other allergies (including nose drops or sprays)

Proper Use of This Medicine

Take this medicine only as directed by your doctor in order to improve your condition as much as possible.

Sometimes this medicine must be taken for up to two or three weeks before you begin to feel better.

If you miss a dose of this medicine and your dosing schedule is:

More than one dose a day—Take the missed dose as soon as possible. Then go back to your regular dosing schedule. However, if it is almost time for your next dose, skip the missed dose and go back to your regular dosing schedule. Do not double doses.

One dose a day at bedtime—Do not take the missed dose in the morning since it may cause disturbing side effects during waking hours. Instead, check with your doctor.

How to store this medicine:

• **Keep out of the reach of children.**

• Store away from heat and direct light.

• Do not store in the bathroom, near the kitchen sink, or in other damp places. Heat or moisture may cause the medicine to break down.

• Do not keep outdated medicine or medicine no longer needed. Be sure that any discarded medicine is out of the reach of children.

Precautions While Using This Medicine

It is very important that your doctor check your progress at regular visits. This will allow your dosage to be changed if necessary.

Do not stop taking this medicine without first checking with your doctor. Your doctor may want you to reduce gradually the amount you are taking before stopping completely. This will allow your body to adjust properly and will reduce the possibility of unwanted effects.

Before having any kind of surgery, dental treatment, or emergency treatment, tell the physician or dentist in charge that you are using this medicine.

This medicine will add to the effects of alcohol and other medicines (CNS depressants) that slow down the nervous system. Some examples of CNS depressants are antihistamines or medicine for hay fever, other allergies, or colds; sedatives, tranquilizers, or sleeping medicine; prescription pain medicine or narcotics; barbiturates; medicine for seizures; or anesthetics, including some dental anesthetics. **Check with your doctor before taking any of the above while you are using this medicine.**

Do not take any other medicine, unless prescribed or approved by your doctor. This especially includes over-the-counter (OTC) or nonprescription medicine such as that for colds, cough, asthma, hay fever, or appetite control.

This medicine may cause some people to become drowsy or less alert than they are normally. **Make sure you know how you react to this medicine before you drive, use machines, or do other jobs that require you to be alert.**

Dizziness, lightheadedness, or fainting may occur, especially when you get up from a lying or sitting position. Getting up slowly may help. If this problem continues or gets worse, check with your doctor.

Maprotiline may cause dryness of the mouth. For temporary relief, use sugarless gum or candy, melt bits of ice in your mouth, or use a saliva substitute. However, if dry mouth continues for more than 2 weeks, check with your physician or dentist. Continuing dryness of the mouth may increase the chance of dental disease, including tooth decay, gum disease, and fungal infections.

Side Effects of This Medicine

Along with its needed effects, a medicine may cause some unwanted effects. Although not all of these side effects may occur, if they do occur they may need medical attention.

Check with your doctor as soon as possible if any of the following side effects occur:

Less common
  Constipation (severe)
  Convulsions (seizures)
  Nausea or vomiting
  Shakiness or trembling
  Unusual excitement

Rare
  Confusion (especially in the elderly)
  Difficulty in urinating
  Fainting
  Hallucinations (seeing, hearing, or feeling things that are not there)
  Irregular heartbeat (pounding, racing, skipping)
  Sore throat and fever
  Yellow eyes or skin

Signs of overdose
  Convulsions (seizures)
  Dizziness (severe)
  Drowsiness (severe)
  Fast or irregular heartbeat
  Fever
  Muscle stiffness or weakness (severe)
  Restlessness or agitation
  Vomiting

Other side effects may occur that usually do not require medical attention. These side effects may go away during treatment as your body adjusts to the medicine. However, check with your doctor if any of the following side effects continue or are bothersome:

More common
  Blurred vision
  Dizziness or lightheadedness (especially in the elderly)
  Drowsiness
  Dry mouth
  Headache
  Skin rash or itching
  Trouble in sleeping
  Unusual tiredness or weakness

Less common
  Constipation (mild)
  Diarrhea
  Heartburn
  Increased sensitivity of skin to sunlight
  Increase in sweating

For elderly patients: The above side effects, especially drowsiness, dizziness, confusion, vision problems, dry mouth, constipation, and problems in urinating are more likely to occur in elderly patients, who are usually more sensitive to the effects of maprotiline.

After you stop taking this medicine, your body will need time to adjust. This usually takes about 3 to 7 days. Continue to follow the precautions listed above during this period of time.

Other side effects not listed above may also occur in some patients. If you notice any other effects, check with your doctor.

December 1987

MEASLES VIRUS VACCINE LIVE
(Systemic)

A commonly used brand name is Attenuvax.

To the Reader: If you do not recognize the names of medical conditions or medicines referred to in this information, check with your doctor, nurse, or pharmacist. Definitions for selected medical terms may be found in the Glossary. Brand names for the generic drug names listed can be found in the Index. In addition, selected brand names commonly associated with the generic name have been included in the text to help you recognize medicine you may be taking. The fact that a brand name product is not mentioned does not mean the information does not apply. It is a good idea for you to learn both the generic and brand names of your medicines and to write them down for future use.

Measles (MEE-zills) Virus Vaccine Live is an immunizing agent given by injection to prevent infection by the measles virus. It works by causing your body to produce its own protection (antibodies) against the virus.

Different types of measles vaccines may be available in countries other than the U.S. The following information applies only to the Enders' attenuated Edmonston strain of measles vaccine.

Measles (also known as coughing measles, hard measles, morbilli, red measles, rubeola, and ten-day measles) is an infection that is easily spread from one person to another. Infection with measles can cause serious problems such as pneumonia, severe ear infections, seizures, brain damage, and possibly death. Except for young infants, the risk of serious complications and death is greater in adults than in children.

Although immunization against measles is recommended for everyone born in or after 1957, it is especially important for:

—all children 15 months of age and older, including school-age children, children of pregnant women who have not yet received their own measles vaccination, and children who have chronic diseases such as cystic fibrosis, heart disease, or asthma.

—women of child-bearing age who are not pregnant.

—persons exposed to measles within the past 72 hours.

—persons vaccinated during the years 1963 through 1967 with either the inactivated (killed) measles vaccine or with an unknown type of measles vaccine.

—persons vaccinated in the past with measles vaccine along with immune globulin.

—employees in medical facilities and persons in colleges, orphanages, and the military.

—persons traveling outside the U.S.

Immunization against measles is not recommended for infants younger than 12 months of age unless the risk of getting a measles infection is high. This is because antibodies they received from the mother before birth may interfere with the effectiveness of the vaccine. Children who were immunized against measles before 12 months of age should be immunized again.

You can be considered to be immune to measles only if you received measles vaccine on or after your first birthday and you have the medical record to prove it, if you have a doctor's diagnosis of a previous measles infection, or if you have had a blood test showing immunity to measles.

Since vaccination with measles vaccine may not provide protection for everyone, you may want to ask your doctor to check your immunity to the measles virus 4 or more weeks following your vaccination. This may be especially important if you plan to travel overseas or if you are a woman of child-bearing age who intends to become pregnant in the future.

This vaccine is available only from your doctor or other authorized health care provider.

Remember:

• **It is very important that you read and understand the following information.** If any of the information causes you special concern, do not decide against receiving this vaccine without first checking with your doctor.

• **If you have any questions** about the following information or if you want more information about this vaccine, **ask your doctor, nurse, or pharmacist.**

Before Receiving This Vaccine

Before you receive measles vaccine, your doctor should be told:

—if you have ever had any unusual or allergic reaction to any form of the antibiotic neomycin. The measles vaccine available in the U.S. contains neomycin; products available in other countries may contain neomycin, streptomycin, or other antibiotics.

—if you have ever had any unusual or allergic reaction to eggs. The measles vaccine available in the U.S. is grown in a chick embryo cell culture.

—if you are **pregnant** or if you may become pregnant within 3 months after receiving this medicine. Although studies have not been done in humans and problems have not been shown to occur, use during pregnancy is not recommended. Since the natural measles infection has been shown to increase the chance of birth defects and other problems, it is thought that the live virus vaccine might also cause similar problems.

—if you are **breast-feeding**, although measles vaccine has not been shown to cause problems in nursing babies.

—if you have any of the following medical problems:
    Brain or head injury
    Convulsions (seizures) due to fever (history of)
    Fever
    Immune deficiency condition (or family history of)
    Tuberculosis

—if you are taking **any** other prescription or nonprescription (OTC) medicine.

—if you have received any other live virus vaccines in the last month or intend to within the next month.

—if you have received any of the following types of products in the last 3 months or intend to within the next 2 weeks:
    Blood transfusions or other blood products
    Gamma globulin or other globulins

—if you have ever been treated with x-rays or cancer medicines.

Precautions After Receiving This Vaccine

Do not become pregnant for 3 months after receiving measles vaccine without first checking with your doctor. There is a chance that this vaccine may cause birth defects.

Tell your doctor that you have received this vaccine:

—if you are to receive blood transfusions or other blood products within 2 weeks after receiving this vaccine.

—if you are to receive gamma globulin or other globulins within 2 weeks after receiving this vaccine.

—if you are to receive any other live virus vaccines within 1 month after receiving this vaccine.

—if you are to receive a tuberculin skin test within 6 weeks after receiving this medicine. The results of the test may be affected by this vaccine.

Side Effects of This Vaccine

Along with its needed effects, a vaccine may cause some unwanted effects. Although not all of these side effects may occur, if they do occur they may need medical attention.

Get emergency help immediately if any of the following side effects occur:

Signs of allergic reaction
Difficulty in breathing or swallowing
Hives
Itching, especially of feet or hands
Reddening of skin, especially around ears
Swelling of eyes, face, or inside of nose
Unusual tiredness or weakness (sudden and severe)

Check with your doctor as soon as possible if any of the following side effects occur:

More common
Fever over 103 °F (39.4 °C)

Rare
Bruising or purple spots on skin
Confusion
Convulsions (seizures)
Double vision
Headache (severe or continuing)
Irritability
Stiff neck
Vomiting

Other side effects may occur that usually do not require medical attention. However, check with your doctor if any of the following side effects continue or are bothersome:

More common
Burning or stinging at the place of injection
Fever of 100 °F (37.7 °C) or less

Less common
Fever between 100 and 103 °F (37.7 and 39.4 °C)
Itching, swelling, redness, tenderness, or hard lump at place of injection
Skin rash

Fever and skin rash may occur from 5 to 12 days after vaccination and usually last 1 or 2 days.

Some side effects, such as fever over 103 °F (39.4 °C) or swelling, blistering, or pain at site of injection, may be more frequent, more severe, or last longer in persons who received inactivated (killed) measles vaccine (available in the U.S. from 1963 to 1967 and in Canada until 1970). If any of these side/adverse effects occur, check with your doctor as soon as possible.

Other side effects not listed above may also occur in some patients. If you notice any other effects, check with your doctor.

December 1987

MEBENDAZOLE (Systemic)

Some commonly used brand names are:

Mebendacin*	Sirben*
Mebutar*	Vermirax*
Nemasole*	Vermox
Pantelmin*	

*Not available in the U.S.

To the Reader: If you do not recognize the names of medical conditions or medicines referred to in this information, check with your doctor, nurse, or pharmacist. Definitions for selected medical terms may be found in the Glossary. Brand names for the generic drug names listed can be found in the Index. In addition, selected brand names commonly associated with the generic name have been included in the text to help you recognize medicine you may be taking. The fact that a brand name product is not mentioned does not mean the information does not apply. It is a good idea for you to learn both the generic and brand names of your medicines and to write them down for future use.

Mebendazole (me-BEN-da-zole) belongs to the family of medicines called anthelmintics (ant-hel-MIN-tiks). Anthelmintics are medicines used in the treatment of worm infections.

Mebendazole is taken by mouth to treat:

—common roundworms (ascariasis);
—hookworms (uncinariasis);
—pinworms (enterobiasis; oxyuriasis);
—whipworms (trichuriasis); and
—more than one worm infection at a time.

This medicine may also be used for other worm infections as determined by your doctor.

Mebendazole works by keeping the worm from absorbing sugar (glucose). This gradually causes loss of energy and death of the worm.

Mebendazole is available only with your doctor's prescription.

Remember:

• **This medicine has been prescribed for your present infection only.** Another infection later on may require a different medicine. Also, even though other people may have the same symptoms as you, they may have a different kind of infection. Your medicine may not work for them and may even cause them harm. Therefore, **your medicine must not be given to other people or used for other infections** unless you are otherwise directed by your doctor.

• **Keep all medicines out of the reach of children.**

• In order for this medicine to work, it must be used as directed.

• **It is very important that you read and understand the following information.** If any of the information causes you special concern, do not decide against using this medicine without first checking with your doctor.

• Before you begin using any new medicine (prescription or nonprescription) or if you develop any new medical problem while you are using this medicine, check with your doctor, nurse, or pharmacist.

• **If you have any questions** about the following information or if you want more information about this medicine or your medical problem, **ask your doctor, nurse, or pharmacist.**

Before Using This Medicine

In order to decide on the best treatment for your medical problem, your doctor should be told:

—if you have ever had any unusual or allergic reaction to mebendazole.

—if you are on a low-salt, low-sugar, or any other special diet, or if you are allergic to any substance, such as foods, sulfites or other preservatives, or dyes. Most medicines contain more than their active ingredient. Your doctor, nurse, or pharmacist can help you avoid products that may cause a problem.

—if you are **pregnant** or if you may become pregnant. Mebendazole has not been shown to cause birth defects or other problems in women who "accidentally" took this medicine during the first 3 months of pregnancy. However, mebendazole is not recommended during pregnancy. It has been shown to cause birth defects and other problems in rats given one dose, which was several times the usual human dose. Be sure you have discussed this with your doctor.

—if you are **breast-feeding**. It is not known whether mebendazole passes into the breast milk. However, this medicine has not been shown to cause problems in nursing babies.

—if you have any of the following medical problems:
Crohn's disease
Liver disease
Ulcerative colitis

—if you are taking **any** other prescription or nonprescription (OTC) medicine.

Proper Use of This Medicine

Mebendazole usually comes with patient directions. Read them carefully before using this medicine.

No special preparations (for example, special diets, fasting, other medicines, laxatives, or enemas) are necessary before, during, or immediately after taking mebendazole.

Mebendazole tablets may be chewed, swallowed whole, or crushed and mixed with food.

For patients taking mebendazole for hookworms, roundworms, or whipworms:

• To help clear up your infection completely, **take this medicine exactly as directed by your doctor for the full time of treatment.** In some patients a second course of this medicine may be required to clear up the infection completely. **Do not miss any doses.**

For patients taking mebendazole for pinworms:

• To help clear up your infection completely, **take this medicine exactly as directed by your doctor.** A second course of this medicine is usually required to clear up the infection completely.

• Pinworms may be easily passed from one person to another, especially in a household. Therefore, all household members may have to be treated at the same time. This helps to prevent infection or reinfection of other household members. Also, all household members may have to be treated again in 2 to 3 weeks to clear up the infection completely.

If you do miss a dose of this medicine, take it as soon as possible. However, if it is almost time for your next dose and your dosing schedule is:

• 2 doses a day—Space the missed dose and the next dose 4 to 5 hours apart or double your next dose.

• 8 doses a day—Space the missed dose and the next dose 1½ hours apart or double your next dose.

Then go back to your regular dosing schedule.

For patients taking mebendazole for infections in which high doses are needed:

• **Mebendazole is best taken with meals, especially fatty ones (for example, whole milk or ice cream).** This helps to clear up the infection by helping your body absorb the medicine better. **However, if you are on a low-fat diet, check with your doctor.**

• If you miss a dose of this medicine, take it as soon as possible. However, if it is almost time for your next dose, skip the missed dose and go back to your regular dosing schedule. Do not double doses.

How to store this medicine:

• **Keep out of the reach of children.**

• Store away from heat and direct light.

• Do not store in the bathroom, near the kitchen sink, or in other damp places. Heat or moisture may cause the medicine to break down.

• Do not keep outdated medicine or medicine no longer needed. Be sure that any discarded medicine is out of the reach of children.

Precautions While Using This Medicine

It is important that your doctor check your progress at regular visits, especially in infections in which high doses are needed. This is to make sure that the infection is cleared up completely and to allow your doctor to check for any unwanted effects.

If your symptoms do not improve within a few days, or if they become worse, check with your doctor.

This medicine may cause some people to become dizzy. **Make sure you know how you react to this medicine before you drive, use machines, or do other jobs that require you to be alert.** If this reaction is especially bothersome, check with your doctor.

For patients taking mebendazole for pinworms:

• In some patients, pinworms may return after treatment with mebendazole. Washing (not shaking) all bedding and nightclothes (pajamas) after treatment may help to prevent this.

• Some doctors may also recommend other measures to help keep your infection from returning. If you have any questions about this, check with your doctor.

Side Effects of This Medicine

Along with its needed effects, a medicine may cause some unwanted effects. The following side effects may go away during treatment as your body adjusts to the medicine. However, check with your doctor if any of the following side effects continue or are bothersome:

Less common or rare
    Abdominal or stomach pain or upset
    Diarrhea
    Dizziness
    Fever
    Headache
    Nausea or vomiting
    Skin rash or itching

For elderly patients: Many medicines have not been tested in older people. Therefore, it is not known whether the medicine acts the same way it does in younger adults. Check with your doctor or pharmacist if you notice any unusual effects while taking this medicine or if you think it is not working as it should.

Other side effects not listed above may also occur in some patients. If you notice any other effects, check with your doctor.

_____

December 1987

Additional Information

In addition to the above information, for patients taking mebendazole for hookworms or whipworms:

• In hookworm and whipworm infections anemia may occur. Therefore, your doctor may want you to take iron supplements to help clear up the anemia. If so, it is important to take iron every day while you are being treated for hookworms or whipworms; do not miss any doses. Your doctor may also want you to keep taking iron supplements for up to 6 months after you stop taking mebendazole. If you have any questions about this, check with your doctor.

MECAMYLAMINE (Systemic)
A commonly used brand name is Inversine.

To the Reader: If you do not recognize the names of medical conditions or medicines referred to in this information, check with your doctor, nurse, or pharmacist. Definitions for selected medical terms may be found in the Glossary. Brand names for the generic drug names listed can be found in the Index. In addition, selected brand names commonly associated with the generic name have been included in the text to help you recognize medicine you may be taking. The fact that a brand name product is not mentioned does not mean the information does not apply. It is a good idea for you to learn both the generic and brand names of your medicines and to write them down for future use.

Mecamylamine (mek-a-MILL-a-meen) belongs to the general class of medicines called antihypertensives. It is taken by mouth to treat high blood pressure.

High blood pressure adds to the workload of the heart and arteries. If it continues for a long time, the heart and arteries may not function properly. This can damage the blood vessels of the brain, heart, and kidneys, resulting in a stroke, heart failure, or kidney failure. High blood pressure may also increase the risk of heart attacks. These problems may be less likely to occur if blood pressure is controlled.

Mecamylamine works by controlling impulses along certain nerve pathways. As a result, it relaxes blood vessels so that blood passes through them more easily. This helps to lower blood pressure.

Mecamylamine is available only with your doctor's prescription.

Remember:
- **This medicine has been prescribed for your current medical problem only.** It must not be given to other people or used for other problems unless you are directed to do so by your doctor.

- **Keep all medicines out of the reach of children.**

- In order for this medicine to work, it must be used as directed.

- **It is very important that you read and understand the following information.** If any of the information causes you special concern, do not decide against using this medicine without first checking with your doctor.

- Before you begin using any new medicine (prescription or nonprescription) or if you develop any new medical problem while you are using this medicine, check with your doctor, nurse, or pharmacist.

- **If you have any questions** about the following information or if you want more information about this medicine or your medical problem, **ask your doctor, nurse, or pharmacist.**

Before Using This Medicine
In order to decide on the best treatment for your medical problem, your doctor should be told:
—if you have ever had any unusual or allergic reaction to mecamylamine.
—if you are on a low-salt, low-sugar, or any other special diet, or if you are allergic to any substance, such as foods, sulfites or other preservatives, or dyes.

Most medicines contain more than their active ingredient. Your doctor, nurse, or pharmacist can help you avoid products that may cause a problem.

—if you are **pregnant** or if you may become pregnant. Mecamylamine may cause bowel problems in the fetus. This medicine has not been shown to cause birth defects. However, in general, use of this medicine during pregnancy is not recommended because pregnant women may be more sensitive to its effects.

—if you are **breast-feeding**. This medicine has not been shown to cause problems in nursing babies.

—if you have any of the following medical problems:
Bladder or prostate problems
Bowel problems
Diarrhea
Fever or infection
Glaucoma
Gout
Heart or blood vessel disease
Kidney disease
Nausea or vomiting

—if you have recently had a heart attack or stroke.

—if you are taking **any** other prescription or nonprescription (OTC) medicine, especially:
Antibiotics
Sulfonamides (sulfa medicine)
Urinary alkalizers (medicine that makes the urine less acid, such as acetazolamide, calcium- and/or magnesium-containing antacids, dichlorphenamide, methazolamide, potassium or sodium citrate and/or citric acid, sodium bicarbonate [baking soda])

Proper Use of This Medicine

Importance of diet—When prescribing medicine for your condition, your doctor may also prescribe a personal diet for you. Such a diet may be low in sodium (salt). Most people eat much more sodium than they need and too much sodium in the diet may increase blood pressure. Some foods that contain large amounts of sodium are canned soup, pickles, ketchup, green and ripe olives, relish, frankfurters, soy sauce, and carbonated beverages. Your doctor may want you to limit the amounts of these and other high-sodium foods in your diet. High blood pressure medicine is usually more effective when such a diet is properly followed.

Also, it may be very important for you to go on a reducing diet. However, check with your doctor before changing your diet.

Many patients who have high blood pressure will not notice any signs of the problem. In fact, many may feel normal. **It is very important that you take your medicine exactly as directed and that you keep your appointments with your doctor** even if you feel well.

Remember that this medicine will not cure your high blood pressure but it does help control it. Therefore, you must continue to take it as directed if you expect to lower your blood pressure and keep it down. **You may have to take high blood pressure medicine for the** rest of your life. If high blood pressure is not treated, it can cause serious problems such as heart failure, blood vessel disease, stroke, or kidney disease.

In order to help remember to take your medicine, try to get into the habit of taking it at the same time each day.

If you do miss a dose of this medicine, take it as soon as possible. Then go back to your regular dosing schedule. **If you miss two or more doses in a row, check with your doctor right away.** If your body goes without this medicine for too long, your blood pressure may go up to a dangerously high level.

How to store this medicine:

- **Keep out of the reach of children.**

- Store away from heat and direct light.

- Do not store in the bathroom, near the kitchen sink, or in other damp places. Heat or moisture may cause the medicine to break down.

- Do not keep outdated medicine or medicine no longer needed. Be sure that any discarded medicine is out of the reach of children.

Precautions While Using This Medicine

It is important that your doctor check your progress at regular visits to make sure that this medicine is working properly.

Check with your doctor before you stop taking this medicine. Your doctor may want you to reduce gradually the amount you are taking before stopping completely.

Make sure that you have enough medicine on hand to last through weekends, holidays, or vacations. You should not miss taking any doses. You may want to ask your doctor for another written prescription for mecamylamine to carry in your wallet or purse. You can then have it filled if you run out of medicine when you are away from home.

Do not take other medicines unless they have been discussed with your doctor. This especially includes over-the-counter (nonprescription) medicines for appetite control, asthma, colds, cough, hay fever, or sinus problems, since they may tend to increase your blood pressure.

Dizziness, lightheadedness, or fainting may occur, especially when you get up from a lying or sitting position. This is more likely to occur in the morning. **Getting up slowly may help.** When you get up from lying down, sit on the edge of the bed with your feet dangling for one or two minutes. Then stand up slowly. If you feel dizzy, sit or lie down. If the problem continues or gets worse, check with your doctor.

The dizziness, lightheadedness, or fainting is also more likely to occur if you drink alcohol, stand for long periods of time, exercise, or if the weather is hot. **While you are taking this medicine, be careful in the amount of alcohol you drink. Also, use extra care during exercise or hot weather or if you must stand for long periods of time.**

Sodium bicarbonate (commonly known as baking soda) may cause you to get a greater than normal effect from this medicine. To prevent problems, check with your doctor or pharmacist before using an antacid or medicine for heartburn since some of these contain sodium bicarbonate.

Tell your doctor if you get a fever or infection since that may change the amount of medicine you have to take.

Mecamylamine may cause dryness of the mouth, nose, and throat. For temporary relief of mouth dryness, use sugarless candy or gum, melt bits of ice in your mouth, or use a saliva substitute. However, if dry mouth continues for more than 2 weeks, check with your physician or dentist. Continuing dryness of the mouth may increase the chance of dental disease, including tooth decay, gum disease, and fungal infections.

Before having any kind of surgery (including dental surgery) or emergency treatment, tell the physician or dentist in charge that you are taking this medicine.

Side Effects of This Medicine

Along with its needed effects, a medicine may cause some unwanted effects. Although not all of these side effects may occur, if they do occur they may need medical attention.

Check with your doctor as soon as possible if any of the following side effects occur:

More common

Dizziness or lightheadedness, especially when getting up from a lying or sitting position

Less common

Difficult urination

Rare

Confusion or excitement
Mental depression
Shortness of breath
Trembling

Other side effects may occur that usually do not require medical attention. These side effects may go away during treatment as your body adjusts to the medicine. However, check with your doctor if any of the following side effects continue or are bothersome:

More common

Constipation
Drowsiness
Tiredness

Less common or rare

Blurred vision
Decreased sexual ability
Dry mouth

    Enlarged pupils
    Loss of appetite
    Nausea and vomiting
    Weakness

For elderly patients: Dizziness or lightheadedness may be more likely to occur in the elderly, who are more sensitive to the effects of mecamylamine.

Other side effects not listed above may also occur in some patients. If you notice any other effects, check with your doctor.

December 1987

MECHLORETHAMINE (Systemic)

Some commonly used brand names or other names are Mustargen and Nitrogen mustard.

To the Reader: If you do not recognize the names of medical conditions or medicines referred to in this information, check with your doctor, nurse, or pharmacist. Definitions for selected medical terms may be found in the Glossary. Brand names for the generic drug names listed can be found in the Index. In addition, selected brand names commonly associated with the generic name have been included in the text to help you recognize medicine you may be taking. The fact that a brand name product is not mentioned does not mean the information does not apply. It is a good idea for you to learn both the generic and brand names of your medicines and to write them down for future use.

Mechlorethamine (me-klor-ETH-a-meen) belongs to the group of medicines called alkylating agents. It is given by injection to treat some kinds of cancer as well as some noncancerous conditions.

Mechlorethamine interferes with the growth of cancer cells, which are eventually destroyed. Since the growth of normal body cells may also be affected by mechlorethamine, other effects will also occur. Some of these may be serious and must be reported to your doctor. Other effects, like hair loss, may not be serious but may cause concern. Some effects may not occur for months or years after the medicine is used.

Before you begin treatment with mechlorethamine, you and your doctor should talk about the good this medicine will do as well as the risks of using it.

Mechlorethamine is to be administered only by or under the immediate supervision of your doctor.

Remember:

• **It is very important that you read and understand the following information.** If any of the information causes you special concern, do not decide against using this medicine without first checking with your doctor.

• Before you begin using any new medicine (prescription or nonprescription) or if you develop any new medical problem while you are using this medicine, check with your doctor, nurse, or pharmacist.

• **If you have any questions** about the following information or if you want more information about this medicine or your medical problem, **ask your doctor, nurse, or pharmacist.**

Before Using This Medicine

In order to decide on the best treatment for your medical problem, your doctor should be told:

—if you have ever had any unusual or allergic reaction to mechlorethamine, including a reaction if it was applied to the skin.

—if you are **pregnant** or if you intend to have children. This medicine may cause birth defects if either the male or female is receiving it at the time of conception or if it is used during pregnancy. In addition, many cancer medicines may cause sterility which could be permanent. This has been reported with mechlorethamine and the possibility should be kept in mind. Be sure that you have discussed this with your doctor before receiving this medicine.

—if you intend to **breast-feed**. Because this medicine may cause serious side effects, breast-feeding is generally not recommended while you are receiving it.

—if you have any of the following medical problems:
Chickenpox (including recent exposure)
Gout
Herpes zoster (shingles)
Infection
Kidney stones

—if you are taking **any** other prescription or nonprescription (OTC) medicine, especially:
Amphotericin B by injection (e.g., Fungizone)
Antithyroid agents (medicine for overactive thyroid)
Azathioprine (e.g., Imuran)
Chloramphenicol (e.g., Chloromycetin)
Colchicine
Flucytosine (e.g., Ancobon)
Interferon (e.g., Intron A; Roferon-A)
Probenecid (e.g., Benemid)
Sulfinpyrazone (e.g., Anturane)

—if you have ever been treated with x-rays or cancer medicines.

Proper Use of This Medicine

Mechlorethamine is sometimes given together with certain other medicines. If you are using a combination of medicines, it is important that you receive each one at the proper time. If you are taking some of these medicines by mouth, ask your doctor, nurse, or pharmacist to help you plan a way to take them at the right times.

While you are using this medicine, your doctor may want you to drink extra fluids so that you will pass more urine. This will help prevent kidney problems and keep your kidneys working well.

Mechlorethamine often causes nausea and vomiting, which usually last only 8 to 24 hours. It is very important that you continue to receive the medicine, even if you begin to feel ill. Ask your doctor, nurse, or pharmacist for ways to lessen these effects.

Precautions While Using This Medicine

It is very important that your doctor check your progress at regular visits to make sure that this medicine is working properly and to check for unwanted effects.

While you are being treated with mechlorethamine, and after you stop treatment with it, **do not have any immunizations without your doctor's approval.** Mechlorethamine lowers your body's resistance and there is a chance you might get the infection the immunization is meant to prevent. In addition, other persons living in your household should not take oral polio vaccine since there is a chance they could pass the polio virus on to you. Also, you should avoid close contact with other persons (for example, at school or work) who have taken oral polio vaccine.

Mechlorethamine can lower the number of white blood cells in your body. This may increase the chance of getting an infection. If you can, avoid people with colds or other infections. If you think you are getting a cold or other infection, check with your doctor.

If mechlorethamine accidentally seeps out of the vein into which it is injected, it may damage some tissues and cause scarring. **Tell the doctor or nurse right away if you notice redness, pain, or swelling at the place of injection**.

Side Effects of This Medicine

Along with their needed effects, medicines like mechlorethamine can sometimes cause blood problems, loss of hair, and other side effects; these are described below. Also, because of the way these medicines act on the body, there is a chance that they might cause other effects that may not occur until months or years after these medicine is used. These delayed effects may include certain types of cancer, such as leukemia. Discuss these possible effects with your doctor.

Although not all of these side effects may occur, if they do occur they may need medical attention.

Check with your doctor or nurse immediately if any of the following side effects occur:

More common
   Fever, chills, or sore throat
   Unusual bleeding or bruising

Less common
   Pain or redness at the place of injection

Rare
   Shortness of breath, itching, wheezing

Check with your doctor or nurse as soon as possible if any of the following side effects occur:

More common
   Missing menstrual periods
   Painful rash

Less common
   Dizziness
   Joint pain
   Loss of hearing

   Lower back, side, or stomach pain
   Ringing in the ears
   Swelling of feet or lower legs

Rare
   Black, tarry stools
   Numbness, tingling, or burning of fingers, toes, or face
   Sores in the mouth and on the lips
   Yellow eyes and skin

Other side effects may occur that usually do not require medical attention. These side effects may go away during treatment as your body adjusts to the medicine. Also, your doctor or nurse may be able to tell you about ways to prevent or reduce some of these side effects. Check with your doctor if any of the following side effects continue or are bothersome or if you have any questions about them:

More common
   Nausea and vomiting (usually lasts only 8 to 24 hours)

Less common
   Confusion
   Diarrhea
   Drowsiness
   Headache
   Loss of appetite
   Metallic taste
   Weakness

This medicine may cause a temporary loss of hair in some people. After treatment with mechlorethamine has ended, normal hair growth should return.

For elderly patients: Many medicines have not been tested in older people. Therefore, it is not known whether the medicine acts the same way it does in younger adults. Check with your doctor or pharmacist if you notice any unusual effects while taking this medicine or if you think it is not working as it should.

After you stop receiving mechlorethamine, it may still produce some side effects that need attention. During this period of time, check with your doctor if you notice any of the following side effects:
   Fever, chills, or sore throat
   Unusual bleeding or bruising

Other side effects not listed above may also occur in some patients. If you notice any other effects, check with your doctor.

December 1987

MECHLORETHAMINE (Topical)*

A commonly used other name is Nitrogen mustard.

*Not commercially available in the U.S.

To the Reader: If you do not recognize the names of medical conditions or medicines referred to in this information, check with your doctor, nurse, or pharmacist. Definitions for selected medical terms may be found in the Glossary. Brand names for the generic drug names listed can be found in the Index. In addition, selected brand names commonly associated with the generic name have been included in the text to help you recognize medicine you may be taking. The fact that a brand name product is not mentioned does not mean the information does not apply. It is a good idea for you to learn both the generic and brand names of your medicines and to write them down for future use.

Mechlorethamine (me-klor-ETH-a-meen) belongs to the group of medicines called alkylating agents. It is applied to the skin to treat certain conditions that could turn to cancer if left untreated.

Mechlorethamine interferes with the growth of problem cells, which are eventually destroyed. However, there is also a chance that mechlorethamine can cause some kinds of skin cancer, especially after it has been used for several years.

Before you begin treatment with mechlorethamine, you and your doctor should talk about the good this medicine will do as well as the risks of using it.

Mechlorethamine is available only with your doctor's prescription.

Remember:
• **This medicine has been prescribed for your current medical problem only.** It must not be given to other people or used for other problems unless you are directed to do so by your doctor.

• **Keep all medicines out of the reach of children.**

• In order for this medicine to work, it must be used as directed.

• **It is very important that you read and understand the following information.** If any of the information causes you special concern, do not decide against using this medicine without first checking with your doctor.

• Before you begin using any new medicine (prescription or nonprescription) or if you develop any new medical problem while you are using this medicine, check with your doctor, nurse, or pharmacist.

• **If you have any questions** about the following information or if you want more information about this medicine or your medical problem, **ask your doctor, nurse, or pharmacist.**

Before Using This Medicine

In order to decide on the best treatment for your medical problem, your doctor should be told:
—if you have ever had any unusual or allergic reaction to mechlorethamine.

—if you are **pregnant** or if you may become pregnant. Although mechlorethamine applied to the skin has not been shown to cause problems in humans, some of it may be absorbed through the skin.

—if you are **breast-feeding**. Although mechlorethamine applied to the skin has not been shown to cause problems in humans, some of it may be absorbed through the skin. Because this medicine can cause serious side effects, breast-feeding is generally not recommended while you are using it.

—if you have any other skin problems.

—if you are using other medicines on your skin.

Proper Use of This Medicine

Mechlorethamine may be used either as a solution or as an ointment. If you are using the solution, it must be mixed just before you use it since it breaks down quickly. **Mix the solution carefully according to your doctor's or pharmacist's directions.**

When preparing the solution, remember:

• Do not use the mechlorethamine if the solution is discolored or if droplets of water appear in the vial.

• Avoid inhaling the powder or any vapors. If some of the powder or solution accidentally gets on your skin, *immediately* wash that area of skin. Use a large amount of water and continue to wash for at least 15 minutes. If eye contact occurs, use an eyewash recommended by your doctor. Keep this eyewash on hand. **Follow carefully any other instructions your doctor may have given you.**

• All equipment used must be neutralized or decontaminated, even if it is to be thrown away. **Follow carefully your doctor's instructions** for doing this, using the special solution recommended.

Take a shower and rinse carefully just before you apply mechlorethamine solution or ointment, unless otherwise directed by your doctor. Make sure your skin is completely dry before applying the ointment. Do not shower again until the next treatment.

Apply the solution or ointment all over the body, until the entire amount for a dose is used up. Wear rubber or plastic gloves if you are using your hands. To apply the solution, a 2-inch-wide soft brush or gauze may be used instead. Let the solution dry.

Mechlorethamine should be applied more lightly to the groin, armpits, inside the bends of the elbows, and behind the knees. These areas are more likely to get irritated.

Avoid contact with the eyes, nose, or mouth, unless otherwise directed by your doctor.

Mechlorethamine is usually applied once a day. However, follow your doctor's instructions. Continue to use the medicine as long as you are told to. This may be months or years. However, do not use this medicine more often or for a longer period of time than ordered. To do so may increase the chance of unwanted effects.

If you miss a dose of this medicine, go back to your regular dosing schedule and check with your doctor. Do not change the amount you are using unless directed to do so by your doctor.

How to store this medicine:

• **Keep out of the reach of children.**

• Store away from heat and direct light. This applies to either the ointment or the vials of mechlorethamine used to make the solution. The solution should not be stored but instead should be freshly made just before it is used.

• Do not store in the bathroom, near the kitchen sink, or in other damp places. Heat or moisture may cause the medicine to break down.

• Do not keep outdated medicine or medicine no longer needed. Be sure that any discarded medicine is out of the reach of children.

Precautions While Using This Medicine

It is very important that your doctor check your progress at regular visits to make sure that mechlorethamine is working properly and to check for unwanted effects.

Side Effects of This Medicine

Along with its needed effects, a medicine may cause some unwanted effects. When mechlorethamine is applied to the skin, it does not usually cause the same effects as when it is given by injection. **However, stop using this medicine and check with your doctor immediately** if the following side effects occur:

Hives
Shortness of breath (sudden)
Skin rash or itching
Sore, reddened skin

Check with your doctor also if you develop dry skin. There may be a lotion or ointment that you can use to help this. However, do not use anything else on your skin unless directed by your doctor.

Your skin color may darken after you have used this medicine for a while. The effect will go away after you have stopped using the medicine.

For elderly patients: Many medicines have not been tested in older people. Therefore, it is not known whether the medicine acts the same way it does in younger adults. Check with your doctor or pharmacist if you notice any unusual effects while using this medicine or if you think it is not working as it should.

Other side effects not listed above may also occur in some patients. If you notice any other effects, check with your doctor.

December 1987

MECLIZINE (Systemic)

This information applies to the following medicines.

Buclizine (BYOO-kli-zeen)
Cyclizine (SYE-kli-zeen)
Meclizine (MEK-li-zeen)

Some commonly used brand names are:	Generic names:
Bucladin-S	Buclizine
Marezine Marzine*	Cyclizine
Antivert Bonamine* Bonine	Meclizine†

*Not available in the U.S.
†Generic name product may also be available in the U.S.

To the Reader: If you do not recognize the names of medical conditions or medicines referred to in this information, check with your doctor, nurse, or pharmacist. Definitions for selected medical terms may be found in the Glossary. Brand names for the generic drug names listed can be found in the Index. In addition, selected brand names commonly associated with the generic name have been included in the text to help you recognize medicine you may be taking. The fact that a brand name product is not mentioned does not mean the information does not apply. It is a good idea for you to learn both the generic and brand names of your medicines and to write them down for future use.

Buclizine, cyclizine, and meclizine are used to prevent motion sickness, nausea, vomiting, and dizziness.

Some of these preparations are available only with your doctor's prescription. Others are available without a prescription; however, your doctor may have special instructions on the proper dose of the medicine for your medical condition.

Remember:

• **Keep all medicines out of the reach of children.**

• In order for this medicine to work, it must be used as directed. **If you are using this medicine without a prescription, it is very important to follow the directions on the label.**

• **It is also very important that you read and understand the following information.** If any of the information causes you special concern, check with your doctor before using this medicine without a prescription.

• Before you begin using any new medicine (prescription or nonprescription) or if you develop any new medical problem while you are using this medicine, check with your doctor, nurse, or pharmacist.

• **If you have any questions** about the following information or if you want more information about this medicine or your medical problem, **ask your doctor, nurse, or pharmacist.**

Before Using This Medicine

Before you use this medicine, check with your doctor, nurse, or pharmacist:

—if you have ever had any unusual or allergic reaction to buclizine, cyclizine, or meclizine.

—if you are on a low-salt, low-sugar, or any other special diet, or if you are allergic to any substance, such as foods, sulfites or other preservatives, or dyes. Most medicines contain more than their active ingredient. Your doctor, nurse, or pharmacist can help you avoid products that may cause a problem.

—if you are **pregnant** or if you may become pregnant. These medicines have not been shown to cause birth defects or other problems in humans. However, studies in animals have shown that buclizine, cyclizine, and meclizine given in doses many times the usual human dose cause birth defects.

—if you are **breast-feeding**. Although these medicines have not been shown to cause problems in nursing babies, the chance always exists since they may pass into the breast milk. In addition, since these medicines tend to decrease the secretions of the body, it is possible that the flow of breast milk may be reduced in some patients.

—if you have any of the following medical problems:
Enlarged prostate
Intestinal blockage
Urinary tract blockage

—if you are taking any of the following medicines or types of medicine:
Aminoglycosides by injection (amikacin, gentamicin, kanamycin, neomycin, netilmicin, streptomycin, tobramycin)
Antimuscarinics (medicine for abdominal or stomach spasms or cramps)
Capreomycin
Chloroquine
Cisplatin
Clonidine
Guanabenz
Hydroxychloroquine
Ipratropium
Maprotiline
Medicine for inflammation or pain (aspirin or other salicylates, diclofenac, diflunisal, fenoprofen, ibuprofen, indomethacin, ketoprofen, meclofenamate, mefenamic acid, naproxen, phenylbutazone, piroxicam, sulindac, suprofen, tolmetin)
Methyldopa
Metyrosine
Minocycline
Paromomycin
Quinine
Trazodone
Tricyclic antidepressants (amitriptyline, amoxapine, clomipramine, desipramine, doxepin, imipramine, nortriptyline, protriptyline, trimipramine)
Vancomycin by injection

—if you are now taking any central nervous system (CNS) depressants, such as:
Anticonvulsants (seizure medicine)
Antihistamines or medicine for hay fever, other allergies, or colds

Barbiturates
Narcotics
Prescription pain medicine
Sedatives, tranquilizers, or sleeping medicine

Proper Use of This Medicine

If necessary, take this medicine with food or a glass of water or milk to lessen stomach irritation.

This medicine is used to relieve or prevent the symptoms of your medical problem. Take it only as directed. Do not take more of it or take it more often than stated on the label or ordered by your doctor. To do so may increase the chance of side effects.

For patients taking this medicine for motion sickness:

• Take buclizine or cyclizine at least 30 minutes before you begin to travel.

• Take meclizine at least 1 hour before you begin to travel.

If you must take this medicine regularly and you miss a dose, take the missed dose as soon as possible. However, if it is almost time for your next dose, skip the missed dose and go back to your regular dosing schedule. Do not double doses.

How to store this medicine:

• Store away from heat and direct light.

• **Keep out of the reach of children.**

• Do not store the tablets in the bathroom medicine cabinet because the heat or moisture may cause the medicine to break down.

• Do not keep outdated medicine or medicine no longer needed. Flush the contents of the container down the toilet, unless otherwise directed.

Precautions While Using This Medicine

Tell the doctor in charge that you are taking this medicine before you have any skin tests for allergies. The results of the test may be affected by this medicine.

Buclizine, cyclizine, or meclizine will add to the effects of alcohol and other CNS depressants (medicines that slow down the nervous system, possibly causing drowsiness). Some examples of CNS depressants are antihistamines or medicine for hay fever, other allergies, or colds; sedatives, tranquilizers, or sleeping medicine; prescription pain medicine or narcotics; barbiturates; medicine for seizures; muscle relaxants; or anesthetics, including some dental anesthetics. **Check with your doctor before taking any of the above while you are using this medicine.**

This medicine may cause some people to become drowsy or less alert than they are normally. **Make sure you know how you react to this medicine before you drive, use machines, or do other jobs that require you to be alert.**

Your mouth may feel very dry while you are taking buclizine, cyclizine, or meclizine. For temporary relief of mouth dryness, use sugarless candy or gum, melt bits of ice in your mouth, or use a saliva substitute.

When taking this medicine on a regular basis, make sure your doctor knows if you are taking large amounts of aspirin at the same time (as in arthritis or rheumatism). Effects of too much aspirin, such as ringing in the ears, may be covered up by this medicine.

Side Effects of This Medicine

Along with its needed effects, a medicine may cause some unwanted effects. The following side effects may go away during treatment as your body adjusts to the medicine; however, check with your doctor if they continue or are bothersome:

More common
    Drowsiness

Less common or rare
    Blurred vision
    Difficult or painful urination
    Dizziness
    Dryness of mouth, nose, and throat
    Headache
    Loss of appetite
    Nervousness, restlessness, or trouble in sleeping
    Skin rash
    Unusually fast heartbeat
    Upset stomach

Although not all of the side effects listed above have been reported for all of these medicines, they have been reported for at least one of them. However, since buclizine, cyclizine, and meclizine are very similar, any of the above side effects may occur with any of these medicines.

Other side effects not listed above may also occur in some patients. If you notice any other effects, check with your doctor.

December 1987

MELPHALAN (Systemic)

Some commonly used brand names or other names are Alkeran, L-PAM, and Phenylalanine mustard.

To the Reader: If you do not recognize the names of medical conditions or medicines referred to in this information, check with your doctor, nurse, or pharmacist. Definitions for selected medical terms may be found in the Glossary. Brand names for the generic drug names listed can be found in the Index. In addition, selected brand names commonly associated with the generic name have been included in the text to help you recognize medicine you may be taking. The fact that a brand name product is not mentioned does not mean the information does not apply. It is a good idea for you to learn both the generic and brand names of your medicines and to write them down for future use.

Melphalan (MEL-fa-lan) belongs to the group of medicines called alkylating agents. It is taken by mouth to treat some kinds of cancer.

Melphalan interferes with the growth of cancer cells, which are eventually destroyed. Since the growth of normal body cells may also be affected by melphalan, other effects will also occur. Some of these may be serious and must be reported to your doctor. Other effects may not be serious but may cause concern. Some effects may not occur for months or years after the medicine is used.

Before you begin treatment with melphalan, you and your doctor should talk about the good this medicine will do as well as the risks of using it.

Melphalan is available only with your doctor's prescription.

Remember:

• **This medicine has been prescribed for your current medical problem only.** It must not be given to other people or used for other problems unless you are directed to do so by your doctor.

• **Keep all medicines out of the reach of children.**

• In order for this medicine to work, it must be used as directed.

• **It is very important that you read and understand the following information.** If any of the information causes you special concern, do not decide against using this medicine without first checking with your doctor.

• Before you begin using any new medicine (prescription or nonprescription) or if you develop any new medical problem while you are using this medicine, check with your doctor, nurse, or pharmacist.

• **If you have any questions** about the following information or if you want more information about this medicine or your medical problem, **ask your doctor, nurse, or pharmacist.**

Before Using This Medicine

In order to decide on the best treatment for your medical problem, your doctor should be told:

—if you have ever had any unusual or allergic reaction to melphalan or chlorambucil.

—if you are **pregnant** or if you intend to have children. There is a chance that this medicine may cause birth defects if either the male or female is taking it at the time of conception or if it is taken during pregnancy. In addition, many cancer medicines may cause sterility which could be permanent. This has been reported with melphalan and the possibility should be kept in mind. Be sure that you have discussed this with your doctor before taking this medicine.

—if you intend to **breast-feed**. Because this medicine may cause serious side effects, breast-feeding is generally not recommended while you are receiving it.

—if you have any of the following medical problems:
   Chickenpox (including recent exposure)
   Gout (history of)
   Herpes zoster (shingles)
   Infection
   Kidney disease
   Kidney stones (history of)

—if you are taking **any** other prescription or nonprescription (OTC) medicine, especially:
   Amphotericin B by injection (e.g., Fungizone)
   Antithyroid agents (medicine for overactive thyroid)
   Azathioprine (e.g., Imuran)
   Chloramphenicol (e.g., Chloromycetin)
   Colchicine
   Flucytosine (e.g., Ancobon)
   Interferon (e.g., Intron A; Roferon-A)
   Probenecid (e.g., Benemid)
   Sulfinpyrazone (e.g., Anturane)

—if you have ever been treated with x-rays or cancer medicines.

Proper Use of This Medicine

Take melphalan only as directed by your doctor. Do not take more or less of it, do not take it more often, and do not take it for a longer period of time than your doctor ordered. The exact amount of medicine you need has been carefully worked out. Taking too much may increase the chance of side effects, while taking too little may not improve your condition.

This medicine is sometimes given together with certain other medicines. If you are using a combination of medicines, make sure that you take each one at the proper time and do not mix them. Ask your doctor, nurse, or pharmacist to help you plan a way to remember to take your medicine at the right times.

While you are using melphalan, your doctor may want you to drink extra fluids so that you will pass more urine. This will help prevent kidney problems and keep your kidneys working well.

This medicine often causes nausea, vomiting, and loss of appetite. However, it may have to be taken for several months to be effective. Even if you begin to feel ill, **do not stop using this medicine without first checking with your doctor.** Ask your doctor, nurse, or pharmacist for ways to lessen these effects.

If you vomit shortly after taking a dose of melphalan, check with your doctor. You may be told to take the dose again or you may have to wait until the next scheduled dose.

If you miss a dose of this medicine, do not take the missed dose at all and do not double the next one. Instead, go back to your regular dosing schedule and check with your doctor.

How to store this medicine:

- **Keep out of the reach of children.**

- Store in the original glass container away from heat and direct light.

- Do not store in the bathroom, near the kitchen sink, or in other damp places. Heat or moisture may cause the medicine to break down.

- Do not keep outdated medicine or medicine no longer needed. Be sure that any discarded medicine is out of the reach of children.

Precautions While Using This Medicine

It is very important that your doctor check your progress at regular visits to make sure that this medicine is working properly and to check for unwanted effects.

While you are being treated with melphalan, and after you stop treatment with it, **do not have any immunizations without your doctor's approval.** Melphalan lowers your body's resistance and there is a chance you might get the infection the immunization is meant to prevent. In addition, other persons living in your household should not take oral polio vaccine since there is a chance they could pass the polio virus on to you. Also, you should avoid close contact with other persons (for example, at school or work) who have taken oral polio vaccine.

Melphalan can lower the number of white blood cells in your body. This may increase the chance of getting an infection. If you can, avoid people with colds or other infections. If you think you are getting a cold or other infection, check with your doctor.

Side Effects of This Medicine

Along with their needed effects, medicines like melphalan can sometimes cause unwanted effects such as blood problems and other side effects; these are described below. Also, because of the way these medicines act on the body, there is a chance that they might cause other unwanted effects that may not occur until months or years after the medicine is used. These delayed effects may include certain types of cancer, such as leukemia. Discuss these possible effects with your doctor.

Although not all of these side effects may occur, if they do occur they may need medical attention.

Check with your doctor immediately if any of the following side effects occur:

More common
    Black tarry stools
    Fever, chills, or sore throat
    Unusual bleeding or bruising

Less common or rare
    Skin rash or itching (sudden)

Check with your doctor as soon as possible if any of the following side effects occur:

Less common or rare
    Joint pain
    Lower back, side, or stomach pain
    Sores in the mouth and on the lips
    Swelling of feet or lower legs

Other side effects may occur that usually do not require medical attention. These side effects may go away during treatment as your body adjusts to the medicine. Also, your doctor or nurse may be able to tell you about ways to prevent or reduce some of these side effects. Check with your doctor if the following side effects continue or are bothersome or if you have any questions about them:

Less common
    Nausea and vomiting

For elderly patients: Many medicines have not been tested in older people. Therefore, it is not known whether the medicine acts the same way it does in younger adults. Check with your doctor or pharmacist if you notice any unusual effects while taking this medicine or if you think it is not working as it should.

After you stop taking melphalan, it may still produce some side effects that need attention. During this period of time, check with your doctor if you notice any of the following side effects:
    Fever, chills, or sore throat
    Unusual bleeding or bruising

Other side effects not listed above may also occur in some patients. If you notice any other effects, check with your doctor.

December 1987

MENOTROPINS (Systemic)

A commonly used brand name is Pergonal.

To the Reader: If you do not recognize the names of medical conditions or medicines referred to in this information, check with your doctor, nurse, or pharmacist. Definitions for selected medical terms may be found in the Glossary. Brand names for the generic drug names listed can be found in the Index. In addition, selected brand names commonly associated with the generic name have been included in the text to help you recognize medicine you may be taking. The fact that a brand name product is not mentioned does not mean the information does not apply. It is a good idea for you to learn both the generic and brand names of your medicines and to write them down for future use.

Menotropins (men-oh-TROE-pins) is used in combination with another medicine to treat infertility. It is used in some women who are unable to become pregnant and to stimulate production of sperm in men.

Menotropins is to be administered only by or under the supervision of your doctor.

Remember:

• **It is very important that you read and understand the following information.** If any of the information causes you special concern, do not decide against using this medicine without first checking with your doctor.

• Before you begin using any new medicine (prescription or nonprescription) or if you develop any new medical problem while you are using this medicine, check with your doctor, nurse, or pharmacist.

• **If you have any questions** about the following information or if you want more information about this medicine or your medical problem, **ask your doctor, nurse, or pharmacist.**

Before Using This Medicine

If you become pregnant as a result of using this medicine, there is a greater chance of a multiple birth (for example, twins, triplets) occurring. If you have any questions about this, check with your doctor.

In order to decide on the best treatment for your medical problem, your doctor should be told:

—if you have ever had any unusual or allergic reaction to menotropins.

—if you are on a low-salt, low-sugar, or any other special diet, or if you are allergic to any substance, such as foods or sulfites or other preservatives. Most medicines contain more than their active ingredient. Your doctor, nurse, or pharmacist can help you avoid products that may cause a problem.

—if you have any of the following medical problems:

For females only
    Cyst on ovary
    Fibroid tumors of the uterus
    Unusual vaginal bleeding
For both males and females
    Asthma
    Epilepsy
    Heart disease

    Kidney disease
    Migraine headaches
    Pituitary disease

—if you are taking **any** other prescription or nonprescription (OTC) medicine.

Precautions While Using This Medicine

It is very important that your doctor check your progress at regular visits to make sure that the medicine is working properly and to check for unwanted effects.

It may take some time for menotropins to work. **It is very important that you continue to receive the medicine.** If you are concerned that it is not working, check with your doctor.

For females only:

• If your doctor has asked you to record your temperature daily, make sure that you do this every day so that you will know if you have begun to ovulate. It is important that intercourse take place at the correct time to give you the best chance of becoming pregnant. **Follow your doctor's instructions carefully.**

Side Effects of This Medicine

Along with its needed effects, a medicine may cause some unwanted effects. Although not all of these side effects may occur, if they do occur they may need medical attention.

Check with your doctor as soon as possible if any of the following side effects occur:

For females only
    More common
        Bloating
        Stomach or pelvic pain

Other side effects may occur that usually do not require medical attention. These side effects may go away during treatment as your body adjusts to the medicine. However, check with your doctor if the following side effect continues or is bothersome:

For males only
    Less common
        Enlargement of breasts

After you stop using this medicine, your body may need time to adjust. The length of time this takes depends on the amount of medicine you were using and how long you used it. During this period of time check with your doctor if you notice any of the following side effects:

For females only
    Bloating
    Stomach or pelvic pain

Other side effects not listed above may also occur in some patients. If you notice any other effects, check with your doctor.

December 1987

© 1988   The United States Pharmacopeial Convention, Inc.

MEPROBAMATE (Systemic)

Some commonly used brand names are:

Apo-Meprobamate*	Neuramate
Equanil	Neurate
Equanil Wyseals	Novomepro*
Meditran*	Sedabamate
Meprospan	SK-Bamate
Miltown	Tranmep
Neo-Tran*	

Generic name product may also be available in the U.S.

*Not available in the U.S.

To the Reader: If you do not recognize the names of medical conditions or medicines referred to in this information, check with your doctor, nurse, or pharmacist. Definitions for selected medical terms may be found in the Glossary. Brand names for the generic drug names listed can be found in the Index. In addition, selected brand names commonly associated with the generic name have been included in the text to help you recognize medicine you may be taking. The fact that a brand name product is not mentioned does not mean the information does not apply. It is a good idea for you to learn both the generic and brand names of your medicines and to write them down for future use.

Meprobamate (me-proe-BA-mate) is taken by mouth to relieve nervousness or tension.

Meprobamate should not be used for nervousness or tension caused by the stress of everyday life.

This medicine is available only with your doctor's prescription.

Remember:

• **This medicine has been prescribed for your current medical problem only.** It must not be given to other people or used for other problems unless you are directed to do so by your doctor.

• **Keep all medicines out of the reach of children.**

• In order for this medicine to work, it must be used as directed.

• **It is very important that you read and understand the following information.** If any of the information causes you special concern, do not decide against using this medicine without first checking with your doctor.

• Before you begin using any new medicine (prescription or nonprescription) or if you develop any new medical problem while you are using this medicine, check with your doctor, nurse, or pharmacist.

• **If you have any questions** about the following information or if you want more information about this medicine or your medical problem, **ask your doctor, nurse, or pharmacist.**

Before Using This Medicine

In order to decide on the best treatment for your medical problem, your doctor should be told:

—if you have ever had any unusual or allergic reaction to meprobamate or to medicines like meprobamate such as carbromal, carisoprodol, mebutamate, or tybamate.

—if you are on a low-salt, low-sugar, or any other special diet, or if you are allergic to any substance, such as foods, sulfites or other preservatives, or dyes.

Most medicines contain more than their active ingredient. Your doctor, nurse, or pharmacist can help you avoid products that may cause a problem.

—if you are **pregnant** or if you may become pregnant. Meprobamate has been reported to increase the chance of birth defects if taken during the first 3 months of pregnancy.

—if you are **breast-feeding.** Meprobamate passes into the breast milk and may cause drowsiness in babies of mothers taking this medicine.

—if you have any of the following medical problems:
Epilepsy
Kidney disease
Liver disease
Porphyria

—if you are taking **any** other prescription or nonprescription (OTC) medicine, especially central nervous system (CNS) depressants.

Proper Use of This Medicine

Take this medicine only as directed by your doctor. Do not take more of it, do not take it more often, and do not take it for a longer period of time than your doctor ordered. If too much is taken, it may become habit-forming.

If you miss a dose of this medicine and remember within an hour or so of the missed dose, take it right away. However, if you do not remember until later, skip the missed dose and go back to your regular dosing schedule. Do not double doses.

How to store this medicine:

• **Keep out of the reach of children.**

• Store away from heat and direct light.

• Do not store in the bathroom, near the kitchen sink, or in other damp places. Heat or moisture may cause the medicine to break down.

• Do not keep outdated medicine or medicine no longer needed. Be sure that any discarded medicine is out of the reach of children.

Precautions While Using This Medicine

If you will be taking this medicine regularly for a long period of time:

• Your doctor should check your progress at regular visits.

• Check with your doctor at least every 4 months to make sure you need to continue taking this medicine.

If you will be taking this medicine in large doses or for a long period of time, do not stop taking it without first checking with your doctor. Your doctor may want you to reduce gradually the amount you are taking before stopping completely.

This medicine will add to the effects of alcohol and other CNS depressants (medicines that slow down the nervous system, possibly causing drowsiness). Some examples of CNS depressants are antihistamines or medicine for hay fever, other allergies, or colds; sedatives, tranquilizers, or sleeping medicine; prescription pain medicine or narcotics; barbiturates; medicine for convulsions (seizures); muscle relaxants; or anesthetics, including some dental anesthetics. **Check with your doctor before taking any of the above while you are taking this medicine.**

If you think you or someone else may have taken an overdose of this medicine, get emergency help at once. Taking an overdose of meprobamate or taking alcohol or other CNS depressants with meprobamate may lead to unconsciousness and possibly death. Some signs of an overdose are severe confusion, drowsiness, or weakness; shortness of breath or slow or troubled breathing; slurred speech; staggering; and slow heartbeat.

This medicine may cause some people to become dizzy, lightheaded, drowsy, or less alert than they are normally. Even if taken at bedtime, it may cause some people to feel drowsy or less alert on arising. **Make sure you know how you react to this medicine before you drive, use machines, or do other jobs that require you to be alert.**

Meprobamate may cause dryness of the mouth. For temporary relief, use sugarless candy or gum, melt bits of ice in your mouth, or use a saliva substitute. However, if dry mouth continues for more than 2 weeks, check with your dentist. Continuing dryness of the mouth may increase the chance of dental disease, including tooth decay, gum disease, and fungal infections.

Side Effects of This Medicine

Along with its needed effects, a medicine may cause some unwanted effects. Although not all of these side effects may occur, if they do occur they may need medical attention.

Check with your doctor as soon as possible if any of the following side effects occur:

Less common
   Skin rash, hives, or itching

Rare
   Confusion
   Fast, pounding, or irregular heartbeat
   Sore throat and fever
   Unusual bleeding or bruising
   Unusual excitement
   Wheezing, shortness of breath, or troubled breathing

Signs of overdose
   Confusion (severe)
   Dizziness or lightheadedness (continuing)
   Drowsiness (severe)
   Shortness of breath or slow or troubled breathing
   Slow heartbeat
   Slurred speech
   Staggering
   Weakness (severe)

Other side effects may occur that usually do not require medical attention. These side effects may go away during treatment as your body adjusts to the medicine. However, check with your doctor if any of the following side effects continue or are bothersome:

More common
   Clumsiness or unsteadiness
   Drowsiness

Less common
   Blurred vision or change in near or distant vision
   Diarrhea
   Dizziness or lightheadedness
   False sense of well-being
   Headache
   Nausea or vomiting
   Unusual tiredness or weakness

For elderly patients: The above side effects are more likely to occur in elderly patients, who are usually more sensitive to the effects of meprobamate.

After you stop using this medicine, your body may need time to adjust. If you took this medicine in high doses or for a long time, this may take about 2 days. During this period of time check with your doctor if you notice any of the following side effects:

   Clumsiness or unsteadiness
   Confusion
   Convulsions (seizures)
   Hallucinations (seeing, hearing, or feeling things that are not there)
   Increased dreaming
   Muscle twitching
   Nausea or vomiting
   Nervousness or restlessness
   Nightmares
   Trembling
   Trouble in sleeping

Other side effects not listed above may also occur in some patients. If you notice any other effects, check with your doctor.

December 1987

MEPROBAMATE AND ASPIRIN (Systemic)

Some commonly used brand names are:

Equagesic‡	Micrainin
Equazine-M	Tranquigesic
Meprogesic Q	

‡In Canada, this product also contains ethoheptazine citrate.

To the Reader: If you do not recognize the names of medical conditions or medicines referred to in this information, check with your doctor, nurse, or pharmacist. Definitions for selected medical terms may be found in the Glossary. Brand names for the generic drug names listed can be found in the Index. In addition, selected brand names commonly associated with the generic name have been included in the text to help you recognize medicine you may be taking. The fact that a brand name product is not mentioned does not mean the information does not apply. It is a good idea for you to learn both the generic and brand names of your medicines and to write them down for future use.

Meprobamate (me-proe-BA-mate) and aspirin (AS-pir-in) combination is taken by mouth to relieve pain, anxiety, and tension in certain disorders or diseases.

This medicine is available only with your doctor's prescription.

Remember:

• **This medicine has been prescribed for your current medical problem only.** It must not be given to other people or used for other problems unless you are directed to do so by your doctor.

• **Keep all medicines out of the reach of children.**

• In order for this medicine to work, it must be used as directed.

• **It is very important that you read and understand the following information.** If any of the information causes you special concern, do not decide against using this medicine without first checking with your doctor.

• Before you begin using any new medicine (prescription or nonprescription) or if you develop any new medical problem while you are using this medicine, check with your doctor, nurse, or pharmacist.

• **If you have any questions** about the following information or if you want more information about this medicine or your medical problem, **ask your doctor, nurse, or pharmacist.**

Before Using This Medicine

In order to decide on the best treatment for your medical problem, your doctor should be told:

—if you have ever had any unusual or allergic reaction to carbromal, carisoprodol, mebutamate, meprobamate, or tybamate; or to aspirin or other salicylates including diflunisal or methyl salicylate (oil of wintergreen); or to any of the following medicines:

Diclofenac
Fenoprofen
Flurbiprofen (oral)
Ibuprofen
Indomethacin
Ketoprofen
Meclofenamate
Mefenamic acid
Naproxen
Phenylbutazone
Piroxicam
Sulindac
Tiaprofenic acid
Tolmetin
Zomepirac

—if you are on a low-salt, low-sugar, or any other special diet, or if you are allergic to any substance, such as foods, sulfites or other preservatives, or dyes. Most medicines contain more than their active ingredient. Your doctor, nurse, or pharmacist can help you avoid products that may cause a problem.

—if you are **pregnant** or if you may become pregnant. Meprobamate (contained in this combination medicine) has been reported to increase the chance of birth defects if taken during the first 3 months of pregnancy. Studies in humans have not shown that aspirin (contained in this combination medicine) causes birth defects. However, studies in animals have shown that aspirin causes birth defects. Some reports have suggested that too much use of aspirin late in pregnancy may cause a decrease in the newborn's weight and possible death of the fetus or newborn infant. However, the mothers in these reports had been taking much larger amounts of aspirin than are usually recommended. Studies of mothers taking aspirin in the doses that are usually recommended did not show these unwanted effects. However, regular use of aspirin late in pregnancy may cause unwanted effects on the heart or blood flow in the fetus or in the newborn infant. Also, use of aspirin during the last 2 weeks of pregnancy may cause bleeding problems in the fetus before or during delivery or in the newborn infant. In addition, too much use of aspirin during the last 3 months of pregnancy may increase the length of pregnancy, prolong labor, cause other problems during delivery, or cause severe bleeding in the mother before, during, or after delivery.

—if you are **breast-feeding**. Meprobamate (contained in this combination medicine) passes into the breast milk and may cause drowsiness in babies of mothers taking this medicine. Although aspirin (contained in this combination medicine) passes into the breast milk, it has not been shown to cause problems in nursing babies.

—if you have any of the following medical problems:
Anemia
Asthma, allergies, and nasal polyps (history of)
Epilepsy
Gout
Hemophilia or other bleeding problems
Kidney disease
Liver disease
Porphyria
Stomach ulcer or other stomach problems

—if you are taking **any** other prescription or nonprescription (OTC) medicine, especially:
Anticoagulants (blood thinners)
Antidiabetic agents, oral (diabetes medicine you take by mouth)
Central nervous system (CNS) depressants

Heparin (e.g., Panheprin)

Medicine for inflammation or pain (aspirin or other salicylates, diclofenac [e.g., Voltaren], diflunisal [e.g., Dolobid], fenoprofen [e.g., Nalfon], flurbiprofen [oral] [e.g., Ansaid], ibuprofen [e.g., Motrin], indomethacin [e.g., Indocin], ketoprofen [e.g., Orudis], meclofenamate [e.g., Meclomen], mefenamic acid [e.g., Ponstel], naproxen [e.g., Naprosyn], phenylbutazone [e.g., Butazolidin], piroxicam [e.g., Feldene], sulindac [e.g., Clinoril], tiaprofenic acid [e.g., Surgam], tolmetin [e.g., Tolectin]

Methotrexate (e.g., Mexate)

Probenecid (e.g., Benemid)

Sulfinpyrazone (e.g., Anturane)

Urinary alkalizers (medicine that makes the urine less acid, such as acetazolamide [e.g., Diamox], calcium- and magnesium-containing antacids, dichlorphenamide [e.g., Daranide], methazolamide [e.g., Neptazane], potassium or sodium citrate and/or citric acid, sodium bicarbonate [baking soda])

Vancomycin [e.g., Vancocin])

Proper Use of This Medicine

Take this medicine with food or a full glass (8 ounces) of water to lessen stomach irritation.

Do not use this medicine if it has a strong vinegar-like odor, since this means the aspirin is breaking down. If you have any questions about this, check with your doctor or pharmacist.

There have been reports suggesting that use of aspirin in children with fever due to a viral infection (especially flu or chickenpox) may cause a serious illness called Reye's syndrome. **Do not give a medicine containing aspirin or other salicylates to a child with flu or chickenpox without first discussing this with your child's doctor.**

Take this medicine only as directed by your doctor. Do not take more of it, do not take it more often, and do not take it for a longer period of time than your doctor ordered. If too much meprobamate is taken, it may become habit-forming. Also, taking too much aspirin may cause stomach problems or lead to medical problems because of an overdose.

How to store this medicine:

• **Keep this medicine out of the reach of children** since overdose is very dangerous in children.

• Store away from heat and direct light.

• Do not store in the bathroom, near the kitchen sink, or in other damp places. Heat or moisture may cause the medicine to break down.

• Do not keep outdated medicine or medicine no longer needed. Be sure that any discarded medicine is out of the reach of children.

Precautions While Using This Medicine

If you will be taking this medicine regularly for a long period of time:

• Your doctor should check your progress at regular visits.

• Check with your doctor at least every 4 months to make sure you need to continue taking this medicine.

If you will be taking this medicine in large doses or for a long period of time, do not stop taking it without first checking with your doctor. Your doctor may want you to reduce gradually the amount you are taking before stopping completely.

Check the labels of all over-the-counter (OTC), nonprescription, and prescription medicines you now take. If any contain aspirin or other salicylates (including diflunisal or bismuth subsalicylate), be especially careful. Taking or using any of these medicines while taking this combination medicine containing aspirin may lead to overdose. If you have any questions about this, check with your doctor or pharmacist.

This medicine will add to the effects of alcohol and other CNS depressants (medicines that slow down the nervous system, possibly causing drowsiness). Some examples of CNS depressants are antihistamines or medicine for hay fever, other allergies, or colds; sedatives, tranquilizers, or sleeping medicine; prescription pain medicine or narcotics; barbiturates; medicine for convulsions (seizures); muscle relaxants; or anesthetics, including some dental anesthetics. **Check with your doctor before taking any of the above while you are taking this medicine.**

Stomach problems may be more likely to occur if you drink alcoholic beverages while being treated with this medicine, especially if you are taking the medicine in high doses or for a long time. Check with your doctor if you have any questions about this.

Too much use of this medicine together with certain other medicines may increase the chance of stomach problems. Therefore, do not regularly take this medicine together with any of the following medicines, unless directed to do so by your physician or dentist:

Diclofenac
Diflunisal
Fenoprofen
Flurbiprofen (oral)
Ibuprofen
Indomethacin
Ketoprofen
Meclofenamate
Mefenamic acid
Phenylbutazone
Piroxicam
Sulindac
Tiaprofenic acid
Tolmetin

If you are taking a laxative containing cellulose, do not take it within 2 hours of taking this medicine. Taking these medicines close together may make this medicine less effective by preventing the aspirin (contained in this combination medicine) from being absorbed by your body.

Diabetics—False urine sugar test results may occur if you take 8 or more 325-mg (5-grain) doses of aspirin (contained in this combination medicine) every day for several days in a row. Smaller doses or occasional use of aspirin usually will not affect urine sugar tests.

If you have any questions about this, check with your doctor, especially if your diabetes is not well controlled.

If you plan to have surgery, including dental surgery, do not take aspirin (contained in this combination medicine) for 5 days before the surgery, unless otherwise directed by your physician or dentist. Taking aspirin during this time may cause bleeding problems.

If you think you or someone else may have taken an overdose of this medicine, get emergency help at once. Taking an overdose of this medicine or taking alcohol or other CNS depressants with it may lead to unconsciousness and possibly death. Some signs of an overdose are continuing ringing or buzzing in ears; any hearing loss; severe confusion, drowsiness, or weakness; shortness of breath or slow or troubled breathing; staggering; and slow heartbeat.

This medicine may cause some people to become dizzy, lightheaded, drowsy, or less alert than they are normally. **Make sure you know how you react to this medicine before you drive, use machines, or do other jobs that require you to be alert.**

Meprobamate (contained in this combination medicine) may cause dryness of the mouth. For temporary relief, use sugarless candy or gum, melt bits of ice in your mouth, or use a saliva substitute. However, if dry mouth continues for more than 2 weeks, check with your dentist. Continuing dryness of the mouth may increase the chance of dental disease, including tooth decay, gum disease, and fungal infections.

Side Effects of This Medicine

Along with its needed effects, a medicine may cause some unwanted effects. Although not all of these side effects may occur, if they do occur they may need medical attention.

Check with your doctor immediately if any of the following side effects occur:

Rare

 Wheezing, shortness of breath, troubled breathing, or tightness in chest

Signs of overdose

 Any loss of hearing
 Bloody urine
 Confusion (severe)
 Convulsions (seizures)
 Diarrhea (severe or continuing)
 Dizziness or lightheadedness (continuing)
 Drowsiness (severe)
 Fast or deep breathing
 Hallucinations (seeing, hearing, or feeling things that are not there)
 Headache (severe or continuing)
 Increase in sweating
 Nausea or vomiting (continuing)
 Nervousness or excitement (severe)
 Ringing or buzzing in ears (continuing)
 Slow heartbeat

 Slurred speech
 Staggering
 Stomach pain (severe or continuing)
 Unexplained fever
 Unusual or uncontrollable flapping movements of the hands, especially in elderly patients
 Unusual thirst
 Vision problems
 Weakness (severe)

Signs of overdose in children

 Changes in behavior
 Drowsiness or tiredness (severe)
 Fast or deep breathing

Also, check with your doctor as soon as possible if any of the following side effects occur:

Rare

 Bloody or black tarry stools
 Confusion
 Skin rash, hives, or itching
 Sore throat and fever
 Unusual bleeding or bruising
 Unusual excitement
 Unusual tiredness or weakness
 Vomiting of blood or material that looks like coffee grounds

Other side effects may occur that usually do not require medical attention. These side effects may go away during treatment as your body adjusts to the medicine. However, check with your doctor if any of the following side effects continue or are bothersome:

More common

 Drowsiness
 Heartburn or indigestion
 Stomach pain (mild)

Less common

 Blurred vision or change in near or distant vision
 Dizziness or lightheadedness
 Headache
 Nausea or vomiting

For children and elderly patients: Some of the above side effects are more likely to occur in children, especially those with fever and who are dehydrated, and elderly patients, who are usually more sensitive to the effects of the meprobamate and aspirin combination.

After you stop using this medicine, your body may need time to adjust. The length of time this takes depends on the amount of medicine you were using and how long you used it. During this period of time check with your doctor if you notice any of the following side effects:

 Clumsiness or unsteadiness
 Confusion
 Convulsions (seizures)

Hallucinations (seeing, hearing, or feeling things that are
not there)
Increased dreaming
Muscle twitching
Nausea or vomiting
Nervousness or restlessness
Nightmares
Trembling
Trouble in sleeping

Other side effects not listed above may also occur in some
patients. If you notice any other effects, check with
your doctor.

December 1987

MERCAPTOPURINE (Systemic)

Some commonly used brand names or other names are Purinethol and 6-MP.

To the Reader: If you do not recognize the names of medical conditions or medicines referred to in this information, check with your doctor, nurse, or pharmacist. Definitions for selected medical terms may be found in the Glossary. Brand names for the generic drug names listed can be found in the Index. In addition, selected brand names commonly associated with the generic name have been included in the text to help you recognize medicine you may be taking. The fact that a brand name product is not mentioned does not mean the information does not apply. It is a good idea for you to learn both the generic and brand names of your medicines and to write them down for future use.

Mercaptopurine (mer-kap-toe-PYOOR-een) belongs to the group of medicines known as antimetabolites. It is taken by mouth to treat some kinds of cancer.

Mercaptopurine interferes with the growth of cancer cells, which are eventually destroyed. Since the growth of normal body cells may also be affected by mercaptopurine, other effects will also occur. Some of these may be serious and must be reported to your doctor. Other effects may not be serious but may cause concern. Some effects may not occur for months or years after the medicine is used.

Before you begin treatment with mercaptopurine, you and your doctor should talk about the good this medicine will do as well as the risks of using it.

Mercaptopurine may also be used for other conditions as determined by your doctor.

Mercaptopurine is available only with your doctor's prescription.

Remember:

• **This medicine has been prescribed for your current medical problem only.** It must not be given to other people or used for other problems unless you are directed to do so by your doctor.

• **Keep all medicines out of the reach of children.**

• In order for this medicine to work, it must be used as directed.

• **It is very important that you read and understand the following information.** If any of the information causes you special concern, do not decide against using this medicine without first checking with your doctor.

• Before you begin using any new medicine (prescription or nonprescription) or if you develop any new medical problem while you are using this medicine, check with your doctor, nurse, or pharmacist.

• **If you have any questions** about the following information or if you want more information about this medicine or your medical problem, **ask your doctor, nurse, or pharmacist.**

Before Using This Medicine

In order to decide on the best treatment for your medical problem, your doctor should be told:

—if you have ever had any unusual or allergic reaction to mercaptopurine.

—if you are **pregnant** or if you intend to have children. There is a chance that this medicine may cause birth defects if either the male or female is taking it at the time of conception or if it is taken during pregnancy. However, studies have not been done in humans. Mercaptopurine has been shown to cause damage to the fetus in rats and increases the risk of miscarriage or premature births in humans. In addition, many cancer medicines may cause sterility which could be permanent. Although this has not been reported with this medicine, the possibility should be kept in mind. Be sure that you have discussed this with your doctor before taking this medicine.

—if you intend to **breast-feed**. Because this medicine may cause serious side effects, breast-feeding is generally not recommended while you are taking it.

—if you have any of the following medical problems:
Chickenpox (including recent exposure)
Gout (history of)
Herpes zoster (shingles)
Infection
Kidney disease
Kidney stones (history of)
Liver disease

—if you are taking **any** other prescription or nonprescription (OTC) medicine, especially:
Acetaminophen (with long-term, high-dose use) (e.g., Tylenol)
Adrenocorticoids (cortisone-like medicines)
Amiodarone (e.g., Cordarone)
Amphotericin B by injection (e.g., Fungizone)
Anabolic steroids (dromostanolone, ethylestrenol, nandrolone, oxandrolone, oxymetholone, stanozolol)
Androgens (male hormones)
Antithyroid agents (medicine for overactive thyroid)
Azathioprine (e.g., Imuran)
Azlocillin (e.g., Azlin)
Carbamazepine (e.g., Tegretol)
Chloramphenicol (e.g., Chloromycetin)
Chloroquine (e.g., Aralen)
Colchicine
Cyclosporine (e.g., Sandimmune)
Dantrolene (e.g., Dantrium)
Disulfiram (e.g., Antabuse)
Divalproex (e.g., Depakote)
Erythromycins
Estrogens (female hormones)
Flucytosine (e.g., Ancobon)
Furazolidone (e.g., Furoxone)
Gold salts
Hydroxychloroquine (e.g., Plaquenil)
Interferon (e.g., Intron A; Roferon-A)
Isoniazid (e.g., Nydrazid)
Ketoconazole (e.g., Nizoral)
Methyldopa (e.g., Aldomet)
Mezlocillin (e.g., Mezlin)
Muromonab-CD3 (monoclonal antibody; e.g., Orthoclone OKT3)
Naltrexone (with long-term, high-dose use) (e.g., Trexan)

Nitrofurantoin (e.g., Furadantin)
Oral contraceptives (birth control pills) containing estrogen
Phenothiazines (acetophenazine, chlorpromazine, fluphenazine, mesoridazine, perphenazine, prochlorperazine, promazine, promethazine, thioridazine, trifluoperazine, triflupromazine, trimeprazine)
Phenytoin (e.g., Dilantin)
Piperacillin (e.g., Pipracil)
Plicamycin (e.g., Mithracin)
Probenecid (e.g., Benemid)
Rifampin (e.g., Rifadin)
Sulfinpyrazone (e.g., Anturane)
Sulfonamides (sulfa medicines)
Valproic acid (e.g., Depakene)

—if you have ever been treated with x-rays or cancer medicines.

Proper Use of This Medicine

Use this medicine only as directed by your doctor. Do not use more or less of it, and do not use it more often than your doctor ordered. The exact amount of medicine you need has been carefully worked out. Taking too much may increase the chance of side effects, while taking too little may not improve your condition.

Mercaptopurine is often given together with certain other medicines. If you are using a combination of medicines, make sure that you take each one at the right time and do not mix them. Ask your doctor, nurse, or pharmacist to help you plan a way to remember to take your medicines at the right times.

While you are using mercaptopurine, your doctor may want you to drink extra fluids so that you will pass more urine. This will help prevent kidney problems and keep your kidneys working well.

If you miss a dose of this medicine, do not take the missed dose at all and do not double the next one. Instead, go back to your regular dosing schedule and check with your doctor.

How to store this medicine:

- **Keep out of the reach of children.**

- Store away from heat and direct light.

- Do not store in the bathroom, near the kitchen sink, or in other damp places. Heat or moisture may cause the medicine to break down.

- Do not keep outdated medicine or medicine no longer needed. Be sure that any discarded medicine is out of the reach of children.

Precautions While Using This Medicine

It is very important that your doctor check your progress at regular visits to make sure that this medicine is working properly and to check for unwanted effects.

Avoid alcoholic beverages until you have discussed their use with your doctor. Alcohol may increase the harmful effects of this medicine.

While you are being treated with mercaptopurine, and after you stop treatment with it, **do not have any immunizations without your doctor's approval**. Mercaptopurine lowers your body's resistance and there is a chance you might get the infection the immunization is meant to prevent. In addition, other persons living in your household should not take oral polio vaccine since there is a chance they could pass the polio virus on to you. Also, you should avoid close contact with other persons (for example, at school or work) who have taken oral polio vaccine.

Mercaptopurine can lower the number of white blood cells in your body. This may increase the chance of getting an infection. If you can, avoid people with colds or other infections. If you think you are getting a cold or other infection, check with your doctor.

Side Effects of This Medicine

Along with their needed effects, medicines like mercaptopurine can sometimes cause unwanted effects such as blood problems, liver problems, and other side effects; these are described below. Also, because of the way these medicines act on the body, there is a chance that they might cause other unwanted effects that may not occur until months or years after the medicine is used. These delayed effects may include certain types of cancer, such as leukemia. Discuss these possible effects with your doctor.

Although not all of these side effects may occur, if they do occur they may need medical attention.

Check with your doctor immediately if any of the following side effects occur:

More common
　　Fever, chills, or sore throat
　　Unusual bleeding or bruising

Check with your doctor as soon as possible if any of the following side effects occur:

More common
　　Unusual tiredness or weakness
　　Yellow eyes and skin

Less common
　　Joint pain
　　Loss of appetite
　　Lower back, side, or stomach pain
　　Nausea and vomiting
　　Swelling of feet or lower legs

Rare
　　Black tarry stools
　　Sores in the mouth and on the lips

Other side effects may occur that usually do not require medical attention. These side effects may go away during treatment as your body adjusts to the medicine. Also, your doctor or nurse may be able to tell you about ways to prevent or reduce some of these side effects. Check with your doctor if any of the following side effects continue or are bothersome or if you have any questions about them:

Less common

    Darkening of skin
    Diarrhea
    Headache
    Skin rash and itching
    Weakness

For elderly patients: Many medicines have not been tested in older people. Therefore, it is not known whether the medicine acts the same way it does in younger adults. Check with your doctor or pharmacist if you notice any unusual effects while taking this medicine or if you think it is not working as it should.

After you stop taking mercaptopurine, it may still produce some side effects that need attention. During this period of time, check with your doctor if you notice any of the following side effects:

    Fever, chills, or sore throat
    Unusual bleeding or bruising
    Yellow eyes and skin

Other side effects not listed above may also occur in some patients. If you notice any other effects, check with your doctor.

December 1987

METHACHOLINE (Inhalation)

A commonly used brand name is Provocholine.

To the Reader: If you do not recognize the names of medical conditions or medicines referred to in this information, check with your doctor, nurse, or pharmacist. Definitions for selected medical terms may be found in the Glossary. Brand names for the generic drug names listed can be found in the Index. In addition, selected brand names commonly associated with the generic name have been included in the text to help you recognize medicine you may be taking. The fact that a brand name product is not mentioned does not mean the information does not apply. It is a good idea for you to learn both the generic and brand names of your medicines and to write them down for future use.

Methacholine (METH-a-koe-leen) is given by inhalation to help find out whether a patient has asthma.

Before the test with methacholine inhalation is given, another test will be done to find out how well your lungs are working.

How test is done: Although there are 5 different strengths of methacholine solution that may be used in this test, not all of them may be necessary. It depends on how you react to each increasing strength of solution during the test. The weakest strength solution is used first. It is placed in a nebulizer and 5 inhalations are taken by mouth. After 3 to 5 minutes, a test will be done to determine what effect the medicine had on your lungs. Each time the test dose is repeated, a stronger solution will be used. During this test, wheezing and difficulty in breathing may occur. If these effects do occur, your doctor may give you a bronchodilator (medicine that opens up the bronchial tubes [air passages] of the lungs) by inhalation to relieve the discomfort.

Methacholine is to be used only by or under the immediate supervision of a doctor.

Remember:
• **It is very important that you read and understand the following information.** If any of the information causes you special concern, do not decide against having this test without first checking with your doctor.

• **If you have any questions** about the following information or if you want more information about this medicine or your medical problem, **ask your doctor, nurse, or pharmacist.**

Before Having This Test

Before this test is given, your doctor should be told:

—if you have ever had any unusual or allergic reaction to methacholine or to similar medicines, such as ambenonium, bethanechol, neostigmine, and pyridostigmine.

—if you are **pregnant** or if you may become pregnant soon after receiving this medicine. Studies on birth defects have not been done in either humans or animals. However, to be safe if the test is necessary, women of child-bearing potential should be given the test within 10 days after the beginning of the last menstrual period or within 2 weeks after a pregnancy test has shown they are not pregnant.

—if you are **breast-feeding**. It is not known whether methacholine passes into the breast milk.

—if you have any of the following medical problems:

Asthma, hay fever, allergic rhinitis, wheezing, chronic lung disease, or respiratory virus illness
Epilepsy
Heart or blood vessel disease
Stomach ulcer
Thyroid disease
Urinary tract blockage

—if any member of your family has asthma.

—if you are taking **any** other prescription or nonprescription (OTC) medicine, especially:

Adrenocorticoids (cortisone-like medicine)
Antimuscarinics (medicine for abdominal or stomach spasms or cramps)
Beta-blockers (acebutolol [e.g., Sectral], atenolol [e.g., Tenormin], esmolol [e.g., Brevibloc], labetalol [e.g., Normodyne], metoprolol [e.g., Lopressor], nadolol [e.g., Corgard], oxprenolol [e.g., Trasicor], pindolol [e.g., Visken], propranolol [e.g., Inderal], sotalol [e.g., Sotacor], timolol [e.g., Blocadren])
Cromolyn (e.g., Intal)
Medicine for breathing problems, colds, sinus problems, or hay fever or other allergies (including nose drops or sprays).

—if you smoke. Smoking may affect the results of this test.

Preparation for This Test

Unless otherwise directed by your doctor:

• **For 24 hours before the test, do not take any extended-release capsule or tablet form of aminophylline, oxtriphylline, or theophylline. For 12 hours before the test, do not use any other medicine**, especially antimuscarinics (medicine for abdominal or stomach spasms or cramps) or medicine for breathing problems, sinus problems, or hay fever or other allergies (including nose drops or sprays). To do so may affect the results of this test.

Side Effects of This Medicine

Along with its needed effects, a medicine may cause some unwanted effects. Although not all of these side effects may occur, if they do occur they may need medical attention.

Check with your doctor or nurse immediately if any of the following side effects occur:

Wheezing, tightness in chest, or difficulty in breathing (continuing or severe)

Other side effects may occur that usually do not require medical attention. These side effects should go away

---

as the effects of the medicine wear off. However, check with your doctor if any of the following side effects continue or are bothersome:

Less common or rare
   Headache or lightheadedness
   Irritation of throat
   Itching

For elderly patients: Many medicines have not been tested in older people. Therefore, it is not known whether the medicine acts the same way it does in younger adults.

Check with your doctor if you notice any unusual effects after receiving this test.

Other side effects not listed above may also occur in some patients. If you notice any other effects, check with your doctor.

_____

December 1987

METHENAMINE (Systemic)

Some commonly used brand names or other names are:	Generic names:
Hexamine	Methenamine†
Hiprex Hip-Rex* Urex	Methenamine Hippurate
Mandelamine	Methenamine Mandelate†

*Not available in the U.S.
†Generic name product may also be available in the U.S.

To the Reader: If you do not recognize the names of medical conditions or medicines referred to in this information, check with your doctor, nurse, or pharmacist. Definitions for selected medical terms may be found in the Glossary. Brand names for the generic drug names listed can be found in the Index. In addition, selected brand names commonly associated with the generic name have been included in the text to help you recognize medicine you may be taking. The fact that a brand name product is not mentioned does not mean the information does not apply. It is a good idea for you to learn both the generic and brand names of your medicines and to write them down for future use.

Methenamine (meth-EN-a-meen) belongs to the general family of medicines called anti-infectives. It is taken by mouth to help prevent and treat infections of the urinary tract.

Methenamine tablets are available without a prescription; however, your doctor may have special instructions on the proper use of this medicine for your medical problem. Methenamine hippurate (HIP-yoo-rate) and methenamine mandelate (MAN-de-late) are available only with your doctor's prescription.

Remember:
• **Methenamine hippurate or methenamine mandelate has been prescribed for your present infection only.** Another infection later on may require a different medicine. Also, even though other people may have the same symptoms as you, they may have a different kind of infection. Your medicine may not work for them and may even cause them harm. Therefore, **your medicine must not be given to other people or used for other infections** unless you are otherwise directed by your doctor.

• **Keep all medicines out of the reach of children.**

• In order for this medicine to work, it must be used as directed. **If you are using this medicine without a prescription, it is very important that you follow the directions on the label.**

• **It is also very important that you read and understand the following information.** If any of the information causes you special concern, check with your doctor or pharmacist.

• Before you begin using any new medicine (prescription or nonprescription) or if you develop any new medical problem while you are using this medicine, check with your doctor, nurse, or pharmacist.

• **If you have any questions** about the following information or if you want more information about this medicine or your medical problem, **ask your doctor, nurse, or pharmacist.**

Before Using This Medicine

Before you use methenamine, check with your doctor or pharmacist:

—if you have ever had any unusual or allergic reaction to methenamine.

—if you are on a low-salt, low-sugar, or any other special diet, or if you are allergic to any substance, such as foods, sulfites or other preservatives, or dyes. Most medicines contain more than their active ingredient, and many liquid medicines contain alcohol. Your doctor, nurse, or pharmacist can help you avoid products that may cause a problem.

—if you are **pregnant** or if you may become pregnant. Studies have not been done in either humans or animals. However, individual case reports on the use of methenamine during pregnancy have not shown that this medicine causes birth defects or other problems in humans.

—if you are **breast-feeding**. Methenamine passes into the breast milk. However, methenamine has not been shown to cause problems in nursing babies.

—if you have either of the following medical problems:
   Kidney disease, severe
   Liver disease, severe

—if you are taking **any** other prescription or nonprescription (OTC) medicine, especially:
   Sulfonamides (sulfa medicine)
   Thiazide diuretics (water pills)
   Urinary alkalizers (medicine that makes the urine less acid, such as acetazolamide, calcium- and/or magnesium-containing antacids, dichlorphenamide, methazolamide, potassium or sodium citrate and/or citric acid, sodium bicarbonate [baking soda])

Proper Use of This Medicine

Before you start taking this medicine, check your urine with phenaphthazine paper or another test to see if it is acid. **Your urine must be acid (pH 5.5 or below) in order for this medicine to work well.** If you have any questions about this, check with your doctor, nurse, or pharmacist.

The following changes in your diet may help make your urine more acid; however, check with your doctor first if you are on a special diet (for example, for diabetes). Avoid most fruits (especially citrus fruits and juices), milk and other dairy products, and other foods that make the urine more alkaline. Also, avoid antacids unless otherwise directed by your doctor. Eating more protein and foods such as cranberries (especially cranberry juice with vitamin C added), plums, or prunes may also help. If your urine is still not acid enough, check with your doctor.

If this medicine causes nausea or upset stomach, it may be taken after meals and at bedtime.

For patients taking the dry granule form of this medicine:
- Dissolve the contents of each packet in 2 to 4 ounces of cold water immediately before taking. Stir well. Be sure to drink all the liquid in order to get the full dose of medicine.

For patients taking the oral liquid form of this medicine:
- Use a specially marked measuring spoon or other device to measure each dose accurately, since the average household teaspoon may not hold the right amount of liquid.

For patients taking the enteric-coated tablet form of this medicine:
- Swallow tablets whole. Do not break, crush, or take if chipped.

To help clear up your infection completely, **keep taking this medicine for the full time of treatment** even if you begin to feel better after a few days; **do not miss any doses.**

If you do miss a dose of this medicine, take it as soon as possible. However, if it is almost time for your next dose and your dosing schedule is:
- 2 doses a day—Space the missed dose and the next dose 5 to 6 hours apart.
- 3 or more doses a day—Space the missed dose and the next dose 2 to 4 hours apart or double your next dose.

Then go back to your regular dosing schedule.

How to store this medicine:
- **Keep out of the reach of children.**
- Store away from heat and direct light.
- Do not store the dry granule or tablet form of this medicine in the bathroom, near the kitchen sink, or in other damp places. Heat or moisture may cause the medicine to break down.
- Keep the oral liquid form of this medicine from freezing.
- Do not keep outdated medicine or medicine no longer needed. Be sure that any discarded medicine is out of the reach of children.

Precautions While Using This Medicine

If your symptoms do not improve within a few days, or if they become worse, check with your doctor.

Side Effects of This Medicine

Along with its needed effects, a medicine may cause some unwanted effects. Although not all of these side effects may occur, if they do occur they may need medical attention.

Check with your doctor immediately if any of the following side effects occur:

Less common
     Blood in urine
     Lower back pain
     Pain or burning while urinating

Other side effects may occur that usually do not require medical attention. These side effects may go away during treatment as your body adjusts to the medicine. However, check with your doctor if any of the following side effects continue or are bothersome:

Less common
     Nausea
     Skin rash
     Stomach upset

For elderly patients: Many medicines have not been tested in older people. Therefore, it is not known whether the medicine acts the same way it does in younger adults. Check with your doctor or pharmacist if you notice any unusual effects while taking this medicine or if you think it is not working as it should.

Other side effects not listed above may also occur in some patients. If you notice any other effects, check with your doctor.

December 1987

METHOTREXATE (Systemic)

Some commonly used brand names are:

Folex	Mexate
Folex PFS	Mexate-AQ

Generic name product may also be available in the U.S. and Canada.

To the Reader: If you do not recognize the names of medical conditions or medicines referred to in this information, check with your doctor, nurse, or pharmacist. Definitions for selected medical terms may be found in the Glossary. Brand names for the generic drug names listed can be found in the Index. In addition, selected brand names commonly associated with the generic name have been included in the text to help you recognize medicine you may be taking. The fact that a brand name product is not mentioned does not mean the information does not apply. It is a good idea for you to learn both the generic and brand names of your medicines and to write them down for future use.

Methotrexate (meth-o-TREX-ate) belongs to the group of medicines known as antimetabolites. It is taken by mouth or given by injection to treat some kinds of cancer.

Methotrexate is also used to treat some medical conditions that are not cancerous, such as psoriasis. It may also be used for other conditions as determined by your doctor.

Methotrexate blocks an enzyme needed by the cell to live. This interferes with the growth of cancer cells, which are eventually destroyed. The way methotrexate works in psoriasis is similar to the way it works against cancer, since skin cells in psoriasis are also growing rapidly. Since the growth of normal body cells may also be affected by methotrexate, other effects will also occur. Some of these may be serious and must be reported to your doctor. Other effects, like hair loss, may not be serious but may cause concern. Some effects may not occur for months or years after the medicine is used.

Before you begin treatment with methotrexate, you and your doctor should talk about the good this medicine will do as well as the risks of using it.

Methotrexate is available only with your doctor's prescription.

Remember:

• **This medicine has been prescribed for your current medical problem only.** It must not be given to other people or used for other problems unless you are directed to do so by your doctor.

• **Keep all medicines out of the reach of children.**

• In order for this medicine to work, it must be used as directed.

• If you are receiving this medicine by injection, some of the information about this medicine may not apply.

• **It is very important that you read and understand the following information.** If any of the information causes you special concern, do not decide against using this medicine without first checking with your doctor.

• Before you begin using any new medicine (prescription or nonprescription) or if you develop any new medical problem while you are using this medicine, check with your doctor, nurse, or pharmacist.

• **If you have any questions** about the following information or if you want more information about this medicine or your medical problem, **ask your doctor, nurse, or pharmacist.**

Before Using This Medicine

In order to decide on the best treatment for your medical problem, your doctor should be told:

—if you have ever had any unusual or allergic reaction to methotrexate.

—if you are **pregnant** or if you intend to have children. There is a good chance that this medicine may cause birth defects if either the male or female is taking it at the time of conception or if it is taken during pregnancy. Methotrexate may cause harm or even death of the fetus. In addition, many cancer medicines may cause sterility which could be permanent. Although this is probably rare with this medicine, the possibility should be kept in mind. Be sure that you have discussed this with your doctor before taking this medicine.

—if you intend to **breast-feed**. Because this medicine may cause serious side effects, breast-feeding is generally not recommended while you are receiving it.

—if you have any of the following medical problems:
Alcoholism
Chickenpox (including recent exposure)
Colitis
Gout (history of)
Herpes zoster (shingles)
Infection
Intestinal blockage
Kidney disease
Kidney stones (or history of)
Liver disease
Mouth sores or inflammation
Stomach ulcer

—if you are taking **any** other prescription or nonprescription (OTC) medicine, especially:
Acetaminophen (with long-term, high-dose use) (e.g., Tylenol)
Amiodarone (e.g., Cordarone)
Amphotericin B (e.g., Fungizone)
Anabolic steroids (dromostanolone, ethylestrenol, nandrolone, oxandrolone, oxymetholone, stanozolol)
Androgens (male hormones)
Antithyroid agents (medicine for overactive thyroid)
Azathioprine (e.g., Imuran)
Azlocillin (e.g., Azlin)
Carbamazepine (e.g., Tegretol)
Chloramphenicol (e.g., Chloromycetin)
Chloroquine (e.g., Aralen)
Colchicine
Dantrolene (e.g., Dantrium)
Disulfiram (e.g., Antabuse)
Divalproex (e.g., Depakote)
Erythromycins
Estrogens (female hormones)
Flucytosine (e.g., Ancobon)
Furazolidone (e.g., Furoxone)
Gold salts
Hydroxychloroquine (e.g., Plaquenil)
Interferon (e.g., Intron A; Roferon-A)
Isoniazid (e.g., Nydrazid)

Ketoconazole (e.g., Nizoral)
Medicine for inflammation or pain (aspirin or other sal-
icylates, diclofenac, diflunisal, fenoprofen, ibuprofen,
indomethacin, ketoprofen, meclofenamate, mefenamic acid, naproxen, phenylbutazone, piroxicam, sul-
indac, suprofen, tolmetin)
Methyldopa (e.g., Aldomet)
Mezlocillin (e.g., Mezlin)
Naltrexone (with long-term, high-dose use) (e.g., Trexan)
Nitrofurantoin (e.g., Furadantin)
Oral contraceptives (birth control pills) containing estro-
gen
Phenothiazines (acetophenazine, chlorpromazine, flu-
phenazine, mesoridazine, perphenazine, prochlorper-
azine, promazine, promethazine, thioridazine, triflu-
operazine, triflupromazine, trimeprazine)
Phenytoin (e.g., Dilantin)
Piperacillin (e.g., Pipracil)
Plicamycin (e.g., Mithracin)
Probenecid (e.g., Benemid)
Rifampin (e.g., Rifadin)
Sulfinpyrazone (e.g., Anturane)
Sulfonamides (sulfa medicines)
Valproic acid (e.g., Depakene)

—if you have ever been treated with x-rays or cancer
medicines.

—if you drink alcohol.

Proper Use of This Medicine

Take this medicine only as directed by your doctor. Do
not take more or less of it, and do not take it more
often than your doctor ordered. The exact amount of
medicine you need has been carefully worked out. Taking too much may increase the chance of side effects
while taking too little may not improve your condition.

Methotrexate is often given together with certain other
medicines. If you are using a combination of medicines, make sure that you take each one at the proper
time and do not mix them. Ask your doctor, nurse, or
pharmacist to help you plan a way to remember to
take your medicines at the right times.

While you are using methotrexate, your doctor may want
you to drink extra fluids so that you will pass more
urine. This will help prevent kidney problems and keep
your kidneys working well.

Methotrexate commonly causes nausea and vomiting.
Even if you begin to feel ill, **do not stop using this
medicine without first checking with your doctor.** Ask
your doctor, nurse, or pharmacist for ways to lessen
these effects.

If you vomit shortly after taking a dose of methotrexate,
check with your doctor. You may be told to take the
dose again or you may have to wait until the next
scheduled dose.

If you miss a dose of this medicine, do not take the missed
dose at all and do not double the next one. Instead,
go back to your regular dosing schedule and check
with your doctor.

How to store this medicine:

• **Keep out of the reach of children**.

• Store away from heat and direct light.

• Do not store in the bathroom, near the kitchen sink,
or in other damp places. Heat or moisture may cause
the medicine to break down.

• Do not keep outdated medicine or medicine no longer
needed. Be sure that any discarded medicine is out of
the reach of children.

Precautions While Using This Medicine

**It is very important that your doctor check your progress
at regular visits** to make sure that this medicine is
working properly and to check for unwanted effects.

Do not drink alcohol while using this medicine. Alcohol
can increase the chance of liver problems.

When you begin to take methotrexate, avoid too much
sun or use of a sunlamp since you may become more
sensitive to sunlight than usual. In case of a severe
burn, check with your doctor. This is especially important if you are taking this medicine for psoriasis
because sunlight can make the psoriasis worse.

**Do not take medicine for inflammation or pain (aspirin
or other salicylates, diclofenac, diflunisal, fenoprofen,
ibuprofen, indomethacin, ketoprofen, meclofenamate,
mefenamic acid, naproxen, phenylbutazone, piroxicam,
sulindac, suprofen, tolmetin) without first checking with
your doctor.** These medicines may increase the effects
of methotrexate.

While you are being treated with methotrexate, and after
you stop treatment with it, **do not have any immunizations without your doctor's approval**. Methotrexate
lowers your body's resistance and there is a chance
you might get the infection the immunization is meant
to prevent. In addition, other persons living in your
household should not take oral polio vaccine since there
is a chance they could pass the polio virus on to you.
Also, you should avoid close contact with other persons
(for example, at school or work) who have taken oral
polio vaccine.

Methotrexate can lower the number of white blood cells
in your body. This may increase the chance of getting
an infection. If you can, avoid people with colds or
other infections. If you think you are getting a cold
or other infection, check with your doctor.

Side Effects of This Medicine

Along with their needed effects, medicines like methotrexate can sometimes cause unwanted effects such as
blood problems, kidney problems, stomach or liver
problems, loss of hair, and other side effects; these are
described below. Also, because of the way these medicines act on the body, there is a chance that they
might cause other unwanted effects that may not occur

until months or years after the medicine is used. These delayed effects may include certain types of cancer, such as leukemia. Discuss these possible effects with your doctor.

Although not all of these side effects may occur, if they do occur they may need medical attention.

Check with your doctor immediately if any of the following side effects occur:

More common
  Black, tarry stools
  Bloody vomit
  Diarrhea
  Fever, chills, or sore throat
  Reddening of skin
  Sores in the mouth and on the lips
  Stomach pain
  Unusual bleeding or bruising

Check with your doctor as soon as possible if any of the following side effects occur:

Less common
  Blood in urine
  Blurred vision
  Confusion
  Convulsions (seizures)
  Cough
  Dark urine
  Dizziness
  Drowsiness
  Headache
  Joint pain
  Shortness of breath
  Swelling of feet or lower legs
  Unusual tiredness or weakness
  Yellow eyes and skin

Other side effects may occur that usually do not require medical attention. These side effects may go away during treatment as your body adjusts to the medicine.

Also, your doctor or nurse may be able to tell you about ways to prevent or reduce some of these side effects. Check with your doctor if any of the following side effects continue or are bothersome or if you have any questions about them:

More common
  Loss of appetite
  Nausea or vomiting

Less common
  Acne
  Boils
  Pale skin
  Skin rash or itching

This medicine may cause a temporary loss of hair in some people. After treatment with methotrexate has ended, normal hair growth should return.

For children and elderly patients: The above side effects may be more likely to occur in very young patients and in the elderly, who are usually more sensitive to the effects of methotrexate.

After you stop using methotrexate, it may still produce some side effects that need attention. During this period of time, check with your doctor as soon as possible if you notice any of the following side effects:
  Blurred vision
  Confusion
  Convulsions (seizures)
  Dizziness
  Drowsiness
  Headache
  Unusual tiredness or weakness

Other side effects not listed above may also occur in some patients. If you notice any other effects, check with your doctor.

———————
December 1987
—————————————————————————

METHOXSALEN (Systemic)

Some commonly used brand names are Oxsoralen, Oxsoralen-Ultra, and UltraMOP*.

*Not available in the U.S.

To the Reader: If you do not recognize the names of medical conditions or medicines referred to in this information, check with your doctor, nurse, or pharmacist. Definitions for selected medical terms may be found in the Glossary. Brand names for the generic drug names listed can be found in the Index. In addition, selected brand names commonly associated with the generic name have been included in the text to help you recognize medicine you may be taking. The fact that a brand name product is not mentioned does not mean the information does not apply. It is a good idea for you to learn both the generic and brand names of your medicines and to write them down for future use.

Methoxsalen (meth-OX-a-len) belongs to the group of medicines called psoralens. It is used along with ultraviolet light (found in sunlight and some special lamps) in a treatment called PUVA to treat vitiligo, a disease in which skin color is lost. It is also used to treat psoriasis. Methoxsalen may also be used for other conditions as determined by your doctor.

This medicine is available only with your doctor's prescription.

Remember:

• **This medicine has been prescribed for your current medical problem only.** It must not be given to other people or used for other problems unless you are directed to do so by your doctor.

• **Keep all medicines out of the reach of children.**

• In order for this medicine to work, it must be used as directed.

• **It is very important that you read and understand the following information.** If any of the information causes you special concern, do not decide against using this medicine without first checking with your doctor.

• Before you begin using any new medicine (prescription or nonprescription) or if you develop any new medical problem while you are using this medicine, check with your doctor, nurse, or pharmacist.

• **If you have any questions** about the following information or if you want more information about this medicine or your medical problem, **ask your doctor, nurse, or pharmacist.**

Before Using This Medicine

Methoxsalen is a very strong medicine that increases the sensitivity of skin to sunlight. In addition to causing serious sunburns if not properly used, it has been reported to increase the chance of skin cancer and cataracts. Also, like too much sunlight, PUVA can cause premature aging of the skin. Therefore, methoxsalen should be used only as directed and it should **not** be used simply for suntanning. Before using this medicine, be sure that you have discussed the use of it with your doctor.

In order to decide on the best treatment for your medical problem, your doctor should be told:

—if you have ever had any unusual or allergic reaction to methoxsalen.

—if you are on a low-salt, low-sugar, or any other special diet, or if you are allergic to any substance, such as foods, sulfites or other preservatives, or dyes. Most medicines contain more than their active ingredient. Your doctor, nurse, or pharmacist can help you avoid products that may cause a problem.

—if you are **pregnant** or if you may become pregnant. Studies have not been done in either humans or animals.

—if you are **breast-feeding**. It is not known whether methoxsalen passes into breast milk. However, this medicine has not been shown to cause problems in nursing babies.

—if you have any of the following medical problems:
  Allergy to sunlight (family history of)
  Eye problems such as cataracts or loss of the lens of the eyes
  Heart or blood vessel disease (severe)
  Infection
  Liver disease
  Lupus erythematosus
  Melanoma or other skin cancer (history of)
  Other skin conditions
  Porphyria
  Stomach problems

—if you are taking **any** other prescription or nonprescription (OTC) medicine.

—if you have recently had x-ray treatment or cancer medicines or plan to have x-rays in the near future.

Proper Use of This Medicine

This medicine may take several weeks or months to really help your condition. **Do not increase the amount of methoxsalen you are taking or spend extra time in the sunlight or under an ultraviolet lamp.** This will not make the medicine act any more quickly and may result in a serious burn.

If this medicine upsets your stomach:

• Patients taking the hard gelatin capsules may take them with food or milk.

• Patients taking the soft gelatin capsules may take them with low fat food or milk.

If you are late in taking, or miss taking, a dose of this medicine, notify your doctor. Remember that exposure to sunlight or ultraviolet light must take place a certain number of hours **after** you take the medicine or it will not work. For patients taking the hard gelatin capsules, this is 2 to 4 hours. For patients taking the soft gelatin capsules, this is 1½ to 2 hours. If you have any questions about this, check with your doctor.

How to store this medicine:

• **Keep out of the reach of children.**

• Store away from heat and direct light.

© 1988   The United States Pharmacopeial Convention, Inc.

• Do not store in the bathroom, near the kitchen sink, or in other damp places. Heat or moisture may cause the medicine to break down.

• Do not keep outdated medicine or medicine no longer needed. Be sure that any discarded medicine is out of the reach of children.

Precautions While Using This Medicine

Your doctor should check your progress at regular visits to make sure this medicine is working and that it does not cause unwanted effects. Eye examinations should be included.

This medicine increases the sensitivity of your skin to sunlight; too much exposure to the sun could cause a serious burn. If you must go out in the sunlight, **cover your skin for at least 24 hours before and 8 hours following treatment.** A special sunscreening lotion may also help.

Your skin may continue to be sensitive to sunlight for some time after treatment with this medicine is stopped. Use extra caution if you plan to spend any time in the sun.

For 24 hours after you take each dose of methoxsalen, your eyes should be protected during daylight hours with special wraparound sunglasses that totally block or absorb ultraviolet light. This is to prevent cataracts. Your doctor will tell you what kind of sunglasses to use. These glasses are needed even in indirect light, such as light coming through a window glass. In addition, protect your lips with a special lipstick that blocks sunlight.

Eating certain foods while you are taking methoxsalen may increase the sensitivity of your skin to sunlight. To help prevent this, avoid eating limes, figs, parsley, parsnips, mustard, carrots, and celery while you are being treated with this medicine.

This medicine may cause your skin to become dry or itchy. **However, check with your doctor before applying anything to your skin to treat this problem.**

Side Effects of This Medicine

Along with its needed effects, a medicine may cause some unwanted effects. Although not all of these side effects may occur, if they do occur they may need medical attention.

Check with your doctor immediately if you think you have taken an overdose or if any of the following side effects occur since they may indicate a serious burn:
Blistering and peeling of skin
Reddened, sore skin
Swelling (especially in feet or lower legs)

Other side effects may occur that usually do not require medical attention. These side effects may go away during treatment as your body adjusts to the medicine. However, check with your doctor if any of the following side effects continue or are bothersome:

More common
Itching of skin
Nausea

Less common
Dizziness
Headache
Mental depression
Nervousness
Trouble in sleeping

Treatment with this medicine usually causes slight reddening of the skin 24 to 48 hours after the treatment. This is an expected effect and is no cause for concern. However, check with your doctor right away if skin becomes sore and red or blistered.

For pediatric patients: Some of the above side effects are more likely to occur in children up to 12 years of age, since these children may be more sensitive to the effects of methoxsalen.

For elderly patients: Many medicines have not been tested in older people. Therefore, it is not known whether the medicine acts the same way it does in younger adults. Check with your doctor or pharmacist if you notice any unusual effects while taking this medicine or if you think it is not working as it should.

Other side effects not listed above may also occur in some patients. If you notice any other effects, check with your doctor.

December 1987

METHOXSALEN (Topical)

A commonly used brand name is Oxsoralen.

To the Reader: If you do not recognize the names of medical conditions or medicines referred to in this information, check with your doctor, nurse, or pharmacist. Definitions for selected medical terms may be found in the Glossary. Brand names for the generic drug names listed can be found in the Index. In addition, selected brand names commonly associated with the generic name have been included in the text to help you recognize medicine you may be taking. The fact that a brand name product is not mentioned does not mean the information does not apply. It is a good idea for you to learn both the generic and brand names of your medicines and to write them down for future use.

Methoxsalen (meth-OX-a-len) belongs to the group of medicines called psoralens. It is used on the skin along with ultraviolet light (found in sunlight and some special lamps) in a treatment called PUVA to treat vitiligo, a disease in which skin color is lost. Methoxsalen may also be used for other conditions as determined by your doctor.

If you want more information about this medicine, ask your doctor, nurse, or pharmacist.

Methoxsalen is available only with a prescription and is to be administered by or under the direct supervision of your doctor.

Remember:

• **It is very important that you read and understand the following information.** If any of the information causes you special concern, do not decide against being treated with this medicine without first checking with your doctor.

• Before you begin using any new medicine (prescription or nonprescription) or if you develop any new medical problem while you are being treated with this medicine, check with your doctor, nurse, or pharmacist.

• **If you have any questions** about the following information or if you want more information about this medicine or your medical problem, **ask your doctor, nurse, or pharmacist.**

Before Using This Medicine

Methoxsalen is a very strong medicine that increases the sensitivity of skin to sunlight. In addition to causing serious sunburns if not properly used, it has been reported to increase the chance of skin cancer. Also, like too much sunlight, PUVA can cause premature aging of the skin. Therefore, methoxsalen should be used only as directed and should **not** be used simply for suntanning. Before using this medicine, be sure that you have discussed the use of it with your doctor.

In order to decide on the best treatment for your medical problem, your doctor should be told:

—if you have ever had any unusual or allergic reaction to methoxsalen.

—if you are allergic to any substance, such as certain preservatives or dyes. Most medicines contain more than their active ingredient. Your doctor, nurse, or pharmacist can help you avoid products that may cause a problem.

—if you are **pregnant** or if you may become pregnant. Studies have not been done in either humans or animals.

—if you are **breast-feeding**, although methoxsalen has not been shown to cause problems in nursing babies.

—if you have any of the following medical problems:

Allergy to sunlight (family history of)
Heart or blood vessel disease (severe)
Infection
Lupus erythematosus
Melanoma or other skin cancer (history of)
Other skin conditions
Porphyria

—if you are taking **any** other prescription or nonprescription (OTC) medicine.

—if you have recently had x-ray treatment or cancer medicines or plan to have x-rays in the near future.

Precautions While Using This Medicine

It is important that you visit your doctor as directed for treatments and to have your progress checked.

This medicine increases the sensitivity of your skin to sunlight; too much exposure to the sun could cause a serious burn. Thoroughly wash the treated areas after the light treatment. If you must go out in the sunlight, **cover the treated areas of your skin for at least 12 to 48 hours following treatment.** A special sunscreening lotion may also help.

Your skin may continue to be sensitive to sunlight for some time after treatment with this medicine is stopped. Use extra caution if you plan to spend any time in the sun.

Eating certain foods while you are using methoxsalen may increase the sensitivity of your skin to sunlight. To help prevent this, avoid eating limes, figs, parsley, parsnips, mustard, carrots, and celery while you are being treated with this medicine.

This medicine may cause your skin to become dry or itchy. **However, check with your doctor before applying anything to your skin to treat this problem.**

Side Effects of This Medicine

Along with its needed effects, a medicine may cause some unwanted effects. Although not all of these side effects may occur, if they do occur they may need medical attention.

Check with your doctor immediately if any of the following side effects occur since they may indicate a serious burn:

    Blistering and peeling of skin
    Reddened, sore skin
    Swelling, especially in the feet or lower legs

For elderly patients: Many medicines have not been tested in older people. Therefore, it is not known whether the medicine acts the same way it does in younger adults.

Check with your doctor or pharmacist if you notice any unusual effects while using this medicine or if you think it is not working as it should.

Other side effects not listed above may also occur in some patients. If you notice any other effects, check with your doctor.

_____

December 1987
_____

METHYLDOPA (Systemic)

Some commonly used brand names are:

Aldomet	Dopamet*
Apo-Methyldopa*	Novomedopa*

Generic name product may also be available in the U.S. and Canada.

---

*Not available in the U.S.

To the Reader: If you do not recognize the names of medical conditions or medicines referred to in this information, check with your doctor, nurse, or pharmacist. Definitions for selected medical terms may be found in the Glossary. Brand names for the generic drug names listed can be found in the Index. In addition, selected brand names commonly associated with the generic name have been included in the text to help you recognize medicine you may be taking. The fact that a brand name product is not mentioned does not mean the information does not apply. It is a good idea for you to learn both the generic and brand names of your medicines and to write them down for future use.

Methyldopa (meth-ill-DOE-pa) belongs to the general class of medicines called antihypertensives. It is used to treat high blood pressure.

High blood pressure adds to the workload of the heart and arteries. If it continues for a long time, the heart and arteries may not function properly. This can damage the blood vessels of the brain, heart, and kidneys, resulting in a stroke, heart failure, or kidney failure. High blood pressure may also increase the risk of heart attacks. These problems may be less likely to occur if blood pressure is controlled.

Methyldopa works by controlling impulses along certain nerve pathways. As a result, it relaxes blood vessels so that blood passes through them more easily. This helps to lower blood pressure.

Methyldopa is available only with your doctor's prescription.

Remember:

• **This medicine has been prescribed for your current medical problem only.** It must not be given to other people or used for other problems unless you are directed to do so by your doctor.

• **Keep all medicines out of the reach of children.**

• In order for this medicine to work, it must be used as directed.

• If you are receiving this medicine by injection, some of the information about this medicine may not apply.

• **It is very important that you read and understand the following information.** If any of the information causes you special concern, do not decide against using this medicine without first checking with your doctor.

• Before you begin using any new medicine (prescription or nonprescription) or if you develop any new medical problem while you are using this medicine, check with your doctor, nurse, or pharmacist.

• **If you have any questions** about the following information or if you want more information about this medicine or your medical problem, **ask your doctor, nurse, or pharmacist.**

Before Using This Medicine

In order to decide on the best treatment for your medical problem, your doctor should be told:

—if you have ever had any unusual or allergic reaction to methyldopa.

—if you are on a low-salt, low-sugar, or any other special diet, or if you are allergic to any substance, such as foods, sulfites or other preservatives, or dyes. Most medicines contain more than their active ingredient and some methyldopa products may contain sulfites. Your doctor, nurse, or pharmacist can help you avoid products that may cause a problem.

—if you are **pregnant** or if you may become pregnant. Studies in humans have not shown that methyldopa causes birth defects or other problems.

—if you are **breast-feeding**. Although methyldopa passes into breast milk, it has not been shown to cause problems in nursing babies.

—if you have any of the following medical problems:
   Angina (chest pain)
   Kidney disease
   Liver disease
   Mental depression (history of)
   Parkinson's disease
   Pheochromocytoma (PCC)

—if you have taken methyldopa in the past and developed liver problems.

—if you are now taking or have taken within the past 2 weeks monoamine oxidase (MAO) inhibitors, such as:
   Furazolidone (e.g., Furoxone)
   Isocarboxazid (e.g., Marplan)
   Pargyline (e.g., Eutonyl)
   Phenelzine (e.g., Nardil)
   Procarbazine (e.g., Matulane)
   Tranylcypromine (e.g., Parnate)

—if you are taking **any** other prescription or nonprescription (OTC) medicine.

Proper Use of This Medicine

Importance of diet—When prescribing medicine for your condition, your doctor may also prescribe a personal diet for you. Such a diet may be low in sodium (salt). Most people eat much more sodium than they need and too much sodium in the diet may increase blood pressure. Some foods that contain large amounts of sodium are canned soup, pickles, ketchup, green and ripe olives, relish, frankfurters, soy sauce, and carbonated beverages. Your doctor may want you to limit the amounts of these and other high-sodium foods in your diet. High blood pressure medicine is usually more effective when such a diet is properly followed.

Also, it may be very important for you to go on a reducing diet. However, check with your doctor before changing your diet.

Many patients who have high blood pressure will not notice any signs of the problem. In fact, many may feel normal. It is very important that you **take your medicine exactly as directed** and that you keep your appointments with your doctor even if you feel well.

Remember that methyldopa will not cure your high blood pressure but it does help control it. Therefore, you must continue to take it as directed if you expect to lower your blood pressure and keep it down. **You may have to take high blood pressure medicine for the rest of your life.** If high blood pressure is not treated, it can cause serious problems such as heart failure, blood vessel disease, stroke, or kidney disease.

In order to help remember to take your medicine, try to get into the habit of taking it at the same time each day.

If you miss a dose of this medicine, take it as soon as possible. However, if it is almost time for your next dose, skip the missed dose and go back to your regular dosing schedule. Do not double doses.

How to store this medicine:

- **Keep out of the reach of children.**
- Store away from heat and direct light.
- Do not store in the bathroom, near the kitchen sink, or in other damp places. Heat or moisture may cause the medicine to break down.
- Keep the oral liquid form of this medicine from freezing.
- Do not keep outdated medicine or medicine no longer needed. Be sure that any discarded medicine is out of the reach of children.

Precautions While Using This Medicine

It is important that your doctor check your progress at regular visits to make sure that this medicine is working properly.

Do not take other medicines unless they have been discussed with your doctor. This especially includes over-the-counter (nonprescription) medicines for appetite control, asthma, colds, cough, hay fever, or sinus problems, since they may tend to increase your blood pressure.

If you have a fever and there seems to be no reason for it, check with your doctor. This is especially important during the first few weeks you take methyldopa, since fever may be a sign of a serious reaction to this medicine.

Before having any kind of surgery (including dental surgery) or emergency treatment, make sure the physician or dentist in charge knows that you are taking this medicine.

Methyldopa may cause some people to become drowsy or less alert than they are normally. This is more likely to happen when you begin to take it or when you increase the amount of medicine you are taking. **Make sure you know how you react to this medicine before you drive, use machines, or do other jobs that require you to be alert.**

Dizziness, lightheadedness, or fainting may occur, especially when you get up from a lying or sitting position. Getting up slowly may help, but if the problem continues or gets worse, check with your doctor.

Methyldopa may cause dryness of the mouth. For temporary relief, use sugarless candy or gum, melt bits of ice in your mouth, or use a saliva substitute. However, if dry mouth continues for more than 2 weeks, check with your physician or dentist. Continuing dryness of the mouth may increase the chance of dental disease, including tooth decay, gum disease, and fungal infections.

Side Effects of This Medicine

Along with its needed effects, a medicine may cause some unwanted effects. Although not all of these side effects may occur, if they do occur they may need medical attention.

Check with your doctor immediately if the following side effect occurs:

Less common
    Fever shortly after starting to take this medicine

Check with your doctor as soon as possible if any of the following side effects occur:

More common
    Swelling of feet or lower legs

Less common
    Mental depression or anxiety
    Nightmares or unusually vivid dreams
    Trouble in sleeping

Rare
    Dark or amber urine
    Diarrhea or stomach cramps (severe or continuing)
    Fever, chills, troubled breathing, and unusually fast
        heartbeat
    Pale stools
    Shakiness or unusual body movements
    Sore throat and fever
    Stomach pain (severe) with nausea and vomiting
    Tiredness or weakness after having taken this medicine
        for several weeks (continuing)
    Unusual bleeding or bruising
    Yellow eyes and skin

Other side effects may occur that usually do not require medical attention. These side effects may go away during treatment as your body adjusts to the medicine. However, check with your doctor if any of the following side effects continue or are bothersome:

More common
    Drowsiness
    Dry mouth
    Headache

Less common
    Decreased sexual ability
    Diarrhea
    Dizziness or lightheadedness when getting up from a lying
        or sitting position
    Fainting
    Nausea or vomiting

Numbness, tingling, pain, or weakness in hands or feet
Skin rash
Slow heartbeat
Stuffy nose
Swelling of the breasts or unusual milk production

For elderly patients: Dizziness or lightheadedness and drowsiness may be more likely to occur in the elderly, who are more sensitive to the effects of methyldopa.

Other side effects not listed above may also occur in some patients. If you notice any other effects, check with your doctor.

December 1987

METHYLDOPA AND THIAZIDE DIURETICS (Systemic)

This information applies to the following medicines:

Methyldopa (meth-ill-DOE-pa) and Chlorothiazide (klor-oh-THYE-a-zide)

Methyldopa and Hydrochlorothiazide (hye-droe-klor-oh-THYE-a-zide)

Some commonly used brand names are:	Generic names:
Aldoclor	Methyldopa and Chlorothiazide
Aldoril Novodoparil* PMS Dopazide*	Methyldopa and Hydrochlorothiazide†

*Not available in the U.S.

†Generic name product may also be available in the U.S.

To the Reader: If you do not recognize the names of medical conditions or medicines referred to in this information, check with your doctor, nurse, or pharmacist. Definitions for selected medical terms may be found in the Glossary. Brand names for the generic drug names listed can be found in the Index. In addition, selected brand names commonly associated with the generic name have been included in the text to help you recognize medicine you may be taking. The fact that a brand name product is not mentioned does not mean the information does not apply. It is a good idea for you to learn both the generic and brand names of your medicines and to write them down for future use.

Combinations of methyldopa and a thiazide diuretic (chlorothiazide or hydrochlorothiazide) are taken by mouth to treat high blood pressure.

High blood pressure adds to the workload of the heart and arteries. If it continues for a long time, the heart and arteries may not function properly. This can damage the blood vessels of the brain, heart, and kidneys, resulting in a stroke, heart failure, or kidney failure. High blood pressure may also increase the risk of heart attacks. These problems may be less likely to occur if blood pressure is controlled.

Methyldopa works by controlling nerve impulses along certain nerve pathways. As a result, it relaxes blood vessels so that blood passes through them more easily. Thiazide diuretics help reduce the amount of water in the body by increasing the flow of urine. These actions help to lower blood pressure.

This medicine is available only with your doctor's prescription.

Remember:

• **This medicine has been prescribed for your current medical problem only.** It must not be given to other people or used for other problems unless you are directed to do so by your doctor.

• **Keep all medicines out of the reach of children.**

• In order for this medicine to work, it must be used as directed.

• **It is very important that you read and understand the following information.** If any of the information causes you special concern, do not decide against using this medicine without first checking with your doctor.

• Before you begin using any new medicine (prescription or nonprescription) or if you develop any new medical problem while you are using this medicine, check with your doctor, nurse, or pharmacist.

• **If you have any questions** about the following information or if you want more information about this medicine or your medical problem, **ask your doctor, nurse, or pharmacist**.

Before Using This Medicine

In order to decide on the best treatment for your medical problem, your doctor should be told:

—if you have ever had any unusual or allergic reaction to methyldopa, sulfonamides (sulfa drugs), or thiazide diuretics (water pills).

—if you are on a low-salt, low-sugar, or any other special diet, or if you are allergic to any substance, such as foods, sulfites or other preservatives, or dyes. Most medicines contain more than their active ingredient. Your doctor, nurse, or pharmacist can help you avoid products that may cause a problem.

—if you are **pregnant** or if you may become pregnant. Studies in humans have not shown that methyldopa causes birth defects or other problems. When thiazide diuretics are used during pregnancy, they may cause side effects including jaundice, blood problems, and low potassium in the newborn infant. Thiazide diuretics have not been shown to cause birth defects.

—if you are **breast-feeding**. Although this medicine passes into breast milk, it has not been shown to cause problems in nursing babies.

—if you have any of the following medical problems:

Angina (chest pain)
Diabetes mellitus (sugar diabetes)
Gout (history of)
Kidney disease
Liver disease
Lupus erythematosus (history of)
Mental depression (history of)
Pancreas disease
Parkinson's disease
Pheochromocytoma (PCC)

—if you have taken methyldopa in the past and developed liver problems.

—if you are taking **any** other prescription or nonprescription (OTC) medicine, especially:

Adrenocorticoids (cortisone-like medicines)
Digitalis glycosides (heart medicine)
Lithium (e.g., Lithane)
Methenamine (e.g., Mandelamine)

—if you are now taking or have taken within the past 2 weeks monoamine oxidase (MAO) inhibitors, such as:

Furazolidone (e.g., Furoxone)
Isocarboxazid (e.g., Marplan)
Pargyline (e.g., Eutonyl)
Phenelzine (e.g., Nardil)
Procarbazine (e.g., Matulane)
Tranylcypromine (e.g., Parnate)

Proper Use of This Medicine

Importance of diet—When prescribing medicine for your condition, your doctor may also prescribe a personal diet for you. Such a diet may be low in sodium (salt). Most people eat much more sodium than they need and too much sodium in the diet may increase blood pressure. Some foods that contain large amounts of sodium are canned soup, pickles, ketchup, green and ripe olives, relish, frankfurters, soy sauce, and carbonated beverages. Your doctor may want you to limit the amounts of these and other high-sodium foods in your diet. High blood pressure medicine is usually more effective when such a diet is properly followed.

Also, it may be very important for you to go on a reducing diet. However, check with your doctor before changing your diet.

Many patients who have high blood pressure will not notice any signs of the problem. In fact, many may feel normal. It is very important **that you take your medicine exactly as directed** and that you keep your appointments with your doctor even if you feel well.

Remember that this medicine will not cure your high blood pressure but it does help control it. Therefore, you must continue to take it as directed if you expect to lower your blood pressure and keep it down. **You may have to take high blood pressure medicine for the rest of your life.** If high blood pressure is not treated, it can cause serious problems such as heart failure, blood vessel disease, stroke, or kidney disease.

This medicine may cause you to have an unusual feeling of tiredness when you begin to take it. You may also notice an increase in the amount of urine or in your frequency of urination. After taking the medicine for a while, these effects should lessen. In general, in order to keep the increase in urine from affecting your sleep:

• If you are to take a single dose a day, take it in the morning after breakfast.

• If you are to take more than one dose a day, take the last dose no later than 6 p.m., unless otherwise directed by your doctor.

However, it is best to plan your dose or doses according to a schedule that will least affect your personal activities and sleep. Ask your doctor, nurse, or pharmacist to help you plan the best time to take this medicine.

In order to help remember to take your medicine, try to get into the habit of taking it at the same time each day.

If you miss a dose of this medicine, take it as soon as possible. However, if it is almost time for your next dose, skip the missed dose and go back to your regular dosing schedule. Do not double doses.

How to store this medicine:

• **Keep out of the reach of children.**

• Store away from heat and direct light.

• Do not store in the bathroom, near the kitchen sink, or in other damp places. Heat or moisture may cause the medicine to break down.

• Do not keep outdated medicine or medicine no longer needed. Be sure that any discarded medicine is out of the reach of children.

Precautions While Using This Medicine

It is important that your doctor check your progress at regular visits to make sure that this medicine is working properly.

Do not take other medicines unless they have been discussed with your doctor. This especially includes over-the-counter (nonprescription) medicines for appetite control, asthma, colds, cough, hay fever, or sinus problems, since they may tend to increase your blood pressure.

This medicine may cause a loss of potassium from your body:

• To help prevent this, your doctor may want you to:

—eat or drink foods that have a high potassium content (for example, orange or other citrus fruit juices), or

—take a potassium supplement, or

—take another medicine to help prevent the loss of the potassium in the first place.

• It is very important to follow these directions. Also, it is important not to change your diet on your own. This is more important if you are already on a special diet (as for diabetes), or if you are taking a potassium supplement or a medicine to reduce potassium loss. Extra potassium may not be necessary and, in some cases, too much potassium could be harmful.

Check with your doctor if you become sick and have severe or continuing vomiting or diarrhea. These problems may cause you to lose additional water and potassium.

Before having any kind of surgery (including dental surgery) or emergency treatment, tell the physician or dentist in charge that you are taking this medicine.

If you have a fever and there seems to be no reason for it, check with your doctor. This is especially important during the first few weeks you take this medicine since fever may be a sign of a serious reaction to methyldopa.

This medicine may cause some people to become drowsy or less alert than they are normally. This is more likely to happen when you begin to take it or when you increase the amount of medicine you are taking. **Make sure you know how you react to this medicine before you drive, use machines, or do other jobs that require you to be alert.**

Dizziness, lightheadedness, or fainting may occur, especially when you get up from a lying or sitting position. Getting up slowly may help, but if the problem continues or gets worse, check with your doctor.

The dizziness, lightheadedness, or fainting is also more likely to occur if you drink alcohol, stand for long periods of time, exercise, or if the weather is hot. Drinking alcoholic beverages may also make the drowsiness worse. **While you are taking this medicine, be careful in the amount of alcohol you drink.** Also, use extra care during exercise or hot weather or if you must stand for long periods of time.

Diabetics—This medicine may raise blood sugar levels. While you are using this medicine, be especially careful in testing for sugar in your urine. If you have any questions about this, check with your doctor.

This medicine may cause dryness of the mouth. For temporary relief, use sugarless candy or gum, melt bits of ice in your mouth, or use a saliva substitute. However, if dry mouth continues for more than 2 weeks, check with your physician or dentist. Continuing dryness of the mouth may increase the chance of dental disease, including tooth decay, gum disease, and fungal infections.

A few people who take this medicine may become more sensitive to sunlight than they are normally. When you begin taking this medicine, avoid too much sun and do not use a sunlamp until you see how you react to the sun, especially if you tend to burn easily. If you have a severe reaction, check with your doctor.

Side Effects of This Medicine

Along with its needed effects, a medicine may cause some unwanted effects. Although not all of these side effects may occur, if they do occur they may need medical attention.

Check with your doctor immediately if the following side effect occurs:

Rare
> Unexplained fever shortly after starting to take this medicine

Check with your doctor as soon as possible if any of the following side effects occur, especially since some of them may mean that your body is losing too much potassium:

Signs of too much potassium loss
> Dryness of mouth
> Increased thirst
> Irregular heartbeats

> Muscle cramps or pain
> Nausea or vomiting
> Unusual tiredness or weakness
> Weak pulse

Less common
> Mental depression or anxiety
> Nightmares or unusually vivid dreams
> Trouble in sleeping

Rare
> Dark or amber urine
> Diarrhea or stomach cramps (severe or continuing)
> Fever, chills, troubled breathing, and fast heartbeat
> Joint pain
> Lower back, side, or stomach pain
> Pale stools
> Shakiness or unusual body movements
> Skin rash or hives
> Sore throat and fever
> Stomach pain (severe) with nausea and vomiting
> Tiredness or weakness after having taken this medicine for several weeks (continuing)
> Unusual bleeding or bruising
> Yellow eyes and skin

Other side effects may occur that usually do not require medical attention. These side effects may go away during treatment as your body adjusts to the medicine. However, check with your doctor if any of the following side effects continue or are bothersome:

More common
> Dizziness or lightheadedness when getting up from a lying or sitting position
> Drowsiness
> Headache

Less common
> Decreased sexual ability
> Diarrhea
> Fainting
> Increased sensitivity to sunlight
> Loss of appetite
> Numbness, tingling, pain, or weakness in hands or feet
> Skin rash
> Slow heartbeat
> Stuffy nose
> Swelling of the breasts or unusual milk production

For elderly patients: Dizziness or lightheadedness, drowsiness, or signs of too much potassium loss may be more likely to occur in the elderly, who are more sensitive to the effects of methyldopa and thiazide diuretics.

Other side effects not listed above may also occur in some patients. If you notice any other effects, check with your doctor.

December 1987

METHYLPHENIDATE (Systemic)

Some commonly used brand names are Ritalin and Ritalin-SR.

Generic name product may also be available.

To the Reader: If you do not recognize the names of medical conditions or medicines referred to in this information, check with your doctor, nurse, or pharmacist. Definitions for selected medical terms may be found in the Glossary. Brand names for the generic drug names listed can be found in the Index. In addition, selected brand names commonly associated with the generic name have been included in the text to help you recognize medicine you may be taking. The fact that a brand name product is not mentioned does not mean the information does not apply. It is a good idea for you to learn both the generic and brand names of your medicines and to write them down for future use.

Methylphenidate (meth-ill-FEN-i-date) belongs to the group of medicines called central stimulants. It is taken by mouth to treat children with attention deficit disorder (ADD).

Methylphenidate works by increasing attention and decreasing restlessness in children who are overactive, cannot concentrate for very long or are easily distracted, and have unstable emotions. This medicine is used as part of a total treatment program that also includes social, educational, and psychological treatment.

Methylphenidate is also used in the treatment of narcolepsy (uncontrollable desire for sleep or sudden attacks of deep sleep).

This medicine is available only with a doctor's prescription. Prescriptions cannot be refilled. A new written prescription must be obtained from your doctor each time you or your child needs this medicine.

Remember:
* **This medicine has been prescribed for your current medical problem only.** It must not be given to other people or used for other problems unless you are directed to do so by your doctor.

* **Keep all medicines out of the reach of children.**

* In order for this medicine to work, it must be used as directed.

* **It is very important that you read and understand the following information.** If any of the information causes you special concern, do not decide against using this medicine without first checking with your doctor.

* Before you begin using any new medicine (prescription or nonprescription) or if you develop any new medical problem while you are using this medicine, check with your doctor, nurse, or pharmacist.

* **If you have any questions** about the following information or if you want more information about this medicine or your medical problem, **ask your doctor, nurse, or pharmacist.**

Before Using This Medicine

In order to decide on the best treatment for your medical problem, your doctor should be told:

—if you have ever had any unusual or allergic reaction to methylphenidate.

—if you are on a low-salt, low-sugar, or any other special diet, or if you are allergic to any substance, such as foods, sulfites or other preservatives, or dyes. Most medicines contain more than their active ingredient. Your doctor, nurse, or pharmacist can help you avoid products that may cause a problem.

—if you are **pregnant** or if you may become pregnant. Studies have not been done in either humans or animals.

—if you are **breast-feeding**. Methylphenidate has not been shown to cause problems in nursing babies.

—if you have any of the following medical problems:
    Drug dependence or alcoholism (or history of)
    Epilepsy or other seizure disorders
    Gilles de la Tourette's disorder (or history of)
    Glaucoma
    High blood pressure
    Psychosis
    Severe anxiety, agitation, tension, or depression
    Tics (other than Tourette's disorder)

—if you are taking **any** other prescription or nonprescription (OTC) medicine, especially:
    Amantadine (e.g., Symmetrel)
    Amphetamines
    Appetite suppressants (diet pills), except fenfluramine
    Caffeine
    Chlophedianol
    Medicine for asthma or other breathing problems
    Medicine for colds, sinus problems, hay fever or other allergies (including nose drops or sprays)
    Pemoline (e.g., Cylert)
    Pimozide (e.g., Orap)

—if you are now taking or have taken within the past 2 weeks monoamine oxidase (MAO) inhibitors, such as:
    Furazolidone (e.g., Furoxone)
    Isocarboxazid (e.g., Marplan)
    Pargyline (e.g., Eutonyl)
    Phenelzine (e.g., Nardil)
    Procarbazine (e.g., Matulane)
    Tranylcypromine (e.g., Parnate)

Proper Use of This Medicine

Take this medicine only as directed by your doctor. Do not take more of it, do not take it more often, and do not take it for a longer period of time than your doctor ordered. If too much is taken, it may become habit-forming.

Take this medicine about a half hour to 45 minutes before meals. To do so will help it to work better.

If you are taking the long-acting form of this medicine:
* These tablets are to be swallowed whole. Do not break, crush, or chew before swallowing.

To help prevent trouble in sleeping, take the last dose of this medicine for each day before 6 p.m., unless otherwise directed by your doctor.

If you think this medicine is not working as well after you have taken it for several weeks, **do not increase the dose.** Instead, check with your doctor.

If you miss a dose of this medicine, take it as soon as possible. Then take any remaining doses for that day at regularly spaced intervals. Do not double doses.

How to store this medicine:

- **Keep out of the reach of children.**

- Store away from heat and direct light.

- Do not store in the bathroom, near the kitchen sink, or in other damp places. Heat or moisture may cause the medicine to break down.

- Do not keep outdated medicine or medicine no longer needed. Be sure that any discarded medicine is out of the reach of children.

Precautions While Using This Medicine

Your doctor should check your progress at regular visits to make sure that this medicine does not cause unwanted effects.

If you will be taking this medicine in large doses for a long period of time, **do not stop taking it without first checking with your doctor.** Your doctor may want you to reduce gradually the amount you are taking before stopping completely.

If you have been using this medicine for a long time and you think you may have become mentally or physically dependent on it, check with your doctor. Some signs of dependence on methylphenidate are:

—a strong desire or need to continue taking the medicine.

—a need to increase the dose to receive the effects of the medicine.

—withdrawal side effects (for example, mental depression, unusual behavior, or unusual tiredness or weakness) occurring after the medicine is stopped.

Side Effects of This Medicine

Along with its needed effects, a medicine may cause some unwanted effects. Although not all of these side effects may occur, if they do occur they may need medical attention.

Check with your doctor as soon as possible if any of the following side effects occur:

More common
Fast heartbeat

Less common
Bruising
Chest pain
Fever

Joint pain
Skin rash or hives
Uncontrolled movements of the body

Rare
Blurred vision or any change in vision
Convulsions (seizures)
Sore throat and fever
Unusual tiredness or weakness

With long-term use
Mood or mental changes
Weight loss

Signs of overdose
Agitation
Confusion
Convulsions (seizures)
Delirium or hallucinations
Dry mouth
False sense of well-being
Fast, pounding, or irregular heartbeat
Fever and sweating
Headache (severe)
Increased blood pressure
Muscle twitching
Trembling or tremors
Vomiting

Other side effects may occur which usually do not require medical attention. These side effects may go away during treatment as your body adjusts to the medicine. However, check with your doctor if any of the following side effects continue or are bothersome:

More common
Loss of appetite
Nervousness
Trouble in sleeping

Less common
Dizziness
Drowsiness
Headache
Nausea
Stomach pain

For children: Some of the side effects listed above, such as loss of appetite, trouble in sleeping, stomach pain, and weight loss, may occur more often in children. Children are usually more sensitive to the effects of methylphenidate.

After you stop using this medicine, your body may need time to adjust. The length of time this takes depends on the amount of medicine you were using and how long you used it. During this period of time check with your doctor if you notice any of the following side effects:

Mental depression (severe)
Unusual behavior
Unusual tiredness or weakness

Other side effects not listed above may also occur in some patients. If you notice any other effects, check with your doctor.

December 1987

METHYPRYLON (Systemic)

A commonly used brand name is Noludar.

To the Reader: If you do not recognize the names of medical conditions or medicines referred to in this information, check with your doctor, nurse, or pharmacist. Definitions for selected medical terms may be found in the Glossary. Brand names for the generic drug names listed can be found in the Index. In addition, selected brand names commonly associated with the generic name have been included in the text to help you recognize medicine you may be taking. The fact that a brand name product is not mentioned does not mean the information does not apply. It is a good idea for you to learn both the generic and brand names of your medicines and to write them down for future use.

Methyprylon (meth-i-PRYE-lon) is taken by mouth to treat insomnia (sleeplessness). It helps patients fall asleep and stay asleep through the night. However, if used regularly (for example, every day) for insomnia, methyprylon may not be effective for more than 1 week.

This medicine is available only with your doctor's prescription.

Remember:

• **This medicine has been prescribed for your current medical problem only.** It must not be given to other people or used for other problems unless you are directed to do so by your doctor.

• **Keep all medicines out of the reach of children.**

• In order for this medicine to work, it must be used as directed.

• **It is very important that you read and understand the following information.** If any of the information causes you special concern, do not decide against using this medicine without first checking with your doctor.

• Before you begin using any new medicine (prescription or nonprescription) or if you develop any new medical problem while you are using this medicine, check with your doctor, nurse, or pharmacist.

• **If you have any questions** about the following information or if you want more information about this medicine or your medical problem, **ask your doctor, nurse, or pharmacist.**

Before Using This Medicine

In order to decide on the best treatment for your medical problem, your doctor should be told:

—if you have ever had any unusual or allergic reaction to methyprylon.

—if you are on a low-salt, low-sugar, or any other special diet, or if you are allergic to any substance, such as foods, sulfites or other preservatives, or dyes. Most medicines contain more than their active ingredient. Your doctor, nurse, or pharmacist can help you avoid products that may cause a problem.

—if you are **pregnant** or if you may become pregnant. Studies have not been done in humans. However, methyprylon has not been shown to cause birth defects or other problems in animal studies.

—if you are **breast-feeding.** It is not known whether methyprylon passes into the breast milk. This medicine has not been shown to cause problems in nursing babies.

—if you have any of the following medical problems:
Kidney disease
Liver disease
Porphyria

—if you are taking **any** other prescription or nonprescription (OTC) medicine, especially central nervous system (CNS) depressants.

Proper Use of This Medicine

Take this medicine only as directed by your doctor. Do not take more of it, do not take it more often, and do not take it for a longer period of time than your doctor ordered. If too much is taken, it may become habit-forming.

How to store this medicine:

• **Keep out of the reach of children** since overdose is especially dangerous in children.

• Store away from heat and direct light.

• Do not store in the bathroom, near the kitchen sink, or in other damp places. Heat or moisture may cause the medicine to break down.

• Do not keep outdated medicine or medicine no longer needed. Be sure that any discarded medicine is out of the reach of children.

Precautions While Using This Medicine

If you will be taking this medicine regularly for a long period of time:

• Your doctor should check your progress at regular visits.

• Do not stop taking it without first checking with your doctor. Your doctor may want you to reduce gradually the amount you are taking before stopping completely.

This medicine will add to the effects of alcohol and other CNS depressants (medicines that slow down the nervous system, possibly causing drowsiness). Some examples of CNS depressants are antihistamines or medicine for hay fever, other allergies, or colds; sedatives, tranquilizers, or sleeping medicine; prescription pain medicine or narcotics; barbiturates; medicine for convulsions (seizures); muscle relaxants; or anesthetics, including some dental anesthetics. **Check with your doctor before taking any of the above while you are taking this medicine.**

If you think you or someone else may have taken an overdose of this medicine, get emergency help at once. Taking an overdose of methyprylon or taking alcohol or other CNS depressants with methyprylon may lead to unconsciousness and possibly death. Some signs of an overdose are confusion, severe weakness, shortness of breath or slow or troubled breathing, staggering, and slow heartbeat.

This medicine may cause some people to become dizzy,
drowsy, or less alert than they are normally. Even if
taken at bedtime, it may cause some people to feel
drowsy or less alert on arising. **Make sure you know
how you react to this medicine before you drive, use
machines, or do other jobs that require you to be alert.**

Side Effects of This Medicine

Along with its needed effects, a medicine may cause some
unwanted effects. Although not all of these side effects
may occur, if they do occur they may need medical
attention.

Check with your doctor as soon as possible if any of the
following side effects occur:

Less common
  Skin rash
  Unusual excitement

Rare
  Ulcers or sores in mouth or throat (continuing)
  Unusual bleeding or bruising

Signs of overdose
  Confusion
  Shortness of breath or slow or troubled breathing
  Slow heartbeat
  Staggering
  Swelling of feet or lower legs
  Weakness (severe)

Other side effects may occur that usually do not require
medical attention. These side effects may go away
during treatment as your body adjusts to the medicine.
However, check with your doctor if any of the following side effects continue or are bothersome:

More common
  Dizziness
  Drowsiness (daytime)
  Headache

Less common
  Diarrhea
  Nausea
  Vomiting

For elderly patients: The above side effects are more
likely to occur in the elderly, who are usually more
sensitive to the effects of methyprylon.

After you stop using this medicine, your body may need
time to adjust. The length of time this takes depends
on the amount of medicine you were using and how
long you used it. During this period of time check with
your doctor if you notice any of the following side
effects:

  Confusion
  Convulsions (seizures)
  Hallucinations (seeing, hearing, or feeling things that are
    not there)
  Increased dreaming
  Increase in sweating
  Nausea or vomiting
  Nightmares
  Restlessness or nervousness
  Stomach cramps
  Trembling
  Trouble in sleeping
  Unusual weakness

Other side effects not listed above may also occur in some
patients. If you notice any other effects, check with
your doctor.

_____

December 1987

METHYSERGIDE (Systemic)

A commonly used brand name is Sansert.

To the Reader: If you do not recognize the names of medical conditions or medicines referred to in this information, check with your doctor, nurse, or pharmacist. Definitions for selected medical terms may be found in the Glossary. Brand names for the generic drug names listed can be found in the Index. In addition, selected brand names commonly associated with the generic name have been included in the text to help you recognize medicine you may be taking. The fact that a brand name product is not mentioned does not mean the information does not apply. It is a good idea for you to learn both the generic and brand names of your medicines and to write them down for future use.

Methysergide (meth-i-SER-jide) belongs to the group of medicines known as ergot alkaloids. It is taken by mouth to prevent migraine headaches and some kinds of throbbing headaches. It is not used to treat an attack once it has started. The exact way methysergide acts on the body is not known.

This medicine is available only with your doctor's prescription.

Remember:

• **This medicine has been prescribed for your current medical problem only.** It must not be given to other people or used for other problems unless you are directed to do so by your doctor.

• **Keep all medicines out of the reach of children.**

• In order for this medicine to work, it must be used as directed.

• **It is very important that you read and understand the following information.** If any of the information causes you special concern, do not decide against using this medicine without first checking with your doctor.

• Before you begin using any new medicine (prescription or nonprescription) or if you develop any new medical problem while you are using this medicine, check with your doctor, nurse, or pharmacist.

• **If you have any questions** about the following information or if you want more information about this medicine or your medical problem, **ask your doctor, nurse, or pharmacist.**

Before Using This Medicine

In order to decide on the best treatment for your medical problem, your doctor should be told:

—if you have ever had any unusual or allergic reaction to methysergide or other ergot medicines.

—if you are on a low-salt, low-sugar, or any other special diet, or if you are allergic to any substance, such as foods, sulfites or other preservatives, or dyes. Most medicines contain more than their active ingredient. Your doctor, nurse, or pharmacist can help you avoid products that may cause a problem.

—if you are **pregnant** or if you may become pregnant. Studies have not been done in either humans or animals.

—if you are **breast-feeding.** This medicine passes into the breast milk and may cause unwanted effects such as vomiting, diarrhea, weak pulse, unstable blood pressure, and convulsions (seizures) in nursing babies.

—if you have any of the following medical problems:
  Arthritis
  Heart or blood vessel disease
  High blood pressure
  Infection
  Itching (severe)
  Kidney disease
  Liver disease
  Lung disease
  Stomach ulcer

—if you are now taking **any** other prescription or non-prescription (OTC) medicine.

—if you smoke.

Proper Use of This Medicine

Take this medicine only as directed by your doctor. If the amount you are to take does not relieve your headache, do not take more than your doctor ordered. Instead, check with your doctor. Taking too much of this medicine or taking it too frequently may cause serious effects such as nausea and vomiting; cold, painful hands or feet; or even gangrene.

If this medicine upsets your stomach, it may be taken with meals or milk. If stomach upset continues or is severe, check with your doctor.

If you miss a dose of this medicine, skip the missed dose and go back to your regular dosing schedule. Do not double doses.

How to store this medicine:

• **Keep out of the reach of children.**

• Store away from heat and direct light.

• Do not store in the bathroom, near the kitchen sink, or in other damp places. Heat or moisture may cause the medicine to break down.

• Do not keep outdated medicine or medicine no longer needed. Be sure that any discarded medicine is out of the reach of children.

Precautions While Using This Medicine

If you have been taking this medicine regularly, **do not stop taking it without first checking with your doctor.** Your doctor may want you to reduce gradually the amount you are using before stopping completely. If you stop taking it suddenly, your headaches may return or worsen.

Your doctor will tell you how long you should take this medicine. Usually it is not taken for longer than 6 months at a time. **If the doctor tells you to stop taking the medicine for a while, do not continue to take it.** If your body does not get a rest from the medicine, it can have harmful effects.

This medicine may cause some people to become dizzy, lightheaded, drowsy, or less alert than they are normally. Even if taken at bedtime, it may cause some people to feel drowsy or less alert on arising. **Make sure you know how you react to this medicine before you drive, use machines, or do other jobs that require you to be alert.**

If dizziness occurs, get up slowly after lying or sitting down. If the problem continues or gets worse, check with your doctor.

Since drinking alcoholic beverages may make headaches worse, it is best to avoid alcohol while you are suffering from them. If you have any questions about this, check with your doctor.

Since smoking may increase some of the harmful effects of this medicine, it is best to avoid smoking while you are using it. If you have any questions about this, check with your doctor.

Avoid prolonged exposure to very cold temperatures while you are using this medicine, since cold may increase the harmful effects of the medicine.

If you have an infection or illness of any kind, check with your doctor before taking this medicine, since you may be more sensitive to the effects of it.

Side Effects of This Medicine

Along with its needed effects, a medicine may cause some unwanted effects. Although not all of these side effects may occur, if they do occur they may need medical attention.

Check with your doctor immediately if any of the following side effects occur:

> Chest pain
> Difficult or painful urination
> Dizziness (severe)
> Fever
> Leg cramps or lower back pain
> Loss of appetite or weight loss
> Lower back, side, or groin pain
> Pale or cold hands or feet
> Shortness of breath
> Swelling of hands or ankles

Check with your doctor as soon as possible if the following side effects occur:

More common

> Itching
> Numbness and tingling of fingers, toes, or face
> Weakness in the legs

Less common or rare

> Changes in vision
> Excitement or difficulty in thinking
> Fast or slow heartbeat
> Feeling of being outside the body
> Hallucinations (seeing, hearing, or feeling things that are not there)
> Nightmares

Other side effects may occur that usually do not require medical attention. These side effects may go away during treatment as your body adjusts to the medicine. However, check with your doctor if any of the following side effects continue or are bothersome:

More common

> Diarrhea
> Dizziness or lightheadedness, especially when getting up from a lying or sitting position
> Drowsiness
> Nausea or vomiting or stomach pain

Less common or rare

> Clumsiness
> Mental depression
> Trouble in sleeping

After you stop using this medicine, your body may need time to adjust. The length of time this takes depends on the amount of medicine you were using and how long you used it. During this period of time check with your doctor if your headaches begin again or worsen.

For elderly patients: Some of the above side effects are more likely to occur in the elderly, who are more likely to already have problems with blood vessels.

Other side effects not listed above may also occur in some patients. If you notice any other effects, check with your doctor.

December 1987

METOCLOPRAMIDE (Systemic)

Some commonly used brand names are:

Clopra	Maxolon
Emex*	Reclomide
Maxeran*	Reglan

Generic name product may also be available in the U.S.

---

*Not available in the U.S.

To the Reader: If you do not recognize the names of medical conditions or medicines referred to in this information, check with your doctor, nurse, or pharmacist. Definitions for selected medical terms may be found in the Glossary. Brand names for the generic drug names listed can be found in the Index. In addition, selected brand names commonly associated with the generic name have been included in the text to help you recognize medicine you may be taking. The fact that a brand name product is not mentioned does not mean the information does not apply. It is a good idea for you to learn both the generic and brand names of your medicines and to write them down for future use.

Metoclopramide (met-oh-KLOE-pra-mide) is a medicine that increases the movements or contractions of the stomach and intestines. When given by injection it is used to help diagnose certain problems of the stomach and/or intestines. It is also used by injection to prevent the nausea and vomiting that may occur after treatment with anticancer medicines.

When taken by mouth, metoclopramide is used to treat the symptoms of a certain type of stomach problem called diabetic gastroparesis. It relieves symptoms such as nausea, vomiting, continued feeling of fullness after meals, and loss of appetite. Metoclopramide is also used, for a short period of time, to treat symptoms such as heartburn in patients who regurgitate food.

Metoclopramide may also be used for other conditions as determined by your doctor.

Metoclopramide is available only with your doctor's prescription.

Remember:

• **This medicine has been prescribed for your current medical problem only.** It must not be given to other people or used for other problems unless you are directed to do so by your doctor.

• **Keep all medicines out of the reach of children.**

• In order for this medicine to work, it must be used as directed.

• If you are receiving this medicine by injection, some of the information about this medicine may not apply.

• **It is very important that you read and understand the following information.** If any of the information causes you special concern, do not decide against using this medicine without first checking with your doctor.

• Before you begin using any new medicine (prescription or nonprescription) or if you develop any new medical problem while you are using this medicine, check with your doctor, nurse, or pharmacist.

• **If you have any questions** about the following information or if you want more information about this medicine or your medical problem, **ask your doctor, nurse, or pharmacist.**

Before Using This Medicine

In order to decide on the best treatment for your medical problem, your doctor should be told:

—if you have ever had any unusual or allergic reaction to metoclopramide, procaine, or procainamide.

—if you are on a low-salt, low-sugar, or any other special diet, or if you are allergic to any substance, such as foods, sulfites or other preservatives, or dyes. Most medicines contain more than their active ingredient. Your doctor, nurse, or pharmacist can help you avoid products that may cause a problem.

—if you are **pregnant** or if you may become pregnant. Not enough studies have been done in humans to determine metoclopramide's safety during pregnancy. However, metoclopramide has not been shown to cause birth defects or other problems in animal studies.

—if you are **breast-feeding**. Although metoclopramide has not been shown to cause problems in nursing babies, the chance always exists since it passes into the breast milk.

—if you have any of the following medical problems:
Abdominal or stomach bleeding
Epilepsy
Intestinal blockage
Kidney disease (severe)
Liver disease (severe)
Parkinson's disease

—if you are now taking any of the following medicines or types of medicine:
Amoxapine
Antimuscarinics (medicine for abdominal or stomach spasms or cramps)
Bromocriptine
Carbamazepine
Chlorprothixene
Digoxin
Droperidol
Guanabenz
Haloperidol
Levodopa
Loxapine
Metyrosine
Mexiletine
Molindone
Pargyline
Phenothiazines (acetophenazine, chlorpromazine, fluphenazine, mesoridazine, perphenazine, prochlorperazine, promazine, promethazine, thioridazine, trifluoperazine, triflupromazine, trimeprazine)
Pimozide
Rauwolfia alkaloids (alseroxylon, deserpidine, rauwolfia serpentina, reserpine)
Thiothixene
Tricyclic antidepressants (amitriptyline, amoxapine, clomipramine, desipramine, doxepin, imipramine, nortriptyline, protriptyline, trimipramine)

—if you are now using central nervous system (CNS) depressants such as:
Anticonvulsants (seizure medicine)
Antihistamines or medicine for hay fever, other allergies, or colds
Barbiturates
Narcotics
Prescription pain medicine
Sedatives, tranquilizers, or sleeping medicine

Proper Use of This Medicine

Take this medicine 30 minutes before meals and at bedtime, unless otherwise directed by your doctor.

Take metoclopramide only as directed. Do not take more of it, do not take it more often, and do not take it for a longer period of time than your doctor ordered. To do so may increase the chance of side effects.

If you miss a dose of this medicine, take it as soon as possible. However, if it is almost time for your next dose, skip the missed dose and go back to your regular dosing schedule. Do not double doses.

How to store this medicine:

• **Keep out of the reach of children.**

• Store away from heat and direct light.

• Do not store the tablet form of this medicine in the bathroom, near the kitchen sink, or in other damp places. Heat or moisture may cause the medicine to break down.

• Keep the syrup form of this medicine from freezing.

• Do not keep outdated medicine or medicine no longer needed. Be sure that any discarded medicine is out of the reach of children.

Precautions While Using This Medicine

This medicine will add to the effects of alcohol and other CNS depressants (medicines that slow down the nervous system, possibly causing drowsiness). Some examples of CNS depressants are antihistamines or medicine for hay fever, other allergies, or colds; sedatives, tranquilizers, or sleeping medicine; prescription pain medicine or narcotics; barbiturates; medicine for seizures; muscle relaxants; or anesthetics, including some dental anesthetics. **Check with your doctor before taking any of the above while you are using this medicine.**

This medicine may cause some people to become dizzy, lightheaded, drowsy, or less alert than they are normally. **Make sure you know how you react to this medicine before you drive, use machines, or do other jobs that require you to be alert.**

Side Effects of This Medicine

Along with its needed effects, a medicine may cause some unwanted effects. Although not all of these side effects may occur, if they do occur they may need medical attention.

Check with your doctor as soon as possible if any of the following side effects occur:

Signs of overdose—may also occur rarely with usual doses, especially in children and young adults, and with high doses used to treat the nausea and vomiting caused by anticancer medicines
    Confusion
    Drowsiness (severe)
    Muscle spasms (especially of jaw, neck, and back)
    Shuffling walk
    Tic-like (jerky) movements of head and face
    Trembling and shaking of hands

Other side effects may occur that usually do not require medical attention. These side effects may go away during treatment as your body adjusts to the medicine. However, check with your doctor if any of the following side effects continue or are bothersome:

More common
    Drowsiness
    Restlessness
    Unusual tiredness or weakness

Less common or rare
    Breast tenderness and swelling
    Changes in menstruation
    Constipation
    Depression
    Diarrhea
    Dizziness
    Headache
    Increased flow of breast milk
    Nausea
    Skin rash
    Trouble in sleeping
    Unusual dryness of mouth
    Unusual irritability

For children: Muscle spasms, especially of the jaw, neck, and back, and tic-like (jerky) movements of the head and face are more likely to occur in children.

For elderly patients: Shuffling walk, trembling, and shaking of hands are more likely to occur in elderly patients, especially after taking metoclopramide over a long period of time.

Other side effects not listed above may also occur in some patients. If you notice any other effects, check with your doctor.

December 1987

METRIZAMIDE (Systemic)

A commonly used brand name is Amipaque.

Read the bold information first. Then go back and read the rest. If you do not recognize the names of medical conditions or medicines included in this information, check with your doctor, nurse, or pharmacist. Brand names for the generic drug names listed can also be found in the index. It is a good idea for you to learn both the generic and brand names of your medicines and to write them down for future use.

Metrizamide (me-TRI-za-mide) is a radiopaque agent. This agent contains iodine, which absorbs x-rays. Depending on how the radiopaque agent is given, it builds up in certain areas of the body. The resulting high level of iodine allows the x-rays to make a "picture" of the area.

Metrizamide is given by injection into the spinal canal before x-ray tests to help diagnose problems or diseases in different areas of the head, spinal canal, and nervous system. It may be injected into a specific vein or artery to help check for problems with the heart and blood vessels.

Metrizamide is to be used only by or under the supervision of a doctor.

Remember:

• **It is very important that you read and understand the following information.** If any of the information causes you special concern, do not decide against taking or receiving this radiopaque agent without first checking with your doctor.

• **If you have any questions** about the following information or if you want more information about this radiopaque agent or your medical problem, **ask your doctor, nurse, or pharmacist.**

Before Having This Test

Before this test is given, your doctor should be told:

—if you have ever had any unusual or allergic reaction to iodine, to products containing iodine (for example, iodine-containing foods, such as seafood, cabbage, kale, rape, turnips, or iodized salt), or to other radiopaque agents.

—if you are allergic to any substance, such as sulfites or other preservatives. Most medicines contain more than their active ingredient. Your doctor can help you avoid products that may cause a problem.

—if you are pregnant or if you suspect that you may be pregnant when you are to receive this radiopaque agent. Studies have not been done in humans; however, metrizamide has not been shown to cause birth defects or other problems in animal studies when given in doses up to many times the usual human dose. Other radiopaque agents containing iodine have caused, on rare occasions, hypothyroidism (underactive thyroid) in the baby. Also, x-rays of the abdomen are usually not recommended during pregnancy. This is to avoid exposing the fetus to radiation. Be sure you have discussed this with your doctor.

—if you are breast-feeding. Although metrizamide has not been shown to cause problems in humans, the chance always exists since it passes into the breast milk.

—if you have any of the following medical problems:
   Asthma, hay fever, or other allergies (history of)
   Diabetes mellitus (sugar diabetes)
   Epilepsy (history of)
   Heart or blood vessel disease
   High blood pressure (severe)
   Kidney disease (severe)
   Liver disease
   Multiple myeloma (bone disease)
   Multiple sclerosis
   Overactive thyroid
   Pheochromocytoma (PCC)
   Sickle cell disease

—if you are taking any of the following medicines or types of medicines:
   Phenothiazines (acetophenazine, chlorpromazine, fluphenazine, mesoridazine, perphenazine, prochlorperazine, promazine, promethazine, thioridazine, trifluoperazine, triflupromazine, trimeprazine)
   Tricyclic antidepressants (amitriptyline, amoxapine, clomipramine, desipramine, doxepin, imipramine, nortriptyline, protriptyline, trimipramine)

—if you are taking **any** other medicines including over-the-counter (OTC) or nonprescription medicines (for example, aspirin). Some medicines increase the chances of metrizamide causing side effects.

Preparation for This Test

Your doctor may have special instructions for you in preparation for your test. If you have not received such instructions or if you do not understand them, check with your doctor in advance.

For patients having this radiopaque agent injected into the spinal canal, unless otherwise directed by your doctor:

• You may eat and drink your usual diet up to 2 hours before the test.

Precautions After Having This Test

Make sure your doctor knows if you are planning to have any future thyroid tests. Even after several weeks or months the results of the thyroid test may be affected by the iodine in this agent.

For patients having this radiopaque agent injected into the spinal canal, unless otherwise directed by your doctor or radiologist:

• Remain still during and for several hours after the test.

• Keep head high as instructed during and after test.

For patients having this radiopaque agent injected into a vein or an artery, unless otherwise directed by your doctor or radiologist:

• Remain still and avoid swallowing during and right after tests of the head and neck.

Side Effects of This Medicine

Along with its needed effects, radiopaque agents like metrizamide can sometimes cause serious effects such as severe allergic reactions or heart problems. These effects may occur almost immediately or a few minutes after the radiopaque agent is given. Although these serious side effects appear only rarely, your doctor or nurse will be prepared to give you immediate medical attention if needed. If you have any questions about this, check with your doctor. Also, check with your doctor as soon as possible if the following side effects occur:

Rare
>   Hallucinations (seeing, hearing, or feeling things that are not there)
>   Paralysis of one side of body or of legs and arms

Some side effects may occur which usually do not require medical attention. These side effects should go away as the effects of the radiopaque agent wear off. However, check with your doctor if any of the following side effects continue or are bothersome:

With injection into the spinal canal, a vein, or an artery
>   *More common*
>>   Nausea and vomiting
>>   Restlessness
>>   Trembling

With injection into the spinal canal
>   *More common*
>>   Headache (mild to moderate)
>   *Less common or rare*
>>   Backache
>>   Blurred or double vision or other changes in vision
>>   Chills
>>   Confusion
>>   Dizziness
>>   Fever (more common in children)
>>   Headache (severe)
>>   Ringing or buzzing sound in ears
>>   Speech difficulty
>>   Stiffness of neck
>>   Unusual sweating
>>   Unusual tiredness or weakness

With injection into a vein or an artery
>   *Less common or rare*
>>   Increase in amount of urine
>>   Unusual warmth and flushing of skin

The above side effects are more likely to occur in children and the elderly, who are usually more sensitive to the effects of metrizamide.

Other side effects not listed above may also occur in some patients. If you notice any other effects, check with your doctor.

_____

December 1987

METRONIDAZOLE (Systemic)

Some commonly used brand names are:

Apo-Metronidazole*	Metryl IV
Flagyl	Neo-Metric*
Flagyl I.V.	Novonidazol*
Flagyl I.V. RTU	PMS Metronidazole*
Metizol	Protostat
Metro I.V.	Satric
Metryl	

Generic name product may also be available in the U.S.

---

*Not available in the U.S.

To the Reader: If you do not recognize the names of medical conditions or medicines referred to in this information, check with your doctor, nurse, or pharmacist. Definitions for selected medical terms may be found in the Glossary. Brand names for the generic drug names listed can be found in the Index. In addition, selected brand names commonly associated with the generic name have been included in the text to help you recognize medicine you may be taking. The fact that a brand name product is not mentioned does not mean the information does not apply. It is a good idea for you to learn both the generic and brand names of your medicines and to write them down for future use.

Metronidazole (me-troe-NI-da-zole) belongs to the general family of medicines called anti-infectives. It is taken by mouth or given by injection to help the body overcome infections and to help some problems such as dysentery. It may also be used for other problems as determined by your doctor. It will not work for colds, flu, or other virus infections.

Metronidazole is available only with your doctor's prescription.

Remember:

• **This medicine has been prescribed for your present medical problem only.** Even though other people may have the same symptoms as you, they may have a different kind of problem. Your medicine may not work for them and may even cause them harm. Therefore, **your medicine must not be given to other people or used for other problems** unless you are otherwise directed by your doctor.

• **Keep all medicines out of the reach of children.**

• In order for this medicine to work, it must be used as directed.

• If you are receiving this medicine by injection, some of the information about this medicine may not apply.

• **It is very important that you read and understand the following information.** If any of the information causes you special concern, do not decide against using this medicine without first checking with your doctor.

• Before you begin using any new medicine (prescription or nonprescription) or if you develop any new medical problem while you are using this medicine, check with your doctor, nurse, or pharmacist.

• **If you have any questions** about the following information or if you want more information about this medicine or your medical problem, **ask your doctor, nurse, or pharmacist.**

Before Using This Medicine

In order to decide on the best treatment for your medical problem, your doctor should be told:

—if you have ever had any unusual or allergic reaction to metronidazole.

—if you are on a low-salt, low-sugar, or any other special diet, or if you are allergic to any substance, such as foods, sulfites or other preservatives, or dyes. Most medicines contain more than their active ingredient. Your doctor, nurse, or pharmacist can help you avoid products that may cause a problem.

—if you are **pregnant** or if you may become pregnant. Studies have not been done in humans. However, metronidazole has not been shown to cause birth defects in animal studies.

—if you are **breast-feeding**. Use is not recommended in nursing mothers since metronidazole passes into the breast milk and may cause unwanted effects in the baby. However, in some infections your doctor may want you to stop breast-feeding and take this medicine for a short time. During this time the breast milk should be squeezed out or sucked out with a breast pump and thrown away. One or two days after you finish taking this medicine, you may go back to breast-feeding.

—if you have any of the following medical problems:
  Blood disease or a history of blood disease
  Central nervous system (CNS) disease, including epilepsy
  Heart disease (injection only)
  Liver disease, severe

—if you are taking **any** other prescription or nonprescription (OTC) medicine, especially:
  Anticoagulants (blood thinners)
  Disulfiram (e.g., Antabuse)

Proper Use of This Medicine

If this medicine upsets your stomach, it may be taken with meals or a snack. If stomach upset (nausea, vomiting, stomach pain, or diarrhea) continues, check with your doctor.

To help clear up your infection completely, **keep taking this medicine for the full time of treatment** even if you begin to feel better after a few days. If you stop taking this medicine too soon, your symptoms may return.

In some kinds of infections, this medicine works best when there is a constant amount in the blood. **To help keep the amount constant, do not miss any doses. Also, it is best to take each dose at evenly spaced times day and night.** For example, if you are to take 4 doses a day, each dose should be spaced about 6 hours apart. If this interferes with your sleep or other daily activities, or if you need help in planning the best times to take your medicine, check with your doctor, nurse, or pharmacist.

If you do miss a dose of this medicine, take it as soon as possible. This will help to keep a constant amount of medicine in the blood. However, if it is almost time for your next dose, skip the missed dose and go back to your regular dosing schedule. Do not double doses.

How to store this medicine:

- **Keep out of the reach of children.**

- Store away from heat and direct light.

- Do not store the capsule or tablet form of this medicine in the bathroom, near the kitchen sink, or in other damp places. Heat or moisture may cause the medicine to break down.

- Do not keep outdated medicine or medicine no longer needed. Be sure that any discarded medicine is out of the reach of children.

Precautions While Using This Medicine

If your symptoms do not improve within a few days, or if they become worse, check with your doctor.

Drinking alcoholic beverages while taking this medicine may cause stomach pain, nausea, vomiting, headache, or flushing or redness of the face. Other alcohol-containing preparations (for example, elixirs, cough syrups, tonics) may also cause problems. Also, this medicine may cause alcoholic beverages to taste different. Therefore, **you should not drink alcoholic beverages or use other alcohol-containing preparations while you are taking this medicine.**

Metronidazole may cause dryness of the mouth, an unpleasant or sharp metallic taste, and a change in taste sensation. For temporary relief of dry mouth, use sugarless candy or gum, melt bits of ice in your mouth, or use a saliva substitute. However, if dry mouth continues for more than 2 weeks, check with your dentist. Continuing dryness of the mouth may increase the chance of dental disease, including tooth decay, gum disease, and fungal infections.

This medicine may also cause some people to become dizzy or lightheaded. **Make sure you know how you react to this medicine before you drive, use machines, or do other jobs that require you to be alert.** If these reactions are especially bothersome, check with your doctor.

If you are taking this medicine for trichomoniasis (a genital infection in males and females), your doctor may want to treat your sexual partner at the same time you are being treated, even if he has no symptoms. Also, it may be desirable for your partner to wear a condom (prophylactic) during intercourse. These measures will help keep you from getting the infection back again from your partner. If you have any questions about this, check with your doctor.

Side Effects of This Medicine

Metronidazole has been shown to cause cancer and/or tumors in some animals. However, this medicine has not been shown to cause cancer in humans. **You and your doctor should discuss the good this medicine will do, as well as the risks of taking it.**

Along with its needed effects, a medicine may cause some unwanted effects. Although not all of these side effects may occur, if they do occur they may need medical attention.

Check with your doctor immediately if any of the following side effects occur:
More common
    Numbness, tingling, pain, or weakness in hands or feet
Less common
    Convulsions (seizures)

Also, check with your doctor as soon as possible if any of the following side effects occur:
Less common
    Any vaginal irritation, discharge, or dryness not present before using this medicine
    Clumsiness or unsteadiness
    Mood or other mental changes
    Skin rash, hives, redness, or itching
    Sore throat and fever
For injection form
    Pain, tenderness, redness, or swelling over vein in which the medicine is given

Other side effects may occur that usually do not require medical attention. These side effects may go away during treatment as your body adjusts to the medicine. However, check with your doctor if any of the following side effects continue or are bothersome:
More common
    Diarrhea
    Dizziness or lightheadedness
    Headache
    Loss of appetite
    Nausea or vomiting
    Stomach pain or cramps
Less common or rare
    Change in taste sensation
    Constipation
    Dryness of mouth
    Unpleasant or sharp metallic taste
    Unusual tiredness or weakness

In some patients metronidazole may cause dark urine. This is only temporary and will go away when you stop taking this medicine.

For elderly patients: Many medicines have not been tested in older people. Therefore, it is not known whether the medicine acts the same way it does in younger adults. Check with your doctor or pharmacist if you notice any unusual effects while taking this medicine or if you think it is not working as it should.

Other side effects not listed above may also occur in some patients. If you notice any other effects, check with your doctor.

—————

December 1987

—————

METYROSINE (Systemic)

A commonly used brand name is Demser.

To the Reader: If you do not recognize the names of medical conditions or medicines referred to in this information, check with your doctor, nurse, or pharmacist. Definitions for selected medical terms may be found in the Glossary. Brand names for the generic drug names listed can be found in the Index. In addition, selected brand names commonly associated with the generic name have been included in the text to help you recognize medicine you may be taking. The fact that a brand name product is not mentioned does not mean the information does not apply. It is a good idea for you to learn both the generic and brand names of your medicines and to write them down for future use.

Metyrosine (me-TYE-roe-seen) belongs to the general class of medicines called antihypertensives. It is taken by mouth to treat high blood pressure caused by a disease called pheochromocytoma.

Metyrosine reduces the amount of certain chemicals in the body. When these chemicals are present in large amounts, they cause high blood pressure.

Metyrosine is available only with your doctor's prescription.

Remember:

• **This medicine has been prescribed for your current medical problem only.** It must not be given to other people or used for other problems unless you are directed to do so by your doctor.

• **Keep all medicines out of the reach of children.**

• In order for this medicine to work, it must be used as directed.

• **It is very important that you read and understand the following information.** If any of the information causes you special concern, do not decide against using this medicine without first checking with your doctor.

• Before you begin using any new medicine (prescription or nonprescription) or if you develop any new medical problem while you are using this medicine, check with your doctor, nurse, or pharmacist.

• **If you have any questions** about the following information or if you want more information about this medicine or your medical problem, **ask your doctor, nurse, or pharmacist.**

Before Using This Medicine

In order to decide on the best treatment for your medical problem, your doctor should be told:

—if you have ever had any unusual or allergic reaction to metyrosine.

—if you are on a low-salt, low-sugar, or any other special diet, or if you are allergic to any substance, such as foods, sulfites or other preservatives, or dyes. Most medicines contain more than their active ingredient. Your doctor, nurse, or pharmacist can help you avoid products that may cause a problem.

—if you are **pregnant** or if you may become pregnant. Studies have not been done in either humans or animals.

—if you are **breast-feeding**. It is not known whether metyrosine passes into the breast milk. This medicine has not been shown to cause problems in nursing babies.

—if you have any of the following medical problems:
Kidney disease
Liver disease
Mental depression (or history of)
Parkinson's disease

—if you are taking **any** other prescription or nonprescription (OTC) medicine.

Proper Use of This Medicine

Take this medicine only as directed by your doctor. Do not take more or less of it than your doctor ordered.

In order to help remember to take your medicine, try to get into the habit of taking it at the same times each day.

If you miss a dose of this medicine, take it as soon as possible. However, if it is almost time for your next dose, skip the missed dose and go back to your regular dosing schedule. Do not double doses.

How to store this medicine:

• **Keep out of the reach of children.**

• Store away from heat and direct light.

• Do not store in the bathroom, near the kitchen sink, or in other damp places. Heat or moisture may cause the medicine to break down.

• Do not keep outdated medicine or medicine no longer needed. Be sure that any discarded medicine is out of the reach of children.

Precautions While Using This Medicine

It is important that your doctor check your progress at regular visits to make sure that this medicine is working properly and to check for unwanted effects.

While taking this medicine, it is important that you drink plenty of fluids and urinate often. This will help prevent kidney problems and keep your kidneys working well. If you have any questions about how much you should drink, check with your doctor.

This medicine may cause most people to become drowsy or less alert than they are normally. **Make sure you know how you react to this medicine before you drive, use machines, or do other jobs that require you to be alert.**

This medicine will add to the effects of alcohol and other CNS depressants (medicines that slow down the nervous system, possibly causing drowsiness). Some examples of CNS depressants are antihistamines or medicine for hay fever, other allergies, or colds; sedatives, tranquilizers, or sleeping medicine; prescription pain

medicine or narcotics; barbiturates; medicine for convulsions (seizures); tricyclic antidepressants (medicine for depression); muscle relaxants; or anesthetics, including some dental anesthetics. **Check with your doctor before taking any of the above while you are taking this medicine.**

Before having any kind of surgery (including dental surgery), tell the physician or dentist in charge that you are taking this medicine.

Side Effects of This Medicine

Along with its needed effects, a medicine may cause some unwanted effects. Although not all of these side effects may occur, if they do occur they may need medical attention.

Check with your doctor as soon as possible if any of the following side effects occur:

More common
> Diarrhea
> Difficulty in speaking
> Drooling
> Trembling and shaking of hands and fingers

Less common
> Anxiety
> Confusion
> Hallucinations (seeing, hearing, or feeling things that are not there)
> Mental depression

Rare
> Blood in urine
> Decrease in urination
> Muscle spasms, especially of neck and back
> Painful urination
> Restlessness

> Shortness of breath
> Shuffling walk
> Skin rash and itching
> Swelling of feet or lower legs
> Tic-like (jerky) movements of head, face, mouth, and neck

Other side effects may occur that usually do not require medical attention. These side effects may go away during treatment as your body adjusts to the medicine. However, check with your doctor if the following side effect continues or is bothersome:
> Drowsiness

For elderly patients: Many medicines have not been tested in older people. Therefore, it is not known whether the medicine acts the same way it does in younger adults. Check with your doctor or pharmacist if you notice any unusual effects while taking this medicine or if you think it is not working as it should.

After you stop taking this medicine, it may still produce some side effects that need attention. During this period of time check with your doctor if you notice the following side effect:
> Diarrhea

Also, after you stop taking this medicine, you may have feelings of increased energy or you may have trouble in sleeping. However, these effects should last only for two or three days.

Other side effects not listed above may also occur in some patients. If you notice any other effects, check with your doctor.

_____

December 1987

MEXILETINE (Systemic)

A commonly used brand name is Mexitil.

To the Reader: If you do not recognize the names of medical conditions or medicines referred to in this information, check with your doctor, nurse, or pharmacist. Definitions for selected medical terms may be found in the Glossary. Brand names for the generic drug names listed can be found in the Index. In addition, selected brand names commonly associated with the generic name have been included in the text to help you recognize medicine you may be taking. The fact that a brand name product is not mentioned does not mean the information does not apply. It is a good idea for you to learn both the generic and brand names of your medicines and to write them down for future use.

Mexiletine (mex-IL-e-teen) belongs to the group of medicines known as antiarrhythmics. It is taken by mouth to change irregular heartbeats to a normal rhythm.

Mexiletine produces its helpful effects by slowing nerve impulses in the heart and making the heart tissue less sensitive.

Mexiletine is available only with your doctor's prescription.

Remember:

• **This medicine has been prescribed for your current medical problem only.** It must not be given to other people or used for other problems unless you are directed to do so by your doctor.

• **Keep all medicines out of the reach of children.**

• In order for this medicine to work, it must be used as directed.

• **It is very important that you read and understand the following information.** If any of the information causes you special concern, do not decide against using this medicine without first checking with your doctor.

• Before you begin using any new medicine (prescription or nonprescription) or if you develop any new medical problem while you are using this medicine, check with your doctor, nurse, or pharmacist.

• **If you have any questions** about the following information or if you want more information about this medicine or your medical problem, **ask your doctor, nurse, or pharmacist.**

Before Using This Medicine

In order to decide on the best treatment for your medical problem, your doctor should be told:

—if you have ever had any unusual or allergic reaction to mexiletine, lidocaine, or tocainide.

—if you are on a low-salt, low-sugar, or any other special diet, or if you are allergic to any substance, such as foods, sulfites or other preservatives, or dyes. Most medicines contain more than their active ingredient. Your doctor, nurse, or pharmacist can help you avoid products that may cause a problem.

—if you are **pregnant** or if you may become pregnant. Studies have not been done in humans. However, studies in mice, rats, and rabbits at doses up to 4 times the human dose found a decrease in successful pregnancies but no birth defects.

—if you are **breast-feeding**. Although mexiletine passes into breast milk, it has not been shown to cause problems in nursing babies. However, because this medicine may cause serious side effects, breast-feeding is generally not recommended while you are receiving it. Be sure you have discussed this with your doctor before taking mexiletine.

—if you have either of the following medical problems:
  Liver disease
  Seizures (history of)

—if you are taking **any** other prescription or nonprescription (OTC) medicine.

—if you smoke.

Proper Use of This Medicine

Take mexiletine exactly as directed by your doctor, even though you may feel well. Do not take more medicine than ordered.

To lessen the possibility of stomach upset, mexiletine should be taken with food or immediately after meals or with milk or an antacid.

This medicine works best when there is a constant amount in the blood. **To help keep this amount constant, do not miss any doses. Also it is best to take each dose at evenly spaced times day and night.** For example, if you are to take 3 doses a day, the doses should be spaced about 8 hours apart. If this interferes with your sleep or other daily activities, or if you need help in planning the best times to take your medicine, check with your doctor, nurse, or pharmacist.

If you miss a dose of this medicine and remember within 4 hours, take it as soon as possible. Then go back to your regular dosing schedule. However, if you do not remember until later, skip the missed dose and go back to your regular dosing schedule. Do not double doses.

How to store this medicine:

• **Keep out of the reach of children.**

• Store away from heat and direct light.

• Do not store in the bathroom, near the kitchen sink, or in other damp places. Heat or moisture may cause the medicine to break down.

• Do not keep outdated medicine or medicine no longer needed. Be sure that any discarded medicine is out of the reach of children.

Precautions While Using This Medicine

It is important that your doctor check your progress at regular visits to make sure the medicine is working properly. This will allow for changes to be made in the amount of medicine you are taking, if necessary.

Your doctor may want you to carry a medical identification card or bracelet stating that you are using this medicine.

Before having any kind of surgery (including dental surgery) or emergency treatment, tell the physician or dentist in charge that you are taking this medicine.

Mexiletine may cause some people to become dizzy, lightheaded, or less alert than they are normally. **Make sure you know how you react to this medicine before you drive, use machines, or do other jobs that require you to be alert.**

Side Effects of This Medicine

Along with its needed effects, a medicine may cause some unwanted effects. Although not all of these side effects may occur, if they do occur they may need medical attention.

Check with your doctor as soon as possible if any of the following side effects occur:

Less common

Chest pain
Fast or irregular heartbeat
Shortness of breath

Rare

Convulsions (seizures)
Fever, chills, or sore throat
Unusual bleeding or bruising

Other side effects may occur that usually do not require medical attention. These side effects may go away during treatment as your body adjusts to the medicine.

However, check with your doctor if any of the following side effects continue or are bothersome:

More common

Dizziness or lightheadedness
Heartburn
Nausea and vomiting
Nervousness
Trembling or shaking of the hands
Unsteadiness or difficulty in walking

Less common

Blurred vision
Confusion
Constipation or diarrhea
Headache
Numbness or tingling of fingers and toes
Ringing in the ears
Skin rash
Slurred speech
Trouble in sleeping
Unusual tiredness or weakness

For elderly patients: Many medicines have not been tested in older people. Therefore, it is not known whether the medicine acts the same way it does in younger adults. Check with your doctor or pharmacist if you notice any unusual effects while taking this medicine or if you think it is not working as it should.

Other side effects not listed above may also occur in some patients. If you notice any other effects, check with your doctor.

December 1987

MICONAZOLE (Systemic)

A commonly used brand name is Monistat I.V.

To the Reader: If you do not recognize the names of medical conditions or medicines referred to in this information, check with your doctor, nurse, or pharmacist. Definitions for selected medical terms may be found in the Glossary. Brand names for the generic drug names listed can be found in the Index. In addition, selected brand names commonly associated with the generic name have been included in the text to help you recognize medicine you may be taking. The fact that a brand name product is not mentioned does not mean the information does not apply. It is a good idea for you to learn both the generic and brand names of your medicines and to write them down for future use.

Miconazole (mi-KON-a-zole) belongs to the group of medicines called antifungals. It is given by injection to treat certain fungal infections.

Miconazole is available only with your doctor's prescription.

Remember:

• **It is very important that you read and understand the following information.** If any of the information causes you special concern, do not decide against using this medicine without first checking with your doctor.

• Before you begin using any new medicine (prescription or nonprescription) or if you develop any new medical problem while you are using this medicine, check with your doctor, nurse, or pharmacist.

• **If you have any questions** about the following information or if you want more information about this medicine or your medical problem, **ask your doctor, nurse, or pharmacist.**

Before Using This Medicine

In order to decide on the best treatment for your medical problem, your doctor should be told:

—if you have ever had any unusual or allergic reaction to miconazole.

—if you are on a low-salt, low-sugar, or any other special diet, or if you are allergic to any substance, such as foods or sulfites or other preservatives. Most medicines contain more than their active ingredient. Your doctor, nurse, or pharmacist can help you avoid products that may cause a problem.

—if you are **pregnant** or if you may become pregnant. Studies have not been done in humans. However, miconazole has not been shown to cause birth defects or other problems in studies in rats and rabbits.

—if you are **breast-feeding**. However, miconazole has not been shown to cause problems in nursing babies.

—if you are taking **any** other prescription or nonprescription (OTC) medicine.

Side Effects of This Medicine

Along with its needed effects, a medicine may cause some unwanted effects. Although not all of these side effects may occur, if they do occur they may need medical attention.

Check with your doctor as soon as possible if any of the following side effects occur:
More common
   Fever and chills
   Redness, swelling, or pain at place of injection
   Skin rash or itching
Less common or rare
   Unusual bleeding or bruising
   Unusual tiredness or weakness
   Wheezing or troubled breathing

Other side effects may occur that usually do not require medical attention. These side effects may go away during treatment as your body adjusts to the medicine. However, check with your doctor if any of the following side effects continue or are bothersome:
More common
   Nausea or vomiting
Less common
   Diarrhea
   Drowsiness
   Flushing or redness of face or skin
   Loss of appetite

For elderly patients: Many medicines have not been tested in older people. Therefore, it is not known whether the medicine acts the same way it does in younger adults. Check with your doctor or pharmacist if you notice any unusual effects while receiving this medicine or if you think it is not working as it should.

Other side effects not listed above may also occur in some patients. If you notice any other effects, check with your doctor.

December 1987

MICONAZOLE (Topical)

Some commonly used brand names are Micatin and Monistat-Derm.

To the Reader: If you do not recognize the names of medical conditions or medicines referred to in this information, check with your doctor, nurse, or pharmacist. Definitions for selected medical terms may be found in the Glossary. Brand names for the generic drug names listed can be found in the Index. In addition, selected brand names commonly associated with the generic name have been included in the text to help you recognize medicine you may be taking. The fact that a brand name product is not mentioned does not mean the information does not apply. It is a good idea for you to learn both the generic and brand names of your medicines and to write them down for future use.

Miconazole (mi-KON-a-zole) belongs to the group of medicines called antifungals. Topical miconazole is used on the skin to treat some types of fungal infections.

One brand of miconazole cream and the aerosol powder, powder, and aerosol solution forms may be available without a prescription; however, your doctor may have special instructions on the proper use of these medicines for your medical problem. The other brand of the cream and the lotion form of miconazole are available only with your doctor's prescription.

Remember:

• **Some forms of this medicine have been prescribed for your present infection only.** Another infection later on may require a different medicine. Also, even though other people may have the same symptoms as you, they may have a different kind of infection. Your medicine may not work for them and may even cause them harm. Therefore, **your medicine must not be given to other people or used for other infections** unless you are otherwise directed by your doctor.

• **Keep all medicines out of the reach of children.**

• In order for this medicine to work, it must be used as directed. **If you are using this medicine without a prescription, it is very important to follow the directions on the label.**

• **It is also very important that you read and understand the following information.** If any of the information causes you special concern, check with your doctor or pharmacist.

• Before you begin using any new medicine (prescription or nonprescription) or if you develop any new medical problem while you are using this medicine, check with your doctor, nurse, or pharmacist.

• **If you have any questions** about the following information or if you want more information about this medicine or your medical problem, **ask your doctor, nurse, or pharmacist.**

Before Using This Medicine

Before you use miconazole, check with your doctor or pharmacist:

—if you have ever had any unusual or allergic reaction to miconazole.

—if you are allergic to any substance, such as certain foods or preservatives or dyes. Most medicines contain more than their active ingredient. Your doctor, nurse, or pharmacist can help you avoid products that may cause a problem.

—if you are **pregnant** or if you may become pregnant. However, miconazole topical preparations have not been shown to cause birth defects or other problems in humans.

—if you are **breast-feeding**. However, miconazole topical preparations have not been shown to cause problems in nursing babies.

Proper Use of This Medicine

Keep this medicine away from the eyes.

Apply enough miconazole to cover the affected area, and rub in gently.

For patients using the aerosol powder form of miconazole:

• Shake well before using.

• From a distance of 6 to 10 inches, spray the powder on the affected areas. If it is used on the feet, spray it between the toes, on the feet, and in the socks and shoes.

• Do not inhale the powder.

• Do not use near heat, near open flame, or while smoking.

For patients using the powder form of miconazole:

• If the powder is used on the feet, sprinkle it between the toes, on the feet, and in the socks and shoes.

For patients using the aerosol solution form of miconazole:

• Shake well before using.

• From a distance of 4 to 6 inches, spray the solution on the affected areas. If it is used on the feet, spray it between the toes and on the feet.

• Do not inhale the vapors from the spray.

• Do not use near heat, near open flame, or while smoking.

When miconazole is used to treat certain types of fungal infections of the skin, an occlusive dressing or airtight covering (for example, kitchen plastic wrap) should *not* be applied over this medicine. To do so may cause irritation of the skin. **Do not apply an occlusive dressing over this medicine unless you have been directed to do so by your doctor.**

To help clear up your infection completely, **keep using this medicine for the full time of treatment** even though your condition may have improved. **Do not miss any doses.**

If you do miss a dose of this medicine, apply it as soon as possible. However, if it is almost time for your next dose, skip the missed dose and go back to your regular dosing schedule.

How to store this medicine:

• **Keep out of the reach of children.**

• Store away from heat and direct light.

• Do not store the powder form of this medicine in the bathroom, near the kitchen sink, or in other damp places. Heat or moisture may cause the medicine to break down.

• Keep the cream, lotion, and aerosol solution forms of this medicine from freezing.

• Do not puncture, break, or burn the aerosol powder or aerosol solution container.

• Do not keep outdated medicine or medicine no longer needed. Be sure that any discarded medicine is out of the reach of children.

Precautions While Using This Medicine

If your skin problem does not improve within 4 weeks, or if it becomes worse, check with your doctor or pharmacist.

Side Effects of This Medicine

Along with its needed effects, a medicine may cause some unwanted effects. Although not all of these side effects may occur, if they do occur they may need medical attention.

Check with your doctor as soon as possible if any of the following side effects occur:

> Skin rash, blistering, burning, redness, or other sign of skin irritation not present before using this medicine

Other side effects not listed above may also occur in some patients. If you notice any other effects, check with your doctor.

December 1987

MICONAZOLE (Vaginal)

Some commonly used brand names are Monistat*, Monistat 3, and Monistat 7.

*Not available in the U.S.

To the Reader: If you do not recognize the names of medical conditions or medicines referred to in this information, check with your doctor, nurse, or pharmacist. Definitions for selected medical terms may be found in the Glossary. Brand names for the generic drug names listed can be found in the Index. In addition, selected brand names commonly associated with the generic name have been included in the text to help you recognize medicine you may be taking. The fact that a brand name product is not mentioned does not mean the information does not apply. It is a good idea for you to learn both the generic and brand names of your medicines and to write them down for future use.

Miconazole (mi-KON-a-zole) belongs to the group of medicines called antifungals. Vaginal miconazole is used in the vagina to treat fungal infections of the vagina.

Miconazole is available only with your doctor's prescription.

Remember:

• **This medicine has been prescribed for your present infection only.** Another infection later on may require a different medicine. Also, even though other people may have the same symptoms as you, they may have a different kind of infection. Your medicine may not work for them and may even cause them harm. Therefore, **your medicine must not be given to other people or used for other infections** unless you are otherwise directed by your doctor.

• **Keep all medicines out of the reach of children.**

• In order for this medicine to work, it must be used as directed.

• **It is very important that you read and understand the following information.** If any of the information causes you special concern, do not decide against using this medicine without first checking with your doctor.

• Before you begin using any new medicine (prescription or nonprescription) or if you develop any new medical problem while you are using this medicine, check with your doctor, nurse, or pharmacist.

• **If you have any questions** about the following information or if you want more information about this medicine or your medical problem, **ask your doctor, nurse, or pharmacist.**

Before Using This Medicine

In order to decide on the best treatment for your medical problem, your doctor should be told:

—if you have ever had any unusual or allergic reaction to miconazole.

—if you are allergic to any substance, such as certain foods or preservatives or dyes. Most medicines contain more than their active ingredient. Your doctor, nurse, or pharmacist can help you avoid products that may cause a problem.

—if you are **pregnant** or if you may become pregnant. However, only a small amount of miconazole is absorbed into the body and this medicine has not been shown to cause birth defects and other problems in humans.

—if you are **breast-feeding**. It is not known whether miconazole passes into the breast milk. However, this medicine has not been shown to cause problems in nursing babies.

Proper Use of This Medicine

Miconazole usually comes with patient directions. Read them carefully before using this medicine.

Use this medicine at bedtime, unless otherwise directed by your doctor.

To help clear up your infection completely, **keep using this medicine for the full time of treatment** even though your condition may have improved. Also, keep using this medicine even if you begin to menstruate or if you have intercourse during the time of treatment. **Do not miss any doses.**

If you do miss a dose of this medicine, insert it as soon as possible. However, if it is almost time for your next dose, skip the missed dose and go back to your regular dosing schedule.

How to store this medicine:

• **Keep out of the reach of children.**

• Store away from heat and direct light.

• Do not store the vaginal suppository form of this medicine in the bathroom, near the kitchen sink, or in other damp places. Heat or moisture may cause the medicine to break down.

• Keep the vaginal cream form of this medicine from freezing.

• Do not keep outdated medicine or medicine no longer needed. Be sure that any discarded medicine is out of the reach of children.

Precautions While Using This Medicine

To help cure the infection and to help prevent reinfection, good health habits are required.

• Wear cotton panties (or panties or pantyhose with cotton crotches) instead of synthetic (for example, nylon, rayon) underclothes.

• Wear freshly laundered underclothes.

If you have any questions about this, check with your doctor, nurse, or pharmacist.

If you have any questions about douching during the time of treatment with this medicine, check with your doctor.

Since there may be some vaginal drainage while you are using this medicine, a sanitary napkin may be worn to protect your clothing.

Side Effects of This Medicine

Along with its needed effects, a medicine may cause some unwanted effects. Although not all of these side effects may occur, if they do occur they may need medical attention.

Check with your doctor as soon as possible if any of the following side effects occur:

More common

Vaginal burning, itching, or irritation not present before using this medicine

Rare

Skin rash or hives

Other side effects may occur that usually do not require medical attention. These side effects may go away during treatment as your body adjusts to the medicine. However, check with your doctor if any of the following side effects continue or are bothersome:

Less common or rare

Headache

Pelvic cramps

Other side effects not listed above may also occur in some patients. If you notice any other effects, check with your doctor.

_____

December 1987

MIDAZOLAM (Systemic)

A commonly used brand name is Versed.

To the Reader: If you do not recognize the names of medical conditions or medicines referred to in this information, check with your doctor, nurse, or pharmacist. Definitions for selected medical terms may be found in the Glossary. Brand names for the generic drug names listed can be found in the Index. In addition, selected brand names commonly associated with the generic name have been included in the text to help you recognize medicine you may be taking. The fact that a brand name product is not mentioned does not mean the information does not apply. It is a good idea for you to learn both the generic and brand names of your medicines and to write them down for future use.

Midazolam (mid-AY-zoe-lam) is given by injection to produce sleepiness or drowsiness and to relieve anxiety before surgery or certain procedures. It is also used to produce loss of consciousness before and during surgery.

Midazolam is given only by or under the immediate supervision of a physician or dentist trained to use this medicine. If you will be receiving midazolam during surgery, your doctor or anesthesiologist will give you the medicine and closely follow your progress.

Remember:

• **It is very important that you read and understand the following information.** If any of the information causes you special concern, do not decide against receiving this medicine without first checking with your doctor.

• **If you have any questions** about the following information or if you want more information about this medicine or your medical problem, **ask your doctor, nurse, or pharmacist.**

Before Receiving This Medicine

In order to decide on the best treatment for your medical problem, your doctor should be told:

—if you have ever had any unusual or allergic reaction to midazolam or other benzodiazepines (such as alprazolam, chlordiazepoxide, clonazepam, diazepam, flurazepam, halazepam, lorazepam, oxazepam, prazepam, temazepam, triazolam).

—if you are on a low-salt, low-sugar, or any other special diet, or if you are allergic to any substance, such as preservatives. Most medicines contain more than their active ingredient.

—if you are **pregnant**. Midazolam is not recommended during pregnancy because it may cause birth defects. Other benzodiazepines such as chlordiazepoxide and diazepam, related chemically and in action to midazolam, have been reported to increase the chance of birth defects when used during the first 3 months of pregnancy. Also, use of midazolam during pregnancy, especially during the last few days, may cause drowsiness, slow heartbeat, shortness of breath, or troubled breathing in the newborn infant. In addition, receiving midazolam just before or during labor may cause weakness in the newborn infant.

—if you are **breast-feeding**. It is not known whether midazolam passes into the breast milk. This medicine has not been shown to cause problems in nursing babies.

—if you have any of the following medical problems:
Heart disease
Kidney disease
Liver disease
Lung disease
Myasthenia gravis

—if you are taking **any** other prescription or nonprescription (OTC) medicine, especially central nervous system (CNS) depressants.

Precautions After Receiving This Medicine

For patients going home within 24 hours after receiving midazolam:

• Midazolam may cause some people to feel drowsy, tired, or weak for one or two days after it has been given. It may also cause problems with coordination and one's ability to think. Therefore, **do not drive, use machines, or do other jobs that require you to be alert** until the effects of the medicine have disappeared or until the day after receiving midazolam, whichever period of time is longer.

• **Do not drink alcoholic beverages or take other CNS depressants (medicines that slow down the nervous system, possibly causing drowsiness) for about 24 hours after you have received midazolam, unless otherwise directed by your doctor.** To do so may add to the effects of the medicine. Some examples of CNS depressants are antihistamines or medicine for hay fever, other allergies, or colds; other sedatives, tranquilizers, or sleeping medicine; prescription pain medicine or narcotics; medicine for convulsions (seizures); and muscle relaxants.

Side Effects of This Medicine

Some side effects may occur that usually do not require medical attention. The following side effects may go away as the effects of midazolam wear off. However, check with your doctor if any of the following side effects continue or are bothersome:

Less common or rare
Blurred vision or other changes in vision
Dizziness, lightheadedness, or feeling faint
Drowsiness (prolonged)
Headache
Nausea or vomiting
Numbness, tingling, pain, or weakness in hands or feet
Redness, pain, lump or hardness, or muscle stiffness at place of injection

Other side effects not listed above may also occur in some patients. If you notice any other effects, check with your doctor.

December 1987

MINOXIDIL (Systemic)

A commonly used brand name is Loniten.

A generic name product may also be available in the U.S.

To the Reader: If you do not recognize the names of medical conditions or medicines referred to in this information, check with your doctor, nurse, or pharmacist. Definitions for selected medical terms may be found in the Glossary. Brand names for the generic drug names listed can be found in the Index. In addition, selected brand names commonly associated with the generic name have been included in the text to help you recognize medicine you may be taking. The fact that a brand name product is not mentioned does not mean the information does not apply. It is a good idea for you to learn both the generic and brand names of your medicines and to write them down for future use.

Minoxidil (mi-NOX-i-dill) belongs to the general class of medicines called antihypertensives. It is taken by mouth to treat high blood pressure.

High blood pressure adds to the workload of the heart and arteries. If it continues for a long time, the heart and arteries may not function properly. This can damage the blood vessels of the brain, heart, and kidneys, resulting in a stroke, heart failure, or kidney failure. High blood pressure may also increase the risk of heart attacks. These problems may be less likely to occur if blood pressure is controlled.

Minoxidil works by relaxing blood vessels so that blood passes through them more easily. This helps to lower blood pressure.

Minoxidil has other effects that could be bothersome for some patients. These include increased hair growth, weight gain, fast heartbeat, and chest pain. Before you take this medicine, be sure that you have discussed the use of it with your doctor.

Minoxidil is being applied to the scalp in liquid form by some balding men to stimulate hair growth. However, improper use of liquids made from minoxidil tablets can result in minoxidil being absorbed into the body, where it may cause unwanted effects on the heart and blood vessels.

Minoxidil is available only with your doctor's prescription.

Remember:

• **This medicine has been prescribed for your current medical problem only.** It must not be given to other people or used for other problems unless you are directed to do so by your doctor.

• **Keep all medicines out of the reach of children.**

• In order for this medicine to work, it must be used as directed.

• **It is very important that you read and understand the following information.** If any of the information causes you special concern, do not decide against using this medicine without first checking with your doctor.

• Before you begin using any new medicine (prescription or nonprescription) or if you develop any new medical problem while you are using this medicine, check with your doctor, nurse, or pharmacist.

• **If you have any questions** about the following information or if you want more information about this medicine or your medical problem, **ask your doctor, nurse, or pharmacist.**

Before Using This Medicine

In order to decide on the best treatment for your medical problem, your doctor should be told:

—if you have ever had any unusual or allergic reaction to minoxidil.

—if you are on a low-salt, low-sugar, or any other special diet, or if you are allergic to any substance, such as foods, sulfites or other preservatives, or dyes. Most medicines contain more than their active ingredient. Your doctor, nurse, or pharmacist can help you avoid products that may cause a problem.

—if you are **pregnant** or if you may become pregnant. Studies have not been done in humans. However, studies in rats found a decreased rate of conception, and studies in rabbits at 5 times the human dose have shown a decrease in successful pregnancies. Minoxidil did not cause birth defects in rats or rabbits.

—if you are **breast-feeding**. Although minoxidil passes into breast milk, it has not been shown to cause problems in nursing babies.

—if you have any of the following medical problems:

Angina (chest pain)
Heart or blood vessel disease
Kidney disease
Pheochromocytoma

—if you have recently had a heart attack or stroke.

—if you are taking **any** other prescription or nonprescription (OTC) medicine, especially:

Guanethidine (e.g., Ismelin)
Nitrates (medicine for angina)

Proper Use of This Medicine

Importance of diet—When prescribing medicine for your condition, your doctor may also prescribe a personal diet for you. Such a diet may be low in sodium (salt). Most people eat much more sodium than they need and too much sodium in the diet may increase blood pressure. Some foods that contain large amounts of sodium are canned soup, pickles, ketchup, green and ripe olives, relish, frankfurters, soy sauce, and carbonated beverages. Your doctor may want you to limit the amounts of these and other high-sodium foods in your diet. High blood pressure medicine is usually more effective when such a diet is properly followed.

Also, it may be very important for you to go on a reducing diet. However, check with your doctor before changing your diet.

Many patients who have high blood pressure will not notice any signs of the problem. In fact, many may feel normal. It is very important that you **take your medicine exactly as directed** and that you keep your appointments with your doctor even if you feel well.

Remember that minoxidil will not cure your high blood pressure but it does help control it. Therefore, you must continue to take it as directed if you expect to lower your blood pressure and keep it down. **You may have to take high blood pressure medicine for the rest of your life.** If high blood pressure is not treated, it can cause serious problems such as heart failure, blood vessel disease, stroke, or kidney disease.

In order to help remember to take your medicine, try to get into the habit of taking it at the same time each day.

This medicine is usually given together with certain other medicines. If you are using a combination of drugs, make sure that you take each medicine at the proper time and do not mix them. Ask your doctor, nurse, or pharmacist to help you plan a way to remember to take your medicines at the right time.

If you miss a dose of this medicine and remember it within a few hours, take it when you remember. However, if you do not remember until the next day, skip the missed dose and go back to your regular dosing schedule. Do not double doses.

How to store this medicine:

- **Keep out of the reach of children.**

- Store away from heat and direct light.

- Do not store in the bathroom, near the kitchen sink, or in other damp places. Heat or moisture may cause the medicine to break down.

- Do not keep outdated medicine or medicine no longer needed. Be sure that any discarded medicine is out of the reach of children.

Precautions While Using This Medicine

It is important that your doctor check your progress at regular visits to make sure that this medicine is working properly.

Ask your doctor about checking your pulse rate before and after taking minoxidil. Then, while you are taking this medicine, **check your pulse regularly while you are resting**. If it increases by 20 beats or more a minute, check with your doctor right away.

While you are taking minoxidil, **weigh yourself every day**. A weight gain of 2 to 3 pounds (about 1 kg) in an adult is normal and should be lost with continued treatment. However, if you suddenly gain 5 pounds (2 kg) or more (for a child, 2 pounds [1 kg] or more) or if you notice swelling of your feet or lower legs, check with your doctor right away.

Do not take other medicines unless they have been discussed with your doctor. This especially includes over-the-counter (nonprescription) medicines for appetite control, asthma, colds, cough, hay fever, or sinus problems, since they may tend to increase your blood pressure.

Side Effects of This Medicine

Along with its needed effects, a medicine may cause some unwanted effects. Although not all of these side effects may occur, if they do occur they may need medical attention.

Check with your doctor immediately if any of the following side effects occur:
More common
Fast or irregular heartbeat
Weight gain (rapid) of more than 5 pounds (2 pounds in children)
Less common
Chest pains
Shortness of breath

Check with your doctor as soon as possible if any of the following side effects occur:
More common
Bloating
Flushing or redness of skin
Swelling of feet or lower legs
Less common
Numbness or tingling of hands, feet, or face
Rare
Skin rash and itching

Other side effects may occur that usually do not require medical attention. These side effects may go away during treatment as your body adjusts to the medicine. However, check with your doctor if any of the following side effects continue or are bothersome:
More common
Increase in hair growth, usually on face, arms, and back
Less common or rare
Breast tenderness in males and females
Headache

This medicine causes a temporary increase in hair growth in most people. Hair may grow longer and darker in both men and women. This may first be noticed on the face several weeks after you start taking minoxidil. Later, new hair growth may be noticed on the back, arms, legs, and scalp. Talk to your doctor about shaving or using a hair remover during this time. After treatment with minoxidil has ended, the hair will stop growing, although it may take several months for the new hair growth to go away.

For elderly patients: Minoxidil may reduce tolerance to cold temperatures in elderly patients.

Other side effects not listed above may also occur in some patients. If you notice any other effects, check with your doctor.

December 1987

MINOXIDIL (Topical)*

A commonly used brand name is Rogaine*.

---

*Not commercially available in the U.S.

To the Reader: If you do not recognize the names of medical conditions or medicines referred to in this information, check with your doctor, nurse, or pharmacist. Definitions for selected medical terms may be found in the Glossary. Brand names for the generic drug names listed can be found in the Index. In addition, selected brand names commonly associated with the generic name have been included in the text to help you recognize medicine you may be taking. The fact that a brand name product is not mentioned does not mean the information does not apply. It is a good idea for you to learn both the generic and brand names of your medicines and to write them down for future use.

Minoxidil (mi-NOX-i-dill) applied to the skin is used to stimulate hair growth in men who are balding. The exact way that it works is not known, but it may stimulate hair growth by improving the blood supply to the hair follicle.

Hair growth from use of minoxidil occurs and lasts only as long as the medicine continues to be used. The new hair will be lost within a few months after minoxidil treatment is stopped.

This medicine is available only with your doctor's prescription.

Remember:

• **This medicine has been prescribed for your current medical problem only.** It must not be given to other people or used for other problems unless you are directed to do so by your doctor.

• **Keep all medicines out of the reach of children.**

• In order for this medicine to work, it must be used as directed.

• **It is very important that you read and understand the following information.** If any of the information causes you special concern, do not decide against using this medicine without first checking with your doctor.

• Before you begin using any new medicine (prescription or nonprescription) or if you develop any new medical problem while you are using this medicine, check with your doctor, nurse, or pharmacist.

• **If you have any questions** about the following information or if you want more information about this medicine or your medical problem, **ask your doctor, nurse, or pharmacist.**

Before Using This Medicine

In order to decide on the best treatment for your medical problem, your doctor should be told:

—if you have ever had any unusual or allergic reaction to minoxidil.

—if you have any other skin problems.

—if you are taking **any** other prescription or nonprescription (OTC) medicine.

Proper Use of This Medicine

It is very important that you use this medicine only as directed. Do not use more of it and do not use it more often than your doctor ordered. To do so may increase the chance of absorption through the skin. Absorption into the body may affect the heart and blood vessels and cause unwanted effects.

How to apply minoxidil solution:

• Shampoo your hair each morning before applying minoxidil. Make sure your hair and scalp are completely dry before applying this medicine.

• Apply the amount prescribed to the area of the scalp being treated, beginning in the center of the area. Follow your doctor's instructions on how to apply the solution, using the applicator provided.

• Immediately after using this medicine, wash your hands to remove any medicine that may be on them.

• Do not use a hairdryer to dry the scalp after you apply minoxidil solution. Blowing with a hairdryer on the scalp may make the treatment less effective.

• If you are using this medicine at bedtime, do not go to bed until at least 30 minutes after you use it. That way, less of the medicine will rub off on the pillowcase.

Keep this medicine away from the eyes, nose, and mouth. If you should accidentally get some in your eyes, nose, or mouth, flush the area thoroughly with water.

If you miss a dose of this medicine, apply it as soon as possible. Then go back to your regular dosing schedule. But if it is almost time for your next dose, do not apply the missed dose at all. Instead, go back to your regular dosing schedule. Do not double the amount used.

How to store this medicine:

• **Keep out of the reach of children.**

• Store away from heat and direct light.

• Keep the medicine from freezing.

• Do not keep outdated medicine or medicine no longer needed. Be sure that any discarded medicine is out of the reach of children.

Precautions While Using This Medicine

It is important that your doctor check your progress at regular visits to make sure that this medicine is working properly and to check for unwanted effects.

Side Effects of This Medicine

Along with its needed effects, a medicine may cause some unwanted effects. Although not all of these side effects may occur, if they do occur they may need medical attention.

Check with your doctor as soon as possible if any of the following side effects occur:

Less common
  Itching

© 1988   The United States Pharmacopeial Convention, Inc.

Rare

  Burning of scalp
  Skin rash
  Swelling of face

Signs of too much medicine being absorbed into the body

  Chest pain
  Dizziness or faintness
  Fast or irregular heartbeat
  Flushing
  Headache
  Numbness or tingling of hands, feet, or face
  Swelling of feet or lower legs
  Weight gain (rapid)

Other side effects may occur that usually do not require medical attention. These side effects may go away during treatment as your body adjusts to the medicine.

However, check with your doctor if either of the following side effects continues or is bothersome:

Less common

  Dry or flaking skin
  Reddened skin

For elderly patients: Many medicines have not been tested in older people. Therefore, it is not known whether the medicine acts the same way it does in younger adults. Check with your doctor or pharmacist if you notice any unusual effects while using this medicine or if you think it is not working as it should.

Other side effects not listed above may also occur in some patients. If you notice any other effects, check with your doctor.

December 1987

MITOMYCIN (Systemic)

A commonly used brand name is Mutamycin.

To the Reader: If you do not recognize the names of medical conditions or medicines referred to in this information, check with your doctor, nurse, or pharmacist. Definitions for selected medical terms may be found in the Glossary. Brand names for the generic drug names listed can be found in the Index. In addition, selected brand names commonly associated with the generic name have been included in the text to help you recognize medicine you may be taking. The fact that a brand name product is not mentioned does not mean the information does not apply. It is a good idea for you to learn both the generic and brand names of your medicines and to write them down for future use.

Mitomycin (mye-toe-MYE-sin) belongs to the group of medicines known as antineoplastics. It is given by injection to treat some kinds of cancer.

Mitomycin interferes with the growth of cancer cells, which are eventually destroyed. Since the growth of normal body cells may also be affected by mitomycin, other effects will also occur. Some of these may be serious and must be reported to your doctor. Other effects, like hair loss, may not be serious but may cause concern. Some effects may not occur for months or years after the medicine is used.

Before you begin treatment with mitomycin, you and your doctor should talk about the good this medicine will do as well as the risks of using it.

Mitomycin is to be administered only by or under the immediate supervision of your doctor.

Remember:

• **It is very important that you read and understand the following information.** If any of the information causes you special concern, do not decide against treatment with this medicine without first checking with your doctor.

• Before you begin treatment with any new medicine (prescription or nonprescription) or if you develop any new medical problem while you are using this medicine, check with your doctor, nurse, or pharmacist.

• **If you have any questions** about the following information or if you want more information about this medicine or your medical problem, **ask your doctor, nurse, or pharmacist.**

Before Using This Medicine

In order to decide on the best treatment for your medical problem, your doctor should be told:

—if you have ever had any unusual or allergic reaction to mitomycin.

—if you are **pregnant** or if you intend to have children. There is a chance that this medicine may cause birth defects if either the male or female is taking it at the time of conception or if it is taken during pregnancy. Studies have shown that mitomycin causes birth defects in animals. In addition, many cancer medicines may cause sterility which could be permanent. Although this has not been reported with this medicine, the possibility should be kept in mind. Be sure that you have discussed this with your doctor before taking this medicine.

—if you intend to **breast-feed**. Because this medicine may cause serious side effects, breast-feeding is generally not recommended while you are receiving it.

—if you have any of the following medical problems:
    Bleeding problems
    Chickenpox (including recent exposure)
    Herpes zoster (shingles)
    Infection
    Kidney disease

—if you are taking **any** other prescription or nonprescription (OTC) medicine, especially:
    Amphotericin B by injection (e.g., Fungizone)
    Antithyroid agents (medicine for overactive thyroid)
    Azathioprine (e.g., Imuran)
    Chloramphenicol (e.g., Chloromycetin)
    Colchicine
    Flucytosine (e.g., Ancobon)
    Interferon (e.g., Intron A; Roferon-A)

—if you have ever been treated with x-rays or cancer medicines.

Proper Use of This Medicine

Mitomycin is usually given together with certain other medicines. If you are using a combination of medicines, it is important that you receive each one at the proper time. If you are taking some of these medicines by mouth, ask your doctor, nurse, or pharmacist to help you plan a way to remember to take them at the right times.

This medicine often causes nausea, vomiting, and loss of appetite. However, it is very important that you continue to receive the medicine, even if you begin to feel ill. Ask your doctor, nurse, or pharmacist for ways to lessen these effects.

Precautions While Using This Medicine

It is very important that your doctor check your progress at regular visits to make sure that this medicine is working properly and to check for unwanted effects.

While you are being treated with mitomycin, and after you stop treatment with it, **do not have any immunizations without your doctor's approval**. Mitomycin lowers your body's resistance and there is a chance you might get the infection the immunization is meant to prevent. In addition, other persons living in your household should not take oral polio vaccine since there is a chance they could pass the polio virus on to you. Also, you should avoid close contact with other persons (for example, at school or work) who have taken oral polio vaccine.

Mitomycin can lower the number of white blood cells in your body. This may increase the chance of getting an infection. If you can, avoid people with colds or other infections. If you think you are getting a cold or other infection, check with your doctor.

If mitomycin accidentally seeps out of the vein into which it is injected, it may damage the skin and cause scarring. **Tell the doctor or nurse right away if you notice redness, pain, or swelling at the place of injection.**

Side Effects of This Medicine

Along with their needed effects medicines like mitomycin can sometimes cause unwanted effects such as blood problems, loss of hair, and other side effects; these are described below. Also, because of the way these medicines act on the body, there is a chance that they might cause other unwanted effects that may not occur until months or years after the medicine is used. These delayed effects may include certain types of cancer, such as leukemia. Discuss these possible effects with your doctor.

Although not all of these side effects may occur, if they do occur they may need medical attention.

Check with your doctor or nurse immediately if any of the following side effects occur:

More common
Fever, chills, or sore throat
Unusual bleeding or bruising

Less common
Blood in urine

Rare
Redness or pain at place of injection

Check with your doctor or nurse as soon as possible if any of the following side effects occur:

Less common
Cough
Decreased urination
Shortness of breath
Sores in the mouth and on the lips
Swelling of feet or lower legs

Rare
Bloody vomit

Other side effects may occur that usually do not require medical attention. These side effects may go away during treatment as your body adjusts to the medicine.

Also, your doctor or nurse may be able to tell you about ways to prevent or reduce some of these side effects. Check with your doctor if any of the following side effects continue or are bothersome or if you have any questions about them:

More common
Loss of appetite
Nausea and vomiting

Less common
Numbness or tingling in fingers and toes
Purple-colored bands on nails
Skin rash
Tiredness or weakness

Mitomycin sometimes causes a temporary loss of hair. After treatment has ended, normal hair growth should return.

For elderly patients: Many medicines have not been tested in older people. Therefore, it is not known whether the medicine acts the same way it does in younger adults. Check with your doctor or pharmacist if you notice any unusual effects while taking this medicine or if you think it is not working as it should.

After you stop receiving mitomycin, it may still produce some side effects that need attention. During this period of time, **check with your doctor immediately** if you notice the following:

Blood in urine

Also, check with your doctor if you notice any of the following:

Decreased urination
Fever, chills, or sore throat
Shortness of breath
Swelling of feet or lower legs
Unusual bleeding or bruising

Other side effects not listed above may also occur in some patients. If you notice any other effects, check with your doctor.

December 1987

MITOTANE (Systemic)

A commonly used brand name is Lysodren.

To the Reader: If you do not recognize the names of medical conditions or medicines referred to in this information, check with your doctor, nurse, or pharmacist. Definitions for selected medical terms may be found in the Glossary. Brand names for the generic drug names listed can be found in the Index. In addition, selected brand names commonly associated with the generic name have been included in the text to help you recognize medicine you may be taking. The fact that a brand name product is not mentioned does not mean the information does not apply. It is a good idea for you to learn both the generic and brand names of your medicines and to write them down for future use.

Mitotane (MYE-toe-tane) is a medicine that acts on a part of the body called the adrenal cortex. It is taken by mouth to treat some kinds of cancer which affect the adrenal cortex. Also, it is sometimes used when the adrenal cortex is overactive without being cancerous.

Mitotane reduces the amounts of adrenocorticoids (cortisone-like hormones) produced by the adrenal cortex. These steroids are important for various functions of the body, including growth. However, too much of these steroids can cause problems.

Mitotane is available only with your doctor's prescription.

Remember:

• **This medicine has been prescribed for your current medical problem only.** It must not be given to other people or used for other problems unless you are directed to do so by your doctor.

• **Keep all medicines out of the reach of children.**

• In order for this medicine to work, it must be used as directed.

• **It is very important that you read and understand the following information.** If any of the information causes you special concern, do not decide against using this medicine without first checking with your doctor.

• Before you begin using any new medicine (prescription or nonprescription) or if you develop any new medical problem while you are using this medicine, check with your doctor, nurse, or pharmacist.

• **If you have any questions** about the following information or if you want more information about this medicine or your medical problem, **ask your doctor, nurse, or pharmacist.**

Before Using This Medicine

In order to decide on the best treatment for your medical problem, your doctor should be told:

—if you have ever had any unusual or allergic reaction to mitotane.

—if you are on a low-salt, low-sugar, or any other special diet, or if you are allergic to any substance, such as foods, sulfites or other preservatives, or dyes. Most medicines contain more than their active ingredient. Your doctor, nurse, or pharmacist can help you avoid products that may cause a problem.

—if you are **pregnant** or if you may become pregnant. Mitotane has not been shown to cause problems in humans.

—if you are **breast-feeding**. It is not known whether mitotane passes into the breast milk. This medicine has not been shown to cause problems in nursing babies.

—if you have either of the following medical problems:
Infection
Liver disease

—if you are taking **any** other prescription or nonprescription (OTC) medicine, especially central nervous system (CNS) depressants.

Proper Use of This Medicine

Take mitotane only as directed by your doctor. Do not take more or less of it, and do not take it more often than your doctor ordered.

Do not stop taking this medicine without first checking with your doctor. To do so may increase the chance of unwanted effects.

If you miss a dose of this medicine, take the missed dose as soon as you remember it. However, if it is almost time for the next dose, skip the missed dose and do not double the next one. Instead, go back to your regular dosing schedule and check with your doctor.

How to store this medicine:

• **Keep out of the reach of children.**

• Store away from heat and direct light.

• Do not store in the bathroom, near the kitchen sink, or in other damp places. Heat or moisture may cause the medicine to break down.

• Do not keep outdated medicine or medicine no longer needed. Be sure that any discarded medicine is out of the reach of children.

Precautions While Using This Medicine

It is very important that your doctor check your progress at regular visits to make sure this medicine is working properly and to check for unwanted effects.

Your doctor may want you to carry an identification card stating that you are taking this medicine.

This medicine will add to the effects of alcohol and other CNS depressants (medicines that slow down the nervous system, possibly causing drowsiness). Some examples of CNS depressants are antihistamines or medicine for hay fever, other allergies, or colds; sedatives, tranquilizers, or sleeping medicine; prescription pain medicine or narcotics; barbiturates; medicine for convulsions (seizures); tricyclic antidepressants (medicine for depression); muscle relaxants; or anesthetics, including some dental anesthetics. **Check with your doctor before taking any of the above while you are using this medicine.**

This medicine may cause some people to become dizzy, drowsy, or less alert than they are normally. **Make sure you know how you react to this medicine before you drive, use machines, or do other jobs that require you to be alert.**

Check with your doctor right away if you get an injury, infection, or illness of any kind. This medicine may weaken your body's defenses against infection or inflammation.

Side Effects of This Medicine

Along with its needed effects, a medicine may cause some unwanted effects. Although not all of these side effects may occur, if they do occur they may need medical attention.

Check with your doctor as soon as possible if any of the following side effects occur:

More common
> Darkening of skin
> Diarrhea
> Dizziness
> Drowsiness
> Loss of appetite
> Mental depression
> Nausea and vomiting
> Skin rash
> Tiredness

Less common
> Blood in urine
> Blurred vision
> Double vision

Rare
> Shortness of breath
> Wheezing

Other side effects may occur that usually do not require medical attention. These side effects may go away during treatment as your body adjusts to the medicine. However, check with your doctor if any of the following side effects continue or are bothersome:

Less common
> Aching muscles
> Dizziness or lightheadedness when getting up from a lying or sitting position
> Fever
> Flushing or redness of skin
> Muscle twitching

For elderly patients: Many medicines have not been tested in older people. Therefore, it is not known whether the medicine acts the same way it does in younger adults. Check with your doctor or pharmacist if you notice any unusual effects while taking this medicine or if you think it is not working as it should.

Other side effects not listed above may also occur in some patients. If you notice any other effects, check with your doctor.

December 1987

MOLINDONE (Systemic)

A commonly used brand name is Moban.

To the Reader: If you do not recognize the names of medical conditions or medicines referred to in this information, check with your doctor, nurse, or pharmacist. Definitions for selected medical terms may be found in the Glossary. Brand names for the generic drug names listed can be found in the Index. In addition, selected brand names commonly associated with the generic name have been included in the text to help you recognize medicine you may be taking. The fact that a brand name product is not mentioned does not mean the information does not apply. It is a good idea for you to learn both the generic and brand names of your medicines and to write them down for future use.

Molindone (moe-LIN-done) is taken by mouth to treat nervous, mental, and emotional conditions.

Molindone is available only with your doctor's prescription.

Remember:

• **This medicine has been prescribed for your current medical problem only.** It must not be given to other people or used for other problems unless you are directed to do so by your doctor.

• **Keep all medicines out of the reach of children.**

• In order for this medicine to work, it must be used as directed.

• **It is very important that you read and understand the following information.** If any of the information causes you special concern, do not decide against using this medicine without first checking with your doctor.

• Before you begin using any new medicine (prescription or nonprescription) or if you develop any new medical problem while you are using this medicine, check with your doctor, nurse, or pharmacist.

• **If you have any questions** about the following information or if you want more information about this medicine or your medical problem, **ask your doctor, nurse, or pharmacist.**

Before Using This Medicine

In order to decide on the best treatment for your medical problem, your doctor should be told:

—if you have ever had any unusual or allergic reaction to molindone, phenothiazines, thioxanthenes, haloperidol, or loxapine.

—if you are on a low-salt, low-sugar, or any other special diet, or if you are allergic to any substance, such as foods, sulfites or other preservatives, or dyes. Most medicines contain more than their active ingredient, and many liquid medicines contain alcohol. Your doctor, nurse, or pharmacist can help you avoid products that may cause a problem.

—if you are **pregnant** or if you may become pregnant. Molindone has not been shown to cause birth defects or other problems in humans. However, studies in mice have shown a slight decrease in successful pregnancies.

—if you are **breast-feeding**. It is not known if molindone passes into breast milk. However, this medicine has not been shown to cause problems in nursing babies.

—if you have any of the following medical problems:
  Brain tumor
  Difficult urination
  Enlarged prostate
  Glaucoma
  Intestinal blockage
  Liver disease
  Parkinson's disease

—if you are taking **any** other prescription or nonprescription (OTC) medicine, especially:
  Amoxapine (e.g., Asendin)
  Central nervous system (CNS) depressants
  Chlorprothixene (e.g., Taractan)
  Haloperidol (e.g., Haldol)
  Lithium (e.g., Eskalith; Lithane)
  Loxapine (e.g., Loxitane)
  Methyldopa (e.g., Aldomet)
  Metoclopramide (e.g., Reglan)
  Metyrosine (e.g., Demser)
  Pemoline
  Phenothiazines (acetophenazine [e.g., Tindal], chlorpromazine [e.g., Thorazine], fluphenazine [e.g., Prolixin], mesoridazine [e.g., Serentil], perphenazine [e.g., Trilafon], prochlorperazine [e.g., Compazine], promazine [e.g., Sparine], promethazine [e.g., Phenergan], thioridazine [e.g., Mellaril], trifluoperazine [e.g., Stelazine], triflupromazine [e.g., Vesprin], trimeprazine [e.g., Temaril])
  Pimozide (e.g., Orap)
  Rauwolfia alkaloids (alseroxylon, deserpidine, rauwolfia serpentina, reserpine)
  Thiothixene (e.g., Navane)

Proper Use of This Medicine

Molindone should be taken with food or a full glass (8 ounces) of water or milk to reduce stomach irritation.

The liquid form of molindone may be taken undiluted or mixed with milk, water, fruit juice, or carbonated beverages.

Take this medicine only as directed by your doctor. Do not take more of it, do not take it more often, and do not take it for a longer period of time than your doctor ordered. To do so may increase the chance of side effects.

Sometimes this medicine must be taken for several weeks before its full effect is reached in the treatment of certain mental and emotional conditions.

If you miss a dose of this medicine, take it as soon as possible. However, if it is within 2 hours of your next dose, skip the missed dose and go back to your regular dosing schedule. Do not double doses.

How to store this medicine:

• **Keep out of the reach of children.**

• Store away from heat and direct light.

• Do not store the tablets in the bathroom, near the kitchen sink, or in other damp places. Heat or moisture may cause the medicine to break down.

• Keep the liquid form of this medicine from freezing

• Do not keep outdated medicine or medicine no longer needed. Be sure that any discarded medicine is out of the reach of children.

Precautions While Using This Medicine

Your doctor should check your progress at regular visits. This will allow the dosage of the medicine to be adjusted when necessary and also will reduce the possibility of side effects.

Do not stop taking this medicine without first checking with your doctor. Your doctor may want you to reduce gradually the amount you are taking before stopping completely.

Do not take molindone within 1 or 2 hours of taking antacids or medicine for diarrhea. Taking them too close together may make molindone less effective.

This medicine will add to the effects of alcohol and other CNS depressants (medicines that slow down the nervous system, possibly causing drowsiness). Some examples of CNS depressants are antihistamines or medicine for hay fever, other allergies, or colds; sedatives, tranquilizers, or sleeping medicine; prescription pain medicine or narcotics; barbiturates; medicine for seizures; muscle relaxants; or anesthetics, including some dental anesthetics. **Check with your doctor before taking any of the above while you are using this medicine.**

Molindone may cause some people to become drowsy or less alert than they are normally, especially during the first few weeks the medicine is being taken. Even if you take this medicine only at bedtime, you may feel drowsy or less alert on arising. **Make sure you know how you react to this medicine before you drive, use machines, or do other jobs that require you to be alert.**

Dizziness or lightheadedness may occur, especially when you get up from a lying or sitting position. Getting up slowly may help. If the problem continues or gets worse, check with your doctor.

This medicine will often make you sweat less, allowing your body temperature to increase. **Use extra care not to become overheated during exercise or hot weather while you are taking this medicine,** since overheating could possibly result in heat stroke. Also, **hot baths or saunas may make you feel dizzy or faint** while you are taking this medicine.

Molindone may cause dryness of the mouth. For temporary relief, use sugarless candy or gum, melt bits of ice in your mouth, or use a saliva substitute. However, if dry mouth continues for more than 2 weeks, check with your physician or dentist. Continuing dryness of the mouth may increase the chance of dental disease, including tooth decay, gum disease, and fungal infection.

Side Effects of This Medicine

Along with its needed effects, a medicine may cause some unwanted effects. Although not all of these side effects may occur, if they do occur they may need medical attention.

Stop taking this medicine and get emergency help immediately if any of the following side effects occur:

Rare

Convulsions (seizures)
Fast heartbeat
Fever
High or low (irregular) blood pressure
Increased sweating
Loss of bladder control
Muscle stiffness (severe)
Troubled breathing
Unusual feeling of tiredness
Unusually pale skin

Also, check with your doctor as soon as possible if any of the following side effects occur:

More common

Difficulty in talking
Loss of balance control
Mask-like face
Restlessness or need to keep moving (severe)
Shuffling walk
Stiffness of arms and legs
Trembling and shaking of hands

Less common

Chewing movements
Lip smacking or puckering
Mental depression
Puffing of cheeks
Rapid or worm-like movements of tongue
Uncontrolled movements of arms and legs

Rare

Difficulty in swallowing
Fixation of eyes
Muscle spasms, especially of neck and back
Skin rash
Twisting movements of body
Yellow eyes or skin

Other side effects may occur that usually do not require medical attention. These side effects may go away during treatment as your body adjusts to the medicine. However, check with your doctor if any of the following side effects continue or are bothersome:

More common

Blurred vision
Constipation
Decreased sweating
Difficult urination
Dizziness or lightheadedness, especially when getting up suddenly from a lying or sitting position
Drowsiness
Dry mouth
Headache
Nausea
Stuffy nose

Less common
    Changes in menstrual periods
    Decreased sexual ability
    False sense of well-being
    Swelling of breasts
    Unusual secretion of milk

Some side effects may occur after you have stopped taking this medicine. Check with your doctor as soon as possible if you notice any of the following effects:
    Chewing movements
    Lip smacking or puckering
    Puffing of cheeks
    Rapid or worm-like movements of tongue
    Uncontrolled movements of arms and legs

For elderly patients: The above side effects, especially constipation, dizziness or lightheadedness, drowsiness, dry mouth, uncontrolled movements of the mouth and tongue, and trembling of hands, are more likely to occur in the elderly. These patients are usually more sensitive to the effects of molindone.

Other side effects not listed above may also occur in some patients. If you notice any other effects, check with your doctor.

December 1987

MONOOCTANOIN (Local)

A commonly used brand name is Moctanin.

Read the bold information first. Then go back and read the rest. If you do not recognize the names of medical conditions or medicines included in this information, check with your doctor, nurse, or pharmacist. Brand names for the generic drug names listed can also be found in the index. It is a good idea for you to learn both the generic and brand names of your medicines and to write them down for future use.

Monooctanoin (mono-OCK-ta-noyn) is used to dissolve cholesterol gallstones. Gallstones, which are found in the gallbladder or bile duct, sometimes remain in the bile duct even after the gallbladder has been removed by surgery. These stones may be too large to pass out of the body on their own. A catheter or tube is used to put the solution of monooctanoin into the bile duct where it will come in contact with the gallstone or gallstones and dissolve them. This is done for a period of 1 to 3 weeks.

Monooctanoin is available only with your doctor's prescription.

Remember:

• **It is very important that you read and understand the following information.** If any of the information causes you special concern, do not decide against receiving this medicine without first checking with your doctor.

• Before you begin using any new medicine (prescription or nonprescription) or if you develop any new medical problem while you are receiving this medicine, check with your doctor, nurse, or pharmacist.

• **If you have any questions** about the following information or if you want more information about this medicine or your medical problem, **ask your doctor, nurse, or pharmacist.**

Before Using This Medicine

In order to decide on the best treatment for your medical problem, your doctor should be told:

—if you have ever had any unusual or allergic reaction to monooctanoin or any vegetable oils.

—if you are pregnant or if you intend to become pregnant while taking this medicine. Studies have not been done in either humans or animals.

—if you are breast-feeding. Although it is not known whether monooctanoin passes into the breast milk and this medicine has not been shown to cause problems in humans, the chance always exists.

—if you have any of the following medical problems:
   Biliary tract problems (other)
   Duodenal ulcer (recent)
   Intestinal problems
   Jaundice
   Liver disease (severe)
   Pancreas disease

Side Effects of This Medicine

Along with its needed effects, a medicine may cause some unwanted effects. Although not all of these side effects appear very often, when they do occur they may require medical attention. Check with your doctor as soon as possible if any of the following side effects occur:

Less common or rare
   Abdominal or stomach pain (severe)
   Back pain (severe)
   Drowsiness (severe)
   Fever, chills, or sore throat
   Nausea (continuing)
   Shortness of breath (severe)

Other side effects may occur which usually do not require medical attention. These side effects may go away during treatment as your body adjusts to the medicine. However, check with your doctor if any of the following side effects continue or are bothersome:

More common
   Abdominal or stomach pain (mild) or burning sensation

Less common or rare
   Back pain (mild)
   Diarrhea
   Flushing or redness of face
   Loss of appetite
   Metallic taste
   Nausea or vomiting

Other side effects not listed above may also occur in some patients. If you notice any other effects, check with your doctor.

December 1987

MUMPS VIRUS VACCINE LIVE (Systemic)

A commonly used brand name is Mumpsvax.

To the Reader: If you do not recognize the names of medical conditions or medicines referred to in this information, check with your doctor, nurse, or pharmacist. Definitions for selected medical terms may be found in the Glossary. Brand names for the generic drug names listed can be found in the Index. In addition, selected brand names commonly associated with the generic name have been included in the text to help you recognize medicine you may be taking. The fact that a brand name product is not mentioned does not mean the information does not apply. It is a good idea for you to learn both the generic and brand names of your medicines and to write them down for future use.

Mumps Virus Vaccine Live is an active immunizing agent given by injection to prevent infection by the mumps virus. It works by causing your body to produce its own protection (antibodies) against the virus.

The following information applies only to the Jeryl Lynn strain of mumps vaccine. Different types of mumps vaccines may be available in countries other than the U.S.

Mumps is an infection that can cause serious problems, such as encephalitis and meningitis, which affect the brain. In addition, adolescent boys and men are very susceptible to a condition called orchitis, which causes pain and swelling in the testicles and scrotum and, in rare cases, sterility. Also, mumps infection can cause spontaneous abortion in women during the first three months of pregnancy.

Although immunization against mumps is recommended for everyone born in or after 1957, it is especially important for:

—children 12 months of age and older, including school-age children, children in day-care centers, and children of pregnant women who have not yet received their own mumps vaccination.

—boys nearing the age of puberty, adolescent boys, and men.

—women of child-bearing age who are not pregnant.

—persons vaccinated during the years 1950 through 1978 (especially during the years 1950 through 1967) with either the inactivated (killed) mumps vaccine or with an unknown type of mumps vaccine.

—persons traveling outside the U.S.

Immunization against mumps is not recommended for infants younger than 12 months of age. The reason is that antibodies they received from their mother before birth may interfere with the effectiveness of the vaccine. Children who were immunized against mumps before 12 months of age should be immunized again.

If the mumps vaccine is going to be given in a combination immunization that includes measles vaccine, the person to be immunized should be at least 15 months old to make sure the vaccine is effective.

You can be considered to be immune to mumps only if you received mumps vaccine on or after your first birthday and you have the medical record to prove it or if you have a doctor's diagnosis of a previous mumps infection.

This vaccine is available only from your doctor or other authorized health care provider.

Remember:

• **It is very important that you read and understand the following information.** If any of the information causes you special concern, do not decide against receiving this vaccine without first checking with your doctor.

• **If you have any questions** about the following information or if you want more information about this vaccine, **ask your doctor, nurse, or pharmacist.**

Before Receiving This Vaccine

Before you receive mumps vaccine, your doctor should be told:

—if you have ever had any unusual or allergic reaction to any form of the antibiotic neomycin. The mumps vaccine available in the U.S. contains neomycin; products available in other countries may contain other antibiotics.

—if you have ever had any unusual or allergic reaction to eggs. The mumps vaccine available in the U.S. is grown in a chick embryo cell culture.

—if you are **pregnant** or if you may become pregnant within 3 months after receiving this medicine. Studies have not been done in either humans or animals; however, use during pregnancy is not recommended. The reason is that mumps vaccine may infect the placenta. However, the vaccine has not been shown to infect the fetus or to cause birth defects. Still, the chance always exists that the vaccine may cause problems during pregnancy.

—if you are **breast-feeding**, although mumps vaccine has not been shown to cause problems in humans.

—if you have any of the following medical problems:
    Fever
    Immune deficiency condition (or family history of)
    Tuberculosis

—if you are taking **any** other prescription or nonprescription (OTC) medicine.

—if you have received any other live virus vaccines in the last month or intend to within the next month.

—if you have received any of the following types of products in the last 3 months or intend to within the next 2 weeks:
    Blood transfusions or other blood products
    Gamma globulin or other globulins

—if you have ever been treated with x-rays or cancer medicines.

Precautions After Receiving This Vaccine

Do not become pregnant for 3 months after receiving mumps vaccine without first checking with your doctor. There is a change that this vaccine may cause problems during pregnancy.

Tell your doctor that you have received this vaccine:

—if you are to receive blood transfusions or other blood products within 2 weeks after receiving this vaccine.

—if you are to receive gamma globulin or other globulins within 2 weeks after receiving this vaccine.

—if you are to receive any other live virus vaccines within 1 month after receiving this vaccine.

—if you are to receive a tuberculin skin test within 6 weeks after receiving this vaccine. The results of the test may be affected by this vaccine.

Side Effects of This Vaccine

Along with its needed effects, a medicine may cause some unwanted effects. Although not all of these side effects may occur, if they do occur they may need medical attention.

Get emergency help immediately if any of the following side effects occur:

Signs of allergic reaction
　　Difficulty in breathing or swallowing
　　Hives
　　Itching, especially of feet or hands
　　Reddening of skin, especially around ears
　　Swelling or eyes, face, or inside of nose
　　Unusual tiredness or weakness (sudden and severe)

Check with your doctor as soon as possible if any of the following side effects occur:

Rare
　　Bruising or purple spots on skin
　　Confusion
　　Convulsions (seizures)

Fever over 103 °F (39.4 °C)
Headache (severe or continuing)
Irritability
Pain, tenderness, or swelling in testicle and scrotum (in adolescent boys and men)
Stiff neck
Vomiting

Other side effects may occur that usually do not require medical attention. However, check with your doctor if any of the following side effects continue or are bothersome:

More common
　　Burning or stinging at place of injection

Less common or rare
　　Fever of 100 °F (37.7 °C) or less
　　Itching, swelling, redness, tenderness, or hard lump at place of injection
　　Skin rash
　　Swollen glands on side of face or neck

Other side effects not listed above may also occur in some patients. If you notice any other effects, check with your doctor.

_____

December 1987

MUROMONAB-CD3 (Systemic)

A commonly used brand name is Orthoclone OKT3.

To the Reader: If you do not recognize the names of medical conditions or medicines referred to in this information, check with your doctor, nurse, or pharmacist. Definitions for selected medical terms may be found in the Glossary. Brand names for the generic drug names listed can be found in the Index. In addition, selected brand names commonly associated with the generic name have been included in the text to help you recognize medicine you may be taking. The fact that a brand name product is not mentioned does not mean the information does not apply. It is a good idea for you to learn both the generic and brand names of your medicines and to write them down for future use.

Muromonab (myoor-oh-MON-ab)-CD3 is a monoclonal antibody. It is used to reduce the body's natural immunity in patients who receive organ (for example, kidney) transplants.

When a patient receives an organ transplant, the body's white blood cells will try to get rid of (reject) the transplanted organ. Muromonab-CD3 works by preventing the white blood cells from doing this.

The effect of muromonab-CD3 on the white blood cells may also reduce the body's ability to fight infections. Before you begin treatment, you and your doctor should talk about the good this medicine will do as well as the risks of using it.

Muromonab-CD3 is to be administered only by or under the immediate supervision of your doctor.

Remember:
• **It is very important that you read and understand the following information.** If any of the information causes you special concern, do not decide against using this medicine without first checking with your doctor.

• Before you begin using any new medicine (prescription or nonprescription) or if you develop any new medical problem while you are receiving this medicine, check with your doctor, nurse, or pharmacist.

• **If you have any questions** about the following information or if you want more information about this medicine or your medical problem, **ask your doctor, nurse, or pharmacist.**

Before Using This Medicine

In order to decide on the best treatment for your medical problem, your doctor should be told:

—if you have ever had any unusual or allergic reaction to muromonab-CD3 or to rodents (such as mice or rats). Muromonab-CD3 is grown in a mouse cell culture.

—if you are on a low-salt, low-sugar, or any other special diet, or if you are allergic to any substance, such as sulfites or other preservatives. Most medicines contain more than their active ingredient.

—if you are **pregnant** or if you may become pregnant. Studies have not been done in either humans or animals.

—if you are **breast-feeding**. Muromonab-CD3 has not been shown to cause problems in nursing babies. However, it may be necessary for you to stop breast-feeding during treatment. Be sure you have discussed the risks and benefits of the medicine with your doctor.

—if you have any of the following medical problems:

Chickenpox (including recent exposure)
Herpes zoster (shingles)
Infection

—if you are taking **any** other prescription or nonprescription (OTC) medicine, especially other immunosuppressants (including adrenocorticoids, azathioprine, chlorambucil, cyclophosphamide, cyclosporine, and mercaptopurine).

Precautions While Using This Medicine

It is very important that your doctor check your progress at regular visits to make sure that this medicine is working properly and to check for unwanted effects.

While you are being treated with muromonab-CD3 and after you stop treatment with it, **do not have any immunizations without your doctor's approval.** Muromonab-CD3 lowers your body's resistance and there is a chance you might get the infection the immunization is meant to prevent. In addition, other persons living in your house should not take oral polio vaccine since there is a chance they could pass the polio virus on to you. Also, you should avoid close contact with other persons (for example, at school or work) who have taken oral polio vaccine.

Treatment with muromonab-CD3 may also increase the chance of getting other infections. If you can, avoid people with colds or other infections. If you think you are getting a cold or other infection, check with your doctor.

This medicine commonly causes chest pain, dizziness, fever and chills, shortness of breath, stomach upset, and trembling within a few hours after the first dose. These effects should be much less after the second dose and should not occur after that. However, **check with your doctor or nurse immediately** if you have severe shortness of breath after the first dose or if the effects continue.

Side Effects of This Medicine

Along with its needed effects, a medicine may cause some unwanted effects. Because of the way that muromonab-CD3 acts on the body, there is a chance that it may cause effects that may not occur until years after the medicine is used. These delayed effects may include certain types of cancer, such as lymphomas. Discuss these possible effects with your doctor.

Although not all of these side effects may occur, if they do occur, they may need medical attention.

Check with your doctor or nurse immediately if the following side effect occurs with the first dose of this medicine:

Rare

Shortness of breath (severe)

Check with your doctor as soon as possible if any of the following side effects occur:

More common

Chest pain
Diarrhea
Dizziness or faintness
Fever and chills
Nausea and vomiting
Shortness of breath or wheezing
Trembling and shaking of hands

For elderly patients: Many medicines have not been tested in older people. Therefore, it is not known whether the medicine acts the same way it does in younger adults. Check with your doctor or pharmacist if you notice any unusual effects while receiving this medicine or if you think it is not working as it should.

After you stop using this medicine, it may still produce some side effects that need medical attention. During this period of time check with your doctor if you notice the following side effects:

Fever and chills

Other side effects not listed above may also occur in some patients. If you notice any other effects, check with your doctor.

December 1987

NALIDIXIC ACID (Systemic)

A commonly used brand name is NegGram.

To the Reader: If you do not recognize the names of medical conditions or medicines referred to in this information, check with your doctor, nurse, or pharmacist. Definitions for selected medical terms may be found in the Glossary. Brand names for the generic drug names listed can be found in the Index. In addition, selected brand names commonly associated with the generic name have been included in the text to help you recognize medicine you may be taking. The fact that a brand name product is not mentioned does not mean the information does not apply. It is a good idea for you to learn both the generic and brand names of your medicines and to write them down for future use.

Nalidixic (nal-i-DIX-ik) acid belongs to the general family of medicines called anti-infectives. It is taken by mouth to help the body overcome infections of the urinary tract.

Nalidixic acid is available only with your doctor's prescription.

Remember:

• **This medicine has been prescribed for your present infection only.** Another infection later on may require a different medicine. Also, even though other people may have the same symptoms as you, they may have a different kind of infection. Your medicine may not work for them and may even cause them harm. Therefore, **your medicine must not be given to other people or used for other infections** unless you are otherwise directed by your doctor.

• **Keep all medicines out of the reach of children.**

• In order for this medicine to work, it must be used as directed.

• **It is very important that you read and understand the following information.** If any of the information causes you special concern, do not decide against using this medicine without first checking with your doctor.

• Before you begin using any new medicine (prescription or nonprescription) or if you develop any new medical problem while you are using this medicine, check with your doctor, nurse, or pharmacist.

• **If you have any questions** about the following information or if you want more information about this medicine or your medical problem, **ask your doctor, nurse, or pharmacist.**

Before Using This Medicine

In order to decide on the best treatment for your medical problem, your doctor should be told:

—if you have ever had any unusual or allergic reaction to this medicine or to any related medicines such as cinoxacin or norfloxacin.

—if you are on a low-salt, low-sugar, or any other special diet, or if you are allergic to any substance, such as foods, sulfites or other preservatives, or dyes. Most medicines contain more than their active ingredient, and many liquid medicines contain alcohol. Your doctor, nurse, or pharmacist can help you avoid products that may cause a problem.

—if you are **pregnant** or if you may become pregnant. Studies have not been done in humans during the first 3 months of pregnancy. However, nalidixic acid has not been shown to cause problems during the last 6 months of pregnancy.

—if you are **breast-feeding**. Nalidixic acid passes into the breast milk and may cause side effects in nursing babies.

—if you have any of the following medical problems:
  Central nervous system (brain or spinal cord) damage
  Convulsive disorders, history of (seizures, epilepsy)
  Hardening of the arteries in the brain (severe)
  Kidney disease (severe)
  Liver disease

—if you are taking **any** other prescription or nonprescription (OTC) medicine, especially anticoagulants (blood thinners).

Proper Use of This Medicine

Do not give this medicine to infants under 3 months of age unless otherwise directed by your doctor.

Nalidixic acid is best taken with a full glass (8 ounces) of water on an empty stomach (either 1 hour before or 2 hours after meals). However, if this medicine causes nausea or upset stomach, it may be taken with food or milk.

For patients taking the oral liquid form of this medicine:

• Use a specially marked measuring spoon or other device to measure each dose accurately since the average household teaspoon may not hold the right amount of liquid.

To help clear up your infection completely, **keep taking this medicine for the full time of treatment** even if you begin to feel better after a few days; **do not miss any doses.**

If you do miss a dose of this medicine, take it as soon as possible. However, if it is almost time for your next dose and your dosing schedule is:

• 3 or more doses a day—Space the missed dose and next dose 2 to 4 hours apart or double your next dose.

Then go back to your regular dosing schedule.

How to store this medicine:

• **Keep out of the reach of children.**

• Store away from heat and direct light.

• Do not store the tablet form of this medicine in the bathroom, near the kitchen sink, or in other damp places. Heat or moisture may cause the medicine to break down.

• Keep the oral liquid form of this medicine from freezing.

• Do not keep outdated medicine or medicine no longer needed. Be sure that any discarded medicine is out of the reach of children.

Precautions While Using This Medicine

If you will be taking this medicine for more than 2 weeks, your doctor should check your progress at regular visits.

If your symptoms do not improve within 2 days, or if they become worse, check with your doctor.

This medicine may cause blurred vision or other vision problems, or it may cause some people to become dizzy, drowsy, or less alert than they are normally. **Make sure you know how you react to this medicine before you drive, use machines, or do other jobs that require you to be alert or to see clearly.** If these reactions are especially bothersome, check with your doctor.

Some people who take nalidixic acid may become more sensitive to sunlight than they are normally. **When you first begin taking this medicine, avoid too much sun and do not use a sunlamp until you see how you react to the sun,** especially if you tend to burn easily. You may still be more sensitive to sunlight or sunlamps for up to 1 year after stopping this medicine. **If you have a severe reaction, check with your doctor.**

Diabetics—This medicine may cause false test results with some urine sugar tests. Check with your doctor before changing your diet or the dosage of your diabetes medicine.

Side Effects of This Medicine

Along with its needed effects, a medicine may cause some unwanted effects. Although not all of these side effects may occur, if they do occur they may need medical attention.

Check with your doctor immediately if any of the following side effects occur:

More common
   Blurred or decreased vision
   Change in color vision
   Double vision
   Halos around lights
   Overbright appearance of lights

Rare
   Convulsions (seizures)
   Dark or amber urine
   Hallucinations (seeing, hearing, or feeling things that are not there)
   Mood or other mental changes
   Pale skin
   Pale stools
   Sore throat and fever
   Stomach pain (severe)
   Unusual bleeding or bruising
   Unusual tiredness or weakness
   Yellow eyes or skin

Other side effects may occur that usually do not require medical attention. These side effects may go away during treatment as your body adjusts to the medicine. However, check with your doctor if any of the following side effects continue or are bothersome:

More common
   Diarrhea
   Headache
   Itching
   Nausea or vomiting
   Skin rash

Less common
   Dizziness
   Drowsiness
   Increased sensitivity of skin to sunlight

For elderly patients: Many medicines have not been tested in older people. Therefore, it is not known whether the medicine acts the same way it does in younger adults. Check with your doctor or pharmacist if you notice any unusual effects while taking this medicine or if you think it is not working as it should.

Other side effects not listed above may also occur in some patients. If you notice any other effects, check with your doctor.

December 1987

NALTREXONE (Systemic)

A commonly used brand name is Trexan.

To the Reader: If you do not recognize the names of medical conditions or medicines referred to in this information, check with your doctor, nurse, or pharmacist. Definitions for selected medical terms may be found in the Glossary. Brand names for the generic drug names listed can be found in the Index. In addition, selected brand names commonly associated with the generic name have been included in the text to help you recognize medicine you may be taking. The fact that a brand name product is not mentioned does not mean the information does not apply. It is a good idea for you to learn both the generic and brand names of your medicines and to write them down for future use.

Naltrexone (nal-TREX-zone) is used to help narcotic addicts who have stopped taking narcotics to stay drug-free. The medicine is not a cure for addiction. It is used as part of an overall program that may include counseling, attending support group meetings, and other treatment recommended by your doctor.

Naltrexone is not a narcotic. It works by blocking the effects of narcotics, especially the "high" feeling that made you want to use them. It will not produce any narcotic-like effects or cause mental or physical dependence.

Naltrexone will cause withdrawal symptoms in people who are physically dependent on narcotics. Therefore, naltrexone treatment is started after you are no longer dependent on narcotics. The length of time this takes may depend on which narcotic you took, the amount you took, and how long you took it.

Naltrexone is available only with your doctor's prescription.

Remember:
- **This medicine has been prescribed for your current medical problem only.** It must not be given to other people or used for other problems unless you are directed to do so by your doctor.

- **Keep all medicines out of the reach of children.**

- In order for this medicine to work, it must be used as directed.

- **It is very important that you read and understand the following information.** If any of the information causes you special concern, do not decide against using this medicine without first checking with your doctor.

- Before you begin using any new medicine (prescription or nonprescription) or if you develop any new medical problem while you are using this medicine, check with your doctor, nurse, or pharmacist.

- **If you have any questions** about the following information or if you want more information about this medicine or your medical problem, **ask your doctor, nurse, or pharmacist**.

Before Using This Medicine

In order to decide on the best treatment for your medical problem, your doctor should be told:

—if you have ever had any unusual or allergic reaction to naltrexone.

—if you are on a low-salt, low-sugar, or any other special diet, or if you are allergic to any substance, such as foods, sulfites or other preservatives, or dyes. Most medicines contain more than their active ingredient. Your doctor, nurse, or pharmacist can help you avoid products that may cause a problem.

—if you are **pregnant** or if you may become pregnant. Studies on birth defects with naltrexone have not been done in humans. Studies in animals have shown that naltrexone causes unwanted effects when given in very large doses.

—if you are **breast-feeding**. It is not known whether naltrexone passes into the breast milk. However, this medicine has not been shown to cause problems in nursing babies.

—if you think that you still may be having any withdrawal symptoms.

—if you now have, or have recently had, hepatitis or other liver disease.

Proper Use of This Medicine

Take naltrexone regularly as ordered by your doctor. It may be helpful to have someone else, such as a family member, doctor, or nurse, give you each dose as scheduled.

If you miss a dose of this medicine, and your regular dosing schedule is:

One tablet every day—
    Take the missed dose as soon as possible. However, if you do not remember until the next day, skip the missed dose and go back to your regular dosing schedule. Do not double the next day's dose.

One tablet every weekday and two tablets on Saturday—
    If you miss a weekday dose, follow the directions for one tablet every day.
    If you miss the Saturday dose, take it as soon as possible. However, if you do not remember until Sunday, take one tablet on Sunday. Then go back to your regular dosing schedule on Monday.

Two tablets every other day—
    Take two tablets as soon as you remember, then skip a day, then go back to taking the medicine every other day; or
    Take two tablets as soon as possible if you remember the same day. However, if you do not remember until the next day, take one tablet the next day. Then go back to your regular dosing schedule.

Two tablets on Monday and Wednesday and three tablets on Friday—

If you miss one of the Monday or Wednesday doses, take it as soon as possible. However, if you do not remember until the next day, take one tablet the next day. Then go back to your regular dosing schedule.

If you miss the Friday dose, take it as soon as possible if you remember the same day. However, if you do not remember until Saturday, take two tablets on Saturday. If you do not remember until Sunday, take one tablet on Sunday. Then go back to your regular dosing schedule on Monday.

Three tablets every three days—

Take three tablets as soon you remember, then skip two days, then go back to taking the medicine every three days; or

Take three tablets as soon as possible if you remember the same day. However, if you do not remember until the next day, take two tablets, then skip a day and go back to your regular dosing schedule. If you do not remember until the second day, take one tablet. Then go back to your regular dosing schedule.

How to store this medicine:

• **Keep out of the reach of children.**

• Store away from heat and direct light.

• Do not store this medicine in the bathroom, near the kitchen sink, or in other damp places. Heat or moisture may cause the medicine to break down.

• Do not keep outdated medicine.

Precautions While Using This Medicine

It is very important that your doctor check your progress at regular visits. Your doctor may want to do certain blood tests to see if the medicine is causing unwanted effects.

Remember that use of naltrexone is only part of your treatment. **Be sure that you follow all of your doctor's orders, including seeing your therapist and/or attending support group meetings on a regular basis.**

Do not try to overcome the effects of naltrexone by taking very large amounts of narcotics. To do so may cause coma or death.

Naltrexone also blocks the useful effects of narcotics. **Always use a non-narcotic medicine to treat pain, diarrhea, or cough.** If you have any questions about the proper medicine to use, check with your doctor, nurse, or pharmacist.

Never share this medicine with anyone else. This is especially important if the other person is using narcotics because naltrexone will cause withdrawal symptoms.

Tell all physicians, dentists, and pharmacists you go to that you are taking naltrexone.

It is recommended that you carry identification stating that you are taking naltrexone. Identification cards may be available from your doctor.

Side Effects of This Medicine

Along with its needed effects, a medicine may cause some unwanted effects. Although not all of these side effects may occur, if they do occur they may need medical attention.

Check with your doctor as soon as possible if any of the following side effects occur:

More common
  Skin rash

Rare
  Abdominal or stomach pain (severe)
  Blurred vision
  Confusion
  Earache
  Fever
  Hallucinations (seeing, hearing, or feeling things that are not there)
  Mental depression or other mood or mental changes
  Nosebleeds (unexplained)
  Pain, tenderness, or color changes in legs or feet
  Ringing or buzzing in ears
  Swelling of face, feet, or lower legs
  Swollen glands
  Weight gain

Other side effects may occur that usually do not require medical attention. These side effects may go away during treatment as your body adjusts to the medicine. However, check with your doctor if any of the following side effects continue or are bothersome:

More common
  Abdominal or stomach cramping or pain (mild or moderate)
  Headache
  Joint or muscle pain
  Nausea or vomiting
  Nervousness or restlessness
  Unusual tiredness

Less common or rare
  Chills
  Constipation
  Diarrhea
  Dizziness
  Fast or pounding heartbeat
  Increased thirst
  Irritability
  Loss of appetite
  Sexual problems in males

Other side effects not listed above, possibly including withdrawal symptoms, may also occur in some patients. If you notice any other effects, check with your doctor.

December 1987

NAPHAZOLINE (Ophthalmic)

Some commonly used brand names are:

Ak-Con	I-Naphline
Albalon	Muro's Opcon
Allerest	Naphcon
Allergy Drops	Naphcon Forte
Clear Eyes	VasoClear
Degest 2	Vasocon

Generic name product may also be available in the U.S.

To the Reader: If you do not recognize the names of medical conditions or medicines referred to in this information, check with your doctor, nurse, or pharmacist. Definitions for selected medical terms may be found in the Glossary. Brand names for the generic drug names listed can be found in the Index. In addition, selected brand names commonly associated with the generic name have been included in the text to help you recognize medicine you may be taking. The fact that a brand name product is not mentioned does not mean the information does not apply. It is a good idea for you to learn both the generic and brand names of your medicines and to write them down for future use.

Naphazoline (naf-AZ-oh-leen) is used in the eye to relieve redness, burning, itching, or other irritation caused by colds, dust, wind, smog, pollen, swimming, wearing contact lenses, or overuse of the eyes in reading, driving, watching television, or close work.

Some of these preparations are available only with your doctor's prescription. Others are available without a prescription; however, your doctor may have special instructions on the proper use of this medicine for your medical problem.

Remember:

• **Keep all medicines out of the reach of children.**

• In order for this medicine to work, it must be used as directed. **If you are using this medicine without a prescription, it is very important to follow the directions on the label.**

• **It is also very important that you read and understand the following information.** If any of the information causes you special concern, check with your doctor before using this medicine without a prescription.

• Before you begin using any new medicine (prescription or nonprescription) or if you develop any new medical problem while you are using this medicine, check with your doctor or pharmacist.

• **If you have any questions** about the following information or if you want more information about this medicine or your medical problem, **ask your doctor, nurse, or pharmacist.**

Before Using This Medicine

Before you use naphazoline ophthalmic solution, check with your doctor or pharmacist:

—if you have ever had any unusual or allergic reaction to naphazoline.

—if you are allergic to any substance, such as certain preservatives. Most medicines contain more than their active ingredient. Your doctor or pharmacist can help you avoid products that may cause a problem.

—if you are **pregnant** or if you may become pregnant, since this medicine may be absorbed into the body. Studies have not been done in either humans or animals.

—if you are **breast-feeding**, since naphazoline may be absorbed into the body. However, it is not known whether naphazoline passes into the breast milk and this medicine has not been shown to cause problems in nursing babies.

—if you have any of the following medical problems:
  Diabetes mellitus (sugar diabetes)
  Eye disease, infection, or injury
  Heart disease
  High blood pressure
  Overactive thyroid

—if you are taking **any** other prescription or nonprescription (OTC) medicine.

Proper Use of This Medicine

Do not use naphazoline ophthalmic solution if it becomes cloudy or changes color.

Naphazoline should not be used in infants and children. It may cause severe slowing down of the central nervous system (CNS), which may lead to unconsciousness. It may also cause a severe decrease in body temperature.

Use this medicine only as directed. Do not use more of it, do not use it more often, and do not use it for more than 4 days, unless otherwise directed by your doctor. To do so may make your eye irritation worse and may also increase the chance of side effects.

How to apply this medicine: First, wash your hands. With the middle finger, apply pressure to the inside corner of the eye (and continue to apply pressure for 1 or 2 minutes after the medicine has been placed in the eye). Tilt the head back and with the index finger of the same hand, pull the lower eyelid away from the eye to form a pouch. Drop the medicine into the pouch and gently close the eyes. Do not blink. Keep the eyes closed for 1 or 2 minutes to allow the medicine to be absorbed.

To prevent contamination of the eye drops, do not touch the applicator tip to any surface (including the eye), and keep the container tightly closed.

How to store this medicine:

• **Keep out of the reach of children.**

• Store away from heat and direct light.

• Keep the medicine from freezing.

• Do not keep outdated medicine or medicine no longer needed. Be sure that any discarded medicine is out of the reach of children.

Precautions While Using This Medicine

If your eye irritation continues or becomes worse, check with your doctor.

Side Effects of This Medicine

Along with its needed effects, a medicine may cause some unwanted effects. Although not all of these side effects may occur, if they do occur they may need medical attention.

When this medicine is used for short periods of time at recommended doses, side effects usually are rare. However, check with your doctor as soon as possible if any of the following occur:

With overuse or long-term use
  Increase in eye irritation

Signs of too much medicine being absorbed into the body
  Dizziness
  Headache
  Increase in sweating
  Nausea
  Nervousness
  Weakness

Signs of overdose
  Decrease in body temperature
  Drowsiness
  Slow heartbeat
  Weakness (severe)

Other side effects may occur that usually do not require medical attention. These side effects may go away during treatment as your body adjusts to the medicine. However, check with your doctor or pharmacist if either of the following side effects continues or is bothersome:

Less common or rare
  Blurred vision
  Large pupils

For elderly patients: Many medicines have not been tested in older people. Therefore, it is not known whether the medicine acts the same way it does in younger adults. Check with your doctor or pharmacist if you notice any unusual effects while using this medicine or if you think it is not working as it should.

Other side effects not listed above may also occur in some patients. If you notice any other effects, check with your doctor or pharmacist.

December 1987

NARCOTIC ANALGESICS
(Systemic—For Pain Relief)

This information applies to the following medicines:

Buprenorphine (byoo-pre-NOR-feen)
Butorphanol (byoo-TOR-fa-nole)
Codeine (KOE-deen)
Hydrocodone (hye-droe-KOE-done)
Hydromorphone (hye-droe-MOR-fone)
Levorphanol (lee-VOR-fa-nole)
Meperidine (me-PER-i-deen)
Methadone (METH-a-done)
Morphine (MOR-feen)
Nalbuphine (NAL-byoo-feen)
Opium Injection (OH-pee-um)
Oxycodone (ox-i-KOE-done)
Oxymorphone (ox-i-MOR-fone)
Pentazocine (pen-TAZ-oh-seen)
Propoxyphene (proe-POX-i-feen)

This information does *not* apply to Opium Tincture or Paregoric.

Some commonly used brand names or other names are:	Generic names:
Buprenex Temgesic*	Buprenorphine
Stadol	Butorphanol
Paveral*	Codeine†
Hycodan§ Robidone*	Hydrocodone†
Dihydromorphinone Dilaudid Dilaudid-HP	Hydromorphone†
Dromoran* Levo-Dromoran Levorphan	Levorphanol
Demerol Pethidine	Meperidine†
Dolophine Methadose Physeptone*	Methadone†
Astramorph Astramorph-PF Duramorph PF Epimorph* Morphitec* M.O.S.* M S Contin MSIR MST Continus* RMS Uniserts Roxanol Roxanol SR Statex*	Morphine†
Nubain	Nalbuphine†
Pantopon	Opium
Roxicodone Supeudol*	Oxycodone
Numorphan	Oxymorphone
Fortral* Talwin Talwin-Nx	Pentazocine

Darvon Darvon-N Dolene Doloxene* Doxaphene Novopropoxyn* Profene 642*	Propoxyphene†

*Not available in the U.S.
†Generic name product may also be available in the U.S.
§For Canadian product only. In the U.S., *Hycodan* also contains homatropine; in Canada, *Hycodan* contains only hydrocodone.

To the Reader: If you do not recognize the names of medical conditions or medicines referred to in this information, check with your doctor, nurse, or pharmacist. Definitions for selected medical terms may be found in the Glossary. Brand names for the generic drug names listed can be found in the Index. In addition, selected brand names commonly associated with the generic name have been included in the text to help you recognize medicine you may be taking. The fact that a brand name product is not mentioned does not mean the information does not apply. It is a good idea for you to learn both the generic and brand names of your medicines and to write them down for future use.

Narcotic (nar-KOT-ik) analgesics (an-al-JEE-zicks) are used to relieve pain. Some of these medicines are also used just before or during an operation to help the anesthetic work better. Codeine and hydrocodone are also used to relieve coughing. Methadone is also used to help some people control their dependence on heroin or other narcotics. Narcotic analgesics may also be used for other conditions as determined by your doctor.

Narcotic analgesics act in the central nervous system (CNS) to relieve pain. Some of their side effects are also caused by actions in the CNS.

If a narcotic is used for a long time, it may become habit-forming (causing mental or physical dependence). Physical dependence may lead to withdrawal side effects when you stop taking the medicine.

These medicines are available only with your physician's or dentist's prescription. For some of them, prescriptions cannot be refilled and you must obtain a new prescription from your physician or dentist each time you need the medicine. In addition, other rules and regulations may apply when methadone is used to treat narcotic dependence.

Remember:
• **This medicine has been prescribed for your current medical problem only.** It must not be given to other people or used for other problems unless you are directed to do so by your doctor.

• **Keep all medicines out of the reach of children.**

• In order for this medicine to work, it must be used as directed.

• If you are receiving this medicine by injection, some of the information about this medicine may not apply.

• **It is very important that you read and understand the following information.** If any of the information causes you special concern, do not decide against using this medicine without first checking with your doctor.

• Before you begin using any new medicine (prescription or nonprescription) or if you develop any new medical problem while you are using this medicine, check with your doctor, nurse, or pharmacist.

• **If you have any questions** about the following information or if you want more information about this medicine or your medical problem, **ask your doctor, nurse, or pharmacist.**

Before Using This Medicine

In order to decide on the best treatment for your medical problem, your physician or dentist should be told:

—if you have ever had any unusual or allergic reaction to this medicine.

—if you are on a low-salt, low-sugar, or any other special diet, or if you are allergic to any substance, such as foods, sulfites or other preservatives, or dyes. Most medicines contain more than their active ingredient, and many liquid medicines contain alcohol. Your doctor, nurse, or pharmacist can help you avoid products that may cause a problem.

—if you are **pregnant** or if you may become pregnant. Although studies on birth defects with narcotic analgesics have not been done in humans, these medicines have not been reported to cause birth defects in humans. However, hydrocodone, hydromorphone, and morphine have been shown to cause birth defects in animals when given in very large doses. Buprenorphine and codeine have not been shown to cause birth defects in animal studies, but they caused other unwanted effects. Butorphanol, nalbuphine, pentazocine, and propoxyphene have not been shown to cause birth defects in animals. There is no information about whether other narcotic analgesics cause birth defects in animals.

Too much use of a narcotic during pregnancy may cause the baby to become dependent on the medicine. This may lead to withdrawal side effects after birth. Also, some of these medicines may cause breathing problems in the newborn infant if taken just before delivery.

—if you are **breast-feeding**. Most narcotic analgesics have not been shown to cause problems in nursing babies. However, when the mother is taking large amounts of methadone (in a methadone maintenance program), the nursing baby may become dependent on the medicine. Also, butorphanol, codeine, meperidine, morphine, opium, and propoxyphene have been shown to pass into the breast milk.

—if you have any of the following medical problems:
   Brain disease or head injury
   Colitis
   Convulsions (seizures), history of
   Emphysema, asthma, or other chronic lung disease
   Enlarged prostate or problems with urination
   Gallbladder disease or gallstones
   Heart disease
   Kidney disease
   Liver disease
   Underactive thyroid

—if you are now taking or have taken within the past 2 weeks monoamine oxidase (MAO) inhibitors, such as:
   Furazolidone (e.g., Furoxone)
   Isocarboxazid (e.g., Marplan)
   Pargyline (e.g., Eutonyl)
   Phenelzine (e.g., Nardil)
   Procarbazine (e.g., Matulane)
   Tranylcypromine (e.g., Parnate)

—if you are taking **any** other prescription or nonprescription (OTC) medicine, especially:
   Carbamazepine (e.g., Tegretol)
   Central nervous system (CNS) depressants
   Naltrexone
   Rifampin (e.g., Rifadin)
   Tricyclic antidepressants (amitriptyline [e.g., Elavil], amoxapine, [e.g., Asendin], clomipramine [e.g., Anafranil], desipramine [e.g., Pertofrane], doxepin [e.g., Sinequan], imipramine [e.g., Tofranil], nortriptyline [e.g., Aventyl], protriptyline [e.g., Vivactil], trimipramine [e.g., Surmontil])

Proper Use of This Medicine

Some narcotic analgesics given by injection may be given at home to patients who do not need to be in the hospital. If you are using an injection form of this medicine at home, **make sure you clearly understand and carefully follow your doctor's instructions.**

For patients taking the syrup form of meperidine:
• Unless otherwise directed by your physician or dentist, **take this medicine mixed with a half glass (4 ounces) of water** to lessen the numbing effect of the medicine on your mouth and throat.

For patients taking the oral liquid form of methadone available only through a methadone treatment center:
• **This medicine may have to be mixed with water or another liquid before you take it.** Read the label carefully for directions. If you have any questions about this, check with your doctor, nurse, or pharmacist.

For patients taking the soluble tablet form of methadone:
• **These tablets must be dissolved in water or fruit juice before taking. Read the label carefully for directions.** If you have any questions about this, check with your doctor, nurse, or pharmacist.

For patients taking an oral liquid form of morphine:
• This medicine may be mixed with a glass of fruit juice just before you take it, if desired, to improve the taste.

For patients taking long-acting morphine tablets:
• **These tablets must be swallowed whole.** Do not break, crush, or chew them before swallowing.

For patients using a suppository form of a narcotic analgesic:
• If the suppository is too soft to insert because of storage in a warm place, before removing the foil wrapper chill the suppository in the refrigerator for 30 minutes or run cold water over it.

• How to insert the suppository: First remove the foil wrapper and moisten the suppository with water. Lie down on your side and push the suppository well up into the rectum with your finger.

Take this medicine only as directed by your physician or dentist. Do not take more of it, do not take it more often, and do not take it for a longer period of time than your physician or dentist ordered. If too much is taken, it may become habit-forming (causing mental or physical dependence) or lead to medical problems because of an overdose.

If you think this medicine is not working as well after you have been taking it for a few weeks, **do not increase the dose.** Instead, check with your doctor.

If your physician or dentist has ordered you to take this medicine according to a regular schedule and you miss a dose, take it as soon as you remember. However, if it is almost time for your next dose, skip the missed dose and go back to your regular dosing schedule. **Do not double doses.**

How to store this medicine:

• **Keep out of the reach of children** because overdose is very dangerous in young children.

• Store away from heat and direct light.

• Do not store tablets or capsules in the bathroom, near the kitchen sink, or in other damp places. Heat or moisture may cause the medicine to break down.

• Store hydromorphone, oxycodone, or oxymorphone suppositories in the refrigerator.

• Keep liquid (including injections) and suppository forms of the medicine from freezing.

• Do not keep outdated medicine or medicine no longer needed. Be sure that any discarded medicine is out of the reach of children.

Precautions While Using This Medicine

If you will be taking this medicine for a long period of time (for example, for several months at a time), your doctor should check your progress at regular visits.

Narcotic analgesics will add to the effects of alcohol and other CNS depressants (medicines that slow down the nervous system, possibly causing drowsiness). Some examples of CNS depressants are antihistamines or medicine for hay fever, other allergies, or colds; sedatives, tranquilizers, or sleeping medicine; other prescription pain medicines including other narcotics; barbiturates; medicine for convulsions (seizures); muscle relaxants; or anesthetics, including some dental anesthetics. **Do not drink alcoholic beverages, and check with your physician or dentist before taking any of the medicines listed above, while you are using this medicine.**

This medicine may cause some people to become drowsy, dizzy, or lightheaded, or to feel a false sense of well-being. **Make sure you know how you react to this medicine before you drive, use machines, or do other jobs that require you to be alert and clearheaded.**

Dizziness, lightheadedness, or fainting may occur, especially when you get up suddenly from a lying or sitting position. Getting up slowly may help lessen this problem.

Nausea or vomiting may occur, especially after the first couple of doses. This effect may go away if you lie down for a while. However, if nausea or vomiting continues, check with your physician or dentist. Lying down for a while may also help relieve some other side effects, such as dizziness or lightheadedness, that may occur.

Before having any kind of surgery (including dental surgery) or emergency treatment, tell the physician or dentist in charge that you are taking this medicine.

Narcotic analgesics may cause dryness of the mouth. For temporary relief, use sugarless candy or gum, melt bits of ice in your mouth, or use a saliva substitute. However, if dry mouth continues for more than 2 weeks, check with your dentist. Continuing dryness of the mouth may increase the chance of dental disease, including tooth decay, gum disease, and fungal infections.

If you have been taking this medicine regularly for several weeks or more, **do not suddenly stop using it without first checking with your doctor.** Your doctor may want you to reduce gradually the amount you are taking before stopping completely, in order to lessen the chance of withdrawal side effects.

If you think you or someone else may have taken an overdose, get emergency help at once. Taking an overdose of this medicine or taking alcohol or CNS depressants with this medicine may lead to unconsciousness or death. Signs of overdose include convulsions (seizures), confusion, severe nervousness or restlessness, severe dizziness, severe drowsiness, slow or troubled breathing, and severe weakness.

Side Effects of This Medicine

Along with its needed effects, a medicine may cause some unwanted effects. Although not all of these side effects may occur, if they do occur they may need medical attention.

Get emergency help immediately if any of the following signs of overdose occur:
Cold, clammy skin
Confusion
Convulsions (seizures)
Dizziness (severe)
Drowsiness (severe)
Low blood pressure
Nervousness or restlessness (severe)
Pinpoint pupils of eyes

Slow heartbeat
Slow or troubled breathing
Weakness (severe)

Also, check with your doctor as soon as possible if any of the following side effects occur:

Less common or rare

Dark urine (for propoxyphene only)
Fast, slow, or pounding heartbeat
Feelings of unreality
Hallucinations (seeing, hearing, or feeling things that are not there)
Hives, itching, or skin rash
Irregular breathing
Mental depression or other mood or mental changes
Pale stools (for propoxyphene only)
Ringing or buzzing in the ears
Shortness of breath or troubled breathing
Swelling of face
Trembling or uncontrolled muscle movements
Unusual excitement (especially in children)
Yellow eyes or skin (for propoxyphene only)

Other side effects may occur that usually do not require medical attention. These side effects may go away during treatment as your body adjusts to the medicine. However, check with your doctor if any of the following side effects continue or are bothersome:

More common

Dizziness, lightheadedness, or feeling faint
Drowsiness
Nausea or vomiting

Less common or rare

Blurred or double vision or other changes in vision
Constipation (more common with long-term use and with codeine)
Decrease in amount of urine
Difficult or painful urination
Dry mouth
False sense of well-being
Frequent urge to urinate
General feeling of discomfort or illness
Headache

Increased sweating (more common with hydrocodone, meperidine, and methadone)
Loss of appetite
Nervousness or restlessness
Nightmares or unusual dreams
Redness or flushing of face (more common with hydrocodone, meperidine, and methadone)
Redness, swelling, pain, or burning at place of injection
Stomach cramps or pain
Trouble in sleeping
Unusual tiredness or weakness

For children or elderly patients: The above side effects, especially breathing problems, are more likely to occur in very young children or in elderly patients, who are usually more sensitive to the effects of these medicines.

After you stop using this medicine, your body may need time to adjust. The length of time this takes depends on the amount of medicine you were using and how long you used it. During this period of time check with your doctor if you notice any of the following side effects:

Body aches
Diarrhea
Fast heartbeat
Fever, runny nose, or sneezing
Gooseflesh
Increased sweating
Increased yawning
Loss of appetite
Nausea or vomiting
Nervousness, restlessness, or irritability
Shivering or trembling
Stomach cramps
Trouble in sleeping
Unusually large pupils of eyes
Weakness

Other side effects not listed above may also occur in some patients. If you notice any other effects, check with your doctor.

_____
December 1987

_____

NARCOTIC ANALGESICS (Systemic—For Surgery and Obstetrics)

This information applies to the following medicines:

Alfentanil (al-FEN-ta-nil)
Fentanyl (FEN-ta-nil)
Meperidine (me-PER-i-deen)
Morphine (MOR-feen)
Sufentanil (soo-FEN-ta-nil)

Some commonly used brand names or other names are:	Generic names:
Alfenta Rapifen*	Alfentanil
Sublimaze	Fentanyl
Demerol Pethidine	Meperidine
Astramorph Astramorph PF Duramorph PF Epimorph*	Morphine
Sufenta	Sufentanil

*Not available in the U.S.

To the Reader: If you do not recognize the names of medical conditions or medicines referred to in this information, check with your doctor, nurse, or pharmacist. Definitions for selected medical terms may be found in the Glossary. Brand names for the generic drug names listed can be found in the Index. In addition, selected brand names commonly associated with the generic name have been included in the text to help you recognize medicine you may be taking. The fact that a brand name product is not mentioned does not mean the information does not apply. It is a good idea for you to learn both the generic and brand names of your medicines and to write them down for future use.

Narcotic analgesics (nar-KOT-ik an-al-JEE-zicks) are given to relieve pain before and during surgery (including dental surgery) or during labor and delivery. These medicines may also be given before or together with an anesthetic (either a general anesthetic or a local anesthetic), even when the patient is not in pain, to help the anesthetic work better.

When a narcotic analgesic is used for surgery or obstetrics (labor and delivery), it will be given by or under the immediate supervision of a physician or dentist, or by a specially trained nurse, in the doctor's office or in a hospital.

The following information applies only to these special uses of narcotic analgesics. If you are taking or receiving a narcotic analgesic to relieve pain after surgery, or for any other reason, ask your doctor, nurse, or pharmacist for additional information about the medicine and its use.

Remember:
- **If you have any questions** about the following information or if you want more information about this medicine or your medical problem, **ask your doctor, nurse, or pharmacist.**

Before Receiving This Medicine

In order to decide on the best medicine for you to receive for surgery or obstetrics, your doctor or nurse should be told:

—if you have ever had any unusual or allergic reaction to a narcotic.

—if you are allergic to any substance, such as sulfites or other preservatives. Your doctor or nurse can help you avoid products that may cause a problem.

—if you are **pregnant** or if you may become pregnant. Although studies on birth defects have not been done in humans, these medicines have not been reported to cause birth defects in humans. However, in animal studies, many narcotics have caused birth defects or other unwanted effects when they were given for a long period of time in amounts that were large enough to cause harmful effects in the mother.

Use of a narcotic during labor and delivery sometimes causes drowsiness or breathing problems in the newborn baby. If this happens, your doctor or nurse can give the baby another medicine that will overcome these effects. However, narcotics are usually not used during the delivery of a premature baby.

—if you are **breast-feeding.** Some narcotics have been shown to pass into the breast milk. However, these medicines have not been shown to cause problems in nursing babies.

—if you have **any** other medical problems.

—if you are taking **any** other prescription or nonprescription (OTC) medicine.

Precautions After Receiving This Medicine

For patients going home within a few hours after surgery:

- Narcotic analgesics and other medicines that may be given with them during surgery may cause some people to feel drowsy, tired, or weak for up to a few days after they have been given. Therefore, for at least 24 hours (or longer if necessary) after receiving this medicine, **do not drive, use machines, or do other jobs that require you to be alert.**

- Unless otherwise directed by your physician or dentist, **do not drink alcoholic beverages or take other CNS depressants (medicines that slow down the nervous system, possibly causing drowsiness) for about 24 hours after you have received this medicine.** To do so may add to the effects of the narcotic analgesic. Some examples of CNS depressants are antihistamines or medicine for hay fever, other allergies, or colds; sedatives, tranquilizers, or sleeping medicine; prescription pain medicine or narcotics; barbiturates; medicine for convulsions (seizures); and muscle relaxants.

Side Effects of This Medicine

Along with its needed effects, a medicine may cause some unwanted effects. Before you leave the hospital or doctor's office, your doctor or nurse will closely follow the effects of this medicine. However, some effects may continue, or may not be noticed until later.

© 1988   The United States Pharmacopeial Convention, Inc.

The following side effects usually do not need medical attention. They will gradually go away as the effects of the medicine wear off. However, check with your doctor if any of the following side effects continue or are bothersome:

More common

Dizziness, lightheadedness, or feeling faint
Drowsiness
Nausea or vomiting
Unusual tiredness or weakness

Less common or rare

Blurred or double vision or other vision problems
Confusion
Constipation
Difficult or painful urination

Dry mouth
General feeling of discomfort or illness
Headache
Mental depression or other mood or mental changes
Nightmares or unusual dreams

For elderly patients: Some of the above side effects may be more likely to occur in the elderly, who are usually more sensitive to the effects of narcotic analgesics.

Other side effects not listed above may also occur in some patients. If you notice any other effects, check with your doctor.

December 1987

NARCOTIC ANALGESICS AND ACETAMINOPHEN (Systemic)

This information applies to the following medicines:

Acetaminophen (a-seat-a-MIN-oh-fen) and Codeine (KOE-deen)

Acetaminophen, Codeine, and Caffeine (kaf-EEN)

Dihydrocodeine (dye-hye-droe-KOE-deen), Acetaminophen, and Caffeine

Hydrocodone (hye-droe-KOE-done) and Acetaminophen

Meperidine (me-PER-i-deen) and Acetaminophen

Oxycodone (ox-i-KOE-done) and Acetaminophen

Pentazocine (pen-TAZ-oh-seen) and Acetaminophen

Propoxyphene (proe-POX-i-feen) and Acetaminophen

Some commonly used brand names and other names are:	Generic names:
Acetaco Aceta with Codeine APAP with codeine Bayapap with Codeine Capital with Codeine Empracet with Codeine Emtec* Phenaphen with Codeine (U.S.) Proval Rounox with Codeine* Stopayne Tylenol with Codeine Ty-Tab with Codeine	Acetaminophen and Codeine†
Atasol with Codeine* Cotabs* Exdol with Codeine* Lenoltec* Tylenol with Codeine (Canada) Tylenol No. 1 Forte*	Acetaminophen, Codeine, and Caffeine*
Compal Drocode, acetaminophen, and caffeine Synalgos-DC-A	Dihydrocodeine, Acetaminophen, and Caffeine
Amacodone Anexsia Bancap-HC Co-gesic Damacet-P Dolacet Dolo-Pap Duradyne DHC Hydrocet Hydrocodone with APAP Hydrogesic HY-PHEN Lorcet-HD Lortab Norcet Propain-HC Vicodin Zydone	Hydrocodone and Acetaminophen†
Demerol-APAP	Meperidine and Acetaminophen
Oxycocet* Oxycodone with APAP Percocet Percocet-Demi* Roxicet Tylox	Oxycodone and Acetaminophen†
Talacen	Pentazocine and Acetaminophen
Darvocet-N Dolene-AP Lorcet Propacet Propoxyphene with APAP Wygesic	Propoxyphene and Acetaminophen†

*Not available in the U.S.

†Generic name product may also be available in the U.S.

To the Reader: If you do not recognize the names of medical conditions or medicines referred to in this information, check with your doctor, nurse, or pharmacist. Definitions for selected medical terms may be found in the Glossary. Brand names for the generic drug names listed can be found in the Index. In addition, selected brand names commonly associated with the generic name have been included in the text to help you recognize medicine you may be taking. The fact that a brand name product is not mentioned does not mean the information does not apply. It is a good idea for you to learn both the generic and brand names of your medicines and to write them down for future use.

Combination medicines containing narcotic (nar-KOT-ik) analgesics (an-al-JEE-zicks) and acetaminophen are used to relieve pain. A narcotic analgesic and acetaminophen used together may provide better pain relief than either medicine used alone. In some cases, relief of pain may come at lower doses of each medicine.

Narcotic analgesics act in the central nervous system (CNS) to relieve pain. Many of their side effects are also caused by actions in the CNS. When narcotics are used for a long time, your body may get used to them so that larger amounts are needed to relieve pain. This is called tolerance to the medicine. Also, when narcotics are used for a long time or in large doses, they may become habit-forming (causing mental or physical dependence). Physical dependence may lead to withdrawal symptoms when you stop taking the medicine.

Acetaminophen does not become habit-forming when taken for a long time or in large doses, but it may cause other unwanted effects, including liver damage, if too much is taken.

In the U.S., these medicines are available only with your physician's or dentist's prescription. In Canada, some of these medicines may be available without a prescription.

Remember:

• **This medicine has been prescribed for your current medical problem only.** It must not be given to other people or used for other problems unless you are directed to do so by your doctor.

• **Keep all medicines out of the reach of children.**

• In order for this medicine to work, it must be used as directed.

• **It is very important that you read and understand the following information.** If any of the information causes you special concern, do not decide against using this medicine without first checking with your doctor.

• Before you begin using any new medicine (prescription or nonprescription) or if you develop any new medical problem while you are using this medicine, check with your doctor, nurse, or pharmacist.

• **If you have any questions** about the following information or if you want more information about this medicine or your medical problem, **ask your doctor, nurse, or pharmacist.**

Before Using This Medicine

In order to decide on the best treatment for your medical problem, your physician or dentist should be told:

—if you have ever had any unusual or allergic reaction to acetaminophen or narcotic analgesics.

—if you are on a low-salt, low-sugar, or any other special diet, or if you are allergic to any substance, such as foods, sulfites or other preservatives, or dyes. Most medicines contain more than their active ingredient, and many liquid medicines contain alcohol. Your doctor, nurse, or pharmacist can help you avoid products that may cause a problem.

—if you are **pregnant** or if you may become pregnant. Although studies on birth defects with narcotic analgesics have not been done in humans, these medicines have not been reported to cause birth defects in humans. However, studies in animals have shown that hydrocodone causes birth defects when given in very large doses. Studies in animals have not shown that codeine causes birth defects, but it may cause slower development of bones and other toxic or harmful effects in the fetus. Pentazocine and propoxyphene have not been shown to cause birth defects in animals. There is no information about whether dihydrocodeine, meperidine, or oxycodone causes birth defects in animals.

Too much use of narcotics during pregnancy may cause the fetus to become dependent on the medicine. This may lead to withdrawal side effects in the newborn baby. Also, some of these medicines may cause breathing problems in the newborn baby if taken just before or during delivery.

Acetaminophen has not been shown to cause birth defects or other problems in humans. However, studies on birth defects with acetaminophen have not been done in humans.

—if you are **breast-feeding.** Acetaminophen, codeine, meperidine, and propoxyphene have been shown to pass into the breast milk. It is not known whether other narcotic analgesics pass into the breast milk. However, these medicines have not been shown to cause problems in nursing babies.

—if you have any of the following medical problems:
Brain disease or head injury
Colitis
Convulsions (seizures), history of
Emotional problems or mental illness
Emphysema, asthma, or other chronic lung disease
Enlarged prostate or problems with urination
Gallbladder disease or gallstones
Hepatitis or other liver disease
Heart disease
Kidney disease
Underactive thyroid

—if you regularly take large amounts of aspirin or other salicylates.

—if you regularly drink large amounts of alcoholic beverages.

—if you are now taking or have taken within the past 2 weeks monoamine oxidase (MAO) inhibitors such as:
Furazolidone (e.g., Furoxone)
Isocarboxazid (e.g., Marplan)
Pargyline (e.g., Eutonyl)
Phenelzine (e.g., Nardil)
Procarbazine (e.g., Matulane)
Tranylcypromine (e.g., Parnate)

—if you are taking **any** other prescription or nonprescription (OTC) medicine, especially:
Carbamazepine (e.g., Tegretol)
Central nervous system (CNS) depressants
Naltrexone (e.g., Trexan)
Tricyclic antidepressants (amitriptyline [e.g., Elavil], amoxapine, [e.g., Asendin], clomipramine [e.g., Anafranil], desipramine [e.g., Pertofrane], doxepin [e.g., Sinequan], imipramine [e.g., Tofranil], nortriptyline [e.g., Aventyl], protriptyline [e.g., Vivactil], trimipramine [e.g., Surmontil])

Proper Use of This Medicine

Take this medicine only as directed by your physician or dentist. Do not take more of it, do not take it more often, and do not take it for a longer period of time than your physician or dentist ordered. If too much of a narcotic analgesic is taken, it may become habit-forming (causing mental or physical dependence) or lead to medical problems because of an overdose. Taking too much acetaminophen may cause liver damage.

If you think that this medicine is not working as well after you have been taking it for a few weeks, **do not increase the dose.** Instead, check with your doctor.

If your physician or dentist has ordered you to take this medicine according to a regular schedule and you miss a dose, take it as soon as you remember. However, if it is almost time for your next dose, skip the missed dose and go back to your regular dosing schedule. **Do not double doses.**

How to store this medicine:

• **Keep out of the reach of children** because overdose is very dangerous in young children.

• Store away from heat and direct light.

• Do not store tablets or capsules in the bathroom, near the kitchen sink, or in other damp places. Heat or moisture may cause the medicine to break down.

• Keep the liquid forms of this medicine from freezing.

• Do not keep outdated medicine or medicine no longer needed. Be sure that any discarded medicine is out of the reach of children.

Precautions While Using This Medicine

If you will be taking this medicine for a long period of time (for example, for several months at a time), or in high doses, your doctor should check your progress at regular visits.

Check the labels of all over-the-counter (OTC), nonprescription, and prescription medicines you now take. If any contain acetaminophen or a narcotic be especially careful, since taking them while taking this medicine may lead to overdose. If you have any questions about this, check with your physician, dentist, or pharmacist.

The narcotic analgesic in this medicine will add to the effects of alcohol and other CNS depressants (medicines that slow down the nervous system, possibly causing drowsiness). Some examples of CNS depressants are antihistamines or medicine for hay fever, other allergies, or colds; sedatives, tranquilizers, or sleeping medicine; other prescription pain medicine or narcotics; barbiturates; medicine for seizures; muscle relaxants; or anesthetics, including some dental anesthetics. Also, there may be a greater risk of liver damage if large amounts of alcoholic beverages are used while you are taking acetaminophen. **Do not drink alcoholic beverages, and check with your physician or dentist before taking any of the medicines listed above, while you are using this medicine.**

Too much use of the acetaminophen in this combination medicine together with certain other medicines may increase the chance of kidney problems. Therefore, do not regularly take this medicine together with any of the following, unless directed to do so by your physician or dentist:

     Aspirin or other salicylates
     Diclofenac (e.g., Voltaren)
     Diflunisal (e.g., Dolobid)
     Fenoprofen (e.g., Nalfon)
     Flurbiprofen, oral (e.g., Ansaid)
     Ibuprofen (e.g., Motrin)
     Indomethacin (e.g., Indocin)
     Ketoprofen (e.g., Orudis)
     Meclofenamate (e.g., Meclomen)
     Mefenamic acid (e.g., Ponstel)
     Naproxen (e.g., Naprosyn)
     Phenylbutazone (e.g., Butazolidin)
     Piroxicam (e.g., Feldene)
     Sulindac (e.g., Clinoril)
     Tiaprofenic acid (e.g., Surgam)
     Tolmetin (e.g., Tolectin)

This medicine may cause some people to become drowsy, dizzy, or lightheaded, or to feel a false sense of well-being. **Make sure you know how you react to this medicine before you drive, use machines, or do other jobs that require you to be alert and clearheaded.**

Dizziness, lightheadedness, or fainting may occur, especially when you get up suddenly from a lying or sitting position. Getting up slowly may help lessen this problem.

Nausea or vomiting may occur, especially after the first couple of doses. This effect may go away if you lie down for a while. However, if nausea or vomiting continues, check with your physician or dentist. Lying down for a while may also help relieve some other side effects, such as dizziness or lightheadedness, that may occur.

Before having any kind of surgery (including dental surgery) or emergency treatment, tell the physician or dentist in charge that you are taking this medicine.

Narcotic analgesics may cause dryness of the mouth. For temporary relief, use sugarless candy or gum, melt bits of ice in your mouth, or use a saliva substitute. However, if dry mouth continues for more than 2 weeks, check with your dentist. Continuing dryness of the mouth may increase the chance of dental disease, including tooth decay, gum disease, and fungal infections.

If you have been taking this medicine regularly for several weeks or more, **do not suddenly stop taking it without first checking with your doctor.** Your doctor may want you to reduce gradually the amount you are taking before stopping completely, in order to lessen the chance of withdrawal side effects. This will depend on which of these medicines you have been taking, and the amount you have been taking every day.

If you think you or someone else may have taken an overdose of this medicine, get emergency help at once. Taking an overdose of this medicine or taking alcohol or CNS depressants with this medicine may lead to unconsciousness or death. Signs of overdose of narcotics include convulsions (seizures), confusion, severe nervousness or restlessness, severe dizziness, severe drowsiness, shortness of breath or troubled breathing, and severe weakness. Signs of severe acetaminophen overdose may not occur until several days after the overdose is taken.

Side Effects of This Medicine

Along with its needed effects, a medicine may cause some unwanted effects. Although not all of these side effects may occur, if they do occur they may need medical attention.

Get emergency help immediately if any of the following signs of overdose occur:
     Cold, clammy skin
     Confusion (severe)
     Convulsions (seizures)
     Diarrhea
     Dizziness (severe)
     Drowsiness (severe)
     Increased sweating
     Low blood pressure
     Nausea or vomiting (continuing)
     Nervousness or restlessness (severe)
     Pinpoint pupils of eyes
     Shortness of breath or unusually slow or troubled breathing
     Slow heartbeat
     Stomach cramps or pain
     Weakness (severe)

Also, check with your doctor as soon as possible if any of the following side effects occur:
Less common or rare
     Bloody or cloudy urine
     Confusion
     Dark urine

Difficult or painful urination
Fast, slow, or pounding heartbeat
Frequent urge to urinate
Hallucinations (seeing, hearing, or feeling things that are not there)
Irregular breathing
Mental depression
Pale stools
Ringing or buzzing in ears
Skin rash, hives, or itching
Sore throat and fever
Sudden decrease in amount of urine
Swelling of face
Trembling or uncontrolled muscle movements
Unusual bleeding or bruising
Unusual excitement (especially in children)
Yellow eyes or skin

Other side effects may occur that usually do not require medical attention. These side effects may go away during treatment as your body adjusts to the medicine. However, check with your physician or dentist if any of the following side effects continue or are bothersome:

More common

Dizziness, lightheadedness, or feeling faint
Drowsiness
Nausea or vomiting
Unusual tiredness or weakness

Less common or rare

Blurred or double vision or other changes in vision
Constipation (more common with long-term use and with codeine or meperidine)
Dry mouth
False sense of well-being
General feeling of discomfort or illness
Headache
Increased sweating
Loss of appetite
Nervousness or restlessness
Nightmares or unusual dreams
Redness or flushing of face (more common with hydrocodone or meperidine)
Trouble in sleeping

For children and elderly patients: The above side effects, especially breathing problems, are more likely to occur in young children and the elderly, who are usually more sensitive to the effects of narcotic analgesics.

Although not all of the side effects listed above have been reported for all of these combination medicines, they have been reported for at least one of them. However, since all of the narcotic analgesics are very similar, any of the above side effects may occur with any of these medicines.

After you stop using this medicine, your body may need time to adjust. The length of time this takes depends on which of these medicines you were taking, the amount of medicine you were using, and how long you used it. During this period of time check with your doctor if you notice any of the following side effects:

Body aches
Diarrhea
Fast heartbeat
Fever, runny nose, or sneezing
Gooseflesh
Increased sweating
Increased yawning
Loss of appetite
Nausea or vomiting
Nervousness, restlessness, or irritability
Shivering or trembling
Stomach cramps
Trouble in sleeping
Weakness

Other side effects not listed above may also occur in some patients. If you notice any other effects, check with your doctor.

_____

December 1987

NARCOTIC ANALGESICS, ACETAMINOPHEN, AND SALICYLATES
(Systemic)

This information applies to the following medicines:

Acetaminophen (a-seat-a-MIN-oh-fen), Aspirin (AS-pir-in), and Codeine (KOE-deen)

Acetaminophen, Aspirin, and Codeine, Buffered

Acetaminophen, Aspirin, Salicylamide (sal-i-SILL-a-mide), Codeine, and Caffeine (kaf-EEN)

Hydrocodone (hye-droe-KOE-done), Acetaminophen, Aspirin, and Caffeine

Some commonly used brand names are:	Generic names:
Veganin*	Acetaminophen, Aspirin§, and Codeine*
Dolprn	Acetaminophen, Aspirin, and Codeine, Buffered
Rid-A-Pain with Codeine	Acetaminophen, Aspirin, Salicylamide, Codeine, and Caffeine
Anodynos DHC Dia-Gesic Hyco-Pap	Hydrocodone, Acetaminophen, Aspirin, and Caffeine

*Not available in the U.S.

§In Canada, *Aspirin* is a brand name. Acetylsalicylic acid is the generic name in Canada. However, ASA (a commonly used synonym for acetylsalicylic acid) is the term that appears on most Canadian product labels.

To the Reader: If you do not recognize the names of medical conditions or medicines referred to in this information, check with your doctor, nurse, or pharmacist. Definitions for selected medical terms may be found in the Glossary. Brand names for the generic drug names listed can be found in the Index. In addition, selected brand names commonly associated with the generic name have been included in the text to help you recognize medicine you may be taking. The fact that a brand name product is not mentioned does not mean the information does not apply. It is a good idea for you to learn both the generic and brand names of your medicines and to write them down for future use.

Combination medicines containing narcotic (nar-KOT-ik) analgesics (an-al-JEE-zicks), acetaminophen, and salicylates are used to relieve pain. A narcotic analgesic, acetaminophen, and a salicylate used together may provide better pain relief than any of these medicines used alone. In some cases, relief of pain may come with lower doses of each medicine.

Narcotic analgesics act in the central nervous system (CNS) to relieve pain. Many of their side effects are also caused by actions in the CNS. When narcotics are used for a long time, your body may get used to them so that larger amounts are needed to relieve pain. This is called tolerance to the medicine. Also, when narcotics are used for a long time or in large doses, they may become habit-forming (causing mental or physical dependence). Physical dependence may lead to withdrawal symptoms when you stop taking the medicine.

Acetaminophen and salicylates do not become habit-forming when taken for a long time or in large doses, but they may cause other unwanted effects if too much is taken.

In the U.S., these medicines are available only with your doctor's prescription. In Canada, some of these medicines may be available without a prescription.

Remember:

• **This medicine has been prescribed for your current medical problem only.** It must not be given to other people or used for other problems unless you are directed to do so by your doctor.

• **Keep all medicines out of the reach of children.**

• In order for this medicine to work, it must be used as directed.

• **It is very important that you read and understand the following information.** If any of the information causes you special concern, do not decide against using this medicine without first checking with your doctor.

• Before you begin using any new medicine (prescription or nonprescription) or if you develop any new medical problem while you are using this medicine, check with your doctor, nurse, or pharmacist.

• **If you have any questions** about the following information or if you want more information about this medicine or your medical problem, **ask your doctor, nurse, or pharmacist**.

Before Using This Medicine

In order to decide on the best treatment for your medical problem, your physician or dentist should be told:

—if you have ever had any unusual or allergic reaction to codeine, hydrocodone, acetaminophen, aspirin or other salicylates including methyl salicylate (oil of wintergreen), or to any of the following medicines:

Diclofenac (e.g., Voltaren)
Diflunisal (e.g., Dolobid)
Fenoprofen (e.g., Nalfon)
Flurbiprofen, oral (e.g., Ansaid)
Ibuprofen (e.g., Motrin)
Indomethacin (e.g., Indocin)
Ketoprofen (e.g., Orudis)
Meclofenamate (e.g., Meclomen)
Mefenamic acid (e.g., Ponstel)
Naproxen (e.g., Naprosyn)
Oxyphenbutazone (e.g., Tandearil)
Phenylbutazone (e.g., Butazolidin)
Piroxicam (e.g., Feldene)
Sulindac (e.g., Clinoril)
Suprofen (e.g., Suprol)
Tiaprofenic acid (e.g., Surgam)
Tolmetin (e.g., Tolectin)
Zomepirac (e.g., Zomax)

—if you are on a low-salt, low-sugar, or any other special diet, or if you are allergic to any substance, such as foods, sulfites or other preservatives, or dyes. Most medicines contain more than their active ingredient. Your doctor, nurse, or pharmacist can help you avoid products that may cause a problem.

—if you are **pregnant** or if you may become pregnant.
For narcotic analgesics
Although studies on birth defects with narcotic analgesics have not been done in humans, these medicines have not been reported to cause birth defects in humans. However, studies in animals have shown that

hydrocodone causes birth defects when given in very large doses. Animal studies have not shown that codeine causes birth defects, but it slowed development of bones and caused a decrease in successful pregnancies.

Too much use of a narcotic during pregnancy may cause the fetus to become dependent on the medicine. This may lead to withdrawal side effects in the newborn baby. Also, some of these medicines may cause breathing problems in the newborn baby if taken just before or during delivery.

For acetaminophen
Acetaminophen has not been shown to cause birth defects or other problems in humans. However, studies on birth defects with acetaminophen have not been done in humans.

For salicylates
Studies in humans have not shown that aspirin causes birth defects. However, studies in animals have shown that salicylates cause birth defects.

Some reports have suggested that too much use of aspirin late in pregnancy may cause a decrease in the newborn's weight and possible death of the fetus or newborn infant. However, the mothers in these reports had been taking much larger amounts of aspirin than are usually recommended. Studies of mothers taking aspirin in the doses that are usually recommended did not show these effects. However, regular use of aspirin late in pregnancy may cause unwanted effects on the heart or blood flow in the fetus or in the newborn infant. Also, use of aspirin during the last 2 weeks of pregnancy may cause bleeding problems in the fetus before or during delivery or in the newborn infant.

Too much use of aspirin during the last 3 months of pregnancy may increase the length of pregnancy, prolong labor, cause other problems during delivery, or cause severe bleeding in the mother before, during, or after delivery.

For caffeine
Studies in humans have not shown that caffeine (contained in some of these combination medicines) causes birth defects. However, studies in animals have shown that caffeine causes birth defects when given in very large doses (amounts equal to those present in 12 to 24 cups of coffee a day).

—if you are **breast-feeding**. These combination medicines have not been shown to cause problems in nursing babies. However, acetaminophen passes into the breast milk in small amounts. Also, aspirin, caffeine, and codeine pass into the breast milk. It is not known whether hydrocodone passes into the breast milk.

—if you have any of the following medical problems:
  Anemia
  Asthma, allergies, and nasal polyps (history of)
  Brain disease or head injury
  Colitis
  Convulsions (seizures), history of
  Emotional problems or mental illness
  Emphysema, asthma, or chronic lung disease
  Enlarged prostate or problems with urination
  Gallbladder disease or gallstones
  Gout

  Heart disease (for combinations containing caffeine only)
  Hemophilia or other bleeding problems
  Hepatitis or other liver disease
  Kidney disease
  Liver disease
  Stomach ulcer or other stomach problems
  Underactive thyroid
  Vitamin K deficiency

—if you regularly drink large amounts of alcoholic beverages.

—if you are taking **any** other prescription or nonprescription (OTC) medicine, especially:
  Anticoagulants (blood thinners)
  Antidiabetic agents, oral (diabetes medicine you take by mouth)
  Central nervous system (CNS) depressants
  Dipyridamole (e.g., Persantine)
  Heparin
  Medicine for pain and/or inflammation
  Methotrexate (e.g., Mexate)
  Naltrexone (e.g., Trexan)
  Probenecid (e.g., Benemid)
  Sulfinpyrazone (e.g., Anturane)
  Tricyclic antidepressants (amitriptyline [e.g., Elavil], amoxapine, [e.g., Asendin], clomipramine [e.g., Anafranil], desipramine [e.g., Pertofrane], doxepin [e.g., Sinequan], imipramine [e.g., Tofranil], nortriptyline [e.g., Aventyl], protriptyline [e.g., Vivactil], trimipramine [e.g., Surmontil])
  Urinary alkalizers (medicine that makes the urine less acid, such as acetazolamide [e.g., Diamox], dichlorphenamide [e.g., Daranide], methazolamide [e.g., Neptazane], potassium or sodium citrate and/or citric acid)
  Vancomycin (e.g., Vancocin)

Proper Use of This Medicine

There is a possibility that use of aspirin (contained in this combination medicine) in children with fever due to a viral infection (especially flu or chickenpox) may cause a serious illness called Reye's syndrome. Do not give this medicine to a child or a teenager with symptoms of flu or chickenpox unless you have first discussed this with your child's doctor.

Take this medicine only as directed by your physician or dentist. Do not take more of it, do not take it more often, and do not take it for a longer period of time than your physician or dentist ordered. If too much of a narcotic analgesic is taken, it may become habit-forming (causing mental or physical dependence) or lead to medical problems because of an overdose. Also, taking too much acetaminophen or aspirin may increase the chance of other unwanted effects, including stomach problems or liver damage, or lead to medical problems because of an overdose.

If you think that this medicine is not working as well after you have been taking it for a few weeks, **do not increase the dose.** Instead, check with your doctor.

Take this medicine with food and a full glass (8 ounces) of water to lessen stomach irritation. Also, do not lie down for about 15 or 30 minutes after swallowing the medicine. This helps to prevent irritation that may lead to trouble in swallowing.

Do not take this medicine if it has a strong vinegar-like odor, since this means the aspirin in it is breaking down. If you have any questions about this, check with your doctor or pharmacist.

If your doctor has ordered you to take this medicine according to a regular schedule and you miss a dose, take it as soon as you remember. However, if it is almost time for your next dose, skip the missed dose and go back to your regular dosing schedule. **Do not double doses.**

How to store this medicine:

• **Keep out of the reach of children** because overdose is very dangerous in young children.

• Store away from heat and direct light.

• Do not store this medicine in the bathroom, near the kitchen sink, or in other damp places. Heat or moisture may cause the medicine to break down.

• Do not keep outdated medicine or medicine no longer needed. Be sure that any discarded medicine is out of the reach of children.

Precautions While Using This Medicine

If you will be taking this medicine for a long period of time (for example, for several months at a time) or in large amounts, your doctor should check your progress at regular visits.

Check the labels of all over-the-counter (OTC), nonprescription, and prescription medicines you now take. If any contain a narcotic, acetaminophen, aspirin, or other salicylates including diflunisal, be especially careful, since taking them while taking this medicine may lead to overdose. If you have any questions about this, check with your doctor or pharmacist.

Too much use of certain other medicines together with the acetaminophen or aspirin contained in this combination medicine may increase the chance of unwanted effects. Therefore, do not regularly take any of the following medicines together with this combination medicine, unless your doctor has directed you to do so:

    Diclofenac (e.g., Voltaren)
    Diflunisal (e.g., Dolobid)
    Fenoprofen (e.g., Nalfon)
    Flurbiprofen, oral (e.g., Ansaid)
    Ibuprofen (e.g., Motrin)
    Indomethacin (e.g., Indocin)
    Ketoprofen (e.g., Orudis)
    Meclofenamate (e.g., Meclomen)
    Mefenamic acid (e.g., Ponstel)
    Naproxen (e.g., Naprosyn)
    Phenylbutazone (e.g., Butazolidin)
    Piroxicam (e.g., Feldene)
    Sulindac (e.g., Clinoril)
    Tiaprofenic acid (e.g., Surgam)
    Tolmetin (e.g., Tolectin)

The narcotic analgesic in this medicine will add to the effects of alcohol and other CNS depressants (medicines that slow down the nervous system, possibly causing drowsiness). Some examples of CNS depressants are antihistamines or medicine for hay fever, other allergies, or colds; sedatives, tranquilizers, or sleeping medicine; other prescription pain medicine or narcotics; barbiturates; medicine for convulsions (seizures); muscle relaxants; or anesthetics, including some dental anesthetics. Also, liver problems may be more likely to occur if you drink large amounts of alcoholic beverages while taking acetaminophen. In addition, stomach problems may be more likely to occur if you drink alcoholic beverages while you are taking aspirin. **Do not drink alcoholic beverages, and check with your doctor before taking any of the medicines listed above, while you are using this medicine.**

This medicine may cause some people to become drowsy, dizzy, or lightheaded, or to feel a false sense of well-being. **Make sure you know how you react to this medicine before you drive, use machines, or do other jobs that require you to be alert and clearheaded.**

Dizziness, lightheadedness, or fainting may occur, especially when you get up suddenly from a lying or sitting position. Getting up slowly may help lessen this problem.

Nausea or vomiting may occur, especially after the first couple of doses. This effect may go away if you lie down for a while. However, if nausea or vomiting continues, check with your doctor. Lying down for a while may also help lessen some other side effects, such as dizziness or lightheadedness.

Before having any kind of surgery, dental work, or emergency treatment, tell the physician or dentist in charge that you are taking this medicine.

Do not take this medicine for 5 days before any surgery, including dental surgery, unless otherwise directed by your physician or dentist. Taking aspirin during this time may cause bleeding problems.

Diabetics—False urine sugar test results may occur if you are regularly taking 8 or more 325-mg (5-grain) or 4 or more 650-mg (10-grain) doses of aspirin a day. Smaller doses or occasional use of aspirin usually will not affect urine sugar tests. However, check with your doctor, nurse, or pharmacist (especially if your diabetes is not well controlled) if:

—you are not sure how much aspirin you are taking every day.

—you notice any change in your urine sugar test results.

—you have any other questions about this.

If you are taking the buffered tablets containing acetaminophen, aspirin, and codeine, and you are also taking a tetracycline antibiotic, do not take the two medicines within one hour of each other. Taking them at the same time may prevent the tetracycline from being absorbed by your body. If you have any questions about this, check with your doctor or pharmacist.

If you are taking a laxative containing cellulose, take this medicine at least 2 hours before or after you take the laxative. Taking these medicines too close together may lessen the effects of the aspirin in this combination medicine.

Narcotic analgesics may cause dryness of the mouth. For temporary relief, use sugarless candy or gum, melt bits of ice in your mouth, or use a saliva substitute. However, if dry mouth continues for more than 2 weeks, check with your dentist. Continuing dryness of the mouth may increase the chance of dental disease, including tooth decay, gum disease, and fungal infections.

If you have been taking this medicine regularly for several weeks or more, **do not suddenly stop taking it without first checking with your doctor.** Depending on which of these medicines you have been taking, and the amount you have been taking every day, your doctor may want you to reduce gradually the amount you are taking before stopping completely, in order to lessen the chance of withdrawal side effects.

If you think you or someone else may have taken an overdose of this medicine, get emergency help at once. Taking an overdose of this medicine or taking alcohol or CNS depressants with this medicine may lead to unconsciousness or death. Signs of overdose of this medicine include convulsions (seizures); hearing loss or ringing or buzzing in the ear; severe confusion, excitement, nervousness, or restlessness; severe dizziness or drowsiness; shortness of breath or troubled breathing; and severe weakness.

Side Effects of This Medicine

Along with its needed effects, a medicine may cause some unwanted effects. Although not all of these side effects may occur, if they do occur they may need medical attention.

Get emergency help immediately if any of the following signs of overdose occur:

Any loss of hearing
Bloody urine
Cold, clammy skin
Confusion (severe)
Convulsions (seizures)
Diarrhea (severe or continuing)
Dizziness or lightheadedness (severe)
Drowsiness (severe)
Excitement, nervousness, or restlessness (severe)
Hallucinations (seeing, hearing, or feeling things that are not there)
Headache (severe or continuing)
Increased sweating
Low blood pressure
Nausea or vomiting (severe or continuing)
Pinpoint pupils of eyes
Ringing or buzzing in the ears
Shortness of breath or troubled breathing
Slow heartbeat
Stomach cramps or pain (severe or continuing)
Swelling or tenderness in the upper abdomen or stomach area

Uncontrollable flapping movements of the hands, especially in elderly patients
Unexplained fever
Unusual thirst
Vision problems
Weakness (severe)

Also, check with your doctor as soon as possible if any of the following side effects occur:

More common

Nausea or vomiting
Stomach pain

Less common or rare

Bloody or black tarry stools
Cloudy urine
Confusion
Difficult, painful, or decreased urination
Fast or pounding heartbeat
Irregular breathing
Mental depression
Skin rash, hives, or itching
Sore throat and fever
Swelling of face
Trembling or uncontrolled muscle movements
Unusual bleeding or bruising
Unusual excitement, especially in children
Unusual tiredness or weakness
Vomiting of blood or material that looks like coffee grounds
Wheezing or tightness in chest
Yellow eyes or skin

Other side effects may occur that usually do not require medical attention. These side effects may go away during treatment as your body adjusts to the medicine. However, check with your doctor if any of the following side effects continue or are bothersome:

More common

Dizziness, lightheadedness, or feeling faint
Drowsiness
Heartburn or indigestion

Less common or rare

Constipation (more common with long-term use and with codeine)
Dry mouth
False sense of well-being
Frequent urge to urinate
General feeling of discomfort or illness
Headache
Loss of appetite
Nervousness or restlessness
Nightmares or unusual dreams
Redness or flushing of face (more common with hydrocodone)
Trouble in sleeping

For children and elderly patients: Some of the above side effects are more likely to occur in children, especially those who have a fever or are dehydrated (those who have lost large amounts of body fluid because of vomiting, diarrhea, or sweating), and in elderly patients (60 years of age or older). These patients are usually more sensitive to the effects of narcotic analgesics (especially the breathing problems they may cause) and aspirin.

After you stop using this medicine, your body may need time to adjust. The length of time this takes depends on which of these medicines you were taking, the amount of medicine you were taking, and how long you took it. During this period of time check with your doctor if you notice any of the following side effects:

Body aches
Diarrhea
Fever, runny nose, or sneezing
Gooseflesh
Increased sweating
Increased yawning
Loss of appetite
Nausea or vomiting
Nervousness, restlessness, or irritability
Shivering or trembling
Stomach cramps
Trouble in sleeping
Unusually large pupils of eyes
Weakness

Other side effects not listed above may also occur in some patients. If you notice any other effects, check with your doctor.

_____

December 1987

_____

NARCOTIC ANALGESICS AND ASPIRIN
(Systemic)

This information applies to the following medicines:
Aspirin (AS-pir-in) and Codeine (KOE-deen)
Aspirin, Codeine, and Caffeine (kaf-EEN)
Aspirin and Codeine, Buffered
Aspirin, Codeine, and Caffeine, Buffered
Dihydrocodeine (dye-hye-droe-KOE-deen) and Aspirin
Hydrocodone (hye-droe-KOE-done), Aspirin, and Caffeine
Oxycodone (ox-i-KOE-done) and Aspirin
Pentazocine (pen-TAZ-oh-seen) and Aspirin
Pentazocine, Aspirin, and Caffeine
Propoxyphene (proe-POX-i-feen) and Aspirin
Propoxyphene, Aspirin, and Caffeine

Some commonly used brand names and other names are:	Generic names:
Coryphen with Codeine* Emcodeine Empirin with Codeine	Aspirin and Codeine†
A.C.&C.* A&C with Codeine* Anacin with Codeine* Ancasal* C2 with Codeine* Instantine Plus* Novo AC&C* 222* 282* 292* 293*	Aspirin, Codeine, and Caffeine*
Ascriptin with Codeine	Aspirin and Codeine, Buffered
C2 Buffered with Codeine*	Aspirin, Codeine, and Caffeine, Buffered*
Drocode, Aspirin, and Caffeine Synalgos-DC	Dihydrocodeine, Aspirin, and Caffeine
Damason-P	Hydrocodone, Aspirin, and Caffeine
Codoxy Oxycodan* Percodan Percodan-Demi	Oxycodone and Aspirin†
Talwin Compound	Pentazocine and Aspirin
Talwin Compound-50*	Pentazocine, Aspirin, and Caffeine*
Darvon with A.S.A. Darvon-N with A.S.A.	Propoxyphene and Aspirin
Bexophene Darvon Compound Darvon-N Compound* Dolene Compound Doxaphene Compound 692*	Propoxyphene, Aspirin, and Caffeine†

*Not available in the U.S.
†Generic name product may also be available in the U.S.

To the Reader: If you do not recognize the names of medical conditions or medicines referred to in this information, check with your doctor, nurse, or pharmacist. Definitions for selected medical terms may be found in the Glossary. Brand names for the generic drug names listed can be found in the Index. In addition, selected brand names commonly associated with the generic name have been included in the text to help you recognize medicine you may be taking. The fact that a brand name product is not mentioned does not mean the information does not apply. It is a good idea for you to learn both the generic and brand names of your medicines and to write them down for future use.

Combination medicines containing narcotic (nar-KOT-ik) analgesics (an-al-JEE-zicks) and aspirin are used to relieve pain. A narcotic analgesic and aspirin used together may provide better pain relief than either medicine used alone. In some cases, relief of pain may come at lower doses of each medicine.

Narcotic analgesics act in the central nervous system (CNS) to relieve pain. Many of their side effects are also caused by actions in the CNS. When narcotics are used for a long time, your body may get used to them so that larger amounts are needed to relieve pain. This is called tolerance to the medicine. Also, when narcotics are used for a long time or in large doses, they may become habit-forming (causing mental or physical dependence). Physical dependence may lead to withdrawal symptoms when you stop taking the medicine.

Aspirin does not become habit-forming when taken for a long time or in large doses, but it may cause other unwanted effects if too much is taken.

In the U.S., these medicines are available only with your physician's or dentist's prescription. In Canada, some of these medicines may be available without a prescription.

Remember:
• **This medicine has been prescribed for your current medical problem only.** It must not be given to other people or used for other problems unless you are directed to do so by your doctor.

• **Keep all medicines out of the reach of children.**

• In order for this medicine to work, it must be used as directed.

• **It is very important that you read and understand the following information.** If any of the information causes you special concern, do not decide against using this medicine without first checking with your doctor.

• Before you begin using any new medicine (prescription or nonprescription) or if you develop any new medical problem while you are using this medicine, check with your doctor, nurse, or pharmacist.

• **If you have any questions** about the following information or if you want more information about this medicine or your medical problem, **ask your doctor, nurse, or pharmacist**.

Before Using This Medicine
In order to decide on the best treatment for your medical problem, your physician or dentist should be told:
—if you have ever had any unusual or allergic reaction to this medicine, to aspirin or other salicylates including methyl salicylate (oil of wintergreen), or to any of the following medicines:
Diclofenac (e.g., Voltaren)
Diflunisal (e.g., Dolobid)
Fenoprofen (e.g., Nalfon)

Flurbiprofen, oral (e.g., Ansaid)
Ibuprofen (e.g., Motrin)
Indomethacin (e.g., Indocin)
Ketoprofen (e.g., Orudis)
Meclofenamate (e.g., Meclomen)
Mefenamic acid (e.g., Ponstel)
Naproxen (e.g., Naprosyn)
Oxyphenbutazone (e.g., Tandearil)
Phenylbutazone (e.g., Butazolidin)
Piroxicam (e.g., Feldene)
Sulindac (e.g., Clinoril)
Suprofen (e.g., Suprol)
Tiaprofenic acid (e.g., Surgam)
Tolmetin (e.g., Tolectin)
Zomepirac (e.g., Zomax)

—if you are on a low-salt, low-sugar, or any other special diet, or if you are allergic to any substance, such as foods, sulfites or other preservatives, or dyes. Most medicines contain more than their active ingredient. Your doctor, nurse, or pharmacist can help you avoid products that may cause a problem.

—if you are **pregnant** or if you may become pregnant. Studies in humans have not shown that aspirin causes birth defects. However, studies in animals have shown that aspirin causes birth defects.

Some reports have suggested that too much use of aspirin late in pregnancy may cause a decrease in the newborn's weight and possible death of the fetus or newborn baby. However, the mothers in these reports had been taking much larger amounts of aspirin than are usually recommended. Studies of mothers taking aspirin in the doses that are usually recommended did not show these effects. However, regular use of aspirin late in pregnancy may cause unwanted effects on the heart or blood flow in the fetus or in the newborn baby. Also, use of aspirin during the last 2 weeks of pregnancy may cause bleeding problems in the fetus before or during delivery or in the newborn baby.

Too much use of aspirin during the last 3 months of pregnancy may increase the length of pregnancy, prolong labor, cause other problems during delivery, or cause severe bleeding in the mother before, during, or after delivery.

Although studies on birth defects with narcotic analgesics have not been done in humans, these medicines have not been reported to cause birth defects in humans. However, studies in animals have shown that hydrocodone causes birth defects when given in very large doses. Studies in animals have not shown that codeine causes birth defects, but it caused slower development of bones and other toxic or harmful effects on the fetus. Pentazocine and propoxyphene have not been shown to cause birth defects in animals. There is no information about whether dihydrocodeine or oxycodone causes birth defects in animals.

Too much use of a narcotic during pregnancy may cause the fetus to become dependent on the medicine. This may lead to withdrawal side effects in the newborn baby. Also, some of these medicines may cause breathing problems in the newborn baby if taken just before or during delivery.

Studies in humans have not shown that caffeine (contained in some of these combination medicines) causes birth defects. However, studies in animals have shown that caffeine causes birth defects when given in very large doses (amounts equal to those present in 12 to 24 cups of coffee a day).

—if you are **breast-feeding**. These combination medicines have not been shown to cause problems in nursing babies. However, aspirin, caffeine, codeine, and propoxyphene pass into the breast milk. It is not known whether dihydrocodeine, hydrocodone, oxycodone, or pentazocine pass into the breast milk.

—if you have any of the following medical problems:
Anemia
Asthma, allergies, and nasal polyps (history of)
Brain disease or head injury
Colitis
Convulsions (seizures), history of
Emotional problems or mental illness
Emphysema, asthma, or other chronic lung disease
Enlarged prostate or problems with urination
Gallbladder disease or gallstones
Gout
Heart disease
Hemophilia or other bleeding problems
Kidney disease
Liver disease
Stomach ulcer or other stomach problems
Vitamin K deficiency
Underactive thyroid

—if you regularly take large amounts of acetaminophen or antacids.

—if you are taking **any** other prescription or nonprescription (OTC) medicine, especially:
Anticoagulants (blood thinners)
Antidiabetic agents, oral (diabetes medicine you take by mouth)
Carbamazepine (e.g., Tegretol)
Central nervous system (CNS) depressants
Diarrhea medicine
Dipyridamole (e.g., Persantine)
Medicine for pain and/or inflammation
Methotrexate (e.g., Mexate)
Naltrexone (e.g., Trexan)
Probenecid (e.g., Benemid)
Sulfinpyrazone (e.g., Anturane)
Tricyclic antidepressants (amitriptyline [e.g., Elavil], amoxapine, [e.g., Asendin], clomipramine [e.g., Anafranil], desipramine [e.g., Pertofrane], doxepin [e.g., Sinequan], imipramine [e.g., Tofranil], nortriptyline [e.g., Aventyl], protriptyline [e.g., Vivactil], trimipramine [e.g., Surmontil])
Urinary alkalizers (medicine that makes the urine less acid, such as acetazolamide [e.g., Diamox], calcium- and/or magnesium-containing antacids, dichlorphenamide [e.g., Daranide], methazolamide [e.g., Neptazane], potassium or sodium citrate and/or citric acid, sodium bicarbonate [baking soda])
Vancomycin (e.g., Vancocin)

Proper Use of This Medicine

There is a possibility that use of aspirin (contained in this combination medicine) in children with fever due to a viral infection (especially flu or chickenpox) may cause

a serious illness called **Reye's syndrome. Do not give this medicine to a child or a teenager with symptoms of flu or chickenpox** unless you have first discussed this with your child's doctor.

Take this medicine with food or a full glass (8 ounces) of water to lessen stomach irritation.

Do not take this medicine if it has a strong vinegar-like odor, since this means the aspirin in it is breaking down. If you have any questions about this, check with your doctor or pharmacist.

Take this medicine only as directed by your physician or dentist. Do not take more of it, do not take it more often, and do not take it for a longer period of time than your physician or dentist ordered. If too much of a narcotic analgesic is taken, it may become habit-forming (causing mental or physical dependence) or lead to medical problems because of an overdose. Also, taking too much aspirin may cause stomach problems or lead to medical problems because of an overdose.

If you think that this medicine is not working as well after you have been taking it for a few weeks, **do not increase the dose.** Instead, check with your doctor.

If your physician or dentist has ordered you to take this medicine according to a regular schedule and you miss a dose, take it as soon as you remember. However, if it is almost time for your next dose, skip the missed dose and go back to your regular dosing schedule. **Do not double doses.**

How to store this medicine:

- **Keep out of the reach of children** because overdose is very dangerous in young children.

- Store away from heat and direct light.

- Do not store this medicine in the bathroom, near the kitchen sink, or in other damp places. Heat or moisture may cause the medicine to break down.

- Do not keep outdated medicine or medicine no longer needed. Be sure that any discarded medicine is out of the reach of children.

Precautions While Using This Medicine

If you will be taking this medicine for a long period of time (for example, for several months at a time), your doctor should check your progress at regular visits.

Check the labels of all over-the-counter (OTC), nonprescription, and prescription medicines you now take. If any contain a narcotic, aspirin, or other salicylates, be especially careful, since taking them while taking this medicine may lead to overdose. If you have any questions about this, check with your physician, dentist, or pharmacist.

This medicine will add to the effects of alcohol and other CNS depressants (medicines that slow down the nervous system, possibly causing drowsiness). Some examples of CNS depressants are antihistamines or medicine for hay fever, other allergies, or colds; sedatives, tranquilizers, or sleeping medicine; other prescription pain medicine or narcotics; barbiturates; medicine for convulsions (seizures); muscle relaxants; or anesthetics, including some dental anesthetics. Also, stomach problems may be more likely to occur if you drink alcoholic beverages while you are taking aspirin. **Do not drink alcoholic beverages, and check with your physician or dentist before taking any of the medicines listed above, while you are using this medicine.**

Too much use of acetaminophen together with the aspirin in this combination medicine may increase the chance of kidney problems. Also, too much use of certain other medicines together with aspirin may increase the chance of unwanted effects. Therefore, do not regularly take acetaminophen or any of the following medicines together with this combination medicine, unless your physician or dentist has directed you to do so:

    Diclofenac (e.g., Voltaren)
    Diflunisal (e.g., Dolobid)
    Fenoprofen (e.g., Nalfon)
    Flurbiprofen, oral (e.g., Ansaid)
    Ibuprofen (e.g., Motrin)
    Indomethacin (e.g., Indocin)
    Ketoprofen (e.g., Orudis)
    Meclofenamate (e.g., Meclomen)
    Mefenamic acid (e.g., Ponstel)
    Naproxen (e.g., Naprosyn)
    Phenylbutazone (e.g., Butazolidin)
    Piroxicam (e.g., Feldene)
    Sulindac (e.g., Clinoril)
    Tiaprofenic acid (e.g., Surgam)
    Tolmetin (e.g., Tolectin)

This medicine may cause some people to become drowsy, dizzy, or lightheaded, or to feel a false sense of well-being. **Make sure you know how you react to this medicine before you drive, use machines, or do other jobs that require you to be alert and clearheaded.**

Dizziness, lightheadedness, or fainting may occur, especially when you get up suddenly from a lying or sitting position. Getting up slowly may help lessen this problem.

Nausea or vomiting may occur, especially after the first couple of doses. This effect may go away if you lie down for a while. However, if nausea or vomiting continues, check with your doctor. Lying down for a while may also help some other side effects, such as dizziness or lightheadedness.

Before having any kind of surgery (including dental surgery) or emergency treatment, tell the physician or dentist in charge that you are taking this medicine.

Do not take this medicine for 5 days before any surgery, including dental surgery, unless otherwise directed by your physician or dentist. Taking aspirin during this time may cause bleeding problems.

If you are taking one of the combination medicines containing buffered aspirin, and you are also taking a tetracycline antibiotic, do not take the two medicines within one hour of each other. Taking them together may prevent the tetracycline from being absorbed by your body. If you have any questions about this, check with your doctor or pharmacist.

Diabetics—False urine sugar test results may occur if you are regularly taking 8 or more 325-mg (5-grain) or 4 or more 650-mg (10-grain) doses of aspirin a day. Smaller doses or occasional use of aspirin usually will not affect urine sugar tests. If you have any questions about this, check with your doctor, nurse, or pharmacist, especially if your diabetes is not well controlled.

Narcotic analgesics may cause dryness of the mouth. For temporary relief, use sugarless candy or gum, melt bits of ice in your mouth, or use a saliva substitute. However, if dry mouth continues for more than 2 weeks, check with your dentist. Continuing dryness of the mouth may increase the chance of dental disease, including tooth decay, gum disease, and fungal infections.

If you have been taking this medicine regularly for several weeks or more, **do not suddenly stop using it without first checking with your doctor.** Depending on which of these medicines you have been taking, and the amount you have been taking every day, your doctor may want you to reduce gradually the amount you are taking before stopping completely, in order to lessen the chance of withdrawal side effects.

If you think you or someone else may have taken an overdose of this medicine, get emergency help at once. Taking an overdose of this medicine or taking alcohol or CNS depressants with this medicine may lead to unconsciousness or death. Signs of overdose of this medicine include convulsions (seizures); hearing loss; confusion; ringing or buzzing in the ears; severe excitement, nervousness, or restlessness; severe dizziness, severe drowsiness, shortness of breath or troubled breathing, and severe weakness.

Side Effects of This Medicine

Along with its needed effects, a medicine may cause some unwanted effects. Although not all of these side effects may occur, if they do occur they may need medical attention.

Get emergency help immediately if any of the following signs of overdose occur:

Any loss of hearing
Bloody urine
Cold, clammy skin
Confusion (severe)
Convulsions (seizures)
Diarrhea (severe or continuing)
Dizziness or lightheadedness (severe)
Drowsiness (severe)
Excitement, nervousness, or restlessness (severe)
Hallucinations (seeing, hearing, or feeling things that are not there)
Headache (severe or continuing)
Increased sweating
Low blood pressure

Nausea or vomiting (severe or continuing)
Pinpoint pupils of eyes
Ringing or buzzing in the ears
Shortness of breath or unusually slow or troubled breathing
Slow heartbeat
Stomach pain (severe or continuing)
Uncontrollable flapping movements of the hands (especially in elderly patients)
Unexplained fever
Unusual thirst
Vision problems
Weakness (severe)

Also, check with your doctor as soon as possible if any of the following side effects occur:

More common

Nausea or vomiting
Stomach pain

Less common or rare

Bloody or black tarry stools
Confusion
Dark urine
Fast, slow, or pounding heartbeat
Irregular breathing
Mental depression
Pale stools
Skin rash, hives, or itching
Stomach pain (severe)
Swelling of face
Tightness in chest or wheezing
Trembling or uncontrolled muscle movements
Unusual excitement (especially in children)
Unusual tiredness or weakness
Vomiting of blood or material that looks like coffee grounds
Yellow eyes or skin

Other side effects may occur that usually do not require medical attention. These side effects may go away during treatment as your body adjusts to the medicine. However, check with your doctor if any of the following side effects continue or are bothersome:

More common

Dizziness, lightheadedness, or feeling faint
Drowsiness
Heartburn or indigestion

Less common or rare

Blurred or double vision or other changes in vision
Constipation (more common with long-term use and with codeine)
Difficult, painful, or decreased urination
Dry mouth
False sense of well-being
Frequent urge to urinate
General feeling of discomfort or illness
Headache
Loss of appetite
Nervousness or restlessness
Nightmares or unusual dreams
Redness or flushing of face (more common with hydrocodone)
Trouble in sleeping
Unusual tiredness
Unusual weakness

For children and elderly patients: Some of the above side effects are more likely to occur in children, especially those with fever or who are dehydrated (those who have lost large amounts of body fluid because of vomiting, diarrhea, or sweating), and in elderly patients (60 years of age or older). These patients are usually more sensitive to the effects of narcotic analgesics (especially the breathing problems they may cause) and aspirin.

Although not all of the side effects listed above have been reported for all of these medicines, they have been reported for at least one of them. However, since all of the narcotic analgesics are very similar, any of the above side effects may occur with any of these medicines.

After you stop using this medicine, your body may need time to adjust. The length of time this takes depends on which of these medicines you were taking, the amount of medicine you were using, and how long you used it. During this period of time check with your doctor if you notice any of the following side effects:

Body aches
Diarrhea
Fever, runny nose, or sneezing
Gooseflesh
Increased sweating
Increased yawning
Loss of appetite
Nausea or vomiting
Nervousness, restlessness, or irritability
Shivering or trembling
Stomach cramps
Trouble in sleeping
Weakness

Other side effects not listed above may also occur in some patients. If you notice any other effects, check with your physician or dentist.

December 1987

NATAMYCIN (Ophthalmic)

Some commonly used brand names or other names are Natacyn and Pimaricin.

To the Reader: If you do not recognize the names of medical conditions or medicines referred to in this information, check with your doctor, nurse, or pharmacist. Definitions for selected medical terms may be found in the Glossary. Brand names for the generic drug names listed can be found in the Index. In addition, selected brand names commonly associated with the generic name have been included in the text to help you recognize medicine you may be taking. The fact that a brand name product is not mentioned does not mean the information does not apply. It is a good idea for you to learn both the generic and brand names of your medicines and to write them down for future use.

Natamycin (na-ta-MYE-sin) belongs to the group of medicines called antifungals. It is used in the eye to treat some types of fungal infections of the eye.

Natamycin is available only with your doctor's prescription.

Remember:

• **This medicine has been prescribed for your present infection only.** Another infection later on may require a different medicine. Also, even though other people may have the same symptoms as you, they may have a different kind of infection. Your medicine may not work for them and may even cause them harm. Therefore, **your medicine must not be given to other people or used for other infections** unless you are otherwise directed by your doctor.

• **Keep all medicines out of the reach of children.**

• In order for this medicine to work, it must be used as directed.

• **It is very important that you read and understand the following information.** If any of the information causes you special concern, do not decide against using this medicine without first checking with your doctor.

• Before you begin using any new medicine (prescription or nonprescription) or if you develop any new medical problem while you are using this medicine, check with your doctor, nurse, or pharmacist.

• **If you have any questions** about the following information or if you want more information about this medicine or your medical problem, **ask your doctor, nurse, or pharmacist.**

Before Using This Medicine

In order to decide on the best treatment for your medical problem, your doctor should be told:

—if you have ever had any unusual or allergic reaction to natamycin.

—if you are allergic to any substance, such as certain foods or preservatives or dyes. Most medicines contain more than their active ingredient. Your doctor, nurse, or pharmacist can help you avoid products that may cause a problem.

—if you are **pregnant** or if you may become pregnant. However, natamycin has not been shown to cause birth defects or other problems in humans.

—if you are **breast-feeding**. However, natamycin has not been shown to cause problems in nursing babies.

Proper Use of This Medicine

The bottle is only partially full to provide proper drop control.

How to apply this medicine: First, wash your hands. Then tilt the head back and pull the lower eyelid away from the eye to form a pouch. Drop the medicine into the pouch and gently close the eyes. Do not blink. Keep the eyes closed for 1 or 2 minutes to allow the medicine to come into contact with the infection.

If you think you did not get the drop of medicine into your eye properly, use another drop.

To prevent contamination of the eye drops, do not touch the applicator tip to any surface (including the eye). Also, keep the container tightly closed.

To help clear up your eye infection completely, **keep using this medicine for the full time of treatment** even though your condition may have improved. **Do not miss any doses.**

If you do miss a dose of this medicine, apply it as soon as possible. Then go back to your regular dosing schedule.

How to store this medicine:

• **Keep out of the reach of children.**

• Do not keep outdated medicine or medicine no longer needed. Be sure that any discarded medicine is out of the reach of children.

Precautions While Using This Medicine

Your doctor should check your progress at regular visits.

If your symptoms do not improve within 7 to 10 days, or if they become worse, check with your doctor.

Side Effects of This Medicine

Along with its needed effects, a medicine may cause some unwanted effects. Although not all of these side effects may occur, if they do occur they may need medical attention.

Check with your doctor as soon as possible if the following side effect occurs:

Eye irritation not present before using this medicine

Other side effects not listed above may also occur in some patients. If you notice any other effects, check with your doctor.

December 1987

NEOMYCIN (Ophthalmic)*

*Not commercially available in the U.S.

To the Reader: If you do not recognize the names of medical conditions or medicines referred to in this information, check with your doctor, nurse, or pharmacist. Definitions for selected medical terms may be found in the Glossary. Brand names for the generic drug names listed can be found in the Index. In addition, selected brand names commonly associated with the generic name have been included in the text to help you recognize medicine you may be taking. The fact that a brand name product is not mentioned does not mean the information does not apply. It is a good idea for you to learn both the generic and brand names of your medicines and to write them down for future use.

Neomycin (nee-oh-MYE-sin) belongs to the general family of medicines called antibiotics. Neomycin ophthalmic preparations are used in the eye to help the body overcome infections of the eye.

Neomycin is available only with your doctor's prescription.

Remember:
• **This medicine has been prescribed for your present infection only.** Another infection later on may require a different medicine. Also, even though other people may have the same symptoms as you, they may have a different kind of infection. Your medicine may not work for them and may even cause them harm. Therefore, **your medicine must not be given to other people or used for other infections** unless you are otherwise directed by your doctor.

• **Keep all medicines out of the reach of children.**

• In order for this medicine to work, it must be used as directed.

• **It is very important that you read and understand the following information.** If any of the information causes you special concern, do not decide against using this medicine without first checking with your doctor.

• Before you begin using any new medicine (prescription or nonprescription) or if you develop any new medical problem while you are using this medicine, check with your doctor, nurse, or pharmacist.

• **If you have any questions** about the following information or if you want more information about this medicine or your medical problem, **ask your doctor, nurse, or pharmacist.**

Before Using This Medicine

In order to decide on the best treatment for your medical problem, your doctor should be told:

—if you have ever had any unusual or allergic reaction to this medicine or to any related antibiotics such as amikacin, gentamicin, kanamycin, neomycin (by mouth or by injection), netilmicin, streptomycin, or tobramycin.

—if you are allergic to any substance, such as certain foods or preservatives or dyes. Most medicines contain more than their active ingredient. Your doctor, nurse, or pharmacist can help you avoid products that may cause a problem.

—if you are **pregnant** or if you may become pregnant. However, neomycin ophthalmic preparations have not been shown to cause birth defects or other problems in humans.

—if you are **breast-feeding**. However, neomycin ophthalmic preparations have not been shown to cause problems in nursing babies.

Proper Use of This Medicine

How to apply this medicine: First, wash your hands. Then pull the lower eyelid away from the eye to form a pouch. Squeeze a thin strip of ointment into the pouch. A 1-cm (approximately ⅓-inch) strip of ointment is usually enough unless otherwise directed by your doctor. Gently close the eyes and keep them closed for 1 or 2 minutes to allow the medicine to come into contact with the infection.

To prevent contamination of the eye ointment, do not touch the applicator tip to any surface (including the eye). After using neomycin eye ointment, wipe the tip of the ointment tube with a clean tissue and keep the tube tightly closed.

To help clear up your infection completely, **keep using this medicine for the full time of treatment,** even though your symptoms may have disappeared; **do not miss any doses.**

If you do miss a dose of this medicine, apply it as soon as possible. However, if it is almost time for your next dose, skip the missed dose and go back to your regular dosing schedule.

How to store this medicine:

• **Keep out of the reach of children.**

• Store away from heat and direct light.

• Keep the medicine from freezing.

• Do not keep outdated medicine or medicine no longer needed. Be sure that any discarded medicine is out of the reach of children.

Precautions While Using This Medicine

If your symptoms do not improve within a few days, or if they become worse, check with your doctor.

Side Effects of This Medicine

Along with its needed effects, a medicine may cause some unwanted effects. Although not all of these side effects may occur, if they do occur they may need medical attention.

Check with your doctor immediately if any of the following side effects occur:
More common
  Itching, rash, redness, swelling, or other sign of irritation not present before using this medicine

Other side effects may occur that usually do not require medical attention. These side effects may go away during treatment as your body adjusts to the medicine. However, check with your doctor if either of the following side effects continues or is bothersome:
Less common
  Burning or stinging

After application, eye ointments may be expected to cause your vision to blur for a few minutes.

Other side effects not listed above may also occur in some patients. If you notice any other effects, check with your doctor.

December 1987

NEOMYCIN (Oral)

A commonly used brand name is Mycifradin.

Generic name product may also be available in the U.S.

To the Reader: If you do not recognize the names of medical conditions or medicines referred to in this information, check with your doctor, nurse, or pharmacist. Definitions for selected medical terms may be found in the Glossary. Brand names for the generic drug names listed can be found in the Index. In addition, selected brand names commonly associated with the generic name have been included in the text to help you recognize medicine you may be taking. The fact that a brand name product is not mentioned does not mean the information does not apply. It is a good idea for you to learn both the generic and brand names of your medicines and to write them down for future use.

Oral neomycin (nee-oh-MYE-sin) belongs to the general family of medicines called antibiotics. It is taken by mouth to help lessen the symptoms of hepatic coma, a complication of liver disease. In addition, it may be used before any surgery affecting the bowels to help prevent infection during surgery. Oral neomycin may also be used for other problems as determined by your doctor.

Neomycin is available only with your doctor's prescription.

Remember:

• **This medicine has been prescribed for your present medical problem only.** Even though other people may have the same symptoms as you, they may have a different kind of problem. Your medicine may not work for them and may even cause them harm. Therefore, **your medicine must not be given to other people or used for other problems** unless you are otherwise directed by your doctor.

• **Keep all medicines out of the reach of children.**

• In order for this medicine to work, it must be used as directed.

• **It is very important that you read and understand the following information.** If any of the information causes you special concern, do not decide against using this medicine without first checking with your doctor.

• Before you begin using any new medicine (prescription or nonprescription) or if you develop any new medical problem while you are using this medicine, check with your doctor, nurse, or pharmacist.

• **If you have any questions** about the following information or if you want more information about this medicine or your medical problem, **ask your doctor, nurse, or pharmacist.**

Before Using This Medicine

In order to decide on the best treatment for your medical problem, your doctor should be told:

—if you have ever had any unusual or allergic reaction to this medicine or to any related antibiotics such as amikacin, gentamicin, kanamycin, neomycin (by injection), netilmicin, streptomycin, or tobramycin.

—if you are on a low-salt, low-sugar, or any other special diet, or if you are allergic to any substance, such as foods, sulfites or other preservatives, or dyes.

Most medicines contain more than their active ingredient, and many liquid medicines contain alcohol. Your doctor, nurse, or pharmacist can help you avoid products that may cause a problem.

—if you are **pregnant** or if you may become pregnant. However, oral neomycin has not been shown to cause birth defects or other problems in humans.

—if you are **breast-feeding.** However, oral neomycin has not been shown to cause problems in nursing babies.

—if you have any of the following medical problems:
   Blockage of the bowel
   Eighth-cranial-nerve disease (loss of hearing and/or balance)
   Kidney disease
   Myasthenia gravis
   Parkinson's disease
   Ulcers of the bowel

—if you are taking **any** other prescription or nonprescription (OTC) medicine.

Proper Use of This Medicine

This medicine may be taken on a full or empty stomach.

For patients taking the oral liquid form of neomycin:

• Use a specially marked measuring spoon or other device to measure each dose accurately since the average household teaspoon may not hold the right amount of liquid.

Keep taking this medicine for the full time of treatment; do not miss any doses.

For patients taking neomycin for hepatic coma:

• If you do miss a dose of this medicine, take it as soon as possible. However, if it is almost time for your next dose, skip the missed dose and go back to your regular dosing schedule. Do not double doses.

For patients taking neomycin before any surgery affecting the bowels:

• If you do miss a dose of this medicine, take it as soon as possible. However, if it is almost time for your next dose and your dosing schedule is:

   —1 dose every hour (for 4 hours): Space the missed dose and the next dose ½ hour apart.

   —3 or more doses a day: Space the missed dose and the next dose 2 to 4 hours apart or double your next dose.

Then go back to your regular dosing schedule.

How to store this medicine:

• **Keep out of the reach of children.**

• Store away from heat and direct light.

• Do not store the tablet form of this medicine in the bathroom, near the kitchen sink, or in other damp places. Heat or moisture may cause the medicine to break down.

- Keep the oral liquid form of this medicine from freezing.

- Do not keep outdated medicine or medicine no longer needed. Be sure that any discarded medicine is out of the reach of children.

Precautions While Using This Medicine

This medicine may cause some people to become dizzy. **Make sure you know how you react to this medicine before you drive, use machines, or do other jobs that require you to be alert.** If this reaction is especially bothersome, check with your doctor.

Side Effects of This Medicine

Along with its needed effects, a medicine may cause some unwanted effects. Although not all of these side effects may occur, if they do occur they may need medical attention.

Check with your doctor immediately if any of the following side effects occur:

Rare
- Any loss of hearing
- Clumsiness
- Dizziness
- Greatly decreased frequency of urination or amount of urine
- Increased thirst
- Ringing or buzzing or a feeling of fullness in the ears
- Unsteadiness

Other side effects may occur that usually do not require medical attention. These side effects may go away during treatment as your body adjusts to the medicine. However, check with your doctor if any of the following side effects continue or are bothersome:

More common
- Irritation or soreness of the mouth or rectal area
- Nausea or vomiting

Rare
- Diarrhea
- Increased amount of gas
- Light-colored, frothy, fatty-appearing stools
- Skin rash

For elderly patients: Many medicines have not been tested in older people. Therefore, it is not known whether the medicine acts the same way it does in younger adults. Check with your doctor or pharmacist if you notice any unusual effects while taking this medicine or if you think it is not working as it should.

Other side effects not listed above may also occur in some patients. If you notice any other effects, check with your doctor.

_____
December 1987

_____

Additional Information

In addition to the above information, for patients taking neomycin to lower the level of cholesterol in the blood:

- Some doctors may prescribe oral neomycin for certain patients who have too much cholesterol in their blood. Your doctor might also want you to follow a special diet while you are taking this medicine. If you have any questions about this, check with your doctor.

- If you do miss a dose of this medicine, take it as soon as possible. However, if it is almost time for your next dose and your dosing schedule is 3 or more doses a day, space the missed dose and the next dose 2 to 4 hours apart or double your next dose. Then go back to your regular dosing schedule.

NEOMYCIN (Topical)

A commonly used brand name is Myciguent.

Generic name product may also be available in the U.S.

To the Reader: If you do not recognize the names of medical conditions or medicines referred to in this information, check with your doctor, nurse, or pharmacist. Definitions for selected medical terms may be found in the Glossary. Brand names for the generic drug names listed can be found in the Index. In addition, selected brand names commonly associated with the generic name have been included in the text to help you recognize medicine you may be taking. The fact that a brand name product is not mentioned does not mean the information does not apply. It is a good idea for you to learn both the generic and brand names of your medicines and to write them down for future use.

Neomycin (nee-oh-MYE-sin) belongs to the general family of medicines called antibiotics. Neomycin topical preparations are used on the skin to help prevent infections of the skin.

Neomycin topical preparations are available without a prescription; however, your doctor may have special instructions on the proper use of topical neomycin for your medical problem.

Remember:

• **Keep all medicines out of the reach of children.**

• In order for this medicine to work, it must be used as directed. **If you are using this medicine without a prescription, it is very important to follow the directions on the label.**

• **It is also very important that you read and understand the following information.** If any of the information causes you special concern, check with your doctor or pharmacist.

• Before you begin using any new medicine (prescription or nonprescription) or if you develop any new medical problem while you are using this medicine, check with your doctor, nurse, or pharmacist.

• **If you have any questions** about the following information or if you want more information about this medicine or your medical problem, **ask your doctor, nurse, or pharmacist.**

Before Using This Medicine

Before you use topical neomycin, check with your doctor or pharmacist:

—if you have ever had any unusual or allergic reaction to this medicine or to any related antibiotics such as amikacin, gentamicin, kanamycin, neomycin (by mouth or by injection), netilmicin, streptomycin, or tobramycin.

—if you are allergic to any substance, such as certain foods or preservatives or dyes. Most medicines contain more than their active ingredient. Your doctor, nurse, or pharmacist can help you avoid products that may cause a problem.

—if you are **pregnant** or if you may become pregnant. However, neomycin topical preparations have not been shown to cause birth defects or other problems in humans.

—if you are **breast-feeding**. However, neomycin topical preparations have not been shown to cause problems in nursing babies.

—if you are taking **any** other prescription or nonprescription (OTC) medicine.

Proper Use of This Medicine

If you are using this medicine without a prescription, do not use it to treat deep wounds, puncture wounds, serious burns, or raw areas without first checking with your doctor or pharmacist.

Do not use this medicine in the eyes.

Before applying this medicine, wash the affected area with soap and water, and dry thoroughly.

For patients using the cream form of this medicine:

• Apply a generous amount of cream to the affected area, and rub in gently until the cream disappears.

For patients using the ointment form of this medicine:

• Apply a generous amount of ointment to the affected area, and rub in gently.

After applying this medicine, the treated area may be covered with a gauze dressing if desired.

To help clear up your infection completely, **keep using this medicine for the full time of treatment,** even though your symptoms may have disappeared. **Do not miss any doses.**

If you do miss a dose of this medicine, apply it as soon as possible. However, if it is almost time for your next dose, skip the missed dose and go back to your regular dosing schedule.

How to store this medicine:

• **Keep out of the reach of children.**

• Store away from heat and direct light.

• Keep the medicine from freezing.

• Do not keep outdated medicine or medicine no longer needed. Be sure that any discarded medicine is out of the reach of children.

Precautions While Using This Medicine

If your skin problem does not improve within 1 week, or if it becomes worse, check with your doctor or pharmacist.

Side Effects of This Medicine

Along with its needed effects, a medicine may cause some unwanted effects. Although not all of these side effects may occur, if they do occur they may need medical attention.

Check with your doctor immediately if any of the following side effects occur:

More common

Itching, rash, redness, swelling, or other sign of irritation not present before using this medicine

Rare

Any loss of hearing

Other side effects not listed above may also occur in some patients. If you notice any other effects, check with your doctor.

_____

December 1987
_____

NEOMYCIN, POLYMYXIN B, AND BACITRACIN (Ophthalmic)

Some commonly used brand names are Mycitracin and Neosporin.

Generic name product may also be available in the U.S.

To the Reader: If you do not recognize the names of medical conditions or medicines referred to in this information, check with your doctor, nurse, or pharmacist. Definitions for selected medical terms may be found in the Glossary. Brand names for the generic drug names listed can be found in the Index. In addition, selected brand names commonly associated with the generic name have been included in the text to help you recognize medicine you may be taking. The fact that a brand name product is not mentioned does not mean the information does not apply. It is a good idea for you to learn both the generic and brand names of your medicines and to write them down for future use.

Neomycin (nee-oh-MYE-sin), polymyxin (pol-i-MIX-in) B, and bacitracin (bass-i-TRAY-sin) is a combination antibiotic medicine used in the eye to help the body overcome infections of the eye.

Neomycin, polymyxin B, and bacitracin combination is available only with your doctor's prescription.

Remember:

• **This medicine has been prescribed for your present infection only.** Another infection later on may require a different medicine. Also, even though other people may have the same symptoms as you, they may have a different kind of infection. Your medicine may not work for them and may even cause them harm. Therefore, **your medicine must not be given to other people or used for other infections** unless you are otherwise directed by your doctor.

• **Keep all medicines out of the reach of children.**

• In order for this medicine to work, it must be used as directed.

• **It is very important that you read and understand the following information.** If any of the information causes you special concern, do not decide against using this medicine without first checking with your doctor.

• Before you begin using any new medicine (prescription or nonprescription) or if you develop any new medical problem while you are using this medicine, check with your doctor, nurse, or pharmacist.

• **If you have any questions** about the following information or if you want more information about this medicine or your medical problem, **ask your doctor, nurse, or pharmacist.**

Before Using This Medicine

In order to decide on the best treatment for your medical problem, your doctor should be told:

—if you have ever had any unusual or allergic reaction to this medicine or to any related antibiotics such as amikacin, colistimethate, colistin, gentamicin, kanamycin, neomycin (by mouth or by injection), netilmicin, paromomycin, polymyxin B (by injection), streptomycin, or tobramycin.

—if you are allergic to any substance, such as certain foods or preservatives or dyes. Most medicines contain more than their active ingredient. Your doctor, nurse, or pharmacist can help you avoid products that may cause a problem.

—if you are **pregnant** or if you may become pregnant. However, neomycin, polymyxin B, and bacitracin ophthalmic preparations have not been shown to cause birth defects or other problems in humans.

—if you are **breast-feeding**. However, neomycin, polymyxin B, and bacitracin ophthalmic preparations have not been shown to cause problems in nursing babies.

Proper Use of This Medicine

How to apply this medicine: First, wash your hands. Then pull the lower eyelid away from the eye to form a pouch. Squeeze a thin strip of ointment into the pouch. A 1-cm (approximately ⅓-inch) strip of ointment is usually enough unless otherwise directed by your doctor. Gently close the eyes and keep them closed for 1 or 2 minutes to allow the medicine to come into contact with the infection.

To prevent contamination of the eye ointment, do not touch the applicator tip to any surface (including the eye). After using neomycin, polymyxin B, and bacitracin eye ointment, wipe the tip of the ointment tube with a clean tissue and keep the tube tightly closed.

To help clear up your infection completely, **keep using this medicine for the full time of treatment,** even though your symptoms may have disappeared. **Do not miss any doses**.

If you do miss a dose of this medicine, apply it as soon as possible. However, if it is almost time for your next dose, skip the missed dose and go back to your regular dosing schedule.

How to store this medicine:

• **Keep out of the reach of children.**

• Store away from heat and direct light.

• Keep the medicine from freezing.

• Do not keep outdated medicine or medicine no longer needed. Be sure that any discarded medicine is out of the reach of children.

Precautions While Using This Medicine

If your symptoms do not improve within a few days, or if they become worse, check with your doctor.

Side Effects of This Medicine

Along with its needed effects, a medicine may cause some unwanted effects. Although not all of these side effects may occur, if they do occur they may need medical attention.

Check with your doctor immediately if any of the following side effects occur:

More common

Itching, rash, redness, swelling, or other sign of irritation not present before using this medicine

After application, eye ointments usually cause your vision to blur for a few minutes.

Other side effects not listed above may also occur in some patients. If you notice any other effects, check with your doctor.

December 1987

NEOMYCIN, POLYMYXIN B, AND BACITRACIN (Topical)

Some commonly used brand names are:

Foille	Neo-Polycin
Mycitracin	Neosporin

Generic name product may also be available in the U.S.

To the Reader: If you do not recognize the names of medical conditions or medicines referred to in this information, check with your doctor, nurse, or pharmacist. Definitions for selected medical terms may be found in the Glossary. Brand names for the generic drug names listed can be found in the Index. In addition, selected brand names commonly associated with the generic name have been included in the text to help you recognize medicine you may be taking. The fact that a brand name product is not mentioned does not mean the information does not apply. It is a good idea for you to learn both the generic and brand names of your medicines and to write them down for future use.

Neomycin (nee-oh-MYE-sin), polymyxin (pol-i-MIX-in) B, and bacitracin (bass-i-TRAY-sin) is a combination antibiotic medicine used on the skin to help prevent infections of the skin.

Neomycin, polymyxin B, and bacitracin combination is available without a prescription; however, your doctor may have special instructions on the proper use of this medicine for your medical problem.

Remember:

• **Keep all medicines out of the reach of children.**

• In order for this medicine to work, it must be used as directed. **If you are using this medicine without a prescription, it is very important to follow the directions on the label.**

• **It is also very important that you read and understand the following information.** If any of the information causes you special concern, check with your doctor or pharmacist.

• Before you begin using any new medicine (prescription or nonprescription) or if you develop any new medical problem while you are using this medicine, check with your doctor, nurse, or pharmacist.

• **If you have any questions** about the following information or if you want more information about this medicine or your medical problem, **ask your doctor, nurse, or pharmacist.**

Before Using This Medicine

Before you use neomycin, polymyxin B, and bacitracin combination, check with your doctor or pharmacist:

—if you have ever had any unusual or allergic reaction to this medicine or to any related antibiotics such as amikacin, colistimethate, colistin, gentamicin, kanamycin, neomycin (by mouth or by injection), netilmicin, paromomycin, polymyxin B (by injection), streptomycin, or tobramycin.

—if you are allergic to any substance, such as certain foods or preservatives or dyes. Most medicines contain more than their active ingredient. Your doctor, nurse, or pharmacist can help you avoid products that may cause a problem.

—if you are **pregnant** or if you may become pregnant. However, neomycin, polymyxin B, and bacitracin topical preparations have not been shown to cause birth defects or other problems in humans.

—if you are **breast-feeding**. However, neomycin, polymyxin B, and bacitracin topical preparations have not been shown to cause problems in nursing babies.

—if you are taking **any** other prescription or nonprescription (OTC) medicine.

Proper Use of This Medicine

If you are using this medicine without a prescription, do not use it to treat deep wounds, puncture wounds, serious burns, or raw areas without first checking with your doctor or pharmacist.

Do not use this medicine in the eyes.

Before applying this medicine, wash the affected area with soap and water, and dry thoroughly.

After applying this medicine, the treated area may be covered with a gauze dressing if desired.

To help clear up your infection completely, **keep using this medicine for the full time of treatment,** even though your symptoms may have disappeared. **Do not miss any doses.**

If you do miss a dose of this medicine, apply it as soon as possible. However, if it is almost time for your next dose, skip the missed dose and go back to your regular dosing schedule.

How to store this medicine:

• **Keep out of the reach of children.**

• Store away from heat and direct light.

• Keep the medicine from freezing.

• Do not keep outdated medicine or medicine no longer needed. Be sure that any discarded medicine is out of the reach of children.

Precautions While Using This Medicine

If your skin problem does not improve within 1 week, or if it becomes worse, check with your doctor or pharmacist.

Side Effects of This Medicine

Along with its needed effects, a medicine may cause some unwanted effects. Although not all of these side effects may occur, if they do occur they may need medical attention.

© 1988   The United States Pharmacopeial Convention, Inc.

Check with your doctor immediately if any of the following side effects occur:

More common

Itching, skin rash, redness, swelling, or other sign of irritation not present before using this medicine

Rare

Any loss of hearing

Other side effects not listed above may also occur in some patients. If you notice any other effects, check with your doctor.

_____

December 1987

NEOMYCIN, POLYMYXIN B, AND GRAMICIDIN (Ophthalmic)

A commonly used brand name is Neosporin.

To the Reader: If you do not recognize the names of medical conditions or medicines referred to in this information, check with your doctor, nurse, or pharmacist. Definitions for selected medical terms may be found in the Glossary. Brand names for the generic drug names listed can be found in the Index. In addition, selected brand names commonly associated with the generic name have been included in the text to help you recognize medicine you may be taking. The fact that a brand name product is not mentioned does not mean the information does not apply. It is a good idea for you to learn both the generic and brand names of your medicines and to write them down for future use.

Neomycin (nee-oh-MYE-sin), polymyxin (pol-i-MIX-in) B, and gramicidin (gram-i-SYE-din) is a combination antibiotic medicine used in the eye to help the body overcome infections of the eye.

Neomycin, polymyxin B, and gramicidin combination is available only with your doctor's prescription.

Remember:

• **This medicine has been prescribed for your present infection only.** Another infection later on may require a different medicine. Also, even though other people may have the same symptoms as you, they may have a different kind of infection. Your medicine may not work for them and may even cause them harm. Therefore, **your medicine must not be given to other people or used for other infections** unless you are otherwise directed by your doctor.

• **Keep all medicines out of the reach of children.**

• In order for this medicine to work, it must be used as directed.

• **It is very important that you read and understand the following information.** If any of the information causes you special concern, do not decide against using this medicine without first checking with your doctor.

• Before you begin using any new medicine (prescription or nonprescription) or if you develop any new medical problem while you are using this medicine, check with your doctor, nurse, or pharmacist.

• **If you have any questions** about the following information or if you want more information about this medicine or your medical problem, **ask your doctor, nurse, or pharmacist.**

Before Using This Medicine

In order to decide on the best treatment for your medical problem, your doctor should be told:

—if you have ever had any unusual or allergic reaction to this medicine or to any related antibiotics such as amikacin, colistimethate, colistin, gentamicin, kanamycin, neomycin (by mouth or by injection), netilmicin, paromomycin, polymyxin B (by injection), streptomycin, or tobramycin.

—if you are allergic to any substance, such as certain foods or preservatives or dyes. Most medicines contain more than their active ingredient. Your doctor, nurse, or pharmacist can help you avoid products that may cause a problem.

—if you are **pregnant** or if you may become pregnant. However, neomycin, polymyxin B, and gramicidin combination has not been shown to cause birth defects or other problems in humans.

—if you are **breast-feeding**. However, neomycin, polymyxin B, and gramicidin combination has not been shown to cause problems in nursing babies.

Proper Use of This Medicine

The bottle is only partially full to provide proper drop control.

How to apply this medicine: First, wash your hands. Then tilt the head back and pull the lower eyelid away from the eye to form a pouch. Drop the medicine into the pouch and gently close the eyes. Do not blink. Keep the eyes closed for 1 or 2 minutes to allow the medicine to come into contact with the infection.

If you think you did not get the drop of medicine into your eye properly, use another drop.

To prevent contamination of the eye drops, do not touch the applicator tip or dropper to any surface (including the eye). Also, keep the container tightly closed.

To help clear up your infection completely, **keep using this medicine for the full time of treatment,** even though your symptoms may have disappeared. **Do not miss any doses.**

If you do miss a dose of this medicine, apply it as soon as possible. However, if it is almost time for your next dose, skip the missed dose and go back to your regular dosing schedule.

How to store this medicine:

• **Keep out of the reach of children.**

• Store away from heat and direct light.

• Keep the medicine from freezing.

• Do not keep outdated medicine or medicine no longer needed. Be sure that any discarded medicine is out of the reach of children.

Precautions While Using This Medicine

If your symptoms do not improve within a few days, or if they become worse, check with your doctor.

Side Effects of This Medicine

Along with its needed effects, a medicine may cause some unwanted effects. Although not all of these side effects may occur, if they do occur they may need medical attention.

Check with your doctor immediately if any of the following side effects occur:

More common

   Itching, rash, redness, swelling, or other sign of irritation not present before using this medicine

Other side effects may occur that usually do not require medical attention. These side effects may go away during treatment as your body adjusts to the medicine.

However, check with your doctor if either of the following side effects continues or is bothersome:
Less common
   Burning or stinging

Other side effects not listed above may also occur in some patients. If you notice any other effects, check with your doctor.

December 1987

NEOMYCIN, POLYMYXIN B, AND HYDROCORTISONE (Ophthalmic)

Some commonly used brand names or other names are Cortisporin and Neomycin, polymyxin B, and cortisol.

To the Reader: If you do not recognize the names of medical conditions or medicines referred to in this information, check with your doctor, nurse, or pharmacist. Definitions for selected medical terms may be found in the Glossary. Brand names for the generic drug names listed can be found in the Index. In addition, selected brand names commonly associated with the generic name have been included in the text to help you recognize medicine you may be taking. The fact that a brand name product is not mentioned does not mean the information does not apply. It is a good idea for you to learn both the generic and brand names of your medicines and to write them down for future use.

Neomycin (nee-oh-MYE-sin), polymyxin (pol-i-MIX-in) B, and hydrocortisone (hye-droe-KOR-ti-sone) is a combination antibiotic and cortisone-like medicine. It is used in the eye to help the body overcome infections of the eye and to help provide relief from redness, irritation, and discomfort of certain eye problems.

Neomycin, polymyxin B, and hydrocortisone combination is available only with your doctor's prescription.

Remember:
- **This medicine has been prescribed for your present medical problem only.** Even though other people may have the same symptoms as you, they may have a different kind of problem. Your medicine may not work for them and may even cause them harm. Therefore, **your medicine must not be given to other people or used for other problems** unless you are otherwise directed by your doctor.

- **Keep all medicines out of the reach of children.**

- In order for this medicine to work, it must be used as directed.

- **It is very important that you read and understand the following information.** If any of the information causes you special concern, do not decide against using this medicine without first checking with your doctor.

- Before you begin using any new medicine (prescription or nonprescription) or if you develop any new medical problem while you are using this medicine, check with your doctor, nurse, or pharmacist.

- **If you have any questions** about the following information or if you want more information about this medicine or your medical problem, **ask your doctor, nurse, or pharmacist.**

Before Using This Medicine

In order to decide on the best treatment for your medical problem, your doctor should be told:

—if you have ever had any unusual or allergic reaction to this medicine or to any related antibiotics such as amikacin, colistimethate, colistin, gentamicin, kanamycin, neomycin (by mouth or by injection), netilmicin, paromomycin, polymyxin B (by injection), streptomycin, or tobramycin.

—if you are allergic to any substance, such as certain foods or preservatives or dyes. Most medicines contain more than their active ingredient. Your doctor, nurse, or pharmacist can help you avoid products that may cause a problem.

—if you are **pregnant** or if you may become pregnant. However, neomycin, polymyxin B, and hydrocortisone ophthalmic drops have not been shown to cause birth defects or other problems in humans.

—if you are **breast-feeding**. However, neomycin, polymyxin B, and hydrocortisone ophthalmic drops have not been shown to cause problems in nursing babies.

—if you have any other eye infection or condition.

Proper Use of This Medicine

The bottle is only partially full to provide proper drop control.

How to apply this medicine: First, wash your hands. Then tilt the head back and pull the lower eyelid away from the eye to form a pouch. Drop the medicine into the pouch and gently close the eyes. Do not blink. Keep the eyes closed for 1 or 2 minutes to allow the medicine to come into contact with the infection.

If you think you did not get the drop of medicine into your eye properly, use another drop.

To prevent contamination of the eye drops, do not touch the applicator tip to any surface (including the eye). Also, keep the container tightly closed.

To help clear up your infection completely, **keep using this medicine for the full time of treatment,** even though your symptoms may have disappeared. **Do not miss any doses.**

If you do miss a dose of this medicine, apply it as soon as possible. However, if it is almost time for your next dose, skip the missed dose and go back to your regular dosing schedule.

Do not use any leftover medicine for future eye problems without checking with your doctor first, since this medicine should not be used on many different kinds of infection.

How to store this medicine:
- **Keep out of the reach of children.**
- Store away from heat and direct light.
- Keep the medicine from freezing.
- Do not keep outdated medicine or medicine no longer needed. Be sure that any discarded medicine is out of the reach of children.

Precautions While Using This Medicine

If you will be using this medicine for a long time (for example, longer than 6 weeks), your doctor should check your eyes at regular visits.

If your symptoms do not improve within a few days, or if they become worse, check with your doctor.

Side Effects of This Medicine

Along with its needed effects, a medicine may cause some unwanted effects. Although not all of these side effects may occur, if they do occur they may need medical attention.

Check with your doctor immediately if any of the following side effects occur:

More common
Itching, rash, redness, swelling, or other sign of irritation not present before using this medicine

Other side effects may occur that usually do not require medical attention. These side effects may go away during treatment as your body adjusts to the medicine. However, check with your doctor if either of the following side effects continues or is bothersome:

Less common
Burning or stinging

Other side effects not listed above may also occur in some patients. If you notice any other effects, check with your doctor.

_____

December 1987

NEOMYCIN, POLYMYXIN B, AND HYDROCORTISONE (Otic)

Some commonly used brand names or other names are:

Cortisporin	Octicair
Drotic	Ortega Otic-M
Neomycin, polymyxin B,	Otocort
and cortisol	Otoreid-HC

Generic name product may also be available in the U.S.

To the Reader: If you do not recognize the names of medical conditions or medicines referred to in this information, check with your doctor, nurse, or pharmacist. Definitions for selected medical terms may be found in the Glossary. Brand names for the generic drug names listed can be found in the Index. In addition, selected brand names commonly associated with the generic name have been included in the text to help you recognize medicine you may be taking. The fact that a brand name product is not mentioned does not mean the information does not apply. It is a good idea for you to learn both the generic and brand names of your medicines and to write them down for future use.

Neomycin (nee-oh-MYE-sin), polymyxin (pol-i-MIX-in) B, and hydrocortisone (hye-droe-KOR-ti-sone) is a combination antibiotic and cortisone-like medicine. It is used in the ear to help the body overcome infections of the ear canal and to help provide relief from redness, irritation, and discomfort of certain ear problems.

Neomycin, polymyxin B, and hydrocortisone combination is available only with your doctor's prescription.

Remember:

• **This medicine has been prescribed for your present medical problem only.** Even though other people may have the same symptoms as you, they may have a different kind of problem. Your medicine may not work for them and may even cause them harm. Therefore, **your medicine must not be given to other people or used for other problems** unless you are otherwise directed by your doctor.

• **Keep all medicines out of the reach of children.**

• In order for this medicine to work, it must be used as directed.

• **It is very important that you read and understand the following information.** If any of the information causes you special concern, do not decide against using this medicine without first checking with your doctor.

• Before you begin using any new medicine (prescription or nonprescription) or if you develop any new medical problem while you are using this medicine, check with your doctor, nurse, or pharmacist.

• **If you have any questions** about the following information or if you want more information about this medicine or your medical problem, **ask your doctor, nurse, or pharmacist.**

Before Using This Medicine

In order to decide on the best treatment for your medical problem, your doctor should be told:

—if you have ever had any unusual or allergic reaction to this medicine or to any related antibiotics such as amikacin, colistimethate, colistin, gentamicin, kanamycin, neomycin (by mouth or by injection), netilmicin, paromomycin, polymyxin B (by injection), streptomycin, or tobramycin.

—if are allergic to any substance, such as certain foods or preservatives or dyes. Most medicines contain more than their active ingredient. Your doctor, nurse, or pharmacist can help you avoid products that may cause a problem.

—if you are **pregnant** or if you may become pregnant. However, neomycin, polymyxin B, and hydrocortisone otic preparations have not been shown to cause birth defects or other problems in humans.

—if you are **breast-feeding**. However, neomycin, polymyxin B, and hydrocortisone otic preparations have not been shown to cause problems in nursing babies.

—if you have any other ear infection or condition (including punctured eardrum).

Proper Use of This Medicine

You may warm the ear drops to body temperature (37 °C or 98.6 °F), but no higher, by holding the bottle in your hand for a few minutes before applying. If the medicine gets too warm, it may break down and not work at all.

How to apply this medicine: Lie down or tilt the head so that the infected ear faces up. Gently pull the earlobe up and back for adults (down and back for children) to straighten the ear canal. Drop the medicine into the ear canal. Keep the ear facing up for about 5 minutes to allow the medicine to come into contact with the infection. A sterile cotton plug may be gently inserted into the ear opening to prevent the medicine from leaking out. However, your doctor may want you to keep a sterile cotton plug moistened with this medicine in your ear for the full time of treatment. If you have any questions about this, check with your doctor.

To prevent contamination of the ear drops, do not touch the dropper to any surface (including the ear). Also, keep the container tightly closed.

To help clear up your infection completely, **keep using this medicine for the full time of treatment,** even though your symptoms may have disappeared. **Do not miss any doses.**

If you do miss a dose of this medicine, apply it as soon as possible. However, if it is almost time for your next dose, skip the missed dose and go back to your regular dosing schedule.

Do not use this medicine for more than 10 days unless otherwise directed by your doctor.

How to store this medicine:

- **Keep out of the reach of children.**

- Store away from heat and direct light.

- Keep the medicine from freezing.

- Do not keep outdated medicine or medicine no longer needed. Be sure that any discarded medicine is out of the reach of children.

Precautions While Using This Medicine

If your symptoms do not improve within 1 week, or if they become worse, check with your doctor.

Side Effects of This Medicine

Along with its needed effects, a medicine may cause some unwanted effects. Although not all of these side effects may occur, if they do occur they may need medical attention.

Check with your doctor immediately if any of the following side effects occur:
More common
  Itching, skin rash, redness, swelling, or other sign of irritation not present before using this medicine

Other side effects not listed above may also occur in some patients. If you notice any other effects, check with your doctor.

December 1987

NIACIN
(Systemic—For High Cholesterol)

Some commonly used brand names are:

Diacin	Nicolar	Span-Niacin
Niac	Nico-Span	Tega-Span
Nico-400	Nicotinex	Tri-B3*
Nicobid		

Generic name product may also be available in the U.S. and Canada.

---

*Not available in the U.S.

To the Reader: If you do not recognize the names of medical conditions or medicines referred to in this information, check with your doctor, nurse, or pharmacist. Definitions for selected medical terms may be found in the Glossary. Brand names for the generic drug names listed can be found in the Index. In addition, selected brand names commonly associated with the generic name have been included in the text to help you recognize medicine you may be taking. The fact that a brand name product is not mentioned does not mean the information does not apply. It is a good idea for you to learn both the generic and brand names of your medicines and to write them down for future use.

Niacin (NYE-a-sin) (also known as nicotinic acid) is taken by mouth to lower high cholesterol and fat levels in the blood. This may help prevent medical problems caused by cholesterol and fat clogging the blood vessels.

Some strengths of niacin are available only with your doctor's prescription. Others are available without a prescription, since niacin is also a vitamin. However, it is best to take it only under your doctor's direction so that you can be sure you are taking the correct dose.

Remember:

• **This medicine has been prescribed for your current medical problem only.** It must not be given to other people or used for other problems unless you are directed to do so by your doctor.

• **Keep all medicines out of the reach of children.**

• In order for this medicine to work, it must be used as directed.

• **It is very important that you read and understand the following information.** If any of the information causes you special concern, do not decide against using this medicine without first checking with your doctor.

• Before you begin using any new medicine (prescription or nonprescription) or if you develop any new medical problem while you are using this medicine, check with your doctor, nurse, or pharmacist.

• **If you have any questions** about the following information or if you want more information about this medicine or your medical problem, **ask your doctor, nurse, or pharmacist.**

Before Using This Medicine

Importance of diet—Before prescribing medicine for your condition, your doctor will probably try to control your condition by prescribing a personal diet for you. Such a diet may be low in fats, sugars, and/or cholesterol. Many people are able to control their condition by carefully following their doctor's orders for proper diet and exercise. Medicine is prescribed only when additional help is needed and is effective only when a schedule of diet and exercise is properly followed.

Also, this medicine is less effective if you are greatly overweight. It may be very important for you to go on a reducing diet. However, check with your doctor before going on any diet.

In order to decide on the best treatment for your medical problem, your doctor should be told:

—if you have ever had any unusual or allergic reaction to niacin or niacinamide.

—if you are on a low-salt, low-sugar, or any other special diet, or if you are allergic to any substance, such as foods, sulfites or other preservatives, or dyes. Most medicines contain more than their active ingredient. Your doctor, nurse, or pharmacist can help you avoid products that may cause a problem.

—if you are **pregnant** or if you may become pregnant. Studies have not been done in either humans or animals.

—if you are **breast-feeding**. Niacin has not been shown to cause problems in nursing babies.

—if you have any of the following medical problems:
  Diabetes mellitus (sugar diabetes)
  Glaucoma
  Gout
  Liver disease
  Stomach ulcer

—if you are taking **any** other prescription or nonprescription (OTC) medicine.

Proper Use of This Medicine

Use this medicine only as directed by your doctor. Do not use more or less of it, do not use it more often, and do not use it for a longer period of time than your doctor ordered. To do so may increase the chance of unwanted effects.

Follow carefully the special diet your doctor gave you. This is the most important part of controlling your condition, and is necessary if the medicine is to work properly.

If this medicine upsets your stomach, it may be taken with meals or milk. If stomach upset (nausea or diarrhea) continues, check with your doctor.

For patients taking the extended-release capsule form of this medicine:

• Swallow the capsule whole.

• Do not crush, break, or chew before swallowing.

• If the capsule is too large to swallow, you may mix the contents of the capsule with jam or jelly and swallow without chewing.

For patients taking the extended-release tablet form of this medicine:

• Swallow the tablet whole.

• Do not break, crush, or chew before swallowing.

If you miss a dose of this medicine, take it as soon as possible. However, if it is almost time for your next dose, skip the missed dose and go back to your regular dosing schedule. Do not double doses.

How to store this medicine:

- **Keep out of the reach of children.**

- Store away from heat and direct light.

- Do not store in the bathroom, near the kitchen sink, or in other damp places. Heat or moisture may cause the medicine to break down.

- Keep the oral solution form of this medicine from freezing.

- Do not keep outdated medicine or medicine no longer needed. Be sure that any discarded medicine is out of the reach of children.

Precautions While Using This Medicine

It is very important that your doctor check your progress at regular visits. This will allow your doctor to see if the medicine is working properly to lower your cholesterol and triglyceride (fat) levels and if you should continue to take it.

This medicine may cause you to feel dizzy or faint, especially when you get up from a lying or sitting position. Getting up slowly may help. This effect should lessen after a week or two as your body gets used to the medicine. However, if the problem continues or gets worse, check with your doctor.

Side Effects of This Medicine

Along with its needed effects, a medicine may cause some unwanted effects. The following side effects may go away during treatment as your body adjusts to the medicine. However, check with your doctor or pharmacist if any of the following side effects continue or are bothersome:

Less common
   Feeling of warmth
   Flushing or redness of skin, especially on face and neck
   Headache

With high doses
   Diarrhea
   Dizziness or faintness
   Dryness of skin
   Nausea or vomiting
   Stomach pain

For elderly patients: Many medicines have not been tested in older people. Therefore, it is not known whether the medicine acts the same way it does in younger adults. Check with your doctor or pharmacist if you notice any unusual effects while taking this medicine or if you think it is not working as it should.

Other side effects not listed above may also occur in some patients. If you notice any other effects, check with your doctor or pharmacist.

December 1987

NIACIN (Vitamin B₃)
(Systemic—Vitamin)

Some commonly used brand names are:

Diacin	Nicolar	Span-Niacin
Niac	Nico-Span	Tega-Span
Nico-400	Nicotinex	Tri-B3*
Nicobid		

Generic name product may also be available in the U.S. and Canada.

*Not available in the U.S.

To the Reader: If you do not recognize the names of medical conditions or medicines referred to in this information, check with your doctor, nurse, or pharmacist. Definitions for selected medical terms may be found in the Glossary. Brand names for the generic drug names listed can be found in the Index. In addition, selected brand names commonly associated with the generic name have been included in the text to help you recognize medicine you may be taking. The fact that a brand name product is not mentioned does not mean the information does not apply. It is a good idea for you to learn both the generic and brand names of your medicines and to write them down for future use.

Vitamins (VYE-ta-mins) are compounds that you *must* have for growth and health. They are needed in small amounts only and are usually available in the foods that you eat. Niacin (NYE-a-sin) (also known as niacinamide [nye-a-SIN-a-mide], nicotinic acid, nicotinamide, or vitamin B₃) is necessary for many normal functions of the body.

Lack of niacin may lead to a condition called pellagra, with diarrhea, stomach problems, skin problems, sores in the mouth, anemia (weak blood), and mental problems. Your doctor may treat this by prescribing niacin for you.

Claims that niacin is effective for treatment of acne, leprosy, motion sickness, poor circulation, and mental problems, and for prevention of heart attacks have not been proven. Many of these treatments involve large and expensive amounts of vitamins.

Some strengths of niacin are available only with your doctor's prescription. Others are available without a prescription. However, it may be a good idea to check with your doctor or pharmacist before taking niacin on your own.

Remember:

• **This medicine has been prescribed for your current medical problem only.** It must not be given to other people or used for other problems unless you are directed to do so by your doctor.

• **Keep all medicines out of the reach of children.**

• In order for this medicine to work, it must be used as directed.

• If you are receiving this medicine by injection, some of the information about this medicine may not apply.

• **It is very important that you read and understand the following information.** If any of the information causes you special concern, do not decide against using this medicine without first checking with your doctor.

• Before you begin using any new medicine (prescription or nonprescription) or if you develop any new medical problem while you are using this medicine, check with your doctor, nurse, or pharmacist.

• **If you have any questions** about the following information or if you want more information about this medicine or your medical problem, **ask your doctor, nurse, or pharmacist**.

Importance of Diet

Vitamin supplements should be taken only if you cannot get enough vitamins in your diet. A balanced diet should provide all the vitamins you normally need.

Nutritionists recommend that you eat:
• Cereal or bread—4 or more servings per day and
• Dairy products (milk, cheese, ice cream, cottage cheese)—3 or more servings per day and
• Meat, fish, or eggs—2 or more servings per day and
• Vegetables and fruits—4 or more servings per day.

If you are not getting all of these foods every day, you may not be getting enough vitamins in your diet. The best way to correct this is to start eating the foods that contain what you need.

Niacin is found in meats, eggs, and milk and dairy products. Little niacin is lost from foods during ordinary cooking.

Vitamins alone will not take the place of a good diet and will not provide energy. Your body also needs other substances found in food such as protein, minerals, carbohydrates, and fat. Vitamins themselves often cannot work without the presence of other foods.

In some cases, it may not be possible for you to get enough food to supply you with the proper vitamins. In other cases, the amount of vitamins you need may be increased above normal. Therefore, a vitamin supplement may be needed.

Experts have developed a list of recommended dietary allowances (RDA) for most of the vitamins. The RDA are not an exact number but a general idea of how much you need. They do not cover amounts needed for problems caused by a serious lack of vitamins.

The RDA for niacin are:

Children 4 to 6 years of age—11 mg per day
Adult males—18 mg per day
Adult females—13 mg per day
Pregnant females—15 mg per day
Breast-feeding females—18 mg per day.

Remember:

• The total amount of each vitamin that you get every day includes what you get from the foods that you eat *and* what you may take as a supplement.

• This total amount should not be greater than the RDA, unless ordered by your doctor. Taking too much niacin over a period of time may cause unwanted effects such as high blood sugar, peptic ulcer, gout, heart problems, or liver problems.

Before Using This Medicine

In deciding whether you need additional niacin, the following should be kept in mind and/or your doctor should be told:

—if you have ever had any unusual or allergic reaction to niacin or niacinamide.

—if you are on a low-salt, low-sugar, or any other special diet, or if you are allergic to any substance, such as foods, sulfites or other preservatives, or dyes. Most medicines contain more than their active ingredient. Your doctor, nurse, or pharmacist can help you avoid products that may cause a problem.

—if you are **pregnant** or if you may become pregnant. It is especially important that you are receiving enough vitamins when you become pregnant and that you continue to receive the right amount of vitamins throughout your pregnancy. The healthy growth and development of the fetus depend on a steady supply of nutrients from the mother.

—if you are **breast-feeding**. It is especially important that you receive the right amounts of vitamins so that your baby will also get the vitamins needed to grow properly.

—if you are not able to get a diet that contains all the vitamins you need. This may occur with rapid weight loss, unusual diets (such as some reducing diets in which choice of foods is very limited), prolonged intravenous feeding, or malnutrition.

—if you have had a large part of your stomach removed.

—if you have been under a lot of stress for a long time, or if you have had a long illness or serious injury.

—if you have any of the following medical problems:
  Alcoholism
  Cancer
  Diabetes mellitus (sugar diabetes)
  Diarrhea (prolonged)
  Glaucoma
  Gout
  Hartnup disease
  Intestinal problems
  Liver disease
  Mouth and throat problems
  Overactive thyroid
  Pancreas disease
  Stomach ulcer

—if you are taking **any** other prescription or nonprescription (OTC) medicine.

Proper Use of This Medicine

Some people believe that taking very large doses of vitamins (called megadoses or megavitamin therapy) is useful for treating certain medical problems. Studies have not proven this. Large doses should be taken only under the direction of your doctor after need has been identified.

If this medicine upsets your stomach, it may be taken with meals or milk. If stomach upset (nausea or diarrhea) continues, check with your doctor.

For patients taking the extended-release capsule form of this medicine:

• Swallow the capsule whole.

• Do not crush, break, or chew before swallowing.

• If the capsule is too large to swallow, you may mix the contents of the capsule with jam or jelly and swallow without chewing.

For patients taking the extended-release tablet form of this medicine:

• Swallow the tablet whole.

• Do not break, crush, or chew before swallowing.

If you miss taking a vitamin for one or more days there is no cause for concern, since it takes some time for your body to become seriously low in vitamins. However, if your doctor has recommended that you take this vitamin, try to remember to take it as directed every day.

How to store this medicine:

• **Keep out of the reach of children.**

• Store away from heat and direct light.

• Do not store in the bathroom, near the kitchen sink, or in other damp places. Heat or moisture may cause the medicine to break down.

• Keep the oral solution form of this medicine from freezing.

• Do not keep outdated medicine or medicine no longer needed. Be sure that any discarded medicine is out of the reach of children.

Precautions While Using This Medicine

This medicine may cause you to feel dizzy or faint, especially when you get up from a lying or sitting position. Getting up slowly may help. This effect should lessen after a week or two as your body gets used to the medicine. However, if the problem continues or gets worse, check with your doctor.

Side Effects of This Medicine

Along with its needed effects, a medicine may cause some unwanted effects. Although not all of these side effects may occur, if they do occur they may need medical attention.

Check with your doctor immediately if any of the following side effects occur shortly after this vitamin is given by injection:

With injection only
  Skin rash or itching
  Wheezing

Other side effects may occur that usually do not require medical attention. These side effects may go away during treatment as your body adjusts to the medicine.

However, check with your doctor or pharmacist if any of the following side effects continue or are bothersome:

Less common—with niacin only
Feeling of warmth
Flushing or redness of skin, especially on face and neck
Headache

With high doses
Diarrhea
Dizziness or faintness

Dryness of skin
Nausea or vomiting
Stomach pain

Other side effects not listed above may also occur in some patients. If you notice any other effects, check with your doctor or pharmacist.

_____

December 1987

NICLOSAMIDE (Oral)

Some commonly used brand names are Niclocide and Yomesan*.

---

*Not available in the U.S.

To the Reader: If you do not recognize the names of medical conditions or medicines referred to in this information, check with your doctor, nurse, or pharmacist. Definitions for selected medical terms may be found in the Glossary. Brand names for the generic drug names listed can be found in the Index. In addition, selected brand names commonly associated with the generic name have been included in the text to help you recognize medicine you may be taking. The fact that a brand name product is not mentioned does not mean the information does not apply. It is a good idea for you to learn both the generic and brand names of your medicines and to write them down for future use.

Niclosamide (ni-KLOE-sa-mide) belongs to the general family of medicines called anthelmintics (ant-hel-MIN-tiks). Anthelmintics are medicines used in the treatment of worm infections.

Niclosamide is taken by mouth to treat broad or fish tapeworm, dwarf tapeworm, and beef tapeworm infections. Niclosamide may also be used for other tapeworm infections as determined by your doctor. It will not work for other types of worm infections (for example, pinworms or roundworms).

Niclosamide works by killing tapeworms on contact. The killed worms are then passed in the stool. However, you may not notice them since they are sometimes destroyed in the intestine.

Niclosamide is available only with your doctor's prescription.

Remember:

• **This medicine has been prescribed for your present infection only.** Another infection later on may require a different medicine. Also, even though other people may have the same symptoms as you, they may have a different kind of infection. Your medicine may not work for them and may even cause them harm. Therefore, **your medicine must not be given to other people or used for other infections** unless you are otherwise directed by your doctor.

• **Keep all medicines out of the reach of children.**

• In order for this medicine to work, it must be used as directed.

• **It is very important that you read and understand the following information.** If any of the information causes you special concern, do not decide against using this medicine without first checking with your doctor.

• Before you begin using any new medicine (prescription or nonprescription) or if you develop any new medical problem while you are using this medicine, check with your doctor, nurse, or pharmacist.

• **If you have any questions** about the following information or if you want more information about this medicine or your medical problem, **ask your doctor, nurse, or pharmacist.**

Before Using This Medicine

In order to decide on the best treatment for your medical problem, your doctor should be told:

—if you have ever had any unusual or allergic reaction to niclosamide.

—if you are on a low-salt, low-sugar, or any other special diet, or if you are allergic to any substance, such as foods, sulfites or other preservatives, or dyes. Most medicines contain more than their active ingredient. Your doctor, nurse, or pharmacist can help you avoid products that may cause a problem.

—if you are **pregnant** or if you may become pregnant. Studies have not been done in humans. However, niclosamide has not been shown to cause birth defects or other problems in rats and rabbits given 25 times the usual human dose or in mice given 12 times the usual human dose.

—if you are **breast-feeding**. It is not known whether niclosamide passes into the breast milk. However, this medicine has not been shown to cause problems in nursing babies. In addition, niclosamide is unlikely to pass into the breast milk in large amounts since not very much is absorbed into the body.

Proper Use of This Medicine

No special preparations (for example, special diets, fasting, other medicines, laxatives, or enemas) are necessary before, during, or immediately after taking niclosamide.

Niclosamide may be taken on an empty stomach (either 1 hour before or 2 hours after a meal). However, to prevent stomach upset, it is best taken after a light meal (for example, breakfast).

Niclosamide tablets should be thoroughly chewed or crushed and then swallowed with a small amount of water. If this medicine is being given to a young child, the tablets should be crushed to a fine powder and mixed with a small amount of water to form a paste.

For patients taking this medicine for beef tapeworms or broad or fish tapeworms:

• To help clear up your infection completely, **take this medicine exactly as directed by your doctor.** Usually one dose is enough. However, in some patients a second dose of this medicine may be required to clear up the infection completely.

For patients taking this medicine for dwarf tapeworms:

• To help clear up your infection completely, **keep taking this medicine for the full time of treatment (usually 7 days),** even if your symptoms begin to clear up after a few days. In some patients, a second course of this medicine may be required to clear up the infection completely. If you stop taking this medicine too soon, your infection may return. **Do not miss any doses.** Some patients with tapeworm infections may not notice any symptoms or may have only mild symptoms.

• If you do miss a dose of this medicine, take it as soon as possible. However, if it is almost time for your next dose, space the missed dose and the next dose 10 to 12 hours apart. Then go back to your regular dosing schedule.

How to store this medicine:

• **Keep out of the reach of children.**

• Store away from heat and direct light.

• Do not store in the bathroom, near the kitchen sink, or in other damp places. Heat or moisture may cause the medicine to break down.

• Do not keep outdated medicine or medicine no longer needed. Be sure that any discarded medicine is out of the reach of children.

Precautions While Using This Medicine

It is important that your doctor check your progress at regular visits. This is to make sure that the infection is cleared up completely.

If your symptoms do not improve within a few days, or if they become worse, check with your doctor.

This medicine may cause some people to become dizzy, lightheaded, drowsy, or less alert than they are normally. **Make sure you know how you react to this medicine before you drive, use machines, or do other jobs that require you to be alert.** If these reactions are especially bothersome, check with your doctor.

Side Effects of This Medicine

Along with its needed effects, a medicine may cause some unwanted effects. The following side effects may go away during treatment as your body adjusts to the medicine. However, check with your doctor if any of the following side effects continue or are bothersome:

More common
Abdominal or stomach cramps or pain
Loss of appetite
Nausea or vomiting

Less common or rare
Bad taste
Diarrhea
Dizziness or lightheadedness
Drowsiness
Itching of the rectal area
Skin rash

For elderly patients: Many medicines have not been tested in older people. Therefore, it is not known whether the medicine acts the same way it does in younger adults. Check with your doctor or pharmacist if you notice any unusual effects while taking this medicine or if you think it is not working as it should.

Other side effects not listed above may also occur in some patients. If you notice any other effects, check with your doctor.

_____

December 1987

NICOTINE (Systemic)

A commonly used brand name is Nicorette.

To the Reader: If you do not recognize the names of medical conditions or medicines referred to in this information, check with your doctor, nurse, or pharmacist. Definitions for selected medical terms may be found in the Glossary. Brand names for the generic drug names listed can be found in the Index. In addition, selected brand names commonly associated with the generic name have been included in the text to help you recognize medicine you may be taking. The fact that a brand name product is not mentioned does not mean the information does not apply. It is a good idea for you to learn both the generic and brand names of your medicines and to write them down for future use.

Nicotine (NIK-o-teen) in a flavored chewing gum is used to help you stop smoking. It is used for up to 3 months as part of a supervised stop-smoking program.

As you chew nicotine gum, nicotine passes through the lining of your mouth and into your body. This nicotine takes the place of nicotine that you would otherwise get from smoking. In this way, the withdrawal effects of not smoking are less severe. Then, as your body adjusts to not smoking, the use of the nicotine gum is decreased gradually. Finally, its use is stopped altogether.

Children, pregnant women, and nonsmokers should not use nicotine gum because of unwanted side effects.

Nicotine gum is available only with your doctor's prescription.

Remember:

- **This medicine has been prescribed for your current medical problem only.** It must not be given to other people or used for other problems unless you are directed to do so by your doctor.

- **Keep all medicines out of the reach of children.**

- In order for this medicine to work, it must be used as directed.

- **It is very important that you read and understand the following information.** If any of the information causes you special concern, do not decide against using this medicine without first checking with your doctor.

- Before you begin using any new medicine (prescription or nonprescription) or if you develop any new medical problem while you are using this medicine, check with your doctor, nurse, or pharmacist.

- **If you have any questions** about the following information or if you want more information about this medicine or your medical problem, **ask your doctor, nurse, or pharmacist.**

Before Using This Medicine

In order to decide on the best treatment for your medical problem, your doctor should be told:

—if you have ever had any unusual or allergic reaction to nicotine.

—if you are **pregnant** or if you may become pregnant. Nicotine, whether from smoking or from the gum, is not recommended during pregnancy. Studies in humans show that nicotine, when used during the last 3 months of pregnancy, causes breathing problems in the fetus.

—if you are **breast-feeding**. Nicotine passes into breast milk and may cause unwanted effects in the baby. It may be necessary for you to stop breast-feeding during treatment.

—if you have any of the following medical problems:
Dental problems
Diabetes mellitus (sugar diabetes)
Heart or blood vessel disease
High blood pressure
Inflammation of mouth or throat
Overactive thyroid
Pheochromocytoma (PCC)
Stomach ulcer
Temperomandibular (jaw) joint disease (TMJ)

—if you are taking **any** other prescription or nonprescription (OTC) medicine, especially:
Aminophylline (e.g., Somophyllin)
Insulin
Oxtriphylline (e.g., Choledyl)
Propoxyphene (e.g., Darvon)
Propranolol (e.g., Inderal)
Theophylline (e.g., Somophyllin-T)

Proper Use of This Medicine

Nicotine gum usually comes with patient directions. **Read the directions carefully before using this medicine.**

When you feel the urge to smoke, chew one piece of gum very slowly until you taste it or feel a slight tingling in your mouth. Stop chewing until the taste or tingling is almost gone. Then chew slowly until you taste it again. Continue chewing and stopping in this way for about 30 minutes in order to get the full dose of nicotine.

Do not chew too fast, do not chew more than one piece at a time, and do not chew a piece of gum too soon after another. To do so may cause unwanted side effects or an overdose. Also, slower chewing will reduce the possibility of belching.

Use nicotine gum exactly as directed by your doctor. Remember that it is also important to participate in a stop-smoking program during treatment. This may make it easier for you to stop smoking.

As your urge to smoke becomes less frequent, **gradually reduce the number of pieces of gum you chew each day** until you are chewing one or two pieces a day. This may be possible within 2 to 3 months.

Remember to carry nicotine gum with you at all times in case you feel the sudden urge to smoke. One cigarette may be enough to start you on the smoking habit again.

Using hard sugarless candy between doses of gum may help to relieve the discomfort in your mouth.

How to store this medicine:

- **Keep out of the reach of children** because children are more sensitive to the unwanted effects of even small doses of nicotine.

- Store away from heat and direct light.

- Do not store in the bathroom, near the kitchen sink, or in other damp places. Heat or moisture may cause the medicine to break down.

- Do not keep outdated medicine or medicine no longer needed. Be sure that any discarded medicine is out of the reach of children.

Precautions While Using This Medicine

Your doctor should check your progress at regular visits to make sure that the nicotine gum is working properly and that possible side effects are avoided.

Do not chew more than 30 pieces of gum a day. Chewing too many pieces may be harmful because of the risk of overdose.

Do not use nicotine gum for longer than 6 months. To do so may result in physical dependence on the nicotine.

Do not smoke during treatment with nicotine gum because of the risk of nicotine overdose.

If the gum sticks to your dental work, stop using it and check with your physician or dentist. Dentures or other dental work may be damaged because nicotine gum is stickier and harder to chew than ordinary gum.

Nicotine should not be used in pregnancy. If there is a possibility you might become pregnant, you may want to use some type of birth control. If you think you may have become pregnant, stop taking this medicine immediately and check with your doctor.

Side Effects of This Medicine

Along with its needed effects, a medicine may cause some unwanted effects. Although not all of these side effects may occur, if they do occur they may need medical attention.

Check with your doctor as soon as possible if any of the following side effects occur:
More common
   Injury to mouth, teeth, or dental work
Rare
   Irregular heartbeat

Signs of overdose (may occur in the following order)
   Nausea or vomiting
   Increased watering of mouth (severe)
   Abdominal or stomach pain (severe)
   Diarrhea
   Cold sweat
   Headache (severe)
   Dizziness (severe)
   Disturbed hearing and vision
   Confusion
   Weakness (severe)
   Fainting
   Difficulty in breathing (severe)
   Fast, weak, or irregular heartbeat
   Convulsions (seizures)

Other side effects may occur that usually do not require medical attention. These side effects may go away during treatment as your body adjusts to the medicine. However, check with your doctor if any of the following side effects continue or are bothersome:
More common
   Belching
   Fast heartbeat
   Headache (mild)
   Increased appetite
   Increased watering of mouth (mild)
   Jaw muscle ache
   Sore mouth or throat
Less common or rare
   Constipation
   Coughing
   Dizziness or lightheadedness (mild)
   Dry mouth
   Hiccups
   Hoarseness
   Irritability
   Laxative effect
   Loss of appetite
   Stomach upset or indigestion (mild)
   Trouble in sleeping

Other side effects not listed above may also occur in some patients. If you notice any other effects, check with your doctor.

December 1987

NICOTINYL ALCOHOL (Systemic)

A commonly used brand name is Roniacol*.

Generic name product may also be available in the U.S.

*Not available in the U.S.

To the Reader: If you do not recognize the names of medical conditions or medicines referred to in this information, check with your doctor, nurse, or pharmacist. Definitions for selected medical terms may be found in the Glossary. Brand names for the generic drug names listed can be found in the Index. In addition, selected brand names commonly associated with the generic name have been included in the text to help you recognize medicine you may be taking. The fact that a brand name product is not mentioned does not mean the information does not apply. It is a good idea for you to learn both the generic and brand names of your medicines and to write them down for future use.

Nicotinyl (nik-oh-TIN-ill) alcohol belongs to the group of medicines called vasodilators. Vasodilators increase the size of blood vessels and are used to treat problems resulting from poor blood circulation.

Nicotinyl alcohol is available only with your doctor's prescription.

Remember:

• **This medicine has been prescribed for your current medical problem only.** It must not be given to other people or used for other problems unless you are directed to do so by your doctor.

• **Keep all medicines out of the reach of children.**

• In order for this medicine to work, it must be used as directed.

• **It is very important that you read and understand the following information.** If any of the information causes you special concern, do not decide against using this medicine without first checking with your doctor.

• Before you begin using any new medicine (prescription or nonprescription) or if you develop any new medical problem while you are using this medicine, check with your doctor, nurse, or pharmacist.

• **If you have any questions** about the following information or if you want more information about this medicine or your medical problem, **ask your doctor, nurse, or pharmacist.**

Before Using This Medicine

In order to decide on the best treatment for your medical problem, your doctor should be told:

—if you have ever had any unusual or allergic reaction to nicotinyl alcohol.

—if you are on a low-salt, low-sugar, or any other special diet, or if you are allergic to any substance, such as foods, sulfites or other preservatives, or dyes. Most medicines contain more than their active ingredient. Your doctor, nurse, or pharmacist can help you avoid products that may cause a problem.

—if you are **pregnant** or if you may become pregnant. Studies have not been done in either humans or animals.

—if you are **breast-feeding**. This medicine has not been shown to cause problems in nursing babies.

—if you have any of the following medical problems:
Angina (chest pain)
Diabetes mellitus (sugar diabetes)
Glaucoma
High cholesterol levels
Stomach ulcer

—if you have recently had a heart attack or stroke.

—if you are taking **any** other prescription or nonprescription (OTC) medicine.

—if you smoke.

Proper Use of This Medicine

If you miss a dose of this medicine, take it as soon as you remember. However, if it is almost time for your next dose, skip the missed dose and go back to your regular dosing schedule. Do not double doses.

How to store this medicine:

• **Keep out of the reach of children.**

• Store away from heat and direct light.

• Do not store in the bathroom, near the kitchen sink, or in other damp places. Heat or moisture may cause the medicine to break down.

• Do not keep outdated medicine or medicine no longer needed. Be sure that any discarded medicine is out of the reach of children.

Precautions While Using This Medicine

It may take some time for this medicine to work. If you feel that the medicine is not working, do not stop taking it on your own. Instead, check with your doctor.

The helpful effects of this medicine may be decreased if you smoke.

Side Effects of This Medicine

Along with its needed effects, a medicine may cause some unwanted effects. Although not all of these side effects may occur, if they do occur they may need medical attention.

Check with your doctor as soon as possible if any of the following side effects occur:
Rare
Swelling of feet or lower legs
Yellow eyes or skin

Other side effects may occur that usually do not require medical attention. These side effects may go away during treatment as your body adjusts to the medicine.

However, check with your doctor if any of the following side effects continue or are bothersome:

More common
    Flushing
    Warmth or tingling

Less common or rare
    Diarrhea
    Dizziness or faintness
    Increased hair loss
    Nausea and vomiting
    Skin rash

For elderly patients: Many medicines have not been tested in older people. Therefore, it is not known whether the medicine acts the same way it does in younger adults. Check with your doctor or pharmacist if you notice any unusual effects while taking this medicine or if you think it is not working as it should. In addition, nicotinyl alcohol may reduce tolerance to cold temperatures in elderly patients.

Other side effects not listed above may also occur in some patients. If you notice any other effects, check with your doctor.

December 1987

NITRATES (Systemic—Lingual Aerosol)

This information applies to nitroglycerin oral spray.

A commonly used brand name is Nitrolingual.

To the Reader: If you do not recognize the names of medical conditions or medicines referred to in this information, check with your doctor, nurse, or pharmacist. Definitions for selected medical terms may be found in the Glossary. Brand names for the generic drug names listed can be found in the Index. In addition, selected brand names commonly associated with the generic name have been included in the text to help you recognize medicine you may be taking. The fact that a brand name product is not mentioned does not mean the information does not apply. It is a good idea for you to learn both the generic and brand names of your medicines and to write them down for future use.

Nitrates (NYE-trates) are used to treat the symptoms of angina (chest pain). Depending on the type of dosage form and how it is taken, nitrates are used to treat angina in three ways:

—to relieve an attack that is occurring by using the medicine when the attack begins;

—to prevent attacks from occurring by using the medicine just before an attack is expected to occur; or

—to reduce the number of attacks that occur by using the medicine regularly on a long-term basis.

When used as a lingual (in the mouth) spray, nitroglycerin is used either to relieve the pain of angina attacks or to prevent an expected angina attack.

Nitroglycerin works by relaxing blood vessels and increasing the supply of blood and oxygen to the heart while reducing its work load.

Nitroglycerin is available only with your doctor's prescription.

Remember:

• **This medicine has been prescribed for your current medical problem only.** It must not be given to other people or used for other problems unless you are directed to do so by your doctor.

• **Keep all medicines out of the reach of children.**

• In order for this medicine to work, it must be used as directed.

• **It is very important that you read and understand the following information.** If any of the information causes you special concern, do not decide against using this medicine without first checking with your doctor.

• Before you begin using any new medicine (prescription or nonprescription) or if you develop any new medical problem while you are using this medicine, check with your doctor, nurse, or pharmacist.

• **If you have any questions** about the following information or if you want more information about this medicine or your medical problem, **ask your doctor, nurse, or pharmacist.**

Before Using This Medicine

In order to decide on the best treatment for your medical problem, your doctor should be told:

—if you have ever had any unusual or allergic reaction to nitrates or nitrites.

—if you are allergic to any substance, such as certain foods or preservatives or dyes. Most medicines contain more than their active ingredient. Your doctor, nurse, or pharmacist can help you avoid products that may cause a problem.

—if you are **pregnant** or if you may become pregnant. Studies have not been done in humans. However, nitroglycerin has not been shown to cause problems.

—if you are **breast-feeding**. This medicine has not been shown to cause problems in nursing babies.

—if you have any of the following medical problems:
Anemia (severe)
Glaucoma
Intestinal problems
Overactive thyroid

—if you have recently had a heart attack, stroke, or head injury.

—if you are taking **any** other prescription or nonprescription (OTC) medicine, especially antihypertensives (high blood pressure medicine).

Proper Use of This Medicine

Use nitroglycerin spray exactly as directed by your doctor. It will work only if used correctly.

This medicine usually comes with patient instructions. Read them carefully before you actually need to use it. Then, if you need it quickly, you will know how to use it.

How to use nitroglycerin lingual spray:

• Remove the plastic cover. **Do not shake the container.**

• Hold the container upright. With the container held close to your mouth, press the button to spray onto or under your tongue. **Do not inhale the spray.**

• Release the button and close your mouth. Avoid swallowing immediately after using the spray.

For patients using nitroglycerin oral spray to relieve the pain of an angina attack:

• **When you begin to feel an attack of angina starting (chest pains or a tightness or squeezing in the chest), sit down. Then use 1 or 2 sprays as directed by your doctor.** This medicine works best when you are standing or sitting. However, since you may become dizzy, lightheaded, or faint soon after using a spray, it is safer to sit rather than stand while the medicine is working. If you become dizzy or faint while sitting, take several deep breaths and bend forward with your head between your knees.

• Remain calm and you should feel better in a few minutes.

- **This medicine usually gives relief in less than 5 minutes.** However, if the pain is not relieved, use a second spray. If the pain continues for another 5 minutes, a third spray may be used. **If you still have the chest pains after a total of 3 sprays in a 15-minute period, contact your doctor or go to a hospital emergency room immediately.**

For patients using nitroglycerin oral spray to prevent an expected angina attack:

- You may prevent anginal chest pains for up to 1 hour by using a spray 5 to 10 minutes before expected emotional stress or physical exertion that in the past seemed to bring on an attack.

How to store this medicine:

- **Keep out of the reach of children.**
- Store away from heat and direct light.
- Keep the medicine from freezing.
- Do not puncture, break, or burn the aerosol container, even after it is empty.
- Do not keep outdated medicine or medicine no longer needed. Be sure that any discarded medicine is out of the reach of children.

Precautions While Using This Medicine

If you have been using this medicine regularly for several weeks, do not suddenly stop using it. Stopping suddenly may bring on attacks of angina. Check with your doctor for the best way to reduce gradually the amount you are using before stopping completely.

Dizziness, lightheadedness, or a fainting feeling may occur, especially when you get up quickly from a lying or sitting position. Getting up slowly may help. If you feel dizzy, sit or lie down.

The dizziness, lightheadedness, or fainting is also more likely to occur if you drink alcohol, stand for long periods of time, exercise, or if the weather is hot. **While you are taking this medicine, be careful in the amount of alcohol you drink. Also, use extra care during exercise or hot weather or if you must stand for long periods of time.**

After using a dose of this medicine you may get a headache that lasts for a short time. This is a common side effect which should become less noticeable after you have used the medicine for a while. If this effect continues or if the headaches are severe, check with your doctor.

Side Effects of This Medicine

Along with its needed effects, a medicine may cause some unwanted effects. Although not all of these side effects may occur, if they do occur they may need medical attention.

Check with your doctor as soon as possible if any of the following side effects occur:

Rare
   Blurred vision
   Dry mouth
   Headache (severe or prolonged)
   Skin rash

Signs of overdose (in the order in which they may occur)
   Bluish-colored lips, fingernails, or palms of hands
   Dizziness (extreme) or fainting
   Feeling of extreme pressure in head
   Shortness of breath
   Unusual tiredness or weakness
   Weak and fast heartbeat
   Fever
   Convulsions (seizures)

Other side effects may occur that usually do not require medical attention. These side effects may go away during treatment as your body adjusts to the medicine. However, check with your doctor if any of the following side effects continue or are bothersome:

More common
   Dizziness or lightheadedness, especially when getting up from a lying or sitting position
   Fast pulse
   Flushing of face and neck
   Headache
   Nausea or vomiting
   Restlessness

For elderly patients: Many medicines have not been tested in older people. Therefore, it is not known whether the medicine acts the same way it does in younger adults. Check with your doctor or pharmacist if you notice any unusual effects while taking this medicine or if you think it is not working as it should.

Other side effects not listed above may also occur in some patients. If you notice any other effects, check with your doctor.

_____

December 1987

NITRATES (Systemic—Oral)

This information applies to the following medicines:

Erythrityl Tetranitrate (e-RI-thri-till tet-ra-NYE-trate)
Isosorbide Dinitrate (eye-soe-SOR-bide dye-NYE-trate)
Nitroglycerin (nye-troe-GLI-ser-in)
Pentaerythritol Tetranitrate (pen-ta-er-ITH-ri-tole tet-ra-NYE-trate)

This information does *not* apply to amyl nitrite or mannitol hexanitrate.

Some commonly used brand names or other names are:	Generic names:
Cardilate Erythritol Tetranitrate	Erythrityl Tetranitrate
Apo-ISDN* Coronex* Dilatrate SR Iso-Bid Isochron Isonate Isonate TR Isordil Isotrate Novosorbide* Sorate Sorbide T.D. Sorbitrate Sorbitrate SA	Isosorbide Dinitrate†
Ang-O-Span Glyceryl Trinitrate Klavikordal N-G-C Niong Nitro-Bid Nitrobon Nitrocap Nitrocap T.D. Nitrocardin Nitroglyn Nitrolin Nitro-Long Nitronet Nitrong Nitrong SR* Nitrospan Nitro-Time	Nitroglycerin†
Duotrate Naptrate Pentol Pentol S.A. Pentraspan SR Pentritol Pentylan Peritrate Peritrate Forte* Peritrate SA P.E.T.N.	Pentaerythritol Tetranitrate†

*Not available in the U.S.
†Generic name product may also be available in the U.S.

To the Reader: If you do not recognize the names of medical conditions or medicines referred to in this information, check with your doctor, nurse, or pharmacist. Definitions for selected medical terms may be found in the Glossary. Brand names for the generic drug names listed can be found in the Index. In addition, selected brand names commonly associated with the generic name have been included in the text to help you recognize medicine you may be taking. The fact that a brand name

product is not mentioned does not mean the information does not apply. It is a good idea for you to learn both the generic and brand names of your medicines and to write them down for future use.

Nitrates (NYE-trates) are used to treat the symptoms of angina (chest pain). Depending on the type of dosage form and how it is taken, nitrates are used to treat angina in three ways:

—to relieve an attack that is occurring by using the medicine when the attack begins;
—to prevent attacks from occurring by using the medicine just before an attack is expected to occur; or
—to reduce the number of attacks that occur by using the medicine regularly on a long-term basis.

Oral nitrates come in the form of regular tablets, chewable tablets, or extended-release capsules or tablets. When taken orally and swallowed, nitrates are used to reduce the number of angina attacks that occur. They do not act fast enough to relieve the pain of an angina attack.

Nitrates work by relaxing blood vessels and increasing the supply of blood and oxygen to the heart while reducing its work load.

Nitrates may also be used for other conditions as determined by your doctor.

Nitrates are available only with your doctor's prescription.

Remember:
• **This medicine has been prescribed for your current medical problem only.** It must not be given to other people or used for other problems unless you are directed to do so by your doctor.

• **Keep all medicines out of the reach of children.**

• In order for this medicine to work, it must be used as directed.

• **It is very important that you read and understand the following information.** If any of the information causes you special concern, do not decide against using this medicine without first checking with your doctor.

• Before you begin using any new medicine (prescription or nonprescription) or if you develop any new medical problem while you are using this medicine, check with your doctor, nurse, or pharmacist.

• **If you have any questions** about the following information or if you want more information about this medicine or your medical problem, **ask your doctor, nurse, or pharmacist**.

Before Using This Medicine

In order to decide on the best treatment for your medical problem, your doctor should be told:

—if you have ever had any unusual or allergic reaction to nitrates or nitrites.

—if you are on a low-salt, low-sugar, or any other special diet, or if you are allergic to any substance, such as foods, sulfites or other preservatives, or dyes. Most medicines contain more than their active ingredient. Your doctor, nurse, or pharmacist can help you avoid products that may cause a problem.

—if you are **pregnant** or if you may become pregnant. Although nitrates have not been shown to cause problems in humans, studies in rabbits given large doses of isosorbide dinitrate have shown adverse effects on the fetus. Studies have not been done with erythrityl tetranitrate, nitroglycerin, or pentaerythrityl tetranitrate.

—if you are **breast-feeding**. This medicine has not been shown to cause problems in nursing babies.

—if you have any of the following medical problems:
    Anemia (severe)
    Glaucoma
    Intestinal problems
    Overactive thyroid

—if you have recently had a heart attack, stroke, or head injury.

—if you are taking **any** other prescription or nonprescription (OTC) medicine, especially antihypertensives (high blood pressure medicine).

Proper Use of This Medicine

Take this medicine exactly as directed by your doctor. It will work only if taken correctly.

This form of nitrate is used to reduce the number of angina attacks. In most cases, it will not relieve an attack that has already started, because it works too slowly (the extended-release form releases medicine gradually over a 6-hour period to provide its effect for 8 to 10 hours). Check with your doctor if you need a fast-acting medicine to relieve the pain of an angina attack.

Take this medicine with a full glass (8 ounces) of water on an empty stomach. If taken either 1 hour before or 2 hours after meals, it will start working sooner.

Extended-release capsules and tablets are not to be broken, crushed, or chewed before they are swallowed. If broken up, they will not release the medicine properly.

If you are taking this medicine regularly and you miss a dose, take it as soon as possible. However, if the next scheduled dose is within 2 hours (or within 6 hours for extended-release capsules or tablets), skip the missed dose and go back to your regular dosing schedule. Do not double doses.

How to store this medicine:

• **Keep out of the reach of children.**

• Store away from heat and direct light.

• Do not store in the bathroom, near the kitchen sink, or in other damp places. Heat or moisture may cause the medicine to break down.

• Do not keep outdated medicine or medicine no longer needed. Be sure that any discarded medicine is out of the reach of children.

Precautions While Using This Medicine

If you have been taking this medicine regularly for several weeks or more, do not suddenly stop using it. Stopping suddenly may bring on attacks of angina. Check with your doctor for the best way to reduce gradually the amount you are taking before stopping completely.

Dizziness, lightheadedness, or a fainting feeling may occur, especially when you get up quickly from a lying or sitting position. Getting up slowly may help. If you feel dizzy, sit or lie down.

The dizziness, lightheadedness, or fainting is also more likely to occur if you drink alcohol, stand for long periods of time, exercise, or if the weather is hot. **While you are taking this medicine, be careful in the amount of alcohol you drink. Also, use extra care during exercise or hot weather or if you must stand for long periods of time.**

After taking a dose of this medicine you may get a headache that lasts for a short time. This is a common side effect which should become less noticeable after you have taken the medicine for a while. If this effect continues, or if the headaches are severe, check with your doctor.

For patients taking the extended-release dosage forms of isosorbide dinitrate or pentaerythritol tetranitrate:

• Partially dissolved tablets have been found in the stools of a few patients taking the extended-release tablets of this medicine. Be alert to this possibility especially if you have frequent bowel movements, diarrhea, or digestive problems. Notify your doctor if any such tablets are discovered. The tablets must be properly digested in order to provide the correct dose of medicine.

Side Effects of This Medicine

Along with its needed effects, a medicine may cause some unwanted effects. Although not all of these side effects may occur, if they do occur they may need medical attention.

Check with your doctor as soon as possible if any of the following side effects occur:
Rare
    Blurred vision
    Dry mouth
    Headache (severe or prolonged)
    Skin rash
Signs of overdose (in the order in which they may occur)
    Bluish-colored lips, fingernails, or palms of hands
    Dizziness (extreme) or fainting
    Feeling of extreme pressure in head
    Shortness of breath
    Unusual tiredness or weakness
    Weak and fast heartbeat
    Fever
    Convulsions (seizures)

Other side effects may occur that usually do not require medical attention. These side effects may go away during treatment as your body adjusts to the medicine. However, check with your doctor if any of the following side effects continue or are bothersome:

More common

    Dizziness or lightheadedness, especially when getting up from a lying or sitting position
    Fast pulse
    Flushing of face and neck
    Headache
    Nausea or vomiting
    Restlessness

For elderly patients: Many medicines have not been tested in older people. Therefore, it is not known whether the medicine acts the same way it does in younger adults. Check with your doctor or pharmacist if you notice any unusual effects while taking this medicine or if you think it is not working as it should.

Other side effects not listed above may also occur in some patients. If you notice any other effects, check with your doctor.

_____

December 1987

NITRATES (Systemic—Sublingual, Chewable, or Buccal)

This information applies to the following medicines:

Erythrityl Tetranitrate (e-RI-thri-till tet-ra-NYE-trate)
Isosorbide Dinitrate (eye-soe-SOR-bide dye-NYE-trate)
Nitroglycerin (nye-troe-GLI-ser-in)

This information does *not* apply to amyl nitrite or pentaerythritol tetranitrate.

Some commonly used brand names or other names are:	Generic names:
Cardilate Erythritol Tetranitrate	Erythrityl Tetranitrate
Apo-ISDN* Coronex* Iso-Bid Isonate Isordil Onset Sorate Sorbitrate	Isosorbide Dinitrate†
Glyceryl Trinitrate Nitrogard Nitrogard SR* Nitrostabilin* Nitrostat	Nitroglycerin†‡

*Not available in the U.S.
†Generic name product may also be available in the U.S.
‡Generic name product may also be available in Canada.

To the Reader: If you do not recognize the names of medical conditions or medicines referred to in this information, check with your doctor, nurse, or pharmacist. Definitions for selected medical terms may be found in the Glossary. Brand names for the generic drug names listed can be found in the Index. In addition, selected brand names commonly associated with the generic name have been included in the text to help you recognize medicine you may be taking. The fact that a brand name product is not mentioned does not mean the information does not apply. It is a good idea for you to learn both the generic and brand names of your medicines and to write them down for future use.

Nitrates (NYE-trates) are used to treat the symptoms of angina (chest pain). Depending on the type of dosage form and how it is taken, nitrates are used to treat angina in three ways:

—to relieve an attack that is occurring by using the medicine when the attack begins;

—to prevent attacks from occurring by using the medicine just before an attack is expected to occur; or

—to reduce the number of attacks that occur by using the medicine regularly on a long-term basis.

Nitrates are available in different forms. Sublingual nitrates are generally placed under the tongue where they dissolve and are absorbed through the lining of the mouth. Some can also be used buccally, being placed under the lip or in the cheek. The chewable dosage forms, after being chewed and held in the mouth before swallowing, are absorbed in the same way. **It is important to remember that each dosage form is different and that the specific directions for each type must be followed if the medicine is to work properly.**

Nitrates that are used *to relieve the pain* of an angina attack include:

—sublingual nitroglycerin;
—buccal nitroglycerin;
—sublingual isosorbide dinitrate; and
—chewable isosorbide dinitrate.

Those that can be used *to prevent expected attacks* of angina include:

—sublingual nitroglycerin;
—buccal nitroglycerin;
—sublingual erythrityl tetranitrate;
—sublingual isosorbide dinitrate; and
—chewable isosorbide dinitrate.

Products that are used regularly on a long-term basis *to reduce the number of attacks* that occur include:

—buccal nitroglycerin;
—oral/sublingual erythrityl tetranitrate; and
—chewable isosorbide dinitrate; and
—sublingual isosorbide dinitrate.

Nitrates work by relaxing blood vessels and increasing the supply of blood and oxygen to the heart while reducing its work load.

Nitrates may also be used for other conditions as determined by your doctor.

Nitrates are available only with your doctor's prescription.

Remember:

• **This medicine has been prescribed for your current medical problem only.** It must not be given to other people or used for other problems unless you are directed to do so by your doctor.

• **Keep all medicines out of the reach of children.**

• In order for this medicine to work, it must be used as directed.

• **It is very important that you read and understand the following information.** If any of the information causes you special concern, do not decide against using this medicine without first checking with your doctor.

• Before you begin using any new medicine (prescription or nonprescription) or if you develop any new medical problem while you are using this medicine, check with your doctor, nurse, or pharmacist.

• **If you have any questions** about the following information or if you want more information about this medicine or your medical problem, **ask your doctor, nurse, or pharmacist**.

Before Using This Medicine

In order to decide on the best treatment for your medical problem, your doctor should be told:

—if you have ever had any unusual or allergic reaction to nitrates or nitrites.

—if you are on a low-salt, low-sugar, or any other special diet, or if you are allergic to any substance, such as foods, sulfites or other preservatives, or dyes. Most medicines contain more than their active ingredient. Your doctor, nurse, or pharmacist can help you avoid products that may cause a problem.

—if you are **pregnant** or if you may become pregnant. Although nitrates have not been shown to cause problems in humans, studies in rabbits given large doses of isosorbide dinitrate have shown adverse effects on the fetus. Studies have not been done with erythrityl tetranitrate or nitroglycerin.

—if you are **breast-feeding**. This medicine has not been shown to cause problems in nursing babies.

—if you have any of the following medical problems:

Anemia (severe)
Glaucoma
Intestinal problems
Overactive thyroid

—if you have recently had a heart attack, stroke, or head injury.

—if you are taking **any** other prescription or nonprescription (OTC) medicine, especially antihypertensives (high blood pressure medicine).

Proper Use of This Medicine

Take this medicine exactly as directed by your doctor. It will work only if taken correctly.

Sublingual tablets should not be chewed, crushed, or swallowed. They work much faster when absorbed through the lining of the mouth. Place the tablet under the tongue, between the lip and gum, or between the cheek and gum and let it dissolve there. Do not eat, drink, smoke, or use chewing tobacco while a tablet is dissolving.

Buccal extended-release tablets should not be chewed, crushed, or swallowed. They are designed to release a dose of nitroglycerin over a period of hours, not all at one time.

• Allow the tablet to dissolve slowly in place between the upper lip and gum (above the front teeth), or between the cheek and upper gum. If food or drink is to be taken during the 3 to 5 hours the tablet is dissolving, place the tablet between the *upper* lip and gum, above the front teeth. If you have dentures, you may place the tablet anywhere between the cheek and gum.

• Touching the tablet with your tongue or drinking hot liquids may cause the tablet to dissolve faster.

• Do not go to sleep while a tablet is dissolving because it could slip down your throat and cause choking.

• If you accidentally swallow the tablet, replace it with another one.

• Do not use chewing tobacco while a tablet is in place.

Chewable tablets must be chewed well and held in the mouth for about 2 minutes before swallowing. This will allow the medicine to be absorbed through the lining of the mouth.

For patients using nitroglycerin or isosorbide dinitrate to relieve the pain of an angina attack:

• **When you begin to feel an attack of angina starting (chest pains or a tightness or squeezing in the chest), sit down. Then place a tablet in your mouth, either sublingually or buccally, or chew a chewable tablet.** This medicine works best when you are standing or sitting. However, since you may become dizzy, light-headed, or faint soon after using a tablet, it is safer to sit rather than stand while the medicine is working. If you become dizzy or faint while sitting, take several deep breaths and bend forward with your head between your knees.

• Remain calm and you should feel better in a few minutes.

• **This medicine usually gives relief in 1 to 5 minutes.** However, if the pain is not relieved, and you are using:

—Sublingual tablets, either sublingually or buccally: Use a second tablet. If the pain continues for another 5 minutes, a third tablet may be used. **If you still have the chest pains after a total of 3 tablets in a 15-minute period, contact your doctor or go to a hospital emergency room immediately.**

—Buccal extended-release tablets: **Use a sublingual (under the tongue) nitroglycerin tablet and check with your doctor.** Do not use another tablet since the effects of a buccal tablet last for several hours.

For patients using nitroglycerin, erythrityl tetranitrate, or isosorbide dinitrate to prevent an expected angina attack:

• You may prevent anginal chest pains for up to 1 hour (6 hours for the extended-release nitroglycerin tablet) by using a buccal or sublingual tablet or chewing a chewable tablet 5 to 10 minutes before expected emotional stress or physical exertion that in the past seemed to bring on an attack.

For patients using isosorbide dinitrate or extended-release buccal nitroglycerin regularly on a long-term basis to reduce the number of angina attacks that occur:

• Chewable or sublingual isosorbide dinitrate and buccal extended-release nitroglycerin tablets can be used either to prevent angina attacks or to help relieve an attack that has already started.

• If you miss a dose of this medicine, use it as soon as possible. However, if the next scheduled dose is within 2 hours, skip the missed dose and go back to your regular dosing schedule. Do not double doses.

Stability and storage of sublingual nitroglycerin:

• When properly stored, sublingual nitroglycerin tablets retain their strength until the expiration date printed on the original label. However, because of patient usage, changing temperature and moisture, shaking, and repeated bottle opening, the tablets may be good for only 3 to 6 months. The "stabilized" sublingual tablets may stay good for a longer period of time but require the same care in storage and use.

- Some people think they should test the strength of their sublingual nitroglycerin tablets by looking for a tingling or burning sensation, a feeling of warmth or flushing, or a headache, after a tablet has been dissolved under the tongue. This kind of testing is not completely reliable since some patients may be unable to detect these effects. In addition, newer, stabilized sublingual nitroglycerin tablets are less likely to produce these detectable effects.

- To help keep the nitroglycerin tablets at full strength:
  —keep the medicine in the original glass, screw-cap bottle. For patients who may wish to carry a small number of tablets with them for emergency use, a specially designed container is available. However, only containers specifically labeled as being suitable for use with nitroglycerin sublingual tablets should be used.

  —remove the cotton plug that comes in the bottle and *do not* put it back.

  —**put the cap on the bottle quickly and tightly after each use.**

  —to select a tablet for use, pour several into the bottle cap, take one, and pour the others back into the bottle. Try not to hold them in the palm of your hand because they may pick up moisture and crumble.

  —do not keep other medicines in the same bottle with the nitroglycerin since they will weaken the nitroglycerin effect.

  —keep the medicine handy at all times but try not to carry the bottle close to the body. Medicine may lose strength because of body warmth. Instead, carry the tightly closed bottle in your purse, jacket pocket, or other loose-fitting clothing whenever possible.

  —store the bottle of nitroglycerin tablets in a cool, dry place. Average room temperature away from direct heat or direct sunlight is best. Do not store in the refrigerator or in a bathroom medicine cabinet because the moisture usually present in these areas may cause the tablets to crumble if the container is not tightly closed. Do not keep the tablets in your automobile glove compartment.

- **Keep out of the reach of children.**

- Do not keep outdated medicine or medicine no longer needed. Be sure that any discarded medicine is out of the reach of children.

Stability and storage of erythrityl tetranitrate, isosorbide dinitrate, and buccal extended-release nitroglycerin:

- These forms of nitrates are more stable than sublingual nitroglycerin.

- **Keep out of the reach of children.**

- Store away from heat and direct light.

- Do not store in the bathroom, near the kitchen sink, or in other damp places. Heat or moisture may cause the medicine to break down.

- Do not keep outdated medicine or medicine no longer needed. Be sure that any discarded medicine is out of the reach of children.

Precautions While Using This Medicine

If you have been taking this medicine regularly for several weeks, do not suddenly stop using it. Stopping suddenly may bring on attacks of angina. Check with your doctor for the best way to reduce gradually the amount you are taking before stopping completely.

Dizziness, lightheadedness, or a fainting feeling may occur, especially when you get up quickly from a lying or sitting position. Getting up slowly may help. If you feel dizzy, sit or lie down.

The dizziness, lightheadedness, or fainting is also more likely to occur if you drink alcohol, stand for long periods of time, exercise, or if the weather is hot. **While you are taking this medicine, be careful in the amount of alcohol you drink. Also, use extra care during exercise or hot weather or if you must stand for long periods of time.**

After taking a dose of this medicine you may get a headache that lasts for a short time. This is a common side effect which should become less noticeable after you have taken the medicine for a while. If this effect continues or if the headaches are severe, check with your doctor.

Side Effects of This Medicine

Along with its needed effects, a medicine may cause some unwanted effects. Although not all of these side effects may occur, if they do occur they may need medical attention.

Check with your doctor as soon as possible if any of the following side effects occur:

Rare
　　Blurred vision
　　Dry mouth
　　Headache (severe or prolonged)
　　Skin rash

Signs of overdose (in the order in which they may occur)
　　Bluish-colored lips, fingernails, or palms of hands
　　Dizziness (extreme) or fainting
　　Feeling of extreme pressure in head
　　Shortness of breath
　　Unusual tiredness or weakness
　　Weak and fast heartbeat
　　Fever
　　Convulsions (seizures)

Other side effects may occur that usually do not require medical attention. These side effects may go away during treatment as your body adjusts to the medicine. However, check with your doctor if any of the following side effects continue or are bothersome:

More common
　　Dizziness or lightheadedness, especially when getting up from a lying or sitting position
　　Fast pulse
　　Flushing of face and neck
　　Headache
　　Nausea or vomiting
　　Restlessness

For elderly patients: Many medicines have not been tested in older people. Therefore, it is not known whether the medicine acts the same way it does in younger adults. Check with your doctor or pharmacist if you notice any unusual effects while taking this medicine or if you think it is not working as it should.

Other side effects not listed above may also occur in some patients. If you notice any other effects, check with your doctor.

December 1987

NITRATES (Systemic—Topical)

This information applies to nitroglycerin ointment and transdermal patches.

Some commonly used brand names or other names are:

Deponit	Nitrol
Glyceryl Trinitrate	Nitrong
Nitro-Bid	Nitrostat
Nitrodisc	NTS
Nitro-Dur	Transderm-Nitro
Nitro-Dur II	

Generic name product may also be available in the U.S.

To the Reader: If you do not recognize the names of medical conditions or medicines referred to in this information, check with your doctor, nurse, or pharmacist. Definitions for selected medical terms may be found in the Glossary. Brand names for the generic drug names listed can be found in the Index. In addition, selected brand names commonly associated with the generic name have been included in the text to help you recognize medicine you may be taking. The fact that a brand name product is not mentioned does not mean the information does not apply. It is a good idea for you to learn both the generic and brand names of your medicines and to write them down for future use.

Nitrates (NYE-trates) are used to treat the symptoms of angina (chest pain). Depending on the type of dosage form and how it is taken, nitrates are used to treat angina in three ways:

—to relieve an attack that is occurring by using the medicine when the attack begins;
—to prevent attacks from occurring by using the medicine just before an attack is expected to occur; or
—to reduce the number of attacks that occur by using the medicine regularly on a long-term basis.

When applied to the skin, nitrates are used to reduce the number of angina attacks that occur. The only nitrate available for this purpose is topical nitroglycerin (nye-troe-GLI-ser-in). It is available either as an ointment or a transdermal (stick-on) patch.

Topical nitroglycerin is absorbed through the skin. It works by relaxing blood vessels and increasing the supply of blood and oxygen to the heart while reducing its work load. This helps prevent future angina attacks from occurring.

Topical nitroglycerin may also be used for other conditions as determined by your doctor.

Nitroglycerin is available only with your doctor's prescription.

Remember:

• **This medicine has been prescribed for your current medical problem only.** It must not be given to other people or used for other problems unless you are directed to do so by your doctor.

• **Keep all medicines out of the reach of children.**

• In order for this medicine to work, it must be used as directed.

• **It is very important that you read and understand the following information.** If any of the information causes you special concern, do not decide against using this medicine without first checking with your doctor.

• Before you begin using any new medicine (prescription or nonprescription) or if you develop any new medical problem while you are using this medicine, check with your doctor, nurse, or pharmacist.

• **If you have any questions** about the following information or if you want more information about this medicine or your medical problem, **ask your doctor, nurse, or pharmacist**.

Before Using This Medicine

In order to decide on the best treatment for your medical problem, your doctor should be told:

—if you have ever had any unusual or allergic reaction to nitrates or nitrites.

—if you are allergic to any substance, such as certain foods or preservatives or dyes. Most medicines contain more than their active ingredient. Your doctor, nurse, or pharmacist can help you avoid products that may cause a problem.

—if you are **pregnant** or if you may become pregnant. Studies have not been done in humans. However, nitroglycerin has not been shown to cause problems.

—if you are **breast-feeding**. This medicine has not been shown to cause problems in nursing babies.

—if you have any of the following medical problems:
   Anemia (severe)
   Glaucoma
   Intestinal problems
   Overactive thyroid

—if you have recently had a heart attack, stroke, or head injury.

—if you are taking **any** other prescription or nonprescription (OTC) medicine, especially antihypertensives (high blood pressure medicine).

Proper Use of This Medicine

Use nitroglycerin exactly as directed by your doctor. It will work only if applied correctly.

The ointment and transdermal forms of nitroglycerin are used to reduce the number of angina attacks. They will not relieve an attack that has already started because they work too slowly. Check with your doctor if you need a fast-acting medicine to relieve the pain of an angina attack.

This medicine usually comes with patient instructions. Read them carefully before using.

For patients using the ointment form of this medicine:

• Before applying a new dose of ointment, remove any ointment remaining on the skin from a previous dose; this will allow the fresh ointment to release the nitroglycerin properly.

• This medicine comes with dose-measuring papers. Use them to measure the length of ointment squeezed from the tube and to apply the ointment to the skin.

© 1988   The United States Pharmacopeial Convention, Inc.

Do not rub or massage the ointment into the skin; just spread in a thin, even layer, covering an area of the same size each time it is applied.

• Apply the ointment to skin that has little or no hair.

• Each dose of ointment is best applied to a different area of skin to prevent irritation or other skin problems.

• If your doctor has ordered an occlusive dressing (for example, kitchen plastic wrap) to be applied over this medicine, make sure you know how to apply it. Since occlusive dressings increase the amount of medicine absorbed through the skin and the possibility of side effects, use them only as directed. If you have any questions about this, check with your doctor, nurse, or pharmacist.

• If you miss a dose of this medicine, apply it as soon as possible unless the next scheduled dose is within 2 hours. Then go back to your regular dosing schedule. Do not increase the amount used.

• How to store this medicine:

—**Keep out of the reach of children.**

—Store the tube of nitroglycerin ointment in a cool place and keep it tightly closed.

—Do not keep outdated medicine or medicine no longer needed. Be sure that any discarded medicine is out of the reach of children.

For patients using the transdermal (stick-on patch) system:

• Do not try to trim or cut the adhesive patch to adjust the dosage. Check with your doctor if you think the medicine is not working as it should.

• Apply the patch to a clean, dry skin area with little or no hair and free of scars, cuts, or irritation. Remove the previous patch before applying a new one.

• Apply a new patch if the first one becomes loose or falls off.

• Each dose is best applied to a different area of skin to prevent skin problems or other irritation.

• If you miss a dose of this medicine, apply it as soon as possible. Then go back to your regular dosing schedule.

• How to store this medicine:

—**Keep out of the reach of children.**

—Store away from heat and direct light.

—Do not store in the bathroom, near the kitchen sink, or in other damp places. Heat or moisture may cause the medicine to break down.

—Do not keep outdated medicine or medicine no longer needed. Be sure that any discarded medicine is out of the reach of children.

Precautions While Using This Medicine

If you have been using nitroglycerin regularly for several weeks or more, do not suddenly stop using it. Stopping suddenly may bring on attacks of angina. Check with your doctor for the best way to reduce gradually the amount you are using before stopping completely.

Dizziness, lightheadedness, or a fainting feeling may occur, especially when you get up quickly from a lying or sitting position. Getting up slowly may help. If you feel dizzy, sit or lie down.

The dizziness, lightheadedness, or fainting is also more likely to occur if you drink alcohol, stand for long periods of time, exercise, or if the weather is hot. **While you are taking this medicine, be careful in the amount of alcohol you drink. Also, use extra care during exercise or hot weather or if you must stand for long periods of time.**

After using a dose of this medicine you may get a headache that lasts for a short time. This is a common side effect, which should become less noticeable after you have used the medicine for a while. If this effect continues, or if the headaches are severe, check with your doctor.

Side Effects of This Medicine

Along with its needed effects, a medicine may cause some unwanted effects. Although not all of these side effects may occur, if they do occur they may need medical attention.

Check with your doctor as soon as possible if any of the following side effects occur:

Rare

Blurred vision
Dry mouth
Headache (severe or prolonged)

Signs of overdose (in the order in which they may occur)

Bluish-colored lips, fingernails, or palms of hands
Dizziness (extreme) or fainting
Feeling of extreme pressure in head
Shortness of breath
Unusual tiredness or weakness
Weak and fast heartbeat
Fever
Convulsions (seizures)

Other side effects may occur that usually do not require medical attention. These side effects may go away during treatment as your body adjusts to the medicine. However, check with your doctor if any of the following side effects continue or are bothersome:

More common

Dizziness or lightheadedness, especially when getting up from a lying or sitting position
Fast pulse
Flushing of face and neck
Headache
Nausea or vomiting
Restlessness

Less common

Sore, reddened skin

For elderly patients: Many medicines have not been tested in older people. Therefore, it is not known whether the medicine acts the same way it does in younger adults. Check with your doctor or pharmacist if you notice any unusual effects while taking this medicine or if you think it is not working as it should.

Other side effects not listed above may also occur in some patients. If you notice any other effects, check with your doctor.

December 1987

NITROFURANTOIN (Systemic)

Some commonly used brand names are:

Apo-Nitrofurantoin*	Macrodantin
Furadantin	Nephronex*
Furalan	Novofuran*

Generic name product may also be available in the U.S.

*Not available in the U.S.

To the Reader: If you do not recognize the names of medical conditions or medicines referred to in this information, check with your doctor, nurse, or pharmacist. Definitions for selected medical terms may be found in the Glossary. Brand names for the generic drug names listed can be found in the Index. In addition, selected brand names commonly associated with the generic name have been included in the text to help you recognize medicine you may be taking. The fact that a brand name product is not mentioned does not mean the information does not apply. It is a good idea for you to learn both the generic and brand names of your medicines and to write them down for future use.

Nitrofurantoin (nye-troe-fyoor-AN-toyn) belongs to the family of medicines called anti-infectives. It is taken by mouth to treat infections of the urinary tract. It may also be used for other problems as determined by your doctor.

Nitrofurantoin is available only with your doctor's prescription.

Remember:

• **This medicine has been prescribed for your present infection only.** Another infection later on may require a different medicine. Also, even though other people may have the same symptoms as you, they may have a different kind of infection. Your medicine may not work for them and may even cause them harm. Therefore, **your medicine must not be given to other people or used for other infections** unless you are otherwise directed by your doctor.

• **Keep all medicines out of the reach of children.**

• In order for this medicine to work, it must be used as directed.

• **It is very important that you read and understand the following information.** If any of the information causes you special concern, do not decide against using this medicine without first checking with your doctor.

• Before you begin using any new medicine (prescription or nonprescription) or if you develop any new medical problem while you are using this medicine, check with your doctor, nurse, or pharmacist.

• **If you have any questions** about the following information or if you want more information about this medicine or your medical problem, **ask your doctor, nurse, or pharmacist.**

Before Using This Medicine

In order to decide on the best treatment for your medical problem, your doctor should be told:

—if you have ever had any unusual or allergic reaction to this medicine or to any related medicines such as furazolidone or nitrofurazone.

—if you are on a low-salt, low-sugar, or any other special diet, or if you are allergic to any substance, such as foods, sulfites or other preservatives, or dyes. Most medicines contain more than their active ingredient, and many liquid medicines contain alcohol. Your doctor, nurse, or pharmacist can help you avoid products that may cause a problem.

—if you are **pregnant** and within a week or two of your delivery date. Nitrofurantoin should not be used at term (start of labor) since it may cause problems in the infant.

—if you are **breast-feeding**. Nitrofurantoin passes into the breast milk in small amounts and may cause problems in nursing babies with glucose-6-phosphate dehydrogenase (G6PD) deficiency.

—if you have any of the following medical problems:

Glucose-6-phosphate dehydrogenase (G6PD) deficiency
Kidney disease (other than infection)
Lung disease
Nerve damage

—if you are taking **any** other prescription or nonprescription (OTC) medicine, especially:

Aminoglycosides by injection or topical application (amikacin, gentamicin, kanamycin, neomycin, netilmicin, streptomycin, tobramycin)
Antidiabetic agents, oral (diabetes medicine you take by mouth)
Capreomycin (e.g., Capastat)
Carbamazepine (e.g., Tegretol)
Chloramphenicol (e.g., Chloromycetin)
Chloroquine (e.g., Aralen)
Cisplatin (e.g., Platinol)
Clindamycin (e.g., Cleocin)
Cycloserine (e.g., Seromycin)
Dapsone
Disulfiram (e.g., Antabuse)
Ethambutol (e.g., Myambutol)
Ethionamide (e.g., Trecator-SC)
Ethotoin (e.g., Peganone)
Furazolidone (e.g., Furoxone)
Hydroxychloroquine (e.g., Plaquenil)
Isoniazid (e.g., INH; Nydrazid)
Lincomycin (e.g., Lincocin)
Lindane (topical) (e.g., Kwell)
Lithium (e.g., Lithane)
Mephenytoin (e.g., Mesantoin)
Methyldopa (e.g., Aldomet)
Metronidazole (e.g., Flagyl)
Mexiletine (e.g., Mexitil)
Moxalactam (e.g., Moxam)
Oxamniquine (e.g., Vansil)
Penicillins by injection
Phenytoin (e.g., Dilantin)
Primaquine
Probenecid (e.g., Benemid)
Procainamide (e.g., Pronestyl)
Quinacrine (e.g., Atabrine)
Quinidine (e.g., Quinidex)
Quinine (e.g., Quinamm)
Sulfinpyrazone (e.g., Anturane)
Sulfonamides (sulfa medicine)

Sulfoxone (e.g., Diasone)
Vincristine (e.g., Oncovin)
Vitamin K (e.g., Aqua MEPHYTON; Synkayvite)

—if you have received within the last 30 days or are going to receive diphtheria, tetanus, and pertussis (DTP) vaccine.

Proper Use of This Medicine

Do not give this medicine to infants under 1 month of age.

Nitrofurantoin is best taken with food or milk. This may lessen stomach upset and help your body absorb the medicine better.

For patients taking the oral liquid form of this medicine:

• Shake the oral liquid forcefully before each dose to help make it pour more smoothly and to be sure the medicine is evenly mixed.

• Use a specially marked measuring spoon or other device to measure each dose accurately since the average household teaspoon may not hold the right amount of liquid.

• May be mixed with water, milk, fruit juices, or infants' formulas. If mixed with other liquids, take immediately after mixing. Be sure to drink all the liquid in order to get the full dose of medicine.

To help clear up your infection completely, **keep taking this medicine for the full time of treatment** even if you begin to feel better after a few days. **Do not miss any doses.**

If you do miss a dose of this medicine, take it as soon as possible. However, if it is almost time for your next dose and your dosing schedule is:

• 3 or more doses a day—Space the missed dose and the next dose 2 to 4 hours apart or double your next dose.

Then go back to your regular dosing schedule.

How to store this medicine:

• **Keep out of the reach of children.**

• Store away from heat and direct light.

• Do not store the capsule or tablet form of this medicine in the bathroom, near the kitchen sink, or in other damp places. Heat or moisture may cause the medicine to break down.

• Keep the oral liquid form of this medicine from freezing.

• Do not keep outdated medicine or medicine no longer needed. Be sure that any discarded medicine is out of the reach of children.

Precautions While Using This Medicine

If your symptoms do not improve within a few days, or if they become worse, check with your doctor.

This medicine may cause some people to become dizzy, drowsy, or less alert than they are normally. **Make sure you know how you react to this medicine before** you drive, use machines, or do other jobs that require you to be alert. If these reactions are especially bothersome, check with your doctor.

Diabetics—This medicine may cause false test results with some urine sugar tests. Check with your doctor before changing your diet or the dosage of your diabetes medicine.

Side Effects of This Medicine

Along with its needed effects, a medicine may cause some unwanted effects. Although not all of these side effects may occur, if they do occur they may need medical attention.

Check with your doctor immediately if any of the following side effects occur:

More common

Chest pain
Chills
Cough
Fever
Troubled breathing

Less common

Dizziness
Drowsiness
Headache
Numbness, tingling, or burning of face or mouth
Pale skin
Unusual tiredness or weakness

Rare

Yellow eyes or skin

Other side effects may occur that usually do not require medical attention. These side effects may go away during treatment as your body adjusts to the medicine. However, check with your doctor if any of the following side effects continue or are bothersome:

More common

Abdominal or stomach pain or upset
Diarrhea
Loss of appetite
Nausea or vomiting

Less common

Itching
Skin rash

This medicine may cause the urine to become rust-yellow to brown. This side effect does not require medical attention.

For elderly patients: Many medicines have not been tested in older people. Therefore, it is not known whether the medicine acts the same way it does in younger adults.

Check with your doctor or pharmacist if you notice any unusual effects while taking this medicine or if you think it is not working as it should.

Other side effects not listed above may also occur in some patients. If you notice any other effects, check with your doctor.

_____

December 1987

Additional Information

In addition to the above information, for patients taking nitrofurantoin to *prevent* infections:

• Nitrofurantoin may also be taken as a single dose at bedtime to help *prevent* infections of the urinary tract.

• If you miss the bedtime dose of this medicine, take it as soon as possible. However, if it is almost time for your next bedtime dose, space the missed dose and the next dose 10 to 12 hours apart. Then go back to your regular dosing schedule.

NORFLOXACIN (Systemic)

A commonly used brand name is Noroxin.

To the Reader: If you do not recognize the names of medical conditions or medicines referred to in this information, check with your doctor, nurse, or pharmacist. Definitions for selected medical terms may be found in the Glossary. Brand names for the generic drug names listed can be found in the Index. In addition, selected brand names commonly associated with the generic name have been included in the text to help you recognize medicine you may be taking. The fact that a brand name product is not mentioned does not mean the information does not apply. It is a good idea for you to learn both the generic and brand names of your medicines and to write them down for future use.

Norfloxacin (nor-FLOX-a-sin) belongs to the family of medicines called anti-infectives. Anti-infectives are used in the treatment of infections caused by bacteria. They work by killing bacteria or preventing their growth. This medicine will not work for colds, flu, or other virus infections.

Norfloxacin is taken by mouth to treat infections of the urinary tract. It may also be used for other problems as determined by your doctor.

This medicine is available only with your doctor's prescription.

Remember:

• **This medicine has been prescribed for your present infection only.** Another infection later on may require a different medicine. Also, even though other people may have the same symptoms as you, they may have a different kind of infection. Your medicine may not work for them and may even cause them harm. Therefore, **your medicine must not be given to other people or used for other infections** unless you are otherwise directed by your doctor.

• **Keep all medicines out of the reach of children.**

• In order for this medicine to work, it must be used as directed.

• **It is very important that you read and understand the following information.** If any of the information causes you special concern, do not decide against using this medicine without first checking with your doctor.

• Before you begin using any new medicine (prescription or nonprescription) or if you develop any new medical problem while you are using this medicine, check with your doctor, nurse, or pharmacist.

• **If you have any questions** about the following information or if you want more information about this medicine or your medical problem, **ask your doctor, nurse, or pharmacist.**

Before Using This Medicine

In order to decide on the best treatment for your medical problem, your doctor should be told:

—if you have ever had any unusual or allergic reaction to norfloxacin or to any related medicines such as cinoxacin or nalidixic acid.

—if you are on a low-salt, low-sugar, or any other special diet, or if you are allergic to any substance, such as foods, sulfites or other preservatives, or dyes.

Most medicines contain more than their active ingredient. Your doctor, nurse, or pharmacist can help you avoid products that may cause a problem.

—if you are **pregnant** or if you may become pregnant. Studies have not been done in humans. However, studies in some monkeys have shown that norfloxacin causes a decrease in successful pregnancies and that it may kill the fetus when given in doses of 10 to 15 times the highest human dose. Studies in rats, rabbits, and mice, and other studies in monkeys have not shown that norfloxacin causes birth defects when given in doses of 6 to 50 times the usual human dose. However, use is not recommended during pregnancy since norfloxacin has been shown to cause lameness in young animals.

—if you are **breast-feeding**. It is not known whether norfloxacin passes into the breast milk. Norfloxacin has not been shown to pass into breast milk when it was given in low doses. However, other related drugs do pass into the breast milk. Also, norfloxacin has been shown to cause lameness in young animals. Therefore, use is not recommended in nursing mothers.

—if you have seizures or a history of seizures.

—if you are taking **any** other prescription or nonprescription (OTC) medicine, especially antacids.

Proper Use of This Medicine

Do not give this medicine to infants or children unless otherwise directed by your doctor.

Norfloxacin is best taken with a full glass (8 ounces) of water on an empty stomach (either 1 hour before or 2 hours after meals). **Several additional glasses of water should be taken every day,** unless otherwise directed by your doctor. Drinking extra water will help to prevent unwanted side effects of norfloxacin, especially if you are taking high doses.

To help clear up your infection completely, **keep taking norfloxacin for the full time of treatment,** even if you begin to feel better after a few days. If you stop taking this medicine too soon, your symptoms may return.

This medicine works best when there is a constant amount in the blood or urine. **To help keep the amount constant, do not miss any doses. Also, it is best to take the doses at evenly spaced times day and night.** For example, if you are to take 2 doses a day, the doses should be spaced about 12 hours apart. If this interferes with your sleep or other daily activities, or if you need help in planning the best times to take your medicine, check with your doctor, nurse, or pharmacist.

If you do miss a dose of this medicine, take it as soon as possible. This will help to keep a constant amount of medicine in the blood or urine. However, if it is almost time for your next dose, skip the missed dose and go back to your regular dosing schedule. Do not double doses.

How to store this medicine:

- **Keep out of the reach of children.**

- Store away from heat and direct light.

- Do not store in the bathroom, near the kitchen sink, or in other damp places. Heat or moisture may cause the medicine to break down.

- Do not keep outdated medicine or medicine no longer needed. Be sure that any discarded medicine is out of the reach of children.

Precautions While Using This Medicine

If your symptoms do not improve within a few days, or if they become worse, check with your doctor.

If you are taking antacids, do not take them at the same time that you take norfloxacin. Antacids may keep norfloxacin from working as well. Take antacids at least 2 hours after you take this medicine.

This medicine may cause your eyes to become more sensitive to light than they are normally. Wearing sunglasses and avoiding too much exposure to bright light may help lessen the discomfort.

This medicine may also cause blurred vision or other vision problems, or it may cause some people to become dizzy, lightheaded, drowsy, or less alert than they are normally. **Make sure you know how you react to this medicine before you drive, use machines, or do other jobs that require you to be alert or to see clearly.** If these reactions occur, check with your doctor.

Norfloxacin may cause dryness of the mouth. For temporary relief, use sugarless candy or gum, melt bits of ice in your mouth, or use a saliva substitute. However, if dry mouth continues for more than 2 weeks, check with your dentist. Continuing dryness of the mouth may increase the chance of dental disease, including tooth decay, gum disease, and fungal infections.

Side Effects of This Medicine

Along with its needed effects, a medicine may cause some unwanted effects. Although not all of these side effects may occur, if they do occur they may need medical attention.

Check with your doctor as soon as possible if any of the following side effects occur:

More common
    Dizziness
    Headache
    Lightheadedness

Less common
    Mental depression

Rare
    Blurred or decreased vision
    Change in color vision
    Double vision
    Halos around lights
    Increased sensitivity of the eyes to light
    Overbright appearance of lights

Other side effects may occur that usually do not require medical attention. These side effects may go away during treatment as your body adjusts to the medicine. However, check with your doctor if any of the following side effects continue or are bothersome:

More common
    Drowsiness
    Loss of appetite
    Nausea or vomiting

Less common or rare
    Abdominal or stomach pain or upset
    Blood in urine
    Constipation
    Diarrhea
    Dry mouth
    Lower back pain
    Pain or burning while urinating
    Skin rash, itching, or redness
    Swollen or inflamed joints or tendons
    Trouble in sleeping

For elderly patients: Many medicines have not been tested in older people. Therefore, it is not known whether the medicine acts the same way it does in younger adults. Check with your doctor or pharmacist if you notice any unusual effects while taking this medicine or if you think it is not working as it should.

Other side effects not listed above may also occur in some patients. If you notice any other effects, check with your doctor.

December 1987

NYLIDRIN (Systemic)

Some commonly used brand names are Arlidin, Arlidin Forte*, and PMS Nylidrin*.

---

*Not available in the U.S.

To the Reader: If you do not recognize the names of medical conditions or medicines referred to in this information, check with your doctor, nurse, or pharmacist. Definitions for selected medical terms may be found in the Glossary. Brand names for the generic drug names listed can be found in the Index. In addition, selected brand names commonly associated with the generic name have been included in the text to help you recognize medicine you may be taking. The fact that a brand name product is not mentioned does not mean the information does not apply. It is a good idea for you to learn both the generic and brand names of your medicines and to write them down for future use.

Nylidrin (NYE-li-drin) belongs to the group of medicines called vasodilators. Vasodilators increase the size of blood vessels. Nylidrin is taken by mouth to treat problems due to poor blood circulation.

Nylidrin is available only with your doctor's prescription.

Remember:
• **This medicine has been prescribed for your current medical problem only.** It must not be given to other people or used for other problems unless you are directed to do so by your doctor.

• **Keep all medicines out of the reach of children.**

• In order for this medicine to work, it must be used as directed.

• **It is very important that you read and understand the following information.** If any of the information causes you special concern, do not decide against using this medicine without first checking with your doctor.

• Before you begin using any new medicine (prescription or nonprescription) or if you develop any new medical problem while you are using this medicine, check with your doctor, nurse, or pharmacist.

• **If you have any questions** about the following information or if you want more information about this medicine or your medical problem, **ask your doctor, nurse, or pharmacist.**

Before Using This Medicine

In order to decide on the best treatment for your medical problem, your doctor should be told:
—if you have ever had any unusual or allergic reaction to nylidrin.

—if you are on a low-salt, low-sugar, or any other special diet, or if you are allergic to any substance, such as foods, sulfites or other preservatives, or dyes. Most medicines contain more than their active ingredient. Your doctor, nurse, or pharmacist can help you avoid products that may cause a problem.

—if you are **pregnant** or if you may become pregnant. Studies have not been done in either humans or animals.

—if you are **breast-feeding**. Nylidrin has not been shown to cause problems in nursing babies.

—if you have any of the following medical problems:
Angina (chest pain)
Heart disease
Stomach ulcer

—if you have recently had a heart attack.

—if you are taking **any** other prescription or nonprescription (OTC) medicine.

—if you smoke.

Proper Use of This Medicine

Nylidrin may cause you to have a rapid or pounding heartbeat. In order to keep this from affecting your nighttime sleep, do not take the last dose of the day at bedtime. However, it is best to plan your dose or doses according to a schedule that will least affect your sleep. Ask your doctor, nurse, or pharmacist to help you plan the best time to take this medicine.

If you miss a dose of this medicine, take the missed dose as soon as you remember. However, if it is almost time for the next dose, skip the missed dose and go back to your regular dosing schedule. Do not double doses.

How to store this medicine:
• **Keep out of the reach of children.**

• Store away from heat and direct light.

• Do not store in the bathroom, near the kitchen sink, or in other damp places. Heat or moisture may cause the medicine to break down.

• Do not keep outdated medicine or medicine no longer needed. Be sure that any discarded medicine is out of the reach of children.

Precautions While Using This Medicine

It may take some time for this medicine to work. If you feel that the medicine is not working, do not stop taking it on your own. Instead, check with your doctor.

The helpful effects of this medicine may be decreased if you smoke. If you have any questions about this, check with your doctor.

Side Effects of This Medicine

Along with its needed effects, a medicine may cause some unwanted effects. Although not all of these side effects may occur, if they do occur they may need medical attention.

Check with your doctor as soon as possible if any of the following side effects occur:
Less common
Dizziness
Fast or irregular heartbeat
Weakness or tiredness (continuing)

Signs of overdose
- Blurred vision
- Chest pain
- Decrease in urination or inability to urinate
- Fever
- Metallic taste

Other side effects may occur that usually do not require medical attention. These side effects may go away during treatment as your body adjusts to the medicine. However, check with your doctor if any of the following side effects continue or are bothersome:

Less common
- Chilliness
- Flushing or redness of face
- Headache
- Nausea and vomiting
- Nervousness
- Trembling

For elderly patients: Many medicines have not been tested in older people. Therefore, it is not known whether the medicine acts the same way it does in younger adults. Check with your doctor or pharmacist if you notice any unusual effects while taking this medicine or if you think it is not working as it should. In addition, nylidrin may reduce tolerance to cold temperatures in elderly patients.

Other side effects not listed above may also occur in some patients. If you notice any other effects, check with your doctor.

_____

December 1987

NYSTATIN (Oral)

Some commonly used brand names are:

Mycostatin	Nilstat
Nadostine*	Nystex

Generic name product may also be available in the U.S.

---

*Not available in the U.S.

To the Reader: If you do not recognize the names of medical conditions or medicines referred to in this information, check with your doctor, nurse, or pharmacist. Definitions for selected medical terms may be found in the Glossary. Brand names for the generic drug names listed can be found in the Index. In addition, selected brand names commonly associated with the generic name have been included in the text to help you recognize medicine you may be taking. The fact that a brand name product is not mentioned does not mean the information does not apply. It is a good idea for you to learn both the generic and brand names of your medicines and to write them down for future use.

Nystatin (nye-STAT-in) belongs to the group of medicines called antifungals. The dry powder, lozenge, and liquid forms of this medicine are used to treat infections in the mouth and the tablet form is used to treat intestinal infections.

Nystatin is available only with your doctor's prescription.

Remember:

• **This medicine has been prescribed for your present infection only.** Another infection later on may require a different medicine. Also, even though other people may have the same symptoms as you, they may have a different kind of infection. Your medicine may not work for them and may even cause them harm. Therefore, **your medicine must not be given to other people or used for other infections** unless you are otherwise directed by your doctor.

• **Keep all medicines out of the reach of children.**

• In order for this medicine to work, it must be used as directed.

• **It is very important that you read and understand the following information.** If any of the information causes you special concern, do not decide against using this medicine without first checking with your doctor.

• Before you begin using any new medicine (prescription or nonprescription) or if you develop any new medical problem while you are using this medicine, check with your doctor, nurse, or pharmacist.

• **If you have any questions** about the following information or if you want more information about this medicine or your medical problem, **ask your doctor, nurse, or pharmacist.**

Before Using This Medicine

In order to decide on the best treatment for your medical problem, your doctor should be told:

—if you have ever had any unusual or allergic reaction to nystatin.

—if you are on a low-salt, low-sugar, or any other special diet, or if you are allergic to any substance, such as foods, sulfites or other preservatives, or dyes.

Most medicines contain more than their active ingredient, and many liquid medicines contain alcohol. Your doctor, nurse, or pharmacist can help you avoid products that may cause a problem.

—if you are **pregnant** or if you may become pregnant. However, studies in humans have not shown that oral nystatin causes birth defects or other problems.

—if you are **breast-feeding.** However, oral nystatin has not been shown to cause problems in nursing babies.

Proper Use of This Medicine

For patients taking the dry powder form of nystatin:

• Add about ⅛ teaspoonful of dry powder to about 4 to 8 ounces of water immediately before taking. Stir well.

• Take this medicine by dividing the whole amount (4 to 8 ounces) into several portions, if necessary. Hold each portion of the medicine in your mouth or swish it around in your mouth for as long as possible before swallowing. Be sure to use all the liquid in order to get the full dose of medicine.

For patients taking the lozenge form of nystatin:

• Nystatin lozenges should be held in the mouth and allowed to dissolve slowly and completely. This may take 15 to 30 minutes. Also, the saliva should be swallowed during this time. **Do not chew or swallow the lozenges whole.**

• **Do not give nystatin lozenges to infants or children under 5 years of age** since they may be too young to use the lozenges safely.

For patients taking the oral liquid form of nystatin:

• This medicine is to be taken by mouth even though it may come in a dropper bottle. If it does come in a dropper bottle, use the specially marked dropper to measure each dose accurately.

• Take this medicine by placing ½ of the dose in each side of your mouth. Hold the medicine in your mouth or swish it around in your mouth for as long as possible before swallowing.

To help clear up your infection completely, **keep taking this medicine for the full time of treatment** even though your condition may have improved; **do not miss any doses.**

If you do miss a dose of this medicine, take it as soon as possible. However, if it is almost time for your next dose, skip the missed dose and go back to your regular dosing schedule. Do not double doses.

How to store this medicine:

• **Keep out of the reach of children.**

• Store away from heat and direct light.

• Do not store the tablet form of this medicine in the bathroom, near the kitchen sink, or in other damp places. Heat or moisture may cause the medicine to break down.

• Store the lozenge form in the refrigerator because heat will cause this medicine to break down.

• Keep the oral liquid form of this medicine from freezing.

• Do not keep outdated medicine or medicine no longer needed. Be sure that any discarded medicine is out of the reach of children.

Side Effects of This Medicine

Along with its needed effects, a medicine may cause some unwanted effects. The following side effects may go away during treatment as your body adjusts to the medicine. However, check with your doctor if any of the following side effects continue or are bothersome:

More common with high doses
    Diarrhea
    Nausea or vomiting
    Stomach pain

For elderly patients: Many medicines have not been tested in older people. Therefore, it is not known whether the medicine acts the same way it does in younger adults. Check with your doctor or pharmacist if you notice any unusual effects while taking this medicine or if you think it is not working as it should.

Other side effects not listed above may also occur in some patients. If you notice any other effects, check with your doctor.

December 1987

NYSTATIN (Topical)

Some commonly used brand names are:

Mycostatin	Nilstat
Mykinac	Nyaderm*
Nadostine*	Nystex

Generic name product may also be available in the U.S.

*Not available in the U.S.

To the Reader: If you do not recognize the names of medical conditions or medicines referred to in this information, check with your doctor, nurse, or pharmacist. Definitions for selected medical terms may be found in the Glossary. Brand names for the generic drug names listed can be found in the Index. In addition, selected brand names commonly associated with the generic name have been included in the text to help you recognize medicine you may be taking. The fact that a brand name product is not mentioned does not mean the information does not apply. It is a good idea for you to learn both the generic and brand names of your medicines and to write them down for future use.

Nystatin (nye-STAT-in) belongs to the group of medicines called antifungals. Topical nystatin is used on the skin to treat some types of fungal infections.

Nystatin is available only with your doctor's prescription.

Remember:
• **This medicine has been prescribed for your present infection only.** Another infection later on may require a different medicine. Also, even though other people may have the same symptoms as you, they may have a different kind of infection. Your medicine may not work for them and may even cause them harm. Therefore, **your medicine must not be given to other people or used for other infections** unless you are otherwise directed by your doctor.

• **Keep all medicines out of the reach of children.**

• In order for this medicine to work, it must be used as directed.

• **It is very important that you read and understand the following information.** If any of the information causes you special concern, do not decide against using this medicine without first checking with your doctor.

• Before you begin using any new medicine (prescription or nonprescription) or if you develop any new medical problem while you are using this medicine, check with your doctor, nurse, or pharmacist.

• **If you have any questions** about the following information or if you want more information about this medicine or your medical problem, **ask your doctor, nurse, or pharmacist.**

Before Using This Medicine

In order to decide on the best treatment for your medical problem, your doctor should be told:

—if you have ever had any unusual or allergic reaction to nystatin.

—if you are allergic to any substance, such as certain foods or preservatives or dyes. Most medicines contain more than their active ingredient. Your doctor, nurse, or pharmacist can help you avoid products that may cause a problem.

—if you are **pregnant** or if you may become pregnant. However, nystatin topical preparations have not been shown to cause birth defects or other problems in humans.

—if you are **breast-feeding**. It is not known whether nystatin passes into the breast milk. However, this medicine has not been shown to cause problems in nursing babies.

Proper Use of This Medicine

Apply enough nystatin to cover the affected area.

For patients using the powder form of this medicine on the feet:

• Sprinkle the powder between the toes, on the feet, and in socks and shoes.

The use of any kind of airtight covering over this medicine may increase the chance of irritation. Therefore, **do not bandage, wrap, or apply any airtight covering or other occlusive dressing (for example, kitchen plastic wrap) over this medicine** unless directed to do so by your doctor. When using this medicine on the diaper area of children, **avoid tight-fitting diapers and plastic pants.**

To help clear up your infection completely, **keep using this medicine for the full time of treatment** even though your condition may have improved. **Do not miss any doses.**

If you do miss a dose of this medicine, apply it as soon as possible. Then go back to your regular dosing schedule.

How to store this medicine:

• **Keep out of the reach of children.**

• Store away from heat and direct light.

• Do not store the powder form of this medicine in the bathroom, near the kitchen sink, or in other damp places. Heat or moisture may cause the medicine to break down.

• Keep the cream and ointment forms of this medicine from freezing.

• Do not keep outdated medicine or medicine no longer needed. Be sure that any discarded medicine is out of the reach of children.

Side Effects of This Medicine

Along with its needed effects, a medicine may cause some unwanted effects. Although not all of these side effects may occur, if they do occur they may need medical attention.

Check with your doctor as soon as possible if the following side effect occurs:

Skin irritation not present before using this medicine

Other side effects not listed above may also occur in some patients. If you notice any other effects, check with your doctor.

—————————

December 1987
—————————————————————————————————

NYSTATIN (Vaginal)

Some commonly used brand names are Mycostatin, Nadostine*, and Nilstat.

Generic name product may also be available in the U.S.

*Not available in the U.S.

To the Reader: If you do not recognize the names of medical conditions or medicines referred to in this information, check with your doctor, nurse, or pharmacist. Definitions for selected medical terms may be found in the Glossary. Brand names for the generic drug names listed can be found in the Index. In addition, selected brand names commonly associated with the generic name have been included in the text to help you recognize medicine you may be taking. The fact that a brand name product is not mentioned does not mean the information does not apply. It is a good idea for you to learn both the generic and brand names of your medicines and to write them down for future use.

Nystatin (nye-STAT-in) belongs to the group of medicines called antifungals. Vaginal nystatin tablets are used in the vagina to treat fungal infections of the vagina. Also, they have been used as lozenges to treat fungal infections of the mouth.

Nystatin is available only with your doctor's prescription.

Remember:

• **This medicine has been prescribed for your present infection only.** Another infection later on may require a different medicine. Also, even though other people may have the same symptoms as you, they may have a different kind of infection. Your medicine may not work for them and may even cause them harm. Therefore, **your medicine must not be given to other people or used for other infections** unless you are otherwise directed by your doctor.

• **Keep all medicines out of the reach of children.**

• In order for this medicine to work, it must be used as directed.

• **It is very important that you read and understand the following information.** If any of the information causes you special concern, do not decide against using this medicine without first checking with your doctor.

• Before you begin using any new medicine (prescription or nonprescription) or if you develop any new medical problem while you are using this medicine, check with your doctor, nurse, or pharmacist.

• **If you have any questions** about the following information or if you want more information about this medicine or your medical problem, **ask your doctor, nurse, or pharmacist.**

Before Using This Medicine

In order to decide on the best treatment for your medical problem, your doctor should be told:

—if you have ever had any unusual or allergic reaction to nystatin.

—if you are allergic to any substance, such as certain foods or preservatives or dyes. Most medicines contain more than their active ingredient. Your doctor, nurse, or pharmacist can help you avoid products that may cause a problem.

—if you are **pregnant** or if you may become pregnant. However, nystatin vaginal tablets have not been shown to cause birth defects or other problems in humans.

—if you are **breast-feeding**. However, nystatin vaginal tablets have not been shown to cause problems in nursing babies.

Proper Use of This Medicine

Nystatin usually comes with patient directions. Read them carefully before using this medicine.

This medicine is usually inserted into the vagina with an applicator. However, if you are pregnant, check with your doctor before using the applicator to insert the vaginal tablet.

To help clear up your infection completely, **keep using this medicine for the full time of treatment** even though your condition may have improved. Also, keep using this medicine even if you begin to menstruate during the time of treatment. **Do not miss any doses.**

If you do miss a dose of this medicine, insert it as soon as possible. However, if it is almost time for your next dose, skip the missed dose and go back to your regular dosing schedule.

How to store this medicine:

• **Keep out of the reach of children.**

• Store away from heat and direct light.

• Do not store in the bathroom, near the kitchen sink, or in other damp places. Heat or moisture may cause the medicine to break down.

• Do not keep outdated medicine or medicine no longer needed. Be sure that any discarded medicine is out of the reach of children.

Precautions While Using This Medicine

To help cure the infection and to help prevent reinfection, good health habits are required.

• Wear cotton panties (or panties or pantyhose with cotton crotches) instead of synthetic (for example, nylon, rayon) underclothes.

• Wear freshly laundered underclothes.

If you have any questions about this, check with your doctor, nurse, or pharmacist.

If you have any questions about douching or intercourse during the time of treatment with nystatin, check with your doctor.

Since there may be some vaginal drainage while you are using this medicine, a sanitary napkin may be worn to protect your clothing.

Side Effects of This Medicine

Along with its needed effects, a medicine may cause some unwanted effects. Although not all of these side effects may occur, if they do occur they may need medical attention.

Check with your doctor as soon as possible if the following side effect occurs:

Vaginal irritation not present before using this medicine

Other side effects not listed above may also occur in some patients. If you notice any other effects, check with your doctor.

_____

December 1987

NYSTATIN AND TRIAMCINOLONE
(Topical)

Some commonly used brand names are:

Mycolog-II	Mykacet
Myco-Triacet II	Mytrex F

Generic name product may also be available in the U.S.

To the Reader: If you do not recognize the names of medical conditions or medicines referred to in this information, check with your doctor, nurse, or pharmacist. Definitions for selected medical terms may be found in the Glossary. Brand names for the generic drug names listed can be found in the Index. In addition, selected brand names commonly associated with the generic name have been included in the text to help you recognize medicine you may be taking. The fact that a brand name product is not mentioned does not mean the information does not apply. It is a good idea for you to learn both the generic and brand names of your medicines and to write them down for future use.

Nystatin (nye-STAT-in) and triamcinolone (trye-am-SIN-oh-lone) combination contains an antifungal and an adrenocorticoid (a-dree-noe-KOR-ti-koid) (cortisone-like medicine).

Antifungals are used to treat infections caused by a fungus. They work by killing the fungus or preventing its growth. This medicine will not work for other kinds of infections. Adrenocorticoids belong to the general family of medicines called steroids. They are used to help relieve redness, swelling, itching, and other discomfort of many skin problems.

This medicine is applied to the skin to treat certain fungal infections, such as Candida (Monilia), and to help relieve the discomfort of the infection.

Topical adrenocorticoids may rarely cause some serious side effects. Some of the side effects may be more likely to occur in children. **Before using this medicine in children, be sure to talk to your doctor about these problems, as well as the good this medicine may do.**

Nystatin and triamcinolone combination is available only with your doctor's prescription.

Remember:

• **This medicine has been prescribed for your present medical problem only.** Even though other people may have the same symptoms as you, they may have a different kind of problem. Your medicine may not work for them and may even cause them harm. Therefore, **your medicine must not be given to other people or used for other problems** unless you are otherwise directed by your doctor.

• **Keep all medicines out of the reach of children.**

• In order for this medicine to work, it must be used as directed.

• **It is very important that you read and understand the following information.** If any of the information causes you special concern, do not decide against using this medicine without first checking with your doctor.

• Before you begin using any new medicine (prescription or nonprescription) or if you develop any new medical problem while you are using this medicine, check with your doctor, nurse, or pharmacist.

• **If you have any questions** about the following information or if you want more information about this medicine or your medical problem, **ask your doctor, nurse, or pharmacist.**

Before Using This Medicine

In order to decide on the best treatment for your medical problem, your doctor should be told:

—if you have ever had any unusual or allergic reaction to nystatin or triamcinolone.

—if you are allergic to any substance, such as certain foods or preservatives or dyes. Most medicines contain more than their active ingredient. Your doctor, nurse, or pharmacist can help you avoid products that may cause a problem.

—if you are **pregnant** or if you may become pregnant. Studies on birth defects with nystatin and triamcinolone combination have not been done in humans. However, studies in animals have shown that adrenocorticoids given by mouth or by injection may cause birth defects, even at low doses. Also, some of the stronger adrenocorticoids have been shown to cause birth defects when applied to the skin of animals. Therefore, this medicine should not be used on large areas of skin, in large amounts, or for long periods of time in pregnant patients.

—if you are **breast-feeding**. It is not known whether nystatin or triamcinolone passes into the breast milk. Also, this combination medicine has not been shown to cause problems in humans. However, topical adrenocorticoids may be absorbed into the body. Also, adrenocorticoids given by mouth or by injection do pass into the breast milk and may cause unwanted effects, such as interfering with nursing babies' growth.

—if you have any of the following medical problems:
Herpes
Tuberculosis (TB) of the skin
Vaccinia (cowpox)
Varicella (chickenpox)
Other viral infections of the skin

Proper Use of This Medicine

Do not use this medicine in or around the eyes.

Check with your doctor before using this medicine on any other skin problems since it should not be used on bacterial, viral, or certain fungal skin infections.

Apply a thin layer of this medicine to the affected area and rub in gently and thoroughly.

The use of any kind of airtight covering over this medicine may increase absorption of the medicine and the chance of irritation and other side effects. Therefore, **do not bandage, wrap, or apply any airtight covering or other occlusive dressing (for example, kitchen plastic wrap) over this medicine** unless directed to do so by your doctor. Also, wear loose-fitting clothing when using this medicine on the groin area. When using this medicine on the diaper area of children, **avoid tight-fitting diapers and plastic pants.**

To help clear up your infection completely, **keep using this medicine for the full time of treatment** even though your symptoms may have disappeared. **Do not miss any doses.** However, **do not use this medicine more often or for a longer period of time than your doctor ordered.** To do so may increase absorption through your skin and the chance of side effects. In addition, too much use, especially on thin skin areas (for example, face, armpits, groin), may result in thinning of the skin and stretch marks.

If you do miss a dose of this medicine, apply it as soon as possible. However, if it is almost time for your next dose, skip the missed dose and go back to your regular dosing schedule.

How to store this medicine:

- **Keep out of the reach of children.**

- Store away from heat and direct light.

- Keep the medicine from freezing.

- Do not keep outdated medicine or medicine no longer needed. Be sure that any discarded medicine is out of the reach of children.

Precautions While Using This Medicine

To help clear up your infection completely and to help make sure it does not return, good health habits are also required. Keep the affected area as cool and dry as possible.

If your skin problem does not improve within 2 or 3 weeks, or if it becomes worse, check with your doctor.

The adrenocorticoid in this medicine may be absorbed through the skin and may be more likely to cause side effects in children. Long-term use may affect growth and development as well. **Children who must use this medicine should be followed closely by their doctor.**

Diabetics—Although rare, the adrenocorticoid in this medicine may cause higher blood and urine sugar levels, especially if you have severe diabetes and are using
large amounts of this medicine. Check with your doctor before changing your diet or the dosage of your diabetes medicine.

Side Effects of This Medicine

Along with its needed effects, a medicine may cause some unwanted effects. Although not all of these side effects may occur, if they do occur they may need medical attention.

Check with your doctor immediately if any of the following side effects occur:
Rare
     Blistering, burning, itching, peeling, dryness, or other sign of irritation not present before using this medicine

Additional side effects may occur if you use this medicine for a long period of time. Check with your doctor as soon as possible if any of the following side effects occur:
     Acne or oily skin
     Increased hair growth, especially on the face
     Increased loss of hair, especially on the scalp
     Reddish purple lines on arms, face, legs, trunk, or groin
     Thinning of skin with easy bruising

Many of the above side effects are more likely to occur in children, who may absorb greater amounts of this medicine.

For elderly patients: Many medicines have not been tested in older people. Therefore, it is not known whether the medicine acts the same way it does in younger adults. Check with your doctor or pharmacist if you notice any unusual effects while using this medicine or if you think it is not working as it should.

Other side effects not listed above may also occur in some patients. If you notice any other effects, check with your doctor.

December 1987

OPIUM PREPARATIONS (Systemic)

This information applies to the following medicines:
Opium Tincture (OH-pee-um)
Paregoric (par-e-GOR-ik)

Some commonly used names are:	Generic names:
Laudanum	Opium Tincture
Camphorated Opium Tincture	Paregoric

To the Reader: If you do not recognize the names of medical conditions or medicines referred to in this information, check with your doctor, nurse, or pharmacist. Definitions for selected medical terms may be found in the Glossary. Brand names for the generic drug names listed can be found in the Index. In addition, selected brand names commonly associated with the generic name have been included in the text to help you recognize medicine you may be taking. The fact that a brand name product is not mentioned does not mean the information does not apply. It is a good idea for you to learn both the generic and brand names of your medicines and to write them down for future use.

Opium preparations are used along with other measures to treat severe diarrhea. These medicines belong to the group of medicines called narcotics. If too much of a narcotic is taken, it may become habit-forming, causing mental or physical dependence. Physical dependence may lead to withdrawal side effects when you stop taking the medicine.

Opium preparations are available only with your doctor's prescription.

Remember:

• **This medicine has been prescribed for your current medical problem only.** It must not be given to other people or used for other problems unless you are directed to do so by your doctor.

• **Keep all medicines out of the reach of children.**

• In order for this medicine to work, it must be used as directed.

• **It is very important that you read and understand the following information.** If any of the information causes you special concern, do not decide against using this medicine without first checking with your doctor.

• Before you begin using any new medicine (prescription or nonprescription) or if you develop any new medical problem while you are using this medicine, check with your doctor, nurse, or pharmacist.

• **If you have any questions** about the following information or if you want more information about this medicine or your medical problem, **ask your doctor, nurse, or pharmacist.**

Before Using This Medicine

In order to decide on the best treatment for your medical problem, your doctor should be told:

—if you have ever used a medicine like morphine, codeine, or papaverine and had an unusual or allergic reaction to it.

—if you are on a low-salt, low-sugar, or any other special diet, or if you are allergic to any substance, such as foods, sulfites or other preservatives, or dyes.

Most medicines contain more than their active ingredient, and this medicine also contains alcohol. Your doctor, nurse, or pharmacist can help you avoid products that may cause a problem.

—if you are **pregnant** or if you may become pregnant. Although studies on birth defects with these medicines have not been done in humans, opium preparations have not been reported to cause birth defects in humans. However, morphine (contained in these medicines) has been shown to cause birth defects in animals when given in very large doses.

Regular use of opium preparations during pregnancy may cause the fetus to become dependent on the medicine. This may lead to withdrawal side effects in the newborn baby. Also, these medicines may cause breathing problems in the newborn baby, especially if they are taken just before delivery.

—if you are **breast-feeding**. Opium preparations have not been shown to cause problems in nursing babies.

—if you have any of the following medical problems:
Alcoholism, active or treated
Brain disease or head injury
Colitis
Convulsions (seizures), history of
Emphysema, asthma, bronchitis, or other chronic lung disease
Enlarged prostate or problems with urination
Gallbladder disease or gallstones
Heart disease
Kidney disease
Liver disease
Underactive thyroid

—if you regularly drink large amounts of alcoholic beverages.

—if you are taking **any** other prescription or nonprescription (OTC) medicine, especially:
Antimuscarinics (medicine for abdominal or stomach spasms or cramps)
Central nervous system (CNS) depressants, especially other narcotics
Naltrexone (e.g., Trexan)
Other diarrhea medicine
Tricyclic antidepressants (amitriptyline [e.g., Elavil], amoxapine, [e.g., Asendin], clomipramine [e.g., Anafranil], desipramine [e.g., Pertofrane], doxepin [e.g., Sinequan], imipramine [e.g., Tofranil], nortriptyline [e.g., Aventyl], protriptyline [e.g., Vivactil], trimipramine [e.g., Surmontil])

Proper Use of This Medicine

This medicine is to be taken by mouth even though it may come in a dropper bottle. The amount you should take is to be measured with the special dropper provided with your prescription and diluted with water just before you take each dose. This will cause the medicine to turn milky in color, but it will still work.

If your prescription is a liquid form but not in a dropper bottle and the directions on the bottle say to take it by the teaspoonful, it is not necessary to dilute it before using.

If this medicine upsets your stomach, your doctor may want you to take it with food.

Take this medicine only as directed by your doctor. Do not take more of it, do not take it more often, and do not take it for a longer period of time than your doctor ordered. If too much is taken, it may become habit-forming (causing mental or physical dependence) or lead to problems because of an overdose.

If you miss a dose of this medicine, take it as soon as you remember. However, if it is almost time for your next dose, skip the missed dose and go back to your regular dosing schedule. **Do not double doses.**

How to store this medicine:

- **Keep out of the reach of children** because overdose is very dangerous in young children.

- Store away from heat and direct light.

- **Keep the container for this medicine tightly closed** to prevent the alcohol from evaporating and the medicine from becoming stronger.

- **Do not store this medicine in the refrigerator** or allow the medicine to freeze. If it does get cold and you notice any solid particles in it, throw it away.

- Do not keep outdated medicine or medicine no longer needed. Be sure that any discarded medicine is out of the reach of children.

Precautions While Using This Medicine

Check with your doctor if your diarrhea does not stop after 1 or 2 days or if you develop a fever.

This medicine will add to the effects of alcohol and other CNS depressants (medicines that slow down the nervous system, possibly causing drowsiness). Some examples of CNS depressants are antihistamines or medicine for hay fever, other allergies, or colds; sedatives, tranquilizers, or sleeping medicine; prescription pain medicine or other narcotics; barbiturates; medicine for convulsions (seizures); muscle relaxants; or anesthetics, including some dental anesthetics. **Do not drink alcoholic beverages, and check with your doctor before taking any of the medicines listed above, while you are taking this medicine.**

This medicine may cause some people to become drowsy, dizzy, lightheaded, or less alert than they are normally. Even if taken at bedtime, it may cause some people to feel drowsy or less alert on arising. **Make sure you know how you react to this medicine before you drive, use machines, or do other jobs that require you to be alert.**

Dizziness, lightheadedness, or fainting may be especially likely to occur when you get up suddenly from a lying or sitting position. Getting up slowly may help lessen this problem. If you feel very dizzy, lightheaded, or faint after taking this medicine, lying down for a while may help.

If you have been taking this medicine regularly for several weeks or more, **do not stop using it without first checking with your doctor.** Your doctor may want you to reduce gradually the amount you are using before stopping completely, in order to lessen the chance of withdrawal side effects.

If you think you or someone else may have taken an overdose, get emergency help at once. Taking an overdose of this medicine or taking alcohol or other CNS depressants with this medicine may lead to unconsciousness and possibly death. Signs of overdose include convulsions (seizures), confusion, severe nervousness or restlessness, severe dizziness, severe drowsiness, slow or irregular breathing, and severe weakness.

Side Effects of This Medicine

Along with its needed effects, a medicine may cause some unwanted effects. Although not all of these side effects may occur, if they do occur they may need medical attention.

Get emergency help immediately if any of the following signs of overdose occur:
    Cold, clammy skin
    Confusion
    Convulsions (seizures)
    Dizziness (severe)
    Drowsiness (severe)
    Low blood pressure
    Nervousness or restlessness (severe)
    Pinpoint pupils of eyes
    Slow heartbeat
    Slow or irregular breathing
    Weakness (severe)

Also, **check with your doctor immediately** if any of the following side effects are severe and occur suddenly since they may indicate a more severe and dangerous problem with your bowels:
Rare
    Bloating
    Constipation
    Loss of appetite
    Nausea or vomiting
    Stomach cramps or pain

In addition, check with your doctor as soon as possible if any of the following side effects occur:
Rare
    Mental depression
    Shortness of breath or troubled breathing
    Skin rash, hives, or itching
    Slow heartbeat

Other side effects may occur that usually do not require medical attention. These side effects may go away during treatment as your body adjusts to the medicine. However, check with your doctor if any of the following side effects continue or are bothersome:
More common with large doses
    Difficult or painful urination
    Dizziness, lightheadedness, or feeling faint
    Drowsiness

Frequent urge to urinate
Increased sweating
Nervousness or restlessness
Redness or flushing of face
Unusual decrease in amount of urine
Unusual tiredness or weakness

For children and elderly patients: Breathing problems may be more likely to occur in young children and in elderly patients, who are usually more sensitive to the effects of opium preparations.

After you stop using this medicine, your body may need time to adjust. The length of time this takes depends on the amount of medicine you were using and how long you used it. During this period of time check with your doctor if you notice any of the following side effects:

Body aches
Diarrhea
Fever, runny nose, or sneezing

Gooseflesh
Increased sweating
Increased yawning
Loss of appetite
Nausea or vomiting
Nervousness, restlessness, or irritability
Shivering or trembling
Stomach cramps
Trouble in sleeping
Unusually large pupils of eyes
Weakness (severe)

Other side effects not listed above may also occur in some patients. If you notice any other effects, check with your doctor.

_____

December 1987

© 1988   The United States Pharmacopeial Convention, Inc.

ORPHENADRINE (Systemic)

Some commonly used brand names are:

Banflex	Myotrol
Disipal	Neocyten
Flexoject	Norflex
Flexon	O-Flex
K-Flex	Orflagen
Myolin	Orphenate

Generic name product may also be available in the U.S.

To the Reader: If you do not recognize the names of medical conditions or medicines referred to in this information, check with your doctor, nurse, or pharmacist. Definitions for selected medical terms may be found in the Glossary. Brand names for the generic drug names listed can be found in the Index. In addition, selected brand names commonly associated with the generic name have been included in the text to help you recognize medicine you may be taking. The fact that a brand name product is not mentioned does not mean the information does not apply. It is a good idea for you to learn both the generic and brand names of your medicines and to write them down for future use.

Orphenadrine (or-FEN-a-dreen) is used to help relax certain muscles in your body and relieve the pain and discomfort caused by strains, sprains, or other injury to your muscles. One form of orphenadrine is also used to relieve trembling caused by Parkinson's disease. However, this medicine does not take the place of rest, exercise or physical therapy, or other treatment that your doctor may recommend for your medical problem.

Orphenadrine acts in the central nervous system (CNS) to produce its muscle relaxant effects. Orphenadrine also has other actions (antimuscarinic) that produce its helpful effects in Parkinson's disease. Orphenadrine's CNS and antimuscarinic actions may also be responsible for some of its side effects.

This medicine is available only with your doctor's prescription.

Remember:

• **This medicine has been prescribed for your current medical problem only.** It must not be given to other people or used for other problems unless you are directed to do so by your doctor.

• **Keep all medicines out of the reach of children.**

• In order for this medicine to work, it must be used as directed.

• If you are receiving this medicine by injection, some of the information about this medicine may not apply.

• **It is very important that you read and understand the following information.** If any of the information causes you special concern, do not decide against using this medicine without first checking with your doctor.

• Before you begin using any new medicine (prescription or nonprescription) or if you develop any new medical problem while you are using this medicine, check with your doctor, nurse, or pharmacist.

• **If you have any questions** about the following information or if you want more information about this medicine or your medical problem, **ask your doctor, nurse, or pharmacist.**

Before Using This Medicine

In order to decide on the best treatment for your medical problem, your doctor should be told:

—if you have ever had any unusual or allergic reaction to orphenadrine.

—if you are on a low-salt, low-sugar, or any other special diet, or if you are allergic to any substance, such as foods, sulfites or other preservatives, or dyes. Most medicines contain more than their active ingredient. Your doctor, nurse, or pharmacist can help you avoid products that may cause a problem.

—if you are **pregnant** or if you may become pregnant. Orphenadrine has not been shown to cause birth defects or other problems in humans.

—if you are **breast-feeding**. It is not known whether orphenadrine passes into the breast milk. However, orphenadrine has not been shown to cause problems in nursing babies.

—if you have any of the following medical problems:

Disease of the digestive tract, especially esophagus disease, stomach ulcer, or intestinal blockage
Enlarged prostate
Fast or irregular heartbeat
Glaucoma
Heart disease
Kidney disease
Liver disease
Myasthenia gravis
Urinary tract blockage

—if you are now taking or have taken within the past 2 weeks monoamine oxidase (MAO) inhibitors, such as:

Furazolidone (e.g., Furoxone)
Isocarboxazid (e.g., Marplan)
Pargyline (e.g., Eutonyl)
Phenelzine (e.g., Nardil)
Procarbazine (e.g., Matulane)
Tranylcypromine (e.g., Parnate)

—if you are taking **any** other prescription or nonprescription (OTC) medicine, especially:

Central nervous system (CNS) depressants
Tricyclic antidepressants (amitriptyline [e.g., Elavil], amoxapine, [e.g., Asendin], clomipramine [e.g., Anafranil], desipramine [e.g., Pertofrane], doxepin [e.g., Sinequan], imipramine [e.g., Tofranil], nortriptyline [e.g., Aventyl], protriptyline [e.g., Vivactil], trimipramine [e.g., Surmontil])

Proper Use of This Medicine

If you miss a dose of this medicine and remember within an hour or so of the missed dose, take it right away. But if you do not remember until later, skip the missed dose and go back to your regular dosing schedule. Do not double doses.

How to store this medicine:

• **Keep out of the reach of children.**

• Store away from heat and direct light.

• Do not store this medicine in the bathroom, near the kitchen sink, or in other damp places. Heat or moisture may cause the medicine to break down.

• Do not keep outdated medicine or medicine no longer needed. Be sure that any discarded medicine is out of the reach of children.

Precautions While Using This Medicine

If you will be taking this medicine for a long period of time (for example, more than a few weeks), your doctor should check your progress at regular visits.

This medicine may add to the effects of alcohol and other CNS depressants (medicines that slow down the nervous system, possibly causing drowsiness). Some examples of CNS depressants are antihistamines or medicine for hay fever, other allergies, or colds; sedatives, tranquilizers, or sleeping medicine; prescription pain medicine or narcotics; barbiturates; medicine for seizures; other muscle relaxants; or anesthetics, including some dental anesthetics. **Do not drink alcoholic beverages, and check with your doctor before taking any of the medicines listed above, while you are using this medicine.**

This medicine may cause some people to have blurred vision or to become drowsy, dizzy, lightheaded, faint, or less alert than they are normally. It may also cause muscle weakness in some people. **Make sure you know how you react to this medicine before you drive, use machines, or do other jobs that require you to be alert.**

Orphenadrine may cause dryness of the mouth. For temporary relief, use sugarless candy or gum, melt bits of ice in your mouth, or use a saliva substitute. However, if dry mouth continues for more than 2 weeks, check with your dentist. Continuing dryness of the mouth may increase the chance of dental disease, including tooth decay, gum disease, and fungal infections.

Side Effects of This Medicine

Along with its needed effects, a medicine may cause some unwanted effects. Although not all of these side effects may occur, if they do occur they may need medical attention.

Check with your doctor as soon as possible if any of the following side effects occur:

Less common
   Fainting
   Fast or pounding heartbeat

Rare
   Hallucinations (seeing, hearing, or feeling things that are not there)
   Skin rash, hives, itching, or redness
   Unusual tiredness or weakness

Other side effects may occur that usually do not require medical attention. These side effects may go away during treatment as your body adjusts to the medicine. However, check with your doctor if any of the following side effects continue or are bothersome:

More common
   Dry mouth

Less common or rare
   Abdominal or stomach cramps or pain
   Blurred or double vision or other vision problems
   Confusion
   Constipation
   Difficult urination
   Dizziness or lightheadedness
   Drowsiness
   Excitement, irritability, nervousness, or restlessness
   Headache
   Muscle weakness
   Nausea or vomiting
   Trembling

For elderly patients: Many medicines have not been tested in older people. Therefore, it is not known whether the medicine acts the same way it does in younger adults. Check with your doctor or pharmacist if you notice any unusual effects while taking this medicine or if you think it is not working as it should.

Other side effects not listed above may also occur in some patients. If you notice any other effects, check with your doctor.

December 1987

ORPHENADRINE AND ASPIRIN
(Systemic)

Some commonly used brand names are Back-Ese*, Norgesic, and Norgesic Forte.

---

*Not available in the U.S.

To the Reader: If you do not recognize the names of medical conditions or medicines referred to in this information, check with your doctor, nurse, or pharmacist. Definitions for selected medical terms may be found in the Glossary. Brand names for the generic drug names listed can be found in the Index. In addition, selected brand names commonly associated with the generic name have been included in the text to help you recognize medicine you may be taking. The fact that a brand name product is not mentioned does not mean the information does not apply. It is a good idea for you to learn both the generic and brand names of your medicines and to write them down for future use.

Orphenadrine (or-FEN-a-dreen) and aspirin (AS-pir-in) combination is used to help relax certain muscles in your body and relieve the pain and discomfort caused by strains, sprains, or other injury to your muscles. However, this medicine does not take the place of rest, exercise, or other treatment that your doctor may recommend for your medical problem.

Orphenadrine acts in the central nervous system (CNS) to produce its muscle relaxant effects. Actions in the CNS may also be responsible for some of its side effects. Orphenadrine also has other actions (antimuscarinic) which may be responsible for some of its side effects.

This combination medicine also contains caffeine (kaf-EEN).

In the U.S., this combination medicine is available only with your doctor's prescription. In Canada, it is available without a prescription.

Remember:

• **This medicine has been prescribed for your current medical problem only.** It must not be given to other people or used for other problems unless you are directed to do so by your doctor.

• **Keep all medicines out of the reach of children.**

• In order for this medicine to work, it must be used as directed.

• **It is very important that you read and understand the following information.** If any of the information causes you special concern, do not decide against using this medicine without first checking with your doctor.

• Before you begin using any new medicine (prescription or nonprescription) or if you develop any new medical problem while you are using this medicine, check with your doctor, nurse, or pharmacist.

• **If you have any questions** about the following information or if you want more information about this medicine or your medical problem, **ask your doctor, nurse, or pharmacist.**

Before Using This Medicine

In order to decide on the best treatment for your medical problem, your doctor should be told:

—if you have ever had any unusual or allergic reaction to orphenadrine, caffeine, aspirin or other salicylates including methyl salicylate (oil of wintergreen), or to any of the following medicines:

Diclofenac (e.g., Voltaren)
Diflunisal (e.g., Dolobid)
Fenoprofen (e.g., Nalfon)
Flurbiprofen, oral (e.g., Ansaid)
Ibuprofen (e.g., Motrin)
Indomethacin (e.g., Indocin)
Ketoprofen (e.g., Orudis)
Meclofenamate (e.g., Meclomen)
Mefenamic acid (e.g., Ponstel)
Naproxen (e.g., Naprosyn)
Oxyphenbutazone (e.g., Tandearil)
Phenylbutazone (e.g., Butazolidin)
Piroxicam (e.g., Feldene)
Sulindac (e.g., Clinoril)
Suprofen (e.g., Suprol)
Tiaprofenic acid (e.g., Surgam)
Tolmetin (e.g., Tolectin)
Zomepirac (e.g., Zomax)

—if you are on a low-salt, low-sugar, or any other special diet, or if you are allergic to any substance, such as foods, sulfites or other preservatives, or dyes. Most medicines contain more than their active ingredient. Your doctor, nurse, or pharmacist can help you avoid products that may cause a problem.

—if you are **pregnant** or if you may become pregnant. Studies in humans have not shown that aspirin causes birth defects. However, studies in animals have shown that aspirin causes birth defects.

Some reports have suggested that too much use of aspirin late in pregnancy may cause a decrease in the newborn's weight and possible death of the fetus or newborn baby. However, the mothers in these reports had been taking much larger amounts of aspirin than are usually recommended. Studies of mothers taking aspirin in the doses that are usually recommended did not show these unwanted effects.

Regular use of aspirin late in pregnancy may cause unwanted effects on the heart or blood flow in the fetus or in the newborn baby. Also, use of aspirin during the last 2 weeks of pregnancy may cause bleeding problems in the fetus before or during delivery or in the newborn baby. In addition, too much use of aspirin during the last 3 months of pregnancy may increase the length of pregnancy, prolong labor, cause other problems during delivery, or cause severe bleeding in the mother before, during, or after delivery.

Orphenadrine has not been shown to cause birth defects or other problems in humans.

—if you are **breast-feeding**. This medicine has not been shown to cause problems in nursing babies. However, aspirin passes into the breast milk. Also, caffeine passes into the breast milk in small amounts. It is not known whether orphenadrine passes into the breast milk.

—if you have any of the following medical problems:

Anemia
Asthma, allergies, and nasal polyps, history of
Disease of the digestive tract, especially esophagus disease or intestinal blockage
Enlarged prostate
Fast or irregular heartbeat or other heart disease
Glaucoma
Gout
Hemophilia or other bleeding problems
Kidney disease
Liver disease
Myasthenia gravis
Stomach ulcer or other stomach problems
Urinary tract blockage
Vitamin K deficiency

—if you regularly take large amounts of acetaminophen or antacids.

—if you are taking **any** other prescription or nonprescription (OTC) medicine, especially:

Anticoagulants (blood thinners)
Antidiabetic agents, oral (diabetes medicine you take by mouth)
Antimuscarinics (medicine for abdominal or stomach spasms or cramps)
Central nervous system (CNS) depressants
Dipyridamole (e.g., Persantine)
Medicine for pain and/or inflammation
Methotrexate (e.g., Mexate)
Probenecid (e.g., Benemid)
Sulfinpyrazone (e.g., Anturane)
Tricyclic antidepressants (amitriptyline [e.g., Elavil], amoxapine, [e.g., Asendin], clomipramine [e.g., Anafranil], desipramine [e.g., Pertofrane], doxepin [e.g., Sinequan], imipramine [e.g., Tofranil], nortriptyline [e.g., Aventyl], protriptyline [e.g., Vivactil], trimipramine [e.g., Surmontil])
Urinary alkalizers (medicine that makes the urine less acid, such as acetazolamide [e.g., Diamox], dichlorphenamide [e.g., Daranide], methazolamide [e.g., Neptazane], potassium or sodium citrate and/or citric acid)
Vancomycin (e.g., Vancocin)

Proper Use of This Medicine

There is a possibility that use of aspirin (contained in this combination medicine) in children with fever due to a viral infection (especially flu or chickenpox) may cause a serious illness called Reye's syndrome. Do not give this medicine to a child or a teenager with symptoms of flu or chickenpox unless you have first discussed this with your child's doctor.

Take this medicine with food or a full glass (8 ounces) of water to lessen stomach irritation.

Do not take this medicine if it has a strong vinegar-like odor, since this means the aspirin in it is breaking down. If you have any questions about this, check with your doctor or pharmacist.

Do not take more of this medicine than your doctor ordered in order to lessen the chance of side effects or overdose.

If you miss a dose of this medicine and remember within an hour or so of the missed dose, take it right away. But if you do not remember until later, skip the missed dose and go back to your regular dosing schedule. Do not double doses.

How to store this medicine:

• **Keep out of the reach of children** because overdose of aspirin is especially dangerous in young children.

• Store away from heat and direct light.

• Do not store this medicine in the bathroom, near the kitchen sink, or in other damp places. Heat or moisture may cause the medicine to break down.

• Do not keep outdated medicine or medicine no longer needed. Be sure that any discarded medicine is out of the reach of children.

Precautions While Using This Medicine

If you will be taking this medicine for a long period of time (for example, more than a few weeks), your doctor should check your progress at regular visits.

Check the labels of all over-the-counter (OTC), nonprescription, and prescription medicines you now take. If any contain orphenadrine or aspirin or other salicylates be especially careful, since taking them while taking this medicine may lead to overdose. If you have any questions about this, check with your doctor or pharmacist.

Too much use of acetaminophen or certain other medicines together with the aspirin in this combination medicine may increase the chance of side effects. Therefore, do not regularly take acetaminophen or any of the following medicines together with this medicine, unless your doctor has directed you to do so:

Diclofenac (e.g., Voltaren)
Diflunisal (e.g., Dolobid)
Fenoprofen (e.g., Nalfon)
Flurbiprofen, oral (e.g., Ansaid)
Ibuprofen (e.g., Motrin)
Indomethacin (e.g., Indocin)
Ketoprofen (e.g., Orudis)
Meclofenamate (e.g., Meclomen)
Mefenamic acid (e.g., Ponstel)
Naproxen (e.g., Naprosyn)
Phenylbutazone (e.g., Butazolidin)
Piroxicam (e.g., Feldene)
Sulindac (e.g., Clinoril)
Tiaprofenic acid (e.g., Surgam)
Tolmetin (e.g., Tolectin)

Diabetics—The aspirin in this combination medicine may cause false urine sugar test results if you are regularly taking 6 or more of the regular-strength tablets or 3 or more of the double-strength tablets of this medicine a day. Smaller doses or occasional use of aspirin usually will not affect urine sugar tests. If you have any questions about this, check with your doctor, nurse, or pharmacist, especially if your diabetes is not well controlled.

© 1988   The United States Pharmacopeial Convention, Inc.

Do not take this medicine for 5 days before any surgery, including dental surgery, unless otherwise directed by your physician or dentist. Taking aspirin during this time may cause bleeding problems.

The orphenadrine in this combination medicine may add to the effects of alcohol and other CNS depressants (medicines that slow down the nervous system, possibly causing drowsiness). Some examples of CNS depressants are antihistamines or medicine for hay fever, other allergies, or colds; sedatives, tranquilizers, or sleeping medicine; prescription pain medicine or narcotics; barbiturates; medicine for convulsions (seizures); other muscle relaxants; or anesthetics, including some dental anesthetics. Also, stomach problems may be more likely to occur if you drink alcoholic beverages while you are taking aspirin. **Do not drink alcoholic beverages, and check with your doctor before taking any of the medicines listed above, while you are using this medicine.**

This medicine may cause some people to have blurred vision or to become drowsy, dizzy, lightheaded, faint, or less alert than they are normally. **Make sure you know how you react to this medicine before you drive, use machines, or do other jobs that require you to be alert.**

Dryness of the mouth may occur while you are taking this medicine. For temporary relief, use sugarless candy or gum, melt bits of ice in your mouth, or use a saliva substitute. However, if dry mouth continues for more than 2 weeks, check with your dentist. Continuing dryness of the mouth may increase the chance of dental disease, including tooth decay, gum disease, and fungal infections.

If you think that you or someone else may have taken an overdose of this medicine, get emergency help at once. Taking an overdose of this medicine may cause unconsciousness or death. Signs of overdose include convulsions (seizures), hearing loss, confusion, ringing or buzzing in the ears, severe drowsiness or tiredness, severe excitement or nervousness, and unusually fast or deep breathing.

Side Effects of This Medicine

Along with its needed effects, a medicine may cause some unwanted effects. Although not all of these side effects may occur, if they do occur they may need medical attention.

Get emergency help immediately if any of the following signs of overdose occur:

Any loss of hearing
Bloody urine
Confusion
Convulsions (seizures)
Diarrhea
Dizziness or lightheadedness (severe)
Drowsiness (severe)
Excitement or nervousness (severe)
Fast or deep breathing

Hallucinations (seeing, hearing, or feeling things that are not there)
Headache (severe or continuing)
Increased sweating
Nausea or vomiting (severe or continuing)
Ringing or buzzing in the ears (continuing)
Uncontrollable flapping movements of the hands, especially in elderly patients
Unexplained fever
Unusual thirst
Vision problems
Signs of overdose in children
Changes in behavior
Drowsiness or tiredness (severe)
Fast or deep breathing

Also, check with your doctor as soon as possible if any of the following side effects occur:
More common
Nausea or vomiting
Stomach pain
Less common or rare
Bloody or black tarry stools
Fainting
Fast or pounding heartbeat
Shortness of breath, troubled breathing, tightness in chest, or wheezing
Skin rash, hives, itching, or redness
Sore throat and fever
Unusual bleeding or bruising
Unusual tiredness or weakness
Vomiting of blood or material that looks like coffee grounds

Other side effects may occur that usually do not require medical attention. These side effects may go away during treatment as your body adjusts to the medicine. However, check with your doctor if any of the following side effects continue or are bothersome:
More common
Dry mouth
Heartburn or indigestion
Less common
Blurred or double vision or other vision problems
Confusion
Constipation
Difficult urination
Dizziness or lightheadedness
Drowsiness
Excitement, nervousness, or restlessness
Headache
Trembling

For children and elderly patients: Some of the above side effects are more likely to occur in children, especially those with fever or who are dehydrated (those who have lost large amounts of body fluid because of vomiting, diarrhea, or sweating), and in elderly patients (60 years of age or older). These patients are usually more sensitive to the effects of the aspirin in this combination medicine.

Other side effects not listed above may also occur in some patients. If you notice any other effects, check with your doctor.

December 1987

OXAMNIQUINE (Systemic)

A commonly used brand name is Vansil.

To the Reader: If you do not recognize the names of medical conditions or medicines referred to in this information, check with your doctor, nurse, or pharmacist. Definitions for selected medical terms may be found in the Glossary. Brand names for the generic drug names listed can be found in the Index. In addition, selected brand names commonly associated with the generic name have been included in the text to help you recognize medicine you may be taking. The fact that a brand name product is not mentioned does not mean the information does not apply. It is a good idea for you to learn both the generic and brand names of your medicines and to write them down for future use.

Oxamniquine (ox-AM-ni-kwin) belongs to the family of medicines called anthelmintics (ant-hel-MIN-tiks). It is taken by mouth to help the body overcome a certain kind of worm infection (blood fluke), also known as Manson's schistosomiasis (shis-toe-soe-MYE-a-siss) or bilharziasis (bil-har-ZYE-a-siss). It will not work for other kinds of worm infections (for example, pinworms or roundworms).

Oxamniquine is available only with your doctor's prescription.

Remember:

• **This medicine has been prescribed for your present infection only.** Another infection later on may require a different medicine. Also, even though other people may have the same symptoms as you, they may have a different kind of infection. Your medicine may not work for them and may even cause them harm. Therefore, **your medicine must not be given to other people or used for other infections** unless you are otherwise directed by your doctor.

• **Keep all medicines out of the reach of children.**

• In order for this medicine to work, it must be used as directed.

• **It is very important that you read and understand the following information.** If any of the information causes you special concern, do not decide against using this medicine without first checking with your doctor.

• Before you begin using any new medicine (prescription or nonprescription) or if you develop any new medical problem while you are using this medicine, check with your doctor, nurse, or pharmacist.

• **If you have any questions** about the following information or if you want more information about this medicine or your medical problem, **ask your doctor, nurse, or pharmacist.**

Before Using This Medicine

In order to decide on the best treatment for your medical problem, your doctor should be told:

—if you have ever had any unusual or allergic reaction to oxamniquine.

—if you are on a low-salt, low-sugar, or any other special diet, or if you are allergic to any substance, such as foods, sulfites or other preservatives, or dyes.

Most medicines contain more than their active ingredient. Your doctor, nurse, or pharmacist can help you avoid products that may cause a problem.

—if you are **pregnant** or if you may become pregnant. Studies have not been done in humans. However, studies in animals have shown that oxamniquine may harm the unborn animal when given in high doses.

—if you are **breast-feeding**. It is not known whether oxamniquine passes into the breast milk. However, this medicine has not been shown to cause problems in nursing babies.

—if you have any of the following medical problems:
History of epilepsy or other medical problem that causes convulsions
Kidney disease
Liver disease

Proper Use of This Medicine

No special preparations (for example, special diets, fasting, other medicines, laxatives, or enemas) are necessary before, during, or immediately after taking oxamniquine.

Take this medicine after meals to lessen the chance of side effects such as stomach upset, drowsiness, or dizziness, unless otherwise directed by your doctor.

To help clear up your infection completely, **take this medicine exactly as directed by your doctor for the full time of treatment. Do not miss any doses.**

If you do miss a dose of this medicine, take it as soon as possible. However, if it is almost time for your next dose, skip the missed dose and go back to your regular dosing schedule. Do not double doses.

How to store this medicine:

• **Keep out of the reach of children.**

• Store away from heat and direct light.

• Do not store in the bathroom, near the kitchen sink, or in other damp places. Heat or moisture may cause the medicine to break down.

• Do not keep outdated medicine or medicine no longer needed. Be sure that any discarded medicine is out of the reach of children.

Precautions While Using This Medicine

It is important that your doctor check your progress at regular visits.

If your symptoms do not improve after you take this medicine for the full time of treatment, or if they become worse, check with your doctor.

This medicine may cause some people to become dizzy, drowsy, or less alert than they are normally. **Make sure you know how you react to this medicine before you drive, use machines, or do other jobs that require you to be alert.** If these reactions are especially bothersome, check with your doctor.

Side Effects of This Medicine

Along with its needed effects, a medicine may cause some unwanted effects. Although not all of these side effects may occur, if they do occur they may need medical attention.

Check with your doctor immediately if any of the following side effects occur:

Rare
> Convulsions (seizures)
> Fever
> Hallucinations (seeing, hearing, or feeling things that are not there)
> Increased excitement

Other side effects may occur that usually do not require medical attention. These side effects may go away during treatment as your body adjusts to the medicine. However, check with your doctor if any of the following side effects continue or are bothersome:

More common
> Dizziness
> Drowsiness

Less common
> Abdominal or stomach pain
> Diarrhea
> Headache
> Loss of appetite
> Nausea or vomiting
> Skin rash or hives

This medicine may cause the urine to turn reddish orange. This side effect does not require medical attention.

For elderly patients: Many medicines have not been tested in older people. Therefore, it is not known whether the medicine acts the same way it does in younger adults. Check with your doctor or pharmacist if you notice any unusual effects while taking this medicine or if you think it is not working as it should.

Other side effects not listed above may also occur in some patients. If you notice any other effects, check with your doctor.

December 1987

OXTRIPHYLLINE AND GUAIFENESIN
(Systemic)

Some commonly used brand names are Brondecon and Brondelate.

To the Reader: If you do not recognize the names of medical conditions or medicines referred to in this information, check with your doctor, nurse, or pharmacist. Definitions for selected medical terms may be found in the Glossary. Brand names for the generic drug names listed can be found in the Index. In addition, selected brand names commonly associated with the generic name have been included in the text to help you recognize medicine you may be taking. The fact that a brand name product is not mentioned does not mean the information does not apply. It is a good idea for you to learn both the generic and brand names of your medicines and to write them down for future use.

Oxtriphylline (ox-TRYE-fi-lin) and guaifenesin (gwye-FEN-e-sin) combination is used to treat the symptoms of bronchial asthma, chronic bronchitis, emphysema, and other lung diseases. This medicine relieves cough, wheezing, shortness of breath, and troubled breathing. It works by opening up the bronchial tubes or air passages of the lungs and increasing the flow of air through them.

This medicine is available only with your doctor's prescription.

Remember:
- **This medicine has been prescribed for your current medical problem only.** It must not be given to other people or used for other problems unless you are directed to do so by your doctor.

- **Keep all medicines out of the reach of children.**

- In order for this medicine to work, it must be used as directed.

- **It is very important that you read and understand the following information.** If any of the information causes you special concern, do not decide against using this medicine without first checking with your doctor.

- Before you begin using any new medicine (prescription or nonprescription) or if you develop any new medical problem while you are using this medicine, check with your doctor, nurse, or pharmacist.

- **If you have any questions** about the following information or if you want more information about this medicine or your medical problem, **ask your doctor, nurse, or pharmacist.**

Before Using This Medicine

In order to decide on the best treatment for your medical problem, your doctor should be told:

—if you have ever had any unusual or allergic reaction to aminophylline, caffeine, dyphylline, oxtriphylline, theobromine, or theophylline.

—if you are on a low-salt, low-sugar, or any other special diet, or if you are allergic to any substance, such as foods, sulfites or other preservatives, or dyes. Most medicines contain more than their active ingredient, and many liquid medicines contain alcohol. Your doctor, nurse, or pharmacist can help you avoid products that may cause a problem.

—if you are **pregnant** or if you may become pregnant. Studies on birth defects have not been done in humans. However, some studies in animals have shown that oxtriphylline (contained in this combination medicine) causes birth defects when given in doses many times the human dose. Also, use of oxtriphylline during pregnancy may cause unwanted effects such as fast heartbeat, jitteriness, irritability, gagging, vomiting, and breathing problems in the newborn infant. Guaifenesin (contained in this combination medicine) has not been shown to cause birth defects or other problems in humans.

—if you are **breast-feeding.** Theophylline passes into the breast milk and may cause irritability, fretfulness, or trouble in sleeping in babies of mothers taking oxtriphylline (contained in this combination medicine). Guaifenesin (contained in this combination medicine) has not been shown to cause problems in nursing babies.

—if you have any of the following medical problems:
    Diarrhea
    Enlarged prostate
    Fever
    Fibrocystic breast disease
    Heart disease
    Liver disease
    Overactive thyroid
    Respiratory infections, such as influenza (flu)
    Stomach ulcer (or history of) or other stomach problems

—if you are using **any** other prescription or nonprescription (OTC) medicine, especially:
    Beta-blockers (acebutolol [e.g., Sectral], atenolol [e.g., Tenormin], betaxolol [e.g., Betoptic], esmolol [e.g., Brevibloc], labetalol [e.g., Normodyne], levobunolol [e.g., Betagan], metoprolol [e.g., Lopressor], nadolol [e.g., Corgard], oxprenolol [e.g., Trasicor], pindolol [e.g., Visken], propranolol [e.g., Inderal], sotalol [e.g., Sotacor], timolol [e.g., Blocadren, Timoptic])
    Cimetidine (e.g., Tagamet)
    Erythromycin (e.g., E-Mycin)
    Phenytoin (e.g., Dilantin)
    Troleandomycin (e.g., TAO)

—if you smoke or have smoked (tobacco or marijuana) regularly within the last 2 years. The amount of medicine you need may vary, depending on how much and how recently you have smoked.

Proper Use of This Medicine

This medicine works best when taken with a glass of water on an empty stomach (either 30 minutes to 1 hour before meals or 2 hours after meals) since that way it will get into the blood sooner. However, in some cases your doctor may want you to take this medicine with meals or right after meals to lessen stomach upset. If you have any questions about how you should be taking this medicine, check with your doctor.

Take this medicine only as directed by your doctor. Do not take more of it, do not take it more often, and do not take it for a longer period of time than your doctor ordered. To do so may increase the chance of serious side effects.

In order for this medicine to help your medical problem, it must be taken every day in regularly spaced doses as ordered by your doctor. This is necessary to keep a constant amount of the medicine in the blood. To help keep the amount constant, do not miss any doses.

If you do miss a dose of this medicine, take it as soon as possible. However, if it is almost time for your next dose, skip the missed dose and go back to your regular dosing schedule. Do not double doses.

How to store this medicine:

- **Keep out of the reach of children.**
- Store away from heat and direct light.
- Do not store the tablet form of this medicine in the bathroom, near the kitchen sink, or in other damp places. Heat or moisture may cause the medicine to break down.
- Keep the liquid form of this medicine from freezing.
- Do not keep outdated medicine or medicine no longer needed. Be sure that any discarded medicine is out of the reach of children.

Precautions While Using This Medicine

Your doctor should check your progress at regular visits, especially for the first few weeks after you begin using this medicine. A blood test may be taken to help your doctor decide whether the dose of this medicine should be changed.

The oxtriphylline in this medicine may add to the central nervous system stimulant effects of caffeine-containing foods or beverages such as chocolate, cocoa, tea, coffee, and cola drinks. **Avoid eating or drinking large amounts of these foods or beverages while taking this medicine.** If you have any questions about this, check with your doctor.

Do not eat charcoal-broiled foods every day while taking this medicine since these foods may keep the medicine from working as well.

Check with your doctor at once if you develop symptoms of influenza (flu) or a fever since either of these may increase the chance of side effects with this medicine.

Also, **check with your doctor if diarrhea occurs** because the dose of this medicine may need to be changed.

Side Effects of This Medicine

Along with its needed effects, a medicine may cause some unwanted effects. Although not all of these side effects may occur, if they do occur they may need medical attention.

Check with your doctor as soon as possible if any of the following side effects occur:

Less common
  Heartburn and/or vomiting

Signs of overdose
  Bloody or black tarry stools
  Confusion or change in behavior
  Convulsions (seizures)
  Diarrhea
  Dizziness or lightheadedness
  Fast breathing
  Fast, pounding, or irregular heartbeat
  Flushing or redness of face
  Headache
  Increased urination
  Irritability
  Loss of appetite
  Muscle twitching
  Nausea (continuing or severe) or vomiting
  Stomach cramps or pain
  Trembling
  Trouble in sleeping
  Unusual tiredness or weakness
  Vomiting blood or material that looks like coffee grounds

Other side effects may occur that usually do not require medical attention. These side effects may go away during treatment as your body adjusts to the medicine. However, check with your doctor if any of the following side effects continue or are bothersome:

More common
  Nausea
  Nervousness or restlessness

For elderly patients and newborn infants: The above side effects are more likely to occur in elderly patients and newborn infants, who are usually more sensitive to the effects of this medicine.

Other side effects not listed above may also occur in some patients. If you notice any other effects, check with your doctor.

December 1987

OXYBUTYNIN (Systemic)

A commonly used brand name is Ditropan.

To the Reader: If you do not recognize the names of medical conditions or medicines referred to in this information, check with your doctor, nurse, or pharmacist. Definitions for selected medical terms may be found in the Glossary. Brand names for the generic drug names listed can be found in the Index. In addition, selected brand names commonly associated with the generic name have been included in the text to help you recognize medicine you may be taking. The fact that a brand name product is not mentioned does not mean the information does not apply. It is a good idea for you to learn both the generic and brand names of your medicines and to write them down for future use.

Oxybutynin (ox-i-BYOO-ti-nin) belongs to the general group of medicines called antispasmodics. It helps decrease muscle spasms of the bladder and the frequent urge to urinate caused by these spasms.

Oxybutynin is available only with your doctor's prescription.

Remember:

• **This medicine has been prescribed for your current medical problem only.** It must not be given to other people or used for other problems unless you are directed to do so by your doctor.

• **Keep all medicines out of the reach of children.**

• In order for this medicine to work, it must be used as directed.

• **It is very important that you read and understand the following information.** If any of the information causes you special concern, do not decide against using this medicine without first checking with your doctor.

• Before you begin using any new medicine (prescription or nonprescription) or if you develop any new medical problem while you are using this medicine, check with your doctor, nurse, or pharmacist.

• **If you have any questions** about the following information or if you want more information about this medicine or your medical problem, **ask your doctor, nurse, or pharmacist.**

Before Using This Medicine

In order to decide on the best treatment for your medical problem, your doctor should be told:

—if you have ever had any unusual or allergic reaction to oxybutynin.

—if you are on a low-salt, low-sugar, or any other special diet, or if you are allergic to any substance, such as foods, sulfites or other preservatives, or dyes. Most medicines contain more than their active ingredient, and many liquid medicines contain alcohol. Your doctor, nurse, or pharmacist can help you avoid products that may cause a problem.

—if you are **pregnant** or if you may become pregnant. Oxybutynin has not been shown to cause birth defects or other problems in humans or in animal studies.

—if you are **breast-feeding**. Oxybutynin has not been shown to cause problems in nursing babies. However, since this medicine tends to decrease the secretions of the body, it is possible that the flow of breast milk may be reduced in some patients.

—if you have any of the following medical problems:
  Bleeding (severe)
  Colitis (severe)
  Dry mouth (severe and continuing)
  Enlarged prostate
  Hiatal hernia
  Heart disease
  High blood pressure
  Intestinal blockage or other intestinal or stomach problems
  Kidney disease
  Liver disease
  Myasthenia gravis
  Overactive thyroid
  Toxemia of pregnancy
  Urinary tract blockage or problems with urination

—if you are taking **any** other prescription or nonprescription (OTC) medicine, especially:
  Central nervous system (CNS) depressants
  Other antimuscarinics (medicine for abdominal or stomach spasms or cramps)

Proper Use of This Medicine

Take this medicine on an empty stomach with water, or with food or milk to lessen stomach upset, unless otherwise directed by your doctor.

Take this medicine only as directed. Do not take more of it, do not take it more often, and do not take it for a longer period of time than your doctor ordered. To do so may increase the chance of side effects.

If you miss a dose of this medicine, take it as soon as possible. However, if it is almost time for your next dose, skip the missed dose and go back to your regular dosing schedule. Do not double doses.

How to store this medicine:

• **Keep out of the reach of children.**

• Store away from heat and direct light.

• Do not store the tablet form of this medicine in the bathroom, near the kitchen sink, or in other damp places. Heat or moisture may cause the medicine to break down.

• Keep the syrup form of this medicine from freezing.

• Do not keep outdated medicine or medicine no longer needed. Be sure that any discarded medicine is out of the reach of children.

Precautions While Using This Medicine

This medicine will add to the effects of alcohol and other CNS depressants (medicines that slow down the nervous system, possibly causing drowsiness). Some examples of CNS depressants are antihistamines or medicine for hay fever, other allergies, or colds; sedatives, tranquilizers, or sleeping medicine; prescription pain

medicine or narcotics; barbiturates; medicine for seizures; muscle relaxants; or anesthetics, including some dental anesthetics. **Check with your doctor before taking any of the above while you are using this medicine.**

This medicine may cause your eyes to become more sensitive to light than they are normally. Wearing sunglasses may help lessen the discomfort from bright light.

This medicine may cause some people to become drowsy or have blurred vision. **Make sure you know how you react to this medicine before you drive, use machines, or do other jobs that require you to be alert or to see well.**

Oxybutynin may make you sweat less, causing your body temperature to increase. **Use extra care not to become overheated during exercise or hot weather while you are taking this medicine,** since overheating may result in heat stroke.

Your mouth, nose, and throat may feel very dry while you are taking this medicine. For temporary relief of mouth dryness, use sugarless candy or gum, melt bits of ice in your mouth, or use a saliva substitute. However, if dry mouth continues for more than 2 weeks, check with your dentist. Continuing dryness of the mouth may increase the chance of dental disease, including tooth decay, gum disease, and fungal infections.

Side Effects of This Medicine

Along with its needed effects, a medicine may cause some unwanted effects. Although not all of these side effects may occur, if they do occur they may need medical attention.

Check with your doctor as soon as possible if any of the following side effects occur:
Rare
  Eye pain
  Skin rash or hives

Signs of overdose
  Clumsiness or unsteadiness
  Confusion
  Dizziness
  Drowsiness (severe)
  Fast heartbeat
  Fever
  Flushing or redness of face
  Hallucinations (seeing, hearing, or feeling things that are not there)
  Shortness of breath or troubled breathing
  Unusual excitement, nervousness, restlessness, or irritability

Other side effects may occur that usually do not require medical attention. These side effects may go away during treatment as your body adjusts to the medicine. However, check with your doctor if any of the following side effects continue or are bothersome:
More common
  Constipation
  Decrease in sweating
  Drowsiness
  Dryness of mouth, nose, and throat
Less common or rare
  Blurred vision
  Decreased flow of breast milk
  Decreased sexual ability
  Difficult urination
  Difficulty in swallowing
  Headache
  Increased sensitivity of eyes to light
  Nausea or vomiting
  Trouble in sleeping
  Unusual tiredness or weakness

For elderly patients: The above side effects are more likely to occur in the elderly, who are usually more sensitive to the effects of oxybutynin.

Other side effects not listed above may also occur in some patients. If you notice any other effects, check with your doctor.

December 1987

OXYMETAZOLINE (Nasal)

Some commonly used brand names are:

Afrin	Neo-Synephrine 12 Hour
Allerest 12-Hour Nasal	Nostrilla
Coricidin Nasal Mist	NTZ Long Acting Nasal
Dristan Long Lasting	Sinarest 12-Hour
Duramist Plus	Sinex Long-Lasting
Duration	4-Way Long-Acting Nasal
Nafrine*	

Generic name product may also be available in the U.S.

*Not available in the U.S.

To the Reader: If you do not recognize the names of medical conditions or medicines referred to in this information, check with your doctor, nurse, or pharmacist. Definitions for selected medical terms may be found in the Glossary. Brand names for the generic drug names listed can be found in the Index. In addition, selected brand names commonly associated with the generic name have been included in the text to help you recognize medicine you may be taking. The fact that a brand name product is not mentioned does not mean the information does not apply. It is a good idea for you to learn both the generic and brand names of your medicines and to write them down for future use.

Oxymetazoline (ox-i-met-AZ-oh-leen) is used for the temporary relief of nasal congestion or stuffiness caused by hay fever or other allergies, colds, or sinus trouble.

This medicine may also be used for other conditions as determined by your doctor.

This medicine is available without a prescription; however, your doctor may have special instructions on the proper use or dose for your medical condition.

Remember:

• **Keep all medicines out of the reach of children.**

• In order for this medicine to work, it must be used as directed. **If you are using this medicine without a prescription, it is very important to follow the directions on the label.**

• **It is also very important that you read and understand the following information.** If any of the information causes you special concern, check with your doctor or pharmacist.

• Before you begin using any new medicine (prescription or nonprescription) or if you develop any new medical problem while you are using this medicine, check with your doctor, nurse, or pharmacist.

• **If you have any questions** about the following information or if you want more information about this medicine or your medical problem, **ask your doctor, nurse, or pharmacist.**

Before Using This Medicine

Before you use oxymetazoline, check with your doctor or pharmacist:

—if you have ever had any unusual or allergic reaction to nasal decongestants.

—if you are allergic to any substance, such as certain preservatives. Most medicines contain more than their active ingredient. Your doctor, nurse, or pharmacist can help you avoid products that may cause a problem.

—if you are **pregnant** or if you may become pregnant, since the medication may be absorbed into the body. However, oxymetazoline has not been shown to cause birth defects or other problems in humans.

—if you are **breast-feeding**, since oxymetazoline may be absorbed into the body. However, oxymetazoline has not been shown to cause problems in nursing babies.

—if you have any of the following medical problems:
  Diabetes mellitus (sugar diabetes)
  Heart or blood vessel disease
  High blood pressure
  Overactive thyroid

—if you are taking **any** other prescription or nonprescription (OTC) medicine.

Proper Use of This Medicine

For patients using the nose drops:

How to use: Blow the nose gently. Tilt the head back while standing or sitting up, or lie down on a bed and hang the head over the side. Place the drops into each nostril and keep the head tilted back for a few minutes to allow the medicine to spread throughout the nose.

For patients using the nose spray:

How to use: Blow the nose gently. With the head upright, spray the medicine into each nostril. Sniff briskly while squeezing the bottle quickly and firmly. For best results, spray once into each nostril, wait 3 to 5 minutes to allow the medicine to work, then blow the nose gently and thoroughly. Repeat until the complete dose is used.

Wipe the tip of the applicator with a clean, damp tissue and replace the cap right after use. To avoid the spread of infection, do not use the bottle for more than one person.

Use this medicine only as directed. Do not use more of it, do not use it more often, and do not use it for longer than 3 days without first checking with your doctor. To do so may make your runny or stuffy nose worse and may also increase the chance of side effects.

If you miss a dose of this medicine and remember within an hour or so of the missed dose, use it right away. However, if you do not remember until later, skip the missed dose and go back to your regular dosing schedule. Do not double doses.

How to store this medicine:

• **Keep out of the reach of children.**

• Store away from heat and direct light.

• Keep the medicine from freezing.

• Do not keep outdated medicine or medicine no longer needed. Be sure that any discarded medicine is out of the reach of children.

Side Effects of This Medicine

Along with its needed effects, a medicine may cause some unwanted effects. Although not all of these side effects may occur, if they do occur they may need medical attention.

When this medicine is used for short periods of time at low doses, side effects usually are rare. However, check with your doctor as soon as possible if any of the following occur:

   Increase in runny or stuffy nose

Signs of too much medicine being absorbed into the body

   Fast, irregular, or pounding heartbeat
   Headache or lightheadedness
   Nervousness
   Trembling
   Trouble in sleeping

The above side effects are more likely to occur in children because there is a greater chance in children that too much of this medicine may be absorbed into the body.

Other side effects may occur that usually do not require medical attention. These side effects may go away during treatment as your body adjusts to the medicine. However, check with your doctor or pharmacist if any of the following side effects continue or are bothersome:

   Burning, dryness, or stinging on inside of nose
   Sneezing

For elderly patients: Many medicines have not been tested in older people. Therefore, it is not known whether the medicine acts the same way it does in younger adults. Check with your doctor or pharmacist if you notice any unusual effects while using this medicine or if you think it is not working as it should.

Other side effects not listed above may also occur in some patients. If you notice any other effects, check with your doctor or pharmacist.

December 1987

OXYMETAZOLINE (Ophthalmic)

A commonly used brand name is OcuClear.

To the Reader: If you do not recognize the names of medical conditions or medicines referred to in this information, check with your doctor, nurse, or pharmacist. Definitions for selected medical terms may be found in the Glossary. Brand names for the generic drug names listed can be found in the Index. In addition, selected brand names commonly associated with the generic name have been included in the text to help you recognize medicine you may be taking. The fact that a brand name product is not mentioned does not mean the information does not apply. It is a good idea for you to learn both the generic and brand names of your medicines and to write them down for future use.

Oxymetazoline (ox-i-met-AZ-oh-leen) is used in the eye to relieve redness, burning, itching, or other irritation caused by colds, dust, wind, smog, pollen, swimming, contact lenses, or eye strain caused by reading, driving, watching television, or close work.

Oxymetazoline is available without a prescription; however, your doctor may have special instructions on the proper use of this medicine for your medical condition.

Remember:
• **Keep all medicines out of the reach of children.**

• In order for this medicine to work, it must be used as directed. **If you are using this medicine without a prescription, it is very important that you follow the directions on the label.**

• **It is also very important that you read and understand the following information.** If any of the information causes you special concern, check with your doctor or pharmacist.

• Before you begin using any new medicine (prescription or nonprescription) or if you develop any new medical problem while you are using this medicine, check with your doctor, nurse, or pharmacist.

• **If you have any questions** about the following information or if you want more information about this medicine or your medical problem, **ask your doctor, nurse, or pharmacist.**

Before Using This Medicine

Before you use oxymetazoline ophthalmic solution, check with your doctor or pharmacist:

—if you have ever had any unusual or allergic reaction to oxymetazoline or to any other decongestant used in the eye.

—if you are allergic to any substance, such as certain preservatives. Most medicines contain more than their active ingredient. Your doctor, nurse, or pharmacist can help you avoid products that may cause a problem.

—if you are **pregnant** or if you may become pregnant. Oxymetazoline has not been shown to cause birth defects or other problems in humans.

—if you are **breast-feeding**, since oxymetazoline may be absorbed into the body. However, oxymetazoline has not been shown to cause problems in nursing babies.

—if you have any of the following medical problems:
Eye disease, infection, or injury
Heart or blood vessel disease
High blood pressure
Overactive thyroid

—if you wear soft contact lenses.

—if you are taking **any** other prescription or nonprescription (OTC) medicine.

Proper Use of This Medicine

Do not use oxymetazoline ophthalmic solution if it becomes cloudy or changes color.

Check with your doctor before using these eye drops in children. Eye redness in children can occur with illnesses, such as allergies, fevers, colds, and measles, that may require medical attention.

How to apply this medicine: First, wash your hands. With the middle finger, apply pressure to the inside corner of the eye (and continue to apply pressure for 1 or 2 minutes after the medicine has been placed in the eye). Tilt the head back and with the index finger of the same hand, pull the lower eyelid away from the eye to form a pouch. Drop the medicine into the pouch and gently close the eyes. Do not blink. Keep the eyes closed for 1 or 2 minutes to allow the medicine to be absorbed.

To prevent contamination of the eye drops, do not touch the applicator tip to any surface (including the eye), and keep the container tightly closed.

Use this medicine only as directed. Do not use more of it, do not use it more often, and do not use it for more than 4 days, unless otherwise directed by your doctor. To do so may make your eye irritation worse and may also increase the chance of side effects.

How to store this medicine:

• **Keep out of the reach of children.**

• Store away from heat and direct light.

• Keep the medicine from freezing.

• Do not keep outdated medicine or medicine no longer needed. Be sure that any discarded medicine is out of the reach of children.

Precautions While Using This Medicine

If your eye irritation continues or becomes worse, stop using this medicine and check with your doctor.

Side Effects of This Medicine

Along with its needed effects, a medicine may cause some unwanted effects. Although not all of these side effects may occur, if they do occur they may need medical attention.

When this medicine is used for short periods of time at low doses, side effects usually are rare.

Check with your doctor as soon as possible if any of the following side effects occur:

With overuse or long-term use

Increase in irritation or redness of eyes

Signs of too much medicine being absorbed into the body

Fast, irregular, or pounding heartbeat
Headache or lightheadedness
Nervousness
Trembling
Trouble in sleeping

For elderly patients: Many medicines have not been tested in older people. Therefore, it is not known whether the medicine acts the same way it does in younger adults. Check with your doctor or pharmacist if you notice any unusual effects while using this medicine or if you do not think it is working as it should.

Other side effects not listed above may also occur in some patients. If you notice any other effects, check with your doctor.

December 1987

OXYTOCIN (Systemic)

Some commonly used brand names are Pitocin and Syntocinon.

To the Reader: If you do not recognize the names of medical conditions or medicines referred to in this information, check with your doctor, nurse, or pharmacist. Definitions for selected medical terms may be found in the Glossary. Brand names for the generic drug names listed can be found in the Index. In addition, selected brand names commonly associated with the generic name have been included in the text to help you recognize medicine you may be taking. The fact that a brand name product is not mentioned does not mean the information does not apply. It is a good idea for you to learn both the generic and brand names of your medicines and to write them down for future use.

Oxytocin (ox-i-TOE-sin) is a hormone used to help start or continue labor and to control bleeding after delivery. It is also sometimes used to help milk secretion in breast-feeding.

Oxytocin is available only with your doctor's prescription.

Remember:

• **This medicine has been prescribed for your current medical problem only.** It must not be given to other people or used for other problems unless you are directed to do so by your doctor.

• **Keep all medicines out of the reach of children.**

• In order for this medicine to work, it must be used as directed.

• If you are receiving this medicine by injection, some of the information about this medicine may not apply.

• **It is very important that you read and understand the following information.** If any of the information causes you special concern, do not decide against using this medicine without first checking with your doctor.

• Before you begin using any new medicine (prescription or nonprescription) or if you develop any new medical problem while you are using this medicine, check with your doctor, nurse, or pharmacist.

• **If you have any questions** about the following information or if you want more information about this medicine or your medical problem, **ask your doctor, nurse, or pharmacist.**

Before Using This Medicine

In order to decide on the best treatment for your medical problem, your doctor should be told:

—if you have ever had any unusual or allergic reaction to oxytocin.

—if you are allergic to any substance, such as certain preservatives or dyes. Most medicines contain more than their active ingredient. Your doctor, nurse, or pharmacist can help you avoid products that may cause a problem.

For use during labor

Oxytocin can be very useful for helping labor. However, there are certain risks associated with its use. Oxytocin causes contractions of the uterus. In women who are unusually sensitive to its effects, these contractions may become too strong. In rare cases, this may lead to tearing of the uterus. Also, if contractions are too strong, the supply of blood and oxygen to the fetus may be decreased.

Oxytocin has been reported to cause irregular heartbeat and increase bleeding after delivery in some women. It has also been reported to cause jaundice in some newborn infants.

In general, oxytocin should not be used to induce labor unless there are specific medical reasons. Be sure you have discussed this with your doctor before receiving this medicine.

Proper Use of This Medicine

For patients using the nasal spray form of this medicine:

• This medicine usually comes with directions for use. Read them carefully before using.

• How to store this medicine:

—**Keep out of the reach of children.**

—Store away from heat and direct light.

—Protect the medicine from freezing.

—Do not keep outdated medicine or medicine no longer needed. Be sure that any discarded medicine is out of the reach of children.

Side Effects of This Medicine

Along with its needed effects, a medicine may cause some unwanted effects. At usual doses, side effects with this medicine are rare. However, check with your doctor if any of the following side effects continue or are bothersome:

Nausea or vomiting
Rapid or irregular heartbeat

Other side effects not listed above may also occur in some patients. If you notice any other effects, check with your doctor.

December 1987

PANCREATIN, PEPSIN, BILE SALTS, HYOSCYAMINE, ATROPINE, SCOPOLAMINE, AND PHENOBARBITAL
(Systemic)

A commonly used brand name is Donnazyme.

Read the bold information first. Then go back and read the rest. If you do not recognize the names of medical conditions or medicines included in this information, check with your doctor, nurse, or pharmacist. Brand names for the generic drug names listed can also be found in the index. It is a good idea for you to learn both the generic and brand names of your medicines and to write them down for future use.

Pancreatin (PAN-kree-a-tin), pepsin (PEP-sin), bile salts, hyoscyamine (hye-oh-SYE-a-meen), atropine (A-troe-peen), scopolamine (skoe-POL-a-meen), and phenobarbital (fee-noe-BAR-bi-tal) combination is taken by mouth to relieve indigestion in certain conditions in which the body does not produce enough of the enzymes needed for the complete digestion of food.

This medicine is available only with your doctor's prescription.

Remember:

• **This medicine has been prescribed for your current medical problem only.** It must not be given to other people or used for other problems unless you are directed to do so by your doctor.

• **Keep all medicines out of the reach of children.**

• In order for this medicine to work, it must be used as directed.

• **It is very important that you read and understand the following information.** If any of the information causes you special concern, do not decide against using this medicine without first checking with your doctor.

• Before you begin using any new medicine (prescription or nonprescription) or if you develop any new medical problem while you are using this medicine, check with your doctor, nurse, or pharmacist.

• **If you have any questions** about the following information or if you want more information about this medicine or your medical problem, **ask your doctor, nurse, or pharmacist.**

Before Using This Medicine

In order to decide on the best treatment for your medical problem, your doctor should be told:

—if you have ever had any unusual or allergic reaction to any of the belladonna alkaloids such as atropine, hyoscyamine, or scopolamine; to pancrelipase, pancreatin, or beef or pork products; or to barbiturates.

—if you are on a low-salt, low-sugar, or any other special diet, or if you are allergic to any substance, such as foods, sulfites or other preservatives, or dyes. Most medicines contain more than their active ingredient. Your doctor, nurse, or pharmacist can help you avoid products that may cause a problem.

—if you are pregnant or if you intend to become pregnant while taking this medicine. Studies have not been done in either humans or animals.

—if you are breast-feeding. Although this medicine has not been shown to cause problems in humans, the chance always exists.

—if you have any of the following medical problems:
  Bleeding (severe)
  Colitis
  Difficult urination or problems with urination
  Dry mouth (severe and continuing)
  Enlarged prostate
  Heart disease
  Hernia
  High blood pressure
  Intestinal blockage or other intestinal or stomach problems
  Kidney disease
  Liver disease
  Myasthenia gravis
  Overactive thyroid
  Porphyria (or history of)
  Rapid heartbeat
  Urinary tract blockage

—if you are now taking any of the following medicines or types of medicine:
  Antacids
  Anticoagulants, coumarin- or indandione-type (blood thinners)
  Diarrhea medicine containing kaolin or attapulgite
  Medicine containing iron
  Other antimuscarinics (medicine for abdominal or stomach spasms or cramps)
  Tricyclic antidepressants (amitriptyline, amoxapine, clomipramine, desipramine, doxepin, imipramine, nortriptyline, protriptyline, trimipramine)

—if you are now using central nervous system (CNS) depressants, such as:
  Anticonvulsants (seizure medicine)
  Antihistamines or medicine for hay fever, other allergies, or colds
  Barbiturates, other
  Muscle relaxants
  Narcotics
  Prescription pain medicine
  Sedatives, tranquilizers, or sleeping medicine

—if you are now taking or have taken within the past 2 weeks monoamine oxidase (MAO) inhibitors, such as:
  Furazolidone
  Isocarboxazid
  Pargyline
  Phenelzine
  Procarbazine
  Tranylcypromine

Proper Use of This Medicine

Take this medicine with or after meals unless otherwise directed by your doctor.

Take this medicine only as directed by your doctor. Do not take more or less of it, do not take it more often, and do not take it for a longer period of time than your doctor ordered. If too much is used, it may increase the chance of side effects and it may also become habit-forming.

Importance of diet— When prescribing this medicine for your condition, your doctor may also prescribe a personal diet for you. Follow carefully the special diet your doctor gave you. This is most important and necessary for the medicine to work properly and to avoid indigestion.

Swallow the tablets without chewing, to avoid mouth irritation.

If you miss a dose of this medicine, take it as soon as possible. However, if it is almost time for your next dose, skip the missed dose and go back to your regular dosing schedule. Do not double doses.

How to store this medicine:

• Store away from heat and direct light.

• **Keep out of the reach of children** since overdose is especially dangerous in young children.

• Do not store the tablet form of this medicine in the bathroom medicine cabinet because the heat or moisture may cause the medicine to break down.

• Do not keep outdated medicine or medicine no longer needed. Flush the contents of the container down the toilet, unless otherwise directed.

Precautions While Using This Medicine

This medicine will add to the effects of alcohol and other CNS depressants (medicines that slow down the nervous system, possibly causing drowsiness). Some examples of CNS depressants are antihistamines or medicine for hay fever, other allergies, or colds; sedatives, tranquilizers, or sleeping medicine; prescription pain medicine or narcotics; barbiturates; medicine for seizures; muscle relaxants; or anesthetics, including some dental anesthetics. **Check with your doctor before taking any of the above while you are using this medicine.**

This medicine may cause your eyes to become more sensitive to light than they are normally. Wearing sunglasses may help lessen the discomfort from bright light.

This medicine may cause some people to have blurred vision or to become drowsy, dizzy, or less alert than they are normally. **Make sure you know how you react to this medicine before you drive, use machines, or do other jobs that require you to be alert.**

Belladonna alkaloids will often make you sweat less, causing your body temperature to increase. **Use extra care not to become overheated during exercise or hot weather while you are taking this medicine,** as overheating could possibly result in heat stroke.

Your mouth, nose, and throat may feel very dry while you are taking this medicine. For temporary relief of mouth dryness, use sugarless candy or gum, melt bits of ice in your mouth, or use a saliva substitute. However, if dry mouth continues for more than 2 weeks, check with your dentist. Continuing dryness of the mouth may increase the chance of dental disease, including tooth decay, gum disease, and fungal infections.

Side Effects of This Medicine

Along with its needed effects, a medicine may cause some unwanted effects. Although not all of these side effects appear very often, when they do occur they may require medical attention. Check with your doctor as soon as possible if any of the following side effects occur:

Rare

Blood in urine
Diarrhea
Eye pain
Joint pain
Nausea or vomiting
Skin rash or hives
Sore throat and fever
Stomach cramps or pain
Swelling of feet or lower legs
Unusual bleeding or bruising
Yellowing of eyes or skin

Signs of overdose

Clumsiness, unsteadiness, or staggering
Confusion (especially in the elderly)
Dizziness
Fever
Flushing or redness of face
Hallucinations (seeing, hearing, or feeling things that are not there)
Shortness of breath or troubled breathing
Unusual excitement, nervousness, restlessness, or irritability
Unusually slow or fast heartbeat

Other side effects may occur which usually do not require medical attention. These side effects may go away during treatment as your body adjusts to the medicine. However, check with your doctor if any of the following side effects continue or are bothersome:

More common

Constipation
Decrease in sweating
Drowsiness
Dryness of mouth, nose, and throat

Less common or rare

Blurred vision
Decreased flow of breast milk
Decreased sexual ability
Difficult urination (especially in older men)
Difficulty in swallowing
Headache
Increased sensitivity of eyes to light
Trouble in sleeping
Unusual tiredness or weakness

The above side effects are more likely to occur in children and the elderly, who are usually more sensitive to the effects of the belladonna alkaloids and barbiturates. Memory loss may also be more likely to occur in elderly patients.

Other side effects not listed above may also occur in some patients. If you notice any other effects, check with your doctor.

December 1987

PANCRELIPASE (Systemic)

Some commonly used brand names and other names are:

Cotazym	Ku-Zyme HP
Cotazym E.C.S.*	Lipancreatin
Cotazym-S	Pancrease
Festal II	Viokase
Ilozyme	

To the Reader: If you do not recognize the names of medical conditions or medicines referred to in this information, check with your doctor, nurse, or pharmacist. Definitions for selected medical terms may be found in the Glossary. Brand names for the generic drug names listed can be found in the Index. In addition, selected brand names commonly associated with the generic name have been included in the text to help you recognize medicine you may be taking. The fact that a brand name product is not mentioned does not mean the information does not apply. It is a good idea for you to learn both the generic and brand names of your medicines and to write them down for future use.

Pancrelipase (pan-kre-LI-pase) is a medicine taken by mouth to help digestion in certain conditions in which the pancreas is not working properly.

Pancrelipase contains the enzymes needed for the digestion of proteins, starches, and fats.

Pancrelipase is available only with your doctor's prescription.

Remember:

• **This medicine has been prescribed for your current medical problem only.** It must not be given to other people or used for other problems unless you are directed to do so by your doctor.

• **Keep all medicines out of the reach of children.**

• In order for this medicine to work, it must be used as directed.

• **It is very important that you read and understand the following information.** If any of the information causes you special concern, do not decide against using this medicine without first checking with your doctor.

• Before you begin using any new medicine (prescription or nonprescription) or if you develop any new medical problem while you are using this medicine, check with your doctor, nurse, or pharmacist.

• **If you have any questions** about the following information or if you want more information about this medicine or your medical problem, **ask your doctor, nurse, or pharmacist.**

Before Using This Medicine

In order to decide on the best treatment for your medical problem, your doctor should be told:

—if you have ever had any unusual or allergic reaction to pancrelipase, pancreatin, or pork products.

—if you are on a low-salt, low-sugar, or any other special diet, or if you are allergic to any substance, such as foods, sulfites or other preservatives, or dyes. Most medicines contain more than their active ingredient. Your doctor, nurse, or pharmacist can help you avoid products that may cause a problem.

—if you are **pregnant** or if you may become pregnant. Studies have not been done in either humans or animals.

—if you are **breast-feeding**. Pancrelipase has not been shown to cause problems in nursing babies.

—if you are now taking any of the following medicines or types of medicine:

Antacids containing calcium carbonate and/or magnesium hydroxide
Medicine containing iron

Proper Use of This Medicine

Take this medicine before or with meals and snacks, unless otherwise directed by your doctor.

Importance of diet—**When prescribing this medicine for your condition, your doctor may also prescribe a personal diet for you. Follow carefully the special diet your doctor gave you.** This is most important and necessary for the medicine to work properly and to avoid indigestion.

For patients taking the tablet form of this medicine:

• **Swallow the tablets quickly with some liquid, without chewing**, to avoid mouth irritation.

For patients taking the capsules containing the enteric-coated spheres:

• Swallow the capsule whole.

• Do not crush, break, or chew before swallowing.

• When given to children, the capsule may be opened and sprinkled on a small amount of liquid or soft food that can be swallowed without chewing, such as applesauce or gelatin. However, it should not be mixed with alkaline foods, such as milk and ice cream, which may reduce its effect.

If you miss a dose of this medicine, take it as soon as possible. However, if it is almost time for your next dose, skip the missed dose and go back to your regular dosing schedule. Do not double doses.

How to store this medicine:

• **Keep out of the reach of children.**

• Store away from heat and direct light.

• Do not store the capsule, powder, or tablet form of this medicine in the bathroom, near the kitchen sink, or in other damp places. Heat or moisture may cause the medicine to break down.

• Do not keep outdated medicine or medicine no longer needed. Be sure that any discarded medicine is out of the reach of children.

Precautions While Using This Medicine

For patients taking the capsules containing the powder:

• If the capsules are opened to mix with food, be careful not to breathe in the powder. To do so may cause harmful effects such as stuffy nose, shortness of breath, troubled breathing, wheezing, or tightness in chest.

For patients taking the powder form of this medicine:

• Avoid breathing in the powder. To do so may cause harmful effects such as stuffy nose, shortness of breath, troubled breathing, wheezing, or tightness in chest.

Side Effects of This Medicine

Along with its needed effects, a medicine may cause some unwanted effects. Although not all of these side effects may occur, if they do occur they may need medical attention.

Check with your doctor as soon as possible if any of the following side effects occur:

Rare

Skin rash or hives

With high doses

Diarrhea

Nausea

Stomach cramps or pain

With very high doses

Blood in urine

Joint pain

Swelling of feet or lower legs

With powder dosage form or powder from opened capsules—if breathed in

Shortness of breath, troubled breathing, wheezing, or tightness in chest

Stuffy nose

With tablets—if held in mouth

Irritation of the mouth

Other side effects not listed above may also occur in some patients. If you notice any other effects, check with your doctor.

December 1987

PANTOTHENIC ACID (Vitamin B₅) (Systemic)

Some commonly used brand names are Dexol T.D., Durasil, and Pantholin.

Generic name product may also be available in the U.S. and Canada.

To the Reader: If you do not recognize the names of medical conditions or medicines referred to in this information, check with your doctor, nurse, or pharmacist. Definitions for selected medical terms may be found in the Glossary. Brand names for the generic drug names listed can be found in the Index. In addition, selected brand names commonly associated with the generic name have been included in the text to help you recognize medicine you may be taking. The fact that a brand name product is not mentioned does not mean the information does not apply. It is a good idea for you to learn both the generic and brand names of your medicines and to write them down for future use.

Vitamins (VYE-ta-mins) are compounds that you *must* have for growth and health. They are needed in only small amounts and are usually available in the foods that you eat. Pantothenic acid (vitamin B₅) is necessary for normal metabolism.

No problems have been found that are due to a lack of pantothenic acid alone. However, a lack of one B vitamin usually goes along with a lack of others, so pantothenic acid is often included in B complex products.

Claims that pantothenic acid is effective for treatment of nerve damage, breathing problems, itching and other skin problems, and poisoning with some other drugs; for getting rid of or preventing gray hair; for preventing arthritis, allergies, and birth defects; or for improving mental ability have not been proven.

Oral forms of pantothenic acid are available without a prescription. However, it may be a good idea to check with your doctor before taking any on your own. If you take more than you need, it will simply be lost from your body.

Remember:

• **Keep all medicines out of the reach of children.**

• In order for this medicine to work, it must be used as directed. **If you are using this medicine without a prescription, it is very important to follow the directions on the label.**

• **It is also very important that you read and understand the following information.** If any of the information causes you special concern, check with your doctor or pharmacist.

• Before you begin using any new medicine (prescription or nonprescription) or if you develop any new medical problem while you are using this medicine, check with your doctor, nurse, or pharmacist.

• **If you have any questions** about the following information or if you want more information about this medicine or your medical problem, **ask your doctor, nurse, or pharmacist.**

Importance of Diet

Vitamin supplements should be taken only if you cannot get enough vitamins in your diet. A balanced diet should provide all the vitamins you normally need.

Nutritionists recommend that you eat:
• Cereal or bread—4 or more servings per day and
• Dairy products (milk, cheese, ice cream, cottage cheese)—3 or more servings per day and
• Meat, fish, or eggs—2 or more servings per day and
• Vegetables and fruits—4 or more servings per day.

If you are not getting all of these foods every day, you may not be getting enough vitamins in your diet. The best way to correct this is to start eating the foods that contain what you need.

Pantothenic acid is found in various foods including organ meats (such as liver or kidney) and whole-grain cereals. Little pantothenic acid is lost from foods with ordinary cooking.

Vitamins alone will not take the place of a good diet and will not provide energy. Your body also needs other substances found in food—protein, minerals, carbohydrates, and fat. In fact, vitamins themselves often cannot work without the presence of other foods.

In some cases, it may not be possible for you to get enough food to supply you with the proper vitamins. In other cases, the amount of vitamins you need may be increased above normal. Therefore, a vitamin supplement may be needed.

Experts have developed a list of recommended dietary allowances (RDA) for most of the vitamins. The RDA are not an exact number but a general idea of how much you need. They do not cover amounts needed for problems caused by a serious lack of vitamins. Because lack of pantothenic acid is so rare, there are no RDA for this vitamin. However, it is thought that 5 to 10 mg of pantothenic acid a day is plenty. This amount is found in most diets.

Remember:

• The total amount of each vitamin that you get every day includes what you get from the foods that you eat *and* what you may take as a supplement.

• This total amount should not be greater than the RDA, unless ordered by your doctor.

Before Using This Medicine

In deciding whether you need additional pantothenic acid, the following should be kept in mind and/or your doctor should be told:

—if you have ever had any unusual or allergic reaction to pantothenic acid.

—if you are on a low-salt, low-sugar, or any other special diet, or if you are allergic to any substance, such as foods, sulfites or other preservatives, or dyes. Most medicines contain more than their active ingredient. Your doctor, nurse, or pharmacist can help you avoid products that may cause a problem.

—if you are **pregnant** or if you may become pregnant. It is especially important that you are receiving enough vitamins when you become pregnant and that you continue to receive the right amount of vitamins throughout your pregnancy. The healthy growth and development of the fetus depend on a steady supply of nutrients from the mother.

—if you are **breast-feeding**. It is especially important that you receive the right amounts of vitamins so that your baby will also get the vitamins needed to grow properly.

—if you are not able to get a diet that contains all of the vitamins you need.

—if you have hemophilia (a disease in which your blood does not clot normally).

—if you are taking **any** other prescription or nonprescription (OTC) medicine.

Proper Use of This Medicine

Some people believe that taking very large doses of vitamins (called megadoses or megavitamin therapy) is useful for treating certain medical problems. Studies have not proven this. Large doses should be taken only under the direction of your doctor after need has been identified.

If you miss taking a vitamin for one or more days there is no cause for concern, since it takes some time for your body to become seriously low in vitamins. However, if your doctor has recommended that you take this vitamin, try to remember to take it as directed every day.

How to store this medicine:

• **Keep out of the reach of children.**

• Store away from heat and direct light.

• Do not store in the bathroom, near the kitchen sink, or in other damp places. Heat or moisture may cause the medicine to break down.

• Do not keep outdated medicine or medicine no longer needed. Be sure that any discarded medicine is out of the reach of children.

Side Effects of This Medicine

Along with its needed effects, a medicine may cause some unwanted effects. Although pantothenic acid does not usually cause any side effects, check with your doctor if you notice any unusual effects while you are taking it.

December 1987

PAPAVERINE (Intracavernosal)

Generic name product available.

To the Reader: If you do not recognize the names of medical conditions or medicines referred to in this information, check with your doctor, nurse, or pharmacist. Definitions for selected medical terms may be found in the Glossary. Brand names for the generic drug names listed can be found in the Index. In addition, selected brand names commonly associated with the generic name have been included in the text to help you recognize medicine you may be taking. The fact that a brand name product is not mentioned does not mean the information does not apply. It is a good idea for you to learn both the generic and brand names of your medicines and to write them down for future use.

Papaverine (pa-PAV-er-een) belongs to the group of medicines called vasodilators. Vasodilators cause blood vessels to expand, thereby increasing blood flow. Papaverine is used to produce erections in some impotent men. When papaverine is injected into the penis (intracavernosal), it increases blood flow to the penis, which results in an erection.

Papaverine injection should not be used as a sexual aid by men who are not impotent. If the medicine is not used properly, permanent damage to the penis could result.

Papaverine is available only with your doctor's prescription.

Remember:

• **This medicine has been prescribed for your current medical problem only.** It must not be given to other people or used for other problems unless you are directed to do so by your doctor.

• **Keep all medicines out of the reach of children.**

• In order for this medicine to work, it must be used as directed.

• **It is very important that you read and understand the following information.** If any of the information causes you special concern, do not decide against using this medicine without first checking with your doctor.

• Before you begin using any new medicine (prescription or nonprescription) or if you develop any new medical problem while you are using this medicine, check with your doctor, nurse, or pharmacist.

• **If you have any questions** about the following information or if you want more information about this medicine or your medical problem, **ask your doctor, nurse, or pharmacist.**

Before Using This Medicine

In order to decide on the best treatment for your medical problem, your doctor should be told:

—if you have ever had any unusual or allergic reaction to papaverine.

—if you are on a low-salt, low-sugar, or any other special diet, or if you are allergic to any substance, such as foods, sulfites or other preservatives, or dyes.

Most medicines contain more than their active ingredient. Your doctor, nurse, or pharmacist can help you avoid products that may cause a problem.

—if you have any of the following medical problems:
   Bleeding problems
   Liver disease
   Priapism (history of)
   Sickle cell disease

—if you are taking **any** other prescription or nonprescription (OTC) medicine.

Proper Use of This Medicine

How to give papaverine injection:

• Cleanse the injection site with alcohol. Using a sterile needle, **inject the medicine slowly and directly into the base of the penis as instructed by your doctor. Papaverine should not be injected under the skin.** The injection is usually not painful, although you may feel some tingling in the tip of your penis. If the injection is very painful or you notice bruising, that means you have been injecting the medicine under the skin. Stop, withdraw the needle, and reposition it properly before continuing with the injection.

• After you have completed the injection, massage your penis as instructed by your doctor. This helps the medicine spread to all parts of the penis, so that it will work better.

This medicine usually begins to work in about 10 minutes. You should attempt intercourse within 2 hours after injecting the medicine.

How to store this medicine:

• **Keep out of the reach of children.**

• Store away from heat and direct light.

• Keep the medicine from freezing.

Precautions While Using This Medicine

Use papaverine injection exactly as directed by your doctor. Do not use more of it and do not use it more often than ordered. If too much is used, the erection may become so strong that it cannot be reversed. This condition is called priapism, and it can be very dangerous. If the effect is not reversed, the blood supply to the penis may be cut off and permanent damage may occur.

Contact your doctor immediately if the erection lasts for longer than 4 hours or if it becomes painful. This may be a sign of priapism and must be treated right away to prevent permanent damage.

If you notice bleeding at the site when you inject papaverine, put pressure on the spot until the bleeding stops. If it doesn't stop, check with your doctor.

It is important for you to examine your penis regularly. Check with your doctor if you find a lump where the medicine has been injected or if you notice that your penis is becoming curved.

© 1988 The United States Pharmacopeial Convention, Inc.

Side Effects of This Medicine

Along with its needed effects, a medicine may cause some unwanted effects. Although not all of these side effects may occur, if they do occur they may need medical attention.

Check with your doctor immediately if the following side effect occurs:

Rare
>   Erection continuing for more than 4 hours, or painful erection

Check with your doctor as soon as possible if the following side effects occur:

Rare
>   Dizziness
>   Lumps in the penis

Other side effects may occur that usually do not require medical attention. These side effects may go away during treatment as your body adjusts to the medicine. However, check with your doctor if any of the following side effects continue or are bothersome:

Less common or rare
>   Bruising or bleeding at place of injection
>   Burning (mild) along penis
>   Difficulty in ejaculating

Papaverine injected into the penis may cause tingling at the tip of the penis. This is no cause for concern.

Other side effects not listed above may also occur in some patients. If you notice any other effects, check with your doctor.

_____

December 1987

_____

PAPAVERINE (Systemic)

Some commonly used brand names are:

Cerespan	Pavacen	Pavased
Genabid	Pavadur	Pavasule
Pavabid	Pavagen	Pavatine
Pavabid HP	Pava-Par	Pavatym
Pavacap	Pavarine	Paverolan

Generic name product may also be available in the U.S. and Canada.

To the Reader: If you do not recognize the names of medical conditions or medicines referred to in this information, check with your doctor, nurse, or pharmacist. Definitions for selected medical terms may be found in the Glossary. Brand names for the generic drug names listed can be found in the Index. In addition, selected brand names commonly associated with the generic name have been included in the text to help you recognize medicine you may be taking. The fact that a brand name product is not mentioned does not mean the information does not apply. It is a good idea for you to learn both the generic and brand names of your medicines and to write them down for future use.

Papaverine (pa-PAV-er-een) belongs to the group of medicines called vasodilators. Vasodilators cause blood vessels to expand, thereby increasing blood flow. This medicine is used to treat problems resulting from poor blood circulation.

It may also be used for other conditions as determined by your doctor.

Papaverine is available only with your doctor's prescription.

Remember:

• **This medicine has been prescribed for your current medical problem only.** It must not be given to other people or used for other problems unless you are directed to do so by your doctor.

• **Keep all medicines out of the reach of children.**

• In order for this medicine to work, it must be used as directed.

• If you are receiving this medicine by injection, some of the information about this medicine may not apply.

• **It is very important that you read and understand the following information.** If any of the information causes you special concern, do not decide against using this medicine without first checking with your doctor.

• Before you begin using any new medicine (prescription or nonprescription) or if you develop any new medical problem while you are using this medicine, check with your doctor, nurse, or pharmacist.

• **If you have any questions** about the following information or if you want more information about this medicine or your medical problem, **ask your doctor, nurse, or pharmacist.**

Before Using This Medicine

In order to decide on the best treatment for your medical problem, your doctor should be told:

—if you have ever had any unusual or allergic reaction to papaverine.

—if you are on a low-salt, low-sugar, or any other special diet, or if you are allergic to any substance, such as foods, sulfites or other preservatives, or dyes.

Most medicines contain more than their active ingredient. Your doctor, nurse, or pharmacist can help you avoid products that may cause a problem.

—if you are **pregnant** or if you may become pregnant. Studies have not been done in either humans or animals.

—if you are **breast-feeding**. It is not known whether papaverine passes into the breast milk. This medicine has not been shown to cause problems in nursing babies.

—if you have any of the following medical problems:
  Angina (chest pain)
  Glaucoma
  Heart disease

—if you have recently had a heart attack or stroke.

—if you are now taking levodopa (e.g., Larodopa).

—if you smoke.

Proper Use of This Medicine

If this medicine upsets your stomach, it may be taken with meals, milk, or antacids.

For patients taking the extended-release capsule form of this medicine:

• The capsules are to be swallowed whole and must not be chewed or crushed. If the capsule is too large to swallow, mix the contents with a little jam and swallow it without chewing.

For patients taking the extended-release tablet form of this medicine:

• The tablets are not to be chewed or crushed before being swallowed.

If you miss a dose of this medicine, take it as soon as you remember. However, if it is almost time for the next dose, skip the missed dose and go back to your regular dosing schedule. Do not double doses.

How to store this medicine:

• **Keep out of the reach of children.**

• Store away from heat and direct light.

• Do not store in the bathroom, near the kitchen sink, or in other damp places. Heat or moisture may cause the medicine to break down.

• Do not keep outdated medicine or medicine no longer needed. Be sure that any discarded medicine is out of the reach of children.

Precautions While Using This Medicine

It may take some time for this medicine to work. If you feel that the medicine is not working, do not stop taking it on your own. Instead, check with your doctor.

The helpful effects of this medicine may be decreased if you smoke. If you have any questions about this, check with your doctor.

© 1988   The United States Pharmacopeial Convention, Inc.

Dizziness may occur, especially when you get up from a lying or sitting position or climb stairs. Getting up slowly may help. If this problem continues or gets worse, check with your doctor.

Side Effects of This Medicine

Along with its needed effects, a medicine may cause some unwanted effects. Although not all of these side effects may occur, if they do occur they may need medical attention.

Check with your doctor as soon as possible if any of the following side effects occur:

Signs of overdose

    Blurred or double vision
    Drowsiness
    Weakness

Rare

    Yellow eyes and skin

For patients having papaverine injected:
- Check with your doctor if any of the following side effects occur:

    Redness, swelling, or pain at the place of injection

- Also, check with your doctor if any of the following side effects continue or are bothersome:

    Deep breathing
    Dizziness
    Fast heartbeat
    Flushing of the face

Other side effects not listed above may also occur in some patients. If you notice any other effects, check with your doctor.

December 1987

PARALDEHYDE (Systemic)

A commonly used brand name is Paral.

Generic name product may also be available in the U.S.

To the Reader: If you do not recognize the names of medical conditions or medicines referred to in this information, check with your doctor, nurse, or pharmacist. Definitions for selected medical terms may be found in the Glossary. Brand names for the generic drug names listed can be found in the Index. In addition, selected brand names commonly associated with the generic name have been included in the text to help you recognize medicine you may be taking. The fact that a brand name product is not mentioned does not mean the information does not apply. It is a good idea for you to learn both the generic and brand names of your medicines and to write them down for future use.

Paraldehyde (par-AL-de-hyde) is taken by mouth, given by injection, or used rectally to treat certain convulsive disorders. It also has been used in the treatment of alcoholism and in the treatment of nervous and mental conditions to calm or relax patients who are nervous or tense and to produce sleep.

This medicine is available only with your doctor's prescription.

Remember:

• **This medicine has been prescribed for your current medical problem only.** It must not be given to other people or used for other problems unless you are directed to do so by your doctor.

• **Keep all medicines out of the reach of children.**

• In order for this medicine to work, it must be used as directed.

• If you are receiving this medicine by injection, some of the information about this medicine may not apply.

• **It is very important that you read and understand the following information.** If any of the information causes you special concern, do not decide against using this medicine without first checking with your doctor.

• Before you begin using any new medicine (prescription or nonprescription) or if you develop any new medical problem while you are using this medicine, check with your doctor, nurse, or pharmacist.

• **If you have any questions** about the following information or if you want more information about this medicine or your medical problem, **ask your doctor, nurse, or pharmacist.**

Before Using This Medicine

In order to decide on the best treatment for your medical problem, your doctor should be told:

—if you have ever had any unusual or allergic reaction to paraldehyde.

—if you are allergic to any substance, such as foods, sulfites or other preservatives, or dyes. Most medicines contain more than their active ingredient. Your doctor, nurse, or pharmacist can help you avoid products that may cause a problem.

—if you are **pregnant** or if you may become pregnant. Studies on birth defects have not been done in either humans or animals. Use of paraldehyde during labor may cause breathing problems in the newborn infant.

—if you are **breast-feeding.** Paraldehyde has not been shown to cause problems in nursing babies.

—if you have any of the following medical problems:
   Emphysema, asthma, bronchitis, or other chronic lung disease
   Liver disease

—if you have gastroenteritis (stomach flu) or stomach ulcer. Your doctor may not want you to take this medicine by mouth since it may make your condition worse.

—if you have colitis. Your doctor may not want you to use the rectal form of this medicine since it may make your condition worse.

—if you are taking **any** other prescription or nonprescription (OTC) medicine, especially:
   Central nervous system (CNS) depressants
   Disulfiram (e.g., Antabuse)

Proper Use of This Medicine

Do not use if liquid turns brownish in color or if it has a strong vinegar-like odor, since this means the paraldehyde is breaking down. If you have any questions about this, check with your doctor or pharmacist.

For patients taking this medicine by mouth:

• **Do not use a plastic spoon, plastic glass, or any other plastic container to take this medicine,** since paraldehyde may react with the plastic. Use a metal spoon or glass container.

• **Take this medicine mixed in a glass of milk or iced fruit juice** to improve the taste and odor and to lessen stomach upset.

For patients using this medicine rectally:

• **Do not use paraldehyde in any plastic container** since it may react with the plastic.

• Before using paraldehyde rectally, make sure you understand exactly how to use it. Paraldehyde may need to be diluted. If you have any questions about this, check with your doctor or pharmacist.

Keep this medicine away from the eyes and avoid getting it on the skin and clothing.

Keep this medicine away from heat, open flame, and sparks.

Use this medicine only as directed by your doctor. Do not use more of it, do not use it more often, and do not use it for a longer period of time than your doctor ordered. If too much is used, the medicine may become habit-forming.

If you are taking this medicine regularly (for example, every day) and you miss a dose, take it right away if you remember within an hour or so of the missed dose.

However, if you do not remember until later, skip the missed dose and go back to your regular dosing schedule. Do not double doses.

How to store this medicine:

- **Keep out of the reach of children.**

- Store away from heat and direct light.

- Keep the medicine from freezing.

- Do not keep outdated medicine or medicine no longer needed. Be sure that any discarded medicine is out of the reach of children.

Precautions While Using This Medicine

If you will be using this medicine regularly for a long period of time:

—your doctor should check your progress at regular visits.

—do not stop using it without first checking with your doctor. Your doctor may want you to reduce gradually the amount you are using before stopping completely.

This medicine will add to the effects of alcohol and other CNS depressants (medicines that slow down the nervous system, possibly causing drowsiness). Some examples of CNS depressants are antihistamines or medicine for hay fever, other allergies, or colds; sedatives, tranquilizers, or sleeping medicine; prescription pain medicine or narcotics; barbiturates; medicine for convulsions (seizures); muscle relaxants; or anesthetics, including some dental anesthetics. **Check with your doctor before taking any of the above while you are using this medicine.**

If you think you or someone else may have taken an overdose of this medicine, get emergency help at once. Taking an overdose of paraldehyde or taking alcohol or other CNS depressants with paraldehyde may lead to unconsciousness and possibly death. Some signs of an overdose are confusion, muscle tremors, nausea or vomiting (continuing or severe), severe stomach cramps, severe weakness, shortness of breath or slow or troubled breathing, and slow heartbeat.

This medicine may cause some people to become drowsy or less alert than they are normally. Even if taken at bedtime, it may cause some people to feel drowsy or less alert on arising. **Make sure you know how you react to this medicine before you drive, use machines, or do other jobs that require you to be alert.**

Side Effects of This Medicine

Along with its needed effects, a medicine may cause some unwanted effects. Although not all of these side effects may occur, if they do occur they may need medical attention.

Check with your doctor as soon as possible if any of the following side effects occur:
More common
Skin rash
With long-term use
Yellow eyes or skin
Signs of overdose
Cloudy urine
Confusion
Decreased urination
Fast and deep breathing
Muscle tremors
Nausea or vomiting (continuing or severe)
Nervousness, restlessness, or irritability
Shortness of breath or slow or troubled breathing
Slow heartbeat
Stomach cramps (severe)
Weakness (severe)

Other side effects may occur that usually do not require medical attention. These side effects may go away during treatment as your body adjusts to the medicine. However, check with your doctor if any of the following side effects continue or are bothersome:
More common
Drowsiness
Nausea or vomiting (when taken by mouth)
Stomach pain (when taken by mouth)
Unpleasant breath odor
Less common
Clumsiness or unsteadiness
Dizziness
"Hangover" effect

For elderly patients: Many medicines have not been tested in older people. Therefore, it is not known whether the medicine acts the same way it does in younger adults. Check with your doctor or pharmacist if you notice any unusual effects while taking this medicine or if you think it is not working as it should.

After you stop using this medicine, your body may need time to adjust. The length of time this takes depends on the amount of medicine you were using and how long you used it. During this period of time check with your doctor if you notice any of the following side effects:
Convulsions (seizures)
Hallucinations (seeing, hearing, or feeling things that are not there)
Increase in sweating
Muscle cramps
Nausea and vomiting
Stomach cramps
Trembling

Paraldehyde will cause your breath to have a strong unpleasant odor. This effect will last until about one day after you have stopped using this medicine.

Other side effects not listed above may also occur in some patients. If you notice any other effects, check with your doctor.

December 1987

PARGYLINE (Systemic)

A commonly used brand name is Eutonyl.

To the Reader: If you do not recognize the names of medical conditions or medicines referred to in this information, check with your doctor, nurse, or pharmacist. Definitions for selected medical terms may be found in the Glossary. Brand names for the generic drug names listed can be found in the Index. In addition, selected brand names commonly associated with the generic name have been included in the text to help you recognize medicine you may be taking. The fact that a brand name product is not mentioned does not mean the information does not apply. It is a good idea for you to learn both the generic and brand names of your medicines and to write them down for future use.

Pargyline (PAR-gi-leen) belongs to the group of medicines called antihypertensives. Specifically, it is a monoamine oxidase (MAO) inhibitor. It is taken by mouth to treat high blood pressure.

High blood pressure adds to the workload of the heart and arteries. If it continues for a long time, the heart and arteries may not function properly. This can damage the blood vessels of the brain, heart, and kidneys, resulting in a stroke, heart failure, or kidney failure. High blood pressure may also increase the risk of heart attacks. These problems may be less likely to occur if blood pressure is controlled.

Pargyline works by blocking the enzyme monoamine oxidase (MAO).

Pargyline is available only with your doctor's prescription.

Remember:

• **This medicine has been prescribed for your current medical problem only.** It must not be given to other people or used for other problems unless you are directed to do so by your doctor.

• **Keep all medicines out of the reach of children.**

• In order for this medicine to work, it must be used as directed.

• **It is very important that you read and understand the following information.** If any of the information causes you special concern, do not decide against using this medicine without first checking with your doctor.

• Before you begin using any new medicine (prescription or nonprescription) or if you develop any new medical problem while you are using this medicine, check with your doctor, nurse, or pharmacist.

• **If you have any questions** about the following information or if you want more information about this medicine or your medical problem, **ask your doctor, nurse, or pharmacist.**

Before Using This Medicine

In order to decide on the best treatment for your medical problem, your doctor should be told:

—if you have ever had any unusual or allergic reaction to pargyline.

—if you are on a low-salt, low-sugar, or any other special diet, or if you are allergic to any substance, such as foods, sulfites or other preservatives, or dyes. Most medicines contain more than their active ingredient. Your doctor, nurse, or pharmacist can help you avoid products that may cause a problem.

—if you are **pregnant** or if you may become pregnant. Studies have not been done in either humans or animals.

—if you are **breast-feeding**. Pargyline has not been shown to cause problems in nursing babies.

—if you have frequent headaches.

—if you have any of the following medical problems:
    Alcoholism (active or treated)
    Angina (chest pain)
    Asthma or bronchitis
    Diabetes mellitus (sugar diabetes)
    Epilepsy
    Fever
    Glaucoma
    Headaches (severe or frequent)
    Heart or blood vessel disease
    Kidney disease
    Liver disease
    Mental illness (or history of)
    Overactive thyroid
    Parkinson's disease
    Pheochromocytoma

—if you have recently had a heart attack or stroke.

—if you are now taking or have taken within the past 2 weeks any of the following medicines or types of medicine:
    Carbamazepine (e.g., Tegretol)
    Cyclobenzaprine (e.g., Flexeril)
    Maprotiline (e.g., Ludiomil)
    Other monoamine oxidase (MAO) inhibitors such as furazolidone, isocarboxazid, phenelzine, procarbazine, or tranylcypromine
    Tricyclic antidepressants (amitriptyline, amoxapine, clomipramine, desipramine, doxepin, imipramine, nortriptyline, protriptyline, trimipramine)

—if you are taking **any** other prescription or nonprescription (OTC) medicine, especially:
    Amphetamines
    Antidiabetic agents, oral (diabetes medicine you take by mouth)
    Antihistamines
    Antimuscarinics (medicine for abdominal or stomach spasms or cramps)
    Appetite suppressants (diet pills)
    Central nervous system (CNS) depressants
    Chlophedianol (e.g., Ulo)
    Dextromethorphan (e.g., Delsym)
    Estrogens (female hormones)
    Guanadrel (e.g., Hylorel)
    Guanethidine (e.g., Ismelin)
    Insulin
    Levodopa (e.g., Dopar)
    Medicine for asthma or other breathing problems
    Medicine for colds, sinus problems, or hay fever or other allergies (including nose drops or sprays)
    Methyldopa (e.g., Aldomet)
    Methylphenidate (e.g., Ritalin)
    Rauwolfia alkaloids (alseroxylon, deserpidine, rauwolfia serpentina, reserpine)

—if you use cocaine. Cocaine use by individuals taking pargyline or other MAO inhibitors may cause a severe increase in blood pressure.

Proper Use of This Medicine

Importance of diet—When prescribing medicine for your condition, your doctor may also prescribe a personal diet for you. Such a diet may be low in sodium (salt). Most people eat much more sodium than they need and too much sodium in the diet may increase blood pressure. Some foods that contain large amounts of sodium are canned soup, pickles, ketchup, green and ripe olives, relish, frankfurters, soy sauce, and carbonated beverages. Your doctor may want you to limit the amounts of these and other high-sodium foods in your diet. High blood pressure medicine is usually more effective when such a diet is properly followed.

Also, it may be very important for you to go on a reducing diet. However, check with your doctor before changing your diet.

Many patients who have high blood pressure will not notice any signs of the problem. In fact, many may feel normal. It is very important that you **take your medicine exactly as directed** and that you keep your appointments with your doctor even if you feel well.

Remember that this medicine will not cure your high blood pressure but it does help control it. Therefore, you must continue to take it as directed if you expect to lower your blood pressure and keep it down. **You may have to take high blood pressure medicine for the rest of your life.** If high blood pressure is not treated, it can cause serious problems such as heart failure, blood vessel disease, stroke, or kidney disease.

In order to help remember to take your medicine, try to get into the habit of taking it at the same time each day.

If you miss a dose of this medicine and remember within 2 hours, take it right away and then go back to your regular dosing schedule. However, if you do not remember until later, skip the missed dose and go back to your regular dosing schedule. Do not double doses.

How to store this medicine:

• **Keep out of the reach of children.**

• Store away from heat and direct light.

• Do not store in the bathroom, near the kitchen sink, or in other damp places. Heat or moisture may cause the medicine to break down.

• Do not keep outdated medicine or medicine no longer needed. Be sure that any discarded medicine is out of the reach of children.

Precautions While Using This Medicine

It is important that your doctor check your progress at regular visits to make sure that this medicine is working properly and to check for unwanted effects.

Check with your doctor or hospital emergency room immediately if severe headache, stiff neck, chest pains, rapid heartbeat, or nausea and vomiting occur while you are taking this medicine. These may be symptoms of a serious reaction which should have a doctor's attention.

When taken with certain foods, drinks, or other medicines, pargyline can cause very dangerous reactions. To avoid such reactions, **obey the following rules of caution:**

• Do not eat foods that have a high tyramine content (most common in foods that are aged or fermented to increase their flavor), such as cheeses, yeast or meat extracts, fava or broad bean pods, smoked or pickled fish, beef or chicken liver, fermented sausage (bologna, pepperoni, salami, and summer sausage) or other unfresh meat, or any overripe fruit. If a list of these foods and beverages is not given to you, ask your doctor, nurse, or pharmacist to provide one.

• Do not drink alcoholic beverages, including beer and wines (especially chianti and other hearty red wines).

• Do not eat or drink excessive amounts of caffeine-containing food or beverages such as chocolate, coffee, tea, or cola.

• Do not take any other medicine unless approved or prescribed by your doctor. This especially includes over-the-counter (OTC) or nonprescription medicine such as that for colds (including nose drops), cough, asthma, hay fever, sinus problems, or appetite control; "keep awake" products; or products that make you sleepy.

After you stop using this medicine you must continue to obey the rules of caution concerning food, drink, and other medicine for at least 2 weeks. This medicine may continue to react with certain foods or other medicines for up to 14 days after you stop taking it.

This medicine will add to the effects of alcohol and other CNS depressants (medicines that slow down the nervous system, possibly causing drowsiness). Some examples of CNS depressants are antihistamines or medicine for hay fever, other allergies, or colds; sedatives, tranquilizers, or sleeping medicine; prescription pain medicine or narcotics; barbiturates; medicine for convulsions (seizures); tricyclic antidepressants (medicine for depression); muscle relaxants; or anesthetics, including some dental anesthetics. **Check with your doctor before taking any of the above while you are using this medicine.**

This medicine may cause some people to become drowsy or less alert than they are normally. **Make sure you know how you react to this medicine before you drive, use machines, or do other jobs that require you to be alert.**

Dizziness, lightheadedness, or fainting may occur, especially when you get up from a lying or sitting position. **Getting up slowly may help.** When you get up from lying down, sit on the edge of the bed with your feet dangling for 1 or 2 minutes. Then stand up slowly. If the problem continues or gets worse, check with your doctor.

Diabetics—This medicine may affect blood sugar levels. While you are using this medicine, be especially careful in testing for sugar in your blood or urine. If you have any questions about this, check with your doctor.

Before having any kind of surgery (including dental surgery) or emergency treatment, tell the physician or dentist in charge that you are using this medicine or have used it within the past 2 weeks.

Your doctor may want you to carry an identification card stating that you are using this medicine.

Tell your doctor if you develop a fever since that may change the amount of medicine you have to take.

Patients with angina (chest pain)—This medicine may cause you to have an unusual feeling of health and energy. However, **do not suddenly increase the amount of exercise you get without discussing it with your doctor.** To do so could bring on an attack of angina.

Side Effects of This Medicine

Along with its needed effects, a medicine may cause some unwanted effects. Although not all of these side effects may occur, if they do occur they may need medical attention.

Check with your doctor immediately if any of the following side effects occur:

Less common

    Fast or pounding heartbeat

Rare

    Chest pain (severe)
    Enlarged pupils
    Headache (severe)
    Increased sensitivity of eyes to light
    Nausea and vomiting
    Stiff or sore neck

Check with your doctor as soon as possible if any of the following side effects occur:

Less common

    Diarrhea
    Fainting
    Swelling of feet and lower legs

Rare

    Dark urine
    Fever
    Hallucinations (seeing, hearing, or feeling things that are not there)
    Yellow eyes and skin

Other side effects may occur that usually do not require medical attention. These side effects may go away during treatment as your body adjusts to the medicine. However, check with your doctor if any of the following side effects continue or are bothersome:

More common

    Constipation
    Difficult urination
    Dizziness or lightheadedness, especially when getting up from a lying or sitting position
    Drowsiness
    Dry mouth
    Tiredness and weakness

Less common or rare

    Chills
    Increase in appetite and weight gain
    Increased sensitivity of skin to sunlight
    Muscle twitching during sleep
    Nightmares
    Restlessness
    Shakiness
    Trouble in sleeping

For elderly patients: Dizziness, lightheadedness, or fainting, as well as other side effects, may be more likely to occur in the elderly, who are more sensitive to the effects of pargyline.

Other side effects not listed above may also occur in some patients. If you notice any other effects, check with your doctor.

December 1987

PARGYLINE AND METHYCLOTHIAZIDE
(Systemic)

A commonly used brand name is Eutron.

To the Reader: If you do not recognize the names of medical conditions or medicines referred to in this information, check with your doctor, nurse, or pharmacist. Definitions for selected medical terms may be found in the Glossary. Brand names for the generic drug names listed can be found in the Index. In addition, selected brand names commonly associated with the generic name have been included in the text to help you recognize medicine you may be taking. The fact that a brand name product is not mentioned does not mean the information does not apply. It is a good idea for you to learn both the generic and brand names of your medicines and to write them down for future use.

Pargyline (PAR-gi-leen) and methyclothiazide (meth-ee-kloe-THYE-a-zide) combination is taken by mouth to treat high blood pressure.

High blood pressure adds to the workload of the heart and arteries. If it continues for a long time, the heart and arteries may not function properly. This can damage the blood vessels of the brain, heart, and kidneys, resulting in a stroke, heart failure, or kidney failure. High blood pressure may also increase the risk of heart attacks. These problems may be less likely to occur if blood pressure is controlled.

Pargyline works by blocking the enzyme monoamine oxidase (MAO). The methyclothiazide in this combination is a thiazide diuretic (water pill) that helps reduce the amount of water in the body by increasing the flow of urine.

Pargyline and methyclothiazide combination is available only with your doctor's prescription.

Remember:

• **This medicine has been prescribed for your current medical problem only.** It must not be given to other people or used for other problems unless you are directed to do so by your doctor.

• **Keep all medicines out of the reach of children.**

• In order for this medicine to work, it must be used as directed.

• **It is very important that you read and understand the following information.** If any of the information causes you special concern, do not decide against using this medicine without first checking with your doctor.

• Before you begin using any new medicine (prescription or nonprescription) or if you develop any new medical problem while you are using this medicine, check with your doctor, nurse, or pharmacist.

• **If you have any questions** about the following information or if you want more information about this medicine or your medical problem, **ask your doctor, nurse, or pharmacist.**

Before Using This Medicine

In order to decide on the best treatment for your medical problem, your doctor should be told:

—if you have ever had any unusual or allergic reaction to pargyline, sulfonamides (sulfa drugs), or methyclothiazide or any other thiazide diuretics (water pills).

—if you are on a low-salt, low-sugar, or any other special diet, or if you are allergic to any substance, such as foods, sulfites or other preservatives, or dyes. Most medicines contain more than their active ingredient. Your doctor, nurse, or pharmacist can help you avoid products that may cause a problem.

—if you are **pregnant** or if you may become pregnant. When methyclothiazide is used during pregnancy, it may cause side effects including jaundice, blood problems, and low potassium in the newborn infant. Studies with pargyline have not been done in either humans or animals.

—if you are **breast-feeding**. This medicine has not been shown to cause problems in nursing babies.

—if you have frequent headaches.

—if you have any of the following medical problems:
   Alcoholism (active or treated)
   Angina (chest pain)
   Asthma or bronchitis
   Diabetes mellitus (sugar diabetes)
   Epilepsy
   Fever
   Glaucoma
   Gout (history of)
   Headaches (severe or frequent)
   Heart or blood vessel disease
   Kidney disease
   Liver disease
   Lupus erythematosus (or history of)
   Mental illness (history of)
   Overactive thyroid
   Pancreas disease
   Parkinson's disease
   Pheochromocytoma

—if you have recently had a heart attack or stroke.

—if you are taking **any** other prescription or nonprescription (OTC) medicine, especially:
   Adrenocorticoids (cortisone-like medicines)
   Antidiabetic agents, oral (diabetes medicine you take by mouth)
   Antihistamines
   Antimuscarinics (medicine for abdominal or stomach spasms or cramps)
   Central nervous system (CNS) depressants
   Chlophedianol (e.g., Ulo)
   Dextromethorphan (e.g., Delsym)
   Digitalis glycosides (heart medicine)
   Estrogens (female hormones)
   Guanadrel (e.g., Hylorel)
   Guanethidine (e.g., Ismelin)
   Insulin
   Levodopa (e.g., Dopar)
   Lithium (e.g., Lithane)
   Medicine for asthma or other breathing problems
   Medicine for colds, sinus problems, or hay fever or other allergies (including nose drops or sprays)
   Methenamine (e.g., Mandelamine)

Methyldopa (e.g., Aldomet)
Methylphenidate (e.g., Ritalin)
Rauwolfia alkaloids (alseroxylon, deserpidine, rauwolfia
serpentina, reserpine)

—if you are now taking or have taken within the past
2 weeks any of the following medicines or types of
medicine:

Carbamazepine (e.g., Tegretol)
Cyclobenzaprine (e.g., Flexeril)
Maprotiline (e.g., Ludiomil)
Other monoamine oxidase (MAO) inhibitors such as furazolidone, isocarboxazid, phenelzine, procarbazine,
or tranylcypromine
Tricyclic antidepressants (amitriptyline, amoxapine,
clomipramine, desipramine, doxepin, imipramine, nortriptyline, protriptyline, trimipramine)

—if you use cocaine. Cocaine use by individuals taking
pargyline (contained in this combination) or other
MAO inhibitors may cause a severe increase in blood
pressure.

Proper Use of This Medicine

Importance of diet—When prescribing medicine for your
condition, your doctor may also prescribe a personal
diet for you. Such a diet may be low in sodium (salt).
Most people eat much more sodium than they need
and too much sodium in the diet may increase blood
pressure. Some foods that contain large amounts of
sodium are canned soup, pickles, ketchup, green and
ripe olives, relish, frankfurters, soy sauce, and carbonated beverages. Your doctor may want you to limit
the amounts of these and other high-sodium foods in
your diet. High blood pressure medicine is usually more
effective when such a diet is properly followed.

Also, it may be very important for you to go on a
reducing diet. However, check with your doctor before
changing your diet.

Many patients who have high blood pressure will not
notice any signs of the problem. In fact, many may
feel normal. It is very important that you **take your
medicine exactly as directed** and that you keep your
appointments with your doctor even if you feel well.

Remember that this medicine will not cure your high
blood pressure but it does help control it. Therefore,
you must continue to take it as directed if you expect
to lower your blood pressure and keep it down. **You
may have to take high blood pressure medicine for the
rest of your life.** If high blood pressure is not treated,
it can cause serious problems such as heart failure,
blood vessel disease, stroke, or kidney disease.

This medicine may cause you to have an unusual feeling
of tiredness when you begin to take it. You may also
notice an increase in the amount of urine or in your
frequency of urination. After taking the medicine for

a while, these effects should lessen. In order to keep
the increase in urine from affecting your nighttime
sleep:

• If you are to take a single dose a day, take it in the
morning after breakfast.

• If you are to take more than one dose a day, take
the last dose no later than 6 p.m., unless otherwise
directed by your doctor.

However, it is best to plan your dose or doses according
to a schedule that will least affect your personal activities and sleep. Ask your doctor, nurse, or pharmacist to help you plan the best time to take this
medicine.

In order to help remember to take your medicine, try to
get into the habit of taking it at the same time each
day.

If you miss a dose of this medicine and remember within
2 hours, take it right away and then go back to your
regular dosing schedule. If you do not remember until
later, skip the missed dose and go back to your regular
dosing schedule. Do not double doses.

How to store this medicine:

• **Keep out of the reach of children.**

• Store away from heat and direct light.

• Do not store in the bathroom, near the kitchen sink,
or in other damp places. Heat or moisture may cause
the medicine to break down.

• Do not keep outdated medicine or medicine no longer
needed. Be sure that any discarded medicine is out of
the reach of children.

Precautions While Using This Medicine

It is important that your doctor check your progress at
regular visits to make sure that this medicine is working properly.

When taken with certain foods, drinks, or other medicines, pargyline and methyclothiazide combination can
cause very dangerous reactions. To avoid such reactions, **obey the following rules of caution:**

• Do not eat foods that have a high tyramine content
(most common in foods that are aged or fermented to
increase their flavor), such as cheeses, yeast or meat
extracts, fava or broad bean pods, smoked or pickled
fish, beef or chicken liver, fermented sausage (bologna, pepperoni, salami, and summer sausage) or other
unfresh meat, or any overripe fruit. If a list of these
foods and beverages is not given to you, ask your doctor, nurse, or pharmacist to provide one.

• Do not drink alcoholic beverages, including beer and
wines (especially chianti and other hearty red wines).

• Do not eat or drink excessive amounts of caffeine-
containing food or beverages such as chocolate, coffee,
tea, or cola.

• Do not take any other medicine unless approved or prescribed by your doctor. This especially includes over-the-counter (OTC) or nonprescription medicine such as that for colds (including nose drops), cough, asthma, hay fever, sinus, or appetite control; "keep awake" products; or products that make you sleepy.

After you stop using this medicine you must continue to obey the rules of caution concerning food, drink, and other medicine for at least 2 weeks. This medicine may continue to react with certain foods or other medicines for up to 14 days after you stop taking it.

This medicine will add to the effects of alcohol and other CNS depressants (medicines that slow down the nervous system, possibly causing drowsiness). Some examples of CNS depressants are antihistamines or medicine for hay fever, other allergies, or colds; sedatives, tranquilizers, or sleeping medicine; prescription pain medicine or narcotics; barbiturates; medicine for seizures; muscle relaxants; or anesthetics, including some dental anesthetics. **Check with your doctor before taking any of the above while you are using this medicine.**

Before having any kind of surgery (including dental surgery) or emergency treatment, tell the physician or dentist in charge that you are using this medicine or have used it within the past 2 weeks.

This medicine may cause a loss of potassium from your body.

• To help prevent this, your doctor may want you to:
—eat or drink foods that have a high potassium content (for example, orange or other citrus fruit juices), or
—take a potassium supplement, or
—take another medicine to help prevent the loss of the potassium in the first place.

• It is very important to follow these directions. Also, it is important not to change your diet on your own. This is more important if you are already on a special diet (as for diabetes), or if you are taking a potassium supplement or a medicine to reduce potassium loss. Extra potassium may not be necessary and, in some cases, too much potassium could be harmful.

Patients with angina (chest pain)—This medicine may cause you to have an unusual feeling of health and energy. However, **do not suddenly increase the amount of exercise you get without discussing it with your doctor** since that could bring on an attack of angina.

Diabetics—This medicine may affect blood sugar levels. While you are using this medicine, be especially careful in testing for sugar in your blood or urine. If you have any questions about this, check with your doctor.

Your doctor may want you to carry an identification card stating that you are using this medicine.

Check with your doctor or hospital emergency room immediately if severe headache, stiff neck, chest pains, rapid heartbeat, or nausea and vomiting occur while

you are taking this medicine. These may be symptoms of a serious side reaction which should have a doctor's attention.

This medicine may cause some people to become drowsy or less alert than they are normally. **Make sure you know how you react to this medicine before you drive, use machines, or do other jobs that require you to be alert.**

Dizziness, lightheadedness, or fainting may occur, especially when you get up from a lying or sitting position. **Getting up slowly may help.** When you get up from lying down, sit on the edge of the bed with your feet dangling for 1 or 2 minutes. Then stand up slowly. If the problem continues or gets worse, check with your doctor.

Tell your doctor if you develop a fever since that may change the amount of medicine you have to take.

Check with your doctor if you become sick and have severe or continuing vomiting or diarrhea. These problems may cause you to lose additional water and potassium.

Some people who take this medicine may become more sensitive to sunlight than they are normally. When you first begin taking this medicine, avoid too much sun and do not use a sunlamp until you see how you react to the sun, especially if you tend to burn easily. If you have a severe reaction, check with your doctor.

Side Effects of This Medicine
Along with its needed effects, a medicine may cause some unwanted effects. Although not all of these side effects may occur, if they do occur they may need medical attention.

Check with your doctor immediately if any of the following side effects occur:
Less common
Fast or pounding heartbeat
Rare
Chest pain (severe)
Enlarged pupils
Headache (severe)
Increased sensitivity of eyes to light
Nausea and vomiting
Stiff or sore neck

Check with your doctor as soon as possible if any of the following side effects occur:
Less common
Fainting
Swelling of feet and lower legs
Rare
Dark urine
Fever
Hallucinations (seeing, hearing, or feeling things that are not there)
Joint, lower back or side, or stomach pain
Skin rash or hives
Sore throat and fever

Stomach pain (severe) with nausea and vomiting
Unusual bleeding or bruising
Yellow eyes or skin

Signs of too much potassium loss
Dryness of mouth
Increased thirst
Irregular heartbeats
Mood or mental changes
Muscle cramps or pain
Nausea or vomiting
Unusual tiredness or weakness
Weak pulse

Other side effects may occur that usually do not require medical attention. These side effects may go away during treatment as your body adjusts to the medicine. However, check with your doctor if any of the following side effects continue or are bothersome:

More common
Constipation
Difficult urination
Dizziness or lightheadedness, especially when getting up from a lying or sitting position
Drowsiness

Less common or rare
Chills
Decreased sexual ability
Increased sensitivity of skin to sunlight
Insomnia
Muscle twitching during sleep
Nightmares
Restlessness
Shakiness

For elderly patients: Dizziness, lightheadedness, or fainting, signs of too much potassium loss, as well as other side effects, may be more likely to occur in the elderly, who are usually more sensitive to the effects of this medicine.

Other side effects not listed above may also occur in some patients. If you notice any other effects, check with your doctor.

—————

December 1987

PEMOLINE (Systemic)

A commonly used brand name is Cylert.

To the Reader: If you do not recognize the names of medical conditions or medicines referred to in this information, check with your doctor, nurse, or pharmacist. Definitions for selected medical terms may be found in the Glossary. Brand names for the generic drug names listed can be found in the Index. In addition, selected brand names commonly associated with the generic name have been included in the text to help you recognize medicine you may be taking. The fact that a brand name product is not mentioned does not mean the information does not apply. It is a good idea for you to learn both the generic and brand names of your medicines and to write them down for future use.

Pemoline (PEM-oh-leen) belongs to the group of medicines called central nervous system (CNS) stimulants. It is taken by mouth to treat children with attention deficit disorder.

Pemoline increases attention and decreases restlessness in children who are overactive, unable to concentrate for very long, or easily distracted, and have unstable emotions. This medicine is used as part of a total treatment program that also includes social, educational, and psychological treatment.

This medicine is available only with your doctor's prescription.

Remember:

• **This medicine has been prescribed for your current medical problem only.** It must not be given to other people or used for other problems unless you are directed to do so by your doctor.

• **Keep all medicines out of the reach of children.**

• In order for this medicine to work, it must be used as directed.

• **It is very important that you read and understand the following information.** If any of the information causes you special concern, do not decide against using this medicine without first checking with your doctor.

• Before you begin using any new medicine (prescription or nonprescription) or if you develop any new medical problem while you are using this medicine, check with your doctor, nurse, or pharmacist.

• **If you have any questions** about the following information or if you want more information about this medicine or your medical problem, **ask your doctor, nurse, or pharmacist**.

Before Using This Medicine

In order to decide on the best treatment for your medical problem, your doctor should be told:

—if you have ever had any unusual or allergic reaction to pemoline.

—if you are on a low-salt, low-sugar, or any other special diet, or if you are allergic to any substance, such as foods, sulfites or other preservatives, or dyes. Most medicines contain more than their active ingredient. Your doctor, nurse, or pharmacist can help you avoid products that may cause a problem.

—if you are **pregnant** or if you may become pregnant. Pemoline has not been shown to cause birth defects or other problems in humans. However, studies in animals given large doses of pemoline have shown that pemoline causes an increase in stillbirths and decreased survival of the offspring after birth.

—if you are **breast-feeding**. It is not known if pemoline is excreted in breast milk. This medicine has not been shown to cause problems in nursing babies.

—if you have any of the following medical problems:
   Gilles de la Tourette's disorder or other tics
   Kidney disease
   Liver disease

—if you are taking **any** other prescription or nonprescription (OTC) medicine.

Proper Use of This Medicine

For patients taking the chewable tablet form of this medicine:

• These tablets must be chewed. Do not swallow whole.

Sometimes this medicine must be taken for 3 to 4 weeks before improvement is noticed.

Take pemoline only as directed by your doctor. Do not take more of it, do not take it more often, and do not take it for a longer period of time than your doctor ordered. If too much is taken, it may become habit-forming.

If you miss a dose of this medicine, take it as soon as possible. Then go back to your regular dosing schedule. But if you do not remember the missed dose until the next day, skip it and go back to your regular dosing schedule. Do not double doses.

How to store this medicine:

• **Keep out of the reach of children.**

• Store away from heat and direct light.

• Do not store in the bathroom, near the kitchen sink, or in other damp places. Heat or moisture may cause the medicine to break down.

• Do not keep outdated medicine or medicine no longer needed. Be sure that any discarded medicine is out of the reach of children.

Precautions While Using This Medicine

Your doctor should check your progress at regular visits to make sure that this medicine does not cause unwanted effects.

If you will be taking this medicine in large doses for a long period of time, do not stop taking it without first checking with your doctor. Your doctor may want you to reduce gradually the amount you are taking before stopping completely.

© 1988   The United States Pharmacopeial Convention, Inc.

This medicine may cause some people to become dizzy or less alert than they are normally. **Make sure you know how you react to this medicine before you drive, use machines, or do other jobs that require you to be alert.**

If you have been using this medicine for a long time and you think you may have become mentally or physically dependent on it, check with your doctor. Some signs of dependence on pemoline are:

—a strong desire or need to continue taking the medicine.

—a need to increase the dose to receive the effects of the medicine.

—withdrawal side effects (for example, mental depression, unusual behavior, or unusual tiredness or weakness) occurring after the medicine is stopped.

Side Effects of This Medicine

Along with its needed effects, a medicine may cause some unwanted effects. Although not all of these side effects may occur, if they do occur they may need medical attention.

Check with your doctor as soon as possible if any of the following side effects occur:

Rare

Yellow eyes or skin

Signs of overdose

Agitation
Confusion
Convulsions (seizures)
False sense of well-being
Fast heartbeat
Hallucinations (seeing, hearing, or feeling things that are not there)
Headache (severe)
High blood pressure
High fever with sweating

Large pupils
Muscle trembling or twitching
Nervousness or restlessness
Uncontrolled movements of the eyes or other parts of the body
Vomiting

Other side effects may occur that usually do not require medical attention. These side effects may go away during treatment as your body adjusts to the medicine. However, check with your doctor if any of the following side effects continue or are bothersome:

More common

Loss of appetite
Trouble in sleeping
Weight loss

Less common

Dizziness
Drowsiness
Increased irritability
Mental depression
Nausea
Skin rash
Stomach ache

After you stop using this medicine, your body may need time to adjust. The length of time this takes depends on the amount of medicine you were using and how long you used it. During this period of time check with your doctor if you notice any of the following side effects:

Mental depression (severe)
Unusual behavior
Unusual tiredness or weakness

Other side effects not listed above may also occur in some patients. If you notice any other effects, check with your doctor.

_____

December 1987

_____

PENICILLAMINE (Systemic)

Some commonly used brand names are:

Cuprimine   Distamine*
Depen   Pendramine*

---

*Not available in the U.S.

To the Reader: If you do not recognize the names of medical conditions or medicines referred to in this information, check with your doctor, nurse, or pharmacist. Definitions for selected medical terms may be found in the Glossary. Brand names for the generic drug names listed can be found in the Index. In addition, selected brand names commonly associated with the generic name have been included in the text to help you recognize medicine you may be taking. The fact that a brand name product is not mentioned does not mean the information does not apply. It is a good idea for you to learn both the generic and brand names of your medicines and to write them down for future use.

Penicillamine (pen-i-SILL-a-meen) is used in the treatment of medical problems such as Wilson's disease (too much copper in the body) and rheumatoid arthritis. Also, it is used to prevent kidney stones. Penicillamine may also be used for other conditions as determined by your doctor.

In addition to the helpful effects of this medicine, it has side effects that can be very serious. Before you take penicillamine, be sure that you have discussed the use of it with your doctor.

This medicine is available only with your doctor's prescription.

Remember:

• **This medicine has been prescribed for your current medical problem only.** It must not be given to other people or used for other problems unless you are directed to do so by your doctor.

• **Keep all medicines out of the reach of children.**

• In order for this medicine to work, it must be used as directed.

• **It is very important that you read and understand the following information.** If any of the information causes you special concern, do not decide against using this medicine without first checking with your doctor.

• Before you begin using any new medicine (prescription or nonprescription) or if you develop any new medical problem while you are using this medicine, check with your doctor, nurse, or pharmacist.

• **If you have any questions** about the following information or if you want more information about this medicine or your medical problem, **ask your doctor, nurse, or pharmacist.**

Before Using This Medicine

In order to decide on the best treatment for your medical problem, your doctor should be told:

—if you have ever had any unusual or allergic reaction to penicillamine or to penicillin, or if you have taken penicillamine before and had a serious side effect from it.

—if you are on a low-salt, low-sugar, or any other special diet, or if you are allergic to any substance, such as foods, sulfites or other preservatives, or dyes. Most medicines contain more than their active ingredient. Your doctor, nurse, or pharmacist can help you avoid products that may cause a problem.

—if you are **pregnant** or if you may become pregnant. Penicillamine may cause birth defects if taken during pregnancy.

—if you are **breast-feeding**. Penicillamine has not been shown to cause problems in nursing babies.

—if you have kidney disease or a history of kidney disease (only for patients with rheumatoid arthritis).

—if you are taking **any** other prescription or nonprescription (OTC) medicine, especially gold compounds.

Proper Use of This Medicine

Since penicillamine is taken in different ways for different medical problems, it is very important that you understand exactly why you are taking this medicine and how to take it. See below for information on specific medical problems. If you have any questions about this, check with your doctor.

For patients taking this medicine to prevent kidney stones:

• You should drink 2 full glasses (8 ounces each) of water at bedtime and another 2 full glasses (8 ounces each) during the night.

• It is very important that you follow any special instructions from your doctor, such as following a low-methionine diet. If you have any questions about this, check with your doctor.

For patients taking this medicine for rheumatoid arthritis:

• Take this medicine on an empty stomach (at least 1 hour before meals or 2 hours after meals) and at least 1 hour before or after any other food, milk, or medicine.

• After you begin taking this medicine, 2 to 3 months may pass before you feel its effects. It is very important that you keep taking the medicine, even if you do not feel better, in order to give it time to work.

For patients taking this medicine for Wilson's disease:

• Take this medicine on an empty stomach (at least ½ to 1 hour before meals or 2 hours after meals).

• It is very important that you follow any special instructions from your doctor, such as following a low-copper diet. If you have any questions about this, check with your doctor.

• After you begin taking this medicine, 1 to 3 months may pass before you notice any improvement in your condition.

For patients taking this medicine for lead poisoning:

• Take this medicine on an empty stomach (2 hours before meals or at least 3 hours after meals).

© 1988   The United States Pharmacopeial Convention, Inc.

For all patients:

- **Take this medicine regularly as directed. Do not stop taking it without first checking with your doctor,** since stopping the medicine and then restarting it may increase the possibility of side effects.

- If you miss a dose of this medicine and your dosing schedule is one dose to be taken:

    Once a day—Take the missed dose as soon as possible. But if you do not remember the missed dose until the next day, skip the missed dose and go back to your regular dosing schedule. Do not double the next day's dose.

    Two times a day—Take the missed dose as soon as possible. However, if it is almost time for your next dose, skip the missed dose and go back to your regular dosing schedule. Do not double doses.

    More than two times a day—If you remember within an hour or so of the missed dose, take it right away. But if you do not remember until later, skip the missed dose and go back to your regular dosing schedule. Do not double doses.

How to store this medicine:

- **Keep out of the reach of children.**

- Store away from heat and direct light.

- Do not store this medicine in the bathroom, near the kitchen sink, or in other damp places. Heat or moisture may cause the medicine to break down.

- Do not keep outdated medicine or medicine no longer needed. Be sure that any discarded medicine is out of the reach of children.

Precautions While Using This Medicine

Your doctor should check your progress at regular visits in order to make sure that this medicine does not cause unwanted effects.

Before having any kind of surgery (including dental surgery), tell the physician or dentist in charge that you are taking this medicine.

If you are taking iron preparations, or vitamin preparations containing iron, do not take them within 2 hours of the time you take this medicine.

Side Effects of This Medicine

Along with its needed effects, a medicine may cause some unwanted effects. Although not all of these side effects may occur, if they do occur they may need medical attention.

Check with your doctor as soon as possible if any of the following side effects occur:

More common

    Fever
    Joint pain
    Skin rash, hives, or itching
    Swelling of lymph glands
    Ulcers, sores, or white spots in mouth

Less common

    Bloody or cloudy urine
    Sore throat, fever, and chills
    Swelling of face, feet, or lower legs
    Unusual bleeding or bruising
    Unusual tiredness or weakness
    Weight gain

Rare

    Abdominal or stomach pain (severe)
    Blisters on skin
    Chest pain
    Darkening of urine
    Difficulty in breathing, chewing, talking, or swallowing
    Eye pain, blurred or double vision, or any change in vision
    General feeling of body discomfort or weakness
    Muscle weakness
    Pale stools
    Redness, tenderness, itching, burning, or peeling of skin
    Red or irritated eyes
    Ringing or buzzing in the ears
    Spitting up blood
    Thickened or scaly skin
    Unexplained coughing, wheezing, or shortness of breath
    Yellow eyes or skin

Other side effects may occur that usually do not require medical attention. These side effects may go away during treatment as your body adjusts to the medicine. However, check with your doctor if any of the following side effects continue or are bothersome:

More common

    Diarrhea
    Lessening or loss of taste sense
    Loss of appetite
    Nausea or vomiting
    Stomach pain (mild)

For elderly patients: Some of the above side effects may be more likely to occur in the elderly, who are usually more sensitive to the effects of penicillamine.

Other side effects not listed above may also occur in some patients. If you notice any other effects, check with your doctor.

December 1987

PENICILLINS (Systemic)

This information applies to the following medicines:

Amdinocillin (am-DEE-noe-sill-in)
Amoxicillin (a-mox-i-SILL-in)
Amoxicillin and Clavulanate (klav-yoo-LAN-ate)
Ampicillin (am-pi-SILL-in)
Azlocillin (az-loe-SILL-in)
Bacampicillin (ba-kam-pi-SILL-in)
Carbenicillin (kar-ben-i-SILL-in)
Cloxacillin (klox-a-SILL-in)
Cyclacillin (sye-kla-SILL-in)
Dicloxacillin (dye-klox-a-SILL-in)
Methicillin (meth-i-SILL-in)
Mezlocillin (mez-loe-SILL-in)
Nafcillin (naf-SILL-in)
Oxacillin (ox-a-SILL-in)
Penicillin G (pen-i-SILL-in)
Penicillin V
Piperacillin (pi-PER-a-sill-in)
Ticarcillin (tye-kar-SILL-in)
Ticarcillin and Clavulanate

Some commonly used brand names or other names are:	Generic names:
Coactin Mecillinam	Amdinocillin
Amoxil Apo-Amoxi* Novamoxin* Polymox Sumox Trimox Utimox Wymox	Amoxicillin†
Augmentin Clavulin*	Amoxicillin and Clavulanate
Amcill Ampicin* Ampilean* Apo-Ampi* NaMPICIL Novoampicillin* Omnipen Omnipen-N Penbritin* Polycillin Polycillin-N Principen Supen Totacillin Totacillin-N	Ampicillin†
Azlin	Azlocillin
Penglobe* Spectrobid	Bacampicillin
Geocillin Geopen Geopen Oral* Pyopen	Carbenicillin
Apo-Cloxi* Cloxapen Novocloxin* Orbenin* Tegopen	Cloxacillin†
Cyclapen-W	Cyclacillin

Dycill Dynapen Pathocil	Dicloxacillin†
Staphcillin	Methicillin
Baypen* Mezlin	Mezlocillin
Nafcil Nallpen Unipen	Nafcillin
Bactocill Prostaphlin	Oxacillin†
Ayercillin* Bicillin Bicillin L-A Crystapen* Crysticillin Duracillin A.S. Megacillin* Novopen-G* P-50* Pentids Permapen Pfizerpen Pfizerpen-AS Wycillin	Penicillin G†
Apo-Pen-VK* Beepen-VK Betapen-VK Ledercillin VK Nadopen-V* Novopen-VK* Penapar VK Pen Vee K PVF K* Robicillin VK V-Cillin K VC-K* Veetids	Penicillin V†
Pipracil	Piperacillin
Ticar	Ticarcillin
Timentin	Ticarcillin and Clavulanate

*Not available in the U.S.
†Generic name product may also be available in the U.S.

To the Reader: If you do not recognize the names of medical conditions or medicines referred to in this information, check with your doctor, nurse, or pharmacist. Definitions for selected medical terms may be found in the Glossary. Brand names for the generic drug names listed can be found in the Index. In addition, selected brand names commonly associated with the generic name have been included in the text to help you recognize medicine you may be taking. The fact that a brand name product is not mentioned does not mean the information does not apply. It is a good idea for you to learn both the generic and brand names of your medicines and to write them down for future use.

Penicillins belong to the family of medicines called antibiotics. Antibiotics are used in the treatment of infections caused by bacteria. They work by killing bacteria or preventing their growth.

There are several different kinds of penicillins. Each is used to treat different kinds of infections. One kind of penicillin usually may not be used in place of another. None of the penicillins will work for colds, flu, or other virus infections.

Penicillins are taken by mouth or given by injection to treat infections in many different parts of the body. They are sometimes given with other antibiotics. Carbenicillin taken by mouth is used only to treat infections of the urinary tract and prostate gland. Penicillin G and penicillin V are also used to prevent "strep" infections in patients with a history of rheumatic heart disease. Piperacillin is also given by injection to prevent infections before, during, and after surgery. Some of the penicillins may also be used for other problems as determined by your doctor.

Penicillins are available only with your doctor's prescription.

Remember:
- **This medicine has been prescribed for your present infection only.** Another infection later on may require a different medicine. Also, even though other people may have the same symptoms as you, they may have a different kind of infection. Your medicine may not work for them and may even cause them harm. Therefore, **your medicine must not be given to other people or used for other infections** unless you are otherwise directed by your doctor.

- **Keep all medicines out of the reach of children.**

- In order for this medicine to work, it must be used as directed.

- If you are receiving this medicine by injection, some of the information about this medicine may not apply.

- **It is very important that you read and understand the following information.** If any of the information causes you special concern, do not decide against using this medicine without first checking with your doctor.

- Before you begin using any new medicine (prescription or nonprescription) or if you develop any new medical problem while you are using this medicine, check with your doctor, nurse, or pharmacist.

- **If you have any questions** about the following information or if you want more information about this medicine or your medical problem, **ask your doctor, nurse, or pharmacist.**

Before Using This Medicine

In order to decide on the best treatment for your medical problem, your doctor should be told:

—if you have ever had any unusual or allergic reaction to any of the penicillins, cephalosporins, griseofulvin, or penicillamine. Serious reactions may occur in patients who are allergic to penicillins.

—if you are receiving penicillin G procaine and have ever had any unusual or allergic reaction to procaine or other "caine-type" anesthetics (medicines that cause numbing).

—if you are on a low-salt, low-sugar, or any other special diet, or if you are allergic to any substance, such as foods, sulfites or other preservatives, or dyes. Most medicines contain more than their active ingredient, and many liquid medicines contain alcohol. Your doctor, nurse, or pharmacist can help you avoid products that may cause a problem.

—if you are **pregnant** or if you may become pregnant. Studies have not been done in humans. However, penicillins have not been shown to cause birth defects or other problems in animals given more than 25 times the usual human dose.

—if you are **breast-feeding**. Most penicillins (except amdinocillin) pass into the breast milk. Even though only small amounts may pass into breast milk, allergic reactions, diarrhea, fungal infections, and skin rash may occur in nursing babies.

—if you have any of the following medical problems (may not apply to all penicillins):
  Allergy, general, history of (such as asthma, eczema, hay fever, hives)
  Bleeding problems, history of
  Kidney disease
  Liver disease
  Mononucleosis, infectious ("mono")
  Stomach or intestinal disease, history of (especially colitis, including colitis caused by antibiotics, or enteritis)

—if you are taking **any** other prescription or nonprescription (OTC) medicine, especially (may not apply to all penicillins):
  Amiloride (e.g., Midamor)
  Anticoagulants (blood thinners)
  Captopril (e.g., Capoten)
  Cefamandole (e.g., Mandol)
  Cefoperazone (e.g., Cefobid)
  Cholestyramine (e.g., Questran)
  Colestipol (e.g., Colestid)
  Dipyridamole (e.g., Persantine)
  Divalproex (e.g., Depakote)
  Enalapril (e.g., Vasotec)
  Heparin (e.g., Panheprin)
  Medicine containing potassium
  Medicine for inflammation or pain (aspirin or other salicylates, diclofenac, diflunisal, fenoprofen, flurbiprofen [oral], ibuprofen, indomethacin, ketoprofen, meclofenamate, mefenamic acid, naproxen, phenylbutazone, piroxicam, sulindac, tiaprofenic acid, tolmetin)
  Moxalactam (e.g., Moxam)
  Oral contraceptives (birth control pills) containing estrogen
  Pentoxifylline (e.g., Trental)
  Plicamycin (e.g., Mithracin)
  Probenecid (e.g., Benemid)
  Spironolactone (e.g., Aldactone)
  Sulfinpyrazone (e.g., Anturane)
  Triamterene (e.g., Dyrenium)
  Valproic acid (e.g., Depakene)

Proper Use of This Medicine

Penicillins (except bacampicillin tablets, amoxicillin, amoxicillin and clavulanate combination, and penicillin V) are best taken with a full glass (8 ounces) of water on an empty stomach (either 1 hour before or 2 hours after meals) unless otherwise directed by your doctor.

For patients taking amoxicillin, amoxicillin and clavulanate combination, and penicillin V:

• Amoxicillin, amoxicillin and clavulanate combination, and penicillin V may be taken on a full or empty stomach.

• The liquid form of amoxicillin may also be taken straight or mixed with formulas, milk, fruit juice, water, ginger ale, or other cold drinks. If mixed with other liquids, take immediately after mixing. Be sure to drink all the liquid in order to get the full dose of medicine.

For patients taking bacampicillin:

• The liquid form of this medicine is best taken with a full glass (8 ounces) of water on an empty stomach (either 1 hour before or 2 hours after meals) unless otherwise directed by your doctor.

• The tablet form of this medicine may be taken on a full or empty stomach.

For patients taking carbenicillin by mouth:

• This medicine usually comes with a drying agent in a small packet to help keep the tablets from taking on water and breaking down. **Do not swallow the drying agent.** Keep it in the bottle with the tablets until they are used up and then throw it away.

For patients taking penicillin G by mouth:

• Do not drink acidic fruit juices (for example, orange or grapefruit juice) or other acidic beverages within 1 hour of taking penicillin G since this may keep the medicine from working as well.

For patients taking the oral liquid form of penicillins:

• This medicine is to be taken by mouth even though it may come in a dropper bottle. If this medicine does not come in a dropper bottle, use a specially marked measuring spoon or other device to measure each dose accurately since the average household teaspoon may not hold the right amount of liquid.

• Do not use after the expiration date on the label since the medicine may not work as well. Check with your pharmacist if you have any questions about this.

For patients taking the chewable tablet form of penicillins:

• Tablets should be chewed or crushed before they are swallowed.

To help clear up your infection completely, **keep taking this medicine for the full time of treatment** even if you begin to feel better after a few days. **If you have a "strep" infection, you should keep taking this medicine for at least 10 days. This is especially important in "strep" infections since serious heart problems could develop later** if your infection is not cleared up completely. Also, if you stop taking this medicine too soon, your symptoms may return.

This medicine works best when there is a constant amount in the blood or urine. **To help keep the amount constant, do not miss any doses. Also, it is best to take the doses at evenly spaced times day and night.** For example, if you are to take 4 doses a day, the doses should be spaced about 6 hours apart. If this interferes with your sleep or other daily activities, or if you need help in planning the best times to take your medicine, check with your doctor, nurse, or pharmacist.

If you do miss a dose of this medicine, take it as soon as possible. This will help to keep a constant amount of medicine in the blood or urine. However, if it is almost time for your next dose and your dosing schedule is:

• 2 doses a day—Space the missed dose and the next dose 5 to 6 hours apart.

• 3 or more doses a day—Space the missed dose and the next dose 2 to 4 hours apart or double your next dose.

Then go back to your regular dosing schedule.

How to store this medicine:

• **Keep out of the reach of children.**

• Store away from heat and direct light.

• Do not store the capsule or tablet form of penicillins in the bathroom, near the kitchen sink, or in other damp places. Heat or moisture may cause the medicine to break down.

• Store the oral liquid form of penicillins in the refrigerator because heat will cause this medicine to break down. However, keep the medicine from freezing. Follow the directions on the label.

• Do not keep outdated medicine or medicine no longer needed. Be sure that any discarded medicine is out of the reach of children.

Precautions While Using This Medicine

If your symptoms do not improve within a few days, or if they become worse, check with your doctor.

If you have ever had an allergic reaction to any of the penicillins, your doctor may want you to carry a medical identification (ID) card or wear a medical ID bracelet stating this.

If diarrhea occurs, do not take any diarrhea medicine without first checking with your doctor or pharmacist. These medicines may make your diarrhea worse or make it last longer.

Oral contraceptives (birth control pills) containing estrogen may not work as well if you take them while you are taking ampicillin, bacampicillin, or penicillin V. Unplanned pregnancies may occur. You should use a different or additional means of birth control while you are taking any of these penicillins. If you have any questions about this, check with your doctor or pharmacist.

Diabetics—Amoxicillin, amoxicillin and clavulanate combination, ampicillin, bacampicillin, and penicillin G may cause false test results with some urine sugar tests. Check with your doctor before changing your diet or the dosage of your diabetes medicine.

Side Effects of This Medicine

Along with its needed effects, a medicine may cause some unwanted effects. Although not all of these side effects may occur, if they do occur they may need medical attention.

Stop taking this medicine and get emergency help immediately if any of the following side effects occur:

More common (may be less common with some penicillins)

Skin rash, hives, itching, or wheezing

Note: Skin rash may occur much more commonly in patients with infectious mononucleosis ("mono") who are taking amoxicillin, ampicillin, or bacampicillin.

In addition to the side effects mentioned above, **check with your doctor immediately** if any of the following side effects occur:

Less common (may be more common with some penicillins)

Blood in urine
Passage of large amounts of light-colored urine
Swelling of the face and ankles
Troubled breathing
Unusual tiredness or weakness

Rare (may be more common with some penicillins)

Abdominal or stomach cramps, pain, and bloating (severe)
Diarrhea (watery and severe), which may also be bloody
Fever
Increased thirst
Increased weight loss
Nausea or vomiting
Unusual tiredness or weakness
(the above side effects may also occur up to several weeks after you stop taking any of these medicines)
Convulsions (seizures)
Unusual bleeding or bruising

For patients receiving azlocillin, mezlocillin, or piperacillin:

• In addition to the side effects mentioned above, **check with your doctor immediately** if any of the following side effects also occur:

Less common

Dark or amber urine
Pale stools
Stomach pain
Yellow eyes or skin

Other side effects may occur that usually do not require medical attention. These side effects may go away during treatment as your body adjusts to the medicine. However, check with your doctor if any of the following side effects continue or are bothersome:

More common (may be less common with some penicillins)

Bitter, unpleasant, or unusual taste (for carbenicillin by mouth and mezlocillin only)
Diarrhea (mild)
Nausea, vomiting, or stomach upset
Sore mouth or tongue (for amoxicillin, amoxicillin and clavulanate combination, ampicillin, azlocillin, and bacampicillin only)

Less common or rare

Changes in sense of taste and smell (for azlocillin and ticarcillin and clavulanate combination only)
Dizziness (for amdinocillin and azlocillin only)
Muscle weakness

In some patients, amoxicillin, amoxicillin and clavulanate combination, ampicillin, bacampicillin, penicillin G, and penicillin V may cause the tongue to become darkened or discolored. These changes are only temporary and will go away when you stop taking these medicines.

Overdose is very unlikely to occur with penicillins. However, if you think that you or someone else, especially a child, has taken too much, check with your doctor. Severe diarrhea, nausea, or vomiting may need to be treated.

For elderly patients: Many medicines have not been tested in older people. Therefore, it is not known whether the medicine acts the same way it does in younger adults. Check with your doctor or pharmacist if you notice any unusual effects while taking this medicine or if you think it is not working as it should.

Other side effects not listed above may also occur in some patients. If you notice any other effects, check with your doctor.

December 1987

PENTAGASTRIN (Systemic)

A commonly used brand name is Peptavlon.

Read the bold information first. Then go back and read the rest. If you do not recognize the names of medical conditions or medicines included in this information, check with your doctor, nurse, or pharmacist. Brand names for the generic drug names listed can also be found in the index. It is a good idea for you to learn both the generic and brand names of your medicines and to write them down for future use.

Pentagastrin (pen-ta-GAS-trin) is used as a test to help diagnose problems or disease of the stomach. This test determines how much acid your stomach produces.

Pentagastrin is to be used only under the supervision of a doctor.

Remember:

• **It is very important that you read and understand the following information.** If any of the information causes you special concern, do not decide against having this test without first checking with your doctor.

• **If you have any questions** about the following information or if you want more information about this test or your medical problem, **ask your doctor, nurse, or pharmacist.**

Before Having This Test

Before this test is given, your doctor should be told:

—if you have ever had any unusual or allergic reaction to pentagastrin.

—if you are allergic to any substance, such as sulfites or other preservatives or dyes. Most medicines contain more than their active ingredient. Your doctor can help you avoid products that may cause a problem.

—if you are pregnant or if you suspect that you may be pregnant. Although pentagastrin has not been shown to cause birth defects or other problems in humans, the chance always exists.

—if you are breast-feeding. Although pentagastrin has not been shown to cause problems in humans, the chance always exists.

—if you have any of the following medical problems:
Gallbladder problems
Liver disease
Pancreas disease (severe)
Stomach ulcer (severe or bleeding)

—if you are now taking any of the following medicines or types of medicines:
Antacids
Antimuscarinics (medicine for abdominal or stomach spasms or cramps)
Cimetidine
Famotidine
Ranitidine

Preparation For This Test

Unless otherwise directed by your doctor:

• Do not eat anything the night before and do not drink anything for at least four hours before the test. Having food or liquid in the stomach may affect the interpretation of the test results.

• Do not take antacids on the morning of the test. To do so may decrease the effect of pentagastrin.

• For 24 hours before the test, do not take any antimuscarinics (medicine for abdominal or stomach spasms or cramps), cimetidine, famotidine, ranitidine, or any other medicine that decreases stomach acid.

Side Effects of This Medicine

Along with its needed effects, pentagastrin may cause some unwanted effects. Although the side effects usually are rare, when they do occur they may require medical attention. **Check with your doctor or nurse immediately** if either of the following side effects occurs:

Rare
Skin rash or hives

Other side effects may occur which usually do not require medical attention. These side effects should go away as the effects of the medicine wear off. However, check with your doctor if any of the following side effects continue or are bothersome:

More common (usually disappear within 15 minutes after injection)
Gas
Nausea or vomiting
Stomach pain
Urge to have bowel movement

Less common or rare
Blurred vision
Chills
Dizziness, faintness, or lightheadedness
Drowsiness
Feeling of heaviness of arms and legs
Headache
Numbness, tingling, pain, or weakness in hands or feet
Shortness of breath
Unusually fast heartbeat
Unusual increase in sweating
Unusual tiredness
Unusual warmth or flushing of skin

Other side effects not listed above may also occur in some patients. If you notice any other effects, check with your doctor.

December 1987

PENTAMIDINE (Systemic)

Some commonly used brand names are Lomidine* and Pentam.

*Not available in the U.S.

To the Reader: If you do not recognize the names of medical conditions or medicines referred to in this information, check with your doctor, nurse, or pharmacist. Definitions for selected medical terms may be found in the Glossary. Brand names for the generic drug names listed can be found in the Index. In addition, selected brand names commonly associated with the generic name have been included in the text to help you recognize medicine you may be taking. The fact that a brand name product is not mentioned does not mean the information does not apply. It is a good idea for you to learn both the generic and brand names of your medicines and to write them down for future use.

Pentamidine (pen-TAM-i-deen) belongs to the family of medicines called antiprotozoals (an-tee-proe-toe-ZOE-als). They work by killing protozoa (tiny, one-celled animals) or preventing their growth. Some protozoa are parasites that can cause many different kinds of infections in the body.

Pentamidine is given by injection into a muscle or vein to treat pneumocystis (noo-moe-SISS-tis) pneumonia, a very serious kind of pneumonia. This particular kind of pneumonia occurs commonly in patients whose immune systems are not working normally, such as patients with acquired immune deficiency syndrome (AIDS). This medicine may also be used for other conditions as determined by your doctor.

Since pentamidine may cause some serious side effects, it is usually used only for serious infections where other medicines may not work.

Pentamidine is to be administered only by or under the immediate supervision of your doctor.

Remember:

• **It is very important that you read and understand the following information.** If any of the information causes you special concern, do not decide against receiving this medicine without first checking with your doctor.

• Before you begin using any new medicine (prescription or nonprescription) or if you develop any new medical problem while you are using this medicine, check with your doctor, nurse, or pharmacist.

• **If you have any questions** about the following information or if you want more information about this medicine or your medical problem, **ask your doctor, nurse, or pharmacist.**

Before Using This Medicine

In order to decide on the best treatment for your medical problem, your doctor should be told:

—if you have ever had any unusual or allergic reaction to pentamidine.

—if you are on a low-salt, low-sugar, or any other special diet, or if you are allergic to any substance, such as foods or sulfites or other preservatives. Most medicines contain more than their active ingredient. Your doctor, nurse, or pharmacist can help you avoid products that may cause a problem.

—if you are **pregnant** or if you may become pregnant. Studies have not been done in either humans or animals.

—if you are **breast-feeding.** However, pentamidine has not been shown to cause problems in nursing babies.

—if you have any of the following medical problems:

    Anemia
    Bleeding disorders (history of)
    Diabetes mellitus (sugar diabetes)
    Heart disease
    Hypoglycemia (low blood sugar)
    Hypotension (low blood pressure)
    Kidney disease
    Liver disease

—if you are taking **any** other prescription or nonprescription (OTC) medicine, especially:

    Aminoglycosides by injection or topical application (amikacin, gentamicin, kanamycin, neomycin, netilmicin, streptomycin, tobramycin)
    Amphotericin B by injection (e.g., Fungizone)
    Capreomycin (e.g., Capastat)
    Captopril (e.g., Capoten)
    Carmustine (e.g., BiCNU)
    Cisplatin (e.g., Platinol)
    Cyclosporine (e.g., Sandimmune)
    Gold salts
    Lithium (e.g., Lithane)
    Medicine for inflammation or pain (diclofenac, diflunisal, fenoprofen, flurbiprofen [oral], ibuprofen, indomethacin, ketoprofen, meclofenamate, mefenamic acid, naproxen, phenylbutazone, piroxicam, sulindac, tiaprofenic acid, tolmetin)
    Methotrexate (e.g., Mexate)
    Neomycin by mouth (e.g., Mycifradin)
    Penicillamine (e.g., Cuprimine)
    Plicamycin (e.g., Mithracin)
    Rifampin (e.g., Rifadin)
    Streptozocin (e.g., Zanosar)
    Sulfonamides (sulfa medicine)
    Tetracyclines, except doxycycline and minocycline
    Vancomycin by injection (e.g., Vancocin)

—if you regularly take large amounts of combination pain medicine containing acetaminophen and aspirin (e.g., Excedrin) or other salicylates.

Proper Use of This Medicine

To help clear up your infection completely, **pentamidine must be given for the full time of treatment** even if you begin to feel better after a few days. Also, it works best when there is a constant amount in the blood. To help keep the amount constant, pentamidine must be given on a regular schedule.

Precautions While Using This Medicine

Some patients may develop sudden, severe low blood pressure after a single dose of pentamidine. Therefore, you should be lying down while you are receiving this medicine. Also, your doctor may want to check your blood pressure while you are receiving pentamidine and several times afterward until your blood pressure is stable.

Side Effects of This Medicine

Pentamidine may cause some serious side effects, including heart problems, low blood pressure, low or high blood sugar, and other blood problems. **You and your doctor should discuss the good this medicine will do as well as the risks of receiving it.**

Along with its needed effects, a medicine may cause some unwanted effects. Although not all of these side effects may occur, if they do occur they may need medical attention.

Check with your doctor or nurse immediately if any of the following side effects occur:

More common
Drowsiness
Flushed, dry skin
Fruit-like breath odor
Increased thirst
Increased urination
Loss of appetite
> Note: The above side effects may also occur up to several months after you stop receiving this medicine.

Anxiety
Chills
Cold sweats
Cool, pale skin
Headache
Increased hunger
Nausea
Nervousness
Rapid or irregular pulse
Shakiness
Unusual tiredness or weakness

In addition to the side effects mentioned above, check with your doctor as soon as possible if any of the following side effects also occur:

More common
Blurred vision
Confusion
Dizziness
Fainting or lightheadedness
Hallucinations (seeing, hearing, or feeling things that are not there)
Skin rash
Sore throat and fever
Unusual bleeding or bruising

Other side effects may occur that usually do not require medical attention. These side effects may go away during treatment as your body adjusts to the medicine.

However, check with your doctor if any of the following side effects continue or are bothersome:

More common
Sore, hardness, or pain at place of injection into a muscle
Vomiting
Less common
Redness or flushing of the face, especially following injection into a vein

Pentamidine may also cause an unpleasant metallic taste. This side effect is to be expected and does not require medical attention.

For elderly patients: Many medicines have not been tested in older people. Therefore, it is not known whether the medicine acts the same way it does in younger adults. Check with your doctor or pharmacist if you notice any unusual effects while receiving this medicine or if you think it is not working as it should.

Other side effects not listed above may also occur in some patients. If you notice any other effects, check with your doctor.

December 1987

Additional Information

In addition to the above information, for patients receiving pentamidine for the prevention of visceral leishmaniasis (black fever; Dumdum fever; kala-azar) or African trypanosomiasis (trypanosome fever; African sleeping sickness):

• If you are living in or will be traveling to an area where there is a chance of getting black fever or African sleeping sickness, the following measures will help to prevent either disease:

—If possible, sleep under fine-mesh netting to avoid being bitten by sandflies (which cause black fever) or tsetse flies (which cause African sleeping sickness).

—Wear long-sleeved shirts or blouses and long trousers to protect arms and legs, especially at dusk or during evening hours when sandflies are out. Since tsetse flies can bite through thin clothing, it is best to wear clothing made from fairly heavy material to protect arms and legs.

—Apply insect repellant to uncovered areas of the skin when sandflies or tsetse flies are out.

PENTOXIFYLLINE (Systemic)

A commonly used brand name is Trental.

To the Reader: If you do not recognize the names of medical conditions or medicines referred to in this information, check with your doctor, nurse, or pharmacist. Definitions for selected medical terms may be found in the Glossary. Brand names for the generic drug names listed can be found in the Index. In addition, selected brand names commonly associated with the generic name have been included in the text to help you recognize medicine you may be taking. The fact that a brand name product is not mentioned does not mean the information does not apply. It is a good idea for you to learn both the generic and brand names of your medicines and to write them down for future use.

Pentoxifylline (pen-tox-IF-i-lin) is a medicine that improves the flow of blood through blood vessels. It is taken by mouth to reduce leg pain caused by poor blood circulation. Pentoxifylline makes it possible to walk farther before having to rest because of leg cramps.

Pentoxifylline is available only with your doctor's prescription.

Remember:
• **This medicine has been prescribed for your current medical problem only.** It must not be given to other people or used for other problems unless you are directed to do so by your doctor.

• **Keep all medicines out of the reach of children.**

• In order for this medicine to work, it must be used as directed.

• **It is very important that you read and understand the following information.** If any of the information causes you special concern, do not decide against using this medicine without first checking with your doctor.

• Before you begin using any new medicine (prescription or nonprescription) or if you develop any new medical problem while you are using this medicine, check with your doctor, nurse, or pharmacist.

• **If you have any questions** about the following information or if you want more information about this medicine or your medical problem, **ask your doctor, nurse, or pharmacist.**

Before Using This Medicine

In order to decide on the best treatment for your medical problem, your doctor should be told:

—if you have ever had any unusual or allergic reaction to pentoxifylline or to other xanthines such as aminophylline, caffeine, dyphylline, ethylenediamine (contained in aminophylline), oxtriphylline, theobromine, or theophylline.

—if you are on a low-salt, low-sugar, or any other special diet, or if you are allergic to any substance, such as foods, sulfites or other preservatives, or dyes. Most medicines contain more than their active ingredient. Your doctor, nurse, or pharmacist can help you avoid products that may cause a problem.

—if you are **pregnant** or if you may become pregnant. Studies have not been done in humans. Although pentoxifylline has not been shown to cause birth defects in animals, it has caused other harmful effects in rats given doses 25 times the maximum human dose.

—if you are **breast-feeding**. It is not known whether pentoxifylline passes into the breast milk. This medicine has not been shown to cause problems in nursing babies.

—if you have kidney disease.

—if you are taking **any** other prescription or nonprescription (OTC) medicine.

—if you smoke tobacco.

Proper Use of This Medicine

Swallow the tablet whole. Do not crush, break, or chew before swallowing.

Pentoxifylline should be taken with meals so that it will not upset your stomach.

If you miss a dose of this medicine, take it as soon as possible. However, if it is almost time for your next dose, skip the missed dose and go back to your regular dosing schedule. Do not double doses.

How to store this medicine:

• **Keep out of the reach of children.**

• Store away from heat and direct light.

• Do not store in the bathroom, near the kitchen sink, or in other damp places. Heat or moisture may cause the medicine to break down.

• Do not keep outdated medicine or medicine no longer needed. Be sure that any discarded medicine is out of the reach of children.

Precautions While Using This Medicine

It may take several weeks for this medicine to work. If you feel that pentoxifylline is not working, do not stop taking it on your own. Instead, check with your doctor.

Smoking tobacco may worsen your condition since nicotine may further narrow your blood vessels. Therefore, it is best to avoid smoking.

Side Effects of This Medicine

Along with its needed effects, a medicine may cause some unwanted effects. Although not all of these side effects may occur, if they do occur they may need medical attention.

Check with your doctor as soon as possible if any of the
following side effects occur:

Rare
    Chest pain
    Irregular heartbeat

*Signs of overdose (in the order in which they may
occur)*
    Drowsiness
    Flushing
    Faintness
    Unusual excitement
    Convulsions (seizures)

Other side effects may occur that usually do not require
    medical attention. These side effects may go away
    during treatment as your body adjusts to the medicine.

However, check with your doctor if any of the following side effects continue or are bothersome:
Less common
    Dizziness
    Headache
    Nausea or vomiting
    Stomach discomfort

For elderly patients: The above side effects may be more
    likely to occur in the elderly, who are usually more
    sensitive to the effects of pentoxifylline.

Other side effects not listed above may also occur in some
    patients. If you notice any other effects, check with
    your doctor.

December 1987

PERMETHRIN (Topical)

A commonly used brand name is Nix.

To the Reader: If you do not recognize the names of medical conditions or medicines referred to in this information, check with your doctor, nurse, or pharmacist. Definitions for selected medical terms may be found in the Glossary. Brand names for the generic drug names listed can be found in the Index. In addition, selected brand names commonly associated with the generic name have been included in the text to help you recognize medicine you may be taking. The fact that a brand name product is not mentioned does not mean the information does not apply. It is a good idea for you to learn both the generic and brand names of your medicines and to write them down for future use.

Permethrin (per-METH-rin) is applied to the hair and scalp to treat head lice infections. It acts by destroying both the lice and their eggs.

This medicine is available only with your doctor's prescription.

Remember:

• **This medicine has been prescribed for your current medical problem only.** It must not be given to other people or used for other problems unless you are directed to do so by your doctor.

• **Keep all medicines out of the reach of children.**

• In order for this medicine to work, it must be used as directed.

• **It is very important that you read and understand the following information.** If any of the information causes you special concern, do not decide against using this medicine without first checking with your doctor.

• Before you begin using any new medicine (prescription or nonprescription) or if you develop any new medical problem while you are using this medicine, check with your doctor, nurse, or pharmacist.

• **If you have any questions** about the following information or if you want more information about this medicine or your medical problem, **ask your doctor, nurse, or pharmacist.**

Before Using This Medicine

In order to decide on the best treatment for your medical problem, your doctor should be told:

—if you have ever had any unusual or allergic reaction to other synthetic pyrethroids, such as those found in household insecticides; to pyrethrins or chrysanthemums; or to veterinary insecticides containing permethrin.

—if you are allergic to any substance, such as sulfites or other preservatives or dyes. Most medicines contain more than their active ingredient. Your doctor, nurse, or pharmacist can help you avoid products that may cause a problem.

—if you are **pregnant** or if you may become pregnant. Studies have not been done in humans. However, permethrin has not been shown to cause birth defects in animal studies.

—if you are **breast-feeding**. Although it is not known whether permethrin passes into the breast milk, some animal studies have shown that permethrin can cause tumors.

—if you have severe inflammation of the scalp.

Proper Use of This Medicine

Keep this medicine away from the eyes. If you should accidentally get some in your eyes, flush them thoroughly with water at once.

Permethrin lotion comes in a container that holds only one treatment. Use as much of the medicine as you need and discard any remaining lotion properly.

How to apply this medicine:

• Shampoo the hair and scalp using regular shampoo.

• Thoroughly rinse and towel dry the hair and scalp.

• Allow hair to air dry for a few minutes.

• Shake the permethrin lotion well before applying.

• Thoroughly wet the hair and scalp with the permethrin lotion and allow it to remain in place for 10 minutes.

• Then, rinse the hair and scalp thoroughly and dry with a clean towel.

• When the hair is dry, you may want to comb the hair with a fine-toothed comb to remove any remaining nits (eggs) or nit shells.

Head lice can be easily transferred from one person to another by direct contact with clothing, hats, scarves, bedding, towels, washcloths, hairbrushes and combs, or hairs from infected persons. Therefore, **all members of your household should be examined for head lice and should receive treatment if they are found to be infected.** If you have any questions about this, check with your doctor.

How to store this medicine:

• **Keep out of the reach of children.**

• Store away from heat and direct light.

• Keep this medicine from freezing. Do not refrigerate.

• Do not keep outdated medicine or medicine no longer needed. Be sure that any discarded medicine is out of the reach of children.

Precautions While Using This Medicine

To prevent reinfection or spreading of the infection to other people, good health habits are required. These include the following:

• Machine wash all clothing (including hats, scarves, and coats), bedding, towels, and washcloths in very hot water and dry them by using the hot cycle of a dryer for at least 20 minutes. Clothing or bedding that cannot be washed should be dry cleaned or sealed in an airtight plastic bag for 2 weeks.

• Shampoo all wigs and hairpieces.

• Wash all hairbrushes and combs in very hot soapy water (above 130 °F) for 5 to 10 minutes and do not share them with other people.

• Clean the house or room by thoroughly vacuuming upholstered furniture, rugs, and floors.

• Wash all toys in very hot soapy water (above 130 °F) for 5 to 10 minutes or seal in an airtight plastic bag for 2 weeks. This is especially important for stuffed toys used on the bed.

Side Effects of This Medicine

Along with its needed effects, a medicine may cause some unwanted effects. Although not all of these side effects may occur, if they do occur they may need medical attention.

Check with your doctor if any of the following side effects continue or are bothersome:

Less common or rare
  Itching, redness, swelling, burning, numbness, rash, stinging, or tingling of the scalp

For elderly patients: Many medicines have not been tested in older people. Therefore, it is not known whether the medicine acts the same way it does in younger adults. Check with your doctor or pharmacist if you notice any unusual effects while using this medicine or if you think it is not working as it should.

Other side effects not listed above may also occur in some patients. If you notice any other effects, check with your doctor.

December 1987

PERPHENAZINE AND AMITRIPTYLINE
(Systemic)

Some commonly used brand names are Etrafon, PMS Levazine*, and Triavil.

Generic name product may also be available.

---

*Not available in the U.S.

To the Reader: If you do not recognize the names of medical conditions or medicines referred to in this information, check with your doctor, nurse, or pharmacist. Definitions for selected medical terms may be found in the Glossary. Brand names for the generic drug names listed can be found in the Index. In addition, selected brand names commonly associated with the generic name have been included in the text to help you recognize medicine you may be taking. The fact that a brand name product is not mentioned does not mean the information does not apply. It is a good idea for you to learn both the generic and brand names of your medicines and to write them down for future use.

Perphenazine (per-FEN-a-zeen) and amitriptyline (a-mee-TRIP-ti-leen) combination is taken by mouth to treat certain mental and emotional conditions.

This combination is available only with your doctor's prescription.

Remember:
- **This medicine has been prescribed for your current medical problem only.** It must not be given to other people or used for other problems unless you are directed to do so by your doctor.

- **Keep all medicines out of the reach of children.**

- In order for this medicine to work, it must be used as directed.

- **It is very important that you read and understand the following information.** If any of the information causes you special concern, do not decide against using this medicine without first checking with your doctor.

- Before you begin using any new medicine (prescription or nonprescription) or if you develop any new medical problem while you are using this medicine, check with your doctor, nurse, or pharmacist.

- **If you have any questions** about the following information or if you want more information about this medicine or your medical problem, **ask your doctor, nurse, or pharmacist.**

Before Using This Medicine

In order to decide on the best treatment for your medical problem, your doctor should be told:

—if you have ever had any unusual or allergic reaction to other phenothiazine medicines (such as acetophenazine, chlorpromazine, fluphenazine, mesoridazine, perphenazine, prochlorperazine, promazine, thioridazine, trifluoperazine, or triflupromazine), other tricyclic antidepressants (such as amoxapine, clomipramine, desipramine, doxepin, imipramine, nortriptyline, protriptyline, or trimipramine), or thioxanthenes (chlorprothixene or thiothixene).

—if you are on a low-salt, low-sugar, or any other special diet, or if you are allergic to any substance, such as foods, sulfites or other preservatives, or dyes. Most medicines contain more than their active ingredient. Your doctor, nurse, or pharmacist can help you avoid products that may cause a problem.

—if you are **pregnant** or if you may become pregnant. Perphenazine and amitriptyline combination has not been shown to cause birth defects. However, some side effects such as jaundice and muscle tremors have occurred in some newborn babies when their mothers received other phenothiazines during pregnancy.

—if you are **breast-feeding**. Perphenazine and amitriptyline combination passes into the breast milk. However, it has not been shown to cause problems in nursing babies.

—if you have any of the following medical problems:
   Alcoholism
   Asthma (history of) or other lung disease
   Blood disease
   Difficult urination
   Enlarged prostate
   Epilepsy or other seizure disorders
   Glaucoma
   Heart or blood vessel disease
   Liver disease
   Overactive thyroid
   Parkinson's disease
   Stomach or intestinal problems

—if you are taking **any** other prescription or nonprescription (OTC) medicine, especially:
   Amoxapine (e.g., Asendin)
   Antithyroid agents (medicine for overactive thyroid)
   Appetite suppressants (diet pills)
   Chlorprothixene (e.g., Taractan)
   Central nervous system (CNS) depressants
   Cimetidine (e.g., Tagamet)
   Ephedrine
   Epinephrine (e.g., Adrenalin)
   Guanadrel (e.g., Hylorel)
   Guanethidine (e.g., Ismelin)
   Haloperidol (e.g., Haldol)
   Isoproterenol (e.g., Isuprel)
   Levodopa (e.g., Dopar)
   Lithium (e.g., Lithane)
   Loxapine (e.g., Loxitane)
   Methyldopa (e.g., Aldomet)
   Metoclopramide (e.g., Reglan)
   Metyrosine (e.g., Demser)
   Molindone (e.g., Moban)
   Pemoline (e.g., Cylert)
   Phenylephrine (e.g., Neo-Synephrine)
   Pimozide (e.g., Orap)
   Rauwolfia alkaloids (alseroxylon, deserpidine, rauwolfia serpentina, reserpine)
   Thiothixene (e.g., Navane)

—if you are planning to have a myelogram.

Proper Use of This Medicine

To lessen stomach upset, take this medicine immediately after meals or with food, unless your doctor has told you to take it on an empty stomach.

Do not take more of this medicine and do not take it more often than your doctor ordered. This is particularly important when it is given to the elderly, since they are more sensitive to the effects of this medicine.

Sometimes perphenazine and amitriptyline combination must be taken for several weeks before its full effect is reached.

If you miss a dose of this medicine, take it as soon as possible. However, if it is within 2 hours of your next dose, skip the missed dose and go back to your regular dosing schedule. Do not double doses.

How to store this medicine:

• **Keep out of the reach of children** since overdose is especially dangerous in young children.

• Store away from heat and direct light.

• Do not store in the bathroom, near the kitchen sink, or in other damp places. Heat or moisture may cause the medicine to break down.

• Do not keep outdated medicine or medicine no longer needed. Be sure that any discarded medicine is out of the reach of children.

Precautions While Using This Medicine

Your doctor should check your progress at regular visits to adjust the dosage and to check for possible unwanted effects of the medicine.

Do not take this medicine within two hours of taking antacids or medicine for diarrhea. Taking them too close together may make this medicine less effective.

Before having any kind of surgery, dental treatment, or emergency treatment, tell the physician or dentist in charge that you are taking this medicine.

This medicine will add to the effects of alcohol and other CNS depressants (medicines that slow down the nervous system, possibly causing drowsiness). Some examples of CNS depressants are antihistamines or medicine for hay fever, other allergies, or colds; sedatives, tranquilizers, or sleeping medicine; prescription pain medicine or narcotics barbiturates; medicine for seizures; or anesthetics, including some dental anesthetics. **Check with your doctor before taking any of the above while you are using this medicine.**

This medicine may cause some people to become drowsy or less alert than they are normally, especially during the first few weeks the medicine is being taken. Even if you take this medicine only at bedtime, you may feel drowsy or less alert on arising. **Make sure you know how you react to this medicine before you drive, use machines, or do other jobs that require you to be alert.**

Dizziness, lightheadedness, or fainting may occur, especially when you get up from a lying or sitting position. Getting up slowly may help. If the problem continues or gets worse, check with your doctor.

Sometimes patients may show signs of restlessness and excitement after taking this medicine. If this occurs, check with your doctor.

This medicine will often cause you to sweat less, allowing your body temperature to increase. **Use extra care not to become overheated during exercise or hot weather while you are taking this medicine,** since overheating could possibly result in heat stroke. Also, **hot baths or saunas may make you feel dizzy or faint** while you are taking this medicine.

Perphenazine and amitriptyline combination may cause dryness of the mouth. For temporary relief, use sugarless gum or candy, melt bits of ice in your mouth, or use a saliva substitute. However, if dry mouth continues for more than 2 weeks, check with your physician or dentist. Continuing dryness of the mouth may increase the chance of dental disease, including tooth decay, gum disease, and fungal infections.

Some people who take this medicine may become more sensitive to sunlight than they are normally. When you first begin taking this medicine, avoid too much sun and do not use a sunlamp, especially if you tend to burn easily. If you have a severe reaction, check with your doctor.

Do not stop taking this medicine without first checking with your doctor. Your doctor may want you to reduce gradually the amount you are taking before stopping completely. This is to prevent side effects and to prevent your condition from becoming worse.

Side Effects of This Medicine

Along with its needed effects, a medicine may cause some unwanted effects. Although not all of these side effects may occur, if they do occur they may need medical attention.

Get emergency help immediately if any of the following side effects occur:

Rare
>   Convulsions (seizures)
>   Difficulty in breathing
>   Fast heartbeat
>   Fever
>   High or low blood pressure
>   Increase in sweating
>   Loss of bladder control
>   Muscle stiffness (severe)
>   Unusual feeling of tiredness or weakness
>   Unusually pale skin

Also, check with your doctor as soon as possible if any of the following side effects occur:

More common
>   Difficulty in speaking or swallowing
>   Eye pain
>   Fainting
>   Fixation of eyes
>   Loss of balance control
>   Mask-like face
>   Muscle spasms, especially of face, neck, and back

Shuffling walk
Stiffness of arms and legs
Trembling and shaking of fingers and hands
Unusual twisting movements of body

Less common

Blurred vision or any change in vision
Confusion
Constipation
Chewing movements
Difficult urination
Hallucinations (seeing, hearing, or feeling things that are
    not there)
Irregular heartbeat
Lip smacking or puckering
Puffing of cheeks
Rapid or fine, worm-like movements of tongue
Nervousness or restlessness or need to keep moving
Shakiness
Uncontrolled movements of arms or legs
Unusually slow pulse

Rare

Skin discoloration
Skin rash and itching
Sore throat and fever
Swelling of face and tongue
Yellow eyes or skin

Other side effects may occur that usually do not require
    medical attention. These side effects may go away
    during treatment as your body adjusts to the medicine.

However, check with your doctor if any of the following side effects continue or are bothersome:

More common

Decreased sweating
Dizziness
Drowsiness
Dry mouth
Headache
Increased appetite for sweets
Increased skin sensitivity to sun
Nasal congestion
Nausea or vomiting

Less common

Changes in menstrual period
Decreased sexual ability
Diarrhea
Swelling of breasts
Trouble in sleeping

For elderly patients: The above side effects, especially
    constipation, dizziness or fainting, drowsiness, dry
    mouth, uncontrolled movements of the mouth and
    tongue, and trembling of fingers and hands are more
    likely to occur in the elderly, who are usually more
    sensitive to the effects of perphenazine and amitrip-
    tyline combination.

Other side effects not listed above may also occur in some
    patients. If you notice any other effects, check with
    your doctor.

December 1987

PHENAZOPYRIDINE (Systemic)

Some commonly used brand names are:

Azo-Standard	Phenazodine
Baridium	Pyridiate
Di-Azo	Pyridium
Phenazo*	Pyronium*

Generic name product may also be available in the U.S.

*Not available in the U.S.

To the Reader: If you do not recognize the names of medical conditions or medicines referred to in this information, check with your doctor, nurse, or pharmacist. Definitions for selected medical terms may be found in the Glossary. Brand names for the generic drug names listed can be found in the Index. In addition, selected brand names commonly associated with the generic name have been included in the text to help you recognize medicine you may be taking. The fact that a brand name product is not mentioned does not mean the information does not apply. It is a good idea for you to learn both the generic and brand names of your medicines and to write them down for future use.

Phenazopyridine (fen-az-oh-PEER-i-deen) is used to relieve the pain, burning, and discomfort caused by infection or irritation of the urinary tract. It is not an antibiotic and will not cure the infection itself.

Phenazopyridine is available only with your doctor's prescription.

Remember:

• **This medicine has been prescribed for your current medical problem only.** It must not be given to other people or used for other problems unless you are directed to do so by your doctor.

• **Keep all medicines out of the reach of children.**

• In order for this medicine to work, it must be used as directed.

• **It is very important that you read and understand the following information.** If any of the information causes you special concern, do not decide against using this medicine without first checking with your doctor.

• Before you begin using any new medicine (prescription or nonprescription) or if you develop any new medical problem while you are using this medicine, check with your doctor, nurse, or pharmacist.

• **If you have any questions** about the following information or if you want more information about this medicine or your medical problem, **ask your doctor, nurse, or pharmacist**.

Before Using This Medicine

In order to decide on the best treatment for your medical problem, your doctor should be told:

—if you have ever had any unusual or allergic reaction to phenazopyridine.

—if you are on a low-salt, low-sugar, or any other special diet, or if you are allergic to any substance, such as foods, sulfites or other preservatives, or dyes.

Most medicines contain more than their active ingredient. Your doctor, nurse, or pharmacist can help you avoid products that may cause a problem.

—if you are **pregnant** or if you may become pregnant. Studies on birth defects with phenazopyridine have not been done in humans. However, the medicine has not been shown to cause birth defects in animal studies.

—if you are **breast-feeding**. Phenazopyridine has not been shown to cause problems in nursing babies.

—if you have either of the following medical problems:
Hepatitis
Kidney disease

Proper Use of This Medicine

This medicine is best taken with food or after eating a meal or a snack to lessen stomach upset.

Do not use any leftover medicine for future urinary tract problems without first checking with your doctor. An infection may require additional medicine.

If you miss a dose of this medicine, take it as soon as you remember. However, if it is almost time for your next dose, skip the missed dose and go back to your regular dosing schedule. Do not double doses.

How to store this medicine:

• **Keep out of the reach of children.**

• Store away from heat and direct light.

• Do not store this medicine in the bathroom, near the kitchen sink, or in other damp places. Heat or moisture may cause the medicine to break down.

• Do not keep outdated medicine or medicine no longer needed. Be sure that any discarded medicine is out of the reach of children.

Precautions While Using This Medicine

Check with your doctor if symptoms such as bloody urine, difficult or painful urination, frequent urge to urinate, or sudden decrease in the amount of urine appear or become worse while you are taking this medicine.

This medicine causes the urine to turn reddish orange. This is to be expected while you are using this medicine. Also, the medicine may stain clothing.

Diabetics—This medicine may cause false test results with urine sugar tests and urine ketone tests. If you have any questions about this, check with your doctor, nurse, or pharmacist, especially if your diabetes is not well controlled.

Side Effects of This Medicine

Along with its needed effects, a medicine may cause some unwanted effects. Although not all of these side effects may occur, if they do occur they may need medical attention.

© 1988   The United States Pharmacopeial Convention, Inc.

Check with your doctor as soon as possible if any of the following side effects occur:

- Blue or blue-purple color of skin
- Skin rash
- Unusual tiredness or weakness
- Yellow eyes or skin

Other side effects may occur that usually do not require medical attention. These side effects may go away during treatment as your body adjusts to the medicine. However, check with your doctor if any of the following side effects continue or are bothersome:

- Dizziness
- Headache
- Indigestion
- Stomach cramps or pain

For elderly patients: Many medicines have not been tested in older people. Therefore, it is not known whether the medicine acts the same way it does in younger adults. Check with your doctor or pharmacist if you notice any unusual effects while taking this medicine or if you think it is not working as it should.

Other side effects not listed above may also occur in some patients. If you notice any other effects, check with your doctor.

December 1987

PHENOLSULFONPHTHALEIN (Systemic)

Some commonly used names are Phenol Red and PSP.

To the Reader: If you do not recognize the names of medical conditions or medicines referred to in this information, check with your doctor, nurse, or pharmacist. Definitions for selected medical terms may be found in the Glossary. Brand names for the generic drug names listed can be found in the Index. In addition, selected brand names commonly associated with the generic name have been included in the text to help you recognize medicine you may be taking. The fact that a brand name product is not mentioned does not mean the information does not apply. It is a good idea for you to learn both the generic and brand names of your medicines and to write them down for future use.

Phenolsulfonphthalein   (fee-nole-sul-fon-THAY-leen) is used as a test to help diagnose problems or disease of the kidneys. This test determines how well your kidneys are working.

Phenolsulfonphthalein passes out of the body almost entirely in the urine. Measuring the amount of phenolsulfonphthalein in the urine can help the doctor determine if the kidneys are working properly.

How test is done: After you have emptied your bladder, phenolsulfonphthalein will be given by injection. Then you will be asked to empty your bladder into a container one or more times after the medicine is given. The amount of this medicine in your urine will be measured. Then the results of the test will be studied.

It is very important that you **empty the bladder completely** and collect all the urine when you are asked to do so. If any urine is left behind or lost, it will change the results of the test.

Phenolsulfonphthalein is to be used only under the supervision of a doctor.

Remember:

• **If you have any questions** about the following information or if you want more information about this test or your medical problem, **ask your doctor, nurse, or pharmacist.**

Before Having This Test

Before this test is given, your doctor should be told:

—if you have ever had any unusual or allergic reaction to phenolsulfonphthalein.

—if you are **pregnant** or if you suspect that you may be pregnant. Studies have not been done in either humans or animals.

—if you are **breast-feeding**. It is not known whether phenolsulfonphthalein passes into the breast milk. This medicine has not been shown to cause problems in nursing babies.

—if you have any of the following medical problems:
   Gout
   Heart or blood vessel disease
   Liver disease
   Multiple myeloma (a kind of cancer)

—if you are taking **any** other prescription or nonprescription (OTC) medicine, especially:
   Aspirin or other salicylates
   Atropine
   Diuretics (water pills)
   Penicillins
   Probenecid (e.g., Benemid)
   Sulfinpyrazone (e.g., Anturane)
   Sulfonamides (sulfa medicine)

Preparation for This Test

Your doctor will ask you to drink a certain amount of water a little while before this test is done. **Follow your doctor's instructions carefully**. Otherwise, this test may not work and may have to be done again.

Side Effects of This Medicine

Along with its needed effects, a medicine may cause some unwanted effects. Although this medicine usually does not cause any side effects, **tell your doctor or nurse immediately if you notice wheezing or skin rash or itching shortly after it is given.**

Other side effects not listed above may also occur in some patients. If you notice any other effects, check with your doctor.

December 1987

PHENOTHIAZINES (Systemic)

This information applies to the following medicines:

Acetophenazine (a-set-oh-FEN-a-zeen)
Chlorpromazine (klor-PROE-ma-zeen)
Fluphenazine (floo-FEN-a-zeen)
Mesoridazine (mez-oh-RID-a-zeen)
Perphenazine (per-FEN-a-zeen)
Prochlorperazine (proe-klor-PAIR-a-zeen)
Promazine (PROE-ma-zeen)
Thioridazine (thye-oh-RID-a-zeen)
Trifluoperazine (trye-floo-oh-PAIR-a-zeen)
Triflupromazine (trye-floo-PROE-ma-zeen)

This information does *not* apply to the following medicines:

Ethopropazine
Methdilazine
Promethazine
Propiomazine
Thiethylperazine
Trimeprazine

Some commonly used brand names are:	Generic names:
Tindal	Acetophenazine
Chlorpromanyl* Clorazine Largactil* Novochlorpromazine* Ormazine Promaz Thorazine	Chlorpromazine†
Apo-Fluphenazine* Modecate* Moditen* Moditen Enanthate* Permitil Prolixin Prolixin Decanoate Prolixin Enanthate	Fluphenazine
Serentil	Mesoridazine
Apo-Perphenazine* Phenazine* Trilafon	Perphenazine
Chlorazine Compazine Stemetil*	Prochlorperazine†
Prozine Sparine	Promazine†
Apo-Thioridazine* Mellaril Mellaril-S Millazine Novoridazine* PMS Thioridazine*	Thioridazine†
Apo-Trifluoperazine* Novoflurazine* Solazine* Stelazine Suprazine Terfluzine*	Trifluoperazine†
Vesprin	Triflupromazine

*Not available in the U.S.
†Generic name product may also be available.

To the Reader: If you do not recognize the names of medical conditions or medicines referred to in this information, check with your doctor, nurse, or pharmacist. Definitions for selected medical terms may be found in the Glossary. Brand names for the generic drug names listed can be found in the Index. In addition, selected brand names commonly associated with the generic name have been included in the text to help you recognize medicine you may be taking. The fact that a brand name product is not mentioned does not mean the information does not apply. It is a good idea for you to learn both the generic and brand names of your medicines and to write them down for future use.

Phenothiazines (FEE-noe-THYE-a-zeens) are used to treat nervous, mental, and emotional conditions. Some are used also to control anxiety, nausea and vomiting, and severe hiccups. Phenothiazines may also be used for other conditions as determined by your doctor.

Phenothiazines are available only with your doctor's prescription.

Remember:

• **This medicine has been prescribed for your current medical problem only.** It must not be given to other people or used for other problems unless you are directed to do so by your doctor.

• **Keep all medicines out of the reach of children.**

• In order for this medicine to work, it must be used as directed.

• If you are receiving this medicine by injection, some of the information about this medicine may not apply.

• **It is very important that you read and understand the following information.** If any of the information causes you special concern, do not decide against using this medicine without first checking with your doctor.

• Before you begin using any new medicine (prescription or nonprescription) or if you develop any new medical problem while you are using this medicine, check with your doctor, nurse, or pharmacist.

• **If you have any questions** about the following information or if you want more information about this medicine or your medical problem, **ask your doctor, nurse, or pharmacist**.

Before Using This Medicine

In order to decide on the best treatment for your medical problem, your doctor should be told:

—if you have ever had any unusual or allergic reaction to phenothiazine medicines.

—if you are on a low-salt, low-sugar, or any other special diet, or if you are allergic to any substance, such as foods, sulfites or other preservatives, or dyes. Most medicines contain more than their active ingredient, and many liquid medicines contain alcohol. Your doctor, nurse, or pharmacist can help you avoid products that may cause a problem.

—if you are **pregnant** or if you may become pregnant. Although phenothiazines have not been shown to cause birth defects, some side effects, such as jaundice and muscle tremors and other movement problems, have occurred in a few newborns whose mothers received phenothiazines during pregnancy close to time of delivery.

—if you are **breast-feeding**. Small amounts of some phenothiazines are known to pass into the breast milk, and they may cause drowsiness in the nursing baby.

—if you have any of the following medical problems:

Alcoholism, active
Blood disease
Difficult urination
Enlarged prostate
Glaucoma
Heart or blood vessel disease
Liver disease
Lung disease
Parkinson's disease
Reye's syndrome
Seizure disorders
Stomach ulcers

—if you are taking **any** other prescription or nonprescription (OTC) medicine, especially:

Amoxapine (e.g., Asendin)
Antithyroid agents (medicine for overactive thyroid)
Chlorprothixene (e.g., Taractan)
Central nervous system (CNS) depressants
Epinephrine (e.g., Adrenalin)
Haloperidol (e.g., Haldol)
Levodopa (e.g., Dopar)
Lithium (e.g., Lithane; Lithizine)
Loxapine (e.g., Loxitane)
Methyldopa (e.g., Aldomet)
Metoclopramide (e.g., Reglan)
Metyrosine (e.g., Demser)
Molindone (e.g., Moban)
Pemoline (e.g., Cylert)
Pimozide (e.g., Orap)
Rauwolfia alkaloids (alseroxylon, deserpidine, rauwolfia serpentina, reserpine)
Thiothixene (e.g., Navane)

—if you are planning to have a myelogram.

Proper Use of This Medicine

For patients taking this medicine by mouth:

• This medicine may be taken with food or a full glass (8 ounces) of water or milk to reduce stomach irritation.

• Do not take this medicine within two hours of taking antacids or medicine for diarrhea. Taking them too close together may make this medicine less effective.

• **If your medicine comes in a dropper bottle,** it must be diluted before you take it. Just before taking, measure each dose with the specially marked dropper and dilute it in ½ glass (4 ounces) of orange or grapefruit juice or distilled water.

• If you are taking the extended-release tablet form of this medicine, each dose should be swallowed whole. Do not break, crush, or chew before swallowing.

For patients using the suppository form of this medicine:

• To insert suppository: First remove the foil wrapper and moisten the suppository with water. Lie down on left side with right knee bent, and push the suppository well up into the rectum with finger.

• If the suppository is too soft to insert because of storage in a warm place, before removing the foil wrapper chill the suppository in the refrigerator for 30 minutes or run cold water over it.

Do not take more of this medicine or take it more often than your doctor ordered. This is particularly important when it is given to children or the elderly, since they may react very strongly to the effects of the medicine.

Sometimes this medicine must be taken for several weeks before its full effect is reached in the treatment of certain mental and emotional conditions.

Do not stop taking this medicine without first checking with your doctor. Your doctor may want you to reduce gradually the amount you are taking before stopping completely. This is to prevent side effects and to prevent your condition from becoming worse.

If you miss a dose of this medicine and your dosing schedule is one dose to be taken:

Once a day—Take the missed dose as soon as possible. Then go back to your regular dosing schedule. However, if you do not remember the missed dose until the next day, skip it and go back to your regular dosing schedule. Do not double doses.

Two times a day—Take the missed dose as soon as possible. Then go back to your regular dosing schedule. However, if it is almost time for your next dose, skip the missed dose and go back to your regular dosing schedule. Do not double doses.

More than two times a day—If you remember within an hour or so of the missed dose, take it right away. However, if you do not remember until later, skip the missed dose and go back to your regular dosing schedule. Do not double doses.

How to store this medicine:

• **Keep out of the reach of children.**

• Store away from heat and direct light.

• Do not store the capsule or tablet form of this medicine in the bathroom, near the kitchen sink, or in other damp places. Heat or moisture may cause the medicine to break down.

• Keep the liquid form of this medicine from freezing.

• Do not keep outdated medicine or medicine no longer needed. Be sure that any discarded medicine is out of the reach of children.

Precautions While Using This Medicine

Your doctor should check your progress at regular visits, especially for the first few months you take this medicine. This will allow your dosage to be changed if necessary to meet your needs.

This medicine will add to the effects of alcohol and other CNS depressants (medicines that slow down the nervous system, possibly causing drowsiness). Some examples of CNS depressants are antihistamines or medicine for hay fever, other allergies, or colds; sedatives,

tranquilizers, or sleeping medicine; prescription pain medicine or narcotics; barbiturates; medicine for seizures; muscle relaxants; or anesthetics, including some dental anesthetics. **Check with your doctor before taking any of the above while you are using this medicine.**

This medicine may cause some people to become drowsy or less alert than they are normally and to have blurred vision, especially during the first few weeks the medicine is being taken. Even if you take this medicine only at bedtime, you may feel drowsy or less alert on arising. **Make sure you know how you react to this medicine before you drive, use machines, or do other jobs that require you to be alert and to see well.**

Dizziness, lightheadedness, or fainting may occur, especially when you get up from a lying or sitting position. Getting up slowly may help. If the problem continues or gets worse, check with your doctor.

Sometimes patients may show signs of restlessness and excitement after taking this medicine. If this occurs, check with your doctor.

This medicine will often make you sweat less, allowing your body temperature to increase. **Use extra care not to become overheated during exercise or hot weather while you are taking this medicine.** Overheating could possibly result in heat stroke. Also, **hot baths or saunas may make you feel dizzy or faint while you are taking this medicine.**

Before having any kind of surgery, dental treatment, or emergency treatment, tell the physician or dentist in charge that you are using this medicine.

Some people who take this medicine may become more sensitive to sunlight than they are normally. When you first begin taking this medicine, avoid too much sun and do not use a sunlamp, especially if you tend to burn easily. **If you have a severe reaction, check with your doctor.**

Phenothiazines may cause dryness of the mouth. For temporary relief, use sugarless candy or gum, melt bits of ice in your mouth, or use a saliva substitute. However, if dry mouth continues for more than 2 weeks, check with your dentist. Continuing dryness of the mouth may increase the chance of dental disease, including tooth decay, gum disease, and fungal infections.

If you are taking a liquid form of this medicine, try to avoid getting it on your skin or clothing because it may cause a skin rash or other irritation.

If you are receiving this medicine by injection:
• The effects of the long-acting injection form of this medicine may last for up to 6 weeks. The precautions and side effects information for this medicine applies during this period of time.

Side Effects of This Medicine

Along with its needed effects, a medicine may cause some unwanted effects. Although not all of these side effects may occur, if they do occur they may need medical attention.

Stop taking this medicine and check with your doctor immediately if any of the following side effects occur:

Rare

Convulsions (seizures)
Difficult or unusually fast breathing
Fast heartbeat or irregular pulse
Fever
High or low blood pressure
Increased sweating
Loss of bladder control
Muscle stiffness (severe)
Unusual feeling of tiredness or weakness
Unusually pale skin

Also, check with your doctor as soon as possible if any of the following side effects occur:

More common

Blurred vision or any change in vision
Difficulty in speaking or swallowing
Fainting
Loss of balance control
Mask-like face
Muscle spasms (especially of face, neck, and back)
Restlessness or need to keep moving
Shuffling walk
Stiffness of arms or legs
Trembling and shaking of hands and fingers
Twisting movements of body

Less common

Chewing movements
Difficult urination
Lip smacking or puckering
Puffing of cheeks
Rapid or fine, worm-like movements of tongue
Skin rash
Uncontrolled movements of arms or legs

Rare

Skin discoloration (after prolonged use)
Sore throat and fever
Yellow eyes or skin

Other side effects may occur that usually do not require medical attention. These side effects may go away during treatment as your body adjusts to the medicine. However, check with your doctor if any of the following side effects continue or are bothersome:

More common

Constipation
Decreased sweating
Dizziness
Drowsiness
Dry mouth
Nasal congestion

Less common

Changes in menstrual period
Decreased sexual ability
Increased sensitivity of skin to sun
Swelling or pain in breasts
Unusual secretion of milk

Some side effects, such as dizziness, stomach pain, nausea or vomiting, trembling of fingers and hands, or uncontrolled movements of the mouth, tongue, and jaw, may occur after you have stopped taking this medicine. If you notice any of these effects, check with your doctor as soon as possible.

Although not all of the side effects listed above have been reported for all of these medicines, they have been reported for at least one of them. However, since all of the phenothiazines are very similar, any of the above side effects may occur with any of these medicines.

For elderly patients: The above side effects, especially constipation, dizziness or fainting, drowsiness, dry mouth, uncontrolled movements of the mouth and tongue, and trembling of fingers and hands are more likely to occur in the elderly, who are usually more sensitive to the effects of phenothiazines.

Other side effects not listed above may also occur in some patients. If you notice any other effects, check with your doctor.

December 1987

PHENOXYBENZAMINE (Systemic)

A commonly used brand name is Dibenzyline.

To the Reader: If you do not recognize the names of medical conditions or medicines referred to in this information, check with your doctor, nurse, or pharmacist. Definitions for selected medical terms may be found in the Glossary. Brand names for the generic drug names listed can be found in the Index. In addition, selected brand names commonly associated with the generic name have been included in the text to help you recognize medicine you may be taking. The fact that a brand name product is not mentioned does not mean the information does not apply. It is a good idea for you to learn both the generic and brand names of your medicines and to write them down for future use.

Phenoxybenzamine (fen-ox-ee-BEN-za-meen) belongs to the general class of medicines called antihypertensives. It is taken by mouth to treat high blood pressure due to a disease called pheochromocytoma. It is also used to treat some problems due to poor blood circulation.

Phenoxybenzamine blocks the effects of certain chemicals in the body. When these chemicals are present in large amounts, they cause high blood pressure.

Phenoxybenzamine is available only with your doctor's prescription.

Remember:
• **This medicine has been prescribed for your current medical problem only.** It must not be given to other people or used for other problems unless you are directed to do so by your doctor.

• **Keep all medicines out of the reach of children.**

• In order for this medicine to work, it must be used as directed.

• **It is very important that you read and understand the following information.** If any of the information causes you special concern, do not decide against using this medicine without first checking with your doctor.

• Before you begin using any new medicine (prescription or nonprescription) or if you develop any new medical problem while you are using this medicine, check with your doctor, nurse, or pharmacist.

• **If you have any questions** about the following information or if you want more information about this medicine or your medical problem, **ask your doctor, nurse, or pharmacist.**

Before Using This Medicine

In order to decide on the best treatment for your medical problem, your doctor should be told:

—if you have ever had any unusual or allergic reaction to phenoxybenzamine.

—if you are on a low-salt, low-sugar, or any other special diet, or if you are allergic to any substance, such as foods, sulfites or other preservatives, or dyes. Most medicines contain more than their active ingredient. Your doctor, nurse, or pharmacist can help you avoid products that may cause a problem.

—if you are **pregnant** or if you may become pregnant. Studies have not been done in either humans or animals.

—if you are **breast-feeding**. Phenoxybenzamine has not been shown to cause problems in nursing babies.

—if you have any of the following medical problems:
Angina (chest pain)
Heart or blood vessel disease
Kidney disease
Lung infection

—if you have recently had a heart attack or stroke.

—if you are taking **any** other prescription or nonprescription (OTC) medicine.

Proper Use of This Medicine

In order to help remember to take your medicine, try to get into the habit of taking it at the same time each day.

If you miss a dose of this medicine, take it as soon as you remember. However, if it is almost time for your next dose, skip the missed dose and go back to your regular dosing schedule. Do not double doses.

How to store this medicine:

• **Keep out of the reach of children.**

• Store away from heat and direct light.

• Do not store in the bathroom, near the kitchen sink, or in other damp places. Heat or moisture may cause the medicine to break down.

• Do not keep outdated medicine or medicine no longer needed. Be sure that any discarded medicine is out of the reach of children.

Precautions While Using This Medicine

It is important that your doctor check your progress at regular visits to make sure that this medicine is working properly and to check for unwanted effects.

Do not take other medicines unless they have been discussed with your doctor. This especially includes over-the-counter (nonprescription) medicines for appetite control, asthma, colds, cough, hay fever, or sinus problems, since they may interfere with the effects of this medicine.

Phenoxybenzamine may cause some people to become dizzy, drowsy, or less alert than they are normally. This is more likely to happen when you begin to take it or when you increase the amount of medicine you are taking. **Make sure you know how you react to this medicine before you drive, use machines, or do other jobs that require you to be alert.**

Dizziness, lightheadedness, or fainting may occur, especially when you get up from a lying or sitting position. Getting up slowly may help, but if the problem continues or gets worse, check with your doctor.

The dizziness, lightheadedness, or fainting is also more likely to occur if you drink alcohol, stand for long periods of time, exercise, or if the weather is hot. **While you are taking this medicine, be careful in the amount of alcohol you drink. Also, use extra care during exercise or hot weather or if you must stand for long periods of time.**

Before having any kind of surgery (including dental surgery) or emergency treatment, **tell the physician or dentist in charge that you are using this medicine.**

Phenoxybenzamine may cause dryness of the mouth, nose, and throat. For temporary relief of mouth dryness, use sugarless candy or gum, melt bits of ice in your mouth, or use a saliva substitute. However, if dry mouth continues for more than 2 weeks, check with your physician or dentist. Continuing dryness of the mouth may increase the chance of dental disease, including tooth decay, gum disease, and fungal infections.

Side Effects of This Medicine

In rats and mice, phenoxybenzamine has been found to increase the risk of development of malignant tumors. It is not known if phenoxybenzamine increases the chance of tumors in humans.

Along with its needed effects, a medicine may cause some unwanted effects. The following side effects may go away as your body adjusts to the medicine. However, check with your doctor if any of these effects continue or are bothersome:

More common
    Dizziness or lightheadedness, especially when getting up from a lying or sitting position
    Fast heartbeat
    Pinpoint pupils
    Stuffy nose

Less common
    Confusion
    Drowsiness
    Dry mouth
    Headache
    Lack of energy
    Sexual problems in males
    Tiredness or weakness

For elderly patients: Dizziness or lightheadedness may be more likely to occur in the elderly, who are more sensitive to the effects of phenoxybenzamine. In addition, phenoxybenzamine may reduce tolerance to cold temperatures in elderly patients.

Other side effects not listed above may also occur in some patients. If you notice any other effects, check with your doctor.

December 1987

PHENTOLAMINE AND PAPAVERINE
(Intracavernosal)

Some commonly used brand names are Regitine and Rogitine*.

---

*Not available in the U.S.

To the Reader: If you do not recognize the names of medical conditions or medicines referred to in this information, check with your doctor, nurse, or pharmacist. Definitions for selected medical terms may be found in the Glossary. Brand names for the generic drug names listed can be found in the Index. In addition, selected brand names commonly associated with the generic name have been included in the text to help you recognize medicine you may be taking. The fact that a brand name product is not mentioned does not mean the information does not apply. It is a good idea for you to learn both the generic and brand names of your medicines and to write them down for future use.

Phentolamine (fen-TOLE-a-meen) given by injection causes blood vessels to expand, thereby increasing blood flow. When it is used in combination with papaverine, another medicine that has this effect, and is injected into the penis (intracavernosal), it increases blood flow to the penis, which results in an erection. This combination is used to treat some men who are impotent.

This medicine should not be used as a sexual aid by men who are not impotent. If the medicine is not used properly, permanent damage to the penis could result.

Phentolamine and papaverine are available only with your doctor's prescription.

Remember:
- **This medicine has been prescribed for your current medical problem only.** It must not be given to other people or used for other problems unless you are directed to do so by your doctor.

- **Keep all medicines out of the reach of children.**

- In order for this medicine to work, it must be used as directed.

- **It is very important that you read and understand the following information.** If any of the information causes you special concern, do not decide against using this medicine without first checking with your doctor.

- Before you begin using any new medicine (prescription or nonprescription) or if you develop any new medical problem while you are using this medicine, check with your doctor, nurse, or pharmacist.

- **If you have any questions** about the following information or if you want more information about this medicine or your medical problem, **ask your doctor, nurse, or pharmacist.**

Before Using This Medicine

In order to decide on the best treatment for your medical problem, your doctor should be told:
  —if you have ever had any unusual or allergic reaction to phentolamine.
  —if you are on a low-salt, low-sugar, or any other special diet, or if you are allergic to any substance, such as foods, sulfites or other preservatives, or dyes.

Most medicines contain more than their active ingredient. Your doctor, nurse, or pharmacist can help you avoid products that may cause a problem.

  —if you have any of the following medical problems:
    Bleeding problems
    Liver disease
    Priapism (history of)
    Sickle cell disease

  —if you are taking **any** other prescription or nonprescription (OTC) medicine.

Proper Use of This Medicine

How to give the injection:
- Cleanse the injection site with alcohol. Using a sterile needle, **inject the medicine slowly and directly into the base of the penis as instructed by your doctor. It should not be injected under the skin.** The injection is usually not painful, although you may feel some tingling in the tip of your penis. If the injection is very painful or you notice bruising, that means you are injecting the medicine under the skin. Stop, withdraw the needle, and reposition it properly before continuing with the injection.

- After you have completed the injection, massage your penis as instructed by your doctor. This helps the medicine spread to all parts of the penis, so that it will work better.

This medicine usually begins to work in about 10 minutes. You should attempt intercourse within 2 hours after injecting the medicine.

How to store this medicine:
- **Keep out of the reach of children.**

- Store away from heat and direct light.

- Keep the medicine from freezing.

Precautions While Using This Medicine

Use the injection exactly as directed by your doctor. Do not use more of it and do not use it more often than ordered. If too much is used, the erection may become so strong that it cannot be reversed. This condition is called priapism, and it can be very dangerous. If the effect is not reversed, the blood supply to the penis may be cut off and permanent damage may occur.

Contact your doctor immediately if the erection lasts for longer than 4 hours or if it becomes painful. This may be a sign of priapism and must be treated right away to prevent permanent damage.

If you notice bleeding at the site when you inject the medicine, put pressure on the spot until the bleeding stops. If it doesn't stop, check with your doctor.

It is important for you to examine your penis regularly. Check with your doctor if you find a lump where the medicine has been injected or if you notice that your penis is becoming curved.

Side Effects of This Medicine

Along with its needed effects, a medicine may cause some unwanted effects. Although not all of these side effects may occur, if they do occur they may need medical attention.

Check with your doctor immediately if the following side effect occurs:

Rare

Erection continuing for more than 4 hours, or painful erection

Check with your doctor as soon as possible if the following side effects occur:

Rare

Dizziness

Lumps in the penis

Other side effects may occur that usually do not require medical attention. These side effects may go away during treatment as your body adjusts to the medicine. However, check with your doctor if any of the following side effects continue or are bothersome:

Less common or rare

Bruising or bleeding at place of injection

Burning (mild) along penis

Difficulty in ejaculating

Phentolamine and papaverine injected into the penis may cause tingling at the tip of the penis. This is no cause for concern.

Other side effects not listed above may also occur in some patients. If you notice any other effects, check with your doctor.

December 1987

PHENYLBUTAZONE (Systemic)

Some commonly used brand names are:	Generic names
Apo-Phenylbutazone*	
Azolid	
Butazolidin	Phenylbutazone†
Neo-Zoline*	
Novobutazone*	
Alka-Butazolidin*	
Alkabutazone*	Phenylbutazone,
Alka-Phenylbutazone*	Buffered*

*Not available in the U.S.
†Generic name product may also be available in the U.S.

To the Reader: If you do not recognize the names of medical conditions or medicines referred to in this information, check with your doctor, nurse, or pharmacist. Definitions for selected medical terms may be found in the Glossary. Brand names for the generic drug names listed can be found in the Index. In addition, selected brand names commonly associated with the generic name have been included in the text to help you recognize medicine you may be taking. The fact that a brand name product is not mentioned does not mean the information does not apply. It is a good idea for you to learn both the generic and brand names of your medicines and to write them down for future use.

Phenylbutazone (fen-ill-BYOO-ta-zone) belongs to the family of medicines known as anti-inflammatory analgesics. It is used to treat the symptoms of certain types of arthritis or rheumatism and to relieve attacks of gout. Phenylbutazone helps relieve inflammation, swelling, stiffness, joint pain, and fever.

Phenylbutazone is a very strong medicine. In addition to its helpful effects in treating your medical problem, it has side effects that can be very serious. Before you take phenylbutazone, be sure that you have discussed its use with your doctor. **Also, do not use this medicine to treat any painful condition other than the one for which it was prescribed by your doctor.**

Phenylbutazone is available only with your doctor's prescription.

Remember:

• **This medicine has been prescribed for your current medical problem only.** It must not be given to other people or used for other problems unless you are directed to do so by your doctor.

• **Keep all medicines out of the reach of children.**

• In order for this medicine to work, it must be used as directed.

• **It is very important that you read and understand the following information.** If any of the information causes you special concern, do not decide against using this medicine without first checking with your doctor.

• Before you begin using any new medicine (prescription or nonprescription) or if you develop any new medical problem while you are using this medicine, check with your doctor, nurse, or pharmacist.

• **If you have any questions** about the following information or if you want more information about this medicine or your medical problem, **ask your doctor, nurse, or pharmacist.**

Before Using This Medicine

In order to decide on the best treatment for your medical problem, your doctor should be told:

—if you have ever had any unusual or allergic reaction to phenylbutazone or to **any** other medicine, especially:

Aspirin or other salicylates
Diclofenac (e.g., Voltaren)
Diflunisal (e.g., Dolobid)
Dipyrone (e.g., Novaldin)
Fenoprofen (e.g., Nalfon)
Flurbiprofen, oral (e.g., Ansaid)
Ibuprofen (e.g., Motrin)
Indomethacin (e.g., Indocin)
Ketoprofen (e.g., Orudis)
Meclofenamate (e.g., Meclomen)
Mefenamic acid (e.g., Ponstel)
Naproxen (e.g., Naprosyn)
Oxyphenbutazone (e.g., Tandearil)
Piroxicam (e.g., Feldene)
Sulfinpyrazone (e.g., Anturane)
Sulindac (e.g., Clinoril)
Suprofen (e.g., Suprol)
Tiaprofenic acid (e.g., Surgam)
Tolmetin (e.g., Tolectin)
Zomepirac (e.g., Zomax)

—if you are on a low-salt, low-sugar, or any other special diet, or if you are allergic to any substance, such as foods, sulfites or other preservatives, or dyes. Most medicines contain more than their active ingredient. Your doctor, nurse, or pharmacist can help you avoid products that may cause a problem.

—if you are **pregnant** or if you may become pregnant. Studies on birth defects have not been done in humans. However, studies in animals have shown that phenylbutazone may cause unwanted effects in the fetus.

—if you are **breast-feeding**. Phenylbutazone passes into the breast milk and may cause unwanted effects, such as blood problems, in nursing babies. It may be necessary for you to take another medicine or to stop breast-feeding during treatment. Be sure that you have discussed the risks and benefits of this medicine with your doctor.

—if you have any of the following medical problems:

Asthma
Blood disease
Edema (swelling of feet or lower legs)
Heart disease
High blood pressure
Kidney disease
Liver disease
Polymyalgia rheumatica
Stomach ulcer, other stomach problems, or colitis
Temporal arteritis
Ulcers, sores, or white spots in mouth

—if you are receiving radiation (x-ray) therapy.

—if you regularly take acetaminophen (e.g., Tylenol).

—if you are taking **any** other prescription or nonprescription (OTC) medicine, especially:

Anticoagulants (blood thinners)
Anticonvulsants (seizure medicine)
Antineoplastics (cancer medicine)

Antithyroid agents (medicine for overactive thyroid)
Azathioprine (e.g., Imuran)
Captopril (e.g., Capoten)
Carbamazepine (e.g., Tegretol)
Chlorambucil (e.g., Leukeran)
Chloramphenicol (e.g., Chloromycetin)
Chlorprothixene (e.g., Taractan)
Colchicine
Cyclophosphamide (e.g., Cytoxan)
Dapsone
Digitalis glycosides (heart medicine)
Enalapril (e.g., Vasotec)
Flecainide (e.g., Tambocor)
Flucytosine (e.g., Ancobon)
Haloperidol (e.g., Haldol)
Interferon (e.g., Intron A; Roferon-A)
Heparin
Loxapine (e.g., Loxitane)
Maprotiline (e.g., Ludiomil)
Mercaptopurine (e.g., Purinethol)
Methotrexate (e.g., Mexate)
Penicillamine (e.g., Cuprimine)
Phenothiazines (acetphenazine [e.g., Tindal], chlorpromazine [e.g., Thorazine], fluphenazine [e.g., Prolixin], mesoridazine [e.g., Serentil], perphenazine [e.g., Trilafon], prochlorperazine [e.g., Compazine], promazine [e.g., Sparine], promethazine [e.g., Phenergan], thioridazine [e.g., Mellaril], trifluoperazine [e.g., Stelazine], triflupromazine [e.g., Vesprin], trimeprazine [e.g., Temaril])
Primaquine
Procainamide (e.g., Pronestyl)
Pyrimethamine (e.g., Daraprim)
Rifampin (e.g., Rifadin)
Sulfonamides (sulfa medicines)
Thiothixene (e.g., Navane)
Tocainide (e.g., Tonocard)
Tricyclic antidepressants (amitriptyline [e.g., Elavil], amoxapine, [e.g., Asendin], clomipramine [e.g., Anafranil], desipramine [e.g., Pertofrane], doxepin [e.g., Sinequan], imipramine [e.g., Tofranil], nortriptyline [e.g., Aventyl], protriptyline [e.g., Vivactil], trimipramine [e.g., Surmontil])
Trimethoprim (e.g., Trimpex)

Proper Use of This Medicine

Take this medicine with meals to lessen stomach upset. If stomach upset (nausea, vomiting, stomach pain, or diarrhea) continues, check with your doctor.

Take phenylbutazone with a full glass (8 ounces) of water. Also, do not lie down for about 15 to 30 minutes after taking this medicine. This helps to prevent irritation that may lead to trouble in swallowing.

This medicine is intended to treat your current medical problem only. **Do not take it for any other aches or pains.**

Take this medicine only as directed by your doctor. Do not take more of it, do not take it more often, and do not take it for a longer period of time than your doctor ordered. To do so may cause serious side effects, especially in patients who are 40 years of age or older.

If you miss a dose of this medicine and your dosing schedule is one dose to be taken:

Once or twice a day—Take the missed dose as soon as possible. But if you do not remember the missed dose until it is almost time for your next dose or until the next day, skip the missed dose and go back to your regular dosing schedule. Do not double doses.

Three or more times a day—If you remember within an hour or so of the missed dose, take it right away. But if you do not remember until later, skip the missed dose and go back to your regular dosing schedule. Do not double doses.

How to store this medicine:

• **Keep out of the reach of children.**

• Store away from heat and direct light.

• Do not store this medicine in the bathroom, near the kitchen sink, or in other damp places. Heat or moisture may cause the medicine to break down.

• Do not keep outdated medicine or medicine no longer needed. Be sure that any discarded medicine is out of the reach of children.

Precautions While Using This Medicine

Your doctor should check your progress at regular visits in order to make sure that this medicine does not cause unwanted effects.

Phenylbutazone may cause some people to become confused, drowsy, or less alert than they are normally. **Make sure you know how you react to this medicine before you drive, use machines, or do other jobs that require you to be alert.**

Stomach problems may be more likely to occur if you drink alcoholic beverages while being treated with this medicine. Also, alcohol may add to the depressant side effects of this medicine. Therefore, **do not drink alcoholic beverages while taking this medicine.**

Too much use of certain other medicines together with phenylbutazone may increase the chance of stomach or kidney problems. Therefore, do not regularly take any of the following medicines together with phenylbutazone, unless your doctor has directed you to do so:

Acetaminophen (e.g., Tylenol)
Aspirin or other salicylates
Diclofenac (e.g., Voltaren)
Diflunisal (e.g., Dolobid)
Fenoprofen (e.g., Nalfon)
Flurbiprofen, oral (e.g., Ansaid)
Ibuprofen (e.g., Motrin)
Indomethacin (e.g., Indocin)
Ketoprofen (e.g., Orudis)
Meclofenamate (e.g., Meclomen)
Mefenamic acid (e.g., Ponstel)
Naproxen (e.g., Naprosyn)
Piroxicam (e.g., Feldene)
Sulindac (e.g., Clinoril)
Tiaprofenic acid (e.g., Surgam)
Tolmetin (e.g., Tolectin)

Check with your doctor immediately if chills, fever, muscle aches or pains, or other influenza-like symptoms occur shortly before, or together with, a skin rash. Very rarely, these effects may be the first signs of a serious reaction to this medicine.

Side Effects of This Medicine

Along with its needed effects, a medicine may cause some unwanted effects. Although not all of these side effects may occur, if they do occur they may need medical attention.

Stop taking this medicine and check with your doctor immediately if any of the following side effects occur:

More common
> Swelling of face, feet, or lower legs
> Weight gain

Rare
> Abdominal or stomach pain (severe)
> Bloody or black, tarry stools
> Shortness of breath, troubled breathing, wheezing, or tightness in chest
> Sore throat and fever
> Ulcers, sores, or white spots in mouth
> Unusual bleeding or bruising
> Unusual tiredness or weakness
> Vomiting of blood or material that looks like coffee grounds

Also, check with your doctor as soon as possible if any of the following side effects occur:

Less common
> Skin rash

Rare
> Bleeding sores on lips
> Bloody or cloudy urine
> Burning feeling in throat, chest, or stomach
> Chest pain
> Confusion
> Difficult, painful, or decreased urination
> Eye pain, blurred vision, or any change in vision
> Fever and joint pain
> Hives or itching of skin
> Mental depression (especially in elderly patients)
> Red eyes
> Redness, tenderness, burning, or peeling of skin
> Ringing or buzzing in ears or any loss of hearing
> Swelling of neck or throat
> Thickened or scaly skin
> Yellow eyes or skin

Signs of overdose
> Bluish color of fingernails, lips, or skin
> Convulsions (seizures), especially in children
> Dizziness or lightheadedness

> Hallucinations (seeing, hearing, or feeling things that are not there)
> Headache (severe and continuing)
> Increase or decrease in blood pressure
> Mood or mental changes
> Nausea, vomiting, or stomach pain (severe)
> Shortness of breath, troubled breathing, or unusually slow, fast, or irregular breathing

Other side effects may occur that usually do not require medical attention. These side effects may go away during treatment as your body adjusts to the medicine. However, check with your doctor if any of the following side effects continue or are bothersome:

More common
> Nausea

Less common or rare
> Bloated feeling or gas
> Constipation
> Diarrhea
> Drowsiness
> Feeling of numbness
> Headache
> Indigestion
> Nervousness, restlessness, or irritability
> Stomach pain (mild)
> Swelling of stomach
> Trembling
> Vomiting

The above side effects are more likely to occur in patients 40 years of age or older. These patients, especially those 60 years of age or older, are usually more sensitive to the effects of phenylbutazone.

Some side effects may occur many days or weeks after you have stopped using this medicine. During this period of time **check with your doctor immediately** if you notice any of the following side effects:

> Sore throat and fever
> Ulcers, sores, or white spots in mouth
> Unusual bleeding or bruising
> Unusual tiredness or weakness

Other side effects not listed above may also occur in some patients. If you notice any other effects, check with your doctor.

December 1987

PHENYLEPHRINE (Nasal)

Some commonly used brand names are:

Alconefrin	Nostril
Allerest Nasal	Rhinall
Coricidin Nasal Mist	Sinarest Nasal
doktors	Sinex
Duration Mild	Sinophen Intranasal
Neo-Synephrine	Vacon

Generic name product may also be available in the U.S.

To the Reader: If you do not recognize the names of medical conditions or medicines referred to in this information, check with your doctor, nurse, or pharmacist. Definitions for selected medical terms may be found in the Glossary. Brand names for the generic drug names listed can be found in the Index. In addition, selected brand names commonly associated with the generic name have been included in the text to help you recognize medicine you may be taking. The fact that a brand name product is not mentioned does not mean the information does not apply. It is a good idea for you to learn both the generic and brand names of your medicines and to write them down for future use.

Phenylephrine (fen-ill-EF-rin) is used for the temporary relief of congestion or stuffiness in the nose caused by hay fever or other allergies, colds, or sinus trouble. It may also be used in ear infections to relieve congestion.

This medicine may also be used for other conditions as determined by your doctor.

This medicine is available without a prescription; however, your doctor may have special instructions on the proper use or dose for your medical condition.

Remember:
- **Keep all medicines out of the reach of children.**

- In order for this medicine to work, it must be used as directed. **If you are using this medicine without a prescription, it is very important to follow the directions on the label.**

- **It is also very important that you read and understand the following information.** If any of the information causes you special concern, check with your doctor or pharmacist.

- Before you begin using any new medicine (prescription or nonprescription) or if you develop any new medical problem while you are using this medicine, check with your doctor, nurse, or pharmacist.

- **If you have any questions** about the following information or if you want more information about this medicine or your medical problem, **ask your doctor, nurse, or pharmacist.**

Before Using This Medicine

Before you use nasal phenylephrine, check with your doctor or pharmacist:

—if you have ever had any unusual or allergic reaction to nasal decongestants.

—if you are **pregnant** or if you may become pregnant, since nasal phenylephrine may be absorbed into the body. However, nasal phenylephrine has not been shown to cause birth defects or other problems in humans.

—if you are **breast-feeding**, since nasal phenylephrine may be absorbed into the body. However, it is not known whether phenylephrine passes into the breast milk and this medicine has not been shown to cause problems in nursing babies.

—if you have any of the following medical problems:
  Diabetes mellitus (sugar diabetes)
  Heart or blood vessel disease
  High blood pressure
  Overactive thyroid

—if you are taking **any** other prescription or nonprescription (OTC) medicine.

Proper Use of This Medicine

For patients using the nose drops:

- How to use: Blow the nose gently. Tilt the head back while standing or sitting up, or lie down on a bed and hang head over the side. Place the drops into each nostril and keep the head tilted back for a few minutes to allow the medicine to spread throughout the nose.

- Rinse the dropper with hot water and dry with a clean tissue. Replace the cap right after use. To avoid the spread of infection, do not use the container for more than one person.

For patients using the nose spray:

- How to use: Blow the nose gently. With the head upright, spray the medicine into each nostril. Sniff briskly while squeezing the bottle quickly and firmly. For best results, spray once or twice into each nostril and wait 3 to 5 minutes to allow the medicine to work. Then, blow the nose gently and thoroughly and repeat the sprays if needed.

- Rinse the tip of the spray bottle with hot water, taking care not to suck water into the bottle, and dry with a clean tissue. Replace the cap right after use. To avoid the spread of infection, do not use the container for more than one person.

For patients using the nose jelly:

- How to use: Blow the nose gently. With your finger, place a small amount of jelly (about the size of a pea) up into each nostril. Sniff it well back into the nose.

- Wipe the tip of the tube with a clean, damp tissue and replace the cap right after use.

Use this medicine only as directed. Do not use more of it, do not use it more often, and do not use it for longer than 3 days without first checking with your doctor. To do so may make your runny or stuffy nose worse and may also increase the chance of side effects.

If you are using this medicine on a regular schedule and you miss a dose, use it right away if you remember within an hour or so of the missed dose. However, if you do not remember until later, skip the missed dose and go back to your regular dosing schedule. Do not double doses.

How to store this medicine:

- **Keep out of the reach of children.**

- Store away from heat and direct light.

- Keep the medicine from freezing.

- Do not keep outdated medicine or medicine no longer needed. Be sure that any discarded medicine is out of the reach of children.

Side Effects of This Medicine

Along with its needed effects, a medicine may cause some unwanted effects. Although not all of these side effects may occur, if they do occur they may need medical attention.

When this medicine is used for short periods of time at low doses, side effects usually are rare. However, check with your doctor as soon as possible if any of the following occur:

> Increase in runny or stuffy nose

> *Signs of too much medicine being absorbed into the body*

> Fast, irregular, or pounding heartbeat
> Headache or dizziness
> Increase in sweating
> Nervousness

> Paleness
> Trembling
> Trouble in sleeping

> Note: The above side effects are more likely to occur in children because there is a greater chance that too much of this medicine may be absorbed into the body.

Other side effects may occur that usually do not require medical attention. These side effects may go away during treatment as your body adjusts to the medicine. However, check with your doctor or pharmacist if any of the following side effects continue or are bothersome:

> Burning, dryness, or stinging of inside of nose

For elderly patients: Many medicines have not been tested in older people. Therefore, it is not known whether the medicine acts the same way it does in younger adults. Check with your doctor or pharmacist if you notice any unusual effects while using this medicine or if you think it is not working as it should.

Other side effects not listed above may also occur in some patients. If you notice any other effects, check with your doctor or pharmacist.

December 1987

PHENYLEPHRINE (Ophthalmic)

Some commonly used brand names are:

Ak-Dilate	Minims Phenylephrine*
Ak-Nefrin	Mydfrin
I-Liqui-Tears Plus	Neo-Synephrine
I-Phrine	Prefrin Liquifilm
Isopto Frin	Relief

Generic name may also be available in the U.S.

*Not available in the U.S.

To the Reader: If you do not recognize the names of medical conditions or medicines referred to in this information, check with your doctor, nurse, or pharmacist. Definitions for selected medical terms may be found in the Glossary. Brand names for the generic drug names listed can be found in the Index. In addition, selected brand names commonly associated with the generic name have been included in the text to help you recognize medicine you may be taking. The fact that a brand name product is not mentioned does not mean the information does not apply. It is a good idea for you to learn both the generic and brand names of your medicines and to write them down for future use.

Ophthalmic phenylephrine (fen-ill-EF-rin) in strengths of 2.5 and 10% is used in the eye to dilate (enlarge) the pupil. It is used before eye examinations, before and after eye surgery, and to treat certain eye conditions. These preparations are available only with your doctor's prescription.

Ophthalmic phenylephrine in strengths of 0.12% and less is used to relieve minor irritation of the eye caused by allergy, dust, smoke, wind, and other irritants. These preparations are available without a prescription; however, your doctor may have special instructions on the proper use of phenylephrine for your eye problem.

Remember:

• **Keep all medicines out of the reach of children.**

• In order for this medicine to work, it must be used as directed. **If you are using this medicine without a prescription, it is very important to follow the directions on the label.**

• **It is also very important that you read and understand the following information.** If any of the information causes you special concern, check with your doctor or pharmacist.

• Before you begin using any new medicine (prescription or nonprescription) or if you develop any new medical problem while you are using this medicine, check with your doctor, nurse, or pharmacist.

• **If you have any questions** about the following information or if you want more information about this medicine or your medical problem, **ask your doctor, nurse, or pharmacist.**

Before Using This Medicine

Before you use phenylephrine ophthalmic solution, check with your doctor or pharmacist:

—if you have ever had any unusual or allergic reaction to phenylephrine.

—if you are allergic to any substance, such as certain preservatives. Most medicines contain more than their active ingredient. Your doctor, nurse, or pharmacist can help you avoid products that may cause a problem.

—if you are **pregnant** or if you may become pregnant, since ophthalmic phenylephrine may be absorbed into the body. Studies on birth defects have not been done in either humans or animals.

—if you are **breast-feeding**, since ophthalmic phenylephrine may be absorbed into the body. However, it is not known whether phenylephrine passes into the breast milk and this medicine has not been shown to cause problems in nursing babies.

—if you have any of the following medical problems:

Diabetes mellitus (sugar diabetes)
Heart or blood vessel disease
High blood pressure

—if you are taking **any** other prescription or nonprescription (OTC) medicine.

Proper Use of This Medicine

Do not use if the solution turns brown or becomes cloudy.

How to apply this medicine: First, wash your hands. With the middle finger, apply pressure to the inside corner of the eye (and continue to apply pressure for 1 or 2 minutes after the medicine has been placed in the eye). Tilt the head back and with the index finger of the same hand, pull the lower eyelid away from eye to form a pouch. Drop the medicine into the pouch and gently close the eyes. Do not blink. Keep the eyes closed for 1 or 2 minutes to allow the medicine to be absorbed.

Immediately after applying the eye drops, wash your hands to remove any medicine that may be on them.

To prevent contamination of the eye drops, do not touch the applicator tip to any surface (including the eye) and keep the container tightly closed.

For patients using the 2.5 or 10% eye drops:

• **It is very important that you use this medicine only as directed.** Do not use more of it and do not use it more often than your doctor ordered. To do so may increase the chance of too much medicine being absorbed into the body and the chance of side effects. **This is especially important when this medicine is used in children or in patients with heart disease or high blood pressure,** since high doses of this medicine may cause an irregular heartbeat and an increase in blood pressure.

• If you miss a dose of this medicine, apply it as soon as possible. However, if it is almost time for your next dose, skip the missed dose and apply your next dose at the regularly scheduled time. Then continue with your regular dosing schedule.

How to store this medicine:

• **Keep out of the reach of children.**

• Store away from heat and direct light.

© 1988   The United States Pharmacopeial Convention, Inc.

• Keep the medicine from freezing.

• Do not keep outdated medicine or medicine no longer needed. Be sure that any discarded medicine is out of the reach of children.

Precautions While Using This Medicine

For patients using the 2.5 or 10% eye drops:

• After you apply this medicine to your eyes, your pupils will become unusually large. This may cause your eyes to become more sensitive to light than they are normally. **Wear sunglasses to protect your eyes from sunlight and other bright lights.** If this effect continues for longer than 12 hours after you have stopped using this medicine, check with your doctor.

Side Effects of This Medicine

Along with its needed effects, a medicine may cause some unwanted effects. Although not all of these side effects may occur, if they do occur they may need medical attention.

Check with your doctor as soon as possible if any of the following side effects occur:

Signs of too much medicine being absorbed into the body—Less common with 10% solution; rare with 2.5% or weaker solution

Dizziness
Fast, irregular, or pounding heartbeat
Increase in blood pressure

Increase in sweating
Paleness
Trembling

Other side effects may occur that usually do not require medical attention. These side effects may go away during treatment as your body adjusts to the medicine. However, check with your doctor if any of the following side effects continue or are bothersome:

More common with 2.5 or 10% solution

Burning or stinging of eyes
Headache or browache
Sensitivity of eyes to light
Watering of eyes

Less common

Eye irritation not present before using this medicine

For elderly patients: Many medicines have not been tested in older people. Therefore, it is not known whether the medicine acts the same way it does in younger adults. Check with your doctor or pharmacist if you notice any unusual effects while using this medicine or if you think it is not working as it should.

Other side effects not listed above may also occur in some patients. If you notice any other effects, check with your doctor.

December 1987

PHENYLPROPANOLAMINE (Systemic)

Some commonly used brand names or other names are:

Acutrim	PPA
Control	Prolamine
Dex-A-Diet	Rhindecon
Dexatrim	Unitrol
Diadax	Westrim
Efed II	Westrim LA

To the Reader: If you do not recognize the names of medical conditions or medicines referred to in this information, check with your doctor, nurse, or pharmacist. Definitions for selected medical terms may be found in the Glossary. Brand names for the generic drug names listed can be found in the Index. In addition, selected brand names commonly associated with the generic name have been included in the text to help you recognize medicine you may be taking. The fact that a brand name product is not mentioned does not mean the information does not apply. It is a good idea for you to learn both the generic and brand names of your medicines and to write them down for future use.

Phenylpropanolamine (fen-ill-proe-pa-NOLE-a-meen) or PPA is used as a nasal decongestant and as an appetite suppressant. It acts on many different parts of the body. PPA's actions produce effects that may be helpful or harmful. This depends on a patient's individual condition and response and the amount of medicine taken.

PPA is taken by mouth. It produces two effects which are used in medicine: constriction of blood vessels and decrease in appetite.

Blood vessel constriction leads to clearing of nasal congestion (stuffy nose). However, the same effect may cause an increase in blood pressure in patients who have hypertension (high blood pressure).

The way PPA and similar medicines decrease appetite is unclear. Stimulation of the central nervous system (CNS) may be a major reason. The decrease in appetite is temporary—no more than a few weeks—and requires a change in diet for best effect. The continuous use of PPA for dieting is not recommended.

PPA has caused serious side effects (even death) when too much was taken.

There are a number of products on the market that contain only phenylpropanolamine. Other products contain PPA along with added ingredients. The information that follows is for PPA alone. There may be additional information for the combination products. Read the label of the product you are using. If you have questions or if you want more information about the other ingredients, check with your doctor or pharmacist.

Some preparations containing PPA are available only with your doctor's prescription. Others are available without a prescription; however, your doctor may have special instructions on the proper use of this medicine.

Remember:

• **This medicine has been prescribed for your current medical problem only.** It must not be given to other people or used for other problems unless you are directed to do so by your doctor.

• **Keep all medicines out of the reach of children.**

• In order for this medicine to work, it must be used as directed.

• **It is very important that you read and understand the following information.** If any of the information causes you special concern, do not decide against using this medicine without first checking with your doctor.

• Before you begin using any new medicine (prescription or nonprescription) or if you develop any new medical problem while you are using this medicine, check with your doctor, nurse, or pharmacist.

• **If you have any questions** about the following information or if you want more information about this medicine or your medical problem, **ask your doctor, nurse, or pharmacist.**

Before Using This Medicine

Before you use phenylpropanolamine, check with your doctor or pharmacist:

—if you have ever had any unusual or allergic reaction to phenylpropanolamine or to amphetamine, dextroamphetamine, ephedrine, epinephrine, isoproterenol, metaproterenol, methamphetamine, norepinephrine, phenylephrine, pseudoephedrine, or terbutaline.

—if you are on a low-salt, low-sugar, or any other special diet, or if you are allergic to any substance, such as foods, sulfites or other preservatives, or dyes. Most medicines contain more than their active ingredient. Your doctor, nurse, or pharmacist can help you avoid products that may cause a problem.

—if you are **pregnant** or if you may become pregnant. Phenylpropanolamine has not been shown to cause birth defects or other problems in humans.

—if you are **breast-feeding**. Phenylpropanolamine has not been shown to cause problems in nursing babies.

—if you have any of the following medical problems:
Diabetes mellitus (sugar diabetes)
Enlarged prostate
Glaucoma
Heart or blood vessel disease
High blood pressure
Overactive thyroid

—if you have suffered a heart attack or stroke.

—if you are taking **any** other prescription or nonprescription (OTC) medicine, especially:
Amantadine (e.g., Symmetrel)
Amphetamines
Beta-blockers (acebutolol [e.g., Sectral], atenolol [e.g., Tenormin], esmolol [e.g., Brevibloc], labetalol [e.g., Normodyne], metoprolol [e.g., Lopressor], nadolol [e.g., Corgard], oxprenolol [e.g., Trasicor], pindolol [e.g., Visken], propranolol [e.g., Inderal], sotalol [e.g., Sotacor], timolol [e.g., Blocadren])
Caffeine (e.g., NoDoz)
Chlophedianol (e.g., Ulo)
Digitalis glycosides (heart medicine)
Medicine for asthma or other breathing problems
Methylphenidate (e.g., Ritalin)
Other appetite suppressants (diet pills)
Other medicine for colds, sinus problems, or hay fever or other allergies (including nose drops or sprays)
Pemoline (e.g., Cylert)
Rauwolfia alkaloids (alseroxylon [e.g., Rauwiloid], deserpidine [e.g., Harmonyl], rauwolfia serpentina [e.g., Raudixin], reserpine [e.g., Serpasil])

—if you are now taking or have taken within the past 2 weeks monoamine oxidase (MAO) inhibitors, such as:

>Furazolidone (e.g., Furoxone)
>Isocarboxazid (e.g., Marplan)
>Pargyline (e.g., Eutonyl)
>Phenelzine (e.g., Nardil)
>Procarbazine (e.g., Matulane)
>Tranylcypromine (e.g., Parnate)

Proper Use of This Medicine

For patients taking an extended-release form of this medicine:

- Swallow the capsule or tablet whole.

- Do not break, crush, or chew before swallowing.

- Take only once a day after breakfast.

Take phenylpropanolamine (PPA) only as directed. Do not take more of it, do not take it more often, and do not take it for a longer period of time than directed. To do so may increase the chance of side effects.

If PPA causes trouble in sleeping, take the last dose for each day a few hours before bedtime. If you are taking an extended-release form of this medicine, take your daily dose at least 12 hours before bedtime.

Phenylpropanolamine should not be used for weight control in children under the age of 12 years. Children 12 to 18 years old should not take phenylpropanolamine for weight control unless its use is ordered and supervised by a doctor.

For patients taking phenylpropanolamine for nasal congestion:

- If you miss a dose, take it as soon as possible. However, if it is within 2 hours (or 12 hours for extended-release forms) of your next dose, skip the missed dose and go back to your regular dosing schedule. Do not double doses.

How to store this medicine:

- **Keep out of the reach of children.**

- Store away from heat and direct light.

- Do not store in the bathroom, near the kitchen sink, or in other damp places. Heat or moisture may cause the medicine to break down.

- Do not keep outdated medicine or medicine no longer needed. Be sure that any discarded medicine is out of the reach of children.

Precautions While Using This Medicine

Do not drink large amounts of caffeine-containing coffee, tea, or colas while you are taking this medicine. To do so may cause unwanted effects.

For patients taking this medicine for nasal congestion:

- **If cold symptoms do not improve within 7 days or if you also have a high fever, check with your doctor.** These signs may mean that you have other medical problems.

Side Effects of This Medicine

Along with its needed effects, a medicine may cause some unwanted effects. Although not all of these side effects may occur, if they do occur they may need medical attention.

Check with your doctor as soon as possible if any of the following side effects occur:

Rare
>Painful or difficult urination
>Tightness in chest

Early signs of overdose
>Abdominal or stomach pain
>Fast, pounding, or irregular heartbeat
>Headache (severe)
>Increased sweating not associated with exercise
>Nausea and vomiting (severe)
>Nervousness (severe)
>Restlessness (severe)

Late signs of overdose
>Confusion
>Convulsions (seizures)
>Fast breathing
>Fast and irregular pulse
>Hallucinations (seeing, hearing, or feeling things that are not there)
>Hostile behavior
>Muscle trembling

Other side effects may occur that usually do not require medical attention. These side effects may go away during treatment as your body adjusts to the medicine. However, check with your doctor if any of the following side effects continue or are bothersome:

Less common—more common with high doses
>Dizziness
>Dryness of nose or mouth
>False sense of well-being
>Headache (mild)
>Nausea (mild)
>Nervousness (mild)
>Restlessness (mild)
>Trouble in sleeping

Other side effects not listed above may also occur in some patients. If you notice any other effects, check with your doctor.

_____

December 1987

_____

PHOSPHATES (Systemic)

This information applies to the following medicines:

Potassium Phosphates (poe-TASS-ee-um FOS-fates)
Potassium Phosphate, Monobasic
Potassium and Sodium (SOE-dee-um) Phosphates
Sodium Phosphates

Some commonly used brand names are:	Generic names:
K-Phos Original	Potassium Phosphate, Monobasic
Neutra-Phos-K	Potassium Phosphates†
K-Phos M. F. K-Phos Neutral K-Phos No. 2 Neutra-Phos Uro-KP-Neutral	Potassium and Sodium Phosphates
	Sodium Phosphates†

†Generic name product may also be available.

To the Reader: If you do not recognize the names of medical conditions or medicines referred to in this information, check with your doctor, nurse, or pharmacist. Definitions for selected medical terms may be found in the Glossary. Brand names for the generic drug names listed can be found in the Index. In addition, selected brand names commonly associated with the generic name have been included in the text to help you recognize medicine you may be taking. The fact that a brand name product is not mentioned does not mean the information does not apply. It is a good idea for you to learn both the generic and brand names of your medicines and to write them down for future use.

Phosphates are taken by mouth or sometimes given by injection. Some are used as dietary supplements for patients who are unable to get enough phosphorus in their regular diet, usually because of certain illnesses or diseases. Some phosphates are used to make the urine more acid to prevent the formation of calcium stones in the urinary tract or to help treat certain urinary tract infections.

Some of these preparations are available only with your doctor's prescription. Others are available without a prescription; however, your doctor may have special instructions on the proper dose of this medicine for your medical condition.

Some phosphates are given only by or under the immediate care of your doctor.

Remember:
• **If this medicine has been prescribed for you, it is to be used for your current medical problem only.** It must not be given to other people or used for other problems unless you are directed to do so by your doctor.

• **Keep all medicines out of the reach of children.**

• In order for this medicine to work, it must be used as directed. **If you are using this medicine without a prescription, it is very important to follow the directions on the label.**

• If you are receiving this medicine by injection, some of the information about this medicine may not apply.

• **It is very important that you read and understand the following information.** If any of the information causes you special concern, do not decide against using this medicine without first checking with your doctor.

• Before you begin using any new medicine (prescription or nonprescription) or if you develop any new medical problem while you are using this medicine, check with your doctor, nurse, or pharmacist.

• **If you have any questions** about the following information or if you want more information about this medicine or your medical problem, **ask your doctor, nurse, or pharmacist.**

Before Using This Medicine

In order to decide on the best treatment for your medical problem, your doctor should be told:

—if you have ever had any unusual or allergic reaction to medicines containing potassium, sodium, or phosphates.

—if you are on a low-salt, low-sugar, or any other special diet, or if you are allergic to any substance, such as foods, sulfites or other preservatives, or dyes. Most medicines contain more than their active ingredient. Your doctor, nurse, or pharmacist can help you avoid products that may cause a problem.

—if you are **pregnant** or if you may become pregnant. Studies have not been done in either humans or animals.

—if you are **breast-feeding**. It is not known whether phosphates pass into the breast milk. However, this medicine has not been shown to cause problems in nursing babies.

—if you have any of the following medical problems:
Edema (swelling in feet or lower legs or fluid in lungs)
Heart disease
High blood pressure
Kidney disease
Liver disease
Myotonia congenita
Pancreatitis (inflammation of the pancreas)
Rickets
Softening of bones
Underactive adrenal glands
Underactive parathyroid glands

—if you are taking **any** other prescription or nonprescription (OTC) medicine, especially:
Adrenocorticoids (cortisone-like medicine)
Calcium-containing medicine, including antacids and calcium supplements
Captopril (e.g., Capoten)
Digitalis glycosides (heart medicine)
Potassium-containing medicine

Proper Use of This Medicine

For patients taking the tablet form of this medicine:

• Do not swallow tablets whole. Before taking, dissolve the tablets in ¾ to 1 glass (6 to 8 ounces) of water. Let the tablets soak in water for 2 to 5 minutes and then stir until completely dissolved.

For patients using the capsules for oral solution form of this medicine:

• Do not swallow capsules whole. Before taking, mix the contents of 1 capsule in ⅓ glass (about 2 ½ ounces) of water or the contents of 2 capsules in ⅔ glass (about 5 ounces) of water and stir well until dissolved.

For patients using the powder for oral solution form of this medicine:

• Add the entire contents of 1 bottle (2 ¼ ounces) to enough warm water to make 1 gallon of solution. Shake the container for 2 or 3 minutes or until all the powder is dissolved.

• Do not dilute solution further.

• This solution may be chilled to improve the flavor; do not allow it to freeze.

• Discard unused solution after 60 days.

Take this medicine immediately after meals or with food to lessen possible stomach upset or laxative action.

To help prevent kidney stones, **drink at least a full glass (8 ounces) of water every hour during waking hours,** unless otherwise directed by your doctor.

Take this medicine only as directed. Do not take more of it and do not take it more often than recommended on the label, unless otherwise directed by your doctor.

If you miss a dose of this medicine, take it as soon as possible. However, if it is within one or two hours of your next dose, skip the missed dose and go back to your regular dosing schedule. Do not double doses.

How to store this medicine:

• **Keep out of the reach of children.**

• Store away from heat and direct light.

• Do not store the capsule, tablet, or powder form of this medicine in the bathroom, near the kitchen sink, or in other damp places. Heat or moisture may cause the medicine to break down.

• Keep the liquid form of this medicine from freezing.

• Do not keep outdated medicine or medicine no longer needed. Be sure that any discarded medicine is out of the reach of children.

Precautions While Using This Medicine

Your doctor should check your progress at regular visits to make sure that this medicine does not cause unwanted effects.

For patients on a potassium- or sodium-restricted diet: This medicine contains a large amount of potassium or sodium or both. If you have any questions about this, check with your doctor or pharmacist.

Side Effects of This Medicine

Along with its needed effects, a medicine may cause some unwanted effects. Although not all of these side effects may occur, if they do occur they may need medical attention.

Check with your doctor as soon as possible if any of the following side effects occur:
Less common or rare
    Confusion
    Convulsions (seizures)
    Decrease in amount of urine or in frequency of urination
    Fast or irregular heartbeat
    Headache or dizziness
    Muscle cramps
    Numbness, tingling, pain, or weakness in hands or feet
    Numbness or tingling around lips
    Shortness of breath or troubled breathing
    Swelling of feet or lower legs
    Unusual thirst
    Unusual tiredness or weakness
    Weakness or heaviness of legs
    Weight gain

Other side effects may occur that usually do not require medical attention. These side effects may go away during treatment as your body adjusts to the medicine. However, check with your doctor if any of the following side effects continue or are bothersome:
    Diarrhea
    Nausea or vomiting
    Stomach pain

Other side effects not listed above may also occur in some patients. If you notice any other effects, check with your doctor.

December 1987

PHYSOSTIGMINE (Ophthalmic)

Some commonly used brand names are Eserine and Isopto Eserine.

Generic name product may also be available in the U.S.

To the Reader: If you do not recognize the names of medical conditions or medicines referred to in this information, check with your doctor, nurse, or pharmacist. Definitions for selected medical terms may be found in the Glossary. Brand names for the generic drug names listed can be found in the Index. In addition, selected brand names commonly associated with the generic name have been included in the text to help you recognize medicine you may be taking. The fact that a brand name product is not mentioned does not mean the information does not apply. It is a good idea for you to learn both the generic and brand names of your medicines and to write them down for future use.

Physostigmine (fi-zoe-STIG-meen) is used in the eye to treat certain types of glaucoma and other eye conditions.

This medicine is available only with your doctor's prescription.

Remember:
- **This medicine has been prescribed for your current medical problem only.** It must not be given to other people or used for other problems unless you are directed to do so by your doctor.

- **Keep all medicines out of the reach of children.**

- In order for this medicine to work, it must be used as directed.

- **It is very important that you read and understand the following information.** If any of the information causes you special concern, do not decide against using this medicine without first checking with your doctor.

- Before you begin using any new medicine (prescription or nonprescription) or if you develop any new medical problem while you are using this medicine, check with your doctor, nurse, or pharmacist.

- **If you have any questions** about the following information or if you want more information about this medicine or your medical problem, **ask your doctor, nurse, or pharmacist.**

Before Using This Medicine

In order to decide on the best treatment for your medical problem, your doctor should be told:
—if you have ever had any unusual or allergic reaction to physostigmine.

—if you are allergic to any substance, such as certain preservatives. Most medicines contain more than their active ingredient. Your doctor, nurse, or pharmacist can help you avoid products that may cause a problem.

—if you are **pregnant** or if you may become pregnant, since ophthalmic physostigmine may be absorbed into the body. Studies on birth defects have not been done in either humans or animals.

—if you are **breast-feeding**, since ophthalmic physostigmine may be absorbed into the body. However, physostigmine has not been shown to cause problems in nursing babies.

—if you are taking **any** other prescription or nonprescription (OTC) medicine.

Proper Use of This Medicine

For patients using the eye drop form of this medicine:
- Do not use if the solution becomes discolored.

- How to apply this medicine: First, wash your hands. With the middle finger, apply pressure to the inside corner of the eye (and continue to apply pressure for 1 or 2 minutes after the medicine has been placed in the eye). Tilt the head back and with the index finger of the same hand, pull the lower eyelid away from the eye to form a pouch. Drop the medicine into the pouch and gently close the eyes. Do not blink. Keep the eyes closed for 1 or 2 minutes to allow the medicine to be absorbed.

- Immediately after applying the eye drops, wash your hands to remove any medicine that may be on them.

- To prevent contamination of the eye drops, do not touch the applicator tip to any surface (including the eye) and keep the container tightly closed.

For patients using the ointment form of this medicine:
- How to apply this medicine: First, wash your hands. Pull the lower eyelid away from the eye to form a pouch. Squeeze a thin strip of ointment into the pouch. A 1-cm (approximately 1/3-inch) strip of ointment is usually enough unless otherwise directed by your doctor. Gently close the eyes and keep them closed for 1 or 2 minutes to allow the medicine to be absorbed.

- Immediately after applying the eye ointment, wash your hands to remove any medicine that may be on them.

- To prevent contamination of the eye ointment, do not touch the applicator tip to any surface (including the eye), wipe the tip of the ointment tube with a clean tissue, and keep the tube tightly closed.

Use this medicine only as directed. Do not use more of it and do not use it more often than your doctor ordered. To do so may increase the chance of too much medicine being absorbed into the body and the chance of side effects.

If you miss a dose of this medicine and your dosing schedule is one dose to be applied:

Once a day—Apply the missed dose as soon as possible. However, if you do not remember the missed dose until the next day, skip it and apply your regularly scheduled dose.

More than once a day—Apply the missed dose as soon as possible. However, if it is almost time for your next dose, skip the missed dose and apply your next dose at the regularly scheduled time. Then continue with your regular dosing schedule.

How to store this medicine:

- **Keep out of the reach of children.**
- Store away from heat and direct light.
- Keep the medicine from freezing.
- Do not keep outdated medicine or medicine no longer needed. Be sure that any discarded medicine is out of the reach of children.

Precautions While Using This Medicine

Your doctor should check your eye pressure at regular visits.

For a short time after you apply this medicine, your vision may be blurred or there may be a change in your near or distant vision, especially at night. **Make sure your vision is clear before you drive or do other jobs that require you to see well.**

Side Effects of This Medicine

Along with its needed effects, a medicine may cause some unwanted effects. Although not all of these side effects may occur, if they do occur they may need medical attention.

Check with your doctor as soon as possible if any of the following side effects occur:

Signs of too much medicine being absorbed into the body

    Increase in sweating
    Loss of bladder control
    Muscle weakness

    Nausea, vomiting, diarrhea, or stomach cramps or pain
    Shortness of breath, tightness in chest, or wheezing
    Slow or irregular heartbeat
    Unusual tiredness or weakness
    Watering of mouth

Other side effects may occur that usually do not require medical attention. These side effects may go away during treatment as your body adjusts to the medicine. However, check with your doctor if any of the following side effects continue or are bothersome:

More common

    Blurred vision or change in near or distant visions
    Eye pain

Less common

    Burning, redness, stinging, or other eye irritation
    Headache or browache
    Twitching of eyelids
    Watering of eyes

For elderly patients: Many medicines have not been tested in older people. Therefore, it is not known whether the medicine acts the same way it does in younger adults. Check with your doctor or pharmacist if you notice any unusual effects while using this medicine or if you think it is not working as it should.

Other side effects not listed above may also occur in some patients. If you notice any other effects, check with your doctor.

December 1987

PILOCARPINE (Ophthalmic)

Some commonly used brand names are:

Adsorbocarpine	Miocarpine*
Akarpine	Ocusert Pilo
Almocarpine	Pilocar
I-Pilopine	Pilokair
Isopto Carpine	Pilopine HS
Minims Pilocarpine*	P. V. Carpine Liquifilm

Generic name product may also be available in the U.S.

---

*Not available in the U.S.

To the Reader: If you do not recognize the names of medical conditions or medicines referred to in this information, check with your doctor, nurse, or pharmacist. Definitions for selected medical terms may be found in the Glossary. Brand names for the generic drug names listed can be found in the Index. In addition, selected brand names commonly associated with the generic name have been included in the text to help you recognize medicine you may be taking. The fact that a brand name product is not mentioned does not mean the information does not apply. It is a good idea for you to learn both the generic and brand names of your medicines and to write them down for future use.

Pilocarpine (pye-loe-KAR-peen) is used in the eye to treat glaucoma and other eye conditions.

This medicine is available only with your doctor's prescription.

Remember:
• **This medicine has been prescribed for your current medical problem only.** It must not be given to other people or used for other problems unless you are directed to do so by your doctor.

• **Keep all medicines out of the reach of children.**

• In order for this medicine to work, it must be used as directed.

• **It is very important that you read and understand the following information.** If any of the information causes you special concern, do not decide against using this medicine without first checking with your doctor.

• Before you begin using any new medicine (prescription or nonprescription) or if you develop any new medical problem while you are using this medicine, check with your doctor, nurse, or pharmacist.

• **If you have any questions** about the following information or if you want more information about this medicine or your medical problem, **ask your doctor, nurse, or pharmacist.**

Before Using This Medicine

In order to decide on the best treatment for your medical problem, your doctor should be told:

—if you have ever had any unusual or allergic reaction to pilocarpine.

—if you are allergic to any substance, such as certain preservatives. Most medicines contain more than their active ingredient. Your doctor, nurse, or pharmacist can help you avoid products that may cause a problem.

—if you are **pregnant** or if you may become pregnant, since ophthalmic pilocarpine may be absorbed into the body. Studies on birth defects have not been done in either humans or animals.

—if you are **breast-feeding**, since ophthalmic pilocarpine may be absorbed into the body. However, it is not known whether pilocarpine passes into the breast milk and this medicine has not been shown to cause problems in nursing babies.

—if you have asthma.

—if you are taking **any** other prescription or nonprescription (OTC) medicine.

Proper Use of This Medicine

For patients using the eye drop form of pilocarpine:

• How to apply this medicine: First, wash your hands. With the middle finger, apply pressure to the inside corner of the eye (and continue to apply pressure for 1 or 2 minutes after the medicine has been placed in the eye). Tilt the head back and with the index finger of the same hand, pull the lower eyelid away from the eye to form a pouch. Drop the medicine into the pouch and gently close the eyes. Do not blink. Keep the eyes closed for 1 or 2 minutes to allow the medicine to be absorbed.

• Immediately after applying the eye drops, wash your hands to remove any medicine that may be on them.

• To prevent contamination of the eye drops, do not touch the applicator tip to any surface (including the eye) and keep the container tightly closed.

• If you miss a dose of this medicine, apply it as soon as possible. However, if it is almost time for your next dose, skip the missed dose and apply your next dose at the regularly scheduled time. Then continue with your regular dosing schedule.

For patients using the eye gel form of pilocarpine:

• How to apply this medicine: First, wash your hands. Pull the lower eyelid away from the eye to form a pouch. Squeeze a thin strip of gel into the pouch. A 1½-cm (approximately ½-inch) strip of gel is usually enough unless otherwise directed by your doctor. Gently close the eyes and keep them closed for 1 or 2 minutes to allow the medicine to be absorbed.

• Immediately after applying the eye gel, wash your hands to remove any medicine that may be on them.

• To prevent contamination of the eye gel, do not touch the applicator tip to any surface (including the eye), wipe the tip of the gel tube with a clean tissue, and keep the tube tightly closed.

• If you miss a dose of this medicine, apply it as soon as possible. However, if you do not remember the missed dose until the next day, skip it and apply your next dose at the regularly scheduled time. Then continue with your regular dosing schedule.

For patients using the eye system form of pilocarpine:

- This medicine usually comes with patient directions. Read them carefully before using this medicine.

- If you think this medicine unit may be damaged, do not use it. If you have any questions about this, check with your doctor or pharmacist.

- If the unit seems to be releasing too much medicine into your eye, remove it and replace with a new unit. If you have any questions about this, check with your doctor.

Use this medicine only as directed. Do not use more of it and do not use it more often than your doctor ordered. To do so may increase the chance of too much medicine being absorbed into the body and the chance of side effects.

How to store this medicine:

- **Keep out of the reach of children.**
- Store away from heat and direct light.
- Store the eye system form of this medicine in the refrigerator. However, keep the medicine from freezing.
- Store the gel form of this medicine in the refrigerator or at room temperature. If stored at room temperature, discard any unused medicine after 8 weeks.
- Keep the gel or solution form of this medicine from freezing.
- Do not keep outdated medicine or medicine no longer needed. Be sure that any discarded medicine is out of the reach of children.

Precautions While Using This Medicine

Your doctor should check your eye pressure at regular visits.

For patients using the eye drop or gel form of this medicine:

- For a short time after you apply this medicine, your vision may be blurred or there may be a change in your near or distant vision, especially at night. **Make sure your vision is clear before you drive or do other jobs that require you to see well.**

For patients using the eye system form of this medicine:

- For the first several hours after inserting this unit in the eye, your vision may be blurred or there may be a change in your near or distant vision, especially at night. Therefore, insert this unit in the eye at bedtime,

unless otherwise directed by your doctor. If this unit is inserted in the eye at any other time of the day, **make sure your vision is clear before you drive or do other jobs that require you to see well.**

Side Effects of This Medicine

Along with its needed effects, a medicine may cause some unwanted effects. Although not all of these side effects may occur, if they do occur they may need medical attention.

Check with your doctor as soon as possible if any of the following side effects occur:

Signs of too much medicine being absorbed into the body

    Increase in sweating
    Muscle tremors
    Nausea, vomiting, or diarrhea
    Troubled breathing or wheezing
    Watering of mouth

Other side effects may occur that usually do not require medical attention. These side effects may go away during treatment as your body adjusts to the medicine. However, check with your doctor if any of the following side effects continue or are bothersome:

More common

    Blurred vision or change in near or distant vision
    Eye pain

Less common

    Eye irritation
    Headache or browache

For elderly patients: Many medicines have not been tested in older people. Therefore, it is not known whether the medicine acts the same way it does in younger adults. Check with your doctor or pharmacist if you notice any unusual effects while using this medicine or if you think it is not working as it should.

Other side effects not listed above may also occur in some patients. If you notice any other effects, check with your doctor.

_____

December 1987

PIMOZIDE (Systemic)

A commonly used brand name is Orap.

To the Reader: If you do not recognize the names of medical conditions or medicines referred to in this information, check with your doctor, nurse, or pharmacist. Definitions for selected medical terms may be found in the Glossary. Brand names for the generic drug names listed can be found in the Index. In addition, selected brand names commonly associated with the generic name have been included in the text to help you recognize medicine you may be taking. The fact that a brand name product is not mentioned does not mean the information does not apply. It is a good idea for you to learn both the generic and brand names of your medicines and to write them down for future use.

Pimozide (PIM-oh-zide) is taken by mouth to treat the symptoms of Gilles de la Tourette's syndrome. It is meant only for patients with severe symptoms who cannot take or have not been helped by other medicine.

Pimozide works in the central nervous system to help control the vocal outbursts and uncontrolled, repeated movements of the body (tics) that interfere with normal life. It will not completely cure the tics, but will help to reduce their number and severity.

Pimozide is available only with your doctor's prescription.

Remember:

• **This medicine has been prescribed for your current medical problem only.** It must not be given to other people or used for other problems unless you are directed to do so by your doctor.

• **Keep all medicines out of the reach of children.**

• In order for this medicine to work, it must be used as directed.

• **It is very important that you read and understand the following information.** If any of the information causes you special concern, do not decide against using this medicine without first checking with your doctor.

• Before you begin using any new medicine (prescription or nonprescription) or if you develop any new medical problem while you are using this medicine, check with your doctor, nurse, or pharmacist.

• **If you have any questions** about the following information or if you want more information about this medicine or your medical problem, **ask your doctor, nurse, or pharmacist.**

Before Using This Medicine

In order to decide on the best treatment for your medical problem, your doctor should be told:

—if you have ever had any unusual or allergic reaction to pimozide, haloperidol, molindone, phenothiazines, or thioxanthenes.

—if you are on a low-salt, low-sugar, or any other special diet, or if you are allergic to any substance, such as foods, sulfites or other preservatives, or dyes. Most medicines contain more than their active ingredient. Your doctor, nurse, or pharmacist can help you avoid products that may cause a problem.

—if you are **pregnant** or if you may become pregnant. Pimozide has not been shown to cause birth defects or other problems in humans. However, studies in rats and rabbits given more than the usual human dose have shown fewer pregnancies, slowed development of the fetus, and toxic effects in the mother and fetus.

—if you are **breast-feeding**. It is not known whether pimozide passes into breast milk. This medicine has not been shown to cause problems in humans.

—if you have any of the following medical problems:
Breast cancer (history of)
Heart disease
Kidney disease
Liver disease
Tics other than those caused by Tourette's syndrome

—if you are taking **any** other prescription or nonprescription (OTC) medicine, especially:
Amphetamines
Antimuscarinics (medicine for abdominal or stomach spasms or cramps)
Central nervous system (CNS) depressants
Chlorprothixene (e.g., Taractan)
Disopyramide (e.g., Norpace)
Haloperidol (e.g., Haldol)
Loxapine (e.g., Loxitane)
Methyldopa (e.g., Aldomet)
Methylphenidate (e.g., Ritalin)
Metoclopramide (e.g., Reglan)
Metyrosine (e.g., Demser)
Molindone (e.g., Moban)
Pemoline (e.g., Cylert)
Phenothiazines (acetophenazine [e.g., Tindal], chlorpromazine [e.g., Thorazine], fluphenazine [e.g., Prolixin], mesoridazine [e.g., Serentil], perphenazine [e.g., Trilafon], prochlorperazine [e.g., Compazine], promazine [e.g., Sparine], promethazine [e.g., Phenergan], thioridazine [e.g., Mellaril], trifluoperazine [e.g., Stelazine], triflupromazine [e.g., Vesprin], trimeprazine [e.g., Temaril])
Procainamide (e.g., Pronestyl)
Quinidine (e.g., Quinidex)
Rauwolfia alkaloids (alseroxylon [e.g., Rauwiloid], deserpidine [e.g., Harmonyl], rauwolfia serpentina [e.g., Raudixin], reserpine [e.g., Serpasil])
Thiothixene (e.g., Navane)
Tricyclic antidepressants (amitriptyline [e.g., Elavil], amoxapine [e.g., Asendin], clomipramine, desipramine [e.g., Pertofrane], doxepin [e.g., Sinequan], imipramine [e.g., Tofranil], nortriptyline [e.g., Aventyl], protriptyline [e.g., Vivactil], trimipramine [e.g., Surmontil])

Proper Use of This Medicine

Use pimozide only as directed by your doctor. Do not use more of it, do not use it more often, and do not use it for a longer period of time than your doctor ordered. To do so may increase the chance of side effects.

If you miss a dose of this medicine, take it as soon as possible. Then take any remaining doses for that day at regularly spaced intervals. Do not double doses.

How to store this medicine:

• **Keep out of the reach of children.**

• Store away from heat and direct light.

- Do not store in the bathroom, near the kitchen sink, or in other damp places. Heat or moisture may cause the medicine to break down.

- Do not keep outdated medicine or medicine no longer needed. Be sure that any discarded medicine is out of the reach of children.

Precautions While Using This Medicine

Your doctor should check your progress at regular visits, especially for the first few months that you take this medicine. The amount of pimozide you take may be changed often to meet the needs of your condition and to help avoid unwanted effects.

Do not suddenly stop taking this medicine without first checking with your doctor. Your doctor may want you to reduce gradually the amount you are taking before stopping completely. This will allow your body time to adjust and help to avoid worsening of your medical condition.

This medicine will add to the effects of alcohol and other CNS depressants (medicines that slow down the nervous system, possibly causing drowsiness). Some examples of CNS depressants are antihistamines or medicine for hay fever, other allergies, or colds; sedatives, tranquilizers, or sleeping medicine; prescription pain medicine or narcotics; barbiturates; medicine for seizures; muscle relaxants; or anesthetics, including some dental anesthetics. **Check with your doctor before taking any of the above while you are using this medicine.**

This medicine may cause some people to become drowsy or less alert or to have blurred vision or muscle stiffness, especially as the amount of medicine is increased. Even if you take pimozide at bedtime, you may feel drowsy or less alert on arising. **Make sure you know how you react to this medicine before you drive, use machines, or do other jobs that require you to see clearly, be alert, and have good muscle control.**

Although not a problem for many patients, dizziness, lightheadedness, or fainting may occur, especially when you get up from a sitting or lying position. Getting up slowly may help. If the problem continues or gets worse, check with your doctor.

Pimozide may cause dryness of the mouth. For temporary relief, use sugarless gum or candy, melt bits of ice in your mouth, or use a saliva substitute. However, if your mouth continues to feel dry for more than 2 weeks, check with your physician or dentist. Continuing dryness of the mouth may increase the chance of dental disease, including tooth decay, gum disease, and fungal infections.

Side Effects of This Medicine

Along with its needed effects, a medicine may cause some unwanted effects. Although not all of these side effects may occur, if they do occur they may need medical attention.

Stop taking this medicine and get emergency help immediately if any of the following side effects occur:

Rare

Convulsions (seizures)
Difficult or unusually fast breathing
Fast heartbeat or irregular pulse
Fever
High or low (irregular) blood pressure
Increased sweating
Loss of bladder control
Muscle stiffness (severe)
Unusual feeling of tiredness or weakness
Unusually pale skin

Signs of overdose

Drowsiness or dizziness (severe)
Muscle trembling, jerking, or stiffness (severe)
Troubled breathing (severe)
Uncontrolled movements (severe)
Unusual tiredness or weakness (severe)

Check with your doctor as soon as possible if any of the following side effects occur:

More common

Difficulty in speaking or swallowing
Loss of balance control
Mask-like face
Mood or behavior changes
Restlessness or need to keep moving
Shuffling walk
Slowed movements
Stiffness of arms and legs
Trembling and shaking of fingers and hands

Less common or rare

Chewing movements
Lip smacking or puckering
Puffing of cheeks
Rapid or worm-like movements of tongue
Uncontrolled movements of arms and legs

Other side effects may occur that usually do not require medical attention. These side effects may go away during treatment as your body adjusts to the medicine. However, check with your doctor if any of the following side effects continue or are bothersome:

More common

Blurred vision or other vision problems
Constipation
Dizziness, lightheadedness, or fainting (especially when getting up from a lying or sitting position)
Drowsiness
Dry mouth

Less common

Decreased sexual ability
Headache
Mental depression

For children and elderly patients: The above side effects are more likely to occur in children and in the elderly, who are usually more sensitive to the effects of pimozide.

After you stop using pimozide, it may still produce some side effects that need attention. During this period of time, check with your doctor as soon as possible if you notice any of the following side effects:

Chewing movements
Lip smacking or puckering
Puffing of cheeks
Rapid or worm-like movements of the tongue
Uncontrolled movements of the arms and legs

Other side effects not listed above may also occur in some patients. If you notice any other effects, check with your doctor.

_____

December 1987

PLICAMYCIN (Systemic)

Some commonly used brand names or other names are Mithracin and Mithramycin.

To the Reader: If you do not recognize the names of medical conditions or medicines referred to in this information, check with your doctor, nurse, or pharmacist. Definitions for selected medical terms may be found in the Glossary. Brand names for the generic drug names listed can be found in the Index. In addition, selected brand names commonly associated with the generic name have been included in the text to help you recognize medicine you may be taking. The fact that a brand name product is not mentioned does not mean the information does not apply. It is a good idea for you to learn both the generic and brand names of your medicines and to write them down for future use.

Plicamycin (plye-ka-MYE-sin) belongs to the group of medicines known as antineoplastics. It is given by injection to treat certain types of cancer. It is also used to treat hypercalcemia or hypercalciuria (too much calcium in the blood or urine) that may occur with some types of cancer.

This medicine is available only with a prescription and is to be administered by or under the immediate care of your doctor.

Remember:
- **It is very important that you read and understand the following information.** If any of the information causes you special concern, do not decide against using this medicine without first checking with your doctor.

- Before you begin using any new medicine (prescription or nonprescription) or if you develop any new medical problem while you are using this medicine, check with your doctor, nurse, or pharmacist.

- **If you have any questions** about the following information or if you want more information about this medicine or your medical problem, **ask your doctor, nurse, or pharmacist.**

Before Using This Medicine

Plicamycin is a very strong medicine. In addition to its helpful effects in treating your medical problem, it has side effects that could be very serious. Before you receive this medicine, be sure that you have discussed the use of it with your doctor.

In order to decide on the best treatment for your medical problem, your doctor should be told:

—if you have ever had any unusual or allergic reaction to plicamycin (mithramycin).

—if you are on a low-salt, low-sugar, or any other special diet, or if you are allergic to any substance, such as foods, sulfites or other preservatives, or dyes. Most medicines contain more than their active ingredient. Your doctor, nurse, or pharmacist can help you avoid products that may cause a problem.

—if you are **pregnant** or if you may become pregnant. Plicamycin has not been shown to cause problems in humans. However, there is a possibility it may be harmful to the fetus.

—if you are **breast-feeding**. Plicamycin has not been shown to cause problems in nursing babies.

—if you have any of the following medical problems:

Bleeding problems
Blood disease
Chickenpox (including recent exposure)
Herpes zoster (shingles)
Kidney disease
Liver disease

—if you are taking **any** other prescription or nonprescription (OTC) medicine, especially:

Acetaminophen (with long-term, high-dose use) (e.g., Tylenol)
Anabolic steroids (dromostanolone, ethylestrenol, nandrolone, oxandrolone, oxymetholone, stanozolol)
Aminoglycosides by injection or topical application (amikacin, gentamicin, kanamycin, neomycin, netilmicin, streptomycin, tobramycin)
Amiodarone (e.g., Cordarone)
Amphotericin B by injection (e.g., Fungizone)
Androgens (male hormones)
Anticoagulants (blood thinners)
Antithyroid agents (medicine for overactive thyroid)
Azlocillin (e.g., Azlin)
Captopril (e.g., Capoten)
Carbamazepine (e.g., Tegretol)
Chloroquine (e.g., Aralen)
Cyclosporine (e.g., Sandimmune)
Dantrolene (e.g., Dantrium)
Dipyridamole (e.g., Persantine)
Disulfiram (e.g., Antabuse)
Divalproex (e.g., Depakote)
Erythromycins
Estrogens (female hormones)
Etretinate (e.g., Tegison)
Furazolidone (e.g., Furoxone)
Gold salts
Hydroxychloroquine (e.g., Plaquenil)
Isoniazid (e.g., INH; Nydrazid)
Ketoconazole by mouth (e.g., Nizoral)
Lithium (e.g., Lithane)
Medicine for inflammation or pain (aspirin or other salicylates, diclofenac, diflunisal, fenoprofen, flurbiprofen [oral], ibuprofen, indomethacin, ketoprofen, meclofenamate, mefenamic acid, naproxen, oxyphenbutazone, phenylbutazone, piroxicam, sulindac, suprofen, tolmetin)
Methyldopa (e.g., Aldomet)
Mezlocillin (e.g., Mezlin)
Naltrexone (with long-term, high-dose use) (e.g., Trexan)
Neomycin by mouth (e.g., Mycifradin)
Nitrofurantoin (e.g., Furadantin)
Oral contraceptives (birth control pills) containing estrogen
Penicillamine (e.g., Cuprimine)
Phenothiazines (acetophenazine, chlorpromazine, fluphenazine, mesoridazine, perphenazine, prochlorperazine, promazine, promethazine, thioridazine, trifluoperazine, triflupromazine, trimeprazine)
Phenytoin (e.g., Dilantin)
Piperacillin (e.g., Pipracil)
Rifampin (e.g., Rifadin)
Streptozocin (e.g., Zanosar)
Sulfinpyrazone (e.g., Anturane)
Sulfonamides (sulfa medicine)

Tetracyclines, except doxycycline and minocycline
Valproic acid (e.g., Depakene)
Vancomycin by injection (e.g., Vancocin)

—if you are now receiving or if you have ever been treated with x-rays or anticancer medicines.

Proper Use of This Medicine

Plicamycin sometimes causes nausea, vomiting, and loss of appetite. However, it is very important that you continue to receive the medicine, even if you begin to feel ill. If you have any questions about this, check with your doctor.

Precautions While Using This Medicine

It is very important that your doctor check your progress daily while you are receiving plicamycin to make sure that this medicine does not cause unwanted effects.

Do not take aspirin or large amounts of any other preparations containing aspirin, other salicylates, or acetaminophen without first checking with your doctor. These medicines may increase the effects of plicamycin.

While you are being treated with plicamycin, and for several weeks after you stop treatment with it, **do not have any immunizations or vaccinations without your doctor's approval.** Plicamycin lowers your resistance and there is a chance you might get the infection the immunization is meant to prevent. Other people living in your household should also avoid immunizations since they could pass the infection on to you.

Plicamycin can lower the number of white blood cells in your body. This may increase the chance of getting an infection. **If you can, avoid people with colds or other infections. If you think you are getting a cold or other infection, check with your doctor.**

Before having any kind of surgery, dental treatment, or emergency treatment, tell the physician or dentist in charge that you are taking this medicine.

Side Effects of This Medicine

Along with its needed effects, a medicine may cause some unwanted effects. Although not all of these side effects may occur, if they do occur they may need medical attention.

Check with your doctor or nurse immediately if any of the following side effects occur:

Signs of overdose
  Bloody or black, tarry stools
  Flushing or redness or swelling of face
  Nosebleed
  Skin rash or small red spots on skin
  Sore throat and fever
  Unusual bleeding or bruising
  Vomiting of blood

Other side effects may occur that usually do not need medical attention. These side effects may go away during treatment as your body adjusts to the medicine. However, check with your doctor if any of the following side effects continue or are bothersome:

More common
  Diarrhea
  Irritation or soreness of mouth
  Loss of appetite
  Nausea or vomiting—may occur 1 to 2 hours after the injection is started and continue for 12 to 24 hours

Less common
  Drowsiness
  Fever
  Headache
  Mental depression
  Pain, redness, soreness, or swelling at place of injection
  Unusual tiredness or weakness

After you stop using plicamycin, it may still produce some side effects that need attention. During this period of time check with your doctor if you notice any of the following side effects:
  Bloody or black, tarry stools
  Nosebleed
  Sore throat and fever
  Unusual bleeding or bruising
  Vomiting of blood

Other side effects not listed above may also occur in some patients. If you notice any other effects, check with your doctor.

December 1987

PNEUMOCOCCAL VACCINE POLYVALENT (Systemic)

Some commonly used brand names are Pneumovax 23 and Pnu-Imune 23.

To the Reader: If you do not recognize the names of medical conditions or medicines referred to in this information, check with your doctor, nurse, or pharmacist. Definitions for selected medical terms may be found in the Glossary. Brand names for the generic drug names listed can be found in the Index. In addition, selected brand names commonly associated with the generic name have been included in the text to help you recognize medicine you may be taking. The fact that a brand name product is not mentioned does not mean the information does not apply. It is a good idea for you to learn both the generic and brand names of your medicines and to write them down for future use.

Pneumococcal (NEU-mo-KOK-al) vaccine polyvalent is an active immunizing agent given by injection to prevent infection by pneumococcal bacteria. It works by causing your body to produce its own protection (antibodies) to the disease.

The following information applies only to the polyvalent 23 pneumococcal vaccine. Other polyvalent pneumococcal vaccines may be available in countries other than the U.S.

Pneumococcal infection can cause serious problems, such as pneumonia, which affects the lungs; meningitis, which affects the brain; bacteremia, which is a severe infection in the blood; and possibly death. These problems are more likely to occur in older adults and persons with certain diseases or conditions that make them more susceptible to a pneumococcal infection or more apt to develop serious problems from a pneumococcal infection.

Immunization against pneumococcal disease is recommended for:

—older adults, especially those 65 years of age and older.

—adults and children 2 years of age or older with chronic illnesses.

—persons without a spleen, with spleen function problems, or who will undergo an operation to remove their spleen.

—persons with sickle cell disease.

—persons who are waiting for an organ transplant.

—persons who will be treated with x-rays or cancer medicines.

—persons in nursing homes and orphanages.

—persons who will be traveling outside the U.S. and who have certain diseases or conditions that make them more susceptible to a pneumococcal infection or more likely to develop serious problems from a pneumococcal infection.

—persons who are bedridden.

Immunization against pneumococcal infection is not recommended for infants and children younger than 2 years of age because these persons cannot produce enough antibodies to the vaccine to protect them against a pneumococcal infection.

Pneumococcal vaccine is usually given only once to each person. Additional injections are not given, except in special cases, because of the possibility of more frequent and more severe side effects.

This vaccine is available only from your doctor or other authorized health care providers.

Remember:

• **It is very important that you read and understand the following information.** If any of the information causes you special concern, do not decide against receiving this vaccine without first checking with your doctor.

• **If you have any questions** about the following information or if you want more information about this vaccine or your medical problem, **ask your doctor, nurse, or pharmacist.**

Before Receiving This Vaccine

Before you receive pneumococcal vaccine, your doctor should be told:

—if you have ever had any unusual or allergic reaction to phenol or thimerosal. The pneumococcal vaccines available in the U.S. contain either phenol or thimerosal as a preservative; products available in other countries may contain other preservatives.

—if you are **pregnant** or if you may become pregnant. Studies have not been done in either humans or animals. However, if the vaccine is needed, it should be given after the first three months of pregnancy and only to women who have certain diseases or conditions that make them more susceptible to a pneumococcal infection or more likely to develop serious problems from a pneumococcal infection.

—if you are **breast-feeding**. However, it is not known whether pneumococcal vaccine passes into the breast milk and this vaccine has not been shown to cause problems in nursing babies.

—if you have any of the following medical problems:
Fever
Hodgkin's disease
Immune deficiency condition
Thrombocytopenic purpura (blood disorder)

—if you have had your spleen removed.

—if you have had an organ transplant within the past 6 months.

—if you have ever been treated with x-rays or cancer medicines.

—if you have had a pneumococcal vaccine injection of any kind in the past.

Precautions After Receiving This Vaccine

If you have more than one doctor, be sure they all know that you have received pneumococcal vaccine polyvalent 23 so that they can put the information in your medical records. This vaccine is usually given only once to each person, except in special cases.

Side Effects of This Medicine

Along with its needed effects, a medicine may cause some unwanted effects. Although not all of these side effects may occur, if they do occur they may need medical attention.

Get emergency help immediately if any of the following side effects occur:

Signs of allergic reaction
Difficulty in breathing or swallowing
Hives
Itching, especially of feet or hands
Reddening of skin, especially around ears
Swelling of eyes, face, or inside of nose
Unusual tiredness or weakness (sudden and severe)

Check with your doctor as soon as possible if the following side effect occurs:

Rare
Fever over 102 °F (39 °C)

Other side effects may occur that usually do not require medical attention. However, check with your doctor if any of the following side effects continue or are bothersome:

More common
Redness, soreness, hard lump, swelling, or pain at place of injection

Less common or rare
Aches or pain in joints or muscles
Fever of 101 °F (38.3 °C) or less
Skin rash

Side effects may be more frequent and more severe if this is not the first time you have received pneumococcal vaccine. Check with your doctor as soon as possible if you do have a severe reaction.

For elderly patients: Many medicines have not been tested in older people. Therefore, it is not known whether the medicine acts the same way it does in younger adults. Check with your doctor or pharmacist if you notice any unusual effects after receiving this vaccine or if you think it is not working as it should.

Other side effects not listed above may also occur in some patients. If you notice any other effects, check with your doctor.

_____

December 1987

PODOPHYLLUM (Topical)

A commonly used brand name is Podofin.

To the Reader: If you do not recognize the names of medical conditions or medicines referred to in this information, check with your doctor, nurse, or pharmacist. Definitions for selected medical terms may be found in the Glossary. Brand names for the generic drug names listed can be found in the Index. In addition, selected brand names commonly associated with the generic name have been included in the text to help you recognize medicine you may be taking. The fact that a brand name product is not mentioned does not mean the information does not apply. It is a good idea for you to learn both the generic and brand names of your medicines and to write them down for future use.

Podophyllum (pode-oh-FILL-um) is used on the skin to remove benign (not cancer) growths, such as certain kinds of warts. It works by destroying the tissue of the growth.

A few hours after podophyllum is applied to a wart, the wart becomes blanched (loses all color). In 24 to 48 hours, the medicine causes death of the tissue. After about 72 hours, the wart begins to slough or come off and gradually disappears.

Podophyllum is usually applied only in a doctor's office because it is a poison and can cause serious side effects if not used properly. However, your doctor may ask you to apply this medicine at home. If you do apply it at home, be sure you understand exactly how to use it.

Podophyllum is available only with your doctor's prescription.

Remember:
- **This medicine has been prescribed for your current medical problem only.** It must not be given to other people or used for other problems unless you are directed to do so by your doctor.
- **Keep all medicines out of the reach of children.**
- In order for this medicine to work, it must be used as directed.
- **It is very important that you read and understand the following information.** If any of the information causes you special concern, do not decide against using this medicine without first checking with your doctor.
- Before you begin using any new medicine (prescription or nonprescription) or if you develop any new medical problem while you are using this medicine, check with your doctor, nurse, or pharmacist.
- **If you have any questions** about the following information or if you want more information about this medicine or your medical problem, **ask your doctor, nurse, or pharmacist**.

Before Using This Medicine

In order to decide on the best treatment for your medical problem, your doctor should be told:
—if you have ever had any unusual or allergic reaction to podophyllum or benzoin.
—if you are allergic to any substance, such as certain preservatives. Most medicines contain more than their active ingredient. Your doctor, nurse, or pharmacist can help you avoid products that may cause a problem.

—if you are **pregnant** or if you may become pregnant. Topical podophyllum is absorbed through the skin. It should not be used during pregnancy, since it may cause birth defects or other harmful effects in the fetus.

—if you are **breast-feeding**. Topical podophyllum is absorbed through the skin. However, it has not been shown to cause problems in nursing babies.

Proper Use of This Medicine

Podophyllum is a poison. Keep it away from the mouth because it is harmful if swallowed.

Also, **keep podophyllum away from the eyes and other mucous membranes,** such as the inside of the nose. This medicine may cause severe irritation. If you get some in your eyes, immediately flush the eyes with water for 15 minutes. If you get some on your normal skin, thoroughly wash the skin with soap and water to remove the medicine. However, if this medicine contains tincture of benzoin, it may be removed more easily from the skin by swabbing with rubbing alcohol.

This medicine may contain alcohol and therefore may be flammable. **Do not use near heat, near open flame, or while smoking**.

Use podophyllum only as directed. Do not use more of it, do not use it more often, and do not use it for a longer period of time than your doctor ordered. To do so may increase the chance of too much medicine being absorbed into the body and the chance of side effects.

Do not use podophyllum on moles or birthmarks. To do so may cause severe irritation.

Also, **do not apply this medicine to crumbling or bleeding warts or to warts that have recently had surgery on them.** To do so may increase the chance of absorption through the skin.

Podophyllum can cause severe irritation of normal skin. Therefore, apply petrolatum around the affected area before you apply podophyllum and/or apply talcum powder to the treated area immediately after you apply podophyllum. This is to prevent the medicine from spreading to the normal skin.

Use a toothpick or a cotton-tipped or glass applicator to apply this medicine. Apply one drop at a time, allowing time for drying between drops, until the affected area is covered.

After podophyllum is applied, allow it to remain on the affected area for 1 to 6 hours as directed by your doctor. Then, remove the medicine by thoroughly washing the affected area with soap and water. If this medicine contains tincture of benzoin, it may be removed more easily by swabbing the affected area with rubbing alcohol. However, this may be more irritating than washing with soap and water.

Immediately after applying this medicine, wash your hands to remove any medicine that may be on them.

If you miss a dose of this medicine, apply it as soon as possible. Then go back to your regular dosing schedule.

How to store this medicine:

- **Keep out of the reach of children.**

- Store away from heat and direct light.

- Do not store in the bathroom, near the kitchen sink, or in other damp places. Heat or moisture may cause the medicine to break down.

- Do not keep outdated medicine or medicine no longer needed. Be sure that any discarded medicine is out of the reach of children.

Side Effects of This Medicine

Along with its needed effects, a medicine may cause some unwanted effects. Although not all of these side effects may occur, if they do occur they may need medical attention.

Check with your doctor immediately if any of the following side effects occur:

Early signs of too much medicine being absorbed into the body

    Abdominal or stomach pain
    Clumsiness or unsteadiness
    Confusion
    Decreased or loss of reflexes
    Diarrhea (may be severe and continuing)
    Excitement, irritability, or nervousness
    Hallucinations (seeing, hearing, or feeling things that are not there)
    Muscle weakness
    Nausea or vomiting
    Sore throat and fever
    Unusual bleeding or bruising

Delayed signs of too much medicine being absorbed into the body

    Constipation
    Convulsions (seizures)
    Difficult or painful urination
    Difficulty in breathing
    Dizziness or lightheadedness, especially when getting up from a lying or sitting position
    Drowsiness
    Fast heartbeat
    Numbness, tingling, pain, or weakness in hands or feet (may not occur for about 2 weeks after medicine is used)
    Pain in upper abdomen or stomach (mild, dull, and continuing)

Also, check with your doctor as soon as possible if any of the following side effects occur:

    Redness, burning, or other irritation of affected area or skin
    Skin rash or itching

For elderly patients: Many medicines have not been tested in older people. Therefore, it is not known whether the medicine acts the same way it does in younger adults. Check with your doctor or pharmacist if you notice any unusual effects while using this medicine or if you think it is not working as it should.

Other side effects not listed above may also occur in some patients. If you notice any other effects, check with your doctor.

December 1987

POSTERIOR PITUITARY (Systemic)

A commonly used brand name is Pituitrin.

To the Reader: If you do not recognize the names of medical conditions or medicines referred to in this information, check with your doctor, nurse, or pharmacist. Definitions for selected medical terms may be found in the Glossary. Brand names for the generic drug names listed can be found in the Index. In addition, selected brand names commonly associated with the generic name have been included in the text to help you recognize medicine you may be taking. The fact that a brand name product is not mentioned does not mean the information does not apply. It is a good idea for you to learn both the generic and brand names of your medicines and to write them down for future use.

Posterior pituitary (poss-TEER-ee-or pi-TOO-i-ter-ee) is a hormone naturally produced by your body. It is used to stop bleeding from the uterus after childbirth. It may be used also to stop bleeding during surgery or to control blockage of the intestine after certain types of surgery.

This medicine is available only with your doctor's prescription.

Remember:
• **It is very important that you read and understand the following information.** If any of the information causes you special concern, do not decide against receiving this medicine without first checking with your doctor.

• Before you begin using any new medicine (prescription or nonprescription) or if you develop any new medical problem while you are receiving this medicine, check with your doctor, nurse, or pharmacist.

• **If you have any questions** about the following information or if you want more information about this medicine or your medical problem, **ask your doctor, nurse, or pharmacist.**

Before Using This Medicine

In order to decide on the best treatment for your medical problem, your doctor should be told:

—if you have ever had any unusual or allergic reaction to posterior pituitary.

—if you are on a low-salt, low-sugar, or any other special diet, or if you are allergic to any substance, such as foods or sulfites or other preservatives. Most medicines contain more than their active ingredient. Your doctor, nurse, or pharmacist can help you avoid products that may cause a problem.

—if you are **pregnant** or if you may become pregnant. Studies have not been done in either humans or animals. However, posterior pituitary has been shown to cause abortions in pregnant women. Also, if used during labor, it may cause harmful side effects to the mother (damage to the uterus) and/or the baby (breathing problems).

—if you are **breast-feeding**. Posterior pituitary has not been shown to cause problems in nursing babies.

—if you have any of the following medical problems:
Epilepsy
Heart or blood vessel disease
High blood pressure
Toxemia of pregnancy

—if you are taking **any** other prescription or nonprescription (OTC) medicine, especially primidone (e.g., Mysoline).

Side Effects of This Medicine

Along with its needed effects, a medicine may cause some unwanted effects. Although not all of these effects may occur, if they do occur they may need medical attention.

Check with your doctor immediately if any of the following side effects occur:
Rare
Chest pain
Skin rash or itching
Wheezing or shortness of breath

Check with your doctor as soon as possible if the following side effects occur:
Less common
Cloudy urine
Loss of eyesight (unexplained, sudden)
Ringing or buzzing sound in ears

Other side effects may occur that usually do not require medical attention. These side effects may go away during treatment as your body adjusts to the medicine. However, check with your doctor if any of the following side effects continue or are bothersome:
More common
Abdominal or stomach cramps
Paleness of face
Uterine cramps

Other side effects not listed above may also occur in some patients. If you notice any other effects, check with your doctor.

December 1987

POTASSIUM IODIDE (Systemic)

Some commonly used brand names or other names are:

Iosat   SSKI
KI   Thyro-Block
Pima

Generic name product may also be available in the U.S.

To the Reader: If you do not recognize the names of medical conditions or medicines referred to in this information, check with your doctor, nurse, or pharmacist. Definitions for selected medical terms may be found in the Glossary. Brand names for the generic drug names listed can be found in the Index. In addition, selected brand names commonly associated with the generic name have been included in the text to help you recognize medicine you may be taking. The fact that a brand name product is not mentioned does not mean the information does not apply. It is a good idea for you to learn both the generic and brand names of your medicines and to write them down for future use.

Potassium iodide (poe-TAS-ee-um EYE-oh-dide) is used to treat overactive thyroid and to protect the thyroid gland from the effects of radiation from radioactive forms of iodine. It may be used before and after administration of a radioactive medicine containing a radioactive form of iodine or accidental exposure to radiation (for example, from nuclear power plant accidents). It may also be used for other problems as determined by your doctor.

Potassium iodide is taken by mouth. It may be taken as an oral solution, syrup, uncoated tablet, or enteric-coated tablet. However, the enteric-coated tablet form may cause serious side effects and its use is generally not recommended.

The lower strength (130 mg) of plain potassium iodide tablets and some brands of the oral solution are available without a prescription. Use them only as directed by state or local public health authorities in case of a radiation emergency. Other forms and strengths of potassium iodide are available only with your doctor's prescription.

Remember:
• **Keep all medicines out of the reach of children.**

• In order for this medicine to work, it must be used as directed. **If you are using this medicine without a prescription, it is very important to follow the directions on the label.**

• **It is also very important that you read and understand the following information.** If any of the information causes you special concern, check with your doctor or pharmacist.

• Before you begin using any new medicine (prescription or nonprescription) or if you develop any new medical problem while you are using this medicine, check with your doctor, nurse, or pharmacist.

• **If you have any questions** about the following information or if you want more information about this medicine or your medical problem, **ask your doctor, nurse, or pharmacist.**

Before Using This Medicine

Before you use potassium iodide, check with your doctor or pharmacist:

—if you have ever had any unusual or allergic reaction to iodine or iodine-containing foods.

—if you are on a low-salt, low-sugar, or any other special diet, or if you are allergic to any substance, such as foods, sulfites or other preservatives, or dyes. Most medicines contain more than their active ingredient, and many liquid medicines contain alcohol. Your doctor, nurse, or pharmacist can help you avoid products that may cause a problem.

—if you are **pregnant** or if you may become pregnant. Taking potassium iodide during pregnancy may cause thyroid problems or goiter in the newborn infant.

—if you are **breast-feeding.** Potassium iodide passes into the breast milk and may cause skin rash and thyroid problems in nursing babies.

—if you have any of the following medical problems:
Kidney disease
Myotonia congenita
Overactive thyroid (unless you are taking this medicine for this medical problem)

—if you are taking **any** other prescription or nonprescription (OTC) medicine, especially:
Amiloride (e.g., Midamor)
Antithyroid agents (medicine for overactive thyroid)
Lithium (e.g., Lithane)
Spironolactone (e.g., Aldactone)
Triamterene (e.g., Dyrenium)

Proper Use of This Medicine

If potassium iodide upsets your stomach, **take it after meals or with food or milk** unless otherwise directed by your doctor. If stomach upset (nausea, vomiting, stomach pain, or diarrhea) continues, check with your doctor.

For patients taking the oral solution form of this medicine:

• Do not use if solution turns brownish yellow.

• Take potassium iodide in a full glass (8 ounces) of water or in fruit juice, milk, or broth to improve the taste and lessen stomach upset. Be sure to drink all of the liquid in order to get the full dose of medicine.

• If crystals form in potassium iodide solution, they may be dissolved by warming the closed container of solution in warm water and then gently shaking the container.

For patients taking the tablet form of this medicine:

• Before taking, dissolve each tablet in ½ glass (4 ounces) of water or milk. Be sure to drink all of the liquid in order to get the full dose of medicine.

If you miss a dose of this medicine, take it as soon as possible. However, if it is almost time for your next dose, skip the missed dose and go back to your regular dosing schedule. Do not double doses.

How to store this medicine:

- **Keep out of the reach of children.**

- Store away from heat and direct light.

- Do not store the tablet form of this medicine in the bathroom, near the kitchen sink, or in other damp places. Heat or moisture may cause the medicine to break down.

- Keep the oral liquid forms of this medicine from freezing. Do not refrigerate.

- Do not keep outdated medicine or medicine no longer needed. Be sure that any discarded medicine is out of the reach of children.

Precautions While Using This Medicine

Your doctor should check your progress at regular visits to make sure that this medicine does not cause unwanted effects.

For patients on a low-potassium diet:

- **This medicine contains potassium.** Check with your doctor or pharmacist before you take this medicine.

Side Effects of This Medicine

Along with its needed effects, a medicine may cause some unwanted effects. Although not all of these side effects may occur, if they do occur they may need medical attention. When this medicine is used for short periods of time at low doses, side effects usually are rare.

Check with your doctor as soon as possible if any of the following side effects occur:

More common
   Skin rash
   Salivary gland swelling or tenderness

Rare
   Bloody or black tarry stools
   Confusion
   Fever
   Irregular heartbeat

   Numbness, tingling, pain, or weakness in hands or feet
   Swelling of neck or throat
   Unusual tiredness
   Weakness or heaviness of legs

With long-term use
   Burning of mouth or throat
   Headache (severe)
   Increase in salivation
   Metallic taste
   Soreness of teeth and gums
   Symptoms of head cold

Other side effects may occur that usually do not require medical attention. These side effects may go away during treatment as your body adjusts to the medicine. However, check with your doctor if any of the following side effects continue or are bothersome:
   Diarrhea
   Nausea or vomiting
   Stomach pain

For elderly patients: Many medicines have not been tested in older people. Therefore, it is not known whether the medicine acts the same way it does in younger adults. Check with your doctor or pharmacist if you notice any unusual effects while taking this medicine or if you think it is not working as it should.

Other side effects not listed above may also occur in some patients. If you notice any other effects, check with your doctor.

December 1987

Additional Information

In addition to the above information, for patients taking this medicine for a fungal infection:

- **Keep taking it for the full course of treatment** even if you begin to feel better after a few days. This will help clear up your infection completely. **Do not miss any doses.**

POTASSIUM SUPPLEMENTS (Systemic)

This information applies to the following medicines:

Potassium Acetate
Potassium Bicarbonate
Potassium Bicarbonate and Potassium Chloride
Potassium Bicarbonate and Potassium Citrate
Potassium Chloride
Potassium Chloride, Potassium Bicarbonate, and Potassium Citrate
Potassium Gluconate
Potassium Gluconate and Potassium Chloride
Potassium Gluconate and Potassium Citrate
Potassium Gluconate, Potassium Citrate, and Ammonium Chloride
Trikates

This information does *not* apply to:
Potassium Citrate
Potassium Iodide
Potassium Permanganate
Potassium Phosphates

Some commonly used brand names and other names are:	Generic names:
	Potassium Acetate†
Klor-Con/EF	Potassium Bicarbonate†
Klorvess K-Lyte/Cl Neo-K* Potassium-Sandoz*	Potassium Bicarbonate and Potassium Chloride
K-Lyte K-Lyte DS	Potassium Bicarbonate and Potassium Citrate
Apo-K* Cena-K K-10* Kalium Durules* Kaochlor Kaochlor S-F Kaon-Cl Kato Kay Ciel KCL* K-Dur K-Long* K-Lor Klor-10% Klor-Con Klor-Con/25 Klorvess Klotrix K-Lyte/Cl Powder K-Tab Micro-K Novolente-K* Potachlor Potage Potasalan Potassine Roychlor* Rum-K Slo-Pot* Slow-K Ten-K	Potassium Chloride†
Kaochlor-Eff	Potassium Chloride, Potassium Bicarbonate, and Potassium Citrate
Bayon Kaon Kao-Nor Kaylixir K-G Elixir Potassium-Rougier* Royonate*	Potassium Gluconate†
Kolyum	Potassium Gluconate and Potassium Chloride
Bi-K Twin-K	Potassium Gluconate and Potassium Citrate
Twin-K-Cl	Potassium Gluconate, Potassium Citrate, and Ammonium Chloride
Potassium triplex Tri-K	Trikates (Potassium Acetate, Potassium Bicarbonate, and Potassium Citrate)

*Not available in the U.S.
†Generic name product available.

To the Reader: If you do not recognize the names of medical conditions or medicines referred to in this information, check with your doctor, nurse, or pharmacist. Definitions for selected medical terms may be found in the Glossary. Brand names for the generic drug names listed can be found in the Index. In addition, selected brand names commonly associated with the generic name have been included in the text to help you recognize medicine you may be taking. The fact that a brand name product is not mentioned does not mean the information does not apply. It is a good idea for you to learn both the generic and brand names of your medicines and to write them down for future use.

Potassium (poe-TASS-ee-um) is needed to maintain good health. Potassium supplements may be needed by patients who do not have enough potassium in their regular diet or have lost too much potassium because of illness or treatment with certain medicines.

Since too much potassium may also cause health problems, most potassium supplements are available only with your doctor's prescription.

Remember:

• **This medicine has been prescribed for your current medical problem only.** It must not be given to other people or used for other problems unless you are directed to do so by your doctor.

• **Keep all medicines out of the reach of children.**

• In order for this medicine to work, it must be used as directed.

• If you are receiving this medicine by injection, some of the information about this medicine may not apply.

• **It is very important that you read and understand the following information.** If any of the information causes you special concern, do not decide against using this medicine without first checking with your doctor.

• Before you begin using any new medicine (prescription or nonprescription) or if you develop any new medical problem while you are using this medicine, check with your doctor, nurse, or pharmacist.

• **If you have any questions** about the following information or if you want more information about this medicine or your medical problem, **ask your doctor, nurse, or pharmacist**.

Before Using This Medicine

In order to decide on the best treatment for your medical problem, your doctor should be told:

—if you have ever had any unusual reaction to potassium preparations.

—if you are on a low-salt, low-sugar, or any other special diet, or if you are allergic to any substance, such as foods, sulfites or other preservatives, or dyes. Most medicines contain more than their active ingredient, and many liquid medicines contain alcohol. Your doctor, nurse, or pharmacist can help you avoid products that may cause a problem.

—if you are **pregnant** or if you may become pregnant. Potassium supplements have not been shown to cause problems in humans.

—if you are **breast-feeding**. Potassium supplements pass into breast milk. However, this medicine has not been shown to cause problems in nursing babies.

—if you have any of the following medical problems:

    Addison's disease (underactive adrenal glands)
    Diarrhea (continuing or severe)
    Heart disease
    Intestinal blockage
    Kidney disease
    Stomach ulcer

—if you are taking **any** other prescription or nonprescription (OTC) medicine, especially:

    Adrenocorticoids (cortisone-like medicine)
    Amiloride (e.g., Midamor)
    Antimuscarinics (medicine for abdominal or stomach spasms or cramps)
    Captopril (e.g., Capoten)
    Digitalis glycosides (heart medicine)
    Enalapril (e.g., Vasotec)
    Other medicines containing potassium
    Spironolactone (e.g., Aldactone)
    Triamterene (e.g., Dyrenium)

—if you are now using salt substitutes or drinking low-salt milk.

Proper Use of This Medicine

For patients taking the liquid form of this medicine:

• This medicine must be diluted in at least ½ glass (4 ounces) of cold water or juice to reduce possible stomach irritation or laxative effect.

• If you are on a salt (sodium)-restricted diet, check with your doctor before using tomato juice to dilute your medicine. Tomato juice has a high salt (sodium) content.

For patients taking the soluble granule, soluble powder, or soluble tablet form of this medicine:

• This medicine must be completely dissolved in at least ½ glass (4 ounces) of cold water or juice to reduce possible stomach irritation or laxative effect.

• Allow any "fizzing" to stop before taking the dissolved medicine.

• If you are on a salt (sodium)-restricted diet, check with your doctor before using tomato juice to dilute your medicine. Tomato juice has a high salt (sodium) content.

For patients taking the extended-release tablet form of this medicine:

• Swallow the tablets whole. Do not chew or suck on the tablet.

• Some tablets may be crushed and sprinkled on apple sauce or other soft food. However, check with your doctor or pharmacist first, since this should not be done for some tablets.

• If you have trouble swallowing tablets or if they seem to stick in your throat, check with your doctor. When this medicine is not properly released, it can cause irritation that may lead to ulcers.

For patients taking the extended-release capsule form of this medicine:

• Do not crush or chew the capsule.

• Some capsules may be opened and the contents sprinkled on apple sauce or other soft food. However, check with your doctor or pharmacist first, since this should not be done for some capsules.

Take this medicine immediately after meals or with food to lessen possible stomach upset or laxative action.

Take this medicine only as directed by your doctor. Do not take more of it, do not take it more often, and do not take it for a longer period of time than your doctor ordered. **This is especially important if you are also taking both diuretics (water pills) and digitalis medicines for your heart.**

If you miss a dose of this medicine and remember within 2 hours, take the missed dose right away with food or liquids. Then go back to your regular dosing schedule. However, if you do not remember until later, skip the missed dose and go back to your regular dosing schedule. Do not double doses.

How to store this medicine:

• **Keep out of the reach of children.**

• Store away from heat and direct light.

• Do not store in the bathroom, near the kitchen sink, or in other damp places. Heat or moisture may cause the medicine to break down.

• Keep the liquid form of this medicine from freezing.

• Do not keep outdated medicine or medicine no longer needed. Be sure that any discarded medicine is out of the reach of children.

Precautions While Using This Medicine

Your doctor should check your progress at regular visits to make sure the medicine is working properly and that possible side effects are avoided. Laboratory tests may be necessary.

Since salt substitutes and low-salt milk may contain potassium, do not use them unless told to do so by your doctor.

Check with your doctor at once if you notice blackish stools or other signs of stomach or intestinal bleeding. This medicine may cause such a condition to become worse, especially when taken in tablet form.

Side Effects of This Medicine

Along with its needed effects, a medicine may cause some unwanted effects. Although not all of these side effects may occur, if they do occur they may need medical attention.

Stop taking this medicine and check with your doctor immediately if any of the following side effects occur:

Rare

    Confusion
    Irregular heartbeat
    Numbness or tingling in hands, feet, or lips
    Shortness of breath or difficult breathing
    Unexplained anxiety
    Unusual tiredness or weakness
    Weakness or heaviness of legs

Also, check with your doctor if any of the following side effects occur:

Rare

    Abdominal or stomach pain, cramping, or soreness (prolonged)
    Chest or throat pain, especially when swallowing
    Stools with signs of blood (red or black color)

Other side effects may occur that usually do not require medical attention. These side effects may go away during treatment as your body adjusts to the medicine. However, check with your doctor if any of the following side effects continue or are bothersome:

More common

    Diarrhea
    Nausea
    Stomach pain or discomfort (mild)
    Vomiting

Sometimes you may see what appears to be a whole tablet in the stool after taking certain extended-release potassium chloride tablets. This is to be expected. Your body has absorbed the potassium from the tablet and the shell is then expelled.

Other side effects not listed above may also occur in some patients. If you notice any other effects, check with your doctor.

December 1987

PRAZIQUANTEL (Systemic)

Some commonly used brand names are Biltricide and Cysticide*.

---

*Not available in the U.S.

To the Reader: If you do not recognize the names of medical conditions or medicines referred to in this information, check with your doctor, nurse, or pharmacist. Definitions for selected medical terms may be found in the Glossary. Brand names for the generic drug names listed can be found in the Index. In addition, selected brand names commonly associated with the generic name have been included in the text to help you recognize medicine you may be taking. The fact that a brand name product is not mentioned does not mean the information does not apply. It is a good idea for you to learn both the generic and brand names of your medicines and to write them down for future use.

Praziquantel (pray-zi-KWON-tel) belongs to the family of medicines called anthelmintics (ant-hel-MIN-tiks). Anthelmintics are used in the treatment of worm infections.

Praziquantel is taken by mouth to treat blood fluke infections. These are also known as snail fever, schistosomiasis (shis-toe-soe-MYE-a-siss), or bilharziasis (bil-har-ZYE-a-siss). Praziquantel may also be used for other worm infections as determined by your doctor. However, it will not work for pinworms or roundworms.

Praziquantel works by causing severe spasms and paralysis of the worms' muscles. Some kinds of worms are then passed in the stool. However, you may not notice them since they are sometimes completely destroyed in the intestine.

Praziquantel is available only with your doctor's prescription.

Remember:
• **This medicine has been prescribed for your present infection only.** Another infection later on may require a different medicine. Also, even though other people may have the same symptoms as you, they may have a different kind of infection. Your medicine may not work for them and may even cause them harm. Therefore, **your medicine must not be given to other people or used for other infections** unless you are otherwise directed by your doctor.

• **Keep all medicines out of the reach of children.**

• In order for this medicine to work, it must be used as directed.

• **It is very important that you read and understand the following information.** If any of the information causes you special concern, do not decide against using this medicine without first checking with your doctor.

• Before you begin using any new medicine (prescription or nonprescription) or if you develop any new medical problem while you are using this medicine, check with your doctor, nurse, or pharmacist.

• **If you have any questions** about the following information or if you want more information about this medicine or your medical problem, **ask your doctor, nurse, or pharmacist.**

Before Using This Medicine

In order to decide on the best treatment for your medical problem, your doctor should be told:

—if you have ever had any unusual or allergic reaction to praziquantel.

—if you are on a low-salt, low-sugar, or any other special diet, or if you are allergic to any substance, such as foods, sulfites or other preservatives, or dyes. Most medicines contain more than their active ingredient. Your doctor, nurse, or pharmacist can help you avoid products that may cause a problem.

—if you are **pregnant** or if you may become pregnant. Studies have not been done in humans. Praziquantel has not been shown to cause birth defects in rats and rabbits given up to 40 times the usual human dose. However, it has been shown to cause a greater chance of abortion in rats given 3 times the human dose.

—if you are **breast-feeding**. Praziquantel passes into the breast milk. You should stop breast-feeding on the day you begin taking praziquantel. Do not restart breast-feeding until 72 hours after treatment is completed. During this time the breast milk should be squeezed out or sucked out with a breast pump and thrown away.

—if you have worm cysts in the eye.

Proper Use of This Medicine

No special preparations (for example, special diets, fasting, other medicines, laxatives, or enemas) are necessary before, during, or immediately after taking praziquantel.

Praziquantel has a bitter taste that may cause gagging or vomiting. The bitter taste may be more noticeable if the tablets are held in the mouth or chewed. Therefore, **do not chew praziquantel tablets.** Swallow them whole with a small amount of liquid during meals.

To help clear up your infection completely, **take this medicine exactly as directed by your doctor for the full time of treatment. Do not miss any doses.**

If you do miss a dose of this medicine, take it as soon as possible. However, if it is almost time for your next dose and your dosing schedule is 3 doses a day (during meals), space the missed dose and the rest of the doses for that day 4 hours apart. Then go back to your regular dosing schedule.

How to store this medicine:

• **Keep out of the reach of children.**

• Store away from heat and direct light.

• Do not store in the bathroom, near the kitchen sink, or in other damp places. Heat or moisture may cause the medicine to break down.

• Do not keep outdated medicine or medicine no longer needed. Be sure that any discarded medicine is out of the reach of children.

Precautions While Using This Medicine

It is important that your doctor check your progress after treatment. This is to make sure that the infection is cleared up completely.

If your symptoms do not improve after you have taken this medicine for the full time of treatment, or if they become worse, check with your doctor.

This medicine may cause some people to become dizzy, drowsy, or less alert than they are normally. If any of these occur, **do not drive, use machines, or do other jobs that require you to be alert** while you are taking praziquantel and for 24 hours after you stop taking it.

Side Effects of This Medicine

Along with its needed effects, a medicine may cause some unwanted effects. The following side effects may go away during treatment as your body adjusts to the medicine. However, check with your doctor if any of the following side effects continue or are bothersome:

More common
   Abdominal or stomach cramps or pain
   Dizziness
   Drowsiness
   Fever
   Headache
   Increased sweating
   Nausea or vomiting

Less common
   Loss of appetite
   Skin rash, hives, or itching

For elderly patients: Many medicines have not been tested in older people. Therefore, it is not known whether the medicine acts the same way it does in younger adults. Check with your doctor or pharmacist if you notice any unusual effects while taking this medicine or if you think it is not working as it should.

Other side effects not listed above may also occur in some patients. If you notice any other effects, check with your doctor.

December 1987

Additional Information

In addition to the above information, for patients taking praziquantel for dwarf tapeworm infections:

• Some patients with tapeworm infections may not notice any symptoms or may have only mild symptoms. Even so, to help clear up your infection completely, **take this medicine exactly as directed by your doctor.** Usually one dose is enough.

PRAZOSIN (Systemic)

A commonly used brand name is Minipress.

To the Reader: If you do not recognize the names of medical conditions or medicines referred to in this information, check with your doctor, nurse, or pharmacist. Definitions for selected medical terms may be found in the Glossary. Brand names for the generic drug names listed can be found in the Index. In addition, selected brand names commonly associated with the generic name have been included in the text to help you recognize medicine you may be taking. The fact that a brand name product is not mentioned does not mean the information does not apply. It is a good idea for you to learn both the generic and brand names of your medicines and to write them down for future use.

Prazosin (PRA-zoe-sin) belongs to the general class of medicines called antihypertensives. It is taken by mouth to treat high blood pressure.

High blood pressure adds to the workload of the heart and arteries. If it continues for a long time, the heart and arteries may not function properly. This can damage the blood vessels of the brain, heart, and kidneys, resulting in a stroke, heart failure, or kidney failure. High blood pressure may also increase the risk of heart attacks. These problems may be less likely to occur if blood pressure is controlled.

Prazosin works by relaxing blood vessels so that blood passes through them more easily. This helps to lower blood pressure.

Prazosin may also be used for other conditions as determined by your doctor.

Prazosin is available only with your doctor's prescription.

Remember:

• **This medicine has been prescribed for your current medical problem only.** It must not be given to other people or used for other problems unless you are directed to do so by your doctor.

• **Keep all medicines out of the reach of children.**

• In order for this medicine to work, it must be used as directed.

• **It is very important that you read and understand the following information.** If any of the information causes you special concern, do not decide against using this medicine without first checking with your doctor.

• Before you begin using any new medicine (prescription or nonprescription) or if you develop any new medical problem while you are using this medicine, check with your doctor, nurse, or pharmacist.

• **If you have any questions** about the following information or if you want more information about this medicine or your medical problem, **ask your doctor, nurse, or pharmacist.**

Before Using This Medicine

In order to decide on the best treatment for your medical problem, your doctor should be told:

—if you have ever had any unusual or allergic reaction to prazosin.

—if you are on a low-salt, low-sugar, or any other special diet, or if you are allergic to any substance, such as foods, sulfites or other preservatives, or dyes. Most medicines contain more than their active ingredient. Your doctor, nurse, or pharmacist can help you avoid products that may cause a problem.

—if you are **pregnant** or if you may become pregnant. Studies have not been done in humans. However, prazosin has not been shown to cause birth defects or other problems in animals.

—if you are **breast-feeding**. Prazosin has not been shown to cause problems in nursing babies.

—if you have any of the following medical problems:
  Angina (chest pain)
  Heart disease
  Kidney disease

—if you are taking **any** other prescription or nonprescription (OTC) medicine.

Proper Use of This Medicine

Importance of diet—When prescribing medicine for your condition, your doctor may also prescribe a personal diet for you. Such a diet may be low in sodium (salt). Most people eat much more sodium than they need and too much sodium in the diet may increase blood pressure. Some foods that contain large amounts of sodium are canned soup, pickles, ketchup, green and ripe olives, relish, frankfurters, soy sauce, and carbonated beverages. Your doctor may want you to limit the amounts of these and other high-sodium foods in your diet. High blood pressure medicine is usually more effective when such a diet is properly followed.

Also, it may be very important for you to go on a reducing diet. However, check with your doctor before changing your diet.

Many patients who have high blood pressure will not notice any signs of the problem. In fact, many may feel normal. It is very important that you **take your medicine exactly as directed** and that you keep your appointments with your doctor even if you feel well.

Remember that prazosin will not cure your high blood pressure but it does help control it. Therefore, you must continue to take it as directed if you expect to lower your blood pressure and keep it down. **You may have to take high blood pressure medicine for the rest of your life.** If high blood pressure is not treated, it can cause serious problems such as heart failure, blood vessel disease, stroke, or kidney disease.

In order to help remember to take your medicine, try to get into the habit of taking it at the same time each day.

If you miss a dose of this medicine, take it as soon as possible. However, if it is almost time for your next dose, skip the missed dose and go back to your regular dosing schedule. Do not double doses.

How to store this medicine:

- **Keep out of the reach of children.**
- Store away from heat and direct light.
- Do not store in the bathroom, near the kitchen sink, or in other damp places. Heat or moisture may cause the medicine to break down.
- Do not keep outdated medicine or medicine no longer needed. Be sure that any discarded medicine is out of the reach of children.

Precautions While Using This Medicine

It is important that your doctor check your progress at regular visits to make sure that this medicine is working properly.

Do not take other medicines unless they have been discussed with your doctor. This especially includes over-the-counter (nonprescription) medicines for appetite control, asthma, colds, cough, hay fever, or sinus problems, since they may tend to increase your blood pressure.

Dizziness and irregular heartbeat may occur after the first dose of this medicine. Taking the first dose at bedtime may prevent problems. However, **be especially careful if you need to get up during the night.** Make sure you know how you react to this medicine before you drive, use machines, or do other jobs that require you to be alert. After you have taken several doses of this medicine, these effects should lessen.

Dizziness, lightheadedness, or fainting may occur, especially when you get up from a lying or sitting position. Getting up slowly may help lessen this problem. **If you begin to feel dizzy, lie down so that you do not faint.** Then sit for a few moments before standing to prevent the dizziness from returning.

The dizziness, lightheadedness, or fainting is also more likely to occur if you drink alcohol, stand for long periods of time, exercise, or if the weather is hot. **While you are taking this medicine, be careful in the amount of alcohol you drink. Also, use extra care during exercise or hot weather or if you must stand for long periods of time.**

Side Effects of This Medicine

Along with its needed effects, a medicine may cause some unwanted effects. Although not all of these side effects may occur, if they do occur they may need medical attention.

Check with your doctor as soon as possible if any of the following side effects occur:

Less common
   Chest pain
   Dizziness or lightheadedness, especially when getting up from a lying or sitting position
   Fainting (sudden)
   Irregular heartbeat
   Shortness of breath
   Swelling of feet or lower legs
   Weight gain

Rare
   Inability to control urination
   Numbness or tingling of hands or feet

Other side effects may occur that usually do not require medical attention. These side effects may go away during treatment as your body adjusts to the medicine. However, check with your doctor if any of the following side effects continue or are bothersome:

Less common
   Drowsiness
   Headache
   Lack of energy
   Nausea and vomiting

For elderly patients: Dizziness, lightheadedness, or fainting may be more likely to occur in the elderly, who are more sensitive to the effects of prazosin. In addition, prazosin may reduce tolerance to cold temperatures in elderly patients.

Other side effects not listed above may also occur in some patients. If you notice any other effects, check with your doctor.

December 1987

PRAZOSIN AND POLYTHIAZIDE
(Systemic)

A commonly used brand name is Minizide.

To the Reader: If you do not recognize the names of medical conditions or medicines referred to in this information, check with your doctor, nurse, or pharmacist. Definitions for selected medical terms may be found in the Glossary. Brand names for the generic drug names listed can be found in the Index. In addition, selected brand names commonly associated with the generic name have been included in the text to help you recognize medicine you may be taking. The fact that a brand name product is not mentioned does not mean the information does not apply. It is a good idea for you to learn both the generic and brand names of your medicines and to write them down for future use.

Prazosin (PRA-zoe-sin) and polythiazide (pol-i-THYE-a-zide) combination is used in the treatment of high blood pressure.

High blood pressure adds to the workload of the heart and arteries. If it continues for a long time, the heart and arteries may not function properly. This can damage the blood vessels of the brain, heart, and kidneys resulting in a stroke, heart failure, or kidney failure. High blood pressure may also increase the risk of heart attacks. These problems may be less likely to occur if blood pressure is controlled.

Prazosin works by relaxing blood vessels so that blood passes through them more easily. The polythiazide in this combination is a thiazide diuretic (water pill) that helps to reduce the amount of water in the body by increasing the flow of urine. Both of these actions help to lower blood pressure.

This medicine is available only with your doctor's prescription.

Remember:

• **This medicine has been prescribed for your current medical problem only.** It must not be given to other people or used for other problems unless you are directed to do so by your doctor.

• **Keep all medicines out of the reach of children.**

• In order for this medicine to work, it must be used as directed.

• **It is very important that you read and understand the following information.** If any of the information causes you special concern, do not decide against using this medicine without first checking with your doctor.

• Before you begin using any new medicine (prescription or nonprescription) or if you develop any new medical problem while you are using this medicine, check with your doctor, nurse, or pharmacist.

• **If you have any questions** about the following information or if you want more information about this medicine or your medical problem, **ask your doctor, nurse, or pharmacist.**

Before Using This Medicine

In order to decide on the best treatment for your medical problem, your doctor should be told:

—if you have ever had any unusual or allergic reaction to prazosin, sulfonamides (sulfa drugs), or any of the thiazide diuretics.

—if you are on a low-salt, low-sugar, or any other special diet, or if you are allergic to any substance, such as foods, sulfites or other preservatives, or dyes. Most medicines contain more than their active ingredient. Your doctor, nurse, or pharmacist can help you avoid products that may cause a problem.

—if you are **pregnant** or if you may become pregnant. When polythiazide (contained in this combination medicine) is used during pregnancy, it may cause side effects including jaundice, blood problems, and low potassium in the newborn infant. The combination of prazosin and polythiazide has not been shown to cause birth defects.

—if you are **breast-feeding**. Polythiazide passes into breast milk. However, prazosin and polythiazide combination has not been shown to cause problems in nursing babies.

—if you have any of the following medical problems:
Angina (chest pain)
Diabetes mellitus (sugar diabetes)
Gout (history of)
Heart disease
Kidney disease
Liver disease
Lupus erythematosus (history of)
Pancreas disease

—if you are taking **any** other prescription or nonprescription (OTC) medicine, especially:
Adrenocorticoids (cortisone-like medicines)
Digitalis glycosides (heart medicine)
Lithium (e.g., Lithane)
Methenamine (e.g., Mandelamine)

Proper Use of This Medicine

Importance of diet—When prescribing medicine for your condition, your doctor may also prescribe a personal diet for you. Such a diet may be low in sodium (salt). Most people eat much more sodium than they need and too much sodium in the diet may increase blood pressure. Some foods that contain large amounts of sodium are canned soup, pickles, ketchup, green and ripe olives, relish, frankfurters, soy sauce, and carbonated beverages. Your doctor may want you to limit the amounts of these and other high-sodium foods in your diet. High blood pressure medicine is usually more effective when such a diet is properly followed.

Also, it may be very important for you to go on a reducing diet. However, check with your doctor before changing your diet.

Many patients who have high blood pressure will not notice any signs of the problem. In fact, many may feel normal. It is very important that you **take your medicine exactly as directed** and that you keep your appointments with your doctor even if you feel well.

Remember that this medicine will not cure your high blood pressure but it does help control it. Therefore, you must continue to take it as directed if you expect to lower your blood pressure and keep it down. **You may have to take high blood pressure medicine for the rest of your life.** If high blood pressure is not treated, it can cause serious problems such as heart failure, blood vessel disease, stroke, or kidney disease.

This medicine may cause you to have an unusual feeling of tiredness when you begin to take it. You may also notice an increase in the amount of urine or in your frequency of urination. After taking the medicine for a while, these effects should lessen. In order to keep the increase in urine from affecting your nighttime sleep:

• If you are to take a single dose a day, take it in the morning after breakfast.

• If you are to take more than one dose a day, take the last dose no later than 6 p.m., unless otherwise directed by your doctor.

However, it is best to plan your dose or doses according to a schedule that will least affect your personal activities and sleep. Ask your doctor, nurse, or pharmacist to help you plan the best time to take this medicine.

In order to help remember to take your medicine, try to get into the habit of taking it at the same time each day.

If you miss a dose of this medicine, take it as soon as possible. However, if it is almost time for your next dose, skip the missed dose and go back to your regular dosing schedule. Do not double doses.

How to store this medicine:

• **Keep out of the reach of children.**

• Store away from heat and direct light.

• Do not store in the bathroom, near the kitchen sink, or in other damp places. Heat or moisture may cause the medicine to break down.

• Do not keep outdated medicine or medicine no longer needed. Be sure that any discarded medicine is out of the reach of children.

Precautions While Using This Medicine

It is important that your doctor check your progress at regular visits to make sure this medicine is working properly.

Do not take other medicines unless they have been discussed with your doctor. This especially includes over-the-counter (nonprescription) medicine for appetite control, asthma, colds, cough, hay fever, or sinus problems, since they may tend to increase your blood pressure.

This medicine may cause a loss of potassium from your body.

• To help prevent this, your doctor may want you to:
—eat or drink foods that have a high potassium content (for example, orange or other citrus fruit juices), or

—take a potassium supplement, or

—take another medicine to help prevent the loss of the potassium in the first place.

• It is very important to follow these directions. Also, it is important not to change your diet on your own. This is more important if you are already on a special diet (as for diabetes), or if you are taking a potassium supplement or a medicine to reduce potassium loss. Extra potassium may not be necessary and, in some cases, too much potassium could be harmful.

Check with your doctor if you become sick and have severe or continuing vomiting or diarrhea. These problems may cause you to lose additional water and potassium.

Dizziness and irregular heartbeat may occur after the first dose of this medicine. Taking the first dose at bedtime may prevent problems. However, **be especially careful if you need to get up during the night. Also, avoid driving or performing hazardous tasks for the first 24 hours after you start taking this medicine or when the dose is increased. Make sure you know how you react to this medicine before you drive, use machines, or do other jobs that require you to be alert.** After you have taken several doses of this medicine, these effects should lessen.

Dizziness, lightheadedness, or fainting may occur, especially when you get up from a lying or sitting position. Getting up slowly may help lessen this problem. **If you begin to feel dizzy, lie down so that you do not faint.** Then sit for a few moments before standing in order to prevent the dizziness from returning.

The dizziness, lightheadedness, or fainting is also more likely to occur if you drink alcohol, stand for long periods of time, exercise, or if the weather is hot. **While you are taking this medicine, be careful in the amount of alcohol you drink. Also, use extra care during exercise or hot weather or if you must stand for long periods of time.**

Diabetics—Polythiazide (contained in this combination medicine) may raise blood sugar levels. While you are using this medicine, be especially careful in testing for sugar in your urine. If you have any questions about this, check with your doctor.

Some people who take this medicine may become more sensitive to sunlight than they are normally. When you first begin taking this medicine, avoid too much sun and do not use a sunlamp until you see how you react to the sun, especially if you tend to burn easily. If you have a severe reaction, check with your doctor.

Side Effects of This Medicine

Along with its needed effects, a medicine may cause some unwanted effects. Although not all of these side effects may occur, if they do occur they may need medical attention.

Check with your doctor as soon as possible if any of the following side effects occur, especially since some of them may mean that your body is losing too much potassium:

Signs of too much potassium loss

Dryness of mouth (severe)
Increased thirst
Irregular heartbeat (continuing)
Mood or mental changes
Muscle cramps or pain
Nausea or vomiting
Unusual tiredness or weakness
Weak pulse

More common

Dizziness or lightheadedness, especially when getting up from a lying or sitting position

Less common

Chest pain
Fainting (sudden)
Irregular heartbeat
Shortness of breath
Swelling of feet or lower legs
Weight gain

Rare

Inability to control urination
Joint, lower back or side, or stomach pain
Numbness or tingling of hands or feet

Skin rash or hives
Sore throat and fever
Stomach pain (severe) with nausea and vomiting
Unusual bleeding or bruising
Yellow eyes or skin

Other side effects may occur that usually do not require medical attention. These side effects may go away during treatment as your body adjusts to the medicine. However, check with your doctor if any of the following side effects continue or are bothersome:

Less common

Decreased sexual ability
Diarrhea
Drowsiness
Headache
Increased sensitivity of skin to sunlight
Lack of energy
Loss of appetite
Stomach upset or pain

For elderly patients: Dizziness, lightheadedness, or fainting or signs of too much potassium loss may be more likely to occur in the elderly, who are more sensitive to the effects of prazosin and polythiazide. In addition, this medicine may reduce tolerance to cold temperatures in elderly patients.

Other side effects not listed above may also occur in some patients. If you notice any other effects, check with your doctor.

_____

December 1987

PRIMAQUINE (Systemic)

To the Reader: If you do not recognize the names of medical conditions or medicines referred to in this information, check with your doctor, nurse, or pharmacist. Definitions for selected medical terms may be found in the Glossary. Brand names for the generic drug names listed can be found in the Index. In addition, selected brand names commonly associated with the generic name have been included in the text to help you recognize medicine you may be taking. The fact that a brand name product is not mentioned does not mean the information does not apply. It is a good idea for you to learn both the generic and brand names of your medicines and to write them down for future use.

Primaquine (PRIM-a-kween) belongs to the group of medicines called antiprotozoals. It is used in the prevention and treatment of malaria.

Primaquine is available only with your doctor's prescription.

Remember:

• **This medicine has been prescribed for your present infection only.** Another infection later on may require a different medicine. Also, even though other people may have the same symptoms as you, they may have a different kind of infection. Your medicine may not work for them and may even cause them harm. Therefore, **your medicine must not be given to other people or used for other infections** unless you are otherwise directed by your doctor.

• **Keep all medicines out of the reach of children.**

• In order for this medicine to work, it must be used as directed.

• **It is very important that you read and understand the following information.** If any of the information causes you special concern, do not decide against using this medicine without first checking with your doctor.

• Before you begin using any new medicine (prescription or nonprescription) or if you develop any new medical problem while you are using this medicine, check with your doctor, nurse, or pharmacist.

• **If you have any questions** about the following information or if you want more information about this medicine or your medical problem, **ask your doctor, nurse, or pharmacist.**

Before Using This Medicine

In order to decide on the best treatment for your medical problem, your doctor should be told:

—if you have ever had any unusual or allergic reaction to primaquine or iodoquinol.

—if you are on a low-salt, low-sugar, or any other special diet, or if you are allergic to any substance, such as foods, sulfites or other preservatives, or dyes. Most medicines contain more than their active ingredient. Your doctor, nurse, or pharmacist can help you avoid products that may cause a problem.

—if you are **pregnant** or if you may become pregnant. However, primaquine has not been shown to cause birth defects or other problems in humans.

—if you are **breast-feeding**. However, primaquine has not been shown to cause problems in nursing babies.

—if you have any of the following medical problems:
  Family or personal history of favism or hemolytic anemia
  Glucose-6-phosphate dehydrogenase (G6PD) deficiency
  Lupus erythematosus
  Nicotinamide adenine dinucleotide (NADH) methemoglobin reductase deficiency
  Rheumatoid arthritis

—if you are taking **any** other prescription or nonprescription (OTC) medicine, especially:
  Antidiabetic agents, oral (diabetes medicine you take by mouth)
  Dapsone
  Furazolidone (e.g., Furoxone)
  Methyldopa (e.g., Aldomet)
  Nitrofurantoin (e.g., Furadantin)
  Procainamide (e.g., Pronestyl)
  Quinacrine (e.g., Atabrine)
  Quinidine (e.g., Quinidex)
  Quinine (e.g., Quinamm)
  Sulfonamides (sulfa medicine)
  Sulfoxone (e.g., Diasone)
  Vitamin K (e.g., AquaMEPHYTON, Synkayvite)

Proper Use of This Medicine

If this medicine upsets your stomach, it may be taken with meals or antacids. If stomach upset (nausea, vomiting, or stomach pain) continues, check with your doctor.

If you are taking primaquine for malaria, **keep taking it for the full time of treatment** to help prevent or completely clear up the infection. Do not miss any doses.

If you do miss a dose of this medicine, take it as soon as possible. However, if it is almost time for your next dose, skip the missed dose and go back to your regular dosing schedule. Do not double doses.

How to store this medicine:

• **Keep out of the reach of children.**

• Store away from heat and direct light.

• Do not store in the bathroom, near the kitchen sink, or in other damp places. Heat or moisture may cause the medicine to break down.

• Do not keep outdated medicine or medicine no longer needed. Be sure that any discarded medicine is out of the reach of children.

Precautions While Using This Medicine

Your doctor should check your progress at regular visits to make sure that primaquine is not causing blood problems.

This medicine may cause some people to become dizzy or lightheaded. **Make sure you know how you react to this medicine before you drive, use machines, or do other jobs that require you to be alert.** If these reactions are especially bothersome, check with your doctor.

Primaquine may cause blood problems. These problems may result in a greater chance of infection, slow healing, and bleeding of the gums. Therefore, you should be careful when using toothbrushes, dental floss, and toothpicks. Dental work should be delayed until your blood counts have returned to normal. Check with your physician or dentist if you have any questions about proper oral hygiene (mouth care) during treatment.

Side Effects of This Medicine

Along with its needed effects, a medicine may cause some unwanted effects. Although not all of these side effects may occur, if they do occur they may need medical attention.

Check with your doctor immediately if any of the following side effects occur:

More common
    Dark urine
    Unusual tiredness or weakness

Less common
    Dizziness or lightheadedness
    Troubled breathing

Rare
    Sore throat and fever

Other side effects may occur that usually do not require medical attention. These side effects may go away during treatment as your body adjusts to the medicine. However, check with your doctor if any of the following side effects continue or are bothersome:

More common
    Nausea or vomiting
    Stomach pain or cramps

Less common
    Headache
    Itching of skin

For elderly patients: Many medicines have not been tested in older people. Therefore, it is not known whether the medicine acts the same way it does in younger adults. Check with your doctor or pharmacist if you notice any unusual effects while taking this medicine or if you think it is not working as it should.

Other side effects not listed above may also occur in some patients. If you notice any other effects, check with your doctor.

December 1987

PRIMIDONE (Systemic)

Some commonly used brand names are:

Apo-Primidone*   Mysoline
Myidone   Sertan*

Generic name product may also be available in the U.S.

*Not available in the U.S.

To the Reader: If you do not recognize the names of medical conditions or medicines referred to in this information, check with your doctor, nurse, or pharmacist. Definitions for selected medical terms may be found in the Glossary. Brand names for the generic drug names listed can be found in the Index. In addition, selected brand names commonly associated with the generic name have been included in the text to help you recognize medicine you may be taking. The fact that a brand name product is not mentioned does not mean the information does not apply. It is a good idea for you to learn both the generic and brand names of your medicines and to write them down for future use.

Primidone (PRI-mi-done) belongs to the group of medicines called anticonvulsants. It is used in the treatment of epilepsy to manage certain types of seizures. Primidone may be used alone or in combination with other anticonvulsants. It acts by controlling nerve impulses in the brain.

Primidone is available only with your doctor's prescription.

Remember:

• **This medicine has been prescribed for your current medical problem only.** It must not be given to other people or used for other problems unless you are directed to do so by your doctor.

• **Keep all medicines out of the reach of children.**

• In order for this medicine to work, it must be used as directed.

• **It is very important that you read and understand the following information.** If any of the information causes you special concern, do not decide against using this medicine without first checking with your doctor.

• Before you begin using any new medicine (prescription or nonprescription) or if you develop any new medical problem while you are using this medicine, check with your doctor, nurse, or pharmacist.

• **If you have any questions** about the following information or if you want more information about this medicine or your medical problem, **ask your doctor, nurse, or pharmacist.**

Before Using This Medicine

In order to decide on the best treatment for your medical problem, your doctor should be told:

—if you have had any unusual or allergic reaction to primidone or to any barbiturate medicine (for example, amobarbital, butabarbital, pentobarbital, phenobarbital, secobarbital).

—if you are on a low-salt, low-sugar, or any other special diet, or if you are allergic to any substance, such as foods, sulfites or other preservatives, or dyes.

Most medicines contain more than their active ingredient, and many liquid medicines contain alcohol. Your doctor, nurse, or pharmacist can help you avoid products that may cause a problem.

—if you are **pregnant** or if you may become pregnant. Although most mothers who take medicine for seizure control deliver normal babies, there are reports of increased birth defects when these medicines are used during pregnancy. Newborns whose mothers were taking primidone during pregnancy have been reported to have bleeding problems. It is not definitely known if any of these medicines are the cause of such problems.

—if you are **breast-feeding**. Primidone passes into the breast milk and may cause unusual drowsiness in nursing babies.

—if you have any of the following medical problems:

Asthma, emphysema, or chronic lung disease
Hyperactivity (in children)
Kidney disease
Liver disease
Porphyria

—if you are taking **any** other prescription or nonprescription (OTC) medicine, especially:

Adrenocorticoids (cortisone-like medicines)
Anticoagulants, coumarin- or indandione-type (blood thinners)
Anticonvulsants (seizure medicine) (other)
Central nervous system (CNS) depressants
Oral contraceptives (birth control pills) containing estrogen

—if you are now taking or have taken within the past 2 weeks monoamine oxidase (MAO) inhibitors, such as:

Furazolidone (e.g., Furoxone)
Isocarboxazid (e.g., Marplan)
Pargyline (e.g., Eutonyl)
Phenelzine (e.g., Nardil)
Procarbazine (e.g., Matulane)
Tranylcypromine (e.g., Parnate)

Proper Use of This Medicine

Take primidone every day in regularly spaced doses as ordered by your doctor. This will provide the proper amount of medicine needed to prevent seizures.

If you miss a dose of this medicine, take it as soon as possible. However, if it is within an hour of your next dose, skip the missed dose and go back to your regular dosing schedule. Do not double doses.

How to store this medicine:

• **Keep out of the reach of children.**

• Store away from heat and direct light.

• Do not store the tablet form of this medicine in the bathroom, near the kitchen sink, or in other damp places. Heat or moisture may cause the medicine to break down.

• Keep the liquid form of this medicine from freezing.

• Do not keep outdated medicine or medicine no longer needed. Be sure that any discarded medicine is out of the reach of children.

Precautions While Using This Medicine

It is very important that your doctor check your progress at regular visits, especially during the first few months you take primidone. This will allow the amount of medicine you are taking to be adjusted to meet your needs.

If you have been taking primidone regularly for several weeks, you should not suddenly stop taking it. Your doctor may want you to reduce gradually the amount you are taking before stopping completely.

Before having any kind of surgery, dental treatment, or emergency treatment, tell the physician or dentist in charge that you are using this medicine.

This medicine will add to the effects of alcohol and other CNS depressants (medicines that slow down the nervous system, possibly causing drowsiness). Some examples of CNS depressants are antihistamines or medicine for hay fever, other allergies, or colds; sedatives, tranquilizers, or sleeping medicine; prescription pain medicine or narcotics; barbiturates; medicine for convulsions (seizures); muscle relaxants; or anesthetics, including some dental anesthetics. **Check with your doctor before taking any of the above while you are using this medicine.**

Primidone may cause some people to become dizzy, lightheaded, drowsy, or less alert than they are normally. Even if taken at bedtime, it may cause some people to feel drowsy or less alert on arising. **Make sure you know how you react to this medicine before you drive, use machines, or do other jobs that require you to be alert.**

Side Effects of This Medicine

Along with its needed effects, a medicine may cause some unwanted effects. Although not all of these side effects may occur, if they do occur they may need medical attention.

Check with your doctor if any of the following side effects occur:
Less common
   Unusual excitement or restlessness (especially in children and sometimes in the elderly)
Rare
   Skin rash or hives
   Swelling of eyelids
   Unusual tiredness or weakness
   Wheezing or tightness in chest
Signs of overdose
   Changes in vision
   Confusion
   Shortness of breath or troubled breathing

Other side effects may occur that usually do not require medical attention. These side effects may go away during treatment as your body adjusts to the medicine. However, check with your doctor if any of the following side effects continue or are bothersome:
More common
   Clumsiness or unsteadiness
   Dizziness
   Drowsiness
Less common
   Decreased sexual ability
   Headache
   Loss of appetite
   Nausea or vomiting

For children and elderly patients: Some side effects, such as unusual excitement or restlessness, are more likely to occur in children and the elderly.

Other side effects not listed above may also occur in some patients. If you notice any other effects, check with your doctor.

December 1987

PROBENECID (Systemic)

Some commonly used brand names are Benemid, Benuryl*, and Probalan

Generic name product may also be available in the U.S.

---

*Not available in the U.S.

To the Reader: If you do not recognize the names of medical conditions or medicines referred to in this information, check with your doctor, nurse, or pharmacist. Definitions for selected medical terms may be found in the Glossary. Brand names for the generic drug names listed can be found in the Index. In addition, selected brand names commonly associated with the generic name have been included in the text to help you recognize medicine you may be taking. The fact that a brand name product is not mentioned does not mean the information does not apply. It is a good idea for you to learn both the generic and brand names of your medicines and to write them down for future use.

Probenecid (proe-BEN-e-sid) is used in the treatment of chronic gout or gouty arthritis. These conditions are caused by too much uric acid in the blood. The medicine works by removing the extra uric acid from the body. Probenecid does not cure gout, but after you have been taking it for a few months it will help prevent gout attacks. This medicine will help prevent gout attacks only as long as you continue to take it.

Probenecid is also used to prevent or treat other medical problems that may occur if too much uric acid is present in the body.

Probenecid is sometimes used with certain kinds of antibiotics to make them more effective in the treatment of infections.

Probenecid is available only with your doctor's prescription.

Remember:

• **This medicine has been prescribed for your current medical problem only.** It must not be given to other people or used for other problems unless you are directed to do so by your doctor.

• **Keep all medicines out of the reach of children.**

• In order for this medicine to work, it must be used as directed.

• **It is very important that you read and understand the following information.** If any of the information causes you special concern, do not decide against using this medicine without first checking with your doctor.

• Before you begin using any new medicine (prescription or nonprescription) or if you develop any new medical problem while you are using this medicine, check with your doctor, nurse, or pharmacist.

• **If you have any questions** about the following information or if you want more information about this medicine or your medical problem, **ask your doctor, nurse, or pharmacist.**

Before Using This Medicine

In order to decide on the best treatment for your medical problem, your doctor should be told:

—if you have ever had any unusual or allergic reaction to probenecid.

—if you are on a low-salt, low-sugar, or any other special diet, or if you are allergic to any substance, such as foods, sulfites or other preservatives, or dyes. Most medicines contain more than their active ingredient. Your doctor, nurse, or pharmacist can help you avoid products that may cause a problem.

—if you are **pregnant** or if you may become pregnant. Probenecid has not been shown to cause problems in humans.

—if you are **breast-feeding**. Probenecid has not been shown to cause problems in nursing babies.

—if you have any of the following medical problems:
   Blood disease
   Kidney disease or stones (or history of)
   Stomach ulcer (history of)

—if you are taking **any** other prescription or nonprescription (OTC) medicine, especially:
   Antineoplastics (cancer medicine)
   Aspirin or other salicylates
   Heparin
   Indomethacin (e.g., Indocin)
   Ketoprofen (e.g., Orudis)
   Medicine for infection, including tuberculosis or virus infection
   Methotrexate (e.g., Mexate)
   Nitrofurantoin (e.g., Furadantin)

Proper Use of This Medicine

If probenecid upsets your stomach, it may be taken with food. If this does not work, an antacid may be taken. If stomach upset (nausea, vomiting, or loss of appetite) continues, check with your doctor.

For patients taking probenecid for gout:

• After you begin to take probenecid, gout attacks may continue to occur for a while. However, if you take this medicine regularly as directed by your doctor, the attacks will gradually become less frequent and less painful than before. After you have been taking probenecid for several months, they may stop completely.

• This medicine will help prevent gout attacks but it will not relieve an attack that has already started. **Even if you take another medicine for gout attacks, continue to take this medicine also.** If you have any questions about this, check with your doctor.

For patients taking probenecid for gout or to help remove uric acid from the body:

• When you first begin taking probenecid, the amount of uric acid in the kidneys is greatly increased. This may cause kidney stones in some people. To help prevent this, your doctor may want you to drink at least 10 to 12 full glasses (8 ounces each) of fluids each day, or to take another medicine to make your urine less acid. It is important that you follow your doctor's instructions very carefully.

If you are taking probenecid regularly and you miss a dose, take the missed dose as soon as possible. However, if you do not remember until it is almost time for the next dose, skip the missed dose and go back to your regular dosing schedule. Do not double doses.

How to store this medicine:

- **Keep out of the reach of children.**

- Store away from heat and direct light.

- Do not store this medicine in the bathroom, near the kitchen sink, or in other damp places. Heat or moisture may cause the medicine to break down.

- Do not keep outdated medicine or medicine no longer needed. Be sure that any discarded medicine is out of the reach of children.

Precautions While Using This Medicine

If you will be taking probenecid for more than a few weeks, your doctor should check your progress at regular visits.

Diabetics—Probenecid may cause false test results with copper sulfate urine sugar tests (Clinitest®), but not with glucose enzymatic urine sugar tests (Clinistix®). If you have any questions about this, check with your doctor or pharmacist.

For patients taking probenecid for gout or to help remove uric acid from the body:

- Taking aspirin or other salicylates will lessen the effects of probenecid. Also, drinking too much alcohol may increase the amount of uric acid in the blood and lessen the effects of this medicine. Therefore, **do not take aspirin or other salicylates or drink alcoholic beverages while taking this medicine**, unless you have first checked with your doctor.

Side Effects of This Medicine

Along with its needed effects, a medicine may cause some unwanted effects. Although not all of these side effects may occur, if they do occur they may need medical attention.

Check with your doctor as soon as possible if any of the following side effects occur:

Less common
    Bloody urine
    Lower back pain
    Painful urination

Rare
    Difficulty in breathing
    Fever
    Skin rash or itching
    Sore throat, fever, and chills
    Sudden decrease in amount of urine
    Swelling of feet, lower legs, or face
    Unusual bleeding or bruising
    Unusual tiredness or weakness
    Weight gain
    Yellow eyes or skin

Signs of overdose
    Convulsions (seizures)
    Vomiting (severe and continuing)

Other side effects may occur that usually do not require medical attention. These side effects may go away during treatment as your body adjusts to the medicine. However, check with your doctor if any of the following side effects continue or are bothersome:

More common
    Headache
    Loss of appetite
    Nausea or vomiting (mild)

Less common
    Dizziness
    Flushing or redness of face
    Frequent urge to urinate
    Sore gums

For elderly patients: Many medicines have not been tested in older people. Therefore, it is not known whether the medicine acts the same way it does in younger adults. Check with your doctor or pharmacist if you notice any unusual effects while taking this medicine or if you think it is not working as it should.

Other side effects not listed above may also occur in some patients. If you notice any other effects, check with your doctor.

December 1987

PROBENECID AND COLCHICINE
(Systemic)

Some commonly used brand names are:

Colabid	Col-Probenecid
ColBenemid	Proben-C

Generic name product may also be available in the U.S.

To the Reader: If you do not recognize the names of medical conditions or medicines referred to in this information, check with your doctor, nurse, or pharmacist. Definitions for selected medical terms may be found in the Glossary. Brand names for the generic drug names listed can be found in the Index. In addition, selected brand names commonly associated with the generic name have been included in the text to help you recognize medicine you may be taking. The fact that a brand name product is not mentioned does not mean the information does not apply. It is a good idea for you to learn both the generic and brand names of your medicines and to write them down for future use.

Probenecid (proe-BEN-e-sid) and colchicine (KOL-chi-seen) combination is used to treat gout or gouty arthritis.

The probenecid in this medicine helps to prevent gout attacks by removing extra uric acid from the body. The colchicine in this medicine also helps to prevent gout attacks. Although colchicine may also be used to relieve an attack of gout, this requires more colchicine than this combination medicine contains. Probenecid and colchicine combination does not cure gout. This medicine will help prevent gout attacks only as long as you continue to take it.

Probenecid and colchicine combination is available only with your doctor's prescription.

Remember:

• **This medicine has been prescribed for your current medical problem only.** It must not be given to other people or used for other problems unless you are directed to do so by your doctor.

• **Keep all medicines out of the reach of children.**

• In order for this medicine to work, it must be used as directed.

• **It is very important that you read and understand the following information.** If any of the information causes you special concern, do not decide against using this medicine without first checking with your doctor.

• Before you begin using any new medicine (prescription or nonprescription) or if you develop any new medical problem while you are using this medicine, check with your doctor, nurse, or pharmacist.

• **If you have any questions** about the following information or if you want more information about this medicine or your medical problem, **ask your doctor, nurse, or pharmacist.**

Before Using This Medicine

In order to decide on the best treatment for your medical problem, your doctor should be told:

—if you have ever had any unusual or allergic reaction to probenecid or colchicine.

—if you are on a low-salt, low-sugar, or any other special diet, or if you are allergic to any substance, such as foods, sulfites or other preservatives, or dyes.

Most medicines contain more than their active ingredient. Your doctor, nurse, or pharmacist can help you avoid products that may cause a problem.

—if you are **pregnant** or if you may become pregnant. Probenecid has not been shown to cause birth defects or other problems in humans. Although studies with colchicine have not been done in humans, some reports have suggested that use of colchicine during pregnancy can cause harm to the fetus. Also, studies in animals have shown that colchicine causes birth defects. Therefore, do not begin taking this medicine during pregnancy, and do not become pregnant while taking it, unless you have first discussed this problem with your doctor. Also, check with your doctor immediately if you suspect that you have become pregnant while taking this medicine.

—if you are **breast-feeding**. Although probenecid and colchicine have not been shown to cause problems in nursing babies, the chance always exists.

—if you have any of the following medical problems:

  Blood disease
  Heart disease
  Intestinal disease
  Kidney disease or stones, or history of
  Liver disease
  Stomach ulcer or other stomach problems (or history of)

—if you are taking **any** other prescription or nonprescription (OTC) medicine, especially:

  Antineoplastics (cancer medicine)
  Antithyroid agents (medicine for overactive thyroid)
  Aspirin or other salicylates
  Azathioprine (e.g., Imuran)
  Chlorambucil (e.g., Leukeran)
  Chloramphenicol (e.g., Chloromycetin)
  Cyclophosphamide (e.g., Cytoxan)
  Flucytosine (e.g., Ancobon)
  Heparin
  Indomethacin (e.g., Indocin)
  Interferon (e.g., Intron A; Roferon-A)
  Ketoprofen (e.g., Orudis)
  Medicine for infection, including tuberculosis or virus infection
  Mercaptopurine (e.g., Purinethol)
  Methotrexate (e.g., Mexate)
  Nitrofurantoin (e.g., Furadantin)

Proper Use of This Medicine

If this medicine upsets your stomach, it may be taken with food. If this does not work, an antacid may be taken. If stomach upset (nausea, vomiting, loss of appetite, or stomach pain) continues, check with your doctor.

Take this medicine only as directed by your doctor. Do not take more of it and do not take it more often than your doctor ordered. The colchicine in this combination medicine may cause serious side effects if too much is taken.

After you begin to take this medicine, gout attacks may continue to occur for a while. However, if you take this medicine regularly as directed by your doctor, the attacks will gradually become less frequent and less painful than before. After you have been taking this medicine for several months, they may stop completely.

This medicine will help prevent gout attacks but it will not relieve an attack that has already started. **Even if you take another medicine for gout attacks, continue to take this medicine also.**

When you first begin taking this medicine, the amount of uric acid in the kidneys is greatly increased. This may cause kidney stones in some people. To help prevent this, your doctor may want you to drink at least 10 to 12 full glasses (8 ounces each) of fluids each day, or to take another medicine to make your urine less acid. It is important that you follow your doctor's instructions very carefully.

If you miss a dose of this medicine, take it as soon as possible. However, if it is almost time for your next dose, skip the missed dose and go back to your regular dosing schedule. Do not double doses.

How to store this medicine:

• **Keep out of the reach of children.**

• Store away from heat and direct light.

• Do not store this medicine in the bathroom, near the kitchen sink, or in other damp places. Heat or moisture may cause the medicine to break down.

• Do not keep outdated medicine or medicine no longer needed. Be sure that any discarded medicine is out of the reach of children.

Precautions While Using This Medicine

Your doctor should check your progress at regular visits while you are taking this medicine.

Diabetics—The probenecid in this combination medicine may cause false test results with copper sulfate urine sugar tests (Clinitest®), but not with glucose enzymatic urine sugar tests (Clinistix®). If you have any questions about this, check with your doctor or pharmacist.

Taking aspirin or other salicylates will lessen the effects of the probenecid in this combination medicine. Also, drinking large amounts of alcoholic beverages may increase the chance of stomach problems and may increase the amount of uric acid in your blood. **Therefore, do not take aspirin or other salicylates or drink alcoholic beverages while you are taking this medicine,** unless you have first checked with your doctor.

For patients taking 4 tablets or more of this medicine a day:

• **Stop taking this medicine immediately and check with your doctor as soon as possible if severe diarrhea, nausea or vomiting, or stomach pain occurs while you are taking this medicine.**

Side Effects of This Medicine

Along with its needed effects, a medicine may cause some unwanted effects. Although not all of these side effects may occur, if they do occur they may need medical attention.

Check with your doctor immediately if any of the following side effects occur:
Signs of overdose
    Bloody urine
    Burning feeling in stomach, throat, or skin
    Convulsions (seizures)
    Diarrhea (severe or bloody)
    Fever
    Mood or mental changes
    Muscle weakness (severe)
    Nausea or vomiting (severe and continuing)
    Sudden decrease in amount of urine
    Troubled or difficult breathing

Also, check with your doctor as soon as possible if any of the following side effects occur:
Rare
    Numbness, tingling, pain, or weakness in hands or feet
    Skin rash or itching
    Sore throat, fever, and chills
    Swelling of feet, lower legs, or face
    Unusual bleeding or bruising
    Unusual tiredness or weakness
    Weight gain
    Yellow eyes or skin
Less common
    Lower back pain
    Painful urination

Other side effects may occur that usually do not require medical attention. These side effects may go away during treatment as your body adjusts to the medicine. However, check with your doctor if any of the following side effects continue or are bothersome:
More common
    Diarrhea (mild)
    Headache
    Loss of appetite
    Nausea or vomiting (mild)
    Stomach pain
Less common
    Dizziness
    Flushing or redness of face
    Frequent urge to urinate
    Sore gums
    Unusual loss of hair

For elderly patients: Some of the above side effects are more likely to occur in the elderly, who are usually more sensitive to the effects of the colchicine in this medicine.

Other side effects not listed above may also occur in some patients. If you notice any other effects, check with your doctor.

_____

December 1987

_____

PROBUCOL (Systemic)

A commonly used brand name is Lorelco.

To the Reader: If you do not recognize the names of medical conditions or medicines referred to in this information, check with your doctor, nurse, or pharmacist. Definitions for selected medical terms may be found in the Glossary. Brand names for the generic drug names listed can be found in the Index. In addition, selected brand names commonly associated with the generic name have been included in the text to help you recognize medicine you may be taking. The fact that a brand name product is not mentioned does not mean the information does not apply. It is a good idea for you to learn both the generic and brand names of your medicines and to write them down for future use.

Probucol (PROE-byoo-kole) is used to lower cholesterol levels in the blood. This may help prevent medical problems caused by cholesterol clogging the blood vessels.

Probucol is available only with your doctor's prescription.

Remember:

• **This medicine has been prescribed for your current medical problem only.** It must not be given to other people or used for other problems unless you are directed to do so by your doctor.

• **Keep all medicines out of the reach of children.**

• In order for this medicine to work, it must be used as directed.

• **It is very important that you read and understand the following information.** If any of the information causes you special concern, do not decide against using this medicine without first checking with your doctor.

• Before you begin using any new medicine (prescription or nonprescription) or if you develop any new medical problem while you are using this medicine, check with your doctor, nurse, or pharmacist.

• **If you have any questions** about the following information or if you want more information about this medicine or your medical problem, **ask your doctor, nurse, or pharmacist.**

Before Using This Medicine

Importance of diet—Before prescribing medicine for your condition, your doctor will probably try to control your condition by prescribing a personal diet for you. Such a diet may be low in fats, sugars, and/or cholesterol. Many people are able to control their condition by carefully following their doctor's orders for proper diet and exercise. Medicine is prescribed only when additional help is needed and is effective only when a schedule of diet and exercise is properly followed.

Also, this medicine is less effective if you are greatly overweight. It may be very important for you to go on a reducing diet. However, check with your doctor before going on any diet.

In order to decide on the best treatment for your medical problem, your doctor should be told:

—if you have ever had any unusual or allergic reaction to probucol.

—if you are on a low-salt, low-sugar, or any other special diet, or if you are allergic to any substance, such as foods, sulfites or other preservatives, or dyes. Most medicines contain more than their active ingredient. Your doctor, nurse, or pharmacist can help you avoid products that may cause a problem.

—if you are **pregnant** or if you may become pregnant up to six months after you stop taking this medicine. Studies have not been done in humans; however, probucol has not been shown to cause birth defects or other problems in rats or rabbits. Small amounts of probucol may stay in your body for up to six months after you stop taking it.

—if you are **breast-feeding**. It is not known whether probucol passes into breast milk in humans and it has not been shown to cause problems in nursing babies. However, probucol does pass into milk in animals.

—if you have any of the following medical problems:
   Gallbladder disease or gallstones
   Heart disease
   Liver disease

—if you are taking **any** other prescription or nonprescription (OTC) medicine.

Proper Use of This Medicine

Many patients who have high cholesterol levels will not notice any signs of the problem. In fact, many may feel normal. **Take this medicine exactly as directed by your doctor, even though you may feel well.** Try not to miss any doses and do not take more medicine than your doctor ordered.

Remember that this medicine will not cure your condition but it does control it. Therefore, you must continue to take it as directed if you expect to keep your cholesterol levels down.

Follow carefully the special diet your doctor gave you. This is the most important part of controlling your condition, and is necessary if the medicine is to work properly.

This medicine works better when taken with meals.

If you miss a dose of this medicine, take it as soon as possible. However, if it is almost time for your next dose, skip the missed dose and go back to your regular dosing schedule. Do not double doses.

How to store this medicine:

• **Keep out of the reach of children.**

• Store away from heat and direct light.

• Do not store in the bathroom, near the kitchen sink, or in other damp places. Heat or moisture may cause the medicine to break down.

• Do not keep outdated medicine or medicine no longer needed. Be sure that any discarded medicine is out of the reach of children.

Precautions While Using This Medicine

It is very important that your doctor check your progress at regular visits. This will allow your doctor to see if the medicine is working properly to lower your cholesterol levels and to decide if you should continue to take it.

Do not stop taking this medicine without first checking with your doctor. When you stop taking this medicine, your blood fat levels may increase again. Your doctor may want you to follow a special diet to help prevent this.

Side Effects of This Medicine

Along with its needed effects, a medicine may cause some unwanted effects. Although not all of these side effects may occur, if they do occur they may need medical attention.

Check with your doctor as soon as possible if any of the following side effects occur:

Rare

   Swellings on face, hands, or feet, or in mouth

Other side effects may occur that usually do not require medical attention. These side effects may go away during treatment as your body adjusts to the medicine. However, check with your doctor if any of the following side effects continue or are bothersome:

More common

   Bloating
   Diarrhea
   Nausea and vomiting
   Stomach pain

Less common

   Dizziness
   Headache
   Numbness or tingling of fingers, toes, or face

For elderly patients: Many medicines have not been tested in older people. Therefore, it is not known whether the medicine acts the same way it does in younger adults. Check with your doctor or pharmacist if you notice any unusual effects while taking this medicine or if you think it is not working as it should.

Other side effects not listed above may also occur in some patients. If you notice any other effects, check with your doctor.

_____

December 1987

PROCAINAMIDE (Systemic)

Some commonly used brand names are:

Procan SR	Pronestyl-SR
Promine	Rhythmin
Pronestyl	

Generic name product may also be available in the U.S.

To the Reader: If you do not recognize the names of medical conditions or medicines referred to in this information, check with your doctor, nurse, or pharmacist. Definitions for selected medical terms may be found in the Glossary. Brand names for the generic drug names listed can be found in the Index. In addition, selected brand names commonly associated with the generic name have been included in the text to help you recognize medicine you may be taking. The fact that a brand name product is not mentioned does not mean the information does not apply. It is a good idea for you to learn both the generic and brand names of your medicines and to write them down for future use.

Procainamide (proe-KANE-a-mide) is used to correct irregular heartbeats to a normal rhythm and to slow an overactive heart. This allows the heart to work more efficiently. Procainamide produces its beneficial effects by slowing nerve impulses in the heart and reducing sensitivity of heart tissues.

Procainamide is taken by mouth in capsules, tablets, or extended-release (long-acting) tablets. It is also given by injection in emergencies or when a rapid effect is needed.

Procainamide is available only with your doctor's prescription.

Remember:
• **This medicine has been prescribed for your current medical problem only.** It must not be given to other people or used for other problems unless you are directed to do so by your doctor.

• **Keep all medicines out of the reach of children.**

• In order for this medicine to work, it must be used as directed.

• If you are receiving this medicine by injection, some of the information about this medicine may not apply.

• **It is very important that you read and understand the following information.** If any of the information causes you special concern, do not decide against using this medicine without first checking with your doctor.

• Before you begin using any new medicine (prescription or nonprescription) or if you develop any new medical problem while you are using this medicine, check with your doctor, nurse, or pharmacist.

• **If you have any questions** about the following information or if you want more information about this medicine or your medical problem, **ask your doctor, nurse, or pharmacist.**

Before Using This Medicine

In order to decide on the best treatment for your medical problem, your doctor should be told:

—if you have ever had any unusual or allergic reaction to procainamide, procaine, or any other "caine-type" medicine.

—if you are on a low-salt, low-sugar, or any other special diet, or if you are allergic to any substance, such as foods, sulfites or other preservatives, or dyes. Most medicines contain more than their active ingredient. Your doctor, nurse, or pharmacist can help you avoid products that may cause a problem.

—if you are **pregnant** or if you may become pregnant. Although procainamide has not been shown to cause problems in humans, it is known to pass from the mother to the fetus.

—if you are **breast-feeding**. Although procainamide passes into breast milk, it has not been shown to cause problems in nursing babies.

—if you have any of the following medical problems:
Asthma
Kidney disease
Liver disease
Lupus erythematosus (history of)
Myasthenia gravis

—if you are taking **any** prescription or nonprescription (OTC) medicine, especially:
Antihypertensives (high blood pressure medicine)
Antimyasthenics (ambenonium, neostigmine, pyridostigmine)
Other heart medicine
Pimozide (e.g., Orap)

Proper Use of This Medicine

Take procainamide exactly as directed by your doctor, even though you may feel well. Do not take more medicine than ordered.

Procainamide should be taken with a glass of water on an empty stomach 1 hour before or 2 hours after meals so that it will be absorbed more quickly. However, to lessen stomach upset, your doctor may want you to take the medicine with food or milk.

For patients taking the extended-release tablets:
• Swallow the tablet whole without breaking, crushing, or chewing it.

This medicine works best when there is a constant amount in the blood. **To help keep this amount constant, do not miss any doses. Also, it is best to take each dose at evenly spaced times day and night.** For example, if you are to take 6 doses a day, each dose should be spaced about 4 hours apart. If this interferes with your sleep or other daily activities, or if you need help in planning the best times to take your medicine, check with your doctor, nurse, or pharmacist.

If you do miss a dose of this medicine and remember within 2 hours (4 hours if you are taking the long-acting tablets), take it as soon as possible. However,

---

© 1988   The United States Pharmacopeial Convention, Inc.

if you do not remember until later, skip the missed dose and go back to your regular dosing schedule. Do not double doses.

How to store this medicine:

- **Keep out of the reach of children.**

- Store away from heat and direct light.

- Do not store in the bathroom, refrigerator, near the kitchen sink, or in other damp places. Moisture usually present in these areas may cause the medicine to break down. Keep the container tightly closed and store in a dry place.

- Do not keep outdated medicine or medicine no longer needed. Be sure that any discarded medicine is out of the reach of children.

Precautions While Using This Medicine

It is important that your doctor check your progress at regular visits to make sure the medicine is working properly. This will allow necessary changes in the amount of medicine you are taking, which also may help reduce side effects.

Do not stop taking this medicine without first checking with your doctor. Stopping it suddenly may cause a serious change in the activity of your heart. Your doctor may want you to reduce gradually the amount you are taking before stopping completely.

Before having any kind of surgery (including dental surgery) or emergency treatment, tell the physician or dentist in charge that you are taking this medicine.

Your doctor may want you to carry a medical identification card or bracelet stating that you are taking this medicine.

Dizziness or lightheadedness may occur, especially in elderly patients and when large doses are used. **Elderly patients should use extra care to avoid falling. Make sure you know how you react to this medicine before you drive, use machines, or do other jobs that require you to be alert.**

Side Effects of This Medicine

Along with its needed effects, a medicine may cause some unwanted effects. Although not all of these side effects may occur, if they do occur they may need medical attention.

Check with your doctor as soon as possible if any of the following side effects occur:

Less common
 Fever and chills
 Joint pain or swelling
 Pains with breathing
 Skin rash or itching
Rare
 Confusion
 Fever or sore mouth, gums, or throat
 Hallucinations (seeing, hearing, or feeling things that are not there)
 Mental depression
 Unusual bleeding or bruising
 Unusual tiredness or weakness
Signs of overdose
 Confusion
 Decrease in urination
 Dizziness (severe) or fainting
 Drowsiness
 Fast or irregular heartbeat
 Nausea and vomiting

Other side effects may occur that usually do not require medical attention. These side effects may go away during treatment as your body adjusts to the medicine. However, check with your doctor if any of the following side effects continue or are bothersome:

More common
 Diarrhea
 Loss of appetite
Less common
 Dizziness or lightheadedness

For elderly patients: Dizziness or lightheadedness are more likely to occur in the elderly, who are usually more sensitive to the effects of this medicine.

The medicine in the extended-release tablets is contained in a special wax form (matrix). The medicine is slowly released, after which the wax matrix passes out of the body. Sometimes it may be seen in the stool. This is normal and is no cause for concern.

Other side effects not listed above may also occur in some patients. If you notice any other effects, check with your doctor.

December 1987

PROCARBAZINE (Systemic)

Some commonly used brand names are Matulane and Natulan*.

---

*Not available in the U.S.

To the Reader: If you do not recognize the names of medical conditions or medicines referred to in this information, check with your doctor, nurse, or pharmacist. Definitions for selected medical terms may be found in the Glossary. Brand names for the generic drug names listed can be found in the Index. In addition, selected brand names commonly associated with the generic name have been included in the text to help you recognize medicine you may be taking. The fact that a brand name product is not mentioned does not mean the information does not apply. It is a good idea for you to learn both the generic and brand names of your medicines and to write them down for future use.

Procarbazine (pro-KAR-ba-zeen) belongs to the group of medicines known as alkylating agents. It is taken by mouth to treat some kinds of cancer.

Procarbazine is thought to interfere with the growth of cancer cells which are eventually destroyed. It also blocks an enzyme in the central nervous system called monoamine oxidase (MAO), but this is probably not related to its effect against cancer. Since the growth of normal body cells may also be affected by procarbazine, other effects will also occur. Some of these may be serious and must be reported to your doctor. Other effects, like hair loss, may not be serious but may cause concern. Some effects may not occur for months or years after the medicine is used.

Before you begin treatment with procarbazine, you and your doctor should talk about the good this medicine will do as well as the risks of using it.

Procarbazine is available only with your doctor's prescription.

Remember:

• **This medicine has been prescribed for your current medical problem only.** It must not be given to other people or used for other problems unless you are directed to do so by your doctor.

• **Keep all medicines out of the reach of children.**

• In order for this medicine to work, it must be used as directed.

• **It is very important that you read and understand the following information.** If any of the information causes you special concern, do not decide against using this medicine without first checking with your doctor.

• Before you begin using any new medicine (prescription or nonprescription) or if you develop any new medical problem while you are using this medicine, check with your doctor, nurse, or pharmacist.

• **If you have any questions** about the following information or if you want more information about this medicine or your medical problem, **ask your doctor, nurse, or pharmacist.**

Before Using This Medicine

In order to decide on the best treatment for your medical problem, your doctor should be told:

—if you have ever had any unusual or allergic reaction to procarbazine.

—if you are **pregnant** or if you intend to have children. This medicine may cause birth defects or premature birth if either the male or female is taking it at the time of conception or if it is taken during pregnancy. Procarbazine causes birth defects frequently in animals. In addition, many cancer medicines may cause sterility which could be permanent. Although this has not been reported with this medicine, procarbazine does affect production of sperm and the possibility should be kept in mind. Be sure that you have discussed this with your doctor before taking this medicine.

—if you intend to **breast-feed.** Because this medicine may cause serious side effects, breast-feeding is generally not recommended while you are taking it.

—if you have any of the following medical problems:
Alcoholism (active or treated)
Angina (chest pain)
Chickenpox (including recent exposure)
Diabetes mellitus (sugar diabetes)
Epilepsy
Headaches (severe or frequent)
Heart or blood vessel disease
Herpes zoster (shingles)
Infection
Kidney disease
Liver disease
Mental illness (or history of)
Overactive thyroid
Parkinson's disease
Pheochromocytoma

—if you have recently had a heart attack or stroke.

—if you have ever been treated with x-rays or cancer medicines.

—if you are now taking or have taken within the past 2 weeks other monoamine oxidase (MAO) inhibitors, such as:
Furazolidone (e.g., Furoxone)
Isocarboxazid (e.g., Marplan)
Pargyline (e.g., Eutonyl)
Phenelzine (e.g., Nardil)
Tranylcypromine (e.g., Parnate)

—if you are now taking or have taken within the past 2 weeks:
Carbamazepine (e.g., Tegretol)
Cyclobenzaprine (e.g., Flexeril)
Maprotiline (e.g., Ludiomil)
Tricyclic antidepressants (amitriptyline, amoxapine, clomipramine, desipramine, doxepin, imipramine, nortriptyline, protriptyline, trimipramine)

—if you are taking **any** other prescription or nonprescription (OTC) medicine, especially:
Amphetamines
Amphotericin B by injection (e.g., Fungizone)
Antidiabetic agents, oral (diabetes medicine you take by mouth)

Antihistamines
Antimuscarinics (medicine for abdominal or stomach spasms or cramps)
Antithyroid agents (medicine for overactive thyroid)
Appetite suppressants (diet pills)
Azathioprine (e.g., Imuran)
Central nervous system (CNS) depressants
Chlophedianol (e.g., Ulo)
Chloramphenicol (e.g., Chloromycetin)
Colchicine
Dextromethorphan (e.g., Delsym)
Flucytosine (e.g., Ancobon)
Guanadrel (e.g., Hylorel)
Guanethidine (e.g., Ismelin)
Insulin
Interferon (e.g., Intron A; Roferon-A)
Levodopa (e.g., Dopar)
Medicine for asthma or other breathing problems
Medicine for colds, sinus problems, or hay fever or other allergies (including nose drops or sprays)
Methyldopa (e.g., Aldomet)
Methylphenidate (e.g., Ritalin)
Rauwolfia alkaloids (alseroxylon, deserpidine, rauwolfia serpentina, reserpine)

—if you use cocaine. Cocaine use by individuals taking procarbazine or other MAO inhibitors may cause a severe increase in blood pressure.

Proper Use of This Medicine

Use this medicine only as directed by your doctor. Do not use more or less of it and do not use it more often than your doctor ordered. The exact amount of medicine you need has been carefully worked out. Taking too much may increase the chance of side effects while taking too little may not improve your condition.

Procarbazine is sometimes given together with certain other medicines. If you are using a combination of medicines, make sure that you take each one at the right time and do not mix them. Ask your doctor, nurse, or pharmacist to help you plan a way to take your medicines at the right times.

Procarbazine commonly causes nausea and vomiting. Even if you begin to feel ill, **do not stop using this medicine without first checking with your doctor.** Ask your doctor, nurse, or pharmacist for ways to lessen these effects.

If you vomit shortly after taking a dose of procarbazine, check with your doctor. You may be told to take the dose again or you may have to wait until the next scheduled dose.

If you miss a dose of this medicine and you remember it within a few hours, take it as soon as you remember it. However, if several hours have passed or if it is almost time for the next dose, skip the missed dose and go back to your regular dosing schedule and check with your doctor. Do not double doses.

How to store this medicine:

• **Keep out of the reach of children.**

• Store away from heat and direct light.

• Do not store in the bathroom, near the kitchen sink, or in other damp places. Heat or moisture may cause the medicine to break down.

• Do not keep outdated medicine or medicine no longer needed. Be sure that any discarded medicine is out of the reach of children.

Precautions While Using This Medicine

It is very important that your doctor check your progress at regular visits to make sure that this medicine is working properly and to check for unwanted effects.

Check with your doctor or hospital emergency room immediately if severe headache, stiff neck, chest pains, rapid heartbeat, or nausea and vomiting occur while you are taking this medicine. These may be symptoms of a serious high blood pressure reaction which should have a doctor's attention.

When taken with certain foods, drinks, or other medicines, procarbazine can cause very dangerous reactions. To avoid such reactions, **obey the following rules of caution:**

• Do not eat foods that have a high tyramine content (most common in foods that are aged or fermented to increase their flavor), such as cheeses, yeast or meat extracts, fava or broad bean pods, smoked or pickled fish, beef or chicken liver, fermented sausage (bologna, pepperoni, salami, and summer sausage) or other unfresh meat, or any overripe fruit. If a list of these foods and beverages is not given to you, ask your doctor, nurse, or pharmacist to provide one.

• Do not drink alcoholic beverages, including beer and wines (especially Chianti and other hearty red wines).

• Do not eat or drink excessive amounts of caffeine-containing food or beverages, such as chocolate, coffee, tea, or cola.

• Do not take any other medicine unless approved or prescribed by your doctor. This especially includes over-the-counter (OTC) or nonprescription medicine such as that for colds (including nose drops), cough, asthma, hay fever, appetite control; "keep awake" products; or products that make you sleepy.

After you stop using this medicine you must continue to obey the rules of caution concerning food, drink, and other medication for at least 2 weeks since procarbazine may continue to react with certain foods or other medicines for up to 14 days after you stop taking it.

This medicine will add to the effects of alcohol and other CNS depressants (medicines that slow down the nervous system, possibly causing drowsiness). Some examples of CNS depressants are antihistamines or medicine for hay fever, other allergies, or colds; sedatives, tranquilizers, or sleeping medicine; prescription pain medicine or narcotics; barbiturates; medicine for convulsions (seizures); muscle relaxants; or anesthetics, including some dental anesthetics. **Check with your doctor before taking any of the above while you are using this medicine.**

This medicine may cause some people to become **drowsy or less alert than they are normally. Make sure you know how you react to this medicine before you drive, use machines, or do other jobs that require you to be alert.**

While you are being treated with procarbazine, and after you stop treatment with it, **do not have any immunizations without your doctor's approval.** Procarbazine lowers your body's resistance and there is a chance you might get the infection the immunization is meant to prevent. In addition, other persons living in your household should not take oral polio vaccine since there is a chance they could pass the polio virus on to you. Also, you should avoid close contact with persons (for example, at school or work) who have taken oral polio vaccine.

Procarbazine can lower the number of white blood cells in your body. This may increase the chance of infection. If you can, avoid people with colds or other infections. If you think you are getting a cold or other infection, check with your doctor.

Diabetics—Procarbazine may affect blood sugar levels. While you are using this medicine, be especially careful in testing for sugar in your blood or urine.

If you are going to have surgery (including dental surgery) or emergency treatment tell the physician or dentist in charge that you are using this medicine or have used it within the past 2 weeks.

Your doctor may want you to carry an identification card stating that you are using this medicine.

Side Effects of This Medicine

Along with their needed effects, medicines like procarbazine can sometimes cause unwanted effects such as blood problems, loss of hair, high blood pressure reactions, and other side effects; these are described below. Also, because of the way these medicines act on the body, there is a chance that they might cause other unwanted effects that may not occur until months or years after the medicine is used. These delayed effects may include certain types of cancer, such as leukemia. Discuss these possible effects with your doctor.

Although not all of these side effects may occur, if they do occur they may need medical attention.

Stop taking this medicine and check with your doctor immediately if the following side effects occur. If your doctor is not available, go to the nearest hospital emergency room.

Rare
  Chest pain (severe)
  Enlarged pupils
  Fast or irregular heartbeat

Headache (severe)
Increased sensitivity of eyes to light
Stiff or sore neck

Check with your doctor immediately if any of the following side effects occur:

More common
  Black tarry stools
  Bloody vomit
  Fever, chills, or sore throat
  Unusual bleeding or bruising

Check with your doctor as soon as possible if any of the following side effects occur:

More common
  Confusion
  Convulsions (seizures)
  Cough
  Hallucinations (seeing, hearing, or feeling things that are not there)
  Missing menstrual periods
  Shortness of breath
  Thickening of bronchial secretions
  Tiredness or weakness (continuing)

Less common
  Diarrhea
  Sores in the mouth and on the lips
  Tingling or numbness of the fingers or toes
  Unsteadiness or awkwardness
  Yellow eyes and skin

Rare
  Fainting
  Skin rash, hives, or itching
  Wheezing

Other side effects may occur that usually do not require medical attention. These side effects may go away during treatment as your body adjusts to the medicine. Also, your doctor or nurse may be able to tell you about ways to prevent or reduce some of these side effects. Check with your doctor if any of the following side effects continue or are bothersome or if you have any questions about them:

More common
  Drowsiness
  Muscle or joint pain
  Muscle twitching
  Nausea and vomiting
  Nervousness
  Nightmares
  Sweating
  Tiredness or weakness
  Trouble in sleeping

Less common
  Constipation
  Darkening of skin
  Difficulty in swallowing
  Dizziness or lightheadedness when getting up from a lying or sitting position
  Dry mouth
  Feeling of warmth and redness in face
  Headache
  Loss of appetite
  Mental depression

This medicine may cause a temporary loss of hair in some people. After treatment with procarbazine has ended, normal hair growth should return.

For elderly patients: The above side effects may be more likely to occur in elderly patients, who are usually more sensitive to the effects of procarbazine.

Other side effects not listed above may also occur in some patients. If you notice any other effects, check with your doctor.

_____

December 1987

PROGESTINS (Systemic)

This information applies to the following medicines:

Hydroxyprogesterone (hye-drox-ee-proe-JESS-te-rone)
Medroxyprogesterone (me-DROX-ee-proe-JESS-te-rone)
Megestrol (me-JESS-trole)
Norethindrone (nor-eth-IN-drone)
Norethindrone Acetate
Norgestrel (nor-JESS-trel)
Progesterone (proe-JESS-ter-one)

Some commonly used brand names are:	Generic names:
Delalutin* Duralutin Gesterol L.A. Hy-Gestrone Hylutin Hyprogest Hyproval P.A. Hyroxon Pro-Depo Prodrox	Hydroxyprogesterone†
Amen Curretab Depo-Provera Provera	Medroxyprogesterone†
Megace	Megestrol
Micronor Norlutin Nor-Q.D.	Norethindrone
Aygestin Norlutate	Norethindrone Acetate
Ovrette	Norgestrel
Femotrone in Oil Gesterol Progestaject Progestilin* Progestronaq-LA	Progesterone†

*Not available in the U.S.
†Generic name product may be available in the U.S.

To the Reader: If you do not recognize the names of medical conditions or medicines referred to in this information, check with your doctor, nurse, or pharmacist. Definitions for selected medical terms may be found in the Glossary. Brand names for the generic drug names listed can be found in the Index. In addition, selected brand names commonly associated with the generic name have been included in the text to help you recognize medicine you may be taking. The fact that a brand name product is not mentioned does not mean the information does not apply. It is a good idea for you to learn both the generic and brand names of your medicines and to write them down for future use.

Progestins (proe-JESS-tins) are sometimes called female hormones. They are produced by the body and are necessary during the childbearing years for the development of the milk-producing glands, and for the proper regulation of the menstrual cycle.

Progestins are prescribed for several reasons:

—for the proper regulation of the menstrual cycle.
—to treat a certain type of disorder of the uterus known as endometriosis.
—to prevent pregnancy, when used in birth-control pills.
—to help treat selected cases of cancer of the breast, kidney, or uterus.
—for testing the body's production of certain hormones.

Progestins may also be used for other conditions as determined by your doctor.

Progestins should not be used in pregnancy tests or in treatment of threatened miscarriage, since if used in the first 4 months of pregnancy they may cause birth defects.

To make the use of a progestin as safe and reliable as possible, you should understand how and when to take it and what effects may be expected. A paper with information for the patient may be given to you with your filled prescription, and will provide many details concerning most uses of this medicine. Read this paper carefully and ask your doctor, nurse, or pharmacist if you need additional information or explanation.

Progestins are taken by mouth in tablet form when possible because of the greater convenience. However, to better suit the individual needs of the patient, they are sometimes given by intramuscular injection, which provides a more constant and longer lasting effect.

Progestins are available only with your doctor's prescription.

Remember:
• **This medicine has been prescribed for your current medical problem only.** It must not be given to other people or used for other problems unless you are directed to do so by your doctor.

• **Keep all medicines out of the reach of children.**

• In order for this medicine to work, it must be used as directed.

• If you are receiving this medicine by injection, some of the information about this medicine may not apply.

• **It is very important that you read and understand the following information.** If any of the information causes you special concern, do not decide against using this medicine without first checking with your doctor.

• Before you begin using any new medicine (prescription or nonprescription) or if you develop any new medical problem while you are using this medicine, check with your doctor, nurse, or pharmacist.

• **If you have any questions** about the following information or if you want more information about this medicine or your medical problem, **ask your doctor, nurse, or pharmacist**.

Before Using This Medicine

In order to decide on the best treatment for your medical problem, your doctor should be told:

—if you have ever had any unusual or allergic reaction to this medicine.

—if you are on a low-salt, low-sugar, or any other special diet, or if you are allergic to any substance, such as foods, sulfites or other preservatives, or dyes. Most medicines contain more than their active ingredient. Your doctor, nurse, or pharmacist can help you avoid products that may cause a problem.

—if you are **pregnant**, if you intend to become pregnant, or if you suspect you are pregnant while using this medicine. Progestins are not recommended during pregnancy since they may cause birth defects if used during the first 4 months.

—if you are **breast-feeding**. Progestins pass into the breast milk and may cause unwanted effects in the nursing baby. It may be necessary for you to take another medicine or to stop breast-feeding during treatment.

—if you have any of the following medical problems:

Asthma
Blood clots (or history of)
Cancer (or history of)
Changes in vaginal bleeding
Diabetes mellitus (sugar diabetes)
Epilepsy
Heart or circulation disease
Kidney disease
Liver or gallbladder disease
Mental depression (or history of)
Migraine headaches
Stroke (or history of)

—if you are taking **any** other prescription or nonprescription (OTC) medicine, especially bromocriptine.

Proper Use of This Medicine

Take this medicine only as directed by your doctor. Do not take more of it and do not take it for a longer period of time than your doctor ordered. To do so may increase the chance of side effects. Try to take the medicine at the same time each day to reduce the possibility of side effects and to allow it to work better. When used for birth control, this medicine should be taken every day of the year, with doses taken 24 hours apart without interruption.

If you miss a dose of this medicine:

• If you are *not* taking this medicine for birth control, take the missed dose as soon as possible. However, if it is almost time for your next dose, skip the missed dose and go back to your regular dosing schedule. Do not double doses.

• **If you are taking this medicine for birth control,** the safest thing to do when you miss 1 day's dose is to stop taking the medicine immediately and use another method of birth control until your period begins or until your doctor determines that you are not pregnant. This procedure is different from the one used after missed doses of birth control tablets that contain more than one hormone.

How to store this medicine:

• **Keep out of the reach of children.**

• Store away from heat and direct light.

• Do not store in the bathroom medicine cabinet because the heat or moisture may cause the medicine to break down.

• Keep the injectable form of this medicine from freezing.

• Do not keep outdated medicine or medicine no longer needed. Be sure that any discarded medicine is out of the reach of children.

Precautions While Using This Medicine

It is very important that your doctor check your progress at regular visits. This will allow your dosage to be adjusted to your changing needs, and will allow any unwanted effects to be detected. These visits will usually be every 6 to 12 months, but some doctors require them more often.

Check with your doctor right away:

—if vaginal bleeding continues for an unusually long time.

—if your menstrual period has not started within 45 days of your last period.

—**if you suspect that you may have become pregnant. You should stop taking this medicine immediately,** since continued use during pregnancy may cause birth defects in the child.

In some patients, tenderness, swelling, or bleeding of the gums may occur. Brushing and flossing your teeth carefully and regularly and massaging your gums may help prevent this. See your dentist regularly to have your teeth cleaned. Check with your physician or dentist if you have any questions about how to take care of your teeth and gums, or if you notice any tenderness, swelling, or bleeding of your gums.

If you are taking this medicine for birth control:

• **When you begin to use birth control tablets** your body will require a period of time to adjust before pregnancy will be prevented; therefore, you should **use a second method of birth control for at least the first 3 weeks to ensure full protection.**

• The hormones in birth control tablets may cause birth defects. Since it takes a while for the effects of this medicine to wear off, birth defects may occur even though the tablets are no longer being used. Therefore, **when you stop using birth control tablets, it is very important that you wait at least 3 months before becoming pregnant. Be sure to use another method of birth control during that time.**

• Since one of the most important factors in the proper use of birth control tablets is taking every dose exactly on schedule, you should never let your tablet supply run out. Therefore, always keep 1 extra month's supply of tablets on hand. To keep the extra month's supply from becoming too old, use it next, after the pills now being used, and replace the extra supply each month on a regular schedule. The tablets will keep well when kept dry and at room temperature (light will fade some tablet colors but will not change the tablets' effect).

• Keep the tablets in the container in which you received them. Most containers aid you in keeping track of dosage schedule.

• Your doctor has prescribed this medicine only for you after studying your health record and the results of your physical examination. Use of the tablets by other persons may be dangerous because of differences in health and body make-up. Therefore, do not give your birth control tablets to anyone else (and do not take tablets prescribed for someone else). Also, check with your doctor before taking any leftover birth control tablets from an old prescription, especially after a pregnancy. This medicine may be dangerous if your health has changed since your last physical examination.

Side Effects of This Medicine

Along with their needed effects, progestins sometimes cause some unwanted effects such as blood clots, heart attack, and stroke, and problems of the liver and eyes. Although these effects are rare, they can be very serious and may cause death.

The following side effects may be caused by blood clots. Although not all of these side effects may occur, if they do occur they need immediate medical attention. **Get emergency help immediately** if any of the following side effects occur:

    Headache (severe or sudden)
    Loss of coordination (sudden)
    Loss of vision or change in vision (sudden)
    Pains in chest, groin, or leg (especially in calf of leg)
    Shortness of breath (sudden)
    Slurred speech (sudden)
    Weakness, numbness, or pain in arm or leg

Also, check with your doctor as soon as possible if any of the following side effects occur:

More common

    Changes in vaginal bleeding (spotting, breakthrough bleeding, prolonged or complete stoppage of bleeding)

Less common or rare

    Bulging eyes
    Discharge from breasts
    Double vision
    Loss of vision (gradual, partial, or complete)
    Mental depression
    Pains in stomach, side, or abdomen
    Skin rash or itching
    Yellow eyes or skin

Other side effects may occur that usually do not require medical attention. These side effects may go away during treatment as your body adjusts to the medicine. However, check with your doctor if any of the following side effects continue or are bothersome:

More common

    Changes in appetite
    Changes in weight
    Pain or irritation at injection site (with progesterone)
    Swelling of ankles and feet
    Unusual tiredness or weakness

Less common or rare

    Acne
    Brown, blotchy spots on exposed skin
    Increased body and facial hair
    Increased breast tenderness
    Nausea
    Some loss of scalp hair

Other side effects not listed above may also occur in some patients. If you notice any other effects, check with your doctor.

December 1987

PROMETHAZINE (Systemic)

Some commonly used brand names are:

Anergan	Phenergan
Baymethazine	Phenergan Fortis
Ganphen	Phenergan Plain
Histantil*	Phenoject-50
K-Phen	PMS Promethazine*
Mallergan	Prometh
Pentazine	Prorex
Phenameth	Prothazine
Phenazine	Prothazine Plain
Phencen-50	Provigan
	Remsed
	V-Gan

Generic name product may also be available in the U.S.

---

*Not available in the U.S.

To the Reader: If you do not recognize the names of medical conditions or medicines referred to in this information, check with your doctor, nurse, or pharmacist. Definitions for selected medical terms may be found in the Glossary. Brand names for the generic drug names listed can be found in the Index. In addition, selected brand names commonly associated with the generic name have been included in the text to help you recognize medicine you may be taking. The fact that a brand name product is not mentioned does not mean the information does not apply. It is a good idea for you to learn both the generic and brand names of your medicines and to write them down for future use.

Promethazine (proe-METH-a-zeen) belongs to the group of medicines called antihistamines. It is used to relieve or prevent the symptoms of hay fever and other types of allergy, and to prevent motion sickness, nausea, vomiting, and dizziness. Since promethazine may cause drowsiness, it is used in some people to help them sleep, and also to produce sedation.

Promethazine is available only with your doctor's prescription.

Remember:

• **This medicine has been prescribed for your current medical problem only.** It must not be given to other people or used for other problems unless you are directed to do so by your doctor.

• **Keep all medicines out of the reach of children.**

• In order for this medicine to work, it must be used as directed.

• If you are receiving this medicine by injection, some of the information about this medicine may not apply.

• **It is very important that you read and understand the following information.** If any of the information causes you special concern, do not decide against using this medicine without first checking with your doctor.

• Before you begin using any new medicine (prescription or nonprescription) or if you develop any new medical problem while you are using this medicine, check with your doctor, nurse, or pharmacist.

• **If you have any questions** about the following information or if you want more information about this medicine or your medical problem, **ask your doctor, nurse, or pharmacist**.

Before Using This Medicine

In order to decide on the best treatment for your medical problem, your doctor should be told:

—if you have ever had any unusual or allergic reaction to promethazine or other phenothiazines.

—if you are on a low-salt, low-sugar, or any other special diet, or if you are allergic to any substance, such as foods, sulfites or other preservatives, or dyes. Most medicines contain more than their active ingredient, and many liquid medicines contain alcohol. Your doctor, nurse, or pharmacist can help you avoid products that may cause a problem.

—if you are **pregnant** or if you may become pregnant. Promethazine has been shown to cause jaundice and muscle tremors in a few newborn babies whose mothers received phenothiazines, such as promethazine, during pregnancy. To avoid these effects, medicines that contain promethazine should be stopped 1 or 2 weeks before the expected delivery date.

—if you are **breast-feeding**. Promethazine has not been shown to cause problems in nursing babies. However, this medicine may pass into the breast milk and cause unwanted effects in the baby.

—if you have any of the following medical problems:
  Blood disease
  Difficult urination
  Emphysema, asthma, or chronic lung disease (especially in children)
  Enlarged prostate
  Heart or bood vessel disease
  High blood pressure
  Intestinal blockage
  Liver disease
  Stomach ulcer
  Urinary tract blockage

—if you have epilepsy or Reye's syndrome. Your doctor may not want you to receive promethazine by injection, since the chance for seizures or uncontrolled movements is greater when these conditions are present.

—if you are now taking or have taken within the past 2 weeks monoamine oxidase (MAO) inhibitors such as:
  Furazolidone (e.g., Furoxone)
  Isocarboxazid (e.g., Marplan)
  Pargyline (e.g., Eutonyl)
  Phenelzine (e.g., Nardil)
  Procarbazine (e.g., Matulane)
  Tranylcypromine (e.g., Parnate)

—if you are taking **any** other prescription or nonprescription (OTC) medicine, especially:
  Amoxapine (e.g., Asendin)
  Antithyroid agents (medicine for overactive thyroid)
  Chlorprothixene (e.g., Taractan)
  Central nervous system (CNS) depressants
  Epinephrine (e.g., Adrenalin)
  Haloperidol (e.g., Haldol)
  Levodopa (e.g., Dopar)
  Loxapine (e.g., Loxitane)
  Methyldopa (e.g., Aldomet)
  Metoclopramide (e.g., Reglan)
  Metyrosine (e.g., Demser)

Molindone (e.g., Moban)
Pemoline (e.g., Cylert)
Phenothiazines (acetophenazine, chlorpromazine, flu-phenazine, mesoridazine, perphenazine, prochlorper-azine, promazine, promethazine, thioridazine, trifluo-perazine, triflupromazine, trimeprazine)
Pimozide (e.g., Orap)
Quinidine (e.g., Quinidex)
Rauwolfia alkaloids (alseroxylon, deserpidine, rauwolfia serpentina, reserpine)
Thiothixene (e.g., Navane)

—if you are having an x-ray test of the head, spinal canal, or nervous system for which you are going to receive an injection into the spinal canal. This medicine may increase the chances of having seizures.

Proper Use of This Medicine

Take promethazine only as directed. Do not take more of it and do not take it more often than directed by your doctor. To do so may increase the chance of side effects.

If you are taking promethazine for motion sickness, take it at least 30 minutes or, even better, 1 to 2 hours before you begin to travel.

For patients taking promethazine by mouth:

• This medicine may be taken with food or a full glass (8 ounces) of water or milk to reduce stomach irritation.

For patients using the suppository form of promethazine:

• To insert suppository: First remove the foil wrapper and moisten the suppository with water. Lie down on side and push the suppository well up into the rectum with finger.

• If the suppository is too soft to insert because of storage in a warm place, before removing the foil wrapper chill the suppository in the refrigerator for 30 minutes or run cold water over it.

If you must take promethazine regularly and you miss a dose, take it as soon as possible. However, if it is almost time for your next dose, skip the missed dose and go back to your regular dosing schedule. Do not double doses.

How to store this medicine:

• **Keep out of the reach of children.**

• Store away from heat and direct light.

• Do not store the tablet form of this medicine in the bathroom, near the kitchen sink, or in other damp places. Heat or moisture may cause the medicine to break down.

• Keep the syrup form of this medicine from freezing.

• Do not keep outdated medicine or medicine no longer needed. Be sure that any discarded medicine is out of the reach of children.

Precautions While Using This Medicine

If you will be using this medicine for a long period of time (for example, for several months at a time), it is important that your doctor check your progress at regular visits. This is to make sure the medicine does not cause unwanted effects.

Tell the doctor in charge that you are taking this medicine before you have any skin tests for allergies. The results of the test may be affected by this medicine.

This medicine will add to the effects of alcohol and other CNS depressants (medicines that slow down the nervous system, possibly causing drowsiness). Some examples of CNS depressants are antihistamines or medicine for hay fever, other allergies, or colds; sedatives, tranquilizers, or sleeping medicine; prescription pain medicine or narcotics; barbiturates; medicine for convulsions (seizures); muscle relaxants; or anesthetics, including some dental anesthetics. **Check with your doctor before taking any of the above while you are using this medicine.**

When taking promethazine on a regular basis, make sure your doctor knows if you are taking large amounts of aspirin (as in arthritis or rheumatism) at the same time. Effects of too much aspirin, such as dizziness or ringing in the ears, may be covered up by this medicine.

This medicine may cause some people to become drowsy or less alert than they are normally. Even if taken at bedtime, it may cause some people to feel drowsy or less alert on arising. **Make sure you know how you react to this medicine before you drive, use machines, or do other jobs that require you to be alert.**

Some people who take promethazine may become more sensitive to sunlight than they are normally. When you first begin taking this medicine, avoid too much sun and do not use a sunlamp until you see how you react to the sun, especially if you tend to burn easily. **If you have a severe reaction, check with your doctor.**

Promethazine may cause dryness of the mouth, nose, and throat. For temporary relief of mouth dryness, use sugarless candy or gum, melt bits of ice in your mouth, or use a saliva substitute. However, if dry mouth continues for more than 2 weeks, check with your dentist. Continuing dryness of the mouth may increase the chance of dental disease, including tooth decay, gum disease, and fungal infections.

Side Effects of This Medicine

Along with its needed effects, a medicine may cause some unwanted effects. Although not all of these side effects may occur, if they do occur they may need medical attention.

Check with your doctor as soon as possible if any of the following side effects occur:

Rare

Increased sensitivity of skin to sun
Nightmares (continuing) (especially in children)
Sore throat and fever
Unusual excitement, nervousness, restlessness, or irritability (continuing) (especially in children)

Signs of overdose

Clumsiness or unsteadiness
Drowsiness (severe)
Fast heartbeat
Flushing or redness of face
Muscle spasms (especially of neck and back)
Restlessness
Shortness of breath or troubled breathing
Shuffling walk
Tic-like (jerky) movements of head and face
Trembling and shaking of hands

Other side effects may occur that usually do not require medical attention. These side effects may go away during treatment as your body adjusts to the medicine. However, check with your doctor if any of the following side effects continue or are bothersome:

More common

Drowsiness

Less common or rare

Blurred vision or any change in vision
Burning or stinging of rectum (with rectal suppository)
Decreased mental alertness (especially with children)
Dizziness or feeling faint
Dryness of mouth, nose, and throat
Nausea or vomiting
Ringing or buzzing in the ears
Skin rash
Stomach upset or pain

For children: Serious side effects are more likely to occur in premature or newborn infants, or in children who are very ill. **Do not give this medicine** to these children.

For elderly patients: Dizziness, drowsiness, confusion, faintness, and uncontrolled movements may be more likely to occur in elderly patients since they are usually more sensitive to the effects of promethazine.

Other side effects not listed above may also occur in some patients. If you notice any other effects, check with your doctor.

December 1987

PROPIOMAZINE (Systemic)

A commonly used brand name is Largon.

To the Reader: If you do not recognize the names of medical conditions or medicines referred to in this information, check with your doctor, nurse, or pharmacist. Definitions for selected medical terms may be found in the Glossary. Brand names for the generic drug names listed can be found in the Index. In addition, selected brand names commonly associated with the generic name have been included in the text to help you recognize medicine you may be taking. The fact that a brand name product is not mentioned does not mean the information does not apply. It is a good idea for you to learn both the generic and brand names of your medicines and to write them down for future use.

Propiomazine (proe-pee-OH-ma-zeen) is given by injection to produce sleepiness or drowsiness and to relieve anxiety before or during surgery or certain procedures. It is also used with analgesics (pain medicine) during labor to produce drowsiness and relieve anxiety.

Propiomazine is given only by or under the immediate supervision of a physician or dentist trained to use this medicine. If you will be receiving propiomazine during surgery, your doctor or anesthesiologist will give you the medicine and closely follow your progress.

Remember:

• **It is very important that you read and understand the following information.** If any of the information causes you special concern, do not decide against receiving this medicine without first checking with your doctor.

• **If you have any questions** about the following information or if you want more information about this medicine or your medical problem, **ask your doctor, nurse, or pharmacist.**

Before Receiving This Medicine

In order to decide on the best treatment for your medical problem, your doctor should be told:

—if you have ever had any unusual or allergic reaction to propiomazine or to other phenothiazines (such as acetophenazine, chlorpromazine, fluphenazine, mesoridazine, perphenazine, prochlorperazine, promazine, promethazine, thioridazine, trifluoperazine, triflupromazine, trimeprazine).

—if you are on a low-salt, low-sugar, or any other special diet, or if you are allergic to any substance, such as preservatives. Most medicines contain more than their active ingredient.

—if you are **pregnant**. Propiomazine has not been shown to cause problems in humans.

—if you are **breast-feeding**. Propiomazine has not been shown to cause problems in nursing babies.

—if you are using **any** other prescription or nonprescription (OTC) medicine, especially:
Central nervous system (CNS) depressants
Epinephrine (e.g., Adrenalin)

Precautions After Receiving This Medicine

For patients going home within 24 hours after receiving propiomazine:

• Propiomazine may cause some people to feel drowsy, tired, or weak for up to one or two days after it has been given. It may also cause problems with coordination and one's ability to think. Therefore, **do not drive, use machines, or do other jobs that require you to be alert** until the effects of the medicine have disappeared or until the day after receiving propiomazine, whichever period of time is longer.

• **Do not drink alcoholic beverages or take other CNS depressants (medicines that slow down the nervous system, possibly causing drowsiness) for about 24 hours after you have received propiomazine, unless otherwise directed by your doctor.** To do so may add to the effects of the medicine. Some examples of CNS depressants are antihistamines or medicine for hay fever, other allergies, or colds; other sedatives, tranquilizers, or sleeping medicine; prescription pain medicine or narcotics; medicine for convulsions (seizures); and muscle relaxants.

Side Effects of This Medicine

Along with its needed effects, a medicine may cause some unwanted effects. Although not all of these side effects may occur, if they do occur they may need medical attention.

Check with your doctor as soon as possible if the following side effect occurs:
Redness, swelling, or pain at place of injection

Other side effects may occur that usually do not require medical attention. The following side effects may go away as the effects of propiomazine wear off. However, check with your doctor if any of the following side effects continue or are bothersome:

More common
Dizziness
Drowsiness (prolonged)

Less common
Confusion
Diarrhea
Nausea or vomiting
Restlessness
Skin rash
Stomach pain

Other side effects not listed above may also occur in some patients. If you notice any other effects, check with your doctor.

December 1987

PROTIRELIN (Systemic)

Some commonly used brand names are Relefact TRH and Thypinone.

To the Reader: If you do not recognize the names of medical conditions or medicines referred to in this information, check with your doctor, nurse, or pharmacist. Definitions for selected medical terms may be found in the Glossary. Brand names for the generic drug names listed can be found in the Index. In addition, selected brand names commonly associated with the generic name have been included in the text to help you recognize medicine you may be taking. The fact that a brand name product is not mentioned does not mean the information does not apply. It is a good idea for you to learn both the generic and brand names of your medicines and to write them down for future use.

Protirelin (proe-TYE-re-lin) is used to test the response of the anterior pituitary gland in people who may have certain medical conditions involving the thyroid gland. Testing with this medicine may help to identify the problem or may ensure that the dose of medicine being used is correct.

Protirelin stimulates release of a hormone called thyroid-stimulating hormone or TSH from the anterior pituitary gland. TSH then stimulates the thyroid gland. By measuring the amount of TSH in the blood after protirelin is given, the doctor can determine how well the anterior pituitary is working.

How test is done: First, a sample of your blood is taken. Then protirelin is given by injection. A little while after it is given, one or more blood samples are taken. Then the results of the test are studied. You will be asked to lie down before, during, and for 15 minutes after the test. This is to prevent dizziness and possible fainting.

Protirelin is to be used only under the supervision of a doctor.

Remember:
• **If you have any questions** about the following information or if you want more information about this test or your medical problem, **ask your doctor, nurse, or pharmacist.**

Before Having This Test

Before this test is given, your doctor should be told:

—if you have ever had any unusual or allergic reaction to protirelin.

—if you are on a low-salt, low-sugar, or any other special diet, or if you are allergic to any substance, such as foods or sulfites or other preservatives. Most medicines contain more than their active ingredient. Your doctor, nurse, or pharmacist can help you avoid products that may cause a problem.

—if you are **pregnant** or if you suspect that you may be pregnant. Studies have not been done in humans. However, studies in rabbits have shown that protirelin increases the chance of death of the fetus when given in doses 1½ to 6 times the human dose.

—if you are **breast-feeding**. Protirelin has not been shown to cause problems in nursing babies. However, it may cause extra swelling of the breasts and leaking of milk for up to 2 or 3 days after it is given.

—if you have any of the following medical problems:
Heart or blood vessel disease
High blood pressure
Kidney disease
Stroke (history of)

—if you are taking **any** other prescription or nonprescription (OTC) medicine.

Preparation for This Test

Your doctor may ask you not to eat for several hours before the test or to eat a low-fat meal before the test. This will not be necessary for all patients. If it is necessary for you, **follow your doctor's instructions carefully.** Otherwise, this test may not work and may have to be done again.

Side Effects of This Medicine

Along with its needed effects, a medicine may cause some unwanted effects. Check with your doctor or nurse as soon as possible if either of the following side effects occurs:

Rare
Fainting
For patients with pituitary tumors—Rare
Loss of vision (temporary)

Protirelin commonly causes some side effects just after it is given. Usually they last for only a few minutes. However, check with your doctor if any of the following side effects continue or are bothersome:

More common
Bad taste in mouth or dry mouth
Flushing or redness of skin
Frequent urge to urinate
Headache (sometimes severe)
Lightheadedness
Nausea
Stomach pain

Less common
Anxiety
Drowsiness
Pressure in the chest or tightness in the throat
Sweating
Tingling

Other side effects not listed above may also occur in some patients. If you notice any other effects, check with your doctor.

December 1987

PSEUDOEPHEDRINE (Systemic)

Some commonly used brand names are:

Afrinol Repetabs	Novafed
Cenafed	PediaCare
Children's Sudafed Liquid	Pseudofrin*
Decofed	Pseudogest
Dorcol Pediatric Formula	Robidrine*
Eltor*	Sinufed
Halofed	Sudafed
NeoFed	Sudafed S.A.
Neo-Synephrinol Day Relief	Sudrin

Generic name product may also be available in the U.S.

---

*Not available in the U.S.

To the Reader: If you do not recognize the names of medical conditions or medicines referred to in this information, check with your doctor, nurse, or pharmacist. Definitions for selected medical terms may be found in the Glossary. Brand names for the generic drug names listed can be found in the Index. In addition, selected brand names commonly associated with the generic name have been included in the text to help you recognize medicine you may be taking. The fact that a brand name product is not mentioned does not mean the information does not apply. It is a good idea for you to learn both the generic and brand names of your medicines and to write them down for future use.

Pseudoephedrine (soo-doe-e-FED-rin) is taken by mouth to relieve nasal or sinus congestion caused by the common cold, sinusitis, and hay fever and other respiratory allergies. It is also used to relieve ear congestion caused by ear inflammation or infection.

Some of these preparations are available only with your doctor's prescription. Others are available without a prescription; however, your doctor may have special instructions on the proper dose of pseudoephedrine for your medical condition.

Remember:

• **Keep all medicines out of the reach of children.**

• In order for this medicine to work, it must be used as directed. **If you are using this medicine without a prescription, it is very important that you follow the directions on the label.**

• **It is also very important that you read and understand the following information.** If any of the information causes you special concern, check with your doctor or pharmacist.

• Before you begin using any new medicine (prescription or nonprescription) or if you develop any new medical problem while you are using this medicine, check with your doctor, nurse, or pharmacist.

• **If you have any questions** about the following information or if you want more information about this medicine or your medical problem, **ask your doctor, nurse, or pharmacist.**

Before Using This Medicine

Before you use pseudoephedrine, check with your doctor or pharmacist:

—if you have ever had any unusual or allergic reaction to medicines like pseudoephedrine, such as albuterol, amphetamines, ephedrine, epinephrine, isoproterenol, metaproterenol, norepinephrine, phenylephrine, phenylpropanolamine, or terbutaline.

—if you are on a low-salt, low-sugar, or any other special diet, or if you are allergic to any substance, such as foods, sulfites or other preservatives, or dyes. Most medicines contain more than their active ingredient, and many liquid medicines contain alcohol. Your doctor, nurse, or pharmacist can help you avoid products that may cause a problem.

—if you are **pregnant** or if you may become pregnant. Studies on birth defects have not been done in humans. However, pseudoephedrine has not been shown to cause birth defects in animal studies. Studies in animals have shown that pseudoephedrine causes a reduction in average weight, length, and rate of bone formation in the animal fetus.

—if you are **breast-feeding**. Pseudoephedrine passes into the breast milk and may cause unwanted side effects in nursing babies (especially newborn and premature babies).

—if you have any of the following medical problems:
  Diabetes mellitus (sugar diabetes)
  Enlarged prostate
  Heart or blood vessel disease
  High blood pressure
  Overactive thyroid

—if you are taking **any** other prescription or nonprescription (OTC) medicine, especially beta-blockers (acebutolol [e.g., Sectral], atenolol [e.g., Tenormin], esmolol [e.g., Brevibloc], labetalol [e.g., Normodyne], metoprolol [e.g., Lopressor], nadolol [e.g., Corgard], oxprenolol [e.g., Trasicor], pindolol [e.g., Visken], propranolol [e.g., Inderal], sotalol [e.g., Sotacor], timolol [e.g., Blocadren]).

—if you are now taking or have taken within the past 2 weeks monoamine oxidase (MAO) inhibitors, such as:

  Furazolidone (e.g., Furoxone)
  Isocarboxazid (e.g., Marplan)
  Pargyline (e.g., Eutonyl)
  Phenelzine (e.g., Nardil)
  Procarbazine (e.g., Matulane)
  Tranylcypromine (e.g., Parnate)

Proper Use of This Medicine

For patients taking the extended-release capsule form of this medicine:

• Swallow the capsule whole. However, if the capsule is too large to swallow, you may mix the contents of the capsule with jam or jelly and swallow without chewing.

• Do not crush, break, or chew before swallowing.

For patients taking the extended-release tablet form of this medicine:

• Swallow the tablet whole.

• Do not break, crush, or chew before swallowing.

To help prevent trouble in sleeping, **take the last dose of pseudoephedrine for each day a few hours before bedtime.** If you have any questions about this, check with your doctor.

Take this medicine only as directed. Do not take more of it and do not take it more often than recommended on the label, unless otherwise directed by your doctor. To do so may increase the chance of side effects.

If you miss a dose of this medicine and you remember within an hour or so of the missed dose, take it right away. However, if you do not remember until later, skip the missed dose and go back to your regular dosing schedule. Do not double doses.

How to store this medicine:

- **Keep out of the reach of children.**

- Store away from heat and direct light.

- Do not store the capsule or tablet form of this medicine in the bathroom, near the kitchen sink, or in other damp places. Heat or moisture may cause the medicine to break down.

- Keep the liquid form of this medicine from freezing.

- Do not keep outdated medicine or medicine no longer needed. Be sure that any discarded medicine is out of the reach of children.

Precautions While Using This Medicine

If symptoms do not improve within 5 days or if you also have a high fever, check with your doctor since these signs may mean that you have other medical problems.

Side Effects of This Medicine

Along with its needed effects, a medicine may cause some unwanted effects. Although not all of these side effects may occur, if they do occur they may need medical attention.

Check with your doctor as soon as possible if any of the following side effects occur:

Rare—more common with high doses
    Convulsions (seizures)
    Hallucinations (seeing, hearing, or feeling things that are not there)
    Irregular or slow heartbeat
    Shortness of breath or troubled breathing

Signs of overdose
    Convulsions (seizures)
    Fast breathing
    Hallucinations (seeing, hearing, or feeling things that are not there)
    Increase in blood pressure
    Irregular heartbeat (continuing)
    Shortness of breath or troubled breathing (severe or continuing)
    Slow or fast heartbeat (severe or continuing)
    Unusual nervousness, restlessness, or excitement

Other side effects may occur that usually do not require medical attention. These side effects may go away during treatment as your body adjusts to the medicine. However, check with your doctor or pharmacist if any of the following side effects continue or are bothersome:

More common
    Nervousness
    Restlessness
    Trouble in sleeping

Less common
    Difficult or painful urination
    Dizziness or lightheadedness
    Fast or pounding heartbeat
    Headache
    Increase in sweating
    Nausea or vomiting
    Trembling
    Troubled breathing
    Unusual paleness
    Weakness

For infants: The above side effects are more likely to occur in infants, especially newborn and premature infants, who are usually more sensitive to the effects of pseudoephedrine.

For elderly patients: Many medicines have not been tested in older people. Therefore, it is not known whether the medicine acts the same way it does in younger adults. Check with your doctor or pharmacist if you notice any unusual effects while taking this medicine or if you think it is not working as it should.

Other side effects not listed above may also occur in some patients. If you notice any other effects, check with your doctor or pharmacist.

December 1987

PYRANTEL (Oral)

Some commonly used brand names are:

Antiminth	Helmex*
Aut*	Lombriareu*
Cobantril*	Trilombrin*
Combantrin*	

*Not commercially available in the U.S.

To the Reader: If you do not recognize the names of medical conditions or medicines referred to in this information, check with your doctor, nurse, or pharmacist. Definitions for selected medical terms may be found in the Glossary. Brand names for the generic drug names listed can be found in the Index. In addition, selected brand names commonly associated with the generic name have been included in the text to help you recognize medicine you may be taking. The fact that a brand name product is not mentioned does not mean the information does not apply. It is a good idea for you to learn both the generic and brand names of your medicines and to write them down for future use.

Pyrantel (pi-RAN-tel) belongs to the family of medicines called anthelmintics (ant-hel-MIN-tiks). Anthelmintics are used in the treatment of worm infections.

Pyrantel is taken by mouth to treat:

—common roundworms (ascariasis);
—pinworms (enterobiasis; oxyuriasis); and
—more than one worm infection at a time.

This medicine may also be used for other worm infections as determined by your doctor.

Pyrantel works by paralyzing the worms. They are then passed in the stool.

Pyrantel is available only with your doctor's prescription.

Remember:

• **This medicine has been prescribed for your present infection only.** Another infection later on may require a different medicine. Also, even though other people may have the same symptoms as you, they may have a different kind of infection. Your medicine may not work for them and may even cause them harm. Therefore, **your medicine must not be given to other people or used for other infections** unless you are otherwise directed by your doctor.

• **Keep all medicines out of the reach of children.**

• In order for this medicine to work, it must be used as directed.

• **It is very important that you read and understand the following information.** If any of the information causes you special concern, do not decide against using this medicine without first checking with your doctor.

• Before you begin using any new medicine (prescription or nonprescription) or if you develop any new medical problem while you are using this medicine, check with your doctor, nurse, or pharmacist.

• **If you have any questions** about the following information or if you want more information about this medicine or your medical problem, **ask your doctor, nurse, or pharmacist.**

Before Using This Medicine

In order to decide on the best treatment for your medical problem, your doctor should be told:

—if you have ever had any unusual or allergic reaction to pyrantel.

—if you are on a low-salt, low-sugar, or any other special diet, or if you are allergic to any substance, such as foods, sulfites or other preservatives, or dyes. Most medicines contain more than their active ingredient, and many liquid medicines contain alcohol. Your doctor, nurse, or pharmacist can help you avoid products that may cause a problem.

—if you are **pregnant** or if you may become pregnant. Studies have not been done in humans. However, pyrantel has not been shown to cause birth defects or other problems in animal studies.

—if you are **breast-feeding**. Pyrantel has not been shown to cause problems in humans. In addition, only small amounts of pyrantel are absorbed into the body. Therefore, pyrantel is unlikely to pass into the breast milk in large amounts and is unlikely to cause serious problems in nursing babies.

—if you have liver disease.

—if you are taking **any** other prescription or nonprescription (OTC) medicine, especially piperazine.

Proper Use of This Medicine

No special preparations (for example, special diets, fasting, other medicines, laxatives, or enemas) are necessary before, during, or immediately after taking pyrantel.

Pyrantel may be taken on a full or empty stomach, with or without beverages (milk or fruit juices), at any time of day.

For patients taking the oral liquid form of pyrantel:

• Use a specially marked measuring spoon or other device to measure each dose accurately since the average household teaspoon may not hold the right amount of liquid.

To help clear up your infection completely, **take this medicine exactly as directed by your doctor.** Usually one dose is enough. However, in some infections a second dose of this medicine may be required to clear up the infection completely.

For patients taking pyrantel for pinworms:

• Pinworms may be easily passed from one person to another, especially among persons in the same household. Therefore, all household members may have to be treated at the same time to prevent their infection or reinfection. Also, all household members may have to be treated again in 2 to 3 weeks to clear up the infection completely.

How to store this medicine:

• **Keep out of the reach of children.**

• Store away from heat and direct light.

• Do not store the tablet form of this medicine in the bathroom, near the kitchen sink, or in other damp places. Heat or moisture may cause the medicine to break down.

• Keep the oral liquid form of this medicine from freezing.

• Do not keep outdated medicine or medicine no longer needed. Be sure that any discarded medicine is out of the reach of children.

Precautions While Using This Medicine

It is important that your doctor check your progress at regular visits. This is to make sure that the infection is cleared up completely.

If your symptoms do not improve within a few days, or if they become worse, check with your doctor.

This medicine may cause some people to become dizzy, drowsy, or less alert than they are normally. **Make sure you know how you react to this medicine before you drive, use machines, or do other jobs that require you to be alert.** If these reactions are especially bothersome, check with your doctor.

For patients taking pyrantel for pinworms:

• In some patients, pinworms may return after treatment with pyrantel. Washing (not shaking) all bedding and nightclothes (pajamas) after treatment may help to prevent this.

• Some doctors may also recommend other measures to help keep your infection from returning. If you have any questions about this, check with your doctor.

Side Effects of This Medicine

Along with its needed effects, a medicine may cause some unwanted effects. Although not all of these side effects may occur, if they do occur they may need medical attention.

Check with your doctor immediately if any of the following side effects occur:

Signs of overdose (may occur in the following order)
Muscle spasms, twitching, or weakness
Lightheadedness
Inability to breathe
Collapse

In addition to the side effects mentioned above, check with your doctor as soon as possible if the following side effect also occurs:

Less common
Skin rash

Other side effects may occur that usually do not require medical attention. These side effects may go away during treatment as your body adjusts to the medicine. However, check with your doctor if any of the following side effects continue or are bothersome:

Less common
Abdominal or stomach cramps or pain
Diarrhea
Dizziness
Drowsiness
Headache
Loss of appetite
Nausea or vomiting
Trouble in sleeping

For elderly patients: Many medicines have not been tested in older people. Therefore, it is not known whether the medicine acts the same way it does in younger adults. Check with your doctor or pharmacist if you notice any unusual effects while taking this medicine or if you think it is not working as it should.

Other side effects not listed above may also occur in some patients. If you notice any other effects, check with your doctor.

_____

December 1987

Additional Information

In addition to the above information, for patients taking pyrantel for hookworms:

• Anemia (iron-poor blood) may occur in patients with hookworm infections. Therefore, your doctor may want you to take iron supplements to help clear up the anemia. If so, it is important to take iron every day while you are being treated for hookworms. Do not miss any doses. Your doctor may also want you to keep taking iron supplements for up to 6 months after you stop taking pyrantel. If you have any questions about this, check with your doctor.

PYRAZINAMIDE (Systemic)

Some commonly used brand names are PMS Pyrazinamide* and Tebrazid*.

Generic name product may also be available in the U.S.

*Not available in the U.S.

To the Reader: If you do not recognize the names of medical conditions or medicines referred to in this information, check with your doctor, nurse, or pharmacist. Definitions for selected medical terms may be found in the Glossary. Brand names for the generic drug names listed can be found in the Index. In addition, selected brand names commonly associated with the generic name have been included in the text to help you recognize medicine you may be taking. The fact that a brand name product is not mentioned does not mean the information does not apply. It is a good idea for you to learn both the generic and brand names of your medicines and to write them down for future use.

Pyrazinamide (peer-a-ZIN-a-mide) belongs to the family of medicines called anti-infectives. It is taken by mouth, along with one or more other medicines, to help the body overcome tuberculosis (TB).

Pyrazinamide is available only with your doctor's prescription.

Remember:

• **This medicine has been prescribed for your present TB infection only.** Another TB infection later on may require a different medicine. Also, even though other people may have the same symptoms as you, they may have a different kind of TB. Your medicine may not work for them and may even cause them harm. Therefore, **your medicine must not be given to other people or used for other infections** unless you are otherwise directed by your doctor.

• **Keep all medicines out of the reach of children.**

• In order for this medicine to work, it must be used as directed.

• **It is very important that you read and understand the following information.** If any of the information causes you special concern, do not decide against using this medicine without first checking with your doctor.

• Before you begin using any new medicine (prescription or nonprescription) or if you develop any new medical problem while you are using this medicine, check with your doctor, nurse, or pharmacist.

• **If you have any questions** about the following information or if you want more information about this medicine or your medical problem, **ask your doctor, nurse, or pharmacist.**

Before Using This Medicine

In order to decide on the best treatment for your medical problem, your doctor should be told:

—if you have ever had any unusual or allergic reaction to this medicine or to ethionamide, isoniazid (INH), or niacin (nicotinic acid).

—if you are on a low-salt, low-sugar, or any other special diet, or if you are allergic to any substance, such as foods, sulfites or other preservatives, or dyes.

Most medicines contain more than their active ingredient. Your doctor, nurse, or pharmacist can help you avoid products that may cause a problem.

—if you are **pregnant** or if you may become pregnant. However, pyrazinamide has not been shown to cause birth defects or other problems in humans. In addition, it is not known whether this medicine causes problems when taken with other TB medicines.

—if you are **breast-feeding**. However, pyrazinamide has not been shown to cause problems in nursing babies.

—if you have any of the following medical problems:
  Diabetes mellitus (sugar diabetes)
  Gout (history of)
  Liver disease (severe)

—if you are taking **any** other prescription or nonprescription (OTC) medicine.

Proper Use of This Medicine

To help clear up your TB completely, **it is important that you keep taking this medicine for the full time of treatment** even if you begin to feel better after a few weeks. You may have to take pyrazinamide every day for up to 1 to 2 years or more. **It is important that you do not miss any doses.**

If you do miss a dose of this medicine, take it as soon as possible. However, if it is almost time for your next dose, skip the missed dose and go back to your regular dosing schedule. Do not double doses.

How to store this medicine:

• **Keep out of the reach of children.**

• Store away from heat and direct light.

• Do not store in the bathroom, near the kitchen sink, or in other damp places. Heat or moisture may cause the medicine to break down.

• Do not keep outdated medicine or medicine no longer needed. Be sure that any discarded medicine is out of the reach of children.

Precautions While Using This Medicine

It is very important that your doctor check your progress at regular visits.

If your symptoms do not improve within 2 to 3 weeks, or if they become worse, check with your doctor.

Some people who take pyrazinamide may become more sensitive to sunlight than they are normally. **When you first begin taking this medicine, avoid too much sun and do not use a sunlamp until you see how you react to the sun,** especially if you tend to burn easily. **If you have a severe reaction, check with your doctor.**

Diabetics—This medicine may cause false test results with urine ketone tests. Check with your doctor before changing your diet or the dosage of your diabetes medicine.

Side Effects of This Medicine

Along with its needed effects, a medicine may cause some unwanted effects. Although not all of these side effects may occur, if they do occur they may need medical attention.

Check with your doctor immediately if any of the following side effects occur:

More common
   Fever
   Loss of appetite
   Unusual tiredness or weakness
   Yellow eyes or skin

Less common
   Chills, pain, and swelling of joints, especially big toe, ankle, and knee
   Tense, hot skin over affected joints

Other side effects may occur that usually do not require medical attention. These side effects may go away during treatment as your body adjusts to the medicine.

However, check with your doctor if any of the following side effects continue or are bothersome:

Less common
   Difficult urination
   Nausea or vomiting

Rare
   Increased sensitivity of skin to sunlight
   Itching
   Skin rash

For elderly patients: Many medicines have not been tested in older people. Therefore, it is not known whether the medicine acts the same way it does in younger adults. Check with your doctor or pharmacist if you notice any unusual effects while taking this medicine or if you think it is not working as it should.

Other side effects not listed above may also occur in some patients. If you notice any other effects, check with your doctor.

_____

December 1987

_____

PYRETHRINS AND PIPERONYL BUTOXIDE (Topical)

Some commonly used brand names are:

A-200 Pyrinate	R & C
Barc	RID
Blue	TISIT
Licetrol	TISIT Blue
Pyrinyl	Triple X

To the Reader: If you do not recognize the names of medical conditions or medicines referred to in this information, check with your doctor, nurse, or pharmacist. Definitions for selected medical terms may be found in the Glossary. Brand names for the generic drug names listed can be found in the Index. In addition, selected brand names commonly associated with the generic name have been included in the text to help you recognize medicine you may be taking. The fact that a brand name product is not mentioned does not mean the information does not apply. It is a good idea for you to learn both the generic and brand names of your medicines and to write them down for future use.

Pyrethrins (pye-REE-thrins)-containing medicine is applied to the hair and scalp or skin to treat head, body, and pubic lice infections. This medicine is absorbed by the lice and destroys them by acting on their nervous systems. It does not affect humans in this way. The piperonyl butoxide (pye-PEER-i-nil byoo-TOX-ide) is included to make the pyrethrins more effective in killing the lice. This combination medicine is known as a pediculicide (pe-DIK-yoo-li-side).

This medicine is available without a prescription; however, your doctor may have special instructions on the proper use of this medicine for your medical condition.

Remember:

• **Keep all medicines out of the reach of children.**

• In order for this medicine to work, it must be used as directed. **If you are using this medicine without a prescription, it is very important to follow the directions on the label.**

• **It is also very important that you read and understand the following information.** If any of the information causes you special concern, check with your doctor or pharmacist.

• Before you begin using any new medicine (prescription or nonprescription) or if you develop any new medical problem while you are using this medicine, check with your doctor, nurse, or pharmacist.

• **If you have any questions** about the following information or if you want more information about this medicine or your medical problem, **ask your doctor, nurse, or pharmacist.**

Before Using This Medicine

Before you use pyrethrins and piperonyl butoxide combination medicine, check with your doctor or pharmacist:

—if you have ever had any unusual or allergic reaction to pyrethrins.

—if you have ever had any unusual or allergic reaction to the ragweed or chrysanthemum plant.

—if you have ever had any unusual or allergic reaction to kerosene or other petroleum products. This medicine contains either kerosene or another petroleum product.

—if you are **pregnant** or if you may become pregnant. Pyrethrins and piperonyl butoxide may be absorbed through the skin. However, this medicine has not been shown to cause birth defects or other problems in humans when used on the skin.

—if you are **breast-feeding**, since pyrethrins and piperonyl butoxide may be absorbed through the skin. However, this medicine has not been shown to cause problems in humans when used on the skin.

—if you have severe inflammation of the skin.

Proper Use of This Medicine

Pyrethrins and piperonyl butoxide combination medicine usually comes with patient directions. Read them carefully before using this medicine.

Use this medicine only as directed. Do not use more of it and do not use it more often than recommended on the label. To do so may increase the chance of absorption through the skin and the chance of side effects.

Keep pyrethrins and piperonyl butoxide combination medicine away from the mouth and do not inhale it. This medicine is harmful if swallowed or inhaled.

To lessen the chance of inhaling this medicine, apply it in a well-ventilated room (for example, one with free flowing air or with a fan turned on).

Keep this medicine away from the eyes and other mucous membranes, such as the inside of the nose, because it may cause irritation. If you accidentally get some in your eyes, flush them thoroughly with water at once.

Do not apply this medicine to the eyelashes or eyebrows. If they become infected with lice, check with your doctor.

For patients using the gel or solution form of this medicine:

• Apply enough medicine to thoroughly wet the dry hair and scalp or skin. Allow the medicine to remain on the affected areas for exactly 10 minutes.

• Then, thoroughly wash the affected areas with warm water and soap or regular shampoo. Rinse thoroughly and dry with a clean towel.

For patients using the shampoo form of this medicine:

• Apply enough medicine to thoroughly wet the dry hair and scalp or skin. Allow the medicine to remain on the affected areas for exactly 10 minutes.

• Then use a small amount of water and work shampoo into the hair and scalp or skin until a lather forms. Rinse thoroughly and dry with a clean towel.

After rinsing and drying, use a nit removal comb (special fine-toothed comb, usually included with this medicine) to remove the dead lice and eggs (nits) from hair.

Immediately after using this medicine, wash your hands to remove any medicine that may be on them.

This medicine should be used again in 7 to 10 days after the first treatment in order to kill any newly hatched lice.

Lice can easily move from one person to another by close body contact. This can happen also by direct contact with such things as clothing, hats, scarves, bedding, towels, washcloths, hairbrushes and combs, or the hair of infected persons. Therefore, **all members of your household should be examined for lice and receive treatment if they are found to be infected.**

For patients using this medicine for pubic (crab) lice:
• Your sexual partner may also need to be treated since the infection may spread to persons in close contact. If your partner is not being treated or if you have any questions about this, check with your doctor.

How to store this medicine:
• **Keep out of the reach of children.**
• Store away from heat and direct light.
• Keep the medicine from freezing.
• Do not keep outdated medicine or medicine no longer needed. Be sure that any discarded medicine is out of the reach of children.

Precautions While Using This Medicine

To prevent reinfection or spreading of the infection to other people, good health habits are also required. These include the following:
• For head lice
    —Machine wash all clothing (including hats, scarves, and coats), bedding, towels, and washcloths in very hot water and dry them by using the hot cycle of a dryer for at least 20 minutes. Clothing or bedding that cannot be washed should be dry cleaned, or sealed in a plastic bag for 2 weeks.
    —Shampoo all wigs and hairpieces.
    —Wash all hairbrushes and combs in very hot soapy water (above 130 °F) for 5 to 10 minutes and do not share them with other people.
    —Clean the house or room by thoroughly vacuuming upholstered furniture, rugs, and floors.

• For body lice
    —Machine wash all clothing, bedding, towels, and washcloths in very hot water and dry them by using the hot cycle of a dryer for at least 20 minutes. Clothing or bedding that cannot be washed should be dry cleaned.
    —Clean the house or room by thoroughly vacuuming upholstered furniture, rugs, and floors.
• For pubic lice
    —Machine wash all clothing (especially underwear), bedding, towels, and washcloths in very hot water and dry them by using the hot cycle of a dryer for at least 20 minutes. Clothing or bedding that cannot be washed should be dry cleaned, or sealed in a plastic bag for 2 weeks.
    —Scrub toilet seats frequently.

Side Effects of This Medicine

Along with its needed effects, a medicine may cause some unwanted effects. Although not all of these side effects may occur, if they do occur they may need medical attention.

Check with your doctor as soon as possible if any of the following side effects occur:
Less common or rare
    Skin irritation not present before using this medicine
    Skin rash or infection
    Sneezing (sudden attacks of)
    Stuffy or runny nose
    Wheezing or difficulty in breathing

For elderly patients: Many medicines have not been tested in older people. Therefore, it is not known whether the medicine acts the same way it does in younger adults. Check with your doctor or pharmacist if you notice any unusual effects while using this medicine or if you think it is not working as it should.

Other side effects not listed above may also occur in some patients. If you notice any other effects, check with your doctor or pharmacist.

December 1987

PYRIDOXINE (VITAMIN B$_6$) (Systemic)

Some commonly used brand names are:

Beesix	Rodex
Hexa-Betalin	TexSix T.R.
Pyroxine	

Generic name product may also be available in the U.S. and Canada.

To the Reader: If you do not recognize the names of medical conditions or medicines referred to in this information, check with your doctor, nurse, or pharmacist. Definitions for selected medical terms may be found in the Glossary. Brand names for the generic drug names listed can be found in the Index. In addition, selected brand names commonly associated with the generic name have been included in the text to help you recognize medicine you may be taking. The fact that a brand name product is not mentioned does not mean the information does not apply. It is a good idea for you to learn both the generic and brand names of your medicines and to write them down for future use.

Vitamins (VYE-ta-mins) are compounds that you *must* have for growth and health. They are needed in small amounts only and are usually available in the foods that you eat. Pyridoxine (peer-i-DOX-een) (vitamin B$_6$) is necessary for normal metabolism.

Lack of pyridoxine may lead to anemia (weak blood), nerve damage, seizures, skin problems, and sores in the mouth. Your doctor may treat this by prescribing pyridoxine for you.

Claims that pyridoxine is effective for treatment of acne and other skin problems, alcohol intoxication, asthma, hemorrhoids, kidney stones, mental problems, migraine headaches, morning sickness, and menstrual problems, or to stimulate appetite or milk production have not been proven.

Oral forms of pyridoxine are available without a prescription. However, it may be a good idea to check with your doctor before taking any on your own.

Remember:

• **Keep all medicines out of the reach of children.**

• In order for this medicine to work, it must be used as directed. **If you are using this medicine without a prescription, it is very important to follow the directions on the label.**

• **It is also very important that you read and understand the following information.** If any of the information causes you special concern, check with your doctor or pharmacist.

• Before you begin using any new medicine (prescription or nonprescription) or if you develop any new medical problem while you are using this medicine, check with your doctor, nurse, or pharmacist.

• **If you have any questions** about the following information or if you want more information about this medicine or your medical problem, **ask your doctor, nurse, or pharmacist.**

Importance of Diet

Vitamin supplements should be taken only if you cannot get enough vitamins in your diet. A balanced diet should provide all the vitamins you normally need.

Nutritionists recommend that you eat:
• Cereal or bread—4 or more servings per day and
• Dairy products (milk, cheese, ice cream, cottage cheese)—3 or more servings per day and
• Meat, fish, or eggs—2 or more servings per day and
• Vegetables and fruits—4 or more servings per day.

If you are not getting all of these foods every day, you may not be getting enough vitamins in your diet. The best way to correct this is to start eating the foods that contain what you need.

Pyridoxine is found in various foods, including meats, bananas, potatoes, lima beans, and whole-grain cereals. Pyridoxine is not lost from food during ordinary cooking, although some other forms of vitamin B$_6$ are.

Vitamins alone will not take the place of a good diet and will not provide energy. Your body also needs other substances found in food such as protein, minerals, carbohydrates, and fat. Vitamins themselves often cannot work without the presence of other foods.

In some cases, it may not be possible for you to get enough food to supply you with the proper vitamins. In other cases, the amount of vitamins you need may be increased above normal. Therefore, a vitamin supplement may be needed.

Experts have developed a list of recommended dietary allowances (RDA) for most of the vitamins. The RDA are not an exact number but a general idea of how much you need. They do not cover amounts needed for problems caused by a serious lack of vitamins.

The RDA for pyridoxine are:

Children 4 to 6 years of age—1.3 mg per day
Adult males—2.2 mg per day
Adult females—2.0 mg per day
Pregnant females—2.6 mg per day
Breast-feeding females—2.5 mg per day.

Remember:

• The total amount of each vitamin that you get every day includes what you get from the foods that you eat *and* what you may take as a supplement.

• This total amount should not be greater than the RDA, unless ordered by your doctor.

Before Using This Medicine

In deciding whether you need additional pyridoxine, the following should be kept in mind and/or your doctor or pharmacist should be told:

—if you have ever had any unusual or allergic reaction to pyridoxine.

—if you are on a low-salt, low-sugar, or any other special diet, or if you are allergic to any substance, such as foods, sulfites or other preservatives, or dyes. Most medicines contain more than their active ingredient. Your doctor, nurse, or pharmacist can help you avoid products that may cause a problem.

—if you are **pregnant** or if you may become pregnant. It is especially important that you are receiving enough vitamins when you become pregnant and that you continue to receive the right amount of vitamins throughout your pregnancy. The healthy growth and development of the fetus depend on a steady supply of nutrients from the mother.

—if you are **breast-feeding**. It is especially important that you receive the right amounts of vitamins so that your baby will also get the vitamins needed to grow properly. You should also check with your doctor if you are giving your baby an unfortified formula. In that case, the baby must get the vitamins needed some other way.

—if you are not able to get a diet that contains all of the vitamins you need. This may occur with rapid weight loss, unusual diets (such as some reducing diets in which choice of foods is very limited), prolonged intravenous feeding, or malnutrition.

—if you have had a large part of your stomach removed.

—if you have been under a lot of stress for a long time, or if you have had a long illness or serious injury.

—if you have any of the following medical problems:
  Alcoholism
  Burns
  Diarrhea (prolonged)
  Heart disease
  Intestinal problems
  Liver disease
  Overactive thyroid
  Parkinson's disease

—if you are taking **any** other prescription or nonprescription (OTC) medicine, especially levodopa (e.g., Larodopa).

Proper Use of This Medicine

Do not take more than the recommended daily amount. Taking too much pyridoxine may cause harmful effects, such as nerve damage, which may appear as clumsiness, or numbness of hands or feet. Some people believe that taking very large doses of vitamins (called megadoses or megavitamin therapy) is useful for treating certain medical problems. Studies have not proven this. Large doses should be taken only under the direction of your doctor after need has been identified.

For patients taking the extended-release capsule form of this medicine:

• Swallow the capsule whole.

• Do not crush, break, or chew before swallowing.

• If the capsule is too large to swallow, you may mix the contents of the capsule with jam or jelly and swallow without chewing.

If you miss taking a vitamin for one or more days there is no cause for concern, since it takes some time for your body to become seriously low in vitamins. However, if your doctor has recommended that you take this vitamin, try to remember to take it as directed every day.

How to store this medicine:

• **Keep out of the reach of children.**

• Store away from heat and direct light.

• Do not store the capsule or tablet form of this medicine in the bathroom, near the kitchen sink, or in other damp places. Heat or moisture may cause the medicine to break down.

• Do not keep outdated medicine or medicine no longer needed. Be sure that any discarded medicine is out of the reach of children.

Side Effects of This Medicine

Along with its needed effects, a medicine may cause some unwanted effects. Although pyridoxine does not usually cause any side effects, check with your doctor as soon as possible if you notice either of the following side effects:

With large doses
  Clumsiness
  Numbness of hands or feet

Also check with your doctor if you notice any other unusual effects while you are taking pyridoxine.

_____

December 1987

PYRIMETHAMINE (Systemic)

A commonly used brand name is Daraprim.

To the Reader: If you do not recognize the names of medical conditions or medicines referred to in this information, check with your doctor, nurse, or pharmacist. Definitions for selected medical terms may be found in the Glossary. Brand names for the generic drug names listed can be found in the Index. In addition, selected brand names commonly associated with the generic name have been included in the text to help you recognize medicine you may be taking. The fact that a brand name product is not mentioned does not mean the information does not apply. It is a good idea for you to learn both the generic and brand names of your medicines and to write them down for future use.

Pyrimethamine (peer-i-METH-a-meen) belongs to the family of medicines called antiprotozoals. Protozoa are tiny, one-celled animals. Some are parasites that can cause many different kinds of infections in the body.

This medicine is taken alone by mouth to prevent one such infection, malaria. It is also taken with one or more other medicines to help the body overcome malaria and toxoplasmosis. This medicine may also be used for other problems as determined by your doctor.

Pyrimethamine is available only with your doctor's prescription.

Remember:

• **This medicine has been prescribed for your present infection only.** Another infection later on may require a different medicine. Also, even though other people may have the same symptoms as you, they may have a different kind of infection. Your medicine may not work for them and may even cause them harm. Therefore, **your medicine must not be given to other people or used for other infections** unless you are otherwise directed by your doctor.

• **Keep all medicines out of the reach of children.**

• In order for this medicine to work, it must be used as directed.

• **It is very important that you read and understand the following information.** If any of the information causes you special concern, do not decide against using this medicine without first checking with your doctor.

• Before you begin using any new medicine (prescription or nonprescription) or if you develop any new medical problem while you are using this medicine, check with your doctor, nurse, or pharmacist.

• **If you have any questions** about the following information or if you want more information about this medicine or your medical problem, **ask your doctor, nurse, or pharmacist.**

Before Using This Medicine

In order to decide on the best treatment for your medical problem, your doctor should be told:

—if you have ever had any unusual or allergic reaction to pyrimethamine.

—if you are on a low-salt, low-sugar, or any other special diet, or if you are allergic to any substance, such as foods, sulfites or other preservatives, or dyes.

Most medicines contain more than their active ingredient. Your doctor, nurse, or pharmacist can help you avoid products that may cause a problem.

—if you are **pregnant** or if you may become pregnant. Studies have not been done in humans. However, use is not recommended during pregnancy since studies in animals have shown that pyrimethamine may cause birth defects, anemia, or other problems.

—if you are **breast-feeding**. Pyrimethamine passes into the breast milk and may cause anemia and other unwanted effects in nursing babies, especially if the baby has glucose-6-phosphate dehydrogenase (G6PD) deficiency.

—if you have any of the following medical problems:
Anemia
Convulsive disorders, such as epilepsy
Glucose-6-phosphate dehydrogenase (G6PD) deficiency
Liver disease

—if you are taking **any** other prescription or nonprescription (OTC) medicine.

Proper Use of This Medicine

Keep this medicine out of the reach of children since overdose is especially dangerous in children.

If this medicine upsets your stomach or causes vomiting, it may be taken with meals or a snack.

For patients taking this medicine to prevent malaria:

• Your doctor may want you to start taking this medicine 2 weeks before you travel to an area where there is a chance of getting malaria. This will build up a supply of medicine in your body so that you will be protected from malaria at the start of your travels. It will also help you to get used to taking the medicine regularly and to see how you react to it.

• Also, you should keep taking this medicine while you are in the area and for 6 weeks after you leave the area. To protect you completely, **it is important that you keep taking this medicine for the full time your doctor ordered.**

If you are taking this medicine to help protect yourself from malaria, **keep taking it for the full time of treatment.** If you already have malaria, you should still keep taking this medicine for the full time of treatment even if you begin to feel better after a few days. This will help to clear up your infection completely. If you stop taking this medicine too soon, your symptoms may return.

This medicine works best when you take it on a regular schedule. For example, if you are to take it once a week to prevent malaria, it is best to take it on the same day each week. If you are to take 2 doses a day, one dose may be taken with breakfast and the other one with the evening meal. **Make sure that you do not miss any doses.** If you have any questions about this, check with your doctor, nurse, or pharmacist.

If you do miss a dose of this medicine, take it as soon as possible. This will help to keep you taking your medicine on a regular schedule. However, if it is almost time for your next dose, skip the missed dose and go back to your regular dosing schedule. Do not double doses.

How to store this medicine:

- **Keep out of the reach of children.**

- Store away from heat and direct light.

- Do not store in the bathroom, near the kitchen sink, or in other damp places. Heat or moisture may cause the medicine to break down.

- Do not keep outdated medicine or medicine no longer needed. Be sure that any discarded medicine is out of the reach of children.

Precautions While Using This Medicine

It is important that your doctor check your progress at regular visits, especially if you will be taking this medicine in high doses for toxoplasmosis. This will allow your doctor to check for any unwanted effects that may be caused by this medicine.

If your symptoms do not improve within a few days (for malaria), or if they become worse, check with your doctor.

If this medicine causes anemia, your doctor may want you to take folinic or folic acid (a vitamin) every day to help clear up the anemia. If so, it is important to take folinic or folic acid every day along with this medicine. Do not miss any doses.

Pyrimethamine, especially in high doses, may cause blood problems. These problems may result in a greater chance of infection, slow healing, and bleeding of the gums. Therefore, you should be careful when using toothbrushes, dental floss, and toothpicks. Dental work should be delayed until your blood counts have returned to normal. Check with your physician or dentist if you have any questions about proper oral hygiene (mouth care) during treatment.

If you are living in or will be traveling to an area where there is a chance of getting malaria, the following measures will help to prevent malaria or malaria reinfection:

- If possible, sleep under mosquito netting to avoid being bitten by malaria-carrying mosquitoes.

- Wear long-sleeved shirts or blouses and long trousers to protect arms and legs, especially at dawn or dusk or during evening hours when mosquitoes are out.

- Apply mosquito repellant to uncovered areas of the skin when mosquitoes are out.

Side Effects of This Medicine

Along with its needed effects, a medicine may cause some unwanted effects. Although not all of these side effects may occur, if they do occur they may need medical attention.

Check with your doctor immediately if any of the following side effects occur:

More common with high doses
    Change in or loss of taste
    Diarrhea
    Irritation of throat or difficulty in swallowing
    Soreness, redness, swelling, burning, or stinging of tongue
    Sore throat and fever
    Ulcers, sores, or white spots in mouth
    Unusual bleeding or bruising
    Unusual tiredness or weakness

Rare
    Skin rash

Signs of overdose
    Clumsiness or unsteadiness
    Convulsions (seizures)
    Trembling

Other side effects may occur that usually do not require medical attention. These side effects may go away during treatment as your body adjusts to the medicine. However, check with your doctor if either of the following side effects continues or is bothersome:

More common with high doses
    Loss of appetite
    Vomiting

For elderly patients: Many medicines have not been tested in older people. Therefore, it is not known whether the medicine acts the same way it does in younger adults. Check with your doctor or pharmacist if you notice any unusual effects while taking this medicine or if you think it is not working as it should.

Other side effects not listed above may also occur in some patients. If you notice any other effects, check with your doctor.

December 1987

PYRITHIONE (Topical)

Some commonly used brand names are:

Danex	Sebex
Dan-Gard*	Sebulon
DHS Zinc	Zincon
Head and Shoulders	ZNP

*Not available in the U.S.

To the Reader: If you do not recognize the names of medical conditions or medicines referred to in this information, check with your doctor, nurse, or pharmacist. Definitions for selected medical terms may be found in the Glossary. Brand names for the generic drug names listed can be found in the Index. In addition, selected brand names commonly associated with the generic name have been included in the text to help you recognize medicine you may be taking. The fact that a brand name product is not mentioned does not mean the information does not apply. It is a good idea for you to learn both the generic and brand names of your medicines and to write them down for future use.

Pyrithione (peer-i-THYE-one) is used as a shampoo to help control dandruff and seborrheic dermatitis of the scalp.

This medicine is available without a prescription; however, your doctor may have special instructions on the proper use of this medicine for your medical condition.

Remember:

• **Keep all medicines out of the reach of children.**

• In order for this medicine to work, it must be used as directed. **If you are using this medicine without a prescription, it is very important to follow the directions on the label.**

• **It is also very important that you read and understand the following information.** If any of the information causes you special concern, check with your doctor or pharmacist.

• Before you begin using any new medicine (prescription or nonprescription) or if you develop any new medical problem while you are using this medicine, check with your doctor, nurse, or pharmacist.

• **If you have any questions** about the following information or if you want more information about this medicine or your medical problem, **ask your doctor, nurse, or pharmacist.**

Before Using This Medicine

Before you use pyrithione, check with your doctor or pharmacist:

—if you have ever had any unusual or allergic reaction to pyrithione.

—if you are allergic to any substance, such as certain preservatives or dyes. Most medicines contain more than their active ingredient, and many liquid medicines contain alcohol. Your doctor or pharmacist can help you avoid products that may cause a problem.

—if you are **pregnant** or if you may become pregnant, although pyrithione has not been shown to cause birth defects or other problems in humans.

—if you are **breast-feeding**, although pyrithione has not been shown to cause problems in nursing babies.

Proper Use of This Medicine

Before applying this shampoo, wet the hair and scalp with lukewarm water. Apply enough shampoo to the scalp to work up a lather and rub in well, then rinse. Apply the shampoo again and rinse thoroughly.

Keep this medicine away from the eyes. If you should accidentally get some in your eyes, flush them thoroughly with water.

How to store this medicine:

• **Keep out of the reach of children.**

• Store away from heat and direct light.

• Keep the medicine from freezing.

• Do not keep outdated medicine or medicine no longer needed. Be sure that any discarded medicine is out of the reach of children.

Side Effects of This Medicine

Along with its needed effects, a medicine may cause some unwanted effects. Although not all of these side effects may occur, if they do occur they may need medical attention.

Check with your doctor as soon as possible if the following side effect occurs:

Irritation of skin

For elderly patients: Many medicines have not been tested in older people. Therefore, it is not known whether the medicine acts the same way it does in younger adults. Check with your doctor or pharmacist if you notice any unusual effects while using this medicine or if you think it is not working as it should.

Other side effects not listed above may also occur in some patients. If you notice any other effects, check with your doctor or pharmacist.

December 1987

PYRVINIUM (Oral)*

Some commonly used brand names or other names are Vanquin* and Viprynium.

*Not commercially available in the U.S.

To the Reader: If you do not recognize the names of medical conditions or medicines referred to in this information, check with your doctor, nurse, or pharmacist. Definitions for selected medical terms may be found in the Glossary. Brand names for the generic drug names listed can be found in the Index. In addition, selected brand names commonly associated with the generic name have been included in the text to help you recognize medicine you may be taking. The fact that a brand name product is not mentioned does not mean the information does not apply. It is a good idea for you to learn both the generic and brand names of your medicines and to write them down for future use.

Pyrvinium (peer-VIN-ee-um) belongs to the family of medicines called anthelmintics (ant-hel-MIN-tiks). Anthelmintics are used in the treatment of worm infections.

Pyrvinium is taken by mouth to treat pinworms (enterobiasis; oxyuriasis). It will not work for other types of worm infections (for example, roundworms or tapeworms).

Pyrvinium is available only with your doctor's prescription.

Remember:

• **This medicine has been prescribed for your present infection only.** Another infection later on may require a different medicine. Also, even though other people may have the same symptoms as you, they may have a different kind of infection. Your medicine may not work for them and may even cause them harm. Therefore, **your medicine must not be given to other people or used for other infections** unless you are otherwise directed by your doctor.

• **Keep all medicines out of the reach of children.**

• In order for this medicine to work, it must be used as directed.

• **It is very important that you read and understand the following information.** If any of the information causes you special concern, do not decide against using this medicine without first checking with your doctor.

• Before you begin using any new medicine (prescription or nonprescription) or if you develop any new medical problem while you are using this medicine, check with your doctor, nurse, or pharmacist.

• **If you have any questions** about the following information or if you want more information about this medicine or your medical problem, **ask your doctor, nurse, or pharmacist.**

Before Using This Medicine

In order to decide on the best treatment for your medical problem, your doctor should be told:

—if you have ever had any unusual or allergic reaction to pyrvinium.

—if you are on a low-salt, low-sugar, or any other special diet, or if you are allergic to any substance, such as foods, sulfites or other preservatives, or dyes.

Most medicines contain more than their active ingredient. Your doctor, nurse, or pharmacist can help you avoid products that may cause a problem.

—if you are **pregnant** or if you may become pregnant. However, pyrvinium has not been shown to cause birth defects or other problems in humans.

—if you are **breast-feeding**. However, pyrvinium has not been shown to cause problems in nursing babies.

—if you have any of the following medical problems:
Inflammatory bowel disease
Kidney disease
Liver disease

Proper Use of This Medicine

No special preparations (for example, special diets, fasting, other medicines, laxatives, or enemas) are necessary before, during, or immediately after you take pyrvinium.

Do not chew or crush the tablets. Swallow them whole. They are coated to prevent staining of your teeth.

Pinworms may be easily passed from one person to another, especially among persons in the same household. Therefore, all household members may have to be treated at the same time to prevent their infection or reinfection. Also, all household members may have to be treated again in 2 to 3 weeks to clear up the infection completely. Make sure each family member takes the correct amount, since the dose may be different for each person.

To help clear up your infection completely, **take this medicine exactly as directed by your doctor.** Read the instructions on the label and follow them carefully. The amount of medicine you need is based on your weight. You must take the exact amount if the medicine is going to work. A second course of pyrvinium is usually required to clear up the infection completely.

How to store this medicine:

• **Keep out of the reach of children.**

• Store away from heat and direct light.

• Do not store in the bathroom, near the kitchen sink, or in other damp places. Heat or moisture may cause the medicine to break down.

• Do not keep outdated medicine or medicine no longer needed. Be sure that any discarded medicine is out of the reach of children.

Precautions While Using This Medicine

If your symptoms do not improve within a few days, or if they become worse, check with your doctor.

Some people who take pyrvinium may become more sensitive to sunlight than they are normally. This reaction usually lasts only a few days. **However, when you first begin taking this medicine, avoid too much sun and do not use a sunlamp until you see how you react to the** sun, especially if you tend to burn easily. **If you have a severe reaction, check with your doctor.**

This medicine may also cause some people to become dizzy. **Make sure you know how you react to this medicine before you drive, use machines, or do other jobs that require you to be alert.** If this reaction is especially bothersome, check with your doctor.

In some patients, pinworms may return after treatment with pyrvinium. Washing (not shaking) all bedding and nightclothes (pajamas) after treatment may help to prevent this. Some doctors may also recommend other measures to help keep your infection from returning. If you have any questions about this, check with your doctor.

Side Effects of This Medicine

Along with its needed effects, a medicine may cause some unwanted effects. Although not all of these side effects may occur, if they do occur they may need medical attention.

Check with your doctor as soon as possible if the following side effect occurs:
Rare
    Skin rash

Other side effects may occur that usually do not require medical attention. These side effects may go away during treatment as your body adjusts to the medicine. However, check with your doctor if any of the following side effects continue or are bothersome:
Rare
    Diarrhea
    Dizziness
    Increased sensitivity of skin to sunlight
    Nausea and vomiting
    Stomach cramps

This medicine is a dye and will color your stools red. This color is not harmful and will disappear in a few days. Pyrvinium may also stain clothing red. If vomiting occurs, the vomit will be red in color.

For elderly patients: Many medicines have not been tested in older people. Therefore, it is not known whether the medicine acts the same way it does in younger adults. Check with your doctor or pharmacist if you notice any unusual effects while taking this medicine or if you think it is not working as it should.

Other side effects not listed above may also occur in some patients. If you notice any other effects, check with your doctor.

December 1987

QUINIDINE (Systemic)

Some commonly used brand names are:

Apo-Quinidine*	Quinaglute Dura-tabs
Cardioquin	Quinalan
Cin-Quin	Quinate*
Duraquin	Quinidex Extentabs
Novoquinidin*	Quinora

Generic name product may also be available in the U.S.

---

*Not available in the U.S.

To the Reader: If you do not recognize the names of medical conditions or medicines referred to in this information, check with your doctor, nurse, or pharmacist. Definitions for selected medical terms may be found in the Glossary. Brand names for the generic drug names listed can be found in the Index. In addition, selected brand names commonly associated with the generic name have been included in the text to help you recognize medicine you may be taking. The fact that a brand name product is not mentioned does not mean the information does not apply. It is a good idea for you to learn both the generic and brand names of your medicines and to write them down for future use.

Quinidine (KWIN-i-deen) is most often used to correct certain irregular heartbeats to a normal rhythm and to slow an overactive heart. It is also sometimes used for other conditions as determined by your doctor.

Quinidine acts directly on the heart tissues to make them less responsive. It also slows impulses along special nerve networks to the heart. This allows the heart to work more efficiently.

Do not confuse this medicine with *quinine*, which, although related, has different medical uses.

Quinidine is available only with your doctor's prescription.

Remember:

• **This medicine has been prescribed for your current medical problem only.** It must not be given to other people or used for other problems unless you are directed to do so by your doctor.

• **Keep all medicines out of the reach of children.**

• In order for this medicine to work, it must be used as directed.

• If you are receiving this medicine by injection, some of the information about this medicine may not apply.

• **It is very important that you read and understand the following information.** If any of the information causes you special concern, do not decide against using this medicine without first checking with your doctor.

• Before you begin using any new medicine (prescription or nonprescription) or if you develop any new medical problem while you are using this medicine, check with your doctor, nurse, or pharmacist.

• **If you have any questions** about the following information or if you want more information about this medicine or your medical problem, **ask your doctor, nurse, or pharmacist.**

Before Using This Medicine

In order to decide on the best treatment for your medical problem, your doctor should be told:

—if you have ever had any unusual or allergic reaction to quinidine or quinine.

—if you are on a low-salt, low-sugar, or any other special diet, or if you are allergic to any substance, such as foods, sulfites or other preservatives, or dyes. Most medicines contain more than their active ingredient. Your doctor, nurse, or pharmacist can help you avoid products that may cause a problem.

—if you are **pregnant** or if you may become pregnant. Although studies have not been done in either humans or animals, a closely related medicine, quinine, has been shown to cause birth defects of the nervous system, fingers, and toes and decreased hearing in the infant. Quinine also may cause contractions of the uterus.

—if you are **breast-feeding**. Although quinidine passes into the breast milk, it has not been reported to cause problems in nursing babies.

—if you have any of the following medical problems:
Asthma or emphysema
Blood disease
Infection
Kidney disease
Liver disease
Myasthenia gravis
Overactive thyroid
Psoriasis

—if you are taking **any** other prescription or nonprescription (OTC) medicine, especially:
Anticoagulants (blood thinners).
Other heart medicine (especially digoxin).
Pimozide (e.g., Orap)
Urinary alkalizers (medicine that makes the urine less acid, such as acetazolamide, calcium- and/or magnesium-containing antacids, dichlorphenamide, methazolamide, potassium or sodium citrate and/or citric acid, sodium bicarbonate [baking soda])

Proper Use of This Medicine

Take quinidine with a full glass (8 ounces) of water on an empty stomach 1 hour before or 2 hours after meals so that it will be absorbed more quickly. However, to lessen stomach upset, your doctor may want you to take the medicine with food or milk.

For patients taking the extended-release tablet form of this medicine:

• These tablets are to be swallowed whole.

• Do not break, crush, or chew before swallowing.

Take quinidine exactly as directed by your doctor even though you may feel well. Do not take more medicine than ordered and do not miss any doses.

If you do miss a dose of this medicine and remember within 2 hours of the missed dose, take it as soon as possible. However, if you do not remember until later, skip the missed dose and go back to your regular dosing schedule. Do not double doses.

How to store this medicine:

- **Keep out of the reach of children.**

- Store away from heat and direct light.

- Do not store in the bathroom, near the kitchen sink, or in other damp places. Heat or moisture may cause the medicine to break down.

- Do not keep outdated medicine or medicine no longer needed. Be sure that any discarded medicine is out of the reach of children.

Precautions While Using This Medicine

It is very important that your doctor check your progress at regular visits to make sure that the quinidine is working properly and does not cause unwanted effects.

Do not stop taking this medicine without first checking with your doctor, in order to avoid possible worsening of your condition.

Before having any kind of surgery (including dental surgery) or emergency treatment, tell the physician or dentist in charge that you are taking this medicine.

Your doctor may want you to carry a medical identification card or bracelet stating that you are using this medicine.

Some people who are unusually sensitive to this medicine may have side effects after the first dose or first few doses. Check with your doctor right away if the following side effects occur: breathing difficulty, changes in vision, dizziness, fever, headache, ringing in ears, or skin rash.

Side Effects of This Medicine

Along with its needed effects, a medicine may cause some unwanted effects. Although not all of these side effects may occur, if they do occur they may need medical attention.

Check with your doctor immediately if any of the following side effects occur:

Less common
Blurred vision or any change in vision
Dizziness, lightheadedness, or fainting
Fever
Headache (severe)
Ringing or buzzing in the ears or any loss of hearing
Skin rash, hives, or itching
Wheezing, shortness of breath, or troubled breathing

Rare
Fast heartbeat
Unusual bleeding or bruising
Unusual tiredness or weakness

Other side effects may occur that usually do not require medical attention. These side effects may go away during treatment as your body adjusts to the medicine. However, check with your doctor if any of the following side effects continue or are bothersome:

More common
Bitter taste
Diarrhea
Flushing of skin with itching
Loss of appetite
Nausea or vomiting
Stomach pain or cramping

Less common
Confusion

For elderly patients: Many medicines have not been tested in older people. Therefore, it is not known whether the medicine acts the same way it does in younger adults. Check with your doctor or pharmacist if you notice any unusual effects while taking this medicine or if you think it is not working as it should.

Other side effects not listed above may also occur in some patients. If you notice any other effects, check with your doctor.

December 1987

QUININE (Systemic)

Some commonly used brand names are Quinamm, Quinite, and Strema.

Generic name product may also be available in the U.S.

To the Reader: If you do not recognize the names of medical conditions or medicines referred to in this information, check with your doctor, nurse, or pharmacist. Definitions for selected medical terms may be found in the Glossary. Brand names for the generic drug names listed can be found in the Index. In addition, selected brand names commonly associated with the generic name have been included in the text to help you recognize medicine you may be taking. The fact that a brand name product is not mentioned does not mean the information does not apply. It is a good idea for you to learn both the generic and brand names of your medicines and to write them down for future use.

Quinine (KWYE-nine) belongs to the group of medicines called antiprotozoals. It is used in the treatment of malaria and to treat and prevent nighttime leg muscle cramps. Quinine may also be used for other conditions as determined by your doctor. Do not confuse this medicine with quinidine, which is a different medicine used for heart problems.

Quinine is available without a prescription; however, your doctor may have special instructions on the proper dose of quinine for your medical condition.

Remember:
• If this medicine has been ordered by your doctor, it has been prescribed for your present medical problem only. Even though other people may have the same symptoms as you, they may have a different kind of problem. Your medicine may not work for them and may even cause them harm. Therefore, **your medicine must not be given to other people or used for other problems** unless you are otherwise directed by your doctor.

• In order for this medicine to work, it must be taken as directed.

• Keep all medicines out of the reach of children.

• If you want more information about this medicine, ask your doctor, nurse, or pharmacist.

• If this medicine has been ordered by your doctor and if any of the following information causes you special concern, do not decide against taking this medicine without first checking with your doctor.

Before Using This Medicine

Before you use quinine, your doctor should be told:

—if you have ever had any unusual or allergic reaction to quinine or quinidine.

—if you are **pregnant** or if you may become pregnant. Quinine may cause birth defects if taken during pregnancy. Also, if too much of this medicine is taken during pregnancy, it may cause hearing problems in the infant.

—if you are **breast-feeding**. Quinine passes into the breast milk. However, this medicine has not been shown to cause problems in nursing babies.

—if you have any of the following medical problems:
    Asthma (or history of)
    Eye disease
    Glucose-6-phosphate dehydrogenase (G6PD) deficiency
    Hearing problems
    Heart disease
    Myasthenia gravis

—if you are taking **any** other prescription or nonprescription (OTC) medicine.

Proper Use of This Medicine

Take this medicine only as directed. Do not take more of it, do not take it more often, and do not take it for a longer period of time than recommended on the label, unless otherwise directed by your doctor. To do so may increase the chance of side effects.

Take this medicine with or after meals to lessen possible stomach upset, unless otherwise directed by your doctor. If you are to take this medicine at bedtime, take it with a snack or with a glass of water, milk, or other beverage.

If you are taking this medicine regularly (for example, every day) and you miss a dose, take it right away if you remember within an hour or so of the missed dose. Then go back to your regular dosing schedule. But if you do not remember until later, do not take the missed dose at all and do not double the next one. Instead, go back to your regular dosing schedule. If you have any questions about this, check with your doctor.

If you are taking this medicine for malaria, **keep taking it for the full time of treatment** to help clear up the infection completely, even if you begin to feel better after a few days.

How to store this medicine:

• **Keep out of the reach of children.**

• Store away from heat and direct light.

• Do not store in the bathroom, near the kitchen sink, or in other damp places. Heat or moisture may cause the medicine to break down.

• Do not keep outdated medicine or medicine no longer needed. Be sure that any discarded medicine is out of the reach of children.

Side Effects of This Medicine

Along with its needed effects, a medicine may cause some unwanted effects. Although not all of these side effects may occur, if they do occur they may need medical attention.

Check with your doctor as soon as possible if any of the following side effects occur:

More common
    Blurred vision or any change in vision
    Dizziness
    Headache (severe)
    Ringing or buzzing in ears or any loss of hearing

Less common

  Skin rash, hives, or itching
  Wheezing, shortness of breath, or troubled breathing

Rare

  Sore throat and fever
  Unusual bleeding or bruising
  Unusual tiredness or weakness

Other side effects may occur that usually do not require medical attention. These side effects may go away during treatment as your body adjusts to the medicine.

However, check with your doctor if any of the following side effects continue or are bothersome:

More common

  Diarrhea
  Nausea or vomiting
  Stomach cramps or pain

Other side effects not listed above may also occur in some patients. If you notice any other effects, check with your doctor.

December 1987

RADIOPHARMACEUTICALS (Diagnostic)

This information applies to the following medicines when used for diagnosis:

Cyanocobalamin Co 57 (sye-an-oh-koe-BAL-a-min)
Cyanocobalamin Co 60
Ferrous Citrate Fe 59 (FER-us SI-trate)
Gallium Citrate Ga 67 (GAL-ee-um)
Indium In 111 Oxyquinoline (IN-dee-um ox-i-KWIN-oh-leen)
Indium In 111 Pentetate (PEN-te-tate)
Iodinated I 131 Albumin (EYE-oh-din-nay-ted al-BYOO-min)
Iodohippurate Sodium I 123 (eye-oh-doe-HIP-yoor-ate SOE-dee-um)
Iodohippurate Sodium I 131
Iothalamate Sodium I 125 (eye-oh-thal-A-mate)
Krypton Kr 81m (KRIP-tonn)
Selenomethionine Se 75 (se-le-noe-me-THYE-oh-neen)
Sodium Chromate Cr 51 (KROE-mate)
Sodium Iodide I 123 (EYE-oh-dyed)
Sodium Iodide I 131
Sodium Pertechnetate Tc 99m (per-TEK-ne-tate)
Sodium Phosphate P 32 (FOS-fate)
Technetium Tc 99m Albumin Aggregated (tek-NEE-see-um)
Technetium Tc 99m Antimony Trisulfide Colloid (AN-ti-moe-nee-try-SUL-fide KOLE-oid)
Technetium Tc 99m Disofenin (DYE-so-fen-in)
Technetium Tc 99m Gluceptate (gloo-SEP-tate)
Technetium Tc 99m Human Serum Albumin
Technetium Tc 99m Lidofenin (lye-doe-FEN-in)
Technetium Tc 99m Mebrofenin (ME-bro-fen-in)
Technetium Tc 99m Medronate (ME-droe-nate)
Technetium Tc 99m Oxidronate (OX-i-dron-ate)
Technetium Tc 99m Pentetate
Technetium Tc 99m Pyrophosphate (peer-oh-FOS-fate)
Technetium Tc 99m Sodium (Pyro- and trimeta-) Phosphates
Technetium Tc 99m Succimer (SUX-sim-mer)
Technetium Tc 99m Sulfur Colloid
Thallous Chloride Tl 201 (THA-luss KLOR-ide)
Xenon Xe 127 (ZEE-non)
Xenon Xe 133

Used in diagnosis of:	Generic names:
Abscess and infection	Gallium Citrate Ga 67 Indium In 111 Oxyquinoline
Biliary tract blockage	Technetium Tc 99m Disofenin Technetium Tc 99m Lidofenin Technetium Tc 99m Mebrofenin
Blood diseases	Technetium Tc 99m Sulfur Colloid
Blood flow and volume studies	Iodinated I 131 Albumin
Blood vessel diseases	Sodium Pertechnetate Tc 99m
Blood vessel diseases of the brain	Xenon Xe 127 Xenon Xe 133
Blood vessel diseases of the heart	Technetium Tc 99m Pyrophosphate Technetium Tc 99m Sodium (Pyro- and trimeta-) Phosphates
Bone diseases	Technetium Tc 99m Medronate Technetium Tc 99m Oxidronate Technetium Tc 99m Pyrophosphate Technetium Tc 99m Sodium (Pyro- and trimeta-) Phosphates
Bone marrow diseases	Technetium Tc 99m Sulfur Colloid
Brain diseases and tumors	Sodium Pertechnetate Tc 99m Technetium Tc 99m Gluceptate Technetium Tc 99m Pentetate
Breast cancer	Technetium Tc 99m Antimony Trisulfide Colloid
Cancer; tumors	Gallium Citrate Ga 67 Technetium Tc 99m Antimony Trisulfide Colloid
Disorders of iron metabolism and absorption	Ferrous Citrate Fe 59
Heart disease	Sodium Pertechnetate Tc 99m Technetium Tc 99m Human Serum Albumin Thallous Chloride Tl 201 Technetium Tc 99m Sodium (Pyro- and trimeta-) Phosphates
Heart infarct	Technetium Tc 99m Pyrophosphate Technetium Tc 99m Sodium (Pyro- and trimeta-) Phosphates
Impaired flow of cerebro-spinal fluid in brain	Indium In 111 Pentetate
Kidney diseases	Iodohippurate Sodium I 123 Iodohippurate Sodium I 131 Iothalamate Sodium I 125 Technetium Tc 99m Gluceptate Technetium Tc 99m Pentetate Technetium Tc 99m Succimer
Liver diseases	Technetium Tc 99m Disofenin Technetium Tc 99m Lidofenin Technetium Tc 99m Mebrofenin Technetium Tc 99m Sulfur Colloid
Lung diseases	Krypton Kr 81m Technetium Tc 99m Albumin Aggregated Xenon Xe 127 Xenon Xe 133
Pancreas diseases	Selenomethionine Se 75
Pernicious anemia; improper absorption of vitamin B_{12} from intestines	Cyanocobalamin Co 57 Cyanocobalamin Co 60
Red blood cell diseases	Sodium Chromate Cr 51
Salivary gland diseases	Sodium Pertechnetate Tc 99m
Spleen diseases	Sodium Chromate Cr 51 Technetium Tc 99m Sulfur Colloid
Stomach and intestinal bleeding	Sodium Chromate Cr 51 Technetium Tc 99m Sodium (Pyro- and trimeta-) Phosphates

Stomach problems	Technetium Tc 99m Sulfur Colloid
Tear duct blockage	Sodium Pertechnetate Tc 99m
Thyroid diseases; thyroid cancer	Sodium Iodide I 123 Sodium Iodide I 131 Sodium Pertechnetate Tc 99m
Urinary bladder diseases	Sodium Pertechnetate Tc 99m

To the Reader: If you do not recognize the names of medical conditions or medicines referred to in this information, check with your doctor, nurse, or pharmacist. Definitions for selected medical terms may be found in the Glossary. Brand names for the generic drug names listed can be found in the Index. In addition, selected brand names commonly associated with the generic name have been included in the text to help you recognize medicine you may be taking. The fact that a brand name product is not mentioned does not mean the information does not apply. It is a good idea for you to learn both the generic and brand names of your medicines and to write them down for future use.

Radiopharmaceuticals (ray-dee-oh-far-ma-SOO-ti-kals) are agents used to diagnose certain medical problems or treat certain diseases. They may be given to the patient in several different ways. For example, some are taken by mouth, given by injection, or placed into the eye or bladder.

Radiopharmaceuticals contain radioactivity. However, when small amounts are used, the radiation your body receives is very low and is considered safe. When larger amounts of these agents are given to treat disease, there may be different effects on the body.

When radiopharmaceuticals are used to help diagnose medical problems, only small amounts are given to the patient. The radioactivity from the radiopharmaceutical is then taken up by an organ of the body (which organ depends on what radiopharmaceutical is used and how it has been given). Then the radioactivity is measured, and readings or pictures are produced by special measuring equipment. These readings or pictures allow the nuclear medicine doctor to study the organ's activity.

Some radiopharmaceuticals are used in larger amounts to treat certain kinds of cancer. In those cases, the radioactive agent is taken up in the cancerous area and destroys the affected tissue. **The information that follows applies only to radiopharmaceuticals when used in small amounts to diagnose medical problems.**

Radiopharmaceuticals are to be given only by or under the direct supervision of a doctor with specialized training in nuclear medicine.

Remember:
• **It is very important that you read and understand the following information.** If any of the information causes you special concern, do not decide against receiving this agent without first checking with your doctor.

• **If you have any questions** about the following information or if you want more information about this agent or your medical problem, **ask your doctor, nuclear medicine physician and/or technologist, nuclear pharmacist, or nurse.**

Before Having This Test

Before this test is given, your doctor should be told:

—if you will be receiving radioactive iodine (iodinated I 131 albumin, iodohippurate sodium I 123, iodohippurate sodium I 131, sodium iodide I 123, or sodium iodide I 131) for your test and you have ever had any unusual or allergic reaction to iodine or to other products containing iodine (for example, seafood, cabbage, kale, rape [turnip-like vegetable] or turnips, or iodized salt).

—if you will be receiving albumin that contains radioactive iodine (iodinated I 131 albumin), technetium Tc 99m albumin aggregated, or technetium Tc 99m human serum albumin for your test and you have ever had any unusual or allergic reaction to products containing human serum albumin.

—if you are allergic to any substance, such as sulfites or other preservatives. Most medicines contain more than their active ingredient. Your doctor can help you avoid products that may cause a problem.

—if you are **pregnant** or if you may become pregnant soon after receiving this agent. Radiopharmaceuticals usually are not recommended for use during pregnancy. This is to avoid exposing the fetus to radiation. Also, radioactive iodine (iodinated I 131 albumin, iodohippurate sodium I 123, iodohippurate sodium I 131, iothalamate sodium I 125, sodium iodide I 123, and sodium iodide I 131) may cause the fetus to have an underactive thyroid gland. However, some tests using radiopharmaceuticals may be needed even during pregnancy. Be sure you have discussed this with your doctor.

—if you are **breast-feeding**. Some radiopharmaceuticals pass into the breast milk and may expose the baby to radiation. If you must receive a radiopharmaceutical, it may be necessary for you to stop breast-feeding for some time after receiving it. Be sure you have discussed this with your doctor.

—if you have any other medical problems.

—if you are also taking any other medicines.

—if you will be receiving radioactive iodine (sodium iodide I 123, sodium iodide I 131) or sodium pertechnetate Tc 99m for your test and you have been taking in iodine through other medicine or foods. For example, the results of your test may be affected if:

• you are taking iodine-containing medicines, including certain multivitamins and cough syrups.

• you eat large amounts of iodine-containing foods, such as iodized salt, seafood, cabbage, kale, rape (turnip-like vegetable) or turnips.

• you have had an x-ray test recently for which you were given a special dye that contained iodine.

Preparation for This Test

The nuclear medicine doctor may have special instructions for you in preparation for your test. For example, before some tests you must fast for several hours, or the results of the test may be affected. For other tests you should drink plenty of liquids and urinate often to lessen the amount of radiation to your bladder. If you do not understand the instructions you receive or if you have not received any instructions, check with the nuclear medicine doctor in advance.

Precautions After Having This Test

There are no special precautions to observe for most of the radiopharmaceuticals, when they are used in small amounts for diagnosis.

Some radiopharmaceuticals may accumulate in your bladder. Therefore, to increase the flow of urine and lessen the amount of radiation to your bladder, your doctor may instruct you to drink plenty of liquids and urinate often after certain tests.

For patients receiving radioactive iodine (iodinated I 131 albumin, iodohippurate sodium I 123, or iodohippurate sodium I 131):
• Make sure your doctor knows if you are planning to have any future thyroid tests. Even after several weeks, the results of the thyroid test may be affected by the iodine present in the Lugol's solution that may be given before the radiopharmaceutical.

For patients receiving sodium pertechnetate Tc 99m for tear duct tests:
• Rinse your eyes and blow your nose often to lessen the amount of radiation to the eyes and nose.

Side Effects of This Medicine

Along with its needed effects, a medicine may cause some unwanted effects. When radiopharmaceuticals are used in very small doses to study an organ of the body, side effects usually are rare. However, on occasion, some radiopharmaceuticals have caused serious side effects such as severe allergic reactions or heart problems. These effects may occur almost immediately or a few minutes after the radiopharmaceutical is given. It may be helpful to note the time when you first notice any side effect. Your doctor, nuclear medicine physician and/or technologist, or nurse will be prepared to give you immediate medical attention if needed.

Check with your doctor or nurse immediately if any of the following side effects occur:

Less common or rare
Chills
Drowsiness (severe)
Fainting
Fast heartbeat
Fever
Flushing or redness of skin
Headache (severe)
Loss of appetite (continuing)
Nausea or vomiting
Skin rash, hives, or itching
Stomach pain
Swelling of throat, hands, or feet

For elderly patients: Many medicines have not been tested in older people. Therefore, it is not known whether the medicine acts the same way it does in younger adults. Check with your doctor if you notice any unusual effects after receiving a radiopharmaceutical.

Other side effects not listed above may also occur in some patients. If you notice any other effects, note the time when they start and check with your doctor.

December 1987

RANITIDINE (Systemic)

A commonly used brand name is Zantac.

To the Reader: If you do not recognize the names of medical conditions or medicines referred to in this information, check with your doctor, nurse, or pharmacist. Definitions for selected medical terms may be found in the Glossary. Brand names for the generic drug names listed can be found in the Index. In addition, selected brand names commonly associated with the generic name have been included in the text to help you recognize medicine you may be taking. The fact that a brand name product is not mentioned does not mean the information does not apply. It is a good idea for you to learn both the generic and brand names of your medicines and to write them down for future use.

Ranitidine (ra-NIT-te-deen) is a medicine used to treat duodenal ulcers and prevent their return. It is also used to treat gastric ulcers. In addition, it is used in some conditions, such as in Zollinger-Ellison disease, in which the stomach produces too much acid. Ranitidine may also be used for other conditions as determined by your doctor.

Ranitidine works by decreasing the amount of acid produced by the stomach.

Ranitidine is available only with your doctor's prescription.

Remember:

• **This medicine has been prescribed for your current medical problem only.** It must not be given to other people or used for other problems unless you are directed to do so by your doctor.

• **Keep all medicines out of the reach of children.**

• In order for this medicine to work, it must be used as directed.

• If you are receiving this medicine by injection, some of the information about this medicine may not apply.

• **It is very important that you read and understand the following information.** If any of the information causes you special concern, do not decide against using this medicine without first checking with your doctor.

• Before you begin using any new medicine (prescription or nonprescription) or if you develop any new medical problem while you are using this medicine, check with your doctor, nurse, or pharmacist.

• **If you have any questions** about the following information or if you want more information about this medicine or your medical problem, **ask your doctor, nurse, or pharmacist.**

Before Using This Medicine

In order to decide on the best treatment for your medical problem, your doctor should be told:

—if you have ever had any unusual or allergic reaction to ranitidine, famotidine, or cimetidine.

—if you are on a low-salt, low-sugar, or any other special diet, or if you are allergic to any substance, such as foods, sulfites or other preservatives, or dyes. Most medicines contain more than their active ingredient. Your doctor, nurse, or pharmacist can help you avoid products that may cause a problem.

—if you are **pregnant** or if you may become pregnant. Studies have not been done in humans; however, ranitidine has not been shown to cause birth defects or other problems in animal studies.

—if you are **breast-feeding**. Although ranitidine has not been shown to cause problems in nursing babies, the chance always exists since this medicine passes into the breast milk.

—if you have any of the following medical problems:
Kidney disease
Liver disease

—if you are taking **any** other prescription or nonprescription (OTC) medicine, especially ketoconazole.

Proper Use of This Medicine

It may take several days for ranitidine to begin to relieve stomach pain. To help relieve this pain antacids may be taken with ranitidine, unless your doctor has told you not to use them. However, one hour should pass between taking the antacid and the ranitidine.

Take this medicine for the full time of treatment, even if you begin to feel better. Also, it is important that you keep your doctor's appointments for check-ups so that your doctor will be better able to tell you when to stop taking ranitidine.

If you miss a dose of this medicine, take it as soon as possible. However, if it is almost time for your next dose, skip the missed dose and go back to your regular dosing schedule. Do not double doses.

How to store this medicine:

• **Keep out of the reach of children.**

• Store away from heat and direct light.

• Do not store the tablet form of this medicine in the bathroom, near the kitchen sink, or in other damp places. Heat or moisture may cause the medicine to break down.

• Do not keep outdated medicine or medicine no longer needed. Be sure that any discarded medicine is out of the reach of children.

Precautions While Using This Medicine

Before you have any skin tests for allergies, tell the doctor in charge that you are taking ranitidine. The results of the tests may be affected by this medicine.

Remember that certain medicines, such as aspirin, and certain foods and drinks that irritate the stomach may make your problem worse.

Cigarette smoking tends to decrease the effect of ranitidine. This is more likely to affect the stomach's nighttime production of acid. While taking ranitidine, stop smoking completely, or at least do not smoke after taking the last dose of the day.

Check with your doctor if your ulcer pain continues or gets worse.

Side Effects of This Medicine

Along with its needed effects, a medicine may cause some unwanted effects. Although not all of these side effects may occur, if they do occur they may need medical attention.

Check with your doctor as soon as possible if any of the following side effects occur:

Rare
   Confusion
   Slow, fast, or irregular heartbeat
   Sore throat and fever
   Unusual bleeding or bruising
   Unusual tiredness or weakness

Other side effects may occur that usually do not require medical attention. These side effects may go away during treatment as your body adjusts to the medicine.

However, check with your doctor if any of the following side effects continue or are bothersome:

Less common or rare
   Constipation
   Dizziness or headache
   Nausea
   Skin rash
   Stomach pain

For elderly patients: Confusion is more likely to occur in very ill elderly patients.

Other side effects not listed above may also occur in some patients. If you notice any other effects, check with your doctor.

_____
December 1987

RAUWOLFIA ALKALOIDS (Systemic)

This information applies to the following medicines:

Alseroxylon (al-ser-OX-i-lon)
Deserpidine (de-SER-pi-deen)
Rauwolfia Serpentina (rah-WOOL-fee-a ser-pen-TEE-na)
Reserpine (re-SER-peen)

Some commonly used brand names are:	Generic names:
Rauwiloid	Alseroxylon
Harmonyl	Deserpidine
Raudixin Rauverid Wolfina	Rauwolfia Serpentina†
Novoreserpine* Releserp-5 Reserfia* Serpasil	Reserpine†‡

*Not available in the U.S.
†Generic name product may also be available in the U.S.
‡Generic name product may also be available in Canada.

To the Reader: If you do not recognize the names of medical conditions or medicines referred to in this information, check with your doctor, nurse, or pharmacist. Definitions for selected medical terms may be found in the Glossary. Brand names for the generic drug names listed can be found in the Index. In addition, selected brand names commonly associated with the generic name have been included in the text to help you recognize medicine you may be taking. The fact that a brand name product is not mentioned does not mean the information does not apply. It is a good idea for you to learn both the generic and brand names of your medicines and to write them down for future use.

Rauwolfia alkaloids belong to the general class of medicines called antihypertensives. They are taken by mouth to treat high blood pressure.

High blood pressure adds to the workload of the heart and arteries. If it continues for a long time, the heart and arteries may not function properly. This can damage the blood vessels of the brain, heart, and kidneys, resulting in a stroke, heart failure, or kidney failure. High blood pressure may also increase the risk of heart attacks. These problems may be less likely to occur if blood pressure is controlled.

Rauwolfia alkaloids work by controlling nerve impulses along certain nerve pathways. As a result, they act on the heart and blood vessels to lower blood pressure.

Rauwolfia alkaloids may also be used to treat other conditions as determined by your doctor.

These medicines are available only with your doctor's prescription.

Remember:

• **This medicine has been prescribed for your current medical problem only.** It must not be given to other people or used for other problems unless you are directed to do so by your doctor.

• **Keep all medicines out of the reach of children.**

• In order for this medicine to work, it must be used as directed.

• **It is very important that you read and understand the following information.** If any of the information causes you special concern, do not decide against using this medicine without first checking with your doctor.

• Before you begin using any new medicine (prescription or nonprescription) or if you develop any new medical problem while you are using this medicine, check with your doctor, nurse, or pharmacist.

• **If you have any questions** about the following information or if you want more information about this medicine or your medical problem, **ask your doctor, nurse, or pharmacist**.

Before Using This Medicine

In order to decide on the best treatment for your medical problem, your doctor should be told:

—if you have ever had any unusual or allergic reaction to rauwolfia alkaloids.

—if you are on a low-salt, low-sugar, or any other special diet, or if you are allergic to any substance, such as foods, sulfites or other preservatives, or dyes. Most medicines contain more than their active ingredient. Your doctor, nurse, or pharmacist can help you avoid products that may cause a problem.

—if you are **pregnant** or if you may become pregnant. Too much use of rauwolfia alkaloids during pregnancy may cause unwanted effects (difficult breathing, low temperature, loss of appetite) in the baby. In rats, use of rauwolfia alkaloids during pregnancy causes birth defects and in guinea pigs decreases newborn survival rates. Be sure you have discussed this with your doctor before taking this medicine.

—if you are **breast-feeding**. Rauwolfia alkaloids pass into the breast milk and may cause unwanted effects (difficult breathing, low temperature, loss of appetite) in infants of mothers taking large doses of this medicine. Be sure you have discussed this with your doctor before taking this medicine.

—if you have any of the following medical problems:
Allergies or other breathing problems such as asthma
Epilepsy
Gallstones
Heart disease
Kidney disease
Mental depression (or history of)
Parkinson's disease
Pheochromocytoma
Stomach ulcer
Ulcerative colitis

—if you are now taking or have taken within the past 2 weeks monoamine oxidase (MAO) inhibitors, such as:
Furazolidone (e.g., Furoxone)
Isocarboxazid (e.g., Marplan)
Pargyline (e.g., Eutonyl)
Phenelzine (e.g., Nardil)
Procarbazine (e.g., Matulane)
Tranylcypromine (e.g., Parnate)

—if you are taking **any** other prescription or nonprescription (OTC) medicine.

Proper Use of This Medicine

Importance of diet—When prescribing medicine for your condition, your doctor may also prescribe a personal diet for you. Such a diet may be low in sodium (salt). Most people eat much more sodium than they need and too much sodium in the diet may increase blood pressure. Some foods that contain large amounts of sodium are canned soup, pickles, ketchup, green and ripe olives, relish, frankfurters, soy sauce, and carbonated beverages. Your doctor may want you to limit the amounts of these and other high-sodium foods in your diet. High blood pressure medicine is usually more effective when such a diet is properly followed.

Also, it may be very important for you to go on a reducing diet. However, check with your doctor before changing your diet.

Many patients who have high blood pressure will not notice any signs of the problem. In fact, many may feel normal. It is very important that you **take your medicine exactly as directed** and that you keep your appointments with your doctor even if you feel well.

Remember that this medicine will not cure your high blood pressure but it does control it. Therefore, you must continue to take it as directed if you expect to lower your blood pressure and keep it down. **You may have to take high blood pressure medicine for the rest of your life.** If high blood pressure is not treated, it can cause serious problems such as heart failure, blood vessel disease, stroke, or kidney disease.

In order to help you remember to take your medicine, try to get into the habit of taking it at the same time each day.

This medicine is sometimes given together with certain other medicines. If you are using a combination of drugs, make sure that you take each medicine at the proper time and do not mix them. Ask your doctor, nurse, or pharmacist to help you plan a way to remember to take your medicines at the right times.

If this medicine upsets your stomach, it may be taken with meals or milk. If stomach upset (nausea, vomiting, stomach cramps or pain) continues or gets worse, check with your doctor.

If you miss a dose of this medicine, do not take the missed dose at all and do not double the next one. Instead, go back to your regular dosing schedule.

How to store this medicine:
- **Keep out of the reach of children.**
- Store away from heat and direct light.
- Do not store in the bathroom, near the kitchen sink, or in other damp places. Heat or moisture may cause the medicine to break down.
- Do not keep outdated medicine or medicine no longer needed. Be sure that any discarded medicine is out of the reach of children.

Precautions While Using This Medicine

It is important that your doctor check your progress at regular visits to make sure that this medicine is working properly.

Do not take other medicines unless they have been discussed with your doctor. This especially includes over-the-counter (nonprescription) medicines for appetite control, asthma, colds, cough, hay fever, or sinus problems, since they may tend to increase your blood pressure.

Before having any kind of surgery (including dental surgery) or emergency treatment, **tell the physician or dentist in charge that you are taking this medicine.**

In some patients, this medicine may cause mental depression. **Tell your doctor right away:**

—if you or anyone else notices unusual changes in your mood.

—if you start having early-morning sleeplessness or unusually vivid dreams or nightmares.

This medicine will add to the effects of alcohol and other CNS depressants (medicines that slow down the nervous system, possibly causing drowsiness). Some examples of CNS depressants are antihistamines or medicine for hay fever, other allergies, or colds; sedatives, tranquilizers, or sleeping medicine; prescription pain medicine or narcotics; barbiturates; medicine for convulsions (seizures); muscle relaxants; or anesthetics, including some dental anesthetics. **Check with your doctor before taking any of the above while you are using this medicine.**

This medicine may cause some people to become drowsy or less alert than they are normally. This is more likely to happen when you begin to take it or when you increase the amount of medicine you are taking. **Make sure you know how you react to this medicine before you drive, use machines, or do other jobs that require you to be alert.**

This medicine may cause dryness of the mouth. For temporary relief, use sugarless candy or gum, melt bits of ice in your mouth, or use a saliva substitute. However, if dry mouth continues for more than 2 weeks, check with your physician or dentist. Continuing dryness of the mouth may increase the chance of dental disease, including tooth decay, gum disease, and fungal infections.

This medicine often causes stuffiness in the nose. However, do not use nasal decongestant medicines without first checking with your doctor or pharmacist.

Side Effects of This Medicine

Suggestions that rauwolfia alkaloids may increase the risk of breast cancer occurring later have not been proven. However, rats and mice given 100 to 300 times the human dose had an increased number of tumors.

Along with its needed effects, a medicine may cause some unwanted effects. Although not all of these side effects may occur, if they do occur they may need medical attention.

Check with your doctor immediately if any of the following side effects occur:

Less common
   Drowsiness or faintness
   Impotence or decreased sexual interest
   Lack of energy or weakness
   Mental depression or inability to concentrate
   Nervousness or anxiety
   Vivid dreams or nightmares or early-morning sleeplessness

Check with your doctor as soon as possible if any of the following side effects occur:

More common
   Dizziness
Less common
   Black tarry stools
   Bloody vomit
   Chest pain
   Headache
   Irregular or slow heartbeat
   Shortness of breath
   Stomach cramps or pain
Rare
   Painful or difficult urination
   Skin rash or itching
   Stiffness
   Trembling and shaking of hands and fingers
   Unusual bleeding or bruising
Signs of overdose
   Dizziness or drowsiness (severe)
   Flushing of skin
   Pinpoint pupils of eyes
   Slow pulse

Other side effects may occur that usually do not require medical attention. These side effects may go away during treatment as your body adjusts to the medicine. However, check with your doctor if any of the following side effects continue or are bothersome:

More common
   Diarrhea
   Dry mouth
   Loss of appetite
   Nausea and vomiting
   Stuffy nose
Less common
   Swelling of feet and lower legs

For elderly patients: Dizziness may be more likely to occur in the elderly, who are more sensitive to the effects of rauwolfia alkaloids.

After you stop using this medicine, it may still produce some side effects that need attention. During this period of time **check with your doctor immediately** if you notice any of the following side effects:

   Drowsiness or faintness
   Impotence or decreased sexual interest
   Irregular or slow heartbeat
   Lack of energy or weakness
   Mental depression or inability to concentrate
   Nervousness or anxiety
   Vivid dreams or nightmares or early-morning sleeplessness

Other side effects not listed above may also occur in some patients. If you notice any other effects, check with your doctor.

December 1987

RAUWOLFIA ALKALOIDS AND THIAZIDE DIURETICS
(Systemic)

This information applies to the following medicines:

Deserpidine (de-SER-pi-deen) and Hydrochlorothiazide (hye-droe-klor-oh-THYE-a-zide)

Deserpidine and Methyclothiazide (meth-i-kloe-THYE-a-zide)

Rauwolfia Serpentina (rah-WOOL-fee-a ser-pen-TEE-na) and Bendroflumethiazide (ben-droe-floo-meth-EYE-a-zide)

Reserpine (re-SER-peen) and Chlorothiazide (klor-oh-THYE-a-zide)

Reserpine and Chlorthalidone (klor-THAL-i-done)

Reserpine and Hydrochlorothiazide

Reserpine and Hydroflumethiazide (hye-droe-floo-meth-EYE-a-zide)

Reserpine and Methyclothiazide

Reserpine and Polythiazide (pol-i-THYE-a-zide)

Reserpine and Quinethazone (kwin-ETH-a-zone)

Reserpine and Trichlormethiazide (trye-klor-meth-EYE-a-zide)

Some commonly used brand names are:	Generic names:
Oreticyl Oreticyl Forte	Deserpidine and Hydrochlorothiazide
Dureticyl* Enduronyl	Deserpidine and Methyclothiazide†
Rauzide	Rauwolfia Serpentina and Bendroflumethiazide
Diupres	Reserpine and Chlorothiazide†
Demi-Regroton Regroton	Reserpine and Chlorthalidone
Hydropres Serpasil-Esidrix	Reserpine and Hydrochlorothiazide†
Salutensin Salutensin-Demi	Reserpine and Hydroflumethiazide†
Diutensen-R	Reserpine and Methyclothiazide
Renese-R	Reserpine and Polythiazide
Hydromox-R	Reserpine and Quinethazone
Metatensin Naquival	Reserpine and Trichlormethiazide†

*Not available in the U.S.

†Generic name product may also be available in the U.S.

To the Reader: If you do not recognize the names of medical conditions or medicines referred to in this information, check with your doctor, nurse, or pharmacist. Definitions for selected medical terms may be found in the Glossary. Brand names for the generic drug names listed can be found in the Index. In addition, selected brand names commonly associated with the generic name have been included in the text to help you recognize medicine you may be taking. The fact that a brand name product is not mentioned does not mean the information does not apply. It is a good idea for you to learn both the generic and brand names of your medicines and to write them down for future use.

Rauwolfia alkaloid and thiazide diuretic combinations are used in the treatment of high blood pressure.

High blood pressure adds to the workload of the heart and arteries. If it continues for a long time, the heart and arteries may not function properly. This can damage the blood vessels of the brain, heart, and kidneys, resulting in a stroke, heart failure, or kidney failure. High blood pressure may also increase the risk of heart attacks. These problems may be less likely to occur if blood pressure is controlled.

Rauwolfia alkaloids work by controlling nerve impulses along certain nerve pathways. As a result, they act on the heart and blood vessels to lower blood pressure. Thiazide diuretics help to reduce the amount of water in the body by increasing the flow of urine. This also helps to lower blood pressure.

These medicines are available only with your doctor's prescription.

Remember:

• **This medicine has been prescribed for your current medical problem only.** It must not be given to other people or used for other problems unless you are directed to do so by your doctor.

• **Keep all medicines out of the reach of children.**

• In order for this medicine to work, it must be used as directed.

• **It is very important that you read and understand the following information.** If any of the information causes you special concern, do not decide against using this medicine without first checking with your doctor.

• Before you begin using any new medicine (prescription or nonprescription) or if you develop any new medical problem while you are using this medicine, check with your doctor, nurse, or pharmacist.

• **If you have any questions** about the following information or if you want more information about this medicine or your medical problem, **ask your doctor, nurse, or pharmacist**.

Before Using This Medicine

In order to decide on the best treatment for your medical problem, your doctor should be told:

—if you have ever had any unusual or allergic reaction to sulfonamides (sulfa drugs), thiazide diuretics (water pills), or rauwolfia alkaloids.

—if you are on a low-salt, low-sugar, or any other special diet, or if you are allergic to any substance, such as foods, sulfites or other preservatives, or dyes. Most medicines contain more than their active ingredient. Your doctor, nurse, or pharmacist can help you avoid products that may cause a problem.

—if you are **pregnant** or if you may become pregnant. Too much use of thiazide diuretics (contained in this combination medicine) during pregnancy may cause unwanted effects including jaundice, blood problems, and low potassium in the baby. Too much use of rauwolfia alkaloids may cause difficult breathing, low temperature, and loss of appetite in the baby. This medicine has not been shown to cause birth defects in humans. In rats, use of rauwolfia alkaloids during

© 1988 The United States Pharmacopeial Convention, Inc.

pregnancy decreases newborn survival rates. Be sure that you have discussed this with your doctor before taking this medicine.

—if you are **breast-feeding**. Rauwolfia alkaloids pass into the breast milk and may cause unwanted effects (difficult breathing, low temperature, loss of appetite) in infants of mothers taking large doses of it. Be sure you have discussed this with your doctor before taking this medicine.

—if you have any of the following medical problems:

Allergies or other breathing problems such as asthma
Diabetes mellitus (sugar diabetes)
Epilepsy
Gallstones
Gout (history of)
Heart disease
Kidney disease
Liver disease
Lupus erythematosus (history of)
Mental depression (or history of)
Pancreas disease
Parkinson's disease
Pheochromocytoma
Stomach ulcer
Ulcerative colitis

—if you are now taking or have taken within the past 2 weeks monoamine oxidase (MAO) inhibitors such as:

Furazolidone (e.g., Furoxone)
Isocarboxazid (e.g., Marplan)
Pargyline (e.g., Eutonyl)
Phenelzine (e.g., Nardil)
Procarbazine (e.g., Matulane)
Tranylcypromine (e.g., Parnate)

—if you are taking **any** other prescription or nonprescription (OTC) medicine, especially:

Adrenocorticoids (cortisone-like medicines)
Digitalis glycosides (heart medicine)
Lithium (e.g., Lithane)
Methenamine (e.g., Mandelamine)

Proper Use of This Medicine

Importance of diet—When prescribing medicine for your condition, your doctor may also prescribe a personal diet for you. Such a diet may be low in sodium (salt). Most people eat much more sodium than they need and too much sodium in the diet may increase blood pressure. Some foods that contain large amounts of sodium are canned soup, pickles, ketchup, green and ripe olives, relish, frankfurters, soy sauce, and carbonated beverages. Your doctor may want you to limit the amounts of these and other high-sodium foods in your diet. High blood pressure medicine is usually more effective when such a diet is properly followed.

Also, it may be very important for you to go on a reducing diet. However, check with your doctor before changing your diet.

Many patients who have high blood pressure will not notice any signs of the problem. In fact, many may feel normal. It is very important that you **take your medicine exactly as directed** and that you keep your appointments with your doctor even if you feel well.

Remember that this medicine will not cure your high blood pressure but it does control it. Therefore, you must continue to take it as directed if you expect to lower your blood pressure and keep it down. **You may have to take high blood pressure medicine for the rest of your life.** If high blood pressure is not treated, it can cause serious problems such as heart failure, blood vessel disease, stroke, or kidney disease.

This medicine may cause you to have an unusual feeling of tiredness when you begin to take it. You may also notice an increase in the amount of urine or in your frequency of urination. After you have taken the medicine for a while, these effects should lessen. In general, in order to keep the increase in urine from affecting your sleep:

• If you are to take a single dose a day, take it in the morning after breakfast.

• If you are to take more than one dose a day, take the last dose no later than 6 p.m., unless otherwise directed by your doctor.

However, it is best to plan your dose or doses according to a schedule that will least affect your personal activities and sleep. Ask your doctor, nurse, or pharmacist to help you plan the best time to take this medicine.

In order to help you remember to take your medicine, try to get into the habit of taking it at the same time each day.

If this medicine upsets your stomach, it may be taken with meals or milk. If stomach upset (nausea, vomiting, stomach pain or cramps) continues, check with your doctor.

If you miss a dose of this medicine, take it as soon as possible. However, if it is almost time for your next dose, skip the missed dose and go back to your regular dosing schedule. Do not double doses.

How to store this medicine:

• **Keep out of the reach of children.**

• Store away from heat and direct light.

• Do not store in the bathroom, near the kitchen sink, or in other damp places. Heat or moisture may cause the medicine to break down.

• Do not keep outdated medicine or medicine no longer needed. Be sure that any discarded medicine is out of the reach of children.

Precautions While Using This Medicine

It is important that your doctor check your progress at regular visits to make sure that this medicine is working properly.

Do not take other medicines unless they have been discussed with your doctor. This especially includes over-the-counter (nonprescription) medicines for appetite control, asthma, colds, cough, hay fever, or sinus problems, since they may tend to increase your blood pressure.

Before having any kind of surgery (including dental surgery), or emergency treatment, **tell the physician or dentist in charge that you are taking this medicine.**

This medicine may cause a loss of potassium from your body.

- To help prevent this, your doctor may want you to:
  —eat or drink foods that have a high potassium content (for example, orange or other citrus fruit juices), or

  —take a potassium supplement, or

  —take another medicine to help prevent the loss of the potassium in the first place.

- It is very important to follow these directions. Also, it is important not to change your diet on your own. This is more important if you are already on a special diet (as for diabetes), or if you are taking a potassium supplement or a medicine to reduce potassium loss. Extra potassium may not be necessary and, in some cases, too much potassium could be harmful.

Check with your doctor if you become sick and have severe or continuing vomiting or diarrhea. These problems may cause you to lose additional water and potassium.

This medicine may cause some people to become drowsy or less alert than they are normally. This is more likely to happen when you begin to take it or when you increase the amount of medicine you are taking. **Make sure you know how you react to this medicine before you drive, use machines, or do other jobs that require you to be alert.**

Dizziness, lightheadedness, or fainting may occur, especially when you get up from a lying or sitting position. Getting up slowly may help but if the problem continues or gets worse, check with your doctor.

In some patients, this medicine may cause mental depression. **Tell your doctor right away:**
  —if you or anyone else notices unusual changes in your moods.

  —if you start having early-morning sleeplessness or unusually vivid dreams or nightmares.

This medicine will add to the effects of alcohol and other CNS depressants (medicines that slow down the nervous system, possibly causing drowsiness). Some examples of CNS depressants are antihistamines or medicine for hay fever, other allergies, or colds; sedatives, tranquilizers, or sleeping medicine; prescription pain medicine or narcotics; barbiturates; medicine for seizures; muscle relaxants; or anesthetics, including dental anesthetics. **Check with your doctor before taking any of the above while you are taking this medicine.**

Diabetics—This medicine may raise blood sugar levels. While you are using this medicine, be especially careful in testing for sugar in your urine. If you have any questions about this, check with your doctor.

A few people who take this medicine may become more sensitive to sunlight than they are normally. When you first begin taking this medicine, avoid too much sun and do not use a sunlamp until you see how you react to the sun, especially if you tend to burn easily. If you have a severe reaction, check with your doctor.

This medicine often causes stuffiness in the nose. However, do not use nasal decongestant medicines without first checking with your doctor or pharmacist.

This medicine may cause dryness of the mouth. For temporary relief, use sugarless candy or gum, melt bits of ice in your mouth, or use a saliva substitute. However, if dry mouth continues for more than 2 weeks, check with your physician or dentist. Continuing dryness of the mouth may increase the chance of dental disease, including tooth decay, gum disease, and fungal infections.

Side Effects of This Medicine

Suggestions that rauwolfia alkaloids may increase the risk of breast cancer occurring later have not been proven. However, rats and mice given 100 to 300 times the human dose had an increased risk of tumors.

Along with its needed effects, a medicine may cause some unwanted effects. Although not all of these side effects may occur, if they do occur they may need medical attention.

Check with your doctor immediately if any of the following side effects occur:

Less common
  Drowsiness or faintness
  Impotence or decreased sexual interest
  Lack of energy or weakness
  Mental depression or inability to concentrate
  Nervousness or anxiety
  Vivid dreams or nightmares or early-morning sleeplessness

Check with your doctor as soon as possible if any of the following side effects occur:

Less common
  Black tarry stools
  Bloody vomit
  Chest pain
  Headache
  Irregular or slow heartbeat
  Joint pain
  Shortness of breath

Rare
  Painful or difficult urination
  Skin rash or itching
  Sore throat and fever
  Stiffness
  Stomach pain (severe) with nausea and vomiting
  Trembling and shaking of hands and fingers
  Unusual bleeding or bruising
  Yellow eyes or skin

Signs of too much potassium loss or overdose

Dry mouth
Increased thirst
Muscle cramps or pain
Nausea or vomiting

Other signs of overdose

Dizziness or drowsiness, severe
Flushing of skin
Pinpoint pupils of eyes
Slow pulse

Other side effects may occur that usually do not require medical attention. These side effects may go away during treatment as your body adjusts to the medicine. However, check with your doctor if any of the following side effects continue or are bothersome:

More common

Diarrhea
Dizziness, especially when getting up from a lying or sitting position
Loss of appetite
Stuffy nose

For elderly patients: Dizziness or faintness or signs of too much potassium loss may be more likely to occur in the elderly, who are more sensitive to the effects of rauwolfia alkaloids and thiazide diuretics.

After you stop using this medicine, it may still produce some side effects that need attention. During this period of time **check with your doctor immediately** if you notice any of the following side effects:

Drowsiness or faintness
Impotence or decreased sexual interest
Irregular or slow heartbeat
Lack of energy or weakness
Mental depression or inability to concentrate
Nervousness or anxiety
Vivid dreams or nightmares or early-morning sleeplessness

Other side effects not listed above may also occur in some patients. If you notice any other effects, check with your doctor.

December 1987

RESERPINE AND HYDRALAZINE
(Systemic)

A commonly used brand name is Serpasil-Apresoline.

To the Reader: If you do not recognize the names of medical conditions or medicines referred to in this information, check with your doctor, nurse, or pharmacist. Definitions for selected medical terms may be found in the Glossary. Brand names for the generic drug names listed can be found in the Index. In addition, selected brand names commonly associated with the generic name have been included in the text to help you recognize medicine you may be taking. The fact that a brand name product is not mentioned does not mean the information does not apply. It is a good idea for you to learn both the generic and brand names of your medicines and to write them down for future use.

The reserpine (re-SER-peen) and hydralazine (hye-DRAL-a-zeen) combination is taken by mouth to treat high blood pressure.

High blood pressure adds to the workload of the heart and arteries. If it continues for a long time, the heart and arteries may not function properly. This can damage the blood vessels of the brain, heart, and kidneys, resulting in a stroke, heart failure, or kidney failure. High blood pressure may also increase the risk of heart attacks. These problems may be less likely to occur if blood pressure is controlled.

Reserpine works by controlling nerve impulses along certain nerve pathways. As a result, it acts on the heart and blood vessels to lower blood pressure. Hydralazine works by relaxing blood vessels and increasing the supply of blood and oxygen to the heart while reducing its work load.

Reserpine and hydralazine combination is available only with your doctor's prescription.

Remember:

• **This medicine has been prescribed for your current medical problem only.** It must not be given to other people or used for other problems unless you are directed to do so by your doctor.

• **Keep all medicines out of the reach of children.**

• In order for this medicine to work, it must be used as directed.

• **It is very important that you read and understand the following information.** If any of the information causes you special concern, do not decide against using this medicine without first checking with your doctor.

• Before you begin using any new medicine (prescription or nonprescription) or if you develop any new medical problem while you are using this medicine, check with your doctor, nurse, or pharmacist.

• **If you have any questions** about the following information or if you want more information about this medicine or your medical problem, **ask your doctor, nurse, or pharmacist.**

Before Using This Medicine

In order to decide on the best treatment for your medical problem, your doctor should be told:

—if you have ever had any unusual or allergic reaction to rauwolfia alkaloids or hydralazine.

—if you are on a low-salt, low-sugar, or any other special diet, or if you are allergic to any substance, such as foods, sulfites or other preservatives, or dyes. Most medicines contain more than their active ingredient. Your doctor, nurse, or pharmacist can help you avoid products that may cause a problem.

—if you are **pregnant** or if you may become pregnant. Too much use of reserpine during pregnancy may cause unwanted effects (difficult breathing, low temperature, loss of appetite) in the baby. In rats, rauwolfia alkaloids decrease the newborn survival rate. Studies in mice have shown that hydralazine causes birth defects (cleft palate, defects in head and face bones); these birth defects may also occur in rabbits, but do not occur in rats; studies have not been done in humans. Be sure that you have discussed this with your doctor before taking this medicine.

—if you are **breast-feeding**. Reserpine passes into the breast milk and may cause unwanted effects (difficult breathing, low temperature, loss of appetite) in infants of mothers taking large doses of it. Hydralazine has not been shown to cause problems in nursing babies. Be sure you have discussed this with your doctor before taking this medicine.

—if you have recently had a stroke.

—if you have any of the following medical problems:
Allergies or other breathing problems, such as asthma
Epilepsy
Gallstones
Heart disease
Kidney disease
Mental depression (or history of)
Parkinson's disease
Pheochromocytoma (PCC)
Stomach ulcer
Ulcerative colitis

—if you are now taking or have taken within the past 2 weeks monoamine oxidase (MAO) inhibitors, such as:
Furazolidone (e.g., Furoxone)
Isocarboxazid (e.g., Marplan)
Pargyline (e.g., Eutonyl)
Phenelzine (e.g., Nardil)
Procarbazine (e.g., Matulane)
Tranylcypromine (e.g., Parnate)

—if you are taking **any** other prescription or nonprescription (OTC) medicine.

Proper Use of This Medicine

Importance of diet—When prescribing medicine for your condition, your doctor may also prescribe a personal diet for you. Such a diet may be low in sodium (salt). Most people eat much more sodium than they need and too much sodium in the diet may increase blood pressure. Some foods that contain large amounts of sodium are canned soup, pickles, ketchup, green and ripe olives, relish, frankfurters, soy sauce, and carbonated beverages. Your doctor may want you to limit the amounts of these and other high-sodium foods in your diet. High blood pressure medicine is usually more effective when such a diet is properly followed.

Also, it may be very important for you to go on a reducing diet. However, check with your doctor before changing your diet.

Many patients who have high blood pressure will not notice any signs of the problem. In fact, many may feel normal. It is very important that you **take your medicine exactly as directed** and that you keep your appointments with your doctor even if you feel well.

Remember that this medicine will not cure your high blood pressure but it does control it. Therefore, you must continue to take it as directed if you expect to lower your blood pressure and keep it down. **You may have to take high blood pressure medicine for the rest of your life.** If high blood pressure is not treated, it can cause serious problems such as heart failure, blood vessel disease, stroke, or kidney disease.

In order to help you remember to take your medicine, try to get into the habit of taking it at the same time each day.

If this medicine upsets your stomach, it may be taken with meals or milk. If stomach upset (nausea, vomiting, stomach pain, or cramps) continues, check with your doctor.

If you miss a dose of this medicine, take it as soon as possible. However, if it is almost time for your next dose, skip the missed dose and go back to your regular dosing schedule. Do not double doses.

How to store this medicine:

• **Keep out of the reach of children.**

• Store away from heat and direct light.

• Do not store in the bathroom, near the kitchen sink, or in other damp places. Heat or moisture may cause the medicine to break down.

• Do not keep outdated medicine or medicine no longer needed. Be sure that any discarded medicine is out of the reach of children.

Precautions While Using This Medicine

It is important that your doctor check your progress at regular visits to make sure that this medicine is working properly.

Do not take other medicines unless they have been discussed with your doctor. This especially includes over-the-counter (nonprescription) medicine for appetite control, asthma, colds, cough, hay fever, or sinus problems, since they may tend to increase your blood pressure.

Before having any kind of surgery (including dental surgery), or emergency treatment, **make sure the physician or dentist in charge knows that you are taking this medicine.**

This medicine may cause some people to have headaches or to feel dizzy or drowsy. **Make sure you know how you react to this medicine before you drive, use machines, or do other jobs that require you to be alert.**

In some patients, this medicine may cause mental depression. **Tell your doctor right away:**
—if you or anyone else notices unusual changes in your mood.
—if you start having early-morning sleeplessness or unusually vivid dreams or nightmares.

This medicine will add to the effects of alcohol and other CNS depressants (medicines that slow down the nervous system, possibly causing drowsiness). Some examples of CNS depressants are antihistamines or medicine for hay fever, other allergies, or cold; sedatives, tranquilizers, or sleeping medicine; prescription pain medicine or narcotics; barbiturates; medicine for convulsions (seizures); muscle relaxants; or anesthetics, including dental anesthetics. **Check with your doctor before taking any of the above while you are taking this medicine.**

This medicine often causes stuffiness in the nose. However, do not use nasal decongestant medicines without first checking with your doctor or pharmacist.

This medicine may cause dryness of the mouth. For temporary relief, use sugarless candy or gum, melt bits of ice in your mouth, or use a saliva substitute. However, if dry mouth continues for more than 2 weeks, check with your physician or dentist. Continuing dryness of the mouth may increase the chance of dental disease, including tooth decay, gum disease, and fungal infections.

Side Effects of This Medicine

Suggestions that rauwolfia alkaloids (like reserpine) may increase the risk of breast cancer occurring later have not been proven. However, rats and mice given 100 to 300 times the human dose had an increased number of tumors.

Along with its needed effects, a medicine may cause some unwanted effects. Although not all of these side effects may occur, if they do occur they may need medical attention.

Check with your doctor immediately if any of the following side effects occur:
More common
General feeling of body discomfort or weakness
Less common
Drowsiness or faintness
Impotence or decreased sexual interest
Mental depression or inability to concentrate
Nervousness or anxiety
Vivid dreams or nightmares or early-morning sleeplessness

© 1988   The United States Pharmacopeial Convention, Inc.

Check with your doctor as soon as possible if any of the following side effects occur:

Less common

Black tarry stools
Blisters on skin
Bloody vomit
Chest pain
Fever and sore throat
Headache
Irregular heartbeat
Joint pain
Numbness, tingling, pain, or weakness in hands or feet
Shortness of breath
Skin rash or itching
Swelling of feet or lower legs
Swelling of the lymph glands

Rare

Painful or difficult urination
Stiffness
Stomach pain (severe) with nausea and vomiting
Trembling and shaking of hands and fingers
Unusual bleeding or bruising

Signs of overdose

Dizziness or drowsiness (severe)
Flushing of skin
Pinpoint pupils of eyes
Slow pulse

Other side effects may occur that usually do not require medical attention. These side effects may go away during treatment as your body adjusts to the medicine.

However, check with your doctor if any of the following side effects continue or are bothersome:

More common

Diarrhea
Dizziness
Dry mouth
Loss of appetite
Nausea or vomiting
Stuffy nose

Less common

Constipation
Flushing or redness of skin
Red, sore eyes

For elderly patients: Dizziness or faintness may be more likely to occur in the elderly, who are more sensitive to the effects of reserpine and hydralazine.

After you stop using this medicine, it may still produce some side effects that need attention. During this period of time **check with your doctor immediately** if you notice any of the following side effects:

Drowsiness or faintness
General feeling of body discomfort or weakness
Impotence or decreased sexual interest
Irregular or slow heartbeat
Mental depression or inability to concentrate
Nervousness or anxiety
Vivid dreams or nightmares or early-morning sleeplessness

Other side effects not listed above may also occur in some patients. If you notice any other effects, check with your doctor.

December 1987

RESERPINE, HYDRALAZINE, AND HYDROCHLOROTHIAZIDE (Systemic)

Some commonly used brand names are:

Hydrap-Es	Ser-Ap-Es
Hyserp	Tri-Hydroserpine
R-HCTZ-H	Unipres

Generic name product may also be available in the U.S.

To the Reader: If you do not recognize the names of medical conditions or medicines referred to in this information, check with your doctor, nurse, or pharmacist. Definitions for selected medical terms may be found in the Glossary. Brand names for the generic drug names listed can be found in the Index. In addition, selected brand names commonly associated with the generic name have been included in the text to help you recognize medicine you may be taking. The fact that a brand name product is not mentioned does not mean the information does not apply. It is a good idea for you to learn both the generic and brand names of your medicines and to write them down for future use.

Reserpine (re-SER-peen), hydralazine (hye-DRAL-a-zeen), and hydrochlorothiazide (hye-droe-KLOR-oh-THYE-a-zide) combinations are taken by mouth to treat high blood pressure.

High blood pressure adds to the workload of the heart and arteries. If it continues for a long time, the heart and arteries may not function properly. This can damage the blood vessels of the brain, heart, and kidneys, resulting in a stroke, heart failure, or kidney failure. High blood pressure may also increase the risk of heart attacks. These problems may be less likely to occur if blood pressure is controlled.

Reserpine works by controlling nerve impulses along certain nerve pathways. As a result, it acts on the heart and blood vessels to lower blood pressure. Hydralazine works by relaxing blood vessels and increasing the supply of blood to the heart while reducing its work load. Hydrochlorothiazide is a thiazide diuretic (water pill) that helps to reduce the amount of water in the body by increasing the flow of urine. This also helps to lower blood pressure.

This medicine is available only with your doctor's prescription.

Remember:

• **This medicine has been prescribed for your current medical problem only.** It must not be given to other people or used for other problems unless you are directed to do so by your doctor.

• **Keep all medicines out of the reach of children.**

• In order for this medicine to work, it must be used as directed.

• **It is very important that you read and understand the following information.** If any of the information causes you special concern, do not decide against using this medicine without first checking with your doctor.

• Before you begin using any new medicine (prescription or nonprescription) or if you develop any new medical problem while you are using this medicine, check with your doctor, nurse, or pharmacist.

• **If you have any questions** about the following information or if you want more information about this medicine or your medical problem, **ask your doctor, nurse, or pharmacist**.

Before Using This Medicine

In order to decide on the best treatment for your medical problem, your doctor should be told:

—if you have ever had any unusual or allergic reaction to hydralazine, sulfonamides (sulfa drugs), thiazide diuretics (water pills), or rauwolfia alkaloids.

—if you are on a low-salt, low-sugar, or any other special diet, or if you are allergic to any substance, such as foods, sulfites or other preservatives, or dyes. Most medicines contain more than their active ingredient. Your doctor, nurse, or pharmacist can help you avoid products that may cause a problem.

—if you are **pregnant** or if you may become pregnant. Too much use of reserpine and hydrochlorothiazide during pregnancy may cause unwanted effects (jaundice, blood problems, low potassium, difficult breathing, low temperatures, and loss of appetite) in the baby. In rats, rauwolfia alkaloids (like reserpine) decrease newborn survival rates. Studies in mice have shown that hydralazine causes birth defects (cleft palate, defects in head and face bones); these birth defects may also occur in rabbits, but do not occur in rats; studies have not been done in humans. Be sure that you have discussed this with your doctor before taking this medicine.

—if you are **breast-feeding**. Reserpine passes into the breast milk and may cause unwanted effects (difficult breathing, low temperature, loss of appetite) in infants of mothers taking large doses of it. Hydrochlorothiazide also passes into breast milk. Be sure you have discussed this with your doctor before taking this medicine.

—if you have any of the following medical problems:
Allergies or other breathing problems such as asthma
Diabetes mellitus (sugar diabetes)
Epilepsy
Gallstones
Gout (history of)
Heart disease
Kidney disease
Liver disease
Lupus erythematosus (history of)
Mental depression (or history of)
Pancreas disease
Parkinson's disease
Pheochromocytoma
Stomach ulcer
Ulcerative colitis

—if you have recently had a stroke.

—if you are now taking or have taken within the past 2 weeks monoamine oxidase (MAO) inhibitors, such as:
Furazolidone (e.g., Furoxone)
Isocarboxazid (e.g., Marplan)
Pargyline (e.g., Eutonyl)

Phenelzine (e.g., Nardil)
Procarbazine (e.g., Matulane)
Tranylcypromine (e.g., Parnate)

—if you are taking **any** other prescription or nonprescription (OTC) medicine, especially:

Adrenocorticoids (cortisone-like medicines)
Digitalis glycosides (heart medicine)
Lithium (e.g., Lithane)
Methenamine (e.g., Mandelamine)

Proper Use of This Medicine

Importance of diet—When prescribing medicine for your condition, your doctor may also prescribe a personal diet for you. Such a diet may be low in sodium (salt). Most people eat much more sodium than they need and too much sodium in the diet may increase blood pressure. Some foods that contain large amounts of sodium are canned soup, pickles, ketchup, green and ripe olives, relish, frankfurters, soy sauce, and carbonated beverages. Your doctor may want you to limit the amounts of these and other high-sodium foods in your diet. High blood pressure medicine is usually more effective when such a diet is properly followed.

Also, it may be very important for you to go on a reducing diet. However, check with your doctor before changing your diet.

Many patients who have high blood pressure will not notice any signs of the problem. In fact, many may feel normal. It is very important that you **take your medicine exactly as directed** and that you keep your appointments with your doctor even if you feel well.

Remember that this medicine will not cure your high blood pressure but it does control it. Therefore, you must continue to take it as directed if you expect to lower your blood pressure and keep it down. **You may have to take high blood pressure medicine for the rest of your life.** If high blood pressure is not treated, it can cause serious problems such as heart failure, blood vessel disease, stroke, or kidney disease.

This medicine may cause you to have an unusual feeling of tiredness when you begin to take it. You may also notice an increase in the amount of urine or in your frequency of urination. After you have taken the medicine for a while, these effects should lessen. In general, in order to keep the increase in urine from affecting your sleep:

• If you are to take a single dose a day, take it in the morning after breakfast.

• If you are to take more than one dose a day, take the last dose no later than 6 p.m., unless otherwise directed by your doctor.

However, it is best to plan your dose or doses according to a schedule that will least affect your personal activities and sleep. Ask your doctor, nurse, or pharmacist to help you plan the best time to take this medicine.

In order to help you remember to take your medicine, try to get into the habit of taking it at the same time each day.

If this medicine upsets your stomach, it may be taken with meals or milk. If stomach upset (nausea, vomiting, stomach pain or cramps) continues, check with your doctor.

If you miss a dose of this medicine, take it as soon as possible. However, if it is almost time for your next dose, skip the missed dose and go back to your regular dosing schedule. Do not double doses.

How to store this medicine:

• **Keep out of the reach of children.**

• Store away from heat and direct light.

• Do not store in the bathroom, near the kitchen sink, or in other damp places. Heat or moisture may cause the medicine to break down.

• Do not keep outdated medicine or medicine no longer needed. Be sure that any discarded medicine is out of the reach of children.

Precautions While Using This Medicine

It is important that your doctor check your progress at regular visits to make sure that this medicine is working properly.

Do not take other medicines unless they have been discussed with your doctor. This especially includes over-the-counter (nonprescription) medicines for appetite control, asthma, colds, cough, hay fever, or sinus problems, since they may tend to increase your blood pressure.

Before having any kind of surgery (including dental surgery), or emergency treatment, **make sure the physician or dentist in charge knows that you are taking this medicine.**

This medicine may cause some people to have headaches or to feel dizzy or drowsy. **Make sure you know how you react to this medicine before you drive, use machines, or do other jobs that require you to be alert.**

Dizziness, lightheadedness, or fainting may occur, especially when you get up from a lying or sitting position. Getting up slowly may help, but if the problem continues or gets worse, check with your doctor.

In some patients, this medicine may cause mental depression. **Tell your doctor right away:**

—if you or anyone else notices unusual changes in your mood.

—if you start having early-morning sleeplessness or unusually vivid dreams or nightmares.

This medicine will add to the effects of alcohol and other CNS depressants (medicines that slow down the nervous system, possibly causing drowsiness). Some examples of CNS depressants are antihistamines or medicine for hay fever, other allergies, or colds; sedatives, tranquilizers, or sleeping medicine; prescription pain medicine or narcotics; barbiturates; medicine for convulsions (seizures); muscle relaxants; or anesthetics, including dental anesthetics. **Check with your doctor before taking any of the above while you are taking this medicine.**

This medicine may cause a loss of potassium from your body.

- To help prevent this, your doctor may want you to:
  - —eat or drink foods that have a high potassium content (for example, orange or other citrus fruit juices), or
  - —take a potassium supplement, or
  - —take another medicine to help prevent the loss of the potassium in the first place.

- It is very important to follow these directions. Also, it is important not to change your diet on your own. This is more important if you are already on a special diet (as for diabetes), or if you are taking a potassium supplement or a medicine to reduce potassium loss. Extra potassium may not be necessary and, in some cases, too much potassium could be harmful.

Diabetics—This medicine may raise blood sugar levels. While you are using this medicine, be especially careful in testing for sugar in your urine. If you have any questions about this, check with your doctor.

A few people who take this medicine may become more sensitive to sunlight than they are normally. When you first begin taking this medicine, avoid too much sun and do not use a sunlamp until you see how you react to the sun, especially if you tend to burn easily. If you have a severe reaction, check with your doctor.

This medicine often causes stuffiness in the nose. However, do not use nasal decongestant medicines without first checking with your doctor or pharmacist.

This medicine may cause dryness of the mouth. For temporary relief, use sugarless candy or gum, melt bits of ice in your mouth, or use a saliva substitute. However, if dry mouth continues for more than 2 weeks, check with your physician or dentist. Continuing dryness of the mouth may increase the chance of dental disease, including tooth decay, gum disease, and fungal infections.

Side Effects of This Medicine

Suggestions that rauwolfia alkaloids may increase the risk of breast cancer occurring later have not been proven. However, rats and mice given 100 to 300 times the human dose had an increased number of tumors.

Along with its needed effects, a medicine may cause some unwanted effects. Although not all of these side effects may occur, if they do occur they may need medical attention.

Check with your doctor immediately if any of the following side effects occur:
More common
    General feeling of body discomfort or weakness
Less common
    Drowsiness or faintness
    Impotence or decreased sexual interest
    Mental depression or inability to concentrate
    Nervousness or anxiety
    Vivid dreams or nightmares or early-morning sleeplessness

Check with your doctor as soon as possible if any of the following side effects occur:
Less common
    Black tarry stools
    Blisters on skin
    Bloody vomit
    Chest pain
    Fever and sore throat
    Headache
    Irregular heartbeat
    Joint pain
    Numbness, tingling, pain, or weakness in hands or feet
    Shortness of breath
    Skin rash or itching
    Swelling of the lymph glands
Rare
    Painful or difficult urination
    Stiffness
    Stomach pain (severe) with nausea and vomiting
    Trembling and shaking of hands and fingers
    Unusual bleeding or bruising
    Yellow eyes or skin
Signs of overdose
    Dizziness or drowsiness (severe)
    Dryness of mouth
    Flushing of skin
    Increased thirst
    Muscle cramps or pain
    Nausea or vomiting (severe)
    Pinpoint pupils of eyes
    Slow pulse

Other side effects may occur that usually do not require medical attention. These side effects may go away during treatment as your body adjusts to the medicine. However, check with your doctor if any of the following side effects continue or are bothersome:
More common
    Diarrhea
    Dizziness, especially when getting up from a lying or sitting position
    Loss of appetite
    Nausea or vomiting
    Stuffy nose
Less common
    Constipation
    Flushing or redness of skin
    Red, sore eyes

For elderly patients: Dizziness or faintness or signs of too much potassium loss may be more likely to occur in the elderly, who are more sensitive to the effects of this medicine.

After you stop using this medicine, it may still produce some side effects that need attention. During this period of time **check with your doctor immediately** if you notice any of the following side effects:

    Drowsiness or faintness
    General feeling of body discomfort or weakness
    Impotence or decreased sexual interest
    Irregular heartbeat

    Mental depression or inability to concentrate
    Nervousness or anxiety
    Vivid dreams or nightmares or early-morning sleeplessness

Other side effects not listed above may also occur in some patients. If you notice any other effects, check with your doctor.

———————

December 1987

RESORCINOL (Topical)

A commonly used brand name is RA.

To the Reader: If you do not recognize the names of medical conditions or medicines referred to in this information, check with your doctor, nurse, or pharmacist. Definitions for selected medical terms may be found in the Glossary. Brand names for the generic drug names listed can be found in the Index. In addition, selected brand names commonly associated with the generic name have been included in the text to help you recognize medicine you may be taking. The fact that a brand name product is not mentioned does not mean the information does not apply. It is a good idea for you to learn both the generic and brand names of your medicines and to write them down for future use.

Resorcinol (re-SOR-si-nole) is applied to the skin to treat acne, seborrhea, and other skin disorders.

Some of these preparations are available only with your doctor's prescription. Others are available without a prescription; however, your doctor may have special instructions on the proper use of resorcinol for your medical condition.

Remember:

• **Keep all medicines out of the reach of children.**

• In order for this medicine to work, it must be used as directed. **If you are using this medicine without a prescription, it is very important that you follow the directions on the label.**

• **It is also very important that you read and understand the following information.** If any of the information causes you special concern, check with your doctor or pharmacist.

• Before you begin using any new medicine (prescription or nonprescription) or if you develop any new medical problem while you are using this medicine, check with your doctor, nurse, or pharmacist.

• **If you have any questions** about the following information or if you want more information about this medicine or your medical problem, **ask your doctor, nurse, or pharmacist.**

Before Using This Medicine

Before you use topical resorcinol, check with your doctor or pharmacist:

—if you have ever had any unusual or allergic reaction to resorcinol.

—if you are allergic to any substance, such as certain preservatives or dyes. Most medicines contain more than their active ingredient. Your doctor, nurse, or pharmacist can help you avoid products that may cause a problem.

—if you are **pregnant** or if you may become pregnant, since resorcinol may be absorbed through the skin. However, topical resorcinol has not been shown to cause birth defects or other problems in humans.

—if you are **breast-feeding**, since this medicine may be absorbed through the skin. However, topical resorcinol has not been shown to cause problems in nursing babies.

—if you are taking **any** other prescription or nonprescription (OTC) medicine.

Proper Use of This Medicine

It is very important that you use this medicine only as directed. Do not use more of it, do not use it more often, and do not use it for a longer period of time than your doctor ordered. To do so may increase the chance of absorption through the skin and the chance of resorcinol poisoning.

Apply enough resorcinol to cover the affected areas, and rub in gently.

Immediately after using this medicine, wash your hands to remove any medicine that may be on them.

Keep this medicine away from the eyes. If you should accidentally get some in your eyes, flush them thoroughly with water.

If you miss a dose of this medicine, apply it as soon as possible. However, if it is almost time for your next dose, skip the missed dose and go back to your regular dosing schedule.

How to store this medicine:

• **Keep out of the reach of children.**

• Store away from heat and direct light.

• Keep the medicine from freezing.

• Do not keep outdated medicine or medicine no longer needed. Be sure that any discarded medicine is out of the reach of children.

Precautions While Using This Medicine

When using resorcinol, do not use any of the following preparations on the same affected area as this medicine, unless otherwise directed by your doctor:

    Abrasive soaps or cleansers
    Alcohol-containing preparations
    Any other topical acne preparation or preparation containing a peeling agent (for example, benzoyl peroxide, salicylic acid, sulfur, or tretinoin [vitamin A acid])
    Cosmetics or soaps that dry the skin
    Medicated cosmetics
    Other topical medicine for the skin

To use any of the above preparations on the same affected area as resorcinol may cause severe irritation of the skin.

This medicine may darken light-colored hair.

Side Effects of This Medicine

Along with its needed effects, a medicine may cause some unwanted effects. Although not all of these side effects may occur, if they do occur they may need medical attention.

Check with your doctor as soon as possible if any of the following side effects occur:

Skin irritation not present before using this medicine

Signs of resorcinol poisoning

Diarrhea, nausea, stomach pain, or vomiting
Dizziness
Drowsiness
Headache (severe or continuing)
Nervousness or restlessness
Slow heartbeat, shortness of breath, or troubled breathing
Sweating
Unusual tiredness or weakness

Other side effects may occur that usually do not require medical attention. These side effects may go away during treatment as your body adjusts to the medicine.

However, check with your doctor if the following side effect continues or is bothersome:

More common

Redness and peeling of skin (may occur after a few days)

For elderly patients: Many medicines have not been tested in older people. Therefore, it is not known whether the medicine acts the same way it does in younger adults. Check with your doctor or pharmacist if you notice any unusual effects while using this medicine or if you think it is not working as it should.

Other side effects not listed above may also occur in some patients. If you notice any other effects, check with your doctor.

_____

December 1987

RESORCINOL AND SULFUR (Topical)

Some commonly used brand names are:

Acne-Aid*   Rezamid
Acnomel   Sulforcin
Clearasil

*Not available in the U.S.

To the Reader: If you do not recognize the names of medical conditions or medicines referred to in this information, check with your doctor, nurse, or pharmacist. Definitions for selected medical terms may be found in the Glossary. Brand names for the generic drug names listed can be found in the Index. In addition, selected brand names commonly associated with the generic name have been included in the text to help you recognize medicine you may be taking. The fact that a brand name product is not mentioned does not mean the information does not apply. It is a good idea for you to learn both the generic and brand names of your medicines and to write them down for future use.

Resorcinol and sulfur (re-SOR-si-nole and SUL-fur) combination is applied to the skin to treat acne and similar skin conditions.

This medicine is available without a prescription; however, your doctor may have special instructions on the proper use of this medicine for your medical condition.

Remember:

• **Keep all medicines out of the reach of children.**

• In order for this medicine to work, it must be used as directed. **If you are using this medicine without a prescription, it is very important to follow the directions on the label.**

• It is also very important that you read and understand the following information. If any of the information causes you special concern, check with your doctor or pharmacist.

• Before you begin using any new medicine (prescription or nonprescription) or if you develop any new medical problem while you are using this medicine, check with your doctor, nurse, or pharmacist.

• **If you have any questions** about the following information or if you want more information about this medicine or your medical problem, **ask your doctor, nurse, or pharmacist.**

Before Using This Medicine

Before you use resorcinol and sulfur combination, check with your doctor or pharmacist:

—if you have ever had any unusual or allergic reaction to resorcinol or sulfur.

—if you are allergic to any substance, such as certain foods or preservatives or dyes. Most medicines contain more than their active ingredient. Your doctor, nurse, or pharmacist can help you avoid products that may cause a problem.

—if you are **pregnant** or if you may become pregnant, since resorcinol (contained in this combination medicine) may be absorbed through the skin. However, topical resorcinol and sulfur combination has not been shown to cause birth defects or other problems in humans.

—if you are **breast-feeding**, since resorcinol (contained in this combination medicine) may be absorbed through the skin. However, topical resorcinol and sulfur combination has not been shown to cause problems in nursing babies.

—if you are taking **any** other prescription or nonprescription (OTC) medicine.

Proper Use of This Medicine

Use this medicine only as directed. Do not use more of it and do not use it more often than recommended on the label, unless otherwise directed by your doctor.

Before using this medicine, wash the affected areas thoroughly and gently pat dry. Then apply a small amount to the affected areas and spread on gently, but do not rub in.

Immediately after using this medicine, wash your hands to remove any medicine that may be on them.

Keep this medicine away from the eyes. If you should accidentally get some in your eyes, flush them thoroughly with water.

If you miss a dose of this medicine, apply it as soon as possible. However, if it is almost time for your next dose, skip the missed dose and go back to your regular dosing schedule.

How to store this medicine:

• **Keep out of the reach of children.**

• Store away from heat and direct light.

• Keep the medicine from freezing.

• Do not keep outdated medicine or medicine no longer needed. Be sure that any discarded medicine is out of the reach of children.

Precautions While Using This Medicine

When using resorcinol and sulfur combination, do not use any of the following preparations on the same affected area as this medicine, unless otherwise directed by your doctor:

Abrasive soaps or cleansers
Alcohol-containing preparations
Any other topical acne preparation or preparation containing a peeling agent (for example, benzoyl peroxide, salicylic acid, or tretinoin [vitamin A acid])
Cosmetics or soaps that dry the skin
Medicated cosmetics
Other topical medicine for the skin

To use any of the above preparations on the same affected area as this medicine may cause severe irritation of the skin.

Do not use any topical mercury-containing preparation, such as ammoniated mercury ointment, on the same affected area as this medicine. To do so may cause a foul odor, be irritating to the skin, and stain the skin black. If you have any questions about this, check with your doctor or pharmacist.

This medicine (depending on the product you are using) may darken light-colored hair. If you have any questions about this, check with your doctor or pharmacist.

Side Effects of This Medicine

Along with its needed effects, a medicine may cause some unwanted effects. Although not all of these side effects may occur, if they do occur they may need medical attention.

Check with your doctor as soon as possible if the following side effect occurs:

  Skin irritation not present before using this medicine

Other side effects may occur that usually do not require medical attention. However, check with your doctor or pharmacist if the following side effects continue or are bothersome:

More common

  Redness and peeling of skin (may occur after a few days)

Less common

  Unusual dryness of skin

For elderly patients: Many medicines have not been tested in older people. Therefore, it is not known whether the medicine acts the same way it does in younger adults. Check with your doctor or pharmacist if you notice any unusual effects while using this medicine or if you think it is not working as it should.

Other side effects not listed above may also occur in some patients. If you notice any other effects, check with your doctor or pharmacist.

_____

December 1987

RIBAVIRIN (Systemic)

Some commonly used brand names or other names are:

Tribavirin	Viramid*
Vilona*	Virazole

*Not available in the U.S.

To the Reader: If you do not recognize the names of medical conditions or medicines referred to in this information, check with your doctor, nurse, or pharmacist. Definitions for selected medical terms may be found in the Glossary. Brand names for the generic drug names listed can be found in the Index. In addition, selected brand names commonly associated with the generic name have been included in the text to help you recognize medicine you may be taking. The fact that a brand name product is not mentioned does not mean the information does not apply. It is a good idea for you to learn both the generic and brand names of your medicines and to write them down for future use.

Ribavirin (rye-ba-VYE-rin) belongs to the family of medicines called antivirals. Antivirals are medicines used to treat infections caused by viruses. They work by killing viruses or preventing their growth.

Ribavirin is used to treat severe viral pneumonia. It is given by oral inhalation (breathing in the medicine as a fine mist through the mouth), using a special nebulizer (sprayer) attached to an oxygen hood or tent or face mask.

This medicine may also be used for other viral infections as determined by your doctor. However, it will not work for certain viruses such as the common cold.

Ribavirin is to be administered only by or under the immediate supervision of your doctor.

Remember:

• **It is very important that you read and understand the following information.** If any of the information causes you special concern, do not decide against using this medicine without first checking with your doctor.

• **If you have any questions** about the following information or if you want more information about this medicine or your medical problem, **ask your doctor, nurse, or pharmacist.**

Before Using This Medicine

In order to decide on the best treatment for your medical problem, your doctor should be told:

—if you have ever had any unusual or allergic reaction to ribavirin.

—if you are on a low-salt, low-sugar, or any other special diet, or if you are allergic to any substance, such as foods or sulfites or other preservatives. Most medicines contain more than their active ingredient. Your doctor, nurse, or pharmacist can help you avoid products that may cause a problem.

—if you are **pregnant** or if you may become pregnant. Ribavirin is not recommended during pregnancy. Although studies have not been done in humans, ribavirin has been shown to cause birth defects and other problems in certain animal studies. Be sure you have discussed this with your doctor.

—if you are **breast-feeding.** Ribavirin passes into the breast milk and has been shown to cause problems in nursing animals and their young. You should stop breast-feeding during treatment with ribavirin. During this time the breast milk should be squeezed out or sucked out with a breast pump and thrown away. After treatment with ribavirin is finished, you may go back to breast-feeding. Be sure you have discussed this with your doctor.

Proper Use of This Medicine

To help clear up your infection completely, **this medicine must be given for the full time of treatment** even if you begin to feel better after a few days. Also, it works best when there is a constant amount in the lungs. To help keep this amount constant, it must be given on a regular or continuous schedule.

Side Effects of This Medicine

In studies in rats, ribavirin given by mouth was shown to cause benign (not cancerous) tumors. It is not known whether ribavirin causes tumors in humans.

Along with its needed effects, a medicine may cause some unwanted effects. The following side effects may go away during treatment as your body adjusts to the medicine. However, check with your doctor if any of the following side effects continue or are bothersome:

Less common
   Blurred vision
   Dizziness
   Faintness or lightheadedness
   Feeling of something in eye
   Increased sensitivity of eyes to light
   Itching, redness, or swelling of eye
   Unusual tiredness or weakness

Other side effects not listed above may also occur in some patients. If you notice any other effects, check with your doctor.

December 1987

RIBOFLAVIN (VITAMIN B₂) (Systemic)

To the Reader: If you do not recognize the names of medical conditions or medicines referred to in this information, check with your doctor, nurse, or pharmacist. Definitions for selected medical terms may be found in the Glossary. Brand names for the generic drug names listed can be found in the Index. In addition, selected brand names commonly associated with the generic name have been included in the text to help you recognize medicine you may be taking. The fact that a brand name product is not mentioned does not mean the information does not apply. It is a good idea for you to learn both the generic and brand names of your medicines and to write them down for future use.

Vitamins (VYE-ta-mins) are compounds that you *must* have for growth and health. They are needed in small amounts only and are usually available in the foods that you eat. Riboflavin (RYE-boe-flay-vin) (vitamin B₂) is necessary for normal metabolism.

Lack of riboflavin may lead to itching and burning eyes, sensitivity of eyes to light, sore tongue, itching and peeling skin on the nose and scrotum, and sores in the mouth. Your doctor may treat this condition by prescribing riboflavin for you.

Claims that riboflavin is effective for treatment of acne, some kinds of anemia (weak blood), migraine headaches, and muscle cramps have not been proven.

Oral forms of riboflavin are available without a prescription. However, it may be a good idea to check with your doctor before taking riboflavin on your own. If you take more than you need, it will simply be lost from your body.

Remember:

• **Keep all medicines out of the reach of children.**

• In order for this medicine to work, it must be used as directed. **If you are using this medicine without a prescription, it is very important to follow the directions on the label.**

• **It is also very important that you read and understand the following information.** If any of the information causes you special concern, check with your doctor before using this medicine without a prescription.

• Before you begin using any new medicine (prescription or nonprescription) or if you develop any new medical problem while you are using this medicine, check with your doctor, nurse, or pharmacist.

• **If you have any questions** about the following information or if you want more information about this medicine or your medical problem, **ask your doctor, nurse, or pharmacist.**

Importance of Diet

Vitamin supplements should be taken only if you cannot get enough vitamins in your diet. A balanced diet should provide all the vitamins you normally need.

Nutritionists recommend that you eat:
• Cereal or bread—4 or more servings per day and
• Dairy products (milk, cheese, ice cream, cottage cheese)—3 or more servings per day and

• Meat, fish, or eggs—2 or more servings per day and
• Vegetables and fruits—4 or more servings per day.

If you are not getting all of these foods every day, you may not be getting enough vitamins in your diet. The best way to correct this is to start eating the foods that contain what you need.

Riboflavin is found in various foods, including milk and dairy products, meats, and green leafy vegetables. It is best to eat fresh fruits and vegetables whenever possible since they contain the most vitamins. Food processing may destroy some of the vitamins, although little riboflavin is lost from foods during ordinary cooking.

Vitamins alone will not take the place of a good diet and will not provide energy. Your body also needs other substances found in food such as protein, minerals, carbohydrates, and fat. Vitamins themselves often cannot work without the presence of other foods.

In some cases it may not be possible for you to get enough food to supply you with the proper vitamins. In other cases, the amount of vitamins you need may be increased above normal. Therefore, a vitamin supplement may be needed.

Experts have developed a list of recommended dietary allowances (RDA) for most of the vitamins. The RDA are not an exact number but a general idea of how much you need. They do not cover amounts needed for problems caused by a serious lack of vitamins.

The RDA for riboflavin are:

Children 4 to 6 years of age—1 mg per day
Adult males—1.6 mg per day
Adult females—1.2 mg per day
Pregnant females—1.5 mg per day
Breast-feeding females—1.7 mg per day.

Remember:

• The total amount of each vitamin that you get every day includes what you get from the foods that you eat *and* what you may take as a supplement.

• This total amount should not be greater than the RDA, unless ordered by your doctor.

Before Using This Medicine

In deciding whether you need additional riboflavin, the following should be kept in mind and/or your doctor or pharmacist should be told:

—if you have ever had any unusual or allergic reaction to riboflavin.

—if you are on a low-salt, low-sugar, or any other special diet, or if you are allergic to any substance, such as foods, sulfites or other preservatives, or dyes. Most medicines contain more than their active ingredient. Your doctor, nurse, or pharmacist can help you avoid products that may cause a problem.

—if you are **pregnant** or if you may become pregnant. It is especially important that you are receiving enough vitamins when you become pregnant and that you continue to receive the right amount of vitamins throughout your pregnancy. The healthy growth and development of the fetus depend on a steady supply of nutrients from the mother.

—if you are **breast-feeding**. It is especially important that you receive the right amounts of vitamins so that your baby will also get the vitamins needed to grow properly.

—if you are not able to get a diet that contains all of the vitamins you need. This may occur with rapid weight loss, unusual diets (such as some reducing diets in which choice of foods is very limited), prolonged intravenous feeding, or malnutrition.

—if you have had a large part of your stomach removed.

—if you have been under a lot of stress for a long time, or if you have had a long illness or serious injury.

—if you have any of the following medical problems:
Alcoholism
Burns
Cancer
Diarrhea (prolonged)
Infection
Intestinal problems
Liver disease
Overactive thyroid

—if you are taking **any** other prescription or nonprescription (OTC) medicine:

Proper Use of This Medicine

Some people believe that taking very large doses of vitamins (called megadoses or megavitamin therapy) is useful for treating certain medical problems. Studies have not proven this. Large doses should be taken only under the direction of your doctor after need has been identified.

If you miss taking a vitamin for one or more days there is no cause for concern, since it takes some time for your body to become seriously low in vitamins. However, if your doctor has recommended that you take this vitamin, try to remember to take it as directed every day.

How to store this medicine:

• **Keep out of the reach of children.**

• Store away from heat and direct light.

• Do not store in the bathroom, near the kitchen sink, or in other damp places. Heat or moisture may cause the medicine to break down.

• Do not keep outdated medicine or medicine no longer needed. Be sure that any discarded medicine is out of the reach of children.

Side Effects of This Medicine

Along with its needed effects, a medicine may cause some unwanted effects. This medicine may cause urine to have a more yellow color than normal. This is to be expected and is no cause for alarm. Usually, however, riboflavin does not cause any side effects. Check with your doctor if you notice any other unusual effects while you are using it.

December 1987

RIFAMPIN (Systemic)

Some commonly used brand names or other names are:

Rifadin	Rimactane
Rifampicin	Rofact*

*Not available in the U.S.

To the Reader: If you do not recognize the names of medical conditions or medicines referred to in this information, check with your doctor, nurse, or pharmacist. Definitions for selected medical terms may be found in the Glossary. Brand names for the generic drug names listed can be found in the Index. In addition, selected brand names commonly associated with the generic name have been included in the text to help you recognize medicine you may be taking. The fact that a brand name product is not mentioned does not mean the information does not apply. It is a good idea for you to learn both the generic and brand names of your medicines and to write them down for future use.

Rifampin (rif-AM-pin) belongs to the family of medicines called antibiotics. It is taken by mouth in combination with one or more other medicines to help the body overcome tuberculosis (TB). Rifampin is also given alone in patients who may carry meningitis bacteria (without feeling sick) and may spread them to others. This medicine may also be used for other problems as determined by your doctor.

Rifampin is available only with your doctor's prescription.

Remember:

• **This medicine has been prescribed for your present infection only.** Another infection later on may require a different medicine. Also, even though other people may have the same symptoms as you, they may have a different kind of infection. Your medicine may not work for them and may even cause them harm. Therefore, **your medicine must not be given to other people or used for other infections** unless you are otherwise directed by your doctor.

• **Keep all medicines out of the reach of children.**

• In order for this medicine to work, it must be used as directed.

• **It is very important that you read and understand the following information.** If any of the information causes you special concern, do not decide against using this medicine without first checking with your doctor.

• Before you begin using any new medicine (prescription or nonprescription) or if you develop any new medical problem while you are using this medicine, check with your doctor, nurse, or pharmacist.

• **If you have any questions** about the following information or if you want more information about this medicine or your medical problem, **ask your doctor, nurse, or pharmacist.**

Before Using This Medicine

In order to decide on the best treatment for your medical problem, your doctor should be told:

—if you have ever had any unusual or allergic reaction to rifampin.

—if you are on a low-salt, low-sugar, or any other special diet, or if you are allergic to any substance, such as sulfites or other preservatives or dyes. Most medicines contain more than their active ingredient. Your doctor, nurse, or pharmacist can help you avoid products that may cause a problem.

—if you are **pregnant** or if you may become pregnant. Rifampin has not been shown to cause birth defects or other problems in humans. However, studies in rodents have shown that rifampin given in high doses causes backbone problems (spina bifida) and cleft palate. In addition, it is not known whether this medicine causes problems when taken with other TB medicines.

—if you are **breast-feeding**. Rifampin passes into the breast milk. However, rifampin has not been shown to cause problems in nursing babies.

—if you have either of the following medical problems:
  Alcoholism (active or treated)
  Liver disease

—if you are taking **any** other prescription or nonprescription (OTC) medicine, especially:
  Adrenocorticoids (cortisone-like medicines)
  Anticoagulants (blood thinners)
  Corticotropin (ACTH)
  Digitalis glycosides (heart medicine)
  Disopyramide (e.g., Norpace)
  Estramustine (e.g., EMCYT)
  Estrogens (female hormones)
  Isoniazid (e.g., INH, Nydrazid)
  Ketoconazole by mouth (e.g., Nizoral)
  Methadone (e.g., Dolophine)
  Miconazole by injection (e.g., Monistat)
  Oral contraceptives (birth control pills) containing estrogen
  Quinidine (e.g., Quinidex)

Proper Use of This Medicine

Rifampin is best taken with a full glass (8 ounces) of water on an empty stomach (either 1 hour before or 2 hours after a meal). However, if this medicine upsets your stomach, your doctor may want you to take it with food.

For patients unable to swallow capsules (for example, children and some adults):

• Contents of the capsules may be mixed with applesauce or jelly. Be sure to take all the food in order to get the full dose of medicine.

• Your pharmacist can prepare an oral liquid form of this medicine if needed. The liquid form should be kept in the refrigerator. Follow the directions on the label and shake the bottle well before using. Do not use after the expiration date on the label since the medicine may not work. In addition, use a specially marked measuring spoon or other device to measure each dose accurately since the average household teaspoon may not hold the right amount of liquid.

To help clear up your tuberculosis (TB) completely, **it is very important that you keep taking this medicine for the full time of treatment** even if you begin to feel better after a few weeks. You may have to take it every day for as long as 1 to 2 years or more. **It is important that you do not miss any doses.**

If you do miss a dose of this medicine, take it as soon as possible. However, if it is almost time for your next dose, skip the missed dose and go back to your regular dosing schedule. Do not double doses. **If this medicine is taken on an irregular schedule, side effects may occur more often and may be more serious than usual.** If you have any questions about this, check with your doctor or pharmacist.

How to store this medicine:

- **Keep out of the reach of children.**

- Store away from heat and direct light.

- Do not store in the bathroom, near the kitchen sink, or in other damp places. Heat or moisture may cause the medicine to break down.

- Do not keep outdated medicine or medicine no longer needed. Be sure that any discarded medicine is out of the reach of children.

Precautions While Using This Medicine

Do not take rifampin within 6 hours of the time you take aminosalicylates (another TB medicine) since they may keep rifampin from working as well.

This medicine will cause the urine, stool, saliva, sputum, sweat, and tears to turn reddish orange to reddish brown. This is to be expected while you are taking this medicine. Since this effect may cause soft contact lenses to become permanently discolored and standard cleaning solutions may not take out all the discoloration, **it is best not to wear soft contact lenses while taking this medicine.** Hard contact lenses are not discolored by this medicine. If you have any questions about this, check with your doctor.

Oral contraceptives (birth control pills) containing estrogen may not work as well if you take them while you are taking rifampin. Unplanned pregnancies may occur. You should use a different means of birth control while you are taking rifampin. If you have any questions about this, check with your doctor or pharmacist.

If your symptoms do not improve within 2 to 3 weeks, or if they become worse, check with your doctor.

It is very important that your doctor check your progress at regular visits.

If this medicine causes you to feel very tired or very weak or causes a loss of appetite, nausea, or vomiting, stop taking it and check with your doctor immediately. These may be early warning signs of more serious problems that could develop later.

Liver problems may be more likely to occur if you drink alcoholic beverages regularly while you are taking this medicine. Also, the regular use of alcohol may keep this medicine from working as well. Therefore, **you should not drink alcoholic beverages while you are taking this medicine.**

Side Effects of This Medicine

Along with its needed effects, a medicine may cause some unwanted effects. Although not all of these side effects may occur, if they do occur they may need medical attention.

Check with your doctor immediately if any of the following side effects occur:

Less common
    Chills
    Difficult breathing
    Dizziness
    Fever
    Headache
    Muscle and bone pain
    Shivering
Rare
    Bloody or cloudy urine
    Greatly decreased frequency of urination or amount of urine
    Loss of appetite
    Nausea or vomiting
    Sore throat
    Unusual bruising or bleeding
    Unusual tiredness or weakness
    Yellow eyes or skin

Other side effects may occur that usually do not require medical attention. These side effects may go away during treatment as your body adjusts to the medicine. However, check with your doctor if any of the following side effects continue or are bothersome:

More common
    Diarrhea
    Reddish orange to reddish brown discoloration of urine, stools, saliva, sputum, sweat, and tears
    Stomach cramps
Less common
    Itching
    Redness
    Skin rash
    Sore mouth or tongue

Other side effects not listed above may also occur in some patients. If you notice any other effects, check with your doctor.

December 1987

RIFAMPIN AND ISONIAZID (Systemic)

A commonly used brand name is Rifamate.

To the Reader: If you do not recognize the names of medical conditions or medicines referred to in this information, check with your doctor, nurse, or pharmacist. Definitions for selected medical terms may be found in the Glossary. Brand names for the generic drug names listed can be found in the Index. In addition, selected brand names commonly associated with the generic name have been included in the text to help you recognize medicine you may be taking. The fact that a brand name product is not mentioned does not mean the information does not apply. It is a good idea for you to learn both the generic and brand names of your medicines and to write them down for future use.

Rifampin (rif-AM-pin) and isoniazid (eye-soe-NYE-a-zid) is a combination antibiotic and anti-infective medicine. It is taken by mouth to help the body overcome tuberculosis (TB). It may be taken alone or with one or more other medicines for TB.

Rifampin and isoniazid combination is available only with your doctor's prescription.

Remember:
• This medicine has been prescribed for your present TB infection only. Another TB infection later on may require a different medicine. Also, even though other people may have the same symptoms as you, they may have a different kind of TB. Your medicine may not work for them and may even cause them harm. Therefore, **your medicine must not be given to other people or used for other infections** unless you are otherwise directed by your doctor.

• In order for this medicine to work, it must be taken as directed.

• If you want more information about this medicine, ask your doctor, nurse, or pharmacist.

• Keep all medicines out of the reach of children.

• If any of the following information causes you special concern, do not decide against taking this medicine without first checking with your doctor.

Before Using This Medicine

In order to decide on the best treatment for your medical problem, your doctor should be told:

—if you have ever had any unusual or allergic reaction to ethionamide, pyrazinamide, niacin (nicotinic acid), rifampin, or isoniazid.

—if you are **pregnant** or if you may become pregnant. Rifampin and isoniazid combination has not been shown to cause birth defects or other problems in humans. However, studies in rodents have shown that rifampin given in high doses causes backbone problems (spina bifida) and cleft palate. Studies in rats and rabbits have shown that isoniazid may kill the fetus. In addition, it is not known whether this medicine causes problems when taken with other TB medicines.

—if you are **breast-feeding**. Rifampin and isoniazid both pass into the breast milk. However, rifampin and isoniazid have not been shown to cause problems in nursing babies.

—if you have any of the following medical problems:

Alcoholism (active or treated)
Convulsive disorders such as seizures or epilepsy
Kidney disease, severe
Liver disease

—if you are taking **any** other prescription or nonprescription (OTC) medicine, especially:

Acetaminophen (e.g., Tylenol) (with long-term, high-dose use)
Adrenocorticoids (cortisone-like medicine)
Amiodarone (e.g., Cordarone)
Anabolic steroids (dromostanolone, ethylestrenol, nandrolone, oxandrolone, oxymetholone, stanozolol)
Androgens (male hormones)
Anticoagulants (blood thinners)
Antithyroid agents (medicine for overactive thyroid)
Azlocillin (e.g., Azlin)
Carbamazepine (e.g., Tegretol)
Carmustine (e.g., BiCNU)
Chloroquine (e.g., Aralen)
Corticotropin (ACTH)
Dantrolene (e.g., Dantrium)
Daunorubicin (e.g., Cerubidine)
Digitalis glycosides (heart medicine)
Disopyramide (e.g., Norpace)
Disulfiram (e.g., Antabuse)
Divalproex (e.g., Depakote)
Doxorubicin (e.g., Adriamycin)
Erythromycins
Estramustine (e.g., EMCYT)
Estrogens (female hormones)
Etretinate (e.g., Tegison)
Furazolidone (e.g., Furoxone)
Gold salts
Hydroxychloroquine (e.g., Plaquenil)
Ketoconazole by mouth (e.g., Nizoral)
Mercaptopurine (e.g., Purinethol)
Methadone (e.g., Dolophine)
Methotrexate (e.g., Mexate)
Methyldopa (e.g., Aldomet)
Mezlocillin (e.g., Mezlin)
Miconazole by injection (e.g., Monistat)
Naltrexone (e.g., Trexan) (with long-term, high-dose use)
Nitrofurantoin (e.g., Furadantin)
Oral contraceptives (birth control pills) containing estrogen
Phenothiazines (acetophenazine, chlorpromazine, fluphenazine, mesoridazine, perphenazine, prochlorperazine, promazine, promethazine, thioridazine, trifluoperazine, triflupromazine, trimeprazine)
Phenytoin (e.g., Dilantin)
Piperacillin (e.g., Pipracil)
Plicamycin (e.g., Mithracin)
Quinidine (e.g., Quinidex)
Sulfonamides (sulfa medicine)
Valproic acid (e.g., Depakene)

—if you have ever had any problems with rifampin or isoniazid.

Proper Use of This Medicine

Rifampin and isoniazid combination is best taken with a full glass (8 ounces) of water on an empty stomach (either 1 hour before or 2 hours after a meal). However, if this medicine upsets your stomach, your doctor may want you to take it with food.

Antacids may also help; but do not take aluminum-containing antacids within 1 hour of the time you take rifampin and isoniazid since they may keep this medicine from working as well.

To help clear up your tuberculosis (TB) completely, **it is very important that you keep taking this medicine for the full time of treatment** even if you begin to feel better after a few weeks. You may have to take it every day for as long as 1 to 2 years or more. **It is important that you do not miss any doses.**

Your doctor may also want you to take pyridoxine (vitamin B$_6$) every day to help prevent or lessen some of the side effects of isoniazid. If so, **it is very important to take pyridoxine every day along with this medicine; do not miss any doses.**

If you do miss a dose of either of these medicines, take it as soon as possible. However, if it is almost time for your next dose, do not take the missed dose or double your next dose. Instead, go back to your regular dosing schedule. **If rifampin and isoniazid is taken on an irregular schedule, side effects may occur more often and may be more serious than usual.** If you have any questions about this, check with your doctor or pharmacist.

How to store this medicine:

• **Keep out of the reach of children.**

• Store away from heat and direct light.

• Do not store in the bathroom, near the kitchen sink, or in other damp places. Heat or moisture may cause the medicine to break down.

• Do not keep outdated medicine or medicine no longer needed. Be sure that any discarded medicine is out of the reach of children.

Precautions While Using This Medicine

Certain foods such as cheese (Swiss or Cheshire) or fish (tuna, skipjack, or Sardinella) may rarely cause reactions in some patients taking isoniazid-containing medicines. Check with your doctor if redness or itching of the skin, hot feeling, rapid or pounding heartbeat, sweating, chills or clammy feeling, headache, or light-headedness occurs while you are taking this medicine.

Do not take rifampin and isoniazid within 6 hours of the time you take aminosalicylates (another TB medicine) since they may keep rifampin and isoniazid from working as well.

This medicine will cause the urine, stool, saliva, sputum, sweat, and tears to turn reddish orange to reddish brown. This is to be expected while you are taking this medicine. Since this effect may cause soft contact lenses to become permanently discolored and standard cleaning solutions may not take out all the discoloration, **it is best not to wear soft contact lenses while taking this medicine.** Hard contact lenses are not discolored by this medicine. If you have any questions about this, check with your doctor.

Oral contraceptives (birth control pills) containing estrogen may not work as well if you take them while you are taking rifampin and isoniazid. Unplanned pregnancies may occur. You should use a different means of birth control while you are taking this medicine. If you have any questions about this, check with your doctor or pharmacist.

If your symptoms do not improve within 2 to 3 weeks, or if they become worse, check with your doctor.

It is very important that your doctor check your progress at regular visits. In addition, you should **check with your doctor immediately if blurred vision or any loss of vision, with or without eye pain, occurs during treatment.** He may want you to have your eyes checked by an ophthalmologist (eye doctor).

If this medicine causes you to feel very tired or very weak; or causes clumsiness; unsteadiness; a loss of appetite; nausea; numbness, tingling, burning, or pain in the hands and feet; or vomiting, stop taking it and check with your doctor immediately. These may be early warning signs of more serious liver or nerve problems that could develop later.

Diabetics—This medicine may cause false test results with some urine sugar tests. Check with your doctor before changing your diet or the dosage of your diabetes medicine.

Liver problems may be more likely to occur if you drink alcoholic beverages regularly while you are taking this medicine. Also, the regular use of alcohol may keep this medicine from working as well. Therefore, **you should not drink alcoholic beverages while you are taking this medicine.**

Side Effects of This Medicine

Along with its needed effects, a medicine may cause some unwanted effects. Although not all of these side effects may occur, if they do occur they may need medical attention.

Check with your doctor immediately if any of the following side effects occur:

More common
   Clumsiness or unsteadiness
   Dark urine
   Loss of appetite
   Nausea or vomiting
   Numbness, tingling, burning, or pain in hands and feet
   Unusual tiredness or weakness
   Yellow eyes or skin

Less common
- Chills
- Difficult breathing
- Dizziness
- Fever
- Headache
- Muscle and bone pain
- Shivering

Rare
- Bloody or cloudy urine
- Blurred vision or any loss of vision, with or without eye pain
- Greatly decreased frequency of urination or amount of urine
- Sore throat
- Unusual bruising or bleeding

Other side effects may occur that usually do not require medical attention. These side effects may go away during treatment as your body adjusts to the medicine.

However, check with your doctor if any of the following side effects continue or are bothersome:

More common
- Diarrhea
- Reddish orange to reddish brown discoloration of urine, stool, saliva, sputum, sweat, and tears
- Stomach cramps or upset

Less common
- Enlargement of the breasts—males
- Itching
- Redness
- Skin rash
- Sore mouth or tongue

Other side effects not listed above may also occur in some patients. If you notice any other effects, check with your doctor.

_____

December 1987

_____

RITODRINE (Systemic)

A commonly used brand name is Yutopar.

To the Reader: If you do not recognize the names of medical conditions or medicines referred to in this information, check with your doctor, nurse, or pharmacist. Definitions for selected medical terms may be found in the Glossary. Brand names for the generic drug names listed can be found in the Index. In addition, selected brand names commonly associated with the generic name have been included in the text to help you recognize medicine you may be taking. The fact that a brand name product is not mentioned does not mean the information does not apply. It is a good idea for you to learn both the generic and brand names of your medicines and to write them down for future use.

Ritodrine (RI-toe-dreen) is a medicine used to stop premature labor. It is available only with your doctor's prescription and is to be administered only by or under the supervision of your doctor.

Remember:

• **This medicine has been prescribed for your current medical problem only.** It must not be given to other people or used for other problems unless you are directed to do so by your doctor.

• **Keep all medicines out of the reach of children.**

• In order for this medicine to work, it must be used as directed.

• If you are receiving this medicine by injection, some of the information about this medicine may not apply.

• **It is very important that you read and understand the following information.** If any of the information causes you special concern, do not decide against using this medicine without first checking with your doctor.

• Before you begin using any new medicine (prescription or nonprescription) or if you develop any new medical problem while you are using this medicine, check with your doctor, nurse, or pharmacist.

• **If you have any questions** about the following information or if you want more information about this medicine or your medical problem, **ask your doctor, nurse, or pharmacist.**

Before Using This Medicine

In order to decide on the best treatment for your medical problem, your doctor should be told:

—if you have ever had any unusual or allergic reaction to ritodrine.

—if you are on a low-salt, low-sugar, or any other special diet, or if you are allergic to any substance, such as foods, sulfites or other preservatives, or dyes. Most medicines contain more than their active ingredient. Your doctor, nurse, or pharmacist can help you avoid products that may cause a problem.

—if you have any of the following medical problems:
    Asthma
    Diabetes mellitus (sugar diabetes)
    Heart disease
    Hypertension (high blood pressure)
    Overactive thyroid

—if you are taking **any** other prescription or nonprescription (OTC) medicine, especially:
    Adrenocorticoids (cortisone-like medicines)
    Beta-blockers (acebutolol, atenolol, labetalol, metoprolol, nadolol, oxprenolol, pindolol, propranolol, sotalol, timolol)

Proper Use of This Medicine

If you miss a dose of this medicine and remember within an hour or so of the missed dose, take it right away. However, if you do not remember until later, skip the missed dose and go back to your regular dosing schedule. Do not double doses.

How to store this medicine:

• **Keep out of the reach of children.**

• Store away from heat and direct light.

• Do not store in the bathroom, near the kitchen sink, or in other damp places. Heat or moisture may cause the medicine to break down.

• Do not keep outdated medicine or medicine no longer needed. Be sure that any discarded medicine is out of the reach of children.

Precautions While Using This Medicine

Check with your doctor right away if your contractions begin again or your water breaks.

Do not take other medicines unless they have been discussed with your doctor. This especially includes over-the-counter (nonprescription) medicines for appetite control, asthma, colds, cough, hay fever, or sinus problems since they may increase the unwanted effects of this medicine.

Side Effects of This Medicine

Along with its needed effects, a medicine may cause some unwanted effects. Although not all of these side effects may occur, if they do occur they may need medical attention.

Tell your doctor or nurse immediately if either of the following side effects occurs while you are receiving this medicine by injection:

Rare
    Chest pain or tightness
    Shortness of breath

Check with your doctor or nurse as soon as possible if the following side effects occur:

More common
    Fast or irregular heartbeat

Signs of overdose
    Fast or irregular heartbeat (severe)
    Nausea or vomiting (severe)
    Nervousness or trembling (severe)
    Shortness of breath (severe)

Other side effects may occur that usually do not require medical attention. These side effects may go away during treatment as your body adjusts to the medicine. However, check with your doctor if any of the following side effects continue or are bothersome:

More common
   Trembling

Less common
   Headache—more common with injection
   Jitteriness, nervousness, or restlessness

Nausea and vomiting
Reddened skin—injection only
Skin rash

Other side effects not listed above may also occur in some patients. If you notice any other effects, check with your doctor.

December 1987

RUBELLA VIRUS VACCINE LIVE
(Systemic)

Some commonly used brand names are Almevax*, Ervevax*, and Meruvax II.

---

*Not available in the U.S.

To the Reader: If you do not recognize the names of medical conditions or medicines referred to in this information, check with your doctor, nurse, or pharmacist. Definitions for selected medical terms may be found in the Glossary. Brand names for the generic drug names listed can be found in the Index. In addition, selected brand names commonly associated with the generic name have been included in the text to help you recognize medicine you may be taking. The fact that a brand name product is not mentioned does not mean the information does not apply. It is a good idea for you to learn both the generic and brand names of your medicines and to write them down for future use.

Rubella (rue-BELL-a) Virus Vaccine Live is an active immunizing agent given by injection to prevent infection by the rubella virus. It works by causing your body to produce its own protection (antibodies) against the virus.

The following information applies only to the Wistar RA 27/3 strain of rubella vaccine. Different types of rubella vaccines may be available in countries other than the U.S.

Rubella (also known as German measles) is a serious infection that causes miscarriages, stillbirths, or birth defects in unborn babies when pregnant women get the disease. While immunization against rubella is recommended for everyone, it is especially important for women of child-bearing age.

Immunization against rubella is also important for employees in medical facilities, persons in colleges and in the military, children of pregnant women who have not yet received their own rubella immunization, and all children 12 months of age and older, including school-age children.

Immunization against rubella is not recommended for infants younger than 12 months of age because antibodies they received from the mother before birth may interfere with the effectiveness of the vaccine. Children who were immunized against rubella before 12 months of age should be immunized again.

If the rubella vaccine is going to be given in a combination immunization that includes measles vaccine, the child to be immunized should be at least 15 months old to make sure the measles vaccine is effective.

You can be considered to be immune to rubella only if you received rubella vaccine on or after your first birthday and you have the medical record to prove it or if you have had a blood test showing immunity to rubella. A past history of having a rubella infection is not used to determine immunity because the signs of rubella infection are not reliable enough to be certain that you have had the disease.

Since vaccination with rubella vaccine may not provide protection for everyone, you may want to ask your doctor to check your immunity to the rubella virus 6 to 8 weeks following your vaccination. This may be especially important if you are a woman of child-bearing age who intends to become pregnant in the future.

This vaccine is available only from your doctor or other authorized health care providers.

Remember:
- **It is very important that you read and understand the following information.** If any of the information causes you special concern, do not decide against receiving this vaccine without first checking with your doctor.

- **If you have any questions** about the following information or if you want more information about this vaccine, **ask your doctor, nurse, or pharmacist.**

Before Receiving This Vaccine

Before you receive rubella vaccine, your doctor should be told:

—if you have ever had any unusual or allergic reaction to any form of the antibiotic neomycin. The rubella vaccine available in the U.S. contains neomycin; products available in other countries may contain neomycin, polymyxin B, or other antibiotics.

—if you are **pregnant** or if you may become pregnant within 3 months after receiving this vaccine. Studies have not been done in either humans or animals; however, use during pregnancy is not recommended because rubella vaccine crosses the placenta. However, the Centers for Disease Control observed over 100 women who received the vaccine within 3 months before or after becoming pregnant and those women gave birth to normal babies.

—if you are **breast-feeding**. Rubella vaccine may pass into the breast milk and may cause mild rubella infection in nursing babies. However, studies have not shown that this infection causes any problems.

—if you have any of the following medical problems:
    Fever
    Immune deficiency condition (or family history of)
    Tuberculosis

—if you are taking **any** other prescription or nonprescription (OTC) medicine.

—if you have received any other live virus vaccines in the last month or intend to within the next month.

—if you have received any of the following types of products in the last 3 months or intend to within the next 2 weeks:
    Blood transfusions or other blood products
    Gamma globulin or other globulins

—if you have ever been treated with x-rays or cancer medicines.

Precautions After Receiving This Vaccine

Do not become pregnant for 3 months after receiving rubella vaccine without first checking with your doctor. There is a chance that this vaccine may cause birth defects.

Tell your doctor that you have received this vaccine:

—if you are to receive blood transfusions or other blood products within 2 weeks after receiving this vaccine.

© 1988   The United States Pharmacopeial Convention, Inc.

—if you are to receive gamma globulin or other glob-ulins within 2 weeks after receiving this vaccine.

—if you are to receive any other live virus vaccines within 1 month after receiving this vaccine.

—if you are to receive a tuberculin skin test within 8 weeks after receiving this vaccine. The results of the test may be affected by this vaccine.

Side Effects of This Vaccine

Along with its needed effects, a vaccine may cause some unwanted effects. Although not all of these side effects may occur, if they do occur they may need medical attention.

Get emergency help immediately if any of the following side effects occur:

Signs of allergic reaction
  Difficulty in breathing or swallowing
  Hives
  Itching, especially of feet or hands
  Reddening of skin, especially around ears
  Swelling of eyes, face, or inside of nose
  Unusual tiredness or weakness (sudden and severe)

Check with your doctor as soon as possible if any of the following side effects occur:

Less common
  Pain or tenderness of eyes

Rare
  Bruising or purple spots on skin
  Confusion
  Convulsions (seizures)
  Headache (severe or continuing)
  Pain, numbness, or tingling of hands, arms, legs, or feet
  Stiff neck
  Unusual irritability
  Vomiting

Other side effects may occur that usually do not require medical attention. However, check with your doctor if any of the following side effects continue or are bothersome:

More common
  Burning or stinging at place of injection
  Skin rash
  Swelling of glands in neck

Less common
  Aches or pain in joints
  Headache (mild), sore throat, runny nose, or fever
  Itching, swelling, redness, tenderness, or hard lump at place of injection
  Vague feeling of body discomfort

The above side effects (especially aches or pain in joints) are more likely to occur in adults, particularly women.

Some of the above side effects may not occur until 1 to 4 weeks after immunization and usually last less than 1 week. Check with your doctor as soon as possible if any of the following side effects occur:
  Pain, numbness, or tingling of hands, arms, legs, or feet
  Pain or tenderness of eyes

In addition, check with your doctor if any of the following side effects continue or are bothersome:
  Headache (mild), sore throat, runny nose, or fever
  Swelling of glands in neck
  Vague feeling of body discomfort

Also, aches or pain in joints may not occur until 1 to 10 weeks after immunization and usually last less than 1 week. Check with your doctor if either of these side effects continues or is bothersome.

Other side effects not listed above may also occur in some patients. If you notice any other effects, check with your doctor.

_____

December 1987

SALICYLATES (Systemic)

This information applies to the following medicines:

Aspirin (AS-pir-in)
Aspirin and Caffeine (kaf-EEN)
Buffered Aspirin
Choline Salicylate (KOE-leen sa-LI-si-late)
Choline and Magnesium (mag-NEE-zhum) Salicylates
Magnesium Salicylate
Salicylamide (sal-i-SILL-a-mide)
Salsalate (SAL-sa-late)
Sodium Salicylate

Some commonly used brand names and other names are:

For Aspirin†§

Acetylsalicylic Acid	Encaprin
Apo-Asen*	Entrophen*
Arthrinol*	Measurin
ASA	Norwich Aspirin
A.S.A.	Novasen*
A.S.A. Enseals	Riphen-10*
Aspergum	Safety Coated APF Arthritis
Astrin*	Pain Formula
Bayer Aspirin	Sal-Adult*
Bayer Timed-Release Arthritic	Sal-Infant*
Pain Formula*	St. Joseph Aspirin for
Coryphen*	Children
8-Hour Bayer Timed-Release	Supasa*
Easprin	Triaphen-10*
Ecotrin	ZORprin
Empirin	

For Aspirin§ and Caffeine

Accurate*	Major-cin
Acotin*	Neo-Tigol*
Alsidol*	Nervine*
Anacin	P-A-C Revised
Asafen*	Formula
C2*	Paradol*
CP-2	T-R-C Regular*
812*	217*
Instantine*	

For Buffered Aspirin†§

Alka-Seltzer Effervescent	Buffex
Pain Reliever and Antacid	Buffinol
Arthritic Pain Formula*#	Buf-Tabs
Arthritis Pain Formula#	Cama Arthritis Reliever
Ascriptin#	Magnaprin#
Ascriptin A/D#	Maprin#
Asperbuf	Maprin I-B#
Buffaprin	Wesprin Buffered#
Bufferin	

For Choline Salicylate
    Arthropan

For Choline and Magnesium Salicylates

Choline Magnesium	Trilisate
Trisalicylate	

For Magnesium Salicylate

Doan's Pills (U.S.)	Mobidin
Magan	

For Salicylamide†
    Uromide

For Salsalate†

Artha-G	Mono-Gesic
Disalcid	Salicylsalicylic Acid

For Sodium Salicylate†
    Uracel

*Not available in the U.S.
†Generic name product may also be available in the U.S.
§In Canada, *Aspirin* is also a brand name. Acetylsalicylic acid is the generic name in Canada. ASA, a synonym for aspirin, is the term that commonly appears on Canadian product labels.
#May be identified on product label as Aspirin, Alumina, and Magnesia.

To the Reader: If you do not recognize the names of medical conditions or medicines referred to in this information, check with your doctor, nurse, or pharmacist. Definitions for selected medical terms may be found in the Glossary. Brand names for the generic drug names listed can be found in the Index. In addition, selected brand names commonly associated with the generic name have been included in the text to help you recognize medicine you may be taking. The fact that a brand name product is not mentioned does not mean the information does not apply. It is a good idea for you to learn both the generic and brand names of your medicines and to write them down for future use.

Salicylates are used to relieve pain and reduce fever. Most salicylates are also used to relieve some symptoms caused by arthritis (rheumatism), such as swelling, stiffness, and joint pain. However, they do not cure arthritis and will help you only as long as you continue to take them. Aspirin may also be used, under the care of a doctor, to lessen the chance of heart attack in patients with certain heart problems and to lessen the chance of stroke in some men.

The caffeine present in some of these products may provide additional relief of headache pain or faster pain relief.

Some salicylates are available only with your physician's or dentist's prescription. Others are available without a prescription; however, your physician or dentist may have special instructions on the proper dose of these medicines for your medical condition.

Remember:
• **Keep all medicines out of the reach of children.**

• In order for this medicine to work, it must be used as directed. **If you are using this medicine without a prescription, it is very important to follow the directions on the label.**

• **It is also very important that you read and understand the following information.** If any of the information causes you special concern, check with your doctor before using this medicine without a prescription.

• Before you begin using any new medicine (prescription or nonprescription) or if you develop any new medical problem while you are using this medicine, check with your doctor, nurse, or pharmacist.

• **If you have any questions** about the following information or if you want more information about this medicine or your medical problem, **ask your doctor, nurse, or pharmacist.**

Before Using This Medicine

Before you take a salicylate, check with your doctor or pharmacist:

—if you have ever had any unusual or allergic reaction to aspirin or other salicylates, including methyl salicylate (oil of wintergreen), or to any of the following medicines:

Diclofenac (e.g., Voltaren)
Diflunisal (e.g., Dolobid)
Fenoprofen (e.g., Nalfon)
Flurbiprofen, oral (e.g., Ansaid)
Ibuprofen (e.g., Motrin)
Indomethacin (e.g., Indocin)
Ketoprofen (e.g., Orudis)
Meclofenamate (e.g., Meclomen)
Mefenamic acid (e.g., Ponstel)
Naproxen (e.g., Naprosyn)
Oxyphenbutazone (e.g., Tandearil)
Phenylbutazone (e.g., Butazolidin)
Piroxicam (e.g., Feldene)
Sulindac (e.g., Clinoril)
Suprofen (e.g., Suprol)
Tiaprofenic acid (e.g., Surgam)
Tolmetin (e.g., Tolectin)
Zomepirac (e.g., Zomax)

—if you are on a low-salt, low-sugar, or any other special diet, or if you are allergic to any substance, such as foods, sulfites or other preservatives, or dyes. Most medicines contain more than their active ingredient, and many liquid medicines contain alcohol. Your doctor, nurse, or pharmacist can help you avoid products that may cause a problem.

—if you are **pregnant** or if you may become pregnant. Salicylates have not been shown to cause birth defects in humans. Studies on birth defects in humans have been done with aspirin but not with other salicylates. However, studies in animals have shown that salicylates cause birth defects.

Some reports have suggested that too much use of aspirin late in pregnancy may cause a decrease in the newborn's weight and possible death of the fetus or newborn infant. However, the mothers in these reports had been taking much larger amounts of aspirin than are usually recommended. Studies of mothers taking aspirin in the doses that are usually recommended did not show these unwanted effects. However, there is a chance that regular use of salicylates late in pregnancy may cause unwanted effects on the heart or blood flow in the fetus or in the newborn infant.

Use of salicylates, especially aspirin, during the last 2 weeks of pregnancy may cause bleeding problems in the fetus before or during delivery or in the newborn infant. Also, too much use of salicylates during the last 3 months of pregnancy may increase the length of pregnancy, prolong labor, cause other problems during delivery, or cause severe bleeding in the mother before, during, or after delivery.

Studies in humans have not shown that caffeine causes birth defects. However, studies in animals have shown that caffeine causes birth defects when given in very large doses (amounts equal to those present in 12 to 24 cups of coffee a day).

—if you are **breast-feeding**. Salicylates pass into the breast milk. Although salicylates have not been shown to cause problems in nursing babies, it is possible that problems may occur if large amounts are taken regularly, as for arthritis (rheumatism).

Caffeine passes into the breast milk in small amounts.

—if you have any of the following medical problems:
Anemia
Asthma, allergies, and nasal polyps (history of)
Glucose-6-phosphate dehydrogenase (G6PD) deficiency
Gout
Heart disease
Hemophilia or other bleeding problems
High blood pressure
Kidney disease
Liver disease
Overactive thyroid
Stomach ulcer or other stomach problems

—if you regularly take large amounts of acetaminophen or antacids, especially calcium- and/or magnesium-containing antacids.

—if you are taking **any** other prescription or nonprescription (OTC) medicine, especially:
Adrenocorticoids (cortisone-like medicines)
Anticoagulants (blood thinners)
Antidiabetic agents, oral (diabetes medicine you take by mouth)
Dipyridamole (e.g., Persantine)
Divalproex (e.g., Depakote)
Heparin
Methotrexate (e.g., Mexate)
Other medicine for pain and/or inflammation
Probenecid (e.g., Benemid)
Sulfinpyrazone (e.g., Anturane)
Urinary alkalizers (medicine that makes the urine less acid, such as acetazolamide [e.g., Diamox], dichlorphenamide [e.g., Daranide], methazolamide [e.g., Neptazane], potassium or sodium citrate and/or citric acid)
Valproic acid (e.g., Depakene)

Proper Use of This Medicine

There have been reports suggesting that use of aspirin in children with fever due to a viral infection (especially flu or chickenpox) may cause a serious illness called Reye's syndrome. **Therefore, do not give aspirin or other salicylates to a child with flu or chickenpox without first discussing this with your child's doctor.**

Take this medicine after meals or with food (except for enteric-coated capsules or tablets and aspirin suppositories) to lessen stomach irritation.

Take tablet or capsule forms of this medicine with a full glass (8 ounces) of water. Also, do not lie down for about 15 to 30 minutes after swallowing the medicine. This helps to prevent irritation that may lead to trouble in swallowing.

For patients taking aspirin or buffered aspirin:

• **Do not use aspirin or buffered aspirin if it has a strong, vinegar-like odor**, since this means the medicine is breaking down. If you have any questions about this, check with your doctor or pharmacist.

• If you are to take aspirin or buffered aspirin within 7 days after having your tonsils removed, a tooth pulled, or other dental or mouth surgery, be sure to swallow the aspirin whole. Do not chew aspirin during this time.

• Do not place aspirin or buffered aspirin tablets directly on a tooth or gum surface. This may cause a burn.

• There are several different forms of aspirin or buffered aspirin. If you are using:

—*chewable aspirin tablets,* they may be chewed, dissolved in liquid, crushed, or swallowed whole.

—*effervescent buffered aspirin tablets,* they must be dissolved in water (between ⅓ and ½ cup of water for each tablet) just before taking. Drink all of the liquid to be sure you are taking the full amount of medicine. It is best to add more water to the glass and drink that also, to make sure that you are taking all of the medicine.

—*enteric-coated aspirin tablets,* they must be swallowed whole. Do not crush them or break them up before taking.

—*extended-release (long-acting) aspirin tablets,* check with your pharmacist as to how they should be taken. Some may be broken up (but must not be crushed) before swallowing if you cannot swallow them whole. Others should not be broken up and must be swallowed whole.

—*aspirin suppositories,* first remove the foil wrapper and moisten the suppository with water. Lie down on your side and push the suppository well up into the rectum with your finger.

For patients taking the liquid form of choline and magnesium salicylates:

• The liquid may be mixed with fruit juice just before taking.

• Drink a full glass (8 ounces) of water after taking the medicine.

For patients taking enteric-coated sodium salicylate tablets:

• The tablets must be swallowed whole. Do not crush them or break them up before taking.

For patients taking enteric-coated (also called safety-coated) tablets of aspirin or sodium salicylate or capsules containing enteric-coated aspirin:

• If you are also taking an antacid, take this medicine at least 1 or 2 hours before or after taking the antacid. Taking the two medicines too close together may cause the enteric coating to dissolve too early. The enteric coating will not be able to help prevent stomach irritation if this occurs.

Unless otherwise directed by your physician or dentist:

• Do not take more of this medicine than recommended on the label, in order to lessen the chance of side effects.

• Children up to 12 years of age should not take this medicine more than 5 times a day or for more than 5 days in a row.

• Adults should not take this medicine for more than 10 days in a row.

• Aspirin chewing gum tablets should not be used for more than 2 days in a row if they are being used to relieve a sore throat.

When used for arthritis (rheumatism), this medicine must be taken regularly as ordered by your doctor in order for it to help you. Up to 2 to 3 weeks or longer may pass before you feel the full effects of this medicine.

If your physician or dentist has ordered you to take this medicine according to a regular schedule and you miss a dose, take it as soon as you remember. However, if it is almost time for your next dose, skip the missed dose and go back to your regular dosing schedule. Do not double doses.

How to store this medicine:

• **Keep out of the reach of children** because overdose is very dangerous in young children.

• Store away from heat and direct light.

• Do not store tablets or capsules in the bathroom, near the kitchen sink, or in other damp places. Heat or moisture may cause the medicine to break down.

• Keep liquid forms of this medicine from freezing.

• Store aspirin suppositories in a cool place. It is usually best to keep them in the refrigerator, but keep them from freezing.

• Do not keep outdated medicine or medicine no longer needed. Be sure that any discarded medicine is out of the reach of children.

Precautions While Using This Medicine

Check the labels of all over-the-counter (OTC), nonprescription, and prescription medicines you now take. If any contain aspirin or other salicylates, including bismuth subsalicylate (e.g., Pepto-Bismol), be especially careful. Also, be especially careful if you regularly use a shampoo or other medicine for your skin that contains salicylic acid. Using other salicylate-containing products while taking this medicine may lead to overdose. If you have any questions about this, check with your doctor or pharmacist.

If you will be taking salicylates for a long time (more than 5 days in a row for children or 10 days in a row for adults) or in large amounts, your doctor should check your progress at regular visits.

Check with your doctor:

—if your symptoms do not improve or if they become worse.

—if you are taking this medicine to bring down a fever, and the fever lasts for more than 3 days or returns.

—if you are taking this medicine regularly, as for arthritis (rheumatism), and you notice a ringing or buzzing in your ears or severe or continuing headaches.

These are often the first signs that too much salicylate is being taken. Your doctor may want to change the amount of medicine you are taking every day.

Too much use of certain other medicines together with a salicylate may increase the chance of unwanted effects. This is especially likely to happen if you are taking large amounts of a salicylate or if you must take it for a long time (as for arthritis). Therefore, **do not regularly take any of the following medicines together with a salicylate** unless your physician or dentist directs you to do so.

Acetaminophen (e.g., Tylenol)
Diclofenac (e.g., Voltaren)
Diflunisal (e.g., Dolobid)
Fenoprofen (e.g., Nalfon)
Flurbiprofen, oral (e.g., Ansaid)
Ibuprofen (e.g., Motrin)
Indomethacin (e.g., Indocin)
Ketoprofen (e.g., Orudis)
Meclofenamate (e.g., Meclomen)
Mefenamic acid (e.g., Ponstel)
Naproxen (e.g., Naprosyn)
Phenylbutazone (e.g., Butazolidin)
Piroxicam (e.g., Feldene)
Sulindac (e.g., Clinoril)
Tiaprofenic acid (e.g., Surgam)
Tolmetin (e.g., Tolectin)

Diabetics: False urine sugar test results may occur if you are regularly taking large amounts of salicylates, such as:

—Aspirin: 8 or more 325-mg (5-grain), or 4 or more 500-mg or 650-mg (10-grain), or 3 or more 800-mg (or higher strength), doses a day.

—Buffered aspirin or
—Sodium salicylate: 8 or more 325-mg (5-grain), or 4 or more 500-mg or 650-mg (10-grain), doses a day.

—Choline salicylate: 4 or more teaspoonful (each teaspoonful containing 870 mg) a day.

—Choline and magnesium salicylates: 5 or more 500-mg tablets or teaspoonsful, 4 or more 750-mg tablets, or 2 or more 1000-mg tablets, a day.

—Magnesium salicylate: 7 or more 325-mg, or 4 or more 480-mg (or higher strength), tablets a day.

—Salsalate: 6 or more 325-mg doses, or 4 or more 500-mg doses, a day.

Smaller doses or occasional use of salicylates usually will not affect urine sugar tests. However, check with your doctor, nurse, or pharmacist (especially if your diabetes is not well-controlled) if:

—you are not sure how much salicylate you are taking every day.

—you notice any change in your urine sugar test results.

—you have any other questions about this possible problem.

Do not take aspirin for 5 days before any surgery, including dental surgery, unless otherwise directed by your physician or dentist. Taking aspirin during this time may cause bleeding problems.

For patients taking buffered aspirin, choline and magnesium salicylates, or magnesium salicylate:

• If you are also taking a tetracycline antibiotic, do not take the two medicines within 1 to 2 hours of each other. Taking them too close together may prevent the tetracycline from being absorbed by your body. If you have any questions about this, check with your doctor or pharmacist.

If you are taking a laxative containing cellulose, take the salicylate at least 2 hours before or after you take the laxative. Taking these medicines too close together may lessen the effects of the salicylate.

For patients on a sodium-restricted (low-salt) diet—Buffered aspirin effervescent tablets (e.g., Alka-Seltzer) and sodium salicylate contain large amounts of sodium. Do not take these medicines without first checking with your doctor or pharmacist.

For patients taking this medicine by mouth:

• Stomach problems may be more likely to occur if you drink alcoholic beverages while being treated with this medicine, especially if you are taking it in high doses or for a long time. Check with your doctor if you have any questions about this.

For patients using aspirin suppositories:

• Too much use of aspirin suppositories may cause irritation of the rectum. Check with your doctor if this occurs.

If you think that you or anyone else may have taken an overdose, get emergency help at once. Taking an overdose of these medicines may cause unconsciousness or death. Signs of overdose include convulsions (seizures), hearing loss, confusion, ringing or buzzing in the ears, severe drowsiness or tiredness, severe excitement or nervousness, and fast or deep breathing.

Side Effects of This Medicine

Along with its needed effects, a medicine may cause some unwanted effects. When this medicine is used for short periods of time at low doses, side effects usually are rare. Although not all of the following side effects may occur, if they do occur they may need medical attention.

Get emergency help immediately if any of the following side effects occur:

Any loss of hearing
Bloody urine
Confusion
Convulsions (seizures)
Diarrhea (severe or continuing)
Dizziness or lightheadedness
Drowsiness (severe)
Excitement or nervousness (severe)
Fast or deep breathing
Hallucinations (seeing, hearing, or feeling things that are not there)
Increased sweating
Nausea or vomiting (severe or continuing)

Shortness of breath, troubled breathing, tightness in chest,
or wheezing
Stomach pain (severe or continuing)
Unexplained fever
Uncontrollable flapping movements of the hands (especially in elderly patients)
Unusual thirst
Vision problems

Signs of overdose in children

Changes in behavior
Drowsiness or tiredness (severe)
Fast or deep breathing

Also, check with your doctor as soon as possible if any
of the following side effects occur:

More common

Nausea or vomiting
Stomach pain

Less common or rare

Bloody or black tarry stools
Headache (severe or continuing)
Ringing or buzzing in ears (continuing)
Skin rash, hives, or itching
Unusual tiredness or weakness
Vomiting of blood or material that looks like coffee grounds

For children and elderly patients: The above side effects
are more likely to occur in children, especially those
who have a fever or are dehydrated (those who have
lost large amounts of body fluid because of vomiting,
diarrhea, or sweating), and in elderly patients (60 years
of age or older). These patients are usually more sensitive to the effects of salicylates.

Other side effects may occur that usually do not require
medical attention. These side effects may go away
during treatment as your body adjusts to the medicine.
However, check with your doctor or pharmacist if any
of the following side effects continue or are bothersome:

Drowsiness (for salicylamide only)
Heartburn or indigestion
Sleeplessness, nervousness, or jitters (only for products
containing caffeine)

Other side effects not listed above may also occur in some
patients. If you notice any other effects, check with
your doctor.

_____

December 1987

_____

SALICYLIC ACID (Topical)

Some commonly used brand names are:

Calicylic	P & S
Compound W	Propa P.H.
Derma-Soft Creme	Salacid
Freezone	Saligel
Hydrisalic	Salonil
Ionil	Sebucare
Keralyt	SalAc
Mediplast	Stri-Dex
Occlusal	Xseb
Oxy Clean	

Generic name product may also be available in the U.S.

To the Reader: If you do not recognize the names of medical conditions or medicines referred to in this information, check with your doctor, nurse, or pharmacist. Definitions for selected medical terms may be found in the Glossary. Brand names for the generic drug names listed can be found in the Index. In addition, selected brand names commonly associated with the generic name have been included in the text to help you recognize medicine you may be taking. The fact that a brand name product is not mentioned does not mean the information does not apply. It is a good idea for you to learn both the generic and brand names of your medicines and to write them down for future use.

Salicylic acid (sal-i-SILL-ik AS-id) is used topically to treat many skin disorders such as acne, psoriasis, seborrheic dermatitis, calluses, corns, and warts, depending on the strength of the preparation.

Some of these preparations are available only with your doctor's prescription. Others are available without a prescription; however, your doctor may have special instructions on the proper use of salicylic acid for your medical condition.

Remember:

• **Keep all medicines out of the reach of children.**

• In order for this medicine to work, it must be used as directed. **If you are using this medicine without a prescription, it is very important to follow the directions on the label.**

• **It is also very important that you read and understand the following information.** If any of the information causes you special concern, check with your doctor or pharmacist.

• Before you begin using any new medicine (prescription or nonprescription) or if you develop any new medical problem while you are using this medicine, check with your doctor, nurse, or pharmacist.

• **If you have any questions** about the following information or if you want more information about this medicine or your medical problem, **ask your doctor, nurse, or pharmacist.**

Before Using This Medicine

Before you use salicylic acid, check with your doctor or pharmacist:

—if you have ever had any unusual or allergic reaction to salicylic acid.

—if you are allergic to any substance, such as certain preservatives. Most medicines contain more than their active ingredient. Your doctor, nurse, or pharmacist can help you avoid products that may cause a problem.

—if you are **pregnant** or if you may become pregnant, since this medicine may be absorbed through the skin. Studies have not been done in humans. However, studies in animals have shown that salicylic acid causes birth defects when given orally in doses about 6 times the maximum daily human dose applied topically over a large body surface.

—if you are **breast-feeding**, since salicylic acid may be absorbed through the skin. However, topical salicylic acid has not been shown to cause problems in nursing babies.

—if you are using either the 25% cream, 25 to 60% ointment, plaster, or topical solution form of salicylic acid and you have either of the following medical problems:

Blood vessel disease
Diabetes mellitus (sugar diabetes)

—if you are taking **any** other prescription or nonprescription (OTC) medicine.

Proper Use of This Medicine

It is very important that you use this medicine only as directed. Do not use more of it, do not use it more often, and do not use it for a longer period of time than recommended on the label, unless otherwise directed by your doctor. To do so may increase the chance of absorption through the skin and the chance of salicylic acid poisoning.

If your doctor has ordered an occlusive dressing (for example, kitchen plastic wrap) to be applied over this medicine, make sure you know how to apply it. Since an occlusive dressing will increase the amount of medicine absorbed through your skin and the possibility of salicylic acid poisoning, use it only as directed. If you have any questions about this, check with your doctor.

Keep this medicine away from the eyes and other mucous membranes such as the mouth and inside of the nose. If you should accidentally get some in your eyes or on other mucous membranes, immediately flush them with water for 15 minutes.

For patients using the cream, lotion, or ointment form of salicylic acid:

• Apply enough medicine to cover the affected area, and rub in gently.

For patients using the gel form of salicylic acid:

• Before using salicylic acid gel, apply wet packs to the affected areas for at least 5 minutes. If you have any questions about this, check with your doctor or pharmacist.

• Apply enough gel to cover the affected areas, and rub in gently.

For patients using the pad form of salicylic acid:

• Wipe the pad over the affected areas.

• Do not rinse off medicine after treatment.

For patients using the plaster form of salicylic acid:

- How to apply the salicylic acid plaster: First, cut off the length of plaster needed to cover only the affected area. Remove the gauze from the plaster before applying. If the gauze sticks to the plaster, dampen with a wet cloth. Then apply the plaster to the affected area. Make sure the plaster does not touch any healthy tissue.

- Do not use this plaster on irritated or infected skin.

For patients using the shampoo form of salicylic acid:

- Before applying this medicine, wet the hair and scalp with lukewarm water. Apply enough medicine to work up a lather and rub well into the scalp for 2 or 3 minutes, then rinse. Apply the medicine again and rinse thoroughly.

For patients using the soap form of salicylic acid:

- Work up a lather with the soap, using hot water, and scrub the entire affected area with a washcloth or facial brush.

- If you are to use this soap in a foot bath, work up rich suds in hot water and soak the feet for 10 to 15 minutes. Then pat dry without rinsing.

For patients using the topical solution form of salicylic acid:

- **This medicine is flammable. Do not use it near heat or open flame or while smoking.**

- **Do not use this medicine on moles, birthmarks, unusual warts with hair growing from them, or warts on the face.** To do so may cause severe irritation.

- Before using salicylic acid topical solution, soak the wart in warm water for 5 minutes. Then remove any loosened tissue by gently rubbing with a brush, washcloth, or emery board. Thoroughly dry the affected area.

- Use the brush applicator provided to apply the medicine. Apply the medicine to the affected area once. Allow it to dry completely. Then, apply the medicine a second time.

- Avoid getting this medicine on the skin surrounding the affected area, since it may cause severe irritation of normal skin.

Unless your hands are being treated, wash them immediately after applying this medicine to remove any medicine that may be on them.

If you miss a dose of this medicine, apply it as soon as possible. However, if it is almost time for your next dose, skip the missed dose and go back to your regular dosing schedule.

How to store this medicine:

- **Keep out of the reach of children.**

- Store away from heat and direct light.

- Keep the medicine from freezing.

- Do not keep outdated medicine or medicine no longer needed. Be sure that any discarded medicine is out of the reach of children.

Precautions While Using This Medicine

When using salicylic acid, do not use any of the following preparations on the same affected area as this medicine, unless otherwise directed by your doctor:

> Abrasive soaps or cleansers
> Alcohol-containing preparations
> Any other topical acne preparation or preparation containing a peeling agent (for example, benzoyl peroxide, resorcinol, sulfur, or tretinoin [vitamin A acid])
> Cosmetics or soaps that dry the skin
> Medicated cosmetics
> Other topical medicine for the skin

To use any of the above preparations on the same affected area as salicylic acid may cause severe irritation of the skin.

Taking large doses of aspirin or other salicylates (including diflunisal) while using topical salicylic acid may lead to overdose. If you have any questions about this, check with your doctor or pharmacist.

Side Effects of This Medicine

Along with its needed effects, a medicine may cause some unwanted effects. Although not all of these side effects may occur, if they do occur they may need medical attention.

Check with your doctor as soon as possible if any of the following side effects occur:

> Skin irritation not present before using this medicine

Signs of salicylic acid poisoning
> Confusion
> Dizziness
> Headache (severe or continuing)
> Rapid breathing
> Ringing or buzzing in ears (continuing)

Other side effects may occur that usually do not require medical attention. However, check with your doctor or pharmacist if the following side effect continues or is bothersome:

More common
> Stinging

For elderly patients: Many medicines have not been tested in older people. Therefore, it is not known whether the medicine acts the same way it does in younger adults. Check with your doctor or pharmacist if you notice any unusual effects while using this medicine or if you think it is not working as it should.

Other side effects not listed above may also occur in some patients. If you notice any other effects, check with your doctor or pharmacist.

_____

December 1987

_____

© 1988   The United States Pharmacopeial Convention, Inc.

SALICYLIC ACID AND SULFUR (Topical)

Some commonly used brand names are:

Acno	Sastid Plain
Acnotex	Sebex
Aknasil*	Sebulex
Cuticura	Sulsal*
Fostex	Therac
Pernox	Vanseb
Sastid	

*Not available in the U.S.

To the Reader: If you do not recognize the names of medical conditions or medicines referred to in this information, check with your doctor, nurse, or pharmacist. Definitions for selected medical terms may be found in the Glossary. Brand names for the generic drug names listed can be found in the Index. In addition, selected brand names commonly associated with the generic name have been included in the text to help you recognize medicine you may be taking. The fact that a brand name product is not mentioned does not mean the information does not apply. It is a good idea for you to learn both the generic and brand names of your medicines and to write them down for future use.

Salicylic acid (sal-i-SILL-ik AS-id) and sulfur (SUL-fur) combination may be applied to the skin to treat acne and other skin disorders or used on the scalp as a shampoo to treat dandruff and other scalp disorders.

This medicine is available without a prescription; however, your doctor may have special instructions on the proper use of this medicine for your medical condition.

Remember:
• **Keep all medicines out of the reach of children.**

• In order for this medicine to work, it must be used as directed. **If you are using this medicine without a prescription, it is very important to follow the directions on the label.**

• **It is also very important that you read and understand the following information.** If any of the information causes you special concern, check with your doctor or pharmacist.

• Before you begin using any new medicine (prescription or nonprescription) or if you develop any new medical problem while you are using this medicine, check with your doctor, nurse, or pharmacist.

• **If you have any questions** about the following information or if you want more information about this medicine or your medical problem, **ask your doctor, nurse, or pharmacist.**

Before Using This Medicine

Before you use salicylic acid and sulfur combination, check with your doctor or pharmacist:

—if you have ever had any unusual or allergic reaction to salicylic acid or sulfur.

—if you are allergic to any substance, such as certain preservatives. Most medicines contain more than their active ingredient. Your doctor, nurse, or pharmacist can help you avoid products that may cause a problem.

—if you are **pregnant** or if you may become pregnant, since salicylic acid (contained in this combination medicine) may be absorbed through the skin. Studies with topical salicylic acid have not been done in humans. However, studies in animals have shown that salicylic acid causes birth defects when given orally in doses about 6 times the maximum daily human dose applied topically over a large body surface. Topical sulfur (contained in this combination medicine) has not been shown to cause birth defects or other problems in humans.

—if you are **breast-feeding**, since salicylic acid (contained in this combination medicine) may be absorbed through the skin. However, topical salicylic acid and sulfur combination has not been shown to cause problems in nursing babies.

—if you are taking **any** other prescription or nonprescription (OTC) medicine.

Proper Use of This Medicine

Use this medicine only as directed. Do not use more of it and do not use it more often than recommended on the label, unless otherwise directed by your doctor.

Immediately after using this medicine, wash your hands to remove any medicine that may be on them.

Keep this medicine away from the eyes. If you should accidentally get some in your eyes, flush them thoroughly with water.

For patients using the skin cleanser form of this medicine:
• After wetting the skin, apply this medicine with your fingertips or a wet sponge and rub in gently to work up a lather. Then rinse thoroughly and pat dry.

For patients using the lotion form of this medicine:
• Apply a small amount of this medicine to the affected areas, and rub in gently.

For patients using the shampoo form of this medicine:
• Wet the hair and scalp with lukewarm water. Then apply enough medicine to work up a lather and rub into the scalp. Continue rubbing the lather into the scalp for several minutes or allow it to remain on the scalp for about 5 minutes, depending on the product being used, then rinse. Apply the medicine again and rinse thoroughly.

For patients using the bar soap form of this medicine:
• After wetting the skin, use this medicine to wash the face and other affected areas. Then rinse thoroughly and pat dry.

If you miss a dose of this medicine, apply or use it as soon as possible. However, if it is almost time for your next dose, skip the missed dose and go back to your regular dosing schedule.

How to store this medicine:
• **Keep out of the reach of children.**
• Store away from heat and direct light.

- Keep the medicine from freezing.
- Do not keep outdated medicine or medicine no longer needed. Be sure that any discarded medicine is out of the reach of children.

Precautions While Using This Medicine

When using salicylic acid and sulfur combination medicine, do not use any of the following preparations on the same affected area as this medicine, unless otherwise directed by your doctor:

> Abrasive soaps or cleansers
> Alcohol-containing preparations
> Any other topical acne preparation or preparation containing a peeling agent (for example, benzoyl peroxide, resorcinol, or tretinoin [vitamin A acid])
> Cosmetics or soaps that dry the skin
> Medicated cosmetics
> Other topical medicine for the skin

To use any of the above preparations on the same affected area as salicylic acid and sulfur combination medicine may cause severe irritation of the skin.

Do not use any topical mercury-containing preparation, such as ammoniated mercury ointment on the same affected area as this medicine. To do so may cause a foul odor, may be irritating to the skin, and may stain the skin black. If you have any questions about this, check with your doctor or pharmacist.

Taking large doses of aspirin or other salicylates (including diflunisal) while using topical salicylic acid (contained in this medicine) may lead to overdose. If you have any questions about this, check with your doctor or pharmacist.

Side Effects of This Medicine

Along with its needed effects, a medicine may cause some unwanted effects. Although not all of these side effects may occur, if they do occur they may need medical attention.

Check with your doctor as soon as possible if the following side effect occurs:

> Skin irritation not present before using this medicine

Other side effects may occur that usually do not require medical attention. However, check with your doctor or pharmacist if the following side effects continue or are bothersome:

> Redness and peeling of skin (may occur after a few days)
> Unusual dryness of skin

For elderly patients: Many medicines have not been tested in older people. Therefore, it is not known whether the medicine acts the same way it does in younger adults. Check with your doctor or pharmacist if you notice any unusual effects while using this medicine or if you think it is not working as it should.

Other side effects not listed above may also occur in some patients. If you notice any other effects, check with your doctor or pharmacist.

_____

December 1987

SALICYLIC ACID, SULFUR, AND COAL TAR (Topical)

Some commonly used brand names are Sebex-T, Sebutone, and Vanseb-T.

To the Reader: If you do not recognize the names of medical conditions or medicines referred to in this information, check with your doctor, nurse, or pharmacist. Definitions for selected medical terms may be found in the Glossary. Brand names for the generic drug names listed can be found in the Index. In addition, selected brand names commonly associated with the generic name have been included in the text to help you recognize medicine you may be taking. The fact that a brand name product is not mentioned does not mean the information does not apply. It is a good idea for you to learn both the generic and brand names of your medicines and to write them down for future use.

Salicylic acid (sal-i-SILL-ik AS-id), sulfur (SUL-fur), and coal tar combination is used as a shampoo to treat dandruff, seborrheic dermatitis, and psoriasis of the scalp.

This medicine is available without a prescription; however, your doctor may have special instructions on the proper use of this medicine for your medical condition.

Remember:
• **Keep all medicines out of the reach of children.**

• In order for this medicine to work, it must be used as directed. **If you are using this medicine without a prescription, it is very important to follow the directions on the label.**

• **It is also very important that you read and understand the following information.** If any of the information causes you special concern, check with your doctor or pharmacist.

• Before you begin using any new medicine (prescription or nonprescription) or if you develop any new medical problem while you are using this medicine, check with your doctor, nurse, or pharmacist.

• **If you have any questions** about the following information or if you want more information about this medicine or your medical problem, **ask your doctor, nurse, or pharmacist.**

Before Using This Medicine

Before you use salicylic acid, sulfur, and coal tar combination, check with your doctor, nurse, or pharmacist:

—if you have ever had any unusual or allergic reaction to salicylic acid, sulfur, or coal tar.

—if you are allergic to any substance, such as certain preservatives or dyes. Most medicines contain more than their active ingredient. Your doctor or pharmacist can help you avoid products that may cause a problem.

—if you are **pregnant** or if you may become pregnant, since salicylic acid (contained in this combination medicine) may be absorbed through the skin. Studies with topical salicylic acid have not been done in humans. However, studies in animals have shown that salicylic acid causes birth defects when given orally in doses about 6 times the maximum daily human dose applied topically over a large body surface. Sulfur (contained in this combination medicine) has not been shown to cause birth defects or other problems in humans. Studies with coal tar (contained in this combination medicine) on birth defects have not been done in either animals or humans.

—if you are **breast-feeding**, since salicylic acid (contained in this combination medicine) may be absorbed through the skin. However, topical salicylic acid, sulfur, and coal tar combination has not been shown to cause problems in nursing babies.

—if you are taking **any** other prescription or nonprescription (OTC) medicine.

Proper Use of This Medicine

Use this medicine only as directed. Do not use it more often than recommended on the label, unless otherwise directed by your doctor.

Before using this medicine, wet the hair and scalp with lukewarm water. Then apply a generous amount to the scalp and work up a rich lather. Rub the lather into the scalp for 5 minutes, then rinse. Apply the medicine again and rinse thoroughly.

Immediately after using this medicine, wash your hands to remove any medicine that may be on them.

Keep this medicine away from the eyes. If you should accidentally get some in your eyes, flush them thoroughly with water.

How to store this medicine:

• **Keep out of the reach of children.**

• Store away from heat and direct light.

• Keep the medicine from freezing.

• Do not keep outdated medicine or medicine no longer needed. Be sure that any discarded medicine is out of the reach of children.

Precautions While Using This Medicine

Do not use any topical mercury-containing preparation, such as ammoniated mercury ointment, on the same affected area as this medicine. To do so may cause a foul odor, may be irritating to the skin, and may stain the skin black. If you have any questions about this, check with your doctor or pharmacist.

This medicine may temporarily discolor blond, bleached, or tinted hair.

Side Effects of This Medicine

In animal studies, coal tar (contained in this combination medicine) has been shown to increase the chance of skin cancer.

Along with its needed effects, a medicine may cause some unwanted effects. Although not all of these side effects may occur, if they do occur they may need medical attention.

Check with your doctor as soon as possible if the following side effect occurs:

Skin irritation not present before using this medicine

For elderly patients: Many medicines have not been tested in older people. Therefore, it is not known whether the medicine acts the same way it does in younger adults. Check with your doctor or pharmacist if you notice any unusual effects while using this medicine or if you think it is not working as it should.

Other side effects not listed above may also occur in some patients. If you notice any other effects, check with your doctor or pharmacist.

_____

December 1987
_____

SELENIUM SULFIDE (Topical)

Some commonly used brand names are:

Exsel	Selsun Blue
Selsun	Sul-Blue

Generic name product may also be available in the U.S.

To the Reader: If you do not recognize the names of medical conditions or medicines referred to in this information, check with your doctor, nurse, or pharmacist. Definitions for selected medical terms may be found in the Glossary. Brand names for the generic drug names listed can be found in the Index. In addition, selected brand names commonly associated with the generic name have been included in the text to help you recognize medicine you may be taking. The fact that a brand name product is not mentioned does not mean the information does not apply. It is a good idea for you to learn both the generic and brand names of your medicines and to write them down for future use.

Selenium sulfide (se-LEE-nee-um SUL-fide) is used as a shampoo to treat dandruff and seborrheic dermatitis of the scalp.

Some of these preparations are available only with your doctor's prescription. Others are available without a prescription; however, your doctor may have special instructions on the proper use of this medicine for your medical problem.

Remember:
- **Keep all medicines out of the reach of children.**
- In order for this medicine to work, it must be used as directed. **If you are using this medicine without a prescription, it is very important to follow the directions on the label.**
- **It is also very important that you read and understand the following information.** If any of the information causes you special concern, check with your doctor or pharmacist.
- Before you begin using any new medicine (prescription or nonprescription) or if you develop any new medical problem while you are using this medicine, check with your doctor, nurse, or pharmacist.
- **If you have any questions** about the following information or if you want more information about this medicine or your medical problem, **ask your doctor, nurse, or pharmacist.**

Before Using This Medicine

Before you use selenium sulfide, check with your doctor or pharmacist:

—if you have ever had any unusual or allergic reaction to selenium sulfide.

—if you are allergic to any substance, such as certain preservatives or dyes. Most medicines contain more than their active ingredient. Your doctor or pharmacist can help you avoid products that may cause a problem.

—if you are **pregnant** or if you may become pregnant. However, selenium sulfide has not been shown to cause birth defects or other problems in humans.

—if you are **breast-feeding**. However, selenium sulfide has not been shown to cause problems in nursing babies.

Proper Use of This Medicine

Use this medicine only as directed. Do not use it more often than recommended on the label, unless otherwise directed by your doctor.

Before using this medicine, wet the hair and scalp with lukewarm water. Then apply enough medicine to the scalp to work up a lather. Allow the lather to remain on the scalp for 2 to 3 minutes, then rinse. Apply the medicine again. Then **rinse thoroughly to lessen the possibility of hair discoloration.**

Also, if you use this medicine before or after bleaching, tinting, or permanent-waving your hair, rinse your hair for at least 5 minutes in cool running water after using the medicine.

Do not use this medicine if blistered, raw, or oozing areas are present on your scalp, unless otherwise directed by your doctor.

Keep this medicine away from the eyes. If you should accidentally get some in your eyes, flush them thoroughly with water.

How to store this medicine:

- **Keep out of the reach of children.**
- Store away from heat and direct light.
- Keep the medicine from freezing.
- Do not keep outdated medicine or medicine no longer needed. Be sure that any discarded medicine is out of the reach of children.

Side Effects of This Medicine

Along with its needed effects, a medicine may cause some unwanted effects. Although not all of these side effects may occur, if they do occur they may need medical attention.

Check with your doctor as soon as possible if the following side effect occurs:

Skin irritation

Other side effects may occur that usually do not require medical attention. Check with your doctor or pharmacist if any of the following side effects continue or are bothersome:

More common

Unusual dryness or oiliness of hair or scalp

Less common

Increase in normal hair loss

For elderly patients: Many medicines have not been tested in older people. Therefore, it is not known whether the medicine acts the same way it does in younger adults. Check with your doctor or pharmacist if you notice any unusual effects while using this medicine or if you think it is not working as it should.

Other side effects not listed above may also occur in some patients. If you notice any other effects, check with your doctor or pharmacist.

December 1987

SIMETHICONE (Oral)

Some commonly used brand names are:

Gas-X	Phazyme
Mylicon	Phazyme 125
Ovol*	Silain

*Not available in the U.S.

To the Reader: If you do not recognize the names of medical conditions or medicines referred to in this information, check with your doctor, nurse, or pharmacist. Definitions for selected medical terms may be found in the Glossary. Brand names for the generic drug names listed can be found in the Index. In addition, selected brand names commonly associated with the generic name have been included in the text to help you recognize medicine you may be taking. The fact that a brand name product is not mentioned does not mean the information does not apply. It is a good idea for you to learn both the generic and brand names of your medicines and to write them down for future use.

Simethicone (si-METH-i-kone) is taken by mouth to relieve the painful symptoms of too much gas in the stomach and intestines.

Simethicone is available without a prescription; however, your doctor may have special instructions on the proper use and dose for your medical problem.

Remember:
• **Keep all medicines out of the reach of children.**

• In order for this medicine to work, it must be used as directed. **If you are using this medicine without a prescription, it is very important to follow the directions on the label.**

• **It is also very important that you read and understand the following information.** If any of the information causes you special concern, check with your doctor before using this medicine without a prescription.

• Before you begin using any new medicine (prescription or nonprescription) or if you develop any new medical problem while you are using this medicine, check with your doctor, nurse, or pharmacist.

• **If you have any questions** about the following information or if you want more information about this medicine or your medical problem, **ask your doctor, nurse, or pharmacist.**

Before Using This Medicine

Importance of proper diet and exercise to prevent gas problem—Avoid foods that seem to increase gas. Chew food thoroughly and slowly. Reduce air swallowing by avoiding fizzy, carbonated drinks. Do not smoke before meals. Develop regular bowel habits and exercise regularly.

Before you use this medicine, check with your doctor or pharmacist:
—if you have ever had any unusual or allergic reaction to simethicone.

—if you are on a low-salt, low-sugar, or any other special diet, or if you are allergic to any substance, such as foods, sulfites or other preservatives, or dyes. Most medicines contain more than their active ingredient. Your doctor, nurse, or pharmacist can help you avoid products that may cause a problem.

—if you are **pregnant** or if you may become pregnant. Simethicone is not absorbed into the body and is not likely to cause problems.

—if you are **breast-feeding**. Simethicone has not been shown to cause problems in nursing babies.

Proper Use of This Medicine

For effective use of simethicone:
• Follow your doctor's instructions if this medicine was prescribed.
• Follow the manufacturer's package directions if you are treating yourself.

Take this medicine after meals and at bedtime for best results.

For patients taking the chewable tablet form of this medicine:
• It is important that you chew the tablets thoroughly before swallowing. This is to allow the medicine to work faster and more completely.

If you must take this medicine regularly and you miss a dose, take it as soon as possible. However, if it is almost time for your next dose, skip the missed dose and go back to your regular dosing schedule. Do not double doses.

How to store this medicine:
• **Keep out of the reach of children.**
• Store away from heat and direct light.
• Do not store the tablet form of this medicine in the bathroom, near the kitchen sink, or in other damp places. Heat or moisture may cause the medicine to break down.
• Keep the liquid form of this medicine from freezing.
• Do not keep outdated medicine or medicine no longer needed. Be sure that any discarded medicine is out of the reach of children.

Side Effects of This Medicine

There have not been any common or important side effects reported with this medicine. However, if you notice any side effects, check with your doctor.

December 1987

SKELETAL MUSCLE RELAXANTS
(Systemic)

This information applies to the following medicines:

Carisoprodol (kar-eye-soe-PROE-dole)
Chlorphenesin (klor-FEN-e-sin)
Chlorzoxazone (klor-ZOX-a-zone)
Metaxalone (me-TAX-a-lone)
Methocarbamol (meth-oh-KAR-ba-mole)

This information does *not* apply to the following medicines: Baclofen, cyclobenzaprine, dantrolene, diazepam, and orphenadrine.

Some commonly used brand names are:	Generic names
Rela Soma Soprodol	Carisoprodol†
Maolate	Chlorphenesin
Paraflex Parafon Forte DSC	Chlorzoxazone†
Skelaxin	Metaxalone
Delaxin Marbaxin Robaxin	Methocarbamol†

†Generic name product may also be available in the U.S.

To the Reader: If you do not recognize the names of medical conditions or medicines referred to in this information, check with your doctor, nurse, or pharmacist. Definitions for selected medical terms may be found in the Glossary. Brand names for the generic drug names listed can be found in the Index. In addition, selected brand names commonly associated with the generic name have been included in the text to help you recognize medicine you may be taking. The fact that a brand name product is not mentioned does not mean the information does not apply. It is a good idea for you to learn both the generic and brand names of your medicines and to write them down for future use.

Skeletal muscle relaxants are used to relax certain muscles in your body and relieve the pain and discomfort caused by strains, sprains, or other injury to your muscles. However, these medicines do not take the place of rest, exercise or physical therapy, or other treatment that your doctor may recommend for your medical problem. Methocarbamol also has been used to relieve some of the muscle problems caused by tetanus.

Skeletal muscle relaxants act in the central nervous system (CNS) to produce their muscle relaxant effects. Their actions in the CNS may also produce some of their side effects.

In the U.S., these medicines are available only with your doctor's prescription. In Canada, some of these medicines are available without a prescription.

Remember:

• **This medicine has been prescribed for your current medical problem only.** It must not be given to other people or used for other problems unless you are directed to do so by your doctor.

• **Keep all medicines out of the reach of children.**

• In order for this medicine to work, it must be used as directed.

• If you are receiving methocarbamol by injection, some of the information about this medicine may not apply.

• **It is very important that you read and understand the following information.** If any of the information causes you special concern, do not decide against using this medicine without first checking with your doctor.

• Before you begin using any new medicine (prescription or nonprescription) or if you develop any new medical problem while you are using this medicine, check with your doctor, nurse, or pharmacist.

• **If you have any questions** about the following information or if you want more information about this medicine or your medical problem, **ask your doctor, nurse, or pharmacist.**

Before Using This Medicine

In order to decide on the best treatment for your medical problem, your doctor should be told:

—if you have ever had any unusual or allergic reaction to this medicine.

—if you are taking carisoprodol and have ever had any unusual or allergic reaction to carbromal, mebutamate, meprobamate (e.g., Equanil), or tybamate.

—if you are on a low-salt, low-sugar, or any other special diet, or if you are allergic to any substance such as foods, sulfites or other preservatives, or dyes. Most medicines contain more than their active ingredient. Your doctor, nurse, or pharmacist can help you avoid products that may cause a problem.

—if you are taking metaxalone and any other medicine you have taken has ever caused an allergy or reaction that affected your blood.

—if you are **pregnant** or if you may become pregnant. Although skeletal muscle relaxants have not been shown to cause birth defects or other problems, studies on birth defects have not been done in humans. Studies in animals with metaxalone have not shown that it causes birth defects.

—if you are **breast-feeding**. Carisoprodol passes into the breast milk and may cause drowsiness or stomach upset in nursing babies. Chlorphenesin, chlorzoxazone, metaxalone, and methocarbamol have not been shown to cause problems in nursing babies. However, methocarbamol passes into the breast milk in small amounts. It is not known whether chlorphenesin, chlorzoxazone, or metaxalone passes into the breast milk.

—if you have any of the following medical problems:
    Allergies, history of
    Epilepsy
    Kidney disease
    Liver disease
    Porphyria

—if you are now taking or have taken within the past 2 weeks monoamine oxidase (MAO) inhibitors, such as:

    Furazolidone (e.g., Furoxone)
    Isocarboxazid (e.g., Marplan)
    Pargyline (e.g., Eutonyl)

Phenelzine (e.g., Nardil)
Procarbazine (e.g., Matulane)
Tranylcypromine (e.g., Parnate)

—if you are taking **any** other prescription or nonprescription (OTC) medicine, especially:

Central nervous system (CNS) depressants.
Tricyclic antidepressants (amitriptyline [e.g., Elavil], amoxapine, [e.g., Asendin], clomipramine [e.g., Anafranil], desipramine [e.g., Pertofrane], doxepin [e.g., Sinequan], imipramine [e.g., Tofranil], nortriptyline [e.g., Aventyl], protriptyline [e.g., Vivactil], trimipramine [e.g., Surmontil])

Proper Use of This Medicine

Chlorzoxazone, metaxalone, or methocarbamol tablets may be crushed and mixed with a little food or liquid if needed to make the tablets easier to swallow.

If you miss a dose of this medicine and remember within an hour or so of the missed dose, take it right away. But if you do not remember until later, skip the missed dose and go back to your regular dosing schedule. Do not double doses.

How to store this medicine:

• **Keep out of the reach of children.**

• Store away from heat and direct light.

• Do not store this medicine in the bathroom, near the kitchen sink, or in other damp places. Heat or moisture may cause the medicine to break down.

• Do not keep outdated medicine or medicine no longer needed. Be sure that any discarded medicine is out of the reach of children.

Precautions While Using This Medicine

If you will be taking this medicine for a long period of time (for example, more than a few weeks), your doctor should check your progress at regular visits.

This medicine will add to the effects of alcohol and other CNS depressants (medicines that slow down the nervous system, possibly causing drowsiness). Some examples of CNS depressants are antihistamines or medicine for hay fever, other allergies, or colds; sedatives, tranquilizers, or sleeping medicine; prescription pain medicine or narcotics; barbiturates; medicine for seizures; other muscle relaxants; or anesthetics, including some dental anesthetics. **Do not drink alcoholic beverages, and check with your doctor before taking any of the medicines listed above, while you are using this medicine.**

Skeletal muscle relaxants may cause blurred vision or clumsiness or unsteadiness in some people. They may also cause some people to feel drowsy, dizzy, lightheaded, faint, or less alert than they are normally. **Make sure you know how you react to this medicine before you drive, use machines, or do other jobs that require you to be alert, well-coordinated, and able to see well.**

Diabetics—Metaxalone may cause false test results with one type of test for sugar in your urine. If your urine sugar test shows an unusually large amount of sugar, or if you have any questions about this, check with your doctor, nurse, or pharmacist. This is especially important if your diabetes is not well controlled.

Side Effects of This Medicine

Along with its needed effects, a medicine may cause some unwanted effects. Although not all of these side effects may occur, if they do occur they may need medical attention.

Check with your doctor as soon as possible if any of the following side effects occur:

Less common
Fainting
Fast, slow, or pounding heartbeat
Fever
Mental depression
Skin rash, hives, itching, or redness
Stinging or burning of eyes
Stuffy nose and red or bloodshot eyes
Swelling of face, lips, or tongue
Wheezing, shortness of breath, or troubled breathing

Rare
Bloody or black tarry stools
Convulsions (seizures) (methocarbamol injection only)
Sore throat and fever
Unusual bruising or bleeding
Unusual tiredness or weakness
Yellow eyes or skin

Other side effects may occur that usually do not require medical attention. These side effects may go away during treatment as your body adjusts to the medicine. However, check with your doctor if any of the following side effects continue or are bothersome:

More common
Blurred or double vision or any change in vision
Dizziness or lightheadedness
Drowsiness

Less common or rare
Abdominal or stomach cramps or pain
Clumsiness or unsteadiness
Constipation
Diarrhea
Excitement, nervousness, restlessness, or irritability
Flushing or redness of face
Headache
Heartburn
Hiccups
Muscle weakness
Nausea or vomiting
Pain or peeling of skin at place of injection (methocarbamol only)
Trembling
Trouble in sleeping
Uncontrolled movements of eyes (methocarbamol injection only)

Although not all of the side effects listed above have been reported for all of these medicines, they have been reported for at least one of them. However, since all of these skeletal muscle relaxants have similar effects, it is possible that any of the above side effects may occur with any of these medicines.

In addition to the other side effects listed above, chlorzoxazone may cause your urine to turn orange or reddish purple. Methocarbamol may cause your urine to turn black, brown, or green. This effect is harmless and will go away when you stop taking the medicine. However, if you have any questions about this, check with your doctor.

For elderly patients: Many medicines have not been tested in older people. Therefore, it is not known whether the medicine acts the same way it does in younger adults.

Check with your doctor or pharmacist if you notice any unusual effects while taking this medicine or if you think it is not working as it should.

Other side effects not listed above may also occur in some patients. If you notice any other effects, check with your doctor.

December 1987

SODIUM BICARBONATE (Systemic)

Some commonly used brand names are:

Arm and Hammer	Citrocarbonate
Baking Soda	Neut
Bell/ans	Soda Mint

To the Reader: If you do not recognize the names of medical conditions or medicines referred to in this information, check with your doctor, nurse, or pharmacist. Definitions for selected medical terms may be found in the Glossary. Brand names for the generic drug names listed can be found in the Index. In addition, selected brand names commonly associated with the generic name have been included in the text to help you recognize medicine you may be taking. The fact that a brand name product is not mentioned does not mean the information does not apply. It is a good idea for you to learn both the generic and brand names of your medicines and to write them down for future use.

Sodium bicarbonate (SOE-dee-um bye-KAR-boe-nate), also known as baking soda, is taken by mouth to relieve heartburn, sour stomach, or acid indigestion by neutralizing excess stomach acid. When used for this purpose, it is said to belong to the group of medicines called antacids. It may be used to treat the symptoms of stomach or duodenal ulcers. Sodium bicarbonate is also used by mouth or by injection to make the blood and urine more alkaline in certain conditions.

Antacids should not be given to young children (up to 6 years of age) unless prescribed by their doctor. Since children cannot usually describe their symptoms very well, a doctor should check the child before giving this medicine. This is to prevent an unknown condition from getting worse and to avoid causing unwanted effects in the child.

Sodium bicarbonate for oral use is available without a prescription; however, your doctor may have special instructions on the proper use and dose for your medical problem.

Remember:
- **Keep all medicines out of the reach of children.**

- In order for this medicine to work, it must be used as directed. **If you are using this medicine without a prescription, it is very important to follow the directions on the label.**

- **It is also very important that you read and understand the following information.** If any of the information causes you special concern, check with your doctor before using this medicine without a prescription.

- If you are receiving this medicine by injection, some of the information about this medicine may not apply.

- Before you begin using any new medicine (prescription or nonprescription) or if you develop any new medical problem while you are using this medicine, check with your doctor, nurse, or pharmacist.

- **If you have any questions** about the following information or if you want more information about this medicine or your medical problem, **ask your doctor, nurse, or pharmacist.**

Before Using This Medicine

Before you use this medicine, check with your doctor or pharmacist:

—if you have ever had any unusual or allergic reaction to sodium bicarbonate.

—if you are on a low-salt, low-sugar, or any other special diet, or if you are allergic to any substance, such as foods, sulfites or other preservatives, or dyes. Most medicines contain more than their active ingredient. Your doctor, nurse, or pharmacist can help you avoid products that may cause a problem.

—if you are **pregnant** or if you may become pregnant. Sodium bicarbonate is absorbed by the body and although it has not been shown to cause problems, the chance always exists. In addition, medicines containing sodium should usually be avoided if you tend to retain (keep) body water.

—if you are **breast-feeding**. Sodium bicarbonate has not been shown to cause problems in nursing babies.

—if you are taking sodium bicarbonate as an antacid and also have any signs of appendicitis or intestinal or rectal bleeding (such as black, tarry stools) of unknown cause.

—if you have any of the following medical problems:
Edema (swelling of feet or lower legs)
Heart disease
High blood pressure
Kidney disease
Liver disease
Problems with urination
Toxemia of pregnancy

—if you are taking **any** other prescription or nonprescription (OTC) medicine, especially:
Adrenocorticoids (cortisone-like medicine)
Ketoconazole (e.g., Nizoral)
Mecamylamine (e.g., Inversine)
Methenamine (e.g., Mandelamine)
Tetracyclines

Proper Use of This Medicine

For safe and effective use of sodium bicarbonate:
- Follow your doctor's instructions if this medicine was prescribed.

- Follow the manufacturer's package directions if you are treating yourself.

For patients taking this medicine for a stomach ulcer:
- **Take it exactly as directed and for the full time of treatment as ordered by your doctor** to obtain maximum relief of your symptoms.

- Take it 1 and 3 hours after meals and at bedtime for best results, unless otherwise directed by your doctor.

If you must take this medicine regularly and you miss a dose, take it as soon as possible. However, if it is almost time for your next dose, skip the missed dose and go back to your regular dosing schedule. Do not double doses.

How to store this medicine:

- **Keep out of the reach of children.**

- Store away from heat and direct light.

- Do not store the powder or tablet form of this medicine in the bathroom, near the kitchen sink, or in other damp places. Heat or moisture may cause the medicine to break down.

- Do not keep outdated medicine or medicine no longer needed. Be sure that any discarded medicine is out of the reach of children.

Precautions While Using This Medicine

If this medicine has been ordered by your doctor and if you will be taking it regularly for a long period of time, your doctor should check your progress at regular visits. This is to make sure the medicine does not cause unwanted effects.

Do not take sodium bicarbonate:

—**within 1 to 2 hours of taking other medicine by mouth.** To do so may keep the other medicine from working as well.

—**for a prolonged period of time.** To do so may increase the chance of side effects.

Patients on a sodium-restricted diet—This medicine contains a large amount of sodium. If you have any questions about this, check with your doctor or pharmacist.

For patients taking this medicine as an antacid:

- **Do not take if you have any signs of appendicitis** (such as stomach or lower abdominal pain, cramping, bloating, soreness, nausea, or vomiting). Instead, check with your doctor as soon as possible.

- **Do not take with large amounts of milk or milk products.** To do so may increase the chance of side effects.

- **Do not take for more than 2 weeks** or if the problem comes back often. Instead, check with your doctor. Antacids should be used only for occasional relief, unless otherwise directed by your doctor.

Side Effects of This Medicine

Along with its needed effects, a medicine may cause some unwanted effects. Although the following side effects occur very rarely when this medicine is taken as recommended, they may be more likely to occur if it is taken:

    —in large doses.
    —for a long period of time.
    —by patients with kidney disease.

Check with your doctor as soon as possible if any of the following side effects occur:
    Frequent urge to urinate
    Headache (continuing)
    Loss of appetite (continuing)
    Mood or mental changes
    Muscle pain or twitching
    Nausea or vomiting
    Nervousness or restlessness
    Slow breathing
    Swelling of feet or lower legs
    Unpleasant taste
    Unusual tiredness or weakness

Other side effects may occur that usually do not require medical attention. These side effects may go away during treatment as your body adjusts to the medicine. However, check with your doctor if any of the following side effects continue or are bothersome:
Less common
    Increased thirst
    Stomach cramps

Other side effects not listed above may also occur in some patients. If you notice any other effects, check with your doctor.

December 1987

SODIUM CHLORIDE (Intra-amniotic)

To the Reader: If you do not recognize the names of medical conditions or medicines referred to in this information, check with your doctor, nurse, or pharmacist. Definitions for selected medical terms may be found in the Glossary. Brand names for the generic drug names listed can be found in the Index. In addition, selected brand names commonly associated with the generic name have been included in the text to help you recognize medicine you may be taking. The fact that a brand name product is not mentioned does not mean the information does not apply. It is a good idea for you to learn both the generic and brand names of your medicines and to write them down for future use.

Sodium chloride (SOE-dee-um KLOR-ide) as a 20% solution is given by injection into the uterus to cause abortion. It is to be administered only by or under the immediate care of your doctor.

Remember:
• **It is very important that you read and understand the following information.** If any of the information causes you special concern, do not decide against receiving this medicine without first checking with your doctor.

• **If you have any questions** about the following information or if you want more information about this medicine or your medical problem, **ask your doctor, nurse, or pharmacist.**

Before Using This Medicine

In order to decide on the best treatment for your medical problem, your doctor should be told:
—if you have any of the following medical problems:
Bleeding problems
Epilepsy
Fibroid tumors of the uterus
Heart or blood vessel disease
Hypertension (high blood pressure)
Kidney disease
Uterus surgery (history of)

Proper Use of This Medicine

Unless otherwise directed by your doctor, drink at least 2 liters (about 2 quarts) of fluids the day that this procedure is to be done.

Side Effects of This Medicine

Along with its needed effects, a medicine may cause some unwanted effects. Although not all of these effects may occur, if they do occur they may need medical attention.

Check with your doctor or nurse immediately if any of the following side effects occur during the time that the injection is being given:

Less common
Burning pain in lower abdomen
Confusion or nervousness
Feeling of heat
Feeling of warmth in lips and tongue
Headache (severe)
Numbness of the fingertips
Pain in lower back, pelvis, or stomach
Ringing in the ears
Thirst (sudden) or salty taste

Other side effects may occur that usually do not require medical attention. These side effects usually go away after the medicine is stopped. However, let the doctor or nurse know if either of the following side effects continues or is bothersome:

More common
Fever
Flushing or redness of face

After the procedure, this medicine may still produce some side effects that need attention. Check with your doctor if you notice any of the following side effects:
Chills or shivering
Fever
Foul-smelling vaginal discharge
Increase in uterine bleeding
Pain in lower abdomen

Other side effects not listed above may also occur in some patients. If you notice any other effects, check with your doctor or nurse.

December 1987

SODIUM FLUORIDE (Systemic)

Some commonly used brand names are:

Denta-FL	Flura	Pediaflor
Flo-Tab	Karidium	Pedi-Dent
Fluor-A-Day*	Luride	Solu-Flur*
Fluorident	Luride-SF	Stay-Flo
Fluoritab	Nafeen	Studaflor
Fluorodex		

*Not available in the U.S.

To the Reader: If you do not recognize the names of medical conditions or medicines referred to in this information, check with your doctor, nurse, or pharmacist. Definitions for selected medical terms may be found in the Glossary. Brand names for the generic drug names listed can be found in the Index. In addition, selected brand names commonly associated with the generic name have been included in the text to help you recognize medicine you may be taking. The fact that a brand name product is not mentioned does not mean the information does not apply. It is a good idea for you to learn both the generic and brand names of your medicines and to write them down for future use.

Fluoride has been found to be helpful in reducing the number of cavities in the teeth. It is usually present naturally in drinking water. However, some areas of the country do not have a high enough level in the water to prevent cavities. To make up for this, extra fluorides may be added to the diet. Some children may require both dietary fluorides and fluoride treatments by the dentist. Use of a fluoride toothpaste or rinse may be helpful as well.

Taking fluorides does not replace good dental habits. These include eating a good diet, brushing teeth often, and having regular dental checkups.

This medicine is available only with your physician's or dentist's prescription.

Remember:

• **This medicine has been prescribed for your use only.** It must not be given to other people or used for other problems unless you are directed to do so by your physician or dentist.

• **Keep all medicines out of the reach of children.**

• In order for this medicine to work, it must be used as directed.

• **It is very important that you read and understand the following information.** If any of the information causes you special concern, do not decide against using this medicine without first checking with your physician or dentist.

• Before you begin using any new medicine (prescription or nonprescription) or if you develop any new medical problem while you are using this medicine, check with your physician, dentist, nurse, or pharmacist.

• **If you have any questions** about the following information or if you want more information about this medicine or your medical problem, **ask your physician, dentist, nurse, or pharmacist.**

Before Using This Medicine

In order to decide on the best treatment for your medical problem, your physician or dentist should be told:

—if you have ever had any unusual reaction to medicines containing fluorides.

—if you are on a low-salt, low-sugar, or any other special diet, or if you are allergic to any substance, such as foods, sulfites or other preservatives, or dyes. Most medicines contain more than their active ingredient, and many liquid medicines contain alcohol. Your doctor, nurse, or pharmacist can help you avoid products that may cause a problem.

—if you are **pregnant** or if you may become pregnant. Sodium fluoride occurs naturally in water and has not been shown to cause problems in infants of mothers who drank fluoridated water or took appropriate doses of supplements.

—if you are **breast-feeding**, although only small amounts of sodium fluoride pass into breast milk.

—if you have an underactive thyroid gland.

—if you are taking **any** other prescription or nonprescription (OTC) medicine.

Proper Use of This Medicine

Take this medicine only as directed by your physician or dentist. Do not take more of it and do not take it more often than ordered. Taking too much fluoride over a period of time may cause unwanted effects.

For patients taking the chewable tablet form of this medicine:

• Tablets should be chewed or crushed before they are swallowed.

• This medicine works best if it is taken at bedtime, after the teeth have been thoroughly brushed. Do not eat or drink for at least 15 minutes after taking sodium fluoride.

For patients taking the oral liquid form of this medicine:

• This medicine is to be taken by mouth even though it comes in a dropper bottle. The amount to be taken is to be measured with the specially marked dropper.

• **Always store this medicine in the original plastic container.** Fluoride will affect glass and should not be stored in glass containers.

• This medicine may be dropped directly into the mouth or mixed with cereal, fruit juice, or other food.

If you miss a dose of this medicine, take it as soon as you remember. However, if it is almost time for the next dose, skip the missed dose and go back to your regular dosing schedule. Do not double doses. If you have any questions about this, check with your physician or dentist.

How to store this medicine:

• **Keep out of the reach of children,** since overdose is especially dangerous in children.

• Store away from heat and direct light.

• Do not store in the bathroom, near the kitchen sink, or in other damp places. Heat or moisture may cause the medicine to break down.

• Protect the oral liquid from freezing.

• Do not keep outdated medicine or medicine no longer needed. Be sure that any discarded medicine is out of the reach of children.

Precautions While Using This Medicine

The level of fluoride present in the water is different in different parts of the country. If you move to another area, check with a physician or dentist in the new area as soon as possible to see if this medicine is still needed or if the dose needs to be changed.

Inform your physician or dentist as soon as possible if you notice white, brown, or black spots on the teeth. These are signs of too much fluoride.

Side Effects of This Medicine

Along with its needed effects, a medicine may cause some unwanted effects. Although not all of these side effects may occur, if they do occur they may need medical attention.

Sodium fluoride in drinking water or taken as a supplement does not usually cause any side effects. However, **taking an overdose of fluoride may cause serious problems.**

Stop taking this medicine and check with your physician immediately if any of the following side effects occur, as they may be signs of severe overdose:
    Black tarry stools
    Bloody vomit
    Diarrhea
    Drowsiness
    Faintness
    Increase in saliva
    Nausea or vomiting
    Shallow breathing
    Stomach cramps or pain
    Tremors
    Unusual excitement
    Watery eyes
    Weakness

Check with your physician or dentist as soon as possible if the following side effects occur, as some may be early signs of possible overdose:
    Constipation
    Loss of appetite
    Pain and aching of bones
    Skin rash
    Sores in the mouth and on the lips
    Stiffness
    Weight loss
    White, brown, or black discoloration of teeth

Other side effects not listed above may also occur in some patients. If you notice any other effects, check with your physician or dentist.

December 1987

SODIUM IODIDE I 131 (Therapeutic)

To the Reader: If you do not recognize the names of medical conditions or medicines referred to in this information, check with your doctor, nurse, or pharmacist. Definitions for selected medical terms may be found in the Glossary. Brand names for the generic drug names listed can be found in the Index. In addition, selected brand names commonly associated with the generic name have been included in the text to help you recognize medicine you may be taking. The fact that a brand name product is not mentioned does not mean the information does not apply. It is a good idea for you to learn both the generic and brand names of your medicines and to write them down for future use.

Sodium iodide (EYE-oh-dyed) I 131 (radioactive iodine) is a radiopharmaceutical (ray-dee-oh-far-ma-SOO-ti-kal). Radiopharmaceuticals are radioactive agents, which may be used to treat certain diseases or to study the activity of the body's organs.

Sodium iodide I 131 is taken by mouth to treat an overactive thyroid gland and certain kinds of thyroid cancer. It builds up mainly in the thyroid gland. Large doses of sodium iodide I 131 are usually used after thyroid cancer surgery to destroy any remaining diseased thyroid tissue.

When very small doses are given, the amount of radioactivity in the gland can then be measured to help study the activity of the thyroid gland. Also, a likeness of the organ on paper or a computer print out can be provided.

The information that follows applies only to sodium iodide I 131 when used in treating an overactive or cancerous thyroid gland.

Sodium iodide I 131 is to be given only by or under the direct supervision of a doctor with specialized training in nuclear medicine.

Remember:

• **It is very important that you read and understand the following information.** If any of the information causes you special concern, do not decide against receiving this medicine without first checking with your doctor.

• **If you have any questions** about the following information or if you want more information about this medicine or your medical problem, **ask your doctor, nuclear medicine physician and/or technologist, nuclear pharmacist, or nurse.**

Before Using This Medicine

In order to decide on the best treatment for your medical problem, your doctor should be told:

—if you have ever had any unusual or allergic reaction to iodine or to products containing iodine (for example, iodine-containing foods, such as seafood, cabbage, kale, rape [turnip-like vegetable] or turnips, or iodized salt).

—if you are allergic to any substance, such as sulfites or other preservatives. Most medicines contain more than their active ingredient. Your doctor can help you avoid products that may cause a problem.

—if you are **pregnant** or if you may become pregnant soon after using this medicine. Sodium iodide I 131 is not recommended during pregnancy. This is to avoid exposing the fetus to radiation. Also, it may cause the fetus to have an underactive thyroid gland. Be sure you have discussed this with your doctor.

—if you are **breast-feeding**. Sodium iodide I 131 passes into the breast milk and may cause unwanted effects, such as underactive thyroid, in the baby. If you must receive this radiopharmaceutical, it may be necessary for you to stop breast-feeding during treatment. Be sure you have discussed this with your doctor.

—if you have any of the following medical problems:
Diarrhea
Iodine deficiency
Kidney disease
Vomiting

—if you have heart disease and you are receiving sodium iodide I 131 to treat an overactive thyroid.

—if you are taking **any** other prescription or nonprescription (OTC) medicine.

—if you eat large amounts of iodine-containing foods, such as iodized salt and seafoods, or cabbage, kale, rape (turnip-like vegetable) or turnips. The iodine contained in these foods will reduce the amount of this radiopharmaceutical that your thyroid gland will accept.

—if you have had an x-ray test recently for which you were given a radiopaque agent that contained iodine.

Proper Use of This Medicine

Your doctor may have special instructions for you in preparation for your test or treatment. If you have not received such instructions or you do not understand them, check with your doctor in advance.

Precautions After Using This Medicine

There are no special precautions when this drug is used in very small doses to help study the activity of the thyroid. However, to help reduce the chance of contaminating other persons, **follow these guidelines for 48 to 72 hours** after receiving sodium iodide I 131 for an overactive thyroid or cancer of the thyroid:

• **Do not kiss anyone or use another person's eating or drinking utensils.**

• **Do not engage in any sexual activities.**

• **Do not sit close to others and do not hold children in your lap for long periods of time.**

• Sleep alone.

• **Wash the tub and sink after each use (including after brushing teeth).**

• **Wash your hands after using the toilet.**

• Use a separate towel and washcloth.

• Wash your clothes, bed linens, and eating utensils separately.

Sodium iodide I 131 is passed into the urine. To prevent contamination of your home environment, **flush the toilet twice after urination.**

Side Effects of This Medicine

Studies have not shown that sodium iodide I 131 increases the chance for cancer or other long-term side effects. When used to treat an overactive thyroid gland or cancer of the thyroid, sodium iodide I 131 may cause the patient to have an underactive thyroid gland after treatment. The younger the patient is at the time of treatment, the greater the chance of later developing an underactive thyroid gland. Before receiving this medicine, be sure you have discussed the use of it with your doctor.

Along with its needed effects, a medicine may cause some unwanted effects. Although not all of these side effects may occur, if they do occur they may need medical attention.

When this drug is used in very small doses to help study the activity of the gland, side effects are rare. However, check with your doctor as soon as possible if any of the following side effects occur after treatment for overactive thyroid or cancer of the thyroid:

Signs of an underactive thyroid
>   Changes in menstrual period
>   Clumsiness
>   Coldness
>   Drowsiness
>   Dry, puffy skin
>   Headache
>   Listlessness
>   Muscle aches
>   Thinning of hair (temporary)—may occur 2 to 3 months
>   after treatment
>   Unusual tiredness or weakness
>   Unusual weight gain

Rare
In treatment of overactive thyroid
>   Unusual irritability
>   Unusual tiredness

In treatment of cancer of the thyroid
>   Fever, chills, and sore throat
>   Unusual bleeding or bruising

Other side effects may occur that usually do not require medical attention. These side effects may go away during treatment as your body adjusts to the medicine. However, check with your doctor if any of the following side effects continue or are bothersome:

Less common
In treatment of overactive thyroid or cancer of the thyroid
>   Neck tenderness or swelling
>   Sore throat

In treatment of cancer of the thyroid
>   Loss of taste (temporary)
>   Nausea and vomiting (temporary)
>   Tenderness of salivary glands

Other side effects not listed above may also occur in some patients. If you notice any other effects, check with your doctor.

_____

December 1987

_____

SODIUM PHOSPHATE P 32
(Therapeutic)

To the Reader: If you do not recognize the names of medical conditions or medicines referred to in this information, check with your doctor, nurse, or pharmacist. Definitions for selected medical terms may be found in the Glossary. Brand names for the generic drug names listed can be found in the Index. In addition, selected brand names commonly associated with the generic name have been included in the text to help you recognize medicine you may be taking. The fact that a brand name product is not mentioned does not mean the information does not apply. It is a good idea for you to learn both the generic and brand names of your medicines and to write them down for future use.

Sodium phosphate (SOE-dee-um FOS-fate) P 32 is a radiopharmaceutical (ray-dee-oh-far-ma-SOO-ti-kal). Radiopharmaceuticals are radioactive agents that may be used to treat certain diseases or to study the activity of the body's organs.

Sodium phosphate P 32 is given by injection to treat certain kinds of cancer. In this case, the radioactive agent builds up in the cancerous area and destroys the affected tissue. This radiopharmaceutical may also be used for other conditions as determined by your doctor.

Sodium phosphate P 32 is to be given only by or under the direct supervision of a doctor with specialized training in nuclear medicine.

Remember:

• **It is very important that you read and understand the following information.** If any of the information causes you special concern, do not decide against taking this medicine without first checking with your doctor.

• **If you have any questions** about the following information or if you want more information about this medicine or your medical problem, **ask your doctor, nuclear medicine physician and/or technologist, nuclear pharmacist, or nurse.**

Before Using This Medicine

In order to decide on the best treatment for your medical problem, your doctor should be told:

—if you are allergic to any substance, such as sulfites or other preservatives. Most medicines contain more than their active ingredient. Your doctor can help you avoid products that may cause a problem.

—if you are **pregnant** or if you may become pregnant. Studies have not been done in either humans or animals. However, to avoid exposing the fetus to radiation, sodium phosphate P 32 is not recommended during pregnancy. Be sure you have discussed this with your doctor.

—if you are **breast-feeding**. Sodium phosphate may pass into the breast milk. If you must receive this radiopharmaceutical, it may be necessary for you to stop breast-feeding during treatment. Be sure you have discussed this with your doctor.

Proper Use of This Medicine

Your doctor may have special instructions for you in preparation for your treatment. If you do not understand them or if you have not received such instructions, check with your doctor in advance.

Side Effects of This Medicine

Along with its needed effects, a medicine may cause some unwanted effects. When used at recommended doses, sodium phosphate P 32 usually does not cause any side effects.

December 1987

SOMATREM (Systemic)

A commonly used brand name is Protropin.

To the Reader: If you do not recognize the names of medical conditions or medicines referred to in this information, check with your doctor, nurse, or pharmacist. Definitions for selected medical terms may be found in the Glossary. Brand names for the generic drug names listed can be found in the Index. In addition, selected brand names commonly associated with the generic name have been included in the text to help you recognize medicine you may be taking. The fact that a brand name product is not mentioned does not mean the information does not apply. It is a good idea for you to learn both the generic and brand names of your medicines and to write them down for future use.

Somatrem (SOE-ma-trem) is a man-made version of human growth hormone (HGH). HGH is naturally produced by the pituitary gland and is necessary to stimulate growth in children. If a child fails to grow normally because its body is not producing enough HGH, somatrem may be given by injection to stimulate growth.

Some individuals believe that since somatrem stimulates growth in children, it will also help athletes build muscle tissue and improve their performance. There is no good medical evidence to support this belief. In addition, such use is not recommended since serious unwanted effects such as diabetes, abnormal growth of bones and internal organs (heart, kidneys, liver), atherosclerosis (hardening of the arteries), and hypertension (high blood pressure) may occur in such individuals.

Somatrem is available only with your doctor's prescription.

Remember:
• **It is very important that you read and understand the following information.** If any of the information causes you special concern, do not decide against using this medicine without first checking with your doctor.

• Before you begin using any new medicine (prescription or nonprescription) or if you develop any new medical problem while you are using this medicine, check with your doctor, nurse, or pharmacist.

• **If you have any questions** about the following information or if you want more information about this medicine or your medical problem, **ask your doctor, nurse, or pharmacist.**

Before Using This Medicine

In order to decide on the best treatment for your medical problem, your doctor should be told:

—if you have ever had any unusual or allergic reaction to somatrem, benzyl alcohol, or somatropin.

—if you have any of the following medical problems:
    Brain tumor or any cancer
    Diabetes mellitus (sugar diabetes)
    Underactive thyroid

—if you are now taking any of the following medicines or types of medicine:
    Adrenocorticoids (cortisone-like medicines)
    Anabolic steroids (dromostanolone, ethylestrenol, nandrolone, oxandrolone, oxymetholone, stanozolol)
    Androgens (male hormones)
    Estrogens (female hormones)
    Thyroid hormones

Precautions While Using This Medicine

It is important that your doctor check your progress at regular visits. This includes checking your blood and/or urine for sugar.

Diabetics—This medicine may affect blood and urine glucose (sugar) levels. If you notice a change in the results of your blood or urine glucose test or if you have any questions about this, check with your doctor.

Side Effects of This Medicine

When somatrem is used to promote growth in children who have a lack of naturally produced human growth hormone, serious side effects do not usually occur. However, if pain or swelling occurs at the place of injection or if any other unusual effects occur, check with your doctor.

If somatrem is given to children who are growing normally or to adults, serious unwanted effects may occur. These effects include the development of diabetes, abnormal growth of bones and internal organs such as the heart, kidneys, and liver, atherosclerosis (hardening of the arteries), and hypertension (high blood pressure).

December 1987

SOMATROPIN (Systemic)

Some commonly used brand names are Grorm*, Humatrope, and Nanormon*.

---

*Not available in the U.S.

To the Reader: If you do not recognize the names of medical conditions or medicines referred to in this information, check with your doctor, nurse, or pharmacist. Definitions for selected medical terms may be found in the Glossary. Brand names for the generic drug names listed can be found in the Index. In addition, selected brand names commonly associated with the generic name have been included in the text to help you recognize medicine you may be taking. The fact that a brand name product is not mentioned does not mean the information does not apply. It is a good idea for you to learn both the generic and brand names of your medicines and to write them down for future use.

Somatropin (soe-ma-TROE-pin), also known as human growth hormone (HGH), is a hormone naturally produced by the pituitary gland and is necessary to stimulate growth in children. Somatropin available in the U.S. is a man-made version of HGH. If a child fails to grow normally because its body is not producing enough HGH, somatropin may be given by injection to stimulate growth.

Some individuals believe that since somatropin stimulates growth in children, it will also help athletes build muscle tissue and improve their performance. There is no good medical evidence to support this belief. In addition, such use is not recommended since serious unwanted effects such as diabetes, abnormal growth of bones and internal organs (heart, kidneys, liver), atherosclerosis (hardening of the arteries), and hypertension (high blood pressure) may occur in such individuals.

Somatropin is available only with your doctor's prescription.

Remember:

• **It is very important that you read and understand the following information.** If any of the information causes you special concern, do not decide against using this medicine without first checking with your doctor.

• Before you begin using any new medicine (prescription or nonprescription) or if you develop any new medical problem while you are using this medicine, check with your doctor, nurse, or pharmacist.

• **If you have any questions** about the following information or if you want more information about this medicine or your medical problem, **ask your doctor, nurse, or pharmacist.**

Before Using This Medicine

In order to decide on the best treatment for your medical problem, your doctor should be told:

—if you have ever had any unusual or allergic reaction to somatropin, somatrem, or benzyl alcohol.

—if you have any of the following medical problems:
  Brain tumor or any cancer
  Diabetes mellitus (sugar diabetes) or family history of
  Underactive thyroid

—if you are now taking any of the following medicines or types of medicine:
  Adrenocorticoids (cortisone-like medicine)
  Anabolic steroids (dromostanolone, ethylestrenol, nandrolone, oxandrolone, oxymetholone, stanozolol)
  Androgens (male hormones)
  Estrogens (female hormones)
  Thyroid hormones

Precautions While Using This Medicine

It is important that your doctor check your progress at regular visits. This includes checking your blood and/or urine for sugar.

Diabetics—This medicine may affect blood and urine glucose (sugar) levels. If you notice a change in the results of your blood or urine glucose test or if you have any questions about this, check with your doctor.

Side Effects of This Medicine

When somatropin is used to promote growth in children who have a lack of naturally produced human growth hormone, serious side effects do not usually occur. However, if pain or swelling occurs at the place of injection or if any other unusual effects occur, check with your doctor.

If somatropin is given to children who are growing normally or to adults, serious unwanted effects may occur. These effects include the development of diabetes, abnormal growth of bones and internal organs (heart, kidneys, and liver), atherosclerosis (hardening of the arteries), and hypertension (high blood pressure).

There have been several patients who developed Creutzfeldt-Jakob disease years after receiving somatropin obtained from human pituitary glands before 1977. This disease is thought to be caused by a virus that affects the brain. Deaths have occurred. However, there have been no reports of this disease in patients who received somatropin from human pituitary glands since 1977, when purification by a different process was begun. Further studies are being done to find out whether this disease was actually caused by the somatropin. This problem has not occurred and should not occur with man-made somatropin. Discuss with your doctor the risks as well as the benefits of receiving somatropin.

December 1987

STREPTOZOCIN (Systemic)

A commonly used brand name is Zanosar.

To the Reader: If you do not recognize the names of medical conditions or medicines referred to in this information, check with your doctor, nurse, or pharmacist. Definitions for selected medical terms may be found in the Glossary. Brand names for the generic drug names listed can be found in the Index. In addition, selected brand names commonly associated with the generic name have been included in the text to help you recognize medicine you may be taking. The fact that a brand name product is not mentioned does not mean the information does not apply. It is a good idea for you to learn both the generic and brand names of your medicines and to write them down for future use.

Streptozocin (strep-toe-ZOE-sin) belongs to the group of medicines known as alkylating agents. It is given by injection to treat cancer of the pancreas.

Streptozocin seems to interfere with the growth of cancer cells, which are eventually destroyed. It also directly affects the way the pancreas works. Since the growth of normal body cells may also be affected by streptozocin, other effects will also occur. Some of these may be serious and must be reported to your doctor. Other effects may not be serious but may cause concern. Some effects may not occur for months or years after the medicine is used.

Before you begin treatment with streptozocin, you and your doctor should talk about the good this medicine will do as well as the risks of using it.

Streptozocin is to be given only by or under the immediate supervision of your doctor.

Remember:

• **It is very important that you read and understand the following information.** If any of the information causes you special concern, do not decide against receiving this medicine without first checking with your doctor.

• Before you begin using any new medicine (prescription or nonprescription) or if you develop any new medical problem while you are receiving this medicine, check with your doctor, nurse, or pharmacist.

• **If you have any questions** about the following information or if you want more information about this medicine or your medical problem, **ask your doctor, nurse, or pharmacist.**

Before Using This Medicine

In order to decide on the best treatment for your medical problem, your doctor should be told:

—if you have ever had any unusual or allergic reaction to streptozocin.

—if you are **pregnant** or if you intend to have children. There is a chance that this medicine may cause birth defects if either the male or the female is receiving it at the time of conception or if it is taken during pregnancy. Studies in rats and rabbits have shown that streptozocin causes birth defects or miscarriage. In addition, many cancer medicines may cause sterility which could be permanent. Although this has not been

reported with this medicine, the possibility should be kept in mind. Be sure that you have discussed this with your doctor before receiving this medicine.

—if you intend to **breast-feed**. Because this medicine may cause serious side effects, breast-feeding is generally not recommended while you are receiving it.

—if you have any of the following medical problems:
   Chickenpox (including recent exposure)
   Diabetes mellitus (sugar diabetes)
   Herpes zoster (shingles)
   Infection
   Kidney disease
   Liver disease

—if you are taking **any** other prescription or nonprescription (OTC) medicine, especially:
   Aminoglycosides by injection or topical application (amikacin, gentamicin, kanamycin, neomycin, netilmicin, streptomycin, tobramycin)
   Amphotericin B by injection (e.g., Fungizone)
   Capreomycin (e.g., Capastat)
   Captopril (e.g., Capoten)
   Cyclosporine (e.g., Sandimmune)
   Enalapril (e.g., Vasotec)
   Gold salts
   Lithium (e.g., Lithane)
   Medicine for inflammation or pain (diclofenac, diflunisal, fenoprofen, flurbiprofen [oral], ibuprofen, indomethacin, ketoprofen, meclofenamate, mefenamic acid, naproxen, phenylbutazone, piroxicam, sulindac, tiaprofenic acid, tolmetin)
   Neomycin by mouth
   Penicillamine (e.g., Cuprimine)
   Phenytoin (e.g., Dilantin)
   Plicamycin (e.g., Mithracin)
   Rifampin (e.g., Rifadin)
   Sulfonamides (sulfa medicine)
   Tetracyclines, except doxycycline and minocycline
   Vancomycin by injection (e.g., Vancocin)

—if you regularly take large amounts of combination pain medicine containing acetaminophen or aspirin or other salicylates.

—if you have ever been treated with x-rays or cancer medicines.

Proper Use of This Medicine

While you are receiving streptozocin, your doctor may want you to drink extra fluids so that you will pass more urine. This will help prevent kidney problems and keep your kidneys working well.

This medicine usually causes nausea and vomiting, which may be severe. However, it is very important that you continue to receive the medicine, even if you begin to feel ill. Ask your doctor, nurse, or pharmacist for ways to lessen these effects.

Precautions While Using This Medicine

It is very important that your doctor check your progress at regular visits to make sure that this medicine is working properly and to check for any unwanted effects.

While you are being treated with streptozocin, and after you stop treatment with it, **do not have any immunizations without your doctor's approval**. Streptozocin lowers your body's resistance and there is a chance you might get the infection the immunization is meant to prevent. In addition, other people living in your household should not take oral polio vaccine since there is a chance they could pass the polio virus on to you. Also, you should avoid close contact with other persons (for example, at school or work) who have taken oral polio vaccine.

If streptozocin accidentally seeps out of the vein into which it is injected, it may damage some tissues and cause scarring. **Tell the doctor or nurse right away if you notice redness, pain, or swelling at the place of injection.**

Side Effects of This Medicine

Along with their needed effects, medicines like streptozocin can sometimes cause unwanted effects such as kidney problems and other side effects; these are described below. Also, because of the way these medicines act on the body, there is a chance that they might cause other unwanted effects that may not occur until months or years after the medicine is used. These delayed effects may include certain types of cancer, such as leukemia. Streptozocin has been shown to cause tumors (some cancerous) in animals. Discuss these possible effects with your doctor.

Although not all of these side effects may occur, if they do occur they may need medical attention.

Check with your doctor or nurse immediately if any of the following side effects occur shortly after the medicine is given:

Less common

    Anxiety, nervousness, or shakiness
    Chills, cold sweats, or cool, pale skin
    Drowsiness or unusual tiredness or weakness
    Fast pulse
    Headache
    Pain or redness at place of injection
    Unusual hunger

Check with your doctor immediately if the following side effects occur any time while you are being treated with this medicine:

Rare

    Fever or sore throat
    Unusual bleeding or bruising

Check with your doctor or nurse as soon as possible if any of the following side effects occur:

More common

    Swelling of feet or lower legs
    Unusual decrease in urination

Rare

    Yellow eyes or skin

Other side effects may occur that usually do not require medical attention. These side effects may go away during treatment as your body adjusts to the medicine. Also, your doctor or nurse may be able to tell you about ways to prevent or reduce some of these side effects. Check with your doctor if any of the following side effects continue or are bothersome or if you have any questions about them:

More common

    Nausea and vomiting (usually occurs within 2 to 4 hours after receiving dose and may be severe)

Less common

    Diarrhea

For elderly patients: Many medicines have not been tested in older people. Therefore, it is not known whether the medicine acts the same way it does in younger adults. Check with your doctor if you notice any unusual effects while taking this medicine or if you think it is not working as it should.

After you stop receiving streptozocin, your body may need time to adjust. The length of time this takes depends on the amount of medicine you were using and how long you used it. During this period of time, check with your doctor if you notice either of the following side effects:

More common

    Decrease in urination
    Swelling of feet or lower legs

Other side effects not listed above may also occur in some patients. If you notice any other effects, check with your doctor.

December 1987

SUCRALFATE (Oral)

Some commonly used brand names are Carafate and Sulcrate*.

*Not available in the U.S.

To the Reader: If you do not recognize the names of medical conditions or medicines referred to in this information, check with your doctor, nurse, or pharmacist. Definitions for selected medical terms may be found in the Glossary. Brand names for the generic drug names listed can be found in the Index. In addition, selected brand names commonly associated with the generic name have been included in the text to help you recognize medicine you may be taking. The fact that a brand name product is not mentioned does not mean the information does not apply. It is a good idea for you to learn both the generic and brand names of your medicines and to write them down for future use.

Sucralfate (soo-KRAL-fate) is taken by mouth to treat duodenal ulcer. This medicine may also be used for other conditions as determined by your doctor.

Sucralfate works by forming a "barrier" or "coating" over the ulcer. This protects the ulcer from the acid of the stomach, allowing it to heal.

This medicine is available only with your doctor's prescription.

Remember:

• **This medicine has been prescribed for your current medical problem only.** It must not be given to other people or used for other problems unless you are directed to do so by your doctor.

• **Keep all medicines out of the reach of children.**

• In order for this medicine to work, it must be used as directed.

• **It is very important that you read and understand the following information.** If any of the information causes you special concern, do not decide against using this medicine without first checking with your doctor.

• Before you begin using any new medicine (prescription or nonprescription) or if you develop any new medical problem while you are using this medicine, check with your doctor, nurse, or pharmacist.

• **If you have any questions** about the following information or if you want more information about this medicine or your medical problem, **ask your doctor, nurse, or pharmacist.**

Before Using This Medicine

In order to decide on the best treatment for your medical problem, your doctor should be told:

—if you have ever had any unusual or allergic reaction to sucralfate.

—if you are on a low-salt, low-sugar, or any other special diet, or if you are allergic to any substance, such as foods, sulfites or other preservatives, or dyes. Most medicines contain more than their active ingredient. Your doctor, nurse, or pharmacist can help you avoid products that may cause a problem.

—if you are **pregnant** or if you may become pregnant. Studies have not been done in humans. However, sucralfate has not been shown to cause birth defects or other problems in animal studies.

—if you are **breast-feeding**. Sucralfate has not been shown to cause problems in nursing babies.

—if you are taking **any** other prescription or nonprescription (OTC) medicine.

Proper Use of This Medicine

Sucralfate is best taken with water on an empty stomach 1 hour before meals and at bedtime, unless otherwise directed by your doctor.

Take this medicine for the full time of treatment, even if you begin to feel better. Also, it is important that you keep your doctor's appointments for check-ups so that your doctor will be better able to tell you when to stop taking this medicine.

Do not take this medicine for more than 8 weeks unless your doctor has prescribed or ordered a special schedule for you.

If you miss a dose of this medicine, take it as soon as possible. However, if it is almost time for your next dose, skip the missed dose and go back to your regular dosing schedule. Do not double doses.

How to store this medicine:

• **Keep out of the reach of children.**

• Store away from heat and direct light.

• Do not store in the bathroom, near the kitchen sink, or in other damp places. Heat or moisture may cause the medicine to break down.

• Do not keep outdated medicine or medicine no longer needed. Be sure that any discarded medicine is out of the reach of children.

Precautions While Using This Medicine

Antacids may be taken with sucralfate to help relieve any stomach pain, unless your doctor has told you not to use them. **However, antacids should not be taken within 30 minutes before or 1 hour after sucralfate.** Taking these medicines too close together may keep sucralfate from working as well.

Side Effects of This Medicine

Along with its needed effects, a medicine may cause some unwanted effects. Some side effects may occur that usually do not need medical attention. These side effects may go away during treatment as your body adjusts to the medicine. However, check with your doctor as soon as possible if any of the following side effects continue or are bothersome:

More common
    Constipation

Less common or rare
Backache
Diarrhea
Dizziness or lightheadedness
Drowsiness
Dryness of mouth
Indigestion
Nausea
Skin rash, hives, or itching
Stomach cramps or pain

Other side effects not listed above may also occur in some patients. If you notice any other effects, check with your doctor.

December 1987

SULFASALAZINE (Systemic)

Some commonly used brand names or other names are:

Azulfidine

Azulfidine EN-Tabs

Salazopyrin*

Salicylazosulfapyridine

Generic name product may also be available in the U.S.

*Not available in the U.S.

To the Reader: If you do not recognize the names of medical conditions or medicines referred to in this information, check with your doctor, nurse, or pharmacist. Definitions for selected medical terms may be found in the Glossary. Brand names for the generic drug names listed can be found in the Index. In addition, selected brand names commonly associated with the generic name have been included in the text to help you recognize medicine you may be taking. The fact that a brand name product is not mentioned does not mean the information does not apply. It is a good idea for you to learn both the generic and brand names of your medicines and to write them down for future use.

Sulfasalazine (sul-fa-SAL-a-zeen), a sulfonamide or sulfa medicine, belongs to the family of medicines called anti-infectives. It is taken by mouth to prevent and treat inflammatory bowel disease such as enteritis or colitis.

Sulfasalazine is available only with your doctor's prescription.

Remember:

• This medicine has been prescribed for your present medical problem only. Even though other people may have the same symptoms as you, they may have a different kind of problem. Your medicine may not work for them and may even cause them harm. Therefore, **your medicine must not be given to other people or used for other problems** unless you are otherwise directed by your doctor.

• In order for this medicine to work, it must be taken as directed.

• Keep all medicines out of the reach of children.

• If you want more information about this medicine, ask your doctor, nurse, or pharmacist.

• If any of the following information causes you special concern, do not decide against taking this medicine without first checking with your doctor.

Before Using This Medicine

In order to decide on the best treatment for your medical problem, your doctor should be told:

—if you have ever had any unusual or allergic reaction to any of the sulfonamides, furosemide or thiazide diuretics (water pills), oral antidiabetic agents (diabetes medicine you take by mouth), glaucoma medicine you take by mouth (for example, acetazolamide, dichlorphenamide, methazolamide), or salicylates (for example, aspirin).

—if you are **pregnant** or if you may become pregnant. However, sulfasalazine has not been shown to cause birth defects and other problems do not usually occur.

—if you are **breast-feeding**. Sulfonamides pass into the breast milk in small amounts and may cause unwanted effects in nursing babies with glucose-6-phosphate dehydrogenase (G6PD) deficiency.

—if you have any of the following medical problems:

Blockage of stomach, intestines, or urinary tract

Blood problems

Glucose-6-phosphate dehydrogenase (G6PD) deficiency

Kidney disease

Liver disease

Porphyria

—if you are taking **any** other prescription or nonprescription (OTC) medicine, especially:

Anticoagulants (blood thinners)

Antidiabetic agents, oral (diabetes medicine you take by mouth)

Dapsone

Ethotoin (e.g., Peganone)

Furazolidone (e.g., Furoxone)

Mephenytoin (e.g., Mesantoin)

Methenamine (e.g., Mandelamine)

Methotrexate (e.g., Mexate)

Methyldopa (e.g., Aldomet)

Nitrofurantoin (e.g., Furadantin)

Phenytoin (e.g., Dilantin)

Primaquine

Procainamide (e.g., Pronestyl)

Quinidine (e.g., Quinidex)

Quinine (e.g., Quinamm)

Sulfoxone (e.g., Diasone)

Vitamin K (e.g., AquaMEPHYTON, Synkayvite)

Proper Use of This Medicine

Sulfasalazine is best taken after meals or with food to lessen stomach upset. If stomach upset continues or is bothersome, check with your doctor.

Each dose of sulfasalazine should also be taken with a full glass (8 ounces) of water. Several additional glasses of water should be taken every day, unless otherwise directed by your doctor. Drinking extra water will help to prevent unwanted side effects of the sulfonamide.

For patients taking the enteric-coated tablet form of this medicine:

• Swallow tablets whole. Do not break or crush.

Keep taking this medicine for the full time of treatment even if you begin to feel better after a few days; **do not miss any doses.**

If you do miss a dose of this medicine, take it as soon as possible. However, if it is almost time for your next dose, do not take the missed dose or double your next dose. Instead, go back to your regular dosing schedule.

Do not give sulfasalazine to infants under 2 years of age unless otherwise directed by your doctor.

How to store this medicine:

• **Keep out of the reach of children.**

• Store away from heat and direct light.

• Do not store the tablet form of this medicine in the bathroom, near the kitchen sink, or in other damp places. Heat or moisture may cause the medicine to break down.

• Keep the oral liquid form of this medicine from freezing.

• Do not keep outdated medicine or medicine no longer needed. Be sure that any discarded medicine is out of the reach of children.

Precautions While Using This Medicine

If your symptoms (including diarrhea) do not improve within a month or two, or if they become worse, check with your doctor.

It is important that your doctor check your progress at regular visits.

Before having any kind of surgery (including dental surgery) with a general anesthetic, tell the physician or dentist in charge that you are taking a sulfonamide.

Some people who take sulfonamides may become more sensitive to sunlight than they are normally. **When you first begin taking this medicine, avoid too much sun and do not use a sunlamp until you see how you react to the sun,** especially if you tend to burn easily. You may still be more sensitive to sunlight or sunlamps for many months after stopping this medicine. **If you have a severe reaction, check with your doctor.**

Side Effects of This Medicine

Along with its needed effects, a medicine may cause some unwanted effects. Although not all of these side effects may occur, if they do occur they may need medical attention.

Check with your doctor immediately if any of the following side effects occur:

More common
    Headache (continuing)
    Itching
    Skin rash

Less common
    Aching of joints and muscles
    Difficulty in swallowing
    Fever
    Pale skin
    Redness, blistering, peeling, or loosening of skin
    Sore throat
    Unusual bleeding or bruising
    Unusual tiredness or weakness
    Yellow eyes or skin

Rare
    Blood in urine
    Lower back pain
    Pain or burning while urinating
    Swelling of front part of neck

Also, check with your doctor as soon as possible if the following side effect occurs:

More common
    Increased sensitivity of skin to sunlight

Other side effects may occur that usually do not require medical attention. These side effects may go away during treatment as your body adjusts to the medicine. However, check with your doctor if any of the following side effects continue or are bothersome:

More common
    Diarrhea
    Dizziness
    Loss of appetite
    Nausea or vomiting

In some patients this medicine may also cause the urine to become orange-yellow. This side effect does not require medical attention.

Other side effects not listed above may also occur in some patients. If you notice any other effects, check with your doctor.

December 1987

SULFINPYRAZONE (Systemic)

Some commonly used brand names are:

Antazone*
Anturan*
Anturane
Apo-Sulfinpyrazone*

Aprazone
Novopyrazone*
Zynol*

Generic name product may also be available in the U.S.

---

*Not available in the U.S.

To the Reader: If you do not recognize the names of medical conditions or medicines referred to in this information, check with your doctor, nurse, or pharmacist. Definitions for selected medical terms may be found in the Glossary. Brand names for the generic drug names listed can be found in the Index. In addition, selected brand names commonly associated with the generic name have been included in the text to help you recognize medicine you may be taking. The fact that a brand name product is not mentioned does not mean the information does not apply. It is a good idea for you to learn both the generic and brand names of your medicines and to write them down for future use.

Sulfinpyrazone (sul-fin-PEER-a-zone) is used in the treatment of chronic gout (gouty arthritis), which is caused by too much uric acid in the blood. The medicine works by removing the extra uric acid from the body. Sulfinpyrazone does not cure gout, but after you have been taking it for a few months it may help prevent gout attacks. This medicine will help prevent gout attacks only as long as you continue to take it.

Sulfinpyrazone is also used to prevent or treat other medical problems that may occur if too much uric acid is present in the body.

Sulfinpyrazone may also be used for other conditions as determined by your doctor.

Sulfinpyrazone is available only with your doctor's prescription.

Remember:

• **This medicine has been prescribed for your current medical problem only.** It must not be given to other people or used for other problems unless you are directed to do so by your doctor.

• **Keep all medicines out of the reach of children.**

• In order for this medicine to work, it must be used as directed.

• **It is very important that you read and understand the following information.** If any of the information causes you special concern, do not decide against using this medicine without first checking with your doctor.

• Before you begin using any new medicine (prescription or nonprescription) or if you develop any new medical problem while you are using this medicine, check with your doctor, nurse, or pharmacist.

• **If you have any questions** about the following information or if you want more information about this medicine or your medical problem, **ask your doctor, nurse, or pharmacist.**

Before Using This Medicine

In order to decide on the best treatment for your medical problem, your doctor should be told:

—if you have ever had any unusual or allergic reaction to sulfinpyrazone or to dipyrone (e.g., Novaldin), oxyphenbutazone (e.g., Tandearil), or phenylbutazone (e.g., Butazolidin).

—if you are on a low-salt, low-sugar, or any other special diet, or if you are allergic to any substance, such as foods, sulfites or other preservatives, or dyes. Most medicines contain more than their active ingredient. Your doctor, nurse, or pharmacist can help you avoid products that may cause a problem.

—if you are **pregnant** or if you may become pregnant. Sulfinpyrazone has not been shown to cause problems in humans.

—if you are **breast-feeding**. Sulfinpyrazone has not been shown to cause problems in nursing babies. However, it is not known whether this medicine passes into the breast milk.

—if you have any of the following medical problems:
Blood disease (or history of)
Kidney stones (or history of) or other kidney disease
Stomach ulcer or other stomach problems (or history of)

—if you are taking **any** other prescription or nonprescription (OTC) medicine, especially:
Anticoagulants (blood thinners)
Antineoplastics (cancer medicine)
Aspirin or other salicylates
Dipyridamole (e.g., Persantine)
Divalproex (e.g., Depakote)
Heparin
Nitrofurantoin (e.g., Furadantin)
Valproic acid (e.g., Depakene)

Proper Use of This Medicine

If sulfinpyrazone upsets your stomach, it may be taken with food. If this does not work, an antacid may be taken. If stomach upset (nausea, vomiting, or stomach pain) continues, check with your doctor.

In order for sulfinpyrazone to help you, it must be taken regularly as ordered by your doctor.

For patients taking sulfinpyrazone for gout:

• After you begin to take sulfinpyrazone, gout attacks may continue to occur for a while. However, if you take this medicine regularly as directed by your doctor, the attacks will gradually become less frequent and less painful. After you have been taking sulfinpyrazone for several months, they may stop completely.

• Sulfinpyrazone helps to prevent gout attacks. It will not relieve an attack that has already started. **Even if you take another medicine for gout attacks, continue to take this medicine also.**

For patients taking sulfinpyrazone for gout or to help remove uric acid from the body:

• When you first begin taking sulfinpyrazone, the amount of uric acid in the kidneys is greatly increased. This may cause kidney stones in some people. To help prevent this, your doctor may want you to drink at least 10 to 12 full glasses (8 ounces each) of fluids each day, or to take another medicine to make your urine less acid. It is important that you follow your doctor's instructions very carefully.

If you miss a dose of this medicine, take it as soon as possible. However, if is almost time for your next dose, skip the missed dose and go back to your regular dosing schedule. Do not double doses.

How to store this medicine:

• **Keep out of the reach of children.**

• Store away from heat and direct light.

• Do not store this medicine in the bathroom, near the kitchen sink, or in other damp places. Heat or moisture may cause the medicine to break down.

• Do not keep outdated medicine or medicine no longer needed. Be sure that any discarded medicine is out of the reach of children.

Precautions While Using This Medicine

Your doctor should check your progress at regular visits to make sure that this medicine does not cause unwanted effects.

For patients taking sulfinpyrazone for gout or to help remove uric acid from the body:

• Taking aspirin or other salicylates may lessen the effects of sulfinpyrazone. Also, drinking too much alcohol may increase the amount of uric acid in the blood and lessen the effects of sulfinpyrazone. Therefore, **do not take aspirin or other salicylates or drink alcoholic beverages while taking this medicine,** unless you have first checked with your doctor.

Side Effects of This Medicine

Along with its needed effects, a medicine may cause some unwanted effects. Although not all of these side effects may occur, if they do occur they may need medical attention.

Check with your doctor immediately if any of the following side effects occur:

Rare

Sore throat and fever
Unusual bleeding or bruising
Unusual tiredness or weakness

Signs of overdose

Clumsiness or unsteadiness
Convulsions (seizures)
Diarrhea
Nausea or vomiting (severe or continuing)
Stomach pain (severe or continuing)
Troubled or difficult breathing

Also, check with your doctor as soon as possible if any of the following side effects occur:

Less common

Skin rash

Rare

Bloody or black tarry stools
Bloody urine
Difficult or painful urination
Fever
Lower back pain

Other side effects may occur that usually do not require medical attention. These side effects may go away during treatment as your body adjusts to the medicine. However, check with your doctor if any of the following side effects continue or are bothersome:

More common

Nausea or vomiting
Stomach pain

For elderly patients: Many medicines have not been tested in older people. Therefore, it is not known whether the medicine acts the same way it does in younger adults. Check with your doctor or pharmacist if you notice any unusual effects while taking this medicine or if you think it is not working as it should.

Other side effects not listed above may also occur in some patients. If you notice any other effects, check with your doctor.

December 1987

SULFONAMIDES (Ophthalmic)

This information applies to the following medicines:

Sulfacetamide (sul-fa-SEE-ta-mide)
Sulfisoxazole (sul-fi-SOX-a-zole)

Some commonly used brand names or other names are:	Generic names:
Bleph-10 Cetamide Isopto Cetamide Sulamyd Sulf-10 Sulfex* Sulten-10	Sulfacetamide†
Gantrisin Sulfafurazole	Sulfisoxazole

*Not available in the U.S.
†Generic name product may also be available in the U.S.

To the Reader: If you do not recognize the names of medical conditions or medicines referred to in this information, check with your doctor, nurse, or pharmacist. Definitions for selected medical terms may be found in the Glossary. Brand names for the generic drug names listed can be found in the Index. In addition, selected brand names commonly associated with the generic name have been included in the text to help you recognize medicine you may be taking. The fact that a brand name product is not mentioned does not mean the information does not apply. It is a good idea for you to learn both the generic and brand names of your medicines and to write them down for future use.

Sulfonamides (sul-FON-a-mides) or sulfa drugs belong to the family of medicines called anti-infectives. Sulfonamide ophthalmic preparations are used in the eye to help the body overcome infections of the eye.

Sulfonamides are available only with your doctor's prescription.

Remember:
• This medicine has been prescribed for your present infection only. Another infection later on may require a different medicine. Also, even though other people may have the same symptoms as you, they may have a different kind of infection. Your medicine may not work for them and may even cause them harm. Therefore, **your medicine must not be given to other people or used for other infections** unless you are otherwise directed by your doctor.

• In order for this medicine to work, it must be used as directed.

• Keep all medicines out of the reach of children.

• If you want more information about this medicine, ask your doctor, nurse, or pharmacist.

• If any of the following information causes you special concern, do not decide against using this medicine without first checking with your doctor.

Before Using This Medicine

In order to decide on the best treatment for your medical problem, your doctor should be told:

—if you have ever had any unusual or allergic reaction to any of the sulfonamides, furosemide or thiazide diuretics (water pills), oral antidiabetic agents (diabetes medicine you take by mouth), or glaucoma medicine you take by mouth (for example, acetazolamide, dichlorphenamide, or methazolamide).

—if you are **pregnant** or if you may become pregnant. However, sulfonamide ophthalmic preparations have not been shown to cause birth defects or other problems in humans.

—if you are **breast-feeding**. However, sulfonamide ophthalmic preparations have not been shown to cause problems in nursing babies.

—if you are using **any** other prescription or nonprescription (OTC) medicine, especially silver preparations such as silver nitrate or mild silver protein in the eye.

Proper Use of This Medicine

For patients using the eye drop form of sulfonamides:

• The bottle is only partially full to provide proper drop control.

• How to apply this medicine: First, wash your hands. Then tilt the head back and pull the lower eyelid away from the eye to form a pouch. Drop the medicine into the pouch and gently close the eyes. Do not blink. Keep the eyes closed for 1 or 2 minutes to allow the medicine to come into contact with the infection.

• If you think you did not get the drop of medicine into your eye properly, use another drop.

• To prevent contamination of the eye drops, do not touch the applicator tip to any surface (including the eye). Also, keep the container tightly closed.

For patients using the eye ointment form of sulfonamides:

• How to apply this medicine: First, wash your hands. Then pull the lower eyelid away from the eye to form a pouch. Squeeze a thin strip of ointment into the pouch. A 1.25- to 2.5-cm (approximately ½- to 1-inch) strip of ointment is usually enough unless otherwise directed by your doctor. Gently close the eyes and keep them closed for 1 or 2 minutes to allow the medicine to come into contact with the infection.

• To prevent contamination of the eye ointment, do not touch the applicator tip to any surface (including the eye). After using sulfonamides eye ointment, wipe the tip of the ointment tube with a clean tissue and keep the tube tightly closed.

To help clear up your infection completely, **keep using this medicine for the full time of treatment,** even though your symptoms may have disappeared. **Do not miss any doses.**

If you do miss a dose of this medicine, apply it as soon as possible. However, if it is almost time for your next application, skip the missed dose and go back to your regular dosing schedule.

How to store this medicine:

- **Keep out of the reach of children.**

- Store away from heat and direct light.

- Keep sulfacetamide eye drops in a cool place. Keep all dosage forms of these medicines from freezing.

- Do not keep outdated medicine or medicine no longer needed. Be sure that any discarded medicine is out of the reach of children.

Precautions While Using This Medicine

After application, eye ointments usually cause your vision to blur for a few minutes.

After application of this medicine to the eye, occasional stinging or burning may be expected.

If your symptoms do not improve within a few days, or if they become worse, check with your doctor.

Side Effects of This Medicine

Along with its needed effects, a medicine may cause some unwanted effects. Although not all of these side effects may occur, if they do occur they may need medical attention.

Check with your doctor as soon as possible if any of the following side effects occur:

More common
    Itching, redness, swelling, or other sign of irritation not present before using this medicine

Other side effects not listed above may also occur in some patients. If you notice any other effects, check with your doctor.

_____

December 1987

SULFONAMIDES (Systemic)

This information applies to the following medicines:
Sulfacytine (sul-fa-SYE-teen)
Sulfamethoxazole (sul-fa-meth-OX-a-zole)
Sulfamethoxazole and Trimethoprim (sul-fa-meth-OX-a-zole and trye-METH-oh-prim)
Sulfisoxazole (sul-fi-SOX-a-zole)

Some commonly used brand names or other names are:	Generic names:
Renoquid	Sulfacytine
Gantanol Methoxanol	Sulfamethoxazole†
Apo-Sulfatrim* Bactrim Cotrim Co-trimoxazole Novotrimel* Protrin* Roubac* Septra SMZ-TMP Sulfamethoprim Sulmeprim	Sulfamethoxazole and Trimethoprim†
Gantrisin Lipo Gantrisin Novosoxazole* SK-Soxazole Sulfafurazole	Sulfisoxazole†

*Not available in the U.S.
†Generic name product may also be available in the U.S.

To the Reader: If you do not recognize the names of medical conditions or medicines referred to in this information, check with your doctor, nurse, or pharmacist. Definitions for selected medical terms may be found in the Glossary. Brand names for the generic drug names listed can be found in the Index. In addition, selected brand names commonly associated with the generic name have been included in the text to help you recognize medicine you may be taking. The fact that a brand name product is not mentioned does not mean the information does not apply. It is a good idea for you to learn both the generic and brand names of your medicines and to write them down for future use.

Sulfonamides (sul-FON-a-mides) or sulfa medicines belong to the family of medicines called anti-infectives. They are taken by mouth or given by injection to help the body overcome infections. They will not work for colds, flu, or other virus infections.

Sulfonamides are available only with your doctor's prescription.

Remember:
• **This medicine has been prescribed for your present infection only.** Another infection later on may require a different medicine. Also, even though other people may have the same symptoms as you, they may have a different kind of infection. Your medicine may not work for them and may even cause them harm. Therefore, **your medicine must not be given to other people or used for other infections** unless you are otherwise directed by your doctor.

• **Keep all medicines out of the reach of children.**

• In order for this medicine to work, it must be used as directed.

• If you are receiving this medicine by injection, some of the information about this medicine may not apply.

• **It is very important that you read and understand the following information.** If any of the information causes you special concern, do not decide against using this medicine without first checking with your doctor.

• Before you begin using any new medicine (prescription or nonprescription) or if you develop any new medical problem while you are using this medicine, check with your doctor, nurse, or pharmacist.

• **If you have any questions** about the following information or if you want more information about this medicine or your medical problem, **ask your doctor, nurse, or pharmacist.**

Before Using This Medicine

In order to decide on the best treatment for your medical problem, your doctor should be told:

—if you have ever had any unusual or allergic reaction to any of the sulfonamides, furosemide or thiazide diuretics (water pills), oral antidiabetic agents (diabetes medicine you take by mouth), or glaucoma medicine you take by mouth (for example, acetazolamide, dichlorphenamide, methazolamide).

—if you are on a low-salt, low-sugar, or any other special diet, or if you are allergic to any substance, such as sulfites or other preservatives or dyes. Most medicines contain more than their active ingredient, and many liquid medicines contain alcohol. Your doctor or pharmacist can help you avoid products that may cause a problem.

—if you are **pregnant** or if you may become pregnant. However, sulfonamides have not been shown to cause birth defects in humans. Liver problems, although possible, do not usually occur.

—if you are **breast-feeding.** Sulfonamides pass into the breast milk in small amounts and may cause unwanted effects in nursing babies with glucose-6-phosphate dehydrogenase (G6PD) deficiency.

—if you have any of the following medical problems:
Glucose-6-phosphate dehydrogenase (G6PD) deficiency
Kidney disease
Liver disease
Porphyria

—if you are taking **any** other prescription or nonprescription (OTC) medicine, especially:
Acetaminophen (e.g., Tylenol) (with long-term, high-dose use)
Aminobenzoic acid (PABA)
Amiodarone (e.g., Cordarone)
Anabolic steroids (dromostanolone, ethylestrenol, nandrolone, oxandrolone, oxymetholone, stanozolol)
Androgens (male hormones)
Anticoagulants (blood thinners)
Antidiabetic agents, oral (diabetes medicine you take by mouth)
Antithyroid agents (medicine for overactive thyroid)
Azlocillin (e.g., Azlin)

© 1988   The United States Pharmacopeial Convention, Inc.

Carbamazepine (e.g., Tegretol)
Carmustine (e.g., BiCNU)
Chloroquine (e.g., Aralen)
Dantrolene (e.g., Dantrium)
Dapsone
Daunorubicin (e.g., Cerubidine)
Disulfiram (e.g., Antabuse)
Divalproex (e.g., Depakote)
Doxorubicin (e.g., Adriamycin)
Erythromycins
Estrogens (female hormones)
Ethotoin (e.g., Peganone)
Etretinate (e.g., Tegison)
Furazolidone (e.g., Furoxone)
Gold salts
Hydroxychloroquine (e.g., Plaquenil)
Isoniazid (e.g., INH, Nydrazid)
Ketoconazole by mouth (e.g., Nizoral)
Mephenytoin (e.g., Mesantoin)
Mercaptopurine (e.g., Purinethol)
Methenamine (e.g., Mandelamine)
Methotrexate (e.g., Mexate)
Methyldopa (e.g., Aldomet)
Mezlocillin (e.g., Mezlin)
Naltrexone (e.g., Trexan) (with long-term, high-dose use)
Nitrofurantoin (e.g., Furadantin)
Oral contraceptives (birth control pills) containing estrogen
Phenothiazines (acetophenazine, chlorpromazine, fluphenazine, mesoridazine, perphenazine, prochlorperazine, promazine, promethazine, thioridazine, trifluoperazine, triflupromazine, trimeprazine)
Phenytoin (e.g., Dilantin)
Piperacillin (e.g., Pipracil)
Plicamycin (e.g., Mithracin)
Primaquine
Procainamide (e.g., Pronestyl)
Quinidine (e.g., Quinidex)
Quinine (e.g., Quinamm)
Rifampin (e.g., Rifadin)
Sulfoxone (e.g., Diasone)
Valproic acid (e.g., Depakene)
Vitamin K (e.g., AquaMEPHYTON, Synkayvite)

Proper Use of This Medicine

Do not give sulfonamides to infants under 1 month of age unless otherwise directed by your doctor. However, sulfacytine should not be given to children under 14 years of age.

Sulfonamides are best taken with a full glass (8 ounces) of water on an empty stomach (either 1 hour before or 2 hours after meals). **Several additional glasses of water should be taken every day,** unless otherwise directed by your doctor. Drinking extra water will help to prevent unwanted side effects of sulfonamides.

For patients taking the oral liquid form of this medicine:
• Use a specially marked measuring spoon or other device to measure each dose accurately since the average household teaspoon may not hold the right amount of liquid.

To help clear up your infection completely, **keep taking this medicine for the full time of treatment** even if you begin to feel better after a few days. If you stop taking this medicine too soon, your symptoms may return.

This medicine works best when there is a constant amount in the blood or urine. **To help keep this amount constant, do not miss any doses. Also, it is best to take each dose at evenly spaced times day and night.** For example, if you are to take 4 doses a day, each dose should be spaced about 6 hours apart. If this interferes with your sleep or other daily activities, or if you need help in planning the best times to take your medicine, check with your doctor, nurse, or pharmacist.

If you do miss a dose of this medicine, take it as soon as possible. This will help to keep a constant amount of medicine in the blood or urine. However, if it is almost time for your next dose and your dosing schedule is:

• 2 doses a day—Space the missed dose and the next dose 5 to 6 hours apart.

• 3 or more doses a day—Space the missed dose and the next dose 2 to 4 hours apart or double your next dose.

Then go back to your regular dosing schedule.

How to store this medicine:
• **Keep out of the reach of children.**

• Store away from heat and direct light.

• Do not store the tablet form of this medicine in the bathroom, near the kitchen sink, or in other damp places. Heat or moisture may cause the medicine to break down.

• Keep the oral liquid forms of this medicine from freezing.

• Do not keep outdated medicine or medicine no longer needed. Be sure that any discarded medicine is out of the reach of children.

Precautions While Using This Medicine

It is important that your doctor check your progress at regular visits if you will be taking this medicine for a long time.

If your symptoms do not improve within a few days, or if they become worse, check with your doctor.

Before having any kind of surgery (including dental surgery) with a general anesthetic, tell the physician or dentist in charge that you are taking a sulfonamide.

Sulfonamides may cause blood problems. These problems may result in a greater chance of infection, slow healing, and bleeding of the gums. Therefore, you should be careful when using toothbrushes, dental floss, and toothpicks. Dental work should be delayed until your blood counts have returned to normal. Check with your physician or dentist if you have any questions about proper oral hygiene (mouth care) during treatment.

Some people who take sulfonamides may become more sensitive to sunlight than they are normally. **When you first begin taking this medicine, avoid too much sun and do not use a sunlamp until you see how you react to the sun,** especially if you tend to burn easily. You may still be more sensitive to sunlight or sunlamps for many months after stopping this medicine. **If you have a severe reaction, check with your doctor.**

Side Effects of This Medicine

Along with its needed effects, a medicine may cause some unwanted effects. Although not all of these side effects may occur, if they do occur they may need medical attention.

Check with your doctor immediately if any of the following side effects occur:

More common
 Itching
 Skin rash

Less common
 Aching of joints and muscles
 Difficulty in swallowing
 Pale skin
 Redness, blistering, peeling, or loosening of skin
 Sore throat and fever
 Unusual bleeding or bruising
 Unusual tiredness or weakness
 Yellow eyes or skin

Rare
 Blood in urine
 Lower back pain
 Pain or burning while urinating
 Swelling of front part of neck

Also, check with your doctor as soon as possible if the following side effect occurs:

More common
 Increased sensitivity of skin to sunlight

Other side effects may occur that usually do not require medical attention. These side effects may go away during treatment as your body adjusts to the medicine. However, check with your doctor if any of the following side effects continue or are bothersome:

More common
 Diarrhea
 Dizziness
 Headache
 Loss of appetite
 Nausea or vomiting

For elderly patients: Many medicines have not been tested in older people. Therefore, it is not known whether the medicine acts the same way it does in younger adults. Check with your doctor or pharmacist if you notice any unusual effects while taking this medicine or if you think it is not working as it should.

Other side effects not listed above may also occur in some patients. If you notice any other effects, check with your doctor.

December 1987

SULFONAMIDES (Vaginal)

This information applies to the following medicines:

Sulfanilamide (sul-fa-NILL-a-mide)
Sulfanilamide, Aminacrine (am-in-AK-rin), and Allantoin (al-AN-toyn)
Sulfisoxazole (sul-fi-SOX-a-zole), Aminacrine, and Allantoin
Triple Sulfa (TRI-pel SUL-fa)

Some commonly used brand names are:	Generic names:
AVC Vagitrol	Sulfanilamide
Deltavac Nil Vagimide	Sulfanilamide, Aminacrine, and Allantoin†
Cantri Vagilia	Sulfisoxazole, Aminacrine, and Allantoin
Sulfa-Gyn Sulnac Sultrin Trysul V.V.S.	Triple Sulfa

†Generic name product may also be available in the U.S.

To the Reader: If you do not recognize the names of medical conditions or medicines referred to in this information, check with your doctor, nurse, or pharmacist. Definitions for selected medical terms may be found in the Glossary. Brand names for the generic drug names listed can be found in the Index. In addition, selected brand names commonly associated with the generic name have been included in the text to help you recognize medicine you may be taking. The fact that a brand name product is not mentioned does not mean the information does not apply. It is a good idea for you to learn both the generic and brand names of your medicines and to write them down for future use.

Sulfonamides (sul-FON-a-mides) or sulfa medicines belong to the family of medicines called anti-infectives. The anti-infectives include the antifungal group and other similar groups of medicines. Vaginal sulfonamides are used in and around the vagina to treat infections in those areas.

Sulfanilamide belongs to the antifungal group of medicines. Antifungals are used to treat infections caused by a fungus. They work by killing the fungus or preventing its growth. Sulfanilamide will not work for other kinds of infections, however. Other vaginal sulfonamides may also be used for other problems as determined by your doctor.

Vaginal sulfonamides are available only with your doctor's prescription.

Remember:

• **This medicine has been prescribed for your present medical problem only.** Even though other people may have the same symptoms as you, they may have a different kind of problem. Your medicine may not work for them and may even cause them harm. Therefore, **your medicine must not be given to other people or used for other problems** unless you are otherwise directed by your doctor.

• **Keep all medicines out of the reach of children.**

• In order for this medicine to work, it must be used as directed.

• **It is very important that you read and understand the following information.** If any of the information causes you special concern, do not decide against using this medicine without first checking with your doctor.

• Before you begin using any new medicine (prescription or nonprescription) or if you develop any new medical problem while you are using this medicine, check with your doctor, nurse, or pharmacist.

• **If you have any questions** about the following information or if you want more information about this medicine or your medical problem, **ask your doctor, nurse, or pharmacist.**

Before Using This Medicine

In order to decide on the best treatment for your medical problem, your doctor should be told:

—if you have ever had any unusual or allergic reaction to any of the sulfonamides, furosemide or thiazide diuretics (water pills), oral antidiabetic agents (diabetes medicine you take by mouth), or glaucoma medicine you take by mouth (for example, acetazolamide, dichlorphenamide, or methazolamide).

—if you are allergic to any substance, such as certain foods or preservatives or dyes. Most medicines contain more than their active ingredient. Your doctor, nurse, or pharmacist can help you avoid products that may cause a problem.

—if you are **pregnant** or if you may become pregnant. Studies have not been done in humans. However, vaginal sulfonamides are absorbed through the vagina into the body and appear in the fetal bloodstream. Studies in rats and mice given high doses by mouth have shown that certain sulfonamides cause birth defects.

—if you are **breast-feeding**. Vaginal sulfonamides are absorbed through the vagina into the body and pass into the breast milk. Use is not recommended in nursing mothers since vaginal sulfonamides may cause liver problems in nursing babies. These medicines may also cause anemia in nursing babies with glucose-6-phosphate dehydrogenase (G6PD) deficiency.

—if you have any of the following medical problems:
  Glucose-6-phosphate dehydrogenase (G6PD) deficiency
  Kidney disease
  Liver disease
  Porphyria

Proper Use of This Medicine

Vaginal sulfonamides usually come with patient directions. Read them carefully before using this medicine.

This medicine is usually inserted into the vagina with an applicator. However, if you are pregnant, check with your doctor before using the applicator.

To help clear up your infection completely, **it is very important that you keep using this medicine for the full time of treatment** even if your symptoms begin to clear up after a few days. If you stop using this medicine too soon, your symptoms may return. **Do not miss any doses.** Also, **do not stop using this medicine if your menstrual period starts during the time of treatment.**

If you do miss a dose of this medicine, insert it as soon as possible. However, if it is almost time for your next dose, skip the missed dose and go back to your regular dosing schedule.

How to store this medicine:

- **Keep out of the reach of children.**

- Store away from heat and direct light.

- Do not store the vaginal tablet or vaginal suppository form of this medicine in the bathroom, near the kitchen sink, or in other damp places. Heat or moisture may cause the medicine to break down.

- Keep the vaginal cream and vaginal suppository forms of this medicine from freezing.

- Do not keep outdated medicine or medicine no longer needed. Be sure that any discarded medicine is out of the reach of children.

Precautions While Using This Medicine

If your symptoms do not improve within a few days, or if they become worse, check with your doctor.

Vaginal medicines usually will slowly work their way out of the vagina during treatment. Also, aminacrine-containing vaginal sulfonamides may stain underclothing. To keep the medicine from soiling or staining your clothing, a sanitary napkin may be worn. Minipads, clean paper tissues, or paper diapers may also be used. However, the use of tampons is not recommended since they may soak up too much of the medicine. In addition, tampons may be more likely to slip out of the vagina if you use them during treatment with this medicine.

To help clear up your infection completely and to help make sure it does not return, good health habits are also required.

- Wear cotton panties (or panties or pantyhose with cotton crotches) instead of synthetic (for example, nylon or rayon) underclothes.

- Wear only freshly washed underclothes.

If you have any questions about this, check with your doctor, nurse, or pharmacist.

Many vaginal infections are spread by sexual intercourse. The male sexual partner may carry the fungus or other organism in his reproductive tract. Therefore, it may be desirable that your partner wear a condom (prophylactic) during intercourse to keep the infection from returning. Also, it may be necessary for your partner to be treated at the same time you are being treated to avoid passing the infection back and forth. In addition, **do not stop using this medicine if you have intercourse during treatment.**

Some patients who use vaginal medicines may prefer to use a douche for cleansing purposes before inserting the next dose of medicine. Some doctors recommend a vinegar and water or other douche. However, others do not recommend douching at all. If you do use a douche, **do not overfill the vagina with douche solution.** To do so may force the solution up into the uterus (womb) and may cause inflammation or infection. Also, **do not douche if you are pregnant since this may harm the fetus.** If you have any questions about this or which douche products are best for you, check with your doctor, nurse, or pharmacist.

Side Effects of This Medicine

Studies in rats have shown that long-term use of sulfonamides may cause cancer of the thyroid gland. In addition, sulfonamides may be more likely to cause goiters (noncancerous tumors of the thyroid gland) in rats.

Along with its needed effects, a medicine may cause some unwanted effects. Although not all of these side effects may occur, if they do occur they may need medical attention.

Check with your doctor immediately if any of the following side effects occur:
Less common
> Itching, burning, skin rash, redness, swelling, or other sign of irritation not present before using this medicine

Other side effects may occur that usually do not require medical attention. These side effects may go away during treatment as your body adjusts to the medicine. However, check with your doctor if either of the following side effects continues or is bothersome:
Less common or rare
> Rash or irritation of penis of sexual partner

Other side effects not listed above may also occur in some patients. If you notice any other effects, check with your doctor.

December 1987

SULFONAMIDES AND PHENAZOPYRIDINE (Systemic)

This information applies to the following medicines:

Sulfamethoxazole (sul-fa-meth-OX-a-zole) and Phenazopyridine (fen-az-oh-PEER-i-deen)

Sulfisoxazole (sul-fi-SOX-a-zole) and Phenazopyridine

Some commonly used brand names or other names are:	Generic names:
Azo Gantanol Azo Sulfamethoxazole Uro Gantanol*	Sulfamethoxazole and Phenazopyridine†
Azo Gantrisin Azo-Soxazole Azo-Sulfisoxazole Suldiazo Sulfafurazole and Phenazopyridine	Sulfisoxazole and Phenazopyridine†

*Not available in the U.S.
†Generic name product may also be available in the U.S.

To the Reader: If you do not recognize the names of medical conditions or medicines referred to in this information, check with your doctor, nurse, or pharmacist. Definitions for selected medical terms may be found in the Glossary. Brand names for the generic drug names listed can be found in the Index. In addition, selected brand names commonly associated with the generic name have been included in the text to help you recognize medicine you may be taking. The fact that a brand name product is not mentioned does not mean the information does not apply. It is a good idea for you to learn both the generic and brand names of your medicines and to write them down for future use.

Sulfonamides and phenazopyridine, combination products containing a sulfa medicine and a urinary pain reliever, belong to the family of medicines called anti-infectives. They are taken by mouth to help the body overcome infections of the urinary tract and to help relieve the pain, burning, and irritation of these infections. Sulfonamides and phenazopyridine combinations are available only with your doctor's prescription.

Remember:

• This medicine has been prescribed for your present infection only. Another infection later on may require a different medicine. Also, even though other people may have the same symptoms as you, they may have a different kind of infection. Your medicine may not work for them and may even cause them harm. Therefore, **your medicine must not be given to other people or used for other infections** unless you are otherwise directed by your doctor.

• In order for this medicine to work, it must be taken as directed.

• Keep all medicines out of the reach of children.

• If you want more information about this medicine, ask your doctor, nurse, or pharmacist.

• If any of the following information causes you special concern, do not decide against taking this medicine without first checking with your doctor.

Before Using This Medicine

In order to decide on the best treatment for your medical problem, your doctor should be told:

—if you have ever had any unusual or allergic reaction to any of the sulfonamides, furosemide or thiazide diuretics (water pills), oral antidiabetic agents (diabetes medicine you take by mouth), or glaucoma medicine you take by mouth (for example, acetazolamide, dichlorphenamide, or methazolamide).

—if you are **pregnant** or if you may become pregnant. However, sulfonamides and phenazopyridine have not been shown to cause birth defects in humans. Liver problems, although possible, do not usually occur.

—if you are **breast-feeding**. Sulfonamides pass into the breast milk in small amounts and may cause unwanted effects in nursing babies with glucose-6-phosphate dehydrogenase (G6PD) deficiency.

—if you have any of the following medical problems:

Glucose-6-phosphate dehydrogenase (G6PD) deficiency
Hepatitis or other liver disease
Kidney disease
Porphyria

—if you are taking **any** other prescription or nonprescription (OTC) medicine, especially:

Acetaminophen (e.g., Tylenol) (with long-term, high-dose use)
Aminobenzoic acid (PABA)
Amiodarone (e.g., Cordarone)
Anabolic steroids (dromostanolone, ethylestrenol, nandrolone, oxandrolone, oxymetholone, stanozolol)
Androgens (male hormones)
Anticoagulants (blood thinners)
Antidiabetic agents, oral (diabetes medicine you take by mouth)
Antithyroid agents (medicine for overactive thyroid)
Azlocillin (e.g., Azlin)
Carbamazepine (e.g., Tegretol)
Carmustine (e.g., BiCNU)
Chloroquine (e.g., Aralen)
Dantrolene (e.g., Dantrium)
Dapsone
Daunorubicin (e.g., Cerubidine)
Disulfiram (e.g., Antabuse)
Divalproex (e.g., Depakote)
Doxorubicin (e.g., Adriamycin)
Erythromycins
Estrogens (female hormones)
Ethotoin (e.g., Peganone)
Etretinate (e.g., Tegison)
Furazolidone (e.g., Furoxone)
Gold salts
Hydroxychloroquine (e.g., Plaquenil)
Isoniazid (e.g., INH, Nydrazid)
Ketoconazole by mouth (e.g., Nizoral)
Mercaptopurine (e.g., Purinethol)
Mephenytoin (e.g., Mesantoin)
Methenamine (e.g., Mandelamine)
Methotrexate (e.g., Mexate)
Methyldopa (e.g., Aldomet)
Mezlocillin (e.g., Mezlin)
Naltrexone (e.g., Trexan) (with long-term, high-dose use)
Nitrofurantoin (e.g., Furadantin)
Oral contraceptives (birth control pills) containing estrogen

Phenothiazines (acetophenazine, chlorpromazine, flu-
phenazine, mesoridazine, perphenazine, prochlorper-
azine, promazine, promethazine, thioridazine, trifluo-
perazine, triflupromazine, trimeprazine)
Phenytoin (e.g., Dilantin)
Piperacillin (e.g., Pipracil)
Plicamycin (e.g., Mithracin)
Primaquine
Procainamide (e.g., Pronestyl)
Quinidine (e.g., Quinidex)
Quinine (e.g., Quinamm)
Rifampin (e.g., Rifadin)
Sulfoxone (e.g., Diasone)
Valproic acid (e.g., Depakene)
Vitamin K (e.g., AquaMEPHYTON, Synkayvite)

Proper Use of This Medicine

**Sulfonamides and phenazopyridine are best taken with a
full glass (8 ounces) of water** on an empty stomach
(either 1 hour before or 2 hours after meals). However,
this medicine may be taken with meals or following
meals if it upsets your stomach.

**Several additional glasses of water should be taken every
day,** unless otherwise directed by your doctor. Drinking extra water will help to prevent unwanted side
effects of the sulfonamide. Also, this will help the
medicine clear up your infection sooner by flushing
out the bacteria.

To help clear up your infection completely, **keep taking
this medicine for the full time of treatment** even if you
begin to feel better after a few days; **do not miss any
doses.**

If you do miss a dose of this medicine, take it as soon as
possible. However, if it is almost time for your next
dose, do not take the missed dose or double your next
dose. Instead, go back to your regular dosing schedule.

**Do not give sulfonamides and phenazopyridine to infants
and children under 12 years of age** unless otherwise
directed by your doctor.

How to store this medicine:

• **Keep out of the reach of children.**

• Store away from heat and direct light.

• Do not store in the bathroom, near the kitchen sink,
or in other damp places. Heat or moisture may cause
the medicine to break down.

• Do not keep outdated medicine or medicine no longer
needed. Be sure that any discarded medicine is out of
the reach of children.

Precautions While Using This Medicine

This medicine causes the urine to turn reddish orange.
This is to be expected while you are using this medicine. Also, the medicine may stain clothing. If you
have any questions about removing the stain, check
with your doctor or pharmacist.

**Diabetics—This medicine may cause false test results with
some urine sugar tests and urine ketone tests.** Check
with your doctor before changing your diet or the dosage of your diabetes medicine.

If your symptoms do not improve within a few days, or
if they become worse, check with your doctor.

Before having any kind of surgery (including dental surgery) with a general anesthetic, tell the physician or
dentist in charge that you are taking a sulfonamide.

Sulfonamides may cause blood problems. These problems
may result in a greater chance of infection, slow healing, and bleeding of the gums. Therefore, you should
be careful when using toothbrushes, dental floss, and
toothpicks. Dental work should be delayed until your
blood counts have returned to normal. Check with your
physician or dentist if you have any questions about
proper oral hygiene (mouth care) during treatment.

Some people who take sulfonamides may become more
sensitive to sunlight than they are normally. **When you
first begin taking this medicine, avoid too much sun
and do not use a sunlamp until you see how you react
to the sun,** especially if you tend to burn easily. You
may still be more sensitive to sunlight or sunlamps for
many months after stopping this medicine. **If you have
a severe reaction, check with your doctor.**

Side Effects of This Medicine

Along with its needed effects, a medicine may cause some
unwanted effects. Although not all of these side effects
may occur, if they do occur they may need medical
attention.

Check with your doctor immediately if any of the following side effects occur:

More common
Itching
Skin rash

Less common
Aching of joints and muscles
Difficulty in swallowing
Pale skin
Redness, blistering, peeling, or loosening of skin
Sore throat and fever
Unusual bleeding or bruising
Unusual tiredness or weakness
Yellow eyes or skin

Rare
Lower back pain
Swelling of front part of neck

In addition to the side effects listed above, check with
your doctor as soon as possible if the following side
effect occurs:

More common
Increased sensitivity of skin to sunlight

Other side effects may occur that usually do not require
medical attention. These side effects may go away
during treatment as your body adjusts to the medicine.

However, check with your doctor if any of the following side effects continue or are bothersome:

More common

Diarrhea
Dizziness
Headache
Loss of appetite
Nausea or vomiting

Less common

Indigestion
Stomach cramps or pain

This medicine causes the urine to become reddish orange. This side effect does not require medical attention.

For elderly patients: Many medicines have not been tested in older people. Therefore, it is not known whether the medicine acts the same way it does in younger adults. Check with your doctor or pharmacist if you notice any unusual effects while taking this medicine or if you think it is not working as it should.

Other side effects not listed above may also occur in some patients. If you notice any other effects, check with your doctor.

December 1987

SULFUR (Topical)

Some commonly used brand names are:

Buf-Bar   Lotio Alsulfa*
Fostex   Postacne*

Generic name product may also be available in the U.S. and Canada.

---

*Not available in the U.S.

To the Reader: If you do not recognize the names of medical conditions or medicines referred to in this information, check with your doctor, nurse, or pharmacist. Definitions for selected medical terms may be found in the Glossary. Brand names for the generic drug names listed can be found in the Index. In addition, selected brand names commonly associated with the generic name have been included in the text to help you recognize medicine you may be taking. The fact that a brand name product is not mentioned does not mean the information does not apply. It is a good idea for you to learn both the generic and brand names of your medicines and to write them down for future use.

Sulfur (SUL-fur) is applied to the skin to treat acne, scabies, seborrheic dermatitis, and other skin disorders.

Some of these preparations are available only with your doctor's prescription. Others are available without a prescription; however, your doctor may have special instructions on the proper use of sulfur for your medical condition.

Remember:

• **Keep all medicines out of the reach of children.**

• In order for this medicine to work, it must be used as directed. **If you are using this medicine without a prescription, it is very important to follow the directions on the label.**

• **It is also very important that you read and understand the following information.** If any of the information causes you special concern, check with your doctor or pharmacist.

• Before you begin using any new medicine (prescription or nonprescription) or if you develop any new medical problem while you are using this medicine, check with your doctor, nurse, or pharmacist.

• **If you have any questions** about the following information or if you want more information about this medicine or your medical problem, **ask your doctor, nurse, or pharmacist.**

Before Using This Medicine

Before you use sulfur, check with your doctor or pharmacist:

—if you have ever had any unusual or allergic reaction to sulfur.

—if you are allergic to any substance, such as certain preservatives or dyes. Most medicines contain more than their active ingredient. Your doctor, nurse, or pharmacist can help you avoid products that may cause a problem.

—if you are **pregnant** or if you may become pregnant. However, topical sulfur has not been shown to cause birth defects or other problems in humans.

—if you are **breast-feeding**. However, topical sulfur has not been shown to cause problems in nursing babies.

—if you are using **any** other prescription or nonprescription (OTC) medicine.

Proper Use of This Medicine

Use this medicine only as directed. Do not use it more often and do not use it for a longer period of time than recommended on the label, unless otherwise directed by your doctor.

Keep this medicine away from the eyes. If you should accidentally get some in your eyes, flush them thoroughly with water.

For patients using the cream, lotion, or ointment form of this medicine:

• Before applying the medicine, wash the affected areas with soap and water and dry thoroughly. Then apply enough medicine to cover the affected areas and rub in gently.

For patients using the soap form of this medicine:

• Work up a rich lather with the soap, using hot water. Wash the affected areas and rinse thoroughly. Apply the lather again, and rub in gently for a few minutes. Remove excess lather with a towel or tissue without rinsing.

If you miss a dose of this medicine, apply or use it as soon as possible. However, if it is almost time for your next dose, skip the missed dose and go back to your regular dosing schedule.

How to store this medicine:

• **Keep out of the reach of children.**

• Store away from heat and direct light.

• Keep the cream, lotion, and ointment forms of this medicine from freezing.

• Do not keep outdated medicine or medicine no longer needed. Be sure that any discarded medicine is out of the reach of children.

Precautions While Using This Medicine

When using sulfur, do not use any of the following preparations on the same affected area as this medicine, unless otherwise directed by your doctor:

Abrasive soaps or cleansers
Alcohol-containing preparations
Any other topical acne preparation or preparation containing a peeling agent (for example, benzoyl peroxide, resorcinol, salicylic acid, or tretinoin [vitamin A acid])
Cosmetics or soaps that dry the skin
Medicated cosmetics
Other topical medicine for the skin

To use any of the above preparations on the same affected area as sulfur may cause severe irritation of the skin.

Do not use any topical mercury-containing preparation, such as ammoniated mercury ointment, on the same affected area as this medicine. To do so may cause a foul odor, may be irritating to the skin, and may stain the skin black. If you have any questions about this, check with your doctor or pharmacist.

Side Effects of This Medicine

Along with its needed effects, a medicine may cause some unwanted effects. Although not all of these side effects may occur, if they do occur they may need medical attention.

Check with your doctor as soon as possible if the following side effect occurs:

Skin irritation not present before using this medicine

Other side effects may occur that usually do not require medical attention. However, check with your doctor or pharmacist if the following side effect continues or is bothersome:

Redness and peeling of skin (may occur after a few days)

For elderly patients: Many medicines have not been tested in older people. Therefore, it is not known whether the medicine acts the same way it does in younger adults. Check with your doctor or pharmacist if you notice any unusual effects while using this medicine or if you think it is not working as it should.

Other side effects not listed above may also occur in some patients. If you notice any other effects, check with your doctor or pharmacist.

December 1987

SULFURATED LIME (Topical)

Some commonly used brand names or other names are Vlemasque and Vleminckx's solution.

Generic name product may also be available in the U.S.

To the Reader: If you do not recognize the names of medical conditions or medicines referred to in this information, check with your doctor, nurse, or pharmacist. Definitions for selected medical terms may be found in the Glossary. Brand names for the generic drug names listed can be found in the Index. In addition, selected brand names commonly associated with the generic name have been included in the text to help you recognize medicine you may be taking. The fact that a brand name product is not mentioned does not mean the information does not apply. It is a good idea for you to learn both the generic and brand names of your medicines and to write them down for future use.

Sulfurated (SUL-fur-ay-ted) lime is applied to the skin to treat acne, scabies, and other skin disorders.

This medicine is available without a prescription; however, your doctor may have special instructions on the proper use of this medicine for your medical problem.

Remember:
• **Keep all medicines out of the reach of children.**

• In order for this medicine to work, it must be used as directed. **If you are using this medicine without a prescription, it is very important to follow the directions on the label.**

• **It is also very important that you read and understand the following information.** If any of the information causes you special concern, check with your doctor or pharmacist.

• Before you begin using any new medicine (prescription or nonprescription) or if you develop any new medical problem while you are using this medicine, check with your doctor, nurse, or pharmacist.

• **If you have any questions** about the following information or if you want more information about this medicine or your medical problem, **ask your doctor, nurse, or pharmacist.**

Before Using This Medicine

Before you use sulfurated lime, check with your doctor or pharmacist:
—if you have ever had any unusual or allergic reaction to sulfurated lime.

—if you are allergic to any substance, such as certain preservatives or dyes. Most medicines contain more than their active ingredient. Your doctor or pharmacist can help you avoid products that may cause a problem.

—if you are **pregnant** or if you may become pregnant. However, sulfurated lime has not been shown to cause birth defects or other problems in humans.

—if you are **breast-feeding**. However, sulfurated lime has not been shown to cause problems in nursing babies.

—if you are taking **any** other prescription or nonprescription (OTC) medicine.

Proper Use of This Medicine

Use this medicine only as directed. Do not use more of it, do not use it more often, and do not use it for a longer period of time than recommended on the label, unless otherwise directed by your doctor.

Keep this medicine away from the eyes. If you should accidentally get some in your eyes, flush them thoroughly with water.

For patients using the solution form of sulfurated lime for wet dressings, as a soak, or in a bath:
• Sulfurated lime solution must be diluted before you use it on your skin for wet dressings, as a soak, or in a bath. Make sure you understand exactly how you should use this solution. If you have any questions about this, check with your doctor or pharmacist.

• Before diluting and/or applying this solution, remove all jewelry and metallic ornaments, since the solution may discolor metals. Also, avoid getting this solution on metal spoons or bath fixtures.

For patients using the mask form of sulfurated lime:
• Apply a generous amount of this medicine over the entire face and neck, unless otherwise directed by your doctor.

• Allow the medicine to remain on the affected areas for 20 to 25 minutes.

• Remove the medicine with lukewarm water, using a gentle circular motion. Then, pat the skin dry.

If you miss a dose of this medicine, apply it as soon as possible. However, if it is almost time for your next dose, skip the missed dose and go back to your regular dosing schedule.

How to store this medicine:
• **Keep out of the reach of children.**

• Store away from heat and direct light.

• Keep the medicine from freezing.

• Do not keep outdated medicine or medicine no longer needed. Be sure that any discarded medicine is out of the reach of children.

Precautions While Using This Medicine

When using sulfurated lime, do not use any of the following preparations on the same affected area as this medicine, unless otherwise directed by your doctor:
Abrasive soaps or cleansers
Alcohol-containing preparations
Any other topical acne preparation or preparation containing a peeling agent (for example, benzoyl peroxide, resorcinol, salicylic acid, sulfur, or tretinoin [vitamin A acid])
Cosmetics or soaps that dry the skin
Medicated cosmetics
Other topical medicine for the skin

To use any of the above preparations on the same affected area as sulfurated lime may cause severe irritation of the skin.

Do not use any topical mercury-containing preparation, such as ammoniated mercury ointment on the same affected area as this medicine. To do so may cause a foul odor, may be irritating to the skin, and may stain the skin black. If you have any questions about this, check with your doctor.

Side Effects of This Medicine

Along with its needed effects, a medicine may cause some unwanted effects. Although not all of these side effects may occur, if they do occur they may need medical attention.

Check with your doctor as soon as possible if the following side effect occurs:

Skin irritation not present before using this medicine

Other side effects may occur that usually do not require medical attention. However, check with your doctor or pharmacist if the following side effects continue or are bothersome:

Redness and peeling of skin (may occur after a few days)
Unusual dryness of skin

For elderly patients: Many medicines have not been tested in older people. Therefore, it is not known whether the medicine acts the same way it does in younger adults. Check with your doctor or pharmacist if you notice any unusual effects while using this medicine or if you think it is not working as it should.

Other side effects not listed above may also occur in some patients. If you notice any other effects, check with your doctor or pharmacist.

_____

December 1987

_____

TAMOXIFEN (Systemic)

Some commonly used brand names are Nolvadex, Nolvadex-D*, and Tamofen*.

*Not available in the U.S.

To the Reader: If you do not recognize the names of medical conditions or medicines referred to in this information, check with your doctor, nurse, or pharmacist. Definitions for selected medical terms may be found in the Glossary. Brand names for the generic drug names listed can be found in the Index. In addition, selected brand names commonly associated with the generic name have been included in the text to help you recognize medicine you may be taking. The fact that a brand name product is not mentioned does not mean the information does not apply. It is a good idea for you to learn both the generic and brand names of your medicines and to write them down for future use.

Tamoxifen (ta-MOX-i-fen) is a medicine that blocks the effects of the hormone estrogen in the body. It is taken by mouth to treat some cases of breast cancer.

The exact way that tamoxifen works against cancer is not known but it may be related to the way it blocks the effects of estrogen on the body.

Tamoxifen is available only with your doctor's prescription.

Remember:

• **This medicine has been prescribed for your current medical problem only.** It must not be given to other people or used for other problems unless you are directed to do so by your doctor.

• **Keep all medicines out of the reach of children.**

• In order for this medicine to work, it must be used as directed.

• **It is very important that you read and understand the following information.** If any of the information causes you special concern, do not decide against using this medicine without first checking with your doctor.

• Before you begin using any new medicine (prescription or nonprescription) or if you develop any new medical problem while you are using this medicine, check with your doctor, nurse, or pharmacist.

• **If you have any questions** about the following information or if you want more information about this medicine or your medical problem, **ask your doctor, nurse, or pharmacist.**

Before Using This Medicine

In order to decide on the best treatment for your medical problem, your doctor should be told:

—if you have ever had any unusual or allergic reaction to tamoxifen.

—if you are **pregnant** or if you intend to become pregnant. Tamoxifen has not been shown to cause problems in humans.

—if you are **breast-feeding**. Because this medicine may cause serious side effects, breast-feeding is generally not recommended while you are taking it.

—if you have cataracts or other eye problems.

—if you are now taking **any** other prescription or non-prescription (OTC) medicine.

Proper Use of This Medicine

Use this medicine only as directed by your doctor. Do not use more or less of it, and do not use it more often than your doctor ordered. The exact amount of medicine you need has been carefully worked out. Taking too much may increase the chance of side effects, while taking too little may not improve your condition.

For patients taking enteric-coated tamoxifen tablets:
• The tablets must be swallowed whole. Do not crush them or break them up before taking.

Tamoxifen commonly causes nausea and vomiting. However, it may have to be taken for several weeks or months to be effective. Even if you begin to feel ill, **do not stop using this medicine without first checking with your doctor.** Ask your doctor, nurse, or pharmacist for ways to lessen these effects.

If you vomit shortly after taking a dose of tamoxifen, check with your doctor. You may be told to take the dose again or you may have to wait until the next scheduled dose.

If you miss a dose of this medicine, do not take the missed dose at all and do not double the next one. Instead, go back to your regular dosing schedule and check with your doctor.

How to store this medicine:

• **Keep out of the reach of children.**

• Store away from heat and direct light.

• Do not store in the bathroom, near the kitchen sink, or in other damp places. Heat or moisture may cause the medicine to break down.

• Do not keep outdated medicine or medicine no longer needed. Be sure that any discarded medicine is out of the reach of children.

Precautions While Using This Medicine

It is very important that your doctor check your progress at regular visits to make sure that this medicine is working properly and to check for unwanted effects.

Tamoxifen may make you more fertile. It is best to use some type of birth control while you are taking it. However, do not use oral contraceptives (the "Pill") since they may change the effects of tamoxifen. Tell your doctor right away if you think you have become pregnant while taking this medicine.

For patients taking enteric-coated tamoxifen tablets:
• If you are also taking an antacid, take this medicine at least 1 or 2 hours before or after taking the antacid. Taking the two medicines too close together may cause the enteric coating to dissolve too early. This may increase the risk of unwanted effects from tamoxifen.

Side Effects of This Medicine

Along with its needed effects, a medicine may cause some unwanted effects. Although not all of these side effects may occur, if they do occur they may need medical attention.

Check with your doctor as soon as possible if any of the following side effects occur:

Rare

    Blurred vision
    Confusion
    Pain or swelling in legs
    Shortness of breath
    Weakness or sleepiness

Other side effects may occur that usually do not require medical attention. These side effects may go away during treatment as your body adjusts to the medicine. Also, your doctor or nurse may be able to tell you about ways to prevent or reduce some of these side effects. Check with your doctor if any of the following side effects continue or are bothersome or if you have any questions about them:

More common

    Hot flashes
    Nausea or vomiting
    Weight gain

Less common

    Bone pain
    Changes in menstrual period
    Headache
    Itching in genital area
    Skin rash or dryness
    Vaginal bleeding or discharge

For elderly patients: Many medicines have not been tested in older people. Therefore, it is not known whether the medicine acts the same way it does in younger adults. Check with your doctor if you notice any unusual effects while taking this medicine or if you think it is not working as it should.

Other side effects not listed above may also occur in some patients. If you notice any other effects, check with your doctor.

December 1987

TERPIN HYDRATE (Systemic)

To the Reader: If you do not recognize the names of medical conditions or medicines referred to in this information, check with your doctor, nurse, or pharmacist. Definitions for selected medical terms may be found in the Glossary. Brand names for the generic drug names listed can be found in the Index. In addition, selected brand names commonly associated with the generic name have been included in the text to help you recognize medicine you may be taking. The fact that a brand name product is not mentioned does not mean the information does not apply. It is a good idea for you to learn both the generic and brand names of your medicines and to write them down for future use.

Terpin hydrate (TER-pin HYE-drate) is taken by mouth to relieve coughs due to colds and mild bronchial irritations. It may also loosen mucus or phlegm (pronounced flem) in the lungs.

This medicine is usually not used for the chronic cough that occurs with smoking, asthma, or emphysema or when there is an unusually large amount of mucus or phlegm with the cough.

Terpin hydrate elixir has a very high alcohol content. Do not give this medicine to children up to 12 years of age without first checking with your doctor.

Terpin hydrate is available without a prescription; however, your doctor may have special instructions on the proper dose of this medicine for your medical condition.

Remember:

• **Keep all medicines out of the reach of children.**

• In order for this medicine to work, it must be used as directed. **If you are using this medicine without a prescription, it is very important to follow the directions on the label.**

• **It is also very important that you read and understand the following information.** If any of the information causes you special concern, check with your doctor before using this medicine without a prescription.

• Before you begin using any new medicine (prescription or nonprescription) or if you develop any new medical problem while you are using this medicine, check with your doctor, nurse, or pharmacist.

• **If you have any questions** about the following information or if you want more information about this medicine or your medical problem, **ask your doctor, nurse, or pharmacist.**

Before Using This Medicine

Before you use this medicine, check with your doctor or pharmacist:

—if you have ever had any unusual or allergic reaction to terpin hydrate.

—if you are on a low-salt, low-sugar, or any other special diet, or if you are allergic to any substance, such as foods, sulfites or other preservatives, or dyes. Most medicines contain more than their active ingredient, and many liquid medicines contain alcohol. Your doctor, nurse, or pharmacist can help you avoid products that may cause a problem.

—if you are **pregnant** or if you may become pregnant. This medicine contains a large amount (42.5%) of alcohol. Too much use of alcohol during pregnancy may cause birth defects. In addition, although terpin hydrate has not been shown to cause birth defects or other problems in humans, the chance always exists.

—if you are **breast-feeding**. The alcohol in this medicine passes into the breast milk. The amount of alcohol in recommended doses of this medicine does not usually cause problems in nursing babies.

—if you are taking **any** other prescription or nonprescription (OTC) medicine, especially central nervous system (CNS) depressants.

Proper Use of This Medicine

Take this medicine only as directed. Do not take more of it and do not take it more often than recommended on the label, unless otherwise directed by your doctor. If too much is taken, it may become habit-forming since this medicine contains a large amount of alcohol.

To help loosen mucus or phlegm in the lungs, **drink a glass of water after each dose of this medicine,** unless otherwise directed by your doctor.

If you must take this medicine regularly and you miss a dose, take it as soon as possible. However, if it is almost time for your next dose, skip the missed dose and go back to your regular dosing schedule. Do not double doses.

How to store this medicine:

• **Keep out of the reach of children.**

• Store away from heat and direct light.

• Keep this medicine from freezing.

• Do not keep outdated medicine or medicine no longer needed. Be sure that any discarded medicine is out of the reach of children.

Precautions While Using This Medicine

If your cough has not improved after 7 days or if you have a high fever, skin rash, continuing headache, or sore throat with the cough, check with your doctor. These signs may mean that you have other medical problems.

If crystals form in this solution, dissolve them by warming the closed container of solution in warm water and then gently shaking it.

The alcohol in this medicine will add to the effects of other alcohol-containing preparations and CNS depressants (medicines that slow down the nervous system, possibly causing drowsiness). Some examples of CNS depressants are antihistamines or medicine for hay fever, other allergies, or colds; sedatives, tranquilizers, or sleeping medicine; prescription pain medicine or narcotics; barbiturates; medicine for convulsions (seizures); muscle relaxants; or anesthetics, including some dental anesthetics. **Check with your doctor before taking any of the above while you are using this medicine.**

Side Effects of This Medicine

Along with its needed effects, a medicine may cause some unwanted effects. The following side effects may go away during treatment as your body adjusts to the medicine. However, check with your doctor if any of these effects continue or are bothersome:

Less common or rare

    Nausea
    Stomach pain
    Vomiting

For elderly patients: Many medicines have not been tested in older people. Therefore, it is not known whether the medicine acts the same way it does in younger adults. Check with your doctor or pharmacist if you notice any unusual effects while taking this medicine or if you think it is not working as it should.

Other side effects not listed above may also occur in some patients. If you notice any other effects, check with your doctor.

December 1987

TESTOLACTONE (Systemic)

A commonly used brand name is Teslac.

To the Reader: If you do not recognize the names of medical conditions or medicines referred to in this information, check with your doctor, nurse, or pharmacist. Definitions for selected medical terms may be found in the Glossary. Brand names for the generic drug names listed can be found in the Index. In addition, selected brand names commonly associated with the generic name have been included in the text to help you recognize medicine you may be taking. The fact that a brand name product is not mentioned does not mean the information does not apply. It is a good idea for you to learn both the generic and brand names of your medicines and to write them down for future use.

Testolactone (tess-toe-LAK-tone) belongs to the general group of medicines called antineoplastics. It is used to treat some cases of breast cancer in females.

Testolactone is available only with your doctor's prescription.

Remember:

• **This medicine has been prescribed for your current medical problem only.** It must not be given to other people or used for other problems unless you are directed to do so by your doctor.

• **Keep all medicines out of the reach of children.**

• In order for this medicine to work, it must be used as directed.

• **It is very important that you read and understand the following information.** If any of the information causes you special concern, do not decide against using this medicine without first checking with your doctor.

• Before you begin using any new medicine (prescription or nonprescription) or if you develop any new medical problem while you are using this medicine, check with your doctor, nurse, or pharmacist.

• **If you have any questions** about the following information or if you want more information about this medicine or your medical problem, **ask your doctor, nurse, or pharmacist.**

Before Using This Medicine

In order to decide on the best treatment for your medical problem, your doctor should be told:

—if you have ever had any unusual or allergic reaction to testolactone.

—if you are **pregnant** or if you may become pregnant. Studies have not been done in either humans or animals.

—if you are **breast-feeding**. It is not known whether testolactone passes into breast milk. This medicine has not been shown to cause problems in nursing babies.

—if you have heart or kidney disease.

—if you are taking **any** other prescription or nonprescription (OTC) medicine.

Proper Use of This Medicine

Use this medicine only as directed by your doctor. Do not use more or less of it, and do not use it more often than your doctor ordered. The exact amount of medicine you need has been carefully worked out. Taking too much may increase the chance of side effects, while taking too little may not improve your condition.

Testolactone sometimes causes nausea and vomiting. However, it may have to be taken for several weeks or months to be effective. Even if you begin to feel ill, **do not stop using this medicine without first checking with your doctor.** Ask your doctor, nurse, or pharmacist for ways to lessen these effects.

If you vomit shortly after taking a dose of testolactone, check with your doctor. You may be told to take the dose again or you may have to wait until the next scheduled dose.

If you miss a dose of this medicine, take it as soon as you remember. However, if it is almost time for the next dose, skip the missed dose and go back to your regular dosing schedule. Do not double doses. If you miss two or more doses in a row, check with your doctor.

How to store this medicine:

• **Keep out of the reach of children.**

• Store away from heat and direct light.

• Do not store in the bathroom, near the kitchen sink, or in other damp places. Heat or moisture may cause the medicine to break down.

• Do not keep outdated medicine or medicine no longer needed. Be sure that any discarded medicine is out of the reach of children.

Precautions While Using This Medicine

It is very important that your doctor check your progress at regular visits to make sure that this medicine is working properly and to check for unwanted effects.

Side Effects of This Medicine

Along with its needed effects, a medicine may cause some unwanted effects. Although not all of these side effects may occur, if they do occur they may need medical attention.

Check with your doctor as soon as possible if the following side effect occurs:

Less common
    Numbness or tingling of fingers, toes, or face

Other side effects may occur that usually do not require medical attention. These side effects may go away during treatment as your body adjusts to the medicine. Also, your doctor or nurse may be able to tell you about ways to prevent or reduce some of these side effects. Check with your doctor if any of the following side effects continue or are bothersome or if you have any questions about them:

Less common

Diarrhea
Loss of appetite
Nausea or vomiting
Pain or swelling in feet or lower legs
Swelling or redness of the tongue

For elderly patients: Many medicines have not been tested in older people. Therefore, it is not known whether the medicine acts the same way it does in younger adults. Check with your doctor if you notice any unusual effects while taking this medicine or if you think it is not working as it should.

Other side effects not listed above may also occur in some patients. If you notice any other effects, check with your doctor.

December 1987

TESTOSTERONE AND ESTRADIOL
(Systemic)

Some commonly used brand names are:	Generic names:
Andro/Fem De-Comberol depAndrogyn Depo-Testadiol Depotestogen Duo-Cyp Duratestrin Menoject-L.A. Testadiate-Depo Test-Estro Cypionate	Testosterone Cypionate and Estradiol Cypionate†
Andrest Andro-Estro Androgyn L.A. Deladumone Deladumone OB Ditate DS Duo-Gen L.A. Duogex LA* Duoval PA Estra-Testrin Estrand* Neo-Pause* Teev Testradiol L.A. Valertest	Testosterone Enanthate and Estradiol Valerate†

*Not available in the U.S.
†Generic name product may also be available in the U.S.

To the Reader: If you do not recognize the names of medical conditions or medicines referred to in this information, check with your doctor, nurse, or pharmacist. Definitions for selected medical terms may be found in the Glossary. Brand names for the generic drug names listed can be found in the Index. In addition, selected brand names commonly associated with the generic name have been included in the text to help you recognize medicine you may be taking. The fact that a brand name product is not mentioned does not mean the information does not apply. It is a good idea for you to learn both the generic and brand names of your medicines and to write them down for future use.

Testosterone (tess-TOSS-te-rone) is a male hormone and estradiol (ess-tra-DYE-ole) is a female hormone. They are used as a combination medicine to prevent fullness of the breasts in females after the birth of a child. The combination is also used to relieve signs of menopause, such as hot flashes and unnecessary sweating, chills, faintness, or dizziness.

Estrogens (contained in this combination medicine) are very useful medicines. However, in addition to their helpful effects in treating your medical problem, they sometimes have side effects that could be very serious. **A paper called "Information for the Patient" is given to you with your prescription. Read this carefully.** Also, before you use an estrogen, you and your doctor should discuss the good that it will do as well as the risks of using it.

There is no medical evidence to support the belief that the use of estrogens will keep the patient feeling young, keep the skin soft, or delay the appearance of wrinkles. Nor has it been proven that the use of estrogens during the menopause will relieve emotional and nervous symptoms, unless these symptoms are associated with other menopausal symptoms, such as hot flashes.

This medicine is available only with your doctor's prescription and is given by injection.

Remember:

• **It is very important that you read and understand the following information.** If any of the information causes you special concern, do not decide against receiving this medicine without first checking with your doctor.

• Before you begin using any new medicine (prescription or nonprescription) or if you develop any new medical problem while you are using this medicine, check with your doctor, nurse, or pharmacist.

• **If you have any questions** about the following information or if you want more information about this medicine or your medical problem, **ask your doctor, nurse, or pharmacist**.

Before Using This Medicine

In order to decide on the best treatment for your medical problem, your doctor should be told:

—if you have ever had any unusual or allergic reaction to estradiol or testosterone.

—if you are on a low-salt, low-sugar, or any other special diet, or if you are allergic to any substance, such as sulfites or other preservatives. Most medicines contain more than their active ingredient. Your doctor, nurse, or pharmacist can help you avoid products that may cause a problem.

—if you are **pregnant** or if you may become pregnant. Estradiol (contained in this combination medicine) may cause birth defects if taken during pregnancy. Also, testosterone (contained in this combination medicine) may cause unwanted effects in a female baby if taken during pregnancy.

—if you are **breast-feeding**. Estradiol and testosterone pass into the breast milk and may cause unwanted effects in nursing babies.

—if you have any of the following medical problems:
Asthma
Blood clots (or history of)
Bone disease
Cancer (or history of)
Changes in vaginal bleeding
Diabetes mellitus (sugar diabetes)
Edema (swelling of face, hands, feet, or lower legs)
Endometriosis
Epilepsy
Gallbladder disease or gallstones (or history of)
Heart or circulation disease
High blood pressure
Jaundice (or history of during pregnancy)
Kidney disease
Liver disease, such as jaundice or porphyria
Migraine headaches
Stroke (or history of)
Too much calcium in the blood
Tumor or growths in uterus (not cancerous, such as fibroids)

—if you are bedridden or if you expect to have surgery in the near future.

—if you are taking **any** other prescription or nonprescription (OTC) medicine, especially:

Acetaminophen (with long-term, high-dose use)
Amiodarone
Anabolic steroids (dromostanolone, ethylestrenol, nandrolone, oxandrolone, oxymetholone, stanozolol)
Androgens (male hormones)
Antithyroid agents (medicine for overactive thyroid)
Azlocillin
Bromocriptine
Carbamazepine
Carmustine
Chloroquine
Dantrolene
Daunorubicin
Disulfiram
Doxorubicin
Erythromycins
Etretinate
Furazolidone
Gold salts
Hydroxychloroquine
Isoniazid
Ketoconazole
Mercaptopurine
Methotrexate
Methyldopa
Mezlocillin
Naltrexone (with long-term, high-dose use)
Nitrofurantoin
Oral contraceptives (birth control pills) containing estrogen
Phenothiazines (acetophenazine, chlorpromazine, fluphenazine, mesoridazine, perphenazine, prochlorperazine, promazine, promethazine, thioridazine, trifluoperazine, triflupromazine, trimeprazine)
Phenytoin
Piperacillin
Plicamycin
Rifampin
Sulfonamides (sulfa medicine)
Valproic acid

—if you smoke.

Precautions While Using This Medicine

It is very important that your doctor check your progress at regular visits to make sure this medicine does not cause unwanted effects. These visits will usually be every 6 to 12 months, but many doctors require them more often.

In some patients using estrogens, tenderness, swelling, or bleeding of the gums may occur. Brushing and flossing your teeth carefully and regularly and massaging your gums may help prevent this. See your dentist regularly to have your teeth cleaned. Check with your physician or dentist if you have any questions about how to take care of your teeth and gums, or if you notice any tenderness, swelling, or bleeding of your gums.

While taking this medicine, use caution during exposure to the sun or sunlamps. Some people may develop brown, blotchy spots on exposed areas of their skin. These spots usually disappear gradually when the medicine is stopped.

Diabetics: This medicine may affect blood sugar levels. If you notice a change in the results of your urine sugar test or if you have any questions about this, check with your doctor.

If you think that you may have become pregnant, check with your doctor immediately. Continued use of this medicine during pregnancy may cause birth defects in the child. It may also increase the risk of vaginal cancer developing in daughters when they reach childbearing age.

Side Effects of This Medicine

Discuss these possible effects with your doctor:

• Tumors of the liver, liver cancer, or peliosis hepatis, a form of liver disease, have occurred during long-term, high-dose therapy with androgens. Although these effects are rare, they can be very serious and may cause death.

• When androgens are used in women, especially in high doses, male-like changes may occur, such as hoarseness or deepening of the voice, unnatural hair growth, or unusual hair loss. Most of these changes will go away if the medicine is stopped as soon as the changes are noticed. However, some changes, such as voice changes, may not go away.

• The prolonged use of estrogens has been reported to increase the risk of endometrial cancer (cancer of the uterus lining) in women after the menopause. The risk seems to increase as the dose and the length of use increase. The risk is greatly reduced when lower doses of estrogens are used for less than 1 year. The risk is also reduced if a progestin is added to, or replaces part of, your estrogen dose. However, if the uterus has been removed by surgery (total hysterectomy), there is no risk of endometrial cancer.

• Cigarette smoking during the time estrogens are taken may cause increased risk of serious side effects affecting the heart and/or blood circulation, such as dangerous blood clots, heart attack, or stroke. The risk increases as the amount of smoking and the age of the smoker increase. Women aged 35 to the age of menopause may be at greater risk when they smoke and use estrogens.

Check with your doctor as soon as possible if any of the following side effects occur:

More common
Acne or oily skin
Enlarged clitoris
Hoarseness or deepening of voice
Unnatural hair growth
Unusual hair loss

Less common or rare
Black, tarry, or light-colored stools
Changes in skin color
Changes in vaginal bleeding
Confusion or mental depression
Dark-colored urine
Dizziness
Feeling of discomfort (continuing)
Flushing or redness of skin

Headaches (frequent or continuing)
Increased blood pressure
Lump in, or discharge from, breast
Nausea or vomiting
Purple- or red-colored spots on body or inside the mouth
   or nose
Shortness of breath (unexplained)
Skin rash, hives, or itching
Sore throat and/or fever
Swelling of feet or lower legs
Swelling, pain, or tenderness in stomach, side, or abdomen
Uncontrolled jerky movements
Unpleasant breath odor (continuing)
Unusual bleeding
Unusual tiredness or drowsiness
Yellow eyes or skin
Vomiting of blood

Other side effects may occur that usually do not require medical attention. These side effects may go away during treatment as your body adjusts to the medicine.

However, check with your doctor if any of the following side effects continue or are bothersome:

More common

Bloating of stomach
Cramps of lower stomach
Loss of appetite
Swelling of breast or breast soreness

Less common

Brown, blotchy spots on exposed skin
Diarrhea (mild)
Increased sensitivity to contact lenses
Redness, pain, or other irritation at place of injection
Trouble in sleeping
Unusual decrease or increase in sexual desire

Other side effects not listed above may also occur in some patients. If you notice any other effects, check with your doctor.

_____

December 1987

TETRACYCLINES (Ophthalmic)

This information applies to the following medicines:

Chlortetracycline (klor-te-tra-SYE-kleen)
Tetracycline (te-tra-SYE-kleen)

Some commonly used brand names are:	Generic names:
Aureomycin	Chlortetracycline
Achromycin	Tetracycline

To the Reader: If you do not recognize the names of medical conditions or medicines referred to in this information, check with your doctor, nurse, or pharmacist. Definitions for selected medical terms may be found in the Glossary. Brand names for the generic drug names listed can be found in the Index. In addition, selected brand names commonly associated with the generic name have been included in the text to help you recognize medicine you may be taking. The fact that a brand name product is not mentioned does not mean the information does not apply. It is a good idea for you to learn both the generic and brand names of your medicines and to write them down for future use.

Tetracyclines belong to the family of medicines called antibiotics. Tetracycline ophthalmic preparations are used in the eye to help the body overcome infections of the eye.

Tetracyclines are available only with your doctor's prescription.

Remember:

• This medicine has been prescribed for your present infection only. Another infection later on may require a different medicine. Also, even though other people may have the same symptoms as you, they may have a different kind of infection. Your medicine may not work for them and may even cause them harm. Therefore, **your medicine must not be given to other people or used for other infections** unless you are otherwise directed by your doctor.

• In order for this medicine to work, it must be used as directed.

• Keep all medicines out of the reach of children.

• If you want more information about this medicine, ask your doctor, nurse, or pharmacist.

• If any of the following information causes you special concern, do not decide against using this medicine without first checking with your doctor.

Before Using This Medicine

In order to decide on the best treatment for your medical problem, your doctor should be told:

—if you have ever had any unusual or allergic reaction to any related antibiotics such as demeclocycline, doxycycline, methacycline, minocycline, oxytetracycline, or tetracycline (by mouth or by injection).

—if you are **pregnant** or if you may become pregnant. However, tetracycline ophthalmic preparations have not been shown to cause birth defects or other problems in humans.

—if you are **breast-feeding**. However, tetracycline ophthalmic preparations have not been shown to cause problems in nursing babies.

Proper Use of This Medicine

For patients using the eye drop form of tetracyclines:

• The bottle is only partially full to provide proper drop control.

• How to apply this medicine: First, wash your hands. Then tilt the head back and pull the lower eyelid away from the eye to form a pouch. Drop the medicine into the pouch and gently close the eyes. Do not blink. Keep the eyes closed for 1 or 2 minutes to allow the medicine to come into contact with the infection.

• If you think you did not get the drop of medicine into your eye properly, use another drop.

• To prevent contamination of the eye drops, do not touch the applicator tip to any surface (including the eye). Also, keep the container tightly closed.

For patients using the eye ointment form of tetracyclines:

• How to apply this medicine: First, wash your hands. Then pull the lower eyelid away from the eye to form a pouch. Squeeze a thin strip of ointment into the pouch. A 1-cm (approximately ⅓-inch) strip of ointment is usually enough unless otherwise directed by your doctor. Gently close the eyes and keep them closed for 1 or 2 minutes to allow the medicine to come into contact with the infection.

• To prevent contamination of the eye ointment, do not touch the applicator tip to any surface (including the eye). After using tetracyclines eye ointment, wipe the tip of the ointment tube with a clean tissue and keep the tube tightly closed.

To help clear up your infection completely, **keep using this medicine for the full time of treatment,** even though your symptoms may have disappeared. **Do not miss any doses.**

If you do miss a dose of this medicine, apply it as soon as possible. However, if it is almost time for your next application, skip the missed dose and go back to your regular dosing schedule.

How to store this medicine:

• **Keep out of the reach of children.**

• Store away from heat and direct light.

• Keep the medicine from freezing.

• Do not keep outdated medicine or medicine no longer needed. Be sure that any discarded medicine is out of the reach of children.

Precautions While Using This Medicine

After application, this medicine usually causes your vision to blur for a few minutes.

If your symptoms do not improve within a few days, or if they become worse, check with your doctor.

Side Effects of This Medicine

There have not been any common or important side effects reported with this medicine. However, if you notice any unusual effects, check with your doctor.

December 1987

TETRACYCLINES (Systemic)

This information applies to the following medicines:

Demeclocycline (dem-e-kloe-SYE-kleen)
Doxycycline (dox-i-SYE-kleen)
Methacycline (meth-a-SYE-kleen)
Minocycline (mi-noe-SYE-kleen)
Oxytetracycline (ox-i-te-tra-SYE-kleen)
Tetracycline (te-tra-SYE-kleen)

Some commonly used brand names are:	Generic names:
Declomycin	Demeclocycline
Doryx
Doxy
Doxy-Caps
Doxychel
Doxy-Tabs
Vibramycin
Vibra-Tabs
Vivox	Doxycycline†
Rondomycin	Methacycline
Minocin	Minocycline
Terramycin	Oxytetracycline†
Achromycin
Achromycin V
Bristacycline
Cefracycline*
Cyclopar
Kesso-Tetra
Medicycline*
Neo-Tetrine*
Novotetra*
Panmycin
Retet-S
Robitet
SK-Tetracycline
Sumycin
Tetracyn
Tetralean*
Tetrex
Tetrex-S	Tetracycline†

*Not available in the U.S.
†Generic name product may also be available in the U.S.

To the Reader: If you do not recognize the names of medical conditions or medicines referred to in this information, check with your doctor, nurse, or pharmacist. Definitions for selected medical terms may be found in the Glossary. Brand names for the generic drug names listed can be found in the Index. In addition, selected brand names commonly associated with the generic name have been included in the text to help you recognize medicine you may be taking. The fact that a brand name product is not mentioned does not mean the information does not apply. It is a good idea for you to learn both the generic and brand names of your medicines and to write them down for future use.

Tetracyclines belong to the family of medicines called antibiotics. They are taken by mouth or given by injection to help the body overcome infections. They are also taken by mouth to help control acne. Demeclocycline and doxycycline may also be used for other problems as determined by your doctor. Tetracyclines will not work for colds, flu, or other virus infections.

Tetracyclines are available only with your doctor's prescription.

Remember:
• This medicine has been prescribed for your present infection only. Another infection later on may require a different medicine. Also, even though other people may have the same symptoms as you, they may have a different kind of infection. Your medicine may not work for them and may even cause them harm. Therefore, **your medicine must not be given to other people or used for other infections** unless you are otherwise directed by your doctor.

• In order for this medicine to work, it must be taken as directed.

• If you want more information about this medicine, ask your doctor, nurse, or pharmacist.

• If any of the following information causes you special concern, do not decide against taking this medicine without first checking with your doctor.

• If you are receiving this medicine by injection (in a hospital or nursing home, for example), some of the following information may not apply. If you have any questions about this, check with your doctor, nurse, or pharmacist.

Before Using This Medicine

In order to decide on the best treatment for your medical problem, your doctor should be told:

—if you have ever had any unusual or allergic reaction to any of the tetracyclines or combination medicines containing a tetracycline.

—if you have ever had any unusual or allergic reaction to lidocaine, procaine, or other "caine-type" anesthetics (medicines which cause numbing) (applies only to oxytetracycline and tetracycline given by injection into the muscle).

—if you are **pregnant** or if you may become pregnant. Use is not recommended during the last half of pregnancy. Tetracyclines may cause the unborn infant's teeth to become discolored and may slow down the growth of the infant's teeth and bones if they are taken during that time. In addition, liver problems may occur in pregnant women, especially those receiving high doses by injection into a vein.

—if you are **breast-feeding**. Use is not recommended since tetracyclines pass into the breast milk. They may cause the nursing baby's teeth to become discolored and may slow down the growth of the baby's teeth and bones. They may also cause increased sensitivity of the baby's skin to sunlight and fungal infections of the mouth and vagina. In addition, minocycline may cause dizziness, lightheadedness, or unsteadiness in nursing babies.

—if you have either of the following medical problems:
  Kidney disease (does not apply to doxycycline or minocycline)
  Liver disease

—if you have diabetes insipidus (water diabetes) and you are taking demeclocycline.

—if you are taking **any** other prescription or nonprescription (OTC) medicine, especially:

    Aminosalicylate calcium
    Antacids
    Calcium supplements such as calcium gluconate, calcium lactate, or dicalcium phosphate
    Choline and magnesium salicylates (e.g., Trilisate)
    Laxatives (magnesium-containing)
    Magnesium salicylate (e.g., Magan)
    Medicine containing iron

Proper Use of This Medicine

To help clear up your infection completely, **keep taking this medicine for the full time of treatment** even if you begin to feel better after a few days. If you stop taking this medicine too soon, your symptoms may return.

This medicine works best when there is a constant amount in the blood or urine. **To help keep this amount constant, do not miss any doses. Also, it is best to take each dose at evenly spaced times day and night.** For example, if you are to take 4 doses a day, each dose should be spaced about 6 hours apart. If this interferes with your sleep or other daily activities, or if you need help in planning the best times to take your medicine, check with your doctor, nurse, or pharmacist.

If you do miss a dose of this medicine, take it as soon as possible. This will help to keep a constant amount of medicine in the blood or urine. However, if it is almost time for your next dose and your dosing schedule is:

• 1 dose a day (for example, for acne)—Space the missed dose and the next dose 10 to 12 hours apart.

• 2 doses a day—Space the missed dose and the next dose 5 to 6 hours apart.

• 3 or more doses a day—Space the missed dose and the next dose 2 to 4 hours apart or double your next dose.

Then go back to your regular dosing schedule.

Do not give tetracyclines to infants or children under 8 years of age unless directed by your doctor since they may cause permanently discolored teeth and other problems.

Tetracyclines should be taken with a full glass (8 ounces) of water to prevent irritation of the esophagus (tube between the throat and stomach) or stomach. In addition, most tetracyclines (except doxycycline and minocycline) are best taken on an empty stomach (either 1 hour before or 2 hours after meals). However, if this medicine still upsets your stomach, your doctor may want you to take it with food.

Do not take milk, milk formulas, or other dairy products within 1 to 2 hours of the time you take tetracyclines (except doxycycline and minocycline) by mouth since they may keep this medicine from working as well.

If this medicine has changed color, taste, or looks different, has become outdated (old), has been stored incorrectly (too warm or too damp), or otherwise appears to have broken down, do not use it. To do so may cause serious side effects. Discard by flushing it down the toilet. If you have any questions about this, check with your doctor or pharmacist.

For patients taking the oral liquid form of this medicine:

• Use a specially marked measuring spoon or other device to measure each dose accurately, since the average household teaspoon may not hold the right amount of liquid.

• Do not use after the expiration date on the label since the medicine may not work as well. Check with your pharmacist if you have any questions about this.

For patients taking doxycycline or minocycline:

• These medicines may be taken with food or milk if they upset your stomach.

• Swallow the capsule (with enteric-coated pellets) form of doxycycline whole. Do not break or crush.

How to store this medicine:

• **Keep out of the reach of children.**

• Store away from heat and direct light.

• Do not store the capsule or tablet form of this medicine in the bathroom, near the kitchen sink, or in other damp places. Heat or moisture may cause the medicine to break down.

• Keep the the oral liquid forms of this medicine from freezing.

• Do not keep outdated medicine or medicine no longer needed. Be sure that any discarded medicine is out of the reach of children.

Precautions While Using This Medicine

If your symptoms do not improve within a few days (or a few weeks or months for acne patients), or if they become worse, check with your doctor.

Do not take aminosalicylate calcium; antacids; calcium supplements such as calcium gluconate, calcium lactate, or dicalcium phosphate; choline and magnesium salicylates combination; magnesium salicylate; magnesium-containing laxatives such as Epsom salt; or sodium bicarbonate (baking soda) within 1 to 2 hours of the time you take any of the tetracyclines by mouth. In addition, do not take iron preparations (included also in some vitamin preparations) within 2 to 3 hours of the time you take tetracyclines by mouth. To do so may keep this medicine from working as well.

Before having surgery (including dental surgery) with a general anesthetic, tell the physician or dentist in charge that you are taking a tetracycline. This does not apply to doxycycline, however.

Some people who take tetracyclines may become more sensitive to sunlight than they are normally. **When you first begin taking this medicine, avoid too much sun and do not use a sunlamp until you see how you react to the sun,** especially if you tend to burn easily. You may still be more sensitive to sunlight or sunlamps for

2 weeks to several months or more after stopping this medicine. **If you have a severe reaction, check with your doctor.**

For patients taking minocycline:

• In addition to the precautions mentioned above, minocycline may cause some people to become dizzy, lightheaded, or unsteady. **Make sure you know how you react to this medicine before you drive, use machines, or do other jobs that require you to be alert.** If these reactions are especially bothersome, check with your doctor.

Side Effects of This Medicine

Along with its needed effects, a medicine may cause some unwanted effects. In some infants and children, tetracyclines may cause the teeth to become discolored. Even though this may not happen right away, check with your doctor as soon as possible if you notice this effect or if you have any questions about it.

Less common with demeclocycline

Greatly increased frequency of urination or amount of urine
Increased thirst
Unusual tiredness or weakness

Less common with minocycline

Pigmentation (darker color or discoloration) of skin and mucous membranes

Other side effects may occur that usually do not require medical attention. These side effects may go away during treatment as your body adjusts to the medicine. However, check with your doctor if any of the following side effects continue or are bothersome:

More common with all tetracyclines

Cramps or burning of the stomach
Diarrhea

Increased sensitivity of skin to sunlight (rare with minocycline)
Itching of the rectal or genital (sex organ) areas
Nausea or vomiting
Sore mouth or tongue

More common with minocycline

Dizziness, lightheadedness, or unsteadiness

In some patients tetracyclines may cause the tongue to become darkened or discolored. This is only temporary and will go away when you stop taking this medicine.

Other side effects not listed above may also occur in some patients. If you notice any other effects, check with your doctor.

December 1987

Additional Information

For patients taking demeclocycline as a diuretic in SIADH syndrome:

• Some doctors may prescribe demeclocycline for certain patients who retain (keep) more body water than usual (SIADH syndrome). Although demeclocycline works like a diuretic (water pill) in these patients, it will not work that way in other patients who may need a diuretic.

For patients taking doxycycline to prevent traveler's diarrhea:

• Some doctors may prescribe doxycycline by mouth to help prevent traveler's diarrhea. It is usually given daily for three weeks for this purpose. If you have any questions about this, check with your doctor.

TETRACYCLINES (Topical)

This information applies to the following medicines:

Chlortetracycline (klor-te-tra-SYE-kleen)
Meclocycline (me-kloe-SYE-kleen)
Tetracycline (te-tra-SYE-kleen)

Some commonly used brand names are:	Generic names:
Aureomycin	Chlortetracycline
Meclan	Meclocycline
Achromycin Topicycline	Tetracycline

To the Reader: If you do not recognize the names of medical conditions or medicines referred to in this information, check with your doctor, nurse, or pharmacist. Definitions for selected medical terms may be found in the Glossary. Brand names for the generic drug names listed can be found in the Index. In addition, selected brand names commonly associated with the generic name have been included in the text to help you recognize medicine you may be taking. The fact that a brand name product is not mentioned does not mean the information does not apply. It is a good idea for you to learn both the generic and brand names of your medicines and to write them down for future use.

Tetracyclines belong to the family of medicines called antibiotics. Tetracycline topical preparations are used on the skin. The topical ointment forms are used to help the body overcome infections of the skin. Meclocycline cream and the topical liquid form of tetracycline are used to help control acne. They may be used alone or with one or more other medicines which are applied to the skin or taken by mouth for acne.

Topical ointment forms of the tetracyclines are available without a prescription; however, your doctor may have special instructions on the proper use of these medicines for your medical problem. Meclocycline cream and the topical liquid form of tetracycline are available only with your doctor's prescription.

Remember:
• If you are using the cream form or topical liquid form of this medicine for acne, it has been prescribed for your acne only. Even though other people may also have acne, they may have a different kind. Your medicine may not work for them and may even cause them harm. Therefore, **your medicine must not be given to other people or used for other problems** unless you are otherwise directed by your doctor.

• In order for this medicine to work, it must be used as directed.

• Keep all medicines out of the reach of children.

• If you want more information about this medicine, ask your doctor, nurse, or pharmacist.

• If this medicine has been ordered by your doctor and any of the following information causes you special concern, do not decide against using this medicine without first checking with your doctor.

Before Using This Medicine

In order to decide on the best treatment for your medical problem, your doctor should be told:

—if you have ever had any unusual or allergic reaction to any related antibiotics such as chlortetracycline (for the eye), demeclocycline, doxycycline, methacycline, minocycline, oxytetracycline, or tetracycline (by mouth or by injection).

—if you have ever had any unusual or allergic reaction to formaldehyde (applies only to meclocycline cream).

—if you are **pregnant** or if you may become pregnant. Chlortetracycline and tetracycline topical preparations have not been shown to cause birth defects or other problems in humans. However, studies in animals have shown that meclocycline causes bone problems. Studies have not been done in humans.

—if you are **breast-feeding**. However, tetracycline topical preparations have not been shown to cause problems in nursing babies.

—if you are using **any** other prescription or nonprescription (OTC) medicine.

Proper Use of This Medicine

For patients using the cream form or topical liquid form of this medicine for acne:

• The cream or topical liquid form of this medicine will not cure your acne. However, to help keep your acne under control, **keep using this medicine for the full time of treatment,** even if your symptoms begin to clear up after a few days. You may have to continue using this medicine every day for months or even longer in some cases. If you stop using this medicine too soon, your symptoms may return. **It is important that you do not miss any doses.**

• If you do miss a dose of this medicine, apply it as soon as possible. However, if it is almost time for your next application, skip the missed dose and go back to your regular dosing schedule.

For patients using the cream form of this medicine for acne:

• Do not get this medicine on your clothing since it may stain.

• Before applying this medicine, thoroughly wash the area to be treated with warm water and soap, rinse well, and pat dry.

• How to apply this medicine:

—Apply a thin film of medicine, using enough to cover the affected area lightly. **You should apply the medicine to the whole area usually affected by acne, not just to the pimples themselves.** This will help keep new pimples from breaking out.

—Do not get this medicine in the eyes, nose, mouth, or on other mucous membranes. Spread the medicine away from these areas when applying.

For patients using the topical liquid form of this medicine for acne:

- Do not get this medicine on your clothing since it may stain.

- This medicine usually comes with patient instructions. Read these instructions carefully before using this medicine.

- The liquid form contains alcohol and is flammable. **Do not use near heat, near open flame, or while smoking.**

- Do not use after the expiration date on the label since the medicine may not work at all. Check with your pharmacist if you have any questions about this.

- The presence of the floating plastic plug in the liquid means that the medicine has been mixed properly. **Do not remove the plastic plug.**

- It is important that you do not use this medicine more often than your doctor ordered since it may cause your skin to become too dry or irritated.

- Before applying this medicine, thoroughly wash the area to be treated with warm water and soap, rinse well, and pat dry. After washing or shaving, it is best to wait 30 minutes before applying this medicine since the alcohol in it may irritate freshly washed or shaved skin.

- However, you should avoid washing the acne-affected areas too often since this may dry your skin and make your acne worse. Washing with a mild, bland soap 2 or 3 times a day should be enough, unless you have oily skin. If you have any questions about this, check with your doctor.

- How to apply this medicine:

—This medicine comes in a bottle with an applicator tip which may be used to apply the medicine directly to the skin. Use the applicator with a dabbing motion instead of a rolling motion (not like a roll-on deodorant, for example). Tilt the bottle and press the tip firmly against your skin. If needed, you can make the medicine flow faster from the applicator tip by slightly increasing the pressure against the skin. If the medicine flows too fast, use less pressure.

—Apply a generous amount of medicine, using enough so that the skin feels wet all over. After applying the medicine with the applicator, use your fingertips to spread the medicine around evenly and rub it into your skin. A second coat may be needed to completely cover the affected areas. Be sure to wash the medicine off your hands afterward.

—**You should apply the medicine to the whole area usually affected by acne, not just to the pimples themselves.** This will help keep new pimples from breaking out.

—Since this medicine contains alcohol, it will sting or burn. Therefore, **do not get this medicine in the eyes, nose, mouth, or on other mucous membranes.** Spread the medicine away from these areas when applying. If this medicine does get in the eyes, wash them out immediately, but carefully, with large amounts of cool tap water. If your eyes still burn or are painful, check with your doctor.

- The bottle contains about an 8-week supply of medicine if used only on the face and neck or about a 4-week supply if used on the face and neck plus other affected areas.

For patients using the topical ointment form of this medicine:

- To help clear up your infection completely, **keep using this medicine for the full time of treatment,** even if your symptoms begin to clear up after a few days. If you stop using this medicine too soon, your symptoms may return. **Do not miss any doses.**

- If you do miss a dose of this medicine, apply it as soon as possible. However, if it is almost time for your next application, skip the missed dose and go back to your regular dosing schedule.

- Do not get this medicine on your clothing since it may stain.

- If you are using this medicine without a prescription, do not use it to treat deep wounds, puncture wounds, or serious burns without first checking with your doctor or pharmacist.

- Do not get this medicine in the eyes.

- Before applying this medicine, thoroughly wash the area to be treated with warm water and soap, rinse well, and dry completely.

- After applying this medicine, you may cover the treated area with a gauze dressing if you wish.

How to store this medicine:

- **Keep out of the reach of children.**

- Store away from heat and direct light.

- Keep the medicine from freezing.

- Do not keep outdated medicine or medicine no longer needed. Be sure that any discarded medicine is out of the reach of children.

Precautions While Using This Medicine

For patients using either the cream form or the topical liquid form of this medicine for acne:

- Some people may notice improvement in their acne within 4 to 6 weeks. However, if there is no improvement in your acne after you have used this medicine for 6 to 8 weeks or if it becomes worse, check with your doctor or pharmacist. The treatment of acne may take up to 8 to 12 weeks before full improvement is seen.

- If your doctor has ordered another medicine to be applied to the skin along with this medicine, it is best to wait at least 1 hour before you apply the second medicine. This may help keep your skin from becoming too irritated. Also, if the medicines are used too close together, they may not work as well.

• The liquid form of this medicine may also cause the skin to become unusually dry, even with normal use. If this occurs, check with your doctor.

• This medicine may cause faint yellowing of the skin, especially around hair roots. This may be more easily seen in people with light complexions. The color may be removed by washing. However, the medicine should be left on the skin as long as possible. Do not wash immediately after applying the medicine since this will keep the medicine from working as well. If the yellow color is bothersome during the daytime, the medicine may be applied after school or work and again at bedtime, unless otherwise directed by your doctor.

• Treated areas of the skin may glow bright yellow under "black" (ultraviolet or UV) light such as that used in some discos. To help reduce or avoid this, apply the medicine later in the evening or wash it off before exposure to "black" light.

• You may continue to use cosmetics (make-up) while you are using this medicine for acne. However, it is best to use only "water-base" cosmetics. Also, it is best not to use cosmetics too heavily or too often since they may make your acne worse. If you have any questions about this, check with your doctor.

For patients using the topical ointment form of this medicine:

• If your skin infection does not improve within 2 weeks, or if it becomes worse, check with your doctor or pharmacist.

Side Effects of This Medicine

Along with its needed effects, a medicine may cause some unwanted effects. Although not all of these side effects may occur, if they do occur they may need medical attention.

Check with your doctor as soon as possible if any of the following side effects occur:
Less common
    Pain, redness, swelling, or other sign of irritation not present before using this medicine

Other side effects may occur that usually do not require medical attention. These side effects may go away during treatment as your body adjusts to the medicine. However, check with your doctor if any of the following side effects continue or are bothersome:
More common—For topical liquid form only
    Dry or scaly skin
    Stinging or burning feeling
More common—For cream and topical liquid forms only
    Faint yellowing of the skin, especially around hair roots

Other side effects not listed above may also occur in some patients. If you notice any other effects, check with your doctor.

December 1987

THEOPHYLLINE, EPHEDRINE, AND BARBITURATES (Systemic)

This information applies to the following medicine:
Theophylline, Ephedrine, and Phenobarbital (fee-noe-BAR-bi-tal)

Some commonly used brand names are:

Azma Aid	Theocord
Ephenyllin	Theodrine
Phedral	Theofed
Primatene "P" Formula	Theofedral
Tedral	Theophenyllin
Tedral SA	Theoral
Tedrigen	

Generic name product may also be available in the U.S.

To the Reader: If you do not recognize the names of medical conditions or medicines referred to in this information, check with your doctor, nurse, or pharmacist. Definitions for selected medical terms may be found in the Glossary. Brand names for the generic drug names listed can be found in the Index. In addition, selected brand names commonly associated with the generic name have been included in the text to help you recognize medicine you may be taking. The fact that a brand name product is not mentioned does not mean the information does not apply. It is a good idea for you to learn both the generic and brand names of your medicines and to write them down for future use.

Theophylline, ephedrine, and barbiturates (bar-BI-tyoo-rates) combination is taken by mouth to treat the symptoms of bronchial asthma, asthmatic bronchitis, and other lung diseases. This medicine relieves cough, wheezing, shortness of breath, and troubled breathing. It works by opening up the bronchial tubes or air passages of the lungs and increasing the flow of air through them.

Some preparations of this medicine are available only with your doctor's prescription. Others are available without a prescription; however, your doctor may have special instructions on the proper dose of this medicine for your medical condition.

Remember:
• **Keep all medicines out of the reach of children.**

• In order for this medicine to work, it must be used as directed. **If you are using this medicine without a prescription, it is very important that you follow the directions on the label.**

• **It is also very important that you read and understand the following information.** If any of the information causes you special concern, check with your doctor or pharmacist.

• Before you begin using any new medicine (prescription or nonprescription) or if you develop any new medical problem while you are using this medicine, check with your doctor, nurse, or pharmacist.

• **If you have any questions** about the following information or if you want more information about this medicine or your medical problem, **ask your doctor, nurse, or pharmacist.**

Before Using This Medicine

Before you use theophylline, ephedrine, and barbiturates combination medicine, check with your doctor or pharmacist:

—if you have ever had any unusual or allergic reaction to aminophylline, caffeine, dyphylline, oxtriphylline, theobromine, or theophylline.

—if you have ever had any unusual or allergic reaction to ephedrine or medicines like ephedrine such as albuterol, amphetamines, epinephrine, isoproterenol, metaproterenol, norepinephrine, phenylephrine, phenylpropanolamine, pseudoephedrine, or terbutaline.

—if you have ever had any unusual or allergic reaction to barbiturates.

—if you are on a low-salt, low-sugar, or any other special diet, or if you are allergic to any substance, such as foods, sulfites or other preservatives, or dyes. Most medicines contain more than their active ingredient, and many liquid medicines contain alcohol. Your doctor, nurse, or pharmacist can help you avoid products that may cause a problem.

—if you are **pregnant** or if you may become pregnant. Studies with theophylline (contained in this combination medicine) on birth defects have not been done in humans. However, some studies in animals have shown that theophylline causes birth defects when given in doses many times the human dose. Also, use of theophylline during pregnancy may cause unwanted effects such as fast heartbeat, jitteriness, irritability, gagging, vomiting, and breathing problems in the newborn infant.

Studies with ephedrine (contained in this combination medicine) on birth defects have not been done in either humans or animals.

Barbiturates (contained in this combination medicine) taken during pregnancy have been shown to increase the chance of birth defects in humans. Also, taking barbiturates regularly during the last 3 months of pregnancy may cause the baby to become dependent on the medicine. This may lead to withdrawal side effects in the baby after birth. In addition, one study in humans has suggested that barbiturates taken during pregnancy may increase the chance of brain tumors in the baby.

—if you are **breast-feeding**. The theophylline and barbiturate in this combination medicine pass into the breast milk and may cause unwanted effects such as drowsiness, irritability, fretfulness, or trouble in sleeping in babies of mothers taking this medicine. It is not known whether ephedrine passes into the breast milk. However, ephedrine has not been shown to cause problems in nursing babies.

—if you have any of the following medical problems:
Diabetes mellitus (sugar diabetes)
Diarrhea
Enlarged prostate
Fever
Fibrocystic breast disease
Heart or blood vessel disease

High blood pressure
Hyperactivity (in children)
Kidney disease
Liver disease
Overactive thyroid
Pain
Porphyria (or history of)
Respiratory infections, such as influenza (flu)
Stomach ulcer (or history of) or other stomach problems
Underactive adrenal gland

—if you are using **any** other prescription or nonprescription (OTC) medicine, especially:

Adrenocorticoids (cortisone-like medicine)
Anticoagulants (blood thinners)
Beta-blockers (acebutolol [e.g., Sectral], atenolol [e.g., Tenormin], betaxolol [e.g., Betoptic], esmolol [e.g., Brevibloc], labetalol [e.g., Normodyne], levobunolol [e.g., Betagan], metoprolol [e.g., Lopressor], nadolol [e.g., Corgard], oxprenolol [e.g., Trasicor], pindolol [e.g., Visken], propranolol [e.g., Inderal], sotalol [e.g., Sotacor], timolol [e.g., Blocadren, Timoptic])
Central nervous system (CNS) depressants
Cimetidine (e.g., Tagamet)
Corticotropin (e.g., ACTH)
Digitalis glycosides (heart medicine)
Ergoloid mesylates (e.g., Hydergine)
Ergotamine (e.g., Gynergen)
Erythromycin (e.g., E-Mycin)
Maprotiline (e.g., Ludiomil)
Oral contraceptives (birth control pills) containing estrogen
Tricyclic antidepressants (amitriptyline [e.g., Elavil], amoxapine [e.g., Asendin], clomipramine, desipramine [e.g., Pertofrane], doxepin [e.g., Sinequan], imipramine [e.g., Tofranil], nortriptyline [e.g., Aventyl], protriptyline [e.g., Vivactil], trimipramine [e.g., Surmontil])
Troleandomycin (e.g., TAO)

—if you are now taking or have taken within the past 2 weeks monoamine oxidase (MAO) inhibitors, such as:

Furazolidone (e.g., Furoxone)
Isocarboxazid (e.g., Marplan)
Pargyline (e.g., Eutonyl)
Phenelzine (e.g., Nardil)
Procarbazine (e.g., Matulane)
Tranylcypromine (e.g., Parnate)

—if you smoke or have smoked (tobacco or marijuana) regularly within the last 2 years. The amount of medicine you need may vary, depending on how much and how recently you have smoked.

Proper Use of This Medicine

For patients taking the extended-release tablet form of this medicine:

• Swallow the tablet whole. Do not crush, break, or chew before swallowing.

This medicine works best when taken with a glass of water on an empty stomach (either 30 minutes to 1 hour before meals or 2 hours after meals) since that way it will get into the blood sooner. However, in some cases your doctor may want you to take this medicine with meals or right after meals to lessen stomach upset. If you have any questions about how you should be taking this medicine, check with your doctor.

Take this medicine only as directed. Do not take more of it and do not take it more often than recommended on the label, unless otherwise directed by your doctor. To do so may increase the chance of serious side effects. Also, if too much is taken, the barbiturate in this medicine may become habit-forming.

In order for this medicine to help your medical problem, it must be taken every day in regularly spaced doses as recommended. This is necessary to keep a constant amount of this medicine in the blood. To help keep the amount constant, do not miss any doses.

If you do miss a dose of this medicine, take it as soon as possible. However, if it is almost time for your next dose, skip the missed dose and go back to your regular dosing schedule. Do not double doses.

How to store this medicine:

• **Keep out of the reach of children.**

• Store away from heat and direct light.

• Do not store the tablet form of this medicine in the bathroom, near the kitchen sink, or in other damp places. Heat or moisture may cause the medicine to break down.

• Keep the liquid form of this medicine from freezing.

• Do not keep outdated medicine or medicine no longer needed. Be sure that any discarded medicine is out of the reach of children.

Precautions While Using This Medicine

The theophylline in this medicine may add to the central nervous system stimulant effects of caffeine-containing foods or beverages such as chocolate, cocoa, tea, coffee, and cola drinks. **Avoid eating or drinking large amounts of these foods or beverages while taking this medicine.** If you have any questions about this, check with your doctor.

The barbiturate in this medicine will add to the effects of alcohol and other CNS depressants (medicines that slow down the nervous system, possibly causing drowsiness). Some examples of CNS depressants are antihistamines or medicine for hay fever, other allergies, or colds; sedatives, tranquilizers, or sleeping medicine; prescription pain medicine or narcotics; barbiturates; medicine for convulsions (seizures); muscle relaxants; or anesthetics, including some dental anesthetics. **Check with your doctor before taking any of the above while you are using this medicine.**

Do not eat charcoal-broiled foods every day while taking this medicine since these foods may keep the medicine from working as well.

Check with your doctor at once if you develop symptoms of influenza (flu) or a fever since either of these may increase the chance of side effects with this medicine.

Also, **check with your doctor if diarrhea occurs** because the dose of this medicine may need to be changed.

This medicine may cause some people to become dizzy, lightheaded, drowsy, or less alert than they are normally. **Make sure you know how you react to this medicine before you drive, use machines, or do other jobs that require you to be alert.**

Side Effects of This Medicine

Along with its needed effects, a medicine may cause some unwanted effects. Although not all of these side effects may occur, if they do occur they may need medical attention.

Check with your doctor as soon as possible if any of the following side effects occur:

Less common

Heartburn and/or vomiting

Signs of overdose

Bloody or black tarry stools
Chest pain
Convulsions (seizures)
Diarrhea
Dizziness or lightheadedness
Fast, pounding, or irregular heartbeat
Hallucinations (seeing, hearing, or feeling things that are not there)
Increase or decrease in blood pressure
Irritability
Loss of appetite
Mood or mental changes
Muscle twitching

Nausea (continuing or severe) or vomiting
Stomach cramps or pain
Trembling
Trouble in sleeping
Unusual tiredness or weakness
Vomiting blood or material that looks like coffee grounds

Other side effects may occur that usually do not require medical attention. These side effects may go away during treatment as your body adjusts to the medicine. However, check with your doctor or pharmacist if any of the following side effects continue or are bothersome:

More common

Drowsiness
Headache
Nausea
Nervousness or restlessness

Less common

Difficult or painful urination
Feeling of warmth
Flushing or redness of face

For elderly patients: The above side effects are more likely to occur in elderly patients, who are usually more sensitive to the effects of this medicine.

Other side effects not listed above may also occur in some patients. If you notice any other effects, check with your doctor.

_____

December 1987

_____

THEOPHYLLINE, EPHEDRINE, GUAIFENESIN, AND BARBITURATES
(Systemic)

This information applies to the following medicines:

Theophylline (thee-OFF-i-lin), Ephedrine (e-FED-rin), Guaifenesin (gwye-FEN-e-sin), and Butabarbital (byoo-ta-BAR-bi-tal)

Theophylline, Ephedrine, Guaifenesin, and Phenobarbital (fee-noe-BAR-bi-tal)

Some commonly used brand names are:

Bronkolixir	Mudrane GG
Bronkotabs	Quibron Plus

Generic name product may also be available in the U.S.

To the Reader: If you do not recognize the names of medical conditions or medicines referred to in this information, check with your doctor, nurse, or pharmacist. Definitions for selected medical terms may be found in the Glossary. Brand names for the generic drug names listed can be found in the Index. In addition, selected brand names commonly associated with the generic name have been included in the text to help you recognize medicine you may be taking. The fact that a brand name product is not mentioned does not mean the information does not apply. It is a good idea for you to learn both the generic and brand names of your medicines and to write them down for future use.

Theophylline, ephedrine, guaifenesin, and barbiturates (bar-BI-tyoo-rates) combination is taken by mouth to treat the symptoms of bronchial asthma, chronic bronchitis, emphysema, and other lung diseases. This medicine relieves cough, wheezing, shortness of breath, and troubled breathing. It works by opening up the bronchial tubes or air passages of the lungs and increasing the flow of air through them.

Some of these preparations are available only with your doctor's prescription. Others are available without a prescription; however, your doctor may have special instructions on the proper use of this medicine for your medical condition.

Remember:

• **Keep all medicines out of the reach of children.**

• In order for this medicine to work, it must be used as directed. **If you are using this medicine without a prescription, it is very important that you follow the directions on the label.**

• **It is also very important that you read and understand the following information.** If any of the information causes you special concern, check with your doctor or pharmacist.

• Before you begin using any new medicine (prescription or nonprescription) or if you develop any new medical problem while you are using this medicine, check with your doctor, nurse, or pharmacist.

• **If you have any questions** about the following information or if you want more information about this medicine or your medical problem, **ask your doctor, nurse, or pharmacist.**

Before Using This Medicine

Before you use theophylline, ephedrine, guaifenesin, and barbiturates combination medicine, check with your doctor or pharmacist:

—if you have ever had any unusual or allergic reaction to aminophylline, caffeine, dyphylline, oxtriphylline, theobromine, or theophylline.

—if you have ever had any unusual or allergic reaction to ephedrine or medicines like ephedrine such as albuterol, amphetamines, epinephrine, isoproterenol, metaproterenol, norepinephrine, phenylephrine, phenylpropanolamine, pseudoephedrine, or terbutaline.

—if you have ever had any unusual or allergic reaction to barbiturates.

—if you are on a low-salt, low-sugar, or any other special diet, or if you are allergic to any substance, such as foods, sulfites or other preservatives, or dyes. Most medicines contain more than their active ingredient, and many liquid medicines contain alcohol. Your doctor, nurse, or pharmacist can help you avoid products that may cause a problem.

—if you are **pregnant** or if you may become pregnant. Studies with theophylline (contained in this combination medicine) on birth defects have not been done in humans. However, some studies in animals have shown that theophylline causes birth defects when given in doses many times the human dose. Also, use of theophylline during pregnancy may cause unwanted effects such as fast heartbeat, jitteriness, irritability, gagging, vomiting, and breathing problems in the newborn infant.

Studies with ephedrine (contained in this combination medicine) on birth defects have not been done in either humans or animals.

Barbiturates (contained in this combination medicine) taken during pregnancy have been shown to increase the chance of birth defects in humans. Also, taking barbiturates regularly during the last 3 months of pregnancy may cause the baby to become dependent on the medicine. This may lead to withdrawal side effects in the baby after birth. In addition, one study in humans has suggested that barbiturates taken during pregnancy may increase the chance of brain tumors in the baby.

Guaifenesin (contained in this combination medicine) has not been shown to cause birth defects or other problems in humans.

—if you are **breast-feeding**. The theophylline and barbiturate in this combination medicine pass into the breast milk and may cause unwanted effects such as drowsiness, irritability, fretfulness, or trouble in sleeping in babies of mothers taking this medicine. Ephedrine and guaifenesin (contained in this combination medicine) have not been shown to cause problems in nursing babies.

—if you have any of the following medical problems:
  Diabetes mellitus (sugar diabetes)
  Diarrhea
  Enlarged prostate

Fever
Fibrocystic breast disease
Heart or blood vessel disease
High blood pressure
Hyperactivity (in children)
Kidney disease
Liver disease
Overactive thyroid
Pain
Porphyria (or history of)
Respiratory infections, such as influenza (flu)
Stomach ulcer (or history of) or other stomach problems
Underactive adrenal gland

—if you are using **any** other prescription or nonprescription (OTC) medicine, especially:

Adrenocorticoids (cortisone-like medicine)
Anticoagulants (blood thinners)
Beta-blockers (acebutolol [e.g., Sectral], atenolol [e.g., Tenormin], betaxolol [e.g., Betoptic], esmolol [e.g., Brevibloc], labetalol [e.g., Normodyne], levobunolol [e.g., Betagan], metoprolol [e.g., Lopressor], nadolol [e.g., Corgard], oxprenolol [e.g., Trasicor], pindolol [e.g., Visken], propranolol [e.g., Inderal], sotalol [e.g., Sotacor], timolol [e.g., Blocadren, Timoptic])
Central nervous system (CNS) depressants
Cimetidine (e.g., Tagamet)
Corticotropin (e.g., ACTH)
Digitalis glycosides (heart medicine)
Ergoloid mesylates (e.g., Hydergine)
Ergotamine (e.g., Gynergen)
Erythromycin (e.g., E-Mycin)
Maprotiline (e.g., Ludiomil)
Oral contraceptives (birth control pills) containing estrogen
Tricyclic antidepressants (amitriptyline [e.g., Elavil], amoxapine [e.g., Asendin], clomipramine, desipramine [e.g., Pertofrane], doxepin [e.g., Sinequan], imipramine [e.g., Tofranil], nortriptyline [e.g., Aventyl], protriptyline [e.g., Vivactil], trimipramine [e.g., Surmontil])
Troleandomycin (e.g., TAO)

—if you are now taking or have taken within the past 2 weeks monoamine oxidase (MAO) inhibitors, such as:

Furazolidone (e.g., Furoxone)
Isocarboxazid (e.g., Marplan)
Pargyline (e.g., Eutonyl)
Phenelzine (e.g., Nardil)
Procarbazine (e.g., Matulane)
Tranylcypromine (e.g., Parnate)

—if you smoke or have smoked (tobacco or marijuana) regularly within the last 2 years. The amount of medicine you need may vary, depending on how much and how recently you have smoked.

Proper Use of This Medicine

This medicine works best when taken with a glass of water on an empty stomach (either 30 minutes to 1 hour before meals or 2 hours after meals) since that way it will get into the blood sooner. However, in some cases your doctor may want you to take this medicine with meals or right after meals to lessen stomach upset. If you have any questions about how you should be taking this medicine, check with your doctor.

Take this medicine only as directed. Do not take more of it and do not take it more often than recommended on the label, unless otherwise directed by your doctor. To do so may increase the chance of serious side effects. Also, if too much is taken, the barbiturate in this medicine may become habit-forming.

In order for this medicine to help your medical problem, it must be taken every day in regularly spaced doses as recommended. This is necessary to keep a constant amount of this medicine in the blood. To help keep the amount constant, do not miss any doses.

If you do miss a dose of this medicine, take it as soon as possible. However, if it is almost time for your next dose, skip the missed dose and go back to your regular dosing schedule. Do not double doses.

How to store this medicine:

• **Keep out of the reach of children.**

• Store away from heat and direct light.

• Do not store the capsule or tablet form of this medicine in the bathroom, near the kitchen sink, or in other damp places. Heat or moisture may cause the medicine to break down.

• Keep the elixir form of this medicine from freezing.

• Do not keep outdated medicine or medicine no longer needed. Be sure that any discarded medicine is out of the reach of children.

Precautions While Using This Medicine

The theophylline in this medicine may add to the central nervous system (CNS) stimulant effects of caffeine-containing foods or beverages such as chocolate, cocoa, tea, coffee, and cola drinks. **Avoid eating or drinking large amounts of these foods or beverages while taking this medicine.** If you have any questions about this, check with your doctor.

The barbiturate in this medicine will add to the effects of alcohol and other CNS depressants (medicines that slow down the nervous system, possibly causing drowsiness). Some examples of CNS depressants are antihistamines or medicine for hay fever, other allergies, or colds; sedatives, tranquilizers, or sleeping medicine; prescription pain medicine or narcotics; barbiturates; medicine for convulsions (seizures); muscle relaxants; or anesthetics, including some dental anesthetics. **Check with your doctor before taking any of the above while you are using this medicine.**

Do not eat charcoal-broiled foods every day while taking this medicine since these foods may keep the medicine from working as well.

Check with your doctor at once if you develop symptoms of influenza (flu) or a fever, since either of these may increase the chance of side effects with this medicine.

Also, **check with your doctor if diarrhea occurs** because the dose of this medicine may need to be changed.

This medicine may cause some people to become dizzy, lightheaded, drowsy, or less alert than they are normally. **Make sure you know how you react to this medicine before you drive, use machines, or do other jobs that require you to be alert.**

Side Effects of This Medicine

Along with its needed effects, a medicine may cause some unwanted effects. Although not all of these side effects may occur, if they do occur they may need medical attention.

Check with your doctor as soon as possible if any of the following side effects occur:

Less common

    Heartburn and/or vomiting

Signs of overdose

    Bloody or black tarry stools
    Chest pain
    Convulsions (seizures)
    Diarrhea
    Dizziness or lightheadedness
    Fast, pounding, or irregular heartbeat
    Hallucinations (seeing, hearing, or feeling things that are
      not there)
    Increase or decrease in blood pressure
    Irritability
    Loss of appetite
    Mood or mental changes
    Muscle twitching
    Nausea (continuing or severe) or vomiting

    Stomach cramps or pain
    Trembling
    Trouble in sleeping
    Unusual tiredness or weakness
    Vomiting blood or material that looks like coffee grounds

Other side effects may occur that usually do not require medical attention. These side effects may go away during treatment as your body adjusts to the medicine. However, check with your doctor or pharmacist if any of the following side effects continue or are bothersome:

More common

    Drowsiness
    Headache
    Nausea
    Nervousness or restlessness

Less common

    Difficult or painful urination
    Feeling of warmth
    Flushing or redness of face

For elderly patients: The above side effects are more likely to occur in elderly patients, who are usually more sensitive to the effects of this medicine.

Other side effects not listed above may also occur in some patients. If you notice any other effects, check with your doctor.

_____

December 1987

_____

THEOPHYLLINE, EPHEDRINE, AND HYDROXYZINE (Systemic)

Some commonly used brand names are:

Brophed	Marax D.F.
Hydrophed	T.E.H. Compound
Hydrophed D.F.	Theozine
Marax	

Generic name product may also be available in the U.S.

To the Reader: If you do not recognize the names of medical conditions or medicines referred to in this information, check with your doctor, nurse, or pharmacist. Definitions for selected medical terms may be found in the Glossary. Brand names for the generic drug names listed can be found in the Index. In addition, selected brand names commonly associated with the generic name have been included in the text to help you recognize medicine you may be taking. The fact that a brand name product is not mentioned does not mean the information does not apply. It is a good idea for you to learn both the generic and brand names of your medicines and to write them down for future use.

Theophylline (thee-OFF-i-lin), ephedrine (e-FED-rin), and hydroxyzine (hye-DROX-i-zeen) combination medicine is taken by mouth to treat the symptoms of bronchial asthma, chronic bronchitis, emphysema, and other lung diseases. This medicine relieves cough, wheezing, shortness of breath, and troubled breathing. It works by opening up the bronchial tubes or air passages of the lungs and increasing the flow of air through them.

This medicine is available only with your doctor's prescription.

Remember:

• **This medicine has been prescribed for your current medical problem only.** It must not be given to other people or used for other problems unless you are directed to do so by your doctor.

• **Keep all medicines out of the reach of children.**

• In order for this medicine to work, it must be used as directed.

• **It is very important that you read and understand the following information.** If any of the information causes you special concern, do not decide against using this medicine without first checking with your doctor.

• Before you begin using any new medicine (prescription or nonprescription) or if you develop any new medical problem while you are using this medicine, check with your doctor, nurse, or pharmacist.

• **If you have any questions** about the following information or if you want more information about this medicine or your medical problem, **ask your doctor, nurse, or pharmacist.**

Before Using This Medicine

In order to decide on the best treatment for your medical problem, your doctor should be told:

—if you have ever had any unusual or allergic reaction to aminophylline, caffeine, dyphylline, oxtriphylline, theobromine, or theophylline.

—if you have ever had any unusual or allergic reaction to ephedrine or medicines like ephedrine such as albuterol, amphetamines, epinephrine, isoproterenol, metaproterenol, norepinephrine, phenylephrine, phenylpropanolamine, pseudoephedrine, or terbutaline.

—if you have ever had any unusual or allergic reaction to hydroxyzine.

—if you are on a low-salt, low-sugar, or any other special diet, or if you are allergic to any substance, such as foods, sulfites or other preservatives, or dyes. Most medicines contain more than their active ingredient, and many liquid medicines contain alcohol. Your doctor, nurse, or pharmacist can help you avoid products that may cause a problem.

—if you are **pregnant** or if you may become pregnant. Studies with theophylline (contained in this combination medicine) on birth defects have not been done in humans. However, some studies in animals have shown that theophylline causes birth defects when given in doses many times the human dose. Also, use of theophylline during pregnancy may cause unwanted effects such as fast heartbeat, jitteriness, irritability, gagging, vomiting, and breathing problems in the newborn infant.

Studies with ephedrine (contained in this combination medicine) on birth defects have not been done in either humans or animals.

Hydroxyzine (contained in this combination medicine) is not recommended during the first months of pregnancy because it has been shown to cause birth defects in rats when given in doses up to many times the usual human dose.

—if you are **breast-feeding**. Theophylline (contained in this combination medicine) passes into the breast milk and may cause unwanted effects such as irritability, fretfulness, or trouble in sleeping in babies of mothers taking this medicine. Ephedrine and hydroxyzine (contained in this combination medicine) have not been shown to cause problems in nursing babies.

—if you have any of the following medical problems:
Diabetes mellitus (sugar diabetes)
Diarrhea
Enlarged prostate
Fever
Fibrocystic breast disease
Heart or blood vessel disease
High blood pressure
Liver disease
Overactive thyroid
Respiratory infections, such as influenza (flu)
Stomach ulcer (or history of) or other stomach problems

—if you are using **any** other prescription or nonprescription (OTC) medicine, especially:
Beta-blockers (acebutolol [e.g., Sectral], atenolol [e.g., Tenormin], betaxolol [e.g., Betoptic], esmolol [e.g., Brevibloc], labetalol [e.g., Normodyne], levobunolol [e.g., Betagan], metoprolol [e.g., Lopressor], nadolol [e.g., Corgard], oxprenolol [e.g., Trasicor], pindolol [e.g., Visken], propranolol [e.g., Inderal], sotalol [e.g., Sotacor], timolol [e.g., Blocadren, Timoptic])
Central nervous system (CNS) depressants

Cimetidine (e.g., Tagamet)
Digitalis glycosides (heart medicine)
Ergoloid mesylates (e.g., Hydergine)
Ergotamine (e.g., Gynergen)
Erythromycin (e.g., E-Mycin)
Maprotiline (e.g., Ludiomil)
Tricyclic antidepressants (amitriptyline [e.g., Elavil], amoxapine [e.g., Asendin], clomipramine, desipramine [e.g., Pertofrane], doxepin [e.g., Sinequan], imipramine [e.g., Tofranil], nortriptyline [e.g., Aventyl], protriptyline [e.g., Vivactil], trimipramine [e.g., Surmontil])
Troleandomycin (e.g., TAO)

—if you are now taking or have taken within the past 2 weeks monoamine oxidase (MAO) inhibitors, such as:

Furazolidone (e.g., Furoxone)
Isocarboxazid (e.g., Marplan)
Pargyline (e.g., Eutonyl)
Phenelzine (e.g., Nardil)
Procarbazine (e.g., Matulane)
Tranylcypromine (e.g., Parnate)

—if you smoke or have smoked (tobacco or marijuana) regularly within the last 2 years. The amount of medicine you need may vary, depending on how much and how recently you have smoked.

Proper Use of This Medicine

This medicine works best when taken with a glass of water on an empty stomach (either 30 minutes to 1 hour before meals or 2 hours after meals) since that way it will get into the blood sooner. However, in some cases your doctor may want you to take this medicine with meals or right after meals to lessen stomach upset. If you have any questions about how you should be taking this medicine, check with your doctor.

Take this medicine only as directed. Do not take more of it and do not take it more often than your doctor ordered. To do so may increase the chance of serious side effects.

In order for this medicine to help your medical problem, it must be taken every day in regularly spaced doses as ordered by your doctor. This is necessary to keep a constant amount of this medicine in the blood. To help keep the amount constant, do not miss any doses.

If you do miss a dose of this medicine, take it as soon as possible. However, if it is almost time for your next dose, skip the missed dose and go back to your regular dosing schedule. Do not double doses.

How to store this medicine:

• **Keep out of the reach of children.**

• Store away from heat and direct light.

• Do not store the tablet form of this medicine in the bathroom, near the kitchen sink, or in other damp places. Heat or moisture may cause the medicine to break down.

• Keep the syrup form of this medicine from freezing.

• Do not keep outdated medicine or medicine no longer needed. Be sure that any discarded medicine is out of the reach of children.

Precautions While Using This Medicine

The theophylline in this medicine may add to the central nervous system stimulant effects of caffeine-containing foods or beverages such as chocolate, cocoa, tea, coffee, and cola drinks. **Avoid eating or drinking large amounts of these foods or beverages while taking this medicine.** If you have any questions about this, check with your doctor.

The hydroxyzine in this medicine will add to the effects of alcohol and CNS depressants (medicines that slow down the nervous system, possibly causing drowsiness). Some examples of CNS depressants are antihistamines or medicine for hay fever, other allergies, or colds; sedatives, tranquilizers, or sleeping medicine; prescription pain medicine or narcotics; barbiturates; medicine for convulsions (seizures); muscle relaxants; or anesthetics, including dental anesthetics. **Check with your doctor before taking any of the above while you are taking this medicine.**

Do not eat charcoal-broiled foods every day while taking this medicine since these foods may keep the medicine from working as well.

Check with your doctor at once if you develop symptoms of influenza (flu) or a fever, since either of these may increase the chance of side effects with this medicine.

Also, **check with your doctor if diarrhea occurs** because the dose of this medicine may need to be changed.

This medicine may cause some people to become dizzy, lightheaded, drowsy, or less alert than they are normally. **Make sure you know how you react to this medicine before you drive, use machines, or do other jobs that require you to be alert.**

Side Effects of This Medicine

Along with its needed effects, a medicine may cause some unwanted effects. Although not all of these side effects may occur, if they do occur they may need medical attention.

Check with your doctor as soon as possible if any of the following side effects occur:
Less common
Heartburn and/or vomiting
Signs of overdose
Bloody or black tarry stools
Chest pain
Convulsions (seizures)
Diarrhea
Dizziness or lightheadedness
Fast, pounding, or irregular heartbeat
Hallucinations (seeing, hearing, or feeling things that are not there)
Increase or decrease in blood pressure

Irritability
Loss of appetite
Mood or mental changes
Muscle twitching
Nausea (continuing or severe) or vomiting
Stomach cramps or pain
Trembling
Trouble in sleeping
Unusual tiredness or weakness
Vomiting blood or material that looks like coffee grounds

Other side effects may occur that usually do not require medical attention. These side effects may go away during treatment as your body adjusts to the medicine. However, check with your doctor if any of the following side effects continue or are bothersome:

More common
Drowsiness
Headache
Nausea
Nervousness or restlessness

Less common
Difficult or painful urination
Feeling of warmth
Flushing or redness of face

For elderly patients: The above side effects are more likely to occur in elderly patients, who are usually more sensitive to the effects of this medicine.

Other side effects not listed above may also occur in some patients. If you notice any other effects, check with your doctor.

December 1987

THEOPHYLLINE AND GUAIFENESIN
(Systemic)

Some commonly used brand names are:

Asbron G	Glyceryl T	Synophylate-GG
Asbron G	Lanophyllin-GG	Theocolate
Inlay-Tabs	Quibron	Theolair-Plus
Bronchial	Quiagen	Theolate
Elixophyllin-GG	Slo-Phyllin GG	

Generic name product may also be available in the U.S.

To the Reader: If you do not recognize the names of medical conditions or medicines referred to in this information, check with your doctor, nurse, or pharmacist. Definitions for selected medical terms may be found in the Glossary. Brand names for the generic drug names listed can be found in the Index. In addition, selected brand names commonly associated with the generic name have been included in the text to help you recognize medicine you may be taking. The fact that a brand name product is not mentioned does not mean the information does not apply. It is a good idea for you to learn both the generic and brand names of your medicines and to write them down for future use.

Theophylline (thee-OFF-i-lin) and guaifenesin (gwye-FEN-e-sin) combination is taken by mouth to treat the symptoms of bronchial asthma, chronic bronchitis, emphysema, and other lung diseases. This medicine relieves cough, wheezing, shortness of breath, and troubled breathing. It works by opening up the bronchial tubes or air passages of the lungs and increasing the flow of air through them.

This medicine is available only with your doctor's prescription.

Remember:

• **This medicine has been prescribed for your current medical problem only.** It must not be given to other people or used for other problems unless you are directed to do so by your doctor.

• **Keep all medicines out of the reach of children.**

• In order for this medicine to work, it must be used as directed.

• **It is very important that you read and understand the following information.** If any of the information causes you special concern, do not decide against using this medicine without first checking with your doctor.

• Before you begin using any new medicine (prescription or nonprescription) or if you develop any new medical problem while you are using this medicine, check with your doctor, nurse, or pharmacist.

• **If you have any questions** about the following information or if you want more information about this medicine or your medical problem, **ask your doctor, nurse, or pharmacist.**

Before Using This Medicine

In order to decide on the best treatment for your medical problem, your doctor should be told:

  —if you have ever had any unusual or allergic reaction to aminophylline, caffeine, dyphylline, oxtriphylline, theobromine, or theophylline.

  —if you are on a low-salt, low-sugar, or any other special diet, or if you are allergic to any substance, such as foods, sulfites or other preservatives, or dyes.

Most medicines contain more than their active ingredient, and many liquid medicines contain alcohol. Your doctor, nurse, or pharmacist can help you avoid products that may cause a problem.

  —if you are **pregnant** or if you may become pregnant. Studies on birth defects have not been done in humans. However, some studies in animals have shown that theophylline (contained in this combination medicine) causes birth defects when given in doses many times the human dose. Also, use of theophylline during pregnancy may cause unwanted effects such as fast heartbeat, jitteriness, irritability, gagging, vomiting, and breathing problems in the newborn infant. Guaifenesin (contained in this combination medicine) has not been shown to cause birth defects or other problems in humans.

  —if you are **breast-feeding**. Theophylline (contained in this combination medicine) passes into the breast milk and may cause irritability, fretfulness, or trouble in sleeping in babies of mothers taking this medicine. Guaifenesin (contained in this combination medicine) has not been shown to cause problems in nursing babies.

  —if you have any of the following medical problems:

> Diarrhea
> Enlarged prostate
> Fever
> Fibrocystic breast disease
> Heart disease
> Liver disease
> Overactive thyroid
> Respiratory infections, such as influenza (flu)
> Stomach ulcer (or history of) or other stomach problems

  —if you are using **any** other prescription or nonprescription (OTC) medicine, especially:

> Beta-blockers (acebutolol [e.g., Sectral], atenolol [e.g., Tenormin], betaxolol [e.g., Betoptic], esmolol [e.g., Brevibloc], labetalol [e.g., Normodyne], levobunolol [e.g., Betagan], metoprolol [e.g., Lopressor], nadolol [e.g., Corgard], oxprenolol [e.g., Trasicor], pindolol [e.g., Visken], propranolol [e.g., Inderal], sotalol [e.g., Sotacor], timolol [e.g., Blocadren, Timoptic])
> Cimetidine (e.g., Tagamet)
> Erythromycin (e.g., E-Mycin)
> Phenytoin (e.g., Dilantin)
> Troleandomycin (e.g., TAO)

  —if you smoke or have smoked (tobacco or marijuana) regularly within the last 2 years. The amount of medicine you need may vary, depending on how much and how recently you have smoked.

Proper Use of This Medicine

This medicine works best when taken with a glass of water on an empty stomach (either 30 minutes to 1 hour before meals or 2 hours after meals) since that way it will get into the blood sooner. However, in some cases your doctor may want you to take this medicine with meals or right after meals to lessen stomach upset. If you have any questions about how you should be taking this medicine, check with your doctor.

Take this medicine only as directed. Do not take more of it, do not take it more often, and do not take it for a longer period of time than your doctor ordered. To do so may increase the chance of serious side effects.

In order for this medicine to help your medical problem, it must be taken every day in regularly spaced doses as ordered by your doctor. This is necessary to keep a constant amount of this medicine in the blood. To help keep the amount constant, do not miss any doses.

If you do miss a dose of this medicine, take it as soon as possible. However, if it is almost time for your next dose, skip the missed dose and go back to your regular dosing schedule. Do not double doses.

How to store this medicine:
- **Keep out of the reach of children.**
- Store away from heat and direct light.
- Do not store the capsule or tablet form of this medicine in the bathroom, near the kitchen sink, or in other damp places. Heat or moisture may cause the medicine to break down.
- Keep the liquid form of this medicine from freezing.
- Do not keep outdated medicine or medicine no longer needed. Be sure that any discarded medicine is out of the reach of children.

Precautions While Using This Medicine

Your doctor should check your progress at regular visits, especially for the first few weeks after you begin taking this medicine. A blood test may be taken to help your doctor decide whether the dose of this medicine should be changed.

The theophylline in this medicine may add to the central nervous system stimulant effects of caffeine-containing foods or beverages such as chocolate, cocoa, tea, coffee, and cola drinks. **Avoid eating or drinking large amounts of these foods or beverages while taking this medicine.** If you have any questions about this, check with your doctor.

Do not eat charcoal-broiled foods every day while taking this medicine since these foods may keep the medicine from working as well.

Check with your doctor at once if you develop symptoms of influenza (flu) or a fever since either of these may increase the chance of side effects with this medicine.

Also, **check with your doctor if diarrhea occurs** because the dose of this medicine may need to be changed.

Side Effects of This Medicine

Along with its needed effects, a medicine may cause some unwanted effects. Although not all of these side effects may occur, if they do occur they may need medical attention.

Check with your doctor as soon as possible if any of the following side effects occur:

Less common
    Heartburn and/or vomiting

Signs of overdose of theophylline
    Bloody or black tarry stools
    Confusion or change in behavior
    Convulsions (seizures)
    Diarrhea
    Dizziness or lightheadedness
    Fast breathing
    Fast, pounding, or irregular heartbeat
    Flushing or redness of face
    Headache
    Increased urination
    Irritability
    Loss of appetite
    Muscle twitching
    Nausea (continuing or severe) or vomiting
    Stomach cramps or pain
    Trembling
    Trouble in sleeping
    Unusual tiredness or weakness
    Vomiting blood or material that looks like coffee grounds

Other side effects may occur that usually do not require medical attention. These side effects may go away during treatment as your body adjusts to the medicine. However, check with your doctor if any of the following side effects continue or are bothersome:

More common
    Nausea
    Nervousness or restlessness

For elderly patients and newborn infants: The above side effects are more likely to occur in elderly patients and newborn infants, who are usually more sensitive to the effects of this medicine.

Other side effects not listed above may also occur in some patients. If you notice any other effects, check with your doctor.

December 1987

THIABENDAZOLE (Systemic)

Some commonly used brand names are:

Foldan*	Minzolum*
Mintezol	Triasox*

*Not available in the U.S.

To the Reader: If you do not recognize the names of medical conditions or medicines referred to in this information, check with your doctor, nurse, or pharmacist. Definitions for selected medical terms may be found in the Glossary. Brand names for the generic drug names listed can be found in the Index. In addition, selected brand names commonly associated with the generic name have been included in the text to help you recognize medicine you may be taking. The fact that a brand name product is not mentioned does not mean the information does not apply. It is a good idea for you to learn both the generic and brand names of your medicines and to write them down for future use.

Thiabendazole (thye-a-BEN-da-zole) belongs to the family of medicines called anthelmintics (ant-hel-MIN-tiks). Anthelmintics are medicines used in the treatment of worm infections.

Thiabendazole is taken by mouth to treat:

— creeping eruption (cutaneous larva migrans);
— pork worms (trichinosis; trichinellosis);
— threadworms (strongyloidiasis); and
— visceral larva migrans (toxocariasis).

This medicine may also be used for other worm infections as determined by your doctor.

Thiabendazole is available only with your doctor's prescription.

Remember:

• This medicine has been prescribed for your present infection only. Another infection later on may require a different medicine. Also, even though other people may have the same symptoms as you, they may have a different kind of infection. Your medicine may not work for them and may even cause them harm. Therefore, **your medicine must not be given to other people or used for other infections** unless you are otherwise directed by your doctor.

• In order for this medicine to work, it must be taken as directed.

• Keep all medicines out of the reach of children.

• If you want more information about this medicine, ask your doctor, nurse, or pharmacist.

• If any of the following information causes you special concern, do not decide against taking this medicine without first checking with your doctor.

Before Using This Medicine

In order to decide on the best treatment for your medical problem, your doctor should be told:

— if you have ever had any unusual or allergic reaction to thiabendazole.

— if you are **pregnant** or if you may become pregnant. Studies have not been done in humans. In addition, thiabendazole has not been shown to cause birth defects or other problems in studies in rabbits, rats, and mice given 2½ to 15 times the usual human dose. However, another study in mice given 10 times the usual human dose has shown that thiabendazole causes cleft palate (a split in the roof of the mouth) and bone defects.

— if you are **breast-feeding**. It is not known whether thiabendazole passes into human breast milk. This medicine has not been shown to cause problems in nursing babies. However, thiabendazole does pass into the milk of cattle.

— if you have either of the following medical problems:
  Kidney disease
  Liver disease

Proper Use of This Medicine

No special preparations (for example, special diets, fasting, other medicines, laxatives, or enemas) are necessary before, during, or immediately after taking thiabendazole.

To help clear up your infection completely, **take this medicine exactly as directed by your doctor for the full time of treatment.** In some patients a second course of this medicine may be required to clear up the infection completely. **Do not miss any doses.**

If you do miss a dose of this medicine, take it as soon as possible. However, if it is almost time for your next dose and your dosing schedule is:

• 1 dose a day (after a meal)—Space the missed dose and the next dose 10 to 12 hours apart.

• 2 doses a day (after meals)—Space the missed dose and the next dose 4 to 5 hours apart.

Then go back to your regular dosing schedule.

Thiabendazole is best taken after meals (breakfast and evening meal). This helps to prevent some common side effects such as nausea, vomiting, dizziness, or loss of appetite.

For patients taking the oral liquid form of thiabendazole:

• Use a specially marked measuring spoon or other device to measure each dose accurately since the average household teaspoon may not hold the right amount of liquid.

For patients taking the chewable tablet form of thiabendazole:

• Tablets should be chewed or crushed before they are swallowed.

How to store this medicine:

• **Keep out of the reach of children.**

• Store away from heat and direct light.

• Do not store the chewable tablet form of this medicine in the bathroom, near the kitchen sink, or in other damp places. Heat or moisture may cause the medicine to break down.

• Keep the oral liquid form of this medicine from freezing.

• Do not keep outdated medicine or medicine no longer needed. Be sure that any discarded medicine is out of the reach of children.

Precautions While Using This Medicine

It is important that your doctor check your progress at regular visits. This is to make sure that the infection is cleared up completely.

This medicine may cause some people to become dizzy, drowsy, or to have blurred vision. If this occurs, **do not drive, use machines, or do other jobs that require you to be alert or to see clearly** while you are taking thiabendazole.

Good health habits are required to help prevent reinfection. These include the following:

• For creeping eruption (cutaneous larva migrans) or visceral larva migrans (toxocariasis):

—Keep dogs and cats off beaches and bathing areas.

—Treat household pets for worms (deworm) regularly.

—Cover children's sandboxes when not being used.

These measures help to prevent contamination of the sand or soil by worm larvae from the animals' wastes. This helps to keep children from picking up the larvae when they put their hands in their mouths after touching contaminated sand or soil.

• For pork worms (trichinosis):

—Cook all pork, pork-containing products, and game at not less than 140 °F (60 °C) until well done (not pink in the center) before eating. This will kill any trichinosis larvae that may be in the meat.

Side Effects of This Medicine

Along with its needed effects, a medicine may cause some unwanted effects. Although not all of these side effects may occur, if they do occur they may need medical attention.

Check with your doctor immediately if any of the following side effects occur:

Less common
   Aching of joints and muscles
   Chills
   Fever
   Redness, blistering, peeling, or loosening of skin
   Skin rash or itching
   Swelling
   Unusual tiredness or weakness

In addition to the side effects mentioned above, check with your doctor as soon as possible if any of the following side effects occur:

Rare
   Blurred or yellow vision
   Numbness or tingling in the hands or feet
   Ringing or buzzing sound in the ears
   Unusual feeling in the eyes

Other side effects may occur that usually do not require medical attention. These side effects may go away during treatment as your body adjusts to the medicine. However, check with your doctor if any of the following side effects continue or are bothersome:

More common
   Dizziness
   Loss of appetite
   Nausea or vomiting

Less common or rare
   Bed-wetting
   Diarrhea
   Drowsiness
   Headache
   Lower back pain
   Pain or burning while urinating
   Stomach cramps or upset

This medicine may cause the urine to have an asparagus-like or other unusual odor while you are taking it and for about 24 hours after you stop taking it. This side effect does not require medical attention.

Other side effects not listed above may also occur in some patients. If you notice any other effects, check with your doctor.

December 1987

Additional Information

For patients taking thiabendazole for pork worms (trichinosis):

• Doctors usually prescribe an adrenocorticoid (a cortisone-like medicine) for pork worms (trichinosis). They may prescribe it along with thiabendazole in certain patients, especially those with severe symptoms. This is to help reduce the reactions (for example, inflammation) to the pork worm larvae. If your doctor prescribes these two medicines, it is important to take the adrenocorticoid along with thiabendazole. Take them exactly as directed by your doctor; do not miss any doses.

THIABENDAZOLE (Topical)

A commonly used brand name is Mintezol.

To the Reader: If you do not recognize the names of medical conditions or medicines referred to in this information, check with your doctor, nurse, or pharmacist. Definitions for selected medical terms may be found in the Glossary. Brand names for the generic drug names listed can be found in the Index. In addition, selected brand names commonly associated with the generic name have been included in the text to help you recognize medicine you may be taking. The fact that a brand name product is not mentioned does not mean the information does not apply. It is a good idea for you to learn both the generic and brand names of your medicines and to write them down for future use.

Thiabendazole (thye-a-BEN-da-zole) belongs to the family of medicines called anthelmintics (ant-hel-MIN-tiks). Anthelmintics are medicines used in the treatment of worm infections.

Thiabendazole topical preparations are used on the skin to treat cutaneous larva migrans (creeping eruption). Cutaneous larva migrans is caused by dog and cat hookworm larvae. These larvae cause slowly moving burrows or tunnels in the skin. This may result in itching, redness, or inflammation around the end of the burrows or tunnels.

Thiabendazole is available only with your doctor's prescription.

Remember:
• This medicine has been prescribed for your present infection only. Another infection later on may require a different medicine. Also, even though other people may have the same symptoms as you, they may have a different kind of infection. Your medicine may not work for them and may even cause them harm. Therefore, **your medicine must not be given to other people or used for other infections** unless you are otherwise directed by your doctor.

• In order for this medicine to work, it must be used as directed.

• Keep all medicines out of the reach of children.

• If you want more information about this medicine, ask your doctor, nurse, or pharmacist.

• If any of the following information causes you special concern, do not decide against using this medicine without first checking with your doctor.

Before Using This Medicine

In order to decide on the best treatment for your medical problem, your doctor should be told:
—if you have ever had any unusual or allergic reaction to thiabendazole.

—if you are **pregnant** or if you may become pregnant. Thiabendazole may be absorbed through the skin. However, thiabendazole topical preparations have not been shown to cause birth defects or other problems in humans.

—if you are **breast-feeding**. Thiabendazole may be absorbed through the skin. However, thiabendazole topical preparations have not been shown to cause problems in nursing babies.

Proper Use of This Medicine

Apply thiabendazole directly to and about 5 to 7.5 cm (2 to 3 inches) around the slowly moving end of each burrow or tunnel being made by the larva of the worm in the skin.

To help clear up your infection completely, **use this medicine exactly as directed by your doctor for the full time of treatment. Do not miss any doses.**

If you do miss a dose of this medicine, apply it as soon as possible. However, if it is almost time for your next dose, skip the missed dose and go back to your regular dosing schedule.

How to store this medicine:
• **Keep out of the reach of children.**
• Store away from heat and direct light.
• Keep the medicine from freezing.
• Do not keep outdated medicine or medicine no longer needed. Be sure that any discarded medicine is out of the reach of children.

Precautions While Using This Medicine

If your skin problem does not improve within a few days, or if the burrow or tunnel continues to get longer, check with your doctor.

Side Effects of This Medicine

There have not been any common or important side effects reported with this medicine when used on the skin. However, if you notice any side effects, check with your doctor.

December 1987

THIAMINE (VITAMIN B₁) (Systemic)

Some commonly used brand names are:

Betalin S	Bewon
Betaxin*	Biamine

Generic name product may also be available in the U.S. and Canada.

---

*Not available in the U.S.

To the Reader: If you do not recognize the names of medical conditions or medicines referred to in this information, check with your doctor, nurse, or pharmacist. Definitions for selected medical terms may be found in the Glossary. Brand names for the generic drug names listed can be found in the Index. In addition, selected brand names commonly associated with the generic name have been included in the text to help you recognize medicine you may be taking. The fact that a brand name product is not mentioned does not mean the information does not apply. It is a good idea for you to learn both the generic and brand names of your medicines and to write them down for future use.

Vitamins (VYE-ta-mins) are compounds that you *must* have for growth and health. They are needed in small amounts only and are usually available in the foods that you eat. Thiamine (THYE-a-min) (vitamin B₁) is necessary for normal metabolism.

Lack of thiamine may lead to a condition called beriberi. Signs of beriberi include loss of appetite, constipation, muscle weakness, pain or tingling in arms or legs, and possible swelling of feet or lower legs. In addition, if severe, lack of thiamine may cause mental depression, memory problems, weakness, shortness of breath, and rapid heartbeat. Your doctor may treat this by prescribing thiamine for you.

Thiamine may also be used for other conditions as determined by your doctor.

Claims that thiamine is effective for treatment of skin problems, chronic diarrhea, tiredness, mental problems, multiple sclerosis, nerve problems, and ulcerative colitis (a disease of the intestines), or as an insect repellant or to stimulate appetite have not been proven.

Oral forms of thiamine are available without a prescription. However, it may be a good idea to check with your doctor before taking thiamine on your own.

Remember:

• **Keep all medicines out of the reach of children.**

• In order for this medicine to work, it must be used as directed. **If you are using this medicine without a prescription, it is very important to follow the directions on the label.**

• **It is also very important that you read and understand the following information.** If any of the information causes you special concern, check with your doctor before using this medicine without a prescription.

• Before you begin using any new medicine (prescription or nonprescription) or if you develop any new medical problem while you are using this medicine, check with your doctor, nurse, or pharmacist.

• **If you have any questions** about the following information or if you want more information about this medicine or your medical problem, **ask your doctor, nurse, or pharmacist.**

Importance of Diet

Vitamin supplements should be taken only if you cannot get enough vitamins in your diet. A balanced diet should provide all the vitamins you normally need.

Nutritionists recommend that you eat:
• Cereal or bread—4 or more servings per day and
• Dairy products (milk, cheese, ice cream, cottage cheese)—3 or more servings per day and
• Meat, fish, or eggs—2 or more servings per day and
• Vegetables and fruits—4 or more servings per day.

If you are not getting all of these foods every day, you may not be getting enough vitamins in your diet. The best way to correct this is to start eating the foods that contain what you need.

Thiamine is found in various foods, including cereals (whole-grain and enriched) and meats (especially pork). Some thiamine in foods is lost with cooking.

Vitamins alone will not take the place of a good diet and will not provide energy. Your body also needs other substances found in food such as protein, minerals, carbohydrates, and fat. Vitamins themselves often cannot work without the presence of other foods.

In some cases, it may not be possible for you to get enough food to supply you with the proper vitamins. In other cases, the amount of vitamins you need may be increased above normal. Therefore, a vitamin supplement may be needed.

Experts have developed a list of recommended dietary allowances (RDA) for most of the vitamins. The RDA are not an exact number but a general idea of how much you need. They do not cover amounts needed for problems caused by a serious lack of vitamins.

The RDA for thiamine are:

Children 4 to 6 years of age—0.9 mg per day
Adult males—1.4 mg per day
Adult females—1 mg per day
Pregnant females—1.4 mg per day
Breast-feeding females—1.5 mg per day.

Remember:

• The total amount of each vitamin that you get every day includes what you get from the foods that you eat *and* what you may take as a supplement.

• This total amount should not be greater than the RDA, unless ordered by your doctor.

Before Using This Medicine

In deciding whether you need additional thiamine, the following should be kept in mind and/or your doctor and pharmacist should be told:

—if you have ever had any unusual or allergic reaction to thiamine.

—if you are on a low-salt, low-sugar, or any other special diet, or if you are allergic to any substance, such as foods, sulfites or other preservatives, or dyes.

Most medicines contain more than their active ingredient. Your doctor, nurse, or pharmacist can help you avoid products that may cause a problem.

—if you are **pregnant** or if you may become pregnant. It is especially important that you are receiving enough vitamins when you become pregnant and that you continue to receive the right amount of vitamins throughout your pregnancy. The healthy growth and development of the fetus depend on a steady supply of nutrients from the mother.

—if you are **breast-feeding**. It is especially important that you receive the right amounts of vitamins so that your baby will also get the vitamins needed to grow properly.

—if you are not able to get a diet that contains all of the vitamins you need. This may occur with rapid weight loss, unusual diets (such as some reducing diets in which choice of foods is very limited), prolonged intravenous feeding, or malnutrition.

—if you do heavy manual labor, since this may increase your need for thiamine.

—if you have had a large part of your stomach or intestine removed.

—if you have been under a lot of stress for a long time, or if you have had a long illness or serious injury.

—if you have any of the following medical problems:
    Alcoholism
    Burns
    Diarrhea (prolonged)
    Intestinal problems
    Liver disease
    Overactive thyroid

—if you are taking **any** other prescription or nonprescription (OTC) medicine.

Proper Use of This Medicine

Some people believe that taking very large doses of vitamins (called megadoses or megavitamin therapy) is useful for treating certain medical problems. Studies have not proven this. Large doses should be taken only under the direction of your doctor after need has been identified.

If you miss taking a vitamin for one or more days there is no cause for concern, since it takes some time for your body to become seriously low in vitamins. However, if your doctor has recommended that you take this vitamin, try to remember to take it as directed every day.

How to store this medicine:

• **Keep out of the reach of children.**

• Store away from heat and direct light.

• Do not store in the bathroom, near the kitchen sink, or in other damp places. Heat or moisture may cause the medicine to break down.

• Keep the oral liquid form of this medicine from freezing.

• Do not keep outdated medicine or medicine no longer needed. Be sure that any discarded medicine is out of the reach of children.

Side Effects of This Medicine

Along with its needed effects, a medicine may cause some unwanted effects. Although not all of these side effects may occur, if they do occur they may need medical attention.

Check with your doctor immediately if any of the following side effects occur:
    Rare—Soon after receiving injection only
        Skin rash or itching
        Wheezing

Other side effects not listed above may also occur in some patients. If you notice any other effects, check with your doctor.

_____

December 1987

THIOGUANINE (Systemic)

A commonly used brand name is Lanvis*.
Generic name product available in the U.S.

*Not available in the U.S.

To the Reader: If you do not recognize the names of medical conditions or medicines referred to in this information, check with your doctor, nurse, or pharmacist. Definitions for selected medical terms may be found in the Glossary. Brand names for the generic drug names listed can be found in the Index. In addition, selected brand names commonly associated with the generic name have been included in the text to help you recognize medicine you may be taking. The fact that a brand name product is not mentioned does not mean the information does not apply. It is a good idea for you to learn both the generic and brand names of your medicines and to write them down for future use.

Thioguanine (thye-oh-GWON-een) belongs to the group of medicines known as antimetabolites. It is taken by mouth to treat some kinds of cancer.

Thioguanine interferes with the growth of cancer cells, which are eventually destroyed. Since the growth of normal body cells may also be affected by thioguanine, other effects will also occur. Some of these may be serious and must be reported to your doctor. Other effects may not be serious but may cause concern. Some effects may not occur for months or years after the medicine is used.

Before you begin treatment with thioguanine, you and your doctor should talk about the good this medicine will do as well as the risks of using it.

Thioguanine is available only with your doctor's prescription.

Remember:

• **This medicine has been prescribed for your current medical problem only.** It must not be given to other people or used for other problems unless you are directed to do so by your doctor.

• **Keep all medicines out of the reach of children.**

• In order for this medicine to work, it must be used as directed.

• **It is very important that you read and understand the following information.** If any of the information causes you special concern, do not decide against using this medicine without first checking with your doctor.

• Before you begin using any new medicine (prescription or nonprescription) or if you develop any new medical problem while you are using this medicine, check with your doctor, nurse, or pharmacist.

• **If you have any questions** about the following information or if you want more information about this medicine or your medical problem, **ask your doctor, nurse, or pharmacist.**

Before Using This Medicine

In order to decide on the best treatment for your medical problem, your doctor should be told:

—if you have ever had any unusual or allergic reaction to thioguanine.

—if you are **pregnant** or if you intend to have children. There is a chance that this medicine may cause birth defects if either the male or female is taking it at the time of conception or if it is taken during pregnancy. In addition, many cancer medicines may cause sterility which could be permanent. Although this has not been reported with this medicine, the possibility should be kept in mind. Be sure that you have discussed this with your doctor before taking this medicine.

—if you intend to **breast-feed**. Because this medicine may cause serious side effects, breast-feeding is generally not recommended while you are receiving it.

—if you have any of the following medical problems:
   Chickenpox (including recent exposure)
   Gout (history of)
   Herpes zoster (shingles)
   Infection
   Kidney disease
   Kidney stones (history of)
   Liver disease

—if you are taking **any** other prescription or nonprescription (OTC) medicine, especially:
   Antithyroid agents (medicine for overactive thyroid)
   Azathioprine (e.g., Imuran)
   Chloramphenicol (e.g., Chloromycetin)
   Colchicine
   Flucytosine (e.g., Ancobon)
   Interferon (e.g., Intron A; Roferon-A)
   Probenecid (e.g., Benemid)
   Sulfinpyrazone (e.g., Anturane)

—if you have ever been treated with x-rays or cancer medicines.

Proper Use of This Medicine

Take this medicine only as directed by your doctor. Do not take more or less of it, and do not take it more often than your doctor ordered. The exact amount of medicine you need has been carefully worked out. Taking too much may increase the chance of side effects, while taking too little may not improve your condition.

Thioguanine is sometimes given together with certain other medicines. If you are using a combination of medicines, make sure that you take each one at the right time and do not mix them. Ask your doctor, nurse, or pharmacist to help you plan a way to take your medicine at the right times.

While you are using thioguanine, your doctor may want you to drink extra fluids so that you will pass more urine. This will help prevent kidney problems and keep your kidneys working well.

Thioguanine sometimes causes nausea and vomiting. However, it is very important that you continue to take this medicine, even if you begin to feel ill. **Do not stop taking this medicine without first checking with your doctor.** Ask your doctor, nurse, or pharmacist for ways to lessen these effects.

If you vomit shortly after taking a dose of thioguanine, check with your doctor. You may be told to take the dose again or you may have to wait until the next scheduled dose.

If you miss a dose of this medicine, do not take the missed dose at all and do not double the next one. Instead, go back to your regular dosing schedule and check with your doctor.

How to store this medicine:

- **Keep out of the reach of children.**

- Store away from heat and direct light.

- Do not store in the bathroom, near the kitchen sink, or in other damp places. Heat or moisture may cause the medicine to break down.

- Do not keep outdated medicine or medicine no longer needed. Be sure that any discarded medicine is out of the reach of children.

Precautions While Using This Medicine

It is very important that your doctor check your progress at regular visits to make sure that this medicine is working properly and to check for unwanted effects.

While you are being treated with thioguanine, and after you stop treatment with it, **do not have any immunizations without your doctor's approval**. Thioguanine lowers your body's resistance and there is a chance you might get the infection the immunization is meant to prevent. Other people living in your household should not take oral polio vaccine since there is a chance they could pass the polio virus on to you. Also, you should avoid close contact with other persons (for example, at school or work) who have taken oral polio vaccine.

Thioguanine can lower the number of white blood cells in your body. This may increase the chance of getting an infection. If you can, avoid people with colds or other infections. If you think you are getting a cold or other infection, check with your doctor.

Side Effects of This Medicine

Along with their needed effects, medicines like thioguanine can sometimes cause unwanted effects such as blood problems and other side effects; these are described below. Also, because of the way these medicines act on the body, there is a chance that they might cause other unwanted effects that may not occur until months or years after the medicine is used. These delayed effects may include certain types of cancer, such as leukemia. Discuss these possible effects with your doctor.

Although not all of these side effects may occur, if they do occur they may need medical attention.

Check with your doctor immediately if any of the following side effects occur:
More common
  Fever, chills, or sore throat
  Unusual bleeding or bruising

Check with your doctor as soon as possible if any of the following side effects occur:
Less common
  Joint pain
  Lower back, side, or stomach pain
  Swelling of feet or lower legs
  Unsteadiness when walking
Rare
  Black tarry stools
  Sores in the mouth and on the lips
  Yellow eyes and skin

Other side effects may occur that usually do not require medical attention. These side effects may go away during treatment as your body adjusts to the medicine. Also, your doctor or nurse may be able to tell you about ways to prevent or reduce some of these side effects. Check with your doctor if any of the following side effects continue or are bothersome or if you have any questions about them:
Less common
  Diarrhea
  Loss of appetite
  Nausea and vomiting
  Skin rash or itching

For elderly patients: Many medicines have not been tested in older people. Therefore, it is not known whether the medicine acts the same way it does in younger adults. Check with your doctor if you notice any unusual effects while taking this medicine or if you think it is not working as it should.

After you stop taking thioguanine, it may still produce some side effects that need attention. During this period of time, check with your doctor if you notice any of the following side effects:
  Fever, chills, or sore throat
  Unusual bleeding or bruising

Other side effects not listed above may also occur in some patients. If you notice any other effects, check with your doctor.

December 1987

THIOTEPA (Systemic)

To the Reader: If you do not recognize the names of medical conditions or medicines referred to in this information, check with your doctor, nurse, or pharmacist. Definitions for selected medical terms may be found in the Glossary. Brand names for the generic drug names listed can be found in the Index. In addition, selected brand names commonly associated with the generic name have been included in the text to help you recognize medicine you may be taking. The fact that a brand name product is not mentioned does not mean the information does not apply. It is a good idea for you to learn both the generic and brand names of your medicines and to write them down for future use.

Thiotepa (thye-oh-TEP-a) belongs to the group of medicines called alkylating agents. It is given by injection to treat some kinds of cancer.

Thiotepa interferes with the growth of cancer cells, which are eventually destroyed. Since the growth of normal body cells may also be affected by thiotepa, other effects will also occur. Some of these may be serious and must be reported to your doctor. Other effects, like hair loss, may not be serious but may cause concern. Some effects do not occur for months or years after the medicine is used.

Before you begin treatment with thiotepa, you and your doctor should talk about the good this medicine will do as well as the risks of using it.

Thiotepa is to be administered only by or under the immediate supervision of your doctor.

Remember:

• **It is very important that you read and understand the following information.** If any of the information causes you special concern, do not decide against receiving this medicine without first checking with your doctor.

• Before you begin using any new medicine (prescription or nonprescription) or if you develop any new medical problem while you are receiving this medicine, check with your doctor, nurse, or pharmacist.

• **If you have any questions** about the following information or if you want more information about this medicine or your medical problem, **ask your doctor, nurse, or pharmacist.**

Before Using This Medicine

In order to decide on the best treatment for your medical problem, your doctor should be told:

—if you have ever had any unusual or allergic reaction to thiotepa.

—if you are **pregnant** or if you intend to have children. There is a chance that this medicine may cause birth defects if either the male or female is using it at the time of conception or if it is used during pregnancy. Studies have shown that thiotepa causes birth defects in humans. In addition, many cancer medicines may cause sterility which could be permanent. Although this is uncommon with this medicine, the possibility should be kept in mind. Be sure that you have discussed this with your doctor before using this medicine.

—if you intend to **breast-feed**. Because this medicine may cause serious side effects, breast-feeding is generally not recommended while you are receiving it. It is not known whether thiotepa passes into the breast milk.

—if you have any of the following medical problems:
   Chickenpox (including recent exposure)
   Gout (history of)
   Herpes zoster (shingles)
   Infection
   Kidney disease
   Kidney stones (history of)
   Liver disease

—if you are taking **any** other prescription or nonprescription (OTC) medicine, especially:
   Antithyroid agents (medicine for overactive thyroid)
   Azathioprine (e.g., Imuran)
   Chloramphenicol (e.g., Chloromycetin)
   Colchicine
   Flucytosine (e.g., Ancobon)
   Interferon (e.g., Intron A, Roferon-A)
   Probenecid (e.g., Benemid)
   Sulfinpyrazone (e.g., Anturane)

—if you have ever been treated with x-rays or cancer medicines.

Proper Use of This Medicine

While you are using thiotepa, your doctor may want you to drink extra fluids so that you will pass more urine. This will help prevent kidney problems and keep your kidneys working well.

Thiotepa sometimes causes nausea, vomiting, and loss of appetite. However, it is very important that you continue to receive the medicine, even if you begin to feel ill. Ask your doctor, nurse, or pharmacist for ways to lessen these effects.

Precautions While Using This Medicine

It is very important that your doctor check your progress at regular visits to make sure that this medicine is working properly and to check for unwanted effects.

Before having any kind of surgery, including dental surgery, make sure the physician or dentist in charge knows that you are taking this medicine.

While you are being treated with thiotepa, and after you stop treatment with it, **do not have any immunizations without your doctor's approval**. Thiotepa lowers your body's resistance and there is a chance you might get the infection the immunization is meant to prevent. Other people living in your household should not take oral polio vaccine since there is a chance they could pass the polio virus on to you. Also, you should avoid close contact with other persons (for example, at school or work) who have taken oral polio vaccine.

Thiotepa can lower the number of white blood cells in your body. This may increase the chance of getting an infection. If you can, avoid people with colds or other infections. If you think you are getting a cold or other infection, check with your doctor.

Side Effects of This Medicine

Along with their needed effects, medicines like thiotepa can sometimes cause unwanted effects such as blood problems, loss of hair, and other side effects; these are described below. Also, because of the way these medicines act on the body, there is a chance that they might cause other unwanted effects that may not occur until months or years after the medicine is used. These delayed effects may include certain types of cancer, such as leukemia. Discuss these possible effects with your doctor.

Although not all of these side effects may occur, if they do occur they may need medical attention.

Check with your doctor or nurse immediately if any of the following side effects occur:

More common
    Fever, chills, or sore throat
    Unusual bleeding or bruising

Rare
    Skin rash
    Tightness of throat
    Wheezing

Check with your doctor or nurse as soon as possible if any of the following side effects occur:

Less common
    Joint pain
    Lower back, side, or stomach pain
    Pain at place of injection or instillation
    Swelling of feet or lower legs

Rare
    Painful or difficult urination
    Sores in the mouth and on the lips

Other side effects may occur that usually do not require medical attention. These side effects may go away during treatment as your body adjusts to the medicine.

Also, your doctor or nurse may be able to tell you about ways to prevent or reduce some of these side effects. Check with your doctor if any of the following side effects continue or are bothersome or if you have any questions about them:

Less common
    Dizziness
    Hives
    Loss of appetite
    Missing menstrual periods
    Nausea and vomiting

This medicine may cause a temporary loss of hair in some people. After treatment with thiotepa has ended, normal hair growth should return.

For elderly patients: Many medicines have not been tested in older people. Therefore, it is not known whether the medicine acts the same way it does in younger adults. Check with your doctor if you notice any unusual effects while taking this medicine or if you think it is not working as it should.

After you stop receiving thiotepa, it may still produce some side effects that need attention. During this period of time, check with your doctor if you notice any of the following:
    Fever, chills, or sore throat
    Unusual bleeding or bruising

Other side effects not listed above may also occur in some patients. If you notice any other effects, check with your doctor.

December 1987

THIOXANTHENES (Systemic)

This information applies to the following medicines:

Chlorprothixene (klor-proe-THIX-een)
Flupenthixol (floo-pen-THIX-ole)
Thiothixene (thye-oh-THIX-een)

Some commonly used brand names are:	Generic names:
Taractan Tarasan*	Chlorprothixene
Fluanxol* Fluanxol Depot*	Flupenthixol*
Navane	Thiothixene

*Not commercially available in the U.S.

To the Reader: If you do not recognize the names of medical conditions or medicines referred to in this information, check with your doctor, nurse, or pharmacist. Definitions for selected medical terms may be found in the Glossary. Brand names for the generic drug names listed can be found in the Index. In addition, selected brand names commonly associated with the generic name have been included in the text to help you recognize medicine you may be taking. The fact that a brand name product is not mentioned does not mean the information does not apply. It is a good idea for you to learn both the generic and brand names of your medicines and to write them down for future use.

This medicine belongs to the general family of medicines known as thioxanthenes. It is used in the treatment of nervous, mental, and emotional conditions. Improvement in such conditions is thought to result from the effect of the medicine on nerve pathways in specific areas of the brain. The thioxanthene medicines are usually taken by mouth, but may be given by injection when necessary.

Thioxanthene medicines are available only with your doctor's prescription.

Remember:
• **This medicine has been prescribed for your current medical problem only.** It must not be given to other people or used for other problems unless you are directed to do so by your doctor.

• **Keep all medicines out of the reach of children.**

• In order for this medicine to work, it must be used as directed.

• If you are receiving this medicine by injection, some of the information about this medicine may not apply.

• **It is very important that you read and understand the following information.** If any of the information causes you special concern, do not decide against using this medicine without first checking with your doctor.

• Before you begin using any new medicine (prescription or nonprescription) or if you develop any new medical problem while you are using this medicine, check with your doctor, nurse, or pharmacist.

• **If you have any questions** about the following information or if you want more information about this medicine or your medical problem, **ask your doctor, nurse, or pharmacist**.

Before Using This Medicine

In order to decide on the best treatment for your medical problem, your doctor should be told:

—if you have ever had any unusual or allergic reaction to this or another thioxanthene or to phenothiazine medicines.

—if you are on a low-salt, low-sugar, or any other special diet, or if you are allergic to any substance, such as foods, sulfites or other preservatives, or dyes. Most medicines contain more than their active ingredient, and many liquid medicines contain alcohol. Your doctor, nurse, or pharmacist can help you avoid products that may cause a problem.

—if you are **pregnant** or if you may become pregnant. Studies have not been done in humans. Although animal studies have not shown thioxanthenes to cause birth defects, the studies have shown that these medicines caused a decrease in fertility and fewer successful pregnancies.

—if you are **breast-feeding**. It is not known if thioxanthenes pass into the breast milk. However, thioxanthenes have not been shown to cause problems in nursing babies.

—if you have any of the following medical problems:
Alcoholism
Blood disease
Enlarged prostate
Glaucoma
Heart or blood vessel disease
Liver disease
Lung disease
Parkinson's disease
Seizure disorders
Stomach ulcers
Urination problems

—if you are taking **any** other prescription or nonprescription (OTC) medicine, especially:
Amoxapine (e.g., Asendin)
Central nervous system (CNS) depressants
Epinephrine (e.g., Adrenalin)
Guanadrel (e.g., Hylorel)
Guanethidine (e.g., Ismelin)
Haloperidol (e.g., Haldol)
Loxapine (e.g., Loxitane)
Methyldopa (e.g., Aldomet)
Metoclopramide (e.g., Reglan)
Metyrosine (e.g., Demser)
Molindone (e.g., Moban)
Pemoline (e.g., Cylert)
Phenothiazines (acetophenazine, chlorpromazine, fluphenazine, mesoridazine, perphenazine, prochlorperazine, promazine, promethazine, thioridazine, trifluoperazine, triflupromazine, trimeprazine)
Pimozide (e.g., Orap)
Quinidine (e.g., Quinidex)
Rauwolfia alkaloids (alseroxylon, deserpidine, rauwolfia serpentina, reserpine)

Proper Use of This Medicine

This medicine may be taken with food or a full glass (8 ounces) of water or milk to reduce stomach irritation.

For patients taking thiothixene oral solution:

- This medicine must be diluted before you take it. Just before taking, measure the dose with the specially marked dropper. Mix the medicine with a full glass of water, milk, tomato or fruit juice, soup, or carbonated beverage.

Do not take more of this medicine or take it more often than your doctor ordered. This is particularly important when this medicine is given to children, since they may react very strongly to its effects.

Sometimes this medicine must be taken for several weeks before its full effect is reached.

If you miss a dose of this medicine, take it as soon as possible. However, if it is within 2 hours of your next dose, skip the missed dose and go back to your regular dosing schedule. Do not double doses.

How to store this medicine:

- **Keep out of the reach of children.**

- Store away from heat and direct light.

- Do not store the capsule or tablet form of this medicine in the bathroom, near the kitchen sink, or in other damp places. Heat or moisture may cause the medicine to break down.

- Keep the liquid form of this medicine from freezing.

- Do not keep outdated medicine or medicine no longer needed. Be sure that any discarded medicine is out of the reach of children.

Precautions While Using This Medicine

Your doctor should check your progress at regular visits. This will allow the dosage of the medicine to be adjusted when necessary and also will reduce the possibility of side effects.

Do not stop taking this medicine without first checking with your doctor. Your doctor may want you to gradually reduce the amount you are taking before stopping completely. This is to prevent side effects and to prevent your condition from becoming worse.

This medicine will add to the effects of alcohol and other CNS depressants (medicines that slow down the nervous system, possibly causing drowsiness). Some examples of CNS depressants are antihistamines or medicine for hay fever, other allergies, or colds; sedatives, tranquilizers, or sleeping medicine; prescription pain medicine or narcotics; barbiturates; medicine for convulsions (seizures); muscle relaxants; or anesthetics, including some dental anesthetics. **Check with your doctor before taking any such depressants while you are using this medicine.**

Do not take this medicine within an hour of taking antacids or medicine for diarrhea. Taking them too close together may make this medicine less effective.

Before having any kind of surgery, dental treatment, or emergency treatment, tell the physician or dentist in charge that you are using this medicine.

This medicine may cause some people to become drowsy or less alert than they are normally, especially during the first few weeks the medicine is being taken. Even if you take this medicine only at bedtime, you may feel drowsy or less alert on arising. **Make sure you know how you react to this medicine before you drive, use machines, or do other jobs that require you to be alert.**

Dizziness, lightheadedness, or fainting may occur while you are taking this medicine, especially when you get up from a lying or sitting position. Getting up slowly may help. If the problem continues or gets worse, check with your doctor.

Sometimes, patients may show signs of restlessness and excitement after taking this medicine. If this occurs, check with your doctor as soon as possible.

This medicine will often make you sweat less, allowing your body temperature to increase. **Use extra care not to become overheated during exercise or hot weather while you are taking this medicine,** since overheating could possibly result in heat stroke. **Also, hot baths or saunas may make you feel dizzy or faint while you are taking this medicine.**

Some people who take this medicine may become more sensitive to sunlight than they are normally. When you first begin taking this medicine, avoid too much sun, wear sunglasses, and do not use a sunlamp until you see how you react, especially if you tend to burn easily. **If you have a severe reaction, check with your doctor.**

This medicine may cause dryness of the mouth. For temporary relief, use sugarless gum or candy, melt bits of ice in your mouth, or use a saliva substitute. However, if dry mouth continues for more than 2 weeks, check with your physician or dentist. Continuing dryness of the mouth may increase the chance of dental disease, including tooth decay, gum disease, and fungal infections.

If you are taking a liquid form of this medicine, **try to avoid spilling it on your skin or clothing.** Skin rash and irritation have been caused by similar medicines.

If you are receiving this medicine by injection:

- The effects of the long-acting injection form of this medicine may last for up to 3 weeks. The precautions and side effects information for this medicine applies during this period of time.

Side Effects of This Medicine

Along with its needed effects, a medicine may cause some unwanted effects. Although not all of these side effects may occur, if they do occur they may require medical attention.

Stop taking this medicine and get emergency help immediately if any of the following side effects occur:

Rare

Convulsions (seizures)
Difficulty in breathing
Fast heartbeat
Fever
High or low (irregular) blood pressure
Increased sweating
Loss of bladder control
Muscle stiffness (severe)
Unusual feeling of tiredness
Unusually pale skin

Also, check with your doctor as soon as possible if any of the following side effects occur:

More common

Blurred vision or other eye problems
Difficulty in talking or swallowing
Fainting
Fixation of eyes
Loss of balance control
Mask-like face
Muscle spasms, especially of the neck and back
Restlessness or need to keep moving (severe)
Shuffling walk
Stiffness of arms and legs
Trembling and shaking of fingers and hands
Twisting movements of body

Less common

Chewing movements
Difficult urination
Lip smacking or puckering
Puffing of cheeks
Rapid or worm-like movements of tongue
Skin discoloration
Skin rash
Uncontrolled movements of the arms and legs

Rare

Sore throat and fever
Yellow eyes or skin

Signs of overdose

Difficulty in breathing (severe)
Dizziness (severe)
Drowsiness (severe)
Muscle trembling, jerking, stiffness, or uncontrolled movements (severe)
Small pupils
Unusual excitement
Unusual tiredness or weakness (severe)

Other side effects may occur that usually do not require medical attention. These side effects may go away during treatment as your body adjusts to the medicine. However, check with your doctor if any of the following side effects continue or are bothersome:

More common

Constipation
Decreased sweating
Dizziness, lightheadedness, or fainting
Drowsiness (mild)
Dry mouth
Increased appetite and weight
Increased sensitivity of skin or eyes to sunlight
Stuffy nose

Less common

Changes in menstrual period
Decreased sexual ability
Swelling of breasts (in males and females)
Unusual secretion of milk

After you stop taking this medicine your body may need time to adjust, especially if you took this medicine in high doses or for a long period of time. If you stop taking it too quickly, the following withdrawal effects may occur and should be reported to your doctor:

Dizziness
Nausea and vomiting
Stomach pain
Trembling of fingers and hands
Uncontrolled, continuing movements of mouth, tongue, or jaw

Although not all of the side effects listed above have been reported for all thioxanthenes, they have been reported for at least one of them. However, since these medicines are very similar, any of the above side effects may occur with any of them.

For children and the elderly: The above side effects, especially constipation, dizziness or fainting, drowsiness, dry mouth, uncontrolled movements of the mouth and tongue, and trembling of fingers and hands are more likely to occur in older children and the elderly, who are usually more sensitive to the effects of thioxanthenes.

Other side effects not listed above may also occur in some patients. If you notice any other effects, check with your doctor.

December 1987

THROMBOLYTIC AGENTS (Systemic)

This information applies to the following medicines:

Streptokinase (strep-toe-KYE-nase)
Urokinase (yoor-oh-KYE-nase)

Some commonly used brand names are:	Generic names:
Kabikinase Streptase	Streptokinase
Abbokinase Ukidan*	Urokinase

*Not available in the U.S.

To the Reader: If you do not recognize the names of medical conditions or medicines referred to in this information, check with your doctor, nurse, or pharmacist. Definitions for selected medical terms may be found in the Glossary. Brand names for the generic drug names listed can be found in the Index. In addition, selected brand names commonly associated with the generic name have been included in the text to help you recognize medicine you may be taking. The fact that a brand name product is not mentioned does not mean the information does not apply. It is a good idea for you to learn both the generic and brand names of your medicines and to write them down for future use.

Thrombolytic agents are used to break up (lyse) or dissolve blood clots that have formed in certain blood vessels. These medicines are most likely to be used when a blood clot seriously lessens the flow of blood to certain parts of the body.

Thrombolytic agents are also used to dissolve blood clots that form in tubes that are placed into the body. The tubes allow treatments (such as dialysis or injections into a vein) to be given over a long period of time. When used to clear these tubes, the medicine is placed directly into the tube. It is not injected into the body. However, some may get into the body and cause unwanted effects.

These medicines are used only in a hospital. They are given by or under the direct supervision of a doctor.

Remember:

• If you want more information about this medicine, ask your doctor, nurse, or pharmacist.

• If any of the following information causes you special concern, discuss the use of this medicine with your doctor before deciding whether or not to receive it.

Before Using This Medicine

In order to decide on the best treatment for your medical problem, your doctor should be told:

—if you have ever had any unusual or allergic reaction to streptokinase or urokinase.

—if you have received streptokinase within the past year.

—if you are **pregnant** or if you have recently delivered a baby. Studies in humans have not shown that streptokinase causes miscarriage or birth defects or other problems in the fetus or newborn baby. However, there is a slight chance that use of a thrombolytic agent during the first 5 months of pregnancy may cause a miscarriage.

Studies on birth defects with urokinase have not been done in humans. However, studies in animals have not shown that urokinase causes birth defects or other problems.

Use of a thrombolytic agent soon after the birth of a baby may cause serious bleeding in the mother.

—if you are **breast-feeding**. Streptokinase or urokinase has not been shown to cause problems in nursing babies. However, it is not known whether these medicines pass into the breast milk.

—if you have recently had a streptococcal ("strep") infection.

—if you have any of the following medical problems:

Blood disease, bleeding problems, or a history of bleeding in any part of the body
Brain disease or tumor
Colitis or stomach ulcer (or history of)
Heart or blood vessel disease
High blood pressure
Stroke (or history of)
Tuberculosis (TB) (active)

—if you have recently had any of the following conditions:

Falls or blows to the body or head or any other injury
Injections into a blood vessel
Placement of any tube into the body
Surgery, including dental surgery

—if you are taking **any** other prescription or nonprescription (OTC) medicine, especially:

Anticoagulants (blood thinners)
Dipyridamole (e.g., Persantine)
Divalproex (e.g., Depakote)
Heparin
Medicine for pain and/or inflammation (aspirin or other salicylates, diclofenac [e.g., Voltaren], diflunisal [e.g., Dolobid], fenoprofen [e.g., Nalfon], flurbiprofen [oral] [e.g., Ansaid], ibuprofen [e.g., Motrin], indomethacin [e.g., Indocin], ketoprofen [e.g., Orudis], meclofenamate [e.g., Meclomen], mefenamic acid [e.g., Ponstel], naproxen [e.g., Naprosyn], phenylbutazone [e.g., Butazolidin], piroxicam [e.g., Feldene], sulindac [e.g., Clinoril], tiaprofenic acid [e.g., Surgam], tolmetin [e.g., Tolectin])
Sulfinpyrazone (e.g., Anturane)
Valproic acid (e.g., Depakene)

Precautions While Using This Medicine

Streptokinase and urokinase can cause bleeding that usually is not serious. However, serious bleeding may occur in some people. **To help prevent serious bleeding, follow any instructions given by your doctor or nurse very carefully. Also, move around as little as possible, and do not get out of bed on your own, while receiving this medicine.**

Side Effects of This Medicine

Along with its needed effects, a medicine may cause some unwanted effects. Although not all of these side effects may occur, if they do occur they may need medical attention.

Tell your doctor or nurse immediately if any of the following side effects occur:

More common

Bleeding or oozing from cuts or around the place of injection

Fast, slow, or irregular heartbeat

Fever

Less common or rare

Flushing or redness of skin

Headache (mild)

Muscle pain (mild)

Nausea

Shortness of breath, troubled breathing, tightness in chest, or wheezing

Skin rash, itching, or hives

Swelling of eyes, face, lips, or tongue

Signs of bleeding inside the body

Abdominal or stomach pain or swelling

Back pain or backaches

Blood in urine

Bloody or black tarry stools

Constipation

Coughing up blood

Dizziness

Headaches (severe or continuing)

Joint pain, stiffness, or swelling

Muscle pain or stiffness (severe or continuing)

Nosebleeds

Unexpected or unusually heavy bleeding from vagina

Vomiting of blood or material that looks like coffee grounds

Other side effects not listed above may also occur in some patients. If you notice any other effects, check with your doctor.

_____

December 1987

_____

THYROID HORMONES (Systemic)

This information applies to the following medicines:

Levothyroxine (lee-voe-thye-ROX-een)
Liothyronine (lye-oh-THYE-roe-neen)
Liotrix (LYE-oh-trix)
Thyroglobulin (thye-roe-GLOB-yoo-lin)
Thyroid (THYE-roid)

This information does not apply to Thyrotropin.

Some commonly used brand names are:	Generic names:
Eltroxin* Levothroid Levoxine Synthroid	Levothyroxine
Cytomel	Liothyronine
Euthroid Thyrolar	Liotrix
Proloid	Thyroglobulin
	Thyroid†

*Not available in the U.S.
†Generic name product may also be available.

To the Reader: If you do not recognize the names of medical conditions or medicines referred to in this information, check with your doctor, nurse, or pharmacist. Definitions for selected medical terms may be found in the Glossary. Brand names for the generic drug names listed can be found in the Index. In addition, selected brand names commonly associated with the generic name have been included in the text to help you recognize medicine you may be taking. The fact that a brand name product is not mentioned does not mean the information does not apply. It is a good idea for you to learn both the generic and brand names of your medicines and to write them down for future use.

Thyroid medicines belong to the general group of medicines called hormones. They are used when the thyroid gland does not produce enough hormone.

These medicines are available only with your doctor's prescription.

Remember:

• **This medicine has been prescribed for your current medical problem only.** It must not be given to other people or used for other problems unless you are directed to do so by your doctor.

• **Keep all medicines out of the reach of children.**

• In order for this medicine to work, it must be used as directed.

• If you are receiving this medicine by injection, some of the information about this medicine may not apply.

• **It is very important that you read and understand the following information.** If any of the information causes you special concern, do not decide against using this medicine without first checking with your doctor.

• Before you begin using any new medicine (prescription or nonprescription) or if you develop any new medical problem while you are using this medicine, check with your doctor, nurse, or pharmacist.

• **If you have any questions** about the following information or if you want more information about this medicine or your medical problem, **ask your doctor, nurse, or pharmacist.**

Before Using This Medicine

In order to decide on the best treatment for your medical problem, your doctor should be told:

—if you have ever had any unusual or allergic reaction to thyroid medicine.

—if you are on a low-salt, low-sugar, or any other special diet, or if you are allergic to any substance, such as foods, sulfites or other preservatives, or dyes. Most medicines contain more than their active ingredient. Your doctor, nurse, or pharmacist can help you avoid products that may cause a problem.

—if you are **pregnant** or if you may become pregnant. It is essential that your baby receive the right amount of thyroid for normal development. You may need to take different amounts while you are pregnant. In addition, you may respond differently than usual to some tests. Your doctor should check your progress at regular visits while you are pregnant.

—if you are **breast-feeding**, although use of proper amounts of thyroid hormones by mothers has not been shown to cause problems in nursing babies.

—if you have any of the following medical problems:
Diabetes mellitus (sugar diabetes)
Hardening of the arteries
Heart disease
High blood pressure
Overactive thyroid (history of)
Underactive adrenal gland
Underactive pituitary gland

—if you are taking **any** other prescription or nonprescription (OTC) medicine, especially:
Amphetamines
Anticoagulants (blood thinners)
Appetite suppressants (diet pills)
Cholestyramine (e.g., Questran)
Colestipol (e.g., Colestid)
Medicine for asthma or other breathing problems
Medicine for colds, sinus problems, or hay fever or other allergies (including nose drops or sprays)

Proper Use of This Medicine

Use this medicine only as directed by your doctor. Do not use more or less of it, and do not use it more often than your doctor ordered. Your doctor has prescribed the exact amount your body needs and if you take different amounts, you may experience symptoms of an overactive or underactive thyroid. Take it at the same time each day to make sure it always has the same effect.

If your condition is due to a lack of thyroid hormone, you may have to take this medicine for the rest of your life. It is very important that you **do not stop taking this medicine without first checking with your doctor.**

If you miss a dose of this medicine, take it as soon as possible. However, if it is almost time for your next dose, skip the missed dose and go back to your regular dosing schedule. Do not double doses. If you miss 2 or more doses in a row or if you have any questions about this, check with your doctor.

How to store this medicine:

• **Keep out of the reach of children.**

• Store away from heat and direct light.

• Do not store in the bathroom, near the kitchen sink, or in other damp places. Heat or moisture may cause the medicine to break down.

• Do not keep outdated medicine or medicine no longer needed. Be sure that any discarded medicine is out of the reach of children.

Precautions While Using This Medicine

It is very important that your doctor check your progress at regular visits, to make sure that this medicine is working properly.

If you have certain kinds of heart disease, this medicine may cause chest pain or shortness of breath when you exert yourself. Do not overdo exercise or physical work. If you have any questions about this, check with your doctor.

Before having any kind of surgery (including dental surgery) or emergency treatment, **tell the physician or dentist in charge that you are taking this medicine.**

Do not take any other medicine unless prescribed by your doctor. Some medicines may increase or decrease the effects of thyroid on your body and cause problems in controlling your condition. Also, thyroid hormones may change the effects of other medicines.

Side Effects of This Medicine

Along with its needed effects, a medicine may cause some unwanted effects. Although not all of these side effects may occur, if they do occur they may need medical attention.

Check with your doctor as soon as possible if any of the following side effects occur since they may indicate an overdose or an allergic reaction:

Rare
  Headache (severe) in children
  Skin rash or hives

Signs of overdose
  Chest pain
  Fast or irregular heartbeat
  Shortness of breath

This medicine may take a few days or weeks to have a noticeable effect on your condition. Until it begins to work, you may experience no change in your symptoms. Check with your doctor if the following symptoms continue:
  Clumsiness
  Coldness
  Constipation
  Dry, puffy skin
  Listlessness
  Muscle aches
  Sleepiness
  Tiredness
  Weakness
  Weight gain

Other effects may occur if the dose of the medicine is not exactly right. These side effects will go away when the dose is corrected. Check with your doctor if any of the following symptoms occur:
  Changes in appetite
  Changes in menstrual periods
  Diarrhea
  Fever
  Hand tremors
  Headache
  Irritability
  Leg cramps
  Nervousness
  Sensitivity to heat
  Sleeplessness
  Sweating
  Vomiting
  Weight loss

For elderly patients: Many medicines have not been tested in older people. Therefore, it is not known whether the medicine acts the same way it does in younger adults. Check with your doctor or pharmacist if you notice any unusual effects while taking this medicine or if you think it is not working as it should.

Other side effects not listed above may also occur in some patients. If you notice any other effects, check with your doctor.

December 1987

THYROTROPIN (Systemic)

A commonly used brand name is Thytropar.

To the Reader: If you do not recognize the names of medical conditions or medicines referred to in this information, check with your doctor, nurse, or pharmacist. Definitions for selected medical terms may be found in the Glossary. Brand names for the generic drug names listed can be found in the Index. In addition, selected brand names commonly associated with the generic name have been included in the text to help you recognize medicine you may be taking. The fact that a brand name product is not mentioned does not mean the information does not apply. It is a good idea for you to learn both the generic and brand names of your medicines and to write them down for future use.

Thyrotropin (thye-roe-TROE-pin) belongs to the general group of medicines called hormones. It is given by injection in a test to determine how well your thyroid is working. It is also sometimes used with other treatment for cancer of the thyroid.

Thyrotropin is to be administered only by or under the immediate supervision of your doctor.

Remember:

• **It is very important that you read and understand the following information.** If any of the information causes you special concern, do not decide against using this medicine without first checking with your doctor.

• Before you begin using any new medicine (prescription or nonprescription) or if you develop any new medical problem while you are using this medicine, check with your doctor, nurse, or pharmacist.

• **If you have any questions** about the following information or if you want more information about this medicine or your medical problem, **ask your doctor, nurse, or pharmacist.**

Before Using This Medicine

In order to decide on the best treatment for your medical problem, your doctor should be told:

—if you have ever had any unusual or allergic reaction to thyrotropin.

—if you are on a low-salt, low-sugar, or any other special diet, or if you are allergic to any substance, such as foods or sulfites or other preservatives. Most medicines contain more than their active ingredient. Your doctor, nurse, or pharmacist can help you avoid products that may cause a problem.

—if you are **pregnant,** or if you may become pregnant. Studies have not been done in either humans or animals.

—if you are **breast-feeding.** It is not known whether thyrotropin passes into breast milk. This medicine has not been shown to cause problems in nursing babies.

—if you have any of the following medical problems:
Hardening of the arteries
Heart disease
High blood pressure
Underactive adrenal gland
Underactive pituitary gland

—if you have been taking thyroid hormones regularly.

—if you are taking **any** other prescription or nonprescription (OTC) medicine.

Proper Use of This Medicine

In order for your doctor to properly treat your medical condition, **you must receive every dose of this medicine.** After the last dose, the doctor may want to perform certain tests that are very important.

Side Effects of This Medicine

Along with its needed effects, a medicine may cause some unwanted effects. Although not all of these side effects may occur, if they do occur they may need medical attention.

Check with your doctor immediately if any of the following side effects occur:
Rare
Faintness
Itching
Redness or swelling at place of injection
Skin rash
Tightness of throat
Wheezing

Other effects may occur if the dose of the medicine is not exactly right. Check with your doctor as soon as possible if any of the following symptoms occur:
Chest pain
Fast or irregular heartbeat
Irritability
Nervousness
Shortness of breath
Sweating

Other side effects may occur that usually do not require medical attention. These side effects may go away during treatment as your body adjusts to the medicine. However, check with your doctor if any of the following side effects continue or are bothersome:
More common
Flushing of face
Frequent urge to urinate
Headache
Nausea and vomiting
Stomach discomfort

For elderly patients: Many medicines have not been tested in older people. Therefore, it is not known whether the medicine acts the same way it does in younger adults. Check with your doctor or pharmacist if you notice any unusual effects while taking this medicine or if you think it is not working as it should.

Other side effects not listed above may also occur in some patients. If you notice any other effects, check with your doctor.

December 1987

TIMOLOL (Ophthalmic)

A commonly used brand name is Timoptic.

To the Reader: If you do not recognize the names of medical conditions or medicines referred to in this information, check with your doctor, nurse, or pharmacist. Definitions for selected medical terms may be found in the Glossary. Brand names for the generic drug names listed can be found in the Index. In addition, selected brand names commonly associated with the generic name have been included in the text to help you recognize medicine you may be taking. The fact that a brand name product is not mentioned does not mean the information does not apply. It is a good idea for you to learn both the generic and brand names of your medicines and to write them down for future use.

Timolol (TIM-oh-lole) is used in the eye to treat certain types of glaucoma. It appears to work by reducing production of fluid in the eye to lower pressure in the eye.

This medicine is available only with your doctor's prescription.

Remember:

• **This medicine has been prescribed for your current medical problem only.** It must not be given to other people or used for other problems unless you are directed to do so by your doctor.

• **Keep all medicines out of the reach of children.**

• In order for this medicine to work, it must be used as directed.

• **It is very important that you read and understand the following information.** If any of the information causes you special concern, do not decide against using this medicine without first checking with your doctor.

• Before you begin using any new medicine (prescription or nonprescription) or if you develop any new medical problem while you are using this medicine, check with your doctor, nurse, or pharmacist.

• **If you have any questions** about the following information or if you want more information about this medicine or your medical problem, **ask your doctor, nurse, or pharmacist**.

Before Using This Medicine

In order to decide on the best treatment for your medical problem, your doctor should be told:

—if you have ever had any unusual or allergic reaction to timolol or other beta-blockers (such as acebutolol, atenolol, betaxolol, labetalol, levobunolol, metoprolol, nadolol, oxprenolol, pindolol, propranolol, or sotalol).

—if you are allergic to any substance, such as certain preservatives. Most medicines contain more than their active ingredient. Your doctor, nurse, or pharmacist can help you avoid products that may cause a problem.

—if you are **pregnant** or if you may become pregnant, since ophthalmic timolol may be absorbed into the body. Studies on birth defects have not been done in humans. However, studies in animals have not shown that timolol causes birth defects. Studies in animals have shown that timolol delays the formation of bone and increases the chance of death in the animal fetus when given in doses many times the maximum recommended human oral dose.

—if you are **breast-feeding**, since this medicine may be absorbed into the body. Although ophthalmic timolol has not been shown to cause problems, this medicine may pass into the breast milk and cause unwanted effects in nursing babies.

—if you have any of the following medical problems:
  Asthma (or history of), chronic bronchitis, emphysema, or other lung disease
  Diabetes mellitus (sugar diabetes)
  Heart or blood vessel disease
  Myasthenia gravis
  Overactive thyroid

—if you are taking **any** other prescription or nonprescription (OTC) medicine.

Proper Use of This Medicine

How to apply timolol eye drops: First, wash your hands. With the middle finger, apply pressure to the inside corner of the eye (and continue to apply pressure for 1 or 2 minutes after the medicine has been placed in the eye). Tilt the head back and with the index finger of the same hand, pull the lower eyelid away from the eye to form a pouch. Drop the medicine into the pouch and gently close the eyes. Do not blink. Keep the eyes closed for 1 or 2 minutes to allow the medicine to be absorbed.

To prevent contamination of the eye drops, do not touch the applicator tip to any surface (including the eye) and keep the container tightly closed.

Use this medicine only as directed. Do not use more of it and do not use it more often than your doctor ordered. To do so may increase the chance of too much medicine being absorbed into the body and the chance of side effects.

If you miss a dose of this medicine and your dosing schedule is one dose to be applied:

Once a day—Apply the missed dose as soon as possible. However, if you do not remember the missed dose until the next day, skip it and apply your regularly scheduled dose.

More than once a day—Apply the missed dose as soon as possible. However, if it is almost time for your next dose, skip the missed dose and apply your next dose at the regularly scheduled time. Then continue with your regular dosing schedule.

How to store this medicine:

• **Keep out of the reach of children.**

• Store away from heat and direct light.

• Keep the medicine from freezing.

• Do not keep outdated medicine or medicine no longer needed. Be sure that any discarded medicine is out of the reach of children.

Precautions While Using This Medicine

Your doctor should check your eye pressure at regular visits in order to make certain that your glaucoma is being controlled.

Before having any kind of surgery (including dental surgery) or emergency treatment, tell the physician or dentist in charge that you are using this medicine.

Diabetics—**This medicine may cause a change in your blood sugar level.** Also, **this medicine may cover up signs of hypoglycemia (low blood sugar),** such as increase in pulse rate or increased blood pressure. However, other signs of low blood sugar, such as dizziness and sweating, are not affected. If you have any questions about this, check with your doctor.

Side Effects of This Medicine

In some animal studies, timolol taken by mouth has been shown to increase the chance of both benign (not cancerous) and malignant (cancerous) tumors when given in doses many times the recommended human dose taken by mouth. However, it is not known if timolol has the same effect in humans when used in the eye in much smaller doses. You should discuss this possible effect with your doctor.

Along with its needed effects, a medicine may cause some unwanted effects. Although not all of these side effects may occur, if they do occur they may need medical attention.

Check with your doctor as soon as possible if any of the following side effects occur:

    Irritation or inflammation of eye (severe)
    Skin rash, hives, or itching
    Vision disturbances

Signs of too much medicine being absorbed into the body

    Anxiety
    Chest pain
    Confusion or mental depression
    Decreased sexual ability
    Diarrhea
    Dizziness or feeling faint
    Hallucinations (seeing, hearing, or feeling things that are not there)
    Headache
    Irregular, slow, or pounding heartbeat
    Nausea or vomiting
    Stomach cramps or pain
    Swelling of feet, ankles, and/or lower legs
    Unusual tiredness or weakness
    Wheezing or troubled breathing

Other side effects may occur that usually do not require medical attention. These side effects may go away during treatment as your body adjusts to the medicine. However, check with your doctor if either of the following side effects continues or is bothersome:

Less common or rare

    Burning or stinging of eye

For elderly patients: Many medicines have not been tested in older people. Therefore, it is not known whether the medicine acts the same way it does in younger adults. Check with your doctor or pharmacist if you notice any unusual effects while using this medicine or if you think it is not working as it should.

Other side effects not listed above may also occur in some patients. If you notice any other effects, check with your doctor.

December 1987

TOCAINIDE (Systemic)

A commonly used brand name is Tonocard.

To the Reader: If you do not recognize the names of medical conditions or medicines referred to in this information, check with your doctor, nurse, or pharmacist. Definitions for selected medical terms may be found in the Glossary. Brand names for the generic drug names listed can be found in the Index. In addition, selected brand names commonly associated with the generic name have been included in the text to help you recognize medicine you may be taking. The fact that a brand name product is not mentioned does not mean the information does not apply. It is a good idea for you to learn both the generic and brand names of your medicines and to write them down for future use.

Tocainide (toe-KAY-nide) belongs to the group of medicines known as antiarrhythmics. It is taken by mouth to correct irregular heartbeats to a normal rhythm.

Tocainide produces its helpful effects by slowing nerve impulses in the heart and making the heart tissue less sensitive.

Tocainide is available only with your doctor's prescription.

Remember:

• **This medicine has been prescribed for your current medical problem only.** It must not be given to other people or used for other problems unless you are directed to do so by your doctor.

• **Keep all medicines out of the reach of children.**

• In order for this medicine to work, it must be used as directed.

• **It is very important that you read and understand the following information.** If any of the information causes you special concern, do not decide against using this medicine without first checking with your doctor.

• Before you begin using any new medicine (prescription or nonprescription) or if you develop any new medical problem while you are using this medicine, check with your doctor, nurse, or pharmacist.

• **If you have any questions** about the following information or if you want more information about this medicine or your medical problem, **ask your doctor, nurse, or pharmacist.**

Before Using This Medicine

In order to decide on the best treatment for your medical problem, your doctor should be told:

—if you have ever had any unusual or allergic reaction to tocainide or anesthetics.

—if you are on a low-salt, low-sugar, or any other special diet, or if you are allergic to any substance, such as foods, sulfites or other preservatives, or dyes. Most medicines contain more than their active ingredient. Your doctor, nurse, or pharmacist can help you avoid products that may cause a problem.

—if you are **pregnant** or if you may become pregnant. Tocainide has not been shown to cause birth defects or other problems in humans. Studies in animals have shown that high doses of tocainide may increase the possibility of death in the animal fetus, although it has not been shown to cause birth defects.

—if you are **breast-feeding**. It is not known whether tocainide passes into breast milk. This medicine has not been shown to cause problems in nursing babies.

—if you have either of the following medical problems:
  Kidney disease
  Liver disease

—if you are taking **any** other prescription or nonprescription (OTC) medicine.

Proper Use of This Medicine

Take tocainide exactly as directed by your doctor, even though you may feel well. Do not take more medicine than ordered.

If tocainide upsets your stomach, your doctor may advise you to take it with food or milk.

This medicine works best when there is a constant amount in the blood. **To help keep this amount constant, do not miss any doses. Also, it is best to take each dose at evenly spaced times day and night.** For example, if you are to take 3 doses a day, the doses should be spaced about 8 hours apart. If this interferes with your sleep or other daily activities, or if you need help in planning the best times to take your medicine, check with your doctor, nurse, or pharmacist.

If you miss a dose of tocainide and remember within 4 hours, take it as soon as possible. Then go back to your regular dosing schedule. However, if you do not remember until later, skip the missed dose and go back to your regular dosing schedule. Do not double doses.

How to store this medicine:

• **Keep out of the reach of children.**

• Store away from heat and direct light.

• Do not store in the bathroom, near the kitchen sink, or in other damp places. Heat or moisture may cause the medicine to break down.

• Do not keep outdated medicine or medicine no longer needed. Be sure that any discarded medicine is out of the reach of children.

Precautions While Using This Medicine

It is important that your doctor check your progress at regular visits to make sure the medicine is working properly. This will allow for changes to be made in the amount of medicine you are taking, if necessary.

Your doctor may want you to carry a medical identification card or bracelet stating that you are using this medicine.

Tocainide may cause some people to become dizzy, lightheaded, or less alert than they are normally. **Make sure you know how you react to this medicine before you drive, use machines, or do other jobs that require you to be alert.**

Before having any kind of surgery (including dental surgery) or emergency treatment, tell the physician or dentist in charge that you are taking this medicine.

Side Effects of This Medicine

Along with its needed effects, a medicine may cause some unwanted effects. Although not all of these side effects may occur, if they do occur they may need medical attention.

Check with your doctor as soon as possible if any of the following side effects occur:

Less common

Trembling or shaking

Rare

Cough or shortness of breath
Fever, chills, or sore throat
Irregular heartbeats
Unusual bleeding or bruising

Other side effects may occur that usually do not require medical attention. These side effects may go away during treatment as your body adjusts to the medicine.

However, check with your doctor if any of the following side effects continue or are bothersome:

More common

Dizziness or lightheadedness
Loss of appetite
Nausea

Less common

Blurred vision
Confusion
Headache
Nervousness
Numbness or tingling of fingers and toes
Skin rash
Sweating
Vomiting

For elderly patients: Dizziness or lightheadedness may be more likely to occur in the elderly, who are usually more sensitive to the effects of tocainide.

Other side effects not listed above may also occur in some patients. If you notice any other effects, check with your doctor.

December 1987

TOLNAFTATE (Topical)

Some commonly used brand names are Aftate, Pitrex*, and Tinactin.

*Not available in the U.S.

To the Reader: If you do not recognize the names of medical conditions or medicines referred to in this information, check with your doctor, nurse, or pharmacist. Definitions for selected medical terms may be found in the Glossary. Brand names for the generic drug names listed can be found in the Index. In addition, selected brand names commonly associated with the generic name have been included in the text to help you recognize medicine you may be taking. The fact that a brand name product is not mentioned does not mean the information does not apply. It is a good idea for you to learn both the generic and brand names of your medicines and to write them down for future use.

Tolnaftate (tole-NAF-tate) belongs to the group of medicines called antifungals. It is used on the skin to treat some types of fungal infections. It may also be used together with medicines taken by mouth for fungal infections.

Tolnaftate is available without a prescription; however, your doctor may have special instructions on the proper use of tolnaftate for your medical problem.

Remember:
• In order for this medicine to work, it must be used as directed.

• Keep all medicines out of the reach of children.

• If you want more information about this medicine, ask your doctor, nurse, or pharmacist.

• If this medicine has been ordered by your doctor and if any of the following information causes you special concern, do not decide against using this medicine without first checking with your doctor.

Before Using This Medicine

Before you use tolnaftate, your doctor should be told:

—if you have ever had any unusual or allergic reaction to tolnaftate.

—if you are **pregnant** or if you may become pregnant. However, tolnaftate topical preparations have not been shown to cause birth defects or other problems in humans.

—if you are **breast-feeding**. However, tolnaftate topical preparations have not been shown to cause problems in nursing babies.

Proper Use of This Medicine

Keep this medicine away from the eyes.

To help clear up your infection completely, **keep using this medicine for 2 weeks after burning, itching, or other symptoms have disappeared,** unless otherwise directed by your doctor. **Do not miss any doses.**

If you do miss a dose of this medicine, apply it as soon as possible. Then go back to your regular dosing schedule.

Before applying tolnaftate, wash the area to be treated and dry thoroughly. Then apply enough medicine to cover the affected area.

For patients using the powder form of this medicine:
• If the powder is used on the feet, sprinkle it between toes, on feet, and in socks and shoes.

For patients using the aerosol powder form of this medicine:
• Shake well before using.

• From a distance of 6 to 10 inches, spray the powder on the affected areas. If it is used on the feet, spray it between toes, on feet, and in socks and shoes.

• Do not inhale the powder.

• Do not use near heat, near open flame, or while smoking.

For patients using the solution form of this medicine:
• If tolnaftate solution becomes a solid, it may be dissolved by warming the closed container of medicine in warm water.

For patients using the aerosol solution form of this medicine:
• Shake well before using.

• From a distance of 6 inches, spray the solution on the affected areas. If it is used on the feet, spray between toes and on feet.

• Do not inhale the vapors from the spray.

• Do not use near heat, near open flame, or while smoking.

For patients using the spray solution form of this medicine:
• From a distance of 4 to 6 inches, spray the solution on the affected areas. If it is used on the feet, spray between toes and on feet.

• Do not use near heat, near open flame, or while smoking.

How to store this medicine:
• **Keep out of the reach of children.**

• Store away from heat and direct light.

• Do not store the powder form of this medicine in the bathroom, near the kitchen sink, or in other damp places. Heat or moisture may cause the medicine to break down.

• Keep the medicine from freezing.

• Do not puncture, break, or burn the aerosol powder or aerosol solution container.

• Do not keep outdated medicine or medicine no longer needed. Be sure that any discarded medicine is out of the reach of children.

Precautions While Using This Medicine

If your skin problem does not improve within 4 weeks, or if it becomes worse, check with your doctor or pharmacist.

To help prevent reinfection after the period of treatment with this medicine, the powder or spray powder form of this medicine may be used each day after bathing and careful drying.

Side Effects of This Medicine

Along with its needed effects, a medicine may cause some unwanted effects. Although not all of these side effects may occur, if they do occur they may need medical attention.

Check with your doctor or pharmacist as soon as possible if the following side effect occurs:

Skin irritation not present before using this medicine

When you apply the spray solution form of this medicine, a mild temporary stinging may be expected.

Other side effects not listed above may also occur in some patients. If you notice any other effects, check with your doctor or pharmacist.

December 1987

TRAZODONE (Systemic)

Some commonly used brand names are Desyrel, Desyrel Dividose, and Trialodine.

Generic name product may also be available in the U.S.

To the Reader: If you do not recognize the names of medical conditions or medicines referred to in this information, check with your doctor, nurse, or pharmacist. Definitions for selected medical terms may be found in the Glossary. Brand names for the generic drug names listed can be found in the Index. In addition, selected brand names commonly associated with the generic name have been included in the text to help you recognize medicine you may be taking. The fact that a brand name product is not mentioned does not mean the information does not apply. It is a good idea for you to learn both the generic and brand names of your medicines and to write them down for future use.

Trazodone (TRAZ-oh-done) belongs to the group of medicines known as antidepressants or "mood elevators." It is taken by mouth to relieve mental depression and depression that sometimes occurs with anxiety.

Trazodone is available only with your doctor's prescription.

Remember:

• **This medicine has been prescribed for your current medical problem only.** It must not be given to other people or used for other problems unless you are directed to do so by your doctor.

• **Keep all medicines out of the reach of children.**

• In order for this medicine to work, it must be used as directed.

• **It is very important that you read and understand the following information.** If any of the information causes you special concern, do not decide against using this medicine without first checking with your doctor.

• Before you begin using any new medicine (prescription or nonprescription) or if you develop any new medical problem while you are using this medicine, check with your doctor, nurse, or pharmacist.

• **If you have any questions** about the following information or if you want more information about this medicine or your medical problem, **ask your doctor, nurse, or pharmacist.**

Before Using This Medicine

In order to decide on the best treatment for your medical problem, your doctor should be told:

—if you have ever had any unusual or allergic reaction to trazodone.

—if you are on a low-salt, low-sugar, or any other special diet, or if you are allergic to any substance, such as foods, sulfites or other preservatives, or dyes. Most medicines contain more than their active ingredient. Your doctor, nurse, or pharmacist can help you avoid products that may cause a problem.

—if you are **pregnant** or if you may become pregnant. Studies have not been done in humans. However, studies in animals have shown that trazodone causes birth defects and fewer successful pregnancies when given in doses up to 50 times the largest recommended human dose.

—if you are **breast-feeding.** It is not known whether trazodone passes into breast milk. However, this medicine has not been shown to cause problems in nursing babies. Trazodone has been found in the milk of test animals.

—if you have any of the following medical problems:
   Alcoholism
   Heart disease
   Kidney disease
   Liver disease

—if you are taking **any** other prescription or nonprescription (OTC) medicine, especially:
   Antihypertensives (high blood pressure medicine)
   Central nervous system (CNS) depressants

Proper Use of This Medicine

To lessen stomach upset and to reduce dizziness and light-headedness, take this medicine with or shortly after a meal or light snack, even for a daily bedtime dose, unless your doctor has told you to take it on an empty stomach.

Take trazodone only as directed by your doctor, to benefit your condition as much as possible.

Sometimes trazodone must be taken for up to 4 weeks before you begin to feel better, although most people notice improvement within 2 weeks.

If you miss a dose of this medicine, take it as soon as possible. However, if it is within 4 hours of your next dose, skip the missed dose and go back to your regular dosing schedule. Do not double doses.

How to store this medicine:

• **Keep out of the reach of children.**

• Store away from heat and direct light.

• Do not store in the bathroom, near the kitchen sink, or in other damp places. Heat or moisture may cause the medicine to break down.

• Do not keep outdated medicine or medicine no longer needed. Be sure that any discarded medicine is out of the reach of children.

Precautions While Using This Medicine

It is very important that your doctor check your progress at regular visits. This will allow your doctor to check the medicine's effects and to change the dose if needed.

Do not stop taking this medicine without first checking with your doctor. Your doctor may want you to reduce gradually the amount you are using before stopping completely, in order to prevent a possible return of your medical problem.

Before having any kind of surgery, dental treatment, or emergency treatment, tell the physician or dentist in charge that you are using this medicine.

This medicine will add to the effects of alcohol and other CNS depressants (medicines that slow down the nervous system, possibly causing drowsiness). Some examples of CNS depressants are antihistamines or medicine for hay fever, other allergies, or colds; sedatives, tranquilizers, or sleeping medicine; prescription pain medicine or narcotics; barbiturates; medicine for convulsions (seizures); muscle relaxants; or anesthetics, including some dental anesthetics. **Check with your doctor before taking any of the above while you are using this medicine.**

This medicine may cause some people to become drowsy or less alert than they are normally. **Make sure you know how you react to this medicine before you drive, use machines, or do other jobs that require you to be alert.**

Dizziness, lightheadedness, or fainting may occur, especially when you get up from a lying or sitting position. Getting up slowly may help. If this problem continues or gets worse, check with your doctor.

Trazodone may cause dryness of the mouth. For temporary relief, use sugarless gum or candy, melt bits of ice in your mouth, or use a saliva substitute. However, if dry mouth continues for more than 2 weeks, check with your physician or dentist. Continuing dryness of the mouth may increase the chance of dental disease, including tooth decay, gum disease, and fungal infections.

Side Effects of This Medicine

Along with its needed effects, a medicine may cause some unwanted effects. Although not all of these side effects may occur, if they do occur they may need medical attention.

Stop taking this medicine and check with your doctor immediately if the following side effect occurs:
Rare
   Prolonged, painful, inappropriate erection of the penis

Also, check with your doctor as soon as possible if any of the following side effects occur:
Less common
   Confusion
   Muscle tremors
Rare
   Fainting
   Fast or slow heartbeat
   Skin rash

Other side effects may occur that usually do not require medical attention. These side effects may go away during treatment as your body adjusts to the medicine. However, check with your doctor if any of the following side effects continue or are bothersome:
More common
   Blurred vision
   Dizziness or lightheadedness
   Drowsiness
   Dry mouth
   Headache
   Nausea and vomiting
Less common
   Constipation
   Diarrhea
   Muscle aches or pains
   Unusual tiredness or weakness

For elderly patients: The above side effects, especially drowsiness, dizziness, confusion, vision problems, dry mouth, and constipation, are more likely to occur in elderly patients, who are usually more sensitive to the effects of trazodone.

Other side effects not listed above may also occur in some patients. If you notice any other effects, check with your doctor.

December 1987

TRETINOIN (Topical)

Some commonly used brand names or other names are:

Retin-A   StieVAA*
Retinoic acid   Vitamin A acid

Generic name product may also be available in the U.S. and Canada.

---

*Not available in the U.S.

To the Reader: If you do not recognize the names of medical conditions or medicines referred to in this information, check with your doctor, nurse, or pharmacist. Definitions for selected medical terms may be found in the Glossary. Brand names for the generic drug names listed can be found in the Index. In addition, selected brand names commonly associated with the generic name have been included in the text to help you recognize medicine you may be taking. The fact that a brand name product is not mentioned does not mean the information does not apply. It is a good idea for you to learn both the generic and brand names of your medicines and to write them down for future use.

Tretinoin (TRET-i-noyn) is applied to the skin to treat certain types of acne. It may also be used to treat other skin diseases as determined by your doctor.

Tretinoin is available only with your doctor's prescription.

Remember:

• **This medicine has been prescribed for your current medical problem only.** It must not be given to other people or used for other problems unless you are directed to do so by your doctor.

• **Keep all medicines out of the reach of children.**

• In order for this medicine to work, it must be used as directed.

• **It is very important that you read and understand the following information.** If any of the information causes you special concern, do not decide against using this medicine without first checking with your doctor.

• Before you begin using any new medicine (prescription or nonprescription) or if you develop any new medical problem while you are using this medicine, check with your doctor, nurse, or pharmacist.

• **If you have any questions** about the following information or if you want more information about this medicine or your medical problem, **ask your doctor, nurse, or pharmacist.**

Before Using This Medicine

In order to decide on the best treatment for your medical problem, your doctor should be told:

—if you have ever had any unusual or allergic reaction to tretinoin or vitamin A–like preparations.

—if you are allergic to any substance, such as certain preservatives. Most medicines contain more than their active ingredient. Your doctor, nurse, or pharmacist can help you avoid products that may cause a problem.

—if you are **pregnant** or if you may become pregnant. Studies on birth defects have not been done in humans.

Although tretinoin has not been shown to cause birth defects in animal studies, it has been shown to slightly increase abnormal skull bone formation in some animal fetuses.

—if you are **breast-feeding**. It is not known whether tretinoin passes into the breast milk; however, this medicine has not been shown to cause problems in nursing babies.

—if you have either of the following medical problems:
Eczema
Sunburn

—if you are taking **any** other prescription or nonprescription (OTC) medicine.

Proper Use of This Medicine

It is very important that you use this medicine only as directed. Do not use more of it, do not use it more often, and do not use it for a longer period of time than your doctor ordered. To do so may cause irritation of the skin.

Do not apply this medicine to windburned or sunburned skin or on open wounds.

Do not use this medicine in or around the eyes or mouth, or inside of the nose. Spread the medicine away from these areas when applying.

This medicine usually comes with patient directions. Read them carefully before using the medicine.

Before applying tretinoin, wash the skin with a mild or nonallergic type of soap and warm water, then gently pat dry. Wait 20 to 30 minutes before applying this medicine to make sure the skin is completely dry.

For patients using the cream or gel form of this medicine:
• Apply enough medicine to cover the affected areas, and rub in gently.

For patients using the solution form of this medicine:
• Using your fingertips, a gauze pad, or a cotton swab, apply enough tretinoin solution to cover the affected areas. If you use a gauze pad or a cotton swab for applying the medicine, avoid getting it too wet, in order to prevent the medicine from running into areas not intended for treatment.

If you miss a dose of this medicine, do not apply the missed dose at all. Instead, apply your next dose at the regularly scheduled time. Then continue with your regular dosing schedule.

How to store this medicine:

• **Keep out of the reach of children.**

• Store away from heat and direct light.

• Keep the medicine from freezing.

• Do not keep outdated medicine or medicine no longer needed. Be sure that any discarded medicine is out of the reach of children.

Precautions While Using This Medicine

During the first 2 or 3 weeks you are using tretinoin, your acne may seem to get worse before it gets better. However, you should not stop using tretinoin unless irritation or other symptoms become severe. If you have any questions about this, check with your doctor.

You should avoid washing your face too often. Washing it with a mild bland soap 2 or 3 times a day should be enough, unless otherwise directed by your doctor.

When using tretinoin, do not use any of the following preparations on the same affected area as this medicine, unless otherwise directed by your doctor:

    Abrasive soaps or cleansers
    Alcohol-containing preparations
    Any other topical acne preparation or preparation containing a peeling agent (for example, benzoyl peroxide, resorcinol, salicylic acid, or sulfur)
    Cosmetics or soaps that dry the skin
    Medicated cosmetics
    Other topical medicine for the skin

To use any of the above preparations on the same affected area as tretinoin may cause severe irritation of the skin.

You may use cosmetics (nonmedicated) while being treated with tretinoin, unless otherwise directed by your doctor. However, the areas to be treated must be washed thoroughly before the medicine is applied.

During treatment with this medicine, **avoid exposing the treated areas to too much sunlight or overuse of a sunlamp,** since the skin may be more prone to sunburn.

If exposure to too much sunlight cannot be avoided while you are using this medicine, sunscreen preparations may be applied or protective clothing worn over the treated areas.

Some people who use this medicine may become more sensitive to wind and cold temperatures than they are normally. **When you first begin using this medicine, use protection against wind or cold until you see how you react.** If you notice severe skin irritation, check with your doctor.

Side Effects of This Medicine

In some animal studies, tretinoin has been shown to cause skin tumors to develop faster when the treated area is exposed to ultraviolet light (sunlight or artificial sunlight of a sunlamp). It is not known if tretinoin causes skin tumors to develop faster in humans.

Along with its needed effects, a medicine may cause some unwanted effects. Although not all of these side effects may occur, if they do occur they may need medical attention.

Check with your doctor as soon as possible if any of the following side effects occur:

    Blistering, crusting, severe burning or redness, or swelling of skin
    Darkening or lightening of the treated skin

Other side effects may occur that usually do not require medical attention. These side effects may go away during treatment as your body adjusts to the medicine. However, check with your doctor if any of the following side effects continue or are bothersome:

    Feeling of warmth on skin
    Peeling of skin (may occur after a few days)
    Stinging (mild) or redness of skin

For elderly patients: Many medicines have not been tested in older people. Therefore, it is not known whether the medicine acts the same way it does in younger adults. Check with your doctor or pharmacist if you notice any unusual effects while using this medicine or if you think it is not working as it should.

Other side effects not listed above may also occur in some patients. If you notice any other effects, check with your doctor.

December 1987

TRIENTINE (Systemic)

A commonly used brand name is Cuprid.

To the Reader: If you do not recognize the names of medical conditions or medicines referred to in this information, check with your doctor, nurse, or pharmacist. Definitions for selected medical terms may be found in the Glossary. Brand names for the generic drug names listed can be found in the Index. In addition, selected brand names commonly associated with the generic name have been included in the text to help you recognize medicine you may be taking. The fact that a brand name product is not mentioned does not mean the information does not apply. It is a good idea for you to learn both the generic and brand names of your medicines and to write them down for future use.

Trientine (TRYE-en-teen) is taken by mouth to treat Wilson's disease, a disease in which there is too much copper in the body.

This medicine combines with excess copper in the body to prevent damage to the liver, brain, and other organs. The combination of copper and trientine is then easily removed from the body through the kidneys into the urine.

Trientine is available only with your doctor's prescription.

Remember:

• **This medicine has been prescribed for your current medical problem only.** It must not be given to other people or used for other problems unless you are directed to do so by your doctor.

• **Keep all medicines out of the reach of children.**

• In order for this medicine to work, it must be used as directed.

• **It is very important that you read and understand the following information.** If any of the information causes you special concern, do not decide against using this medicine without first checking with your doctor.

• Before you begin using any new medicine (prescription or nonprescription) or if you develop any new medical problem while you are using this medicine, check with your doctor, nurse, or pharmacist.

• **If you have any questions** about the following information or if you want more information about this medicine or your medical problem, **ask your doctor, nurse, or pharmacist.**

Before Using This Medicine

In order to decide on the best treatment for your medical problem, your doctor should be told:

—if you have ever had any unusual or allergic reaction to trientine.

—if you are on a low-salt, low-sugar, or any other special diet, or if you are allergic to any substance, such as foods, sulfites or other preservatives, or dyes. Most medicines contain more than their active ingredient. Your doctor, nurse, or pharmacist can help you avoid products that may cause a problem.

—if you are **pregnant** or if you may become pregnant. Trientine has not been shown to cause birth defects or other problems in humans. However, it has been shown to cause birth defects in rats.

—if you are **breast-feeding**. It is not known whether trientine passes into the breast milk. This medicine has not been shown to cause problems in nursing babies.

—if you have iron-deficiency anemia.

—if you are now taking iron supplements or other medicine containing minerals (contained in some vitamin combination products).

Proper Use of This Medicine

Take trientine with water. The capsule should be swallowed whole. It must not be opened, crushed, or chewed.

Take this medicine on an empty stomach (at least 1 hour before or 2 hours after meals) and at least 1 hour before or after any other medicine, food, or milk. This will allow trientine to be better absorbed by your body.

Trientine will not cure Wilson's disease, but it will help remove the excess copper from your body. Therefore, **you must continue to take this medicine regularly, as directed. You may have to take trientine for the rest of your life.** If Wilson's disease is not treated continually, it can cause severe liver damage and can cause death. **Do not stop taking this medicine without first checking with your doctor.**

It is very important for you to follow any special instructions from your doctor, such as following a low-copper diet. You may need to avoid foods known to be high in copper, such as chocolate, mushrooms, liver, molasses, broccoli, cereals enriched with copper, shellfish, organ meats, and nuts. If you have any questions about this, check with your doctor.

Take this medicine only as directed by your doctor. Do not take more or less of it and do not take it more often than your doctor ordered. If too much is used, it may increase the chance of side effects.

If you miss a dose of this medicine, double the next dose. Do not make up more than one missed dose at a time.

How to store this medicine:

• **Keep out of the reach of children.**

• Store sealed, unopened bottles of trientine in the refrigerator, but not in the freezer. Before opening a sealed bottle, let it stand at room temperature for about 6 hours. Keep it at room temperature after opening it.

• Do not store in the bathroom, near the kitchen sink, or in other damp places. Heat or moisture may cause the medicine to break down.

• Do not keep outdated medicine or medicine no longer needed. Be sure that any discarded medicine is out of the reach of children.

Precautions While Using This Medicine

Your doctor should check your progress at regular visits to make sure trientine is working properly and to check for unwanted effects. Laboratory tests may be needed. This will allow your doctor to change your dose, if necessary.

During the first month of treatment, your doctor may want you to take your temperature each night. **Tell your doctor if you develop a fever or skin rash.**

Do not take iron preparations or any other mineral supplements within 2 hours of taking trientine. This includes any vitamin preparation that contains minerals.

If a capsule breaks open and the contents touch your skin, wash the area right away with water. Trientine may cause a rash.

Side Effects of This Medicine

Along with its needed effects, a medicine may cause some unwanted effects. Although not all of these side effects may occur, if they do occur they may need medical attention.

Check with your doctor as soon as possible if any of the following side effects occur:

More common—Signs of anemia
> Tiredness
> Unusually pale skin

Rare
> Fever
> General feeling of bodily discomfort or weakness
> Joint pain
> Skin rash, blisters, hives, or itching
> Swelling of the lymph glands

The above signs of anemia are more likely to occur in children, menstruating women, and pregnant women, who usually need more iron than other patients. If these signs appear during trientine treatment, your doctor will need to do some tests.

For elderly patients: Many medicines have not been tested in older people. Therefore, it is not known if the medicine acts the same way it does in younger adults. Check with your doctor or pharmacist if you notice any unusual effects while taking this medicine or if you do not think it is working as it should.

Other side effects not listed above may also occur in some patients. If you notice any other effects, check with your doctor.

—————————

December 1987

—————————————————————————————

TRIFLURIDINE (Ophthalmic)

A commonly used brand name is Viroptic.

To the Reader: If you do not recognize the names of medical conditions or medicines referred to in this information, check with your doctor, nurse, or pharmacist. Definitions for selected medical terms may be found in the Glossary. Brand names for the generic drug names listed can be found in the Index. In addition, selected brand names commonly associated with the generic name have been included in the text to help you recognize medicine you may be taking. The fact that a brand name product is not mentioned does not mean the information does not apply. It is a good idea for you to learn both the generic and brand names of your medicines and to write them down for future use.

Trifluridine (trye-FLURE-i-deen) belongs to the family of medicines called antivirals. Trifluridine ophthalmic preparations are used in the eye to help the body overcome virus infections of the eye.

Trifluridine is available only with your doctor's prescription.

Remember:

• This medicine has been prescribed for your present infection only. Another infection later on may require a different medicine. Also, even though other people may have the same symptoms as you, they may have a different kind of infection. Your medicine may not work for them and may even cause them harm. Therefore, **your medicine must not be given to other people or used for other infections** unless you are otherwise directed by your doctor.

• In order for this medicine to work, it must be used as directed.

• Keep all medicines out of the reach of children.

• If you want more information about this medicine, ask your doctor, nurse, or pharmacist.

• If any of the following information causes you special concern, do not decide against using this medicine without first checking with your doctor.

Before Using This Medicine

In order to decide on the best treatment for your medical problem, your doctor should be told:

—if you have ever had any unusual or allergic reaction to trifluridine.

—if you are **pregnant** or if you may become pregnant. However, trifluridine has not been shown to cause birth defects or other problems in humans.

—if you are **breast-feeding**. However, trifluridine has not been shown to cause problems in nursing babies.

Proper Use of This Medicine

The bottle is only partially full to provide proper drop control.

How to apply this medicine: First, wash your hands. Then tilt the head back and pull the lower eyelid away from the eye to form a pouch. Drop the medicine into the pouch and gently close the eyes. Do not blink. Keep the eyes closed for 1 or 2 minutes to allow the medicine to come into contact with the infection.

If you think you did not get the drop of medicine into your eye properly, use another drop.

To prevent contamination of the eye drops, do not touch the applicator tip to any surface (including the eye). Also, keep the container tightly closed.

Do not use this medicine more often or for a longer time than your doctor ordered. To do so may cause problems in the eyes. If you have any questions about this, check with your doctor.

To help clear up your infection completely, **keep using this medicine for the full time of treatment,** even though your symptoms may have disappeared; **do not miss any doses.**

If you do miss a dose of this medicine, apply it as soon as possible. However, if it is almost time for your next application, skip the missed dose and go back to your regular dosing schedule.

How to store this medicine:

• **Keep out of the reach of children.**

• Store in the refrigerator because heat will cause this medicine to break down. However, keep the medicine from freezing. Follow the directions on the label.

• Do not keep outdated medicine or medicine no longer needed. Be sure that any discarded medicine is out of the reach of children.

Precautions While Using This Medicine

After application of this medicine to the eye, occasional stinging or burning may be expected.

It is very important that you keep your appointment with your doctor. If your symptoms become worse, check with your doctor sooner.

Side Effects of This Medicine

Along with its needed effects, a medicine may cause some unwanted effects. Although not all of these side effects may occur, if they do occur they may need medical attention.

Check with your doctor as soon as possible if any of the following side effects occur:

Rare

Itching, redness, swelling, or other sign of irritation not present before using this medicine

---

Other side effects may occur that usually do not require medical attention. These side effects may go away during treatment as your body adjusts to the medicine. However, check with your doctor if either of the following side effects continues or is bothersome:

More common

Burning or stinging

Other side effects not listed above may also occur in some patients. If you notice any other effects, check with your doctor.

_____

December 1987

_____

TRILOSTANE (Systemic)

A commonly used brand name is Modrastane.

To the Reader: If you do not recognize the names of medical conditions or medicines referred to in this information, check with your doctor, nurse, or pharmacist. Definitions for selected medical terms may be found in the Glossary. Brand names for the generic drug names listed can be found in the Index. In addition, selected brand names commonly associated with the generic name have been included in the text to help you recognize medicine you may be taking. The fact that a brand name product is not mentioned does not mean the information does not apply. It is a good idea for you to learn both the generic and brand names of your medicines and to write them down for future use.

Trilostane (TRYE-loe-stane) is used in the treatment of Cushing's syndrome. It is normally used in short-term treatment until permanent therapy is possible.

In Cushing's syndrome, the adrenal gland overproduces steroids. Although steroids are important for various functions of the body, too much can cause problems. Trilostane reduces the amount of steroids produced by the adrenal gland.

Trilostane is available only with your doctor's prescription.

Remember:
- **This medicine has been prescribed for your current medical problem only.** It must not be given to other people or used for other problems unless you are directed to do so by your doctor.
- **Keep all medicines out of the reach of children.**
- In order for this medicine to work, it must be used as directed.
- **It is very important that you read and understand the following information.** If any of the information causes you special concern, do not decide against using this medicine without first checking with your doctor.
- Before you begin using any new medicine (prescription or nonprescription) or if you develop any new medical problem while you are using this medicine, check with your doctor, nurse, or pharmacist.
- **If you have any questions** about the following information or if you want more information about this medicine or your medical problem, **ask your doctor, nurse, or pharmacist.**

Before Using This Medicine

In order to decide on the best treatment for your medical problem, your doctor should be told:
—if you have ever had any unusual or allergic reaction to trilostane.
—if you are on a low-salt, low-sugar, or any other special diet, or if you are allergic to any substance, such as foods, sulfites, or yellow dye. Most medicines contain more than their active ingredient.
—if you are **pregnant** or if you may become pregnant. Use of trilostane is not recommended during pregnancy. It has been shown to cause serious problems, including miscarriage, in humans. Trilostane has also been shown to cause birth defects in animals.

—if you are **breast-feeding**. It is not known whether trilostane passes into breast milk. This medicine has not been shown to cause problems in nursing babies.

—if you have any of the following medical problems:
Infection
Injury (sudden)
Kidney disease
Liver disease

—if you are taking **any** other prescription or nonprescription (OTC) medicine.

Proper Use of This Medicine

Take trilostane only as directed by your doctor. Do not take more or less of it, and do not take it more often than your doctor ordered.

If you miss a dose of this medicine, take it as soon as possible. However, if it is almost time for your next dose, skip the missed dose and go back to your regular dosing schedule. Do not double doses.

How to store this medicine:
- **Keep out of the reach of children.**
- Store away from heat and direct light.
- Do not store in the bathroom, near the kitchen sink, or in other damp places. Heat or moisture may cause the medicine to break down.
- Do not keep outdated medicine or medicine no longer needed. Be sure that any discarded medicine is out of the reach of children.

Precautions While Using This Medicine

It is very important that your doctor check your progress at regular visits to make sure that trilostane is working properly and does not cause unwanted effects.

Check with your doctor right away if you get an injury, infection, or illness of any kind. This medicine may weaken your body's normal defenses.

Before having any kind of surgery (including dental surgery) or emergency treatment, tell the physician or dentist in charge that you are taking trilostane.

Your doctor may want you to carry a medical identification card or wear a bracelet stating that you are taking this medicine.

Side Effects of This Medicine

Along with its needed effects, a medicine may cause some unwanted effects. Although not all of these side effects may occur, if they do occur they may need medical attention.

Check with your doctor as soon as possible if any of the following side effects occur:
Rare
Darkening of skin
Drowsiness or tiredness
Loss of appetite

Mental depression
Skin rash
Vomiting

Other side effects may occur that usually do not require medical attention. These side effects may go away during treatment as your body adjusts to the medicine. However, check with your doctor if any of the following side effects continue or are bothersome:

More common

Diarrhea
Stomach pain or cramps

Less common

Aching muscles
Belching or bloating
Burning mouth or nose
Dizziness or lightheadedness
Fever
Flushing

Headache
Increase in salivation
Nausea
Watery eyes

For elderly patients: Many medicines have not been tested in older people. Therefore, it is not known whether the medicine acts the same way it does in younger adults. Check with your doctor or pharmacist if you notice any unusual effects while taking this medicine or if you think it is not working as it should.

Other side effects not listed above may also occur in some patients. If you notice any other effects, check with your doctor.

_____

December 1987

_____

TRIMEPRAZINE (Systemic)

Some commonly used brand names are Panectyl* and Temaril.

Generic name product may also be available in the U.S.

---

*Not available in the U.S.

To the Reader: If you do not recognize the names of medical conditions or medicines referred to in this information, check with your doctor, nurse, or pharmacist. Definitions for selected medical terms may be found in the Glossary. Brand names for the generic drug names listed can be found in the Index. In addition, selected brand names commonly associated with the generic name have been included in the text to help you recognize medicine you may be taking. The fact that a brand name product is not mentioned does not mean the information does not apply. It is a good idea for you to learn both the generic and brand names of your medicines and to write them down for future use.

Trimeprazine (trye-MEP-ra-zeen) belongs to the general group of medicines called antihistamines. It is also related to the phenothiazine medicines and shares their properties. Trimeprazine is taken by mouth to relieve itching of skin rash or hives and other skin conditions. It may also be used for other conditions as determined by your doctor.

Use of this medicine is not recommended in premature or newborn infants since serious side effects are more likely to occur in very young children. Also, **use is not recommended in children who have a history of difficulty in breathing while sleeping, or a family history of sudden infant death syndrome (SIDS).**

Trimeprazine is available only with your doctor's prescription.

Remember:

• **This medicine has been prescribed for your current medical problem only.** It must not be given to other people or used for other problems unless you are directed to do so by your doctor.

• **Keep all medicines out of the reach of children.**

• In order for this medicine to work, it must be used as directed.

• **It is very important that you read and understand the following information.** If any of the information causes you special concern, do not decide against using this medicine without first checking with your doctor.

• Before you begin using any new medicine (prescription or nonprescription) or if you develop any new medical problem while you are using this medicine, check with your doctor, nurse, or pharmacist.

• **If you have any questions** about the following information or if you want more information about this medicine or your medical problem, **ask your doctor, nurse, or pharmacist.**

Before Using This Medicine

In order to decide on the best treatment for your medical problem, your doctor should be told:

—if you have ever had any unusual or allergic reaction to trimeprazine or other phenothiazines.

—if you are on a low-salt, low-sugar, or any other special diet, or if you are allergic to any substance, such as foods, sulfites or other preservatives, or dyes. Most medicines contain more than their active ingredient, and many liquid medicines contain alcohol. Your doctor, nurse, or pharmacist can help you avoid products that may cause a problem.

—if you are **pregnant** or if you may become pregnant. Phenothiazines such as trimeprazine have been shown to cause jaundice (yellowing of skin and eyes) and muscle tremors in a few newborn babies whose mothers received phenothiazines during pregnancy.

—if you are **breast-feeding**. This medicine has not been shown to cause problems in nursing babies. However, this medicine may pass into the breast milk and cause unwanted effects in the baby, such as unusual excitement or irritability.

—if you have any of the following medical problems:

Emphysema, asthma, or chronic lung disease (especially in children)
Enlarged prostate
Heart or blood vessel disease
High blood pressure
Intestinal blockage
Liver disease
Stomach ulcer (or history of)
Urinary tract blockage

—if you are taking **any** other prescription or nonprescription (OTC) medicine, especially:

Amoxapine (e.g., Asendin)
Central nervous system (CNS) depressants
Chlorprothixene (e.g., Taractan)
Epinephrine (e.g., Adrenalin)
Haloperidol (e.g., Haldol)
Levodopa (e.g., Dopar)
Loxapine (e.g., Loxitane)
Methyldopa (e.g., Aldomet)
Metoclopramide (e.g., Reglan)
Metyrosine (e.g., Demser)
Molindone (e.g., Moban)
Pemoline (e.g., Cylert)
Phenothiazines (acetophenazine [e.g., Tindal], chlorpromazine [e.g., Thorazine], fluphenazine [e.g., Prolixin], mesoridazine [e.g., Serentil], perphenazine [e.g., Trilafon], prochlorperazine [e.g., Compazine], promazine [e.g., Sparine], promethazine [e.g., Phenergan], thioridazine [e.g., Mellaril], trifluoperazine [e.g., Stelazine], triflupromazine [e.g., Vesprin], trimeprazine [e.g., Temaril])
Pimozide (e.g., Orap)
Quinidine (e.g., Quinidex)
Rauwolfia alkaloids (alseroxylon [e.g., Rauwiloid], deserpidine [e.g., Harmonyl], rauwolfia serpentina [e.g., Raudixin], reserpine [e.g., Serpasil])
Thiothixene (e.g., Navane)

—if you are now taking or have taken within the past 2 weeks monoamine oxidase (MAO) inhibitors, such as:

    Furazolidone (e.g., Furoxone)
    Isocarboxazid (e.g., Marplan)
    Pargyline (e.g., Eutonyl)
    Phenelzine (e.g., Nardil)
    Procarbazine (e.g., Matulane)
    Tranylcypromine (e.g., Parnate)

—if you are having an x-ray test of the head, spinal canal, or nervous system for which you are going to receive an injection into the spinal canal. This medicine may increase the chances of having seizures.

Proper Use of This Medicine

This medicine may be taken with food or a full glass (8 ounces) of water or milk to reduce stomach irritation.

Trimeprazine is used to relieve the symptoms of your medical problem. Take it only as directed. Do not take more of it and do not take it more often than your doctor ordered. To do so may increase the chance of side effects.

If you must take this medicine regularly and you miss a dose, take it as soon as possible. However, if it is almost time for your next dose, skip the missed dose and go back to your regular dosing schedule. Do not double doses.

How to store this medicine:

• **Keep out of the reach of children.**

• Store away from heat and direct light.

• Do not store the capsule or tablet form of this medicine in the bathroom, near the kitchen sink, or in other damp places. Heat or moisture may cause the medicine to break down.

• Keep the liquid form of this medicine from freezing.

• Do not keep outdated medicine or medicine no longer needed. Be sure that any discarded medicine is out of the reach of children.

Precautions While Using This Medicine

Tell the doctor in charge that you are taking this medicine before you have any skin tests for allergies. The results of the tests may be affected by this medicine.

If you will be taking this medicine for a long period of time (for example, for several months at a time), it is important that your doctor check your progress at regular visits. This is to make sure that this medicine does not cause unwanted effects.

When taking trimeprazine on a regular basis, make sure your doctor knows if you are taking large amounts of aspirin (as for arthritis or rheumatism) at the same time. Effects of too much aspirin, such as dizziness or ringing in the ears, may be covered up by this medicine.

This medicine will add to the effects of alcohol and other CNS depressants (medicines that slow down the nervous system, possibly causing drowsiness). Some examples of CNS depressants are antihistamines or medicine for hay fever, other allergies, or colds; sedatives, tranquilizers, or sleeping medicine; prescription pain medicine or narcotics; barbiturates; medicine for convulsions (seizures); muscle relaxants; or anesthetics, including some dental anesthetics. **Check with your doctor before taking any of the above while you are using this medicine.**

If you think you or anyone else may have taken an overdose, get emergency help at once. Taking an overdose may lead to unconsciousness and possibly death. Some signs of an overdose are clumsiness or unsteadiness; severe drowsiness; muscle spasms (especially of neck and back); shortness of breath or troubled breathing; shuffling walk; tic-like (jerky) movements of head and face; trembling and shaking the hands.

This medicine may cause some people to become drowsy or less alert than they are normally. Even if taken at bedtime, it may cause some people to feel drowsy or less alert on arising. **Make sure you know how you react to this medicine before you drive, use machines, or do other jobs that require you to be alert.**

Side Effects of This Medicine

Along with its needed effects, a medicine may cause some unwanted effects. Although not all of these side effects may occur, if they do occur they may need medical attention.

Check with your doctor as soon as possible if any of the following side effects occur:

Rare

    Sore throat and fever

Signs of overdose

    Clumsiness or unsteadiness
    Drowsiness (severe)
    Fast heartbeat
    Flushing or redness of face
    Muscle spasms (especially of the neck and back)
    Shortness of breath or troubled breathing
    Shuffling walk
    Tic-like (jerky) movements of head and face
    Trembling and shaking of the hands

Other side effects may occur that usually do not require medical attention. These side effects may go away during treatment as your body adjusts to the medicine. However, check with your doctor if any of the following side effects continue or are bothersome:

More common

    Drowsiness
    Feeling faint
    Lightheadedness
    Thickening of bronchial secretions
    Unusual tiredness or weakness

Less common or rare

Blurred vision or any change in vision
Confusion
Decreased mental alertness
Difficult or painful urination
Dizziness
Dryness of mouth, nose, and throat
Increased appetite or weight gain
Increased sensitivity of skin to sun
Nausea or vomiting
Nightmares, continuing
Ringing or buzzing in the ears
Skin rash
Stomach upset or pain
Unusual excitement, nervousness, restlessness, or irritability, continuing

For children: Decreased mental alertness; nightmares; and unusual excitement, nervousness, restlessness, or irritability may be more likely to occur in children.

For elderly patients: Dizziness, severe drowsiness, confusion, faintness, and uncontrolled movements may be more likely to occur in elderly patients, who are usually more sensitive to the effects of trimeprazine.

Other side effects not listed above may also occur in some patients. If you notice any other effects, check with your doctor.

December 1987

TRIMETHOBENZAMIDE (Systemic)

Some commonly used brand names are:

Tegamide	Tigan
Ticon	Tiject-20

To the Reader: If you do not recognize the names of medical conditions or medicines referred to in this information, check with your doctor, nurse, or pharmacist. Definitions for selected medical terms may be found in the Glossary. Brand names for the generic drug names listed can be found in the Index. In addition, selected brand names commonly associated with the generic name have been included in the text to help you recognize medicine you may be taking. The fact that a brand name product is not mentioned does not mean the information does not apply. It is a good idea for you to learn both the generic and brand names of your medicines and to write them down for future use.

Trimethobenzamide (trye-meth-oh-BEN-za-mide) is used to treat nausea and vomiting.

This medicine is available only with your doctor's prescription.

Remember:

• **This medicine has been prescribed for your current medical problem only.** It must not be given to other people or used for other problems unless you are directed to do so by your doctor.

• **Keep all medicines out of the reach of children.**

• In order for this medicine to work, it must be used as directed.

• If you are receiving this medicine by injection, some of the information about this medicine may not apply.

• **It is very important that you read and understand the following information.** If any of the information causes you special concern, do not decide against using this medicine without first checking with your doctor.

• Before you begin using any new medicine (prescription or nonprescription) or if you develop any new medical problem while you are using this medicine, check with your doctor, nurse, or pharmacist.

• **If you have any questions** about the following information or if you want more information about this medicine or your medical problem, **ask your doctor, nurse, or pharmacist.**

Before Using This Medicine

In order to decide on the best treatment for your medical problem, your doctor should be told:

—if you have ever had any unusual or allergic reaction to trimethobenzamide.

—if you are allergic or sensitive to benzocaine or other local anesthetics (the suppository form of this medicine contains benzocaine), or if you are allergic to any substance, such as foods, sulfites or other preservatives, or dyes. Most medicines contain more than their active ingredient. Your doctor, nurse, or pharmacist can help you avoid products that may cause a problem.

—if you are **pregnant** or if you may become pregnant. Studies have not been done in humans. However, although studies in animals have not shown that trimethobenzamide causes birth defects, it has been shown to increase the chance of a miscarriage.

—if you are **breast-feeding.** Trimethobenzamide has not been shown to cause problems in nursing babies.

—if you have either of the following medical problems:
High fever
Intestinal infection

—if you are taking **any** other prescription or nonprescription (OTC) medicine, especially central nervous system (CNS) depressants.

Proper Use of This Medicine

Do not use this medicine to treat nausea and vomiting in children unless otherwise directed by your doctor. If you are giving this medicine to a child, be especially careful not to give more than is prescribed since side effects may be more serious in children.

Trimethobenzamide is used only to relieve or prevent nausea and vomiting. Use it only as directed. Do not use more of it and do not use it more often than your doctor ordered. To do so may increase the chance of side effects.

For patients using the rectal suppository form of this medicine:

• How to insert suppository: First, remove foil wrapper and moisten the suppository with water. Lie down on your side and push the suppository well up into the rectum with your finger. If the suppository is too soft to insert because of storage in a warm place, before removing the foil wrapper chill the suppository in the refrigerator for 30 minutes or run cold water over it.

If you must use this medicine regularly and you miss a dose, use it as soon as possible. However, if it is almost time for your next dose, skip the missed dose and go back to your regular dosing schedule. Do not double doses.

How to store this medicine:

• **Keep out of the reach of children.**

• Store away from heat and direct light.

• Do not store the capsule form of this medicine in the bathroom, near the kitchen sink, or in other damp places. Heat or moisture may cause the medicine to break down.

• Do not keep outdated medicine or medicine no longer needed. Be sure that any discarded medicine is out of the reach of children.

Precautions While Using This Medicine

Trimethobenzamide will add to the effects of alcohol and other CNS depressants (medicines that slow down the nervous system, possibly causing drowsiness). Some examples of CNS depressants are antihistamines or medicine for hay fever, other allergies, or colds; sedatives, tranquilizers, or sleeping medicine; prescription pain medicine or narcotics; barbiturates; medicine for convulsions (seizures); muscle relaxants; or anesthetics, including some dental anesthetics. **Check with your doctor before taking any of the above while you are using this medicine.**

This medicine may cause some people to become dizzy, lightheaded, drowsy, or less alert than they are normally. **Make sure you know how you react to this medicine before you drive, use machines, or do other jobs that require you to be alert.**

When using trimethobenzamide on a regular basis, make sure your doctor knows if you are taking large amounts of aspirin or other salicylates at the same time (as for arthritis or rheumatism). Effects of too much aspirin, such as ringing in the ears, may be covered up by this medicine.

Side Effects of This Medicine

Along with its needed effects, a medicine may cause some unwanted effects. Although not all of these side effects may occur, if they do occur they may need medical attention.

Check with your doctor as soon as possible if any of the following side effects occur:

Rare
   Back pain
   Convulsions (seizures)
   Mental depression
   Shakiness or tremors
   Sore throat and fever
   Unusual feeling of tiredness
   Vomiting (severe or continuing)
   Yellow eyes and skin

Other side effects may occur that usually do not require medical attention. These side effects may go away during treatment as your body adjusts to the medicine. However, check with your doctor if any of the following side effects continue or are bothersome:

More common
   Drowsiness
Less common
   Blurred vision
   Diarrhea
   Dizziness
   Headache
   Muscle cramps

Other side effects not listed above may also occur in some patients. If you notice any other effects, check with your doctor.

December 1987

TRIMETHOPRIM (Systemic)

Some commonly used brand names are Proloprim and Trimpex.

Generic name product may also be available in the U.S.

To the Reader: If you do not recognize the names of medical conditions or medicines referred to in this information, check with your doctor, nurse, or pharmacist. Definitions for selected medical terms may be found in the Glossary. Brand names for the generic drug names listed can be found in the Index. In addition, selected brand names commonly associated with the generic name have been included in the text to help you recognize medicine you may be taking. The fact that a brand name product is not mentioned does not mean the information does not apply. It is a good idea for you to learn both the generic and brand names of your medicines and to write them down for future use.

Trimethoprim (trye-METH-oh-prim) belongs to the family of medicines called anti-infectives. It is taken by mouth to help the body overcome infections of the urinary tract. It may also be used for other problems as determined by your doctor. It will not work for colds, flu, or other virus infections.

Trimethoprim is available only with your doctor's prescription.

Remember:
• This medicine has been prescribed for your present infection only. Another infection later on may require a different medicine. Also, even though other people may have the same symptoms as you, they may have a different kind of infection. Your medicine may not work for them and may even cause them harm. Therefore, **your medicine must not be given to other people or used for other infections** unless you are otherwise directed by your doctor.

• In order for this medicine to work, it must be taken as directed.

• Keep all medicines out of the reach of children.

• If you want more information about this medicine, ask your doctor, nurse, or pharmacist.

• If any of the following information causes you special concern, do not decide against taking this medicine without first checking with your doctor.

Before Using This Medicine

In order to decide on the best treatment for your medical problem, your doctor should be told:
—if you have ever had any unusual or allergic reaction to trimethoprim.

—if you are **pregnant** or if you may become pregnant. Trimethoprim has not been shown to cause birth defects or other problems in humans. However, trimethoprim has been shown to cause birth defects in rats and rabbits given large doses.

—if you are **breast-feeding.** Trimethoprim passes into the breast milk and may cause unwanted effects in nursing babies.

—if you have any of the following medical problems:
  Anemia
  Kidney disease
  Liver disease

—if you are taking **any** other prescription or nonprescription (OTC) medicine.

Proper Use of This Medicine

To help clear up your infection completely, **keep taking this medicine for the full time of treatment** even if you begin to feel better after a few days. If you stop taking this medicine too soon, your symptoms may return.

This medicine works best when there is a constant amount in the urine. **To help keep the amount constant, do not miss any doses. Also, it is best to take each dose at evenly spaced times day and night.** For example, if you are to take 2 doses a day, each dose should be spaced about 12 hours apart. If this interferes with your sleep or other daily activities, or if you need help in planning the best times to take your medicine, check with your doctor, nurse, or pharmacist.

If you do miss a dose of this medicine, take it as soon as possible. This will help to keep a constant amount of medicine in the urine. However, if it is almost time for your next dose and your dosing schedule is:
• 1 dose a day—Space the missed dose and next dose 10 to 12 hours apart.
• 2 doses a day—Space the missed dose and the next dose 5 to 6 hours apart.
Then go back to your regular dosing schedule.

Trimethoprim may be taken on an empty stomach or, if it upsets your stomach, it may be taken with food.

Do not give this medicine to infants or children under 12 years of age unless otherwise directed by your doctor.

How to store this medicine:
• **Keep out of the reach of children.**
• Store away from heat and direct light.
• Do not store in the bathroom, near the kitchen sink, or in other damp places. Heat or moisture may cause the medicine to break down.
• Do not keep outdated medicine or medicine no longer needed. Be sure that any discarded medicine is out of the reach of children.

Precautions While Using This Medicine

It is important that your doctor check your progress at regular visits if you will be taking this medicine for a long time. This will allow your doctor to check for any unwanted effects that may be caused by this medicine.

If your symptoms do not improve within a few days, or if they become worse, check with your doctor.

Trimethoprim may cause blood problems. These problems may result in a greater chance of infection, slow healing, and bleeding of the gums. Therefore, you should be careful when using toothbrushes, dental floss, and toothpicks. Dental work should be delayed until your blood counts have returned to normal. Check with your physician or dentist if you have any questions about proper oral hygiene (mouth care) during treatment.

If this medicine causes anemia, your doctor may want you to take folic acid (a vitamin) every day to help clear up the anemia. If so, it is important to take folic acid every day along with this medicine; do not miss any doses.

Side Effects of This Medicine

Along with its needed effects, a medicine may cause some unwanted effects. Although not all of these side effects may occur, if they do occur they may need medical attention.

Check with your doctor immediately if any of the following side effects occur:

Rare
    Bluish fingernails, lips, or skin
    Difficult breathing
    Pale skin
    Sore throat and fever
    Unusual bleeding or bruising
    Unusual tiredness or weakness

Other side effects may occur that usually do not require medical attention. These side effects may go away during treatment as your body adjusts to the medicine.

However, check with your doctor if any of the following side effects continue or are bothersome:

More common
    Headache
    Skin rash or itching
    Unusual taste
Less common
    Diarrhea
    Loss of appetite
    Nausea or vomiting
    Sore mouth or tongue
    Stomach cramps or pain

Other side effects not listed above may also occur in some patients. If you notice any other effects, check with your doctor.

December 1987

Additional Information

For patients taking trimethoprim to *prevent* infections of the urinary tract:

• Although trimethoprim is used mainly to help the body *overcome* infections of the urinary tract, your doctor may have prescribed this medicine to help *prevent* infections of the urinary tract. It is usually given once a day and may be given for a long time for this purpose. If you have any questions about this, check with your doctor.

• If you miss a dose of this medicine, take it as soon as possible. However, if it is almost time for your next dose, space the missed dose and the next dose 10 to 12 hours apart. Then go back to your regular dosing schedule.

TRIOXSALEN (Systemic)

A commonly used brand name is Trisoralen.

To the Reader: If you do not recognize the names of medical conditions or medicines referred to in this information, check with your doctor, nurse, or pharmacist. Definitions for selected medical terms may be found in the Glossary. Brand names for the generic drug names listed can be found in the Index. In addition, selected brand names commonly associated with the generic name have been included in the text to help you recognize medicine you may be taking. The fact that a brand name product is not mentioned does not mean the information does not apply. It is a good idea for you to learn both the generic and brand names of your medicines and to write them down for future use.

Trioxsalen (trye-OX-sa-len) belongs to the group of medicines called psoralens. It is used along with ultraviolet light (found in sunlight and some special lamps) in a treatment called PUVA to treat vitiligo, a disease in which skin color is lost. Trioxsalen may also be used for other conditions as determined by your doctor.

Trioxsalen is available only with your doctor's prescription.

Remember:

• **This medicine has been prescribed for your current medical problem only.** It must not be given to other people or used for other problems unless you are directed to do so by your doctor.

• **Keep all medicines out of the reach of children.**

• In order for this medicine to work, it must be used as directed.

• **It is very important that you read and understand the following information.** If any of the information causes you special concern, do not decide against using this medicine without first checking with your doctor.

• Before you begin using any new medicine (prescription or nonprescription) or if you develop any new medical problem while you are using this medicine, check with your doctor, nurse, or pharmacist.

• **If you have any questions** about the following information or if you want more information about this medicine or your medical problem, **ask your doctor, nurse, or pharmacist.**

Before Using This Medicine

Trioxsalen is a very strong medicine that increases the sensitivity of skin to sunlight. In addition to causing serious sunburns if not properly used, it has been reported to increase the chance of skin cancer and cataracts. Also, like too much sunlight, PUVA can cause premature aging of the skin. Therefore, trioxsalen should be used only as directed and it should **not** be used simply for suntanning. Before using this medicine, be sure that you have discussed the use of it with your doctor.

In order to decide on the best treatment for your medical problem, your doctor should be told:

—if you have ever had any unusual or allergic reaction to trioxsalen.

—if you are on a low-salt, low-sugar, or any other special diet, or if you are allergic to any substance, such as foods, sulfites or other preservatives, or dyes. Most medicines contain more than their active ingredient. Your doctor, nurse, or pharmacist can help you avoid products that may cause a problem.

—if you are **pregnant** or if you may become pregnant. Studies have not been done in either humans or animals.

—if you are **breast-feeding.** However, trioxsalen has not been shown to cause problems in nursing babies.

—if you have any of the following medical problems:
  Allergy to sunlight (family history of)
  Eye problems such as cataracts or loss of the lens of the eyes
  Heart or blood vessel disease (severe)
  Infection
  Lupus erythematosus
  Melanoma or other skin cancer (history of)
  Other skin conditions
  Porphyria
  Stomach problems

—if you are using **any** other prescription or nonprescription (OTC) medicine.

—if you have recently had x-ray treatment or cancer medicines or plan to have x-rays in the near future.

Proper Use of This Medicine

This medicine may take several weeks or months to really help your condition. **Do not increase the amount of trioxsalen you are taking or spend extra time in the sunlight or under an ultraviolet lamp.** This will not make the medicine act any more quickly and may result in a serious burn.

If this medicine upsets your stomach, it may be taken with meals or milk.

If you are late in taking, or miss taking, a dose of this medicine, notify your doctor. Remember that exposure to sunlight or ultraviolet light must take place 2 to 4 hours **after** you take the medicine or it will not work. If you have any questions about this, check with your doctor.

How to store this medicine:

• **Keep out of the reach of children.**

• Store away from heat and direct light.

• Do not store in the bathroom, near the kitchen sink, or in other damp places. Heat or moisture may cause the medicine to break down.

• Do not keep outdated medicine or medicine no longer needed. Be sure that any discarded medicine is out of the reach of children.

© 1988 The United States Pharmacopeial Convention, Inc.

Precautions While Using This Medicine

Your doctor should check your progress at regular visits to make sure this medicine is working and that it does not cause unwanted effects. Eye examinations should be included.

This medicine increases the sensitivity of your skin to sunlight; too much exposure could cause a serious burn. If you must go out in the sunlight, **cover your skin for at least 24 hours before and 8 hours following treatment.** A special sunscreening lotion may also help.

Your skin may continue to be sensitive to sunlight for some time after treatment with this medicine is stopped. Use extra caution if you plan to spend any time in the sun.

For 24 hours after you take each dose of trioxsalen, your eyes should be protected during daylight hours with special wraparound sunglasses that totally block or absorb ultraviolet light. This is to prevent cataracts. Your doctor will tell you what kind of sunglasses to use. These glasses are needed even in indirect light, such as light coming through a window glass. In addition, protect your lips with a special lipstick that blocks sunlight.

Eating certain foods while you are taking trixosalen may increase the sensitivity of your skin to sunlight. To help prevent this, avoid eating limes, figs, parsley, parsnips, mustard, carrots, and celery while you are being treated with this medicine.

This medicine may cause your skin to become dry or itchy. **However, check with your doctor before applying anything to your skin to treat this problem.**

Side Effects of This Medicine

Along with its needed effects, a medicine may cause some unwanted effects. Although not all of these side effects may occur, if they do occur they may need medical attention.

Check with your doctor immediately if you think you have taken an overdose or if any of the following side effects occur since they may indicate a serious burn:

Blistering and peeling of skin
Reddened, sore skin
Swelling, especially in feet or lower legs

Other side effects may occur that usually do not require medical attention. These side effects may go away during treatment as your body adjusts to the medicine. However, check with your doctor if any of the following side effects continue or are bothersome:

More common

Itching of skin
Nausea

Less common

Dizziness
Headache
Mental depression
Nervousness
Trouble in sleeping

For elderly patients: Many medicines have not been tested in older people. Therefore, it is not known whether the medicine acts the same way it does in younger adults. Check with your doctor or pharmacist if you notice any unusual effects while taking this medicine or if you think it is not working as it should.

Other side effects not listed above may also occur in some patients. If you notice any other effects, check with your doctor.

December 1987

TROPICAMIDE (Ophthalmic)

Some commonly used brand names are:

I-Picamide   Mydriacyl
Minims Tropicamide*   Tropicacyl

Generic name product may also be available in the U.S.

*Not available in the U.S.

To the Reader: If you do not recognize the names of medical conditions or medicines referred to in this information, check with your doctor, nurse, or pharmacist. Definitions for selected medical terms may be found in the Glossary. Brand names for the generic drug names listed can be found in the Index. In addition, selected brand names commonly associated with the generic name have been included in the text to help you recognize medicine you may be taking. The fact that a brand name product is not mentioned does not mean the information does not apply. It is a good idea for you to learn both the generic and brand names of your medicines and to write them down for future use.

Tropicamide (troe-PIK-a-mide) is used in the eye to dilate (enlarge) the pupil. It is used before eye examinations. Tropicamide may also be used before and after eye surgery.

This medicine is available only with your doctor's prescription.

Remember:

• **It is very important that you read and understand the following information.** If any of the information causes you special concern, do not decide against receiving this medicine without first checking with your doctor.

• **If you have any questions** about the following information or if you want more information about this medicine or your medical problem, **ask your doctor, nurse, or pharmacist**.

Before Using This Medicine

In order to decide on the best treatment for your medical problem, your doctor should be told:

—if you have ever had any unusual or allergic reaction to tropicamide.

—if you are allergic to any substance, such as certain preservatives. Most medicines contain more than their active ingredient.

—if you are **pregnant** or if you may become pregnant. Studies have not been done in either humans or animals.

—if you are **breast-feeding**. However, tropicamide has not been shown to cause problems in nursing babies.

—if you have any of the following medical problems:
  Brain damage (in children)
  Down's syndrome (mongolism)
  Spastic paralysis (in children)

Side Effects of This Medicine

When this medicine is applied, some stinging of the eye may be expected.

After this medicine is applied to your eyes, your pupils will become unusually large and you will have blurring of vision, especially for close objects. **Make sure your vision is clear before you drive or do other jobs that require you to see well.** This medicine will also cause your eyes to become more sensitive to light than they are normally. **Wear sunglasses to protect your eyes from sunlight and other bright lights.** If these effects continue for longer than 24 hours after the medicine is used, check with your doctor.

For elderly patients: Many medicines have not been tested in older people. Therefore, it is not known whether the medicine acts the same way it does in younger adults. Check with your doctor or pharmacist if you notice any unusual effects while using this medicine or if you think it is not working as it should.

Other side effects not listed above may also occur in some patients. If you notice any other effects, check with your doctor.

December 1987

UNDECYLENIC ACID, COMPOUND
(Topical)

Some commonly used brand names are:

Cruex	Quinsana Plus
Decylenes	Ting
Desenex	Undoguent

To the Reader: If you do not recognize the names of medical conditions or medicines referred to in this information, check with your doctor, nurse, or pharmacist. Definitions for selected medical terms may be found in the Glossary. Brand names for the generic drug names listed can be found in the Index. In addition, selected brand names commonly associated with the generic name have been included in the text to help you recognize medicine you may be taking. The fact that a brand name product is not mentioned does not mean the information does not apply. It is a good idea for you to learn both the generic and brand names of your medicines and to write them down for future use.

Compound undecylenic acid (un-de-sill-ENN-ik AS-id) belongs to the group of medicines called antifungals. It is used on the skin to treat some types of fungal infections.

Compound undecylenic acid is available without a prescription; however, your doctor may have special instructions on the proper use of this medicine for your medical condition.

Remember:

• In order for this medicine to work, it must be used as directed.

• Keep all medicines out of the reach of children.

• If you want more information about this medicine, ask your doctor, nurse, or pharmacist.

• If this medicine has been ordered by your doctor and if any of the following information causes you special concern, do not decide against using this medicine without first checking with your doctor.

Before Using This Medicine

Before you use compound undecylenic acid, your doctor should be told:

—if you have ever had any unusual or allergic reaction to compound undecylenic acid.

—if you are **pregnant** or if you may become pregnant. However, compound undecylenic acid topical preparations have not been shown to cause birth defects or other problems in humans.

—if you are **breast-feeding**. However, compound undecylenic acid topical preparations have not been shown to cause problems in nursing babies.

Proper Use of This Medicine

Keep this medicine away from the eyes.

To help clear up your infection completely, **keep using this medicine for 2 weeks after burning, itching, or other symptoms have disappeared,** unless otherwise directed by your doctor. **Do not miss any doses.**

If you do miss a dose of this medicine, apply it as soon as possible. Then go back to your regular dosing schedule. If you have any questions about this, check with your doctor or pharmacist.

Before applying compound undecylenic acid, wash the area to be treated and surrounding areas, and dry thoroughly. Then apply enough medicine to cover the affected area.

For patients using the cream form of this medicine:

• Apply cream generously to affected area. Rub in well.

• Do not use on pus-containing sores or on badly broken skin.

For patients using the powder form of this medicine:

• If the powder is used on the feet, sprinkle it between toes, on feet, and in socks and shoes.

For patients using the aerosol powder form of this medicine:

• From a distance of 4 to 6 inches, spray the powder on the affected areas. If it is used on the feet, spray it between toes, on feet, and in socks and shoes.

• Do not use this medicine around the eyes, nose, or mouth.

• Do not inhale the powder.

• Do not use near heat, near open flame, or while smoking.

How to store this medicine:

• **Keep out of the reach of children.**

• Store away from heat and direct light.

• Do not store the powder form of this medicine in the bathroom, near the kitchen sink, or in other damp places. Heat or moisture may cause the medicine to break down.

• Keep the medicine from freezing.

• Do not puncture, break, or burn the aerosol powder container.

• Do not keep outdated medicine or medicine no longer needed. Be sure that any discarded medicine is out of the reach of children.

Precautions While Using This Medicine

If your skin problem does not improve within 4 weeks, or if it becomes worse, check with your doctor or pharmacist.

To help prevent reinfection after the period of treatment with this medicine, the powder or spray powder form of this medicine may be used each day after bathing and careful drying.

Side Effects of This Medicine

Along with its needed effects, a medicine may cause some unwanted effects. Although not all of these side effects may occur, if they do occur they may need medical attention.

Check with your doctor or pharmacist as soon as possible if the following side effect occurs:

Skin irritation not present before using this medicine

Other side effects not listed above may also occur in some patients. If you notice any other effects, check with your doctor or pharmacist.

December 1987

URACIL MUSTARD (Systemic)

To the Reader: If you do not recognize the names of medical conditions or medicines referred to in this information, check with your doctor, nurse, or pharmacist. Definitions for selected medical terms may be found in the Glossary. Brand names for the generic drug names listed can be found in the Index. In addition, selected brand names commonly associated with the generic name have been included in the text to help you recognize medicine you may be taking. The fact that a brand name product is not mentioned does not mean the information does not apply. It is a good idea for you to learn both the generic and brand names of your medicines and to write them down for future use.

Uracil (YOOR-a-sill) mustard belongs to the group of medicines known as alkylating agents. It is taken by mouth to treat some kinds of cancer as well as some noncancerous conditions.

Uracil mustard interferes with the growth of cancer cells, which are eventually destroyed. Since the growth of normal body cells may also be affected by uracil mustard, other effects will also occur. Some of these may be serious and must be reported to your doctor. Other effects, such as hair loss, may not be serious but may cause concern. Some effects may not occur for months or years after the medicine is used.

Before you begin treatment with uracil mustard, you and your doctor should talk about the good this medicine will do as well as the risks of using it.

Uracil mustard is available only with your doctor's prescription.

Remember:

• **This medicine has been prescribed for your current medical problem only.** It must not be given to other people or used for other problems unless you are directed to do so by your doctor.

• **Keep all medicines out of the reach of children.**

• In order for this medicine to work, it must be used as directed.

• **It is very important that you read and understand the following information.** If any of the information causes you special concern, do not decide against using this medicine without first checking with your doctor.

• Before you begin using any new medicine (prescription or nonprescription) or if you develop any new medical problem while you are using this medicine, check with your doctor, nurse, or pharmacist.

• **If you have any questions** about the following information or if you want more information about this medicine or your medical problem, **ask your doctor, nurse, or pharmacist.**

Before Using This Medicine

In order to decide on the best treatment for your medical problem, your doctor should be told:

—if you have ever had any unusual or allergic reaction to uracil mustard.

—if you are **pregnant** or if you intend to have children. This medicine may cause birth defects if either the male or female is taking it at the time of conception

or if it is taken during pregnancy. In addition, many cancer medicines may cause sterility which could be permanent. Although this has not been reported with this medicine, the possibility should be kept in mind. Be sure that you have discussed this with your doctor before taking this medicine.

—if you intend to **breast-feed.** Because this medicine may cause serious side effects, breast-feeding is generally not recommended while you are receiving it.

—if you have any of the following medical problems:
Chickenpox (including recent exposure)
Gout (history of)
Herpes zoster (shingles)
Infection
Kidney disease
Kidney stones
Liver disease

—if you are taking **any** other prescription or nonprescription (OTC) medicine, especially:
Antithyroid agents (medicine for overactive thyroid)
Azathioprine (e.g., Imuran)
Chloramphenicol (e.g., Chloromycetin)
Colchicine
Flucytosine (e.g., Ancobon)
Interferon (e.g., Intron A, Roferon-A)
Probenecid (e.g., Benemid)
Sulfinpyrazone (e.g., Anturane)

—if you have ever been treated with x-rays or cancer medicines.

Proper Use of This Medicine

Use this medicine only as directed by your doctor. Do not use more or less of it, and do not use it more often than your doctor ordered. The exact amount of medicine you need has been carefully worked out. Taking too much may increase the chance of side effects, while taking too little may not improve your condition.

While you are using this medicine, your doctor may want you to drink extra fluids so that you will pass more urine. This will help prevent kidney problems and keep your kidneys working well.

Uracil mustard often causes nausea and vomiting. Even if you begin to feel ill, **do not stop using this medicine without first checking with your doctor.** Ask your doctor, nurse, or pharmacist for ways to lessen these effects.

If you vomit shortly after taking a dose of uracil mustard, check with your doctor. You may be told to take the dose again or you may have to wait until the next scheduled dose.

If you miss a dose of this medicine, skip the missed dose and go back to your regular dosing schedule. Do not double doses.

How to store this medicine:

• **Keep out of the reach of children.**

• Store away from heat and direct light.

- Do not store in the bathroom, near the kitchen sink, or in other damp places. Heat or moisture may cause the medicine to break down.

- Do not keep outdated medicine or medicine no longer needed. Be sure that any discarded medicine is out of the reach of children.

Precautions While Using This Medicine

It is very important that your doctor check your progress at regular visits to make sure that this medicine is working properly and to check for unwanted effects.

While you are being treated with uracil mustard, and after you stop treatment with it, **do not have any immunizations without your doctor's approval**. Uracil mustard lowers your body's resistance and there is a chance you might get the infection the immunization is meant to prevent. Other people living in your household should not take oral polio vaccine since there is a chance they could pass the polio virus on to you. Also, you should avoid close contact with other persons (for example, at school or work) who have taken oral polio vaccine.

Uracil mustard can lower the number of white blood cells in your body. This may increase the chance of getting an infection. If you can, avoid people with colds or other infections. If you think you are getting a cold or other infection, check with your doctor.

Side Effects of This Medicine

Along with their needed effects medicines like uracil mustard can sometimes cause unwanted effects such as blood problems, loss of hair, and other side effects; these are described below. Also, because of the way these medicines act on the body, there is a chance that they might cause other unwanted effects that may not occur until months or years after the medicine is used. These delayed effects may include certain types of cancer, such as leukemia. Discuss these possible effects with your doctor.

Although not all of the side effects may occur, if they do occur they may need medical attention.

Check with your doctor immediately if any of the following side effects occur:
More common
　　Fever, chills, or sore throat
　　Unusual bleeding or bruising

Check with your doctor as soon as possible if any of the following side effects occur:
Less common
　　Joint pain
　　Lower back, side, or stomach pain
　　Swelling of feet or lower legs
Rare
　　Sores in the mouth and on the lips
　　Yellow eyes and skin

Other side effects may occur that usually do not require medical attention. These side effects may go away during treatment as your body adjusts to the medicine. Also, your doctor or nurse may be able to tell you about ways to prevent or reduce some of these side effects. Check with your doctor if any of the following side effects continue or are bothersome or if you have any questions about them:
More common
　　Diarrhea
　　Nausea or vomiting
Less common
　　Darkening of the skin
　　Irritability
　　Mental depression
　　Nervousness
　　Skin rash and itching

This medicine may cause a temporary loss of hair in some people. After treatment with uracil mustard has ended, normal hair growth should return.

For elderly patients: Many medicines have not been tested in older people. Therefore, it is not known whether the medicine acts the same way it does in younger adults. Check with your doctor if you notice any unusual effects while taking this medicine or if you think it is not working as it should.

After you stop taking uracil mustard, it may still produce some side effects that need attention. During this period of time, check with your doctor if you notice any of the following:
　　Fever, chills, or sore throat
　　Unusual bleeding or bruising

Other side effects not listed above may also occur in some patients. If you notice any other effects, check with your doctor.

December 1987

UREA (Intra-amniotic)

To the Reader: If you do not recognize the names of medical conditions or medicines referred to in this information, check with your doctor, nurse, or pharmacist. Definitions for selected medical terms may be found in the Glossary. Brand names for the generic drug names listed can be found in the Index. In addition, selected brand names commonly associated with the generic name have been included in the text to help you recognize medicine you may be taking. The fact that a brand name product is not mentioned does not mean the information does not apply. It is a good idea for you to learn both the generic and brand names of your medicines and to write them down for future use.

Intra-amniotic urea (yoor-EE-a) is given by injection into the uterus to cause abortion. It is to be administered only by or under the immediate care of your doctor.

Remember:

• **It is very important that you read and understand the following information.** If any of the information causes you special concern, do not decide against receiving this medicine without first checking with your doctor.

• Before you begin using any new medicine (prescription or nonprescription) or if you develop any new medical problem while you are receiving this medicine, check with your doctor, nurse, or pharmacist.

• **If you have any questions** about the following information or if you want more information about this medicine or your medical problem, **ask your doctor, nurse, or pharmacist**.

Before Using This Medicine

In order to decide on the best treatment for your medical problem, your doctor should be told:

—if you have ever had any unusual or allergic reaction to urea.

—if you have any of the following medical problems:
Diabetes mellitus (sugar diabetes)
Fibroid tumors of the uterus
Kidney disease
Liver disease
Pelvic adhesions (history of)
Sickle cell disease
Uterus surgery (history of)

Proper Use of This Medicine

During the abortion procedure, you should drink fluids to help prevent your body from losing too much water.

Side Effects of This Medicine

Along with its needed effects, a medicine may cause some unwanted effects. Although not all of these side effects may occur, if they do occur they may need medical attention.

Check with your doctor or nurse immediately if either of the following side effects occurs during the time that the injection is being given:
Pain in lower abdomen
Weakness

Check with your doctor or nurse as soon as possible if any of the following side effects occur:
Rare
Confusion
Irregular heartbeat
Muscle cramps or pain
Numbness, tingling, pain, or weakness in hands or feet
Unusual tiredness or weakness
Weakness and heaviness of legs

Other side effects may occur that usually do not require medical attention. However, check with your doctor or nurse if any of the following side effects continue or are bothersome:
More common
Nausea or vomiting
Less common or rare
Headache

After the procedure, this medicine may still produce some side effects that need attention. Check with your doctor if you notice any of the following side effects:
Chills or shivering
Fever
Foul-smelling vaginal discharge
Increase in uterine bleeding
Pain in lower abdomen

Other side effects not listed above may also occur in some patients. If you notice any other effects, check with your doctor or nurse.

December 1987

UROFOLLITROPIN (Systemic)

A commonly used brand name is Metrodin.

To the Reader: If you do not recognize the names of medical conditions or medicines referred to in this information, check with your doctor, nurse, or pharmacist. Definitions for selected medical terms may be found in the Glossary. Brand names for the generic drug names listed can be found in the Index. In addition, selected brand names commonly associated with the generic name have been included in the text to help you recognize medicine you may be taking. The fact that a brand name product is not mentioned does not mean the information does not apply. It is a good idea for you to learn both the generic and brand names of your medicines and to write them down for future use.

Urofollitropin (YOO-roe-fall-ee-troe-pin) is used in combination with another medicine, chorionic gonadotropin, to treat infertility. It is used in some women who are unable to become pregnant because of polycystic ovary disease.

Urofollitropin is to be administered only by or under the supervision of your doctor.

Remember:

• **It is very important that you read and understand the following information.** If any of the information causes you special concern, do not decide against using this medicine without first checking with your doctor.

• Before you begin using any new medicine (prescription or nonprescription) or if you develop any new medical problem while you are using this medicine, check with your doctor, nurse, or pharmacist.

• **If you have any questions** about the following information or if you want more information about this medicine or your medical problem, **ask your doctor, nurse, or pharmacist.**

Before Using This Medicine

If you become pregnant as a result of using this medicine, there is a chance of a multiple birth (for example, twins, triplets) occurring. If you have any questions about this, check with your doctor.

In order to decide on the best treatment for your medical problem, your doctor should be told:

—if you have ever had any unusual or allergic reaction to urofollitropin.

—if you are on a low-salt, low-sugar, or any other special diet, or if you are allergic to any substance, such as foods, sulfites or other preservatives, or dyes. Most medicines contain more than their active ingredient. Your doctor or pharmacist can help you avoid products that may cause a problem.

—if you have any of the following medical problems:
Adrenal gland disease
Cyst on ovary
Fibroid tumors of the uterus
Pituitary disease
Thyroid disease
Unusual vaginal bleeding

Precautions While Using This Medicine

It is very important that your doctor check your progress at regular visits to make sure that the medicine is working properly and to check for unwanted effects.

It may take some time for urofollitropin to work. **It is very important that you continue to receive this medicine.** If you are concerned that it is not working, check with your doctor.

If your doctor has asked you to record your temperature daily, make sure that you do this every day so that you will know if you have begun to ovulate. It is also important that intercourse take place at the correct time to give you the best chance of becoming pregnant. **Follow your doctor's instructions carefully.**

Side Effects of This Medicine

Along with its needed effects, a medicine may cause some unwanted effects. Although not all of these side effects may occur, if they do occur they may need medical attention. Check with your doctor as soon as possible if any of the following side effects occur:

More common
Bloating
Redness, pain, or swelling at the place of injection
Stomach or pelvic pain

Rare
Fever and chills

Other side effects may occur that usually do not require medical attention. These side effects may go away during treatment as your body adjusts to the medicine. However, check with your doctor if any of the following side effects continue or are bothersome:

Less common or rare
Nausea, vomiting, or diarrhea
Skin rash or hives
Sore breasts

After you stop using this medicine, your body may need time to adjust. The length of time this takes depends on the amount of medicine you were using and how long you used it. During this period of time check with your doctor if you notice any of the following side effects:

Bloating
Stomach or pelvic pain

Other side effects not listed above may also occur in some patients. If you notice any other effects, check with your doctor.

December 1987

VALPROIC ACID (Systemic)

This information applies to the following medicines:

Divalproex (dye-VAL-pro-ex)
Valproic Acid (val-PRO-ic acid)

Some commonly used brand names are:	Generic names:
Depakote Epival*	Divalproex
Depakene Myproic Acid	Valproic Acid†

*Not available in the U.S.
†Generic name product may also be available in the U.S.

To the Reader: If you do not recognize the names of medical conditions or medicines referred to in this information, check with your doctor, nurse, or pharmacist. Definitions for selected medical terms may be found in the Glossary. Brand names for the generic drug names listed can be found in the Index. In addition, selected brand names commonly associated with the generic name have been included in the text to help you recognize medicine you may be taking. The fact that a brand name product is not mentioned does not mean the information does not apply. It is a good idea for you to learn both the generic and brand names of your medicines and to write them down for future use.

Valproic acid and divalproex belong to the group of medicines called anticonvulsants. They are taken by mouth to control certain types of seizures in the treatment of epilepsy. Valproic acid and divalproex may be used alone or with other seizure medicine.

Divalproex forms valproic acid in the body. Therefore, the following information applies to both medicines.

This medicine is available only with your doctor's prescription.

Remember:
• **This medicine has been prescribed for your current medical problem only.** It must not be given to other people or used for other problems unless you are directed to do so by your doctor.

• **Keep all medicines out of the reach of children.**

• In order for this medicine to work, it must be used as directed.

• **It is very important that you read and understand the following information.** If any of the information causes you special concern, do not decide against using this medicine without first checking with your doctor.

• Before you begin using any new medicine (prescription or nonprescription) or if you develop any new medical problem while you are using this medicine, check with your doctor, nurse, or pharmacist.

• **If you have any questions** about the following information or if you want more information about this medicine or your medical problem, **ask your doctor, nurse, or pharmacist**.

Before Using This Medicine

In order to decide on the best treatment for your medical problem, your doctor should be told:

—if you have ever had any unusual or allergic reaction to divalproex or valproic acid.

—if you are on a low-salt, low-sugar, or any other special diet, or if you are allergic to any substance, such as foods, sulfites or other preservatives, or dyes. Most medicines contain more than their active ingredient, and many liquid medicines contain alcohol. Your doctor, nurse, or pharmacist can help you avoid products that may cause a problem.

—if you are **pregnant** or if you may become pregnant. Valproic acid has been reported to cause birth defects when taken by the mother during the first three months of pregnancy. Also, animal studies have shown that valproic acid causes birth defects when taken in doses several times greater than doses used in humans. However, this medicine may be necessary to control seizures in some pregnant patients. Be sure you have discussed this with your doctor.

—if you are **breast-feeding**. Valproic acid passes into the breast milk, but its effect on the nursing baby is not known. It may be necessary for you to take another medicine or to stop breast-feeding during treatment with valproic acid. Be sure you have discussed the risks and benefits of this medicine with your doctor.

—if you have any of the following medical problems:
  Blood disease
  Brain disease
  Kidney disease
  Liver disease

—if you are taking **any** other prescription or nonprescription (OTC) medicine, especially:
  Acetaminophen (with long-term, high-dose use)
  Amiodarone (e.g., Cordarone)
  Anabolic steroids (dromostanolone, ethylestrenol, nandrolone, oxymetholone, stanozolol)
  Androgens (male hormones)
  Antithyroid agents (medicine for overactive thyroid)
  Azlocillin (e.g., Azlin)
  Aspirin and other salicylates
  Carbamazepine (e.g., Tegretol)
  Carmustine (e.g., BiCNU)
  Central nervous system (CNS) depressants
  Chloroquine (e.g., Aralen)
  Dantrolene (e.g., Dantrium)
  Daunorubicin (e.g., Cerubidine)
  Dipyridamole (e.g., Persantine)
  Disulfiram (e.g., Antabuse)
  Doxorubicin (e.g., Adriamycin)
  Erythromycins
  Estrogens (female hormones)
  Etretinate (e.g., Tegison)
  Furazolidone (e.g., Furoxone)
  Gold salts
  Hydroxychloroquine (e.g., Plaquenil)
  Isoniazid (e.g., INH)
  Ketoconazole (e.g., Nizoral)
  Mercaptopurine (e.g., Purinethol)
  Methotrexate (e.g., Mexate)
  Methyldopa (e.g., Aldomet)
  Mezlocillin (e.g., Mezlin)

Naltrexone (e.g., Trexan) (with long-term, high-dose use)
Nitrofurantoin (e.g., Furadantin)
Oral contraceptives (birth control pills) containing estrogen
Phenobarbital (e.g., Luminal)
Phenothiazines (acetophenazine, chlorpromazine, fluphenazine, mesoridazine, perphenazine, prochlorperazine, promazine, promethazine, thioridazine, trifluoperazine, triflupromazine, trimeprazine)
Phenytoin (e.g., Dilantin)
Piperacillin (e.g., Pipracil)
Plicamycin (e.g., Mithracin)
Primidone (e.g., Mysoline)
Rifampin (e.g., Rifadin)
Sulfonamides (sulfa medicine)
Sulfinpyrazone (e.g., Anturane)

Proper Use of This Medicine

For patients taking the capsule form of valproic acid:
• Swallow the capsule whole without chewing or breaking. This is to prevent irritation of the mouth or throat.

For patients taking the tablet form of this medicine:
• Take the tablet with water, not milk, and swallow it whole without chewing, breaking, or crushing. This is to prevent damaging the special coating that helps lessen irritation of the stomach.

For patients taking the syrup form of this medicine:
• The syrup may be mixed with any liquid or added to food for a better taste.

This medicine may be taken with meals or snacks to reduce stomach upset.

This medicine must be taken exactly as directed by your doctor in order to prevent seizures and lessen the possibility of side effects.

If you miss a dose of this medicine, and you are to take it:
Once a day—Take the missed dose as soon as possible. However, if you do not remember until the next day, skip the missed dose and go back to your regular dosing schedule. Do not double doses.
Two or more times a day—If you remember within 6 hours of the missed dose, take it right away. Then take the rest of the doses for that day at equally spaced time periods. Do not double doses.

How to store this medicine:
• **Keep out of the reach of children.**
• Store away from heat and direct light.
• Do not store the capsule or tablet form of this medicine in the bathroom, near the kitchen sink, or in other damp places. Heat or moisture may cause the medicine to break down.
• Keep the syrup form of this medicine from freezing.
• Do not keep outdated medicine or medicine no longer needed. Be sure that any discarded medicine is out of the reach of children.

Precautions While Using This Medicine

Your doctor should check your progress at regular visits, especially for the first few months you take this medicine. This is necessary to allow dose adjustments and to reduce any unwanted effects.

Do not stop taking valproic acid without first checking with your doctor. Your doctor may want you to gradually reduce the amount you are taking before stopping completely. Stopping the medicine suddenly may cause you to have seizures again.

Before having any kind of surgery, dental treatment, or emergency treatment, tell the physician or dentist in charge that you are taking this medicine.

Valproic acid will add to the effects of alcohol and other CNS depressants (medicines that slow down the nervous system, possibly causing drowsiness). Some examples of CNS depressants are antihistamines or medicine for hay fever, other allergies, or colds; sedatives, tranquilizers, or sleeping medicine; prescription pain medicine or narcotics; barbiturates; medicine for convulsions (seizures); muscle relaxants; or anesthetics, including some dental anesthetics. **Check with your doctor before taking any of the above while you are using this medicine.**

Diabetic patients: This medicine may interfere with urine tests for ketones and give false-positive results.

Your doctor may want you to carry a medical identification card or bracelet stating that you are taking this medicine.

This medicine may cause some people to become drowsy or less alert than they are normally. **Make sure you know how you react to this medicine before you drive, use machines, or do other jobs that require you to be alert.**

Side Effects of This Medicine

Along with its needed effects, a medicine may cause some unwanted effects. Although not all of these side effects may occur, if they do occur they may need medical attention.

Check with your doctor as soon as possible if any of the following side effects occur:
Less common
Abdominal or stomach cramps (severe)
Increase in seizures
Lack of coordination
Loss of appetite
Nausea or vomiting
Skin rash
Swelling of face
Tiredness and weakness
Unusual bleeding or bruising
Yellow eyes or skin

Other side effects may occur that usually do not require medical attention. These side effects may go away during treatment as your body adjusts to the medicine.

However, check with your doctor if any of the following side effects continue or are bothersome:

More common

Abdominal or stomach cramps (mild)
Change in menstrual periods
Diarrhea
Indigestion
Trembling of hands and arms
Weight gain

Less common or rare

Constipation
Dizziness
Drowsiness
Hair loss (usually slight and temporary)
Headache
Mental depression
Unusual excitement, restlessness, or irritability

For children: Some of the above side effects, especially abdominal or stomach cramps, loss of appetite, nausea or vomiting, tiredness or weakness, and yellow eyes or skin, are more likely to occur in young children.

For elderly patients: Many medicines have not been tested in older people. Therefore, it is not known whether the medicine acts the same way it does in younger adults. Check with your doctor or pharmacist if you notice any unusual effects while taking this medicine or if you think it is not working as it should.

Other side effects not listed above may also occur in some patients. If you notice any other effects, check with your doctor.

_____
December 1987

VANCOMYCIN (Oral)

Some commonly used brand names are Diatracin* and Vancocin.

*Not available in the U.S.

To the Reader: If you do not recognize the names of medical conditions or medicines referred to in this information, check with your doctor, nurse, or pharmacist. Definitions for selected medical terms may be found in the Glossary. Brand names for the generic drug names listed can be found in the Index. In addition, selected brand names commonly associated with the generic name have been included in the text to help you recognize medicine you may be taking. The fact that a brand name product is not mentioned does not mean the information does not apply. It is a good idea for you to learn both the generic and brand names of your medicines and to write them down for future use.

Vancomycin (van-koe-MYE-sin) belongs to the family of medicines called antibiotics. Antibiotics are medicines used in the treatment of infections caused by bacteria. They work by killing bacteria or preventing their growth. Vancomycin will not work for colds, flu, or other virus infections.

Oral vancomycin is taken by mouth. However, the injection form of vancomycin may also be taken by mouth when the oral liquid is not available. When this medicine is taken by mouth, it is not absorbed very much and works inside the intestinal tract to treat colitis. Colitis is an inflammation of the small or large intestine and may be caused by other antibiotics (for example, cephalosporins, lincomycins, penicillins) or "staph" bacteria. This medicine may be taken alone by mouth or given by injection and by mouth at the same time for colitis. Vancomycin may also be used for other conditions as determined by your doctor.

Vancomycin is available only with your doctor's prescription.

Remember:

• This medicine has been prescribed for your present medical problem only. Even though other people may have the same symptoms as you, they may have a different kind of problem. Your medicine may not work for them and may even cause them harm. Therefore, **your medicine must not be given to other people or used for other problems** unless you are otherwise directed by your doctor.

• In order for this medicine to work, it must be taken as directed.

• Keep all medicines out of the reach of children.

• If you want more information about this medicine, ask your doctor, nurse, or pharmacist.

• If any of the following information causes you special concern, do not decide against taking this medicine without first checking with your doctor.

Before Using This Medicine

In order to decide on the best treatment for your medical problem, your doctor should be told:

—if you have ever had any unusual or allergic reaction to vancomycin.

—if you are **pregnant** or if you may become pregnant. However, oral vancomycin has not been shown to cause birth defects or other problems in humans.

—if you are **breast-feeding**. However, oral vancomycin has not been shown to cause problems in nursing babies. When taken by mouth only small amounts of vancomycin are absorbed into the body and it is unlikely to pass into the breast milk in large amounts. In addition, vancomycin is not absorbed very much from the digestive tract (stomach and intestines) of the nursing infant. Therefore, this medicine is unlikely to cause serious problems in nursing babies.

—if you have any of the following medical problems:
Blockage of the bowel
Kidney disease, severe
Loss of hearing, or deafness, history of

—if you are taking **any** other prescription or nonprescription (OTC) medicine, especially:
Aminoglycosides (amikacin, gentamicin, kanamycin, neomycin, netilmicin, streptomycin, tobramycin)
Amphotericin B by injection (e.g., Fungizone)
Bacitracin by injection
Bumetanide by injection (e.g., Bumex)
Capreomycin (e.g., Capastat)
Cholestyramine (e.g., Questran)
Cisplatin (e.g., Platinol)
Colestipol (e.g., Colestid)
Colistin (e.g., Coly-Mycin)
Cyclosporine (e.g., Sandimmune)
Ethacrynic acid by injection (e.g., Edecrin)
Furosemide by injection (e.g., Lasix)
Paromomycin (e.g., Humatin)
Streptozocin (e.g., Zanosar)

Proper Use of This Medicine

To help clear up your colitis completely, **keep taking this medicine for the full time of treatment** even if you begin to feel better after a few days. If you stop taking this medicine too soon, your symptoms may return. **Do not miss any doses.**

If you do miss a dose of this medicine, take it as soon as possible. However, if it is almost time for your next dose, skip the missed dose and go back to your regular dosing schedule. Do not double doses.

For patients taking the oral liquid form of vancomycin:

• Use a specially marked measuring spoon or other device to measure each dose accurately since the average household teaspoon may not hold the right amount of liquid.

• Do not use after the expiration date on the label since the medicine may not work as well. Check with your pharmacist if you have any questions about this.

For patients taking the injection form of vancomycin by mouth:

- The powder in each vial is dissolved in about 1 ounce of water and taken straight. It may also be given through a nasogastric (NG) tube (tube which passes through the nose, down the throat, and into the stomach) to help prevent or lessen the unpleasant taste and nausea caused by this medicine.

How to store this medicine:

- **Keep out of the reach of children.**

- Store away from heat and direct light.

- Do not store the capsule form of this medicine in the bathroom, near the kitchen sink, or in other damp places. Heat or moisture may cause the medicine to break down.

- Store the oral liquid form of vancomycin in the refrigerator because heat will cause this medicine to break down. However, keep the medicine from freezing. Follow the directions on the label.

- Do not keep outdated medicine or medicine no longer needed. Be sure that any discarded medicine is out of the reach of children.

Precautions While Using This Medicine

It is important that your doctor check your progress during and after treatment. This is to make sure that the colitis is cleared up completely.

If the symptoms of your colitis do not improve within a few days, or if they become worse, check with your doctor.

If you are taking this medicine for diarrhea caused by other antibiotics, do not take any other diarrhea medicine without first checking with your doctor or pharmacist. These medicines may make your diarrhea worse or make it last longer.

If your doctor orders cholestyramine or colestipol for your colitis, do not take vancomycin by mouth within 3 to 4 hours of the time you take either of these medicines. To do so may keep vancomycin from working as well.

Side Effects of This Medicine

Along with its needed effects, a medicine may cause some unwanted effects. The following side effects may go away during treatment as your body adjusts to the medicine. However, check with your doctor if any of the following side effects continue or are bothersome:

More common
    Bitter or unpleasant taste
    Nausea or vomiting

Other side effects not listed above may also occur in some patients. If you notice any other effects, check with your doctor.

December 1987

VANCOMYCIN (Systemic)

Some commonly used brand names are Diatracin*, Vancocin I.V., and Vancoled.

*Not available in the U.S.

To the Reader: If you do not recognize the names of medical conditions or medicines referred to in this information, check with your doctor, nurse, or pharmacist. Definitions for selected medical terms may be found in the Glossary. Brand names for the generic drug names listed can be found in the Index. In addition, selected brand names commonly associated with the generic name have been included in the text to help you recognize medicine you may be taking. The fact that a brand name product is not mentioned does not mean the information does not apply. It is a good idea for you to learn both the generic and brand names of your medicines and to write them down for future use.

Vancomycin (van-koe-MYE-sin) belongs to the family of medicines called antibiotics. Antibiotics are medicines used in the treatment of infections caused by bacteria. They work by killing bacteria or preventing their growth. Vancomycin will not work for colds, flu, or other virus infections.

Vancomycin is given by injection into a vein to treat infections in many different parts of the body. It is sometimes given with other antibiotics. Vancomycin may also be used for other conditions as determined by your doctor.

Vancomycin given by injection is usually used for serious infections in which other medicines may not work. However, this medicine may also cause some serious side effects, including damage to your hearing and kidneys. These side effects may be more likely to occur in elderly patients. You and your doctor should talk about the good this medicine will do as well as the risks of receiving it.

Vancomycin may also be taken by mouth. It is not absorbed very much and works inside the intestinal tract to treat colitis. Colitis is an inflammation of the small or large intestine and may be caused by other antibiotics (for example, cephalosporins, lincomycins, penicillins) or "staph" bacteria. The injection form of this medicine may be taken alone by mouth or given by injection and by mouth at the same time for colitis.

Vancomycin is available only with your doctor's prescription.

Remember:
- If you want more information about this medicine, ask your doctor, nurse, or pharmacist.
- Keep all medicines out of the reach of children.
- If any of the following information causes you special concern, do not decide against receiving this medicine without first checking with your doctor.

Before Using This Medicine

In order to decide on the best treatment for your medical problem, your doctor should be told:

—if you have ever had any unusual or allergic reaction to vancomycin.

—if you are **pregnant** or if you may become pregnant. Vancomycin has been shown to damage the infant's hearing. However, this medicine may be needed in serious diseases or other situations which threaten the mother's life. Be sure you have discussed this with your doctor.

—if you are **breast-feeding**. Vancomycin has not been shown to cause problems in nursing babies. Vancomycin may pass into the breast milk when given by injection. However, vancomycin is not absorbed very much from the digestive tract (stomach and intestines) of the nursing infant. Therefore, this medicine is unlikely to cause serious problems in nursing babies.

—if you have any of the following medical problems:
Kidney disease
Loss of hearing, or deafness, history of

—if you are receiving **any** other prescription or non-prescription (OTC) medicine, especially:
Aminoglycosides (amikacin, gentamicin, kanamycin, neomycin, netilmicin, streptomycin, tobramycin)
Amphotericin B by injection (e.g., Fungizone)
Bacitracin by injection
Bumetanide by injection (e.g., Bumex)
Capreomycin (e.g., Capastat)
Cisplatin (e.g., Platinol)
Colistin (e.g., Coly-Mycin)
Cyclosporine (e.g., Sandimmune)
Ethacrynic acid by injection (e.g., Edecrin)
Furosemide by injection (e.g., Lasix)
Paromomycin (e.g., Humatin)
Streptozocin (e.g., Zanosar)

Proper Use of This Medicine

Some medicines given by injection may sometimes be given at home to patients who do not need to be in the hospital for the full time of treatment. If you are using this medicine at home, **make sure you clearly understand and carefully follow your doctor's instructions.**

To help clear up your infection completely, **this medicine must be given for the full time of treatment** even if you begin to feel better after a few days. Also, it works best when there is a constant amount in the blood or stool. To help keep this amount constant, it is given on a regular schedule.

Side Effects of This Medicine

Along with its needed effects, a medicine may cause some unwanted effects. Although not all of these side effects may occur, if they do occur they may need medical attention.

Check with your doctor or nurse immediately if any of the following side effects occur:

Less common
Any loss of hearing
Blood in urine
Difficulty in breathing
Drowsiness
Greatly increased or decreased frequency of urination or amount of urine
Increased thirst
Loss of appetite

Nausea or vomiting
Ringing or buzzing or a feeling of fullness in the ears
Weakness

> Note: The above side effects may also occur up to several weeks after you stop receiving this medicine.

Signs of "red-neck syndrome"—Rare

Bad taste
Chills or fever
Fainting
Fast heartbeat
Itching
Nausea or vomiting
Rash or redness of the face, base of neck, upper body, back, and arms
Tingling

> Note: Signs of the "red-neck syndrome" are more common when vancomycin is given by direct or rapid injection.

The above side effects, except the "red-neck syndrome," are more likely to occur in the elderly, who are usually more sensitive to the effects of vancomycin.

Other side effects not listed above may also occur in some patients. If you notice any other effects, check with your doctor.

December 1987

Additional Information

For patients receiving vancomycin to prevent endocarditis (inflammation of the lining of the heart):

• Some doctors may prescribe vancomycin by injection in patients with heart valve disease or prosthetic (artificial) heart valves who are allergic to penicillin. Vancomycin is used to prevent endocarditis in these patients who are having dental work, surgery, or procedures done on the upper respiratory tract (for example, nose or throat). It is also used with other antibiotics in patients who are having procedures done on the gastrointestinal or GI tract (stomach and intestines) or genitourinary or GU tract (sex organs and urinary tract). Vancomycin is usually given once about an hour before the procedure begins and again 8 hours later. If you have any questions about this, check with your doctor.

VASOPRESSIN (Systemic)

A commonly used brand name is Pitressin.

To the Reader: If you do not recognize the names of medical conditions or medicines referred to in this information, check with your doctor, nurse, or pharmacist. Definitions for selected medical terms may be found in the Glossary. Brand names for the generic drug names listed can be found in the Index. In addition, selected brand names commonly associated with the generic name have been included in the text to help you recognize medicine you may be taking. The fact that a brand name product is not mentioned does not mean the information does not apply. It is a good idea for you to learn both the generic and brand names of your medicines and to write them down for future use.

Vasopressin (vay-soe-PRESS-in) is a hormone naturally produced by your body. It is necessary to maintain good health. Lack of vasopressin causes your body to lose too much water.

Vasopressin is used by injection to control the frequent urination, increased thirst, and loss of water associated with diabetes insipidus (water diabetes).

This medicine is also given by injection to prevent and treat stomach swelling caused by too much gas. It is also used to break up gas bubbles before a stomach x-ray is taken.

Vasopressin also may be used for other conditions as determined by your doctor.

This medicine is available only with your doctor's prescription.

Remember:

• **This medicine has been prescribed for your current medical problem only.** It must not be given to other people or used for other problems unless you are directed to do so by your doctor.

• **Keep all medicines out of the reach of children.**

• In order for this medicine to work, it must be used as directed.

• **It is very important that you read and understand the following information.** If any of the information causes you special concern, do not decide against using this medicine without first checking with your doctor.

• Before you begin using any new medicine (prescription or nonprescription) or if you develop any new medical problem while you are using this medicine, check with your doctor, nurse, or pharmacist.

• **If you have any questions** about the following information or if you want more information about this medicine or your medical problem, **ask your doctor, nurse, or pharmacist.**

Before Using This Medicine

In order to decide on the best treatment for your medical problem, your doctor should be told:

—if you have ever had any unusual or allergic reaction to vasopressin.

—if you are on a low-salt, low-sugar, or any other special diet, or if you are allergic to any substance, such as foods or sulfites or other preservatives. Most medicines contain more than their active ingredient. Your doctor, nurse, or pharmacist can help you avoid products that may cause a problem.

—if you are **pregnant** or if you may become pregnant. Vasopressin has not been shown to cause birth defects or other problems in humans.

—if you are **breast-feeding**. Vasopressin has not been shown to cause problems in nursing babies.

—if you have any of the following medical problems:
Asthma
Epilepsy
Heart or blood vessel disease
Kidney disease
Migraine headaches

—if you are taking **any** other prescription or nonprescription (OTC) medicine.

Proper Use of This Medicine

For patients using vasopressin tannate in oil injection:

• Before drawing the solution for injection up into the needle, **it is very important that you warm the vial in your hands and shake it vigorously.** This is done to mix in the medicine, which appears as a brown speck in the bottom of the vial.

Use this medicine only as directed. Do not use more of it and do not use it more often than your doctor ordered. To do so may increase the chance of side effects.

Drink 1 or 2 glasses of water at the time you use vasopressin. This will help reduce the chance of side effects such as unusual paleness, nausea, abdominal or stomach cramps, or vomiting. If these side effects do occur, they are not serious and will usually disappear within a few minutes.

If you miss a dose of this medicine, use it as soon as possible. However, if it is almost time for your next dose, skip the missed dose and go back to your regular dosing schedule. Do not double doses.

How to store this medicine:

• **Keep out of the reach of children.**

• Store away from heat and direct light.

• Keep from freezing.

• Do not keep outdated medicine or medicine no longer needed. Be sure that any discarded medicine is out of the reach of children.

Side Effects of This Medicine

Along with its needed effects, a medicine may cause some unwanted effects. Although not all of these effects may occur, if they do occur they may need medical attention.

Check with your doctor immediately if any of the following side effects occur since they may be signs of an allergic reaction or overdose:
Rare
Chest pain
Coma
Confusion

Convulsions (seizures)
Drowsiness
Fever
Headache (continuing)
Problems with urination
Redness of skin
Skin rash, hives, or itching
Swelling of face, feet, hands, or mouth
Weight gain
Wheezing or troubled breathing

Other side effects may occur that usually do not require medical attention. These side effects may go away during treatment as your body adjusts to the medicine. However, check with your doctor if any of the following side effects continue or are bothersome:

More common

Pain at the site of injection

Less common

Abdominal or stomach cramps
Belching
Diarrhea

Dizziness or lightheadedness
Increased urge for bowel movement
Increase in sweating
Nausea or vomiting
Paleness
Passage of gas
"Pounding" in head
Trembling
White-colored area around mouth

For elderly patients: Many medicines have not been tested in older people. Therefore, it is not known whether the medicine acts the same way it does in younger adults. Check with your doctor or pharmacist if you notice any unusual effects while taking this medicine or if you think it is not working as it should.

Other side effects not listed above may also occur in some patients. If you notice any other effects, check with your doctor.

_____

December 1987

VIDARABINE (Ophthalmic)

Some commonly used brand names or other names are Adenine arabinoside, Ara-A, and Vira-A.

To the Reader: If you do not recognize the names of medical conditions or medicines referred to in this information, check with your doctor, nurse, or pharmacist. Definitions for selected medical terms may be found in the Glossary. Brand names for the generic drug names listed can be found in the Index. In addition, selected brand names commonly associated with the generic name have been included in the text to help you recognize medicine you may be taking. The fact that a brand name product is not mentioned does not mean the information does not apply. It is a good idea for you to learn both the generic and brand names of your medicines and to write them down for future use.

Vidarabine (vye-DARE-a-been) belongs to the family of medicines called antivirals. Vidarabine ophthalmic preparations are used in the eye to help the body overcome virus infections of the eye.

Vidarabine is available only with your doctor's prescription.

Remember:

• This medicine has been prescribed for your present infection only. Another infection later on may require a different medicine. Also, even though other people may have the same symptoms as you, they may have a different kind of infection. Your medicine may not work for them and may even cause them harm. Therefore, **your medicine must not be given to other people or used for other infections** unless you are otherwise directed by your doctor.

• In order for this medicine to work, it must be used as directed.

• If you want more information about this medicine, ask your doctor, nurse, or pharmacist.

• If any of the following information causes you special concern, do not decide against using this medicine without first checking with your doctor.

Before Using This Medicine

In order to decide on the best treatment for your medical problem, your doctor should be told:

—if you have ever had any unusual or allergic reaction to vidarabine.

—if you are **pregnant** or if you may become pregnant. However, vidarabine ophthalmic ointment has not been shown to cause birth defects or other problems in humans.

—if you are **breast-feeding.** However, vidarabine ophthalmic ointment has not been shown to cause problems in nursing babies.

Proper Use of This Medicine

How to apply this medicine: First, wash your hands. Then pull the lower eyelid away from the eye to form a pouch. Squeeze a thin strip of ointment into the pouch. A 1.25-cm (approximately ½-inch) strip of ointment is usually enough unless otherwise directed by your

doctor. Gently close the eyes and keep them closed for 1 or 2 minutes to allow the medicine to come into contact with the infection.

To prevent contamination of the eye ointment, do not touch the applicator tip to any surface (including the eye). After using vidarabine eye ointment, wipe the tip of the ointment tube with a clean tissue and keep the tube tightly closed.

Do not use this medicine more often or for a longer time than your doctor ordered. To do so may cause problems in the eyes. If you have any questions about this, check with your doctor.

To help clear up your infection completely, **keep using this medicine for the full time of treatment,** even though your symptoms may have disappeared; **do not miss any doses.**

If you do miss a dose of this medicine, apply it as soon as possible. However, if it is almost time for your next application, skip the missed dose and go back to your regular dosing schedule.

How to store this medicine:

• **Keep out of the reach of children.**

• Store away from heat and direct light.

• Keep the medicine from freezing.

• Do not keep outdated medicine or medicine no longer needed. Be sure that any discarded medicine is out of the reach of children.

Precautions While Using This Medicine

After application, eye ointments usually cause your vision to blur for a few minutes.

It is very important that you keep your appointment with your doctor. If your symptoms become worse, check with your doctor sooner.

This medicine may cause your eyes to become more sensitive to light than they are normally. Wearing sunglasses and avoiding too much exposure to bright light may help lessen the discomfort.

Side Effects of This Medicine

Along with its needed effects, a medicine may cause some unwanted effects. Although not all of these side effects may occur, if they do occur they may need medical attention.

Check with your doctor as soon as possible if any of the following side effects occur:

Increased sensitivity of eyes to light
Itching, redness, swelling, pain, burning, or other sign of irritation not present before using this medicine

Other side effects may occur that usually do not require medical attention. These side effects may go away during treatment as your body adjusts to the medicine. However, check with your doctor if either of the following side effects continues or is bothersome:

   Excess flow of tears
   Feeling of something in the eye

Other side effects not listed above may also occur in some patients. If you notice any other effects, check with your doctor.

December 1987

VINBLASTINE (Systemic)

Some commonly used brand names are Velban and Velbe*.

Generic name product may also be available in the U.S.

*Not available in the U.S.

To the Reader: If you do not recognize the names of medical conditions or medicines referred to in this information, check with your doctor, nurse, or pharmacist. Definitions for selected medical terms may be found in the Glossary. Brand names for the generic drug names listed can be found in the Index. In addition, selected brand names commonly associated with the generic name have been included in the text to help you recognize medicine you may be taking. The fact that a brand name product is not mentioned does not mean the information does not apply. It is a good idea for you to learn both the generic and brand names of your medicines and to write them down for future use.

Vinblastine (vin-BLAS-teen) belongs to the group of medicines known as antineoplastic agents. It is given by injection to treat some kinds of cancer as well as some noncancerous conditions.

Vinblastine interferes with the growth of cancer cells, which are eventually destroyed. Since the growth of normal body cells may also be affected by vinblastine, other effects will also occur. Some of these may be serious and must be reported to your doctor. Other effects, such as hair loss, may not be serious but may cause concern. Some effects do not occur for months or years after the medicine is used.

Before you begin treatment with vinblastine, you and your doctor should talk about the good this medicine will do as well as the risks of using it.

Vinblastine is to be administered only by or under the immediate supervision of your doctor.

Remember:

• **It is very important that you read and understand the following information.** If any of the information causes you special concern, do not decide against receiving this medicine without first checking with your doctor.

• Before you begin using any new medicine (prescription or nonprescription) or if you develop any new medical problem while you are receiving this medicine, check with your doctor, nurse, or pharmacist.

• **If you have any questions** about the following information or if you want more information about this medicine or your medical problem, **ask your doctor, nurse, or pharmacist.**

Before Using This Medicine

In order to decide on the best treatment for your medical problem, your doctor should be told:

—if you have ever had any unusual or allergic reaction to vinblastine.

—if you are **pregnant** or if you intend to have children. This medicine may cause birth defects if either the male or female is taking it at the time of conception or if it is taken during pregnancy. In addition, many cancer medicines may cause sterility which could be permanent. Although this has not been reported with this medicine, vinblastine may interfere with production of sperm and the possibility should be kept in mind. Be sure that you have discussed this with your doctor before receiving this medicine.

—if you intend to **breast-feed**. Because this medicine may cause serious side effects, breast-feeding is generally not recommended while you are receiving it.

—if you have any of the following medical problems:
   Chickenpox (including recent exposure)
   Gout (history of)
   Herpes zoster (shingles)
   Infection
   Kidney stones
   Liver disease

—if you are taking **any** other prescription or nonprescription (OTC) medicine, especially:
   Antithyroid agents (medicine for overactive thyroid)
   Azathioprine (e.g., Imuran)
   Chloramphenicol (e.g., Chloromycetin)
   Colchicine
   Flucytosine (e.g., Ancobon)
   Interferon (e.g., Intron A, Roferon-A)
   Probenecid (e.g., Benemid)
   Sulfinpyrazone (e.g., Anturane)

—if you have ever been treated with x-rays or cancer medicines.

Proper Use of This Medicine

Vinblastine is sometimes given together with certain other medicines. If you are using a combination of medicines, it is important that you receive each one at the proper time. If you are taking some of these medicines by mouth, ask your doctor, nurse, or pharmacist to help you plan a way to take them at the right times.

While you are using this medicine, your doctor may want you to drink extra fluids so that you will pass more urine. This will help prevent kidney problems and keep your kidneys working well.

Vinblastine sometimes causes nausea and vomiting. However, it is very important that you continue to receive the medicine, even if you begin to feel ill. Ask your doctor, nurse, or pharmacist for ways to lessen these effects.

Precautions While Using This Medicine

It is very important that your doctor check your progress at regular visits to make sure that this medicine is working properly and to check for unwanted effects.

While you are being treated with vinblastine, and after you stop treatment with it, **do not have any immunizations without your doctor's approval**. Vinblastine lowers your body's resistance and there is a chance you might get the infection the immunization is meant to prevent. Other people living in your household should not take oral polio vaccine since there is a chance they could pass the polio virus on to you. Also, you should avoid close contact with other persons (for example, at school or work) who have taken oral polio vaccine.

Vinblastine can lower the number of white blood cells in your body. This may increase the chance of getting an infection. If you can, avoid people with colds or other infections. If you think you are getting a cold or other infection, check with your doctor.

If vinblastine accidentally seeps out of the vein into which it is injected, it may damage the skin and cause some scarring. **Tell the doctor or nurse right away if you notice redness, pain, or swelling at the place of injection.**

Side Effects of This Medicine

Along with their needed effects medicines like vinblastine can sometimes cause unwanted effects such as blood problems, loss of hair, and other side effects; these are described below. Also, because of the way these medicines act on the body, there is a chance that they might cause other unwanted effects that may not occur until months or years after the medicine is used. These delayed effects may include certain types of cancer, such as leukemia. Discuss these possible effects with your doctor.

Although not all of these side effects may occur, if they do occur they may need medical attention.

Check with your doctor or nurse immediately if any of the following side effects occur:

More common
    Fever, chills, or sore throat

Less common
    Pain or redness at place of injection
    Unusual bleeding or bruising

Check with your doctor or nurse as soon as possible if any of the following side effects occur:

Less common
    Joint pain
    Lower back, side or stomach pain
    Sores in the mouth and on the lips
    Swelling of feet or lower legs

Rare
    Black tarry stools
    Difficulty in walking
    Dizziness
    Double vision
    Drooping eyelids
    Headache
    Jaw pain
    Mental depression
    Numbness or tingling in fingers and toes
    Pain in fingers and toes
    Pain in testicles
    Weakness

Other side effects may occur that usually do not require medical attention. These side effects may go away during treatment as your body adjusts to the medicine. Also, your doctor or nurse may be able to tell you about ways to prevent or reduce some of these side effects. Check with your doctor if any of the following side effects continue or are bothersome or if you have any questions about them:

Less common
    Muscle pain
    Nausea and vomiting

This medicine often causes a temporary loss of hair. After treatment with vinblastine has ended, or sometimes even during treatment, normal hair growth should return.

For elderly patients: Many medicines have not been tested in older people. Therefore, it is not known whether the medicine acts the same way it does in younger adults. Check with your doctor if you notice any unusual effects while taking this medicine or if you think it is not working as it should.

Other side effects not listed above may also occur in some patients. If you notice any other effects, check with your doctor.

———————
December 1987

VINCRISTINE (Systemic)

Some commonly used brand names are Oncovin and Vincasar PFS.

Generic name product may also be available in the U.S.

To the Reader: If you do not recognize the names of medical conditions or medicines referred to in this information, check with your doctor, nurse, or pharmacist. Definitions for selected medical terms may be found in the Glossary. Brand names for the generic drug names listed can be found in the Index. In addition, selected brand names commonly associated with the generic name have been included in the text to help you recognize medicine you may be taking. The fact that a brand name product is not mentioned does not mean the information does not apply. It is a good idea for you to learn both the generic and brand names of your medicines and to write them down for future use.

Vincristine (vin-KRIS-teen) belongs to the group of medicines known as antineoplastic agents. It is given by injection to treat some kinds of cancer as well as some noncancerous conditions.

Vincristine interferes with the growth of cancer cells, which are eventually destroyed. Since the growth of normal body cells may also be affected by vincristine, other effects will also occur. Some of these may be serious and must be reported to your doctor. Other effects, such as hair loss, may not be serious but may cause concern. Some effects may not occur for months or years after the medicine is used.

Before you begin treatment with vincristine, you and your doctor should talk about the good this medicine will do as well as the risks of using it.

Vincristine is to be administered only by or under the immediate supervision of your doctor.

Remember:

• **It is very important that you read and understand the following information.** If any of the information causes you special concern, do not decide against receiving this medicine without first checking with your doctor.

• Before you begin using any new medicine (prescription or nonprescription) or if you develop any new medical problem while you are receiving this medicine, check with your doctor, nurse, or pharmacist.

• **If you have any questions** about the following information or if you want more information about this medicine or your medical problem, **ask your doctor, nurse, or pharmacist.**

Before Using This Medicine

In order to decide on the best treatment for your medical problem, your doctor should be told:

—if you have ever had any unusual or allergic reaction to vincristine.

—if you are **pregnant** or if you intend to have children. There is a chance that this medicine may cause birth defects if either the male or female is taking it at the time of conception or if it is taken during pregnancy. In addition, many cancer medicines may cause sterility, which could be permanent. Although this has not

been reported with this medicine, the possibility should be kept in mind. Be sure that you have discussed this with your doctor before receiving this medicine.

—if you intend to **breast-feed**. Because this medicine may cause serious side effects, breast-feeding is generally not recommended while you are receiving it.

—if you have any of the following medical problems:
Chickenpox (including recent exposure)
Gout (history of)
Herpes zoster (shingles)
Infection
Kidney stones
Liver disease
Nerve or muscle disease

—if you are taking **any** other prescription or nonprescription (OTC) medicine, especially:
Probenecid (e.g., Benemid)
Sulfinpyrazone (e.g., Anturane)

—if you have ever been treated with x-rays or cancer medicines.

Proper Use of This Medicine

Vincristine is often given together with certain other medicines. If you are using a combination of medicines, it is important that you receive each one at the proper time. If you are taking some of these medicines by mouth, ask your doctor, nurse, or pharmacist to help you plan a way to take them at the right times.

While you are using this medicine, it may be necessary to drink extra fluids so that you will pass more urine. This will help prevent kidney problems and keep your kidneys working well. Ask your doctor if this is necessary for you.

This medicine sometimes causes nausea and vomiting. However, it is very important that you continue to receive the medicine, even if you begin to feel ill. Ask your doctor, nurse, or pharmacist for ways to lessen these effects.

Vincristine frequently causes constipation and stomach cramps. Your doctor may want you to take a laxative or stool softener. However, do not decide to take these medicines on your own without first checking with your doctor.

Precautions While Using This Medicine

It is very important that your doctor check your progress at regular visits to make sure that vincristine is working properly and to check for unwanted effects.

While you are being treated with vincristine, and after you stop treatment with it, **do not have any immunizations without your doctor's approval.** Vincristine lowers your body's resistance and there is a chance you might get the infection the immunization is meant to prevent. Other people living in your household should not take oral polio vaccine since there is a chance they could pass the polio virus on to you. Also, you should avoid close contact with other persons (for example, at school or work) who have taken oral polio vaccine.

If vincristine accidentally seeps out of the vein into which it is injected, it may damage some tissues and cause scarring. **Tell the doctor or nurse right away if you notice redness, pain, or swelling at the place of injection.**

Side Effects of This Medicine

Along with their needed effects, medicines like vincristine can sometimes cause unwanted effects such as blood problems, nervous system problems, loss of hair, and other side effects; these are described below. Also, because of the way these medicines act on the body, there is a chance that they might cause other unwanted effects that may not occur until months or years after the medicine is used. These delayed effects may include certain types of cancer, such as leukemia. Discuss these possible effects with your doctor.

Although not all of these side effects may occur, if they do occur they may need medical attention.

Check with your doctor or nurse immediately if the following side effects occur:

Less common
      Pain or redness at place of injection

Rare
      Fever, chills, or sore throat
      Unusual bleeding or bruising

Check with your doctor or nurse as soon as possible if any of the following side effects occur:

More common
      Blurred or double vision
      Constipation
      Difficulty in walking
      Drooping eyelids
      Flank or stomach pain
      Headache
      Jaw pain
      Joint pain
      Numbness or tingling in fingers and toes
      Pain in fingers and toes
      Pain in testicles
      Stomach cramps
      Swelling of feet or lower legs
      Weakness

Less common
      Agitation
      Bed-wetting
      Confusion
      Convulsions (seizures)
      Decrease or increase in urination
      Dizziness or lightheadedness when getting up from a lying or sitting position
      Hallucinations (seeing, hearing, or feeling things that are not there)
      Lack of sweating
      Loss of appetite
      Mental depression
      Painful or difficult urination
      Trouble in sleeping
      Unconsciousness

Rare
      Sores in the mouth and on the lips

Other side effects may occur that usually do not require medical attention. These side effects may go away during treatment as your body adjusts to the medicine. Also, your doctor or nurse may be able to tell you about ways to prevent or reduce some of these side effects. Check with your doctor if any of the following side effects continue or are bothersome or if you have any questions about them:

Less common
      Bloating
      Diarrhea
      Loss of weight
      Nausea and vomiting
      Skin rash

For elderly patients: Nervous system effects may be more likely to occur in the elderly, who are usually more sensitive to the effects of vincristine.

This medicine often causes a temporary loss of hair. After treatment with vincristine has ended, or sometimes even during treatment, normal hair growth should return.

Other side effects not listed above may also occur in some patients. If you notice any other effects, check with your doctor.

_____

December 1987

VITAMIN A (Systemic)

Some commonly used brand names are Alphalin and Aquasol A.

Generic name product may also be available in the U.S. and Canada.

To the Reader: If you do not recognize the names of medical conditions or medicines referred to in this information, check with your doctor, nurse, or pharmacist. Definitions for selected medical terms may be found in the Glossary. Brand names for the generic drug names listed can be found in the Index. In addition, selected brand names commonly associated with the generic name have been included in the text to help you recognize medicine you may be taking. The fact that a brand name product is not mentioned does not mean the information does not apply. It is a good idea for you to learn both the generic and brand names of your medicines and to write them down for future use.

Vitamins (VYE-ta-mins) are compounds that you *must* have for growth and health. They are needed in small amounts only and are usually available in the foods that you eat. Vitamin A is necessary for normal growth and health and for healthy eyes and skin.

Lack of vitamin A may lead to a rare condition called night blindness (problems seeing in the dark), as well as dry eyes, eye infections, skin problems, and slowed growth. Your doctor may treat this by prescribing vitamin A for you.

Claims that vitamin A is effective for treatment of conditions such as acne, cancer, or lung diseases, or for treatment of eye problems, wounds, or dry or wrinkled skin not caused by lack of vitamin A have not been proven.

Some strengths of vitamin A are available without a prescription. However, it may be a good idea to check with your doctor before taking vitamin A on your own. **Taking large amounts over prolonged periods may cause serious unwanted effects.**

Remember:
- **Keep all medicines out of the reach of children.**

- In order for this medicine to work, it must be used as directed. **If you are using this medicine without a prescription, it is very important to follow the directions on the label.**

- **It is also very important that you read and understand the following information.** If any of the information causes you special concern, check with your doctor before using this medicine without a prescription.

- Before you begin using any new medicine (prescription or nonprescription) or if you develop any new medical problem while you are using this medicine, check with your doctor, nurse, or pharmacist.

- **If you have any questions** about the following information or if you want more information about this medicine or your medical problem, **ask your doctor, nurse, or pharmacist.**

Importance of Diet

Vitamin supplements should be taken only if you cannot get enough vitamins in your diet. A balanced diet should provide all the vitamins you normally need.

Nutritionists recommend that you eat:
- Cereal or bread—4 or more servings per day and
- Dairy products (milk, cheese, ice cream, cottage cheese)—3 or more servings per day and
- Meat, fish, or eggs—2 or more servings per day and
- Vegetables and fruits—4 or more servings per day.

If you are not getting all of these foods every day, you may not be getting enough vitamins in your diet. The best way to correct this is to start eating the foods that contain what you need.

Vitamin A is found in various foods including liver; yellow-orange fruits and vegetables; dark green, leafy vegetables; whole milk; fortified skim milk; butter; margarine; fish liver oils; and egg yolks. Vitamin A comes in different forms. Retinols are a kind of vitamin A found in foods that come from animals (meat, milk, eggs). The form of vitamin A found in plants is called beta-carotene. It is best to eat fresh fruits and vegetables whenever possible since they contain the most vitamins. Food processing may destroy some of the vitamins. For example, freezing may reduce the amount of vitamin A in foods.

Vitamins alone will not take the place of a good diet and will not provide energy. Your body needs other substances found in food, such as protein, minerals, carbohydrates, and fat. Vitamins themselves often cannot work without the presence of other foods. For example, fat is needed so that vitamin A can be absorbed into the body.

In some cases, it may not be possible for you to get enough food to supply you with the proper vitamins. In other cases, the amount of vitamins you need may be increased above normal. Therefore, a vitamin supplement may be needed.

Experts have developed a list of recommended dietary allowances (RDA) for most of the vitamins. The RDA are not an exact number but a general idea of how much you need. They do not cover amounts needed for problems caused by a serious lack of vitamins.

The RDA for vitamin A are:

Children 4 to 6 years of age—2500 Units per day
Adult males—5000 Units per day
Adult females—4000 Units per day
Pregnant females—5000 Units per day
Breast-feeding females—6000 Units per day.

Remember:
- The total amount of each vitamin that you get every day includes what you get from the foods that you eat *and* what you may take as a supplement.

- This total amount should not be greater than the RDA, unless ordered by your doctor. **Taking too much vitamin A over a period of time may cause harmful effects.**

Before Using This Medicine

In deciding whether you need additional vitamin A, the following should be kept in mind and/or your doctor should be told:

—if you have ever had any unusual or allergic reaction to vitamin A.

—if you are on a low-salt, low-sugar, or any other special diet, or if you are allergic to any substance, such as foods, sulfites or other preservatives, or dyes. Most medicines contain more than their active ingredient, and many liquid medicines contain alcohol. Your doctor, nurse, or pharmacist can help you avoid products that may cause a problem.

—if you are **pregnant** or if you may become pregnant. It is especially important that you are receiving enough vitamins when you become pregnant and that you continue to receive the right amount of vitamins throughout your pregnancy. The healthy growth and development of the fetus depend on a steady supply of nutrients from the mother.

However, taking too much vitamin A during pregnancy can also cause harmful effects such as birth defects or slow or reduced growth in the child.

—if you are **breast-feeding**. It is especially important that you receive the right amounts of vitamins so that your baby will also get the vitamins needed to grow properly.

—if you are not able to get a diet that contains all of the vitamins you need. This may occur with rapid weight loss, unusual diets (such as some reducing diets in which choice of foods is very limited), prolonged intravenous feeding, or malnutrition.

—if you have had a large part of your stomach removed.

—if you have been under a lot of stress for a long time, or if you have had a long illness or a serious injury.

—if you have any of the following medical problems:
Cystic fibrosis
Diabetes mellitus (sugar diabetes)
Diarrhea (prolonged)
Intestine problems
Kidney disease
Liver disease
Overactive thyroid
Pancreas disease

—if you are taking **any** other prescription or nonprescription (OTC) medicine, especially isotretinoin (e.g., Accutane).

Proper Use of This Medicine

Do not take more than the recommended daily amount. Vitamin A is stored in the body and **taking too much over a period of time can cause poisoning and even death.** Some people believe that taking very large doses of vitamins (called megadoses or megavitamin therapy) is useful for treating certain medical problems. Studies have not proven this. Large doses should be taken only under the direction of your doctor after need has been identified.

For patients taking the oral liquid form of vitamin A:

• This preparation is to be taken by mouth even though it comes in a dropper bottle.

• This medicine may be dropped directly into the mouth or mixed with cereal, fruit juice, or other food.

If you miss taking a vitamin for one or more days there is no cause for concern, since it takes some time for your body to become seriously low in vitamins. However, if your doctor has recommended that you take this vitamin, try to remember to take it as directed every day.

How to store this medicine:

• **Keep out of the reach of children.**

• Store away from heat and direct light.

• Do not store in the bathroom, near the kitchen sink or in other damp places. Heat or moisture may cause the medicine to break down.

• Keep the oral liquid form of this medicine from freezing.

• Do not keep outdated medicine or medicine no longer needed. Be sure that any discarded medicine is out of the reach of children.

Side Effects of This Medicine

Along with its needed effects, a medicine may cause some unwanted effects. Vitamin A does not usually cause any side effects. **However, taking large amounts of vitamin A over a period of time may cause some unwanted effects which can be serious. Check with your doctor immediately** if any of the following side effects occur, since they may be signs of sudden overdose:

Bleeding from gums or sore mouth
Bulging soft spot on head (in babies)
Confusion or unusual excitement
Convulsions (seizures)
Diarrhea
Dizziness or drowsiness
Double vision
Headache (severe)
Irritability (severe)
Peeling of skin, especially on lips and palms
Vomiting (severe)

Check with your doctor as soon as possible if any of the following side effects occur, since they may also be signs of gradual overdose:

Bone or joint pain
Drying or cracking of skin or lips
Fever
General feeling of body discomfort or weakness
Headache
Increased sensitivity of skin to sunlight
Increase in frequency of urination, especially at night, or in amount of urine
Irritability
Loss of appetite
Loss of hair
Stomach pain

Tiredness
Vomiting
Yellow-orange patches on soles of feet, palms of hands, or skin around nose and lips

For children: The above side effects are more likely to occur in young children, who are usually more sensitive to the effects of vitamin A.

Other side effects not listed above may also occur in some patients. If you notice any other effects, check with your doctor or pharmacist.

December 1987

VITAMIN B₁₂ (Systemic)

This information applies to the following medicines:

Cyanocobalamin (sye-an-oh-koe-BAL-a-min)
Hydroxocobalamin (hye-drox-oh-koe-BAL-a-min)

Some commonly used brand names are:	Generic names:
Anacobin*	
Bedoz*	
Berubigen	
Betalin 12	
Cyanabin*	
Kaybovite	Cyanocobalamin†
Kaybovite-1000	
Redisol	
Rubion*	
Rubramin*	
Rubramin PC	

Acti-B₁₂*	
alphaREDISOL	
Codroxomin	Hydroxocobalamin†
Droxomin	

*Not available in the U.S.
†Generic name product may also be available in the U.S. and Canada.

To the Reader: If you do not recognize the names of medical conditions or medicines referred to in this information, check with your doctor, nurse, or pharmacist. Definitions for selected medical terms may be found in the Glossary. Brand names for the generic drug names listed can be found in the Index. In addition, selected brand names commonly associated with the generic name have been included in the text to help you recognize medicine you may be taking. The fact that a brand name product is not mentioned does not mean the information does not apply. It is a good idea for you to learn both the generic and brand names of your medicines and to write them down for future use.

Vitamins (VYE-ta-mins) are compounds that you *must* have for growth and health. They are needed in small amounts only and are usually available in the foods that you eat. Vitamin B₁₂ is necessary for healthy blood. Cyanocobalamin and hydroxocobalamin are man-made forms of vitamin B₁₂.

Some people have a medical problem called pernicious anemia in which vitamin B₁₂ is not absorbed from the intestine. Others may have a badly diseased intestine or have had a large part of their stomach or intestine removed, so that vitamin B₁₂ cannot be absorbed. These people need to receive vitamin B₁₂ by injection.

Lack of vitamin B₁₂ may lead to anemia (weak blood), stomach problems, and nerve damage. Your doctor may treat this by prescribing vitamin B₁₂ for you.

Claims that vitamin B₁₂ is effective for treatment of various conditions such as aging, allergies, eye problems, slow growth, poor appetite or malnutrition, skin problems, tiredness, mental problems, sterility, thyroid disease, and nerve diseases have not been proven. Many of these treatments involve large and expensive amounts of vitamins.

Some strengths of the B vitamins are available only with your doctor's prescription. Others are available without a prescription. However, it may be a good idea to check with your doctor before taking vitamin B₁₂ on your own.

Remember:

• **If your doctor has prescribed this medicine, it has been prescribed for your current medical problem only.** It must not be given to other people or used for other problems unless you are directed to do so by your doctor.

• **Keep all medicines out of the reach of children.**

• In order for this medicine to work, it must be used as directed.

• If you are receiving this medicine by injection, some of the information about this medicine may not apply.

• **It is very important that you read and understand the following information.** If your doctor has ordered this medicine and if any of the information causes you special concern, do not decide against using this medicine without first checking with your doctor.

• Before you begin using any new medicine (prescription or nonprescription) or if you develop any new medical problem while you are using this medicine, check with your doctor, nurse, or pharmacist.

• **If you have any questions** about the following information or if you want more information about this medicine or your medical problem, **ask your doctor, nurse, or pharmacist.**

Importance of Diet

Vitamin supplements should be taken only if you cannot get enough vitamins in your diet. A balanced diet should provide all the vitamins you normally need.

Nutritionists recommend that you eat:
• Cereal or bread—4 or more servings per day and
• Dairy products (milk, cheese, ice cream, cottage cheese)—3 or more servings per day and
• Meat, fish, or eggs—2 or more servings per day and
• Vegetables and fruits—4 or more servings per day.

If you are not getting all of these foods every day, you may not be getting enough vitamins in your diet. The best way to correct this is to start eating the foods that contain what you need.

Vitamin B₁₂ is found in various foods, including meat, fish, egg yolk, milk, and fermented cheeses. It is *not* found in any vegetables. Ordinary cooking probably does not destroy the vitamin B₁₂ in food.

Vitamins alone will not take the place of a good diet and will not provide energy. Your body also needs other substances found in food such as protein, minerals, carbohydrates, and fat. Vitamins themselves often cannot work without the presence of other foods.

In some cases, it may not be possible for you to get enough food to supply you with the proper vitamins. In other cases, the amount of vitamins you need may be increased above normal. Therefore, a vitamin supplement may be needed.

Experts have developed a list of recommended dietary allowances (RDA) for most of the vitamins. The RDA are not an exact number but a general idea of how much you need. They do not cover amounts needed for problems caused by a serious lack of vitamins.

The RDA for vitamin B$_{12}$ are:

Children 4 to 6 years of age—2.5 mcg (micrograms) per day
Adult males—3 mcg per day
Adult females—3 mcg per day
Pregnant females—4 mcg per day
Breast-feeding females—4 mcg per day.

Remember:

• The total amount of each vitamin that you get every day includes what you get from the foods that you eat *and* what you may take as a supplement.

• This total amount should not be greater than the RDA, unless ordered by your doctor.

Before Using This Medicine

In deciding whether you need additional vitamin B$_{12}$, the following should be kept in mind and/or your doctor should be told:

—if you have ever had any unusual or allergic reaction to vitamin B$_{12}$ or other cobalamins.

—if you are on a low-salt, low-sugar, or any other special diet, or if you are allergic to any substance, such as foods, sulfites or other preservatives, or dyes. Most medicines contain more than their active ingredient. Your doctor, nurse, or pharmacist can help you avoid products that may cause a problem.

—if you are **pregnant** or if you may become pregnant. It is especially important that you are receiving enough vitamins when you become pregnant and that you continue to receive the right amount of vitamins throughout your pregnancy. Healthy fetal growth and development depend on a steady supply of nutrients from mother to fetus. Too little vitamin B$_{12}$ can cause harmful effects such as anemia or nervous system injury.

—if you are **breast-feeding**. It is especially important that you receive the right amounts of vitamins so that your baby will also get the vitamins needed to grow properly. If you are a strict vegetarian, your baby will not be getting the vitamin B$_{12}$ needed.

—if you are not able to get a diet that contains all of the vitamins you need. This may occur with rapid weight loss, unusual diets (such as strict vegetarian or macrobiotic diets, or some reducing diets in which choice of foods is very limited), prolonged intravenous feeding, or malnutrition.

—if you have had a large part of your stomach or intestine removed.

—if you have been under a lot of stress for a long time, or if you have had a long illness or serious injury.

—if you have any of the following medical problems:

Alcoholism
Cancer of the pancreas or bowel
Diarrhea (prolonged)
Fish tapeworm
Gout (history of)
Kidney disease
Leber's disease (an eye disease)
Liver disease
Overactive thyroid
Stomach or intestinal problems

—if you are taking **any** other prescription or nonprescription (OTC) medicine.

Proper Use of This Medicine

Some people believe that taking very large doses of vitamins (called megadoses or megavitamin therapy) is useful for treating certain medical problems. Studies have not proven this. Large doses should be taken only under the direction of your doctor after need has been identified.

For patients receiving vitamin B$_{12}$ by injection for pernicious anemia or if part of the stomach or intestine has been removed:

• You will have to receive treatment for the rest of your life. You must continue to receive this medicine even if you feel well in order to prevent future problems.

If you miss taking a vitamin for one or more days there is no cause for concern, since it takes some time for your body to become seriously low in vitamins. However, if your doctor has recommended that you take this vitamin, try to remember to take it as directed.

How to store this medicine:

• **Keep out of the reach of children.**

• Store away from heat and direct light.

• Do not store in the bathroom, near the kitchen sink, or in other damp places. Heat or moisture may cause the medicine to break down.

• Do not keep outdated medicine or medicine no longer needed. Be sure that any discarded medicine is out of the reach of children.

Side Effects of This Medicine

Along with its needed effects, a medicine may cause some unwanted effects. Cyanocobalamin does not usually cause any side effects. **However, check with your doctor immediately** if any of the following side effects occur:

Rare—Soon after receiving injection only
Skin rash or itching
Wheezing

Check with your doctor as soon as possible if either of the following side effects continues or is bothersome:

Less common
Diarrhea
Itching of skin

Other side effects not listed above may also occur in some patients. If you notice any other effects, check with your doctor or pharmacist.

December 1987

VITAMIN D (Systemic)

Some commonly used brand names and other names are:

Calciferol	Ostoforte*
Deltalin	Radiostol*
Drisdol	Radiostol Forte*
Ergocalciferol	

Generic name product may also be available in the U.S. and Canada.

---

*Not available in the U.S.

To the Reader: If you do not recognize the names of medical conditions or medicines referred to in this information, check with your doctor, nurse, or pharmacist. Definitions for selected medical terms may be found in the Glossary. Brand names for the generic drug names listed can be found in the Index. In addition, selected brand names commonly associated with the generic name have been included in the text to help you recognize medicine you may be taking. The fact that a brand name product is not mentioned does not mean the information does not apply. It is a good idea for you to learn both the generic and brand names of your medicines and to write them down for future use.

Vitamins (VYE-ta-mins) are compounds that you *must* have for growth and health. They are needed in only small amounts and are available in the foods that you eat. Vitamin D is necessary for strong bones and teeth.

Ergocalciferol (er-goe-kal-SIF-e-role) is the form of vitamin D found in vitamin supplements.

Lack of vitamin D may lead to a condition called rickets, especially in children, in which bones and teeth are weak. In adults it may cause a condition called osteomalacia, in which calcium is lost from bones so that they become weak. Your doctor may treat this by prescribing vitamin D for you. Vitamin D is also sometimes used to treat other diseases in which calcium is not used properly by the body.

Claims that vitamin D is effective for treatment of arthritis and prevention of nearsightedness or nerve problems have not been proven.

Some strengths of vitamin D are available only with your doctor's prescription. Others are available without a prescription. However, it may be a good idea to check with your doctor before taking vitamin D on your own. **Taking large amounts over prolonged periods may cause serious unwanted effects.**

Remember:

• **If your doctor has ordered this medicine, it has been prescribed for your current medical problem only.** It must not be given to other people or used for other problems unless you are directed to do so by your doctor.

• **Keep all medicines out of the reach of children.**

• In order for this medicine to work, it must be used as directed.

• If you are receiving this medicine by injection, some of the information about this medicine may not apply.

• **It is very important that you read and understand the following information.** If your doctor has ordered this medicine and if any of the information causes you special concern, do not decide against using this medicine without first checking with your doctor.

• Before you begin using any new medicine (prescription or nonprescription) or if you develop any new medical problem while you are using this medicine, check with your doctor, nurse, or pharmacist.

• **If you have any questions** about the following information or if you want more information about this medicine or your medical problem, **ask your doctor, nurse, or pharmacist.**

Importance of Diet

Vitamin supplements should be taken only if you cannot get enough vitamins in your diet. A balanced diet should provide all the vitamins you normally need.

Nutritionists recommend that you eat:

• Cereal or bread—4 or more servings per day and
• Dairy products (milk, cheese, ice cream, cottage cheese)—3 or more servings per day and
• Meat, fish, or eggs—2 or more servings per day and
• Vegetables and fruits—4 or more servings per day.

If you are not getting all of these foods every day, you may not be getting enough vitamins in your diet. The best way to correct this is to start eating the foods that contain what you need.

Vitamin D is found naturally only in fish and fish-liver oils. It is also found in vitamin D–fortified milk and bread. Cooking does not affect the vitamin D in foods. Vitamin D is sometimes called the "sunshine vitamin" since it is made in your skin when you are exposed to sunlight. If you eat a balanced diet and get outside in the sunshine, you should be getting all the vitamin D you need.

Vitamins alone will not take the place of a good diet and will not provide energy. Your body also needs other substances found in food such as protein, minerals, carbohydrates, and fat. Vitamins themselves often cannot work without the presence of other foods. For example, fat is needed so that vitamin D can be absorbed into the body.

In some cases, it may not be possible for you to get enough food to supply you with the proper vitamins. In other cases, the amount of vitamins you need may be increased above normal.

Experts have developed a list of recommended dietary allowances (RDA) for most of the vitamins. The RDA are not an exact number but a general idea of how much you need. They do not cover amounts needed for problems caused by a serious lack of vitamins.

The RDA for vitamin D are:

Children and adults less than 19 years of age—400 Units per day

Adult males (23 years of age and over)—200 Units per day

Adult females (23 years of age and over)—200 Units per day

Pregnant females—400 Units per day (500 Units if 19 to 22 years of age)

Breast-feeding females—400 Units per day (500 Units if 19 to 22 years of age).

Remember:

• The total amount of each vitamin that you get every day includes what you get from the foods that you eat *and* what you may take as a supplement.

• This total amount should not be greater than the RDA, unless ordered by your doctor. **Taking too much vitamin D over a period of time may cause harmful effects.**

Before Using This Medicine

In deciding whether you need additional vitamin D, the following should be kept in mind and/or your doctor should be told:

—if you have ever had any unusual or allergic reaction to vitamin D, including calcifediol, calcitriol, or dihydrotachysterol.

—if you are on a low-salt, low-sugar, or any other special diet, or if you are allergic to any substance, such as foods, sulfites or other preservatives, or dyes. Most medicines contain more than their active ingredient, and many liquid medicines contain alcohol. Your doctor, nurse, or pharmacist can help you avoid products that may cause a problem.

—if you are **pregnant** or if you may become pregnant. It is especially important that you are receiving enough vitamins when you become pregnant and that you continue to receive the right amount of vitamins throughout your pregnancy. The healthy growth and development of the fetus depend on a steady supply of nutrients from the mother.

However, taking too much vitamin D can also be harmful to the fetus. Taking too much vitamin D can cause your baby to be more sensitive than usual to its effects, can cause problems with a gland called the parathyroid, and can cause a defect in the baby's heart.

—if you are **breast-feeding**. It is especially important that you receive the right amounts of vitamins so that your baby will also get the vitamins needed to grow properly.

—if you have any of the following medical problems:

Diarrhea (continuing)
Heart or blood vessel disease
Intestinal problems
Kidney disease
Liver disease
Pancreas disease
Sarcoidosis

—if you are taking **any** other prescription or nonprescription (OTC) medicine, especially other forms of vitamin D.

—if you are not able to get a diet that contains all of the vitamins you need. This may occur with rapid weight loss, unusual diets (such as strict vegetarian or macrobiotic diets which do not include milk, or some reducing diets in which choice of foods is very limited), prolonged intravenous feeding, or malnutrition.

—if you have had a large part of your stomach removed.

Proper Use of This Medicine

Do not take more than the recommended daily amount. Vitamin D is stored in the body and taking too much over a period of time can cause poisoning and even death. Some people believe that taking very large doses of vitamins (called megadoses or megavitamin therapy) is useful for treating certain medical problems. Studies have not proven this. Large doses should be taken only under the direction of your doctor after need has been identified.

For patients taking the oral liquid form:

• This preparation is to be taken by mouth even though it comes in a dropper bottle.

• This medicine may be dropped directly into the mouth or mixed with cereal, fruit juice, or other food.

If you miss taking a vitamin for one or more days there is no cause for concern, since it takes some time for your body to become seriously low in vitamins. However, if your doctor has recommended that you take this vitamin, try to remember to take it as directed every day.

How to store this medicine:

• **Keep out of the reach of children.**

• Store away from heat and direct light.

• Do not store in the bathroom, near the kitchen sink, or in other damp places. Heat or moisture may cause the medicine to break down.

• Keep the oral liquid form of the medicine from freezing.

• Do not keep outdated medicine or medicine no longer needed. Be sure that any discarded medicine is out of the reach of children.

Side Effects of This Medicine

Along with its needed effects, a medicine may cause some unwanted effects. Vitamin D does not usually cause any side effects. However, **taking large amounts of vitamin D over a period of time may cause some unwanted effects that can be serious.**

Check with your doctor immediately if any of the following effects occur:

Late signs of severe overdose
Convulsions (seizures)
High blood pressure
Irregular heartbeat
Stomach pain (severe)

Check with your doctor as soon as possible if any of the following effects occur:

Early signs of overdose
Constipation (especially in children or adolescents)
Diarrhea
Dry mouth
Headache (continuing)
Increase in thirst
Loss of appetite

Metallic taste
Nausea or vomiting (especially in children or adolescents)
Unusual tiredness or weakness

Late signs of overdose

Bone pain
Cloudy urine
Increased sensitivity of eyes to light or irritation of eyes
Increase in frequency of urination, especially at night, or
    in amount of urine
Itching of skin
Mood or mental changes
Muscle pain
Nausea or vomiting (severe)
Weight loss

For children: Some of the above early signs of overdose, such as constipation and nausea or vomiting, are more likely to occur in children and adolescents. Also, children may show slowed growth when receiving vitamin D for a long time.

Other side effects not listed above may also occur in some patients. If you notice any other effects, check with your doctor.

_____

December 1987

VITAMIN E (Systemic)

Some commonly used brand names are:

Aquasol E	Epsilan-M
Chew-E	Pheryl-E
E-Ferol	Viterra E
Eprolin	

Generic name product may also be available in the U.S. and Canada.

To the Reader: If you do not recognize the names of medical conditions or medicines referred to in this information, check with your doctor, nurse, or pharmacist. Definitions for selected medical terms may be found in the Glossary. Brand names for the generic drug names listed can be found in the Index. In addition, selected brand names commonly associated with the generic name have been included in the text to help you recognize medicine you may be taking. The fact that a brand name product is not mentioned does not mean the information does not apply. It is a good idea for you to learn both the generic and brand names of your medicines and to write them down for future use.

Vitamins (VYE-ta-mins) are compounds that you *must* have for growth and health. They are needed in only small amounts and are available in the foods that you eat. Vitamin E prevents a chemical reaction called oxidation, which can sometimes result in harmful effects in your body.

Claims that vitamin E is effective for prevention or treatment of acne, aging, loss of hair, bee stings, cancer, liver spots on the hands, bursitis, diaper rash, frostbite, stomach ulcer, heart attacks, labor pains, miscarriage, muscular dystrophy, poor posture, sexual impotence, sterility, infertility, menopause, sunburn, and lung damage from air pollution have not been proven.

Vitamin E is available without a prescription. However, it may be a good idea to check with your doctor before taking vitamin E on your own. Lack of vitamin E is extremely rare, except in people who have a disease in which it is not absorbed into the body.

Vitamin E is also sometimes used for other conditions as determined by your doctor. If you are using vitamin E for reasons other than as a vitamin supplement, most of the following information will not apply to you.

Remember:

• **Keep all medicines out of the reach of children.**

• In order for this medicine to work, it must be used as directed. **If you are using this medicine without a prescription, it is very important to follow the directions on the label.**

• **It is also very important that you read and understand the following information.** If any of the information causes you special concern, check with your doctor before using this medicine without a prescription.

• Before you begin using any new medicine (prescription or nonprescription) or if you develop any new medical problem while you are using this medicine, check with your doctor, nurse, or pharmacist.

• **If you have any questions** about the following information or if you want more information about this medicine or your medical problem, **ask your doctor, nurse, or pharmacist.**

Importance of Diet

Vitamin supplements should be taken only if you cannot get enough vitamins in your diet. A balanced diet should provide all the vitamins you normally need.

Nutritionists recommend that you eat:
• Cereal or bread—4 or more servings per day and
• Dairy products (milk, cheese, ice cream, cottage cheese—3 or more servings per day and
• Meat, fish, or eggs—2 or more servings per day and
• Vegetables and fruits—4 or more servings per day.

If you are not getting all of these foods every day, you may not be getting enough vitamins in your diet. The best way to correct this is to start eating the foods that contain what you need.

Vitamin E is found in various foods including vegetable oils (corn, cottonseed, soybean, safflower), wheat germ, whole-grain cereals, egg yolk, and liver. It is best to eat fresh fruits and vegetables whenever possible since they contain the most vitamins. Food processing may destroy some of the vitamins, although cooking does not affect the vitamin E in foods.

Vitamins alone will not take the place of a good diet and will not provide energy. Your body also needs other substances found in food such as protein, minerals, carbohydrates, and fat. Vitamins themselves often cannot work without the presence of other foods. For example, fat is needed so that vitamin E can be absorbed into the body.

In some cases, it may not be possible for you to get enough food to supply you with the proper vitamins. In other cases, the amount of vitamins you need may be increased above normal. Therefore, a vitamin supplement may be needed. However, lack of vitamin E is very rare.

Experts have developed a list of recommended dietary allowances (RDA) for most of the vitamins. The RDA are not an exact number but a general idea of how much you need. They do not cover amounts needed for problems caused by a serious lack of vitamins.

The RDA for vitamin E are:

Babies (up to 1 year of age)—4 to 6 Units per day
Children 1 to 10 years of age—7 to 10 Units per day
Adult males—15 Units per day
Adult females—12 Units per day
Pregnant females—15 Units per day
Breast-feeding females—16 Units per day.

Remember:
• The total amount of each vitamin that you get every day includes what you get from the foods that you eat *and* what you may take as a supplement.

• This total amount should not be greater than the RDA, unless ordered by your doctor. Taking too much vitamin E over a period of time may cause unwanted effects.

Before Using This Medicine

In deciding whether you need additional vitamin E, the following should be kept in mind and/or your doctor should be told:

—if you have ever had any unusual or allergic reaction to vitamin E.

—if you are on a low-salt, low-sugar, or any other special diet, or if you are allergic to any substance, such as foods, sulfites or other preservatives, or dyes. Most medicines contain more than their active ingredient, and many liquid medicines contain alcohol. Your doctor, nurse, or pharmacist can help you avoid products that may cause a problem.

—if you are **pregnant** or if you may become pregnant. It is especially important that you are receiving enough vitamins when you become pregnant and that you continue to receive the right amount of vitamins throughout your pregnancy. The healthy growth and development of the fetus depend on a steady supply of nutrients from the mother.

—if you are **breast-feeding**. It is especially important that you receive the right amounts of vitamins so that your baby will also get the vitamins needed to grow properly. You should also check with your doctor if you are giving your baby an unfortified formula. In that case, the baby must get the vitamins needed some other way.

—if you are not able to get a diet that contains all of the vitamins you need. This may occur with rapid weight loss, unusual diets (such as some reducing diets in which choice of foods is very limited), prolonged intravenous feeding, or malnutrition.

—if you have had a large part of your stomach removed.

—if you have any of the following medical problems:
Anemia caused by low iron
Bleeding problems
Cystic fibrosis
Intestinal problems
Liver disease
Overactive thyroid

—if you are taking **any** other prescription or nonprescription (OTC) medicine, especially iron supplements.

Proper Use of This Medicine

Do not take more than the recommended daily amount. Vitamin E is stored in the body and taking too much over a period of time may cause harmful effects. Some of these effects are described below. Some people believe that taking very large doses of vitamins (called megadoses or megavitamin therapy) is useful for treating certain medical problems. Studies have not proven this. Large doses should be taken only under the direction of your doctor after need has been identified.

For patients taking the oral liquid form:
• This preparation is to be taken by mouth even though it comes in a dropper bottle.

• This medicine may be dropped directly into the mouth or mixed with cereal, fruit juice, or other food.

If you miss taking a vitamin for one or more days there is no cause for concern, since it takes some time for your body to become seriously low in vitamins. However, if your doctor has recommended that you take this vitamin, try to remember to take it as directed every day.

How to store this medicine:
• **Keep out of the reach of children.**

• Store away from heat and direct light.

• Do not store in the bathroom, near the kitchen sink, or in other damp places. Heat or moisture may cause the medicine to break down.

• Keep the oral liquid form of this medicine from freezing.

• Do not keep outdated medicine or medicine no longer needed. Be sure that any discarded medicine is out of the reach of children.

Side Effects of This Medicine

Along with its needed effects, a medicine may cause some unwanted effects. When used for short periods of time at recommended doses, vitamin E usually does not cause any side effects. However, check with your doctor as soon as possible if any of the following side effects occur:

With large doses and long-term use
Blurred vision
Breast enlargement in males and females
Diarrhea
Dizziness
Flu-like symptoms
Headache
Nausea or stomach cramps
Tiredness or weakness (severe)

Other side effects not listed above may also occur in some patients. If you notice any other effects, check with your doctor.

December 1987

VITAMIN K (Systemic)

This information applies to the following medicines:

Menadiol (men-a-DYE-ole)
Phytonadione (fye-toe-na-DYE-one)

Some commonly used brand names or other names are:	Generic names:
Synkayvite	Menadiol
AquaMEPHYTON Konakion Mephyton Phytomenadione	Phytonadione

To the Reader: If you do not recognize the names of medical conditions or medicines referred to in this information, check with your doctor, nurse, or pharmacist. Definitions for selected medical terms may be found in the Glossary. Brand names for the generic drug names listed can be found in the Index. In addition, selected brand names commonly associated with the generic name have been included in the text to help you recognize medicine you may be taking. The fact that a brand name product is not mentioned does not mean the information does not apply. It is a good idea for you to learn both the generic and brand names of your medicines and to write them down for future use.

Vitamins (VYE-ta-mins) are compounds that you *must* have for growth and health. They are needed in only small amounts and are usually available in the foods that you eat. Vitamin K is necessary for normal clotting of the blood.

Vitamin K is found in various foods including green leafy vegetables, meat, and dairy products. If you eat a balanced diet containing these foods, you should be getting all the vitamin K you need. Little vitamin K is lost from foods with ordinary cooking.

Lack of vitamin K is rare but may lead to problems with blood clotting and increased bleeding. Your doctor may treat this by prescribing vitamin K for you.

Vitamin K is routinely given to newborn infants to prevent bleeding problems.

This medicine is available only with your doctor's prescription.

Remember:

• **This medicine has been prescribed for your current medical problem only.** It must not be given to other people or used for other problems unless you are directed to do so by your doctor.

• **Keep all medicines out of the reach of children.**

• In order for this medicine to work, it must be used as directed.

• If you are receiving this medicine by injection, some of the information about this medicine may not apply.

• **It is very important that you read and understand the following information.** If any of the information causes you special concern, do not decide against using this medicine without first checking with your doctor.

• Before you begin using any new medicine (prescription or nonprescription) or if you develop any new medical problem while you are using this medicine, check with your doctor, nurse, or pharmacist.

• **If you have any questions** about the following information or if you want more information about this medicine or your medical problem, **ask your doctor, nurse, or pharmacist.**

Before Using This Medicine

In order to decide on the best treatment for your medical problem, your doctor should be told:

—if you have ever had any unusual or allergic reaction to vitamin K.

—if you are on a low-salt, low-sugar, or any other special diet, or if you are allergic to any substance, such as foods, sulfites or other preservatives, or dyes. Most medicines contain more than their active ingredient. Your doctor, nurse, or pharmacist can help you avoid products that may cause a problem.

—if you are **pregnant**. Vitamin K has not been shown to cause birth defects or other problems in humans.

—if you are **breast-feeding**. Vitamin K taken by the mother has not been shown to cause problems in nursing babies. You should also check with your doctor if you are giving your baby an unfortified formula. In that case, the baby must get the vitamins needed some other way.

—if you have any of the following medical problems:

Cystic fibrosis
Diarrhea (prolonged)
Glucose-6-phosphate dehydrogenase (G6PD) deficiency
Intestinal problems
Liver disease

—if you are taking **any** other prescription or nonprescription (OTC) medicine, especially:

Anticoagulants (blood thinners)
Primaquine

Proper Use of This Medicine

Take this medicine only as directed by your doctor. Do not take more or less of it, do not take it more often, and do not take it for a longer period of time than your doctor ordered. To do so may cause serious unwanted effects such as blood clotting problems.

Your doctor should check your progress at regular visits. A blood test must be taken regularly to see how fast your blood is clotting. This will help your doctor decide how much medicine you need.

If you miss a dose of this medicine, take it as soon as possible. However, if it is almost time for your next dose, skip the missed dose and go back to your regular dosing schedule. Do not double doses. **Tell your doctor about any doses you miss.**

© 1988 The United States Pharmacopeial Convention, Inc.

How to store this medicine:

- **Keep out of the reach of children.**

- Store away from heat and direct light.

- Do not store in the bathroom, near the kitchen sink, or in other damp places. Heat or moisture may cause the medicine to break down.

- Do not keep outdated medicine or medicine no longer needed. Be sure that any discarded medicine is out of the reach of children.

Precautions While Using This Medicine

Tell all physicians and dentists you go to that you are taking this medicine.

Always check with your doctor, nurse, or pharmacist before you start or stop taking any other medicine. This includes any over-the-counter (OTC) or nonprescription medicine, even aspirin. Other medicines may change the way this medicine affects your body.

Side Effects of This Medicine

Along with its needed effects, a medicine may cause some unwanted effects. Although vitamin K does not usually cause side effects that need medical attention, check with your doctor if any of the following side effects continue or are bothersome:

Less common
    Flushing of face
    Redness, pain, or swelling at place of injection
    Unusual taste

Other side effects not listed above may also occur in some patients. If you notice any other effects, check with your doctor.

December 1987

VITAMINS AND FLUORIDE (Systemic)

This information applies to the following medicines:
Multiple Vitamins and Fluoride
Vitamins A, D, and C and Fluoride

Some commonly used brand names are§:	Generic names:
Adeflor Mulvidren-F Poly-Vi-Flor Vi-Daylin/F Vi-Penta F	Multiple Vitamins and Fluoride
Cari-Tab Tri-Vi-Flor	Vitamins A, D, and C and Fluoride

§Specific vitamin content varies among products.

To the Reader: If you do not recognize the names of medical conditions or medicines referred to in this information, check with your doctor, nurse, or pharmacist. Definitions for selected medical terms may be found in the Glossary. Brand names for the generic drug names listed can be found in the Index. In addition, selected brand names commonly associated with the generic name have been included in the text to help you recognize medicine you may be taking. The fact that a brand name product is not mentioned does not mean the information does not apply. It is a good idea for you to learn both the generic and brand names of your medicines and to write them down for future use.

This medicine is a combination of vitamins and fluoride. Vitamins are used when the daily diet does not include enough of the vitamins needed for good health.

Fluoride has been found to be helpful in reducing the number of cavities in the teeth. It is usually present naturally in drinking water. However, some areas of the country do not have a high enough level of fluoride in the water. To make up for this, extra fluorides may be added to the diet. Some children may require both dietary fluorides and fluoride treatments by the dentist. Use of a fluoride toothpaste or rinse may be helpful, as well.

Taking fluorides does not replace good dental habits. These include eating a good diet, brushing teeth frequently, and having regular dental checkups.

This medicine is available only with your physician's or dentist's prescription.

Remember:

• **This medicine has been prescribed for your use only.** It must not be given to other people or used for other problems unless you are directed to do so by your physician or dentist.

• **Keep all medicines out of the reach of children.**

• In order for this medicine to work, it must be used as directed.

• **It is very important that you read and understand the following information.** If any of the information causes you special concern, do not decide against using this medicine without first checking with your physician or dentist.

• Before you begin using any new medicine (prescription or nonprescription) or if you develop any new medical problem while you are using this medicine, check with your physician, dentist, nurse, or pharmacist.

• **If you have any questions** about the following information or if you want more information about this medicine or your medical problem, **ask your physician, dentist, nurse, or pharmacist**.

Before Using This Medicine

In order to decide on the best treatment for your medical problem, your physician or dentist should be told:

—if you have ever had any unusual reaction to medicines containing fluorides.

—if you are on a low-salt, low-sugar, or any other special diet, or if you are allergic to any substance, such as foods, sulfites or other preservatives, or dyes. Most medicines contain more than their active ingredient, and many liquid medicines contain alcohol. Your doctor, nurse, or pharmacist can help you avoid products that may cause a problem.

—if you have an underactive thyroid gland.

—if you are taking **any** other prescription or nonprescription (OTC) medicine, especially

Anticoagulants (blood thinners)
Iron supplements
Vitamin supplements, other

Proper Use of This Medicine

Take this medicine only as directed by your physician or dentist. Do not take more of it and do not take it more often than ordered. Taking too much fluoride and some vitamins (especially vitamins A and D) over a period of time may cause unwanted effects.

For patients taking the chewable tablet form of this medicine:

• Tablets should be chewed or crushed before they are swallowed.

• This medicine works best if it is taken at bedtime, after the teeth have been thoroughly brushed.

For patients taking the oral liquid form of this medicine:

• This medicine is to be taken by mouth even though it comes in a dropper bottle. The amount to be taken is to be measured with the specially marked dropper.

• **Always store this medicine in the original plastic container.** It has been designed to give you the correct dose. Also, fluoride will interact with glass and should not be stored in glass containers.

• This medicine may be dropped directly into the mouth or mixed with cereal, fruit juice, or other food.

If you miss a dose of this medicine, take it as soon as you remember. However, if it is almost time for the next dose, skip the missed dose and go back to your regular dosing schedule. Do not double doses.

How to store this medicine:

• **Keep this medicine out of the reach of children,** since overdose is especially dangerous in children.

• Store away from heat and direct light.

• Do not store in the bathroom, near the kitchen sink, or in other damp places. Heat or moisture may cause the medicine to break down.

• Protect the oral solution from freezing.

• Do not keep outdated medicine or medicine no longer needed. Be sure that any discarded medicine is out of the reach of children.

Precautions While Using This Medicine

The level of fluoride present in the water is different in different parts of the country. If you move to another area, check with a physician or dentist in the new area as soon as possible to see if this medicine is still needed or if the dose needs to be changed.

Inform your physician or dentist as soon as possible if you notice white, brown, or black spots on the teeth. These are signs of too much fluoride.

Side Effects of This Medicine

Along with its needed effects, a medicine may cause some unwanted effects. Although not all of these side effects may occur, if they do occur they may need medical attention.

When the correct amount of this medicine is used, side effects usually are rare. However, **taking an overdose of fluoride may cause serious problems.**

Stop taking this medicine and check with your physician immediately if any of the following side effects occur, as they may be signs of severe fluoride overdose:

Black tarry stools
Bloody vomit
Diarrhea

Drowsiness
Faintness
Increase in saliva
Nausea or vomiting
Shallow breathing
Stomach cramps or pain
Tremors
Unusual excitement
Watery eyes
Weakness

Check with your physician or dentist as soon as possible if the following side effects occur, as some may be early signs of possible fluoride overdose:

Constipation
Loss of appetite
Pain and aching of bones
Skin rash
Sores in the mouth and on the lips
Stiffness
Weight loss
White, brown, or black discoloration of teeth

Other side effects not listed above may also occur in some patients. If you notice any other effects, check with your physician or dentist.

December 1987

XYLOMETAZOLINE (Nasal)

Some commonly used brand names are:

Chlorohist-LA	Otrivin
Neo-Spray Long Acting	Sinutab*
Neo-Synephrine II	Sustaine*
Long Acting	

Generic name product may also be available in the U.S.

---

*Not available in the U.S.

To the Reader: If you do not recognize the names of medical conditions or medicines referred to in this information, check with your doctor, nurse, or pharmacist. Definitions for selected medical terms may be found in the Glossary. Brand names for the generic drug names listed can be found in the Index. In addition, selected brand names commonly associated with the generic name have been included in the text to help you recognize medicine you may be taking. The fact that a brand name product is not mentioned does not mean the information does not apply. It is a good idea for you to learn both the generic and brand names of your medicines and to write them down for future use.

Xylometazoline (zye-loe-met-AZ-oh-leen) is used for the temporary relief of congestion or stuffiness in the nose caused by hay fever or other allergies, colds, or sinus trouble.

This medicine may also be used for other conditions as determined by your doctor.

This medicine is available without a prescription; however, your doctor may have special instructions on the proper use or dose for your medical condition.

Remember:

• **Keep all medicines out of the reach of children.**

• In order for this medicine to work, it must be used as directed. **If you are using this medicine without a prescription, it is very important to follow the directions on the label.**

• **It is also very important that you read and understand the following information.** If any of the information causes you special concern, check with your doctor or pharmacist.

• Before you begin using any new medicine (prescription or nonprescription) or if you develop any new medical problem while you are using this medicine, check with your doctor, nurse, or pharmacist.

• **If you have any questions** about the following information or if you want more information about this medicine or your medical problem, **ask your doctor, nurse, or pharmacist.**

Before Using This Medicine

Before you use xylometazoline, check with your doctor or pharmacist:

—if you have ever had any unusual or allergic reaction to xylometazoline.

—if you are allergic to any substance, such as certain preservatives. Most medicines contain more than their active ingredient. Your doctor, nurse, or pharmacist can help you avoid products that may cause a problem.

—if you are **pregnant** or if you may become pregnant, since xylometazoline may be absorbed into the body. However, xylometazoline has not been shown to cause birth defects or other problems in humans.

—if you are **breast-feeding**, since xylometazoline may be absorbed into the body. However, xylometazoline has not been shown to cause problems in nursing babies.

—if you have any of the following medical problems:
   Diabetes mellitus (sugar diabetes)
   Heart or blood vessel disease
   High blood pressure
   Overactive thyroid

—if you are taking **any** other prescription or nonprescription (OTC) medicine.

Proper Use of This Medicine

For patients using the nose drops:

• How to use: Blow the nose gently. Tilt the head back while standing or sitting up, or lie down on a bed and hang head over the side. Place the drops into each nostril and keep the head tilted back for a few minutes to allow the medicine to spread throughout the nose.

Rinse the dropper with hot water and dry with a clean tissue. Replace the cap right after use.

For patients using the nose spray:

• How to use: Blow the nose gently. With the head upright, spray the medicine into each nostril. Sniff briskly while squeezing the bottle quickly and firmly. For best results, spray once into each nostril, wait 3 to 5 minutes to allow the medicine to work, then blow the nose gently and thoroughly. Repeat until the complete dose is used.

Rinse the tip of the spray bottle with hot water taking care not to suck water into the bottle, and dry with a clean tissue. Replace the cap right after use.

To avoid the spread of infection, do not use the container for more than one person.

Use this medicine only as directed. Do not use more of it, do not use it more often, and do not use it for longer than 3 days, unless otherwise directed by your doctor. To do so may make your runny or stuffy nose worse and may also increase the chance of side effects.

If you miss a dose of this medicine and you remember within an hour or so of the missed dose, use it right away. However, if you do not remember until later, skip the missed dose and go back to your regular dosing schedule. Do not double doses.

How to store this medicine:

• **Keep out of the reach of children.**

• Store away from heat and direct light.

• Keep the medicine from freezing.

• Do not keep outdated medicine or medicine no longer needed. Be sure that any discarded medicine is out of the reach of children.

Side Effects of This Medicine

Along with its needed effects, a medicine may cause some unwanted effects. Although not all of these side effects may occur, if they do occur they may need medical attention.

When this medicine is used for short periods of time at low doses, side effects usually are rare. However, check with your doctor as soon as possible if any of the following occur:

Increase in runny or stuffy nose

Signs of too much medicine being absorbed into the body

Blurred vision
Headache or lightheadedness
Nervousness
Pounding, irregular, or fast heartbeat
Trouble in sleeping

Other side effects may occur that usually do not require medical attention. These side effects may go away during treatment as your body adjusts to the medicine.

However, check with your doctor or pharmacist if any of the following side effects continue or are bothersome:

Burning, dryness, or stinging of inside of nose
Sneezing

For pediatric patients: The above side effects are more likely to occur in children because there is a greater chance in children that too much of this medicine may be absorbed into the body.

For elderly patients: Many medicines have not been tested in older people. Therefore, it is not known whether the medicine acts the same way it does in younger adults. Check with your doctor or pharmacist if you notice any unusual effects while using this medicine or if you think it is not working as it should.

Other side effects not listed above may also occur in some patients. If you notice any other effects, check with your doctor or pharmacist.

December 1987

ZIDOVUDINE (Systemic)

Some commonly used brand names or other names are Azidothymidine, AZT, and Retrovir.

To the Reader: If you do not recognize the names of medical conditions or medicines referred to in this information, check with your doctor, nurse, or pharmacist. Definitions for selected medical terms may be found in the Glossary. Brand names for the generic drug names listed can be found in the Index. In addition, selected brand names commonly associated with the generic name have been included in the text to help you recognize medicine you may be taking. The fact that a brand name product is not mentioned does not mean the information does not apply. It is a good idea for you to learn both the generic and brand names of your medicines and to write them down for future use.

Zidovudine (zye-DOE-vue-deen) belongs to the family of medicines called antivirals. Antivirals are used to treat infections caused by viruses. They work by killing viruses or preventing their growth.

This medicine is taken by mouth to treat certain patients with acquired immune deficiency syndrome (AIDS) and AIDS-related complex (ARC). It will not work for colds, flu, or other virus infections.

AIDS is a very serious, often fatal, disease. Up to 80% of people with AIDS may die. When a person is infected with the AIDS virus, the virus attacks certain cells in the body and breaks down the body's immune system. When this happens, the person may get other serious diseases as well. These include serious fungal infections and pneumocystis (noo-moe-SISS-tis) pneumonia (PCP), a very serious kind of pneumonia caused by a parasite. Other diseases include certain kinds of cancer, such as Kaposi's sarcoma, a rare form of cancer usually involving reddish blue or brownish, soft nodules and tumors of the skin. People with normal immune systems don't usually get these diseases.

AIDS is currently more common in homosexual (gay) and bisexual males, intravenous drug abusers, and hemophiliacs (bleeders). However, AIDS may be increasing in other (e.g., heterosexual [straight]) groups and may occur in anyone, male or female. This disease is spread from person to person through infected body fluids, such as blood, feces, semen, or urine. It may be spread by sexual contact, transfusions of blood products or clotting factor concentrates, sharing of contaminated needles during drug use, or from an infected mother to her newborn child. It is not spread by casual contact, such as hand shaking or talking face-to-face.

The symptoms of AIDS or ARC may take several months or years to appear after a person has been infected by the virus. During this time a person may spread the infection to others without knowing it. The symptoms of AIDS or ARC may include fever; night sweats; swollen glands in the neck, armpit, or groin; unexplained weight loss; yeast infections; diarrhea; continuing cough; weakness; or loss of appetite.

Zidovudine will not cure or prevent AIDS or ARC. Also, it will not keep you from spreading AIDS to other people. People who receive this medicine may continue to have the problems usually related to AIDS or ARC. This medicine may be given with other medicines to treat these problems.

This medicine may cause some serious side effects, including bone marrow problems. Symptoms of bone marrow problems include fever, chills, or sore throat; pale skin; unusual bleeding or bruising; and unusual tiredness or weakness. These problems may require blood transfusions. **Check with your doctor if any new health problems or symptoms occur while you are taking zidovudine.**

Zidovudine is available only with your doctor's prescription.

Remember:
- **This medicine has been prescribed for your present infection only.** Another infection later on may require a different medicine. Also, even though other people may have the same symptoms as you, they may have a different kind of infection. Your medicine may not work for them and may even cause them harm. Therefore, **your medicine must not be given to other people or used for other infections** unless you are otherwise directed by your doctor.

- **Keep all medicines out of the reach of children.**

- In order for this medicine to work, it must be used as directed.

- **It is very important that you read and understand the following information.** If any of the information causes you special concern, do not decide against using this medicine without first checking with your doctor.

- Before you begin using any new medicine (prescription or nonprescription) or if you develop any new medical problem while you are using this medicine, check with your doctor, nurse, or pharmacist.

- **If you have any questions** about the following information or if you want more information about this medicine or your medical problem, **ask your doctor, nurse, or pharmacist.**

Before Using This Medicine

In order to decide on the best treatment for your medical problem, your doctor should be told:

—if you have ever had any unusual or allergic reaction to zidovudine.

—if you are on a low-salt, low-sugar, or any other special diet, or if you are allergic to any substance, such as foods, sulfites or other preservatives, or dyes. Most medicines contain more than their active ingredient.

—if you are **pregnant** or if you may become pregnant. Studies have not been done in humans. However, zidovudine has not been shown to cause birth defects or other problems in studies in rats given this medicine by mouth in doses of up to 20 times the human dose. Other studies in animals have not been completed.

—if you are **breast-feeding**. It is not known whether zidovudine passes into the breast milk. However, many medicines do pass into breast milk. Because of the chance of serious side effects in the nursing baby, you should stop breast-feeding when you begin taking this medicine.

—if you have any of the following medical problems:
Anemia, bleeding, or other blood problems
Kidney disease
Liver disease
Low amounts of folic acid or vitamin B_{12} in the blood

—if you are taking **any** other prescription or nonprescription (OTC) medicine, especially:
Acetaminophen (e.g., Tylenol)
Amphotericin B by injection (e.g., Fungizone)
Antineoplastics (cancer medicine)
Antithyroid agents (medicine for overactive thyroid)
Aspirin
Azathioprine (e.g., Imuran)
Benzodiazepines (alprazolam, chlordiazepoxide, clonazepam, clorazepate, diazepam, flurazepam, halazepam, lorazepam, midazolam, oxazepam, prazepam, temazepam, triazolam)
Chlorambucil (e.g., Leukeran)
Chloramphenicol (e.g., Chloromycetin)
Cimetidine (e.g., Tagamet)
Colchicine
Cyclophosphamide (e.g., Cytoxan)
Flucytosine (e.g., Ancobon)
Indomethacin (e.g., Indocin)
Interferon (e.g., Intron A, Roferon-A)
Mercaptopurine (e.g., Purinethol)
Methotrexate (e.g., Mexate)
Morphine
Sulfonamides (sulfa medicine)

—if you have ever been treated with x-rays.

Proper Use of This Medicine

Patient information sheets about zidovudine are available. Read this information carefully.

Take this medicine exactly as directed by your doctor. Do not take more of it, do not take it more often, and do not take it for a longer period of time than your doctor ordered. Also, do not stop taking this medicine without checking with your doctor first.

Keep taking zidovudine for the full time of treatment, even if you begin to feel better.

This medicine works best when there is a constant amount in the blood. **To help keep the amount constant, do not miss any doses. Also, take the doses at evenly spaced times day and night,** even if this interferes with your sleep or other daily activities. For example, if you are to take 6 doses a day, the doses should be spaced 4 hours apart. If you need help in planning the best times to take your medicine, check with your doctor, nurse, or pharmacist.

If you do miss a dose of this medicine, take it as soon as possible. However, if it is almost time for your next dose, skip the missed dose and go back to your regular dosing schedule. Do not double doses.

How to store this medicine:

• **Keep out of the reach of children.**

• Store away from heat and direct light.

• Do not store in the bathroom, near the kitchen sink, or in other damp places. Heat or moisture may cause the medicine to break down.

• Do not keep outdated medicine or medicine no longer needed. Be sure that any discarded medicine is out of the reach of children.

Precautions While Using This Medicine

It is very important that your doctor check you at regular visits for any blood problems that may be caused by this medicine.

Do not take any other medicines without checking with your doctor first. To do so may increase the chance of side effects from zidovudine.

This medicine may cause some people to faint or become dizzy. **Make sure you know how you react to this medicine before you drive, use machines, or do other jobs that require you to be alert.** If these reactions occur or are especially bothersome, check with your doctor.

Zidovudine may cause bone marrow problems. These problems may result in a greater chance of infection, slow healing, and bleeding of the gums. Therefore, you should be careful when using toothbrushes, dental floss, and toothpicks. Dental work, whenever possible, should be done before you begin taking this medicine or delayed until your blood counts have returned to normal. Check with your dentist if you have any questions about proper oral hygiene (mouth care) during treatment.

The AIDS virus can be caught from or spread to other people through infected body fluids, including blood or semen. **It is best to avoid any sexual activity,** although the use of a condom (prophylactic) may help prevent the spread of the AIDS virus to others. In addition, **do not share needles with anyone.** If you have any questions about this, check with your doctor, nurse, or pharmacist.

Side Effects of This Medicine

Along with its needed effects, a medicine may cause some unwanted effects. Although not all of these side effects may occur, if they do occur they may need medical attention.

Check with your doctor immediately if any of the following side effects occur:
More common
Fever, chills, or sore throat
Pale skin
Unusual bleeding or bruising
Unusual tiredness or weakness
(the above side effects may also occur up to weeks or months after you stop taking this medicine)

Other side effects may occur that usually do not require medical attention. These side effects may go away during treatment as your body adjusts to the medicine.

However, check with your doctor if any of the following side effects continue or are bothersome:

More common

Changes in taste
Diarrhea
Dizziness
Headache
Loss of appetite
Nausea
Skin rash

Less common

Abdominal or stomach pain or upset
Agitation, nervousness, or restlessness
Anxiety
Confusion
Fainting
Itching

Sores in the mouth
Swelling of lips or tongue
Trouble in sleeping
Vomiting

For elderly patients: Many medicines have not been tested in older people. Therefore, it is not known whether the medicine acts the same way it does in younger adults. Check with your doctor or pharmacist if you notice any unusual effects while taking this medicine or if you think it is not working as it should.

Other side effects not listed above may also occur in some patients. If you notice any other effects, check with your doctor.

_____

December 1987

Glossary

Abortifacient—Medicine used to cause abortion.

Abraded—Scraped.

Achlorhydria—Absence of acid in the stomach.

Acidifier, urinary—Medicine used to make the urine more acid.

Acidosis—Condition in which body fluids and tissues are more acidic than normal.

Acromegaly—Increase in size of the face, hands, and feet because of too much growth hormone.

Addison's disease—Disease caused by not enough secretion of hormones by the adrenal glands.

Adhesion—Union of two normally separate surfaces, such as the parts of a joint, by connective tissue formed in an injured area.

Adjunct medicine—Medicine always used with another medicine or procedure for treatment of a particular condition; not effective for that condition if used alone.

Adrenal cortex—Outer part of the adrenal gland.

Adrenal glands—Two triangle-shaped organs located next to the kidneys. They produce several important substances necessary for healthy body functioning.

Adrenocorticoid—Hormone produced naturally by the adrenal glands and necessary to maintain good health. Certain adrenocorticoids also are used to provide relief for inflamed areas of the body and as part of the treatment for a number of different diseases, such as severe allergies or skin problems, asthma, or arthritis. Some of the adrenocorticoids used as medicine are the same as those produced naturally by the body.

Agoraphobia—Fear of public places or open spaces.

AIDS (acquired immune deficiency syndrome)—Disease, caused by the AIDS virus, which results in a breakdown of the body's immune system, thereby making a person more susceptible to other infections and some forms of cancer.

Alcohol-abuse deterrent—Medicine used to help alcoholics avoid the use of alcohol.

Alkalizer, urinary—Medicine used to make the urine more alkaline.

Altitude sickness agent—Medicine used to prevent or lessen some of the effects of high altitude on the body.

Alzheimer's disease—Progressive disorder of thinking and other mental processes, usually associated with age.

Aminoglycoside—A class of chemically related antibiotics used to treat some serious types of bacterial infections.

Analgesic—Medicine used to relieve pain.

Anaphylaxis—Sudden, severe allergic reaction.

Androgen—Male hormone.

Anemia—Too little hemoglobin in the blood, resulting in tiredness, breathlessness, and poor resistance to infection.

Anesthesiologist—A physician who is qualified to give an anesthetic and other medicines to a patient before and during surgery.

Anesthetic—Medicine used to cause loss of consciousness, feeling, or sensation, especially sensation of pain.

Angina—Pain, tightness, or feeling of heaviness in the chest, sometimes accompanied by difficulty in breathing. The pain may be felt in the left shoulder and arm instead of or in addition to the chest. These symptoms often occur during exercise.

Angioedema—Allergic condition marked by continuing swelling and severe itching of areas of the skin.

Antacid—Medicine used to neutralize excess acid in the stomach.

Anthelmintic—Medicine used to treat infections caused by worms.

Antiacne agent—Medicine used to treat acne.

Antiadrenal—Medicine used to prevent an overactive adrenal gland (adrenal cortex) from producing too much cortisone-like hormone.

Antianemic—Medicine to treat anemia.

Antianginal—Medicine used to prevent or treat angina attacks.

Antianxiety agent—Medicine used for the treatment of nervousness, tension, or excessive anxiety.

Antiarrhythmic—Medicine used to treat irregular heartbeats.

Antiasthmatic—Medicine used to treat asthma.

Antibacterial—Medicine used to treat infections caused by bacteria.

Antibiotic—Medicine produced by micro-organisms and used to treat various types of infections.

Antibody—Special kind of blood protein that helps the body fight infection.

Anticholelithic—Medicine used to dissolve gallstones.

Anticoagulant—Medicine used to prevent blood clots from being formed in the blood vessels.

Anticonvulsant—Medicine used to prevent or treat convulsions (seizures).

Antidepressant—Medicine used to treat mental depression.

Antidiabetic agent—Medicine used to control blood sugar levels in patients with diabetes mellitus (sugar diabetes).

Antidiarrheal—Medicine used to treat diarrhea.

Antidiuretic—Medicine used to help hold water in the body (for example, in patients with diabetes insipidus [water diabetes]).

Antidote—Medicine used for preventing or treating harmful effects of another medicine or a poison.

Antidyskinetic—Medicine used in the treatment of certain diseases that cause a loss of muscle control.

Antidysmenorrheal—Medicine used to treat menstrual cramps.

Antiemetic—Medicine used to prevent or treat nausea and vomiting.

Antienuretic—Medicine used to help prevent bedwetting.

Antifibrotic—Medicine used to treat fibrosis.

Antiflatulent—Medicine used to help relieve excess gas in the stomach or intestines.

Antifungal—Medicine used to treat infections caused by a fungus.

Antiglaucoma agent—Medicine used to treat glaucoma.

Antigout agent—Medicine used to prevent or relieve gout attacks.

Antihemorrhagic—Medicine used to prevent or help stop serious bleeding.

Antihistaminic, H_1-receptor—Medicine used to prevent or relieve the symptoms of allergies (such as hay fever).

Antihypercalcemic—Medicine used to help lower the amount of calcium in the blood.

Antihyperlipidemic—Medicine used to help lower the amount of cholesterol or other fat-like substances in the blood.

Antihypertensive—Medicine used in the treatment of high blood pressure.

Antihyperuricemic—Medicine used to prevent or treat gout or other medical problems caused by too much uric acid in the blood.

Antihypocalcemic—Medicine used to increase calcium levels in patients with too little calcium.

Antihypoglycemic—Medicine used to increase blood sugar levels in patients with low blood sugar.

Antihypokalemic—Medicine used to increase potassium levels in patients with too little potassium.

Antihypoparathyroid—Medicine used to treat the effects of an underactive parathyroid gland.

Anti-infective—Medicine that fights infection.

Anti-inflammatory—Medicine used to relieve pain, swelling, and other symptoms caused by inflammation.

Anti-inflammatory, nonsteroidal—An anti-inflammatory medicine that is not a cortisone-like medicine.

Anti-inflammatory, steroidal—A cortisone-like anti-inflammatory medicine.

Antimanic—Medicine used to treat manic-depressive mental illness.

Antimetabolite—Medicine that interferes with the normal processes within cells, preventing their growth.

Antimuscarinic—Medicine used to block the effects of a certain chemical in the body; often used to reduce smooth muscle spasms, especially abdominal or stomach cramps or spasms. It is also used to help reduce the amount of stomach acid.

Antimyasthenic—Medicine used in the treatment of myasthenia gravis.

Antimyotonic—Medicine used to prevent or relieve nighttime leg cramps or muscle spasms.

Antineoplastic—Medicine that is used to treat cancer.

Antineuralgic—Medicine used to treat neuralgia.

Antiprotozoal—Medicine used to treat infections caused by protozoa (tiny, one-celled animals).

Antipsoriatic—Medicine used to treat psoriasis.

Antipsychotic—Medicine used to treat certain nervous, mental, and emotional conditions.

Antipyretic—Medicine used to reduce high fever.

Antirheumatic—Medicine used to treat arthritis (rheumatism).

Antiseborrheic—Medicine used to treat dandruff and seborrhea.

Antiseptic—Medicine that fights bacteria and is used to clean objects or surfaces and thereby prevent infections.

Antispasmodic—Medicine used to reduce smooth muscle spasms (for example, stomach, intestinal, or urinary tract spasms).

Antispastic—Medicine used to treat muscle spasms.

Antithyroid agent—Medicine used to treat the effects of an overactive thyroid gland.

Antitremor agent—Medicine used to treat tremors (trembling or shaking).

Antitubercular—Medicine used to treat tuberculosis (TB).

Antitussive—Medicine used to relieve cough.

Antiulcer agent—Medicine used in the treatment of stomach and duodenal ulcers.

Antivertigo agent—Medicine used to prevent dizziness.

Antiviral—Medicine used to treat infections caused by a virus.

Appendicitis—Inflammation of the appendix.

Appetite stimulant—Medicine used to help increase the appetite.

Appetite suppressant—Medicine used in weight control programs to help decrease the desire for food.

ARC (AIDS-related complex)—Thought to be a forerunner of AIDS. Refers to certain conditions caused by the AIDS virus. Although not AIDS itself, the symptoms of ARC are usually the same as those for AIDS.

Arteritis, temporal—Inflammatory disease of the blood vessels, usually of the scalp, occurring in the elderly.

Arthritis, rheumatoid—Chronic disease of the joints, marked by pain and swelling at the sites.

Bacterium—Tiny, one-celled organism. Many types of bacteria are responsible for a number of diseases and infections.

Beriberi—Disorder caused by too little vitamin B_1 (thiamine), marked by an accumulation of fluid in the body, extreme weight loss, inflammation of nerves, or paralysis.

Bile—Thick fluid made by the liver and stored in the gallbladder. Bile helps the digestive process.

Bile duct—Duct through which bile passes from the liver to the gallbladder.

Biliary—Relating to the bile duct.

Bipolar disorder—Also called manic-depressive illness. Severe mental illness marked by repeated episodes of depression, mania, or both.

Bone resorption inhibitor—Medicine used to prevent or treat certain types of bone disorders, such as Paget's disease of the bone.

Bowel disease, inflammatory, suppressant—Medicine used to treat certain types of intestinal disorders, such as colitis.

Bradycardia—Slowing of the heart rate to less than 50 beats per minute.

Bronchitis—Inflammation of the bronchial tubes (air passages).

Bronchodilator—Medicine used to open up the bronchial tubes (air passages) of the lungs to increase the flow of air through them.

Bursa—Small sac of tissue present where body parts move over one another (such as a joint) to help reduce friction.

Bursitis—Inflammation of a bursa.

Cardiac—Related to the heart.

Cardiac load–reducing agent—Medicine used to ease the workload of the heart by allowing the blood to flow through the body more easily.

Cardiotonic—Medicine used to improve the strength and efficiency of the heart.

Caries, dental—Also called "cavities." Tooth decay leading to pain and crumbling of the tooth.

Cataracts—Areas in the lens of the eye that become opaque (cloudy, not transparent), resulting in blurred vision.

Catheter—Tube to be inserted into a small opening in the body so that fluids can be put in or taken out.

Caustic—Medicine applied the skin to help remove calluses, corns, and warts.

Cerebral palsy—Brain condition resulting in weakness and poor coordination of the limbs.

Cholelitholytic—Medicine used to dissolve gallstones.

Cholesterol—Fat-like material found in the blood and most tissues. Too much cholesterol is associated with several potential health risks, especially atherosclerosis (hardening of the arteries).

Chronic—Describing a condition of long duration, involving very slow changes, and often of gradual onset. Note that the term "chronic" has nothing to do with how serious the condition is.

Cirrhosis—Liver disease marked by abnormal cell growth, which may in turn lead to other serious conditions.

Colitis—Inflammation of the colon (bowel).

Colostomy—Operation in which part of the colon (bowel) is brought through the abdominal wall and opened so as to drain the intestine, thus bypassing the rest of the intestines.

Coma—State of unconsciousness from which the patient cannot be aroused.

Coma, hepatic—Disturbances in mental function and the nervous system caused by severe liver disease.

Conjunctiva—Delicate mucous membrane covering the front of the eye and the inside of the eyelid.

Conjunctivitis—Inflammation of the conjunctiva.

Contraceptive—Medicine or device used to prevent pregnancy.

Creutzfeldt-Jakob disease—Rare disease, probably caused by a slow-acting virus that affects the brain and nervous system.

Crohn's disease—Condition in which parts of the digestive tract become thick and inflamed.

Croup—Inflammation and blockage of the larynx (voice box) in young children.

Cushing's syndrome—Condition in which the adrenal gland produces too much cortisone-like hormone, leading to weight gain, round face, and high blood pressure.

Cycloplegia—Paralysis of certain eye muscles, which can be useful in resting the muscles.

Cycloplegic—Medicine used to induce cycloplegia.

Cyst—Abnormal sac or closed cavity filled with liquid or semisolid matter.

Cystic—Marked by cysts.

Cystitis, interstitial—Inflammation of the bladder, with frequent urge to urinate, and painful urination.

Decongestant, nasal—Medicine used to help relieve nasal congestion (stuffy nose).

Decongestant, ophthalmic—Medicine used in the eye to relieve redness, burning, itching, or other irritation.

Dental—Related to the teeth or gums.

Depression, mental—Deep sadness and difficulty in performing day-to-day tasks. Other symptoms include disturbances in sleep, appetite, and concentration.

Dermatitis herpetiformis—Skin disease marked by sores and itching.

Dermatitis, seborrheic—Type of eczema found on the scalp and face.

Dermatomyositis—Inflammatory disorder of the skin and underlying tissues, including breakdown of muscle fibers.

Diabetes insipidus—Also called water diabetes. Disorder in which the patient produces large amounts of urine and is constantly thirsty.

Diabetes mellitus—Also called sugar diabetes. Disorder in which the body cannot process sugars to produce energy, due to lack of the hormone called insulin. This leads to too much sugar in the blood (hyperglycemia).

Dialysis, renal—Artificial technique for removing waste materials or poisons from the blood when the kidneys are not working properly.

Digestant—Medicine used to help the stomach digest food.

Diuretic—Also called water pill. Medicine that increases the amount of urine produced, by helping the kidneys get rid of water and salt.

Diverticulitis—Inflammation of a diverticulum (sac or pouch formed at weak points in the digestive tract).

Down's syndrome—Also called mongolism. Mental retardation caused by a defect in the genes. Patients with Down's syndrome are marked physically by a round head, flat nose, slightly slanted eyes, and short stature.

Duodenum—First of the three parts of the small intestine.

Eczema—Inflammation of the skin, marked by itching and rash.

Edema—Swelling of feet or lower legs due to accumulation of fluids.

Eighth-cranial-nerve disease—Disease of the eighth cranial (brain) nerve, resulting in dizziness, loss of balance, loss of hearing, nausea, or vomiting.

Emollient—Substance that soothes and softens an irritated surface, such as the skin.

Emphysema—Lung condition in which too much air accumulates in lung tissue because of blockage or narrowing of the bronchial tubes (air passages), leading to troubled breathing and heart problems.

Encephalitis—Inflammation of the brain.

Encephalopathy—Any of a group of diseases that affect the brain.

Endocarditis—Inflammation of the lining of the heart, leading to fever, heart murmurs, and heart failure.

Endometriosis—Condition in which material similar to the lining of the womb appears at other sites within the pelvic cavity, causing pain and bleeding.

Enteric-coated—Tablets coated with a substance that lets them pass through the stomach unchanged before breaking up in the intestine and being absorbed; used to protect the stomach from the drug and/or the drug from the stomach's acid.

Enteritis—Inflammation of the small intestine, usually causing diarrhea.

Enuresis—Urinating while asleep (bedwetting).

Enzyme—Type of protein produced by living cells that is important for normal chemical reactions in the body.

Epilepsy—Any of a group of brain disorders featuring sudden attacks of seizures and other symptoms.

Ergot alkaloids—Medicines that cause narrowing of blood vessels; used to treat migraine headaches, and to reduce bleeding in childbirth.

Estrogen—Female hormone necessary for the normal sexual development of the female and for the regulation of the menstrual cycle during the childbearing years.

Expectorant—Medicine used to relieve cough by loosening and thinning the mucus or phlegm in the lungs so that it may be coughed up.

Familial Mediterranean fever—Also called polyserositis. Inherited condition involving inflammation of the lining of the chest, abdomen, and joints.

Favism—Inherited allergy to broad beans.

Fibrocystic—Having benign (noncancerous) tumors of connective tissue.

Fibrosis—Condition in which the skin and underlying tissues tighten and become less flexible.

Fibrosis, cystic—Disease in which abnormally thick mucus is produced, which interferes with a number of important organs, and often leads to infections of the lungs.

Gamma globulin—Type of protein important in immunity that is found in the blood.

Gastric—Related to the stomach.

Gastric acid secretion inhibitor—Medicine used to decrease the amount of acid formed by the stomach.

Gastroenteritis—Inflammation of the stomach and intestine.

Gastroparesis, diabetic—Condition brought on by diabetes in which the stomach does not function as it should.

Gingival hyperplasia—Enlargement of the gums.

Gingivitis—Inflammation of the gums.

Glaucoma—Condition in which loss of vision may occur because of abnormally high pressure in the eye.

Glucose-6-phosphate dehydrogenase (G6PD) deficiency—Lack of or reduced amounts of an enzyme (glucose-6-phosphate dehydrogenase) that breaks down certain sugar compounds in the body.

Gluten—Type of protein found especially in wheat and rye.

Goiter—Swelling of the neck because of a swollen thyroid gland resulting from a lack of iodine or thyroid hormone.

Gonadotropin—Hormone that simulates the actions of the sex organs.

Gout—Disease in which too much uric acid builds up in the blood and joints, leading to painful swelling.

Graves' disease—Disorder in which too much thyroid hormone is present in the blood.

Guillain-Barré syndrome—Nerve disease marked by sudden numbness and weakness in the limbs that may progress to complete paralysis.

Hair follicle—Sheath of tissue surrounding a hair root.

Hartnup disease—Hereditary disease in which the body has trouble processing certain chemicals, leading to mental retardation, rough skin, and problems with muscle coordination.

Hemoglobin—Iron-containing substance found in red blood cells that transports oxygen from the lungs to the tissues of the body.

Hemolytic anemia—Type of anemia caused by destruction of red blood cells.

Hemophilia—Hereditary blood disease in males in which blood clotting is delayed, leading to excessive and uncontrolled bleeding even after minor injuries.

Hemorrhoids—Also called piles. Enlarged veins in the walls of the anus.

Hepatic—Related to the liver.

Hepatitis—Inflammation of the liver.

Hernia, hiatal—Condition in which the stomach passes partly into the chest through the opening for the esophagus in the diaphragm.

Herpes simplex—Also called cold sores. Inflammation of the skin, caused by a virus, resulting in groups of small, painful blisters. They may occur either around the mouth or, in the case of genital herpes, around the genitals (sex organs).

Herpes zoster—Also called shingles. Inflammation of the nerves, caused by a virus, usually marked by pain and blisters on the face, chest, or stomach. The virus that causes herpes zoster also causes chickenpox.

Hodgkin's disease—Malignant condition marked by swelling of the lymph glands, with weight loss and fever.

Hormone—Substance produced in one part of the body (such as a gland) which then passes into the bloodstream and is carried to other organs or tissues, where it helps them to function.

Hyperactivity—Abnormally increased activity.

Hypercalcemia—Too much calcium in the blood.

Hypercalciuria—Too much calcium in the urine.

Hyperglycemia—High blood sugar.

Hyperphosphatemia—Too much phosphate in the blood.

Hypertension—Also called high blood pressure. Blood pressure in the arteries (blood vessels) that is higher than normal for the patient's age group. Hypertension often shows no signs or symptoms but may lead to a number of serious health problems.

Hyperthermia—Very high body temperature.

Hypocalcemia—Too little calcium in the blood.

Hypoglycemia—Low blood sugar.

Hypothalamus—Area of the brain that controls a number of body functions, including temperature, thirst, hunger, sexual and emotional activity, and sleep.

Ileostomy—Operation in which the ileum is brought through the abdominal wall to create an artificial opening through which the contents of the intestine can be discharged, thus bypassing the colon (bowel).

Ileum—Lowest of the three portions of the small intestine.

Immunizing agent, active—Agent given to cause the body to produce its own protection (antibodies) against certain infections.

Immunosuppressant—Medicine that reduces the body's natural immunity.

Infertility—Inability to become pregnant or, for a man, to cause pregnancy.

Inflammation—Pain, redness, swelling, and heat in a part of the body, usually in response to injury or illness.

Influenza—Also called flu. Highly contagious virus infection of the lungs, marked by coughing and sneezing, headache, chills, fever, muscle pain, and general weakness.

Inhalation—Medicine used by being breathed in (inhaled) into the lungs. Some inhalations work locally in the lungs, while others produce their effects elsewhere in the body.

Inhibitor—Substance that prevents a process or reaction.

Intra-amniotic—Within the sac that contains the fetus and amniotic fluid.

Intracavernosal—Into the corpus cavernosa (cavities in the penis that, when filled with blood, produce an erection).

Intramuscular—Into a muscle.

Intrauterine device (IUD)—Small plastic or metal device placed in the uterus (womb) to prevent pregnancy.

Intravenous—Into a vein.

Irrigation—Washing out a body cavity or wound with a solution of a medicine.

Jaundice—Yellowing of the eyes and skin due to too much of a certain pigment in the bile.

Keratolytic—Medicine used to soften hardened areas of the skin (e.g., warts).

Ketoacidosis—Type of acidosis (too much acid in the body fluids and tissues) associated with diabetes.

Lactation—Secretion of milk by the mammary glands (breasts).

Larvae—Young or immature insects.

Laxative—Medicine taken to encourage bowel movements.

Laxative, bulk-forming—Laxative that acts by absorbing liquid in the intestines and swelling to form a soft, bulky stool. The bowel is then stimulated normally by the presence of the bulky mass.

Laxative, hyperosmotic—Laxative that acts by drawing water into the bowel from surrounding body tissues. This provides a soft stool mass and increased bowel action.

Laxative, lubricant—Laxative that acts by coating the bowel and the stool mass with a waterproof film. This keeps moisture in the stool. The stool remains soft and its passage is made easier.

Laxative, stimulant—Also called contact laxative. Laxative that acts directly on the intestinal wall. The direct stimulation increases the muscle contractions that move along the stool mass.

Laxative, stool softener—Also called emollient laxative. Laxative that acts by helping liquids mix into the stool and prevent dry, hard stool masses. The stool remains soft and its passage is made easier.

Legionnaires' disease—Lung infection caused by a certain bacterium.

Leishmaniasis, visceral—Also called black fever, Dumdum fever, or kala-azar. Tropical disease, transmitted by sandfly bites, which causes liver and spleen enlargement, anemia, weight loss, and fever.

Leprosy—Also called Hansen's disease. Chronic disease affecting the skin, mucous membranes, and nerves. Symptoms include severe numbness, weakness, and paralysis leading to disfigurement and deformity.

Leukemia—Disease of the blood and bone marrow in which too many white blood cells are produced, resulting in anemia, bleeding, and low resistance to infections.

Lugol's solution—Transparent, deep brown liquid containing iodine and potassium iodide, which may be given before a radiopharmaceutical medicine.

Lupus erythematosus—Also called lupus, or SLE. Chronic inflammatory disease affecting the skin and various internal organs.

Lymph—Fluid that bathes the tissues. It is derived from blood and circulated by the lymphatic system.

Lymphatic system—Network of vessels that conveys lymph from the tissue fluids to the bloodstream.

Lymph node—Filter through which lymph passes as it circulates throughout the lymphatic system.

Macrobiotic—Vegetarian diet consisting mostly of whole grains.

Malignant—Describing a condition that becomes continually worse if untreated; also used to mean cancerous.

Malnutrition—Condition caused by a lack of food or of certain necessary substances obtained from food.

Mammogram—X-ray picture of the breast, usually taken to check for abnormal growths.

Mania—Mental state of unusual cheerfulness and activity, but marked by illogical thought and speech, and overbearing, often violent behavior.

Manson's schistosomiasis—Also called blood fluke or bilharziasis. Tropical worm infection in which worms enter the body from contaminated water and settle in the intestines, causing anemia and inflammation.

Mast cell—Large cell that releases certain substances that cause allergic reactions.

Mastocytosis—Accumulation of too many mast cells in the tissues in infants, resulting in a distinctive skin rash.

Megavitamin therapy—Taking very large doses of vitamins to prevent or treat certain medical problems. Studies have not proven this to be useful.

Melanoma—Highly malignant cancer tumor, usually occurring on the skin.

Meningitis—Inflammation of the tissues that line the brain and spinal cord.

Migraine headache—Throbbing headache caused by enlarged blood vessels, usually affecting one side of the head.

Miotic—Medicine used in the eye that causes the pupil to constrict (become smaller).

Monoclonal—Derived from a single cell; related to production of drugs by genetic engineering (e.g., monoclonal antibodies).

Mononucleosis—Also called "mono" or glandular fever. Infectious virus disease, mostly of adolescents and young adults, marked by swelling of the lymph nodes in the neck, armpits, and groin and associated with extreme fatigue.

Mucolytic—Medicine that breaks down or dissolves mucus.

Mucosal—For local effects when applied directly to mucous membranes (for example, the inside of the mouth).

Mucous membrane—Moist layer of tissue surrounding or lining many body structures and cavities, including the mouth, lips, and inside of nose.

Mucus—Thick fluid produced by the body as a protective barrier, as a lubricant, and as a carrier of enzymes.

Multiple sclerosis (MS)—Chronic, progressive nerve disease marked by unsteadiness, shakiness, and problems in speech.

Myasthenia gravis—Chronic disease marked by abnormal weakness, and sometimes paralysis, of certain muscles.

Mydriatic—Medicine used in the eye that causes the pupil to dilate (become larger).

Myelogram—X-ray picture of the spinal cord.

Myeloma, multiple—Cancerous bone marrow disease.

Myocardial infarction—Also called heart attack. Interruption of blood supply to the heart, leading to sudden, severe chest pain, and damage to the heart muscle.

Myocardial reinfarction prophylactic—Medicine used to help prevent additional heart attacks in patients who have already had one attack.

Myotonia congenita—Hereditary muscle disorder marked by difficulty in relaxing a movement, or letting go a grip, after any strong effort.

Narcolepsy—Extreme tendency to fall asleep suddenly.

Nasal—Related to the nose.

Nasogastric (NG) tube—Tube that is inserted through the nose, down the throat, and into the stomach, so that medicine may be administered to patients who cannot swallow.

Nebulizer—Instrument that applies liquid in the form of a fine spray.

Neuralgia—Pain along the course of one or more nerves, occurring suddenly and intensely.

Neuralgia, trigeminal—Also called tic douloureux. Severe burning or stabbing pain along the nerves in the face.

Neuritis, optic—Disease of the nerves in the eye.

Nicotinamide adenine dinucleotide (NADH) methemoglobin reductase deficiency—Lack of or reduced amounts of an enzyme, resulting in reduced ability of the blood to carry oxygen.

Nonsuppurative—Not discharging pus.

Obesity—Accumulation of excess fat.

Obstetrics—Area of medicine concerned with the care of women during pregnancy and childbirth.

Occlusive dressing—Dressing (such as plastic kitchen wrap) that completely cuts off air to the skin.

Ophthalmic—Related to the eyes.

Orchitis—Inflammation of the testis.

Osteomalacia—Softening of the bones due to lack of vitamin D.

Osteoporosis—Loss of bone tissue, resulting in bones that are brittle and easily fractured.

Otic—Related to the ear.

Paget's disease—Also called osteitis deformans. Chronic bone disease, marked by thickening of the bones and severe pain.

Pancreatitis—Inflammation of the pancreas.

Parkinson's disease—Also called Parkinsonism, paralysis agitans, or shaking palsy. Brain disease marked by tremor (shaking), stiffness, and difficulty in moving.

Patent ductus arteriosus (PDA)—Condition in newborn babies in which an important blood vessel in the heart fails to close as it should, resulting in serious health problems.

Pediculicide—Medicine that kills lice.

Pellagra—Disease caused by too little vitamin B_3 (niacin), resulting in scaly skin, diarrhea, and mental depression.

Pemphigus—Skin disease marked by successive outbreaks of blisters.

Peritoneum—Sac that contains the liver, stomach, and intestines.

Peyronie's disease—Dense, fiber-like growth in the penis, which can be felt as an irregular hard lump, and which usually causes bending and pain when the penis is erect.

Phenol—Substance used as a preservative for injections.

Pheochromocytoma (PCC)—Small tumor of the adrenal gland.

Phlebitis—Inflammation of a vein.

Pituitary gland—Pea-sized body located at the base of the skull. It produces a number of hormones that are essential to normal body growth and functioning.

Placebo—Also called "sugar pill." Medicine that has no actual effect on the patient but may help to relieve a condition because the patient believes it will.

Plaque—Mixture of saliva, bacteria, and carbohydrates that forms on the teeth, leading to caries (cavities) and other dental problems.

Platelet—Disc-shaped structure in the blood which performs several functions having to do with blood clotting.

Platelet aggregation inhibitor—Medicine used to help prevent the platelets in the blood from clumping together. This effect reduces the chance of heart attack or stroke in certain patients.

Pleura—Membrane covering the lungs.

Pneumococcal—Having to do with certain bacteria that cause pneumonia.

Pneumocystis pneumonia—Also called interstitial plasma cell pneumonia. A very serious type of pneumonia usually affecting infants and patients in a weakened condition.

Polymorphous light eruption suppressant—Medicine used to help relieve the symptoms of polymorphous light eruption, a type of skin problem.

Polymyalgia rheumatica—Rheumatic disease, most common in the elderly, causing aching and stiffness of the shoulders and hips.

Polyps—Swollen or tumorous tissues; may or may not be cancerous.

Porphyria—Rare, inherited blood disease.

Priapism—Prolonged abnormal, painful erection of the penis.

Proctitis—Inflammation of the rectum.

Progestin—Female hormone necessary during the childbearing years for the development of the milk-producing glands, and for the proper regulation of the menstrual cycle.

Prolactinoma—Pituitary tumor.

Prophylactic—1. Used to prevent the occurrence of a specific condition. 2. Condom.

Prosthesis—Any artificial device attached to the body to help it function.

Protozoa—Tiny, one-celled animals, some of which are important disease-causing parasites in man.

Psoralen—Chemical found in plants and used in certain perfumes and medicines. Exposure to a psoralen and then to sunlight may increase the risk of severe burning.

Psoriasis—Chronic skin disease marked by itchy, scaly, red patches.

Psychosis—Severe mental illness marked by loss of contact with reality, often involving delusions, hallucinations, and disordered thinking.

PUVA—The combination of a psoralen, such as methoxsalen or trioxsalen, and ultraviolet light A; used to treat psoriasis and some other skin conditions.

Radiopaque agent—Iodine-containing substance that makes it easier to see an area of the body with x-rays. Radiopaque agents are used to help diagnose a variety of medical problems.

Radiopharmaceutical—Radioactive agent used to diagnose certain medical problems or treat certain diseases.

Raynaud's syndrome—Condition marked by paleness, numbness, and discomfort in the fingers when they are exposed to cold.

Rectal—Related to the rectum.

Renal—Related to the kidneys.

Reye's syndrome—Serious disease affecting the liver and brain that sometimes occurs after a virus infection such as flu or chickenpox. It occurs most often in young children and teenagers. The first sign of Reye's syndrome is usually severe, prolonged vomiting.

Rheumatic heart disease—Heart disease marked by scarring and chronic inflammation of the heart and its valves, occurring after rheumatic fever.

Rhinitis—Inflammation of the mucous membrane inside the nose.

Rickets—Bone disease caused by too little vitamin D, in which the bones are soft and malformed.

Sarcoidosis—Chronic disorder in which the lymph nodes in many parts of the body are enlarged, and small fleshy swellings develop in the lungs, liver, and spleen.

Scabicide—Medicine used to treat scabies (itch mite) infection.

Scabies—Skin infection caused by a mite, resulting in severe itching and redness.

Schizophrenia—Severe mental disorder marked by a breakdown of the thinking process, of contact with reality, and of normal emotional responses.

Scleroderma—Persistent hardening and shrinking of the body's connective tissue.

Scrotum—Sac that holds the testes (male sex glands).

Scurvy—Disease caused by too little vitamin C (ascorbic acid), marked by bleeding gums, bleeding beneath the skin, and impaired healing of wounds.

Secretion—1. Process in which a gland releases a substance into the body for use. 2. The substance released by the gland.

Sedative-hypnotic—Medicine used to treat nervousness, restlessness, or insomnia (sleeplessness).

Shunt—Surgical tube used to transfer blood from one part of the body to another.

SIADH (secretion of inappropriate antidiuretic hormone) syndrome—Disease in which the body retains (keeps) more fluid and loses more sodium than usual.

Sickle cell anemia—Hereditary blood disease that affects blacks; the name comes from the sickle-shaped red blood cells found in the blood of patients.

Sinusitis—Inflammation of a sinus.

Sjögren's syndrome—Condition marked by swollen salivary glands and dryness of the mouth.

Skeletal muscle relaxant—Medicine used to relax certain muscles and help relieve the pain and discomfort caused by strains, sprains, or other injury to the muscles.

Spastic paralysis—Weakness of a limb because of too much reflex response.

Spina bifida—Also called rachischisis. Birth defect in which the infant's spinal cord is partially exposed through a hole in the backbone.

Stimulant, respiratory—Medicine used to stimulate breathing.

Stroke—Also called apoplexy. Sudden weakness or paralysis, usually affecting one side of the body. Stroke occurs because the flow of blood to an area of the brain is interrupted.

Subcutaneous—Under the skin.

Sudden infant death syndrome (SIDS)—Also called crib death or cot death. Death of a baby, usually while asleep, from an unknown cause.

Sulfite—Type of preservative; causes allergic reactions, such as asthma, in some sensitive patients.

Sulfone—Type of medicine that acts against the bacteria causing leprosy and tuberculosis.

Suppository—Solid but meltable cone or cylinder of medicated material for insertion into the rectum or vagina.

Systemic—For general effects throughout the body; applies to most medicines when taken by mouth or given by injection.

Temporomandibular joint (TMJ)—Hinge that connects the lower jaw to the skull.

Tendinitis—Inflammation of a tendon.

Testosterone—Principal male sex hormone.

Therapeutic—Relating to the treatment of a specific condition.

Thimerosal—Chemical used as a preservative in some medicines, and as an antiseptic and disinfectant.

Thrombocytopenic purpura—Blood disease marked by skin rash.

Thrush—Also called white mouth or candidiasis of the mouth. Mild fungal infection of the mouth marked by white patches on the tongue or insides of cheeks.

Thyroid gland—Large gland in the base of the neck. It releases thyroid hormone, which is important for normal body functioning.

Tics—Condition marked by repeated involuntary movements or spasms of muscles.

Tinea—Also called ringworm. Fungus infection of the surface of the skin, particularly the scalp, feet, and nails.

Topical—For local effects when applied directly to the skin.

Tourette's disorder—Also called Gilles de la Tourette's syndrome. Condition of severe tics, including vocal tics and involuntary obscene speech.

Toxemia—Blood poisoning caused by bacteria growing in a site of infection.

Toxic—Poisonous; potentially deadly.

Toxoplasmosis—Disease caused by a protozoan; generally the symptoms are mild but a severe lymph node infection can result.

Tracheostomy—A surgical opening through the throat into the trachea (main passage from the lungs to the mouth) to permit a patient to breathe easily.

Transdermal disk—Patch applied to the skin as a means of administering medicine; medicine contained in the patch is absorbed into the body through the skin.

Triglyceride—Substance formed in the body from fat in foods, and used to store fats in blood and tissues.

Trypanosomiasis, African—Also called trypanosome fever or African sleeping sickness. Tropical disease, transmitted by tsetse fly bites, which causes fever, headache, and chills, followed by enlarged lymph nodes, anemia, and painful limbs and joints. Months or even years later, the disease affects the central nervous system, causing drowsiness and lethargy.

Tuberculosis (TB)—Infectious disease, usually of the lungs, marked by fever, night sweats, weight loss, and spitting up blood.

Ureters—Pair of tubes through which urine passes from the kidneys to the bladder.

Vaccinia—Also called cowpox. Mild virus infection causing symptoms similar to smallpox.

Vaginal—Related to the vagina.

Varicella—Also called chickenpox. Very infectious virus disease marked by fever and itchy rash that develops into blisters and then scabs.

Vascular—Relating to the blood vessels.

Vasodilator—Medicine that relaxes the blood vessels and thus increases blood flow through them.

Veterinary—Concerning medical care of animals.

Vitiligo—Also called leukoderma. Condition in which some areas of skin lose their color and turn white.

von Willebrand's disease—Hereditary blood disease in which blood clotting is delayed, leading to excessive and uncontrolled bleeding even after minor injuries.

Wilson's disease—Inborn defect in the body's ability to process copper. Too much copper may lead to jaundice, cirrhosis, mental retardation, or symptoms like those of Parkinson's disease.

Zollinger-Ellison syndrome—Disorder in which the stomach produces too much acid, leading to ulcers.

Appendix I

THE MEDICINE CHART

The Medicine Chart presents photographs of the most frequently prescribed medicines in the United States. In general, commonly used brand name products and a representative sampling of generic products have been included. The pictorial listing is not intended to be inclusive and does not represent all products on the market. Only selected solid oral dosage forms (capsules and tablets) have been included. The inclusion of a product does not mean the USPC has any particular knowledge that the product included has properties different from other products, nor should it be interpreted as an endorsement by USPC. Similarly, the fact that a particular product has not been included does not indicate that the product has been judged by the USPC to be unsatisfactory or unacceptable.

The drug products in *The Medicine Chart* are listed alphabetically by generic name of active ingredient(s). To quickly locate a particular medicine, check the product listing index that follows. This listing provides brand and generic names and directs the user to the appropriate page and chart location. In addition, any unique identifying code found on the surface of a capsule or tablet that might be useful in making a correct identification is included in the parentheses that follow the product's index entry. Please note that these codes may change as manufacturers reformulate or redesign their products. In addition, some companies may not manufacture all of their own products. In some of these cases, the imprinting on the tablet or capsule may be that of the actual manufacturer and not of the company marketing the product.

Brand names are in *italics*. An asterisk in the chart identifies those products that are available from a single source with no generic equivalents currently being available in the United States. Where multiple source products are shown, it must be kept in mind that other products may also be available. To learn the names of other companies that supply the same product, check with your pharmacist.

The size and color of the products shown are intended to match the actual product as closely as possible; however, there may be some differences due to variations caused by the photographic process. Also, manufacturers may occasionally change the color, imprinting, or shape of their products, and for a period of time both the "old" and the newly changed dosage form may be on the market. Such changes may not occur uniformly thoughout the different dosages of the product. These types of changes will be incorporated in subsequent versions of the chart as they are brought to our attention. If you have *any* questions about the medicine you are taking, check with your pharmacist.

Bentyl
  Capsules—
    10 mg (10) . . . . IV, D2
  Tablets—
    20 mg (20) . . . . IV, D3
Benztropine. II, D1
Blocadren Tablets—
  5 mg (59) . . . . XVI, A6
  10 mg (136) . . . . XVI, A6
Brethine Tablets—
  2.5 mg (72) . . . . XV, B4
  5 mg (05) . . . . XV, B4
Bumetanide. II, D2
Bumex Tablets—
  0.5 mg (0.5) . . . . II, D2
  1 mg (1) . . . . II, D2
  2 mg (2) . . . . II, D2
Butalbital, Aspirin, and
  Caffeine. II, D3–D4
Butalbital, Aspirin, Codeine, and
  Caffeine. II, D5–D6
Cafergot Tablets—
  1/100 mg . . . . VI, B1
Cafergot-PB Tablets—
  1/0.125/100 mg (78-36) . . . . VI, B2
Calan
  Tablets
    80 mg (80) . . . . XVI, D3
    120 mg (120) . . . . XVI, D3
  Extended-release Tablets—
    240 mg (240) . . . . XVI, D4
Capoten Tablets—
  12.5 mg (450) . . . . III, A1
  25 mg (452) . . . . III, A1
  50 mg (482) . . . . III, A2
  100 mg (485) . . . . III, A2
Capozide Tablets—
  25/15 mg (338) . . . . III, A3
  25/25 mg (349) . . . . III, A3
  50/15 mg (384) . . . . III, A4
  50/25 mg (390) . . . . III, A4
Captopril. . . . . III, A1–A2
Captopril and
  Hydrochlorothiazide. . . . . III, A3–A4
Carafate Tablets—
  1 gram (1712). . . . . XIV, D4
Carbamazepine. . . . . III, A5–A6
Carbidopa and Levodopa . . . . III, B1
Cardizem Tablets—
  30 mg (1771) . . . . V, A4
  60 mg (1772) . . . . V, A4
  90 mg (90 mg) . . . . V, A5
  120 mg (120 mg) . . . . V, A5
Catapres Tablets—
  0.1 mg (BI6) . . . . IV, A6
  0.2 mg (BI7) . . . . IV, A6
  0.3 mg (BI11) . . . . IV, A6
Ceclor Capsules—
  250 mg (3061) . . . . III, B2
  500 mg (3062) . . . . III, B2
Cefaclor. . . . . III, B2
Cefadroxil . . . . III, B3–B4
Centrax
  Capsules—
    5 mg (552) . . . . XIII, B5
    10 mg (553) . . . . XIII, B5
    20 mg (554) . . . . XIII, B5
  Tablets—
    10 mg (276) . . . . XIII, B6
Cephalexin . . . . III, B5–C1
  Warner-Chilcott Capsules—
    250 mg (938) . . . . III, C1
    500 mg (939) . . . . III, C1
Cephradine . . . . III, C2
Chlordiazepoxide . . . . III, C3–C5
  Purepac Capsules—
    5 mg (832 5) . . . . III, C3
    10 mg (832 10) . . . . III, C3
    25 mg (064) . . . . III, C3
Chlordiazepoxide and
  Clidinium . . . . III, C6–D1
  Purepac Capsules—
    5/2.5 mg (214) . . . . III, C6
Chlorpheniramine and
  Pseudoephedrine. . . . . III, D2–D3

Chlorpropamide . . . . III, D4–D6
  Geneva Tablets—
    100 mg (GG61) . . . . III, D5
    250 mg (GG144) . . . . III, D5
  Purepac Tablets—
    100 mg (882 G198) . . . . III, D6
    250 mg (882 G197) . . . . III, D6
Chlorthalidone . . . . IV, A1
Chlorzoxazone. . . . . IV, A2
Cimetidine. . . . . IV, A3–A4
Clemastine and
  Phenylpropanolamine. . . . . IV, A5
Clinoril Tablets—
  150 mg (941) . . . . XV, B2
  200 mg (942) . . . . XV, B2
Clonidine . . . . IV, A6
Clonidine and Chlorthalidone. . . . . . IV, B1
Clorazepate . . . . IV, B2–B3
Cogentin Tablets—
  0.5 mg (21) . . . . II, D1
  1 mg (635) . . . . II, D1
  2 mg (60) . . . . II, D1
Combipres Tablets—
  0.1/15 mg (BI8) . . . . IV, B1
  0.2/15 mg (BI9) . . . . IV, B1
  0.3/15 mg (BI10) . . . . IV, B1
Compazine
  Extended-release Capsules—
    10 mg (C44) . . . . XIII, D5
    15 mg (C46) . . . . XIII, D5
    30 mg (C47) . . . . XIII, D5
  Tablets—
    5 mg (C66) . . . . XIII, D6
    10 mg (C67) . . . . XIII, D6
    25 mg (C69) . . . . XIII, D6
Corgard Tablets—
  20 mg (232) . . . . XI, A4
  40 mg (207) . . . . XI, A4
  80 mg (241) . . . . XI, A4
  120 mg (208) . . . . XI, A5
  160 mg (246) . . . . XI, A5
Corzide Tablets—
  40/5 mg (283) . . . . XI, A6
  80/5 mg (284) . . . . XI, A6
Coumadin Tablets—
  2 mg (2) . . . . XVI, D5
  2.5 mg (2½) . . . . XVI, D5
  5 mg (5) . . . . XVI, D5
  7.5 mg (7½) . . . . XVI, D6
  10 mg (10) . . . . XVI, D6
Cyclobenzaprine . . . . IV, B4
Dalmane Capsules—
  15 mg (15) . . . . VII, A4
  30 mg (30) . . . . VII, A4
Darvocet-N Tablets—
  50/325 mg (50) . . . . XIV, A2
  100/650 mg (100) . . . . XIV, A2
Decadron Tablets—
  0.5 mg (41) . . . . IV, C1
  0.75 mg (63) . . . . IV, C1
  1.5 mg (95) . . . . IV, C2
  4 mg (97) . . . . IV, C2
Deconamine Tablets—
  4/60 mg (184) . . . . III, D3
Deconamine SR Extended-release Capsules—
  8/120 mg (181) . . . . III, D2
Deltasone Tablets—
  2.5 mg (32) . . . . XIII, C5
  5 mg (5) . . . . XIII, C5
  20 mg (20) . . . . XIII, C5
Demerol Tablets—
  50 mg (D35) . . . . X, A5
  100 mg (D37) . . . . X, A5
Desipramine . . . . IV, B5–B6
Desyrel Tablets—
  50 mg (MJ775) . . . . XVI, B4
  100 mg (MJ776) . . . . XVI, B4
Desyrel Dividose Tablets—
  150 mg (778) . . . . XVI, B5
Dexamethasone. . . . . IV, C1–C2
DiaBeta Tablets—
  1.25 mg . . . . VII, B5
  2.5 mg . . . . VII, B5
  5 mg . . . . VII, B5

Diabinese Tablets—
  100 mg (393) . . . . III, D4
  250 mg (394) . . . . III, D4
Diazepam . . . . IV, C4–D1
  PD Tablets—
    2 mg (141) . . . . IV, C4
    5 mg (142) . . . . IV, C4
    10 mg (143) . . . . IV, C4
  Purepac Tablets—
    2 mg (051) . . . . IV, C5
    5 mg (052) . . . . IV, C5
    10 mg (053) . . . . IV, C5
Dicyclomine . . . . IV, D2–D3
Diethylpropion . . . . IV, D4–D5
Diflunisal. IV, D6
Digoxin . . . . V, A1–A2
Dihydrocodeine, Aspirin, and
  Caffeine. . . . . V, A3
Dilantin Infatabs Chewable Tablets—
  50 mg (007) . . . . XIII, A2
Dilantin Kapseals Capsules—
  30 mg (365) . . . . XIII, A3
  100 mg (362) . . . . XIII, A3
Diltiazem . . . . V, A4–A5
Diphenhydramine. . . . . V, A6
Diphenoxylate and Atropine. . . . . . V, B1
Dipyridamole . . . . V, B2–B6
  Barr Tablets—
    25 mg (252) . . . . V, B2
    50 mg (285) . . . . V, B2
    75 mg (286) . . . . V, B2
  Geneva Tablets—
    25 mg (GG49) . . . . V, B4
    50 mg (GG45) . . . . V, B4
    75 mg (GG464) . . . . V, B4
  Purepac Tablets—
    25 mg (193) . . . . V, B5
    50 mg (2976) . . . . V, B5
    75 mg (2977) . . . . V, B5
  Rugby Tablets—
    25 mg (70) . . . . V, B6
    50 mg (3571) . . . . V, B6
    75 mg (3572) . . . . V, B6
Dolobid Tablets
  250 mg (675) . . . . IV, D6
  500 mg (697) . . . . IV, D6
Donnatal
  Capsules—
    0.0194/0.1037/0.0065/16.2 mg
     (4207) . . . . II, C3
  Tablets—
    0.0194/0.1037/0.0065/16.2 mg
     (4250) . . . . II, C4
  Extended-release Tablets—
    0.0582/0.3111/0.0195/48.6 mg . . II, C5
Doxepin. . . . . V, C1–C4
Doxycycline. . . . . V, C5–VI, A4
  Barr
    Capsules—
     50 mg (296) . . . . V, C5
     100 mg (297) . . . . V, C5
    Tablets—
     100 mg (295) . . . . V, C6
  Geneva
    Capsules—
     50 mg (5535) . . . . V, D1
     100 mg (5440) . . . . V, D1
    Tablets—
     100 mg (5553) . . . . V, D2
  Lederle
    Capsules—
     50 mg (D22) . . . . V, D3
     100 mg (D25) . . . . V, D3
    Tablets—
     100 mg (D41) . . . . V, D4
  Rugby
    Capsules—
     50 mg (0280) . . . . VI, A1
     100 mg (0230) . . . . VI, A1
    Tablets—
     100 mg (0340) . . . . VI, A2

In addition to USP headquarters staff, the following are acknowledged for their contribution to *The Medicine Chart*: Diana M. Blais, Project Coordinator; Hazleton/Webb Design, Graphics; Thomas H. Humphrey, Photography; and Salvatore A. Saleme, Robert Borgatti, Jr., Robert Borgatti, Sr., Pharmacy Consultants.

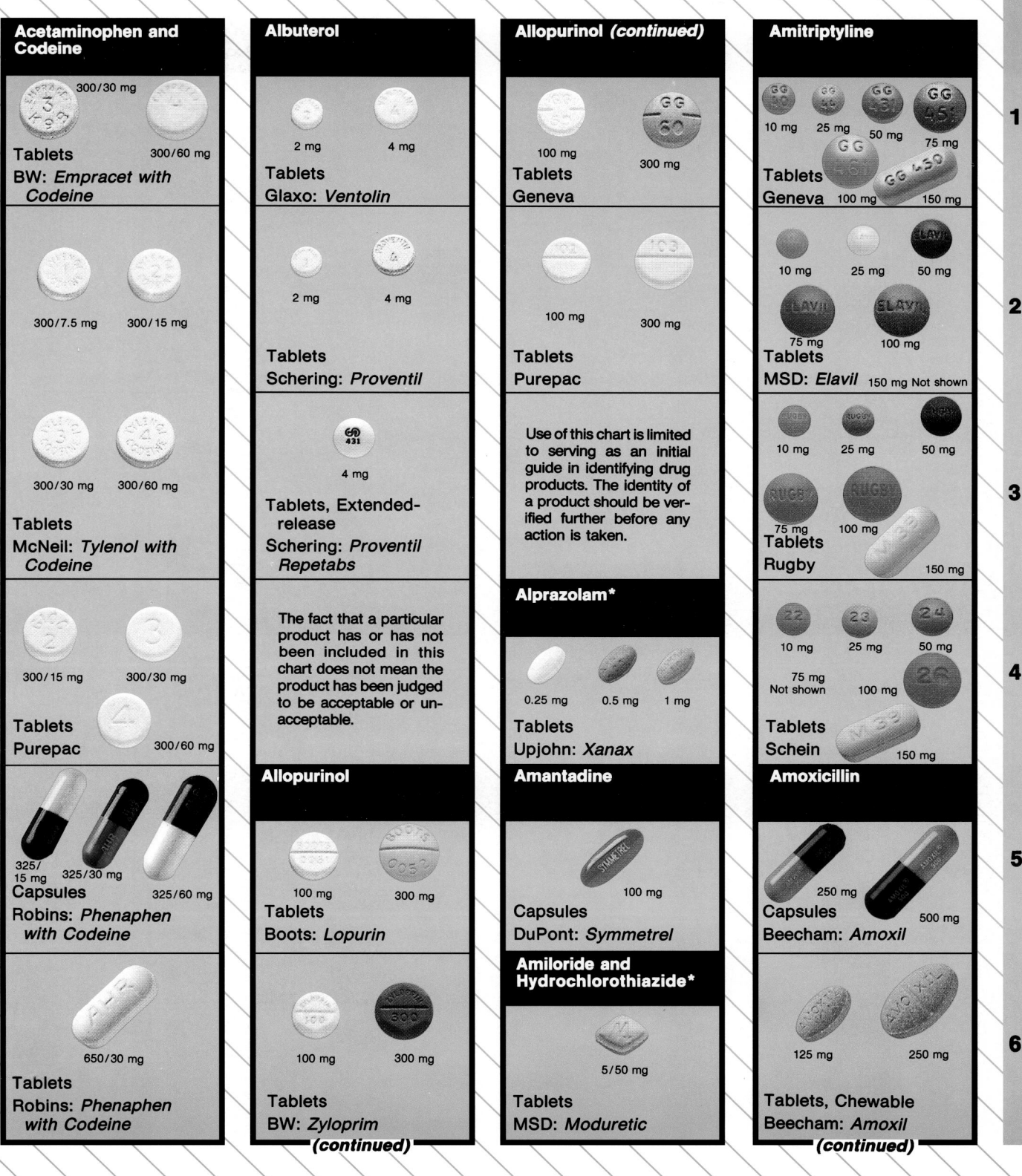

A

Acetaminophen and Codeine

300/30 mg
300/60 mg

Tablets
BW: *Empracet with Codeine*

300/7.5 mg
300/15 mg

300/30 mg
300/60 mg

Tablets
McNeil: *Tylenol with Codeine*

300/15 mg
300/30 mg

Tablets
Purepac
300/60 mg

325/15 mg
325/30 mg
325/60 mg

Capsules
Robins: *Phenaphen with Codeine*

650/30 mg

Tablets
Robins: *Phenaphen with Codeine*

B

Albuterol

2 mg
4 mg

Tablets
Glaxo: *Ventolin*

2 mg
4 mg

Tablets
Schering: *Proventil*

431
4 mg

Tablets, Extended-release
Schering: *Proventil Repetabs*

The fact that a particular product has or has not been included in this chart does not mean the product has been judged to be acceptable or unacceptable.

Allopurinol

100 mg
300 mg

Tablets
Boots: *Lopurin*

100 mg
300 mg

Tablets
BW: *Zyloprim*
(continued)

C

Allopurinol *(continued)*

100 mg
GG 60
300 mg

Tablets
Geneva

100 mg
300 mg

Tablets
Purepac

Use of this chart is limited to serving as an initial guide in identifying drug products. The identity of a product should be verified further before any action is taken.

Alprazolam*

0.25 mg
0.5 mg
1 mg

Tablets
Upjohn: *Xanax*

Amantadine

100 mg

Capsules
DuPont: *Symmetrel*

Amiloride and Hydrochlorothiazide*

5/50 mg

Tablets
MSD: *Moduretic*

D

Amitriptyline

10 mg
25 mg
50 mg
75 mg
100 mg
150 mg

Tablets
Geneva

10 mg
25 mg
50 mg
75 mg
100 mg

Tablets
MSD: *Elavil*   150 mg Not shown

10 mg
25 mg
50 mg
75 mg
100 mg
150 mg

Tablets
Rugby

10 mg
25 mg
50 mg
75 mg Not shown
100 mg
150 mg

Tablets
Schein

Amoxicillin

250 mg
500 mg

Capsules
Beecham: *Amoxil*

125 mg
250 mg

Tablets, Chewable
Beecham: *Amoxil*
(continued)

*Single source product.

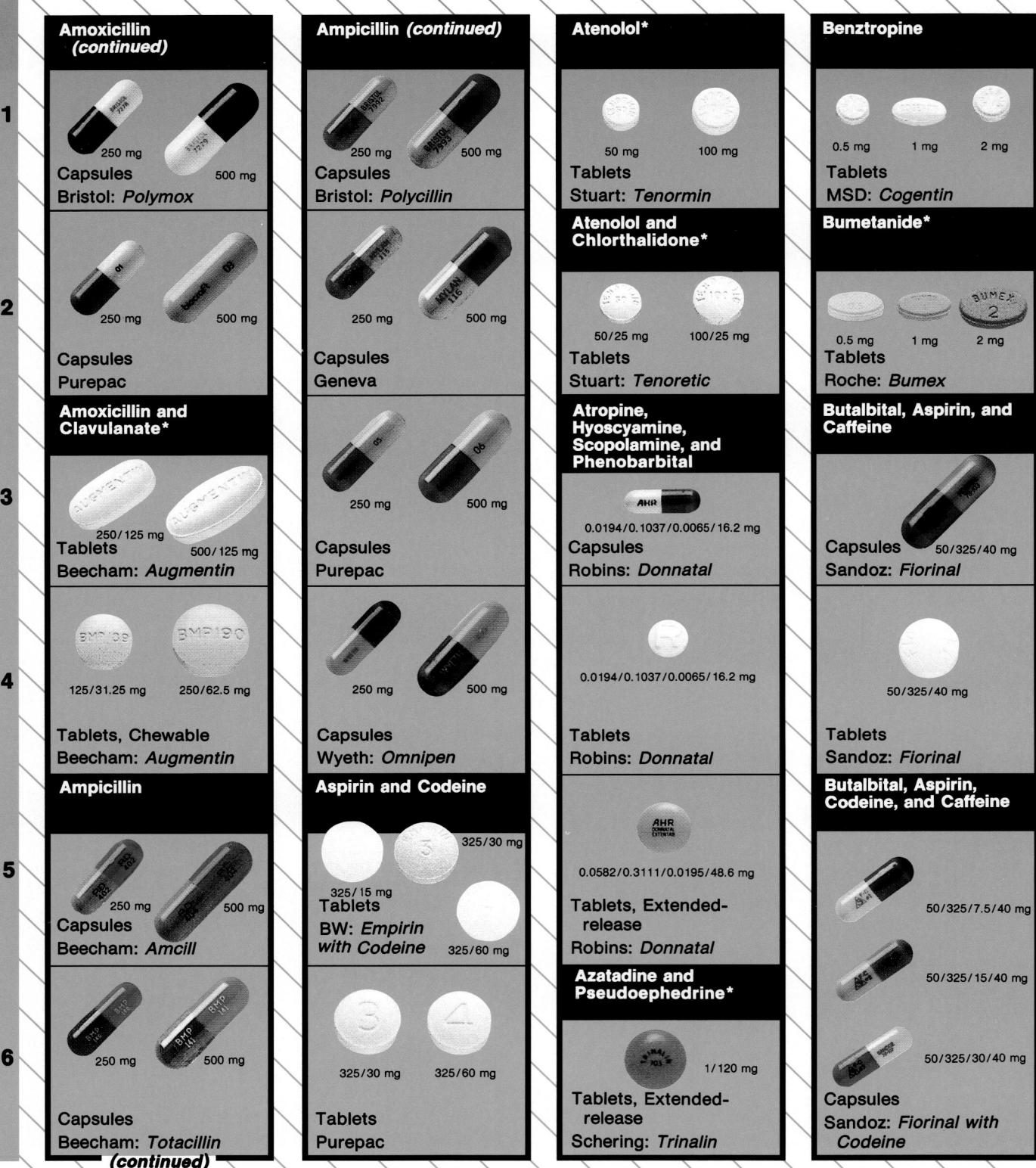

A

Amoxicillin (continued)

1
250 mg 500 mg
Capsules
Bristol: *Polymox*

2
250 mg 500 mg
Capsules
Purepac

Amoxicillin and Clavulanate*

3
250/125 mg 500/125 mg
Tablets
Beecham: *Augmentin*

4
125/31.25 mg 250/62.5 mg
Tablets, Chewable
Beecham: *Augmentin*

Ampicillin

5
250 mg 500 mg
Capsules
Beecham: *Amcill*

6
250 mg 500 mg
Capsules
Beecham: *Totacillin* (continued)

B

Ampicillin (continued)

1
250 mg 500 mg
Capsules
Bristol: *Polycillin*

2
250 mg 500 mg
Capsules
Geneva

3
250 mg 500 mg
Capsules
Purepac

4
250 mg 500 mg
Capsules
Wyeth: *Omnipen*

Aspirin and Codeine

5
325/15 mg 325/30 mg 325/60 mg
Tablets
BW: *Empirin with Codeine*

6
325/30 mg 325/60 mg
Tablets
Purepac

C

Atenolol*

1
50 mg 100 mg
Tablets
Stuart: *Tenormin*

Atenolol and Chlorthalidone*

2
50/25 mg 100/25 mg
Tablets
Stuart: *Tenoretic*

Atropine, Hyoscyamine, Scopolamine, and Phenobarbital

3
0.0194/0.1037/0.0065/16.2 mg
Capsules
Robins: *Donnatal*

4
0.0194/0.1037/0.0065/16.2 mg
Tablets
Robins: *Donnatal*

5
0.0582/0.3111/0.0195/48.6 mg
Tablets, Extended-release
Robins: *Donnatal*

Azatadine and Pseudoephedrine*

6
1/120 mg
Tablets, Extended-release
Schering: *Trinalin*

D

Benztropine

1
0.5 mg 1 mg 2 mg
Tablets
MSD: *Cogentin*

Bumetanide*

2
0.5 mg 1 mg 2 mg
Tablets
Roche: *Bumex*

Butalbital, Aspirin, and Caffeine

3
50/325/40 mg
Capsules
Sandoz: *Fiorinal*

4
50/325/40 mg
Tablets
Sandoz: *Fiorinal*

Butalbital, Aspirin, Codeine, and Caffeine

5
50/325/7.5/40 mg
50/325/15/40 mg

6
50/325/30/40 mg
Capsules
Sandoz: *Fiorinal with Codeine*

*Single source product.

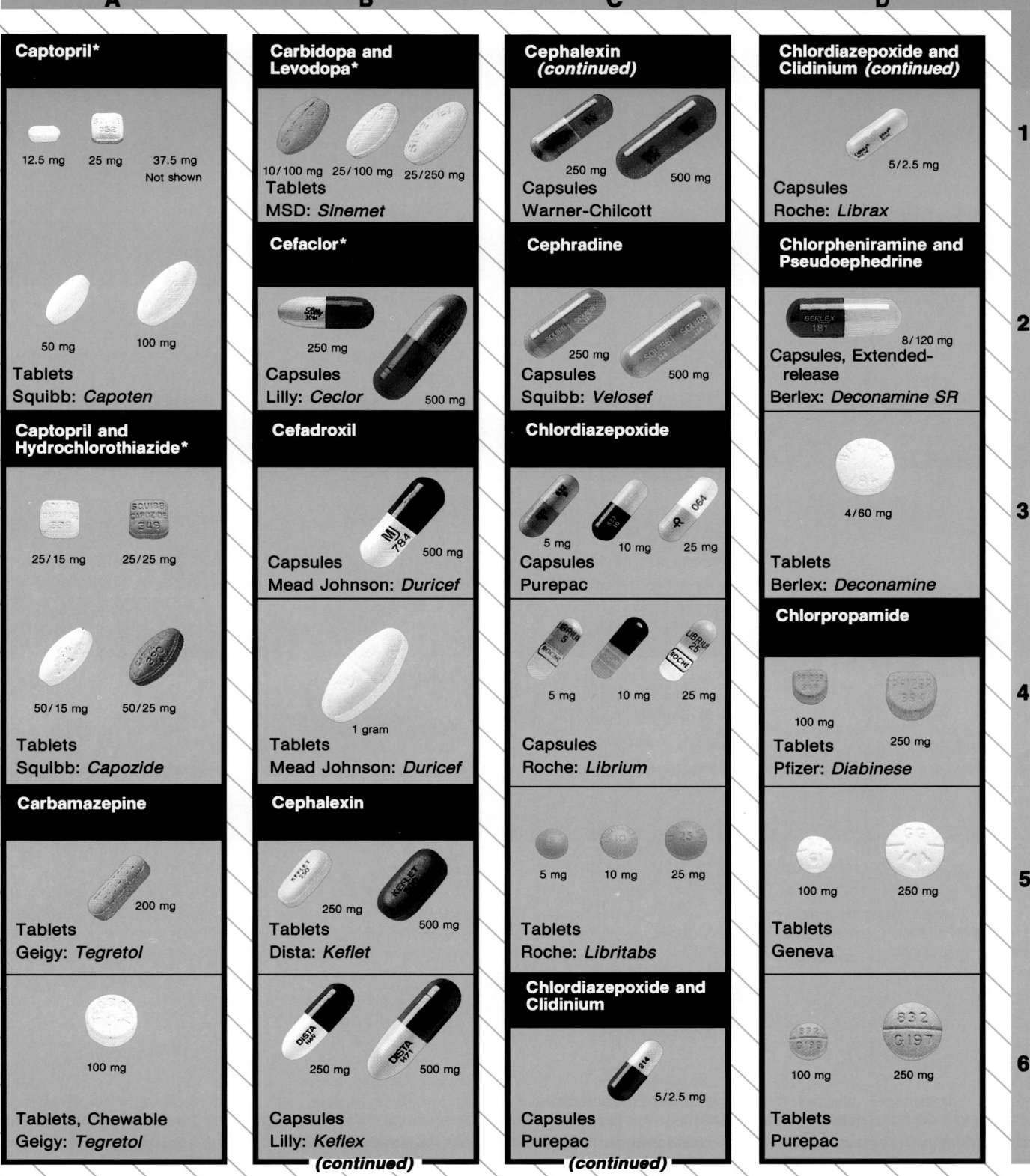

A

Captopril*

12.5 mg   25 mg   37.5 mg
Not shown

50 mg   100 mg

Tablets
Squibb: *Capoten*

Captopril and Hydrochlorothiazide*

25/15 mg   25/25 mg

50/15 mg   50/25 mg

Tablets
Squibb: *Capozide*

Carbamazepine

200 mg

Tablets
Geigy: *Tegretol*

100 mg

Tablets, Chewable
Geigy: *Tegretol*

B

Carbidopa and Levodopa*

10/100 mg 25/100 mg 25/250 mg
Tablets
MSD: *Sinemet*

Cefaclor*

250 mg

Capsules
Lilly: *Ceclor*
500 mg

Cefadroxil

500 mg

Capsules
Mead Johnson: *Duricef*

1 gram

Tablets
Mead Johnson: *Duricef*

Cephalexin

250 mg
Tablets
Dista: *Keflet*
500 mg

250 mg   500 mg

Capsules
Lilly: *Keflex*

(continued)

C

Cephalexin *(continued)*

250 mg
500 mg

Capsules
Warner-Chilcott

Cephradine

250 mg

Capsules
Squibb: *Velosef*
500 mg

Chlordiazepoxide

5 mg 10 mg 25 mg

Capsules
Purepac

5 mg 10 mg 25 mg

Capsules
Roche: *Librium*

5 mg 10 mg 25 mg

Tablets
Roche: *Libritabs*

Chlordiazepoxide and Clidinium

5/2.5 mg

Capsules
Purepac

(continued)

D

Chlordiazepoxide and Clidinium *(continued)*

5/2.5 mg

Capsules
Roche: *Librax*

Chlorpheniramine and Pseudoephedrine

8/120 mg

Capsules, Extended-release
Berlex: *Deconamine SR*

4/60 mg

Tablets
Berlex: *Deconamine*

Chlorpropamide

100 mg   250 mg
Tablets
Pfizer: *Diabinese*

100 mg   250 mg

Tablets
Geneva

100 mg   250 mg

Tablets
Purepac

1
2
3
4
5
6

*Single source product.

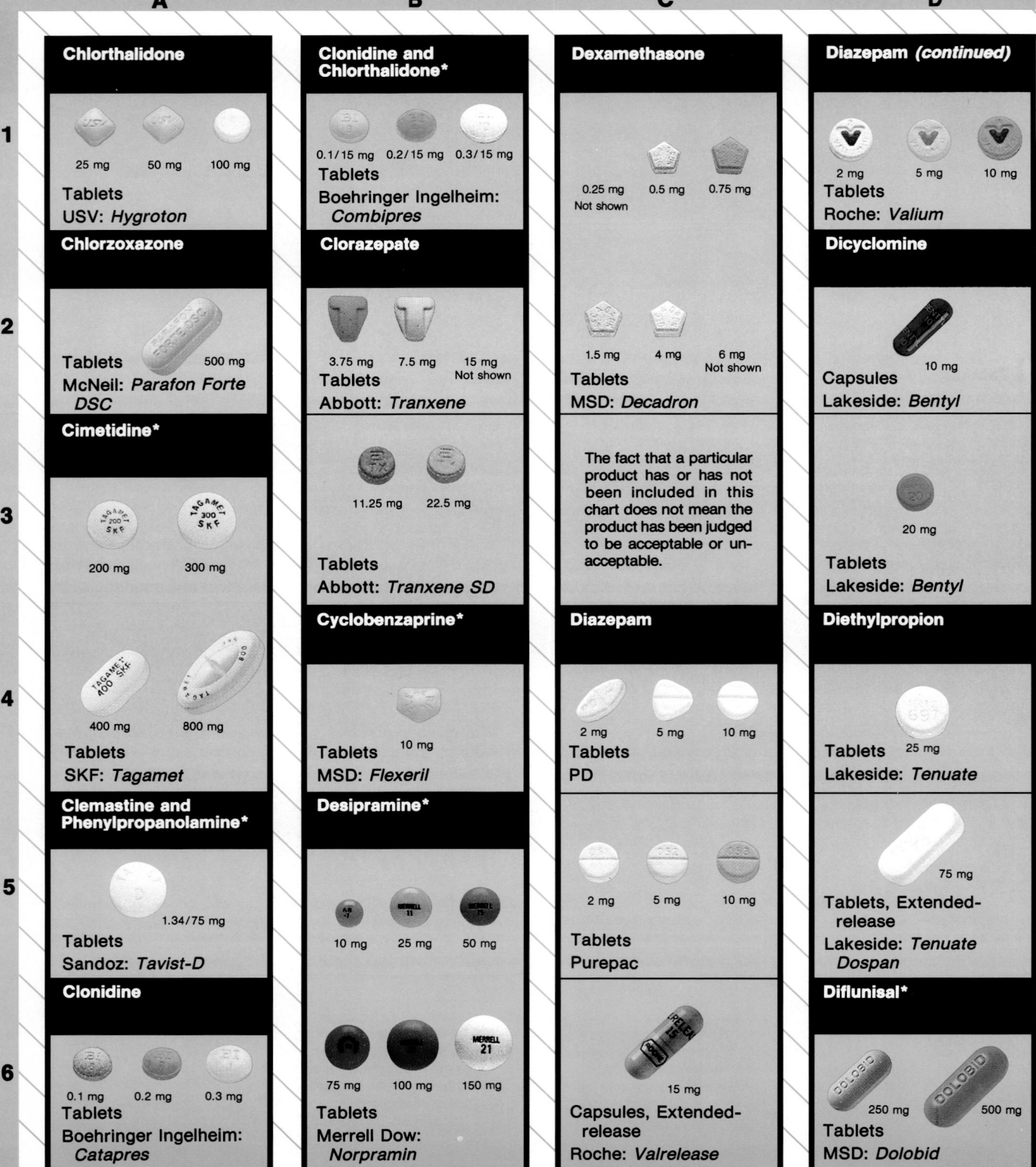

A

Chlorthalidone
25 mg · 50 mg · 100 mg
Tablets
USV: *Hygroton*

Chlorzoxazone
Tablets · 500 mg
McNeil: *Parafon Forte DSC*

Cimetidine*
200 mg · 300 mg · 400 mg · 800 mg
Tablets
SKF: *Tagamet*

Clemastine and Phenylpropanolamine*
1.34/75 mg
Tablets
Sandoz: *Tavist-D*

Clonidine
0.1 mg · 0.2 mg · 0.3 mg
Tablets
Boehringer Ingelheim: *Catapres*

B

Clonidine and Chlorthalidone*
0.1/15 mg · 0.2/15 mg · 0.3/15 mg
Tablets
Boehringer Ingelheim: *Combipres*

Clorazepate
3.75 mg · 7.5 mg · 15 mg Not shown
Tablets
Abbott: *Tranxene*

11.25 mg · 22.5 mg
Tablets
Abbott: *Tranxene SD*

Cyclobenzaprine*
10 mg
Tablets
MSD: *Flexeril*

Desipramine*
10 mg · 25 mg · 50 mg
75 mg · 100 mg · 150 mg
Tablets
Merrell Dow: *Norpramin*

C

Dexamethasone
0.25 mg Not shown · 0.5 mg · 0.75 mg
1.5 mg · 4 mg · 6 mg Not shown
Tablets
MSD: *Decadron*

The fact that a particular product has or has not been included in this chart does not mean the product has been judged to be acceptable or unacceptable.

Diazepam
2 mg · 5 mg · 10 mg
Tablets
PD

2 mg · 5 mg · 10 mg
Tablets
Purepac

15 mg
Capsules, Extended-release
Roche: *Valrelease*
(continued)

D

Diazepam *(continued)*
2 mg · 5 mg · 10 mg
Tablets
Roche: *Valium*

Dicyclomine
10 mg
Capsules
Lakeside: *Bentyl*

20 mg
Tablets
Lakeside: *Bentyl*

Diethylpropion
25 mg
Tablets
Lakeside: *Tenuate*

75 mg
Tablets, Extended-release
Lakeside: *Tenuate Dospan*

Diflunisal*
250 mg · 500 mg
Tablets
MSD: *Dolobid*

*Single source product.

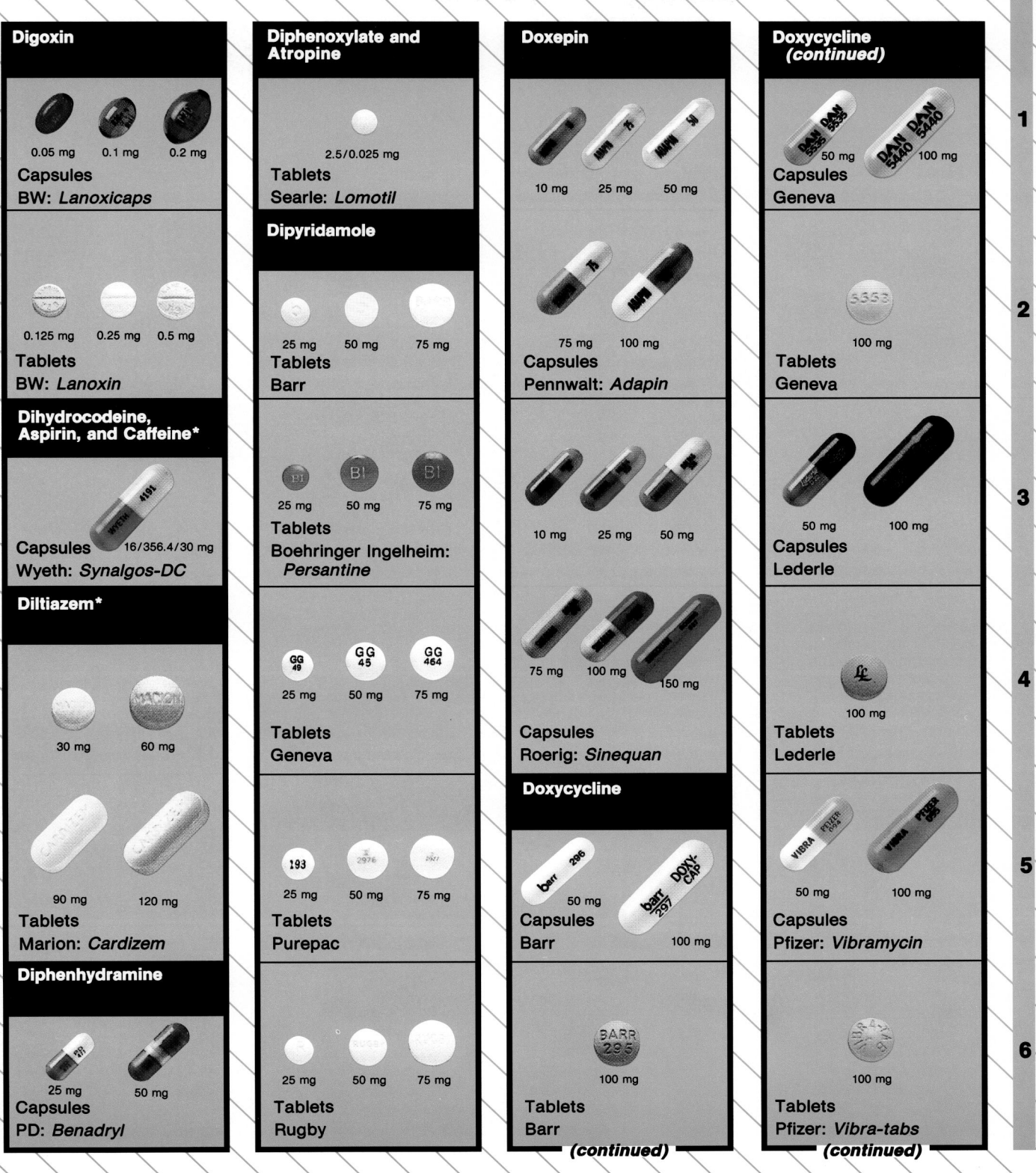

A

Digoxin

0.05 mg   0.1 mg   0.2 mg

Capsules
BW: *Lanoxicaps*

0.125 mg   0.25 mg   0.5 mg

Tablets
BW: *Lanoxin*

Dihydrocodeine, Aspirin, and Caffeine*

Capsules   16/356.4/30 mg
Wyeth: *Synalgos-DC*

Diltiazem*

30 mg   60 mg

90 mg   120 mg

Tablets
Marion: *Cardizem*

Diphenhydramine

25 mg   50 mg

Capsules
PD: *Benadryl*

B

Diphenoxylate and Atropine

2.5/0.025 mg

Tablets
Searle: *Lomotil*

Dipyridamole

25 mg   50 mg   75 mg

Tablets
Barr

25 mg   50 mg   75 mg

Tablets
Boehringer Ingelheim:
Persantine

GG 49   GG 45   GG 464
25 mg   50 mg   75 mg

Tablets
Geneva

193   2976   2977
25 mg   50 mg   75 mg

Tablets
Purepac

25 mg   50 mg   75 mg

Tablets
Rugby

C

Doxepin

10 mg   25 mg   50 mg

75 mg   100 mg

Capsules
Pennwalt: *Adapin*

10 mg   25 mg   50 mg

75 mg   100 mg   150 mg

Capsules
Roerig: *Sinequan*

Doxycycline

barr 296   barr 297 DOXY-CAP
50 mg   100 mg

Capsules
Barr

BARR 295
100 mg

Tablets
Barr

(continued)

D

Doxycycline
(continued)

DAN 5535   DAN 5440
50 mg   100 mg

Capsules
Geneva

5553
100 mg

Tablets
Geneva

50 mg   100 mg

Capsules
Lederle

100 mg

Tablets
Lederle

VIBRA PFIZER 1044   VIBRA PFIZER 093
50 mg   100 mg

Capsules
Pfizer: *Vibramycin*

100 mg

Tablets
Pfizer: *Vibra-tabs*

(continued)

1

2

3

4

5

6

*Single source product.

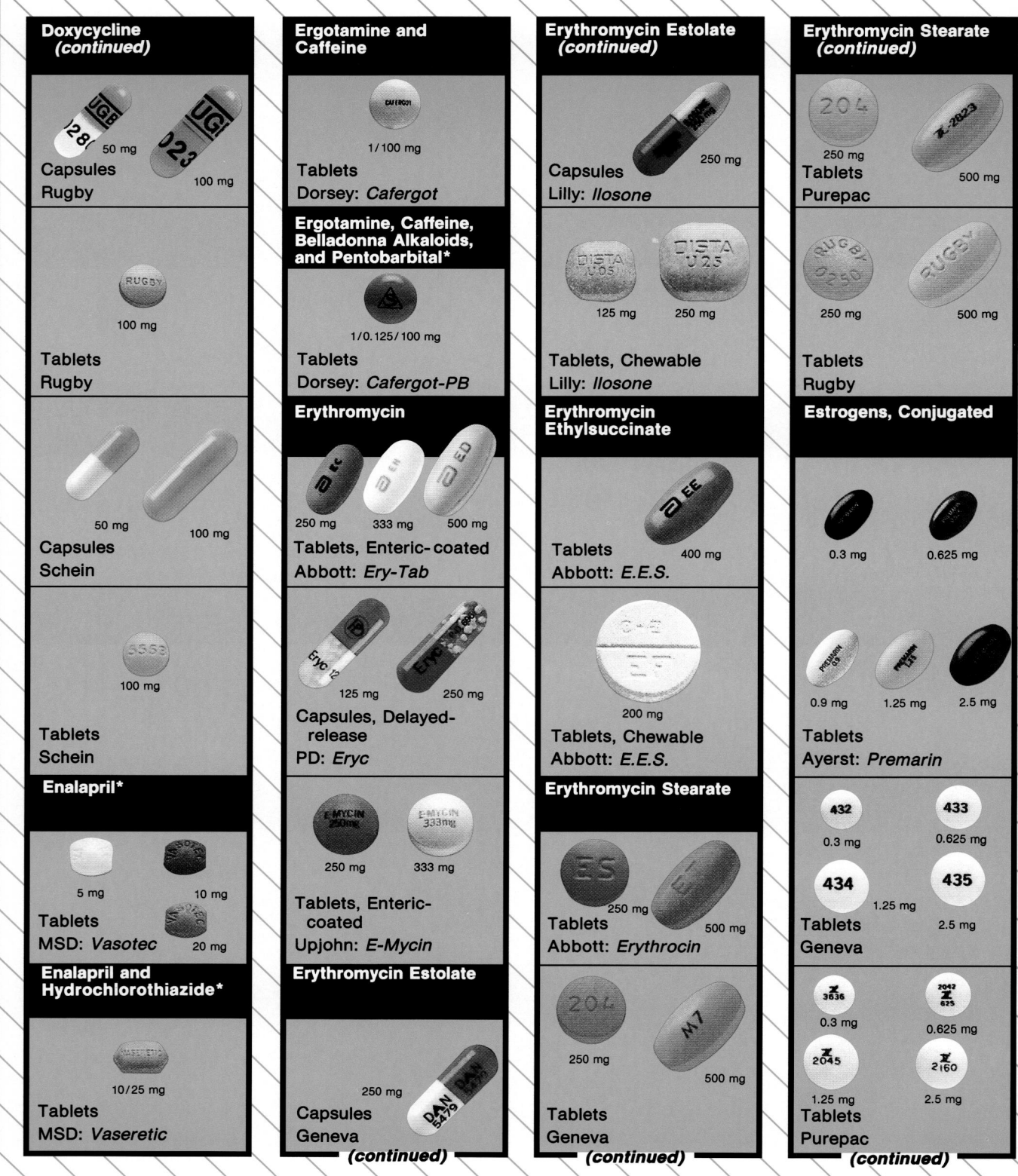

A

Doxycycline (continued)

Capsules
Rugby
50 mg
100 mg

100 mg
Tablets
Rugby

50 mg
100 mg
Capsules
Schein

100 mg
Tablets
Schein

Enalapril*

5 mg
10 mg
20 mg
Tablets
MSD: *Vasotec*

Enalapril and Hydrochlorothiazide*

10/25 mg
Tablets
MSD: *Vaseretic*

B

Ergotamine and Caffeine

1/100 mg
Tablets
Dorsey: *Cafergot*

Ergotamine, Caffeine, Belladonna Alkaloids, and Pentobarbital*

1/0.125/100 mg
Tablets
Dorsey: *Cafergot-PB*

Erythromycin

250 mg
333 mg
500 mg
Tablets, Enteric-coated
Abbott: *Ery-Tab*

125 mg
250 mg
Capsules, Delayed-release
PD: *Eryc*

250 mg
333 mg
Tablets, Enteric-coated
Upjohn: *E-Mycin*

Erythromycin Estolate

250 mg
Capsules
Geneva
(continued)

C

Erythromycin Estolate (continued)

Capsules
Lilly: *Ilosone*
250 mg

125 mg
250 mg
Tablets, Chewable
Lilly: *Ilosone*

Erythromycin Ethylsuccinate

Tablets
Abbott: *E.E.S.*
400 mg

200 mg
Tablets, Chewable
Abbott: *E.E.S.*

Erythromycin Stearate

250 mg
500 mg
Tablets
Abbott: *Erythrocin*

250 mg
500 mg
Tablets
Geneva
(continued)

D

Erythromycin Stearate (continued)

204
250 mg
Z-2823
500 mg
Tablets
Purepac

250 mg
500 mg
Tablets
Rugby

Estrogens, Conjugated

0.3 mg
0.625 mg

0.9 mg
1.25 mg
2.5 mg
Tablets
Ayerst: *Premarin*

432 0.3 mg
433 0.625 mg
434 1.25 mg
435 2.5 mg
Tablets
Geneva

3636 0.3 mg
2042 625 0.625 mg
2045 1.25 mg
2160 2.5 mg
Tablets
Purepac
(continued)

*Single source product.

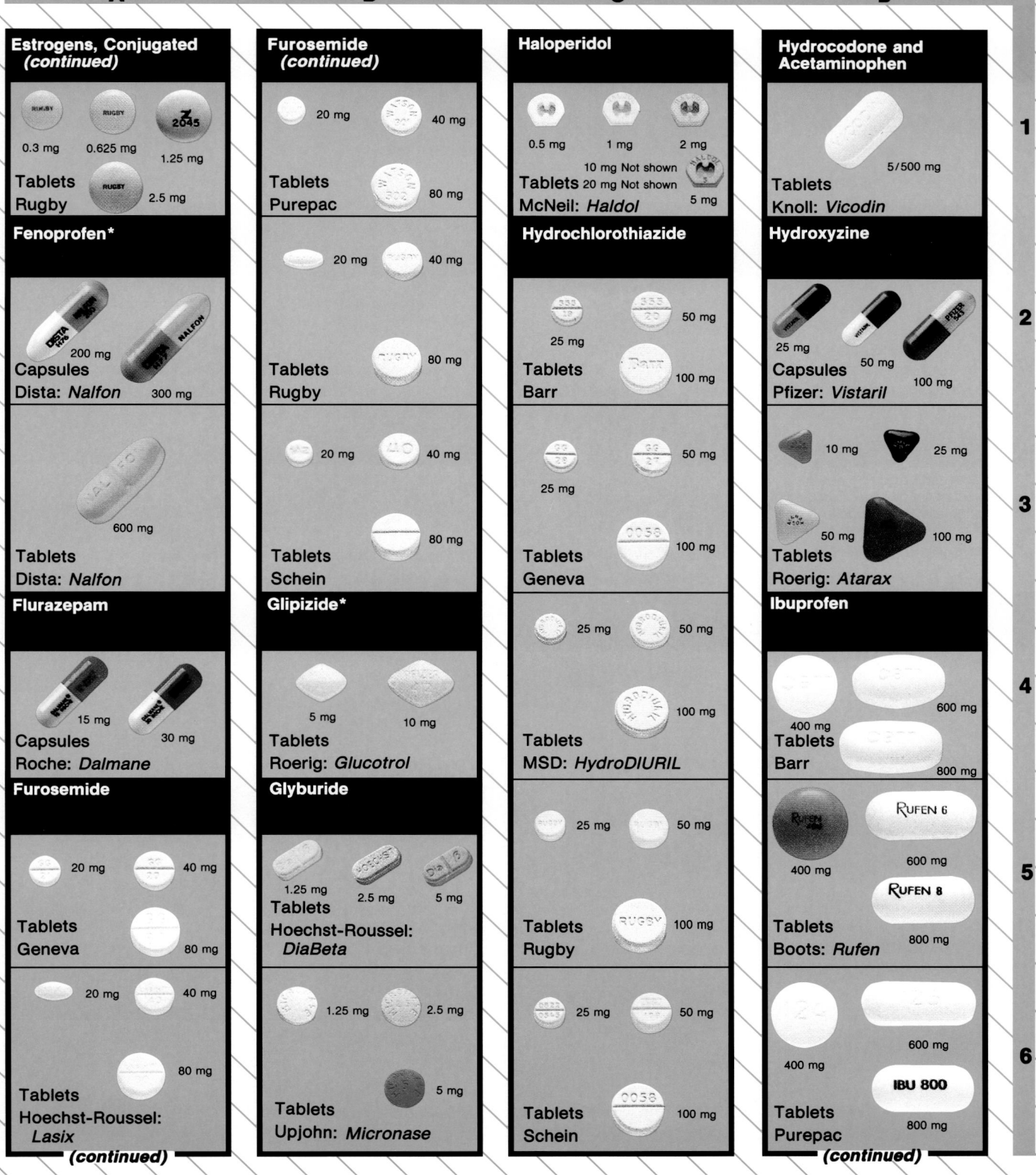

A

Estrogens, Conjugated
(continued)

0.3 mg   0.625 mg   1.25 mg

Tablets
Rugby   2.5 mg

Fenoprofen*

200 mg   NALFON
Capsules
Dista: *Nalfon*   300 mg

600 mg
Tablets
Dista: *Nalfon*

Flurazepam

15 mg   30 mg
Capsules
Roche: *Dalmane*

Furosemide

20 mg   40 mg
Tablets
Geneva   80 mg

20 mg   40 mg
80 mg
Tablets
Hoechst-Roussel:
Lasix
(continued)

B

Furosemide
(continued)

20 mg   40 mg
Tablets
Purepac   80 mg

20 mg   40 mg
Tablets
Rugby   80 mg

20 mg   40 mg
Tablets
Schein   80 mg

Glipizide*

5 mg   10 mg
Tablets
Roerig: *Glucotrol*

Glyburide

1.25 mg   2.5 mg   5 mg
Tablets
Hoechst-Roussel:
DiaBeta

1.25 mg   2.5 mg
5 mg
Tablets
Upjohn: *Micronase*

C

Haloperidol

0.5 mg   1 mg   2 mg
10 mg 20 mg Not shown
Tablets 20 mg Not shown
McNeil: *Haldol*   5 mg

Hydrochlorothiazide

25 mg   50 mg
Tablets
Barr   100 mg

25 mg   50 mg
25 mg
Tablets
Geneva   100 mg

25 mg   50 mg
100 mg
Tablets
MSD: *HydroDIURIL*

25 mg   50 mg
Tablets
Rugby   100 mg

25 mg   50 mg
Tablets
Schein   100 mg

D

Hydrocodone and
Acetaminophen

5/500 mg
Tablets
Knoll: *Vicodin*

Hydroxyzine

25 mg   50 mg
Capsules
Pfizer: *Vistaril*   100 mg

10 mg   25 mg
50 mg   100 mg
Tablets
Roerig: *Atarax*

Ibuprofen

400 mg   600 mg
Tablets
Barr   800 mg

RUFEN 6
400 mg   600 mg
RUFEN 8
Tablets
Boots: *Rufen*   800 mg

400 mg   600 mg
IBU 800
Tablets
Purepac   800 mg
(continued)

1
2
3
4
5
6

*Single source product.

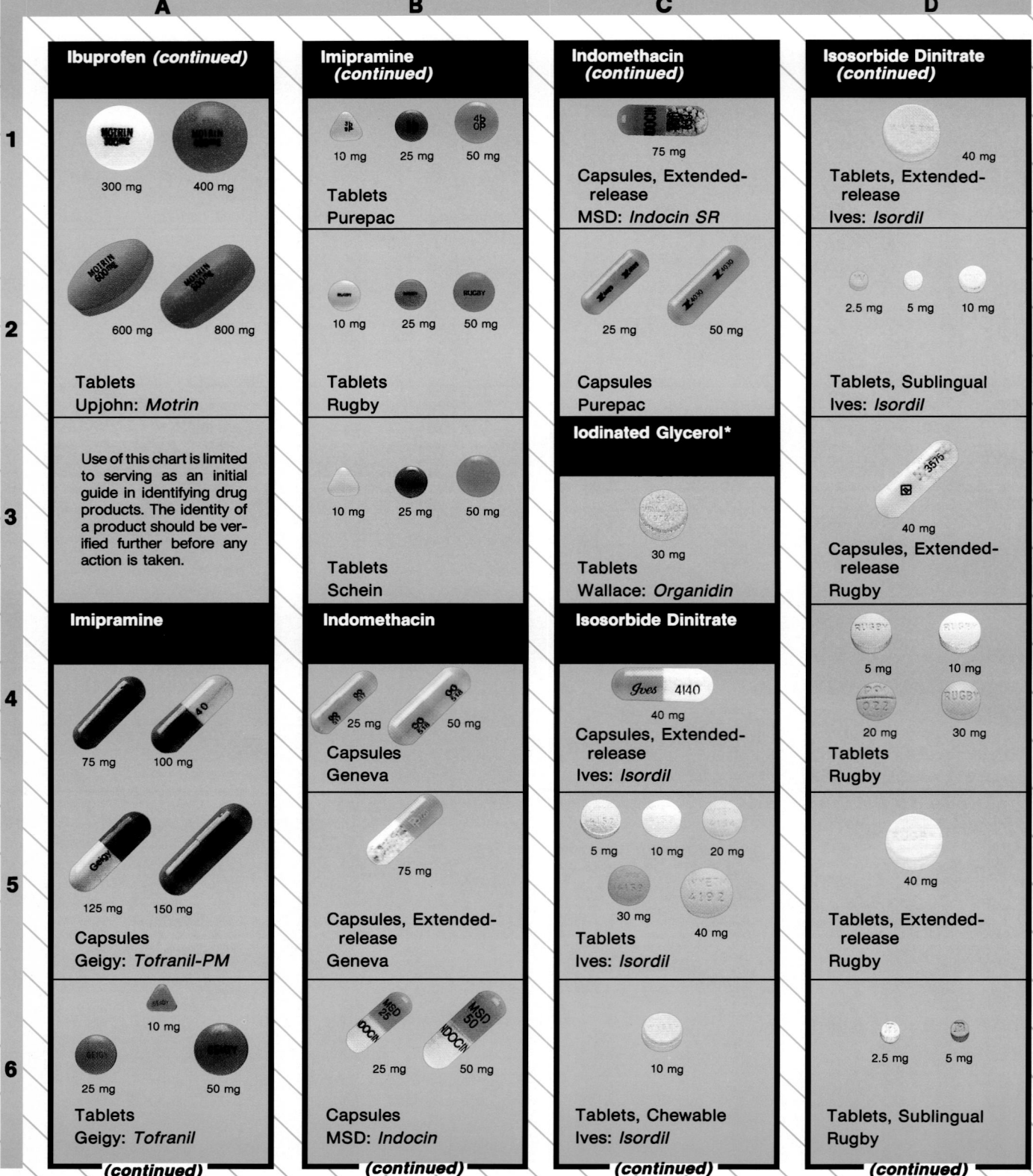

A

Ibuprofen (continued)

300 mg 400 mg

600 mg 800 mg

Tablets
Upjohn: *Motrin*

Use of this chart is limited to serving as an initial guide in identifying drug products. The identity of a product should be verified further before any action is taken.

Imipramine

75 mg 100 mg

125 mg 150 mg

Capsules
Geigy: *Tofranil-PM*

10 mg

25 mg 50 mg

Tablets
Geigy: *Tofranil*

(continued)

B

Imipramine (continued)

10 mg 25 mg 50 mg

Tablets
Purepac

10 mg 25 mg 50 mg

Tablets
Rugby

10 mg 25 mg 50 mg

Tablets
Schein

Indomethacin

25 mg 50 mg

Capsules
Geneva

75 mg

Capsules, Extended-release
Geneva

25 mg 50 mg

Capsules
MSD: *Indocin*

(continued)

C

Indomethacin (continued)

75 mg

Capsules, Extended-release
MSD: *Indocin SR*

25 mg 50 mg

Capsules
Purepac

Iodinated Glycerol*

30 mg

Tablets
Wallace: *Organidin*

Isosorbide Dinitrate

40 mg

Capsules, Extended-release
Ives: *Isordil*

5 mg 10 mg 20 mg

30 mg 40 mg

Tablets
Ives: *Isordil*

10 mg

Tablets, Chewable
Ives: *Isordil*

(continued)

D

Isosorbide Dinitrate (continued)

40 mg

Tablets, Extended-release
Ives: *Isordil*

2.5 mg 5 mg 10 mg

Tablets, Sublingual
Ives: *Isordil*

40 mg

Capsules, Extended-release
Rugby

5 mg 10 mg

20 mg 30 mg

Tablets
Rugby

40 mg

Tablets, Extended-release
Rugby

2.5 mg 5 mg

Tablets, Sublingual
Rugby

(continued)

*Single source product.

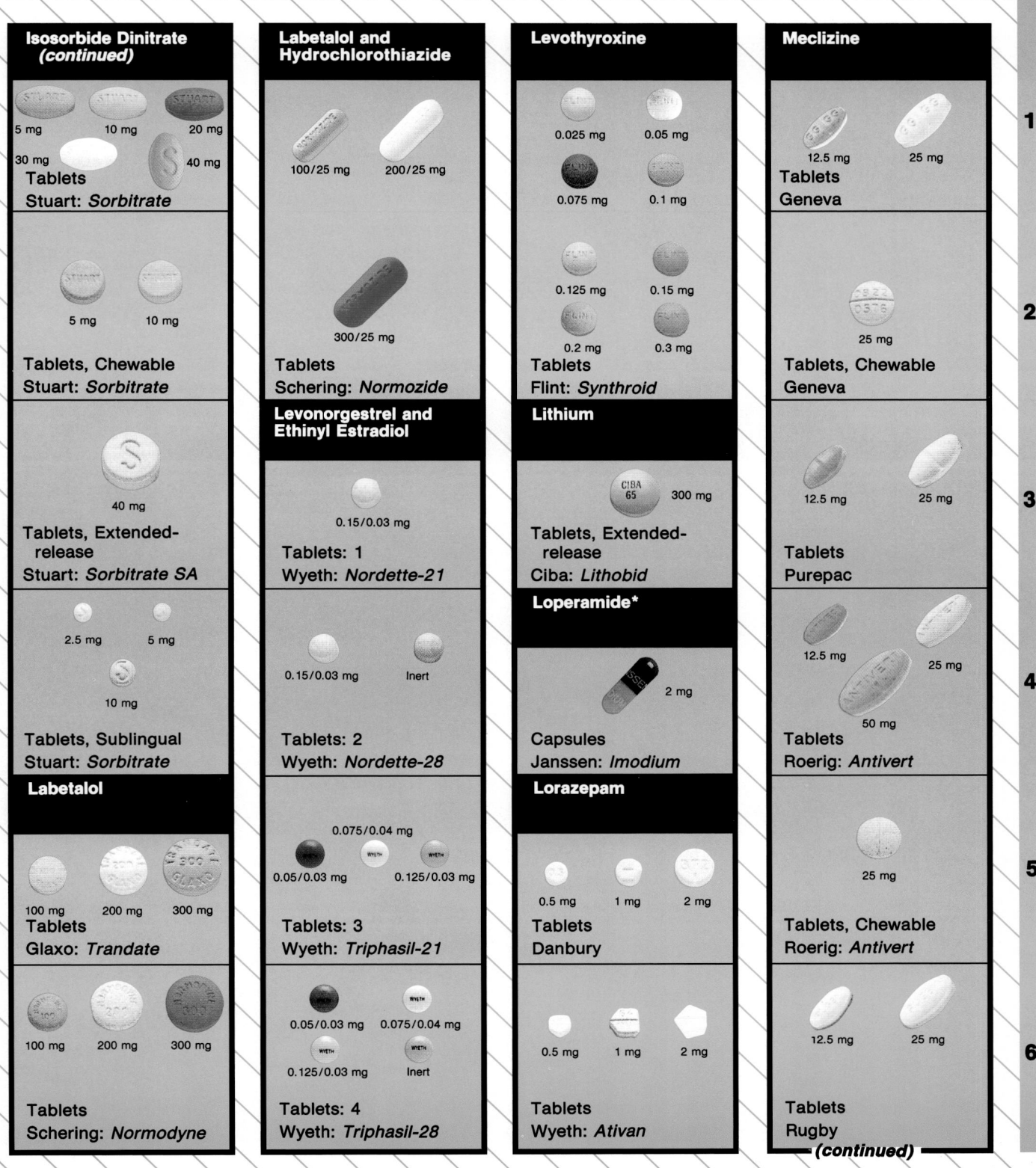

A

Isosorbide Dinitrate (continued)

5 mg 10 mg 20 mg
30 mg 40 mg
Tablets
Stuart: *Sorbitrate*

5 mg 10 mg
Tablets, Chewable
Stuart: *Sorbitrate*

40 mg
Tablets, Extended-release
Stuart: *Sorbitrate SA*

2.5 mg 5 mg
10 mg
Tablets, Sublingual
Stuart: *Sorbitrate*

Labetalol

100 mg 200 mg 300 mg
Tablets
Glaxo: *Trandate*

100 mg 200 mg 300 mg
Tablets
Schering: *Normodyne*

B

Labetalol and Hydrochlorothiazide

100/25 mg 200/25 mg
300/25 mg
Tablets
Schering: *Normozide*

Levonorgestrel and Ethinyl Estradiol

0.15/0.03 mg
Tablets: 1
Wyeth: *Nordette-21*

0.15/0.03 mg Inert
Tablets: 2
Wyeth: *Nordette-28*

0.075/0.04 mg
0.05/0.03 mg 0.125/0.03 mg
Tablets: 3
Wyeth: *Triphasil-21*

0.05/0.03 mg 0.075/0.04 mg
0.125/0.03 mg Inert
Tablets: 4
Wyeth: *Triphasil-28*

C

Levothyroxine

0.025 mg 0.05 mg
0.075 mg 0.1 mg
0.125 mg 0.15 mg
0.2 mg 0.3 mg
Tablets
Flint: *Synthroid*

Lithium

300 mg
Tablets, Extended-release
Ciba: *Lithobid*

Loperamide*

2 mg
Capsules
Janssen: *Imodium*

Lorazepam

0.5 mg 1 mg 2 mg
Tablets
Danbury

0.5 mg 1 mg 2 mg
Tablets
Wyeth: *Ativan*

D

Meclizine

12.5 mg 25 mg
Tablets
Geneva

25 mg
Tablets, Chewable
Geneva

12.5 mg 25 mg
Tablets
Purepac

12.5 mg 25 mg
50 mg
Tablets
Roerig: *Antivert*

25 mg
Tablets, Chewable
Roerig: *Antivert*

12.5 mg 25 mg
Tablets
Rugby

— *(continued)* —

1
2
3
4
5
6

*Single source product.

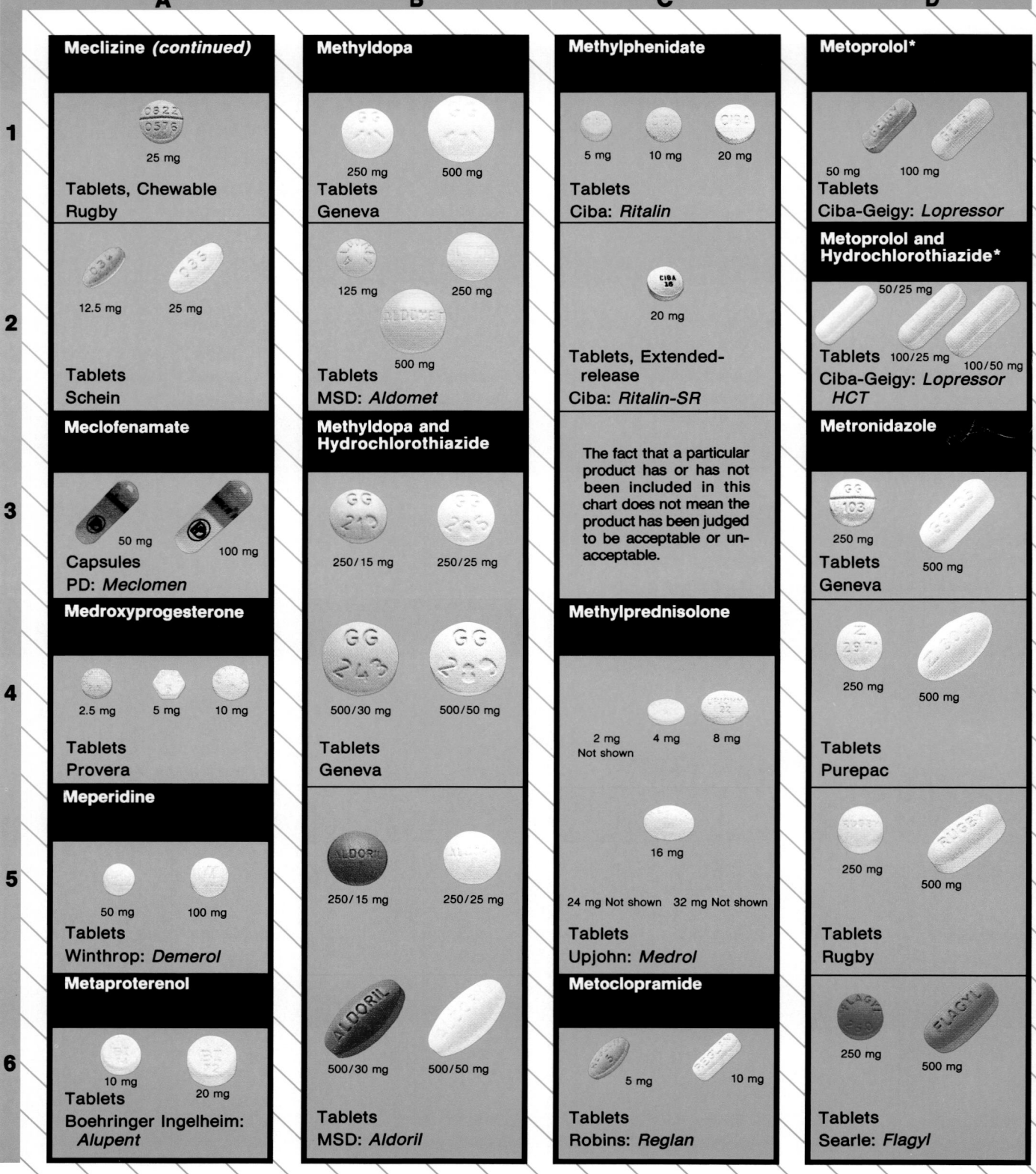

	A	**B**	**C**	**D**
1	**Meclizine** *(continued)* 25 mg Tablets, Chewable Rugby	**Methyldopa** 250 mg / 500 mg Tablets Geneva	**Methylphenidate** 5 mg / 10 mg / 20 mg Tablets Ciba: *Ritalin*	**Metoprolol*** 50 mg / 100 mg Tablets Ciba-Geigy: *Lopressor*
2	12.5 mg / 25 mg Tablets Schein	125 mg / 250 mg 500 mg Tablets MSD: *Aldomet*	20 mg Tablets, Extended-release Ciba: *Ritalin-SR*	**Metoprolol and Hydrochlorothiazide*** 50/25 mg 100/25 mg / 100/50 mg Tablets Ciba-Geigy: *Lopressor HCT*
3	**Meclofenamate** 50 mg / 100 mg Capsules PD: *Meclomen*	**Methyldopa and Hydrochlorothiazide** 250/15 mg / 250/25 mg 500/30 mg / 500/50 mg	The fact that a particular product has or has not been included in this chart does not mean the product has been judged to be acceptable or unacceptable.	**Metronidazole** 250 mg / 500 mg Tablets Geneva
4	**Medroxyprogesterone** 2.5 mg / 5 mg / 10 mg Tablets Provera	Tablets Geneva	**Methylprednisolone** 2 mg Not shown / 4 mg / 8 mg	250 mg / 500 mg Tablets Purepac
5	**Meperidine** 50 mg / 100 mg Tablets Winthrop: *Demerol*	250/15 mg / 250/25 mg	16 mg 24 mg Not shown 32 mg Not shown Tablets Upjohn: *Medrol*	250 mg / 500 mg Tablets Rugby
6	**Metaproterenol** 10 mg / 20 mg Tablets Boehringer Ingelheim: *Alupent*	500/30 mg / 500/50 mg Tablets MSD: *Aldoril*	**Metoclopramide** 5 mg / 10 mg Tablets Robins: *Reglan*	250 mg / 500 mg Tablets Searle: *Flagyl*

*Single source product.

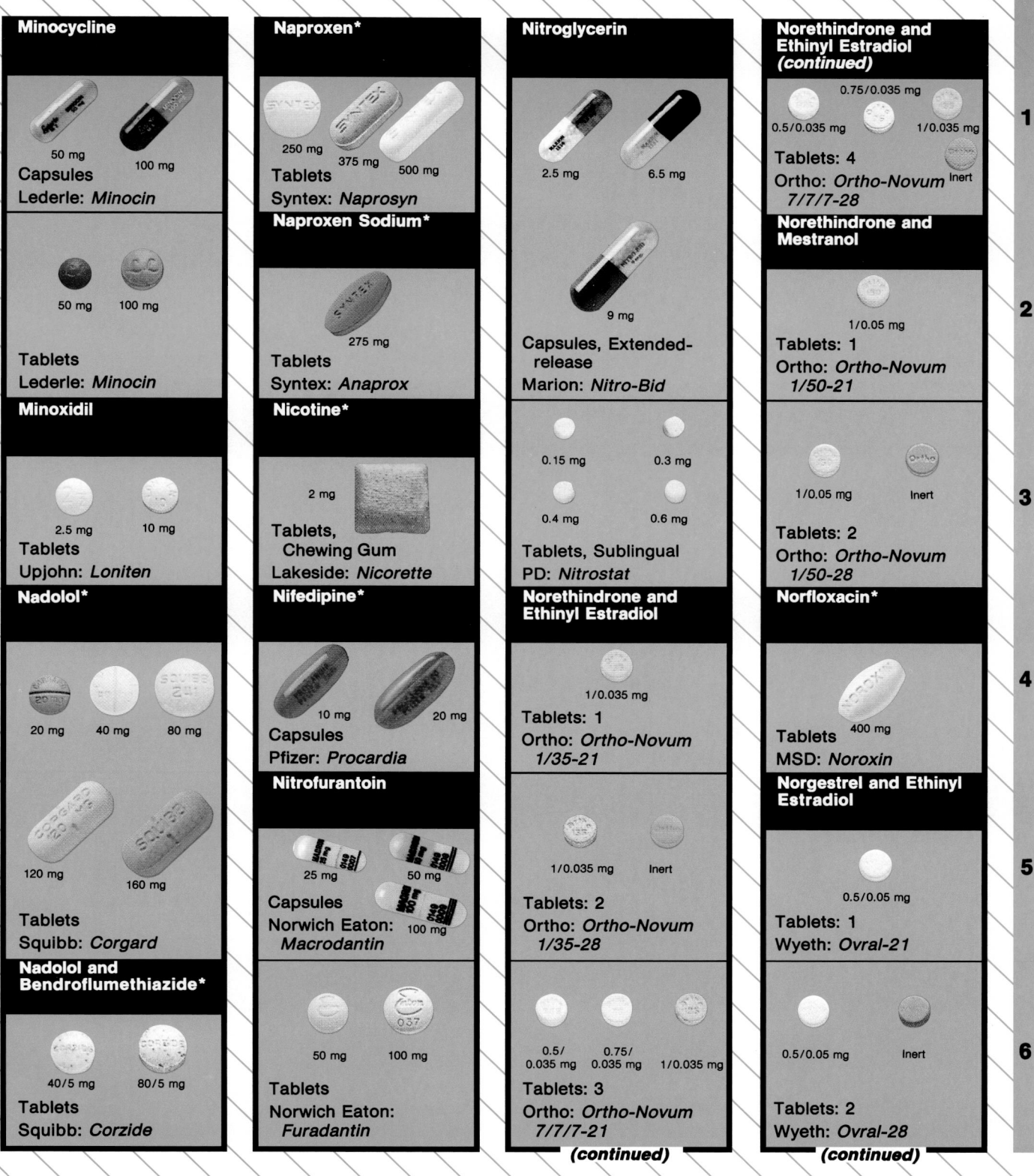

A

Minocycline

50 mg   100 mg

Capsules
Lederle: *Minocin*

50 mg   100 mg

Tablets
Lederle: *Minocin*

Minoxidil

2.5 mg   10 mg

Tablets
Upjohn: *Loniten*

Nadolol*

20 mg   40 mg   80 mg

120 mg   160 mg

Tablets
Squibb: *Corgard*

Nadolol and Bendroflumethiazide*

40/5 mg   80/5 mg

Tablets
Squibb: *Corzide*

B

Naproxen*

250 mg   375 mg   500 mg

Tablets
Syntex: *Naprosyn*

Naproxen Sodium*

275 mg

Tablets
Syntex: *Anaprox*

Nicotine*

2 mg

Tablets, Chewing Gum
Lakeside: *Nicorette*

Nifedipine*

10 mg   20 mg

Capsules
Pfizer: *Procardia*

Nitrofurantoin

25 mg   50 mg
100 mg

Capsules
Norwich Eaton: *Macrodantin*

50 mg   100 mg

Tablets
Norwich Eaton: *Furadantin*

C

Nitroglycerin

2.5 mg   6.5 mg

9 mg

Capsules, Extended-release
Marion: *Nitro-Bid*

0.15 mg   0.3 mg

0.4 mg   0.6 mg

Tablets, Sublingual
PD: *Nitrostat*

Norethindrone and Ethinyl Estradiol

1/0.035 mg

Tablets: 1
Ortho: *Ortho-Novum 1/35-21*

1/0.035 mg   Inert

Tablets: 2
Ortho: *Ortho-Novum 1/35-28*

0.5/ 0.035 mg   0.75/ 0.035 mg   1/0.035 mg

Tablets: 3
Ortho: *Ortho-Novum 7/7/7-21*

(continued)

D

Norethindrone and Ethinyl Estradiol *(continued)*

0.75/0.035 mg
0.5/0.035 mg   1/0.035 mg
Inert

Tablets: 4
Ortho: *Ortho-Novum 7/7/7-28*

Norethindrone and Mestranol

1/0.05 mg

Tablets: 1
Ortho: *Ortho-Novum 1/50-21*

1/0.05 mg   Inert

Tablets: 2
Ortho: *Ortho-Novum 1/50-28*

Norfloxacin*

400 mg

Tablets
MSD: *Noroxin*

Norgestrel and Ethinyl Estradiol

0.5/0.05 mg

Tablets: 1
Wyeth: *Ovral-21*

0.5/0.05 mg   Inert

Tablets: 2
Wyeth: *Ovral-28*

(continued)

*Single source product.

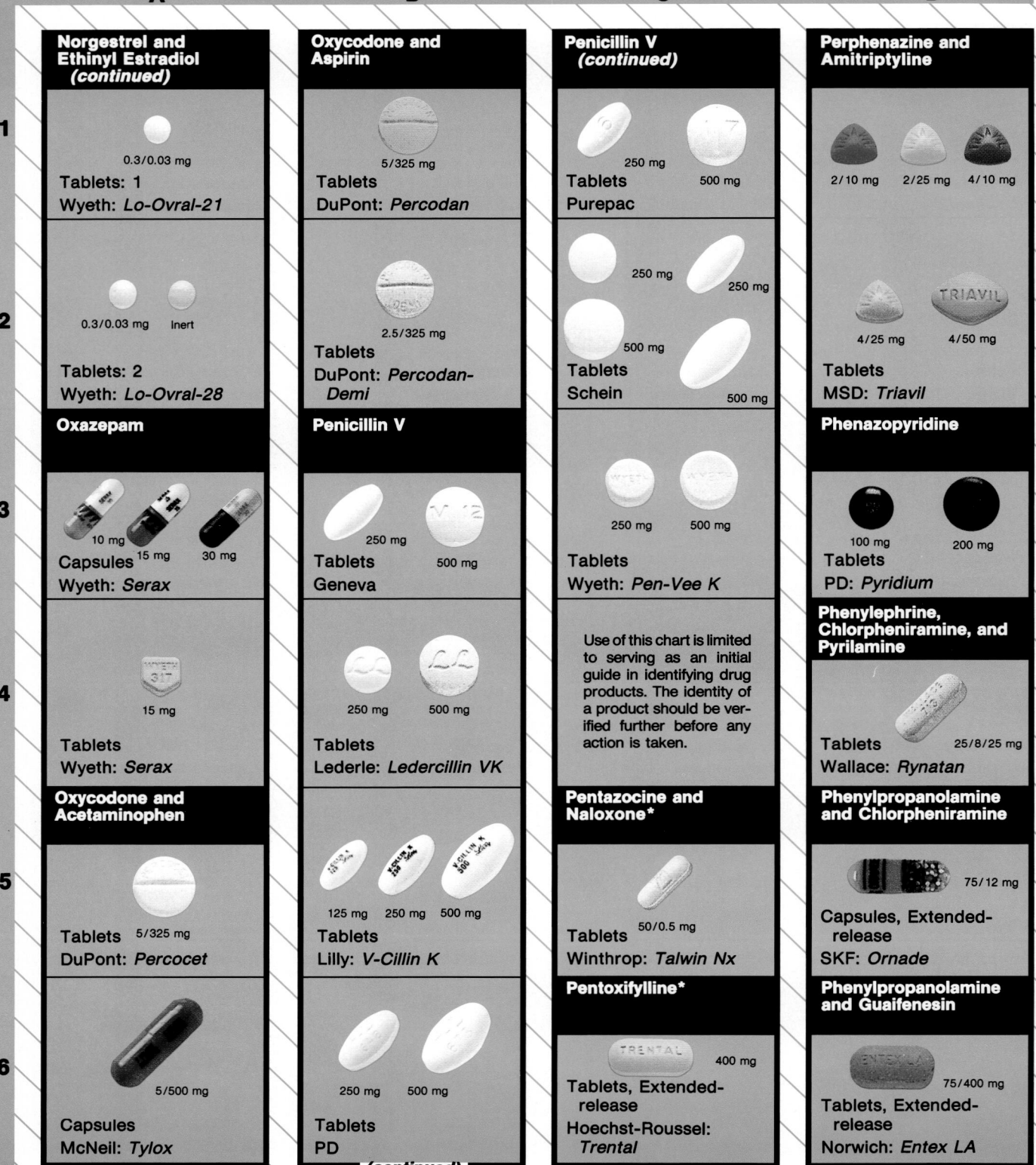

	A	B	C	D

A

Norgestrel and Ethinyl Estradiol *(continued)*

1
0.3/0.03 mg
Tablets: 1
Wyeth: *Lo-Ovral-21*

2
0.3/0.03 mg   Inert
Tablets: 2
Wyeth: *Lo-Ovral-28*

Oxazepam

3
10 mg   15 mg   30 mg
Capsules
Wyeth: *Serax*

4
15 mg
Tablets
Wyeth: *Serax*

Oxycodone and Acetaminophen

5
5/325 mg
Tablets
DuPont: *Percocet*

6
5/500 mg
Capsules
McNeil: *Tylox*

B

Oxycodone and Aspirin

1
5/325 mg
Tablets
DuPont: *Percodan*

2
2.5/325 mg
Tablets
DuPont: *Percodan-Demi*

Penicillin V

3
250 mg   500 mg
Tablets
Geneva

4
250 mg   500 mg
Tablets
Lederle: *Ledercillin VK*

5
125 mg   250 mg   500 mg
Tablets
Lilly: *V-Cillin K*

6
250 mg   500 mg
Tablets
PD

(continued)

C

Penicillin V *(continued)*

1
250 mg   500 mg
Tablets
Purepac

2
250 mg   250 mg
500 mg   500 mg
Tablets
Schein

3
250 mg   500 mg
Tablets
Wyeth: *Pen-Vee K*

Use of this chart is limited to serving as an initial guide in identifying drug products. The identity of a product should be verified further before any action is taken.

Pentazocine and Naloxone*

5
50/0.5 mg
Tablets
Winthrop: *Talwin Nx*

Pentoxifylline*

6
TRENTAL   400 mg
Tablets, Extended-release
Hoechst-Roussel: *Trental*

D

Perphenazine and Amitriptyline

1
2/10 mg   2/25 mg   4/10 mg

2
4/25 mg   4/50 mg
Tablets
MSD: *Triavil*

Phenazopyridine

3
100 mg   200 mg
Tablets
PD: *Pyridium*

Phenylephrine, Chlorpheniramine, and Pyrilamine

4
25/8/25 mg
Tablets
Wallace: *Rynatan*

Phenylpropanolamine and Chlorpheniramine

5
75/12 mg
Capsules, Extended-release
SKF: *Ornade*

Phenylpropanolamine and Guaifenesin

6
75/400 mg
Tablets, Extended-release
Norwich: *Entex LA*

*Single source product.

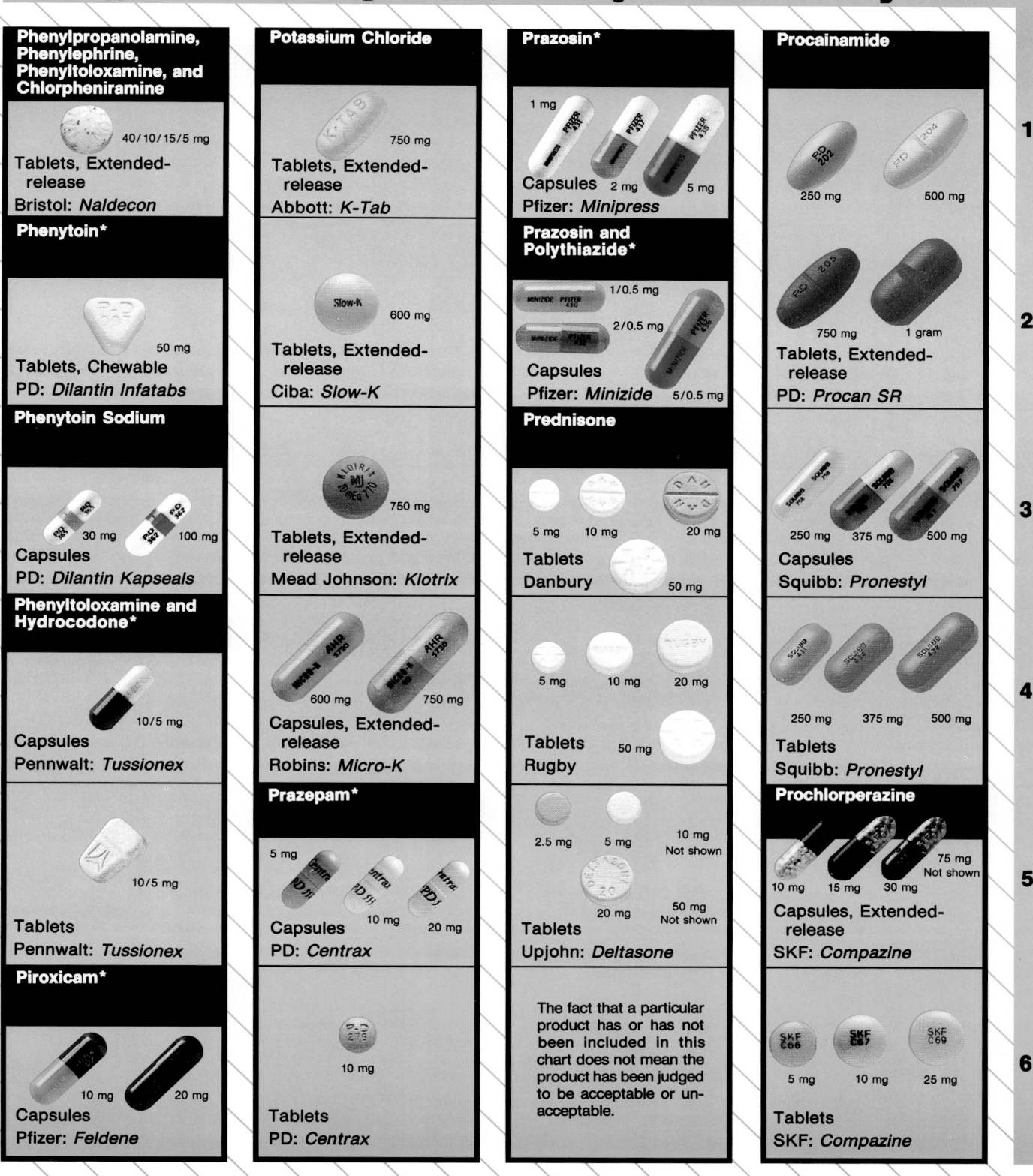

A

Phenylpropanolamine, Phenylephrine, Phenyltoloxamine, and Chlorpheniramine

40/10/15/5 mg

Tablets, Extended-release

Bristol: *Naldecon*

Phenytoin*

50 mg

Tablets, Chewable

PD: *Dilantin Infatabs*

Phenytoin Sodium

30 mg   100 mg

Capsules

PD: *Dilantin Kapseals*

Phenyltoloxamine and Hydrocodone*

10/5 mg

Capsules

Pennwalt: *Tussionex*

10/5 mg

Tablets

Pennwalt: *Tussionex*

Piroxicam*

10 mg   20 mg

Capsules

Pfizer: *Feldene*

B

Potassium Chloride

750 mg

Tablets, Extended-release

Abbott: *K-Tab*

600 mg

Tablets, Extended-release

Ciba: *Slow-K*

750 mg

Tablets, Extended-release

Mead Johnson: *Klotrix*

600 mg   750 mg

Capsules, Extended-release

Robins: *Micro-K*

Prazepam*

5 mg

10 mg   20 mg

Capsules

PD: *Centrax*

10 mg

Tablets

PD: *Centrax*

C

Prazosin*

1 mg

2 mg   5 mg

Capsules

Pfizer: *Minipress*

Prazosin and Polythiazide*

1/0.5 mg

2/0.5 mg

Capsules

Pfizer: *Minizide*   5/0.5 mg

Prednisone

5 mg   10 mg   20 mg

Tablets

Danbury   50 mg

5 mg   10 mg   20 mg

Tablets   50 mg

Rugby

2.5 mg   5 mg   10 mg
Not shown

20 mg   50 mg
Not shown

Tablets

Upjohn: *Deltasone*

The fact that a particular product has or has not been included in this chart does not mean the product has been judged to be acceptable or unacceptable.

D

Procainamide

250 mg   500 mg

750 mg   1 gram

Tablets, Extended-release

PD: *Procan SR*

250 mg   375 mg   500 mg

Capsules

Squibb: *Pronestyl*

250 mg   375 mg   500 mg

Tablets

Squibb: *Pronestyl*

Prochlorperazine

75 mg
Not shown

10 mg   15 mg   30 mg

Capsules, Extended-release

SKF: *Compazine*

5 mg   10 mg   25 mg

Tablets

SKF: *Compazine*

1

2

3

4

5

6

*Single source product.

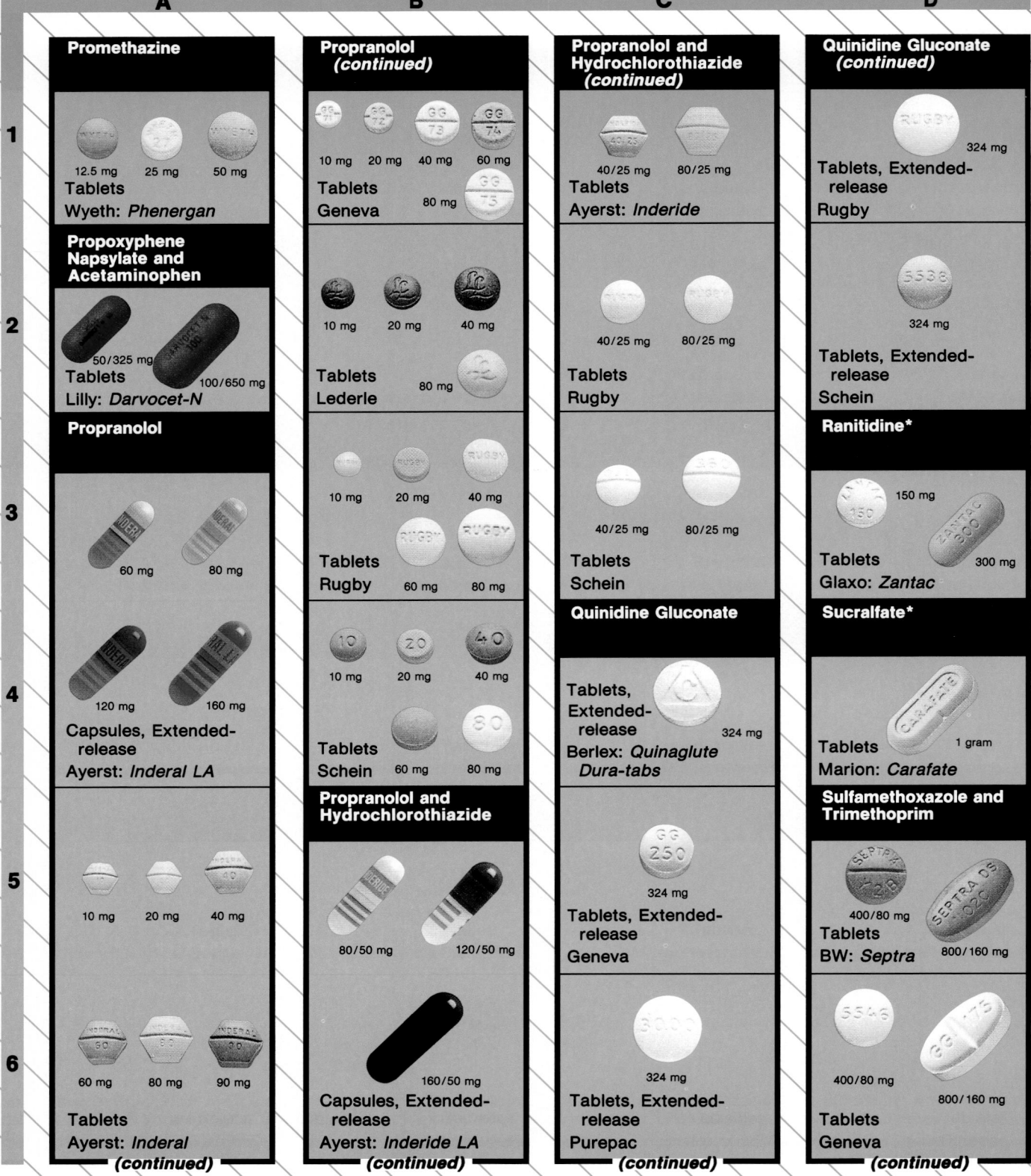

	A	**B**	**C**	**D**

Promethazine

12.5 mg   25 mg   50 mg
Tablets
Wyeth: *Phenergan*

Propoxyphene Napsylate and Acetaminophen

50/325 mg   100/650 mg
Tablets
Lilly: *Darvocet-N*

Propranolol

60 mg   80 mg
120 mg   160 mg
Capsules, Extended-release
Ayerst: *Inderal LA*

10 mg   20 mg   40 mg
60 mg   80 mg   90 mg
Tablets
Ayerst: *Inderal*
(continued)

Propranolol
(continued)

10 mg   20 mg   40 mg   60 mg
80 mg
Tablets
Geneva

10 mg   20 mg   40 mg
80 mg
Tablets
Lederle

10 mg   20 mg   40 mg
60 mg   80 mg
Tablets
Rugby

10 mg   20 mg   40 mg
60 mg   80 mg
Tablets
Schein

Propranolol and Hydrochlorothiazide

80/50 mg   120/50 mg
160/50 mg
Capsules, Extended-release
Ayerst: *Inderide LA*
(continued)

Propranolol and Hydrochlorothiazide
(continued)

40/25 mg   80/25 mg
Tablets
Ayerst: *Inderide*

40/25 mg   80/25 mg
Tablets
Rugby

40/25 mg   80/25 mg
Tablets
Schein

Quinidine Gluconate

324 mg
Tablets, Extended-release
Berlex: *Quinaglute Dura-tabs*

GG 250
324 mg
Tablets, Extended-release
Geneva

324 mg
Tablets, Extended-release
Purepac
(continued)

Quinidine Gluconate
(continued)

324 mg
Tablets, Extended-release
Rugby

5538
324 mg
Tablets, Extended-release
Schein

Ranitidine*

150 mg   300 mg
Tablets
Glaxo: *Zantac*

Sucralfate*

1 gram
Tablets
Marion: *Carafate*

Sulfamethoxazole and Trimethoprim

400/80 mg   800/160 mg
Tablets
BW: *Septra*

400/80 mg   800/160 mg
Tablets
Geneva
(continued)

*Single source product.

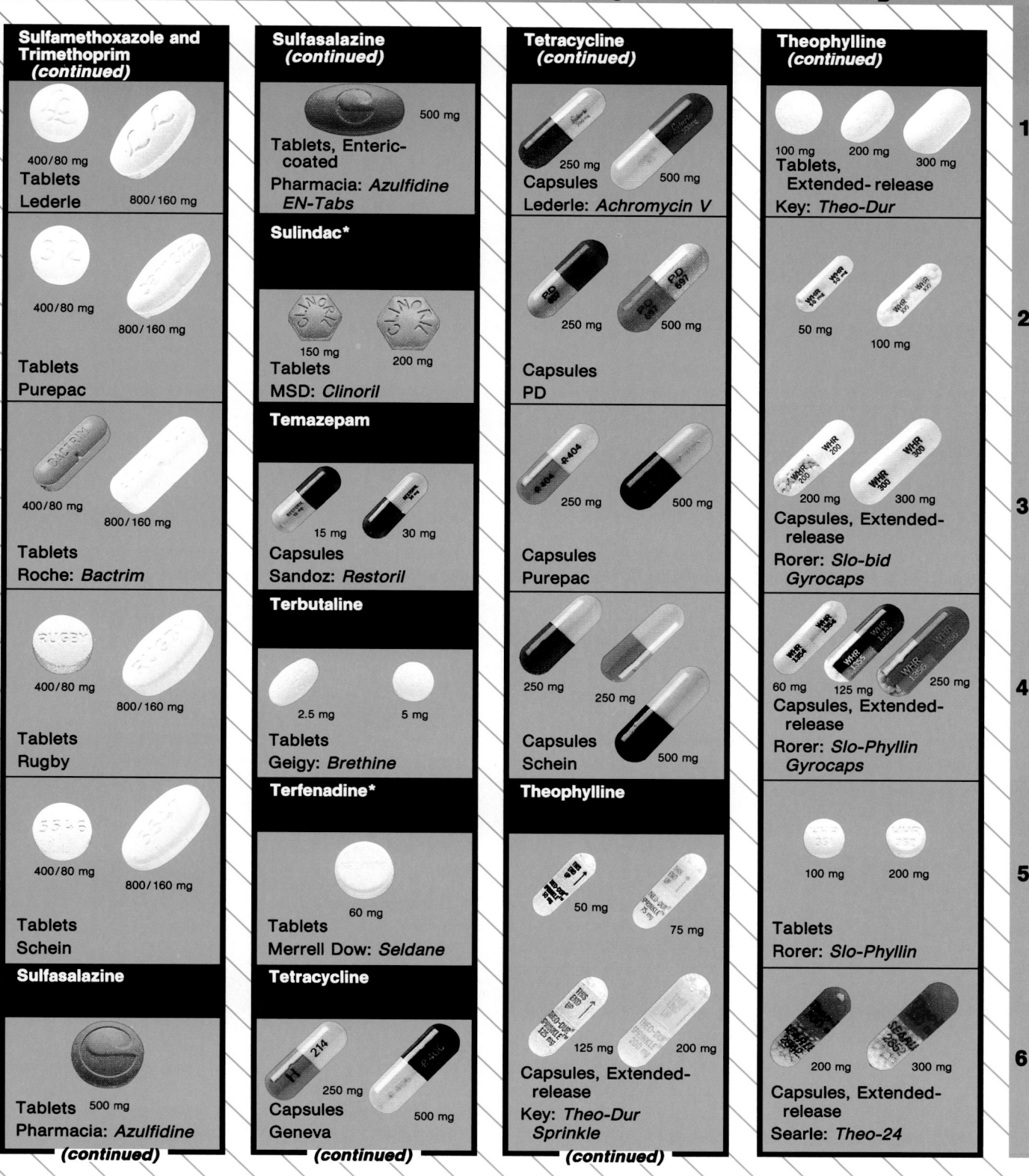

Column A

Sulfamethoxazole and Trimethoprim (continued)

400/80 mg — 800/160 mg
Tablets
Lederle

400/80 mg — 800/160 mg
Tablets
Purepac

400/80 mg — 800/160 mg
Tablets
Roche: *Bactrim*

400/80 mg — 800/160 mg
Tablets
Rugby

400/80 mg — 800/160 mg
Tablets
Schein

Sulfasalazine

Tablets 500 mg
Pharmacia: *Azulfidine*

(continued)

Column B

Sulfasalazine (continued)

500 mg
Tablets, Enteric-coated
Pharmacia: *Azulfidine EN-Tabs*

Sulindac*

150 mg — 200 mg
Tablets
MSD: *Clinoril*

Temazepam

15 mg — 30 mg
Capsules
Sandoz: *Restoril*

Terbutaline

2.5 mg — 5 mg
Tablets
Geigy: *Brethine*

Terfenadine*

60 mg
Tablets
Merrell Dow: *Seldane*

Tetracycline

250 mg — 500 mg
Capsules
Geneva

(continued)

Column C

Tetracycline (continued)

250 mg — 500 mg
Capsules
Lederle: *Achromycin V*

250 mg — 500 mg
Capsules
PD

250 mg — 500 mg
Capsules
Purepac

250 mg — 250 mg — 500 mg
Capsules
Schein

Theophylline

50 mg — 75 mg
125 mg — 200 mg
Capsules, Extended-release
Key: *Theo-Dur Sprinkle*

(continued)

Column D

Theophylline (continued)

100 mg — 200 mg — 300 mg
Tablets, Extended-release
Key: *Theo-Dur*

50 mg — 100 mg
200 mg — 300 mg
Capsules, Extended-release
Rorer: *Slo-bid Gyrocaps*

60 mg — 125 mg — 250 mg
Capsules, Extended-release
Rorer: *Slo-Phyllin Gyrocaps*

100 mg — 200 mg
Tablets
Rorer: *Slo-Phyllin*

200 mg — 300 mg
Capsules, Extended-release
Searle: *Theo-24*

*Single source product.

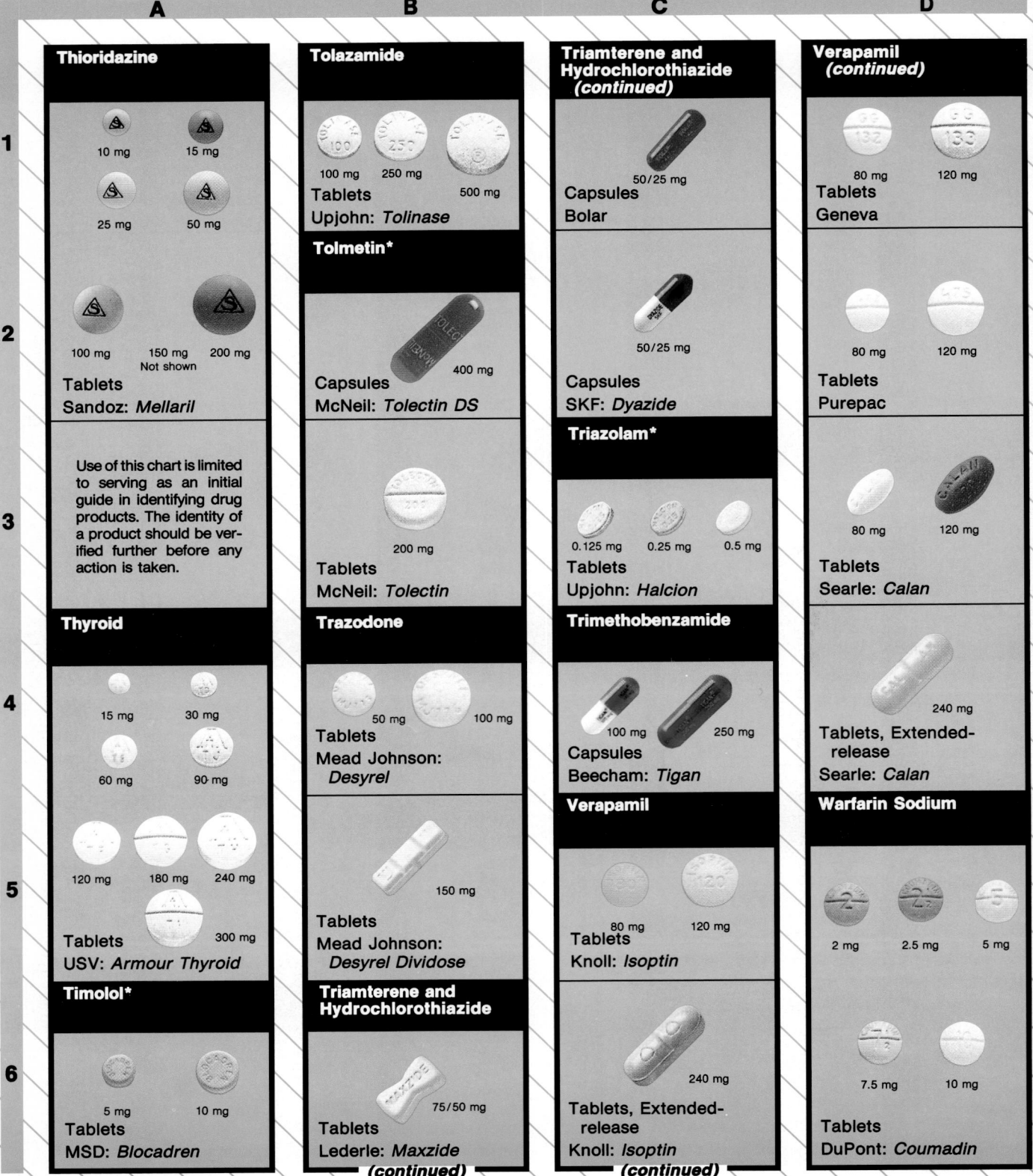

A

1

Thioridazine

10 mg   15 mg

25 mg   50 mg

2

100 mg   150 mg Not shown   200 mg

Tablets
Sandoz: *Mellaril*

Use of this chart is limited to serving as an initial guide in identifying drug products. The identity of a product should be verified further before any action is taken.

Thyroid

4

15 mg   30 mg

60 mg   90 mg

5

120 mg   180 mg   240 mg

300 mg

Tablets
USV: *Armour Thyroid*

Timolol*

6

5 mg   10 mg

Tablets
MSD: *Blocadren*

B

Tolazamide

1

100 mg   250 mg   500 mg

Tablets
Upjohn: *Tolinase*

Tolmetin*

2

400 mg

Capsules
McNeil: *Tolectin DS*

3

200 mg

Tablets
McNeil: *Tolectin*

Trazodone

4

50 mg   100 mg

Tablets
Mead Johnson:
Desyrel

5

150 mg

Tablets
Mead Johnson:
Desyrel Dividose

Triamterene and Hydrochlorothiazide

75/50 mg

Tablets
Lederle: *Maxzide*
(continued)

C

Triamterene and Hydrochlorothiazide (continued)

1

50/25 mg

Capsules
Bolar

2

50/25 mg

Capsules
SKF: *Dyazide*

Triazolam*

3

0.125 mg   0.25 mg   0.5 mg

Tablets
Upjohn: *Halcion*

Trimethobenzamide

4

100 mg   250 mg

Capsules
Beecham: *Tigan*

Verapamil

5

80 mg   120 mg

Tablets
Knoll: *Isoptin*

6

240 mg

Tablets, Extended-release
Knoll: *Isoptin*
(continued)

D

Verapamil (continued)

1

80 mg   120 mg

Tablets
Geneva

2

80 mg   120 mg

Tablets
Purepac

3

80 mg   120 mg

Tablets
Searle: *Calan*

4

240 mg

Tablets, Extended-release
Searle: *Calan*

Warfarin Sodium

5

2 mg   2.5 mg   5 mg

7.5 mg   10 mg

Tablets
DuPont: *Coumadin*

*Single source product.

Appendix II

GENERAL INFORMATION ABOUT USE OF MEDICINES

Information about the proper use of medicines is of two types. One type is drug specific and applies to a certain medicine or group of medicines only. The other type is general in nature and applies to the use of any medicine.

The information that follows is general in nature. For your own safety, health, and well-being, however, it is important that you learn about the proper use of your specific medicines as well. You can get this information from your doctor, nurse, or pharmacist, or find it in the individual listings of this book.

Before Using Your Medicine

Before you use any medicine, your doctor, nurse, and pharmacist should be told:

—if you have ever had an allergic or unusual reaction to any medicine, food, or other substance, such as yellow dye or sulfites.

—if you are on a low-salt, low-sugar, or any other special diet. Most medicines contain more than their active ingredient, and many liquid medicines contain alcohol.

—if you are pregnant or if you plan to become pregnant. Certain medicines may cause birth defects or other problems in the unborn child. For other medicines, safe use during pregnancy has not been established. **The use of any medicine during pregnancy must be carefully considered.**

—if you are breast-feeding. Some medicines may pass into the breast milk and cause unwanted effects in the baby.

—if you have any medical problems.

—if you are now taking or have taken any medicines in the past few weeks. Don't forget over-the-counter (nonprescription) medicines such as aspirin, laxatives, and antacids.

Proper Use of Your Medicine

Take medicine exactly as directed, at the right time, and for the full length of time prescribed by your doctor. If you are using an over-the-counter (nonprescription) medicine, follow the directions on the label, unless otherwise directed by your doctor. If you feel that your medicine is not working for you, check with your doctor.

To avoid mistakes, do not take medicine in the dark. Always read the label before taking, noting especially the expiration date, if any, of the contents.

Child-proof caps on medicines for oral use have greatly decreased the number of accidental poisonings and are required by law. However, if there are no children in your home, and you find it hard to open such caps, you may ask your pharmacist for a regular, easier-to-open cap. He or she is authorized by law to furnish you with a regular cap if you request it.

Different medicines should never be mixed in one container. Always keep your medicine tightly capped in its original container, when not in use. Do not remove the label since directions for use and other special information appear there.

It is important to store your medicines properly. Guidelines for proper storage include:

- **Keep out of the reach of children.**
- Store away from heat and direct light.
- Do not store capsules or tablets in the bathroom, near the kitchen sink, or in other damp places. Heat or moisture may cause the medicine to break down.
- Keep liquid medicines from freezing.
- Do not store medicines in the refrigerator unless directed to do so.
- Do not keep outdated medicine or medicine no longer needed. Be sure that any discarded medicine is out of the reach of children.

Precautions While Using Your Medicine

Never give your medicine to anyone else. It has been prescribed for your personal medical problem and may not be the correct treatment for another person.

Don't take medicines that show even the slightest evidence of tampering or don't seem quite right. If you have any questions, check with your pharmacist.

Before having any kind of surgery (including dental surgery) or emergency treatment, tell the physician or dentist in charge about any medicine you are taking.

If you think you have taken an overdose of any medicine or if a child has taken a medicine by accident: Call your poison control center or your doctor or pharmacist at once. Keep those telephone numbers handy. Also, keep a bottle of Ipecac Syrup safely stored in your home in case you are told to cause vomiting. Read the directions on the label of Ipecac Syrup before using.

Side Effects of Your Medicine

Along with its intended effects, a medicine may cause some unwanted effects. Some of these side effects may need medical attention, while others may not. It is important for you to know what side effects may occur and what you should do if you notice signs of them. If you notice any unusual reactions or side effects that you were not told about, check with your doctor, nurse, or pharmacist.

Tips Against Tampering

Manufacturers of over-the-counter (OTC) medicines now package their products so that any evidence of tampering can be more readily noticed by the consumer. Manufacturers may use one or more different ways of packaging their products to make them tamper-resistant. These may include:

• Wrapping the dosage form and/or its container in a plastic film wrapper or bubble pack.

• Sealing each individual dosing unit in a foil, paper, or plastic pouch or in a blister or strip pack.

• Placing a shrink seal or band which fits tightly around the cap and container.

• Sealing the bottle mouth under the cap or the carton flaps with paper or foil seals or tape.

• Placing a breakable metal or plastic cap over the bottle opening.

General common sense suggestions to help you detect possible signs of tampering include the following:

• Take a few seconds to visually inspect the outer packaging of the drug product before you buy it and again as you open it. When you open the outer package after purchase, also check inner packaging features.

• If the medicine has a protective packaging feature, it should be intact. If it is not, do not buy the product or, if already purchased, return it to the store or manufacturer.

• Don't take medicines that show even the slightest evidence of tampering or that don't seem quite right.

• Never take medicines in the dark or in poor lighting. Look at the label and each dose of medicine *every time* you take a dose.

Additional Information

It is a good idea for you to learn both the generic and brand names of your medicine and even to write them down and keep them for future use.

Many prescriptions may not be refilled unless your pharmacist has first checked with your doctor. To save time, do not wait until you have run out of medicine before requesting a refill. This is especially important if you must take your medicine every day.

If you want more information about your medicines, ask your doctor, nurse, or pharmacist. Do not be embarrassed to ask questions about any medicine you are taking. To help you remember, it may be helpful to write down any questions you have and bring these questions with you on your next visit to your doctor or pharmacist.

Appendix III

PREGNANCY PRECAUTION LISTING

The following medicines, selected from those included in this publication, have specific precautions in regard to use during pregnancy. You will find such precautions in the individual monographs; look in the index for the page number.

The use of any medicine during pregnancy must be carefully considered. The physician and the patient must balance the expected benefits against the possible risks.

Absence of a drug from the list is not meant to imply that it is safe for use in pregnant patients. For many drugs, it is not known whether a problem exists; experimentation on pregnant women is generally not done. Knowledge is usually gained only from the accumulated experience over many years in giving a drug to pregnant women who really needed its benefits. Also, well-planned studies in pregnant animals may reveal problems, although the relation of such findings to pregnant humans and their babies may not be known. Problems suggested by animal studies are often included in the warnings in this book.

Readers are reminded that the information in this text is selected and not considered to be complete.

A

Acebutolol (Systemic)
Acetaminophen and Aspirin (Systemic)
Acetaminophen, Aspirin, and Caffeine (Systemic)
Acetaminophen, Aspirin, and Caffeine, Buffered (Systemic)
Acetaminophen, Aspirin, and Codeine (Systemic)
Acetaminophen, Aspirin, and Codeine, Buffered (Systemic)
Acetaminophen, Aspirin, and Salicylamide (Systemic)
Acetaminophen, Aspirin, and Salicylamide, Buffered (Systemic)
Acetaminophen, Aspirin, Salicylamide, and Caffeine (Systemic)
Acetaminophen, Aspirin, Salicylamide, Codeine, and Caffeine (Systemic)
Acetaminophen and Codeine (Systemic)
Acetaminophen, Codeine, and Caffeine (Systemic)
Acetaminophen and Salicylamide (Systemic)
Acetaminophen, Salicylamide, and Caffeine (Systemic)
Acetaminophen, Sodium Salicylate, and Caffeine (Systemic)
Acetazolamide (Systemic)
Acetohexamide (Systemic)
Acetohydroxamic Acid (Systemic)
Acetophenazine (Systemic)
Acyclovir (Systemic)
Acyclovir (Topical)
Albuterol (Systemic)
Alfentanil (Systemic)
Allopurinol (Systemic)
Alprazolam (Systemic)
Alseroxylon (Systemic)
Alumina and Magnesia (Oral)
Alumina, Magnesia, and Calcium Carbonate (Oral)
Alumina, Magnesia, and Simethicone (Oral)
Alumina and Magnesium Carbonate (Oral)
Alumina, Magnesium Carbonate, and Calcium Carbonate (Oral)
Alumina and Magnesium Trisilicate (Oral)
Alumina, Magnesium Trisilicate, and Sodium Bicarbonate (Oral)
Aluminum Carbonate, Basic (Oral)

Aluminum Hydroxide (Oral)
Amantadine (Systemic)
Ambenonium (Systemic)
Amcinonide (Topical)
Amikacin (Systemic)
Amiloride (Systemic)
Amiloride and Hydrochlorothiazide (Systemic)
Aminoglutethimide (Systemic)
Aminophylline (Systemic)
Amiodarone (Systemic)
Amitriptyline (Systemic)
Amobarbital (Systemic)
Amoxapine (Systemic)
Amphetamine (Systemic)
Amyl Nitrite (Systemic)
Anisindione (Systemic)
Aprobarbital (Systemic)
Ascorbic Acid (Systemic)
Ascorbic Acid and Sodium Ascorbate (Systemic)
Asparaginase (Systemic)
Aspirin (Systemic)
Aspirin, Buffered (Systemic)
Aspirin and Caffeine (Systemic)
Aspirin and Codeine (Systemic)
Aspirin, Codeine, Alumina, and Magnesia (Systemic)
Aspirin, Codeine, and Caffeine (Systemic)
Aspirin, Codeine, Caffeine, Alumina, and Magnesia (Systemic)
Atenolol (Systemic)
Atenolol and Chlorthalidone (Systemic)
Atropine (Systemic)
Atropine, Hyoscyamine, Scopolamine, and Butabarbital (Systemic)
Atropine, Hyoscyamine, Scopolamine, and Phenobarbital (Systemic)
Atropine and Phenobarbital (Systemic)
Auranofin (Systemic)
Aurothioglucose (Systemic)
Azatadine and Pseudoephedrine (Systemic)
Azathioprine (Systemic)

B

Baclofen (Systemic)
Beclomethasone (Inhalation)

Beclomethasone (Nasal)
Belladonna and Butabarbital (Systemic)
Belladonna and Phenobarbital (Systemic)
Bendroflumethiazide (Systemic)
Benzphetamine (Systemic)
Benzthiazide (Systemic)
Betamethasone (Systemic)
Betamethasone (Topical)
Betaxolol (Ophthalmic)
Bethanechol (Systemic)
Bitolterol (Systemic)
Bleomycin (Systemic)
Bromocriptine (Systemic)
Bromodiphenhydramine and Codeine (Systemic)
Bromodiphenhydramine, Diphenhydramine, Codeine, Ammonium Chloride, and Potassium Guaiacolsulfonate (Systemic)
Brompheniramine, Phenylephrine, and Phenylpropanolamine (Systemic)
Brompheniramine, Phenylephrine, Phenylpropanolamine, and Codeine (Systemic)
Brompheniramine, Phenylephrine, Phenylpropanolamine, Codeine, and Guaifenesin (Systemic)
Brompheniramine, Phenylephrine, Phenylpropanolamine, Hydrocodone, and Guaifenesin (Systemic)
Brompheniramine and Phenylpropanolamine (Systemic)
Brompheniramine, Phenylpropanolamine, and Codeine (Systemic)
Brompheniramine and Pseudoephedrine (Systemic)
Brompheniramine, Pseudoephedrine, and Dextromethorphan (Systemic)
Buclizine (Systemic)
Bumetanide (Systemic)
Buprenorphine (Systemic)
Busulfan (Systemic)
Butabarbital (Systemic)
Butalbital and Acetaminophen (Systemic)
Butalbital, Acetaminophen, and Caffeine (Systemic)

Butalbital, Acetaminophen, and Codeine (Systemic)
Butalbital, Acetaminophen, Codeine, and Caffeine (Systemic)
Butalbital, Acetaminophen, Hydrocodone, and Caffeine (Systemic)
Butalbital and Aspirin (Systemic)
Butalbital, Aspirin, and Caffeine (Systemic)
Butalbital, Aspirin, and Codeine (Systemic)
Butorphanol (Systemic)

C

Caffeine (Systemic)
Caffeine, Citrated (Systemic)
Caffeine and Sodium Benzoate (Systemic)
Calcifediol (Systemic)
Calcitonin-Human (Systemic)
Calcitonin-Salmon (Systemic)
Calcitriol (Systemic)
Calcium Carbonate (Oral)
Calcium Carbonate and Magnesia (Oral)
Calcium Carbonate, Magnesia, and Simethicone (Oral)
Calcium and Magnesium Carbonates (Oral)
Calcium and Magnesium Carbonates and Magnesium Oxide (Oral)
Capreomycin (Systemic)
Captopril (Systemic)
Captopril and Hydrochlorothiazide (Systemic)
Carbamazepine (Systemic)
Carbidopa and Levodopa (Systemic)
Carbinoxamine and Pseudoephedrine (Systemic)
Carbinoxamine, Pseudoephedrine, and Dextromethorphan (Systemic)
Carbinoxamine, Pseudoephedrine, and Guaifenesin (Systemic)
Carmustine (Systemic)
Castor Oil (Oral)
Cellulose Sodium Phosphate (Systemic)
Chenodiol (Systemic)
Chloral Hydrate (Systemic)
Chlorambucil (Systemic)
Chloramphenicol (Systemic)
Chlordiazepoxide (Systemic)
Chlordiazepoxide and Amitriptyline (Systemic)
Chlordiazepoxide and Clidinium (Systemic)
Chloroquine (Systemic)
Chlorothiazide (Systemic)
Chlorotrianisene (Systemic)
Chlorpheniramine and Codeine (Systemic)
Chlorpheniramine, Codeine, Aspirin, and Caffeine (Systemic)
Chlorpheniramine, Codeine, Carbetapentane, Guaifenesin, Sodium Citrate, and Citric Acid (Systemic)
Chlorpheniramine, Phenindamine, Phenylephrine, Dextromethorphan, Acetaminophen, Salicylamide, Caffeine, and Ascorbic Acid (Systemic)
Chlorpheniramine, Phenindamine, Pyrilamine, Phenylephrine, Hydrocodone, and Ammonium Chloride (Systemic)
Chlorpheniramine, Phenindamine, Pyrilamine, Phenylephrine, Hydrocodone, Salicylamide, Caffeine, and Ascorbic Acid (Systemic)
Chlorpheniramine, Phenylephrine, Codeine, and Acetaminophen (Systemic)
Chlorpheniramine, Phenylephrine, Codeine, and Ammonium Chloride (Systemic)
Chlorpheniramine, Phenylephrine, Codeine, Ammonium Chloride, Potassium Guaiacolsulfonate, and Sodium Citrate (Systemic)
Chlorpheniramine, Phenylephrine, Codeine, and Potassium Iodide (Systemic)

Chlorpheniramine, Phenylephrine, Dextromethorphan, Acetaminophen, and Salicylamide (Systemic)
Chlorpheniramine, Phenylephrine, and Hydrocodone (Systemic)
Chlorpheniramine, Phenylephrine, Hydrocodone, Acetaminophen, and Caffeine (Systemic)
Chlorpheniramine, Phenylephrine, Phenylpropanolamine, and Codeine (Systemic)
Chlorpheniramine, Phenylephrine, Phenylpropanolamine, and Dihydrocodeine (Systemic)
Chlorpheniramine, Phenylpropanolamine, Codeine, Guaifenesin, and Acetaminophen (Systemic)
Chlorpheniramine, Phenylpropanolamine, Dextromethorphan, Acetaminophen, and Caffeine (Systemic)
Chlorpheniramine, Phenylpropanolamine, Hydrocodone, Guaifenesin, and Salicylamide (Systemic)
Chlorpheniramine, Phenyltoloxamine, Ephedrine, Codeine, and Guaiacol Carbonate (Systemic)
Chlorpheniramine and Pseudoephedrine (Systemic)
Chlorpheniramine, Pseudoephedrine, and Codeine (Systemic)
Chlorpheniramine, Pseudoephedrine, and Dextromethorphan (Systemic)
Chlorpheniramine, Pseudoephedrine, Dextromethorphan, and Acetaminophen (Systemic)
Chlorpheniramine, Pseudoephedrine, Dextromethorphan, Guaifenesin, and Aspirin (Systemic)
Chlorpheniramine, Pseudoephedrine, and Guaifenesin (Systemic)
Chlorpheniramine, Pseudoephedrine, and Hydrocodone (Systemic)
Chlorpheniramine, Pyrilamine, and Phenylpropanolamine (Systemic)
Chlorpheniramine, Tripelennamine, Phenylpropanolamine, and Phenylephrine (Systemic)
Chlorpromazine (Systemic)
Chlorpropamide (Systemic)
Chlorprothixene (Systemic)
Chlorthalidone (Systemic)
Chlorzoxazone and Acetaminophen (Systemic)
Cholestyramine (Systemic)
Choline Salicylate (Systemic)
Choline and Magnesium Salicylates (Systemic)
Chromic Phosphate P 32 (Therapeutic)
Cimetidine (Systemic)
Cinoxacin (Systemic)
Cisplatin (Systemic)
Clemastine and Phenylpropanolamine (Systemic)
Clioquinol and Hydrocortisone (Topical)
Clobetasol (Topical)
Clocortolone (Topical)
Clofazimine (Systemic)
Clofibrate (Systemic)
Clomiphene (Systemic)
Clomipramine (Systemic)
Clonazepam (Systemic)
Clonidine (Systemic)
Clonidine and Chlorthalidone (Systemic)
Clorazepate (Systemic)
Clotrimazole (Oral)
Codeine (Systemic)
Codeine and Calcium Iodide (Systemic)
Codeine and Guaifenesin (Systemic)
Codeine and Iodinated Glycerol (Systemic)
Codeine and Terpin Hydrate (Systemic)
Colchicine (Systemic)
Colestipol (Systemic)
Corticotropin (Systemic)
Cortisone (Systemic)

Cromolyn (Inhalation)
Cromolyn (Nasal)
Cromolyn (Ophthalmic)
Cromolyn (Oral)
Cyanocobalamin Co 57 (Diagnostic)
Cyclizine (Systemic)
Cyclophosphamide (Systemic)
Cyclosporine (Systemic)
Cyclothiazide (Systemic)
Cytarabine (Systemic)

D

Dacarbazine (Systemic)
Dactinomycin (Systemic)
Danazol (Systemic)
Daunorubicin (Systemic)
Deferoxamine (Systemic)
Demeclocycline (Systemic)
Deserpidine (Systemic)
Deserpidine and Hydrochlorothiazide (Systemic)
Deserpidine and Methyclothiazide (Systemic)
Desipramine (Systemic)
Desonide (Topical)
Desoximetasone (Topical)
Desoxycorticosterone (Systemic)
Dexamethasone (Inhalation)
Dexamethasone (Nasal)
Dexamethasone (Ophthalmic)
Dexamethasone (Systemic)
Dexamethasone (Topical)
Dexbrompheniramine and Pseudoephedrine (Systemic)
Dexchlorpheniramine, Pseudoephedrine, and Guaifenesin (Systemic)
Dextroamphetamine (Systemic)
Dextromethorphan and Iodinated Glycerol (Systemic)
Diatrizoate Meglumine (Systemic)
Diatrizoate Meglumine and Diatrizoate Sodium (Systemic)
Diatrizoate Meglumine and Iodipamide Meglumine (Mucosal)
Diatrizoates (Mucosal)
Diatrizoate Sodium (Systemic)
Diazepam (Systemic)
Diazoxide (Oral)
Dichlorphenamide (Systemic)
Dicumarol (Systemic)
Dicyclomine (Systemic)
Dienestrol (Vaginal)
Diethylstilbestrol (Systemic)
Difenoxin and Atropine (Systemic)
Diflorasone (Topical)
Diflunisal (Systemic)
Dihydrocodeine, Acetaminophen, and Caffeine (Systemic)
Dihydrocodeine, Aspirin, and Caffeine (Systemic)
Dihydroergotamine (Systemic)
Dihydrotachysterol (Systemic)
Dihydroxyaluminum Aminoacetate (Oral)
Dihydroxyaluminum Aminoacetate, Magnesia, and Alumina (Oral)
Dihydroxyaluminum Sodium Carbonate (Oral)
Diltiazem (Systemic)
Dimethyl Sulfoxide (Mucosal)
Diphenhydramine, Codeine, and Ammonium Chloride (Systemic)

Diphenhydramine and Pseudoephedrine (Systemic)
Diphenylpyraline, Phenylephrine, and Codeine (Systemic)
Diphenylpyraline, Phenylephrine, and Hydrocodone (Systemic)
Diphenylpyraline, Phenylephrine, Hydrocodone, and Guaifenesin (Systemic)
Diphenoxylate and Atropine (Systemic)
Disopyramide (Systemic)
Divalproex (Systemic)
Docusate and Mineral Oil (Oral)
Doxepin (Systemic)
Doxorubicin (Systemic)
Doxycycline (Systemic)
Doxylamine (Systemic)
Doxylamine, Pseudoephedrine, Dextromethorphan, and Acetaminophen (Systemic)
Dromostanolone (Systemic)
Dronabinol (Systemic)

E–K

Econazole (Topical)
Enalapril (Systemic)
Enalapril and Hydrochlorothiazide (Systemic)
Enflurane (Systemic)
Ephedrine (Systemic)
Ephedrine and Potassium Iodide (Systemic)
Epinephrine (Systemic)
Ergocalciferol (Systemic)
Ergonovine (Systemic)
Ergotamine (Systemic)
Ergotamine, Belladonna Alkaloids, and Phenobarbital (Systemic)
Ergotamine and Caffeine (Systemic)
Ergotamine, Caffeine, Belladonna Alkaloids, and Pentobarbital (Systemic)
Erythromycin and Sulfisoxazole (Systemic)
Estradiol (Systemic)
Estradiol (Vaginal)
Estramustine (Systemic)
Estrogens, Conjugated (Systemic)
Estrogens, Conjugated (Vaginal)
Estrogens, Esterified (Systemic)
Estrone (Systemic)
Estrone (Vaginal)
Estropipate (Systemic)
Estropipate (Vaginal)
Ethacrynic Acid (Systemic)
Ethambutol (Systemic)
Ethchlorvynol (Systemic)
Ethinyl Estradiol (Systemic)
Ethionamide (Systemic)
Ethosuximide (Systemic)
Ethotoin (Systemic)
Ethylestrenol (Systemic)
Ethynodiol Diacetate and Ethinyl Estradiol (Systemic)
Ethynodiol Diacetate and Mestranol (Systemic)
Etidronate (Systemic)
Etoposide (Systemic)
Etretinate (Systemic)
Fenfluramine (Systemic)
Fenoprofen (Systemic)
Ferrous Citrate Fe 59 (Diagnostic)
Flecainide (Systemic)
Floxuridine (Systemic)
Flucytosine (Systemic)
Fludrocortisone (Systemic)
Flumethasone (Topical)
Flunisolide (Inhalation)
Flunisolide (Nasal)
Fluocinolone (Topical)
Fluocinonide (Topical)
Fluorometholone (Ophthalmic)
Fluorouracil (Systemic)
Fluorouracil (Topical)
Fluoxymesterone (Systemic)

Flupenthixol (Systemic)
Fluphenazine (Systemic)
Flurandrenolide (Topical)
Flurazepam (Systemic)
Furosemide (Systemic)
Gallium Citrate Ga 67 (Diagnostic)
Gemfibrozil (Systemic)
Gentamicin (Systemic)
Glipizide (Systemic)
Glutethimide (Systemic)
Glyburide (Systemic)
Glycopyrrolate (Systemic)
Gold Sodium Thiomalate (Systemic)
Gonadorelin (Systemic)
Gonadotropin, Chorionic (Systemic)
Griseofulvin (Systemic)
Guanabenz (Systemic)
Guanethidine and Hydrochlorothiazide (Systemic)
Guanfacine (Systemic)
Halazepam (Systemic)
Halcinonide (Topical)
Haloperidol (Systemic)
Halothane (Systemic)
Heparin (Systemic)
Hexocyclium (Systemic)
Hydralazine (Systemic)
Hydralazine and Hydrochlorothiazide (Systemic)
Hydrochlorothiazide (Systemic)
Hydrocodone (Systemic)
Hydrocodone and Acetaminophen (Systemic)
Hydrocodone, Acetaminophen, Aspirin, and Caffeine (Systemic)
Hydrocodone, Aspirin, and Caffeine (Systemic)
Hydrocodone and Guaifenesin (Systemic)
Hydrocodone and Homatropine (Systemic)
Hydrocodone and Potassium Guaiacolsulfonate (Systemic)
Hydrocortisone (Ophthalmic)
Hydrocortisone (Systemic)
Hydrocortisone (Topical)
Hydrocortisone, Bismuth, Benzyl Benzoate, Peruvian Balsam, and Zinc Oxide (Rectal)
Hydroflumethiazide (Systemic)
Hydromorphone (Systemic)
Hydromorphone and Guaifenesin (Systemic)
Hydroxychloroquine (Systemic)
Hydroxyprogesterone (Systemic)
Hydroxyurea (Systemic)
Hydroxyzine (Systemic)
Hyoscyamine (Systemic)
Hyoscyamine and Phenobarbital (Systemic)
Hyoscyamine and Scopolamine (Systemic)
Hyoscyamine, Scopolamine, and Phenobarbital (Systemic)
Ibuprofen (Systemic)
Idoxuridine (Ophthalmic)
Imipenem and Cilastatin (Systemic)
Imipramine (Systemic)
Indapamide (Systemic)
Indium In 111 Oxyquinoline (Diagnostic)
Indium In 111 Pentetate (Diagnostic)
Indomethacin (Systemic—Anti-inflammatory, Nonsteroidal)
Interferon Alfa-2a, Recombinant (Systemic)
Interferon Alfa-2b, Recombinant (Systemic)
Inulin (Systemic)
Iocetamic Acid (Systemic)
Iodinated Glycerol (Systemic)
Iodinated I 131 Albumin (Diagnostic)
Iodipamide (Systemic)
Iodohippurate Sodium I 123 (Diagnostic)
Iodohippurate Sodium I 131 (Diagnostic)
Iohexol (Systemic)
Iopamidol (Systemic)
Iopanoic Acid (Systemic)
Iophendylate (Systemic)
Iothalamate (Mucosal)
Iothalamate Meglumine (Systemic)

Iothalamate Meglumine and Iothalamate Sodium (Systemic)
Iothalamate Sodium (Systemic)
Ioxaglate (Systemic)
Ipodate (Systemic)
Ipratropium (Inhalation)
Iron Dextran (Systemic)
Isocarboxazid (Systemic)
Isoflurane (Systemic)
Isoniazid (Systemic)
Isoproterenol and Phenylephrine (Systemic)
Isosorbide Dinitrate (Systemic)
Isotretinoin (Systemic)
Isoxsuprine (Systemic)
Kanamycin (Systemic)
Kaolin, Pectin, Belladonna Alkaloids, and Opium (Systemic)
Kaolin, Pectin, and Paregoric (Systemic)
Ketoconazole (Systemic)
Ketoconazole (Topical)
Ketoprofen (Systemic)
Krypton Kr 81m (Diagnostic)

L–O

Labetalol (Systemic)
Labetalol and Hydrochlorothiazide (Systemic)
Leuprolide (Systemic)
Levobunolol (Ophthalmic)
Levodopa (Systemic)
Levonorgestrel and Ethinyl Estradiol (Systemic)
Levorphanol (Systemic)
Lindane (Topical)
Lithium (Systemic)
Lomustine (Systemic)
Loperamide (Oral)
Lorazepam (Systemic)
Loxapine (Systemic)
Magaldrate (Oral)
Magaldrate and Simethicone (Oral)
Magnesium Carbonate and Sodium Bicarbonate (Oral)
Magnesium Citrate (Oral)
Magnesium Hydroxide (Oral)
Magnesium Hydroxide and Mineral Oil (Oral)
Magnesium Oxide (Oral)
Magnesium Salicylate (Systemic)
Magnesium Sulfate (Oral)
Magnesium Sulfate (Systemic)
Magnesium Trisilicate (Oral)
Magnesium Trisilicate, Alumina, and Magnesia (Oral)
Magnesium Trisilicate, Alumina, and Magnesium Carbonate (Oral)
Mazindol (Systemic)
Measles Virus Vaccine Live (Systemic)
Mebendazole (Systemic)
Mecamylamine (Systemic)
Mechlorethamine (Systemic)
Mechlorethamine (Topical)
Meclizine (Systemic)
Meclocycline (Topical)
Meclofenamate (Systemic)
Medroxyprogesterone (Systemic)
Medrysone (Ophthalmic)
Mefenamic Acid (Systemic)
Megestrol (Systemic)
Melphalan (Systemic)
Menadiol (Systemic)

Menotropins (Systemic)
Meperidine (Systemic)
Meperidine and Acetaminophen (Systemic)
Mephenytoin (Systemic)
Mephobarbital (Systemic)
Meprobamate (Systemic)
Meprobamate and Aspirin (Systemic)
Mercaptopurine (Systemic)
Mesoridazine (Systemic)
Metaproterenol (Systemic)
Methacycline (Systemic)
Methadone (Systemic)
Methamphetamine (Systemic)
Metharbital (Systemic)
Methazolamide (Systemic)
Methimazole (Systemic)
Methohexital (Systemic)
Methotrexate (Systemic)
Methoxyflurane (Systemic)
Methsuximide (Systemic)
Methyclothiazide (Systemic)
Methyldopa and Chlorothiazide (Systemic)
Methyldopa and Hydrochlorothiazide (Systemic)
Methylergonovine (Systemic)
Methylprednisolone (Systemic)
Methylprednisolone (Topical)
Methyltestosterone (Systemic)
Metolazone (Systemic)
Metoprolol (Systemic)
Metoprolol and Hydrochlorothiazide (Systemic)
Metrizamide (Systemic)
Metronidazole (Systemic)
Mexiletine (Systemic)
Midazolam (Systemic)
Mineral Oil (Oral)
Mineral Oil and Cascara Sagrada (Oral)
Mineral Oil, Glycerin, and Phenolphthalein (Oral)
Mineral Oil and Phenolphthalein (Oral)
Minocycline (Systemic)
Minoxidil (Systemic)
Mitomycin (Systemic)
Mitotane (Systemic)
Molindone (Systemic)
Morphine (Systemic)
Moxalactam (Systemic)
Mumps Virus Vaccine Live (Systemic)
Nadolol (Systemic)
Nadolol and Bendroflumethiazide (Systemic)
Nalbuphine (Systemic)
Naltrexone (Systemic)
Nandrolone (Systemic)
Naproxen (Systemic)
Neomycin (Systemic)
Neostigmine (Systemic)
Netilmicin (Systemic)
Nicotine (Systemic)
Nifedipine (Systemic)
Nitrofurantoin (Systemic)
Nitrous Oxide (Systemic)
Norethindrone (Systemic)
Norethindrone Acetate and Ethinyl Estradiol (Systemic)
Norethindrone and Ethinyl Estradiol (Systemic)
Norethindrone and Mestranol (Systemic)
Norethynodrel and Mestranol (Systemic)
Norfloxacin (Systemic)
Norgestrel (Systemic)
Norgestrel and Ethinyl Estradiol (Systemic)
Nortriptyline (Systemic)
Nystatin and Triamcinolone (Topical)
Opium (Systemic)
Orphenadrine, Aspirin, and Caffeine (Systemic)
Oxamniquine (Systemic)
Oxandrolone (Systemic)
Oxazepam (Systemic)
Oxprenolol (Systemic)
Oxtriphylline (Systemic)
Oxtriphylline and Guaifenesin (Systemic)

Oxycodone (Systemic)
Oxycodone and Acetaminophen (Systemic)
Oxycodone and Aspirin (Systemic)
Oxymetholone (Systemic)
Oxymorphone (Systemic)
Oxytetracycline (Systemic)
Oxytocin (Systemic)

P

Paraldehyde (Systemic)
Paramethadione (Systemic)
Paramethasone (Systemic)
Paregoric (Systemic)
Pargyline and Methyclothiazide (Systemic)
Pemoline (Systemic)
Penicillamine (Systemic)
Pentazocine (Systemic)
Pentazocine and Acetaminophen (Systemic)
Pentazocine and Aspirin (Systemic)
Pentazocine, Aspirin, and Caffeine (Systemic)
Pentazocine and Naloxone (Systemic)
Pentobarbital (Systemic)
Pentoxifylline (Systemic)
Perphenazine (Systemic)
Perphenazine and Amitriptyline (Systemic)
Phendimetrazine (Systemic)
Phenelzine (Systemic)
Phenindamine, Chlorpheniramine, and Phenylpropanolamine (Systemic)
Phenindamine, Hydrocodone, and Guaifenesin (Systemic)
Pheniramine, Codeine, and Guaifenesin (Systemic)
Pheniramine, Phenylephrine, Codeine, Sodium Citrate, Sodium Salicylate, and Caffeine (Systemic)
Pheniramine, Pyrilamine, Hydrocodone, and Potassium Citrate (Systemic)
Pheniramine, Pyrilamine, Phenylephrine, Phenylpropanolamine, and Hydrocodone (Systemic)
Pheniramine, Pyrilamine, Phenylpropanolamine, Codeine, Acetaminophen, and Caffeine (Systemic)
Pheniramine, Pyrilamine, Phenylpropanolamine, and Hydrocodone (Systemic)
Pheniramine, Pyrilamine, Phenylpropanolamine, Hydrocodone, and Guaifenesin (Systemic)
Phenmetrazine (Systemic)
Phenobarbital (Systemic)
Phensuximide (Systemic)
Phentermine (Systemic)
Phenylbutazone (Systemic)
Phenylephrine and Brompheniramine (Systemic)
Phenylephrine and Chlorpheniramine (Systemic)
Phenylephrine, Chlorpheniramine, and Pyrilamine (Systemic)
Phenylephrine, Hydrocodone, and Guaifenesin (Systemic)
Phenylephrine, Phenylpropanolamine, and Chlorpheniramine (Systemic)
Phenylephrine, Phenylpropanolamine, Pyrilamine, and Chlorpheniramine (Systemic)
Phenylpropanolamine and Chlorpheniramine (Systemic)
Phenylpropanolamine, Codeine, and Guaifenesin (Systemic)
Phenylpropanolamine and Hydrocodone (Systemic)
Phenylpropanolamine, Pheniramine, and Pyrilamine (Systemic)
Phenylpropanolamine, Phenylephrine, Phenyltoloxamine, and Chlorpheniramine (Systemic)
Phenylpropanolamine, Phenyltoloxamine, Pyrilamine, and Pheniramine (Systemic)

Phenyltoloxamine and Hydrocodone (Systemic)
Phenytoin (Systemic)
Phytonadione (Systemic)
Pimozide (Systemic)
Pindolol (Systemic)
Pindolol and Hydrochlorothiazide (Systemic)
Piroxicam (Systemic)
Plicamycin (Systemic)
Pneumococcal Vaccine Polyvalent (Systemic)
Podophyllum (Topical)
Polythiazide (Systemic)
Posterior Pituitary (Systemic)
Potassium Iodide (Systemic)
Prazepam (Systemic)
Praziquantel (Systemic)
Prazosin and Polythiazide (Systemic)
Prednisolone (Ophthalmic)
Prednisolone (Systemic)
Prednisone (Systemic)
Primidone (Systemic)
Probenecid and Colchicine (Systemic)
Procarbazine (Systemic)
Prochlorperazine (Systemic)
Progesterone (Systemic)
Promazine (Systemic)
Promethazine (Systemic)
Promethazine and Codeine (Systemic)
Promethazine and Phenylephrine (Systemic)
Promethazine, Phenylephrine, and Codeine (Systemic)
Promethazine and Pseudoephedrine (Systemic)
Propoxyphene (Systemic)
Propoxyphene and Acetaminophen (Systemic)
Propoxyphene and Aspirin (Systemic)
Propoxyphene, Aspirin, and Caffeine (Systemic)
Propranolol (Systemic)
Propranolol and Hydrochlorothiazide (Systemic)
Propylthiouracil (Systemic)
Protirelin (Systemic)
Protriptyline (Systemic)
Pseudoephedrine (Systemic)
Pseudoephedrine and Chlorcyclizine (Systemic)
Pseudoephedrine and Codeine (Systemic)
Pseudoephedrine, Codeine, and Guaifenesin (Systemic)
Pseudoephedrine and Dextromethorphan (Systemic)
Pseudoephedrine, Dextromethorphan, and Guaifenesin (Systemic)
Pseudoephedrine, Dextromethorphan, Guaifenesin, and Acetaminophen (Systemic)
Pseudoephedrine and Guaifenesin (Systemic)
Pseudoephedrine and Hydrocodone (Systemic)
Pseudoephedrine, Hydrocodone, and Guaifenesin (Systemic)
Pyridostigmine (Systemic)
Pyridoxine (Systemic)
Pyrilamine, Codeine, and Terpin Hydrate (Systemic)
Pyrilamine, Phenylephrine, and Codeine (Systemic)
Pyrilamine, Phenylephrine, and Hydrocodone (Systemic)
Pyrilamine, Phenylephrine, Hydrocodone, and Ammonium Chloride (Systemic)

Pyrilamine, Phenylpropanolamine, Dextromethorphan, and Sodium Salicylate (Systemic)
Pyrimethamine (Systemic)

Q–S

Quinestrol (Systemic)
Quinethazone (Systemic)
Quinidine (Systemic)
Quinine (Systemic)
Rauwolfia Serpentina (Systemic)
Rauwolfia Serpentina and Bendroflumethiazide (Systemic)
Reserpine (Systemic)
Reserpine and Chlorothiazide (Systemic)
Reserpine and Chlorthalidone (Systemic)
Reserpine and Hydralazine (Systemic)
Reserpine, Hydralazine, and Hydrochlorothiazide (Systemic)
Reserpine and Hydrochlorothiazide (Systemic)
Reserpine and Hydroflumethiazide (Systemic)
Reserpine and Methyclothiazide (Systemic)
Reserpine and Polythiazide (Systemic)
Reserpine and Quinethazone (Systemic)
Reserpine and Trichlormethiazide (Systemic)
Ribavirin (Systemic)
Rifampin (Systemic)
Rifampin and Isoniazid (Systemic)
Ritodrine (Systemic)
Rubella Virus Vaccine Live (Systemic)
Salicylamide (Systemic)
Salicylic Acid (Topical)
Salicylic Acid and Sulfur (Topical)
Salicylic Acid, Sulfur, and Coal Tar (Topical)
Salsalate (Systemic)
Scopolamine (Systemic)
Secobarbital (Systemic)
Secobarbital and Amobarbital (Systemic)
Selenomethionine Se 75 (Diagnostic)
Simethicone, Alumina, Calcium Carbonate, and Magnesia (Oral)
Simethicone, Alumina, Magnesium Carbonate and Magnesia (Oral)
Sodium Ascorbate (Systemic)
Sodium Bicarbonate (Systemic)
Sodium Chromate Cr 51 (Diagnostic)
Sodium Iodide I 123 (Diagnostic)
Sodium Iodide I 131 (Diagnostic)
Sodium Iodide I 131 (Therapeutic)
Sodium Pertechnetate Tc 99m (Diagnostic)
Sodium Phosphate (Oral)
Sodium Phosphate P 32 (Therapeutic)
Sodium Salicylate (Systemic)
Sotalol (Systemic)
Spironolactone (Systemic)
Spironolactone and Hydrochlorothiazide (Systemic)

Stanozolol (Systemic)
Streptokinase (Systemic)
Streptomycin (Systemic)
Streptozocin (Systemic)
Sufentanil (Systemic)
Sulfacytine (Systemic)
Sulfamethoxazole (Systemic)
Sulfamethoxazole and Phenazopyridine (Systemic)
Sulfamethoxazole and Trimethoprim (Systemic)
Sulfanilamide (Vaginal)
Sulfanilamide, Aminacrine, and Allantoin (Vaginal)
Sulfasalazine (Systemic)
Sulfisoxazole (Systemic)
Sulfisoxazole, Aminacrine, and Allantoin (Vaginal)
Sulfisoxazole and Phenazopyridine (Systemic)
Sulindac (Systemic)

T–Z

Talbutal (Systemic)
Tamoxifen (Systemic)
Technetium Tc 99m Albumin Aggregated (Diagnostic)
Technetium Tc 99m Antimony Trisulfide Colloid (Diagnostic)
Technetium Tc 99m Disofenin (Diagnostic)
Technetium Tc 99m Gluceptate (Diagnostic)
Technetium Tc 99m Human Serum Albumin (Diagnostic)
Technetium Tc 99m Lidofenin (Diagnostic)
Technetium Tc 99m Mebrofenin (Diagnostic)
Technetium Tc 99m Medronate (Diagnostic)
Technetium Tc 99m Oxidronate (Diagnostic)
Technetium Tc 99m Pentetate (Diagnostic)
Technetium Tc 99m Pyrophosphate (Diagnostic)
Technetium Tc 99m (Pyro- and trimeta-) Phosphates (Diagnostic)
Technetium Tc 99m Succimer (Diagnostic)
Technetium Tc 99m Sulfur Colloid (Diagnostic)
Temazepam (Systemic)
Terbutaline (Systemic)
Terfenadine (Systemic)
Terpin Hydrate (Systemic)
Testosterone (Systemic)
Testosterone and Estradiol (Systemic)
Tetracycline (Systemic)
Thallous Chloride Tl 201 (Diagnostic)
Theophylline (Systemic)
Theophylline, Ephedrine, Guaifenesin, and Butabarbital (Systemic)
Theophylline, Ephedrine, Guaifenesin, and Phenobarbital (Systemic)

Theophylline, Ephedrine, and Hydroxyzine (Systemic)
Theophylline, Ephedrine, and Phenobarbital (Systemic)
Theophylline and Guaifenesin (Systemic)
Thiabendazole (Systemic)
Thiamylal (Systemic)
Thioguanine (Systemic)
Thiopental (Systemic)
Thioridazine (Systemic)
Thiotepa (Systemic)
Thiothixene (Systemic)
Timolol (Ophthalmic)
Timolol (Systemic)
Timolol and Hydrochlorothiazide (Systemic)
Tobramycin (Systemic)
Tocainide (Systemic)
Tolazamide (Systemic)
Tolbutamide (Systemic)
Tolmetin (Systemic)
Tranylcypromine (Systemic)
Trazodone (Systemic)
Tretinoin (Topical)
Triamcinolone (Inhalation)
Triamcinolone (Systemic)
Triamcinolone (Topical)
Triamterene (Systemic)
Triamterene and Hydrochlorothiazide (Systemic)
Triazolam (Systemic)
Trichlormethiazide (Systemic)
Trientine (Systemic)
Trifluoperazine (Systemic)
Triflupromazine (Systemic)
Trilostane (Systemic)
Trimeprazine (Systemic)
Trimethadione (Systemic)
Trimethobenzamide (Systemic)
Trimethoprim (Systemic)
Trimipramine (Systemic)
Triple Sulfa (Vaginal)
Triprolidine and Pseudoephedrine (Systemic)
Triprolidine, Pseudoephedrine, and Codeine (Systemic)
Triprolidine, Pseudoephedrine, Codeine, and Guaifenesin (Systemic)
Triprolidine, Pseudoephedrine, and Dextromethorphan (Systemic)
Tyropanoate (Systemic)
Uracil Mustard (Systemic)
Urofollitropin (Systemic)
Urokinase (Systemic)
Valproic Acid (Systemic)
Vancomycin (Systemic)
Vasopressin (Systemic)
Verapamil (Systemic)
Vidarabine (Ophthalmic)
Vinblastine (Systemic)
Vincristine (Systemic)
Vitamin A (Systemic)
Vitamin E (Systemic)
Warfarin (Systemic)
Xenon Xe 133 (Diagnostic)

Appendix IV

BREAST-FEEDING PRECAUTION LISTING

The following medicines, selected from those included in this publication, have specific precautions in regard to use while breast-feeding. You will find such precautions in the individual monographs; look in the index for the page number.

The use of any medicine while breast-feeding must be carefully considered. The physician and the patient must balance the expected benefits against the possible risks.

Absence of a drug from this list is not meant to imply that it is safe for use while breast-feeding. For many drugs, it is not known whether a problem exists; experimentation on women who are breast-feeding is generally not done. Knowledge is usually gained only from the accumulated experience over many years in giving a drug to breast-feeding women who really needed its benefits. Also, well-planned studies in breast-feeding animals may reveal problems, although the relation of such findings to humans may not be known. Problems suggested by animal studies are often included in the warnings in this book.

Readers are reminded that the information in this text is selected and not considered to be complete.

A

Acebutolol (Systemic)
Acetaminophen, Aspirin, and Codeine (Systemic)
Acetaminophen, Aspirin, and Codeine, Buffered (Systemic)
Acetaminophen, Aspirin, Salicylamide, Codeine, and Caffeine (Systemic)
Acetohexamide (Systemic)
Acetohydroxamic Acid (Systemic)
Acetophenazine (Systemic)
Albuterol (Systemic)
Allopurinol (Systemic)
Alprazolam (Systemic)
Alseroxylon (Systemic)
Amantadine (Systemic)
Amcinonide (Topical)
Amdinocillin (Systemic)
Aminophylline (Systemic)
Amiodarone (Systemic)
Amobarbital (Systemic)
Amoxicillin (Systemic)
Amoxicillin and Clavulanate (Systemic)
Ampicillin (Systemic)
Anisindione (Systemic)
Anisotropine (Systemic)
Aprobarbital (Systemic)
Asparaginase (Systemic)
Aspirin (Systemic)
Aspirin, Buffered (Systemic)
Aspirin and Caffeine (Systemic)
Atenolol (Systemic)
Atenolol and Chlorthalidone (Systemic)
Atropine (Ophthalmic)
Atropine (Systemic)
Atropine, Hyoscyamine, Scopolamine, and Butabarbital (Systemic)
Atropine, Hyoscyamine, Scopolamine, and Phenobarbital (Systemic)
Atropine and Phenobarbital (Systemic)
Auranofin (Systemic)
Aurothioglucose (Systemic)
Azatadine (Systemic)
Azatadine and Pseudoephedrine (Systemic)
Azathioprine (Systemic)
Azlocillin (Systemic)

B

Bacampicillin (Systemic)
Beclomethasone (Inhalation)
Beclomethasone (Nasal)
Belladonna (Systemic)
Belladonna and Butabarbital (Systemic)
Belladonna and Phenobarbital (Systemic)
Benztropine (Systemic)
Betamethasone (Systemic)
Betamethasone (Topical)
Biperiden (Systemic)
Bleomycin (Systemic)
Bromocriptine (Systemic)
Bromodiphenhydramine (Systemic)
Bromodiphenhydramine and Codeine (Systemic)
Bromodiphenhydramine, Diphenhydramine, Codeine, Ammonium Chloride, and Potassium Guaiacolsulfonate (Systemic)
Brompheniramine (Systemic)
Brompheniramine, Phenylephrine, and Phenylpropanolamine (Systemic)
Brompheniramine, Phenylephrine, Phenylpropanolamine, and Codeine (Systemic)
Brompheniramine, Phenylephrine, Phenylpropanolamine, Codeine, and Guaifenesin (Systemic)
Brompheniramine, Phenylephrine, Phenylpropanolamine, and Dextromethorphan (Systemic)
Brompheniramine, Phenylephrine, Phenylpropanolamine, and Guaifenesin (Systemic)
Brompheniramine, Phenylephrine, Phenylpropanolamine, Hydrocodone, and Guaifenesin (Systemic)
Brompheniramine and Phenylpropanolamine (Systemic)
Brompheniramine, Phenylpropanolamine, and Codeine (Systemic)
Brompheniramine, Phenylpropanolamine, and Dextromethorphan (Systemic)
Brompheniramine and Pseudoephedrine (Systemic)
Brompheniramine, Pseudoephedrine, and Dextromethorphan (Systemic)
Buclizine (Systemic)
Buprenorphine (Systemic)

Busulfan (Systemic)
Butabarbital (Systemic)
Butalbital and Acetaminophen (Systemic)
Butalbital, Acetaminophen, and Caffeine (Systemic)
Butalbital, Acetaminophen, and Codeine (Systemic)
Butalbital, Acetaminophen, Codeine, and Caffeine (Systemic)
Butalbital, Acetaminophen, Hydrocodone, and Caffeine (Systemic)
Butalbital and Aspirin (Systemic)
Butalbital, Aspirin, and Caffeine (Systemic)
Butalbital, Aspirin, and Codeine (Systemic)

C

Caffeine (Systemic)
Caffeine, Citrated (Systemic)
Caffeine and Sodium Benzoate (Systemic)
Calcitonin-Human (Systemic)
Calcitonin-Salmon (Systemic)
Carbamazepine (Systemic)
Carbenicillin (Systemic)
Carbidopa and Levodopa (Systemic)
Carbinoxamine (Systemic)
Carbinoxamine and Pseudoephedrine (Systemic)
Carbinoxamine, Pseudoephedrine, and Dextromethorphan (Systemic)
Carbinoxamine, Pseudoephedrine, and Guaifenesin (Systemic)
Carisoprodol (Systemic)
Carmustine (Systemic)
Casanthranol (Oral)
Cascara Sagrada (Oral)
Cascara Sagrada and Aloe (Oral)

Cascara Sagrada and Phenolphthalein (Oral)
Chloral Hydrate (Systemic)
Chlorambucil (Systemic)
Chloramphenicol (Systemic)
Chlordiazepoxide (Systemic)
Chlordiazepoxide and Amitriptyline (Systemic)
Chlordiazepoxide and Clidinium (Systemic)
Chloroquine (Systemic)
Chlorotrianisene (Systemic)
Chlorpheniramine (Systemic)
Chlorpheniramine and Codeine (Systemic)
Chlorpheniramine, Codeine, Aspirin, and Caffeine (Systemic)
Chlorpheniramine, Codeine, Carbetapentane, Guaifenesin, Sodium Citrate, and Citric Acid (Systemic)
Chlorpheniramine and Dextromethorphan (Systemic)
Chlorpheniramine, Dextromethorphan, and Acetaminophen (Systemic)
Chlorpheniramine, Ephedrine, and Guaifenesin (Systemic)
Chlorpheniramine, Ephedrine, Phenylephrine, and Carbetapentane (Systemic)
Chlorpheniramine, Ephedrine, Phenylephrine, Dextromethorphan, Ammonium Chloride, and Ipecac (Systemic)
Chlorpheniramine, Phenindamine, Phenylephrine, Dextromethorphan, Acetaminophen, Salicylamide, Caffeine, and Ascorbic Acid (Systemic)
Chlorpheniramine, Phenindamine, Pyrilamine, Phenylephrine, Hydrocodone, and Ammonium Chloride (Systemic)
Chlorpheniramine, Pheniramine, Pyrilamine, Phenylephrine, Hydrocodone, Salicylamide, Caffeine, and Ascorbic Acid (Systemic)
Chlorpheniramine, Phenylephrine, Codeine, and Acetaminophen (Systemic)
Chlorpheniramine, Phenylephrine, Codeine, and Ammonium Chloride (Systemic)
Chlorpheniramine, Phenylephrine, Codeine, Ammonium Chloride, Potassium Guaiacolsulfonate, and Sodium Citrate (Systemic)
Chlorpheniramine, Phenylephrine, Codeine, and Potassium Iodide (Systemic)
Chlorpheniramine, Phenylephrine, and Dextromethorphan (Systemic)
Chlorpheniramine, Phenylephrine, Dextromethorphan, Acetaminophen, and Salicylamide (Systemic)
Chlorpheniramine, Phenylephrine, Dextromethorphan, and Guaifenesin (Systemic)
Chlorpheniramine, Phenylephrine, Dextromethorphan, Guaifenesin, and Ammonium Chloride (Systemic)
Chlorpheniramine, Phenylephrine, and Guaifenesin (Systemic)
Chlorpheniramine, Phenylephrine, and Hydrocodone (Systemic)
Chlorpheniramine, Phenylephrine, Hydrocodone, Acetaminophen, and Caffeine (Systemic)
Chlorpheniramine, Phenylephrine, Phenylpropanolamine, Carbetapentane, and Potassium Guaiacolsulfonate (Systemic)
Chlorpheniramine, Phenylephrine, Phenylpropanolamine, and Codeine (Systemic)
Chlorpheniramine, Phenylephrine, Phenylpropanolamine, and Dextromethorphan (Systemic)
Chlorpheniramine, Phenylephrine, Phenylpropanolamine, Dextromethorphan, Guaifenesin, and Acetaminophen (Systemic)
Chlorpheniramine, Phenylephrine, Phenylpropanolamine, and Dihydrocodeine (Systemic)
Chlorpheniramine, Phenylpropanolamine, and Caramiphen (Systemic)

Chlorpheniramine, Phenylpropanolamine, Codeine, Guaifenesin, and Acetaminophen (Systemic)
Chlorpheniramine, Phenylpropanolamine, and Dextromethorphan (Systemic)
Chlorpheniramine, Phenylpropanolamine, Dextromethorphan, and Acetaminophen (Systemic)
Chlorpheniramine, Phenylpropanolamine, Dextromethorphan, Acetaminophen, and Caffeine (Systemic)
Chlorpheniramine, Phenylpropanolamine, Dextromethorphan, and Ammonium Chloride (Systemic)
Chlorpheniramine, Phenylpropanolamine, Dextromethorphan, Ammonium Chloride, Terpin Hydrate, and Sodium Citrate (Systemic)
Chlorpheniramine, Phenylpropanolamine, and Guaifenesin (Systemic)
Chlorpheniramine, Phenylpropanolamine, Guaifenesin, Sodium Citrate, and Citric Acid (Systemic)
Chlorpheniramine, Phenylpropanolamine, Hydrocodone, Guaifenesin, and Salicylamide (Systemic)
Chlorpheniramine, Phenyltoloxamine, Ephedrine, Codeine, and Guaiacol Carbonate (Systemic)
Chlorpheniramine and Pseudoephedrine (Systemic)
Chlorpheniramine, Pseudoephedrine, and Codeine (Systemic)
Chlorpheniramine, Pseudoephedrine, and Dextromethorphan (Systemic)
Chlorpheniramine, Pseudoephedrine, Dextromethorphan, and Acetaminophen (Systemic)
Chlorpheniramine, Pseudoephedrine, Dextromethorphan, Guaifenesin, and Aspirin (Systemic)
Chlorpheniramine, Pseudoephedrine, and Guaifenesin (Systemic)
Chlorpheniramine, Pseudoephedrine, and Hydrocodone (Systemic)
Chlorpheniramine, Pyrilamine, and Phenylpropanolamine (Systemic)
Chlorpheniramine, Tripelennamine, Phenylpropanolamine, and Phenylephrine (Systemic)
Chlorpromazine (Systemic)
Chlorpropamide (Systemic)
Choline Salicylate (Systemic)
Choline and Magnesium Salicylates (Systemic)
Chromic Phosphate P 32 (Therapeutic)
Cimetidine (Systemic)
Cinoxacin (Systemic)
Cisplatin (Systemic)
Clemastine (Systemic)
Clemastine and Phenylpropanolamine (Systemic)
Clidinium (Systemic)
Clobetasol (Topical)
Clocortolone (Topical)
Clofazimine (Systemic)
Clonazepam (Systemic)
Clorazepate (Systemic)
Cloxacillin (Systemic)
Codeine and Calcium Iodide (Systemic)
Codeine and Guaifenesin (Systemic)
Codeine and Iodinated Glycerol (Systemic)
Codeine and Terpin Hydrate (Systemic)
Cortisone (Systemic)
Cyanocobalamin Co 57 (Diagnostic)
Cyclacillin (Systemic)
Cyclizine (Systemic)
Cyclophosphamide (Systemic)
Cyclosporine (Systemic)
Cyproheptadine (Systemic)
Cytarabine (Systemic)

D

Dacarbazine (Systemic)
Dactinomycin (Systemic)
Danazol (Systemic)
Danthron (Oral)
Danthron and Docusate (Oral)
Danthron and Poloxamer 188 (Oral)
Dapsone (Systemic)
Daunorubicin (Systemic)
Demeclocycline (Systemic)
Deserpidine (Systemic)
Deserpidine and Hydrochlorothiazide (Systemic)
Deserpidine and Methyclothiazide (Systemic)
Desonide (Topical)
Desoximetasone (Topical)
Desoxycorticosterone (Systemic)
Dexamethasone (Nasal)
Dexamethasone (Inhalation)
Dexamethasone (Systemic)
Dexamethasone (Topical)
Dexbrompheniramine and Pseudoephedrine (Systemic)
Dexchlorpheniramine (Systemic)
Dexchlorpheniramine, Pseudoephedrine, and Guaifenesin (Systemic)
Dextromethorphan and Iodinated Glycerol (Systemic)
Diazepam (Systemic)
Dicloxacillin (Systemic)
Dicumarol (Systemic)
Dicyclomine (Systemic)
Dienestrol (Vaginal)
Diethylstilbestrol (Systemic)
Diflorasone (Topical)
Dihydroergotamine (Systemic)
Dimenhydrinate (Systemic)
Diphenhydramine (Systemic)
Diphenhydramine, Codeine, and Ammonium Chloride (Systemic)
Diphenhydramine, Dextromethorphan, and Ammonium Chloride (Systemic)
Diphenhydramine and Pseudoephedrine (Systemic)
Diphenylpyraline, Phenylephrine, and Codeine (Systemic)
Diphenylpyraline, Phenylephrine, and Dextromethorphan (Systemic)
Diphenylpyraline, Phenylephrine, and Hydrocodone (Systemic)
Diphenylpyraline, Phenylephrine, Hydrocodone, and Guaifenesin (Systemic)
Diphenylpyraline (Systemic)
Doxorubicin (Systemic)
Doxycycline (Systemic)
Doxylamine (Systemic)
Doxylamine, Pseudoephedrine, Dextromethorphan, and Acetaminophen (Systemic)
Dronabinol (Systemic)

E–K

Econazole (Topical)
Epinephrine (Systemic)
Ephedrine and Potassium Iodide (Systemic)
Ergonovine (Systemic)
Ergotamine (Systemic)
Ergotamine, Belladonna Alkaloids, and Phenobarbital (Systemic)
Ergotamine and Caffeine (Systemic)

Ergotamine, Caffeine, Belladonna Alkaloids, and Pentobarbital (Systemic)
Erythromycin and Sulfisoxazole (Systemic)
Estradiol (Systemic)
Estradiol (Vaginal)
Estrogens, Conjugated (Systemic)
Estrogens, Conjugated (Vaginal)
Estrogens, Esterified (Systemic)
Estrone (Systemic)
Estrone (Vaginal)
Estropipate (Systemic)
Estropipate (Vaginal)
Ethinyl Estradiol (Systemic)
Ethopropazine (Systemic)
Ethynodiol Diacetate and Ethinyl Estradiol (Systemic)
Ethynodiol Diacetate and Mestranol (Systemic)
Etoposide (Systemic)
Etretinate (Systemic)
Ferrous Citrate Fe 59 (Diagnostic)
Floxuridine (Systemic)
Fludrocortisone (Systemic)
Flumethasone (Topical)
Flunisolide (Inhalation)
Flunisolide (Nasal)
Fluocinolone (Topical)
Fluocinonide (Topical)
Fluorouracil (Systemic)
Fluoxymesterone (Systemic)
Fluphenazine (Systemic)
Flurandrenolide (Topical)
Flurazepam (Systemic)
Gallium Citrate Ga 67 (Diagnostic)
Gemfibrozil (Systemic)
Glipizide (Systemic)
Glutethimide (Systemic)
Glyburide (Systemic)
Glycopyrrolate (Systemic)
Gold Sodium Thiomalate (Systemic)
Halazepam (Systemic)
Halcinonide (Topical)
Haloperidol (Systemic)
Heparin (Systemic)
Hexocyclium (Systemic)
Homatropine (Systemic)
Hydrocodone, Acetaminophen, Aspirin, and Caffeine (Systemic)
Hydrocodone and Guaifenesin (Systemic)
Hydrocodone and Homatropine (Systemic)
Hydrocodone and Potassium Guaiacolsulfonate (Systemic)
Hydrocortisone (Systemic)
Hydrocortisone (Topical)
Hydromorphone and Guaifenesin (Systemic)
Hydroxychloroquine (Systemic)
Hydroxyprogesterone (Systemic)
Hydroxyurea (Systemic)
Hyoscyamine (Systemic)
Hyoscyamine and Phenobarbital (Systemic)
Hyoscyamine and Scopolamine (Systemic)
Hyoscyamine, Scopolamine, and Phenobarbital (Systemic)
Indium In 111 Oxyquinoline (Diagnostic)
Indomethacin (Systemic—Anti-inflammatory, Nonsteroidal)
Interferon Alfa-2a, Recombinant (Systemic)
Interferon Alfa-2b, Recombinant (Systemic)
Iodinated Glycerol (Systemic)
Iodinated I 131 Albumin (Diagnostic)
Iodohippurate Sodium I 123 (Diagnostic)
Iodohippurate Sodium I 131 (Diagnostic)
Iohexol (Systemic)
Iopamidol (Systemic)
Iothalamate Meglumine (Systemic)
Iothalamate Meglumine and Iothalamate Sodium (Systemic)
Iothalamate Sodium (Systemic)
Ioxaglate (Systemic)
Isopropamide (Systemic)
Isotretinoin (Systemic)
Ketoconazole (Systemic)
Krypton Kr 81m (Diagnostic)

L–O

Labetalol (Systemic)
Labetalol and Hydrochlorothiazide (Systemic)
Levodopa (Systemic)
Levonorgestrel and Ethinyl Estradiol (Systemic)
Lindane (Topical)
Lithium (Systemic)
Lomustine (Systemic)
Lorazepam (Systemic)
Magnesium Salicylate (Systemic)
Mechlorethamine (Systemic)
Mechlorethamine (Topical)
Meclizine (Systemic)
Meclofenamate (Systemic)
Medroxyprogesterone (Systemic)
Megestrol (Systemic)
Melphalan (Systemic)
Mepenzolate (Systemic)
Mephobarbital (Systemic)
Meprobamate (Systemic)
Meprobamate and Aspirin (Systemic)
Mercaptopurine (Systemic)
Mesoridazine (Systemic)
Methacycline (Systemic)
Methadone (Systemic)
Methantheline (Systemic)
Metharbital (Systemic)
Methicillin (Systemic)
Methimazole (Systemic)
Methotrexate (Systemic)
Methscopolamine (Systemic)
Methylergonovine (Systemic)
Methylprednisolone (Systemic)
Methylprednisolone (Topical)
Methyltestosterone (Systemic)
Methysergide (Systemic)
Metoprolol (Systemic)
Metoprolol and Hydrochlorothiazide (Systemic)
Metrizamide (Systemic)
Metronidazole (Systemic)
Mexiletine (Systemic)
Mezlocillin (Systemic)
Mineral Oil and Cascara Sagrada (Oral)
Minocycline (Systemic)
Mitomycin (Systemic)
Muromonab-CD3 (Systemic)
Nadolol (Systemic)
Nadolol and Bendroflumethiazide (Systemic)
Nafcillin (Systemic)
Nalidixic Acid (Systemic)
Nicotine (Systemic)
Nitrofurantoin (Systemic)
Norethindrone (Systemic)
Norethindrone Acetate and Ethinyl Estradiol (Systemic)
Norethindrone and Ethinyl Estradiol (Systemic)
Norethindrone and Mestranol (Systemic)
Norethynodrel and Mestranol (Systemic)
Norfloxacin (Systemic)
Norgestrel (Systemic)
Norgestrel and Ethinyl Estradiol (Systemic)
Nystatin and Triamcinolone (Topical)
Orphenadrine, Aspirin, and Caffeine (Systemic)
Oxacillin (Systemic)
Oxazepam (Systemic)
Oxprenolol (Systemic)
Oxtriphylline (Systemic)
Oxtriphylline and Guaifenesin (Systemic)
Oxybutynin (Systemic)
Oxyphencyclimine (Systemic)
Oxyphenonium (Systemic)
Oxytetracycline (Systemic)

P

Pancreatin, Pepsin, Bile Salts, Hyoscyamine, Atropine, Scopolamine, and Phenobarbital (Systemic)
Paramethasone (Systemic)
Penicillin G (Systemic)
Penicillin V (Systemic)
Pentobarbital (Systemic)
Permethrin (Topical)
Perphenazine (Systemic)
Phenindamine (Systemic)
Phenindamine, Chlorpheniramine, and Phenylpropanolamine (Systemic)
Phenindamine, Hydrocodone, and Guaifenesin (Systemic)
Pheniramine, Codeine, and Guaifenesin (Systemic)
Pheniramine, Phenylephrine, Codeine, Sodium Citrate, Sodium Salicylate, and Caffeine (Systemic)
Pheniramine, Pyrilamine, Hydrocodone, and Potassium Citrate (Systemic)
Pheniramine, Pyrilamine, Phenylephrine, Phenylpropanolamine, and Hydrocodone (Systemic)
Pheniramine, Pyrilamine, Phenylpropanolamine, Codeine, Acetaminophen, and Caffeine (Systemic)
Pheniramine, Pyrilamine, Phenylpropanolamine, and Dextromethorphan (Systemic)
Pheniramine, Pyrilamine, Phenylpropanolamine, Dextromethorphan, and Ammonium Chloride (Systemic)
Pheniramine, Pyrilamine, Phenylpropanolamine, Dextromethorphan, and Guaifenesin (Systemic)
Pheniramine, Pyrilamine, Phenylpropanolamine, Dextromethorphan, Terpin Hydrate, and Acetaminophen (Systemic)
Pheniramine, Pyrilamine, Phenylpropanolamine, and Guaifenesin (Systemic)
Pheniramine, Pyrilamine, Phenylpropanolamine, and Hydrocodone (Systemic)
Pheniramine, Pyrilamine, Phenylpropanolamine, Hydrocodone, and Guaifenesin (Systemic)
Phenobarbital (Systemic)
Phenylbutazone (Systemic)
Phenylephrine and Brompheniramine (Systemic)
Phenylephrine and Chlorpheniramine (Systemic)
Phenylephrine, Chlorpheniramine, and Pyrilamine (Systemic)
Phenylephrine, Hydrocodone, and Guaifenesin (Systemic)
Phenylephrine, Phenylpropanolamine, and Chlorpheniramine (Systemic)
Phenylephrine, Phenylpropanolamine, Pyrilamine, and Chlorpheniramine (Systemic)
Phenylpropanolamine and Chlorpheniramine (Systemic)
Phenylpropanolamine, Codeine, and Guaifenesin (Systemic)
Phenylpropanolamine and Hydrocodone (Systemic)
Phenylpropanolamine, Pheniramine, and Pyrilamine (Systemic)
Phenylpropanolamine, Phenylephrine, Phenyltoloxamine, and Chlorpheniramine (Systemic)

Phenylpropanolamine, Phenyltoloxamine, Pyrilamine, and Pheniramine (Systemic)
Phenyltoloxamine and Hydrocodone (Systemic)
Phenytoin (Systemic)
Pimozide (Systemic)
Pindolol (Systemic)
Pindolol and Hydrochlorothiazide (Systemic)
Piperacillin (Systemic)
Pirenzepine (Systemic)
Piroxicam (Systemic)
Potassium Iodide (Systemic)
Prazepam (Systemic)
Praziquantel (Systemic)
Prednisolone (Systemic)
Prednisone (Systemic)
Primidone (Systemic)
Procarbazine (Systemic)
Prochlorperazine (Systemic)
Procyclidine (Systemic)
Progesterone (Systemic)
Promazine (Systemic)
Promethazine (Systemic)
Promethazine and Codeine (Systemic)
Promethazine and Dextromethorphan (Systemic)
Promethazine and Phenylephrine (Systemic)
Promethazine, Phenylephrine, and Codeine (Systemic)
Promethazine and Pseudoephedrine (Systemic)
Propantheline (Systemic)
Propranolol (Systemic)
Propranolol and Hydrochlorothiazide (Systemic)
Propylthiouracil (Systemic)
Protirelin (Systemic)
Pseudoephedrine (Systemic)
Pseudoephedrine and Chlorcyclizine (Systemic)
Pseudoephedrine and Codeine (Systemic)
Pseudoephedrine, Codeine, and Guaifenesin (Systemic)
Pseudoephedrine and Dextromethorphan (Systemic)
Pseudoephedrine, Dextromethorphan, and Guaifenesin (Systemic)
Pseudoephedrine, Dextromethorphan, Guaifenesin, and Acetaminophen (Systemic)
Pseudoephedrine and Guaifenesin (Systemic)
Pseudoephedrine and Hydrocodone (Systemic)
Pseudoephedrine, Hydrocodone, and Guaifenesin (Systemic)
Pyrilamine (Systemic)
Pyrilamine, Codeine, and Terpin Hydrate (Systemic)
Pyrilamine, Phenylephrine, and Codeine (Systemic)
Pyrilamine, Phenylephrine, and Dextromethorphan (Systemic)
Pyrilamine, Phenylephrine, Dextromethorphan, and Acetaminophen (Systemic)
Pyrilamine, Phenylephrine, and Hydrocodone (Systemic)
Pyrilamine, Phenylephrine, Hydrocodone, and Ammonium Chloride (Systemic)
Pyrilamine, Phenylpropanolamine, Dextromethorphan, and Sodium Salicylate (Systemic)
Pyrimethamine (Systemic)

Q–Z

Quinestrol (Systemic)
Rauwolfia Serpentina (Systemic)
Rauwolfia Serpentina and Bendroflumethiazide (Systemic)
Reserpine (Systemic)
Reserpine and Chlorothiazide (Systemic)
Reserpine and Chlorthalidone (Systemic)
Reserpine and Hydralazine (Systemic)
Reserpine, Hydralazine, and Hydrochlorothiazide (Systemic)
Reserpine and Hydrochlorothiazide (Systemic)
Reserpine and Hydroflumethiazide (Systemic)
Reserpine and Methyclothiazide (Systemic)
Reserpine and Polythiazide (Systemic)
Reserpine and Quinethazone (Systemic)
Reserpine and Trichlormethiazide (Systemic)
Ribavirin (Systemic)
Rifampin (Systemic)
Rifampin and Isoniazid (Systemic)
Salicylamide (Systemic)
Salicylic Acid (Topical)
Salicylic Acid and Sulfur (Topical)
Salicylic Acid, Sulfur, and Coal Tar (Topical)
Salsalate (Systemic)
Scopolamine (Systemic)
Secobarbital (Systemic)
Secobarbital and Amobarbital (Systemic)
Selenomethionine Se 75 (Diagnostic)
Sodium Chromate Cr 51 (Diagnostic)
Sodium Iodide I 123 (Diagnostic)
Sodium Iodide I 131 (Diagnostic)
Sodium Iodide I 131 (Therapeutic)
Sodium Pertechnetate Tc 99m (Diagnostic)
Sodium Phosphate P 32 (Therapeutic)
Sodium Salicylate (Systemic)
Sotalol (Systemic)
Streptozocin (Systemic)
Sulfacytine (Systemic)
Sulfamethoxazole (Systemic)
Sulfamethoxazole and Phenazopyridine (Systemic)
Sulfamethoxazole and Trimethoprim (Systemic)
Sulfanilamide (Vaginal)
Sulfanilamide, Aminacrine, and Allantoin (Vaginal)
Sulfasalazine (Systemic)
Sulfisoxazole (Systemic)
Sulfisoxazole, Aminacrine, and Allantoin (Vaginal)
Sulfisoxazole and Phenazopyridine (Systemic)
Talbutal (Systemic)
Tamoxifen (Systemic)
Technetium Tc 99m Albumin Aggregated (Diagnostic)
Technetium Tc 99m Antimony Trisulfide Colloid (Diagnostic)
Technetium Tc 99m Disofenin (Diagnostic)
Technetium Tc 99m Gluceptate (Diagnostic)
Technetium Tc 99m Human Serum Albumin (Diagnostic)
Technetium Tc 99m Lidofenin (Diagnostic)

Technetium Tc 99m Mebrofenin (Diagnostic)
Technetium Tc 99m Medronate (Diagnostic)
Technetium Tc 99m Oxidronate (Diagnostic)
Technetium Tc 99m Pentetate (Diagnostic)
Technetium Tc 99m Pyrophosphate (Diagnostic)
Technetium Tc 99m (Pyro- and trimeta-) Phosphates (Diagnostic)
Technetium Tc 99m Succimer (Diagnostic)
Technetium Tc 99m Sulfur Colloid (Diagnostic)
Temazepam (Systemic)
Terbutaline (Systemic)
Terfenadine (Systemic)
Terpin Hydrate (Systemic)
Testosterone (Systemic)
Testosterone and Estradiol (Systemic)
Tetracycline (Systemic)
Thallous Chloride Tl 201 (Diagnostic)
Theophylline (Systemic)
Theophylline, Ephedrine, Guaifenesin, and Butabarbital (Systemic)
Theophylline, Ephedrine, Guaifenesin, and Phenobarbital (Systemic)
Theophylline, Ephedrine, and Hydroxyzine (Systemic)
Theophylline, Ephedrine, and Phenobarbital (Systemic)
Theophylline and Guaifenesin (Systemic)
Thioguanine (Systemic)
Thioridazine (Systemic)
Thiotepa (Systemic)
Ticarcillin (Systemic)
Ticarcillin and Clavulanate (Systemic)
Timolol (Ophthalmic)
Timolol (Systemic)
Timolol and Hydrochlorothiazide (Systemic)
Tolazamide (Systemic)
Tolbutamide (Systemic)
Triamcinolone (Inhalation)
Triamcinolone (Systemic)
Triamcinolone (Topical)
Triazolam (Systemic)
Tridihexethyl (Systemic)
Trifluoperazine (Systemic)
Triflupromazine (Systemic)
Trihexyphenidyl (Systemic)
Trimeprazine (Systemic)
Trimethoprim (Systemic)
Tripelennamine (Systemic)
Triple Sulfa (Vaginal)
Triprolidine (Systemic)
Triprolidine and Pseudoephedrine (Systemic)
Triprolidine, Pseudoephedrine, and Codeine (Systemic)
Triprolidine, Pseudoephedrine, Codeine, and Guaifenesin (Systemic)
Triprolidine, Pseudoephedrine, and Dextromethorphan (Systemic)
Uracil Mustard (Systemic)
Vinblastine (Systemic)
Vincristine (Systemic)
Warfarin (Systemic)
Xenon Xe 133 (Diagnostic)
Zidovudine (Systemic)

Appendix V

CATEGORIES OF USE

The following categories of use and the specific drugs listed under each entry are intended only as a useful reference for the consumer and should not be used to make decisions concerning the appropriateness of therapy. The drugs included under each entry should not be considered interchangeable for any given patient. In many instances, the drugs differ significantly with regard to effectiveness, seriousness of side effects, and other critical considerations.

You can find specific information for each drug in the individual monographs; look in the index for the appropriate page number. A glossary of terms can be found on page 1197. Should you desire additional information or if you have any questions as to how this information may relate to you in particular, ask your doctor, nurse, pharmacist, or other health care provider.

The information for this listing has been extracted from the USP DI data base. The category terminology used is intentionally broad in scope, and each entry may cover a wide range of specific indications. These specific indications may not be readily apparent to the reader. In addition, certain uses for some of the drugs listed may not have been specifically included in the manufacturer's product information, but they may be considered appropriate therapy in selected patients as defined by current medical practice.

Readers are reminded that the information in this text is selected and not considered to be complete. Absence of a drug from a category of use listing is not meant to imply that it is inappropriate for such use. On the other hand, presence of a drug in a category of use listing does not necessarily mean that the drug is appropriate for use in a particular patient.

A

Abortifacient
    Carboprost (Systemic)
    Dinoprost (Intra-amniotic)
    Dinoprostone (Vaginal)
    Sodium Chloride (Intra-amniotic)
    Urea (Intra-amniotic)
Acidifier, urinary
    Ascorbic Acid (Systemic)
    Potassium Phosphate, Monobasic (Systemic)
    Potassium and Sodium Phosphates (Systemic)
Adrenocorticoid-antiseptic, otic
    Desonide and Acetic Acid (Otic)
    Hydrocortisone and Acetic Acid (Otic)
Adrenocorticoid-emollient, rectal
    Hydrocortisone, Bismuth, Benzyl Benzoate, Peruvian Balsam, and Zinc Oxide (Rectal)
Adrenocorticoid, glucocorticoid
    Betamethasone (Systemic)
    Cortisone (Systemic)
    Dexamethasone (Systemic)
    Hydrocortisone (Systemic)
    Methylprednisolone (Systemic)
    Paramethasone (Systemic)
    Prednisolone (Systemic)
    Prednisone (Systemic)
    Triamcinolone (Systemic)
Adrenocorticoid, inhalation
    Beclomethasone (Inhalation)
    Dexamethasone (Inhalation)
    Flunisolide (Inhalation)
    Triamcinolone (Inhalation)
Adrenocorticoid, mineralocorticoid
    Desoxycorticosterone (Systemic)
    Fludrocortisone (Systemic)
Adrenocorticoid, nasal
    Beclomethasone (Nasal)
    Dexamethasone (Nasal)
    Flunisolide (Nasal)
Adrenocorticoid, ophthalmic
    Betamethasone (Ophthalmic)
    Dexamethasone (Ophthalmic)
    Fluorometholone (Ophthalmic)

Adrenocorticoid, ophthalmic *(continued)*
    Hydrocortisone (Ophthalmic)
    Medrysone (Ophthalmic)
    Prednisolone (Ophthalmic)
Adrenocorticoid, otic
    Betamethasone (Otic)
    Dexamethasone (Otic)
    Hydrocortisone (Otic)
    Prednisolone (Otic)
Adrenocorticoid, topical
    Amcinonide (Topical)
    Betamethasone (Topical)
    Clobetasol (Topical)
    Clocortolone (Topical)
    Desonide (Topical)
    Desoximetasone (Topical)
    Dexamethasone (Topical)
    Diflorasone (Topical)
    Flumethasone (Topical)
    Fluocinolone (Topical)
    Fluocinonide (Topical)
    Flurandrenolide (Topical)
    Halcinonide (Topical)
    Hydrocortisone (Topical)
    Methylprednisolone (Topical)
    Triamcinolone (Topical)
Adrenocorticotropic hormone
    Corticotropin (Systemic)
Alcohol-abuse deterrent
    Disulfiram (Systemic)
Aldosterone antagonist
    Spironolactone (Systemic)
Alkalizer, systemic
    Potassium Citrate and Citric Acid (Systemic)
    Sodium Bicarbonate (Systemic)
    Sodium Citrate and Citric Acid (Systemic)
    Tricitrates (Systemic)
Alkalizer, urinary
    Potassium Citrate (Systemic)
    Potassium Citrate and Citric Acid (Systemic)
    Potassium Citrate and Sodium Citrate (Systemic)

Alkalizer, urinary *(continued)*
    Sodium Bicarbonate (Systemic)
    Sodium Citrate and Citric Acid (Systemic)
    Tricitrates (Systemic)
Altitude sickness, acute, agent
    Acetazolamide (Systemic)
Amnestic
    Diazepam, Parenteral (Systemic)
    Lorazepam, Parenteral (Systemic)
Amyloidosis suppressant
    Colchicine (Systemic)
Anabolic steroid
    Dromostanolone (Systemic)
    Ethylestrenol (Systemic)
    Nandrolone (Systemic)
    Oxandrolone (Systemic)
    Oxymetholone (Systemic)
    Stanozolol (Systemic)
Analgesia adjunct
    Caffeine (Systemic)
Analgesic
    Acetaminophen (Systemic)
    Acetaminophen and Aspirin (Systemic)
    Acetaminophen, Aspirin, and Caffeine (Systemic)
    Acetaminophen, Aspirin, and Caffeine, Buffered (Systemic)
    Acetaminophen, Aspirin, and Codeine (Systemic)
    Acetaminophen, Aspirin, and Salicylamide (Systemic)
    Acetaminophen, Aspirin, and Salicylamide, Buffered (Systemic)
    Acetaminophen, Aspirin, Salicylamide, and Caffeine (Systemic)
    Acetaminophen, Aspirin, Salicylamide, and Codeine (Systemic)
    Acetaminophen, Buffered (Systemic)
    Acetaminophen and Codeine (Systemic)
    Acetaminophen and Salicylamide (Systemic)
    Acetaminophen, Salicylamide, and Caffeine (Systemic)
    Acetaminophen, Sodium Salicylate, and Caffeine (Systemic)

Analgesic (continued)
  Aspirin (Systemic)
  Aspirin, Buffered (Systemic)
  Aspirin and Codeine (Systemic)
  Aspirin, Codeine, Alumina, and Magnesia (Systemic)
  Buprenorphine (Systemic)
  Butalbital and Acetaminophen (Systemic)
  Butalbital, Acetaminophen, and Caffeine (Systemic)
  Butalbital, Acetaminophen, and Codeine (Systemic)
  Butalbital, Acetaminophen, Codeine, and Caffeine (Systemic)
  Butalbital, Acetaminophen, Hydrocodone, and Caffeine (Systemic)
  Butalbital and Aspirin (Systemic)
  Butalbital, Aspirin, and Caffeine (Systemic)
  Butalbital, Aspirin, and Codeine (Systemic)
  Butorphanol (Systemic)
  Choline Salicylate (Systemic)
  Choline and Magnesium Salicylates (Systemic)
  Codeine (Systemic)
  Diflunisal (Systemic)
  Dihydrocodeine and Acetaminophen (Systemic)
  Dihydrocodeine and Aspirin (Systemic)
  Fenoprofen (Systemic)
  Fentanyl (Systemic)
  Hydrocodone (Systemic)
  Hydrocodone and Acetaminophen (Systemic)
  Hydrocodone, Acetaminophen, and Aspirin (Systemic)
  Hydrocodone and Aspirin (Systemic)
  Hydromorphone (Systemic)
  Ibuprofen (Systemic)
  Levorphanol (Systemic)
  Magnesium Salicylate (Systemic)
  Mefenamic Acid (Systemic)
  Meperidine (Systemic)
  Meperidine and Acetaminophen (Systemic)
  Meprobamate and Aspirin (Systemic)
  Methadone (Systemic)
  Morphine (Systemic)
  Nalbuphine (Systemic)
  Naproxen (Systemic)
  Opium, Parenteral (Systemic)
  Oxycodone (Systemic)
  Oxycodone and Acetaminophen (Systemic)
  Oxycodone and Aspirin (Systemic)
  Oxymorphone (Systemic)
  Pentazocine (Systemic)
  Pentazocine and Acetaminophen (Systemic)
  Pentazocine and Aspirin (Systemic)
  Pentazocine and Naloxone (Systemic)
  Propoxyphene (Systemic)
  Propoxyphene and Acetaminophen (Systemic)
  Propoxyphene and Aspirin (Systemic)
  Salicylamide (Systemic)
  Salsalate (Systemic)
  Sodium Salicylate (Systemic)
Analgesic-anesthetic, otic
  Antipyrine and Benzocaine (Otic)
Analgesic-antacid
  Acetaminophen, Buffered (Systemic)
  Aspirin Tablets, Buffered, Effervescent (Systemic)
Analgesic–skeletal muscle relaxant
  Chlorzoxazone and Acetaminophen (Systemic)
  Orphenadrine, Aspirin, and Caffeine (Systemic)
Analgesic, specific in trigeminal neuralgia
  Baclofen (Systemic)
Analgesic, urinary
  Phenazopyridine (Systemic)

Androgen
  Fluoxymesterone (Systemic)
  Methyltestosterone (Systemic)
  Testosterone (Systemic)
Androgen-estrogen
  Testosterone and Estradiol (Systemic)
Anesthesia adjunct
  Buprenorphine (Systemic)
  Etomidate (Systemic)
  Scopolamine, Parenteral (Systemic)
Anesthesia adjunct, opioid analgesic
  Alfentanil (Systemic)
  Butorphanol (Systemic)
  Fentanyl (Systemic)
  Hydromorphone, Parenteral (Systemic)
  Levorphanol, Parenteral (Systemic)
  Meperidine, Parenteral (Systemic)
  Morphine, Parenteral (Systemic)
  Nalbuphine (Systemic)
  Oxymorphone, Parenteral (Systemic)
  Pentazocine, Parenteral (Systemic)
  Sufentanil (Systemic)
Anesthetic, general
  Enflurane (Systemic)
  Etomidate (Systemic)
  Halothane (Systemic)
  Isoflurane (Systemic)
  Ketamine (Systemic)
  Methohexital (Systemic)
  Methoxyflurane (Systemic)
  Nitrous Oxide (Systemic)
  Thiamylal (Systemic)
  Thiopental (Systemic)
Anesthetic, general, adjunct
  Midazolam (Systemic)
Anesthetic, local, adjunct
  Epinephrine Injection (Systemic)
  Midazolam (Systemic)
Anesthetic, local, dental
  Benzocaine (Dental)
  Butacaine (Dental)
  Lidocaine (Dental)
Anesthetic, local, ophthalmic
  Proparacaine (Ophthalmic)
  Tetracaine (Ophthalmic)
Anesthetic, local, rectal
  Benzocaine (Rectal)
  Dibucaine (Rectal)
  Pramoxine (Rectal)
  Tetracaine (Rectal)
  Tetracaine and Menthol (Rectal)
Anesthetic, local, topical
  Benzocaine (Topical)
  Butamben (Topical)
  Dibucaine (Topical)
  Lidocaine (Topical)
  Pramoxine (Topical)
  Tetracaine (Topical)
  Tetracaine and Menthol (Topical)
Angioedema, hereditary, prophylactic
  Danazol (Systemic)
  Stanozolol (Systemic)
Antacid
  Alumina and Magnesia (Oral)
  Alumina, Magnesia, and Calcium Carbonate (Oral)
  Alumina, Magnesia, and Simethicone (Oral)
  Alumina and Magnesium Carbonate (Oral)
  Alumina, Magnesium Carbonate, and Calcium Carbonate (Oral)
  Alumina and Magnesium Trisilicate (Oral)
  Alumina, Magnesium Trisilicate, and Sodium Bicarbonate (Oral)
  Aluminum Carbonate, Basic (Oral)
  Aluminum Hydroxide (Oral)
  Calcium Carbonate (Oral)
  Calcium Carbonate (Oral)
  Calcium Carbonate and Magnesia (Oral)
  Calcium Carbonate, Magnesia, and Simethicone (Oral)
  Calcium and Magnesium Carbonates (Oral)

Antacid (continued)
  Calcium and Magnesium Carbonates and Magnesium Oxide (Oral)
  Dihydroxyaluminum Aminoacetate (Oral)
  Dihydroxyaluminum Aminoacetate, Magnesia, and Alumina (Oral)
  Dihydroxyaluminum Sodium Carbonate (Oral)
  Magaldrate (Oral)
  Magaldrate and Simethicone (Oral)
  Magnesium Carbonate and Sodium Bicarbonate (Oral)
  Magnesium Hydroxide (Oral)
  Magnesium Oxide (Oral)
  Magnesium Trisilicate (Oral)
  Magnesium Trisilicate, Alumina, and Magnesia (Oral)
  Magnesium Trisilicate, Alumina, and Magnesium Carbonate (Oral)
  Simethicone, Alumina, Calcium Carbonate, and Magnesia (Oral)
  Simethicone, Alumina, Magnesium Carbonate, and Magnesia (Oral)
  Sodium Bicarbonate (Oral)
Anthelmintic
  Mebendazole (Systemic)
  Metronidazole (Systemic)
  Niclosamide (Oral)
  Oxamniquine (Systemic)
  Praziquantel (Systemic)
  Pyrantel (Oral)
  Pyrvinium (Oral)
  Thiabendazole (Systemic)
Anthelmintic, topical
  Thiabendazole (Topical)
Antiacne agent, systemic
  Erythromycin, Oral (Systemic)
  Isotretinoin (Systemic)
  Minocycline, Oral (Systemic)
  Tetracycline, Oral (Systemic)
Antiacne agent, topical
  Alcohol and Acetone (Topical)
  Alcohol and Sulfur (Topical)
  Benzoyl Peroxide (Topical)
  Clindamycin (Topical)
  Erythromycin (Topical)
  Meclocycline (Topical)
  Resorcinol and Sulfur (Topical)
  Salicylic Acid (Topical)
  Salicylic Acid and Sulfur (Topical)
  Sulfur (Topical)
  Sulfurated Lime (Topical)
  Tetracycline (Topical)
  Tretinoin (Topical)
Antiadrenal
  Aminoglutethimide (Systemic)
  Ketoconazole (Systemic)
  Mitotane (Systemic)
  Trilostane (Systemic)
Antiallergic, gastrointestinal allergy
  Cromolyn (Oral)
Antiallergic, inhalation
  Cromolyn (Inhalation)
Antiallergic, nasal
  Cromolyn (Nasal)
Antiallergic, ophthalmic
  Cromolyn (Ophthalmic)
Antianemic
  Cyanocobalamin (Systemic)
  Ethylestrenol (Systemic)
  Ferrous Fumarate (Systemic)
  Ferrous Gluconate (Systemic)
  Ferrous Sulfate (Systemic)
  Fluoxymesterone (Systemic)
  Hydroxocobalamin (Systemic)
  Iron Dextran (Systemic)
  Iron-Polysaccharide (Systemic)
  Leucovorin (Systemic)
  Nandrolone Decanoate (Systemic)
  Oxymetholone (Systemic)
  Testosterone Enanthate (Systemic)
Antianginal
  Acebutolol (Systemic)
  Amyl Nitrite (Systemic)
  Atenolol (Systemic)

Antianginal *(continued)*
    Diltiazem (Systemic)
    Erythrityl Tetranitrate (Systemic)
    Isosorbide Dinitrate (Systemic)
    Labetalol (Systemic)
    Metoprolol (Systemic)
    Nadolol (Systemic)
    Nifedipine (Systemic)
    Nitroglycerin (Systemic)
    Oxprenolol (Systemic)
    Pentaerythritol Tetranitrate (Systemic)
    Pindolol (Systemic)
    Propranolol (Systemic)
    Sotalol (Systemic)
    Timolol (Systemic)
    Verapamil (Systemic)
Antianxiety agent
    Alprazolam (Systemic)
    Buspirone (Systemic)
    Chlordiazepoxide (Systemic)
    Chlorpromazine (Systemic)
    Clomipramine (Systemic)
    Clorazepate (Systemic)
    Diazepam (Systemic)
    Halazepam (Systemic)
    Hydroxyzine (Systemic)
    Imipramine (Systemic)
    Lorazepam (Systemic)
    Meprobamate (Systemic)
    Mesoridazine (Systemic)
    Prochlorperazine (Systemic)
    Thioridazine (Systemic)
    Trifluoperazine (Systemic)
    Oxazepam (Systemic)
    Prazepam (Systemic)
Antianxiety agent–antidepressant
    Chlordiazepoxide and Amitriptyline (Systemic)
    Loxapine (Systemic)
Antianxiety therapy adjunct
    Acebutolol (Systemic)
    Metoprolol (Systemic)
    Oxprenolol (Systemic)
    Propranolol (Systemic)
Antiarrhythmic
    Acebutolol (Systemic)
    Amiodarone (Systemic)
    Atenolol (Systemic)
    Atropine, Parenteral (Systemic)
    Deslanoside (Systemic)
    Digitalis (Systemic)
    Digitoxin (Systemic)
    Digoxin (Systemic)
    Disopyramide (Systemic)
    Encainide (Systemic)
    Esmolol (Systemic)
    Flecainide (Systemic)
    Glycopyrrolate, Parenteral (Systemic)
    Hyoscyamine, Parenteral (Systemic)
    Lidocaine (Systemic)
    Metoprolol (Systemic)
    Mexiletine (Systemic)
    Nadolol (Systemic)
    Oxprenolol (Systemic)
    Phenytoin (Systemic)
    Procainamide (Systemic)
    Propranolol (Systemic)
    Quinidine (Systemic)
    Scopolamine, Parenteral (Systemic)
    Sotalol (Systemic)
    Timolol (Systemic)
    Tocainide (Systemic)
    Verapamil (Systemic)
Antiasthmatic
    Beclomethasone (Inhalation)
    Dexamethasone (Inhalation)
    Flunisolide (Inhalation)
    Triamcinolone (Inhalation)
Antibacterial-adrenocorticoid, ophthalmic
    Neomycin, Polymyxin B, and Hydrocortisone (Ophthalmic)

Antibacterial-adrenocorticoid, otic
    Colistin, Neomycin, and Hydrocortisone (Otic)
    Neomycin, Polymyxin B, and Hydrocortisone (Otic)
Antibacterial-analgesic, urinary tract
    Sulfamethoxazole and Phenazopyridine (Systemic)
    Sulfisoxazole and Phenazopyridine (Systemic)
Antibacterial-antifungal-adrenocorticoid, topical
    Clioquinol and Hydrocortisone (Topical)
Antibacterial, antileprosy agent
    Dapsone (Systemic)
    Ethionamide (Systemic)
    Rifampin (Systemic)
Antibacterial, antimycobacterial
    Clofazimine (Systemic)
    Cycloserine (Systemic)
    Ethambutol (Systemic)
    Ethionamide (Systemic)
    Isoniazid (Systemic)
    Rifampin (Systemic)
    Streptomycin (Systemic)
Antibacterial, antitubercular
    Aminosalicylate (Systemic)
    Aminosalicylic Acid (Systemic)
    Capreomycin (Systemic)
    Pyrazinamide (Systemic)
    Rifampin and Isoniazid (Systemic)
Antibacterial, dental
    Chlorhexidine (Dental)
Antibacterial, ophthalmic
    Chloramphenicol (Ophthalmic)
    Chlortetracycline (Ophthalmic)
    Erythromycin (Ophthalmic)
    Gentamicin (Ophthalmic)
    Neomycin (Ophthalmic)
    Neomycin, Polymyxin B, and Bacitracin (Ophthalmic)
    Neomycin, Polymyxin B, and Gramicidin (Ophthalmic)
    Sulfacetamide (Ophthalmic)
    Sulfisoxazole (Ophthalmic)
    Tetracycline (Ophthalmic)
Antibacterial, otic
    Chloramphenicol (Otic)
    Gentamicin (Otic)
Antibacterial, systemic
    Amdinocillin (Systemic)
    Amikacin (Systemic)
    Amoxicillin (Systemic)
    Amoxicillin and Clavulanate (Systemic)
    Ampicillin (Systemic)
    Azlocillin (Systemic)
    Aztreonam (Systemic)
    Bacampicillin (Systemic)
    Carbenicillin (Systemic)
    Cefaclor (Systemic)
    Cefadroxil (Systemic)
    Cefamandole (Systemic)
    Cefazolin (Systemic)
    Cefonicid (Systemic)
    Cefoperazone (Systemic)
    Ceforanide (Systemic)
    Cefotaxime (Systemic)
    Cefotetan (Systemic)
    Cefoxitin (Systemic)
    Ceftazidime (Systemic)
    Ceftizoxime (Systemic)
    Ceftriaxone (Systemic)
    Cefuroxime (Systemic)
    Cephalexin (Systemic)
    Cephalothin (Systemic)
    Cephapirin (Systemic)
    Cephradine (Systemic)
    Chloramphenicol (Systemic)
    Cinoxacin (Systemic)
    Clindamycin (Systemic)
    Cloxacillin (Systemic)
    Cyclacillin (Systemic)
    Cycloserine (Systemic)
    Demeclocycline (Systemic)
    Dicloxacillin (Systemic)

Antibacterial, systemic *(continued)*
    Doxycycline (Systemic)
    Erythromycin (Systemic)
    Erythromycin and Sulfisoxazole (Systemic)
    Gentamicin (Systemic)
    Imipenem and Cilastatin (Systemic)
    Kanamycin (Systemic)
    Lincomycin (Systemic)
    Methacycline (Systemic)
    Methenamine (Systemic)
    Methicillin (Systemic)
    Metronidazole (Systemic)
    Mezlocillin (Systemic)
    Minocycline (Systemic)
    Moxalactam (Systemic)
    Nafcillin (Systemic)
    Nalidixic Acid (Systemic)
    Netilmicin (Systemic)
    Nitrofurantoin (Systemic)
    Norfloxacin (Systemic)
    Oxacillin (Systemic)
    Oxytetracycline (Systemic)
    Penicillin G (Systemic)
    Penicillin V (Systemic)
    Piperacillin (Systemic)
    Rifampin (Systemic)
    Streptomycin (Systemic)
    Sulfacytine (Systemic)
    Sulfamethoxazole (Systemic)
    Sulfamethoxazole and Trimethoprim (Systemic)
    Sulfisoxazole (Systemic)
    Tetracycline (Systemic)
    Ticarcillin (Systemic)
    Ticarcillin and Clavulanate (Systemic)
    Tobramycin (Systemic)
    Trimethoprim (Systemic)
    Vancomycin (Oral)
    Vancomycin (Systemic)
Antibacterial, topical
    Chloramphenicol (Topical)
    Chlortetracycline (Topical)
    Clindamycin (Topical)
    Clioquinol (Topical)
    Erythromycin (Topical)
    Gentamicin (Topical)
    Neomycin (Topical)
    Neomycin, Polymyxin B, and Bacitracin (Topical)
    Tetracycline (Topical)
Antibiotic therapy adjunct
    Probenecid (Systemic)
Anticholelithic
    Chenodiol (Systemic)
Anticoagulant
    Anisindione (Systemic)
    Dicumarol (Systemic)
    Heparin (Systemic)
    Warfarin (Systemic)
Anticonvulsant
    Acetazolamide (Systemic)
    Amobarbital, Parenteral (Systemic)
    Carbamazepine (Systemic)
    Clonazepam (Systemic)
    Clorazepate (Systemic)
    Diazepam (Systemic)
    Divalproex (Systemic)
    Ethosuximide (Systemic)
    Ethotoin (Systemic)
    Lorazepam, Parenteral (Systemic)
    Magnesium Sulfate (Systemic)
    Mephenytoin (Systemic)
    Mephobarbital (Systemic)
    Metharbital (Systemic)
    Methsuximide (Systemic)
    Paraldehyde (Systemic)
    Paramethadione (Systemic)
    Pentobarbital, Parenteral (Systemic)
    Phenobarbital (Systemic)
    Phensuximide (Systemic)
    Phenytoin (Systemic)
    Primidone (Systemic)

Anticonvulsant *(continued)*
  Secobarbital, Parenteral (Systemic)
  Trimethadione (Systemic)
  Valproic Acid (Systemic)
Anticonvulsant, specific in juvenile my-
  oclonic seizures
  Corticotropin (Systemic)
Antidepressant
  Amitriptyline (Systemic)
  Amoxapine (Systemic)
  Clomipramine (Systemic)
  Desipramine (Systemic)
  Doxepin (Systemic)
  Imipramine (Systemic)
  Isocarboxazid (Systemic)
  Maprotiline (Systemic)
  Nortriptyline (Systemic)
  Phenelzine (Systemic)
  Protriptyline (Systemic)
  Tranylcypromine (Systemic)
  Trazodone (Systemic)
  Trimipramine (Systemic)
Antidepressant therapy adjunct
  Lithium (Systemic)
Antidiabetic
  Acetohexamide (Systemic)
  Chlorpropamide (Systemic)
  Glipizide (Systemic)
  Glyburide (Systemic)
  Insulin (Systemic)
  Tolazamide (Systemic)
  Tolbutamide (Systemic)
Antidiarrheal
  Aluminum Hydroxide (Oral)
  Charcoal, Activated (Oral)
  Codeine (Systemic)
  Difenoxin and Atropine (Systemic)
  Diphenoxylate and Atropine (Systemic)
  Glycopyrrolate (Systemic)
  Kaolin and Pectin (Oral)
  Kaolin, Pectin, Belladonna Alkaloids, and
    Kaolin, Pectin, and Paregoric (Sys-
    temic)
  Loperamide (Oral)
  Opium (Systemic)
  Opium Tincture (Systemic)
  Paregoric (Systemic)
  Polycarbophil (Oral)
  Psyllium Hydrophilic Mucilloid (Oral)
Antidiarrheal, postoperative colonic bile acids
  Cholestyramine (Systemic)
  Colestipol (Systemic)
Antidiuretic
  Carbamazepine (Systemic)
  Chlorpropamide (Systemic)
Antidiuretic, central diabetes insipidus
  Clofibrate (Systemic)
  Desmopressin (Systemic)
  Lypressin (Systemic)
  Vasopressin (Systemic)
Antidiuretic, central and nephrogenic diabe-
  tes insipidus
  Bendroflumethiazide (Systemic)
  Benzthiazide (Systemic)
  Chlorothiazide (Systemic)
  Chlorthalidone (Systemic)
  Cyclothiazide (Systemic)
  Hydrochlorothiazide (Systemic)
  Hydroflumethiazide (Systemic)
  Methyclothiazide (Systemic)
  Metolazone (Systemic)
  Polythiazide (Systemic)
  Quinethazone (Systemic)
  Trichlormethiazide (Systemic)
Antidote adjunct, to tricyclic antidepressants
  Glucagon (Systemic)
Antidote, adsorbent
  Charcoal, Activated (Oral)
Antidote, anion-exchange resin
  Cholestyramine (Systemic)
  Colestipol (Systemic)
Antidote, to beta-adrenergic blocking agents
  Glucagon (Systemic)

Antidote, to cholinesterase inhibitors
  Atropine, Parenteral (Systemic)
  Hyoscyamine, Parenteral (Systemic)
Antidote, to curariform block
  Neostigmine, Parenteral (Systemic)
  Pyridostigmine, Parenteral (Systemic)
Antidote, to cyanide poisoning
  Amyl Nitrite (Systemic)
Antidote, to cycloserine poisoning
  Pyridoxine (Systemic)
Antidote, to drug-induced hypoprothrombine-
  mia
  Menadiol (Systemic)
  Phytonadione (Systemic)
Antidote, to ergot alkaloid poisoning
  Prazosin (Systemic)
Antidote, to folic acid antagonists
  Leucovorin (Systemic)
Antidote, to heavy metals
  Penicillamine (Systemic)
Antidote, to heparin
  Protamine (Systemic)
Antidote, to isoniazid poisoning
  Pyridoxine (Systemic)
Antidote, to muscarine
  Atropine, Parenteral (Systemic)
  Hyoscyamine, Parenteral (Systemic)
Antidote, to organophosphate pesticides
  Atropine, Parenteral (Systemic)
Antidote, to quinidine
  Glucagon (Systemic)
Antidyskinetic
  Amantadine (Systemic)
  Benztropine (Systemic)
  Biperiden (Systemic)
  Bromocriptine (Systemic)
  Carbidopa and Levodopa (Systemic)
  Diphenhydramine (Systemic)
  Ethopropazine (Systemic)
  Levodopa (Systemic)
  Procyclidine (Systemic)
  Trihexyphenidyl (Systemic)
Antidyskinetic, Gilles de la Tourette's syn-
  drome
  Haloperidol (Systemic)
  Pimozide (Systemic)
Antidysmenorrheal
  Belladonna (Systemic)
  Clonidine (Systemic)
  Fenoprofen (Systemic)
  Hyoscyamine and Scopolamine (Sys-
    temic)
  Ibuprofen (Systemic)
  Indomethacin (Systemic—Anti-inflamma-
    tory, Nonsteroidal)
  Isoxsuprine (Systemic)
  Ketoprofen (Systemic)
  Mefenamic Acid (Systemic)
  Naproxen (Systemic)
Antiemetic
  Buclizine (Systemic)
  Chlorpromazine (Systemic)
  Cyclizine (Systemic)
  Dimenhydrinate (Systemic)
  Diphenhydramine (Systemic)
  Diphenidol (Systemic)
  Dronabinol (Systemic)
  Haloperidol (Systemic)
  Hydroxyzine, Parenteral (Systemic)
  Meclizine (Systemic)
  Metoclopramide (Systemic)
  Perphenazine (Systemic)
  Prochlorperazine (Systemic)
  Promethazine (Systemic)
  Scopolamine (Systemic)
  Triflupromazine (Systemic)
  Trimethobenzamide (Systemic)
Antiemetic, in cancer chemotherapy
  Corticotropin (Systemic)
  Dexamethasone (Systemic)
  Hydrocortisone (Systemic)
  Prednisone (Systemic)
Antienuretic
  Imipramine Hydrochloride (Systemic)

Antifibrotic
  Aminobenzoate Potassium (Systemic)
Antiflatulent
  Charcoal, Activated (Oral)
  Simethicone (Oral)
Antifungal-adrenocorticoid, topical
  Nystatin and Triamcinolone (Topical)
Antifungal, ophthalmic
  Natamycin (Ophthalmic)
Antifungal, systemic
  Amphotericin B (Systemic)
  Clotrimazole (Oral)
  Flucytosine (Systemic)
  Griseofulvin (Systemic)
  Ketoconazole (Systemic)
  Miconazole (Systemic)
  Nystatin (Oral)
  Potassium Iodide (Systemic)
Antifungal, topical
  Carbol-Fuchsin (Topical)
  Ciclopirox (Topical)
  Clioquinol (Topical)
  Clotrimazole (Topical)
  Econazole (Topical)
  Haloprogin (Topical)
  Ketoconazole (Topical)
  Nystatin (Topical)
  Miconazole (Topical)
  Tolnaftate (Topical)
Antifungal, vaginal
  Clotrimazole (Vaginal)
  Gentian Violet (Vaginal)
  Miconazole (Vaginal)
  Nystatin (Vaginal)
Antiglaucoma agent, ophthalmic
  Betaxolol (Ophthalmic)
  Carbachol (Ophthalmic)
  Demecarium (Ophthalmic)
  Dipivefrin (Ophthalmic)
  Echothiophate (Ophthalmic)
  Epinephrine (Ophthalmic)
  Epinephrine Bitartrate (Ophthalmic)
  Epinephryl Borate (Ophthalmic)
  Isoflurophate (Ophthalmic)
  Levobunolol (Ophthalmic)
  Physostigmine (Ophthalmic)
  Pilocarpine (Ophthalmic)
  Timolol (Ophthalmic)
Antiglaucoma agent, systemic
  Acetazolamide (Systemic)
  Dichlorphenamide (Systemic)
  Glycerin (Systemic)
  Methazolamide (Systemic)
  Timolol (Systemic)
Antigout agent
  Allopurinol (Systemic)
  Colchicine (Systemic)
  Fenoprofen (Systemic)
  Ibuprofen (Systemic)
  Indomethacin (Systemic—Anti-inflamma-
    tory, Nonsteroidal)
  Ketoprofen (Systemic)
  Naproxen (Systemic)
  Phenylbutazone (Systemic)
  Piroxicam (Systemic)
  Probenecid (Systemic)
  Probenecid and Colchicine (Systemic)
  Sulfinpyrazone (Systemic)
  Sulindac (Systemic)
Antihemorrhagic
  Desmopressin, Parenteral (Systemic)
  Phytonadione (Systemic)
Antihemorrhagic, postpartum and postabor-
  tal uterine bleeding
  Carboprost (Systemic)
  Dinoprostone (Vaginal)
  Oxytocin, Parenteral (Systemic)
Antihemorrhagic, topical
  Epinephrine Injection (Systemic)
Antihistaminic, H_1-receptor
  Azatadine (Systemic)
  Bromodiphenhydramine (Systemic)
  Brompheniramine (Systemic)
  Carbinoxamine (Systemic)
  Chlorpheniramine (Systemic)

Antihistaminic, H₁-receptor *(continued)*
    Clemastine (Systemic)
    Cyproheptadine (Systemic)
    Dexchlorpheniramine (Systemic)
    Dimenhydrinate (Systemic)
    Diphenhydramine (Systemic)
    Diphenylpyraline (Systemic)
    Doxylamine (Systemic)
    Hydroxyzine (Systemic)
    Phenindamine (Systemic)
    Promethazine (Systemic)
    Pyrilamine (Systemic)
    Terfenadine (Systemic)
    Trimeprazine (Systemic)
    Tripelennamine (Systemic)
    Triprolidine (Systemic)
Antihistaminic (H₁-receptor)-antitussive
    Bromodiphenhydramine and Codeine (Systemic)
    Chlorpheniramine and Codeine (Systemic)
    Chlorpheniramine and Dextromethorphan (Systemic)
    Phenyltoloxamine and Hydrocodone (Systemic)
    Promethazine and Codeine (Systemic)
    Promethazine and Dextromethorphan (Systemic)
Antihistaminic (H₁-receptor)-antitussive-analgesic
    Chlorpheniramine, Codeine, Aspirin, and Caffeine (Systemic)
    Chlorpheniramine, Dextromethorphan, and Acetaminophen (Systemic)
Antihistaminic (H₁-receptor)-antitussive-expectorant
    Bromodiphenhydramine, Diphenhydramine, Codeine, Ammonium Chloride, and Potassium Guaiacolsulfonate (Systemic)
    Chlorpheniramine, Codeine, Carbetapentane, Guaifenesin, Sodium Citrate, and Citric Acid (Systemic)
    Diphenhydramine, Codeine, and Ammonium Chloride (Systemic)
    Diphenhydramine, Dextromethorphan, and Ammonium Chloride (Systemic)
    Phenindamine, Hydrocodone, and Guaifenesin (Systemic)
    Pheniramine, Codeine, and Guaifenesin (Systemic)
    Pheniramine, Pyrilamine, Hydrocodone, and Potassium Citrate (Systemic)
    Pyrilamine, Codeine, and Terpin Hydrate (Systemic)
Antihistaminic (H₁-receptor)-decongestant
    Azatadine and Pseudoephedrine (Systemic)
    Brompheniramine, Phenylephrine, and Phenylpropanolamine (Systemic)
    Brompheniramine and Phenylpropanolamine (Systemic)
    Brompheniramine and Pseudoephedrine (Systemic)
    Carbinoxamine and Pseudoephedrine (Systemic)
    Chlorpheniramine and Pseudoephedrine (Systemic)
    Chlorpheniramine, Pyrilamine, and Phenylpropanolamine (Systemic)
    Chlorpheniramine, Tripelennamine, Phenylpropanolamine, and Phenylephrine (Systemic)
    Clemastine and Phenylpropanolamine (Systemic)
    Dexbrompheniramine and Pseudoephedrine (Systemic)
    Diphenhydramine and Pseudoephedrine (Systemic)
    Phenindamine, Chlorpheniramine, and Phenylpropanolamine (Systemic)
    Phenylephrine and Brompheniramine (Systemic)
    Phenylephrine and Chlorpheniramine (Systemic)

Antihistaminic (H₁-receptor)-decongestant *(continued)*
    Phenylephrine, Chlorpheniramine, and Pyrilamine (Systemic)
    Phenylephrine, Phenylpropanolamine, and Chlorpheniramine (Systemic)
    Phenylephrine, Phenylpropanolamine, Pyrilamine, and Chlorpheniramine (Systemic)
    Phenylpropanolamine and Chlorpheniramine (Systemic)
    Phenylpropanolamine, Pheniramine, and Pyrilamine (Systemic)
    Phenylpropanolamine, Phenylephrine, Phenyltoloxamine, and Chlorpheniramine (Systemic)
    Phenylpropanolamine, Phenyltoloxamine, Pyrilamine, and Pheniramine (Systemic)
    Promethazine and Phenylephrine (Systemic)
    Promethazine and Pseudoephedrine (Systemic)
    Pseudoephedrine and Chlorcyclizine (Systemic)
    Triprolidine and Pseudoephedrine (Systemic)
Antihistaminic (H₁-receptor)-decongestant-antitussive
    Brompheniramine, Phenylephrine, Phenylpropanolamine, and Codeine (Systemic)
    Brompheniramine, Phenylephrine, Phenylpropanolamine, and Dextromethorphan (Systemic)
    Brompheniramine, Phenylpropanolamine, and Codeine (Systemic)
    Brompheniramine, Phenylpropanolamine, and Dextromethorphan (Systemic)
    Brompheniramine, Pseudoephedrine, and Dextromethorphan (Systemic)
    Carbinoxamine, Pseudoephedrine, and Dextromethorphan (Systemic)
    Chlorpheniramine, Ephedrine, Phenylephrine, and Carbetapentane (Systemic)
    Chlorpheniramine, Phenylephrine, and Dextromethorphan (Systemic)
    Chlorpheniramine, Phenylephrine, and Hydrocodone (Systemic)
    Chlorpheniramine, Phenylephrine, Phenylpropanolamine, and Codeine (Systemic)
    Chlorpheniramine, Phenylephrine, Phenylpropanolamine, and Dextromethorphan (Systemic)
    Chlorpheniramine, Phenylephrine, Phenylpropanolamine, and Dihydrocodeine (Systemic)
    Chlorpheniramine, Phenylpropanolamine, and Caramiphen (Systemic)
    Chlorpheniramine, Phenylpropanolamine, and Dextromethorphan (Systemic)
    Chlorpheniramine, Pseudoephedrine, and Codeine (Systemic)
    Chlorpheniramine, Pseudoephedrine, and Dextromethorphan (Systemic)
    Chlorpheniramine, Pseudoephedrine, and Hydrocodone (Systemic)
    Diphenylpyraline, Phenylephrine, and Codeine (Systemic)
    Diphenylpyraline, Phenylephrine, and Dextromethorphan (Systemic)
    Diphenylpyraline, Phenylephrine, and Hydrocodone (Systemic)
    Pheniramine, Pyrilamine, Phenylephrine, Phenylpropanolamine, and Hydrocodone (Systemic)
    Pheniramine, Pyrilamine, Phenylpropanolamine, and Dextromethorphan (Systemic)
    Pheniramine, Pyrilamine, Phenylpropanolamine, and Hydrocodone (Systemic)
    Promethazine, Phenylephrine, and Codeine (Systemic)
    Pyrilamine, Phenylephrine, and Codeine (Systemic)

Antihistaminic (H₁-receptor)-decongestant-antitussive *(continued)*
    Pyrilamine, Phenylephrine, and Dextromethorphan (Systemic)
    Pyrilamine, Phenylephrine, and Hydrocodone (Systemic)
    Triprolidine, Pseudoephedrine, and Codeine (Systemic)
    Triprolidine, Pseudoephedrine, and Dextromethorphan (Systemic)
Antihistaminic (H₁-receptor)-decongestant-antitussive-analgesic
    Chlorpheniramine, Phenindamine, Phenylephrine, Dextromethorphan, Acetaminophen, Salicylamide, Caffeine, and Ascorbic Acid (Systemic)
    Chlorpheniramine, Pheniramine, Pyrilamine, Phenylephrine, Hydrocodone, Salicylamide, Caffeine, and Ascorbic Acid (Systemic)
    Chlorpheniramine, Phenylephrine, Codeine, and Acetaminophen (Systemic)
    Chlorpheniramine, Phenylephrine, Dextromethorphan, Acetaminophen, and Salicylamide (Systemic)
    Chlorpheniramine, Phenylephrine, Hydrocodone, Acetaminophen, and Caffeine (Systemic)
    Chlorpheniramine, Phenylpropanolamine, Dextromethorphan, and Acetaminophen (Systemic)
    Chlorpheniramine, Phenylpropanolamine, Dextromethorphan, Acetaminophen, and Caffeine (Systemic)
    Chlorpheniramine, Pseudoephedrine, Dextromethorphan, and Acetaminophen (Systemic)
    Doxylamine, Pseudoephedrine, Dextromethorphan, and Acetaminophen (Systemic)
    Pheniramine, Pyrilamine, Phenylpropanolamine, Codeine, Acetaminophen, and Caffeine (Systemic)
    Pyrilamine, Phenylephrine, Dextromethorphan, and Acetaminophen (Systemic)
    Pyrilamine, Phenylpropanolamine, Dextromethorphan, and Sodium Salicylate (Systemic)
Antihistaminic (H₁-receptor)-decongestant-antitussive-expectorant
    Brompheniramine, Phenylephrine, Phenylpropanolamine, Codeine, and Guaifenesin (Systemic)
    Brompheniramine, Phenylephrine, Phenylpropanolamine, Hydrocodone, and Guaifenesin (Systemic)
    Chlorpheniramine, Ephedrine, Phenylephrine, Dextromethorphan, Ammonium Chloride, and Ipecac (Systemic)
    Chlorpheniramine, Phenindamine, Pyrilamine, Phenylephrine, Hydrocodone, and Ammonium Chloride (Systemic)
    Chlorpheniramine, Phenylephrine, Codeine, and Ammonium Chloride (Systemic)
    Chlorpheniramine, Phenylephrine, Codeine, Ammonium Chloride, Potassium Guaiacolsulfonate, and Sodium Citrate (Systemic)
    Chlorpheniramine, Phenylephrine, Codeine, and Potassium Iodide (Systemic)
    Chlorpheniramine, Phenylephrine, Dextromethorphan, and Guaifenesin (Systemic)
    Chlorpheniramine, Phenylephrine, Dextromethorphan, Guaifenesin, and Ammonium Chloride (Systemic)
    Chlorpheniramine, Phenylephrine, Phenylpropanolamine, Carbetapentane, and Potassium Guaiacolsulfonate (Systemic)
    Chlorpheniramine, Phenylpropanolamine, Dextromethorphan, and Ammonium Chloride (Systemic)

Antihistaminic (H₁-receptor)-decongestant-
antitussive-expectorant *(continued)*
  Chlorpheniramine, Phenylpropanolamine,
    Dextromethorphan, Ammonium Chlo-
    ride, Terpin Hydrate, and Sodium Ci-
    trate (Systemic)
  Chlorpheniramine, Phenyltoloxamine,
    Ephedrine, Codeine, and Guaiacol
    Carbonate (Systemic)
  Diphenylpyraline, Phenylephrine, Hydro-
    codone, and Guaifenesin (Systemic)
  Pheniramine, Pyrilamine, Phenylpropa-
    nolamine, Dextromethorphan, and
    Ammonium Chloride (Systemic)
  Pheniramine, Pyrilamine, Phenylpropa-
    nolamine, Dextromethorphan, and
    Guaifenesin (Systemic)
  Pheniramine, Pyrilamine, Phenylpropa-
    nolamine, Hydrocodone, and Guai-
    fenesin (Systemic)
  Pyrilamine, Phenylephrine, Hydrocodone,
    and Ammonium Chloride (Systemic)
  Triprolidine, Pseudoephedrine, Codeine,
    and Guaifenesin (Systemic)
Antihistaminic (H₁-receptor)-decongestant-
antitussive-expectorant-analgesic
  Chlorpheniramine, Phenylephrine,
    Phenylpropanolamine, Dextromethor-
    phan, Guaifenesin, and Acetamino-
    phen (Systemic)
  Chlorpheniramine, Phenylpropanolamine,
    Codeine, Guaifenesin, and Acetami-
    nophen (Systemic)
  Chlorpheniramine, Phenylpropanolamine,
    Hydrocodone, Guaifenesin, and Sali-
    cylamide (Systemic)
  Chlorpheniramine, Pseudoephedrine,
    Dextromethorphan, Guaifenesin, and
    Aspirin (Systemic)
  Pheniramine, Phenylephrine, Codeine,
    Sodium Citrate, Sodium Salicylate,
    and Caffeine (Systemic)
  Pheniramine, Pyrilamine, Phenylpropanol-
    amine, Dextromethorphan, Terpin Hy-
    drate, and Acetaminophen (Systemic)
Antihistaminic (H₁-receptor)-decongestant-
expectorant
  Brompheniramine, Phenylephrine,
    Phenylpropanolamine, and Guaifene-
    sin (Systemic)
  Carbinoxamine, Pseudoephedrine, and
    Guaifenesin (Systemic)
  Chlorpheniramine, Ephedrine, and Guai-
    fenesin (Systemic)
  Chlorpheniramine, Phenylephrine, and
    Guaifenesin (Systemic)
  Chlorpheniramine, Phenylpropanolamine,
    and Guaifenesin (Systemic)
  Chlorpheniramine, Phenylpropanolamine,
    Guaifenesin, Sodium Citrate, and Cit-
    ric Acid (Systemic)
  Chlorpheniramine, Pseudoephedrine, and
    Guaifenesin (Systemic)
  Dexchlorpheniramine, Pseudoephedrine,
    and Guaifenesin (Systemic)
  Pheniramine, Pyrilamine, Phenylpropa-
    nolamine, and Guaifenesin (Systemic)
Antihyperammonemic
  Lactulose (Oral)
Antihyperbilirubinemic
  Phenobarbital (Systemic)
Antihypercalcemic
  Bumetanide (Systemic)
  Calcitonin-Human (Systemic)
  Calcitonin-Salmon (Systemic)
  Ethacrynic Acid (Systemic)
  Etidronate (Systemic)
  Furosemide (Systemic)
  Plicamycin (Systemic)
Antihypercalciuric
  Plicamycin (Systemic)
Antihyperkalemic
  Calcium Chloride (Systemic)
  Calcium Gluconate, Parenteral (Systemic)

Antihyperlipidemic
  Cholestyramine (Systemic)
  Clofibrate (Systemic)
  Colestipol (Systemic)
  Dextrothyroxine (Systemic)
  Gemfibrozil (Systemic)
  Neomycin (Oral)
  Niacin (Systemic)
  Nicotinyl Alcohol (Systemic)
  Probucol (Systemic)
Antihypermagnesemic
  Calcium Chloride (Systemic)
  Calcium Gluceptate (Systemic)
  Calcium Gluconate, Parenteral (Sys-
    temic)
Antihyperoxaluric
  Cholestyramine (Systemic)
  Colestipol (Systemic)
Antihyperphosphatemic
  Aluminum Carbonate (Oral)
  Aluminum Hydroxide (Oral)
  Calcium Carbonate (Oral)
  Calcium Carbonate (Systemic)
  Calcium Citrate (Systemic)
Antihyperprolactinemic
  Bromocriptine (Systemic)
Antihypertensive
  Acebutolol (Systemic)
  Alseroxylon (Systemic)
  Amiloride (Systemic)
  Amiloride and Hydrochlorothiazide (Sys-
    temic)
  Atenolol (Systemic)
  Atenolol and Chlorthalidone (Systemic)
  Bendroflumethiazide (Systemic)
  Benzthiazide (Systemic)
  Bumetanide (Systemic)
  Captopril (Systemic)
  Captopril and Hydrochlorothiazide (Sys-
    temic)
  Chlorothiazide (Systemic)
  Chlorthalidone (Systemic)
  Clonidine (Systemic)
  Clonidine and Chlorthalidone (Systemic)
  Cyclothiazide (Systemic)
  Deserpidine (Systemic)
  Deserpidine and Hydrochlorothiazide
    (Systemic)
  Deserpidine and Methyclothiazide (Sys-
    temic)
  Diltiazem (Systemic)
  Enalapril (Systemic)
  Enalapril and Hydrochlorothiazide (Sys-
    temic)
  Ethacrynic Acid (Systemic)
  Furosemide (Systemic)
  Guanabenz (Systemic)
  Guanadrel (Systemic)
  Guanethidine (Systemic)
  Guanethidine and Hydrochlorothiazide
    (Systemic)
  Guanfacine (Systemic)
  Hydralazine (Systemic)
  Hydralazine and Hydrochlorothiazide
    (Systemic)
  Hydrochlorothiazide (Systemic)
  Hydroflumethiazide (Systemic)
  Indapamide (Systemic)
  Labetalol (Systemic)
  Labetalol and Hydrochlorothiazide (Sys-
    temic)
  Mecamylamine (Systemic)
  Methyclothiazide (Systemic)
  Methyldopa (Systemic)
  Methyldopa and Chlorothiazide (Sys-
    temic)
  Methyldopa and Hydrochlorothiazide
    (Systemic)
  Metolazone (Systemic)
  Metoprolol (Systemic)
  Metoprolol and Hydrochlorothiazide
    (Systemic)
  Minoxidil (Systemic)
  Nadolol (Systemic)

Antihypertensive *(continued)*
  Nadolol and Bendroflumethiazide (Sys-
    temic)
  Nifedipine (Systemic)
  Oxprenolol (Systemic)
  Pargyline (Systemic)
  Pargyline and Methyclothiazide (Sys-
    temic)
  Pindolol (Systemic)
  Pindolol and Hydrochlorothiazide (Sys-
    temic)
  Polythiazide (Systemic)
  Prazosin (Systemic)
  Prazosin and Polythiazide (Systemic)
  Propranolol (Systemic)
  Propranolol and Hydrochlorothiazide
    (Systemic)
  Quinethazone (Systemic)
  Rauwolfia Serpentina (Systemic)
  Rauwolfia Serpentina and Bendroflume-
    thiazide (Systemic)
  Reserpine (Systemic)
  Reserpine and Chlorothiazide (Systemic)
  Reserpine and Chlorthalidone (Systemic)
  Reserpine and Hydralazine (Systemic)
  Reserpine, Hydralazine, and Hydrochlo-
    rothiazide (Systemic)
  Reserpine and Hydrochlorothiazide (Sys-
    temic)
  Reserpine and Hydroflumethiazide (Sys-
    temic)
  Reserpine and Methyclothiazide (Sys-
    temic)
  Reserpine and Polythiazide (Systemic)
  Reserpine and Quinethazone (Systemic)
  Reserpine and Trichlormethiazide (Sys-
    temic)
  Sotalol (Systemic)
  Spironolactone (Systemic)
  Spironolactone and Hydrochlorothiazide
    (Systemic)
  Timolol (Systemic)
  Timolol and Hydrochlorothiazide (Sys-
    temic)
  Triamterene (Systemic)
  Triamterene and Hydrochlorothiazide
    (Systemic)
  Trichlormethiazide (Systemic)
  Verapamil (Systemic)
Antihypertensive, pheochromocytoma
  Metyrosine (Systemic)
  Phenoxybenzamine (Systemic)
Antihyperthyroid agent
  Ipodate (Systemic)
  Methimazole (Systemic)
  Potassium Iodide (Systemic)
  Propylthiouracil (Systemic)
  Sodium Iodide I 131 (Therapeutic)
Antihyperuricemic
  Allopurinol (Systemic)
  Probenecid (Systemic)
  Sulfinpyrazone (Systemic)
Antihypocalcemic
  Aluminum Hydroxide (Oral)
  Calcifediol (Systemic)
  Calcitriol (Systemic)
  Calcium Carbonate (Oral)
  Calcium Carbonate (Systemic)
  Calcium Chloride (Systemic)
  Calcium Citrate (Systemic)
  Calcium Glubionate (Systemic)
  Calcium Gluceptate (Systemic)
  Calcium Gluconate (Systemic)
  Calcium Lactate (Systemic)
  Calcium Phosphate, Dibasic (Systemic)
  Calcium Phosphate, Tribasic (Systemic)
  Diazoxide (Oral)
  Dihydrotachysterol (Systemic)
  Ergocalciferol (Systemic)
  Glucagon (Systemic)
Antihypokalemic
  Amiloride (Systemic)
  Amiloride and Hydrochlorothiazide (Sys-
    temic)
  Spironolactone (Systemic)

Antihypokalemic *(continued)*
  Spironolactone and Hydrochlorothiazide (Systemic)
  Triamterene (Systemic)
  Triamterene and Hydrochlorothiazide (Systemic)
Antihypoparathyroid
  Calcifediol (Systemic)
  Calcitriol (Systemic)
  Dihydrotachysterol (Systemic)
  Ergocalciferol (Systemic)
Antihypotensive
  Dihydroergotamine (Systemic)
Antihypotensive, idiopathic orthostatic hypotension
  Fludrocortisone (Systemic)
Anti-inflammatory, local, interstitial cystitis
  Dimethyl Sulfoxide (Mucosal)
Anti-inflammatory, nonsteroidal
  Aspirin (Systemic)
  Aspirin, Alumina, and Magnesia (Systemic)
  Aspirin, Buffered (Systemic)
  Choline Salicylate (Systemic)
  Choline and Magnesium Salicylates (Systemic)
  Diflunisal (Systemic)
  Fenoprofen (Systemic)
  Flurbiprofen (Ophthalmic)
  Ibuprofen (Systemic)
  Indomethacin (Systemic—Anti-inflammatory, Nonsteroidal)
  Ketoprofen (Systemic)
  Magnesium Salicylate (Systemic)
  Meclofenamate (Systemic)
  Naproxen (Systemic)
  Piroxicam (Systemic)
  Salsalate (Systemic)
  Sodium Salicylate (Systemic)
  Sulindac (Systemic)
  Tolmetin (Systemic)
Anti-inflammatory, steroidal, nasal
  Beclomethasone (Nasal)
  Dexamethasone (Nasal)
  Flunisolide (Nasal)
Anti-inflammatory, steroidal, ophthalmic
  Betamethasone (Ophthalmic)
  Dexamethasone (Ophthalmic)
  Fluorometholone (Ophthalmic)
  Hydrocortisone (Ophthalmic)
  Medrysone (Ophthalmic)
  Prednisolone (Ophthalmic)
Anti-inflammatory, steroidal, otic
  Betamethasone (Otic)
  Desonide and Acetic Acid (Otic)
  Dexamethasone (Otic)
  Hydrocortisone (Otic)
  Hydrocortisone and Acetic Acid (Otic)
  Prednisolone (Otic)
Anti-inflammatory, steroidal, systemic
  Betamethasone (Systemic)
  Cortisone (Systemic)
  Dexamethasone (Systemic)
  Hydrocortisone (Systemic)
  Methylprednisolone (Systemic)
  Paramethasone (Systemic)
  Prednisolone (Systemic)
  Prednisone (Systemic)
  Triamcinolone (Systemic)
Anti-inflammatory, steroidal, topical
  Amcinonide (Topical)
  Betamethasone (Topical)
  Clobetasol (Topical)
  Clocortolone (Topical)
  Desonide (Topical)
  Desoximetasone (Topical)
  Dexamethasone (Topical)
  Diflorasone (Topical)
  Flumethasone (Topical)
  Fluocinolone (Topical)
  Fluocinonide (Topical)
  Flurandrenolide (Topical)
  Halcinonide (Topical)

Anti-inflammatory, steroidal, topical *(continued)*
  Hydrocortisone (Topical)
  Methylprednisolone (Topical)
  Triamcinolone (Topical)
Antimanic
  Carbamazepine (Systemic)
  Lithium (Systemic)
Antimuscarinic
  Anisotropine (Systemic)
  Atropine (Systemic)
  Belladonna (Systemic)
  Clidinium (Systemic)
  Dicyclomine (Systemic)
  Glycopyrrolate (Systemic)
  Hexocyclium (Systemic)
  Homatropine (Systemic)
  Hyoscyamine (Systemic)
  Hyoscyamine and Scopolamine (Systemic)
  Isopropamide (Systemic)
  Mepenzolate (Systemic)
  Methantheline (Systemic)
  Methscopolamine (Systemic)
  Oxyphencyclimine (Systemic)
  Oxyphenonium (Systemic)
  Pirenzepine (Systemic)
  Propantheline (Systemic)
  Scopolamine (Systemic)
  Tridihexethyl (Systemic)
Antimuscarinic-antibacterial-analgesic, urinary tract
  Atropine, Hyoscyamine, Methenamine, Methylene Blue, Phenyl Salicylate, and Benzoic Acid (Systemic)
Antimuscarinic-sedative
  Atropine, Hyoscyamine, Scopolamine, and Butabarbital (Systemic)
  Atropine, Hyoscyamine, Scopolamine, and Phenobarbital (Systemic)
  Atropine and Phenobarbital (Systemic)
  Belladonna and Butabarbital (Systemic)
  Belladonna and Phenobarbital (Systemic)
  Chlordiazepoxide and Clidinium (Systemic)
  Hyoscyamine and Phenobarbital (Systemic)
  Hyoscyamine, Scopolamine, and Phenobarbital (Systemic)
Antimyasthenic
  Ambenonium (Systemic)
  Neostigmine (Systemic)
  Pyridostigmine (Systemic)
Antimyotonic
  Quinine (Systemic)
Antineoplastic, systemic
  Aminoglutethimide (Systemic)
  Asparaginase (Systemic)
  Bleomycin (Systemic)
  Busulfan (Systemic)
  Carmustine (Systemic)
  Chlorambucil (Systemic)
  Chlorotrianisene (Systemic)
  Chromic Phosphate P 32 (Therapeutic)
  Cisplatin (Systemic)
  Cyclophosphamide (Systemic)
  Cytarabine (Systemic)
  Dacarbazine (Systemic)
  Dactinomycin (Systemic)
  Daunorubicin (Systemic)
  Diethylstilbestrol (Systemic)
  Doxorubicin (Systemic)
  Dromostanolone (Systemic)
  Estradiol (Systemic)
  Estradiol Valerate (Systemic)
  Estramustine (Systemic)
  Estrogens, Conjugated (Systemic)
  Estrogens, Esterified (Systemic)
  Estrone (Systemic)
  Ethinyl Estradiol (Systemic)
  Etoposide (Systemic)
  Floxuridine (Systemic)
  Fluorouracil (Systemic)
  Fluoxymesterone (Systemic)
  Hydroxyprogesterone (Systemic)

Antineoplastic, systemic *(continued)*
  Hydroxyurea (Systemic)
  Interferon Alfa-2a, Recombinant (Systemic)
  Interferon Alfa-2b, Recombinant (Systemic)
  Ketoconazole (Systemic)
  Leuprolide (Systemic)
  Levothyroxine (Systemic)
  Liothyronine (Systemic)
  Liotrix (Systemic)
  Lomustine (Systemic)
  Mechlorethamine (Systemic)
  Medroxyprogesterone, Parenteral (Systemic)
  Megestrol (Systemic)
  Melphalan (Systemic)
  Mercaptopurine (Systemic)
  Methotrexate (Systemic)
  Methyltestosterone (Systemic)
  Mitomycin (Systemic)
  Mitotane (Systemic)
  Nandrolone Phenpropionate (Systemic)
  Plicamycin (Systemic)
  Procarbazine (Systemic)
  Sodium Iodide I 131 (Therapeutic)
  Sodium Phosphate P 32 (Therapeutic)
  Streptozocin (Systemic)
  Tamoxifen (Systemic)
  Testolactone (Systemic)
  Testosterone (Systemic)
  Thioguanine (Systemic)
  Thiotepa (Systemic)
  Thyroglobulin (Systemic)
  Thyroid (Systemic)
  Thyrotropin (Systemic)
  Uracil Mustard (Systemic)
  Vinblastine (Systemic)
  Vincristine (Systemic)
Antineoplastic, topical
  Fluorouracil (Topical)
  Mechlorethamine (Topical)
Antineuralgia adjunct
  Chlorpromazine (Systemic)
  Fluphenazine (Systemic)
Antineuralgic
  Amitriptyline (Systemic)
  Doxepin (Systemic)
  Imipramine (Systemic)
  Nortriptyline (Systemic)
  Phenytoin (Systemic)
  Trazodone (Systemic)
Antineuralgic, specific pain syndromes
  Carbamazepine (Systemic)
Antiosteolytic
  Colchicine (Systemic)
Antiosteoporotic
  Ethylestrenol (Systemic)
  Oxandrolone (Systemic)
Antiparalytic, familial periodic paralysis
  Acetazolamide (Systemic)
Antiprotozoal
  Amphotericin B (Systemic)
  Chloroquine (Systemic)
  Dapsone (Systemic)
  Demeclocycline (Systemic)
  Doxycycline (Systemic)
  Hydroxychloroquine (Systemic)
  Iodoquinol (Oral)
  Methacycline (Systemic)
  Metronidazole (Systemic)
  Minocycline (Systemic)
  Oxytetracycline (Systemic)
  Pentamidine (Systemic)
  Primaquine (Systemic)
  Pyrimethamine (Systemic)
  Quinine (Systemic)
  Sulfamethoxazole (Systemic)
  Sulfamethoxazole and Trimethoprim (Systemic)
  Sulfisoxazole (Systemic)
  Tetracycline (Systemic)
Antipruritic
  Doxepin (Systemic)

Antipruritic, cholestasis
  Cholestyramine (Systemic)
  Colestipol (Systemic)
Antipsoriatic, systemic
  Etretinate (Systemic)
  Methotrexate (Systemic)
  Methoxsalen (Systemic)
  Trioxsalen (Systemic)
Antipsoriatic, topical
  Anthralin (Topical)
  Coal Tar (Topical)
  Methoxsalen (Topical)
  Salicylic Acid (Topical)
  Salicylic Acid, Sulfur, and Coal Tar
    (Topical)
Antipsychotic
  Acetophenazine (Systemic)
  Carbamazepine (Systemic)
  Chlorpromazine (Systemic)
  Chlorprothixene (Systemic)
  Flupenthixol (Systemic)
  Fluphenazine (Systemic)
  Haloperidol (Systemic)
  Loxapine (Systemic)
  Mesoridazine (Systemic)
  Molindone (Systemic)
  Perphenazine (Systemic)
  Prochlorperazine (Systemic)
  Promazine (Systemic)
  Thioridazine (Systemic)
  Thiothixene (Systemic)
  Trifluoperazine (Systemic)
  Triflupromazine (Systemic)
Antipsychotic-antidepressant
  Perphenazine and Amitriptyline (Systemic)
Antipyretic
  Acetaminophen (Systemic)
  Acetaminophen and Aspirin (Systemic)
  Acetaminophen, Aspirin, and Caffeine
    (Systemic)
  Acetaminophen, Aspirin, and Caffeine,
    Buffered (Systemic)
  Acetaminophen, Aspirin, and Salicyla-
    mide (Systemic)
  Acetaminophen, Aspirin, and Salicyla-
    mide, Buffered (Systemic)
  Acetaminophen, Aspirin, Salicylamide,
    and Caffeine (Systemic)
  Acetaminophen and Salicylamide (Sys-
    temic)
  Acetaminophen, Salicylamide, and Caf-
    feine (Systemic)
  Acetaminophen, Sodium Salicylate, and
    Caffeine (Systemic)
  Aspirin (Systemic)
  Aspirin, Alumina, and Magnesia (Sys-
    temic)
  Aspirin, Buffered (Systemic)
  Choline Salicylate (Systemic)
  Choline and Magnesium Salicylates (Sys-
    temic)
  Ibuprofen (Systemic)
  Indomethacin (Systemic—Anti-inflamma-
    tory, Nonsteroidal)
  Magnesium Salicylate (Systemic)
  Salsalate (Systemic)
  Sodium Salicylate (Systemic)
Antirheumatic, disease-modifying
  Auranofin (Systemic)
  Aurothioglucose (Systemic)
  Azathioprine (Systemic)
  Chloroquine (Systemic)
  Gold Sodium Thiomalate (Systemic)
  Hydroxychloroquine (Systemic)
  Methotrexate (Systemic)
  Penicillamine (Systemic)
Antirheumatic, nonsteroidal anti-inflammatory
  Aspirin (Systemic)
  Aspirin, Alumina, and Magnesia (Sys-
    temic)
  Aspirin, Buffered (Systemic)
  Choline Salicylate (Systemic)
  Choline and Magnesium Salicylates (Sys-
    temic)
  Diflunisal (Systemic)

Antirheumatic, nonsteroidal anti-inflamma-
  tory *(continued)*
  Fenoprofen (Systemic)
  Ibuprofen (Systemic)
  Indomethacin (Systemic—Anti-inflamma-
    tory, Nonsteroidal)
  Ketoprofen (Systemic)
  Magnesium Salicylate (Systemic)
  Meclofenamate (Systemic)
  Naproxen (Systemic)
  Phenylbutazone (Systemic)
  Piroxicam (Systemic)
  Salsalate (Systemic)
  Sodium Salicylate (Systemic)
  Sulindac (Systemic)
  Tolmetin (Systemic)
Antiseborrheic
  Chloroxine (Topical)
  Coal Tar (Topical)
  Pyrithione (Topical)
  Salicylic Acid (Topical)
  Salicylic Acid and Sulfur (Topical)
  Salicylic Acid, Sulfur, and Coal Tar
    (Topical)
  Selenium Sulfide (Topical)
  Sulfur (Topical)
Antispasmodic, gastrointestinal
  Dicyclomine (Systemic)
  Oxyphencyclimine (Systemic)
Antispasmodic, urinary tract
  Flavoxate (Systemic)
  Oxybutynin (Systemic)
Antispastic
  Baclofen (Systemic)
  Dantrolene (Systemic)
Antitremor agent
  Chlordiazepoxide, Oral (Systemic)
  Diazepam, Oral (Systemic)
  Lorazepam, Oral (Systemic)
  Metoprolol (Systemic)
  Propranolol (Systemic)
Antitussive
  Chlophedianol (Systemic)
  Codeine, Oral (Systemic)
  Dextromethorphan (Systemic)
  Diphenhydramine (Systemic)
  Hydrocodone (Systemic)
  Hydromorphone (Systemic)
  Methadone (Systemic)
  Morphine (Systemic)
Antitussive-antimuscarinic
  Hydrocodone and Homatropine (Sys-
    temic)
Antitussive-bronchodilator
  Dextromethorphan and Methoxyphen-
    amine (Systemic)
Antitussive-expectorant
  Codeine and Calcium Iodide (Systemic)
  Codeine and Guaifenesin (Systemic)
  Codeine and Iodinated Glycerol (Sys-
    temic)
  Codeine and Terpin Hydrate (Systemic)
  Dextromethorphan and Guaifenesin (Sys-
    temic)
  Dextromethorphan and Iodinated Gly-
    cerol (Systemic)
  Dextromethorphan and Terpin Hydrate
    (Systemic)
  Hydrocodone and Guaifenesin (Systemic)
  Hydrocodone and Potassium Guaiacolsul-
    fonate (Systemic)
  Hydromorphone and Guaifenesin (Sys-
    temic)
Antiulcer agent
  Cimetidine (Systemic)
  Doxepin (Systemic)
  Famotidine (Systemic)
  Ranitidine (Systemic)
  Sucralfate (Oral)
  Trimipramine (Systemic)
Antiurolithic, calcium calculi
  Bendroflumethiazide (Systemic)
  Benzthiazide (Systemic)
  Cellulose Sodium Phosphate (Systemic)
  Chlorothiazide (Systemic)

Antiurolithic, calcium calculi *(continued)*
  Chlorthalidone (Systemic)
  Cyclothiazide (Systemic)
  Hydrochlorothiazide (Systemic)
  Hydroflumethiazide (Systemic)
  Magnesium Hydroxide (Oral)
  Methyclothiazide (Systemic)
  Metolazone (Systemic)
  Polythiazide (Systemic)
  Potassium Phosphate, Monobasic (Sys-
    temic)
  Potassium and Sodium Phosphates (Sys-
    temic)
  Quinethazone (Systemic)
  Trichlormethiazide (Systemic)
Antiurolithic, calcium oxalate calculi
  Allopurinol (Systemic)
  Potassium Citrate (Systemic)
  Potassium Citrate and Citric Acid (Sys-
    temic)
Antiurolithic, calcium phosphate calculi
  Potassium Citrate (Systemic)
  Potassium Citrate and Citric Acid (Sys-
    temic)
Antiurolithic, cystine calculi
  Acetazolamide (Systemic)
  Penicillamine (Systemic)
  Potassium Citrate (Systemic)
  Potassium Citrate and Citric Acid (Sys-
    temic)
  Potassium Citrate and Sodium Citrate
    (Systemic)
  Sodium Citrate and Citric Acid (Sys-
    temic)
  Tricitrates (Systemic)
Antiurolithic, phosphate calculi
  Aluminum Carbonate (Oral)
  Aluminum Hydroxide (Oral)
Antiurolithic, struvite calculi
  Acetohydroxamic Acid (Systemic)
Antiurolithic, uric acid calculi
  Acetazolamide (Systemic)
  Allopurinol (Systemic)
  Potassium Citrate (Systemic)
  Potassium Citrate and Citric Acid (Sys-
    temic)
  Potassium Citrate and Sodium Citrate
    (Systemic)
  Sodium Citrate and Citric Acid (Sys-
    temic)
  Tricitrates (Systemic)
Antivertigo agent
  Belladonna (Systemic)
  Dimenhydrinate (Systemic)
  Diphenhydramine (Systemic)
  Diphenidol (Systemic)
  Hyoscyamine and Scopolamine (Sys-
    temic)
  Meclizine (Systemic)
  Promethazine (Systemic)
  Scopolamine (Systemic)
Antiviral, ophthalmic
  Idoxuridine (Ophthalmic)
  Trifluridine (Ophthalmic)
  Vidarabine (Ophthalmic)
Antiviral, systemic
  Acyclovir (Systemic)
  Amantadine (Systemic)
  Ribavirin (Systemic)
  Zidovudine (Systemic)
Antiviral, topical
  Acyclovir (Topical)
Appetite stimulant
  Cyproheptadine (Systemic)
Appetite suppressant
  Benzphetamine (Systemic)
  Diethylpropion (Systemic)
  Fenfluramine (Systemic)
  Mazindol (Systemic)
  Phendimetrazine (Systemic)
  Phenmetrazine (Systemic)
  Phentermine (Systemic)
  Phenylpropanolamine (Systemic)
Asthma prophylactic
  Cromolyn (Inhalation)

B–C

Bartter's syndrome therapy adjunct
Indomethacin (Systemic—Anti-inflammatory, Nonsteroidal)
Biological response modifier
Interferon Alfa-2a, Recombinant (Systemic)
Interferon Alfa-2b, Recombinant (Systemic)
Bone resorption inhibitor
Calcitonin-Human (Systemic)
Calcitonin-Salmon (Systemic)
Etidronate (Systemic)
Bowel disease, inflammatory, suppressant
Azathioprine (Systemic)
Metronidazole (Systemic)
Sulfasalazine (Systemic)
Bowel preparation, preoperative, adjunct
Kanamycin (Oral)
Neomycin (Oral)
Bronchodilator
Albuterol (Systemic)
Aminophylline (Systemic)
Bitolterol (Systemic)
Dyphylline (Systemic)
Ephedrine (Systemic)
Epinephrine (Systemic)
Ethylnorepinephrine (Systemic)
Fenoterol (Systemic)
Ipratropium (Inhalation)
Isoetharine (Systemic)
Isoproterenol (Systemic)
Metaproterenol (Systemic)
Oxtriphylline (Systemic)
Oxtriphylline and Guaifenesin (Systemic)
Terbutaline (Systemic)
Theophylline (Systemic)
Theophylline and Guaifenesin (Systemic)
Bronchodilator-decongestant
Isoproterenol and Phenylephrine (Systemic)
Buffer, neutralizing
Sodium Citrate and Citric Acid (Systemic)
Tricitrates (Systemic)
Calcium pyrophosphate deposition disease suppressant
Colchicine (Systemic)
Cardiac load–reducing agent
Captopril (Systemic)
Captopril and Hydrochlorothiazide (Systemic)
Enalapril (Systemic)
Enalapril and Hydrochlorothiazide (Systemic)
Erythrityl Tetranitrate (Systemic)
Hydralazine (Systemic)
Isosorbide Dinitrate (Systemic)
Nitroglycerin (Systemic)
Pentaerythritol Tetranitrate (Systemic)
Prazosin (Systemic)
Cardiac stimulant
Epinephrine Injection (Systemic)
Isoproterenol, Oral (Systemic)
Isoproterenol, Parenteral (Systemic)
Cardiotonic
Calcium Chloride (Systemic)
Calcium Gluconate, Parenteral (Systemic)
Deslanoside (Systemic)
Digitalis (Systemic)
Digitoxin (Systemic)
Digoxin (Systemic)
Caustic
Salicylic Acid (Topical)
Cerumen removal adjunct
Antipyrine and Benzocaine (Otic)
Chelating agent
Deferoxamine (Systemic)
Penicillamine (Systemic)
Trientine (Systemic)
Chemonucleolytic, herniated lumbar intervertebral disc therapy
Chymopapain (Parenteral-Local)

Chemotherapy adjunct
Technetium Tc 99m Albumin Aggregated (Diagnostic)
Cholelitholytic
Monooctanoin (Local)
Cholinergic
Bethanechol (Systemic)
Cholinergic adjunct, curariform block
Atropine, Parenteral (Systemic)
Glycopyrrolate, Parenteral (Systemic)
Hyoscyamine, Parenteral (Systemic)
Cleansing agent, astringent
Alcohol and Acetone (Topical)
Cleansing agent, astringent-keratolytic
Alcohol and Sulfur (Topical)
Cleansing agent, defatting
Alcohol and Acetone (Topical)
Cleansing agent, defatting-keratolytic
Alcohol and Sulfur (Topical)
Collagenase synthesis inhibitor
Phenytoin (Systemic)
Contraceptive, postcoital, systemic
Diethylstilbestrol (Systemic)
Estrogens, Conjugated (Systemic)
Ethinyl Estradiol (Systemic)
Norgestrel and Ethinyl Estradiol (Systemic)
Contraceptive, systemic
Ethynodiol Diacetate and Ethinyl Estradiol (Systemic)
Ethynodiol Diacetate and Mestranol (Systemic)
Levonorgestrel and Ethinyl Estradiol (Systemic)
Medroxyprogesterone, Parenteral (Systemic)
Norethindrone (Systemic)
Norethindrone Acetate and Ethinyl Estradiol (Systemic)
Norethindrone and Ethinyl Estradiol (Systemic)
Norethindrone and Mestranol (Systemic)
Norethynodrel and Mestranol (Systemic)
Norgestrel (Systemic)
Norgestrel and Ethinyl Estradiol (Systemic)
Cryptorchidism therapy adjunct
Gonadotropin, Chorionic (Systemic)
Cycloplegic
Atropine (Ophthalmic)
Cyclopentolate (Ophthalmic)
Homatropine (Ophthalmic)
Scopolamine (Ophthalmic)
Tropicamide (Ophthalmic)
Cyclostimulant, accommodative esotropia
Demecarium (Ophthalmic)
Echothiophate (Ophthalmic)
Isoflurophate (Ophthalmic)
Cytotoxic, topical
Podophyllum (Topical)

D

Decongestant-antitussive
Phenylephrine and Dextromethorphan (Systemic)
Phenylpropanolamine and Caramiphen (Systemic)
Phenylpropanolamine and Dextromethorphan (Systemic)
Phenylpropanolamine and Hydrocodone (Systemic)
Pseudoephedrine and Codeine (Systemic)
Pseudoephedrine and Dextromethorphan (Systemic)
Pseudoephedrine and Hydrocodone (Systemic)
Decongestant-antitussive-analgesic
Phenylpropanolamine, Dextromethorphan, and Acetaminophen (Systemic)

Decongestant-antitussive-expectorant
Phenylephrine, Dextromethorphan, and Guaifenesin (Systemic)
Phenylephrine, Hydrocodone, and Guaifenesin (Systemic)
Phenylpropanolamine, Codeine, and Guaifenesin (Systemic)
Phenylpropanolamine, Dextromethorphan, and Guaifenesin (Systemic)
Pseudoephedrine, Codeine, and Guaifenesin (Systemic)
Pseudoephedrine, Dextromethorphan, and Guaifenesin (Systemic)
Pseudoephedrine, Hydrocodone, and Guaifenesin (Systemic)
Decongestant-antitussive-expectorant-analgesic
Phenylephrine, Dextromethorphan, Guaifenesin, and Acetaminophen (Systemic)
Pseudoephedrine, Dextromethorphan, Guaifenesin, and Acetaminophen (Systemic)
Decongestant-expectorant
Ephedrine and Guaifenesin (Systemic)
Ephedrine and Potassium Iodide (Systemic)
Phenylephrine, Phenylpropanolamine, and Guaifenesin (Systemic)
Phenylpropanolamine and Guaifenesin (Systemic)
Pseudoephedrine and Guaifenesin (Systemic)
Decongestant, nasal, systemic
Ephedrine, Oral (Systemic)
Phenylpropanolamine (Systemic)
Pseudoephedrine (Systemic)
Decongestant, ophthalmic
Naphazoline (Ophthalmic)
Oxymetazoline (Ophthalmic)
Phenylephrine (Ophthalmic)
Decongestant, topical
Oxymetazoline (Nasal)
Phenylephrine (Nasal)
Xylometazoline (Nasal)
Deferoxamine adjunct, chronic iron overdose
Ascorbic Acid (Systemic)
Sodium Ascorbate (Systemic)
Dental caries prophylactic
Sodium Fluoride (Systemic)
Dermatitis herpetiformis suppressant
Colchicine (Systemic)
Dapsone (Systemic)
Diagnostic aid, abdominal computed tomographic (CT) scanning
Glucagon (Systemic)
Diagnostic aid, abdominal digital angiography
Glucagon (Systemic)
Diagnostic aid, accommodative esotropia
Demecarium (Ophthalmic)
Echothiophate (Ophthalmic)
Isoflurophate (Ophthalmic)
Diagnostic aid, adrenal-pituitary function
Cosyntropin (Systemic)
Diagnostic aid, adrenocortical function
Corticotropin (Systemic)
Diagnostic aid, bone disease
Technetium Tc 99m Medronate (Diagnostic)
Technetium Tc 99m Oxidronate (Diagnostic)
Technetium Tc 99m Pyrophosphate (Diagnostic)
Technetium Tc 99m (Pyro- and trimeta-) Phosphates (Diagnostic)
Diagnostic aid, brain disorders
Sodium Pertechnetate Tc 99m (Diagnostic)
Diagnostic aid, breast carcinoma
Technetium Tc 99m Antimony Trisulfide Colloid (Diagnostic)
Diagnostic aid, bronchial airway hyperreactivity
Methacholine (Inhalation)

Diagnostic aid, bronchial studies
Acetylcysteine (Inhalation)
Diagnostic aid, cardiac disease
Technetium Tc 99m Human Serum Albumin (Diagnostic)
Technetium Tc 99m Pyrophosphate (Diagnostic)
Technetium Tc 99m (Pyro- and trimeta-) Phosphates (Diagnostic)
Diagnostic aid, cardiac disorders
Sodium Pertechnetate Tc 99m (Diagnostic)
Diagnostic aid, cardiac function
Amyl Nitrite (Systemic)
Diagnostic aid, cerebral disorders
Technetium Tc 99m Gluceptate (Diagnostic)
Diagnostic aid, cerebrospinal fluid flow disorders
Indium In 111 Pentetate (Diagnostic)
Diagnostic aid, cerebrovascular disease
Xenon Xe 133 (Diagnostic)
Diagnostic aid, contact lens procedures
Hydroxypropyl Methylcellulose (Ophthalmic)
Diagnostic aid, coronary vasospasm
Ergonovine (Systemic)
Diagnostic aid, Cushing's syndrome
Dexamethasone (Systemic)
Diagnostic aid, cyanocobalamin malabsorption syndromes
Cyanocobalamin Co 57 (Diagnostic)
Diagnostic aid, cycloplegic
Tropicamide (Ophthalmic)
Diagnostic aid, diabetes insipidus
Vasopressin (Systemic)
Diagnostic aid, endogenous depression
Dexamethasone, Oral (Systemic)
Diagnostic aid, fetal respiratory function
Oxytocin, Parenteral (Systemic)
Diagnostic aid, fluid and blood loss
Iodinated I 131 Albumin (Diagnostic)
Diagnostic aid, focal inflammatory lesions
Gallium Citrate Ga 67 (Diagnostic)
Diagnostic aid, folate deficiency
Folate Sodium (Systemic)
Folic Acid (Systemic)
Diagnostic aid, gastric function
Histamine (Systemic)
Pentagastrin (Systemic)
Diagnostic aid, gastroesophageal disorders
Technetium Tc 99m Sulfur Colloid (Diagnostic)
Diagnostic aid, gastrointestinal bleeding
Sodium Chromate Cr 51 (Diagnostic)
Technetium Tc 99m (Pyro- and trimeta-) Phosphates (unlabeled) (Diagnostic)
Diagnostic aid, gastrointestinal disorders
Sodium Pertechnetate Tc 99m (Diagnostic)
Technetium Tc 99m Sulfur Colloid (Diagnostic)
Diagnostic aid, gastroscopy
Simethicone (Oral)
Diagnostic aid, gonioscopy
Hydroxypropyl Methylcellulose (Ophthalmic)
Diagnostic aid, hematological disease
Technetium Tc 99m Sulfur Colloid (Diagnostic)
Diagnostic aid, hepatic disease
Technetium Tc 99m Sulfur Colloid (Diagnostic)
Diagnostic aid, hepatobiliary disorders
Technetium Tc 99m Disofenin (Diagnostic)
Technetium Tc 99m Lidofenin (Diagnostic)
Technetium Tc 99m Mebrofenin (Diagnostic)
Diagnostic aid, hypogonadism
Gonadotropin, Chorionic (Systemic)
Diagnostic aid, hypothalamic-pituitary-gonadal axis function
Clomiphene (Systemic)
Gonadorelin (Systemic)
Diagnostic aid, hypotonic radiography
Glucagon (Systemic)

Diagnostic aid, inflammatory lesions
Indium In 111 Oxyquinoline (Diagnostic)
Diagnostic aid, intracranial lesions
Technetium Tc 99m Gluceptate (Diagnostic)
Technetium Tc 99m Pentetate (Diagnostic)
Diagnostic aid, iron absorption
Ferrous Citrate Fe 59 (Diagnostic)
Diagnostic aid, iron metabolism
Ferrous Citrate Fe 59 (Diagnostic)
Diagnostic aid, ischemic heart disease
Thallous Chloride Tl 201 (Diagnostic)
Diagnostic aid, malignant melanoma
Technetium Tc 99m Antimony Trisulfide Colloid (Diagnostic)
Diagnostic aid, myasthenia gravis
Neostigmine, Parenteral (Systemic)
Diagnostic aid, mydriatic
Phenylephrine (Ophthalmic)
Tropicamide (Ophthalmic)
Diagnostic aid, myocardial infarction
Thallous Chloride Tl 201 (Diagnostic)
Diagnostic aid, nasolacrimal disorders
Sodium Pertechnetate Tc 99m (Diagnostic)
Diagnostic aid, neoplastic disease
Gallium Citrate Ga 67 (Diagnostic)
Diagnostic aid, ovarian function
Clomiphene (Systemic)
Diagnostic aid, pancreas disease
Selenomethionine Se 75 (Diagnostic)
Diagnostic aid, pancreatic function
Bentiromide (Systemic)
Pancrelipase (Systemic)
Diagnostic aid, placental reserve
Oxytocin, Parenteral (Systemic)
Diagnostic aid, platelet survival
Sodium Chromate Cr 51 (Diagnostic)
Diagnostic aid, primary hyperaldosteronism
Spironolactone (Systemic)
Diagnostic aid, pulmonary disease
Krypton Kr 81m (Diagnostic)
Technetium Tc 99m Albumin Aggregated (Diagnostic)
Xenon Xe 133 (Diagnostic)
Diagnostic aid, pulmonary emboli
Krypton Kr 81m (Diagnostic)
Diagnostic aid, radiography of the bowel
Simethicone (Oral)
Diagnostic aid, radiopaque, biliary tract disorders
Diatrizoate Meglumine, Parenteral (Systemic)
Diatrizoate Meglumine and Diatrizoate Sodium, Parenteral (Systemic)
Diatrizoate Sodium, Parenteral (Systemic)
Iodipamide (Systemic)
Iopanoic Acid (Systemic)
Iothalamate Meglumine (Systemic)
Ipodate (Systemic)
Diagnostic aid, radiopaque, brain disorders
Diatrizoate Meglumine, Parenteral (Systemic)
Diatrizoate Meglumine and Diatrizoate Sodium, Parenteral (Systemic)
Diatrizoate Sodium, Parenteral (Systemic)
Iopamidol (Systemic)
Iothalamate Meglumine (Systemic)
Iothalamate Meglumine and Iothalamate Sodium (Systemic)
Iothalamate Sodium (Systemic)
Ioxaglate (Systemic)
Metrizamide (Systemic)
Diagnostic aid, radiopaque, cardiac disease
Diatrizoate Meglumine, Parenteral (Systemic)
Diatrizoate Meglumine and Diatrizoate Sodium, Parenteral (Systemic)
Iohexol (Systemic)
Iopamidol (Systemic)
Iothalamate Meglumine and Iothalamate Sodium (Systemic)

Diagnostic aid, radiopaque, cardiac disease
(continued)
Iothalamate Sodium (Systemic)
Ioxaglate (Systemic)
Metrizamide (Systemic)
Diagnostic aid, radiopaque, central nervous system disorders
Iohexol (Systemic)
Iopamidol (Systemic)
Iophendylate (Systemic)
Metrizamide (Systemic)
Diagnostic aid, radiopaque, cerebrospinal fluid disorders
Iohexol (Systemic)
Iopamidol (Systemic)
Iophendylate (Systemic)
Metrizamide (Systemic)
Diagnostic aid, radiopaque contrast enhancer in computed tomography
Diatrizoate Meglumine, Parenteral (Systemic)
Diatrizoate Meglumine and Diatrizoate Sodium, Parenteral (Systemic)
Iopamidol (Systemic)
Iothalamate Meglumine (Systemic)
Iothalamate Meglumine and Iothalamate Sodium (Systemic)
Iothalamate Sodium (Systemic)
Ioxaglate (Systemic)
Diagnostic aid, radiopaque, disk disease
Diatrizoate Meglumine, Parenteral (Systemic)
Diatrizoate Meglumine and Diatrizoate Sodium, Parenteral (Systemic)
Diagnostic aid, radiopaque, gallbladder disorders
Iocetamic Acid (Systemic)
Iodipamide (Systemic)
Iopanoic Acid (Systemic)
Ipodate (Systemic)
Tyropanoate (Systemic)
Diagnostic aid, radiopaque, gastrointestinal disorders
Diatrizoate Meglumine and Diatrizoate Sodium, Oral or Rectal (Systemic)
Diatrizoate Sodium, Oral or Rectal (Systemic)
Diagnostic aid, radiopaque, joint disease
Diatrizoate Meglumine, Parenteral (Systemic)
Diatrizoate Meglumine and Diatrizoate Sodium, Parenteral (Systemic)
Ioxaglate (Systemic)
Diagnostic aid, radiopaque, pancreas disease
Iothalamate Meglumine (Systemic)
Diagnostic aid, radiopaque, pregnancy disorders
Diatrizoate Meglumine, Parenteral (Systemic)
Diagnostic aid, radiopaque, splenic and portal vein disorders
Diatrizoate Meglumine, Parenteral (Systemic)
Diatrizoate Meglumine and Diatrizoate Sodium, Parenteral (Systemic)
Diatrizoate Sodium, Parenteral (Systemic)
Diagnostic aid, radiopaque, urinary tract disorders
Diatrizoate Meglumine, Parenteral (Systemic)
Diatrizoate Meglumine and Diatrizoate Sodium, Parenteral (Systemic)
Diatrizoates (Mucosal)
Diatrizoate Sodium, Parenteral (Systemic)
Iohexol (Systemic)
Iothalamate (Mucosal)
Iothalamate Meglumine (Systemic)
Iothalamate Meglumine and Iothalamate Sodium (Systemic)
Iothalamate Sodium (Systemic)
Ioxaglate (Systemic)

Diagnostic aid, radiopaque, uterus and fallopian tube disorders
 Diatrizoate Meglumine and Diatrizoate Sodium, Parenteral (Systemic)
 Diatrizoate Meglumine and Iodipamide Meglumine (Mucosal)
 Diatrizoate Sodium, Parenteral (Systemic)
 Ioxaglate (Systemic)
Diagnostic aid, radiopaque, vascular disease
 Diatrizoate Meglumine, Parenteral (Systemic)
 Diatrizoate Meglumine and Diatrizoate Sodium, Parenteral (Systemic)
 Diatrizoate Sodium, Parenteral (Systemic)
 Iohexol (Systemic)
 Iopamidol (Systemic)
 Iothalamate Meglumine (Systemic)
 Iothalamate Meglumine and Iothalamate Sodium (Systemic)
 Iothalamate Sodium (Systemic)
 Ioxaglate (Systemic)
 Metrizamide (Systemic)
Diagnostic aid, red blood cell disease
 Sodium Chromate Cr 51 (Diagnostic)
Diagnostic aid, renal disorders
 Iodohippurate Sodium I 123 (Diagnostic)
 Iodohippurate Sodium I 131 (Diagnostic)
 Technetium Tc 99m Gluceptate (Diagnostic)
 Technetium Tc 99m Pentetate (Diagnostic)
 Technetium Tc 99m Succimer (Diagnostic)
Diagnostic aid, renal function
 Inulin (Systemic)
 Phenolsulfonphthalein (Systemic)
 Vasopressin (Systemic)
Diagnostic aid, renal tubular acidosis
 Fludrocortisone (Systemic)
Diagnostic aid, residual bladder urine
 Phenolsulfonphthalein (Systemic)
Diagnostic aid, salivary gland disorders
 Sodium Pertechnetate Tc 99m (Diagnostic)
Diagnostic aid, small bowel scintigraphy
 Glucagon (Systemic)
Diagnostic aid, spleen disease
 Technetium Tc 99m Sulfur Colloid (Diagnostic)
Diagnostic aid, thrombosis
 Indium In 111 Oxyquinoline (Diagnostic)
Diagnostic aid, thyroid disorders
 Levothyroxine (Systemic)
 Liothyronine (Systemic)
 Protirelin (Systemic)
 Sodium Iodide I 123 (Diagnostic)
 Sodium Iodide I 131 (Diagnostic)
 Sodium Pertechnetate Tc 99m (Diagnostic)
 Thyrotropin (Systemic)
Diagnostic aid, urinary bladder disorders
 Iodohippurate Sodium I 123 (Diagnostic)
 Iodohippurate Sodium I 131 (Diagnostic)
 Sodium Pertechnetate Tc 99m (Diagnostic)
Diagnostic aid, vascular disorders
 Sodium Pertechnetate Tc 99m (Diagnostic)
 Technetium Tc 99m Albumin Aggregated (Diagnostic)
Diagnostic aid, vitamin deficiency
 Cyanocobalamin (Systemic)
 Hydroxocobalamin (Systemic)
Digestant
 Pancrelipase (Systemic)
Digestant-antimuscarinic-sedative
 Pancreatin, Pepsin, Bile Salts, Hyoscyamine, Atropine, Scopolamine, and Phenobarbital (Systemic)
Diuretic
 Amiloride (Systemic)
 Amiloride and Hydrochlorothiazide (Systemic)
 Bendroflumethiazide (Systemic)
 Benzthiazide (Systemic)

Diuretic *(continued)*
 Bumetanide (Systemic)
 Chlorothiazide (Systemic)
 Chlorthalidone (Systemic)
 Cyclothiazide (Systemic)
 Ethacrynic Acid (Systemic)
 Furosemide (Systemic)
 Glycerin (Systemic)
 Hydrochlorothiazide (Systemic)
 Hydroflumethiazide (Systemic)
 Indapamide (Systemic)
 Methyclothiazide (Systemic)
 Metolazone (Systemic)
 Polythiazide (Systemic)
 Quinethazone (Systemic)
 Spironolactone (Systemic)
 Spironolactone and Hydrochlorothiazide (Systemic)
 Triamterene (Systemic)
 Triamterene and Hydrochlorothiazide (Systemic)
 Trichlormethiazide (Systemic)
Diuretic, syndrome of inappropriate ADH secretion
 Demeclocycline (Systemic)
Diuretic, urinary alkalinizing
 Acetazolamide (Systemic)
Dopaminergic blocker
 Metoclopramide (Systemic)
Drying agent, topical
 Carbol-Fuchsin (Topical)
Duchenne muscular dystrophy therapy adjunct
 Dantrolene (Systemic)

E–H

Electrolyte replenisher
 Calcium Chloride (Systemic)
 Calcium Gluceptate (Systemic)
 Calcium Gluconate, Parenteral (Systemic)
 Potassium Acetate (Systemic)
 Potassium Bicarbonate (Systemic)
 Potassium Bicarbonate and Potassium Chloride (Systemic)
 Potassium Bicarbonate and Potassium Citrate (Systemic)
 Potassium Chloride (Systemic)
 Potassium Chloride, Potassium Bicarbonate, and Potassium Citrate (Systemic)
 Potassium Gluconate (Systemic)
 Potassium Gluconate and Potassium Chloride (Systemic)
 Potassium Gluconate and Potassium Citrate (Systemic)
 Potassium Gluconate, Potassium Citrate, and Ammonium Chloride (Systemic)
 Potassium Phosphates (Systemic)
 Potassium and Sodium Phosphates (Systemic)
 Sodium Bicarbonate (Systemic)
 Sodium Phosphates (Systemic)
 Trikates (Systemic)
Emetic
 Apomorphine (Systemic)
 Ipecac (Oral)
Enzyme, pancreatic, replenisher
 Pancrelipase (Systemic)
Estrogen-progestin
 Ethynodiol Diacetate and Ethinyl Estradiol (Systemic)
 Ethynodiol Diacetate and Mestranol (Systemic)
 Levonorgestrel and Ethinyl Estradiol (Systemic)
 Norethindrone Acetate and Ethinyl Estradiol (Systemic)
 Norethindrone and Ethinyl Estradiol (Systemic)
 Norethindrone and Mestranol (Systemic)
 Norethynodrel and Mestranol (Systemic)
 Norgestrel and Ethinyl Estradiol (Systemic)

Estrogen, systemic
 Chlorotrianisene (Systemic)
 Diethylstilbestrol (Systemic)
 Estradiol (Systemic)
 Estrogens, Conjugated (Systemic)
 Estrogens, Esterified (Systemic)
 Estrone (Systemic)
 Estropipate (Systemic)
 Ethinyl Estradiol (Systemic)
 Quinestrol (Systemic)
Estrogen, vaginal
 Dienestrol (Vaginal)
 Estradiol (Vaginal)
 Estrogens, Conjugated (Vaginal)
 Estrone (Vaginal)
 Estropipate (Vaginal)
Expectorant
 Guaifenesin (Systemic)
Familial Mediterranean fever suppressant
 Colchicine (Systemic)
Gastric acid secretion inhibitor
 Cimetidine (Systemic)
 Famotidine (Systemic)
 Ranitidine (Systemic)
Gastric mucosa protectant
 Sucralfate (Oral)
Gastrointestinal emptying, delayed, adjunct
 Metoclopramide (Systemic)
Gonadotropic principle
 Clomiphene (Systemic)
 Gonadotropin, Chorionic (Systemic)
 Menotropins (Systemic)
 Urofollitropin (Systemic)
Gonadotropin inhibitor
 Danazol (Systemic)
Gonad-stimulating principle
 Gonadorelin (Systemic)
Granulopoietic
 Lithium (Systemic)
Growth hormone suppressant, acromegaly
 Bromocriptine (Systemic)
Hair growth stimulant
 Minoxidil (Topical)
Hair growth stimulant, alopecia areata, systemic
 Methoxsalen (Systemic)
Hair growth stimulant, alopecia areata, topical
 Anthralin (Topical)
 Methoxsalen (Topical)
Hemorrheologic agent
 Pentoxifylline (Systemic)
Hepatic encephalopathy therapy adjunct
 Kanamycin (Oral)
 Neomycin (Oral)
Histamine H_2-receptor antagonist
 Cimetidine (Systemic)
 Famotidine (Systemic)
 Ranitidine (Systemic)
Hormone, growth, human
 Somatrem (Systemic)
 Somatropin, Pituitary-derived (Systemic)
 Somatropin, Recombinant (Systemic)
Hydrocholeretic
 Dehydrocholic Acid (Oral)
Hypertrophic cardiomyopathy therapy adjunct
 Verapamil (Systemic)
Hypertrophic subaortic stenosis therapy adjunct
 Acebutolol (Systemic)
 Atenolol (Systemic)
 Metoprolol (Systemic)
 Nadolol (Systemic)
 Oxprenolol (Systemic)
 Pindolol (Systemic)
 Propranolol (Systemic)
 Sotalol (Systemic)
 Timolol (Systemic)

I–L

Immunizing agent, active
  Diphtheria and Tetanus Toxoids and Pertussis Vaccine Adsorbed (Systemic)
  Measles Virus Vaccine Live (Systemic)
  Mumps Virus Vaccine Live (Systemic)
  Pneumococcal Vaccine Polyvalent (Systemic)
  Rubella Virus Vaccine Live (Systemic)
Immunosuppressant
  Azathioprine (Systemic)
  Betamethasone (Systemic)
  Chlorambucil (Systemic)
  Corticotropin (Systemic)
  Cortisone (Systemic)
  Cyclophosphamide (Systemic)
  Cyclosporine (Systemic)
  Dexamethasone (Systemic)
  Hydrocortisone (Systemic)
  Mercaptopurine (Systemic)
  Methylprednisolone (Systemic)
  Muromonab-CD3 (Systemic)
  Paramethasone (Systemic)
  Prednisolone (Systemic)
  Prednisone (Systemic)
  Triamcinolone (Systemic)
Impotence therapy
  Papaverine (Intracavernosal)
Impotence therapy adjunct
  Phentolamine (Intracavernosal)
Infertility therapy adjunct
  Bromocriptine (Systemic)
  Clomiphene (Systemic)
  Gonadotropin, Chorionic (Systemic)
  Menotropins (Systemic)
  Urofollitropin (Systemic)
Iodine replenisher
  Potassium Iodide (Systemic)
Keratinization stabilizer
  Isotretinoin (Systemic)
Keratolytic, topical
  Benzoyl Peroxide (Topical)
  Coal Tar (Topical)
  Resorcinol (Topical)
  Resorcinol and Sulfur (Topical)
  Salicylic Acid (Topical)
  Salicylic Acid and Sulfur (Topical)
  Salicylic Acid, Sulfur, and Coal Tar (Topical)
  Sulfur (Topical)
  Sulfurated Lime (Topical)
  Tretinoin (Topical)
Labor, premature, inhibitor
  Isoxsuprine (Systemic)
  Ritodrine (Systemic)
  Terbutaline, Oral (Systemic)
  Terbutaline, Parenteral (Systemic)
Lactation inhibitor
  Bromocriptine (Systemic)
Lactation stimulant
  Oxytocin, Nasal (Systemic)
Laxative
  Magnesium Hydroxide (Oral)
  Magnesium Oxide (Oral)
Laxative, bulk-forming
  Malt Soup Extract (Oral)
  Malt Soup Extract and Psyllium (Oral)
  Methylcellulose (Oral)
  Polycarbophil (Oral)
  Psyllium (Oral)
  Psyllium Hydrophilic Mucilloid (Oral)
  Psyllium Hydrophilic Mucilloid and Carboxymethylcellulose (Oral)
Laxative, bulk-forming, and stimulant
  Psyllium Hydrophilic Mucilloid and Senna (Oral)
  Psyllium Hydrophilic Mucilloid and Sennosides (Oral)
  Psyllium and Senna (Oral)
Laxative, bulk-forming, stimulant, and stool softener
  Docusate, Carboxymethylcellulose, and Casanthranol (Oral)

Laxative, bulk-forming and stool softener
  Carboxymethylcellulose and Docusate (Oral)
Laxative, carbon dioxide–releasing
  Potassium Bitartrate and Sodium Bicarbonate (Rectal)
Laxative, hyperosmotic
  Glycerin (Rectal)
  Lactulose (Oral)
Laxative, hyperosmotic and lubricant
  Magnesium Hydroxide and Mineral Oil (Oral)
Laxative, hyperosmotic, lubricant, and stimulant
  Mineral Oil, Glycerin, and Phenolphthalein (Oral)
Laxative, hyperosmotic, saline
  Magnesium Citrate (Oral)
  Magnesium Hydroxide (Oral)
  Magnesium Oxide (Oral)
  Magnesium Sulfate (Oral)
  Sodium Phosphate (Oral)
  Sodium Phosphate (Rectal)
Laxative, lubricant
  Mineral Oil (Oral)
  Mineral Oil (Rectal)
Laxative, lubricant and stimulant
  Mineral Oil and Cascara Sagrada (Oral)
  Mineral Oil and Phenolphthalein (Oral)
Laxative, lubricant and stool softener
  Docusate and Mineral Oil (Oral)
Laxative, stimulant or contact
  Bisacodyl (Oral)
  Bisacodyl (Rectal)
  Casanthranol (Oral)
  Cascara Sagrada (Oral)
  Cascara Sagrada and Aloe (Oral)
  Cascara Sagrada and Phenolphthalein (Oral)
  Castor Oil (Oral)
  Danthron (Oral)
  Dehydrocholic Acid (Oral)
  Phenolphthalein (Oral)
  Senna (Oral)
  Senna (Rectal)
  Sennosides (Oral)
Laxative, stimulant and stool softener
  Bisacodyl and Docusate (Oral)
  Casanthranol and Docusate (Oral)
  Danthron and Docusate (Oral)
  Danthron and Poloxamer 188 (Oral)
  Dehydrocholic Acid and Docusate (Oral)
  Dehydrocholic Acid, Docusate, and Phenolphthalein (Oral)
  Docusate and Phenolphthalein (Oral)
  Senna and Docusate (Oral)
Laxative, stool softener or emollient
  Docusate (Oral)
  Docusate (Rectal)
  Poloxamer 188 (Oral)
Lubricant, ophthalmic
  Hydroxypropyl Methylcellulose (Ophthalmic)
Lupus erythematosus suppressant
  Azathioprine (Systemic)
  Chloroquine (Systemic)
  Hydroxychloroquine (Systemic)

M–O

Malignant hyperthermia therapy adjunct
  Dantrolene (Systemic)
Mast cell stabilizer
  Cromolyn (Inhalation)
  Cromolyn (Oral)
Mast cell stabilizer, ophthalmic
  Cromolyn (Ophthalmic)
Menopausal syndrome therapy adjunct
  Clonidine (Systemic)
Methemoglobinemia (idiopathic) therapy adjunct
  Ascorbic Acid (Systemic)

Miotic
  Carbachol (Ophthalmic)
  Physostigmine (Ophthalmic)
  Pilocarpine (Ophthalmic)
Monoclonal antibody
  Muromonab-CD3 (Systemic)
Mucolytic
  Acetylcysteine (Inhalation)
Muscle phosphorylase deficiency therapy adjunct
  Dantrolene (Systemic)
Mydriatic
  Atropine (Ophthalmic)
  Cyclopentolate (Ophthalmic)
  Homatropine (Ophthalmic)
  Phenylephrine (Ophthalmic)
  Scopolamine (Ophthalmic)
  Tropicamide (Ophthalmic)
Myocardial reinfarction prophylactic
  Acebutolol (Systemic)
  Aspirin (Systemic)
  Aspirin, Buffered (Systemic)
  Atenolol (Systemic)
  Dipyridamole (Systemic)
  Metoprolol (Systemic)
  Nadolol (Systemic)
  Oxprenolol (Systemic)
  Propranolol (Systemic)
  Sulfinpyrazone (Systemic)
  Timolol (Systemic)
Neuroleptic malignant syndrome therapy adjunct
  Dantrolene (Systemic)
Nutritional supplement, mineral
  Calcium Carbonate (Systemic)
  Calcium Citrate (Systemic)
  Calcium Glubionate (Systemic)
  Calcium Gluconate, (Systemic)
  Calcium Lactate (Systemic)
  Calcium Phosphate, Dibasic (Systemic)
  Calcium Phosphate, Tribasic (Systemic)
  Sodium Fluoride (Systemic)
Nutritional supplement, other
  Levocarnitine (Systemic)
Nutritional supplement, vitamin
  Ascorbic Acid (Systemic)
  Ascorbic Acid and Sodium Ascorbate (Systemic)
  Calcifediol (Systemic)
  Calcitriol (Systemic)
  Calcium Pantothenate (Systemic)
  Cyanocobalamin (Systemic)
  Dihydrotachysterol (Systemic)
  Ergocalciferol (Systemic)
  Folate Sodium (Systemic)
  Folic Acid (Systemic)
  Hydroxocobalamin (Systemic)
  Menadiol (Systemic)
  Niacin (Systemic)
  Niacinamide (Systemic)
  Pantothenic Acid (Systemic)
  Phytonadione (Systemic)
  Pyridoxine (Systemic)
  Riboflavin (Systemic)
  Sodium Ascorbate (Systemic)
  Thiamine (Systemic)
  Vitamin A (Systemic)
  Vitamin E (Systemic)
Opioid (narcotic) abuse therapy adjunct
  Naltrexone (Systemic)
Opioid (narcotic) antagonist
  Naltrexone (Systemic)
Opioid withdrawal syndrome suppressant
  Clonidine (Systemic)
Osmotic agent, meconium ileus
  Diatrizoate Meglumine and Diatrizoate Sodium, Rectal (Systemic)
  Diatrizoate Sodium, Rectal (Systemic)
Osteoporosis prophylactic
  Diethylstilbestrol (Systemic)
  Estradiol (Systemic)
  Estrogens, Conjugated (Systemic)
  Estrogens, Esterified (Systemic)
  Estropipate (Systemic)
  Ethinyl Estradiol (Systemic)

Osteoporosis therapy adjunct
  Calcitonin-Human (Systemic)
  Calcitonin-Salmon (Systemic)

P–S

Parkinsonism therapy adjunct
  Orphenadrine Hydrochloride (Systemic)
Pediculicide
  Lindane Shampoo (Topical)
  Malathion (Topical)
  Permethrin (Topical)
  Pyrethrins and Piperonyl Butoxide (Topical)
Peristaltic stimulant
  Metoclopramide (Systemic)
  Vasopressin Injection (Systemic)
Pheochromocytoma therapy adjunct
  Acebutolol (Systemic)
  Atenolol (Systemic)
  Labetalol (Systemic)
  Metoprolol (Systemic)
  Nadolol (Systemic)
  Oxprenolol (Systemic)
  Propranolol (Systemic)
  Sotalol (Systemic)
  Timolol (Systemic)
Pituitary, anterior, hormone
  Corticotropin (Systemic)
Pituitary, posterior, hormone
  Posterior Pituitary (Systemic)
  Vasopressin (Systemic)
Platelet aggregation inhibitor
  Aspirin (Systemic)
  Aspirin, Buffered (Systemic)
  Dipyridamole (Systemic)
  Sulfinpyrazone (Systemic)
Polymorphous light eruption suppressant
  Chloroquine (Systemic)
  Hydroxychloroquine (Systemic)
Porphyria cutanea tarda suppressant
  Chloroquine (Systemic)
  Hydroxychloroquine (Systemic)
Progestin
  Hydroxyprogesterone (Systemic)
  Medroxyprogesterone, Oral (Systemic)
  Norethindrone (Systemic)
  Norgestrel (Systemic)
  Progesterone (Systemic)
Prostaglandin synthesis inhibitor
  Flurbiprofen (Ophthalmic)
Protectant, ophthalmic
  Hydroxypropyl Cellulose (Ophthalmic)
  Hydroxypropyl Methylcellulose (Ophthalmic)
Pulmonary edema therapy adjunct
  Morphine (Systemic)
Radiation protectant, thyroid gland
  Potassium Iodide (Systemic)
Repigmenting agent, systemic
  Methoxsalen (Systemic)
  Trioxsalen (Systemic)
Repigmenting agent, topical
  Methoxsalen (Topical)
Respiratory stimulant
  Aminophylline (Systemic)
  Aminophylline and Sodium Chloride Injection (Systemic)
  Theophylline (Systemic)
  Theophylline and Dextrose Injection (Systemic)
Respiratory stimulant adjunct
  Caffeine (Systemic)
  Caffeine, Citrated (Systemic)
Scabicide
  Crotamiton (Topical)
  Lindane Cream (Topical)
  Lindane Lotion (Topical)
  Sulfurated Lime (Topical)
  Sulfur (Topical)

Sedative-hypnotic
  Amobarbital (Systemic)
  Aprobarbital (Systemic)
  Butabarbital (Systemic)
  Chloral Hydrate (Systemic)
  Chlordiazepoxide (Systemic)
  Clorazepate (Systemic)
  Diazepam (Systemic)
  Diphenhydramine (Systemic)
  Doxylamine (Systemic)
  Ethchlorvynol (Systemic)
  Ethinamate (Systemic)
  Flurazepam (Systemic)
  Glutethimide (Systemic)
  Hydroxyzine (Systemic)
  Lorazepam (Systemic)
  Methyprylon (Systemic)
  Midazolam (Systemic)
  Oxazepam (Systemic)
  Pentobarbital (Systemic)
  Phenobarbital (Systemic)
  Promethazine (Systemic)
  Propiomazine (Systemic)
  Pyrilamine (Systemic)
  Secobarbital (Systemic)
  Secobarbital and Amobarbital (Systemic)
  Talbutal (Systemic)
  Temazepam (Systemic)
  Triazolam (Systemic)
  Trimeprazine (Systemic)
Senility symptoms treatment adjunct
  Cyclandelate (Systemic)
  Ergoloid Mesylates (Systemic)
  Isoxsuprine (Systemic)
Skeletal muscle relaxant
  Carisoprodol (Systemic)
  Chlorphenesin (Systemic)
  Chlorzoxazone (Systemic)
  Cyclobenzaprine (Systemic)
  Diazepam (Systemic)
  Lorazepam (Systemic)
  Metaxalone (Systemic)
  Methocarbamol (Systemic)
  Orphenadrine Citrate (Systemic)
  Phenytoin (Systemic)
Smoking deterrent
  Nicotine (Systemic)
Solubilizing agent, cholesterol
  Monooctanoin (Local)
Stimulant, central nervous system
  Amphetamine (Systemic)
  Caffeine (Systemic)
  Caffeine, Citrated (Systemic)
  Caffeine and Sodium Benzoate (Systemic)
  Dextroamphetamine (Systemic)
  Ephedrine, Oral (Systemic)
  Methamphetamine (Systemic)
  Methylphenidate (Systemic)
  Pemoline (Systemic)
Suppressant, narcotic abstinence syndrome
  Methadone (Systemic)
  Opium Tincture (Systemic)
Surgical aid, antihemorrhagic
  Epinephrine (Ophthalmic)
  Epinephrine Injection (Systemic)
Surgical aid, decongestant
  Epinephrine Injection (Systemic)
Surgical aid, mydriatic
  Epinephrine (Ophthalmic)
  Epinephrine Injection (Systemic)

T–Z

Tears, artificial
  Hydroxypropyl Cellulose (Ophthalmic)
  Hydroxypropyl Methylcellulose (Ophthalmic)
Thrombolytic
  Streptokinase (Systemic)
  Urokinase (Systemic)

Thyroid hormone
  Levothyroxine (Systemic)
  Liothyronine (Systemic)
  Liotrix (Systemic)
  Thyroglobulin (Systemic)
  Thyroid (Systemic)
Thyroid inhibitor
  Potassium Iodide (Systemic)
Thyrotoxicosis therapy adjunct
  Acebutolol (Systemic)
  Atenolol (Systemic)
  Metoprolol (Systemic)
  Nadolol (Systemic)
  Oxprenolol (Systemic)
  Propranolol (Systemic)
  Sotalol (Systemic)
  Timolol (Systemic)
Thyrotropic hormone
  Thyrotropin (Systemic)
Urinary tract infection treatment adjunct
  Acetohydroxamic Acid (Systemic)
Urticaria therapy adjunct
  Ephedrine (Systemic)
Uterine stimulant
  Carboprost (Systemic)
  Dinoprost (Intra-amniotic)
  Dinoprostone (Vaginal)
  Ergonovine (Systemic)
  Methylergonovine (Systemic)
  Oxytocin, Parenteral (Systemic)
Vascular headache prophylactic
  Atenolol (Systemic)
  Clonidine (Systemic)
  Ergotamine, Belladonna Alkaloids, and Phenobarbital (Systemic)
  Fenoprofen (Systemic)
  Ibuprofen (Systemic)
  Indomethacin (Systemic—Anti-inflammatory, Nonsteroidal)
  Lithium (Systemic)
  Mefenamic Acid (Systemic)
  Methysergide (Systemic)
  Metoprolol (Systemic)
  Nadolol (Systemic)
  Naproxen (Systemic)
  Propranolol (Systemic)
  Timolol (Systemic)
Vascular headache suppressant
  Dihydroergotamine (Systemic)
  Ergotamine (Systemic)
  Ergotamine and Caffeine (Systemic)
  Ergotamine, Caffeine, Belladonna Alkaloids, and Pentobarbital (Systemic)
  Fenoprofen (Systemic)
  Ibuprofen (Systemic)
  Indomethacin (Systemic—Anti-inflammatory, Nonsteroidal)
  Isometheptene, Dichloralphenazone, and Acetaminophen (Systemic)
  Naproxen (Systemic)
Vasospastic therapy adjunct
  Alseroxylon (Systemic)
  Cyclandelate (Systemic)
  Deserpidine (Systemic)
  Isoxsuprine (Systemic)
  Nicotinyl Alcohol (Systemic)
  Nylidrin (Systemic)
  Rauwolfia Serpentina (Systemic)
  Reserpine (Systemic)
Vitamin—See Nutritional supplement, vitamin
Vitamin replenisher–dental caries prophylactic
  Vitamins A, D, and C and Potassium Fluoride (Systemic)
  Vitamins A, D, and C and Sodium Fluoride (Systemic)
  Vitamins, Multiple, and Potassium Fluoride (Systemic)
  Vitamins, Multiple, and Sodium Fluoride (Systemic)

Index

Brand names are in *italics*. There are many brands and different manufacturers of drugs and the listing of selected American and Canadian brand names and manufacturers is intended only for ease of reference. There are additional brands and manufacturers that have not been included. Asterisks indicate those brands not available in the United States. The inclusion of a brand name does not mean the USPC has any particular knowledge that the brand listed has properties different from other brands of the same drug, nor should it be interpreted as an endorsement by the USPC. Similarly, the fact that a particular brand has not been included does not indicate that the product has been judged to be unsatisfactory or unacceptable. Page numbers in **bold-faced type** refer the user to the product identification photographs in The Medicine Chart (Appendix I).

A

Abbokinase—Abbott (U.S.) brand of Urokinase (Systemic), 1125

ABC Compound with Codeine—Zenith (U.S.) brand of Butalbital, Aspirin, Codeine, and Caffeine (Systemic), 226

A.C.&C.*—Wampole (Canada) brand of Aspirin, Codeine, and Caffeine (Systemic)*, 794

A&C with Codeine*—Drug Trading (Canada) brand of Aspirin, Codeine, and Caffeine (Systemic)*, 794

Accurate*—Accurate (Canada) brand of Aspirin and Caffeine (Systemic), 1036

Accurate Forte*—Accurate (Canada) brand of Acetaminophen, Salicylamide, and Caffeine (Systemic), 4

Accurbron—Merrell Dow (U.S.) brand of Theophylline (Systemic), 208

Accutane—Roche (U.S. and Canada) brand of Isotretinoin (Systemic), 633

Acebutolol (Systemic), 185

ACE Inhibitors—See Angiotensin-converting Enzyme (ACE) Inhibitors (Systemic), 93

ACE Inhibitors and Hydrochlorothiazide—See Angiotensin-converting Enzyme (ACE) Inhibitors and Hydrochlorothiazide (Systemic), 96

A'Cenol—Kay (U.S.) brand of Acetaminophen (Systemic), 1

Acephen—G & W (U.S.) brand of Acetaminophen (Systemic), 1

Aceta—Century (U.S.) brand of Acetaminophen (Systemic), 1

Ace-Tabs*—Accurate (Canada) brand of Acetaminophen (Systemic), 1

Acetaco—Legere (U.S.) brand of Acetaminophen and Codeine (Systemic), 785

Aceta with Codeine—Century (U.S.) brand of Acetaminophen and Codeine (Systemic), 785

Acetaminophen (Systemic), 1

Acetaminophen and Aspirin (Systemic), 4

Acetaminophen, Aspirin, and Caffeine (Systemic), 4

Acetaminophen, Aspirin, and Caffeine, Buffered (Systemic), 4

Acetaminophen, Aspirin, and Codeine (Systemic), 789

Acetaminophen, Aspirin, and Codeine, Buffered (Systemic), 789

Acetaminophen, Aspirin, and Salicylamide (Systemic), 4

Acetaminophen, Aspirin, and Salicylamide, Buffered (Systemic), 4

Acetaminophen, Aspirin, Salicylamide, and Caffeine (Systemic), 4

Acetaminophen, Aspirin, Salicylamide, Codeine, and Caffeine (Systemic), 789

Acetaminophen, Buffered (Systemic), 1

Acetaminophen and Caffeine (Systemic), 1

Acetaminophen and Codeine (Systemic), 785, **1205**

Acetaminophen, Codeine, and Caffeine (Systemic)*, 785

Acetaminophen and Salicylamide (Systemic), 4

Acetaminophen, Salicylamide, and Caffeine (Systemic), 4

Acetaminophen and Salicylates (Systemic), 4

Acetaminophen, Sodium Salicylate, and Caffeine (Systemic), 4

Acetaminophen Uniserts—Upsher-Smith (U.S.) brand of Acetaminophen (Systemic), 1

Acetazolam*—ICN (Canada) brand of Acetazolamide (Systemic), 253

Acetazolamide (Systemic), 253

Acetohexamide (Systemic), 121

Acetohydroxamic Acid (Systemic), 8

Acetophenazine (Systemic), 913

Acetoxyl*—Stiefel (Canada) brand of Benzoyl Peroxide (Topical), 183

Acetylcysteine (Inhalation), 10

Acetylsalicylic acid—See Aspirin (Systemic), 1036

Achromycin—Lederle (U.S.) brand of Tetracycline (Ophthalmic), 1094; (Systemic), 1096; (Topical), 1099

Achromycin V—Lederle (U.S.) brand of Tetracycline (Systemic), 1096, **1205**

Acne-Aid—Stiefel (U.S.) brand of Benzoyl Peroxide (Topical), 183; Stiefel (Canada) brand of Resorcinol and Sulfur (Topical), 1022

Acno—Baker/Cummins (U.S.) brand of Salicylic Acid and Sulfur (Topical), 1043

Acnomel—Menley & James (U.S.) and SKF (Canada) brand of Resorcinol and Sulfur (Topical), 1022

Acnotex—C & M (U.S.) brand of Salicylic Acid and Sulfur (Topical), 1043

Acotin*—Watkins (Canada) brand of Aspirin and Caffeine (Systemic), 1036

Acrisorcin (Topical)*, 12

Acta-Char—Med-Corp (U.S.) brand of Charcoal, Activated (Oral), 264

Actacin—Vangard (U.S.) brand of Triprolidine and Pseudoephedrine (Systemic), 134

Actagen—Generix (U.S.) brand of Triprolidine and Pseudoephedrine (Systemic), 134

Actamin—Buffington (U.S.) brand of Acetaminophen (Systemic), 1

Actamine—H. L. Moore (U.S.) brand of Triprolidine and Pseudoephedrine (Systemic), 134

ACTH—See Corticotropin (Systemic—Glucocorticoid Effects), 38

Acthar—Armour (U.S. and U.K.) and Rorer (Canada) brand of Corticotropin (Systemic—Glucocorticoid Effects), 38

Acti-B₁₂*—Charton (Canada) brand of Hydroxocobalamin (Systemic), 1180

Acticort—Baker/Cummins (U.S.) brand of Hydrocortisone (Topical), 33

Actidil—BW (U.S.) brand of Triprolidine (Systemic), 130

Actidose-Aqua—Paddock (U.S.) brand of Charcoal, Activated (Oral), 264

Bromodiphenhydramine (Systemic), 130

Bromodiphenhydramine and Codeine (Systemic), 342

Bromodiphenhydramine, Diphenhydramine, Codeine, Ammonium Chloride, and Potassium Guaiacolsulfonate (Systemic), 342

Bromophen—Rugby (U.S.) brand of Brompheniramine and Phenylpropanolamine (Systemic), 134

Bromophen T.D.—Rugby (U.S.) brand of Brompheniramine, Phenylephrine, and Phenylpropanolamine (Systemic), 134

Bromo-Seltzer—Warner-Lambert (U.S.) brand of Acetaminophen, Buffered (Systemic), 1

Bromphen—Schein (U.S.) brand of Brompheniramine (Systemic), 130

Bromphen Compound T.D.—Rugby (U.S.) brand of Brompheniramine, Phenylephrine, and Phenylpropanolamine (Systemic), 134

Brompheniramine (Systemic), 130

Brompheniramine, Phenylephrine, and Phenylpropanolamine (Systemic), 134

Brompheniramine, Phenylephrine, Phenylpropanolamine, and Codeine (Systemic)*, 342

Brompheniramine, Phenylephrine, Phenylpropanolamine, Codeine, and Guaifenesin (Systemic)*, 342

Brompheniramine, Phenylephrine, Phenylpropanolamine, and Dextromethorphan (Systemic)*, 342

Brompheniramine, Phenylephrine, Phenylpropanolamine, and Guaifenesin (Systemic)*, 342

Brompheniramine, Phenylephrine, Phenylpropanolamine, Hydrocodone, and Guaifenesin (Systemic)*, 342

Brompheniramine and Phenylpropanolamine (Systemic), 134

Brompheniramine, Phenylpropanolamine, and Codeine (Systemic), 342

Brompheniramine, Phenylpropanolamine, and Dextromethorphan (Systemic), 342

Brompheniramine and Pseudoephedrine (Systemic), 134

Brompheniramine, Pseudoephedrine, and Dextromethorphan (Systemic), 342

Brompheril—Copley (U.S.) brand of Dexbrompheniramine and Pseudoephedrine (Systemic), 134

Bronchial—Geneva Generics (U.S.) brand of Theophylline and Guaifenesin (Systemic), 1111

Bronchodilators, Adrenergic (Inhalation), 201; (Oral/Injection), 204

Bronchodilators, Xanthine-derivative (Systemic), 208

*Broncho-Grippol-DM**—Charton (Canada) brand of Dextromethorphan (Systemic), 393

Broncholate—Bock (U.S.) brand of Ephedrine and Guaifenesin (Systemic), 342

Brondecon—PD (U.S.) brand of Oxtriphylline and Guaifenesin (Systemic), 864

Brondelate—Balan (U.S.); Barre (U.S.); Bioline (U.S.); CMC (U.S.); Cooper (U.S.); Dixon-Shane (U.S.); Gen-King (U.S.); Harber (U.S.); Moore (U.S.); Murray (U.S.); Schein (U.S.); and Williams (U.S.) brand of Oxtriphylline and Guaifenesin (Systemic), 864

Bronitin Mist—Whitehall (U.S.) brand of Epinephrine (Inhalation), 201

Bronkaid Mist—Winthrop (U.S.) brand of Epinephrine (Inhalation), 201

*Bronkaid Mistometer**—Winthrop (Canada) brand of Epinephrine (Inhalation), 201

Bronkaid Mist Suspension—Winthrop (U.S.) brand of Epinephrine (Inhalation), 201

Bronkephrine—Winthrop (U.S.) brand of Ethylnorepinephrine (Oral/Injection), 204

Bronkodyl—Winthrop (U.S.) brand of Theophylline (Systemic), 208

Bronkolixir—Winthrop (U.S.) brand of Theophylline, Ephedrine, Guaifenesin, and Phenobarbital (Systemic), 1105

Bronkometer—Winthrop (U.S.) brand of Isoetharine (Inhalation), 201

Bronkosol—Winthrop (U.S.) brand of Isoetharine (Inhalation), 201

Bronkotabs—Winthrop (U.S.) brand of Theophylline, Ephedrine, Guaifenesin, and Phenobarbital (Systemic), 1105

Bronkotuss Expectorant—Hyrex (U.S.) brand of Chlorpheniramine, Ephedrine, and Guaifenesin (Systemic), 342

Brophed—Cord (U.S.) brand of Theophylline, Ephedrine, and Hydroxyzine (Systemic), 1108

*Brufen**—Boots (U.K.) brand of Ibuprofen (Systemic), 138

B-S-P—Legere (U.S.) brand of Betamethasone (Systemic—Glucocorticoid Effects), 38

Bucet—UAD (U.S.) brand of Butalbital and Acetaminophen (Systemic), 215

Bucladin-S—Stuart (U.S.) brand of Buclizine (Systemic), 704

Buclizine (Systemic), 704

Buf-Bar—3M Personal Care (U.S.) brand of sulfur (Topical), 1081

Buffaprin—Buffington (U.S.) brand of Aspirin, Buffered (Systemic), 1036

Bufferin—Bristol-Myers (U.S. and Canada) brand of Aspirin, Buffered (Systemic), 1036

Buffets II—Bowman (U.S.) brand of Acetaminophen, Aspirin, and Caffeine, Buffered (Systemic), 4

Buffex—Mayrand (U.S.) brand of Aspirin, Buffered (Systemic), 1036

Buffinol—Otis Clapp (U.S.) brand of Aspirin, Buffered (Systemic), 1036

Buf-Oxal—3M Personal Care (U.S.) brand of Benzoyl Peroxide (Topical), 183

Buf-Tabs—Halsey (U.S.) brand of Aspirin, Buffered (Systemic), 1036

Bumetanide (Systemic), 429, **1205**

Bumex—Roche (U.S.) brand of Bumetanide (Systemic), 429, **1205**

Buprenex—Norwich Eaton (U.S.) brand of Buprenorphine (Systemic—For Pain Relief), 779

Buprenorphine (Systemic—For Pain Relief), 779

Burntame—Otis Clapp (U.S.) brand containing Benzocaine (Topical), 88

BuSpar—Mead Johnson (U.S.) brand of Buspirone (Systemic), 211

Buspirone (Systemic), 211

Busulfan (Systemic), 213

Butabarbital (Systemic), 170

Butacaine (Dental), 82

Butace—American Urologicals (U.S.) brand of Butalbital, Acetaminophen, and Caffeine (Systemic), 215

Butalan—Lannett (U.S.) brand of Butabarbital (Systemic), 170

Butalbital A-C—See Butalbital, Aspirin, and Caffeine (Systemic), 222

Butalbital and Acetaminophen (Systemic), 215

Butalbital, Acetaminophen, and Caffeine (Systemic), 215

Butalbital, Acetaminophen, and Codeine (Systemic), 218

Butalbital, Acetaminophen, Codeine, and Caffeine (Systemic), 218

Butalbital, Acetaminophen, Hydrocodone, and Caffeine (Systemic), 218

Butalbital, Acetaminophen, and Narcotic Analgesics (Systemic), 218

Butalbital and Aspirin (Systemic), 222

Butalbital, Aspirin, and Caffeine (Systemic), 222, **1205**

Butalbital, Aspirin, and Codeine (Systemic), 226

Butalbital, Aspirin, Codeine, and Caffeine (Systemic), 226, **1205**

Butalbital Compound—See Butalbital, Aspirin, and Caffeine (Systemic), 222

Butal Compound—Cord (U.S.) brand of Butalbital, Aspirin, and Caffeine (Systemic), 222

Butamben (Topical), 88

C

Compound W—Whitehall (U.S. and Canada) brand of Salicylic Acid (Topical), 1041

Compoz—Jeffrey Martin (U.S.) brand of Diphenhydramine (Systemic), 130

Comtrex Multi-Symptom Cold Reliever—Bristol-Myers (U.S.) brand of Chlorpheniramine, Phenylpropanolamine, Dextromethorphan, and Acetaminophen (Systemic), 342

Conacetol—CMC (U.S.) brand of Acetaminophen (Systemic), 1

Conar—Beecham (U.S.) brand of Phenylephrine and Dextromethorphan (Systemic), 342

Conar-A—Beecham (U.S.) brand of Phenylephrine, Dextromethorphan, Guaifenesin, and Acetaminophen (Systemic), 342

Conar Expectorant—Beecham (U.S.) brand of Phenylephrine, Dextromethorphan, and Guaifenesin (Systemic), 342

Concentrin—PD (U.S.) brand of Pseudoephedrine, Dextromethorphan, and Guaifenesin (Systemic), 342

Condrin-LA—Mallard (U.S.) brand of Phenylpropanolamine and Chlorpheniramine (Systemic), 134

Conex—Forest (U.S.) brand of Phenylpropanolamine and Guaifenesin (Systemic), 342

Conex with Codeine Liquid—Forest (U.S.) brand of Phenylpropanolamine, Codeine, and Guaifenesin (Systemic), 342

Conex D.A.—Forest (U.S.) brand of Phenylpropanolamine and Chlorpheniramine (Systemic), 134

Congespirin—Bristol-Myers (U.S.) brand of Dextromethorphan (Systemic), 393

Congess JR—Fleming (U.S.) brand of Pseudoephedrine and Guaifenesin (Systemic), 342

Congess SR—Fleming (U.S.) brand of Pseudoephedrine and Guaifenesin (Systemic), 342

Conjugated Estrogens (Vaginal), 480

Conjugated Estrogens C.S.D.*—Pharmascience (Canada) brand of Conjugated Estrogens (Systemic), 476

Conray—Mallinckrodt (U.S.) brand of Iothalamate (Systemic), 615

Conray-400—Mallinckrodt (U.S.) brand of Iothalamate (Systemic), 615

Constant-T—Geigy (U.S.) brand of Theophylline (Systemic), 208

Contac—Menley & James (U.S.) brand of Phenylpropanolamine and Chlorpheniramine (Systemic), 134

Contac-C*—SKF (Canada) brand of Phenylpropanolamine and Chlorpheniramine (Systemic), 134

Contac Jr. Children's Cold Medicine—Menley & James (U.S.) brand of Phenylpropanolamine, Dextromethorphan, and Acetaminophen (Systemic), 342

Contac Severe Cold Formula—Menley & James (U.S.) brand of Chlorpheniramine, Pseudoephedrine, Dextromethorphan, and Acetaminophen (Systemic), 342

Contac Severe Cold Formula Night Strength—Menley & James (U.S.) brand of Doxylamine, Pseudoephedrine, Dextromethorphan, and Acetaminophen (Systemic), 342

Control—Thompson (U.S.) brand of Phenylpropanolamine (Systemic), 928

Cophene No.2—Dunhall (U.S.) brand of Phenylephrine, Phenylpropanolamine, and Chlorpheniramine (Systemic), 134

Cophene-S—Dunhall (U.S.) brand of Chlorpheniramine, Phenylephrine, Phenylpropanolamine, and Dihydrocodeine (Systemic), 342

Cophene-X—Dunhall (U.S.) brand of Chlorpheniramine, Phenylephrine, Phenylpropanolamine, Carbetapentane, and Potassium Guaiacolsulfonate (Systemic), 342

Cophene-XP—Dunhall (U.S.) brand of Chlorpheniramine, Phenylephrine, Phenylpropanolamine, Carbetapentane, and Potassium Guaiacolsulfonate (Systemic), 342

Co-Pyronil 2—Dista (U.S.) brand of Chlorpheniramine and Pseudoephedrine (Systemic), 134

Cordamine-PA—Cord (U.S.) brand of Brompheniramine, Phenylephrine, and Phenylpropanolamine (Systemic), 134

Cordarone—Wyeth (U.S. and Canada) brand of Amiodarone (Systemic), 63

Cordran—Dista (U.S.) brand of Flurandrenolide (Topical), 33

Cordran SP—Dista (U.S.) brand of Flurandrenolide (Topical), 33

Corgard—Squibb (U.S. and Canada) brand of Nadolol (Systemic), 185, **1205**

Coricidin with Codeine*—Schering (Canada) brand of Chlorpheniramine, Codeine, Aspirin, and Caffeine (Systemic)*, 342

Coricidin Cough—Schering (U.S.) brand of Phenylpropanolamine, Dextromethorphan, and Guaifenesin (Systemic), 342

Coricidin Nasal Mist—Schering (U.S.) brand of Oxymetazoline (Nasal), 868; Phenylephrine (Nasal), 924

Coristex-DH*—Technilab (Canada) brand of Diphenylpyraline, Phenylephrine, and Hydrocodone (Systemic)*, 342

Corium*—ICN (Canada) brand of Chlordiazepoxide and Clidinium (Systemic), 285

Coronex*—Ayerst (Canada) brand of Isosorbide Dinitrate (Systemic—Oral), 829; (Systemic—Sublingual, Chewable, or Buccal), 832

Corophyllin*—Beecham (Canada) brand of Aminophylline (Systemic), 208

Correctol—Plough (U.S.) brand of Phenolphthalein (Oral), 654

Corsym—Pennwalt (U.S. and Canada) brand of Phenylpropanolamine and Chlorpheniramine (Systemic), 134

Cortaid—Upjohn (U.S.) brand of Hydrocortisone (Topical), 33

Cortalone—Halsey (U.S.) brand of Prednisolone (Systemic—Glucocorticoid Effects), 38

Cortamed*—Berlex (Canada) brand of Hydrocortisone (Ophthalmic), 26; (Otic), 29

Cortate*—Schering (Canada) brand of Hydrocortisone (Topical), 33

Cort-Dome—Miles (U.S.) brand of Hydrocortisone (Rectal), 575; (Topical), 33

Cortef—Upjohn (U.S. and Canada) brand of Hydrocortisone (Systemic—Glucocorticoid Effects), 38; Upjohn (U.S.) brand of Hydrocortisone (Topical), 33

Cortelan*—Glaxo (U.K.) brand of Cortisone (Systemic—Glucocorticoid Effects), 38

Cortenema—Reid-Rowell (U.S.) and Bengué (U.K.) brand of Hydrocortisone (Systemic—Glucocorticoid Effects), 38

Corticaine—Glaxo (U.S.) brand of Hydrocortisone (Rectal), 575; (Topical), 33

Corticotropin (Systemic—Glucocorticoid Effects), 38

Corticreme*—Rougier (Canada) brand of Hydrocortisone (Topical), 33

Cortifoam—Reed & Carnrick (U.S. and Canada) brand of Hydrocortisone (Systemic—Glucocorticoid Effects), 38

Cortiment*—Nordic (Canada) brand of Hydrocortisone (Rectal), 575; (Topical), 33

Cortisol—See Hydrocortisone (Ophthalmic), 26; (Otic), 29; (Systemic—Glucorticoid Effects), 38; (Topical), 33

Cortisone (Systemic—Glucocorticoid Effects), 38

Cortisporin—BW (U.S.) brand of Neomycin, Polymyxin B, and Hydrocortisone (Ophthalmic), 812; (Otic), 814

Cortistab*—Boots (U.K.) brand of Cortisone (Systemic—Glucocorticoid Effects), 38

Cortizone—Thompson (U.S.) brand of Hydrocortisone (Topical), 33

Cortoderm*—K-Line (Canada) brand of Hydrocortisone (Topical), 33

Cortone—MSD (U.S. and Canada) brand of Cortisone, 38

Cortril—Pfipharmecs (U.S.) brand of Hydrocortisone (Topical), 33

Cortrophin Zinc—Organon (U.S.) brand of Corticotropin (Systemic—Glucocorticoid Effects), 38

Deltastab*—Boots (U.K.) brand of Prednisolone (Systemic—Glucocorticoid Effects), 38

Deltavac—Trimen (U.S.) brand of Sulfanilamide, Aminacrine, and Allantoin (Vaginal), 1076

Demazin—Schering (U.S.) brand of Phenylephrine and Chlorpheniramine (Systemic), 134

Demazin Repetabs—Schering (U.S.) brand of Phenylpropanolamine and Chlorpheniramine (Systemic), 134

Demecarium (Ophthalmic), 127

Demeclocycline (Systemic), 1096

Demerol—Winthrop (U.S. and Canada) brand of Meperidine (Systemic—For Pain Relief), 779, **1205**; (Systemic—For Surgery and Obstetrics), 783, **1205**

Demerol-APAP—Winthrop (U.S.) brand of Meperidine and Acetaminophen (Systemic), 785

Demi-Regroton—Rorer (U.S.) brand of Reserpine and Chlorthalidone (Systemic), 1009

Demo-Cineol*—Sabex (Canada) brand of Dextromethorphan (Systemic), 393

Demser—MSD (U.S.) brand of Metyrosine (Systemic), 747

Demulen—Searle (U.S. and Canada) brand of Ethynodiol Diacetate and Ethinyl Estradiol (Systemic), 483

Denorex—Whitehall (U.S.) brand of Coal Tar (Topical), 334

Denta-FL—Saron (U.S.) brand of Sodium Fluoride (Systemic), 1056

Depakene—Abbott (U.S. and Canada) brand of Valproic Acid (Systemic), 1162

Depakote—Abbott (U.S.) brand of Divalproex (Systemic), 1162

Depanate—Western Research (U.S.) brand of Estradiol (Systemic), 476

depAndro—Forest (U.S.) brand of Testosterone (Systemic), 79

depAndrogyn—Forest (U.S.) brand of Testosterone and Estradiol (Systemic), 1091

Depen—Wallace (U.S.) and Horner (Canada) brand of Penicillamine (Systemic) 894

Depestro—Kay (U.S.) brand of Estradiol (Systemic), 476

depGynogen—Forest (U.S.) brand of Estradiol (Systemic), 476

depMedalone—Forest (U.S.) brand of Methylprednisolone (Systemic—Glucocorticoid Effects), 38

Depo-Estradiol—Upjohn (U.S.) brand of Estradiol (Systemic), 476

Depogen—Hyrex (U.S.) brand of Estradiol (Systemic), 476

Depoject—Mayrand (U.S.) brand of Methylprednisolone (Systemic—Glucocorticoid Effects), 38

Depo-Medrol—Upjohn (U.S. and Canada) brand of Methylprednisolone (Systemic—Glucocorticoid Effects), 38

Depo-Medrone*—Upjohn (U.K.) brand of Methylprednisolone (Systemic—Glucocorticoid Effects), 38

Deponit—Wyeth (U.S.) brand of Nitroglycerin (Systemic—Topical), 836

Depopred—Hyrex (U.S.) brand of Methylprednisolone (Systemic—Glucocorticoid Effects), 38

Depo-Predate—Legere (U.S.) brand of Methylprednisolone (Systemic—Glucocorticoid Effects), 38

Depo-Provera—Upjohn (U.S. and Canada) brand of Medroxyprogesterone (Systemic), 974

Depotest—Hyrex (U.S.) brand of Testosterone (Systemic), 79

Depo-Testadiol—Upjohn (U.S.) brand of Testosterone and Estradiol (Systemic), 1091

Depotestogen—Hyrex (U.S.) brand of Testosterone and Estradiol (Systemic), 1091

Depo-Testosterone—Upjohn (U.S. and Canada) brand of Testosterone (Systemic), 79

Deproist Expectorant with Codeine—Geneva Generics (U.S.) brand of Pseudoephedrine, Codeine, and Guaifenesin (Systemic), 342

Derbac*—Bengue (U.K.) brand of Malathion (Topical)*, 689

Dermacoat—Century (U.S.) brand containing Benzocaine (Topical), 88

Dermacort—Reid-Rowell (U.S.) brand of Hydrocortisone (Topical), 33

Derma Medicone—Medicone (U.S.) brand containing Benzocaine (Topical), 88

Derma-Soft Creme—Ex-Lax (U.S.) brand of Salicylic Acid (Topical), 1041

Dermatologic Shower System—L'Aimee (U.S.) brand of Coal Tar (Topical), 334

DermiCort—Republic (U.S.) brand of Hydrocortisone (Topical), 33

Dermolate—Schering (U.S.) brand of Hydrocortisone (Rectal), 575; (Topical), 33

Dermoplast—Ayerst (U.S. and Canada) brand containing Benzocaine (Topical), 88

Dermovate*—Glaxo (Canada and U.K.) brand of Clobetasol (Topical), 33

Dermovate Scalp Application*—Glaxo (U.K.) brand of Clobetasol (Topical), 33

Dermoxyl*—ICN (Canada) brand of Benzoyl Peroxide (Topical), 183

Dermoxyl Aqua*—ICN (Canada) brand of Benzoyl Peroxide (Topical), 183

Dermtex HC—Pfeiffer (U.S.) brand of Hydrocortisone (Topical), 33

Deronil*—Schering (Canada) brand of Dexamethasone (Systemic—Glucocorticoid Effects), 38

DES—See Diethylstilbestrol (Systemic), 476

Desenex—Pennwalt (U.S.) brand of Undecylenic Acid, Compound (Topical), 1156

Deserpidine (Systemic), 1006

Deserpidine and Hydrochlorothiazide (Systemic), 1009

Deserpidine and Methyclothiazide (Systemic), 1009

Desferal—Ciba (U.S. and Canada) brand of Deferoxamine (Systemic), 389

Desferrioxamine—See Deferoxamine (Systemic), 389

Desipramine (Systemic), 117, **1205**

Deslanoside (Systemic), 406

Desmopressin (Systemic), 391

Desonide (Topical), 33

Desonide and Acetic Acid (Otic), 36

DesOwen—Owen/Allercreme (U.S.) brand of Desonide (Topical), 33

Desoximetasone (Topical), 33

Desoxycorticosterone (Systemic—Mineralocorticoid Effects), 31

Desoxyn—Abbott (U.S.) brand of Methamphetamine (Systemic), 67

Desquam-E—Westwood (U.S.) brand of Benzoyl Peroxide (Topical), 183

Desquam-X—Westwood (U.S. and Canada) brand of Benzoyl Peroxide (Topical), 183

Desyrel—Mead Johnson (U.S.) and Bristol (Canada) brand of Trazodone (Systemic), 1136, **1205**

Desyrel Dividose—Mead Johnson (U.S.) brand of Trazodone (Systemic), 1136, **1205**

Detensol*—Desbergers (Canada) brand of Propranolol (Systemic), 185

De-Tuss—H. L. Moore (U.S.) brand of Pseudoephedrine and Hydrocodone (Systemic), 342

Detussin Expectorant—Barre (U.S.); Bioline (U.S.); Cooper (U.S.); Dixon-Shane (U.S.); Euclid (U.S.); H. L. Moore (U.S.); Murray (U.S.); Parmed (U.S.); Schein (U.S.); Spencer-Mead (U.S.); Veratrex (U.S.); and Vita-Rx (U.S.) brand of Pseudoephedrine, Hydrocodone, and Guaifenesin (Systemic), 342

Detussin Liquid—Barre (U.S.); Bioline (U.S.); CMC (U.S.); Cooper (U.S.); Dixon-Shane (U.S.); Interstate (U.S.); H. L. Moore (U.S.); Murray (U.S.); Parmed (U.S.); Schein (U.S.); Spencer-Mead (U.S.); Veratrex (U.S.); and Vita-Rx (U.S.) brand of Pseudoephedrine and Hydrocodone (Systemic), 342

Dilaudid Cough—Knoll (U.S.) brand of Hydromorphone and Guaifenesin (Systemic), 342

Dilaudid-HP—Knoll (U.S. and Canada) brand of Hydromorphone (Systemic—For Pain Relief), 779

Dilomine—Kay (U.S.) brand of Dicyclomine (Systemic), 142

Dilor—Savage (U.S.) brand of Dyphylline (Systemic), 208

Diltiazem (Systemic), 238, **1205**

Dimelor*—Lilly (Canada) brand of Acetohexamide (Systemic), 121

Dimacol—Robins (U.S.) brand of Pseudoephedrine, Dextromethorphan, and Guaifenesin (Systemic), 342

Dimenhydrinate (Systemic), 130

Dimentabs—Bowman (U.S.) brand of Dimenhydrinate (Systemic), 130

Dimetane—Robins (U.S. and Canada) brand of Brompheniramine (Systemic), 130

Dimetane-DC Cough—Robins (U.S.) brand of Brompheniramine, Phenylpropanolamine, and Codeine (Systemic), 342

Dimetane Decongestant—Robins (U.S.) brand of Phenylephrine and Brompheniramine (Systemic), 134

Dimetane-DX Cough—Robins (U.S.) brand of Brompheniramine, Pseudoephedrine, and Dextromethorphan (Systemic), 342

Dimetane Expectorant*—Robins (Canada) brand of Brompheniramine, Phenylephrine, Phenylpropanolamine, and Guaifenesin (Systemic)*, 342

Dimetane Expectorant-C*—Robins (Canada) brand of Brompheniramine, Phenylephrine, Phenylpropanolamine, Codeine, and Guaifenesin (Systemic)*, 342

Dimetane Expectorant-DC*—Robins (Canada) brand of Brompheniramine, Phenylephrine, Phenylpropanolamine, Hydrocodone, and Guaifenesin (Systemic)*, 342

Dimetane Extentabs—Robins (U.S.) brand of Brompheniramine (Systemic), 130

Dimetane-Ten—Robins (U.S.) brand of Brompheniramine (Systemic), 130

Dimetapp—Robins (Canada) brand of Brompheniramine, Phenylephrine, and Phenylpropanolamine (Systemic); Robins (U.S.) brand of Brompheniramine and Phenylpropanolamine (Systemic), 134

Dimetapp with Codeine*—Robins (Canada) brand of Brompheniramine, Phenylephrine, Phenylpropanolamine, and Codeine (Systemic)*, 342

Dimetapp-DM*—Robins (Canada) brand of Brompheniramine, Phenylephrine, Phenylpropanolamine, and Dextromethorphan (Systemic)*, 342

Dimetapp Extentabs—Robins (Canada) brand of Brompheniramine, Phenylephrine, and Phenylpropanolamine (Systemic); Robins (U.S.) brand of Brompheniramine and Phenylpropanolamine (Systemic), 134

Dimethyl Sulfoxide (Mucosal), 412

Dinate—Seatrace (U.S.) brand of Dimenhydrinate (Systemic), 130

Dinoprost (Intra-amniotic), 413

Dinoprostone (Vaginal), 414

Diocto—Barre-National (U.S.); Bioline (U.S.); Cooper (U.S.); Dixon-Shane (U.S.); Goldline (U.S.); Moore (U.S.); Rugby (U.S.); Schein (U.S.); Unit Dose (U.S.); and United Research (U.S.) brand of Docusate (Oral), 654

Diocto-C—Rugby (U.S.) brand of Casanthranol and Docusate (Oral), 654

Diocto-K—Rugby (U.S.) brand of Docusate (Oral), 654

Diocto-K Plus—Rugby (U.S.) brand of Casanthranol and Docusate (Oral), 654

Diocto Plus—Rugby (U.S.) brand of Docusate, Carboxymethylcellulose, and Casanthranol (Oral), 654

Dioctyl sodium sulfosuccinate—See Docusate (Oral), 654

Dioderm*—Dermal (U.K.) brand of Hydrocortisone (Topical), 33

Diodoquin*—Searle (Canada) brand of Iodoquinol (Oral), 607

Dioeze—Century (U.S.) brand of Docusate (Oral), 654

Diolax—Century (U.S.) brand of Casanthranol and Docusate (Oral), 654

Diosuccin—CMC (U.S.) brand of Docusate (Oral), 654

Dio-Sul—Vortech (U.S.) brand of Docusate (Oral), 654

Diothron—Vortech (U.S.) brand of Casanthranol and Docusate (Oral), 654

Dioval—Keene (U.S.) brand of Estradiol (Systemic), 476

Diovol*—Horner (Canada) brand of Alumina, Magnesia, and Simethicone (Oral), 99

Diovol Ex*—Horner (Canada) brand of Alumina and Magnesia (Oral), 99

Diphen—Bay (U.S.) brand of Diphenhydramine (Systemic), 130

Diphenacen—Central (U.S.) brand of Diphenhydramine (Systemic), 130

Diphenadril—Vitarine (U.S.) brand of Diphenhydramine (Systemic), 130

Diphenatol—Rugby (U.S.) brand of Diphenoxylate and Atropine (Systemic), 417

Diphenhydramine (Systemic), 130, **1205**

Diphenhydramine, Codeine, and Ammonium Chloride (Systemic)*, 342

Diphenhydramine, Dextromethorphan, and Ammonium Chloride (Systemic)*, 342

Diphenhydramine and Pseudoephedrine (Systemic), 134

Diphenidol (Systemic), 415

Diphenoxylate and Atropine (Systemic), 417, **1205**

Diphenylan—Lannett (U.S.) brand of Phenytoin (Systemic), 109

Diphenylhydantoin—See Phenytoin (Systemic), 109

Diphenylpyraline (Systemic), 130

Diphenylpyraline, Phenylephrine, and Codeine (Systemic)*, 342

Diphenylpyraline, Phenylephrine, and Dextromethorphan (Systemic)*, 342

Diphenylpyraline, Phenylephrine, and Hydrocodone (Systemic)*, 342

Diphenylpyraline, Phenylephrine, Hydrocodone, and Guaifenesin (Systemic)*, 342

Diphtheria and Tetanus Toxoids and Pertussis Vaccine Adsorbed (Systemic), 419

Dipivefrin (Ophthalmic), 421

Diprolene—Schering (U.S. and Canada) brand of Betamethasone (Topical), 33

Diprosone—Schering (U.S. and Canada) and Kirby-Warrick (U.K.) brand of Betamethasone (Topical), 33

Dipyridamole (Systemic), 423, **1205**

Diquinol—CMC (U.S.) brand of Iodoquinol (Oral), 607

Disalcid—Riker (U.S.) brand of Salsalate (Systemic), 1036

Disanthrol—Lannett (U.S.) brand of Casanthranol and Docusate (Oral), 654

Discase*—Flint (Canada) brand of Chymopapain (Parenteral-Local), 298

Disipal—Riker (U.S.) and Brocades (U.K.) brand of Orphenadrine (Systemic), 857

Disolan—Lannett (U.S.) brand of Docusate and Phenolphthalein (Oral), 654

Disolan Forte—Lannett (U.S.) brand of Carboxymethylcellulose, Casanthranol, and Docusate (Oral), 654

Disonate—Lannett (U.S.) brand of Docusate (Oral), 654

Disophrol—Schering (U.S.) brand of Dexbrompheniramine and Pseudoephedrine (Systemic), 134

Disophrol Chronotabs—Schering (U.S.) brand of Dexbrompheniramine and Pseudoephedrine (Systemic), 134

Disoplex—Lannett (U.S.) brand of Carboxymethylcellulose and Docusate (Oral), 654

Disopyramide (Systemic), 425

Di-Sosul—Drug Industries (U.S.) brand of Docusate (Oral), 654

Di-Sosul Forte—Drug Industries (U.S.) brand of Casanthranol and Docusate (Oral), 654

Di-Spaz—Vortech (U.S.) brand of Dicyclomine (Systemic), 142

Dispos-a-Med Isoetharine—PD (U.S.) brand of Isoetharine (Inhalation), 201

Dispos-a-Med Isoproterenol—PD (U.S.) brand of Isoproterenol (Inhalation), 201

Distamine*—Dista (U.K.) brand of Penicillamine (Systemic) 894

Disulfiram (Systemic), 427

Ditate DS—Savage (U.S.) brand of Testosterone and Estradiol (Systemic), 1091

Dithranol—See Anthralin (Topical), 102

Ditropan—Marion (U.S.) and Norwich Eaton (Canada) brand of Oxybutynin (Systemic), 866

Diucardin—Ayerst (U.S.) brand of Hydroflumethiazide (Systemic), 438

Diuchlor H*—Medic (Canada) brand of Hydrochlorothiazide (Systemic), 438

Diulo—Searle (U.S.) brand of Metolazone (Systemic), 438

Diupres—MSD (U.S.) brand of Reserpine and Chlorothiazide (Systemic), 1009

Diuretics, Loop (Systemic), 429

Diuretics, Potassium-sparing (Systemic), 432

Diuretics, Potassium-sparing, and Hydrochlorothiazide (Systemic), 435

Diuretics, Thiazide (Systemic), 438

Diuril—MSD (U.S.) brand of Chlorothiazide (Systemic), 438

Diutensen-R—Wallace (U.S.) brand of Reserpine and Methyclothiazide (Systemic), 1009

Divalproex (Systemic), 1162

Dixarit*—Boehringer Ingelheim (Canada) brand of Clonidine (Systemic), 322

DM Cough—Bay (U.S.) brand of Dextromethorphan (Systemic), 393

DMSO—See Dimethyl Sulfoxide (Mucosal), 412

DM Syrup*—PD (Canada) brand of Dextromethorphan (Systemic), 393

Doak Oil—Doak (U.S.) and TCD (Canada) brand of Coal Tar (Topical), 334

Doak Oil Forte—Doak (U.S.) and TCD (Canada) brand of Coal Tar (Topical), 334

Doak Tar—Doak (U.S.) brand of Coal Tar (Topical), 334

Doan's Pills—DEP (U.S.) brand of Magnesium Salicylate, 1036; Fulford (Canada) brand of Acetaminophen and Salicylamide (Systemic), 4

DOCA—See Desoxycorticosterone (Systemic—Mineralocorticoid Effects), 31

Docu-K Plus—Newtron (U.S.) brand of Casanthranol and Docusate (Oral), 654

Docusate (Oral), 654; (Rectal), 659

Docusate, Carboxymethylcellulose, and Casanthranol (Oral), 654

Docusate and Mineral Oil (Oral), 654

Docusate and Phenolphthalein (Oral), 654

doktors—Scherer (U.S.) brand of Phenylephrine (Nasal), 924

Dolacet—Hauck (U.S.) brand of Hydrocodone and Acetaminophen (Systemic), 785

Dolanex—Lannett (U.S.) brand of Acetaminophen (Systemic), 1

Dolene—Lederle (U.S.) brand of Propoxyphene (Systemic—For Pain Relief), 779

Dolene-AP—Lederle (U.S.) brand of Propoxyphene and Acetaminophen (Systemic), 785

Dolene Compound—Lederle (U.S.) brand of Propoxyphene, Aspirin, and Caffeine (Systemic), 794

Dolobid—MSD (U.S.); Frosst (Canada); and Thomas Morson (U.K.) brand of Diflunisal (Systemic), 138, **1205**

Dolo-Pap—T.E. Williams (U.S.) brand of Hydrocodone and Acetaminophen (Systemic), 785

Dolophine—Lilly (U.S.) brand of Methadone (Systemic—For Pain Relief), 779

Doloxene*—Lilly (U.K.) brand of Propoxyphene (Systemic—For Pain Relief), 779

Dolprn—Bock (U.S.) brand of Acetaminophen, Aspirin, and Codeine, Buffered (Systemic), 789

Dolsed—American Urologicals (U.S.) brand of Atropine, Hyoscyamine, Methenamine, Methylene Blue, Phenyl Salicylate, and Benzoic Acid (Systemic), 163

Dommanate—Forest (U.S.) brand of Dimenhydrinate (Systemic), 130

Donatussin—Laser (U.S.) brand of Chlorpheniramine, Phenylephrine, Dextromethorphan, and Guaifenesin (Systemic), 342

Donatussin DC—Laser (U.S.) brand of Phenylephrine, Hydrocodone, and Guaifenesin (Systemic), 342

Donatussin Drops—Laser (U.S.) brand of Chlorpheniramine, Phenylephrine, and Guaifenesin (Systemic), 342

Dondril—Whitehall (U.S.) brand of Chlorpheniramine, Phenylephrine, and Dextromethorphan (Systemic), 342

Donnagel-MB*—Robins (Canada) brand of Kaolin and Pectin (Oral), 639

Donnagel-PG—Robins (U.S.) brand of Kaolin, Pectin, Belladonna Alkaloids, and Opium (Systemic), 641; Robins (Canada) brand of Kaolin, Pectin, and Paregoric (Systemic), 644

Donnapine—Major (U.S.) brand of Atropine, Hyoscyamine, Scopolamine, and Phenobarbital (Systemic), 174

Donna-Sed—Vortech (U.S.) brand of Atropine, Hyoscyamine, Scopolamine, and Phenobarbital (Systemic), 174

Donnatal—Robins (U.S. and Canada) brand of Atropine, Hyoscyamine, Scopolamine, and Phenobarbital (Systemic), 174, **1205**

Donnatal Extentabs—Robins (U.S. and Canada) brand of Atropine, Hyoscyamine, Scopolamine, and Phenobarbital (Systemic), 174

Donnazyme—Robins (U.S. and Canada) brand of Pancreatin, Pepsin, Bile Salts, Hyoscyamine, Atropine, Scopolamine, and Phenobarbital (Systemic) 873

Donphen—Lemmon (U.S.) brand of Atropine, Hyoscyamine, Scopolamine, and Phenobarbital (Systemic), 174

Dopamet*—ICN (Canada) brand of Methyldopa (Systemic), 729

Dopar—Norwich Eaton (U.S.) brand of Levodopa (Systemic), 668

Dorbanex*—Riker (Canada) brand of Danthron and Poloxamer 188 (Oral)*, 654

Dorcol Children's Cough—Dorsey (U.S.) brand of Pseudoephrine, Dextromethorphan, and Guaifenesin (Systemic), 342

Dorcol Children's Fever and Pain Reducer—Dorsey (U.S.) brand of Acetaminophen (Systemic), 1

Dorcol Liquid Cold Formula—Sandoz (U.S.) brand of Chlorpheniramine and Pseudoephedrine (Systemic), 134

Dorcol Pediatric Formula—Dorsey (U.S.) brand of Pseudoephedrine (Systemic), 982

Doriden—Rorer (U.S.) brand of Glutethimide (Systemic), 536

Dormarex—Republic (U.S.) brand of Pyrilamine (Systemic), 130

Doryx—PD (U.S.) brand of Doxycycline (Systemic), 1096

Doss—Bay (U.S.) brand of Docusate (Oral); Beecham (Canada) brand of Danthron and Docusate (Oral), 654

DOW-Isoniazid—Merrell Dow (U.S.) brand of Isoniazid (Systemic), 628

Doxaphene—Major (U.S.) brand of Propoxyphene (Systemic—For Pain Relief), 779

Doxaphene Compound—Major (U.S.) brand of Propoxyphene, Aspirin, and Caffeine (Systemic), 794

Doxepin (Systemic), 117, **1205**

Doxidan—Hoechst-Roussel (U.S.) brand of Docusate and Phenolphthalein (Oral), 654

Doxinate—Hoechst-Roussel (U.S.) brand of Docusate (Oral), 654

Dura-Vent—Dura (U.S.) brand of Phenylpropanolamine and Guaifenesin (Systemic), 342

Duretic*—Abbott (Canada) brand of Methyclothiazide (Systemic), 438

Dureticyl*—Abbott (Canada) brand of Deserpidine and Methyclothiazide (Systemic), 1009

Duricef—Mead Johnson (U.S.) and Bristol (Canada) brand of Cefadroxil (Systemic), 261, **1205**

Durrax—Dermik (U.S.) brand of Hydroxyzine (Systemic), 585

Duvoid—Norwich Eaton (U.S. and Canada) brand of Bethanechol (Systemic), 195

DV—Merrell Dow (U.S. and Canada) brand of Dienestrol (Vaginal), 480

Dyazide—SKF (U.S. and Canada) brand of Triamterene and Hydrochlorothiazide (Systemic), 435, **1205**

Dycill—Beecham (U.S.) brand of Dicloxacillin (Systemic), 896

Dyflex—Econo Med (U.S.) brand of Dyphylline (Systemic), 208

Dylline—Kay (U.S.) brand of Dyphylline (Systemic), 208

Dymelor—Lilly (U.S.) brand of Acetohexamide (Systemic), 121

Dymenate—Keene (U.S.) brand of Dimenhydrinate (Systemic), 130

Dynapen—Bristol (U.S. and Canada) brand of Dicloxacillin (Systemic), 896

Dy-Phyl-Lin—Foy (U.S.) brand of Dyphylline (Systemic), 208

Dyphylline (Systemic), 208

Dyrenium—SKF (U.S. and Canada) brand of Triamterene (Systemic), 432

Dyrexan-OD—Trimen Laboratories (U.S.) brand of Phendimetrazine (Systemic), 153

Dysne-Inhal*—Rougier (Canada) brand of Epinephrine (Inhalation), 201

E

812*—AMC (Canada) brand of Aspirin and Caffeine (Systemic), 1036

8-Hour Bayer Timed-Release—Glenbrook (U.S.) brand of Aspirin (Systemic), 1036

Easprin—PD (U.S.) brand of Aspirin (Systemic), 1036

Echothiophate (Ophthalmic), 127

Econazole (Topical), 445

Econopred—Alcon (U.S.) brand of Prednisolone (Ophthalmic), 26

Econopred Plus—Alcon (U.S.) brand of Prednisolone (Ophthalmic), 26

Ecostatin*—Squibb (Canada) brand of Econazole (Topical), 445

Ecotrin—Menley & James (U.S.) and SKF (Canada) brand of Aspirin (Systemic), 1036

Ectosone*—Technilab (Canada) brand of Betamethasone (Topical), 33

Ectosone Scalp Lotion*—Technilab (Canada) brand of Betamethasone (Topical), 33

E-Cypionate—Legere (U.S.) brand of Estradiol (Systemic), 476

Edecrin—MSD (U.S. and Canada) brand of Ethacrynic Acid (Systemic), 429

E.E.S.—Abbott (U.S. and Canada) brand of Erythromycin Ethylsuccinate (Systemic), 468

Efcortelan*—Glaxo (U.K.) brand of Hydrocortisone (Systemic—Glucocorticoid Effects), 38; (Topical), 33

Efcortesol*—Glaxo (U.K.) brand of Hydrocortisone (Systemic—Glucocorticoid Effects), 38

Efed II—Alto (U.S.) brand of Phenylpropanolamine (Systemic), 928

Efedra P.A.—Cord (U.S.) brand of Dexbrompheniramine and Pseudoephedrine (Systemic), 134

E-Ferol—Forest (U.S.) brand of Vitamin E (Systemic), 1185

Effer-syllium—Stuart (U.S.) brand of Psyllium Hydrophilic Mucilloid (Oral), 654

Efficol Cough Whip (Cough Suppressant/Decongestant)—Block (U.S.) brand of Phenylpropanolamine and Dextromethorphan (Systemic), 342

Efficol Cough Whip (Cough Suppressant/Decongestant/Antihistamine)—Block (U.S.) brand of Chlorpheniramine, Phenylpropanolamine, and Dextromethorphan (Systemic), 342

Efficol Cough Whip (Cough Suppressant/Expectorant)—Block (U.S.) brand of Dextromethorphan and Guaifenesin (Systemic), 342

Efricon Expectorant Liquid—Lannett (U.S.) brand of Chlorpheniramine, Phenylephrine, Codeine, Ammonium Chloride, Potassium Guaiacolsulfonate, and Sodium Citrate (Systemic), 342

Efudex—Roche (U.S. and Canada) brand of Fluorouracil (Topical), 518

E-Ionate P.A.—Reid-Rowell (U.S.) brand of Estradiol (Systemic), 476

Elavil—MSD (U.S. and Canada) brand of Amitriptyline (Systemic), 117, **1205**

Elixicon—Berlex (U.S.) brand of Theophylline (Systemic), 208

Elixomin—Cenci (U.S.) brand of Theophylline (Systemic), 208

Elixophyllin—Berlex (U.S.) and Pentagone (Canada) brand of Theophylline (Systemic), 208

Elixophyllin-GG—Berlex (U.S.) brand of Theophylline and Guaifenesin (Systemic), 1111

Elixophyllin SR—Berlex (U.S.) brand of Theophylline (Systemic), 208

Elspar—MSD (U.S.) brand of Asparaginase (Systemic), 159

Eltor*—Dow (Canada) brand of Pseudoephedrine (Systemic), 982

Eltroxin*—Glaxo (Canada) brand of Levothyroxine (Systemic), 1127

Emcodeine—Major (U.S.) brand of Aspirin and Codeine (Systemic), 794

Emcyt—Roche (U.S. and Canada) brand of Estramustine (Systemic), 474

Emex*—Beecham (Canada) brand of Metoclopramide (Systemic), 741

Emitrip—Major (U.S.) brand of Amitriptyline (Systemic), 117

Emo-Cort*—TCD (Canada) brand of Hydrocortisone (Topical), 33

Empirin—BW (U.S.) brand of Aspirin (Systemic), 1036

Empirin with Codeine—BW (U.S.) brand of Aspirin and Codeine (Systemic), 794, **1205**

Empracet with Codeine—BW (U.S. and Canada) brand of Acetaminophen and Codeine (Systemic), 785, **1205**

Emtec*—Technilab (Canada) brand of Acetaminophen and Codeine (Systemic), 785

Emulsoil—Paddock (U.S.) brand of Castor Oil (Oral), 654

E-Mycin—Upjohn (U.S. and Canada) brand of Erythromycin (Systemic), 468, **1205**

E-Mycin E—Upjohn (U.S.) brand of Erythromycin Ethylsuccinate (Systemic), 468

Enalapril (Systemic), 93, **1205**

Enalapril and Hydrochlorothiazide (Systemic), 96, **1205**

Encainide (Systemic), 447

Encaprin—Vicks Health Care (U.S.) brand of Aspirin (Systemic), 1036

Endep—Roche (U.S.) brand of Amitriptyline (Systemic), 117

Endolor—Keene (U.S.) brand of Butalbital, Acetaminophen, and Caffeine (Systemic), 215

Enduron—Abbott (U.S.) brand of Methyclothiazide (Systemic), 438

F

Feminone—Upjohn (U.S.) brand of Ethinyl Estradiol (Systemic), 476

Femiron—Beecham (U.S.) brand of Ferrous Fumarate (Systemic), 623

Femogen*—Stickley (Canada) brand of Estrone (Systemic), 476

Femogex*—Stickley (Canada) brand of Estradiol (Systemic), 476

Femotrone in Oil—Bluco (U.S.) brand of Progesterone (Systemic), 974

Fenfluramine (Systemic), 505

Fenicol*—Alcon (Canada) brand of Chloramphenicol (Ophthalmic), 275

Fenoprofen (Systemic), 138, **1205**

Fenopron*—Dista (U.K.) brand of Fenoprofen (Systemic), 138

Fenoterol (Inhalation)*, 201; (Oral/Injection)*, 204

Fentanyl (Systemic—For Surgery and Obstetrics), 783

Fenylhist—Mallard (U.S.) brand of Diphenhydramine (Systemic), 130

Feosol—Menley & James (U.S.) brand of Ferrous Sulfate (Systemic), 623

Feostat—Forest (U.S.) brand of Ferrous Fumarate (Systemic); Iron Dextran (Systemic), 623

Fergon—Winthrop (U.S. and Canada) brand of Ferrous Gluconate (Systemic), 623

Fer-In-Sol—Mead Johnson (U.S. and Canada) brand of Ferrous Sulfate (Systemic), 623

Fer-Iron—Bay (U.S.); Interstate (U.S.); My-K (U.S.); Rugby (U.S.) brand of Ferrous Sulfate (Systemic), 623

Ferndex—Ferndale (U.S.) brand of Dextroamphetamine (Systemic), 67

Fero-Grad*—Abbott (Canada) brand of Ferrous Sulfate (Systemic), 623

Fero-Gradumet—Abbott (U.S.) brand of Ferrous Sulfate (Systemic), 623

Feronim—Pasadena (U.S.) brand of Iron Dextran (Systemic), 623

Ferralet—Mission (U.S.) brand of Ferrous Gluconate (Systemic), 623

Ferralyn—Lannett (U.S.) brand of Ferrous Sulfate (Systemic), 623

Ferra-TD—Goldline (U.S.) brand of Ferrous Sulfate (Systemic), 623

Ferrous Citrate Fe 59 (Diagnostic), 1001

Ferrous Fumarate (Systemic), 623

Ferrous Gluconate (Systemic), 623

Ferrous Sulfate (Systemic), 623

Ferrous Sulfate Exsiccated—See Ferrous Sulfate (Systemic), 623

Fertinic*—Desbergers (Canada) brand of Ferrous Gluconate (Systemic), 623

Fesofor*—SKF (Canada) brand of Ferrous Sulfate (Systemic), 623

Festal II—Hoechst-Roussel (U.S.) brand of Pancrelipase (Systemic), 875

Fiberall—Rydelle (U.S.) brand of Psyllium Hydrophilic Mucilloid (Oral), 654

FiberCon—Lederle (U.S.) brand of Polycarbophil (Oral), 654

Fiorgen with Codeine—Goldline (U.S.) brand of Butalbital, Aspirin, Codeine, and Caffeine (Systemic), 226

Fiorgen PF—Goldline (U.S.) brand of Butalbital, Aspirin, and Caffeine (Systemic), 222

Fioricet—Sandoz (U.S.) brand of Butalbital, Acetaminophen, and Caffeine (Systemic), 215

Fiorinal—Sandoz (U.S. and Canada) brand of Butalbital, Aspirin, and Caffeine (Systemic), 222, **1205**

Fiorinal with Codeine—Sandoz (U.S. and Canada) brand of Butalbital, Aspirin, Codeine, and Caffeine (Systemic), 226, **1205**

First Aid Cream*—Watkins (Canada) brand containing Benzocaine (Topical), 88

Fivent*—Fisons (Canada) brand of Cromolyn (Inhalation), 351

Flagyl—Searle (U.S.) and Rhone-Poulenc (Canada) brand of Metronidazole (Systemic), 745, **1205**

Flagyl I.V.—Searle (U.S.) brand of Metronidazole (Systemic), 745

Flagyl I.V. RTU—Searle (U.S.) brand of Metronidazole (Systemic), 745

Flavorcee—Hudson (U.S.) brand of Ascorbic Acid (Systemic), 156

Flavoxate (Systemic), 508

Flecainide (Systemic), 510

Fleet Babylax—Fleet (U.S.) brand of Glycerin (Rectal), 659

Fleet Bisacodyl—Fleet (U.S.) brand of Bisacodyl (Oral), 654; (Rectal), 659

Fleet Bisacodyl Prep—Fleet (U.S.) brand of Bisacodyl (Rectal), 659

Fleet Enema—Fleet (U.S.) brand of Sodium Phosphates (Rectal), 659

Fleet Flavored Castor Oil—Fleet (U.S.) brand of Castor Oil (Oral), 654

Fleet Mineral Oil—Fleet (U.S.) brand of Mineral Oil (Rectal), 659

Fleet Phospho-Soda—Fleet (U.S.) brand of Sodium Phosphates (Oral), 654

Fleet Relief—Fleet (U.S.) brand of Pramoxine (Rectal), 86

Fletcher's Castoria—Glenbrook (U.S.) brand of Senna (Oral), 654

Flexaphen—Trimen (U.S.) brand of Chlorzoxazone and Acetaminophen (Systemic), 291

Flexeril—MSD (U.S. and Canada) brand of Cyclobenzaprine (Systemic), 363, **1205**

Flexoject—Mayrand (U.S.) brand of Orphenadrine (Systemic), 857

Flexon—Keene (U.S.) and Wesley (U.S.) brand of Orphenadrine (Systemic), 857

Florinef—Squibb (U.S., Canada, and U.K.) brand of Fludrocortisone (Systemic—Mineralocorticoid Effects), 31

Florone—Dermik (U.S.) and Upjohn (Canada) brand of Diflorasone (Topical), 33

Floropryl—MSD (U.S.) brand of Isoflurophate (Ophthalmic), 127

Flo-Tab—Misemer (U.S.) brand of Sodium Fluoride (Systemic), 1056

Floxuridine (Systemic), 512

Fluanxol*—Merrell (Canada) brand of Flupenthixol (Systemic)*, 1122

Fluanxol Depot*—Merrell (Canada) brand of Flupenthixol (Systemic)*, 1122

Flucytosine (Systemic), 514

Fludrocortisone (Systemic—Mineralocorticoid Effects), 31

Fluidil—Adria (U.S.) brand of Cyclothiazide (Systemic), 438

Flumethasone (Topical), 33

Flunisolide (Inhalation), 21; (Nasal), 24

Fluocinolone (Topical), 33

Fluocinonide (Topical), 33

Fluoderm*—K-Line (Canada) brand of Fluocinolone (Topical), 33

Fluolar*—Riva (Canada) brand of Fluocinolone (Topical), 33

Fluonid—Herbert (U.S.) brand of Fluocinolone (Topical), 33

Fluonide*—Technilab (Canada) brand of Fluocinolone (Topical), 33

Fluor-A-Day*—Pharmascience (Canada) brand of Sodium Fluoride (Systemic), 1056

Fluorident—Zemmer (U.S.) brand of Sodium Fluoride (Systemic), 1056

Fluoritab—Fluoritab (U.S.) brand of Sodium Fluoride (Systemic), 1056

5-Fluorocytosine—See Flucytosine (Systemic), 514

G

Gynogen—Forest (U.S.) brand of Estrone (Systemic), 476
Gynogen L.A.—Forest (U.S.) brand of Estradiol (Systemic), 476

H

Halazepam (Systemic), 179
Hal-Chlor—Halsom (U.S.) brand of Chlorpheniramine (Systemic), 130
Halciderm*—Squibb (U.K.) brand of Halcinonide (Topical), 33
Halcinonide (Topical), 33
Halcion—Upjohn (U.S. and Canada) brand of Triazolam (Systemic), 179, **1205**
Haldol—McNeil (U.S. and Canada) brand of Haloperidol (Systemic), 561, **1205**
Haldol Decanoate—McNeil (U.S.) brand of Haloperidol Decanoate (Systemic), 561
Haldol LA*—McNeil (Canada) brand of Haloperidol Decanoate (Systemic), 561
Haldrone—Lilly (U.S.) brand of Paramethasone (Systemic—Glucocorticoid Effects), 38
Halenol—Halsey (U.S.) brand of Acetaminophen (Systemic), 1
Haley's M-O—Winthrop (U.S.) brand of Magnesium Hydroxide and Mineral Oil (Oral), 654
Halls Mentho-Lyptus Decongestant Cough Formula—Warner-Lambert (U.S.) brand of Phenylpropanolamine and Dextromethorphan (Systemic), 342
Halofed—Halsey (U.S.) brand of Pseudoephedrine (Systemic), 982
Halog—Squibb (U.S. and Canada) brand of Halcinonide (Topical), 33
Halog-E—Squibb (U.S.) brand of Halcinonide (Topical), 33
Haloperidol (Systemic), 561, **1205**
Haloprogin (Topical), 564
Halotestin—Upjohn (U.S. and Canada) brand of Fluoxymesterone (Systemic), 79
Halotex—Westwood (U.S. and Canada) brand of Haloprogin (Topical), 564
Halothane (Systemic), 91
Halotussin—Halsey (U.S.) brand of Guaifenesin (Systemic), 547
Halotussin-DM Expectorant—Halsey (U.S.) brand of Dextromethorphan and Guaifenesin (Systemic), 342
Haltran—Upjohn (U.S.) brand of Ibuprofen (Systemic), 138
Harmonyl—Abbott (U.S.) brand of Deserpidine (Systemic), 1006
HCG—See Gonadotropin, Chorionic (Systemic), 543
HC-Jel—Recsei (U.S.) brand of Hydrocortisone (Topical), 33
H₂ Cort—Vangard (U.S.) brand of Hydrocortisone (Topical), 33
HCV—Saron (U.S.) brand of Clioquinol and Hydrocortisone (Topical), 314
Head & Chest—Procter & Gamble (U.S.) brand of Phenylpropanolamine and Guaifenesin (Systemic), 342
Head and Shoulders—Procter & Gamble (U.S.) brand of Pyrithione (Topical), 994
Helmex*—Pfizer (Germany) brand of Pyrantel (Oral), 984
Hematran—Hauck (U.S.) brand of Iron Dextran (Systemic), 623
Hemocyte—U.S. Pharmaceutical (U.S.) brand of Ferrous Fumarate (Systemic), 623
Hepahydrin—Great Southern (U.S.) brand of Dehydrocholic Acid (Oral), 654
Hepalean*—Organon (Canada) brand of Heparin (Systemic), 565
Heparin (Systemic), 565
Hepsal*—CP Pharmaceuticals (U.K.) brand of Heparin (Systemic), 565

Herplex—Allergan (U.S. and Canada) brand of Idoxuridine (Ophthalmic), 587
Hexa-Betalin—Lilly (U.S. and Canada) brand of Pyridoxine (Systemic), 990
Hexabrix—Mallinckrodt (U.S.) brand of Ioxaglate (Systemic), 617
Hexadrol—Organon (U.S. and Canada) brand of Dexamethasone (Systemic—Glucocorticoid Effects), 38
Hexalol—Central (U.S.) brand of Atropine, Hyoscyamine, Methenamine, Methylene Blue, Phenyl Salicylate, and Benzoic Acid (Systemic), 163
Hexamine—See Methenamine (Systemic), 720
Hexocyclium (Systemic), 142
Hi-Cor—C&M (U.S.) brand of Hydrocortisone (Topical), 33
Hiprex—Merrell Dow (U.S.) brand of Methenamine (Systemic), 720
Hip-Rex*—Riker (Canada) brand of Methenamine (Systemic), 720
Hispril—SKF (U.S.) brand of Diphenylpyraline (Systemic), 130
Histabid Duracaps—Glaxo (U.S.) brand of Phenylpropanolamine and Chlorpheniramine (Systemic), 134
Histadyl E.C.—Lilly (U.S.) brand of Chlorpheniramine, Ephedrine, Codeine, and Ammonium Chloride (Systemic), 342
Histafed C—Life (U.S.) brand of Triprolidine, Pseudoephedrine, and Codeine (Systemic), 342
Histaject Modified—Mayrand (U.S.) brand of Brompheniramine (Systemic), 130
Histalet—Reid-Rowell (U.S.) brand of Chlorpheniramine and Pseudoephedrine (Systemic), 134
Histalet-DM—Reid-Rowell (U.S.) brand of Chlorpheniramine, Pseudoephedrine, and Dextromethorphan (Systemic), 342
Histalet Forte—Reid-Rowell (U.S.) brand of Phenylephrine, Phenylpropanolamine, Pyrilamine, and Chlorpheniramine (Systemic), 134
Histalet X—Reid-Rowell (U.S.) brand of Pseudoephedrine and Guaifenesin (Systemic), 342
Histamic—Metro Med (U.S.) brand of Phenylpropanolamine, Phenylephrine, Phenyltoloxamine, and Chlorpheniramine (Systemic), 134
Histamine, 568
Histantil*—Pharmascience (Canada) brand of Promethazine (Systemic), 977
Histarall—H. L. Moore (U.S.) brand of Dexbrompheniramine and Pseudoephedrine (Systemic), 134
Histaspan-P*—Rorer (Canada) brand of Phenylephrine and Chlorpheniramine (Systemic), 134
Histaspan-Plus—Rorer (U.S.) brand of Phenylephrine and Chlorpheniramine (Systemic), 134
Histatab Plus—Century (U.S.) brand of Phenylephrine and Chlorpheniramine (Systemic), 134
Histatapp—Upsher-Smith (U.S.) brand of Brompheniramine and Phenylpropanolamine (Systemic), 134
Hista-Vadrin—Scherer (U.S.) brand of Phenylephrine, Phenylpropanolamine, and Chlorpheniramine (Systemic), 134
Histerone—Hauck (U.S.) brand of Testosterone (Systemic), 79
Histocaine*—Dow (Canada) brand containing Benzocaine (Topical), 88
Histor-D—Hauck (U.S.) brand of Phenylephrine and Chlorpheniramine (Systemic), 134
Histrey—Bowman (U.S.) brand of Chlorpheniramine (Systemic), 130
HMS Liquifilm—Allergan (U.S. and Canada) brand of Medrysone (Ophthalmic), 26
Hold—Beecham (U.S.) brand of Dextromethorphan (Systemic), 393

I

L

Magmalin—Vale (U.S.) brand of Alumina and Magnesia (Oral), 99

Magnacef*—Ayerst (Canada) brand of Ceftazidime (Systemic), 261

Magnagel—Mallard (U.S.) brand of Alumina and Magnesium Carbonate (Oral), 99

Magnaprin—Rugby (U.S.) brand of Aspirin, Buffered (Systemic), 1036

Magnatril—Lannett (U.S.) brand of Magnesium Trisilicate, Alumina, and Magnesia (Oral), 99

Magnesium Carbonate and Sodium Bicarbonate (Oral), 99

Magnesium Citrate (Oral), 654

Magnesium Hydroxide (Oral), 99, 654

Magnesium Hydroxide and Mineral Oil (Oral), 654

Magnesium Oxide (Oral), 99, 654

Magnesium Salicylate (Systemic), 1036

Magnesium Sulfate (Oral), 654

Magnesium Trisilicate (Oral), 99

Magnesium Trisilicate, Alumina, and Magnesia (Oral), 99

Magnesium Trisilicate, Alumina, and Magnesium Carbonate (Oral), 99

Mag-Ox 400—Blaine (U.S.) brand of Magnesium Oxide (Oral), 99, 654

Major-cin—Major (U.S.) brand of Aspirin and Caffeine (Systemic), 1036

Malatal—Mallard (U.S.) brand of Atropine, Hyoscyamine, Scopolamine, and Phenobarbital (Systemic), 174

Malathion (Topical)*, 689

Mallergan—Mallard (U.S.) brand of Promethazine (Systemic), 977

Malogen*—Stickley (Canada) brand of Testosterone (Systemic), 79

Malogex*—Stickley (Canada) brand of Testosterone (Systemic), 79

Malotuss—Mallard (U.S.) brand of Guaifenesin (Systemic), 547

Malt Soup Extract (Oral), 654

Malt Soup Extract and Psyllium (Oral), 654

Maltsupex—Wallace (U.S.) brand of Malt Soup Extract (Oral), 654

Mandelamine—PD (U.S. and Canada) brand of Methenamine (Systemic), 720

Mandol—Lilly (U.S. and Canada) brand of Cefamandole (Systemic), 261

Maolate—Upjohn (U.S.) brand of Chlorphenesin (Systemic), 1050

Maox—Kenneth A. Manne (U.S.) brand of Magnesium Oxide (Oral), 99, 654

Maprin—Quantum (U.S.) brand of Aspirin, Buffered (Systemic), 1036

Maprin I-B—Quantum (U.S.) brand of Aspirin, Buffered (Systemic), 1036

Maprotiline (Systemic), 691

Marax—Roerig (U.S.) brand of Theophylline, Ephedrine, and Hydroxyzine (Systemic), 1108

Marax D.F.—Roerig (U.S.) brand of Theophylline, Ephedrine, and Hydroxyzine (Systemic), 1108

Marbaxin—Vortech (U.S.) brand of Methocarbamol (Systemic), 1050

Marblen—Fleming (U.S.) brand of Calcium and Magnesium Carbonates (Oral), 99

Marevan*—Duncan, Flockhart (U.K.) brand of Warfarin (Systemic), 104

Marezine—BW (U.S.) brand of Cyclizine (Systemic), 704

Marinol—Roxane (U.S.) brand of Dronabinol (Systemic), 443

Marmine—Vortech (U.S.) brand of Dimenhydrinate (Systemic), 130

Marnal—Vortech (U.S.) brand of Butalbital, Aspirin, and Caffeine (Systemic), 222

Marplan—Roche (U.S. and Canada) brand of Isocarboxazid (Systemic), 114

Marzine*—BW (Canada) brand of Cyclizine (Systemic), 704

Matulane—Roche (U.S.) brand of Procarbazine (Systemic), 970

Maxeran*—Nordic (Canada) brand of Metoclopramide (Systemic), 741

Maxibolin—Organon (U.S. and Canada) brand of Ethylestrenol (Systemic), 76

Maxidex—Alcon (U.S., Canada, and U.K.) brand of Dexamethasone (Ophthalmic), 26

Maxiflor—Herbert (U.S.) brand of Diflorasone (Topical), 33

Maxolon—Beecham (U.S.) brand of Metoclopramide (Systemic), 741

Maxzide—Lederle (U.S.) brand of Triamterene and Hydrochlorothiazide (Systemic), 435, **1205**

Mazanor—Wyeth (U.S.) brand of Mazindol (Systemic), 153

Mazepine*—ICN (Canada) brand of Carbamazepine (Systemic), 248

Mazindol (Systemic), 153

MD-Gastroview—Mallinckrodt (U.S.) brand of Diatrizoate (Systemic), 399

Measles Virus Vaccine Live (Systemic), 693

Measurin—Winthrop (U.S.) brand of Aspirin (Systemic), 1036

Mebaral—Winthrop (U.S. and Canada) brand of Mephobarbital (Systemic), 170

Mebendacin*—See Mebendazole (Systemic), 695

Mebendazole (Systemic), 695

Mebutar*—See Mebendazole (Systemic), 695

Mecamylamine (Systemic), 697

Mechlorethamine (Systemic), 700; (Topical)*, 702

Mecillinam—See Amdinocillin (Systemic), 896

Meclan—Ortho (U.S.) brand of Meclocycline (Topical), 1099

Meclizine (Systemic), 704, **1205**

Meclocycline (Topical), 1099

Meclofenamate (Systemic), 138, **1205**

Meclomen—PD (U.S.) brand of Meclofenamate (Systemic), 138, **1205**

Meda Cap—Circle (U.S.) brand of Acetaminophen (Systemic), 1

Meda Tab—Circle (U.S.) brand of Acetaminophen (Systemic), 1

Medicone Dressing—Medicone (U.S.) brand containing Benzocaine (Topical), 88

Medicycline*—Medic (Canada) brand of Tetracycline (Systemic), 1096

Medigesic Plus—U.S. Chemical (U.S.) brand of Butalbital, Acetaminophen, and Caffeine (Systemic), 215

Medihaler-Epi—Riker (U.S. and Canada) brand of Epinephrine (Inhalation), 201

Medihaler Ergotamine—Riker (U.S. and Canada) brand of Ergotamine (Systemic), 455

Medihaler-Iso—Riker (U.S. and Canada) brand of Isoproterenol (Inhalation), 201

Medilium*—Medic (Canada) brand of Chlordiazepoxide (Systemic), 179

Mediplast—Beiersdorf (U.S.) brand of Salicylic Acid (Topical), 1041

Medipren—McNeil (U.S.) brand of Ibuprofen (Systemic), 138

Mediquell—Warner-Lambert (U.S.) brand of Dextromethorphan (Systemic), 393

Mediquell Decongestant Formula—Warner-Lambert (U.S.) brand of Pseudoephedrine and Dextromethorphan (Systemic), 342

Medi-Quick—Mentholatum (U.S.) brand containing Lidocaine (Topical), 88

Meditran*—Medic (Canada) brand of Meprobamate (Systemic), 709

Medotar—Medco Lab (U.S.) brand of Coal Tar (Topical), 334

Medralone—Keene (U.S.) brand of Methylprednisolone (Systemic—Glucocorticoid Effects), 38

N

Nadolol (Systemic), 185, **1205**

Nadolol and Bendroflumethiazide (Systemic), 189, **1205**

Nadopen-V*—Nadeau (Canada) brand of Penicillin V (Systemic), 896

Nadostine*—Nadeau (Canada) brand of Nystatin (Oral), 846; (Topical), 848; (Vaginal), 850

Nafcil—Bristol (U.S.) brand of Nafcillin (Systemic), 896

Nafcillin (Systemic), 896

Nafeen—Pacemaker (U.S.) brand of Sodium Fluoride (Systemic), 1056

Nafrine*—Schering (Canada) brand of Oxymetazoline (Nasal), 868

Nalbuphine (Systemic—For Pain Relief), 779

Nalcrom*—Fisons (Canada) brand of Cromolyn (Oral)*, 357

Naldecon—Bristol (U.S.) brand of Phenylpropanolamine, Phenylephrine, Phenyltoloxamine, and Chlorpheniramine (Systemic), 134, **1205**

Naldecon-CX—Bristol (U.S.) brand of Phenylpropanolamine, Codeine, and Guaifenesin (Systemic), 342

Naldecon-DX—Bristol (U.S.) brand of Phenylpropanolamine, Dextromethorphan, and Guaifenesin (Systemic), 342

Naldecon-EX—Bristol (U.S.) brand of Phenylpropanolamine and Guaifenesin (Systemic), 342

Naldelate—Columbia Medical (U.S.); Consolidated Midland (U.S.); Dixon-Shane (U.S.); Moore (U.S.); Parmed (U.S.); and United Research (U.S.) brand of Phenylpropanolamine, Phenylephrine, Phenyltoloxamine, and Chlorpheniramine (Systemic), 134

Nalfon—Dista (U.S.) and Lilly (Canada) brand of Fenoprofen (Systemic), 138, **1205**

Nalidixic Acid (Systemic), 773

Nallpen—Beecham (U.S.) brand of Nafcillin (Systemic), 896

Naltrexone (Systemic), 775

NaMPICIL—Pharma-Tek (U.S.) brand of Ampicillin (Systemic), 896

Nandrobolic—Forest (U.S.) brand of Nandrolone (Systemic), 76

Nandrobolic L.A.—Forest (U.S.) brand of Nandrolone (Systemic), 76

Nandrolone (Systemic), 76

Nanormon*—Nordisk (Europe) brand of Somatropin (Systemic), 1062

Naphazoline (Ophthalmic), 777

Naphcon—Alcon (U.S.) brand of Naphazoline (Ophthalmic), 777

Naphcon Forte—Alcon (U.S. and Canada) brand of Naphazoline (Ophthalmic), 777

Napril Plateau—MiLance (U.S.) brand of Phenylephrine, Phenylpropanolamine, Pyrilamine, and Chlorpheniramine (Systemic), 134

Naprosyn—Syntex (U.S., Canada, and U.K.) brand of Naproxen (Systemic), 138, **1205**

Naproxen (Systemic), 138, **1205**

Naptrate—Vortech (U.S.) brand of Pentaerythritol Tetranitrate (Systemic—Oral), 829

Naqua—Schering (U.S.) brand of Trichlormethiazide (Systemic), 438

Naquival—Schering (U.S.) brand of Reserpine and Trichlormethiazide (Systemic), 1009

Narcotic Analgesics (Systemic—For Pain Relief), 779; (Systemic—For Surgery and Obstetrics), 783

Narcotic Analgesics and Acetaminophen (Systemic), 785

Narcotic Analgesics, Acetaminophen, and Salicylates (Systemic), 789

Narcotic Analgesics and Aspirin (Systemic), 794

Nardil—PD (U.S. and Canada) brand of Phenelzine (Systemic), 114

Nasahist—Keene (U.S.) brand of Phenylephrine, Phenylpropanolamine, and Chlorpheniramine (Systemic), 134

Nasahist B—Keene (U.S.) brand of Brompheniramine (Systemic), 130

Nasalcrom—Fisons (U.S. and Canada) brand of Cromolyn (Nasal), 353

Nasalide—Syntex (U.S.) brand of Flunisolide (Nasal), 24

Natacyn—Alcon (U.S.) brand of Natamycin (Ophthalmic), 799

Natamycin (Ophthalmic), 799

Natrimax*—Trianon (Canada) brand of Hydrochlorothiazide (Systemic), 438

Natulan*—Roche (Canada) brand of Procarbazine (Systemic), 970

Naturacil—Mead Johnson (U.S.) brand of Psyllium (Oral), 654

Nature's Remedy—Norcliff Thayer (U.S.) brand of Cascara Sagrada and Aloe (Oral), 654

Naturetin—Squibb (U.S. and Canada) brand of Bendroflumethiazide (Systemic), 438

Nauseatol*—Sabex (Canada) brand of Dimenhydrinate (Systemic), 130

Navane—Roerig (U.S.) and Pfizer (Canada) brand of Thiothixene (Systemic), 1122

Naxen*—SynCare (Canada) brand of Naproxen (Systemic), 138

ND Clear T.D.—Seatrace (U.S.) brand of Chlorpheniramine and Pseudoephedrine (Systemic), 134

ND-Hist—Hyrex (U.S.) brand of Phenylephrine, Phenylpropanolamine, and Chlorpheniramine (Systemic), 134

ND-Stat Revised—Hyrex (U.S.) brand of Brompheniramine (Systemic), 130

Nebcin—Lilly (U.S. and Canada) brand of Tobramycin (Systemic), 55

NegGram—Winthrop (U.S. and Canada) brand of Nalidixic Acid (Systemic), 773

Nemasol*—ICN (Canada) brand of Aminosalicylate (Systemic), 60

Nemasole*—See Mebendazole (Systemic), 695

Nembutal—Abbott (U.S. and Canada) brand of Pentobarbital (Systemic), 170

Neo-Barb*—Neolab (Canada) brand of Butabarbital (Systemic), 170

Neo-Calglucon—Sandoz (U.S.) brand of Calcium Glubionate (Systemic), 241

Neo-Calme*—Neolab (Canada) brand of Diazepam (Systemic), 179

Neo-Codema*—Neolab (Canada) brand of Hydrochlorothiazide (Systemic), 438

Neo-Cultol—Fisons (U.S.) brand of Mineral Oil (Oral), 654

Neocyten—Central (U.S.) brand of Orphenadrine (Systemic), 857

Neo-DM*—Neolab (Canada) brand of Dextromethorphan (Systemic), 393

Neo-Durabolic—Hauck (U.S.) brand of Nandrolone (Systemic), 76

Neo-Estrone*—Neolab (Canada) brand of Esterified Estrogens (Systemic), 476

NeoFed—Vale (U.S.) brand of Pseudoephedrine (Systemic), 982

Neo-Fer*—Neolab (Canada) brand of Ferrous Fumarate (Systemic), 623

Neo-IM—Pharma-Tek (U.S.) brand of Neomycin (Systemic), 55

Neo-K*—Neolab (Canada) brand of Potassium Bicarbonate and Potassium Chloride (Systemic), 948

Neolax—Central (U.S.) brand of Dehydrocholic Acid and Docusate (Oral), 654

Neoloid—Lederle (U.S. and Canada) brand of Castor Oil (Oral), 654

Neo-Metric*—Neolab (Canada) brand of Metronidazole (Systemic), 745

Neomycin (Ophthalmic)*, 800; (Oral), 802; (Systemic), 55; (Topical), 804

O

Oxalactam*—Lilly (Austria, Belgium) brand of Moxalactam (Systemic), 261

Oxamniquine (Systemic), 862

Oxandrolone (Systemic), 76

Oxazepam (Systemic), 179, **1205**

Ox-Pam*—ICN (Canada) brand of Oxazepam (Systemic), 179

Oxprenolol (Systemic)*, 185

Oxsoralen—Elder (U.S. and Canada) brand of Methoxsalen (Systemic), 725; (Topical), 727

Oxsoralen-Ultra—Elder (U.S.) brand of Methoxsalen (Systemic), 725

Oxtriphylline (Systemic), 208

Oxtriphylline and Guaifenesin (Systemic), 864

Oxy—Norcliff Thayer (U.S.) brand of Benzoyl Peroxide (Topical), 183

Oxybutynin (Systemic), 866

Oxy Clean—Norcliff Thayer (U.S.) brand of Salicylic Acid (Topical), 1041

Oxycocet*—Technilab (Canada) brand of Oxycodone and Acetaminophen (Systemic), 785

Oxycodan*—Technilab (Canada) brand of Oxycodone and Aspirin (Systemic), 794

Oxycodone (Systemic—For Pain Relief), 779

Oxycodone and Acetaminophen (Systemic), 785, **1205**

Oxycodone with APAP—See Oxycodone and Acetaminophen (Systemic), 785

Oxycodone and Aspirin (Systemic), 794, **1205**

Oxyderm*—ICN (Canada) brand of Benzoyl Peroxide (Topical), 183

Oxydess II—Vortech (U.S.) brand of Dextroamphetamine (Systemic), 67

Oxymetazoline (Nasal), 868; (Ophthalmic), 870

Oxymetholone (Systemic), 76

Oxymorphone (Systemic—For Pain Relief), 779

Oxyphencyclimine (Systemic), 142

Oxyphenonium (Systemic), 142

Oxytetracycline (Systemic), 1096

Oxytocin (Systemic), 872

P

P-50*—Horner (Canada) brand of Penicillin G (Systemic), 896

[32]P—See Chromic Phosphate P 32 (Therapeutic), 297

Pacaps—La Salle (U.S.) brand of Butalbital, Acetaminophen, and Caffeine (Systemic), 215

P-A-C Revised Formula—Upjohn (U.S.) brand of Aspirin and Caffeine (Systemic), 1036

Pain Reliever—Rugby (U.S.) brand of Acetaminophen, Aspirin, and Caffeine (Systemic), 4

Palafer*—Beecham (Canada) brand of Ferrous Fumarate (Systemic), 623

Palaron*—Fisons (Canada) brand of Aminophylline (Systemic), 208

Palbar No. 2—Hauck (U.S.) brand of Atropine, Hyoscyamine, Scopolamine, and Butabarbital (Systemic), 174

Palmiron—Hauck (U.S.) brand of Ferrous Fumarate (Systemic), 623

Pama No.1—North American (U.S.) brand of Calcium Carbonate (Oral), 99

Pamelor—Sandoz (U.S.) brand of Nortriptyline (Systemic), 117

Pamine—Upjohn (U.S.) brand of Methscopolamine (Systemic), 142

Pamprin IB—Chettem (U.S.) brand of Ibuprofen (Systemic), 138

Panadol—Glenbrook (U.S.); Sterling (Canada); and Winthrop (U.K.) brand of Acetaminophen (Systemic), 1

Panadyl—Misemer (U.S.) brand of Phenylpropanolamine, Pheniramine, and Pyrilamine (Systemic), 134

Panasol—Seatrace (U.S.) brand of Prednisone (Systemic—Glucocorticoid Effects), 38

Panasorb*—Winthrop (U.K.) brand of Acetaminophen (Systemic), 1

Pancrease—McNeil (U.S. and Canada) brand of Pancrelipase (Systemic), 875

Pancreatin, Pepsin, Bile Salts, Hyoscyamine, Atropine, Scopolamine, and Phenobarbital (Systemic), 873

Pancrelipase (Systemic), 875

Panectyl*—Rhone-Poulenc (Canada) brand of Trimeprazine (Systemic), 1146

Panex—Mallard (U.S.) brand of Acetaminophen (Systemic), 1

Panmycin—Upjohn (U.S.) brand of Tetracycline (Systemic), 1096

PanOxyl—Stiefel (U.S. and Canada) brand of Benzoyl Peroxide (Topical), 183

PanOxyl AQ—Stiefel (U.S.) brand of Benzoyl Peroxide (Topical), 183

Pantelmin*—See Mebendazole (Systemic), 695

Pantholin—Lilly (U.S.) brand of Pantothenic Acid (Systemic), 877

Pantopaque—Lafayette (U.S.) brand of Iophendylate (Systemic), 613

Pantopon—Roche (U.S. and Canada) brand of Opium (Systemic—For Pain Relief), 779

Pantothenic Acid (Systemic), 877

Panwarfin—Abbott (U.S.) brand of Warfarin (Systemic), 104

Papaverine (Intracavernosal), 879; (Systemic), 881

Paracetamol—See Acetaminophen (Systemic), 1

Paracet Forte—Major (U.S.) brand of Chlorzoxazone and Acetaminophen (Systemic), 291

Paradione—Abbott (U.S. and Canada) brand of Paramethadione (Systemic), 107

Paradol*—Chase (Canada) brand of Aspirin and Caffeine (Systemic), 1036

Paraflex—McNeil (U.S.) brand of Chlorzoxazone (Systemic), 1050

Parafon Forte—McNeil (U.S. and Canada) brand of Chlorzoxazone and Acetaminophen (Systemic), 291

Parafon Forte DSC—McNeil (U.S.) brand of Chlorzoxazone (Systemic), 1050, **1205**

Paral—Forest (U.S.) brand of Paraldehyde (Systemic), 883

Paraldehyde (Systemic), 883

Paramethadione (Systemic), 107

Paramethasone (Systemic—Glucocorticoid Effects), 38

Paraphen*—Pharmavite (Canada) brand of Acetaminophen (Systemic), 1

Paregoric (Systemic), 854

Parepectolin—Rorer (U.S.) brand of Kaolin, Pectin, and Paregoric (Systemic), 644

Pargyline (Systemic), 885

Pargyline and Methyclothiazide (Systemic), 888

Parlodel—Sandoz (U.S.) and Anca (Canada) brand of Bromocriptine (Systemic), 199

Par-Mag—Parmed (U.S.) brand of Magnesium Oxide (Oral), 99

Parmine—Parmed (U.S.) brand of Phentermine (Systemic), 153

Parnate—SKF (U.S. and Canada) brand of Tranylcypromine (Systemic), 114

Parsidol—PD (U.S.) brand of Ethopropazine (Systemic), 124

Parsitan*—Rhône-Poulenc (Canada) brand of Ethopropazine (Systemic), 124

P.A.S.—Lannett (U.S.) brand of Aminosalicylate (Systemic), 60

Pathilon—Lederle (U.S.) brand of Tridihexethyl (Systemic), 142

Pathocil—Wyeth (U.S.) brand of Dicloxacillin (Systemic), 896

Pavabid—Marion (U.S.) brand of Papaverine (Systemic), 881

Pavabid HP—Marion (U.S.) brand of Papaverine (Systemic), 881

Pavacap—Reid-Rowell (U.S.) brand of Papaverine (Systemic), 881

Pavacen—Central (U.S.) brand of Papaverine (Systemic), 881

Pyrimethamine (Systemic), 992

Pyrinyl—Barre-National (U.S.); Bioline (U.S.); CMC (U.S.); DeWitt (U.S.); Dixon-Shane (U.S.); Goldline (U.S.); Moore (U.S.); Murray (U.S.); Parmed (U.S.); Rugby (U.S.); Schein (U.S.); Spencer-Mead (U.S.); Vangard (U.S.); Veratex (U.S.); and Williams (U.S.) brand of Pyrethrins and Piperonyl Butoxide (Topical), 988

Pyrithione (Topical), 994

Pyronium*—Pro Doc (Canada) brand of Phenazopyridine (Systemic), 910

Pyroxine—Kay (U.S.) brand of Pyridoxine (Systemic), 990

Pyrvinium (Oral)*, 995

PZI insulin—See Insulin, Protamine Zinc (Systemic), 596

Q

Q-Pam—Quantum Pharmics (U.S.) brand of Diazepam (Systemic), 179

Quadra Hist—Schein (U.S.) brand of Phenylpropanolamine, Phenylephrine, Phenyltoloxamine, and Chlorpheniramine (Systemic), 134

Quarzan—Roche (U.S.) brand of Clidinium (Systemic), 142

Quelidrine Cough—Abbott (U.S.) brand of Chlorpheniramine, Ephedrine, Phenylephrine, Dextromethorphan, Ammonium Chloride, and Ipecac (Systemic), 342

Queltuss—Forest (U.S.) brand of Dextromethorphan and Guaifenesin (Systemic), 342

Questran—Mead Johnson (U.S.) and Bristol (Canada) brand of Cholestyramine (Systemic), 295

Quiagel PG—Rugby (U.S.) brand of Kaolin, Pectin, Belladonna Alkaloids, and Opium (Systemic), 641

Quiagen—Goldline (U.S.) brand of Theophylline and Guaifenesin (Systemic), 1111

Quibron—Mead Johnson (U.S.) brand of Theophylline and Guaifenesin (Systemic), 1111

Quibron Plus—Mead Johnson (U.S.) brand of Theophylline, Ephedrine, Guaifenesin, and Butabarbital (Systemic), 1105

Quibron-T*—Bristol (Canada) brand of Theophylline (Systemic), 208

Quibron-T Dividose—Mead Johnson (U.S.) and Bristol (Canada) brand of Theophylline (Systemic), 208

Quibron-T/SR Dividose—Mead Johnson (U.S.) and Bristol (Canada) brand of Theophylline (Systemic), 208

Quick Pep—Thompson (U.S.) brand of Caffeine (Systemic), 230

Quiess—Forest (U.S.) brand of Hydroxyzine (Systemic), 585

Quinaglute Dura-tabs—Berlex (U.S. and Canada) brand of Quinidine (Systemic), 997, **1205**

Quinalan—Lannett (U.S.) brand of Quinidine (Systemic), 997

Quinamm—Merrell-National (U.S.) brand of Quinine (Systemic), 999

Quinate*—Rougier (Canada) brand of Quinidine (Systemic), 997

Quinestrol (Systemic), 476

Quinethazone (Systemic), 438

Quinidex Extentabs—Robins (U.S. and Canada) brand of Quinidine (Systemic), 997

Quinidine (Systemic), 997, **1205**

Quinine (Systemic), 999

Quinite—Reid-Rowell (U.S.) brand of Quinine (Systemic), 999

Quinora—Key (U.S.) brand of Quinidine (Systemic), 997

Quinsana Plus—Mennen (U.S.) brand of Undecylenic Acid, Compound (Topical), 1156

R

RA—Medco Lab (U.S.) brand of Resorcinol (Topical), 1020

Racepinephrine (Inhalation), 201

Racet—Lemmon (U.S.) brand of Clioquinol and Hydrocortisone (Topical), 314

Racet-SE—Lemmon (U.S.) brand of Hydrocortisone (Topical), 33

Radiopharmaceuticals (Diagnostic), 1001

Radiostol*—Allen & Hanburys (Canada) brand of Vitamin D (Systemic), 1182

Radiostol Forte*—Allen & Hanburys (Canada) brand of Vitamin D (Systemic), 1182

Ranitidine (Systemic), 1004, **1205**

Rapifen*—Janssen (U.K.) brand of Alfentanil (Systemic—For Surgery and Obstetrics), 783

Raudixin—Princeton (U.S.) and Squibb (Canada) brand of Rauwolfia Serpentina (Systemic), 1006

Rauverid—Forest (U.S.) brand of Rauwolfia Serpentina (Systemic), 1006

Rauwiloid—Riker (U.S.) brand of Alseroxylon (Systemic), 1006

Rauwolfia Alkaloids (Systemic), 1006

Rauwolfia Alkaloids and Thiazide Diuretics (Systemic), 1009

Rauwolfia Serpentina (Systemic), 1006

Rauwolfia Serpentina and Bendroflumethiazide (Systemic), 1009

Rauzide—Princeton (U.S.) brand of Rauwolfia Serpentina and Bendroflumethiazide (Systemic), 1009

Razepam—Major (U.S.) brand of Temazepam (Systemic), 179

R & C—Reed & Carnrick (U.S.) brand of Pyrethrins and Piperonyl Butoxide (Topical), 988

Reclomide—Ultra (U.S.) brand of Metoclopramide (Systemic), 741

Rectocort*—Welcker-Lyster (Canada) brand of Hydrocortisone (Rectal), 575; (Topical), 33

Redisol—MSD (U.S.) brand of Cyanocobalamin (Systemic), 1180

Redoxon*—Roche (Canada) brand of Ascorbic Acid (Systemic); Sodium Ascorbate (Systemic), 156

Regibon*—Medic (Canada) brand of Diethylpropion (Systemic), 153

Regitine—Ciba (U.S.) brand of Phentolamine and Papaverine (Intracavernosal), 919

Reglan—Robins (U.S. and Canada) brand of Metoclopramide (Systemic), 741, **1205**

Regonol—Organon (U.S. and Canada) brand of Pyridostigmine (Systemic), 146

Regroton—Rorer (U.S.) brand of Reserpine and Chlorthalidone (Systemic), 1009

Regulace—Republic (U.S.) brand of Casanthranol and Docusate (Oral), 654

Regular—Squibb-Novo (U.S.) brand of Insulin (Systemic), 596

Regular (Concentrated) Iletin II, U-500—Lilly (U.S.) brand of Insulin (Systemic), 596

Regular Iletin I—Lilly (U.S.) brand of Insulin (Systemic), 596

Regular Iletin II—Lilly (U.S.) brand of Insulin (Systemic), 596

Regular insulin—See Insulin (Systemic), 596

Regulax SS—Republic (U.S.) brand of Docusate (Oral), 654

Regulex*—Ayerst (Canada) brand of Docusate (Oral), 654

Regulex-D*—Ayerst (Canada) brand of Danthron and Docusate (Oral)*, 654

Reguloid Natural—Rugby (U.S.) brand of Psyllium Hydrophilic Mucilloid (Oral), 654

Reguloid Orange—Rugby (U.S.) brand of Psyllium Hydrophilic Mucilloid (Oral), 654

Regutol—Plough (U.S.) brand of Docusate (Oral), 654

Riphen-10*—Riva (Canada) brand of Aspirin (Systemic), 1036

Ritalin—Ciba (U.S. and Canada) brand of Methylphenidate (Systemic), 735, **1205**

Ritalin-SR—Ciba (U.S. and Canada) brand of Methylphenidate (Systemic), 735, **1205**

Ritodrine (Systemic), 1032

Rival*—Riva (Canada) brand of Diazepam (Systemic), 179

Rivotril*—Roche (Canada) brand of Clonazepam (Systemic), 179

RMS Uniserts—Upsher-Smith (U.S.) brand of Morphine (Systemic—For Pain Relief), 779

Robafen—Major (U.S.) brand of Guaifenesin (Systemic), 547

Robalate*—Robins (Canada) brand of Dihydroxyaluminum Aminoacetate (Oral), 99

Robalyn—Three P (U.S.) brand of Diphenhydramine (Systemic), 130

Robaxin—Robins (U.S., Canada, and U.K.) brand of Methocarbamol (Systemic), 1050

Robicillin VK—Robins (U.S.) brand of Penicillin V (Systemic), 896

Robidex*—Robins (Canada) brand of Dextromethorphan (Systemic), 393

Robidone*—Robins (Canada) brand of Hydrocodone (Systemic—For Pain Relief), 779

Robidrine*—Robins (Canada) brand of Pseudoephedrine (Systemic), 982

Robigesic*—Robins (Canada) brand of Acetaminophen (Systemic), 1

Robimycin—Robins (U.S.) brand of Erythromycin (Systemic), 468

Robinul—Robins (U.S. and Canada) brand of Glycopyrrolate (Systemic), 142

Robinul Forte—Robins (U.S. and Canada) brand of Glycopyrrolate (Systemic), 142

Robitet—Robins (U.S.) brand of Tetracycline (Systemic), 1096

Robitussin—Robins (U.S. and Canada) brand of Guaifenesin (Systemic), 547

Robitussin A-C—Robins (U.S.) brand of Codeine and Guaifenesin (Systemic); Robins (Canada) brand of Pheniramine, Codeine, and Guaifenesin (Systemic)*, 342

Robitussin-CF—Robins (U.S.) brand of Phenylpropanolamine, Dextromethorphan, and Guaifenesin (Systemic), 342

Robitussin with Codeine*—Robins (Canada) brand of Pheniramine, Codeine, and Guaifenesin (Systemic)*, 342

Robitussin-DAC—Robins (U.S.) brand of Pseudoephedrine, Codeine, and Guaifenesin (Systemic), 342

Robitussin-DM—Robins (U.S. and Canada) brand of Dextromethorphan and Guaifenesin (Systemic), 342

Robitussin-DM Cough Calmers—Robins (U.S.) brand of Dextromethorphan and Guaifenesin (Systemic), 342

Robitussin Night Relief Colds Formula Liquid—Robins (U.S.) brand of Pyrilamine, Phenylephrine, Dextromethorphan, and Acetaminophen (Systemic), 342

Robitussin-PE—Robins (U.S. and Canada) brand of Pseudoephedrine and Guaifenesin (Systemic), 342

Rocaltrol—Roche (U.S. and Canada) brand of Calcitriol (Systemic), 236

Rocephin—Roche (U.S.) brand of Ceftriaxone (Systemic), 261

Rodex—Legere (U.S.) brand of Pyridoxine (Systemic), 990

Rofact*—ICN (Canada) brand of Rifampin (Systemic), 1027

Roferon-A—Roche (U.S.) brand of Interferon Alfa-2a, Recombinant (Systemic), 601

Rogaine*—Upjohn (Canada) brand of Minoxidil (Topical)*, 759

Rogitine*—Ciba (Canada) brand of Phentolamine and Papaverine (Intracavernosal), 919

Rolaids—Warner-Lambert (U.S.) brand of Dihydroxyaluminum Sodium Carbonate (Oral), 99

Rolox—Purepac (U.S.) brand of Alumina and Magnesia (Oral), 99

Ronase—Reid-Rowell (U.S.) brand of Tolazamide (Systemic), 121

Rondec—Ross (U.S.) brand of Carbinoxamine and Pseudoephedrine (Systemic), 134

Rondec-DM—Ross (U.S.) brand of Carbinoxamine, Pseudoephedrine, and Dextromethorphan (Systemic), 342

Rondec-DM Drops—Ross (U.S.) brand of Carbinoxamine, Pseudoephedrine, and Dextromethorphan (Systemic), 342

Rondec-TR—Ross (U.S.) brand of Carbinoxamine and Pseudoephedrine (Systemic), 134

Rondomycin—Wallace (U.S.) brand of Methacycline (Systemic), 1096

Roniacol*—Roche (Canada) brand of Nicotinyl Alcohol (Systemic), 825

Roubac*—Rougier (Canada) brand of Sulfamethoxazole and Trimethoprim (Systemic), 1073

Roucol*—Rougier (Canada) brand of Allopurinol (Systemic), 46

Rounox*—Rougier (Canada) brand of Acetaminophen (Systemic), 1

Rounox with Codeine*—Rougier (Canada) brand of Acetaminophen and Codeine (Systemic), 785

Roxanol—Roxane (U.S.) and Organon (Canada) brand of Morphine (Systemic—For Pain Relief), 779

Roxanol SR—Roxane (U.S.) brand of Morphine (Systemic—For Pain Relief), 779

Roxicet—Roxane (U.S.) brand of Oxycodone and Acetaminophen (Systemic), 785

Roxicodone—Roxane (U.S.) brand of Oxycodone (Systemic—For Pain Relief), 779

Roychlor*—Roy (Canada) brand of Potassium Chloride (Systemic), 948

Roydan*—Roy (Canada) brand of Danthron (Oral)*, 654

Roydan Mild*—Roy (Canada) brand of Danthron (Oral)*, 654

Royonate*—Roy (Canada) brand of Potassium Gluconate (Systemic), 948

RP-Mycin—Reid-Rowell (U.S.) brand of Erythromycin (Systemic), 468

Rubella Virus Vaccine Live (Systemic), 1034

Rubion*—Desbergers (Canada) brand of Cyanocobalamin (Systemic), 1180

Rubramin*—Squibb (Canada) brand of Cyanocobalamin (Systemic), 1180

Rubramin PC—Squibb (U.S.) brand of Cyanocobalamin (Systemic), 1180

Rufen—Boots brand of Ibuprofen (Systemic), 138, **1205**

Rulox—Rugby (U.S.) brand of Alumina and Magnesia (Oral), 99

Rulox No. 1—Rugby (U.S.) brand of Alumina and Magnesia (Oral), 99

Rulox No. 2—Rugby (U.S.) brand of Alumina and Magnesia (Oral), 99

Rum-K—Fleming (U.S.) brand of Potassium Chloride (Systemic), 948

Ru-Tuss II—Boots (U.S.) brand of Phenylpropanolamine and Chlorpheniramine (Systemic), 134

Ru-Tuss Expectorant—Boots (U.S.) brand of Chlorpheniramine, Phenylephrine, Codeine, and Ammonium Chloride (Systemic), 342

Ru-Tuss with Hydrocodone Liquid—Boots (U.S.) brand of Pheniramine, Pyrilamine, Phenylephrine, Phenylpropanolamine, and Hydrocodone (Systemic), 342

Rymed—Edwards (U.S.) brand of Phenylephrine, Phenylpropanolamine, and Guaifenesin (Systemic), 342

Rymed-Jr—Edwards (U.S.) brand of Phenylephrine, Phenylpropanolamine, and Guaifenesin (Systemic), 342

U

W

Wehdryl—Hauck (U.S.) brand of Diphenhydramine (Systemic), 130

Wehgen—Hauck (U.S.) brand of Estrone (Systemic), 476

Wehless—Hauck (U.S.) brand of Phendimetrazine (Systemic), 153

Weightrol—Vortech (U.S.) brand of Phendimetrazine (Systemic), 153

Wellcovorin—BW (U.S.) brand of Leucovorin (Systemic), 662

Wesprin Buffered—Wesley (U.S.) brand of Aspirin, Buffered (Systemic), 1036

Westapp—Western (U.S.) brand of Brompheniramine, Phenylephrine, and Phenylpropanolamine (Systemic), 134

Westcort—Westwood (U.S. and Canada) brand of Hydrocortisone (Topical), 33

Westrim—Western (U.S.) brand of Phenylpropanolamine (Systemic), 928

Westrim LA—Western (U.S.) brand of Phenylpropanolamine (Systemic), 928

Wigraine—Organon (U.S.) brand of Ergotamine and Caffeine (Systemic), 460

Wigrettes—Organon (U.S.) brand of Ergotamine (Systemic), 455

Wilpowr—Foy (U.S.) brand of Phentermine (Systemic), 153

WinGel—Winthrop (U.S.) brand of Alumina and Magnesia (Oral), 99

Winpred*—ICN (Canada) brand of Prednisone (Systemic—Glucocorticoid Effects), 38

Winstrol—Winthrop (U.S. and Canada) brand of Stanozolol (Systemic), 76

Wolfina—Forest (U.S.) brand of Rauwolfia Serpentina (Systemic), 1006

Wyamycin E—Wyeth (U.S.) brand of Erythromycin Ethylsuccinate (Systemic), 468

Wyamycin S—Wyeth (U.S.) brand of Erythromycin Stearate (Systemic), 468

Wycillin—Wyeth (U.S. and Canada) brand of Penicillin G (Systemic), 896

Wygesic—Wyeth (U.S.) brand of Propoxyphene and Acetaminophen (Systemic), 785

Wymox—Wyeth (U.S.) brand of Amoxicillin (Systemic), 896

Wytensin—Wyeth (U.S.) brand of Guanabenz (Systemic), 549

X

Xanax—Upjohn (U.S. and Canada) brand of Alprazolam (Systemic), 179, **1205**

Xenon Xe 127 (Diagnostic), 1001

Xenon Xe 133 (Diagnostic), 1001

Xerac—Person & Covey (U.S.) brand of Alcohol and Sulfur (Topical), 44

Xerac BP—Person & Covey (U.S.) brand of Benzoyl Peroxide (Topical), 183

X-Prep Liquid—Gray (U.S.) brand of Senna (Oral), 654

Xseb—Baker/Cummins (U.S.) brand of Salicylic Acid (Topical), 1041

X-Trozine—Obetrol (U.S.) brand of Phendimetrazine (Systemic), 153

X-Trozine LA—Obetrol (U.S.) brand of Phendimetrazine (Systemic), 153

Xylocaine—Astra (U.S., Canada, and U.K.) brand of Lidocaine (Dental), 82; (Topical), 88

Xylocaine Viscous—Astra (U.S., Canada, and U.K.) brand of Lidocaine (Dental), 82

Xylometazoline (Nasal), 1191

Y

Yodoxin—Glenwood (U.S.) brand of Iodoquinol (Oral), 607

Yomesan*—See Niclosamide (Oral), 821

Yutopar—Astra (U.S.) and Bristol (Canada) brand of Ritodrine (Systemic), 1032

Z

Zanosar—Upjohn (U.S. and Canada) brand of Streptozocin (Systemic), 1063

Zantac—Glaxo (U.S. and Canada) brand of Ranitidine (Systemic), 1004, **1205**

Zapex*—Riva (Canada) brand of Oxazepam (Systemic), 179

Zarontin—PD (U.S. and Canada) brand of Ethosuximide (Systemic), 112

Zeroxin—Syossett (U.S.) brand of Benzoyl Peroxide (Topical), 183

Zaroxolyn—Pennwalt (U.S. and Canada) brand of Metolazone (Systemic), 438

Zendole—Zenith (U.S.) brand of Indomethacin (Systemic—Anti-inflammatory), 593

Zephrex—Bock (U.S.) brand of Pseudoephedrine and Guaifenesin (Systemic), 342

Zephrex-LA—Bock (U.S.) brand of Pseudoephedrine and Guaifenesin (Systemic), 342

Zetar—Dermik (U.S.) brand of Coal Tar (Topical), 334

Zetar Emulsion—Dermik (U.S.) and Rorer (Canada) brand of Coal Tar (Topical), 334

Zidovudine (Systemic), 1193

Zienam*—See Imipenem and Cilastatin (Systemic), 589

Zinacef—Glaxo (U.S. and Canada) brand of Cefuroxime (Systemic), 261

Zincon—Lederle (U.S.) brand of Pyrithione (Topical), 994

ZNP—Stiefel (U.S.) brand of Pyrithione (Topical), 994

ZORprin—Boots (U.S.) brand of Aspirin (Systemic), 1036

Zovirax—BW (U.S. and Canada) brand of Acyclovir (Systemic), 14; (Topical), 17

Zoxaphen—Mallard (U.S.) brand of Chlorzoxazone and Acetaminophen (Systemic), 291

Zurinol—Major (U.S.) brand of Allopurinol (Systemic), 46

Zydone—Du Pont (U.S.) brand of Hydrocodone and Acetaminophen (Systemic), 785

Zyloprim—BW (U.S. and Canada) brand of Allopurinol (Systemic), 46, **1205**

Zyloric*—Calmic (U.K.) brand of Allopurinol (Systemic), 46

Zymenol—Houser (U.S.) brand of Mineral Oil (Oral), 654

Zynol*—Horner (Canada) brand of Sulfinpyrazone (Systemic), 1069